D0151103

Fundamentals of Nursing
Standards & Practice

Fourth Edition

Fundamentals of Nursing
Standards & Practice

Fourth Edition

Sue C. DeLaune, MN, RN

Assistant Professor
RN-BSN Coordinator
William Carey University
School of Nursing
New Orleans, Louisiana

President and Education Director
SDeLaune Consulting
Mandeville, Louisiana

Patricia K. Ladner, RN, MS, MN

Former Consultant for Nursing Practice
Louisiana State Board of Nursing
New Orleans, Louisiana?

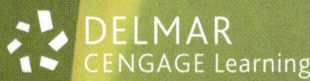
DELMAR
CENGAGE Learning™

Australia • Brazil • Japan • Korea • Mexico • Singapore • Spain • United Kingdom • United States

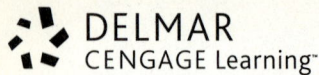
DELMAR
CENGAGE Learning™

**Fundamentals of Nursing: Standards and Practice
Fourth Edition**

By Sue C. DeLaune and Patricia K. Ladner

Vice President, Career and Professional
Editorial: Dave Garza

Director of Learning Solutions: Matthew Kane

Executive Editor: Stephen Helba

Managing Editor: Marah Bellegarde

Senior Product Manager: Patricia Gaworecki

Editorial Assistant: Meghan Orvis

Vice President, Career and Professional Marketing:
Jennifer McAvey

Marketing Director: Wendy E. Mapstone

Senior Marketing Manager: Michele McTighe

Marketing Coordinator: Scott Chrysler

Production Director: Carolyn Miller

Production Manager: Andrew Crouth

Senior Content Project Manager: Kenneth McGrath

Senior Art Director: Jack Pendleton

© 2011, 2006, 2002, 1998, Delmar, Cengage Learning

ALL RIGHTS RESERVED. No part of this work covered by the copyright herein may be reproduced, transmitted, stored, or used in any form or by any means graphic, electronic, or mechanical, including but not limited to photocopying, recording, scanning, digitizing, taping, Web distribution, information networks, or information storage and retrieval systems, except as permitted under Section 107 or 108 of the 1976 United States Copyright Act, without the prior written permission of the publisher.

For product information and technology assistance, contact us at
Cengage Learning Customer & Sales Support, 1-800-354-9706
For permission to use material from this text or product, submit all requests online at **cengage.com/permissions**.
Further permissions questions can be e-mailed to
permissionrequest@cengage.com.

Library of Congress Control Number: 2009937406
ISBN-13: 978-1-4354-8067-4
ISBN-10: 1-4354-8067-8

Delmar
5 Maxwell Drive
Clifton Park, NY 12065-2919
USA

Cengage Learning is a leading provider of customized learning solutions with office locations around the globe, including Singapore, the United Kingdom, Australia, Mexico, Brazil, and Japan. Locate your local office at:
international.cengage.com/region

Cengage Learning products are represented in Canada by Nelson Education, Ltd.

For your lifelong learning solutions, visit **delmar.cengage.com**
Visit our corporate website at **cengage.com**.
Purchase any of our products at your local college store or at our preferred online store **www.CengageBrain.com**.

Notice to the Reader

Publisher does not warrant or guarantee any of the products described herein or perform any independent analysis in connection with any of the product information contained herein. Publisher does not assume, and expressly disclaims, any obligation to obtain and include information other than that provided to it by the manufacturer. The reader is expressly warned to consider and adopt all safety precautions that might be indicated by the activities described herein and to avoid all potential hazards. By following the instructions contained herein, the reader willingly assumes all risks in connection with such instructions. The publisher makes no representations or warranties of any kind, including but not limited to, the warranties of fitness for particular purpose or merchantability, nor are any such representations implied with respect to the material set forth herein, and the publisher takes no responsibility with respect to such material. The publisher shall not be liable for any special, consequential, or exemplary damages resulting, in whole or part, from the readers' use of, or reliance upon, this material.

Printed in the United States of America
1 2 3 4 5 6 7 12 11 10

o Jennifer and Ryan Cardinal, Katie and Jacob Segrave, and Sarabeth and Jay Accardo.
especially want to thank my husband and best friend, Jay, for his continued support and
elief in me. I want to acknowledge my father, Glynn Edward Carter, for unending
pport and encouragement, especially for my academic endeavors.

CD

o Wayne, Kelly, Wayne Jr., Gretchen, and Michael.

KL

e dedicate this book to our grandchildren: Camille Anna Cardinal, Caroline Alexa
ardinal, Leah Marie Ladner, Charles Thomas Lee, Michael and Joshua Ladner, and
ooper and Paige Ladner.
ou are our future. "G" and "Mimi"

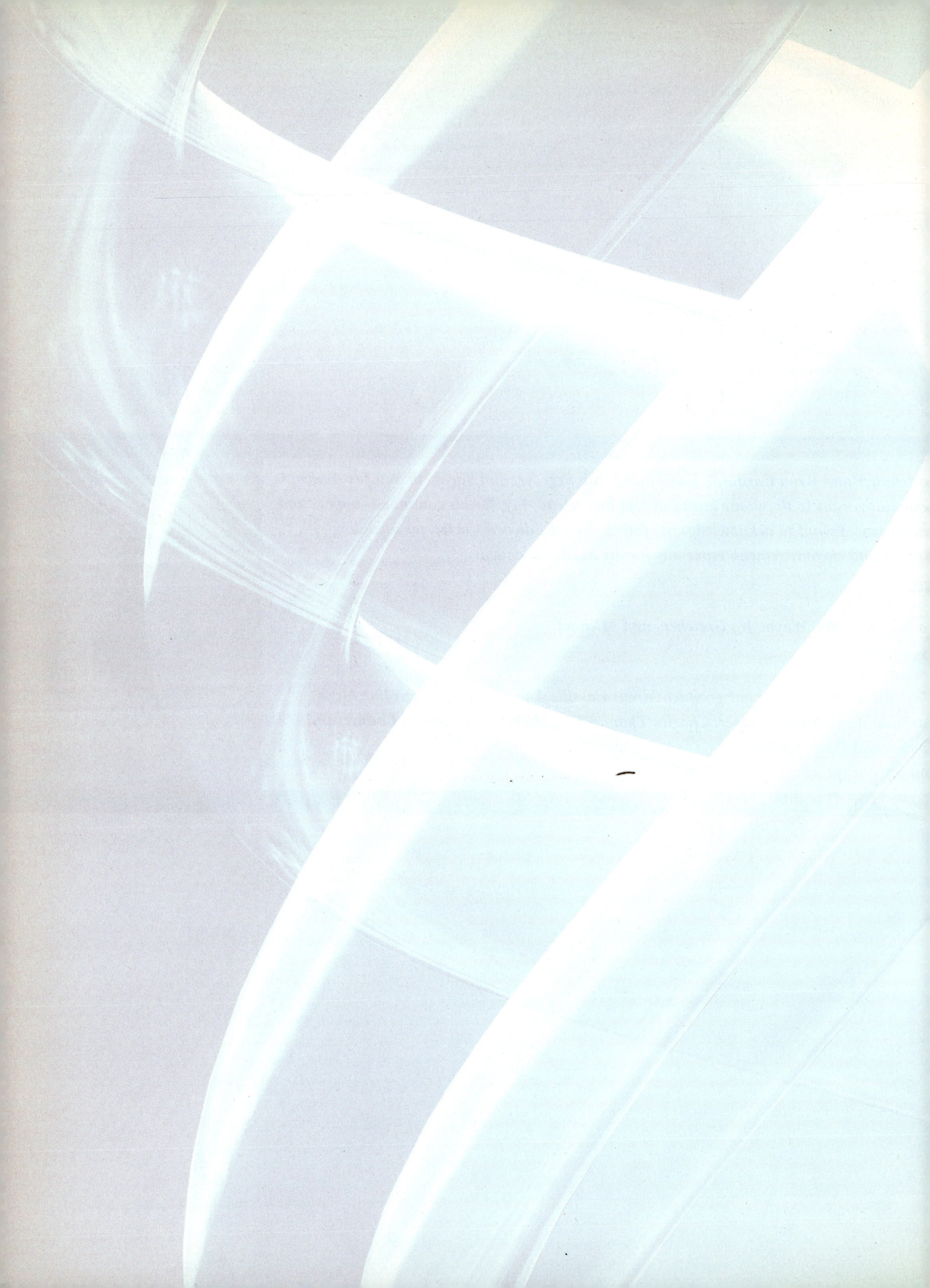

TABLE OF CONTENTS

CHAPTER 29

SAFETY, INFECTION CONTROL, AND HYGIENE / 653

CHAPTER 30

MEDICATION ADMINISTRATION / 749

LIST OF PROCEDURES

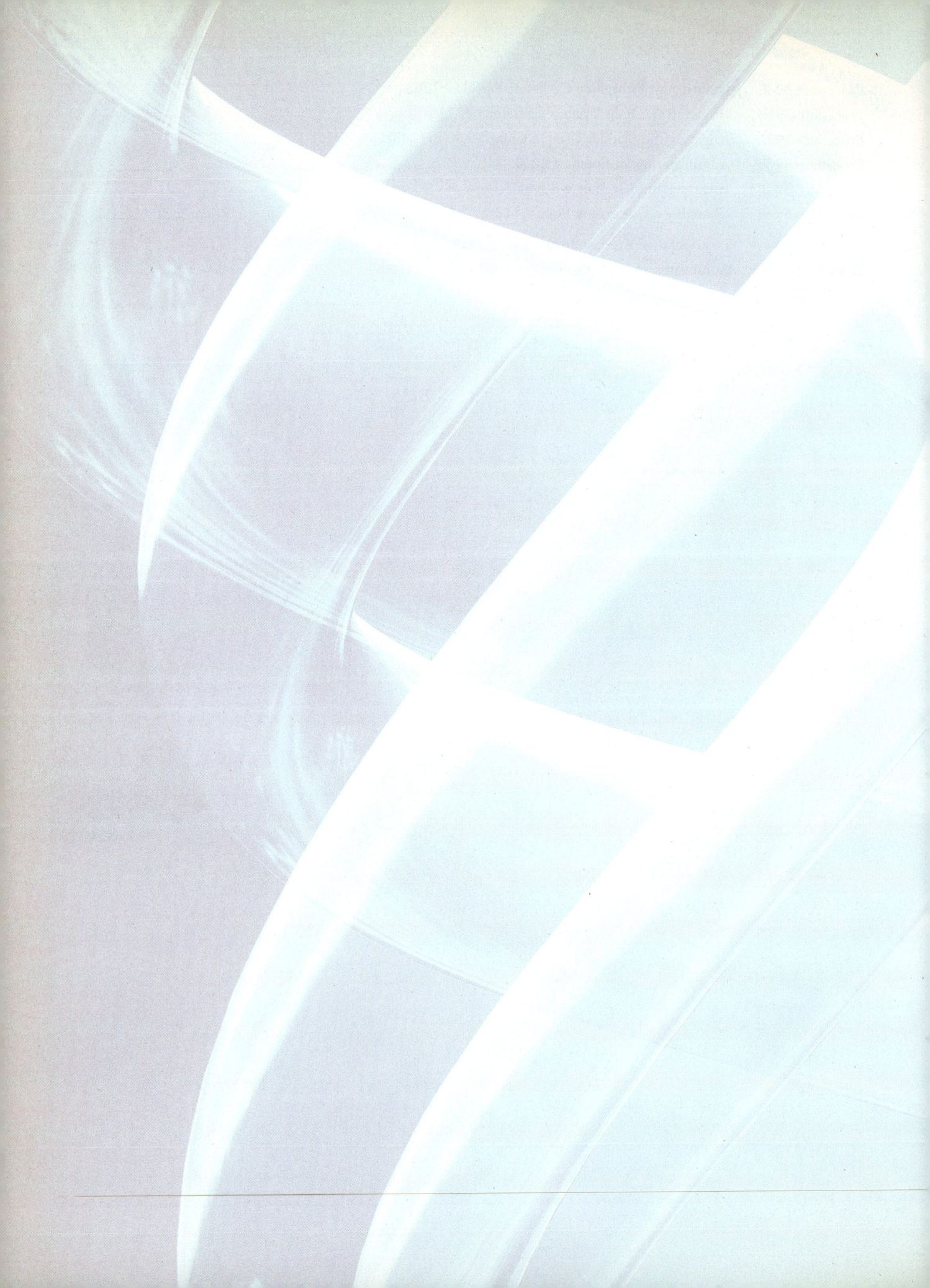

CONTRIBUTORS

Sheila L. Allen, BSN, RN, CNOR, CRNFA
Executive Board Member
International Federation of Perioperative Nurses
President
Association of Operating Room Nurses
Nashville, Tennessee

Carma Andrus, MN, RN, CNS
Dauterive Primary Care Clinic
St. Martinville, Louisiana

Billie Barringer, RN, CS, APRN
School of Nursing
Northeast Louisiana University
Monroe, Louisiana

Barbara Bihm, DNS, RN
Associate Professor of Nursing
Loyola University
New Orleans, Louisiana

Barbara Brillhart, PhD, RN, CRRN, FNP-C
College of Nursing
Arizona State University
Tempe, Arizona

Ali Brown, MSN, RN
Assistant Professor
College of Nursing
University of Tennessee
Knoxville, Tennessee

Virginia Burggraf, MSN, RN
Gerontological Nurse Consultant
Kensington, Maryland

Ann H. Cary, PhD, MPH, RN, A-CCC
Director, School of Nursing
Loyola University
New Orleans, Louisiana

Lissa A. Cash, MSN, RN, CCRN, CEN
Sentara Healthcare CU
Norfolk, Virginia

Beth Christensen, MN, RN, CCRN
Touro Infirmary
New Orleans, Louisiana

Jan Corder, DNS, RN
Dean, School of Nursing
Northeast Louisiana University
Monroe, Louisiana

Julie Coy, MS, RN
Pain Consultation Service
The Children's Hospital
Denver, Colorado

Mary Ellen Zator Estes, MSN, RN, CCRN
Assistant Professor
School of Nursing
Marymount University
Arlington, Virginia

Mary Frost, MS, RN, HNC, CHTP/I, CHt
Healing Touch Practitioner and Instructor
Covington, Louisiana

Norma Fujise, MS, RN, C
School of Nursing
University of Hawaii
Honolulu, Hawaii

Mikel Gray, PhD, FNP-BC, PNP-BC, CUNP, CCCN, FAANP, FAAN
Clinical Professor
University of Virginia School of Nursing
Charlottesville, Virginia

Janet Kula Harden, MSN, RN
Faculty
Wayne State University College of Nursing
Detroit, Michigan

T. Heather Herdman, PhD, RN
Executive Director
North American Nursing Diagnosis Association International

Lucille Joel, EdD, RN, FAAN
Professor
College of Nursing
Rutgers—State University of New Jersey
Newark, New Jersey

Georgia Johnson, MS, RN, CNAA, CPHQ
Director of Nursing
Southeast Louisiana Hospital
Mandeville, Louisiana

Claire Lincoln, MN, RN, CS
West Jefferson Mental Health Clinic
Marrero, Louisiana

Tina M. Liske, MSN, RN, CCRN, CNS, NP
SCCM, National AACN, Local AACN
Smithfield, Virginia

JoAnna Magee, MN, RN, FNP
Metairie, Louisiana

Judy Martin, MS, JD, RN
Nurse Attorney
Louisiana Department of Health and Hospitals
Health Standards Section
Baton Rouge, Louisiana

Linda McCuistion, PhD, RN
Assistant Professor
School of Nursing
Our Lady of Holy Cross College
New Orleans, Louisiana

Elizabeth "Betty" Hauck Miller, MPH, BSN, RN
Director of Education
Ochsner Hospital, Westbank
Gretna, Louisiana

Mary Anne Modrcin, PhD, RN
Dean and Professor
Caylor School of Nursing
Lincoln Memorial University
Knoxville, Tennessee

Barbara S. Moffett, PhD, RN
Director
School of Nursing
Southeastern Louisiana University
Hammond, Louisiana

Barbara Morvant, MN, RN
Executive Director
Louisiana State Board of Nursing
Baton Rouge, Louisiana

Cathy O'Byrne, MN, RN
Tulane University Hospital and Clinic
New Orleans, Louisiana

Brenda Owens, PhD, RN
Associate Professor
School of Nursing
Louisiana State University Medical Center
New Orleans, Louisiana

Roxanne Perucca, MS, RN, CRNI
Infusion Nurse Manager, Clinical Nurse Specialist
University of Kansas Hospital
Kansas City, Kansas

Demetrius Porche, DNS, RN, CCRN
Dean
School of Nursing
Louisiana State University Health Sciences Center
New Orleans, Louisiana

Suzanne Riche, MS, RN, C
Associate Professor
Delgado Community College
New Orleans, Louisiana

Mary W. Surman, BSN, RN, CNOR, CHT, CETN
Wound and Ostomy Unit, Our Lady of the Lake Regional
Medical Center
Baton Rouge, Louisiana

Cheryl Taylor, PhD, RN
Associate Professor of Nursing
Southern University
Baton Rouge, Louisiansa

Lorrie Wong, MS, RN
Instructor
Director for Simulation Learning
School of Nursing and Dental Hygiene
University of Hawaii at Manoa
Honolulu, Hawaii

Martha Yager, RN
Assistant Director of Nurses
Bennington Health and Rehabilitation Center
Bennington, Vermont

Rothlyn Zahourek, MS, RN, CS
Certified Clinical Nurse Specialist
Amherst, Massachusetts

REVIEWERS

Marie Ahrens, MS, RN
University of Tulsa
Tulsa, Oklahoma

Kay Baker, MSN, BSN
Pima Community College
Tucson, Arizona

Katie Ball, MSN, RN
Bellin College of Nursing
Green Bay, Wisconsin

Beth A. Beaudet, MS ed., MSN, FNP
Family Nurse Practitioner
Bassett Healthcare
Oneonta, New York

Mary Bliesmer, DNSc, MPH, BS, RN
Mankato State University
Mankato, Minnesota

Billie Bodo
Associate Professor of Nursing
Lakeland Community College
Mentor, Ohio

Lou Ann Boose, BSN, MSN, RN
Assistant Professor
Harrisburg Area Community College
Harrisburg, Pennsylvania

Bonita Cavanaugh, PhD, RN
University of Colorado
Denver, Colorado

Susan K. R. Collins, MSN, RN
Clinical Assistant Professor
Course Chair, Nursing Fundamentals
University of North Carolina at Greensboro
Greensboro, North Carolina

Dauna L. Crooks, DNS, RN
McMaster University
Hamilton, Ontario, Canada

Ernestine Currier
UCLA Center for the Health Sciences
Los Angeles, California

Debbie Dalrymple, MSN, RN, CRNI
Montgomery County Community College
Blue Bell, Pennsylvania

Sharon Decker, MSN, RN, CS, CCRN
Associate Professor of Clinical Nursing
School of Nursing
Texas Tech University Health Sciences Center
Lubbock, Texas

Toni S. Doherty, MSN, RN
Associate Professor
Department Head, Nursing
Dutchess Community College
Poughkeepsie, New York

Colleen Duggan, MSN, RN
Johnson County Community College
Overland Park, Kansas

Mary Lou Elder, MS, RN
Instructor of Nursing
Central Community College
Grand Island, Nebraska

Joanne M. Flanders, MS, RN
Midwestern State University
Wichita Falls, Texas

Kathy Frey, MSN, RN
University of South Alabama
Mobile, Alabama

Marcia Gellin, EdD, RN
Erie Community College
Buffalo, New York

Marilyn C. Handley, MSN, PhDc, RN
Instructor
University of Alabama
Capstone College of Nursing
Tuscaloosa, Alabama

Renee Harrison, MS, RN
Tulsa Junior College
Tulsa, Oklahoma

Susan Hauser, MSN, BA, RN
Mansfield General Hospital
Mansfield, Ohio

Judith W. Herrman, PhD, RN
Assistant Chair, Department of Nursing
University of Delaware
Newark, Delaware

Franklin Hicks, MSN, RN, CCRN
Marcella Niehoff School of Nursing
Loyola University
Chicago, Illinois

Kathleen Jarvis, MSN, BSN, RN
School of Nursing
California State University—Sacramento
Sacramento, California

Cecilia Jimenez, MSN, PhD, RN
Marymount University
Arlington, Virginia

Joan Jinks, MSN, RN
Eastern Kentucky University
Richmond, Kentucky

Patricia Jones, MSN, RN
Indiana State University
Terre Haute, Indiana

Jan Kinman, RN
Lane Community College
Eugene, Oregon

Anita G. Kinser, EdD, RN, BC
Assistant Professor
California State University at San Bernardino
San Bernardino, California

Marjorie Knox, MA, RN, MPA
Community College of Rhode Island
Lincoln, Rhode Island

Anne M. Larson, PhD, RN, C
Associate Professor of Nursing
Midland Lutheran College
Fremont, Nebraska

Hope B. Laughlin, BSN, MEd, EdD, MSN
Coordinator of Fundamentals of Nursing Courses
Pensacola Junior College
Pensacola, Florida

Patty Leary, MEd, RN
Mecosta Osceola Career Center
Big Rapids, Michigan

Denise LeBlanc
Humber College
Etobicoke, Ontario, Canada

Patricia M. Lester, MSN, RN
Associate Professor
Cumberland Valley Technical College
Pineville, Kentucky

Sharon Little-Stoetzel, MS, RN
Assistant Professor of Nursing
Graceland University
Independence, Missouri

Patricia Kaiser McCloud, BSN, MS, RN
University of Michigan
Ann Arbor, Michigan

Suzanne McDevitt, MSN, RN, CCRN
University of Michigan
Ann Arbor, Michigan

Chris McGeever
School of Nursing
St. Xavier University
Chicago, Illinois

Myrtle Miller, BSN, MA, RN
Assistant Professor
DeKalb College
Clarkson, Georgia

Maureen P. Mitchell, BScN, MN, RN
Center for Health Studies
Mount Royal College
Calgary, Alberta, Canada

Pertice Moffitt, BSN, RN
Aurora College
Yellowknife, Northwest Territories, Canada

Regina Nicholson, RN
Hospital for Joint Diseases
New York, New York

Katherine Bordelon Pearson, FNP, RN, CS
A. D. N. Department Faculty
Temple College
Temple, Texas

Edith Prichett, MSN, RN
Asheville-Buncombe Technical Community College
Asheville, North Carolina

Carol Rafferty, PhD, RN
Northeast Wisconsin Technical College
Green Bay, Wisconsin

Margaret P. Rancourt, MS, RN
School of Nursing
Quincy College
Quincy, Massachusetts

Anita K. Reed, MSN, RN
Instructor of Nursing
St. Elizabeth School of Nursing
Lafayette, Indiana

Neil Rheiner, MSN, EdD, RN
University of Nebraska
Omaha, Nebraska

Julia Robinson, RN, MS, FNP-C
Associate Professor
California State University
Bakersfield, California

Donna Roddy, BSN, MSN, RN
Chattanooga State Practical Nursing and Surgical
Technological Programs
Chattanooga, Tennessee

Julie Sanford, DNS, RN
Assistant Professor of Nursing
Spring Hill College
Mobile, Alabama

Ruth Schaffler, MSN, MA, RN, ARNP
Pacific Lutheran University
Tacoma, Washington

Barbara Scheirer, MSN, RN
Assistant Professor of Nursing
Grambling State University
Grambling, Louisiana

Sandy J. Shortridge, MSN, RN
Southwest Virginia Community College
Keenmtu, Virginia

Gail Smith, MSN, RN
Department of Nursing
Miami-Dade Community College
Miami, Florida

Maria A. Smith, DSN, RN, CCRN
School of Nursing
Middle Tennessee State University
Murfreesboro, Tennessee

Sharon Staib, MS, RN
Assistant Professor
Ohio University
Zanesville, Ohio

Janic Tazbir, RN, MS, CS, CCRN
Associate Professor of Nursing
Purdue University Calumet
Hammond, Indiana

Paula P. Thompson, BSN, RN
Educator
Carilion Roanoke Memorial Hospital
School of Practical Nursing
Roanoke, Virginia

Anita Thorne, MA, RN
Arizona State University
Tempe, Arizona

Elizabeth K. Whitbeck, MS, RN
Assistant Professor of Nursing
Maria College
Albany, New York

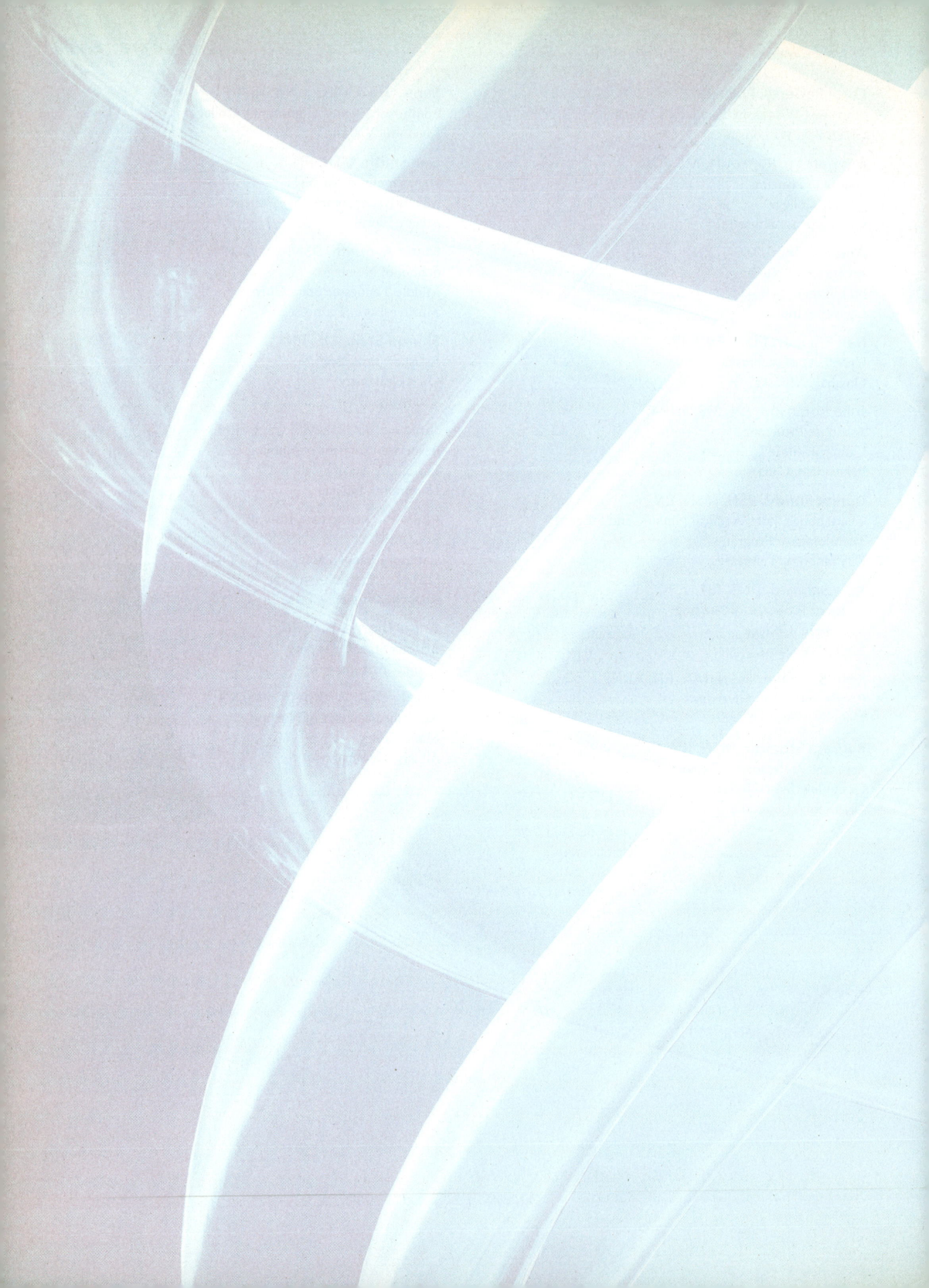

PREFACE

We are very excited to share the fourth edition of *Fundamentals of Nursing: Standards and Practice* with you! It is hoped that this text will encourage the student to develop an inquiring stance based on the joy of discovery and a love of learning.

Nursing is facing new challenges in delivering quality care to clients in a variety of settings. The settings for delivery of care are rapidly expanding and challenge nurses to think outside the box in applying best practices based on current research. This edition presents the most current advances in nursing care, nursing education, and research relative to the demands of delivering care across a continuum of settings. Multiple theories of nursing are embraced, and nursing's metaparadigm elements of theory—human beings, environment, health, and nursing—are threaded throughout this text. The organization of units and chapters is sequential; however, every effort has been made to allow for varying needs of diverse curricula and students. Each chapter may be used independently of the others according to the specific curriculum design.

This comprehensive edition addresses fundamental concepts and skills to help prepare novice graduate nurses to apply an understanding of human behavior to issues encountered in clinical settings. Physiological and psychosocial responses of both client and nurse are addressed in a holistic manner. Integrative modalities are presented in an environment that encourages clients to participate in determining their care.

Up-to-date clinical information is based on sound theoretical concepts and provides a rationale for practice. Scientific evidence is applied to the implementation of nursing interventions.

CONCEPTUAL APPROACH

This edition presents in-depth material in a clear, concise manner using language that is easy to read, by linking related concepts. Nursing knowledge is formulated on the basic concepts of scientific and discipline-specific theory, health and health promotion, the environment, holism, client teaching, spirituality, research and evidence-based practice, and the continuum of care. Emphasis is placed on cultural diversity, care of the older adult, and ethical and legal principles.

The nursing process provides a consistent approach for presenting information. Assessment tools specific to selected topics are presented to assist students with pertinent data collection. Therapeutic nursing interventions reflect standards of practice and emphasize safety, communication skills, interdisciplinary collaboration, and effective delegation in delivering nursing care. Critical thinking and reflective reasoning skills are integrated throughout the text. The safe and appropriate use of technology has been incorporated throughout the text to reflect contemporary nursing practice.

The conceptual approach used as an organizational framework for the fourth edition falls into four categories:

- **Individuals:** Viewed as holistic beings with multiple needs and strengths and the abilities to meet those needs. Holism implies that individuals are treated as whole entities rather than fragmented parts or problems. Each person is a complex entity who is influenced by cultural values, including spiritual beliefs and practices. Every person has the right to be treated with dignity and respect regardless of race, ethnicity, age, religion, socioeconomic status, or health status.
- **Environment:** A complex interrelationship of internal and external variables. Internal variables include one's self-concept, self-efficacy, cognitive development, and psychological traits. The external environment affects an individual's health status by facilitating or hindering the person's achievement of needs.
- **Health:** Viewed as a dynamic force that occurs on a continuum ranging from wellness to death. An individual's actions and choices affect changes in health status. Individuals who are experiencing illness have strengths that

may improve their health status. On the other hand, individuals who are experiencing a high degree of health generally have areas that can be improved.

- **Nursing:** An active, interpersonal, professional practice that seeks to improve the health status of individuals. Nursing's focus is person-centered and communicates a caring intent. Caring and compassion are demonstrated through nursing interventions. Nursing is a professional practice based on scientific knowledge and delivered in an artful manner.

Other important conceptual threads used to direct the development of this book include the following:

- **Health promotion** encourages individuals to engage in behaviors and lifestyles that facilitate wellness.
- **Standards of practice** are discussed, with information from national and specialty organizations incorporated into each chapter as appropriate.
- **Critical thinking** is an essential skill for blending science with the art of nursing.
- **Evidence-based practice,** which is derived from scientific research, is emphasized across chapters.
- **Cultural diversity** is defined as individual differences among people resulting from racial, ethnic, and cultural variables.
- **Continuum of care** is viewed as a process for providing health care services in order to ensure consistent care across practice settings.
- **Community,** as both an aggregate client and as the setting for delivery of care, is evidenced in Chapter 17 and in the Community Considerations critical thinking boxes threaded throughout the text.
- **Holism** recognizes the bodymind connection and views the client as a whole person rather than fragmented parts.
- **Spirituality**—one's relationship with one's self, a sense of connection with others, and a relationship with a higher power or divine source—is discussed in depth in Chapter 24.
- **Caring,** a universal value that directs nursing practice, is incorporated throughout the text, as well as described in depth in a separate chapter.
- **Alternative and complementary modalities** are treatment approaches that can be used in conjunction with conventional medical therapies. Chapter 31 is dedicated to this integrative approach, and related information featuring integrative concepts is included throughout the text.

ORGANIZATION OF TEXT

This textbook provides student nurses with a bridge that connects theory with clinical practice. The intent of the authors is to help students become proficient critical thinkers who are able to use the nursing process with diverse clients in a variety of settings. Research-based knowledge and clinical skills that reflect contemporary practice are presented in a reader-friendly, practical manner.

Features that challenge students to use critical thinking skills are incorporated into each chapter, and critical thinking questions appear at the end of each chapter. Critical information is highlighted throughout the text in a format that is easily accessed and understood. Similar concepts have been grouped together to encourage students to learn through association; this method of presentation also prevents duplication of content.

Fundamentals of Nursing: Standards and Practice, Fourth Edition, presents 40 chapters organized in six units:

- **Unit 1: Nursing's Perspective: Past, Present, and Future** provides a comprehensive discussion of nursing's evolution as a profession and its contributions to health care based on standards of practice. The theoretical frameworks for guiding professional practice and the significance of incorporating research into nursing practice are emphasized. Chapters are reflective of the parallel evolution of nursing and nursing education. Examples showing the incorporation of theory into the nursing process are provided. The concept of evidence-based practice is emphasized along with research utilization. Quality is discussed from the perspective of health care delivery and the continuum of care.
- **Unit 2: Nursing Process: The Standard of Care** discusses standards of care established by the American Nurses Association as well as nursing specialty organizations. Each stage of the nursing process is discussed with an emphasis on critical thinking.
- **Unit 3: Professional Accountability** describes the nurse's responsibilities to the client, the community, and the profession. The legal aspects of delegation are discussed in Chapter 11, and "Delegation Tips" are incorporated into each clinical procedure. Chapter 12 combines legal and ethical aspects of nursing practice to reflect the interfacing of these concepts. An in-depth discussion of informatics has been added to Chapter 13 on documentation.
- **Unit 4: Promoting Client Health** was created to integrate information on health promotion, consumer demand, and client empowerment. Chapter 14 provides nursing theoretical perspectives on caring. Chapter 16 emphasizes the nurse's role in empowering clients to assume more personal accountability for their health-related behaviors. Chapter 17 addresses the health needs of families and communities.
- **Unit 5: Responding to Basic Psychosocial Needs** stresses the importance of the holistic nature of nursing. Spirituality is spotlighted in order to emphasize its impact on individuals' health.
- **Unit 6: Responding to Basic Physiological Needs** discusses aspects of nursing care that are common to every area of nursing practice. Concepts such as safety and infection control, mobility, fluid and electrolyte balance, skin integrity, nutrition, and elimination are described within the nursing process framework.

NEW TO THIS EDITION

- Chapter 13, Documentation and Informatics, has an expanded discussion of the history and impact of technology on nursing practice.

- Free StudyWARE™ CD—with 3-D animations, NCLEX-style chapter quizzes, heart and lung sounds, and a medical terminology audio library—is included.
- NCLEX-style review questions have been added at the end of every chapter. Answers and rationales are located in the instructor's manual.
- Spotlight On is a new feature that focuses attention on issues relating to the caring, compassion, legal, ethical, and professional components of nursing practice.
- Safety First identifies critical health and safety situations and highlights strategies for the appropriate nursing response and management.
- Uncovering the Evidence emphasizes the importance of clinical research by linking theory to practice.
- Respecting Our Differences challenges the student to consider approaches to respectful and appropriate care for clients who may differ in a variety of ways including culture, gender, age, and developmental level.
- Evidence-based practice is highlighted across chapters as appropriate.

EXTENSIVE TEACHING/ LEARNING PACKAGE

The complete supplements package was developed to achieve two goals:

1. To assist students in learning the essential skills and competencies needed to secure a career in the area of nursing
2. To assist instructors in planning and implementing their programs for the most efficient use of time and other resources

ONLINE COMPANION

Delmar offers a series of Online Companions™ through the Delmar Web site: **www.delmarlearning.com/companions/ index.asp?isbn=1401859186**. The DeLaune/Ladner Online Companion enables users of *Fundamentals of Nursing: Standards and Practice,* Fourth Edition, to access a wealth of information designed to enhance the book. Included in the Online Companion are:

- Healthy People 2020 Guidelines
- Appendices, Educational Resources for Caregivers, and Recommended Dietary Allowances
- Concept maps
- HIPAA information

To access the site for *Fundamentals of Nursing: Standards and Practice,* Fourth Edition, simply point your browser to **www.delmar.cengage.com**. Click on Online Companions, and then select the nursing discipline.

STUDY GUIDE
ISBN 10: 1-4354-8068-6
ISBN 13: 978-1-4354-8068-6
Containing 500 sample questions in an easy-to-use format, this study aid builds on and reinforces the content presented

in the text. Students have an avenue to learn key concepts at a pace that is comfortable for them. Features include:

- Discussion Questions and Critical Thinking Challenges added to every chapter
- Various levels of difficulty
- Questions built upon the key concepts on a chapter-by-chapter basis

SKILLS CHECKLIST
ISBN 10: 1-4354-8069-4
ISBN 13: 978-1-4354-8069-8
This teaching/learning tool contains key steps for every procedure in *Fundamentals of Nursing: Standards and Practice,* Fourth Edition, by Sue C. DeLaune and Patricia K. Ladner. These checklists may be used to help students evaluate their comprehension and execution of the procedures. Key features include:

- Three categories to document performance: able to perform, able to perform with assistance, and unable to perform
- Comments section at each step for constructive feedback
- Easy-to-follow format

INSTRUCTOR RESOURCES
ISBN 10: 1-4354-8070-8
ISBN 13: 978-1-4354-8070-4
Free to all instructors who adopt *Fundamentals of Nursing: Standards and Practice,* Fourth Edition, in their courses, this comprehensive resource includes the following:

Instructor's Guide

- **Instructional Strategies**—Centered around the competencies at the beginning of each chapter, critical thinking questions, followed by a student activity (group and/or individual), are provided to enhance student comprehension and critical thinking skills.
- **Additional Resource Aids**—Additional audiovisual material, computer software, and Web sites are included to increase student awareness of current issues, trends, and skills.
- **Evaluation Strategies**—Discussion questions are provided for each chapter to enhance student writing and thinking skills.

Computerized Test Bank with Electronic Gradebook

- **Test Bank**—Computerized test bank includes over 1200 questions and reflects an NCLEX style of review, including rationales, cognitive level, and text reference.

PowerPoint Presentation

A vital resource for instructors, the slides created in Power-Point parallel the content found in the book, serving as a foundation on which instructors may customize their own unique presentations.

Image Library

The Image Library is a software tool that includes an organized digital library of more than 700 illustrations and photographs from the text. With the Image Library you can:

- Create additional libraries
- Set up electronic pointers to actual image files or collections
- Sort art by desired categories
- Print selected pieces

WebTutor Advantage

ISBN 10: 1-4354-8071-6
ISBN 13: 978-1-4354-8071-1

This online resource delivered on Blackboard offers value as a standard component to any fundamentals course. Correlated to the text, the WebTutor Advantage includes quizzes and discussion questions, 3-D animations, concept maps, a glossary, and instructor resources.

HOW TO USE THIS TEXT

The following suggests how you can use the features of this text to gain competence and confidence in your assessment and nursing skills.

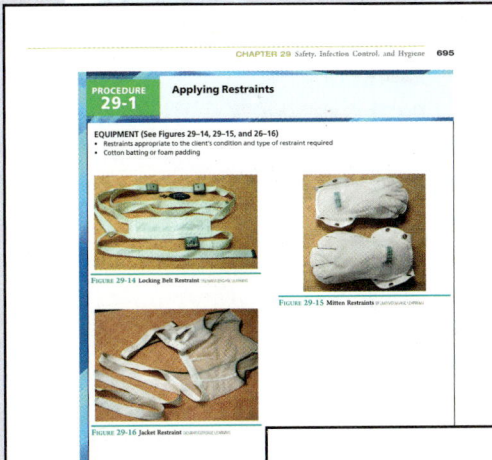

PROCEDURES

Procedure boxes are step-by-step guides to performing basic clinical nursing skills. This feature will help you gain competence in nursing skills. Use this feature as a study tool to help you understand the rationale behind the nursing interventions, as a guide for mastery of procedures, and as a review aid for future reference.

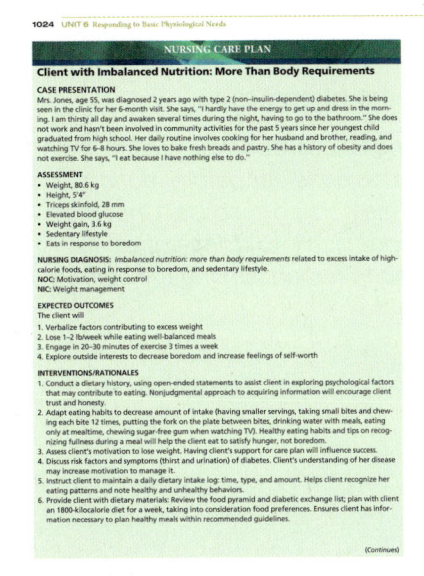

NURSING CARE PLAN

The Nursing Care Plan guides you through the process of planning care, performing interventions, and evaluating the outcomes of your plan of care. These are very helpful in strengthening your understanding of the nursing process in "live" nursing situations, in exercising your critical thinking skills, and for use as a blueprint from which to develop your own complete plans of care.

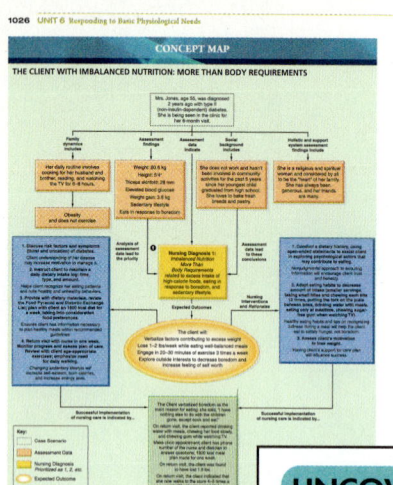

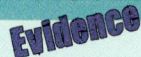

CONCEPT MAPS

Concept maps are used in this edition to visually illustrate five of the nursing care plans included in the text. The mapping process provides the learner with a non-linear option for problem-solving learning.

UNCOVERING THE Evidence

TITLE OF STUDY

"Patterns of Nursing Intervention Use across 6 Days of Acute Care Hospitalization for Three Older Patient Populations"

AUTHORS

L. L. Shever, M. Titler, J. Dochterman, Q. Fei, and D. M. Picone

PURPOSE

The purpose of this study was twofold: (1) to identify frequently used nursing interventions and (2) to describe patterns of interventions used for each of the three selected groups of clients.

METHODS

This secondary data analysis study used data from a medical center in which the Nursing Interventions Classification (NIC) was used to electronically document nursing care. Statistics were examined to determine the types, frequencies, and patterns of interventions used in providing care to older care recipients.

UNCOVERING THE EVIDENCE BOXES

These boxes emphasize the importance of clinical research in nursing by linking theory to practice. As a learning tool, they focus attention on current issues and trends in nursing.

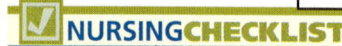

✓ NURSINGCHECKLIST

Critical Thinking

The following questions should be considered by the nurse in the development of a nursing diagnosis:

- Do I have enough data to formulate a nursing diagnosis?
- Are any data missing?
- Is there any information in my database that seems incomplete or uncertain?
- Should I talk to the client and family again?
- What data fit together or have something in common?
- What specific cues from the client made me form this conclusion?
- What elements of this situation, condition, or problem can be enhanced or resolved by therapeutic nursing interventions?
- What elements need to be referred to another discipline (e.g., medicine, social services, dietary)?

NURSING CHECKLIST

Nursing Checklist boxes outline important points for you to consider before, during, and after utilizing the nursing process. Checklists are your reference guide to using critical thinking in nursing and to understanding the steps in the nursing process.

▼ SAFETY FIRST ▼

It is absolutely critical to client safety that nursing students verbalize any questions or concerns relative to their assignments before instituting care. Students must ask for directions if unsure of their abilities.

👁 SPOTLIGHT ON...

Legal

Student Accountability

You are working as a nursing assistant (unlicensed personnel) during your school break. What would be your appropriate response if asked to perform a nursing procedure such as medication administration? Would the fact that you have performed the procedure previously as a nursing student affect your response?

✓ CLIENT TEACHING CHECKLIST

Actions of Parents to Promote Positive Self-Concept in Children

- Encourage expression of feelings.
- Promote mutual respect and trust by establishing and maintaining open lines of communication
- Demonstrate a willingness to talk about any subject.
- Listen carefully to children, and use words they understand.
- Use examples and anecdotes to promote learning.
- Teach by example. Role-model problem solving and coping skills.
- Encourage children's talents and accept their limitations. Be realistic in your expectations, and avoid comparing one child to another.
- Celebrate children's accomplishments.
- Demonstrate confidence in their abilities.
- Provide children with unconditional love.

COMMUNITY CONSIDERATIONS

Belief System

Culturally competent care requires the nurse to work within the client's cultural belief system to resolve health problems. This means that the nurse needs to hear the client and consider the client's world and daily experiences.

SAFETY FIRST

As a professional, you will need to be able to react immediately in some situations in order to ensure the health and safety of your patients. Pay careful attention to this feature as it will help you to begin to identify and respond to critical situations on your own, both efficiently and effectively.

SPOTLIGHT ON

This feature helps you to develop sensitivity to issues about the caring and compassion, legal/ethical, and professional components of nursing practice. You may choose to read through each one and explore the issues before reading the chapter. Then as you read through the chapter, readdress each Spotlight On and reevaluate your original thoughts. If you choose to read them as you go through the chapter, perhaps write your thoughts down, then go back and look at them at a later date.

CLIENT TEACHING CHECKLIST

As a nurse, you will often be a client's main link to health care. The Client Teaching Checklist is a great resource for ensuring success in teaching exercises and procedures and in relaying critical information to clients.

COMMUNITY CONSIDERATIONS

Community Considerations spotlight client care in the community environment. Guidelines for care, current trends and issues, and professional protocols are addressed throughout the text.

ACKNOWLEDGMENTS

This textbook is the product of many dedicated, knowledgeable, and conscientious individuals. First, we would like to thank Carol Ren Kneisl for initiating our work on this text. We would like to thank all the contributors who persevered to produce an outstanding contribution to the nursing literature. Your clinical expertise is evident in this final product.

Likewise, we need to thank all the reviewers who critically read and commented on the manuscript. Your clinical and academic expertise provided valuable suggestions that strengthened the text.

Our friends and professional colleagues provided encouragement throughout the development of this manuscript. A special thank you to Paulette Watts, BSN, RN, CNOR, of Mandeville, Louisiana, who served as a content specialist for Chapter 36, "Mobility." Thank you for sharing so many of your resources and support with us.

Our families deserve recognition for their daily queries relative to the book, which often stimulated humor, easing a sometimes tedious task. Special thanks to the DeLaune family: Jay; Jennifer, Ryan, Camille, and Caroline Cardinal; Katie and Jacob Segrave; and Sarabeth and Jay Accardo. Thanks also to Wayne, Kelly, Wayne Jr., Gretchen, and Michael for demonstrating daily understanding and support when the book had to be given priority.

ABOUT THE AUTHOR

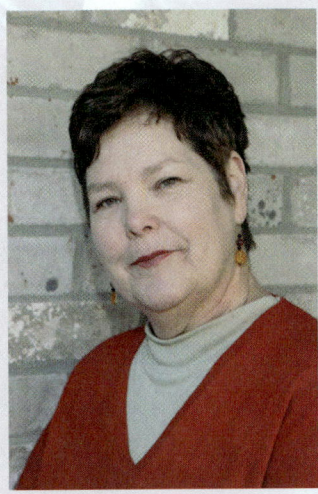

Sue Carter DeLaune earned a bachelor of science in nursing from Northwestern State University, Natchitoches, Louisiana, and a master's degree in nursing from Louisiana State University Medical Center, New Orleans. She has taught nursing in diploma, associate degree, and baccalaureate schools of nursing as well as in RN degree-completion programs. With over 35 years of experience as an educator, clinician, and administrator, Sue has taught fundamentals of nursing, psychiatric–mental health nursing, professionalism, and nursing leadership in a variety of programs. She also presents seminars and workshops across the country that assist nurses to maintain competency in areas of communication, leadership skills, client education, and stress management.

Sue is a member of Sigma Theta Tau, the National League for Nursing, and the American Nurses Association. She has been recognized as one of the "Great 100 Nurses" by the New Orleans District Nurses Association. Sue is a prolific author, having written several professional journal articles and textbook chapters in the areas of nursing education and mental health nursing.

Currently, Sue is an Associate Professor and RN-to-BSN Coordinator at William Carey University School of Nursing, New Orleans. She also is President of SDeLaune Consulting, an independent education consulting business based in Mandeville, Louisiana.

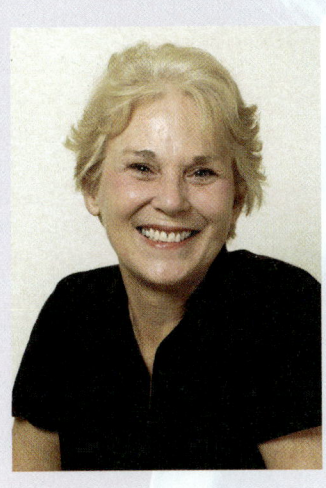

Patricia Ann Kelly Ladner obtained an associate degree in science from Mercy Junior College, St. Louis, Missouri; a bachelor of science in nursing from Marillac College, St. Louis, Missouri; a master of science in counseling and guidance from Troy State University, Troy, Alabama; and a master's degree in nursing from Louisiana State Medical Center, New Orleans, Louisiana.

She has taught at George C. Wallace Junior Community College, Dothan, Alabama; Sampson Technical Institute, Clinton, North Carolina; and Touro Infirmary School of Nursing and Charity/Delgado School of Nursing in New Orleans, Louisiana. She has also been the Director of Touro Infirmary School of Nursing and a Director of Nursing at Tulane University Medical Center in New Orleans. With 35 years as a clinician and academician, Ms. Ladner has taught fundamentals of nursing, medical-surgical nursing, and nursing seminars while maintaining clinical competency in various critical care and medical-surgical settings. Her professional career has provided her with the necessary knowledge and skills to be an effective lecturer and community leader.

Ms. Ladner received a governor's appointment to serve on an Advisory Committee of the Louisiana State Board of Medical Examiners, and she also served on an Advisory Committee for Loyola University in New Orleans. She maintains membership in Sigma Theta Tau, the American Nurses Association, and the Louisiana Organization of Nurse Executives. She served for over 10 years on the Louisiana State Nurses Association's Continuing Education Committee. She is the recipient of the New Orleans District Nurses Association Community Service Award and has been recognized as one of the "Great 100 Nurses" by the New Orleans District Nurses Association.

Ms. Ladner has been listed in *Who's Who in American Nursing*. She is a former Nursing Practice Consultant for the Louisiana State Board of Nursing.

Since Hurricane Katrina in 2004, Ms. Ladner has coordinated the volunteer services for the Catholic Church in DeLisle, Mississippi, and presented in-service education programs on such topics as hygiene, infection control, and grief and loss.

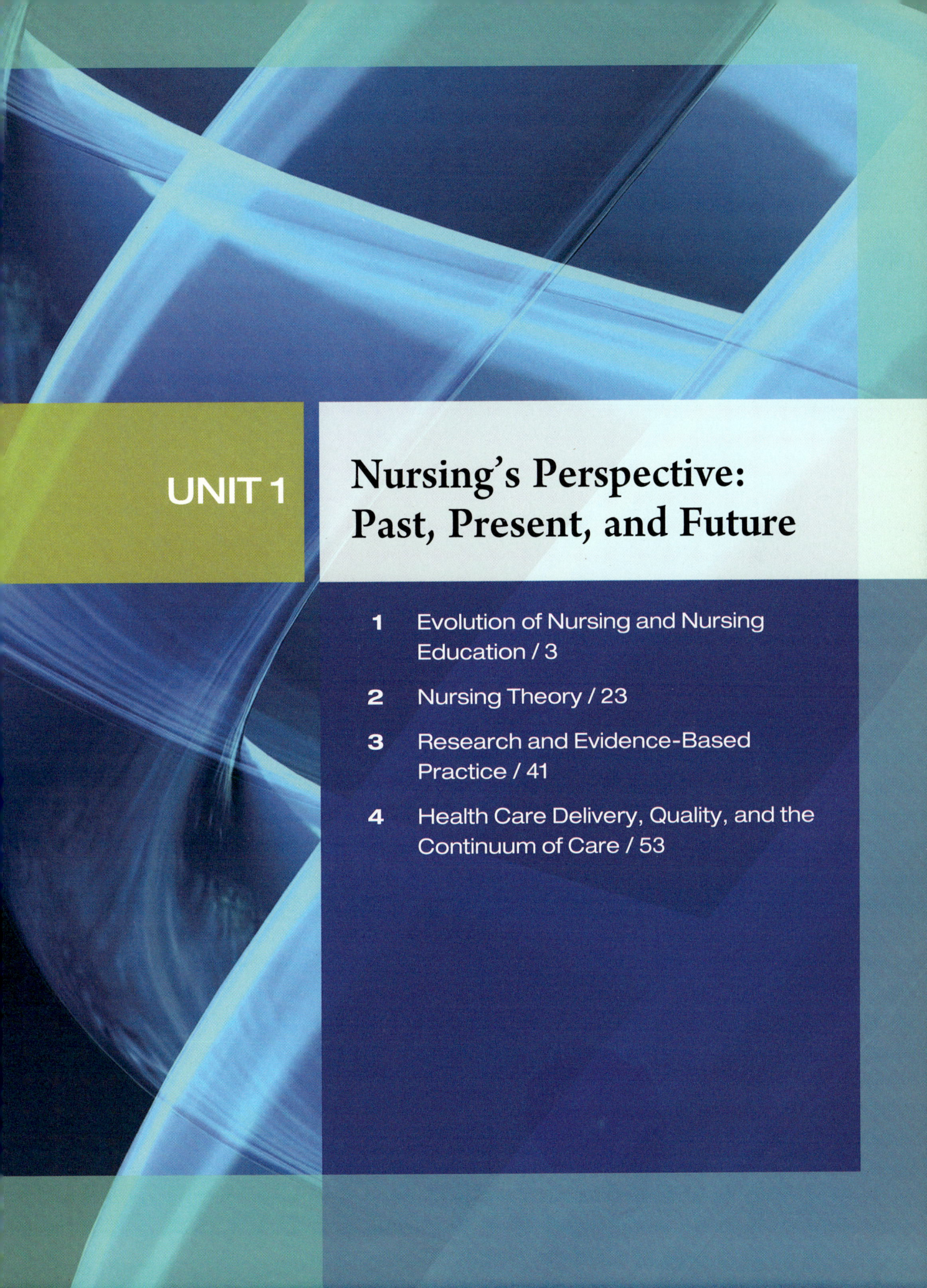

UNIT 1

Nursing's Perspective:
Past, Present, and Future

All history is modern history.

—WALLACE STEVENS,
AMERICAN POET AND AUTHOR (1879–1955)

CHAPTER 1

Evolution of Nursing and Nursing Education

COMPETENCIES

1. Define nursing as an art and a science.
2. Identify major historical and social events that have shaped current nursing practice.
3. Describe Florence Nightingale's impact on current nursing practice.
4. Discuss the contributions of early leaders in American nursing.
5. Discuss the impact of selected landmark reports on nursing education and practice.
6. Describe the characteristics of each of the educational programs for entry-level nursing practice.
7. Discuss the Health Care Professionals' Competencies document and the strategies proposed by the Pew Health Professions Commission for nursing education reform.
8. Describe the trends in nursing education that specifically relate to the issues of competency development and delivery of care.

KEY TERMS

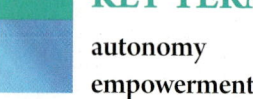

autonomy   history
empowerment   nurse

Nursing is an art and a science by which people are assisted in learning to care for themselves whenever possible and cared for by others when they are unable to meet their own needs.

Nursing has evolved from an unstructured method of caring for the ill to a scientific profession. The result has been movement from the mystical beliefs of primitive times to a "high-tech, high-touch" era. Nursing combines art and science. Using scientific knowledge in a humane manner, nursing combines critical thinking skills with caring behaviors.

Nursing requires a delicate balance of promoting clients' independence and dependence. Nursing focuses not on illness but rather on the client's *response* to illness.

Nursing promotes health and helps clients move to a higher level of wellness. This aspect of nursing also includes assisting a client with a terminal illness to maintain comfort and dignity in the final stage of life.

This chapter traces the evolution of nursing by exploring its rich heritage. Social forces that have affected the development of nursing and nursing education are examined. The various educational programs of the United States and Canada are presented in terms of their characteristics and the graduate's nursing role in health care delivery.

To understand the present status of nursing, it is necessary to have a base of historical knowledge about the profession. By studying nursing history, the nurse is better able to understand such issues as autonomy (being self-directed), unity within the profession, supply and demand, salary, education, and current practice. History is a study of the past that includes events, situations, and individuals (see Figure 1-1). By learning from historical role models, nurses can enhance their abilities to create positive change in the present and set a course for the future.

The study of nursing history offers another advantage—learning where the profession has been and its advancements. Empowerment is the process of enabling others to do for themselves. Only when nurses are empowered are they truly autonomous. Autonomy has historically been difficult for nurses to achieve. Empowerment and autonomy go together and are necessary for nursing to bring about positive changes in health care today (see Figure 1-2).

Learning from the past is the major reason for studying history. Ignoring nursing's history can be detrimental to the future of the profession. By applying the lessons gained from a historical review, nurses will indeed be a vital force in the new millennium.

EVOLUTION OF NURSING

Nursing has evolved with the development of the civilization of mankind. The term nurse stems from the Latin word *nutrix* or *nutrio,* which means to nourish. Primitive humans (cave dwellers) demonstrated knowledge regarding the medicinal value of plants and herbs and the therapeutic use of water and heat. Refer to Table 1-1 on page 5 and the following for a discussion of nursing from early civilizations to the present era of advanced nursing practice and health care reform.

ORIGINS OF NURSING

The evolution of nursing dates back to 4000 BC, to primitive societies in which mother-nurses worked with priests.

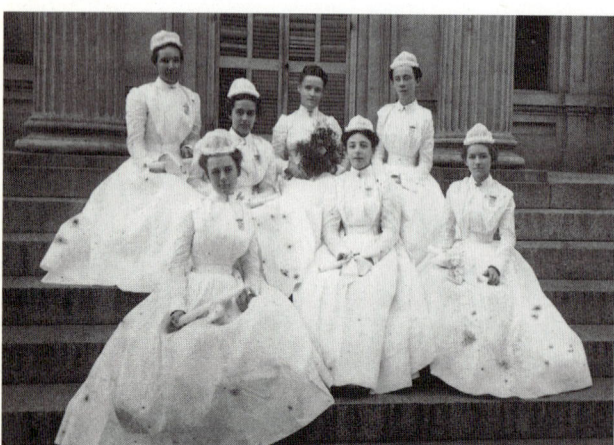

FIGURE 1-1 Graduating class (1900) of Touro Infirmary Training School for Nurses PHOTO COURTESY OF TOURO INFIRMARY ARCHIVES, NEW ORLEANS, LA

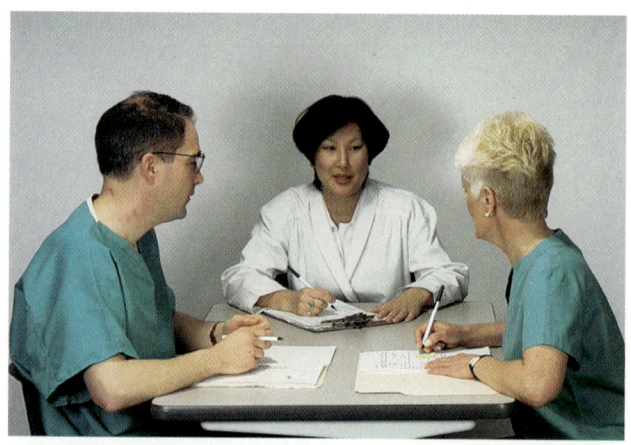

FIGURE 1-2 Through consultation and exchange of information, nurses demonstrate their roles as autonomous professionals. How important are the qualities of autonomy and empowerment to a nurse's career goals? DELMAR/CENGAGE LEARNING

TABLE 1-1 Historical Events Influencing the Evolution of Nursing

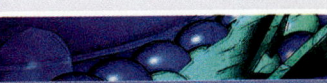

DATE	EVENT
4000 BC	Primitive societies
2000 BC	Babylonia and Assyria
800–600 BC	Health religions of India
700 BC	Greece: source of modern medical science
460 BC	Hippocrates
3 BC	Ireland: pre-Christian nursing
AD 390	Fabiola: founded first hospital
390–407	Early Christianity, deaconesses
711	Field hospital with nursing, Spain
1100	Ambulatory clinics, Spain (Moslems)
1440	First Chairs of Medicine, Oxford and Cambridge
1522	Military nursing orders
1600–1752	Deterioration of hospitals and nursing
1633	Founded: Daughters of Charity
1820	Florence Nightingale born
1826	Kaiserwerth deaconesses reestablished
1837	First American college for women, Mount Holyoke
1841	Founded: Nursing Sisters of the Holy Cross
1848	Women's Rights Convention, Seneca Falls, New York
1854–1856	Crimean War
1859	*Nightingale's Notes on Nursing* published in England
1860	First Nightingale School of Nursing, St. Thomas's Hospital, London
1861–1865	Civil War, United States
1863	Charter granted to the New England Hospital for Women, Boston
1871	New York State Training School for Nurses, Brooklyn Maternity, Brooklyn, New York
1872	New England Hospital for Women: 1-year program for nurses
	America's first trained nurse, Linda Richards
1873	First three Nightingale schools in United States: Bellevue (New York City), Connecticut, and Massachusetts General
1881	Founded: American Red Cross
1882	Founded: American Association of University Women
1888	Founded: International Council of Women (ICW)
	Founded: National Council of Women (NCW)
1893	First Nurses' Settlement House, New York City, founded by Lillian Wald and Mary Brewster
	Founded: first American Nursing Society, American Society of Superintendents of Training Schools for Nurses (Superintendents' Society)
1896	Founded: National Association of Colored Women
1896–1911	Founded: Nurses' Associated Alumnae of the United States and Canada (Associated Alumnae)
1899	Founded: International Council of Nurses (ICN)
	First postgraduate courses for nurses at Teachers College, Columbia University
1900	*American Journal of Nursing (AJN)*
1901–1912	Founded: American Federation of Nurses (Federation)
	Federation joined NCW and ICW
1903	New York: efforts failed to pass a nurse licensing law
	North Carolina: passed first state nurse registration law
	Founded: Army Nurse Corps
1905	Federation withdrew from NCW and joined ICN
1908	National Association of Colored Graduate Nurses (NACGN)
	Founded: Navy Nurse Corps
1909	Founded: first 3-year diploma school in a university setting at University of Minnesota
1910	Flexner report
1911	Founded: American Nurses Association (ANA), formerly the Associated Alumnae

(continues)

TABLE 1-1 (Continued)

DATE	EVENT
1912	Founded: National Organization of Public Health Nursing (NOPHN)
	Founded: National League of Nursing Education (NLN), formerly the Superintendents' Society
	ANA represented American nurses at ICN
	Nutting report: *Educational Status of Nursing*
	Developments in preventive medicine
	Founded: Town and Country Rural Nursing Service
1913	Founded: National Women's Party
1916	Founded: National Association of Deans of Women
1920	Founded: National League of Women Voters
	Congress passed the federal suffrage amendment
1920s	Depression: social programs and health insurance
	First prepaid medical plan, Pacific Northwest
	Founded: Bureaus of Medical Services
	Hospitals offered a prepaid plan
	Baylor Plan (prototype of Blue Cross)
	Goldmark report
1921	Women earned right to vote
1922	Studies of institutional nursing
1923	Studies of nursing education
	Founded: Yale University School of Nursing
1926	Burgess report
1933	American Hospital Association endorsed Blue Cross
1938	American Medical Association endorsed Blue Shield
	Economic Security Program for Nurses
1940	Cost studies of nursing education and service
1943	Founded: Federal Cadet Nurse Corps
1948	Brown report: *Future of Nursing*
1953	U.S. Public Health Services Studies in Nursing Education
1955	Practical Nursing (Title III) Health Amendment Act
1956	Hughes study: *20,000 Nurses Tell Their Stories*
1960s	Created: Medicare and Medicaid
1961	Surgeon General's Consultant Group
1964	Nurse Training Act
1965	First nurse practitioner program, pediatric
	ANA position paper on entry into practice
1966	Educational opportunity grants for nurses
1970	Secretary's commission to study extended roles for nurses
1973	Health Maintenance Organization Act
1977	Rural Health Clinic Service Act
	National Commission for Manpower Policy Study
1979	U.S. surgeon general report: *Healthy People*
1980	Omnibus Budget Reconciliation Act
1982	Budget cut to Health Maintenance Organization Act
	Tax Equity Fiscal Responsibility Act (TEFRA)
1983	Institute of Medicine Committee on Nursing and Nursing Education study
1987	Secretary's Commission on Nursing
1990s	Health care reform
1991	U.S. Department of Health and Human Services Healthy People 2000
1997	Agency for Health Care Policy and Research, now known as the Agency for Healthcare Research and Quality, established 12 evidence-based practice centers
2000	U.S. Department of Health and Human Services Healthy People 2010
2008	Centers for Medicare & Medicaid Services' "Never Events"

The first nurse to be recorded in history is Deborah. Deborah, referred to as a nurse, accompanied Rebekah when she left home to marry Isaac (Holy Bible, Gen. 24). In 2000 BC, the use of wet nurses is recorded in Babylonia and Assyria.

The ancient Greeks built temples to honor Hygiea, the goddess of health. These temples were more like health spas rather than hospitals in that they were religious institutions governed by priests. Priestesses (who were not nurses) attended to those housed in the temples. The nursing that was done by women was performed in the home.

Around 500 BC, Gautama, later known as Buddha, was born in India. Buddha founded many religious orders that later supported King Asoka in the establishment of homes that provided care. The basic nursing care was provided by male nurses.

The spread of Christianity had a profound influence upon nursing. The followers of Jesus spread Christianity throughout the entire world, and men and women who were committed to love of both the church and the poor and infirm dedicated their lives to caring for the ill.

Hospitals were first established in the Eastern Roman (Byzantine) Empire. St. Jerome was responsible, through one of his disciples, Fabiola, for introducing hospitals in the West. Western hospitals were primarily religious and charitable institutions housed in monasteries and convents. The caregivers had no formal training in therapeutic modalities and volunteered their time to nurse the sick.

The fall of the Roman Empire in 476 AD ushered in the Middles Ages, or medieval period (500–1450 AD), which was characterized by the growth of the Christian church. The Crusaders and religious orders traveled throughout Europe and the Near East with the mission of civilization and conversion. Because of their travels, commercial trade flourished and industries were developed to provide for trade in the world market. Universities were established, and monasteries provided impetus and leadership for the restructuring of the Western world.

Hospitals in large Byzantine cities were staffed primarily by paid male assistants and male nurses. During the medieval era, these hospitals were established primarily as almshouses, with care of the sick being secondary.

Medical practices in Western Europe remained basically unchanged until the eleventh and twelfth centuries, when formal medical education for physicians was required in a university setting. Although there were not enough physicians to care for all the sick, other caregivers were not required to receive any formal training. The dominant caregivers in the Byzantine setting were men; however, this was not true in the rural parts of the Eastern Roman Empire and in the West. In these societies, nursing was viewed as a natural nurturing job for women.

During the Renaissance (1400–1550 AD), interest in the arts and sciences emerged. This was also the time of many geographic explorations by Europeans. As a result, the world literally expanded.

Because of renewed interest in science, universities were established, but no formal nursing schools were founded. Because of social status and customs, women were not encouraged to leave their homes; they continued to fulfill the traditional role of nurturer and caregiver in the home.

The Industrial Revolution introduced technology that led to a proliferation of factories. Conditions for the factory workers were deplorable. Long hours, grueling work, and unsafe conditions prevailed in the workplace. The health status of laborers received little, if any, attention.

Medical schools were founded, including the Royal College of Surgeons in London in 1800. In France, men who were barbers also functioned as surgeons by performing procedures such as leeching, giving enemas, and extracting teeth.

At the end of the eighteenth century, there were no standards for nurses who worked in hospitals. In the early to mid-1800s, nursing was considered unseemly for women even though some hospitals (almshouses) relied on women to make beds, scrub floors, and bathe the poor. Most nursing care was still performed in the home by female relatives of the ill.

RELIGIOUS INFLUENCES

The strong influence of religions on the development of nursing started in India (800–600 BC) and flourished in Greece and Ireland in 3 BC with male nurse-priests. The Crusades of the medieval era led to the formation of three primary military orders: the Knights of St. John, the Teutonic Knights, and the Knights of Lazarus. These military orders cared for their wounded peers and built hospitals. The Knights of St. John, also called Knights Hospitalers, still have a viable organization in England today; because of their involvement in the International Red Cross, the insignia of their order was adopted for use by the Red Cross. The Teutonic Knights were established in the early twelfth century in a German hospital in Jerusalem; only men could be full members of the order, though women were granted sisterhood. The Knights of Lazarus was founded to care for the lepers in Jerusalem; when leprosy began to abate, the order was taken over by the Knights of St. John.

In 1836, Theodor Fleidner revived the Church Order of Deaconesses to care for those in a hospital he had founded. These deaconesses of Kaiserwerth became famous because they were the only ones formally trained in nursing. Pastor Fleidner had a profound influence on nursing because Florence Nightingale received her nurse's training at the Kaiserwerth Institute.

The Nursing Sisters of the Holy Cross was founded in LeMans, France, by Father Bassil Moreau in 1841. Father Sorin brought four sisters to Notre Dame in South Bend, Indiana, in 1841. In 1844, these sisters established St. Mary's Academy in Bertrand, Michigan. In 1855, the school was moved to Notre Dame and became known as Saint Mary's College, which became influential on the emerging role of women.

DEMANDS OF WAR

Historically, the demand for nurses has increased during wartime. During the Crimean War (1854–1856) orders of nursing sisters provided care to French and Russian soldiers, but there were no organized services to care for the wounded and sick British soldiers. When the British people learned of their soldiers' poor care, it led to public outcry. The secretary of war, Sir Sidney Herbert, contacted Florence Nightingale for assistance. Nightingale and the recruits were assigned to a barrack hospital in Scutari, Turkey. Using her own private allowance, Nightingale purchased needed supplies, made changes, and within 6 months lowered the death rate from 50%–60% to 2%.

America's need for nurses increased dramatically during the Civil War (1861–1865). The sisters of the Holy Cross were the first to respond to the need for nurses during that war. Answering a request of Indiana's governor, 12 sisters started caring for wounded soldiers. By the end of the war, 80 sisters had cared for soldiers in Illinois, Missouri, Kentucky, and Tennessee.

During the Civil War, nursing care was provided by the Sisters of Mercy, Daughters of Charity, Dominican Sisters, and Franciscan Sisters of the Poor. The sisters were influenced by the roles assigned to women during the nineteenth century. Although they were submissive to authority, they were willing to take risks when human rights were threatened. Women volunteered to care for the soldiers of both the Union and Confederate armies (see Figure 1-3). These women performed various duties, including the implementation of sanitary conditions in field hospitals.

Several individuals are recognized for their nursing contributions during the Civil War: Clara Barton, Dorothea Dix, Harriet Tubman, and Sojourner Truth. Clara Barton, a schoolteacher who volunteered as a nurse during the war, was referred to as the "Angel of the Battlefield" for rendering care in field hospitals. In 1881, Clara Barton established the American Association of the Red Cross and served as its first president. Dorothea Dix (1802–1887), a change agent in government reforms for humane treatment in mental hospitals, volunteered as a nurse when the Civil War began and was appointed the Superintendent of Women Nurses for all military hospitals, the first U.S. Army Nurse Corps.

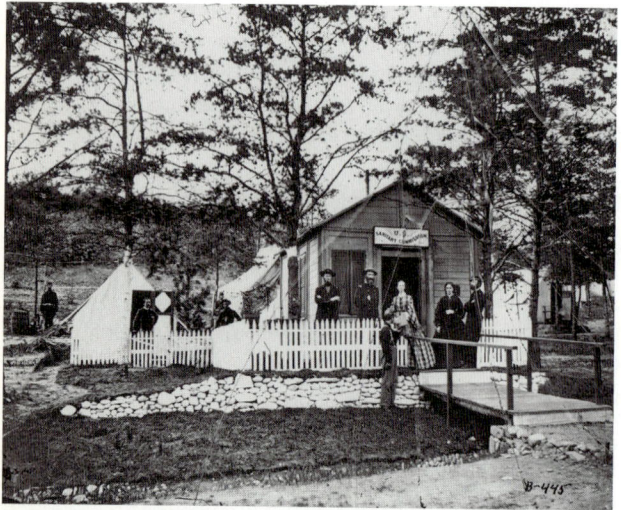

FIGURE 1-3 During the Civil War, women were instrumental in the effort to minimize the risk of spreading contagious diseases among wounded soldiers. PHOTO COURTESY OF CORBIS-BETTMANN

Harriet Tubman (1820–1913) was known as the "Moses of Her People" for her work with the underground railroad; during the Civil War, she served as a nurse for people of her own race. Sojourner Truth (1797–1883), underground railroad agent, preacher, and women's rights advocate, was a nurse during the Civil War and after the war for the Freedmen's Relief Association.

Following the Civil War, nurse training in the United States and Canada began to use curricula patterned after that of the Nightingale School. The first nursing program in Canada, St. Catherine's in Ontario, was founded in 1874.

Again war entered the picture. The casualties of World War II (1939–1945) created an acute nursing shortage. The Cadet Nurse Corps was established during World War II to provide additional nurses to meet both military and civilian needs. The Corps' training for nurses was shorter than the typical civilian education of 3 years. During this time, auxiliary workers such as licensed practical nurses were created to work under the supervision of registered nurses.

During early wars, nurses often found themselves on the front lines administering physical and spiritual care to wounded soldiers with limited supplies and medicine. The nurse would apply pressure to stop the bleeding, assure the soldier someone would stay at his side, pray with the soldier, or write a letter for the soldier. How would a nurse demonstrate caring in a situation such as September 11?

FLORENCE NIGHTINGALE (1820–1910)

Florence Nightingale is considered the founder of modern nursing. She grew up in a wealthy upper-class family in England during the mid-1800s. Unlike other young women of her era, Nightingale received a thorough education including Greek, Latin, history, mathematics, and philosophy. She had always been interested in relieving suffering and caring for the sick. Social mores of the time made it impossible for her to consider caring for others because she was not a member of a religious order. She became a nurse over the objections of society and her family.

After completing the three-month course of study at Kaiserwerth Institute, Nightingale became active in reforming health care. The advent of Britain's war in the Crimea presented the stage for Nightingale to further develop the public's awareness of the need for educated nurses (see Figure 1-4 on page 9). The implementation of her principles in the areas of nursing practice and environmental modifications resulted in reduced morbidity and mortality rates during the war.

Nightingale forged the future of nursing education as a result of her experiences in training nurses to care for British soldiers. In 1860 she opened the Training School of Nurses at St. Thomas's Hospital in London. This was the first school for nurses that provided both theory-based knowledge and clinical skills. Nightingale revolutionized not only the public's perception of nursing but also the method for educating nurses. Some of her novel beliefs about nursing education were:

- A holistic framework inclusive of illness and health
- The need for a theoretical basis for nursing practice

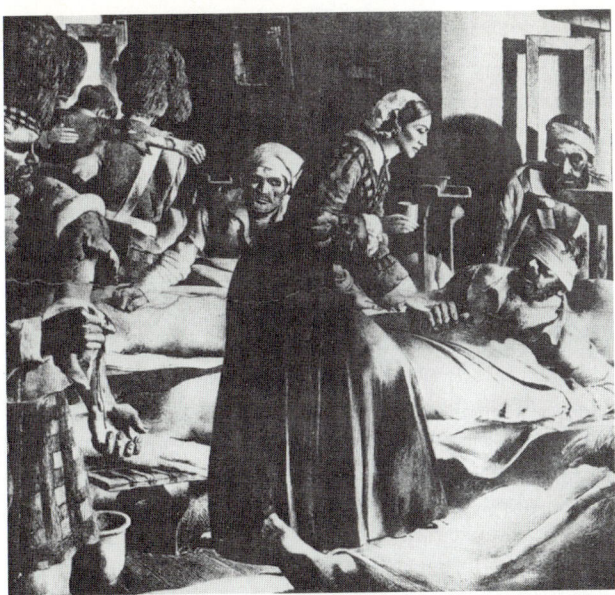

FIGURE 1-4 **Florence Nightingale in the Crimea** PHOTO COURTESY OF PFIZER, INC.

- A liberal education as a foundation for nursing practice
- The importance of creating an environment that promotes healing
- The need for a body of nursing knowledge distinct from medical knowledge (Nightingale, 1969)

Nightingale introduced many other concepts that, though unique in her time, are still used today; for example, she advocated (1) having a systematic method of assessing clients, (2) individualizing care on the basis of the client's needs and preferences, and (3) maintaining confidentiality.

Nightingale also recognized the influence of environmental factors on health. She advocated that nurses provide clean surroundings with fresh air and light to improve the quality of care (Nightingale, 1969). Nightingale believed that nurses should be formally educated and should function as client advocates.

NURSING PIONEERS AND LEADERS

In 1848, the Women's Rights Convention in Seneca Falls, New York, signaled the beginnings of social unrest. Women were not considered equal to men, society did not value education for women, and women did not have the right to vote. With suffrage, not only were the rights of women advocated but also the nursing profession itself advanced. By the mid-1900s, more women were being accepted into colleges and universities, even though only limited numbers of university-based nursing programs were available.

Modern nursing was forged by the contributions of many outstanding nurses through the years. The establishment of public health nursing, the provision of rural health care services, and the advancement of nursing education occurred as a result of the works of nurse pioneers, who are discussed in the text that follows. Note that the term *trained nurse* was used historically as the predecessor of *registered nurse*.

Lillian Wald

Lillian Wald spent her life providing nursing care to the indigent population. In 1893, as the first community health nurse, she founded public health nursing with the establishment of the Henry Street Settlement Service (see Figure 1-5) in New York City. Wald was a tireless reformer who:

- Improved housing conditions in tenement districts
- Supported education for the mentally challenged
- Advocated passage of more lenient immigration regulations
- Initiated change of child labor laws and founded the Children's Bureau of the U.S. Department of Labor

In addition to initiating public health nursing, Wald also established a school of nursing.

Isabel Hampton Robb

Isabel Hampton Robb was responsible for founding several nursing organizations, namely, the Superintendents' Society in 1893 and the Nurses' Associated Alumnae of the United States and Canada in 1896. She recognized the necessity of nurses participating in professional organizations to establish unity throughout nursing on positions and issues. She was instrumental in establishing both the American Nurses Association (ANA) and the National League of Nursing Education. Robb was also an early supporter of the rights of

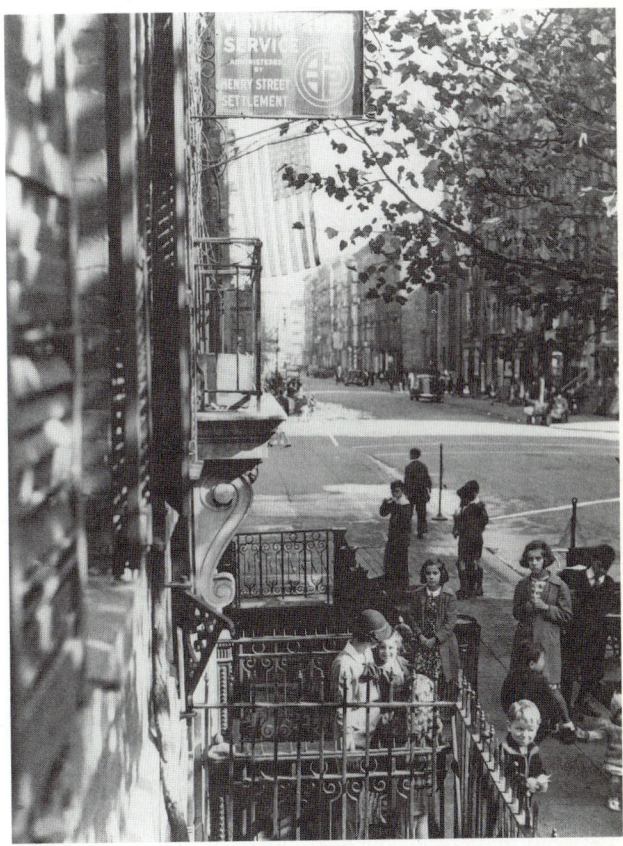

FIGURE 1-5 **Nurses at the Henry Street Settlement in New York City** PHOTO COURTESY OF VISITING NURSES SERVICE OF NEW YORK

nursing students. She called for shorter working hours and emphasized the role of the nursing student as learner instead of employee.

Jane Delano

During World War I, Jane Delano, a graduate of Bellevue School of Nursing and former ANA president, took one of the first stances that created a division among nursing leaders. In 1912, physicians wanted the Red Cross to put untrained nursing aides at their sides to assist with war casualties. Physicians, not nurses, would train the aides in caring for the sick.

Delano was opposed to the aide education plan because it violated the educational standards already established by nursing. This position pitted Delano against Annie Goodrich and Adelaide Nutting. The Red Cross recognized Delano's leadership abilities and dropped the aide plan. Delano was active in the Army Nurse Corps until she resigned her Army position in 1912 to work full time with the Red Cross. She died during wartime service in Europe.

Annie Goodrich

Annie Goodrich was influential in national and international nursing issues. During World War I, the supply of civilian nurses was greatly depleted because of the army's need for trained nurses. Goodrich pushed for the establishment of an army training school for nurses, which she envisioned as a model for other schools of nursing. She then was appointed dean of the Army School of Nursing. As an advocate of college-based educational nursing programs, Goodrich became the first dean of Yale University School of Nursing.

Adelaide Nutting

Adelaide Nutting was a nursing educator, historian, and scholar. She actively campaigned for nurses being educated in university settings and was the first nurse to be appointed to a university professorship. In 1910, Nutting was appointed to direct the newly established Department of Nursing and Health at Teachers College, Columbia University, in New York City. This department was established to prepare nurses for teaching and supervision in nurse training schools, for administration in hospitals, and for work in preventive and social aspects of nursing.

Lavinia Dock

An influential leader in American nursing education was Lavinia Dock, who graduated from Bellevue Training School for Nurses in 1886. In her early nursing practice, she worked at the Henry Street Settlement House in New York City providing visiting nursing services to the indigent. She wrote one of the first nursing textbooks, *Materia Medica for Nurses*. Dock wrote many other books and was the first editor of the *American Journal of Nursing (AJN)*. Dock was a political activist who in 1914 encouraged nurses to unite when physicians objected to reforming labor laws to include nursing students.

Mary Breckinridge

In 1925, Mary Breckinridge introduced a system for delivering health care to rural America. She created a decentralized system for primary nursing care services in the Kentucky Appalachian Mountains. This system, the Frontier Nursing Service, lowered the childbirth mortality rate in Leslie County, Kentucky, from the highest in the nation to below the national average.

Martha Franklin

Martha Franklin was one of the first people to advocate racial equality in nursing. She was the only African American graduate of her class at Women's Hospital Training School for Nurses in Philadelphia. In 1908, Franklin organized the National Association of Colored Graduate Nurses (NACGN), which advocated that black nurses meet the same standards required of other nurses to prevent a double standard based on race. In 1951, the NACGN merged with the ANA.

Amelia Greenwald

Amelia Greenwald was a pioneer in public health nursing on the international scene. In 1908, she entered the Touro Infirmary Training School for Nurses in New Orleans, Louisiana. After graduation, Greenwald studied psychiatric and public health nursing. She served as chief nurse in several field hospitals during World War I. In 1923, she accepted the challenge of establishing a school of nursing in Poland. She received the Polish Golden Cross of Merit for her contributions to the welfare of the people. Greenwald was a catalyst for international public health nursing.

Mamie Hale

In 1942, Mamie Hale was hired by the Arkansas Health Department to upgrade the educational programs for midwives (see Figure 1-6 on page 11). Hale, a graduate of the Tuskegee School of Nurse-Midwifery, gained the support of granny midwives, public health nurses, and obstetricians. Through education, Hale decreased the superstition and illiteracy of those functioning as midwives. Hale's efforts resulted in improved mortality rates for both mothers and infants.

Mary Mahoney

America's first African American professional nurse, Mary Mahoney, was a noted nursing leader who encouraged a respect for cultural diversity. Today, the ANA bestows the Mary Mahoney Award in recognition of individuals who make significant contributions toward improving relationships among multicultural groups.

Harriet Neuton Phillips

Harriet Neuton Phillips was the first known graduate of the Women's Hospital of Philadelphia. A six-month training course for nurses had been established by Dr. Ann Preston in 1861. Although no formal diplomas were awarded, the graduate nurses worked in the hospital and did private duty

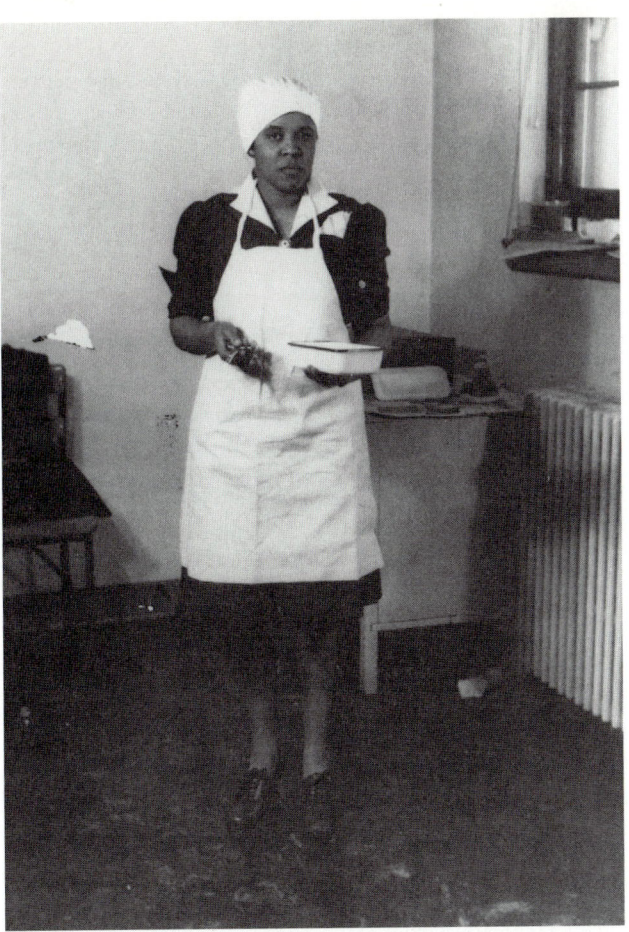

FIGURE 1-6 Mamie Hale PHOTO COURTESY OF HISTORICAL RESEARCH CENTER, UNIVERSITY OF ARKANSAS FOR MEDICAL SCIENCES LIBRARY, LITTLE ROCK

nursing in homes. Thus, Harriet Phillips can claim the title of the first American nurse to receive a training certificate. As a pioneer in community nursing, she worked with Chinese immigrants in San Francisco and with Native Americans in Wisconsin.

Linda Richards

In 1873, the first diploma from an American training school for nurses was awarded to Linda Richards. Richards founded or reorganized 10 hospital-based training schools for nurses. She introduced the practice of keeping nurses' notes and physicians' orders as part of medical records. Also, Richards began the practice of nurses wearing uniforms. As the first superintendent of nurses at Massachusetts General Hospital, she demonstrated that trained nurses gave better care than those without formal nursing education.

Margaret Sanger

In 1912, Margaret Sanger, a nurse living in New York City, became concerned with women who had too many children to support. She coined the phrase "birth control" and began writing about contraceptive measures. Sanger fought to revise legislation that prohibited dissemination of information about contraception.

Sanger was not afraid of controversy and spent 1 month in jail for distributing information on birth control. As a true activist, Sanger made birth control an issue and fought for the rights of poor women. She understood the relationship between poverty, overpopulation, and high infant and maternal mortality rates. Sanger founded the American Birth Control League and was the first president of the International Planned Parenthood Federation.

Adah Belle Thoms

Adah Belle Thoms was a crusader for improved relationships among persons of all races. In the early 1900s, she became acting director of nursing of the Lincoln School for Nurses in New York when African Americans rarely held high-level positions (Chinn, 1994). Thoms was one of the first to recognize public health as a field of nursing. She campaigned for equal rights for black nurses in the American Red Cross and the Army Nurse Corps.

NURSING IN THE TWENTIETH CENTURY

The beginning of the twentieth century brought about changes that have influenced contemporary nursing. Several landmark reports about medical and nursing education, as well as some contemporary reports, are discussed in the following text. The establishment of visiting nurse associations and their use of protocols are discussed.

Flexner Report

With the support of a Carnegie grant in 1910, Abraham Flexner visited the 155 medical schools throughout the United States and Canada to assess the level of accountability in medical education and to bring about necessary reforms. The Flexner report brought about the following changes: closure of inadequate medical schools, consolidation of schools with limited resources, creation of nonprofit status for the remaining schools, and establishment of medical education in university settings based on standards and strong economic resources.

Adalaide Nutting saw the value and impact of the Flexner report on medical education and, in 1911, together with other colleagues of the Superintendents' Society, presented a proposal to the Carnegie Foundation to study nursing education. This foundation never allocated monies to study nursing education, but it supported educational studies in other disciplines such as law, dentistry, and teaching.

Although the efforts of Nutting and other nursing leaders went unheeded, in 1906 Richard Olding Beard successfully established a three-year diploma school of nursing at the University of Minnesota under the College of Medicine.

Early Insurance Plans

At the turn of the twentieth century, there were more than 4,000 hospitals and 1,000 schools of nursing. During this time, the concepts of third-party payments and prepaid health insurance were instituted. Third-party payments refer to situations in which someone other than the recipient of health care (usually an insurance company) pays for the health care services provided. Prepaid medical plans were started in Pacific Northwest lumber and mining camps, where employers contracted for and paid a monthly fee for medical services. This led to the establishment of the Bureau of Medical Services, where the employer contracted for medical services and the subscriber selected one of the physicians in the bureau.

BLUE CROSS AND BLUE SHIELD.   The Depression provided the main impetus for the growth of insurance plans. In addition, the American philosophy of health care for all contributed to the growth of insurance plans. In 1920, American hospitals offered a prepaid hospital plan that led to the "Baylor Plan," which eventually became the prototype of Blue Cross.

Blue Cross was the result of a joint venture between hospitals, physicians, and the general public. The American Hospital Association (AHA) pioneered the development of an insurance company to provide benefits to subscribers who were hospitalized. Blue Shield was developed by the American Medical Association (AMA) to provide reimbursement for medical services provided to subscribers. In 1933, the AHA endorsed Blue Cross, and in 1938 the AMA endorsed Blue Shield.

The federal government became more involved in health care delivery in 1935 with the passage of the Social Security Act, which provided for (among other things) benefits for the elderly, child welfare, and federal funding for training of health care personnel. During World War II, the U.S. government extended the benefits for military services to include health care for veterans and their dependents.

VISITING NURSES ASSOCIATIONS.   In 1901, at the suggestion of Lillian Wald, the Metropolitan Life Insurance Company, which provided visiting nursing services to its policyholders, entered into an agreement with the Henry Street Settlement. Wald worked with Metropolitan to expand the services of the Henry Street Settlement to other cities; thus, one form of managed care began.

Nurses providing care in the home environment experienced greater autonomy of practice than hospital-based nurses (see Figure 1-7). This led to conflicts with some physicians regarding the scope of medical practice versus nursing practice parameters. Some physicians thought nurses were taking over their practice, whereas other physicians encouraged nurses to do whatever was necessary to care for the sick at home.

In 1912, in an effort to provide direction to home health staff nurses, the Chicago Visiting Nurse Association developed a list of standing orders for nurses to follow in providing home care. These orders were to direct the nursing care of clients when the nurse did not have specific orders from a physician. Thus, the groundwork for nursing protocols was established.

Landmark Reports in Nursing Education

During the first half of the twentieth century, a number of reports were issued concerning nursing education and practice. Three of them, the Goldmark, the Brown, and the Institute of Research and Service in Nursing Education reports, are discussed here.

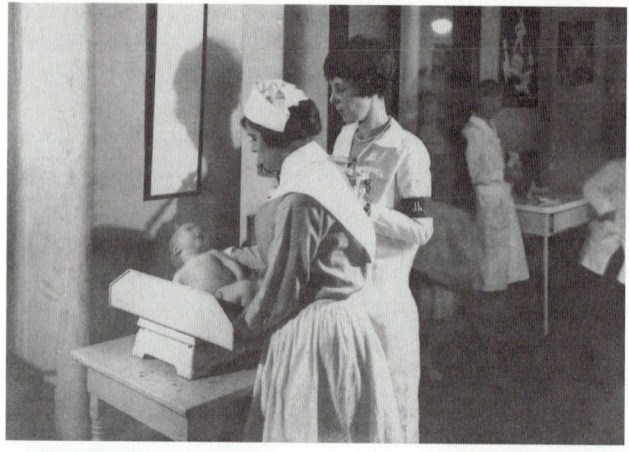

FIGURE 1-7 A baby being weighed by a student nurse and a Junior League volunteer in 1929 PHOTO COURTESY OF TOURO INFIRMARY ARCHIVES, NEW ORLEANS, LA

GOLDMARK REPORT.   In 1918, Adelaide Nutting, relentless in her efforts to document the need for nursing education reform, approached the Rockefeller Foundation for support. Funding was provided and, in 1919, the Committee for the Study of Nursing Education was established to investigate the training of public health nurses. E. A. Winslow, professor of public health, Yale University, chaired the committee, composed of 10 physicians, two lay persons, and six nurses: Adelaide Nutting, Mary Beard, Lillian Clay, Annie Goodrich, Lillian Wald, and Helen Wood. Josephine Goldmark, a social worker, served as the secretary to the committee.

As secretary, Goldmark developed the methodology of data collection and analysis for a small sampling of the 1,800 schools of nursing in existence. The study of 23 of the best nursing schools across the nation represented a cross-sample of schools—small and large, public and private.

The Goldmark report, entitled *Nursing and Nursing Education in the United States,* was published in 1923. Goldmark identified the major weakness of the hospital-based training programs as that of putting the needs of the institution (service delivery) before the needs of the student (education). Nursing tradition and the apprenticeship form of education reinforced putting the needs of the client before the learning needs of the student.

Some major inadequacies identified in nursing education by the study were limited resources, low admission standards, lack of supervision, poorly trained instructors, and failure to correlate clinical practice with theory. The report concluded that for nursing to be on equal footing with other disciplines, nursing education should occur in the university setting.

BROWN REPORT.   In 1948, Esther Lucille Brown, a social anthropologist, published *Nursing for the Future and Nursing Reconsidered: A Study for Change.* Several recommendations were put forth in this study, including the need for nurses to demonstrate greater professional competence by moving nursing education from the hospital to the university setting.

Although published 20 years after the Goldmark report, the Brown report identified many of the same problems in diploma education—nursing students were still being used for service by the hospitals, and inadequate resources and authoritarianism in hospitals still prevailed in nursing education.

Brown recognized that nursing education in the university setting would provide the proper intellectual climate for the professional. Visionary nurse educators were securing necessary learning resources: libraries, laboratories, and clinical facilities. Professional endeavors such as research and publication were being implemented by nurse leaders.

INSTITUTE OF RESEARCH AND SERVICE IN NURSING EDUCATION REPORT.   During the 1950s, there was a deficit in the supply of nurses as the post–World War II demand for nursing services increased. Some contributing factors to the dearth of nurses were the low esteem of nursing as a profession, long hours with a heavy workload, and low salaries.

The Institute of Research and Service in Nursing Education report resulted in the establishment of practical nursing under Title III of the Health Amendment Act of 1955. There was a proliferation of practical nursing schools in the United States to increase the supply of nurses.

CANADIAN REPORTS.   Through the joint efforts of the Canadian Nurses Association and the Canadian Medical Association, a nationwide study of nursing education in Canada was established in 1929. Under the leadership of George M. Weir, MD, the study pointed out serious weaknesses that existed in the hospital schools of nursing. The *Survey of Nursing Education in Canada (1932),* also known as *The Weir Report,* recommended the following reforms: a higher education standard, increased affiliations between schools, increased employment of graduate nurses, student tuition, and qualified faculty (Donahue, 1985).

In 1936 the National Curriculum Committee of the Canadian Nurses Association published *The Proposed Curriculum for Schools of Nursing in Canada.* "The study and the later *Supplement* became valuable guides to assist with the establishment of a sounder educational foundation for nursing in Canada" (Donahue, 1985, p. 391).

Contemporary Reports

During the 1980s, several important studies were commissioned to examine the areas of nursing education and practice.

NATIONAL COMMISSION ON NURSING.   The National Commission on Nursing was created in 1980 by the AHA, the Hospital Research and Education Trust, and the American Hospital Supply Corporation to study nursing education and related issues in hospital management, nursing practice, and nursing education. The commission's conclusions addressed the need for:

- Adequate clinical education for students
- Baccalaureate education and educational mobility
- Involvement of nurses in collaborative institutional and clinical decision making
- Improved working conditions, specifically, salaries, flexible scheduling, and differentiated practice

As a result of the commission's study, attention was given to the need for prescribing practitioners and nurses to enter into collaborative practice.

INSTITUTE OF MEDICINE.   Concurrent with the National Commission on Nursing study, another study was initiated by Congress in 1979 and conducted by the Institute of Medicine (IOM). The study, Nursing and Nursing Education: Public Policies and Private Actions, focused on the need for continued federal funding to nursing education. The findings indicated that there was not a shortage in the general supply of nurses, but there was a serious shortage of nurses in research, teaching, administration, and advanced clinical practice. A significant nursing shortage existed in preventive and primary care for older adults and disadvantaged people in inner cities and rural areas.

SECRETARY'S COMMISSION ON NURSING.   Although the IOM study indicated that there were sufficient numbers of staff nurses, based on supply and demand, hospitals continued to report severe shortages. As a response to hospitals' recruitment and retention challenges, Health and Human Services Secretary Otis R. Brown, MD, established the Secretary's Commission on Nursing, which made the following recommendations related to nursing practice:

- Nurse compensation
- Health care financing
- Nurse decision making
- Development, use, and maintenance of nursing resources

This commission recognized that the federal government alone could not correct the problems facing nursing and health care but rather that the concerted efforts of health care organizations were needed for the implementation of the report's recommendations.

HEALTHY PEOPLE INITIATIVES.   Healthy People initiatives have become the nation's health agenda. These initiatives began with a report entitled *Healthy People: The Surgeon General's Report on Health Promotion and Disease Prevention in 1979.* The report described Healthy People as the nation's health agenda to guide policy on public health initiatives for health promotion and disease prevention activities during the decade 1980–1990. See Chapter 16 for a complete discussion of Healthy People initiatives.

PEW HEALTH PROFESSIONS COMMISSION.   The scientific base for nursing practice demands competencies (the ability to function in a particular way) from multiple sources: philosophy and ethics; physical, economic, behavioral, and social sciences; nursing science; and biomedicine. Additional competencies in collaboration, coordination, and the interdisciplinary practice activities of exchanging knowledge and techniques are critical to nursing practice and health care delivery. These competencies raise questions about the single, discipline-specific method of educating the nursing workforce and offer alternative scenarios for nursing education.

The Pew Health Professions Commission (O'Neil, 1993; Pew Health Professions Commission, 1995; Shugars,

HEALTH CARE PROFESSIONALS' COMPETENCIES

- Care for the community's health
- Expand access to effective care
- Provide contemporary clinical care
- Emphasize primary care
- Participate in coordinated care
- Ensure cost-effective, appropriate care
- Practice prevention
- Involve clients and families in the decision-making process
- Promote healthy lifestyles
- Assess and use technology appropriately
- Improve the health care system
- Manage information
- Understand the role of the environment in mitigating the impact of environmental hazards on health
- Provide counseling on ethical issues
- Accommodate expanded accountability
- Participate in a racially and culturally diverse society
- Continue to learn

From Shugars, D. A., O'Neil, E. H., & Bader, J. D. (Eds.). (1991). *Healthy America: Practitioners for 2005: An agenda for action for U.S. health professional schools* (pp. 18–20). Durham, NC: Pew Health Professions Commission.

O'Neil, & Bader, 1991), in its widely referenced and distributed reports, has recommended that academic institutions investigate whether the providers of educational experiences in health care are addressing the needs of clients. See the accompanying display that lists the Pew Health Professions Commission's Health Care Professionals' Competencies.

Nursing leaders have embraced these competencies as consistent with the values and issues raised in *Nursing's Agenda for Health Care Reform* (ANA, 1991). To ensure that the nursing workforce is educated sufficiently to demonstrate these competencies, schools are being challenged to redefine their educational core. To accomplish this goal, schools of nursing, health science centers, and institutions of higher education are refining mission statements, developing strategic plans and implementation activities, and examining curriculum activities, faculty competencies, educational methods and technologies, and sites and populations for clinical experiences.

SOCIAL FORCES AFFECTING NURSING

From the earliest recordings of nursing, 4000 BC through the Christian era, women were allowed to perform the nurse role only in the home. Nursing's links with the church caused nursing to be viewed as a "service," not a profession such as medicine. The Crimean and Civil wars had a significant impact on nursing's future by focusing on women as nurse providers and on the need for nurse training.

During the twentieth century, the evolution of medical education as an established profession had far advanced that of nursing. The Flexner report carved the destiny for physicians. The Goldmark and Brown reports created havoc for nurses as they debated the issue of nursing education in the university setting.

The Depression and World War II brought social reform and created health and medical insurance that strengthened the organized power base of both physician and hospital. Nursing—almost exclusively a female profession—had little power and, therefore, did not exert much influence on the social forces at play. The greatest advances for nurses were seen in the realm of public health and preventive health care.

As physicians were released from military service after World War II, the era of specialized medicine began. Physicians used their veterans' educational entitlement benefits to take residency training in one or more specialty areas. By 1966, more than 70% of the prescribing practitioners in practice were specialists.

The 1960s was a decade of growth and change. As technologic advances increased the scope of practice of medicine and nursing, other social forces were at play: access to health care services enhanced by Medicare and Medicaid, prescribing practitioner and nurse shortages, the feminist movement, the inception of nurse practitioners, and a focus on health maintenance.

The economic recession of the 1970s saw health care costs escalating along with unemployment. Professional autonomy was being debated, nursing theories were being developed, and nursing education was being integrated into the university setting. Nurses were becoming more politically astute in that they were working through professional organizations to affect health care legislation.

During the 1980s, nursing became more specialized and autonomous. The rapid technologic advances in medicine required more specialization in nursing. Nurse practitioners were being more widely accepted by the general public and other health care providers. Expanded roles of nurses were developing in response to greater demands for nursing services. One factor that led to an increased need for nursing was the proliferation of health maintenance organizations in the early 1980s.

During the 1990s, nurses were actively assuming more responsibilities for the delivery of health care. Evolving technology mandated nurses to continue to advance their knowledge base and skills. The aging of the population called for more nursing involvement with the elderly. Nurses, as individuals and as members of professional organizations, were involved in shaping policies for health care reform. Nursing was a stronger advocate for vulnerable populations: older adults, those living in poverty, the homeless, and those with human immunodeficiency virus (HIV) and acquired immunodeficiency syndrome (AIDS).

In today's society, nurses need to understand how advances in technology, worldwide communication, and globalization and the increasing threat of natural disasters and bioterrorism are constantly evolving and reshaping the practice of nursing. Advancements in technology such as sophisticated client monitoring equipment and the Internet influence where and how nurses increase their knowledge and provide care. Inherent in these changes are cultural, legal, and ethical issues regarding the health and welfare of the population. For example, as a result of globalization and technology, nurses and other health care providers are practicing across state and national boundaries. Today's health care climate requires the nurse to acquire knowledge, skills, and values and to work collaboratively with other health care professionals when delivering safe, competent client care. Although worldwide communication and globalization make health care accessible to larger populations, there are legal issues regarding licensure that the provider must consider.

Many health care institutions, schools, and communities have educational programs to prepare for natural disasters or nuclear, chemical, or biological attack. Nurses play a critical role in participating in disaster preparedness. These roles may include participation in vaccine research, decontamination in the event of biological attack, triage for natural disaster and mass casualty, or membership in a crisis response unit. In order to meet the challenges of these ongoing changes, nurses must achieve educational competencies such as those addressed by the Pew Commission's strategies for change.

NURSING EDUCATION OVERVIEW

Educational programs that prepare graduates to write a licensing examination must be approved by a state or provincial (Canada) board of nursing. Boards approve entry-level programs to ensure the safe practice of nursing by setting minimum educational requirements and guaranteeing the graduate of the program is an eligible candidate to write a licensing examination. In the United States, candidates must pass the National Council Licensure Examination (NCLEX) to obtain a license to practice nursing. In Canada, the licensure examination is administered by the Canadian Nurses Association Testing Service (CNATS).

Two types of entry-level nursing programs are available in the United States: licensed practical or vocational nurse (LPN or LVN) and registered nurse (RN). An *entry-level educational program* means that the program prepares graduates to write a licensing examination. Graduates of the licensed practical or vocational programs write the NCLEX for practical nurses (NCLEX-PN), and graduates of RN programs write the NCLEX for RNs (NCLEX-RN).

Postgraduate programs prepare nurses to practice in various roles as advanced practice registered nurses (APRNs). Individual states have varying statutory provisions for APRNs. For instance, some states recognize the APRN's credentials to practice, whereas others require licensure.

An LPN or LVN is trained in basic nursing skills to provide client care under the guidance of an RN or other licensed provider, for example, a prescribing practitioner or dentist. In the United States, these programs are 9 to 18 months in length and exist in a variety of settings: high schools, community colleges, vocational schools, hospitals, and other health care agencies. The Canadian equivalent to the LPN is a registered nurse's assistant (RNA). RNAs usually receive 12 months of education in a community college or hospital setting.

Practical nursing programs provide the graduate with didactic learning and clinical skills to perform selected nursing skills. Once licensed, practical nurses are prepared to work in structured settings, such as hospital and long-term care facilities, under RN supervision.

RN candidates are graduates from programs that are state approved and, in many cases, accredited by national accrediting organizations. In the United States, the National League for Nursing Accrediting Commission (NLNAC) accredits nursing programs; in Canada, the Canadian Association of University Schools of Nursing (CAUSN) accredits baccalaureate programs. The Commission on Collegiate Nursing Education (CCNE) was established in 1996 as an accrediting agency of the American Association of Colleges of Nursing (AACN) to evaluate the quality and integrity of baccalaureate and graduate degree nursing education programs. A variety of nursing education programs are available for entry into professional registered nursing: diploma, associate degree (AD), baccalaureate of science in nursing (BSN), master's degrees, and a few professional doctorate programs for beginning practitioners. Table 1-2 on page 16 provides a summary of educational programs that prepare graduates for entry into professional nursing practice.

Educational preparation for entry into practice has been an ongoing debate in nursing since the 1930s and 1940s, when the Brown and Goldmark reports recommended two levels of educational preparation for nurses. The ANA's 1965 Position Statement identified two entry levels of educational preparation: minimum preparation for professional practice, baccalaureate degree; and minimum preparation for technical practice, AD. Again in 1985, the ANA adopted a resolution regarding titles: professional nurse, a nurse possessing the baccalaureate degree in nursing; and associate nurse, a nurse prepared in an AD program. Although the AACN, CAUSN, and professional nursing organizations in the United States (ANA) and Canada (Canadian Nurses Association) have supported the baccalaureate degree to be the minimum entry level for professional practice, the authority to enforce this requirement rests with the individual states and provinces.

The CAUSN's mission is to promote health and wellness by advancing nursing education and nursing research. Although the CAUSN supports baccalaureate education as the required educational preparation for beginning practitioners, the association established a Task Force for Collaborative Nursing Education Models to foster collaboration between diploma and university schools in Canada (CAUSN Position Statement on Education, November 1998).

DIPLOMA EDUCATION

Florence Nightingale established the first diploma program at St. Thomas's Hospital, London, in 1860. Nightingale's basic principles of nursing education were:

- Placement of the program in an institution supported by public funds and associated with a medical school

TABLE 1-2 **Educational Programs That Prepare Graduates to Write the National Council Licensure Examination for Registered Nurses (NCLEX-RN)**

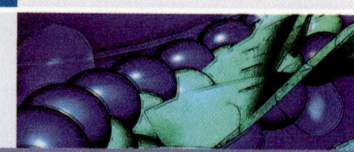

	DIPLOMA PROGRAMS	ASSOCIATE DEGREE PROGRAMS	BACCALAUREATE PROGRAMS	MASTER'S PROGRAMS	DOCTORAL PROGRAMS	NURSE DOCTORATE PROGRAMS
Origin	1873 Hospitals	1952 Community colleges and universities	1909 Universities and colleges	1950s Universities and colleges	1960s Universities and colleges	1979 Universities and colleges
Length	2–3 years	2 years	4 years	18–24 months	3–5 years postmaster's	4 years post-baccalaureate
Graduate outcomes	Clinically competent to plan, direct, and implement care for individuals and groups in collaboration with other health care providers in acute care and community-based settings	Technically competent to plan and implement care in hospitals and long-term care settings with other health care providers	Professionally prepared to plan, implement, and coordinate care, health promotion, and illness prevention for individuals, families, and communities in a variety of settings	Advanced practice nurse prepared in a specific area of specialization, such as education, administration, or clinical practice	Leaders for education, administration, clinical practice, and research	Leaders for advanced clinical practice
Articulation or acceleration placement	LPNs or LVNs	LPNs or LVNs	LPNs or LVNs, diploma, and ADN nurses	RNs without degrees, RNs with degrees in other fields, and nonnurse degree graduates	BSNs	Nonnurse degree graduates

Delmar/Cengage Learning

- Affiliation with a teaching hospital but also independent of it
- A program directed by and staffed with professional nurses
- A residency to teach students discipline and character

The nursing curriculum was based on Nightingale's scientific principles of the need for fresh air, medications, quiet, mobility, piped hot water, a call-bell system for patients, cleanliness and comfort in hospitals, as well as education of the public concerning principles of health and disease.

United States

After the Civil War in 1869, the AMA established a committee, headed by Samuel Gross, to study the training of nurses. The outcome of this study had an impact on nurse training that lasted for a century. In opposition to Nightingale's educational principle of an independent school under the direction of nursing leaders, the AMA's committee recom- mended that all large hospitals have their own nursing schools under the direction of local medical agencies, with the medical staff being responsible for teaching.

Early diploma programs were established based upon the AMA's recommendations, and nurse training was largely of the apprenticeship type. Although there were some formal classes, students learned by doing, and in the process, they provided the majority of the nursing care for the hospitals' clients. The size of the hospital influenced the students' clinical experiences and learning. Standardization of diploma education did not occur until the 1940s following the efforts of the National League for Nursing (NLN), formerly known as the National League for Nursing Education, and the Goldmark report of 1923.

From 1872 until the mid-1960s, the hospital program was the predominant type of nursing program with graduates receiving a diploma in nursing. Refer to Table 1-2 for the general characteristics of diploma programs. By the 1960s, the majority of diploma programs were associated with colleges or universities where students received college credit for their nonnursing courses. Some of the current diploma programs have evolved into what is called a *single-purpose institution,* having baccalaureate-degree-granting privileges for nursing.

ASSOCIATE DEGREE PROGRAMS

In 1951 Mildred Montag developed the blueprint for AD programs that would produce a nursing technician whose scope of practice was narrower than that of the professional nurse and broader than the PN's scope. Montag envisioned the AD as a terminal degree that prepared nurses to function at the bedside. The AD curriculum focused on preparing graduates to:

- Provide general nursing care under the supervision of baccalaureate nurses
- Assist in the planning of nursing care for clients
- Assist in the evaluation of nursing care

Montag's 5-year research project showed that AD nursing graduates could perform the intended nursing functions to work as technicians under the guidance of professional nurses. In 2000, the *National League for Nursing Educational Competencies for Graduates of Associate Degree Nursing Programs* updated the AD competencies, requiring evidence of professional behaviors, communication and assessment skills, caring interventions, teaching and learning, collaboration, and managing care (Coxwell & Gillerman, 2000). Refer to Table 1-2 for the general characteristics of AD programs.

AD programs have attracted a more diverse group of students to nursing. Traditional diploma nursing students were composed mainly of single, white females, approximately 18 years old, from middle-class families. The AD programs have attracted older, mature, goal-oriented students; minorities; males; and married women. The flexible scheduling patterns of community colleges that allow students to attend classes part-time have attributed to the increased numbers of individuals with baccalaureate and higher degrees in other fields seeking admission to AD programs.

BACCALAUREATE PROGRAMS

The first baccalaureate program in nursing was established at the University of Minnesota in 1909 through the efforts of Dr. Richard Olding Beard. There were only 8 baccalaureate programs by 1919. Colleges and universities were reluctant to establish baccalaureate programs in nursing because of the lack of qualified faculty. Following World War II and the passage of the Nurse Training Act in 1943, baccalaureate nursing programs began to increase slowly. In 1983 there were 420 programs, and by 2000 there were 695 programs. Most graduates of baccalaureate programs receive a bachelor of science degree in nursing (BSN). Refer to Table 1-2 for the general characteristics of baccalaureate programs.

The BSN curricula contain courses in general education, liberal arts, and the sciences related to nursing as well as nursing courses. According to the AACN's essential components of baccalaureate education, all programs must include a liberal education, professional values, core competencies, core knowledge, and role development (AACN, 1998). Emphasis is placed on developing critical decision-making skills, exercising independent nursing judgment, and acquiring professional values and research skills. Although nursing research, nursing management, and community health are often cited as skills germane to BSN programs, these educational components also may be found in some diploma and AD programs.

MASTER'S PROGRAMS

The first master's education in nursing program began in 1899 at Teachers College in New York; however, it was not until the late 1950s and early 1960s that the number of master's programs began to escalate. The growth in graduate education was first driven by the need to educate qualified faculty for BSN and other types of entry-level programs. The first graduate programs emphasized role preparation. In response to the need for graduates prepared as administrative personnel for management and clinical positions, the content was expanded to include advanced practice components. As the content for advanced nursing became more defined, graduate programs began to prepare the clinical nurse specialist and advanced nurse practitioner in various areas of specialization such as neonatal, pediatric, and adult and family practice. By 1990, there were 231 nursing master's programs in the United States.

Nontraditional Graduate Programs Leading to RN Licensure

Several types of educational programs at the graduate level serve to prepare graduates to write the NCLEX-RN. These nontraditional paths for entry into nursing practice at the graduate level began at Yale University, the University of Texas at Austin, and the University of Tennessee. The impetus for allowing admission of individuals other than BSN graduates came from the significant numbers of degree-prepared nonnurses seeking admission to AD and BSN programs. These nontraditional programs admit nonnurse college graduates and RNs without the baccalaureate degree. The curricula provide for both groups to complete whatever undergraduate or graduate prerequisite courses are needed to acquire the equivalent of a baccalaureate degree in nursing. Following this component, nonnurses are eligible to the take the NCLEX-RN examination. See Table 1-2 for the general characteristics of master's programs.

DOCTORAL PROGRAMS

There are various doctoral degrees awarded to nurses: the doctor of philosophy (PhD), doctor of nursing science (DNSc), doctor of science in nursing (DNS), doctor of education (EdD), and doctor of public health (DPH). Graduates of these programs are often prepared as researchers and educators to advance the discipline and profession of nursing. Although there were only 2 programs in 1946, the number of programs increased to 27 in 1983 and 50 in 1990.

Nontraditional Doctoral Programs Leading to RN Licensure

In the 1970s, Schlotfeldt developed the first nontraditional nursing doctorate (ND) program at the Frances Payne Bolton School of Nursing at Case Western Reserve University. Nontraditional programs usually provide curricula containing components of both basic and advanced nursing courses. Upon completion of the program, the graduate is eligible to write the NCLEX-RN examination. See Table 1-2 for the general characteristics of doctoral and nurse doctorate programs.

STAFF DEVELOPMENT AND CONTINUING EDUCATION

Once nurses are in practice, both staff development and continuing education are used to maintain the requisite knowledge and skill needed for contemporary practice in addition to a formal academic degree. Staff development typically occurs in the setting of employment and is described as the delivery of instruction to assist the nurse to achieve the goals of the employer. According to the ANA (1990):

nursing staff development is a process of orientation, in-service education and continuing education for the purpose of promoting the development of personnel within any employment setting, consistent with the goals and responsibilities of the employer. (p. 3)

Orientation is an important organizational tool for recruitment and retention. Orientation sessions typically occur at the initiation of employment and whenever positions and roles change. Content in orientation education unique to the institution of employment includes philosophy, goals, policies and procedures, role expectations, facilities, resources and special services, and assessment and development of competency with equipment and supplies used in the work setting (ANA, 1990).

In-service education is that phase of the staff development process that occurs after orientation and supports the nurse in acquiring, maintaining, and increasing skills to fulfill assigned responsibilities. Challenging learning opportunities in the employment setting include:

- Technology development
- Changing nature of health care and nursing science
- Interdisciplinary practice
- Changing delivery systems
- New equipment and supplies
- Enlarging roles of nursing related to leadership, management, delegation, supervision, and legal and ethical demands on practice

Active orientation and in-service development for nurses is a critical element of a delivery system that holds high standards for quality of care delivery in a cost-effective manner. Staff development is guided by the accreditation standards of the Joint Commission on Accreditation of Healthcare Organizations (JCAHO) and the ANA's (1990) *Standards for Nursing Staff Development.*

Professional nurses are responsible for their own continuing education. Continuing education offers both personal and professional growth to the nurse and may serve as an incentive to pursue an academic degree. Continuing education builds on acquired knowledge, attitudes, and skills and constitutes an essential dimension of lifelong learning.

Although half the boards of nursing require continuing education units (CEUs) as part of the licensure renewal process to document the RN's competency, increasing evidence supports the assertion that "CE [continuing education] requirements do not guarantee continuing competence" (Pew Health Professions Commission, 1995, p. 1).

Lifelong learning is essential to career development and competency achievement in nursing practice. Technology has expanded the delivery and scheduling flexibility of continuing education for nurses in different geographic sites. Accessibility to continuing education will continue to improve the ability of the nurse to be flexible, factual, futuristic, and functional. The nurse of the future will be the professional who knows how to obtain and use evidence-based knowledge to achieve quality outcomes for health care.

PREPARING NURSES FOR TOMORROW'S CHALLENGES

The dynamic changes occurring in society and the health care arena are challenging professional nurses to focus on client outcomes and safety (see Chapter 29). When an aging population that requires more specialized nursing care is coupled with the increasing number of faculty members who are retiring, the reasons for the projected nursing shortage are clearly understood. A new nursing paradigm must be developed and educational programs must be willing to change in order to provide society with an adequate number of safe, competent nurses.

Some educational programs have demonstrated their ability to change, but are these changes sufficient to meet current and future challenges? Diploma education, which evolved with the history of nursing and the creation of hospitals in the United States, produced the nursing workforce for almost a century. The lack of nursing faculty prepared to teach at the baccalaureate level and the cost of a college education contributed to the slow growth of BSN programs. The availability and low cost of AD programs in the community college setting created a more diverse group of students and a phenomenal growth of these programs. This growth, in turn, challenged graduate programs to develop nontraditional programs to capture adult learners from diverse backgrounds by admitting RNs without baccalaureate degrees and degree graduates from nonnursing fields.

Nurse educators are facing real educational challenges. With hospital downsizing and shorter client stays, there are fewer opportunities for clinical learning. When one adds into the picture the aging population of nurse faculty, the decreased enrollment of nurses seeking graduate teaching degrees, and the reduced number of acute-care learning experiences, one has to question the viability of the traditional education models used to prepare nursing graduates.

The nursing curriculum is the student's first introduction to the process of socialization into the profession. The process of socialization is based on professional values, which are taught by exposing students to learning opportunities that support compassionate, sensitive, empathic care for individuals, groups, and communities.

For the nursing profession to advance, and for nursing education to remain responsive to the changes that occur in society and health care, nursing programs must adjust their methods of teaching to provide for graduate competencies that are responsive to the health care challenges of the twenty-first century. A discussion of some of the most critical challenges follows.

DIFFERENTIATED PRACTICE

One of the major challenges facing professional nursing is the task of describing and differentiating the competencies and the scope of practice of nurses with multiple entry-level nursing programs. As discussed previously, all nurse graduates write the same licensing examination (NCLEX-RN), which is designed to ensure minimum standards of safe practice. One must ask if all graduates are created equal. Yet the curricula and accreditation requirements for graduate competencies differ for each program, and research documents different skill levels based on educational preparation.

Differentiated nursing practice refers to the practice of structuring nursing roles based on the expected competencies of graduates from different kinds of education programs. The Pew Health Professions Commission (1995) recommended that nursing distinguish between the different levels of nursing:

- AD for the entry-level hospital-based setting and nursing home
- BSN for hospital-based care management and community-based practice
- Master's degree preparation for specialty practice in the hospital and independent practice as a primary provider

Several leading organizations support the need for differentiated practice: the National Commission Nursing Implementation Project (NCNIP), the AACN, and the American Organization of Nurse Executives (AONE). Funds from the Robert Wood Johnson Foundation created a demonstration project, the Task Force on Differentiated Competencies for Nursing Practice under the auspices of the AACN and AONE, to develop a value-neutral language to describe differentiated nursing practice and education. This task force is still collecting data. The Council of Associate Degree Programs is working with the NLN to redefine their statement "Educational Outcomes of Associate Degree Nursing Programs: Roles and Competencies." The NCSBN has conducted studies regarding role delineation and job analysis of entry-level nurses.

The final report of the Pew Health Professions Commission identified 21 professional competencies for health care providers for the twenty-first century. These professional competencies stress the need for providers to work as a team in providing culturally sensitive care that is evidence-based and incorporates preventive health care.

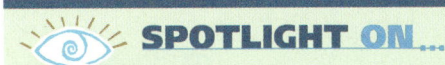

SPOTLIGHT ON...

Professional
With multiple entry-level nursing programs, how would you differentiate the competencies of the graduates of each program?

Should graduates seek employment in settings appropriate to their educational preparation?

If practice settings employed and utilized graduates based on differentiated educational competencies, would this be a strong enough impetus for the NCSBN and state boards of nursing to differentiate licensure?

ACCELERATED DEGREE PROGRAMS

The accelerated degree program for nonnursing students is one innovative educational approach to meet the projected need for a million additional nurses by the year 2010. These programs, at both the baccalaureate and master's degree levels, build on previous learning experiences and transition students with undergraduate degrees in other disciplines into nursing.

Accelerated programs have proliferated over the past 10 years. The growth of these programs can be attributed to their graduates. Employers value the many layers of skill and education these graduates bring to the workplace and are partnering with schools and offering tuition repayment to graduates as a mechanism to recruit highly qualified nurses.

TECHNOLOGY CHANGES IN NURSING EDUCATION

Over the past 10 years, computer technology has been incorporated into all aspects of teaching and learning in nursing programs. Some nursing programs provide distance learning by offering specific courses online, while other programs offer nursing degrees through online courses. Nursing programs have incorporated computer technology into the classroom and learning laboratory, offering a variety of approaches to instruction that appeal to a diverse student population. Computer-assisted instruction (CAI) augments classroom lectures and presentations in the form of interactive and linear video programs, client simulations, and drill and practice routines to promote problem solving, critical thinking, and clinical skills. Electronic mail between faculty members and students provides a mode for reflective learning; faculty members also use handheld computers for student record keeping and evaluation. Other learning management systems, such as Blackboard and WebCT, are an integral part of many nursing programs, whether the programs are online or campus-based.

UNCOVERING THE
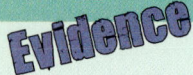

TITLE OF STUDY
"Video Recording in Clinical Research Mapping the Ethical Terrain"

AUTHOR
L. Broyles

PURPOSE
To determine the ethical issues (informed consent, confidentiality and privacy, and participant burden and safety) of video-recorded clients and clinician research participants.

METHOD
The researcher used the Study of Patient-Nurse Effectiveness With Assisted Communication Strategies to show how these ethical issues can be managed in a clinical trial.

FINDINGS
The ethical issues inherent in video recording in acute care research can be adequately addressed through existing universal human subjects protection strategies when the precise nature of the ethical issues is defined clearly.

IMPLICATIONS
Videography is used often for data collection in clinical research, which requires the securing of institutional review board approval, confidentiality and privacy, safety, and informed consent. It is an effective way to conduct research when the ethical issues are determined and managed during the study.

Broyles, L. (2008). Video recording in clinical research: Mapping the ethical terrain. *Nursing Research, 57*(1), 59–63.

In health care, computers are used in a variety of ways, for example, in voice-activated point-of-care charting, developing nursing care plans, communicating with other health care providers, and regulating the administration of medications. See Chapter 13 for a detailed discussion regarding nursing informatics such as electronic medical records and order entry.

Other innovations in technology, such as virtual reality (VR), also help to bridge the education gap between knowledge and application by providing students with the opportunity to practice essential nursing skills. With VR, computers and multimedia peripherals (visual display units and speakers) produce a simulated environment that users perceive as comparable to real-world objects and events. With multimedia simulation, students can practice procedures on the computer, assimilate clinical data, and make decisions independently in order to increase their critical thinking skills.

SERVICE LEARNING

Service learning is an educational method that uses community services with explicit learning objectives, preparation, and intentional reflective activities. Service learning is not a new educational method. The early 1900s educators, such as Dewey, recognized the importance of connecting service to educational goals. The need for educators to incorporate service learning into academic coursework is addressed in the following reports: *Healthy People 2010: Understanding and Improving Health,* the Pew Health Professions Commission report, the *National League for Nursing Educational Competencies for Graduates of Associate Degree Nursing Programs,* and the AACN and the NLN BSN competencies. The incorporation of this methodology into the nursing curriculum requires extensive preparation of faculty and collaborative partnership between the nursing program, students, and community agencies. The four critical components of service learning:

- Are experimental in nature
- Allow students to engage in activities that address human and community needs through structured opportunities for learning
- Incorporate reflection
- Embrace the concept of reciprocity between the learner and the person being served

Reflection is the link between the students' performance of service and the learning outcomes of that service.

From *Nightingale's Notes on Nursing,* to the core competencies of graduates as defined by accrediting bodies, to the Pew report and *Nursing's Educational Agenda for the 21st Century,* caring, teaching, research, social justice, service, and community are recurring concepts that link nursing education to a profession that is responsive to societal and individual health care needs.

KEY CONCEPTS

- Nursing is an art and a science in which people are assisted in learning to care for themselves whenever possible and cared for when they are unable to meet their own needs.

- Nurses will understand such issues as autonomy, unity within the profession, supply and demand, salary, education, and current practice and the empowerment of the profession by studying nursing's history.

- Nursing's early history was heavily influenced by religious organizations and the need for nurses to care for soldiers during wartime.
- Florence Nightingale forged the future of nursing practice and education as a result of her experiences in training nurses to care for soldiers.
- Nursing's early American leaders, professional organizations, and landmark reports have influenced the infrastructure of current nursing practice.
- Influential nursing leaders, such as Lillian Wald, Jane Delano, Isabel Hampton Robb, Annie Goodrich, Adelaide Nutting, and Lavinia Dock, were instrumental in the advancement of nursing education and practice.
- Other nursing pioneers, such as Amelia Greenwald, Mary Breckinridge, Mamie Hale, Mary Mahoney, Linda Richards, and Margaret Sanger, made important contributions to both nursing education and the fields of rural, public health, maternity, and multicultural nursing.
- In 1923, the Goldmark report concluded that for nursing to be on equal footing with other disciplines, nursing education should occur in the university setting.
- The Brown report (1948) addressed the need for nurses to demonstrate greater professional competence by moving nursing education to the university setting.
- The Health Maintenance Organization Act of 1973 provided an alternative to the private health insurance industry.
- Contemporary reports issued by the National Commission on Nursing, the IOM, and the Secretary's Commission on Nursing focused on the areas of nursing education, practice, and nursing's role in health care financing policies.
- The three types of programs that currently prepare nurses for entry-level practice are diploma, AD, and baccalaureate degree nursing programs.
- To achieve the competencies established for health care professionals, several strategies for nursing education reform have been proposed in the areas of institutional, governmental, and federal involvement with the nursing profession.
- As the nursing profession continues to evolve and respond to the challenges within the health care system, nurses will remain responsive to societal needs.

REVIEW QUESTIONS

1. Which of the following are some of Florence Nightingale's beliefs regarding nursing? Select all that apply:
   a. A holistic framework inclusive of illness and health
   b. The need for a theoretical basis for nursing practice
   c. The importance of creating an environment that promotes healing
   d. The need for fresh air and light
   e. The need to support the individual's adaptation to stimuli
   f. The need to assist persons attain a higher degree of harmony

2. During World War I, which nursing leader opposed physician training aides to care for the sick?
   a. Isabel Hampton Robb
   b. Jane Delano
   c. Annie Goodrich
   d. Margaret Sanger

3. Which educational program prepares the nurse for advanced practice?
   a. Associate degree
   b. Baccalaureate
   c. Master's
   d. Licensed practical

4. Which social forces have the greatest impact on the supply and demand for nurses?
   a. Aging and faculty attrition
   b. Economics and technology
   c. Faculty attrition and economics
   d. Science and technology

5. Which is an example of continuing education?
   a. Attending an orientation program
   b. Meeting with a representative regarding a new piece of monitoring equipment
   c. Completing a workshop of legal aspects of nursing
   d. Obtaining information regarding a new computer charting system

online companion

Visit the DeLaune and Ladner online companion resource at **www.delmar.cengage.com** for additional content and study aids. Click on Online Companions, then select the Nursing discipline.

Theory is the poetry of Science.

—Levine

CHAPTER 2

Nursing Theory

COMPETENCIES

1. Explain the relationships of concepts and propositions to theory.
2. Discuss the purpose of theory.
3. Describe the link between nursing theory and the continuing development of the nursing profession.
4. Explain the interdependent roles of nursing practice, nursing theory, and nursing research.
5. Identify the three categories relating to the scope of theories.
6. Describe the metaparadigm concepts in nursing and how they differ from the metaparadigm concepts in medicine.
7. Discuss the process of paradigm revolution and paradigm shift in nursing and relate it to the current paradigms in nursing.
8. Apply the principles of selected nursing theories, such as the conservation theory, the self-care deficit theory of nursing, the Roy adaptation model, the theory of human caring, the science of unitary human beings, and man-living-health, to nursing practice.

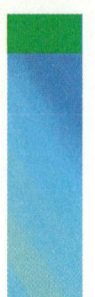

This chapter explores the theoretical foundation on which the knowledge base of the nursing profession has been and is being built. Nursing theory provides a perspective from which to define the *what* of nursing, to describe the *who* of nursing (who is the client) and *when* nursing is needed, and to identify the boundaries and goals of nursing's therapeutic activities. Theory is fundamental to effective nursing practice and research. The professionalization of nursing has been and is being brought about through the development and use of nursing theory.

This chapter first addresses basic ideas about the meaning of nursing theory and its relevance to professional nursing. Issues related to the purpose, use, and diversity of nursing theories are discussed. It then presents a broad overview of selected nursing theories. The major ideas of selected nursing theories are explained, and examples of their use in nursing situations are provided.

COMPONENTS OF THE THEORETICAL FOUNDATION

The basic elements that structure a nursing theory are concepts and propositions. In a theory, propositions represent how concepts affect each other.

WHAT IS A CONCEPT?

A concept is the basic building block of a theory. A **concept** is a vehicle of thought. According to Chinn and Kramer (1999), concepts are complex mental formulations of one's perceptions of the world. A concept labels or names a **phenomenon**, an observable fact that can be perceived through the senses and explained. A concept assists us in formulating a mental image about an object or situation. Concepts help us to name things and occurrences in the world around us and assist us in communicating with each other about the world. Independence, self-care, and caring are just a few examples of concepts frequently encountered in health care. Theories are formulated by linking concepts together. A **conceptual framework** is a structure that links global concepts together and represents the unified whole of a larger reality. The specifics about phenomena within the global whole are better explained by theory.

By its nature, a concept is a socially constructed label that may represent more than a single phenomenon. For example, when you hear the word *chair,* a mental image that probably comes to mind is an item of furniture used for sitting. The word *chair* could represent many different kinds of furniture for sitting, such as a desk chair, a high chair, or an easy chair. Further, the word *chair* could also represent the leader of a committee or the head of a corporation. The meaning of the word chair depends on the context in which it is used.

In health care, the concept of *wandering* may be represented by words such as aimless and random movement, disorganized thought processes, and conversation that is difficult to follow. To be useful, the multiple meanings that often underlie a concept must be thoroughly understood and clearly defined within the context in which it is used.

It is important to remember that the same concept may be used differently in various theories. For example, one nursing theory may use the concept of *environment* to mean all that surrounds a human being (the external environment), whereas another theory may use this concept to mean the external environment *and* all the biological and psychological components of the person (the internal environment).

WHAT IS A PROPOSITION?

A **proposition** (another structural element of a theory) is a statement that proposes a relationship between concepts. An example of a nonnursing proposition might be the statement "people seem to be happier in the springtime." This proposition establishes a relationship between the concept of happiness and the time of the year. A nursing propositional statement linking the concept of helplessness and the concept of loss might be stated as "multiple and rapid losses predispose one to feelings of helplessness." Propositional statements in a theory represent the theorist's particular view of which concepts fit together and, in most theories, establish how concepts affect one another.

WHAT IS A THEORY?

A **theory** is a set of concepts and propositions that provide an orderly way to view phenomena. In the scientific literature, *theory* may be defined in many different ways, with subtle nuances specific to the particular author's viewpoint.

These various explanations share a common notion of the purpose of the theory, that being description, explanation, and prediction. "A theory, by traditional definition, is an organized, coherent set of concepts and their relationship to each other that offers descriptions, explanations, and predictions about phenomena" (Parker, 2001, p. 4). A theory not only helps us to organize our thoughts and ideas but also may help direct us in what to do and when and how to do it.

The use of the term *theory* is not restricted to the scientific world, however. It is often used in daily life and conversation. For example, when telling a friend about a mystery novel you are reading, you may have said, "I have a theory about who committed the crime." Or you may have heard a Little League coach saying to the players, "I have a theory about how to improve our performance." The way in which this term is used in these statements is a useful way to think about the meaning of theory.

USE OF THEORIES FROM OTHER DISCIPLINES

In addition to using theories specifically constructed to describe, explain, and predict the phenomena of concern to nursing, the nursing profession has long used theories from other disciplines. A **discipline** is a field of study. Theories from biological, physical, and behavioral sciences are commonly used in the practice of nursing. For example, nonnursing theories such as Maslow's hierarchy of basic human needs, Erikson's theory of human development, and Selye's general adaptation syndrome theory have been and continue to be useful in nursing practice.

These nonnursing theories are often incorporated into nursing practice together with specific nursing theories. When used in conjunction with a nursing theory, a nonnursing theory is transformed by the unique approach of the nursing perspective. This perspective provides the specific framework or viewpoint within which to use theories and knowledge from other disciplines.

IMPORTANCE OF NURSING THEORIES

Why do we have nursing theories? In the early part of nursing's history, knowledge was extremely limited and almost entirely task oriented. The knowledge explosion that occurred in health care in the 1950s produced the need to systematically organize the tremendous volume of new information being generated. From the very beginnings of nursing education, there was a need to categorize knowledge and to analyze client care situations in order to communicate in coherent and meaningful ways. Nursing practice knowledge is generated by theory. According to McEwen and Willis (2007), the integration of theory into practice is the basis for professional nursing.

The literature about the relationship between theory and nursing care yields many interpretations in terms of the role each component plays in the health care environment. According to Barnum (1994, p. 1), "a theory is a construct that accounts for or organizes some phenomenon." Chinn and Kramer (1999, p. 71) viewed theory as a "creative and rigorous structuring of ideas that projects a tentative purposeful and systematic view of phenomena." Meleis (1997, p. 12) stated that a theory is a "conceptualization of some aspect of reality (invented or discovered) that pertains to nursing. The conceptualization is articulated for the purpose of describing, explaining, predicting or prescribing nursing care." Similarly, Parse (1998, p. 4) defined a theory as a "general term that is a notion or an idea that explains experience, interprets observation, describes relationships, and projects outcomes. Theories are mental powers or constructs created to help understand and find meaning from experience, organize and articulate our knowing, and ask questions leading to new insights."

Nursing theories provide a framework for thought in which to examine situations. As new situations are encountered, this framework provides a structure for organization, analysis, and decision making. In addition, nursing theories provide a structure for communicating with other nurses and with other members of the health care team. Nursing theories assist the discipline of nursing in clarifying beliefs, values, and goals, and they help to define the unique contribution of nursing in the care of clients. When the focus of nursing's contribution is clear, then greater professional autonomy and, ultimately, control of certain aspects of practice are achieved.

In the broadest sense, nursing theory is necessary for the continued development and evolution of the discipline of nursing. Because the world of health care changes virtually on a daily basis, nursing needs to continue to expand its knowledge base to proactively respond to changes in societal needs. Knowledge for nursing practice is developed through nursing research that, in turn, is used to either test existing theories or generate new theories. **Nursing research** is the systematic application of formalized methods for generating valid and dependable information about the phenomena of concern to the discipline of nursing (Chinn & Kramer, 1999).

The relationship between nursing practice, theory, and research is depicted in Figure 2-1. These processes are so

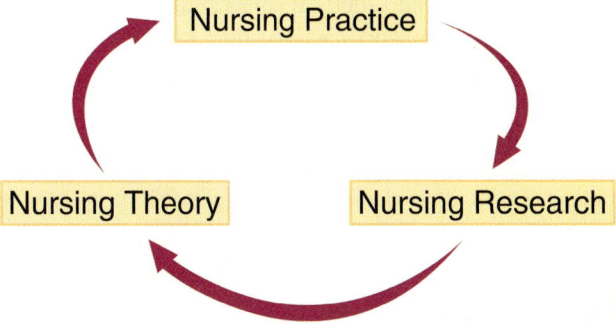

FIGURE 2-1 Process of knowledge development. Nursing practice, theory, and research are interdependent. Nursing theory development and nursing research activities are directed toward developing nursing practice standards. DELMAR/CENGAGE LEARNING

closely related that to consider one aspect without considering the other two aspects would be the same as seeing only a part of the whole. Nursing practice is the focal point of the relationship between practice, theory, and research. It provides the raw material for the ideas that are systematically developed and organized in the form of nursing theory. The ideas proposed by nursing theory must be tested and validated through nursing research. In turn, new knowledge that results from nursing research is used to transform and inform nursing practice. Alternatively, nursing practice generates questions that serve as the basis for nursing research. Nursing research, then, influences the development of nursing theory that, in turn, transforms nursing practice. For example, the Neuman systems model, explained later in this chapter, provides clear direction for the researcher who is interested in describing stressors; explaining the factors that influence reactions to those stressors; and testing the effects of primary, secondary, and tertiary prevention on stressor reactions within the context of a holistic, open system perspective (Fawcett & Gigliotti, 2001).

When nurses explore various nursing theories, they gain new insights into patient care, open new options otherwise hidden, and stimulate innovative interventions (Woodward, 2003). Theoretical thinking enhances and strengthens the nurse's role and helps one to actually *think* nursing. As nurses learn more about specific nursing theories, it may be discovered that they can relate more to one theory than another or that they can appreciate the ideas contained in several different theories. Nurses may use a specific nursing theory to help guide their practice or may choose a more eclectic approach and adopt ideas from several theories. Both of these approaches are valid. Furthermore, nurses may find some theories more appropriate for certain situations. In that case, one theory can be used with a client in a home health care setting, whereas another theory may be more applicable to a client in an acute care environment. Regardless of the approach chosen, nurses will recognize the value and usefulness of nursing theory as a tool for effective nursing practice.

SCOPE OF THEORIES

According to Fawcett (2000), theories address relatively specific and concrete phenomena, but they vary in scope; *scope* refers to the relative level of substantive specificity of a theory and the concreteness of its concepts and propositions. Essentially, three different categories relate to the scope of theories: grand theories, middle-range theories, and micro-range theories. This classification is applicable to both nursing and nonnursing theories.

GRAND THEORIES

A grand theory is composed of concepts representing global and extremely complex phenomena. It is the broadest in scope, represents the most abstract level of development, and addresses the broad phenomena of concern within the discipline. Typically, a grand theory is not intended to provide guidance for the formation of specific nursing interventions, but rather provides an overall framework for structuring broad, abstract ideas (Fawcett, 2005). An example of a grand theory is Orem's self-care deficit theory of nursing.

MIDDLE-RANGE THEORIES

A theory that addresses more concrete and more narrowly defined phenomena than a grand theory is known as a middle-range theory. Descriptions, explanations, and predictions put forth in a middle-range theory are intended to answer questions about nursing phenomena, yet they do not cover the full range of phenomena of concern to the discipline. A middle-range theory provides a perspective from which to view complex situations and a direction for interventions (Fawcett, 2005). An example of a middle-range theory is Peplau's theory of interpersonal relations.

MICRO-RANGE THEORIES

A micro-range theory is the most concrete and narrow in scope. A micro-range theory explains a specific phenomenon of concern to the discipline (Fawcett, 2005), such as the effect of social supports on grieving, and establishes nursing care guidelines to address the problem.

EVOLUTION OF NURSING THEORY

The work of early nursing theorists in the 1950s focused on the tasks of nursing practice from a somewhat mechanistic viewpoint. Because of this emphasis, much of the art of nursing—the value of caring, the relationship aspects of nursing, and the esthetics of practice—was diminished. During the decades of the 1960s, 1970s, and 1980s, many nursing theorists struggled with making nursing practice, theory, and research fit into the then prevailing view of science. Table 2-1 on page 27 provides a chronological summary of the development of nursing's theory base through the contributions of noted theorists and influential leaders in nursing.

Reflecting changes in global awareness of health care needs, several contemporary nursing theorists have projected a new perspective for nursing that truly unifies the notion of nursing as both an art and a science. Noted nursing theorists such as Leininger, Watson, Rogers, Parse, and Newman have been urging the discipline of nursing to embrace this new emerging view that is seen as more holistic, humanistic, client focused, and grounded in the notion of caring as the core of nursing.

Since the early 1950s, many nursing theories have been systematically developed to help describe, explain, and predict the phenomena of concern to nursing. Each of these established theories provides a unique perspective, and each is distinct and separate from other nursing theories in its particular view of nursing phenomena. An overview of several nursing theories is presented later in the chapter.

TABLE 2-1 Chronology of Nursing Theory Development

DATE	THEORIST	THEORY/PUBLICATIONS
1859	Florence Nightingale	*Notes on Nursing: What It Is and What It Is Not*
1952	Hildegard Peplau	*Interpersonal Relations in Nursing*
1964		*Basic Principles of Patient Counseling*
1992		"Interpersonal Relations: A Theoretical Framework for Application in Nursing Practice" (in *Nursing Science Quarterly*)
1955	Virginia Henderson	(with B. Harmer) *Textbook for the Principles and Practice of Nursing*
1966		*The Nature of Nursing: A Definition and Its Implication for Practice, Research and Education*
1991		*The Nature of Nursing: Reflections after 20 Years*
1960, 1968, 1973	Faye Abdelleh	(with Beland, Martin, and Matheney) *Patient-Centered Approaches to Care*
1961, 1990	Ida Jean Orlando (Pelletier)	*The Dynamic Nurse-Patient Relationship*
1964	Ernestine Wiedenbach	*Clinical Nursing: A Helping Art*
1966, 1971	Joyce Travelbee	*Interpersonal Aspects of Nursing*
1969, 1973	Myra Levine	*Introduction to Clinical Nursing*
1989		"The Four Conservation Principles: Twenty Years Later"
1991		"The Conservation Principles: A Model for Health"
1970	Martha Rogers	*An Introduction to the Theoretical Basis of Nursing*
1980		"Nursing: A science of Unitary Humans"
1989		"Nursing: A science of Unitary Human Beings"
1971	Imogene King	*Toward a Theory of Nursing: General Concepts of Human Behavior*
1981		"A Theory for Nursing: Systems, Concepts, and Process"
1989		"King's General Systems Framework and Theory"
1971, 1980, 1988, 1991	Dorothea Orem	*Nursing Concepts of Practice*
1976	Dorothy Johnson	*Behavioral Systems and Nursing*
1980		"The Behavioral Systems Model for Nursing"
1976, 1984	Callista Roy	*Introduction to Nursing: An Adaptation Model*
1979	Callista Roy and Heather Andrews	*The Roy Adaptation Model*
1980		*The Roy Adaptation Model*
1987		*Theory Construction in Nursing: An Adaptation Model*
1991		*The Roy Adaptation Model: The Definitive Statement*
1976	Josephine Paterson and Loretta Zderad	*Humanistic Nursing*
1978	Madeline Leininger	*Transcultural Nursing, Concepts, Theories and Practice*
1980		*Caring: A Central Focus of Nursing*
1988		*Leininger's Theory of Nursing: Culture Care Diversity and Universality*
1979	Jean Watson	*Nursing: The Philosophy and Science of Caring*
1985		*Nursing: Human Science and Human Care*
1988		"New Dimensions of Human Caring Theory"
1989		"Watson's Philosophy and Theory of Human Caring in Nursing"
1979	Margaret Newman	*Theory Development in Nursing*
1983		"Newman's Health Theory"
1986		*Health as Expanding Consciousness*
1972	Betty Neuman	"The Betty Neuman Health Care Systems Model: A Total Person Approach to Patient Problems"
1982, 1989, 1995		*The Neuman Systems Model*

(continues)

TABLE 2-1 (Continued)

DATE	THEORIST	THEORY/PUBLICATIONS
1981, 1989	Rosemarie Parse	*Man-Living-Health: A Theory of Nursing*
1998		"The Human Becoming School of Thought: A Perspective for Nurses and Other Health Professionals"
1983	Joyce Fitzpatrick	"Fitzpatrick's Rhythm Model: Analysis for Nursing Science"
1984	Patricia Benner	*From Novice to Expert: Excellence and Power in Clinical Nursing Practice*
1989	Patricia Benner and Judith Wrubel	*The Primacy of Caring: Stress and Coping in Health and Illness*

Delmar/Cengage Learning

KNOWLEDGE DEVELOPMENT IN NURSING

The knowledge in a particular discipline can be arranged in a hierarchical structure that ranges from abstract to concrete. Theories represent the most concrete component of a discipline. Several theories that share a common view of the world can be grouped together to form a paradigm. A **paradigm** is a particular viewpoint or perspective. Each discipline has a defined metaparadigm, which is the most abstract component of knowledge and which can consist of more than one paradigm (Fawcett, 2005). A **metaparadigm** is the unifying force in a discipline that names the phenomena of concern to that discipline.

METAPARADIGM OF NURSING

What is it that distinguishes nursing from any other discipline such as biology, sociology, or psychology? Each of these other disciplines—biology, sociology, and psychology—is concerned with specific aspects of the human being. Every discipline singles out certain phenomena that it will deal with in a unique manner (Fawcett, 2005). The field of biology (the study of living organisms) has defined limits and boundaries that do not extend into psychology. Similarly, psychology (which is concerned with the behavior of individuals) does not extend its concerns into the domain of sociology, which has as its main focus the social behavior of human beings.

The broadly identified concerns of a discipline are defined in its metaparadigm. The metaparadigm concepts provide the boundaries and limitations of a discipline, identify the common viewpoint that all members of a discipline share, and help to focus the activities of the members of that discipline. Disciplines are distinguished from each other by differing metaparadigm concepts. Most metaparadigms consist of several major concepts.

Initial consensus on the metaparadigm concepts in nursing was achieved in 1984. According to Fawcett (2005), the major concepts that provide structure to the domain of nursing are *person, environment, health,* and *nursing.* These metaparadigm elements name the overall areas of concern for the nursing discipline. Each nursing theory presents a slightly different view of the metaparadigm concepts. Refer to the section later in this chapter entitled "Selected Nursing Theories" for a discussion of how various theorists address and link the metaparadigm concepts.

Consider for a moment the practice of nursing by a school nurse, an emergency room nurse, and a psychiatric nurse. What is the unifying thread among these various nurses? Although each nurse's practice is obviously different, they all consider their work as part of the profession of nursing because all share the same major concerns. Regardless of the setting or the type of client involved, each nurse is concerned with person, environment, health, and nursing. Nursing's metaparadigm is shared by all nurses despite differences in their individual practices.

How is nursing's metaparadigm different from that of other helping professions? The metaparadigm of medicine focuses on pathophysiology and the curing of disease. Nursing's metaparadigm is broader and focuses on the person, health, and the environment. Consider a prescribing practitioner's and a nurse's view of a client who is newly diagnosed with diabetes. The prescribing practitioner is concerned with reducing the client's abnormal blood glucose values to normal levels, if possible. The prescribing practitioner prescribes medications, an exercise regime, and nutritional counseling in an effort to control blood sugar levels. In dealing with the same client situation, the nurse is concerned with such issues as the client's ability to cope with a chronic condition, the effect of the diagnosis on the client's family, and teaching about the need for changes in the client's daily living patterns. The nurse is concerned with the impact of the diagnosis on all aspects of the client's life. Although both health care providers are viewing the same client situation, each has a different perspective or focus. Each discipline's metaparadigm provides a viewpoint that leads to the development of knowledge as seen within that viewpoint.

Despite the fact that person, health, environment, and nursing are the generally accepted metaparadigm elements in nursing, there is growing discontent with the limitation of these elements. As dialogue continues and as clarity emerges, the metaparadigm elements will change to reflect contemporary thought and practice.

One example of this evolution in the discipline of nursing is the inclusion of caring as a basic core concept, central to the practice of nursing. Nurse scholars have urged a reconsideration of the identified metaparadigm elements. Watson stated that "care is the essence of nursing and the most central and unifying focus for nursing practice (1985, p. 35). Watson further stated, "I see the value of human caring theory as a foundational ethic and philosophy for any health professional. Though my work comes from nursing, the current momentum for a focus on caring in several health disciplines is congruent with the caring stance that nursing has had across time" (as cited in Fawcett, 2002a, p. 215).

PARADIGMS IN NURSING

The metaparadigm of a discipline identifies common areas of concern. A paradigm is a particular way of viewing the phenomena of concern that have been delineated by the metaparadigm of the discipline. The term *paradigm* stems from the work of Kuhn (1970), who referred to a paradigm as "worldview" about the phenomena of concern in a discipline.

Two individuals with different paradigmatic views can look at precisely the same phenomenon and each will "see" or view the phenomenon differently. For example, consider the viewpoints of a mother and father who are watching their daughter at T-ball practice. The mother looks at her daughter and sees a graceful, yet somewhat shy child who has shown improvement in her ability to make new friends. On the other hand, the father sees a strong runner who needs help with batting drills. Each parent is looking at the same phenomenon (their daughter), but each is seeing the phenomenon from a completely different perspective. Each parent is operating from a different paradigm.

The prevailing paradigm in a discipline represents the dominant viewpoint of particular concepts. This viewpoint is supported by theories and research that for the time being adequately address the concerns of the discipline. By consensus, the community of scholars in a discipline accepts and agrees on a particular viewpoint or worldview. When new theories and research surface that challenge the prevailing paradigm, a new paradigm emerges to compete with the prevailing worldview. The competition between the paradigms results in what Kuhn (1970) refers to as a paradigm revolution. A **paradigm revolution** is the turmoil and conflict that occur in a discipline when a competing paradigm gains acceptance over the dominant paradigm. If the competing paradigm answers more questions and solves more problems for the discipline than the prevailing paradigm, then a paradigm shift occurs. A **paradigm shift** refers to the acceptance of the competing paradigm over the prevailing paradigm or a shifting away from one worldview toward another worldview. Again, by consensus the competing paradigm becomes the dominant paradigm and the process begins again (Kuhn, 1970).

The notion of paradigm revolution can be likened to the revolution that might occur in a country where the ruling government is overthrown by a competing group who

proposed to have more and better solutions to the country's problems. In this situation, power shifts from one ruling body to another. In another example, a paradigm shift occurred when people began to view the world as round rather than flat. Once it was agreed on by the community of scholars that the world was round (now the prevailing paradigm), all other views about the world also changed. Paradigms can be mutually exclusive. Members of a discipline cannot subscribe to two competing paradigms at the same time. One cannot believe at the same time that the world is flat *and* that the world is round.

Several nursing scholars have proposed that the discipline of nursing is in the midst of a paradigm revolution. The implication is that there are at least two paradigms in competition with each other. Although the scholarly literature in nursing reflects the views of several authors who present and name different paradigms in nursing, the work of Parse is highlighted here. According to Parse (1987), there are currently two paradigms in nursing: the *totality paradigm* and the *simultaneity paradigm* (see Figure 2-2). Each of these paradigms is composed of various nursing theories that are similar in their worldview of the metaparadigm concepts. However, each theory, which is grouped within a particular paradigm, has different definitions of concepts and propositions that state how these concepts are related.

In the **totality paradigm**, the person, who is a combination of biological, psychological, social, and spiritual features, is in constant interaction with the environment to accomplish goals and maintain balance. "The goals of nursing in the totality paradigm focus on health promotion, care

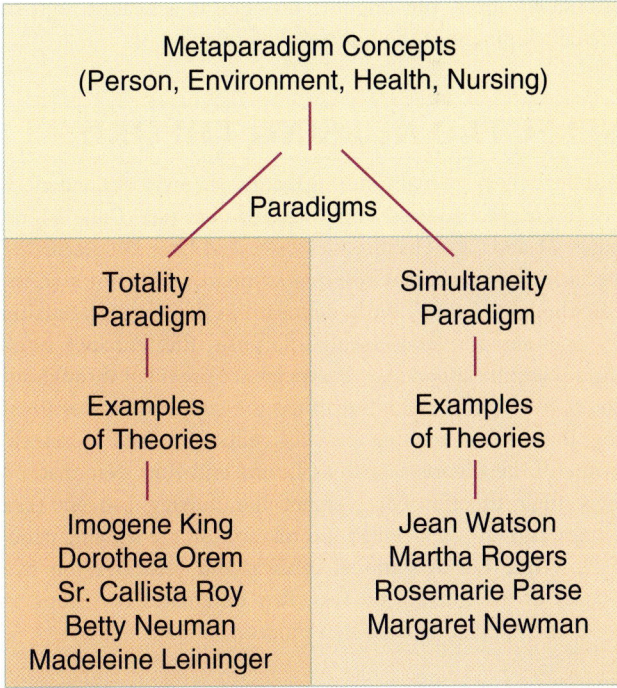

FIGURE 2-2 Hierarchy of knowledge development in nursing. In the hierarchical arrangement of knowledge development in a discipline, the metaparadigm concepts are the most abstract. Theories represent the most concrete level in this hierarchy.
DELMAR/CENGAGE LEARNING

and cure of the sick, and prevention of illness. Those receiving nursing care are persons designated as ill by societal norms" (Parse, 1987, p. 32). Identification with the totality paradigm is understandable because it has been and is the prevailing paradigm in nursing. Many of the nursing theories developed to date have a view of the discipline of nursing that fits the totality paradigm.

In the competing paradigm, the simultaneity paradigm, the person-environment interaction is viewed very differently. In the simultaneity paradigm, *whole* means unitary, and the unitary human has characteristics that are different from the parts and cannot be understood by a knowledge of the parts. Moreover, the human cannot be separated from the entirety of the universe, as both change continuously in innovated, unpredictable ways and together create health, a value defined by people for themselves (Parse, 2000). Nursing's goals in the simultaneity paradigm focus on the quality of life from the person's perspective. Designation of illness by societal norms is not a significant factor. The authority and prime decision maker in regard to nursing is the person, not the nurse (Parse, 2000).

Clearly, these two paradigms represent very different viewpoints. These differences give rise to different methods of inquiry and practice and provide sufficient scope to encompass all disciplinary activities.

Debate, dialogue, discussion, theory development, and research continue within the discipline of nursing. Some nursing scholars argue about the structural elements of the discipline; some debate the value of competing paradigms; and some present alternative metaparadigm elements. Yet with all the uncertainty that is created by these questions and alternative ideas, the ongoing dialogue is a healthy sign of the development of the nursing profession.

SELECTED NURSING THEORIES

Although there are many nursing theories, frameworks, and models, this chapter addresses only selected ones (see Table 2-2 on pages 31 and 32). The theories discussed have been selected because they represent the development of nursing's scientific thought. As previously discussed in this chapter, nursing theories serve several essential purposes that enhance nursing's scientific knowledge. Examples are provided throughout the following discussion regarding the contributions of nursing theories to nursing practice, education, and research. Some of the theorists, such as Levine and Roy, demonstrate how their theories complement the nursing process (see Chapters 5–10 for detailed information on the nursing process). While Levine's model relabels and redefines the five phases of the nursing process, Roy designates two steps to assessment, creating a six-step process.

FLORENCE NIGHTINGALE

Nightingale did not develop a theory of nursing as theory is defined today, but she provided the nursing profession with the philosophical basis from which other theories have emerged and developed. Nightingale's ideas about nursing

have guided both theoretical thought and actual nursing practice throughout the history of modern nursing.

Nightingale considered nursing similar to a religious calling to be answered only by women with an all-consuming and passionate response. She considered nursing to be both an art and a science and believed that nurses should be formally educated.

Her writings did not focus on the nature of the person but did stress the importance of caring for the ill person rather than caring for the illness. In Nightingale's view, the person was a passive recipient of care, and nursing's primary focus was on the manipulation of the person's environment to maintain or achieve a state of health.

Despite the fact that she did not believe in the germ theory, her experiences in the Crimean War magnified her interest in the principles of sanitation and the relationship between environment and health. A person's health was the direct result of environmental influences, specifically, cleanliness, light, pure air, pure water, and efficient drainage. Through manipulating the environment, nursing "aims to discover the laws of nature that would assist in putting the patient in the best possible condition so that nature can effect a cure" (Nightingale, 1859/1946, p. 6). Nursing's main focus was health, and health was closely related to nursing. Nursing was concerned with the healthy as well as the sick (Nightingale, 1859/1946).

Nightingale's principles regarding environment-health-nursing were implemented in America at the turn of the twentieth century. With the development of hospital-based schools of nursing, Nightingale's principles of sanitation were used to clean up the rat-infested, dirty hospitals of the day. With the use of Nightingale's ideas, hospitals became a place for people to recover rather than a place to die. When, for a variety of reasons, hospitals did not hire their own nursing graduates, nurses applied Nightingale's principles in the community in the development of public health nursing. The Henry Street Settlement founded by Lillian Wald is an excellent example of Nightingale's theory in practice.

Private duty nursing and public health nursing remained the primary focus of nursing practice until World War II. At this time, there was a tremendous increase in scientific knowledge and technology affecting health care. As the practice of medicine became more scientifically based, more clients were cared for in hospital settings. Nursing practice likewise became centered in the hospital rather than the home. With this development, it became clear that nursing did not have an adequate theory base to organize new knowledge and guide nursing practice. Nursing began to further develop its knowledge base by incorporating the principles of Nightingale into modern nursing theory.

EARLY NURSING THEORIES

By its very nature, the development of nursing's theoretical base has progressed in a methodical and systematic, albeit slow, fashion. Knowledge development is an ongoing process that is often influenced by driving forces outside the discipline of nursing. The early nurse theorists were not attempting to

TABLE 2-2 Summary of Selected Nursing Theorists' Major Concepts

THEORIST AND MODEL	PERSON	ENVIRONMENT	HEALTH	NURSING
Nightingale (1859) Environmental Theory	Physical, intellectual, and spiritual being unable to manipulate the environment to promote health	Physical elements that affect the healing process: cleanliness, light, pure air and water, comfort	State of well-being using one's powers to the fullest extent	To facilitate healing and restore health by manipulating the person's environment
Peplau (1952) Interpersonal Process	Developing organism living in an unstable equilibrium and striving to reduce anxiety	External factors and significant others	Interpersonal processes that facilitate forward movement of the personality	To develop interaction between the nurse and the person
Henderson (1955) Basic Needs	Biological being, oneness of mind and body, who has 14 fundamental needs	The aggregate of all external conditions affecting life and development	Wholeness, the ability to function independently in relation to 14 needs	To assist the person (well and sick) to perform the 14 essential functions
Levine (1969) Conservation Theory	Who the person knows himself or herself to be	Context in which the person lives his or her life	Response of the person to the environment	To use conversation activities aimed at optimizing the person's resources
Rogers (1970) Science of Unitary Beings	A unified irreducible whole; more than the sum of the parts	Pandimensional energy field integral with the human energy field	Patterns of living in harmony with the environment; defined by the culture or individual	Science and art; the art of nursing is the creative use of science for human betterment
King (1971) Goal Attainment Theory	Open system who exhibits characteristics common to others	Internal and external elements involving temporal and spatial reality	Ability to adjust to stressors to achieve maximum potential for daily living	A process of action, reaction, and interaction
Orem (1971) Self-Care Deficit Theory	A unity who functions biologically, symbolically, and socially and whose functioning is linked with the environment	Linked to the individual, forming an integrated system	State in which the individual is structurally and functionally whole	A triad of interrelated action systems
Roy (1976) Adaptation Model	Biopsychosocial being interacting with a dynamic environment	Internal and external conditions that surround and affect individuals	State or process of being or becoming an integrated and whole person through adaptation	To support the individual's adaptation to stimuli
Paterson & Zderad (1976) Humanistic Nursing	Process of becoming in an environment of time and space	Awareness of the individual's uniqueness and commonality with others	State of becoming, well-being, rather than freedom from disease	To respond to human needs and build humanistic nursing science

(continues)

TABLE 2-2 (Continued)

THEORIST AND MODEL	PERSON	ENVIRONMENT	HEALTH	NURSING
Leininger (1978) Transcultural Caring Theory	Caring, cultural beings	Interrelated, interdependent systems of a society	State of well-being that is culturally defined	To provide care; caring is the central, unifying domain for nursing knowledge and practice
Neuman (1972/1995) Systems Model	Wholistic client, dynamic composite of interrelationships among physiological, psychological, sociocultural, developmental, and spiritual variables	Internal and external factors affecting and affected by the system	Health and wellness is a condition or degree of system stability	To assist client adjustments required for an optimal wellness level through accuracy in the assessment of effects and possible effects of environmental stressors
Watson (1979/1989) Human Caring Theory	Person possesses three spheres: mind, body, and soul; strives to actualize the higher self	Internal and external variables	Unity and harmony within the mind, body, and soul	To assist persons attain a higher degree of harmony by offering caring relationships that clients can use for personal growth and development
Parse (1981/1995) Human Becoming Theory	An open being, coexisting with the environment	Inseparable from the individual; humans and the environment interchange energy, and influence one another's rhythmical patterns of relating	An open process of becoming that emcompasses a lived experience, synthesis of values, and rhythmic process of being or becoming	A discipline, the practice of which is a performing art

Delmar/Cengage Learning

address the metaparadigm concepts because initial consensus on these had not yet been achieved. Rather, these theories were attempting to answer the question "What is nursing?"

Hildegard Peplau

Hildegard Peplau, a psychiatric nurse, combined her research and experience in the development of a theory of psychodynamic nursing, published in *Interpersonal Relations in Nursing* (1952). Drawing from her own knowledge and that from other disciplines, Peplau defined the concepts and stages involved in the development of the nurse-client relationship. From that relationship, she identified the roles of the nurse as stranger, resource person, teacher, leader, surrogate, and counselor. Peplau developed a middle-range theory with a focus on both nursing and the person and did not

incorporate all aspects of the metaparadigm into her theory. Although other theories may view the nurse-client relationship differently, the primacy of this relationship in nursing has remained.

Virginia Henderson

Virginia Henderson's definition of nursing, considered to be a classic, first appeared in 1955.

The unique function of the nurse is to assist the individual, sick or well, in the performance of those activities contributing to health or its recovery (or to a peaceful death) that he would perform unaided if he had the necessary strength, will, or knowledge. And to do this in such a way as to help him gain independence as rapidly as possible. (Henderson, 1966, p. 15)

Together with Bertha Harmer, Henderson attempted to identify those basic human needs viewed as the basis of nursing care. These needs include the need to maintain physiologic balance, to adjust to the environment, to communicate and participate in social interaction, and to worship according to one's faith. Henderson's 14 basic needs were published in the *Textbook of the Principles and Practice of Nursing,* one of the first nursing textbooks. Henderson viewed the nursing role as helping the client from dependence to independence. As an early nursing theorist, she did not intend to develop a theory of nursing but rather attempted to define the unique focus of nursing. Henderson's emphasis on basic human needs as the central focus of nursing practice has led to further theory development regarding the needs of the person and how nursing can assist in meeting those needs.

Faye Abdellah

Faye Abdellah, acknowledging the influence of Henderson, expanded Henderson's 14 needs into 21 problems that she believed would serve as a knowledge base for nursing. Throughout her career, she strongly supported the idea that nursing research would be the key factor in helping nursing to emerge as a true profession. The research that was done regarding these common needs or problems has served as a foundation for the development of what we now know as nursing diagnoses.

Joyce Travelbee

Joyce Travelbee, an educator and psychiatric nurse, was influenced by the philosophy of existentialism, a movement that is centered on individual existence in an incomprehensible world, the role that free will plays in it, and the search to find meaning in life's experiences. She extensively developed the ideas of sympathy, empathy, and rapport in which the nurse could begin to comprehend and relate to the uniqueness of others. Her work focused on the human-to-human relationship and on finding meaning in experiences such as pain, illness, and distress. Travelbee based most of her theory on her own experiences and readings and first published her work in *Interpersonal Aspects of Nursing* in 1966.

Josephine Paterson and Loretta Zderad

The work of Josephine Paterson and Loretta Zderad was similar to that of Travelbee in that it emphasized the humanistic and existential basis of nursing practice. According to Paterson and Zderad, theory developed from the practice of nursing. Although the models proposed by Travelbee and Paterson and Zderad had some impact at the time of their initial introduction, they did not gain wide popularity and application in nursing. The work of Travelbee and Paterson and Zderad most appropriately fits the simultaneity paradigm. Current theorists—such as Watson, Rogers, Parse, Fitzpatrick, and Newman—who have an existential orientation, are rediscovering the merits of Travelbee and Paterson and Zderad.

CONTEMPORARY NURSING THEORIES

Although early nursing theorists attempted to answer the question "What is nursing?" contemporary theorists have addressed the metaparadigm concepts in more depth, focused more specifically on nursing actions, and tried to answer the question "When is nursing needed?" The work of contemporary theorists such as Levine, Orem, and Roy form the theoretical basis for many interventions in current nursing practice.

Myra Levine

Myra Levine's conservation theory is directly grounded in nursing practice. In her attempt to describe, explain, and predict the phenomena of concern to nursing, Levine published the four conservation principles in 1969 in *Introduction to Clinical Nursing.* Conservation is derived from a Latin word meaning "to keep together." Levine believed in the wholeness of the human being, and the primary focus of conservation is to maintain that wholeness. Levine viewed nursing as assisting clients with the conservation of their uniqueness by helping clients to adapt appropriately. Conservation principles are universal principles designed to link concepts into a cohesive framework within which nursing practice in different environments can be performed (Levine, 1990).

According to Levine, the four principles of conservation are:

1. *Conservation of energy:* "The individual requires a balance of energy and a constant renewal of energy to maintain life activities" (Levine, 1990, p. 197).
2. *Conservation of structural integrity:* "Structural integrity is concerned with the processes of healing … to restore wholeness and continuity after injury or illness" (Levine, 1989, p. 333).
3. *Conservation of personal integrity:* "Everyone seeks to defend his or her identity as a self, in both that hidden, intensely private person that dwells within and in the public faces assumed as individuals move through their relationships with others" (Levine, 1989, p. 334).
4. *Conservation of social integrity:* "No diagnosis should be made that does not include the other persons whose lives are entwined with that of the individual" (Levine, 1989, p. 336).

In Levine's view, the *person* is who the person knows himself or herself to be, and the *environment* is the context in which the person lives his or her life. In addition, health is socially defined and the goal of nursing is based on the four conservation principles. Levine did not operationally define and relate the metaparadigm concepts in her theory because her original work was initially intended to be a medical-surgical nursing textbook and not a developed nursing theory. In reevaluating her theory 20 years later, Levine stated that she has "grown in [her] conviction that they [the conservation principles] continue to offer an approach to nursing that is scientific, research oriented, and above all suitable in daily practice in many environments" (Levine, 1989, p. 331). Levine's conservation model is used in a variety of settings with clients across the life span, such as in the emergency and operating rooms; in critical care, acute care, primary care, and long-term care units; with the homeless; and in the community.

Levine's four conservation principles can also be useful in a home setting in which the family rather than a single individual is the client. The nurse recognizes that energy within the family needs to be maintained to keep the family whole. In caring for the family, the nurse needs to maintain the structural, social, and personal integrity of the family and of each individual while dealing with the illness of a specific family member. Consider, for example, the nurse who makes a home health visit to see a child with cystic fibrosis. In this situation, the nurse's attention needs to be directed toward conservation of energy for the child. To help conserve the child's energy for breathing, exercises must be taught to and done by others. The nurse directs strategies toward conserving the child's structural integrity while recognizing that the child is a unique individual and is a member of a social group, the family. Conservation of social integrity would be accomplished through maintaining interest in and monitoring the family dynamics.

Levine's theory is pragmatic, and the conservation principles can be applied to most nursing situations. Her theory, which is congruent with the characteristics of the totality paradigm, is appropriate for use in situations in which the nurse has had a long-term relationship with the client yet is also useful for short-term relationships.

Dorothea Orem

In attempting to plan a nursing curriculum for licensed practical nurses, Dorothea Orem was searching for a pragmatic framework to organize nursing knowledge. She focused on the questions "What is nursing?" and "When do people need nursing care?" and from this she derived that people need nursing when they are unable to care for themselves. In 1971, she presented the self-care deficit theory of nursing (S-CDTN) in the book *Nursing Concepts of Practice* and has continually revised and updated her theory.

Orem's theory incorporates the medical model rather than rejects it, centers on the individual, is problem oriented, and is easily adaptable in varied clinical situations. As a grand theory, the S-CDTN has three interconnecting theories: theory of self-care, theory of self-care deficit, and theory of nursing systems. Each one is discussed in the following text.

THEORY OF SELF-CARE.
According to this theory, **self-care** is a learned behavior and a deliberate action in response to a need. Orem identified three categories of self-care requisites: universal self-care requisites, developmental self-care requisites, and health-deviation self-care requisites. Universal self-care requisites are common to all human beings and include both physiological and social interaction needs. Developmental self-care requisites are the needs that arise as the individual grows and develops. Health-deviation self-care requisites result from the needs produced by disease or illness states. Self-care is performed by mature and maturing individuals. When someone else must perform a self-care need, it is termed dependent care.

THEORY OF SELF-CARE DEFICIT.
This theory purports that nursing care is needed when people are affected by limitations that do not allow them to meet their self-care needs. The relationship between the nurse and the client is established when a self-care deficit is present. Self-care deficits, not medical diagnosis, determine the need for nursing care. According to Orem, the only legitimate need for nursing care is when a self-care deficit exists.

THEORY OF NURSING SYSTEMS.
This is the unifying theory that "subsumes the theory of self-care deficit which subsumes the theory of self-care" (Orem, 1991, p. 66). The theory of nursing systems attempts to answer the question "What do nurses do?" This was the original question that prompted the development of Orem's theory.

The nurse determines whether or not there is a legitimate need for nursing care. Is a person able to meet self-care needs? Does a deficit exist? If a deficit exists, then the nurse plans care that identifies what is to be done by whom: the nurse, the client, or other (family or significant other). Collectively, the actions of all these people are called the nursing system. Orem identified three types of nursing systems: wholly compensatory, partly compensatory, and supportive-educative.

In the wholly compensatory nursing system, the nurse supports and protects the client, compensates for the client's inability to care for himself or herself, and attempts to provide care for the client. The nurse would use the wholly compensatory nursing system when caring for a newborn or with a client in a postanesthesia care unit who is recovering from surgery. Both of these clients are completely unable to provide self-care.

In the partly compensatory nursing system, both the nurse and client perform care measures. For example, the nurse can assist the postoperative client to ambulate. The nurse may bring in a meal tray for the client who is able to feed himself or herself. The nurse compensates for what the client cannot do. The client is able to perform selected self-care activities but also accepts care performed by the nurse for needs the client is unable to meet independently.

In the supportive-educative nursing system, the nurse's actions are to help clients develop their own self-care abilities through knowledge, support, and encouragement. Clients must learn and perform their own self-care activities. The supportive-educative nursing system is being used when a nurse guides a new mother to breastfeed her baby. Counseling a psychiatric client on more adaptive coping strategies is another example of the use of the supportive-educative nursing system.

Orem focused primarily on the needs of the person and the action of nursing to meet those needs. Lesser emphasis was given to defining health and the environment. The S-CDTN is useful in determining the kind of nursing assistance needed by the client and, therefore, has merit as a theory that guides nursing practice. Orem's theory is consistent with the characteristics of the totality paradigm.

Betty Neuman

Betty Neuman was motivated to develop a model to respond to the expressed needs of graduate students at the School of Nursing, University of California, Los Angeles, for course content that would present nursing problems prior to content emphasizing nursing problem areas. The Neuman systems model was first published in 1972 as a teaching approach to patient problems. Refinements in the Neuman system model are evident in the three editions of Neuman's book *The Neuman Systems Model* (1982, 1989, and 1995).

The Neuman systems model focuses on the wellness of the client system in relation to environmental stressors and reactions to stressors. Stressors are categorized as follows:

1. *Intrapersonal stressors:* Those that occur within
2. *Interpersonal stressors:* Those that occur between individuals
3. *Extrapersonal stressors:* Those that occur outside the person (Neuman, 1995)

Nursing interventions focus on retaining or maintaining system stability on three preventive levels:

1. *Primary prevention:* Protecting the normal line of defense and strengthening the flexible line of defense
2. *Secondary prevention:* Strengthening internal lines of resistance, reducing the reaction, and increasing resistance factors
3. *Tertiary prevention:* Readapting, stabilizing, and protecting the **reconstitution** (adaptation to a stressor) or return to wellness following treatment

The Neuman systems model is consistent with the characteristics of the totality paradigm.

Madeleine Leininger

Madeleine Leininger first published her theory of cultural care diversity and universality in 1978, *Transcultural Nursing: Concepts, Theories, and Practices.* Leininger credits the development of her early clinical work with mildly disturbed children as the catalyst for her idea of transcultural nursing. The central purpose of the theory of cultural care diversity and universality is "to discover, document, interpret, and explain the phenomenon of cultural care as a synthesized construct" (Leininger, 1996, p. 72). The theory provides for specific nursing interventions to assist people of diverse cultures:

1. *Cultural care preservation or maintenance:* The nurse accepts and complies with the client's cultural beliefs.
2. *Cultural care accommodation or negotiation:* The nurse plans, negotiates, and accommodates the client's culturally specific food preferences, religious practices, kinship needs, child care practices, and treatment practices.
3. *Cultural care repatterning or restructuring:* The nurse is knowledgeable about cultural care and develops ways to repattern or restructure nursing care. (Leininger, 1991, pp. 41–42)

Transcultural nursing is different from the medical model and traditional nursing knowledge and practice, as it is both

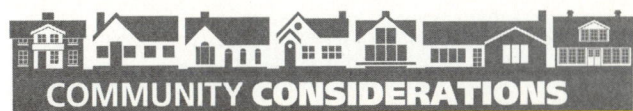

COMMUNITY CONSIDERATIONS

Belief System

Culturally competent care requires the nurse to work within the client's cultural belief system to resolve health problems. This means that the nurse needs to hear the client and consider the client's world and daily experiences.

a discipline and practice profession to understand and serve people worldwide (Leininger, as cited in Fawcett, 2002b); see the accompanying Community Considerations display. Also see Chapter 20 for detailed information on cultural diversity.

The publication of the third edition of *Transcultural Nursing* (Leininger & McFarland, 2002) documents use of the theory-based research findings in practice. Leininger (as cited in Fawcett, 2002b, p. 132) states that "transcultural nursing has contributed a large, unique, and distinct growing body of knowledge that is meaningful and beneficial to cultural consumers. Transcultural nursing also has been a breakthrough to nurses, showing that culturally based care contributes to healing (health), well-being, and helping clients face dying or death as the essence of nursing." Leininger's theory is consistent with the characteristics of the totality paradigm.

Sister Callista Roy

Sister Callista Roy combined general systems theory with adaptation theory to produce the Roy adaptation model. Roy was greatly influenced by her teacher and mentor, Dorothy E. Johnson, a nursing theorist who developed the behavioral systems model. Roy first published her model in the 1970s and has continued to further refine and develop the theory. As a contemporary theorist, Roy worked with the metaparadigm concepts to define and relate these concepts.

Roy defines a person as "an adaptive system ... a whole comprised of parts that function as a unity for some purpose" (Andrews & Roy, 1991, p. 4). The person is a biopsychosocial being in constant interaction with a changing internal and external environment. Nursing attempts to alter the environment when the person is not adapting well or has ineffective coping responses.

"The world around and within (the person as an adaptive system) is called the environment" and "includes all conditions, circumstances, and influences that surround and affect the development and behavior of the person" (Andrews & Roy, 1991, p. 18). The environmental stimuli can be classified as either focal, residual, or contextual. Focal stimuli are those that are immediately present in the person's environment. Focal stimuli are the objects or events that most attract one's attention. Most stimuli never become focal. Residual stimuli are those attitudes that are

UNCOVERING THE

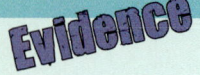

TITLE OF STUDY
"Prayer Warriors: A Grounded Theory Study of American Indians Receiving Hemodialysis"

AUTHOR
J. Walton

PURPOSE
The purpose of this classic grounded theory study was to explore what spirituality means to individuals who are American Indians receiving hemodialysis.

METHODS
Twelve women and nine men, ages 24 to 62, volunteered for this study. Informed consent was obtained, and in-depth interviews, field notes, and theoretical memos were completed. The metaphor "Prayer warriors" described the core category of this study.

FINDINGS
The results of this study indicate that spirituality is a way of "being in the world" and involves all aspects of living for individuals who are American Indians, including honoring spirit, resisting hemodialysis, healing old wounds, and connecting with family and community. The concept of spirituality for American Indians blends new ways with old cultural traditions. Praying played a major role in the following categories: (a) suffering, (b) honoring spirit, (c) healing old wounds, and (d) connecting with community. Praying involved hard work, suffering, sweating, hunger, and passion and was a powerful way to cope with the stress of hemodialysis.

IMPLICATIONS
Although the study was limited to individuals who were American Indians receiving hemodialysis in rural northwestern United States, the study demonstrates the complexity of the participants and that a cultural approach may help individuals who are American Indians prepare for dialysis. Future studies in this area are recommended since the goal of grounded theory research is for nurses to use what "fits" in clinical practice, while continuing to build and revise the theory with evidence-based nursing practice.

Walton, J. (2007). Prayer warriors: A grounded theory study of American Indians receiving hemodialysis. *Nephrology Nursing Journal, 34,* 347–356.

that which is a focal stimulus one minute can become a residual stimulus the next.

According to the Roy adaptation model, the person has coping mechanisms that are broadly categorized in either the regulator or cognator subsystem. Adaptation is accomplished through these coping mechanisms that are innate, "genetically determined … and automatic processes" (Andrews & Roy, 1991, p. 13). The regulator subsystem functions through the autonomic nervous system, which "responds automatically through neural, chemical, and endocrine coping processes" (Andrews & Roy, 1991, p. 14). The cognator subsystem enables the person to respond to stimuli through processing stimuli, learning, judgment, and emotion. All input into the system (the person) is channeled through the regulator and cognator subsystems. If the regulator or cognator subsystem fails, there is ineffective adaptation.

Neither the regulator nor the cognator subsystem can be observed directly. Only the responses that each produces are observable. Roy categorized these responses into four adaptive modes: physiologic, self-concept, role function, and interdependence. The physiologic mode allows individuals to respond physiologically to their environment. The self-concept mode "focuses on psychologic and spiritual aspects of the person" (Andrews & Roy, 1991, p. 16). The basic underlying need of the self-concept mode is psychologic integrity. The role function mode focuses on the need to know who one is. The emphasis of the interdependence mode is affectional adequacy or the feeling of security in nurturing relationships (Andrews & Roy, 1991).

The purposes of adaptation are survival, growth, reproduction, and mastery. Adaptive responses contribute to these goals, whereas ineffective responses may threaten the person's survival, growth, reproduction, or mastery (Andrew & Roy, 1991). Roy's new definition of adaptation is "The process and outcome whereby thinking and feeling persons, as individuals or in groups, use conscious awareness and choice to create human and environmental integration" (Roy & Andrews, 1999, p. 30).

The goal of nursing is "the promotion of adaptation in each of the four modes, thereby contributing to the person's health, quality of life, and dying with dignity" (Andrews & Roy, 1991, p. 20). Nursing care needs to be provided when a person has unusual stressors or when usual coping mechanisms are ineffective. Basically, the nurse attempts to manipulate stimuli in such a way as to allow the client to cope effectively. Roy defines health as "a state and a process of being and becoming an integrated and whole person," and a "lack of integration represents lack of health" (Andrews & Roy, 1991, p. 419).

In Roy's view, the nurse must first assess how the client behaves in each adaptive mode and then determine what can be altered in that mode to produce more efficient and effective adaptive responses. The nurse then either alters the environment directly or helps the person to alter the environment for better adaptive responses.

In the physiological mode, problems may arise in areas such as exercise, nutrition, elimination, fluid and electrolytes, temperature regulation, and oxygenation. For example, in

developed during previous experiences in one's life whose effects on the current situation are unclear. Contextual stimuli are "all the other stimuli present in the situation that contribute to the effect of the focal stimulus" (Andrews & Roy, 1991, p. 9). Because stimuli are constantly changing,

caring for a client with a fever, the nurse helps the client to adapt by administering medications to lower the temperature, administering cool baths, and providing adequate fluids. Through these interventions, the nurse is attempting to alter both the internal and external environments of the person.

In the self-concept mode, the term *self-concept* refers to both the physical and the personal self. The physical self is affected or threatened during invasive procedures such as surgery. Anxiety, guilt, and distress are responses within the personal self to physical or emotional stressors. For example, in caring for an obese person who feels guilty about developing diabetes at an early age, a nurse can help reframe the client's thinking to work through the guilt and anxiety. Through the use of counseling techniques, the nurse can teach the client how to adapt to the present situation and learn how to cope with it in the future.

Within the framework of the role function mode, the nurse would help a woman disabled with arthritis to identify adaptive approaches to maintain the roles of wife and homemaker. Nursing actions might include referral to occupational therapy for needed adaptive devices that could assist the client in maintenance of roles.

In the interdependence mode, problems may include feelings of alienation, disengagement, loneliness, or disenfranchisement that are experienced in various relationships. Examples of clients with problems in interdependence may include a grieving widow or a person with an abusive spouse.

The Roy adaptation model has gained wide acceptance in nursing practice, research, and education and is part of the dominant worldview of nursing. Roy's views of the person and the person-environment interaction clearly represent characteristics of the totality paradigm.

THEORIES FOR THE NEW WORLDVIEW OF NURSING

Theories for the new worldview of nursing describe, explain, and predict the phenomena of concern to nursing from a unique, more holistic perspective. In this new worldview, the client has primacy and the client-environment interaction is of utmost importance. Theories by Jean Watson, Martha Rogers, and Rosemarie Parse exemplify the new worldview.

Jean Watson

In the 1980s, Jean Watson developed the theory of human caring, which focuses on the art and science of human caring. According to Watson (1985, p. 33), "caring is the essence of nursing and the most central and unifying focus of nursing practice." This theory offers a new way of conceptualizing and maximizing human-to-human transactions that occur daily in nursing practice. Watson's theory is influenced by Eastern philosophy and is "based on a metaphysical, spiritual-existential, and phenomenological orientation" (Fawcett, 1993, p. 220). These influences link Watson's theory to the work of early theorists such as Travelbee and Paterson and Zderad.

The theory of human caring evolved from Watson's beliefs, values, and assumptions about caring. In Watson's view (1985), care and love comprise the primal universal psychic energy and are the basis for our humanity. Watson noted that, throughout its history, nursing has been involved in caring and has actually evolved out of caring. Furthermore, she stated that caring will determine nursing's contribution to the humanizing of the world.

Watson's theory is composed of 10 carative factors, which are classified as nursing actions or caring processes. See Chapter 14 for Watson's carative factors. The first three carative factors serve as the philosophical foundation for the science of caring. The remaining seven provide more specific direction for nursing actions.

Watson stated that "health refers to unity and harmony within the mind, body, and soul. Health is also associated with the degree of congruence between the self as perceived and the self as experienced" (Watson, 1985, p. 48). In Watson's (1985, p. 49) view, the goal of nursing "is to help persons gain a higher degree of harmony with the mind, body, and soul." The nurse uses the carative factors to accomplish the goal of nursing. Watson's theory clearly fits within the principles of the simultaneity paradigm.

"Evidence suggests that caring-healing behaviors are the currency that buys patient, family, and coworker satisfaction" (Felgen, 2003, p. 213). The challenge of nursing is to create moments of caring through human-to-human interaction in the fast-paced world of health care.

Martha Rogers

Martha Rogers, a visionary leader and pioneer in the development of nursing's unique knowledge base, developed the highly abstract theory of the science of unitary human beings. According to Rogers, "nursing is a learned profession: a science and an art. A science is an organized body of abstract knowledge. The art involved in nursing is the creative use of science for human betterment" (Rogers, 1990, p. 198). Rogers's contribution to the discipline of nursing was revolutionary and provided new directions for the practice of nursing. Rogers first presented her ideas in the book *An*

👁 **SPOTLIGHT ON...**

Caring and Nurturance

Recall the last time that you were sick with the flu. Reflect on what it means to you "to be cared about," "to be cared for," and "to be taken care of."

How are these the same? How are these different? As the recipient of care, what kinds of behaviors did you identify as "caring behaviors"? How could these behaviors be different for another person who grew up in a different family? A different culture?

Introduction to the Theoretical Basis of Nursing (1970). Her ideas regarding the person and the environment as energy fields were not considered to be consistent with the dominant paradigm of the 1970s but are more applicable to the principles of the simultaneity paradigm of the late 1980s.

According to Rogers (1990, p. 108), "the uniqueness of nursing is identified in the phenomena of concern. Nursing is the study of unitary, irreducible human beings and their respective environments." The unitary person is an irreducible pandimensional energy field characterized by a pattern and expressing qualities that are unique to the whole and cannot be foreseen from knowledge of the parts. Environment is defined as "an irreducible pandimensional energy field identified by pattern and integral with a given human field" (Rogers, 1990, p. 109).

Within the viewpoint of the science of unitary human beings, the person is a unified whole and seen as greater than and different from the sum of the parts. The whole person cannot be known by examining any particular aspect or dimension of the person because all aspects together combine to form an entity different from the collection of parts. It is the characterization of the person as a human energy field that unites all aspects of the person into a unified whole. The whole of the person's energy field interacts with the whole of the environmental energy field, which results in the process of life. There is a constant exchange of matter and energy between the person-environment unit, yet the uniqueness of each person is maintained through rhythmic patterns and relationships.

Nursing identifies the patterns and organization of the person-environment unit and aims to repattern the rhythm and organization of these energy fields so that the person's integrity is heightened. Rogers's theory provides for maintenance and promotion of health, prevention of disease, nursing diagnosis, intervention, and rehabilitation to encompass the scope of nursing goals.

Changes have been made in Rogers's conceptual system as it has evolved over the years. "The concepts of the conceptual system currently are labeled energy fields, openness, pattern, and pandimensionality. The principles of hemodynamics now are labeled helicy, resonancy, and integrality" (Fawcett, 2003, p. 44). The changes in the science of unitary human beings reflect Rogers's concern with language and the insights gained over the years from new knowledge. "The development of a science of unitary human beings is a never-ending process. This abstract system first presented some years ago has continued to gain substance. Concomitantly, early errors have undergone correction, definitions have been revised for greater clarity and accuracy, and updating of content is ongoing" (Rogers, 1992, p. 28). Martha Rogers died on March 13, 1994. The Society of Rogerian Scholars continues to refine Rogers's theory.

Rosemarie Parse

Rosemarie Rizzo Parse (1981) began her work to create a theory grounded in the human sciences that would enhance nursing knowledge; the initial result of Parse's effort was the theory of man-living-health, which was first published in 1982, *Man-Living-Health: A Theory of Nursing*. The theory was renamed the theory of human becoming in 1990. Parse refined her theory to include a school of thought in the second edition of her book (1998) newly titled *The Human Becoming School of Thought: A Perspective for Nurses and Other Health Professionals*. The theory of human becoming and the human becoming school of thought focus on the human-universe-health process. The goal of nursing from the human becoming perspective is quality of life (Parse, 2006). The principles of the theory of human becoming are as follows:

1. Structuring meaning multidimensionally (i.e., based on the belief that we live at many realms of the universe all at once) is cocreating reality through the language of valuing and imaging.
2. Cocreating rhythmic patterns of relating is living the paradoxical unity of revealing-concealing and enabling-limiting while connecting-separating.
3. Cotranscending with the possibles is powering unique ways of originating in the process of transforming.

Clearly, Parse's theory is consistent with the principles of the simultaneity paradigm.

Similar to the work of Parse, Joyce Fitzpatrick's life perspective rhythm model (1989) and Margaret Newman's model of health (1986) are current developing theories within the simultaneity paradigm.

CONTINUING EVOLUTION OF NURSING THEORY

The world of health care changes on a daily basis. Client needs and problems often change on a minute-by-minute basis. Knowledge, information, and technology in both health care and nursing are growing at unprecedented rates. In the face of these advances, nursing strives to preserve *the notion of caring* in health care. Theories are needed to organize knowledge and to guide nursing practice and nursing research.

Nurses encounter a variety of clinical situations in which application of nursing theory is needed. The nursing process has been integrated into many nursing frameworks and theories. In these occurrences, nurses may discover that specific theories will be more appropriate for certain clinical situations than others. Knowledge of specific theories should expand as nurses gain experience in nursing practice. In all cases, theories that are selected for application in practice should be congruent with the nurse's own beliefs and values. Parse (1998, p. 74) defines research as "the formal process of seeking knowledge and understanding through use of rigorous methodologies." Nursing frameworks and theories have provided numerous research instruments to measures constructs operationally defined to provide consistency with the particular framework or theory; such instrumentation is essential to advanced nursing knowledge (Barrett, 2002). Advances have been made in the development of unique research methodologies such as Carboni's Rogerian process of inquiry; Leininger's ethnonursing research method; Newman's praxis method; and Parse's method of basic research.

Current emphasis has shifted from developing new theories to applying existing theories to practice and expanding existing nursing theories by including such concepts as cultural diversity, spirituality, family, and social change. For example, Mendyka and Bloom have expanded King's model by adding a cultural perspective. According to Catalano (2006), the theories that are flexible and adaptable to new discoveries while being realistic and usable in practice will continue to thrive and remain the cornerstones of professional nursing; those theories that are too theoretical or rigid will gradually disappear.

KEY CONCEPTS

- Concepts are abstract vehicles of thought and are the building blocks of theory.
- Propositions are relational statements that link concepts together.
- Theories help to show how things fit together. The function of theory is to provide a framework for explaining, predicting, and sometimes controlling situations.
- Nursing uses theories from other disciplines in conjunction with nursing theory.
- The development, use, and testing of nursing theory are necessary for the professionalization of the discipline of nursing.
- The relationship between nursing theory, practice, and research is an interdependent one. As a practice-oriented discipline, nursing theory and research inform and transform nursing practice.
- Theories range in scope from grand theories to middle-range theories to micro-range theories.

- The metaparadigm names the phenomena of concern to a discipline and distinguishes one discipline from another.
- The currently accepted metaparadigm concepts in nursing are person, environment, health, and nursing.
- The metaparadigm may be composed of more than one paradigm. Parse purports that there are two paradigms in nursing: the totality paradigm and the simultaneity paradigm.
- Early nursing theorists were attempting to answer questions related to the "what" and "how" of nursing.
- The theories developed by Levine, Orem, and Roy are useful in guiding nursing practice.
- A new worldview of nursing is emerging in the work of such theorists as Watson, Rogers, and Parse.

REVIEW QUESTIONS

1. Nursing's metaparadigm includes:
   a. Concepts, theory, health, and environment
   b. Health, person, environment, and nursing
   c. Providers, standards, models, and clients
   d. The person, environment, health, and nursing
2. "An organized, coherent set of concepts and their relationship to each other that is proposed to explain a given phenomenon" best defines which of the following?
   a. A concept
   b. A proposition
   c. A theory
   d. A discipline
3. Which theories are examples of the totality paradigm? Select all that apply.
   a. Martha Rogers
   b. Rosemarie Parse
   c. Sr. Callista Roy
   d. Dorothea Orem
   e. Jean Watson
   f. Madeleine Leininger
4. A caring, cultural being best defines "person" by which theorist?
   a. King
   b. Leininger
   c. Neuman
   d. Watson
5. Why are nursing theories needed? Select all that apply.
   a. To organize knowledge
   b. To guide nursing practice
   c. To promote nursing diagnosis
   d. To guide nursing research
   e. To develop a language for nurses
   f. To define professional nursing practice

online companion

Visit the DeLaune and Ladner online companion resource at **www.delmar.cengage.com** for additional content and study aids. Click on Online Companions, then select the Nursing discipline.

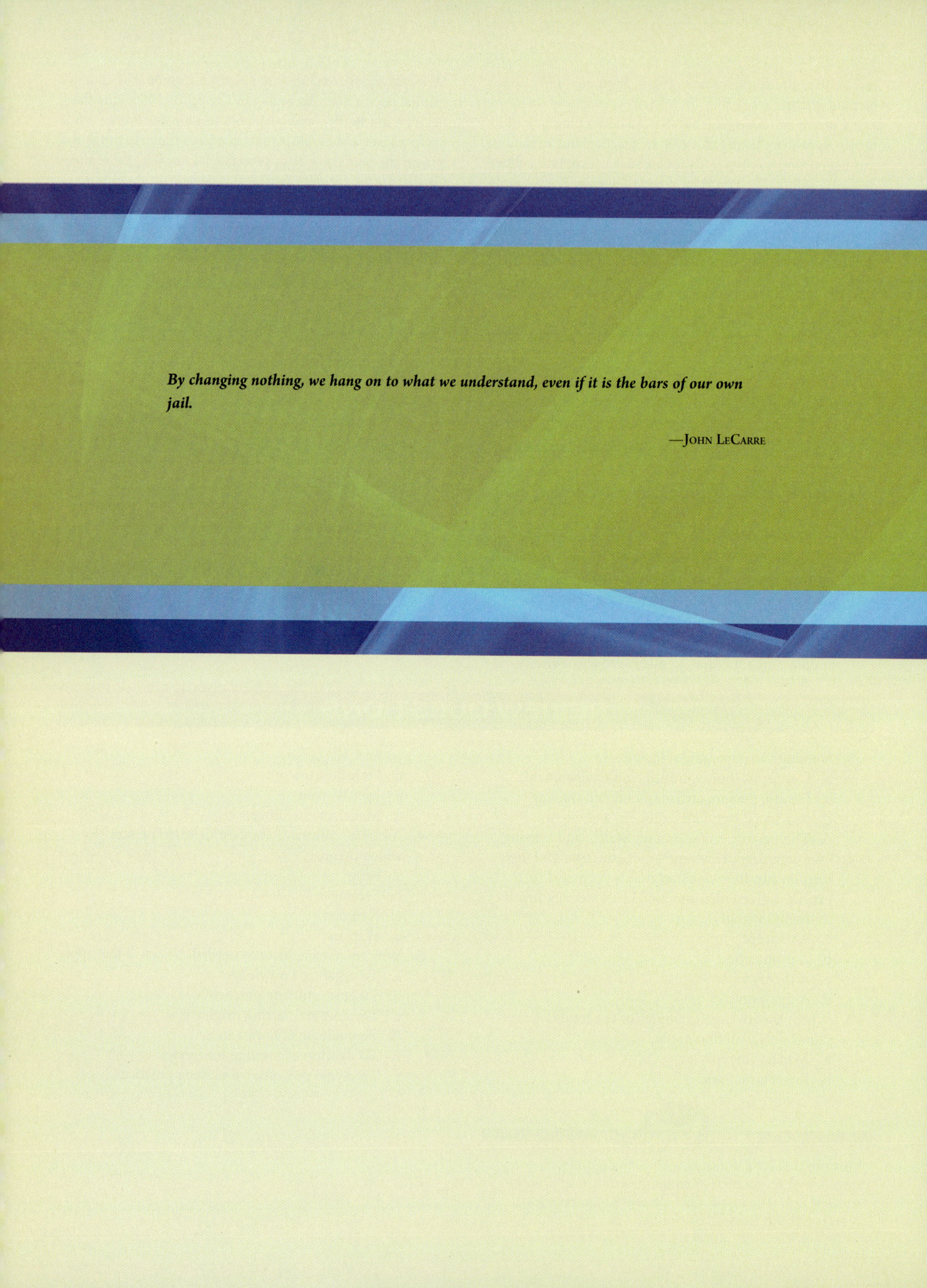

By changing nothing, we hang on to what we understand, even if it is the bars of our own jail.

—John LeCarre

CHAPTER 3

Research and Evidence-Based Practice

COMPETENCIES

1. Explain the basis for research and knowledge development in nursing.
2. Describe the steps in the research process.
3. Explain the responsibilities of the researcher in guarding the rights of research participants and others who assist in the research study.
4. Identify the various applications of nursing research in nursing practice.
5. Describe how evidence-based practice is used to guide clinical decision making.
6. Describe the key elements of evidence reports.

KEY TERMS

abstract	hypothesis	recontextualizing
concepts	independent variable	research
conceptual framework	informed consent	research design
conceptualization	nursing research	secondary source
construct	primary source	theory
dependent variable	qualitative analysis	value
evidence-based practice	qualitative research	variable
full disclosure	quantitative research	

This chapter explores the scientific foundation on which the knowledge base of the profession has been and is being built. **Nursing research** is a "scientific process that validates and refines existing knowledge and generates new knowledge that directly and indirectly influences nursing practice" (Burns & Grove, 2004, p. 4). **Evidence-based practice** (EBP) is using the best evidence available to guide clinical decision making. Research is critical in nursing because the use of research is inherent in the definition of a professional, nurses are accountable for client outcomes, and consumers are demanding evidence-based care (Houser, 2008). The identification of the knowledge base for nursing practice contributes to achieving client outcomes and making nursing practice credible. The emphasis on quality care based on evidence and research is an increasing focus in all areas of health care. The challenge to nurses is to determine the interrelatedness of nursing research to EBP: Does a solid research base exist that will provide evidence of the nursing actions that are effective in promoting positive client outcomes?

RESEARCH: SUBSTANTIATING THE SCIENCE OF NURSING

Nursing is a profession characterized by educational standards, autonomy, socialization, an established knowledge base, licensure, formal entry examinations, a code of ethics, technical expertise, professional standards, altruistic service, and public trust. The main characteristics of a profession are established, specialized training in a body of abstract knowledge and a collectivity of service orientation.

The science of nursing knowledge is established by the same systematic, investigative process used by all science-based disciplines, the research process. **Research** is a systematic method of exploring, describing, explaining, relating, or establishing the existence of a phenomenon, the factors that cause changes in the phenomenon, and how the phenomenon influences other phenomena. Nursing practice activities are substantiated as predicting valid and reliable outcomes for clients (the individual, family, group, or community) only after a body of knowledge has been established and confirmed by numerous research efforts.

HISTORICAL DEVELOPMENT

Nursing research is aligned with the founder of modern nursing, Florence Nightingale. Nightingale "believed that through observation, nurses could best determine care for patients. This early emphasis on systematic observation, as opposed to a trial-and-error approach in providing patient care, planted the seeds for the evolution of nursing science—a unique body of nursing knowledge" (Brockopp & Hastings-Tolsma, 2003, p. 5). The groundwork established by Nightingale for using research to direct client care was not sustained by subsequent nursing leaders because of two forces that had a direct impact on nursing's future. First, societal norms basically excluded women from becoming scientists; therefore, initiating or participating in scientific discovery (research) was not an option for women. The second force dealt with the "training" as opposed to the "education" of nurses.

In 1923 Teachers College at Columbia University offered the first educational doctoral program for nurses. The first master's of nursing degree was offered at Yale University in 1929. The placement of nursing education in the university setting is credited to three key studies that addressed educational reform in nursing: the Nutting report, 1912; the Goldmark report, 1923; and the Burgess report, 1926. In 1932 the Association of Collegiate Schools of Nursing (ACSN) was organized to promote the conduct of research to improve education and practice. The ACSN established the first research journal in nursing, *Nursing Research*, in 1952.

Research activities during the 1940s and early 1950s focused on the organization and delivery of nursing services: staffing patterns, nursing personnel and client satisfaction, and client classification systems. Care delivery systems such as comprehensive care, home care, and progressive care were evaluated. Results of these evaluations laid the foundation for the development of self-study manuals that were the precursors of today's quality assurance manuals.

The American Nurses Association (ANA) contributed to the advancement of nursing research. In 1950 the ANA sponsored a five-year study on nursing functions and activities; the findings were reported in a document entitled *Twenty Thousand Nurses Tell Their Story*. This study benchmarked the development of ANA statements on functions, standards, and qualifications for professional nurses in 1959.

Concurrently, clinical research began expanding as nursing specialty groups developed standards of care.

Nursing research in the late 1950s and early 1960s focused on the effective educational preparation of professional nurses. One outcome was the development of a two-year associate degree nursing program in the junior college setting by Montag. During this era several organizations were established that furthered nursing research by either promoting, expanding, or disseminating study findings: the Institute for Research and Service in Nursing Education at Teachers College, 1952; the American Nurse's Foundation, 1955; the ANA Committee on Research and Studies, 1956; the Department of Nursing Research, Walter Reed Army Hospital, 1957; the Southern Regional Educational Board, 1957; the Western Interstate Commission for Higher Education (WICHE), 1957; and the New England Board of Higher Education, 1957. The *Nursing Research* journal was established in 1952 to communicate nurses' research and scholarly activity.

During the late 1960s and 1970s the nursing profession initiated many scholarly endeavors: the development of conceptual models and theories; clinical studies on quality care, primary client care, and the nursing process; educational studies that evaluated teaching methods and student learning experiences; and the first Nursing Diagnosis Conference in 1973. The ANA established the Commission on Nursing Education in 1970 and the Council of Nurse Researchers in 1972. As enrollments in graduate nursing programs increased at both the master's and doctoral levels, the dissemination of research findings was an issue in the 1970s.

Sigma Theta Tau, the international honor society in nursing, was founded in 1922 and began publishing *Image: Journal of Nursing Scholarship* in 1967 to communicate research findings. The society's purpose is to advance scholarship in nursing by promoting the conduct, communication, and utilization of research in nursing.

The movement of the 1980s and 1990s focused on clinical nursing research as many nurses obtained master's and doctoral degrees, and postdoctoral education was encouraged for nurse researchers. The number of nursing research journals increased during the 1970s and 1980s to include journals such as *Research in Nursing and Health, Advances in Nursing Science, Applied Nursing Research,* and *Nursing Science Quarterly.*

Federal involvement in nursing research dates back to 1946 with the establishment of the Division of Nursing within the Office of the Surgeon General. In 1955, the first extramural nursing research program was established in the Research Grants and Fellowship Branch of the Division of Nursing Resources, and the National Institutes of Health (NIH) established the Nursing Research Section within the Division of Research Grants to conduct scientific review in the field of nursing. The impetus for establishing the National Institute of Nursing Research (NINR) came from the findings of two federal studies:

1. The 1983 report by the Institute of Medicine recommended that nursing research be included in the mainstream of biomedical and behavioral science.

2. The 1984 NIH Task Force study found nursing research activities to be relevant to the NIH mission.

In 1986 these findings led to legislative action that established the National Center for Nursing Research (NCNR) at the NIH. The NIH Revitalization Act of 1993 was signed into law and changed the NCNR to the NINR. The NINR (2003) supports clinical and basic research to establish a scientific basis for the care of individuals across the life span and may include families within a community context. According to its mandate, the institute seeks to understand and ease the symptoms of acute and chronic illness, to prevent or delay the onset of disease or disability or slow its progression, to find effective approaches to achieving and sustaining good health, and to improve the clinical settings in which care is provided. Research involves clinical care in a variety of settings including the community and home in addition to more traditional health care sites.

The current initiative of the NIH is twofold: the Public Trust Initiative (PTI) and Partners in Research. The purpose of the PTI is to support studies of innovative programs designed to improve public understanding of health care research and promote collaboration between scientists and community organizations to increase public awareness and trust in both the role of the NIH and the importance of new directions of research for advancing the public health. The NIH Partners in Research program is intended to engage a diverse group of scientists, community leaders, members of the public, and client advocacy groups to develop partnerships between scientific or research institutions and community organizations and to evaluate a variety of approaches in a range of target audiences or communities. The goals of the program are to:

- Identify and implement new ways to increase science literacy.
- Communicate the research needs and interests of communities.
- Encourage understanding of biomedical and behavioral research by partnering with community-sanctioned organizations, such as voluntary and professional organizations, health groups, faith-based groups, and housing organizations. (NINR, 2008)

FRAMEWORK

Knowledge gained from both nursing research and practice is necessary to support the predictable outcomes of nursing care. Research used in nursing comes from nursing as well as other disciplines such as psychology, education, sociology, biology, and anthropology. Nursing research explores the many pathways through which scientific and practical knowledge regarding nursing care is established.

Research Process

The person conducting the research is called a *researcher, investigator,* or *scientist.* When a researcher poses a problem or answers a question using the *scientific approach,* it is called a study, an investigation, or a research project. The people who are being studied are called *subjects* or *study participants.*

Scientific research is mainly concerned with vehicles of thought defined as **concepts**. The process of developing and refining concepts is referred to as **conceptualization**. A **construct** is an abstraction or mental representation inferred from situations, events, or behaviors. Constructs are different from concepts in that the constructs are deliberately invented (or constructed) by researchers for a specific scientific purpose. These concepts or constructs are ideas that formulate a **theory**, a set of concepts and propositions that provide an orderly way to view phenomena. "In a theory, concepts (or constructs) are knitted together into an orderly system to explain the way in which our world and the people in it function" (Polit, Beck, & Hungler, 2005, p. 22).

Nurse researchers can use one of two broad approaches to gather and analyze scientific information:

- **Quantitative research**: The systematic collection of numerical information, often under conditions of considerable control, and the analysis of the information using statistical procedures
- **Qualitative research**: The systematic collection and analysis of more subjective narrative materials, using procedures in which there tends to be a minimum of researcher-imposed control. (Polit et al., 2005, p. 26)

See Table 3-1 for a comparison of the major characteristics of quantitative and qualitative research.

The scientific method requires an exact, orderly, and objective approach of acquiring knowledge. Controlled methods are used to study problems and test the **hypothesis**, a statement of an asserted relationship between two or more variables. A **variable** is anything that may differ from the norm. The two types of variables are independent and dependent.

The **independent variable** (criterion variable) is the variable that is believed to cause or influence the **dependent variable**, which is the outcome variable of interest and is the variable that is hypothesized to depend on or be caused by or predicted by the independent variable (Polit et al., 2005). For example, if the question reads "To what extent does age predict recovery from surgical anesthesia relative to when perioperative instructions were first given?" the independent variable is age and the dependent variable is recovery from surgical anesthesia relative to when perioperative instructions were first given. **Value** is the variation of the variable. The values of the independent variable are actual ages of surgical clients, and the values of the dependent variable are when instructions were first given.

There are multiple ways in which nurses establish the sources and the realm of knowledge about nursing, human responses, diagnoses, and treatments. Burns and Grove (2004) describe how nursing has historically acquired knowledge:

- *Traditions:* basing practice on customs and past trends
- *Authority:* crediting another person as the source of information
- *Borrowing:* using knowledge from other disciplines to guide nursing practice
- *Trial and error:* using unknown outcomes in a situation of uncertainty
- *Personal experience:* gaining knowledge by being personally involved in an event, situation, or circumstance
- *Role modeling and mentorship:* imitating the behaviors of an exemplar

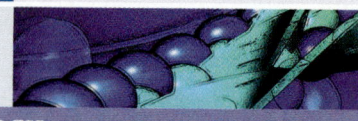

TABLE 3-1 Major Characteristics: Quantitative and Qualitative Research

QUANTITATIVE RESEARCH	QUALITATIVE RESEARCH
Purpose: test theory	Purpose: develop sensitizing concepts, create theory
Focus: concise and narrow	Focus: complete and broad
Reasoning: deductive	Reasoning: inductive
Design: reductionist	Design: holistic
Data collection: control; instruments	Data collection: shared interpretation; communication and observation
Basic element of analysis: numbers; statistical analysis	Basic element of analysis: words; individual interpretation
Reporting of findings: generalization; objective; formal style	Reporting of findings: uniqueness; subjective; rich narrative; expressive language

Adapted from Burns, N., & Grove, S. K. (2004). *The practice of nursing research* (5th ed.). Philadelphia: W. B. Saunders.

- *Intuition:* being guided by a feeling or sense that cannot be logically explained
- *Reasoning:* processing and organizing ideas in order to reach conclusions
- *Research:* validating and refining existing knowledge and generating new knowledge

Carper (1978, 1992) describes four fundamental patterns of knowing:

- *Empirical:* using research to explain, describe, and predict
- *Ethical:* extending knowledge of valuing, clarifying, and advocating
- *Personal:* encountering and focusing on self and others
- *Esthetic:* interpreting, engaging, and envisioning clues to knowledge

The research process is based on sequential, interrelated steps; see the accompanying display on the steps in the research process.

Once the researcher has developed the conceptual framework, the research literature is reviewed to provide a foundation on which to base new knowledge. In selecting a research design, the researcher determines the methods to be used to address the research question and test the hypothesis, the specific population to be studied, and how the data will be collected; see the accompanying display on types of research design.

Clearly, the contemporary thought on knowledge generation incorporates a variety of sources of data collection, each with its own strengths and weaknesses. However, knowledge in nursing is developed and used most effectively through the combination of nursing theory, research, and practice.

TYPES OF RESEARCH DESIGN

- *Historical:* Systematic investigation of a past event using relevant sources to describe or explain the event
- *Exploratory:* Preliminary investigation designed to develop or refine hypotheses or to test the data collection methods
- *Evaluative:* Systematic investigation of how well a program, practice, or policy is working
- *Descriptive:* Investigations that have as their main objective the accurate portrayal of the characteristics of persons, groups, or situations and the frequency with which certain phenomena occur
- *Experimental:* Research studies in which the investigator controls (manipulates) the independent variable and randomly assigns subjects to different conditions
- *Quasi-experimental:* Studies that deviate from the methods of the experimental component in that subjects cannot be randomly assigned to treatment conditions even though the researcher manipulates the independent variable and exercises certain controls to enhance the internal validity of the results

Adapted from Polit, D. F., & Hungler, B. P. (2005). *Nursing research: Principles and methods* (7th ed.). Philadelphia: Lippincott.

STEPS IN THE RESEARCH PROCESS

- Formulating a research question or problem
- Defining the purpose of the study
- Reviewing relevant literature
- Developing a **conceptual framework** (structure that links global concepts together to form a unified whole)
- Developing research objectives, questions, and hypotheses
- Defining research variables
- Selecting a **research design** (overall plan used to conduct the research; see the accompanying display for types of research design)
- Defining the population, sample, and setting
- Conducting a pilot study
- Collecting data
- Analyzing data
- Communicating research findings, their implications, and the limitations of the study

Following data collection, the researcher subjects the data to analysis in an orderly fashion so that patterns and relationships can be discerned. Qualitative analysis involves "four types of intellectual processes: comprehending, synthesizing, theorizing, and recontextualizing (exploration of the developed theory in terms of its applicability to other settings or groups)" (Polit et al., 2005, p. 400), whereas quantitative information is usually analyzed through statistical procedures. If the data support the research hypothesis, the findings are reported in a straightforward fashion; however, if the results fail to support the hypothesis, the researcher must explain the possible reasons for this failure, for example, problems with the research method (use of inappropriate tools for data collection). The research findings can be communicated in various forms such as dissertations and journal articles. Usually, research reports discuss how the findings can be incorporated into the practice of nursing.

Roles

Becoming a nurse researcher requires education and experience in the process of scientific inquiry. That process is then combined with the nurse's already established clinical experience and expertise. A nurse scientist is a registered nurse with

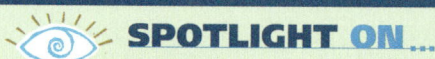

SPOTLIGHT ON...

Ways of Knowing

Nurses use scientific and "other ways of knowing" to measure the effectiveness of nursing interventions.

Name and describe three other ways of knowing that you use in your personal life to solve problems.

What are the advantages and disadvantages of each method you use?

How can other ways of knowing be used by nurses to measure the client's situation or the outcome of the nursing activity applied to the situation?

PROTECTING HUMAN RIGHTS IN RESEARCH

- *Self-determination:* The person has the right to control his or her own destiny.
- *Privacy:* The person has to determine the time, extent, and general circumstances under which private information will be shared with or withheld from others.
- *Anonymity:* Data collected will be kept confidential.
- *Fair treatment:* The person should be treated fairly and should receive what he or she is due or owed.
- *Protection from discomfort and harm:* Based on the principle of beneficence (one should do good and, above all, do no harm), the person should be protected from physical, emotional, social, and economic discomfort and harm.
- *Informed consent:* The person understands the reason for the proposed intervention and its benefits and risks, and he or she agrees to the treatment by signing a consent form.

Adapted from Burns, N., & Grove, S. K. (2004). *The practice of nursing research* (5th ed.). Philadelphia: W. B. Saunders.

a strong clinical background who has also been educated at the doctoral level to conduct research. However, nurses participate as consumers and critics of research by conducting the important work of translating, applying, and evaluating the new knowledge with clients and systems. Nurses also participate on research teams or with research protocols to plan, apply, collect data, and evaluate the process.

Each of these roles (nurse scientist, principal investigator, research team member, research consumer, and advocate for research clients) offers a substantial contribution to the process of scientific knowledge development in nursing and health care. Interdisciplinary experiences can further enrich the nurse's understanding of the concept or phenomenon and add to the research team's perspective of the research project.

Rights

During the research design phase of the process, the researcher must determine how to safeguard the rights of the research participants. An important role of the nurse researcher is that of advocate for the clients' rights during the process; see the accompanying display regarding the human rights that require protection during research.

Obtaining **informed consent** requires that the researcher provide **full disclosure**, the communication of complete information to potential research subjects regarding the nature of the study, the subject's right to refuse participation, and the likely risks and benefits that would be incurred (Polit et al., 2005). The nature, seriousness, and likelihood of risks (physical, psychological, social, and legal) are explained to the participants. The researcher must also identify what precautions will be taken to minimize the risks. Protection of subjects requires that the potential benefits outweigh potential risks. To give informed consent in research, persons must be mentally capable of understanding the study, risks, and benefits (Nokes & Nwakeze, 2007).

Nurses have an obligation to collaborate in the research, provided the researcher has followed proper protocols. The researcher must obtain permission from the agency to use its

facility as part of the research setting. Staff nurses who are expected to participate in the research process must have an adequate understanding of the nature of the study. Likewise, the staff nurse has the right to refuse to participate in the study.

SPOTLIGHT ON...

Legal and Ethical

What should a nurse do when a risk factor has not been fully explained to a client who has agreed to participate in a study?

You are a staff nurse working at a medical center where it is common practice for the nurses to participate in research studies that use investigational drugs. In reading the accompanying literature on the investigational drug being used in this particular study, you discover that the risk for infertility has not been addressed in the informed consent. Although you realize that you do not have to participate in the research, what should you do to protect the client's rights?

RESEARCH UTILIZATION

Research utilization refers to the use of research findings in practice to improve care. Research utilization occurs at three levels—instrumental, conceptual, and symbolic:

1. *Instrumental* utilization is the direct, explicit application of knowledge gained from research to change practice.
2. *Conceptual* utilization refers to the use of findings to enhance one's understanding of a problem or issue in nursing.
3. *Symbolic* utilization is the use of evidence to change the minds of other people, usually decision makers.

Instrumental research utilization allows the nurse to change nursing practice, for example, by adopting new nursing interventions, procedures, clinical protocols, or guidelines. In conceptual research utilization, the nurse uses the knowledge by thinking about a situation, problem, or phenomenon to provide different alternatives and possibilities in nursing situations. With symbolic research utilization, the nurse uses research findings to influence others to make changes in conditions, policies, or practices relevant to nurses and clients or to the health of clients.

To bridge the gap between nursing research and nursing practice, several research utilization models have been developed to promote quality care. The WICHE Regional Program for Nursing Research Development was the first federally funded research utilization project. The six-year WICHE project studied the feasibility of fostering research activities through regional collaborative activities. There are five components of this model:

1. Definition of nursing care problem
2. Retrieval of relevant research
3. Critical review of the research
4. Development of research-based plan of care
5. Evaluation of the effects of change

The final report from the WICHE project indicated that the project was successful in increasing research utilization; however, there were a limited number of scientifically sound, reliable nursing studies with clearly identified implications for nursing care.

A five-year project, awarded to the Michigan Nurses Association by the Division of Nursing in the 1970s, was the Conduct and Utilization of Research in Nursing (CURN). The purpose of this federally funded project was to develop research-based protocols for clinical practice. The five components of the CURN model include:

1. Identification of research studies and establishment of a research base
2. Transformation of findings into research-based protocols
3. Transformation of protocols into specific nursing interventions
4. Clinical trials in the practice setting
5. Evaluation of the research-based practice

The CURN project concluded that research utilization by practicing nurses is feasible, but only if it is relevant to practice and the results are broadly disseminated.

Over the past decade other utilization projects have been undertaken such as the Iowa model, the Nursing Child Assessment Satellite Training model, the Dracup-Breu model, the Stetler model, and the Horne model. In the 1990s California developed the Orange County Research Utilization in Nursing (OCRUN) project to focus on building organizational capacity as a tool for increasing research utilization. Over a three-year period, nearly 400 nurses participated in continuing education courses that focused on the development of research utilization competency (Rutledge & Donaldson, 1995).

Barriers to Utilizing Nursing Research

Polit and colleagues (2005) identify the following barriers to utilizing nursing research:

- Research itself: inadequate scientific base
- Practicing nurses: educational preparation with limited exposure to research utilization and resistance to change
- Organizational settings: unfavorable organizational climates and resource constraints
- Nursing profession: limited communication and collaboration between practitioners and researchers

Cacchione (2008) addressed another barrier, nurse participation in interprofessional research, citing a nursing intervention study in a long-term care setting that failed because the concerned nurses were not involved in the development of the study.

In 1992, the Agency for Health Care Policy and Research within the U.S. Department of Health and Human Services, renamed the Agency for Healthcare Research and Quality (AHRQ), convened a panel of experts to summarize the state-of-the-art research on certain topics and to develop clinical practice guidelines. Guidelines have been published on such topics as pain management in infants and children, prediction and prevention of pressure sores in adults, and identification and treatment of urinary incontinence. These guidelines, which are based on evidence and provide the consumer with information directly related to the clinical practice guidelines, are available at AHRQ's Web site. The future of nursing research utilization will require commitment and collaboration among researchers, practicing nurses, organizations that train and employ nurses, and the leadership of the nursing profession. See the Uncovering the Evidence box.

NURSING STUDENTS

Accessing nursing research can be a challenge to students. "Nursing students are often intimidated by the research process" (Morse, Oleson, Duffy, Patek, & Sohr, 1996, p. 148). Nursing students are exposed to research in varying degrees as determined by the program's curriculum.

Nursing students need to familiarize themselves with a few general terms before they read and analyze research studies. When an article is written by one or more researchers, it is called a **primary source**. When an author addresses the research of someone else, it is referred to as a **secondary source**.

Research articles usually begin with an **abstract**, a summary statement that identifies the purpose, methodology (inclusive of subject population), findings, and conclusions. Some authors also include implications for further study within the abstract; see the accompanying display for the major elements in the content of an abstract.

UNCOVERING THE
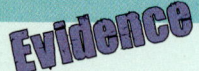

TITLE OF STUDY
"Nurses' Perceptions of Research Utilization in a Corporate Health Care System"

AUTHOR
D. McCloskey

PURPOSE
To explore selected characteristics of nurses based on educational level, years of experience, and hospital position that might affect perceived availability of research resources, attitude toward research, support, and the use of research in practice.

METHODS
A descriptive nonexperimental mailed survey was sent to nurses in five hospitals within a corporate hospital system using the Research Utilization Questionnaire (RUQ). The RUQ was used to measure nurses' perception of research utilization regarding four dimensions: perceived use of research, attitude toward research, availability of research resources, and perceived support for research activities.

FINDINGS
Statistically significant differences ($p < .001$) were found regarding perceived use of research, attitude toward research, availability of research resources, and perceived support for research activities based on educational level and organizational position. No significant differences were found for the nurses' perceptions based on years of experience.

IMPLICATIONS
The results of this study have implications for staff nurses, administrators, advanced practice nurses, hospital educations, and nursing practice. The different nurses' perceptions that were found based on educational level and hospital position can be positively integrated and used to promote research utilization and evidence-based practice initiatives within the organization system.

McCloskey, D. (2008). Nurses' perceptions of research utilization in a corporate health care system. *Journal of Nursing Scholarship, 40*(1), 39–45.

ABSTRACT CONTENTS

Title of the Study

Introduction of the Scientific Problem
- Statement of the problem and purpose
- Identification of the framework

Methodology
- Design
- Sample size
- Identification of data analysis methods

Results
- Major findings
- Conclusions
- Implications for nursing
- Recommendations for further research

During the career of a nurse, many clinical and practice questions will be raised that will require research methods to answer confidently. By pursuing and applying research in the area of choice, nurses acquire valid and reliable information that enables them to provide quality care.

EVIDENCED-BASED PRACTICE

The goal of client care is to provide quality nursing services that are effective in promoting health and wellness and

---

COMMUNITY CONSIDERATIONS

Nursing Research

Research in community health practice is challenging. The variables can be difficult to identify and measure. Consider ways that you might structure your research to answer the following:

How might you measure the "health" or "wellness" of your community?

You have decided to implement a teaching project on stress management to a group of well older adults. What criteria might you use to measure the effectiveness of your nursing interventions?

You are a new occupational health nurse at a local plastics factory. What questions might you ask the employees to better understand their need for and interest in health-promotion topics?

alleviating the discomforts of illness. The need for improved client outcomes, decreased health care costs, and client satisfaction are driving forces for the use of scientific data in the decision-making process of client care (Boswell, 2007). In EBP the nurse integrates research findings with clinical experience, the client's preferences, and available resources in planning and implementing cost-effective, individualized nursing care. Although EBP has been emphasized in medicine for years, nursing is in the initial stages of developing an EBP. "However, for the goals of evidence-based practice to be met, a culture of practice must be developed in which all clinicians from every discipline are expected to justify their practices from the best evidence currently available" (Burns & Grove, 2004, p. 296). Nurses must rely on the best evidence available to justify their practice until a solid scientific knowledge base evolves into EBP. Nursing as a profession has always recognized the importance of research as an essential basis for its development. The identification of the knowledge base for nursing practice contributes to achieving client outcomes and making nursing practice credible.

Although the terms *best practices* and *evidence-based practice* are often used interchangeably, these terms have different meanings. EBP can be a best practice, but a best practice is not necessarily evidence-based; best practices are simply ideas and strategies that work, such as programs, services, or interventions that produce positive client outcomes or reduce costs. Nurses need to base their clinical practice on empirical evidence to optimize client outcomes, to provide cost-effective safe practice, and to enhance the credibility of nursing care.

Nurses draw from their experience by selecting specific nursing interventions that influence client outcomes; however, there is little scientific evidence to support nurses' clinical decision making and expected outcomes. Early efforts to study client outcomes arose from quality assurance or quality improvement studies with nurse involvement in the development of interdisciplinary care plans such as critical pathways and care maps. However, critical pathways and care maps are not necessarily EBPs. According to Burns and Grove, "Outcomes research methods will be an important means to document the effect that nursing practice has on patient outcomes and to build the scientific base for evidence-based practice in nursing" (2004, p. 297). Outcomes studies will allow nurses the opportunity to explain the impact of their care through measures of outcomes of client care that reflect nursing practice. Although nurses are well placed to contribute toward more clinically effective and cost-effective client care, nurses need skills and resources to appraise, synthesize, and implement the best evidence in practice.

Benefield (2002) defines EBP as using the best evidence available to guide clinical decision making. This definition shifts the provision of health care away from opinion, past practice, and precedent toward a more scientific basis. "To use research-based interventions, nurses need to learn how to evaluate research reports, describe the level of evidence that exists on a particular topic, and identify the strength of the association for the research evidence that does exist" (Brockopp & Hastings-Tolsma, 2003, p. 40). Health care

providers use evidence reports that have been developed and disseminated by government programs, such as the AHRQ's National Guideline Clearinghouse that serves as a public resource for evidence-based clinical practice guidelines, or private entities like the Cochrane Collaboration.

EVIDENCE REPORTS

"Evidence reports include knowledge synthesis, review, and documentation of how evidence-based practices are used in the clinical area, and can include discussion of the clinical relevance and utility of such practices" (Benefield, 2002, p. 803). The evidence report usually contains four distinct parts: statement, analysis, evidence, and recommendations (see Figure 3-1). Once the nurse becomes aware of the need for information, EBP requires the development of the *question* or problem statement that best defines the need. Once the question is defined, the nurse systematically reviews what research has been done on the particular topic. Systematic reviews differ from literature reviews. Systematic reviews use all relevant literature from multiple sources, published and unpublished, and there is a more rigorous and systematic appraisal and evaluation.

Following the review and analysis of the systemic data, the nurse must determine what the research demonstrates and decide the level of evidence in order to make recommendations to promote EBP. A structured research summary statement succinctly describes what the evidence reports. The analysis of the scientific data describes a review of the various published and unpublished research, the details of the analysis, target populations that were studied, the type of clinical interventions that were investigated, and the strength of individual and collective study results (Benefield, 2002). The level of evidence ranks the strength and quality of the study results. Research findings should be evaluated within the context of actual or potential usefulness in practice; if the evidence deems it appropriate, the end product is a recommendation in the form of a practice-focused guideline or clinical intervention. EBP promotes quality care that has been demonstrated to be effective; see the accompanying display on page 50 on determining evidence-based nursing practice

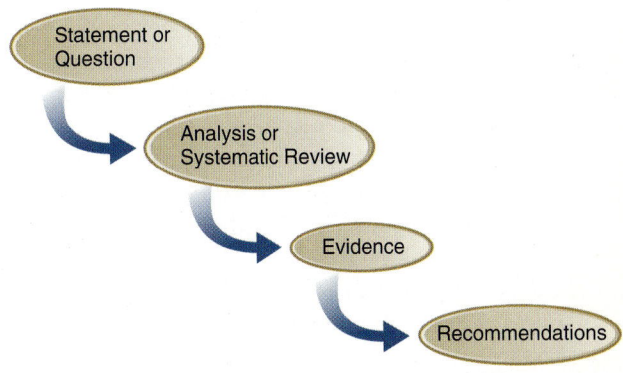

FIGURE 3-1 Evidence reports identify the need for information, analysis of scientific data, level of evidence, and recommendations for practice. DELMAR/CENGAGE LEARNING

for an example of how nurses may utilize research findings to make recommendations to promote EBP. If practice guidelines do not exist for a specific problem, the nurse needs to search for relevant evidence in studies, integrate reviews and analyses, and assess the quality of the evidence.

TRENDS IN RESEARCH AND EVIDENCE-BASED PRACTICE

The following trends in health care will have a definite impact on future nursing research and EBP:

1. Heightened focus on EBP: Nurses will be encouraged to engage in EBP; therefore, improvements are needed in both the quality of nursing studies and in nurses' skills in understanding, critiquing, and utilizing study results.
2. Stronger scientific knowledge base: Nurses should deliberately replicate, or repeat, studies with different populations, settings, and times to ensure that findings are solid.
3. Greater stress on integrative reviews of nursing knowledge: Nurses should amass comprehensive research information on the topic, weigh pieces of evidence, and integrate information to draw conclusions about the state of knowledge.
4. Increased emphases on multidisciplinary collaboration: Collaboration of nurses with researchers in related fields should lead nurses to a more prominent role in creating national and international health care policies.
5. Expanded dissemination of findings: The Internet and other modes of electronic communication, such as the *Online Journal of Knowledge Synthesis for Nursing* and the *Online Journal of Clinical Innovation*, will assist in promoting EBP.
6. Increased interest in outcomes research: Nurses will assess and document the effectiveness of health care

DETERMINING EVIDENCE-BASED NURSING PRACTICE

A nurse working on an oncology unit is interested in the relationship of oral contraceptives and the development of ovarian cancer.

- Step 1. Review and critique research reports related to oral contraceptives and the development of ovarian cancer.
- Step 2. Based on the critique of the literature on oral contraceptives and the development of ovarian cancer, identify the level and strength of the evidence: good, fair, or insufficient to support or reject a cause-and-effect interpretation of the association.
- Step 3. Make specific recommendations regarding the use of oral contraceptives and the development of ovarian cancer based on the critiqued research and the level and strength of the evidence found in the research.

Adapted from Brockopp, D., & Hastings-Tolsma, M. (2003). *Fundamentals of nursing research* (3rd ed.). Sudbury, MA: Jones & Bartlett.

services that are both cost-effective and still achieve outcomes without compromising care (Polit & Beck, 2006).

By identifying clear, significant priorities for study, striving for excellence in the evolving knowledge base, and confirming study findings, nursing researchers are providing a creditable scientific position from which to address societal health care issues and guide nursing practice.

KEY CONCEPTS

- The science of nursing is established by the same systematic, investigative process used by all science-based disciplines, the research process.
- Knowledge and nursing science are predicated on many ways of knowing, such as tradition, systematic inquiry, esthetics, and empiricism, and are influenced by gender perspectives.
- The five steps of the research process are statement of the research problem, delineation of a conceptual framework and review of the literature, selection of a research design, analysis and interpretation of the findings, and communication of the results of the research study.
- Research, education, and practice constitute the required integrated approach to the daily practice of all nurses.

- Obtaining informed consent for clients participating in the research process requires that the researcher provide full disclosure of the nature of the study, the subject's right to refuse participation, and the likely risks and benefits that would be incurred by the study.
- The various applications of nursing research to education and practice can significantly influence the quality and delivery of nursing care.
- The importance of nursing research will increase as the result of trends occurring in educational programs, interdisciplinary collaboration, interrelationships between nursing practice and research, and nurse-client involvement in research activities.
- To bridge the gap between nursing research and nursing practice, several research utilization models

have been developed to promote quality care (e.g., the WICHE, CURN, and OCRUN models).

- EBP promotes quality care that has been demonstrated to be effective.

- Researchers, educators, and practitioners need to work collaboratively to ensure that nursing establishes an evidence base for nursing practice.

REVIEW QUESTIONS

1. Which of the following best describes the foundation of research?
   a. Evidence
   b. Experience
   c. Critical thinking
   d. Scientific method

2. "The systematic collection of numerical information, often under conditions of considerable control, and the analysis of the information using statistical procedures" best defines:
   a. Quantitative research
   b. Qualitative research
   c. Experimental research
   d. Evidence-based practice

3. Informed consent requires that the researcher communicate which of the following to the participant? Select all that apply.
   a. The nature of the study
   b. The subject's right to refuse participation
   c. That the data will be shared with all health care providers

   d. The expected outcomes, risks and benefits, of the study
   e. That the family and the prescribing practitioner determine the client's rights to participate
   f. That the agency has the right to use the data freely

4. Which of the following are obstacles to moving research rapidly into client care?
   a. Inadequate scientific base
   b. Unfavorable organizational climates
   c. Lack of access to a health care library
   d. Limited communication and collaboration between researchers and practitioners

5. Number the following steps of evidence-based reports in the appropriate order.
   a. Level of evidence
   b. Ask the clinical question
   c. Analysis of scientific data
   d. Recommendations for practice

online companion

Visit the DeLaune and Ladner online companion resource at **www.delmar.cengage.com** for additional content and study aids. Click on Online Companions, then select the Nursing discipline.

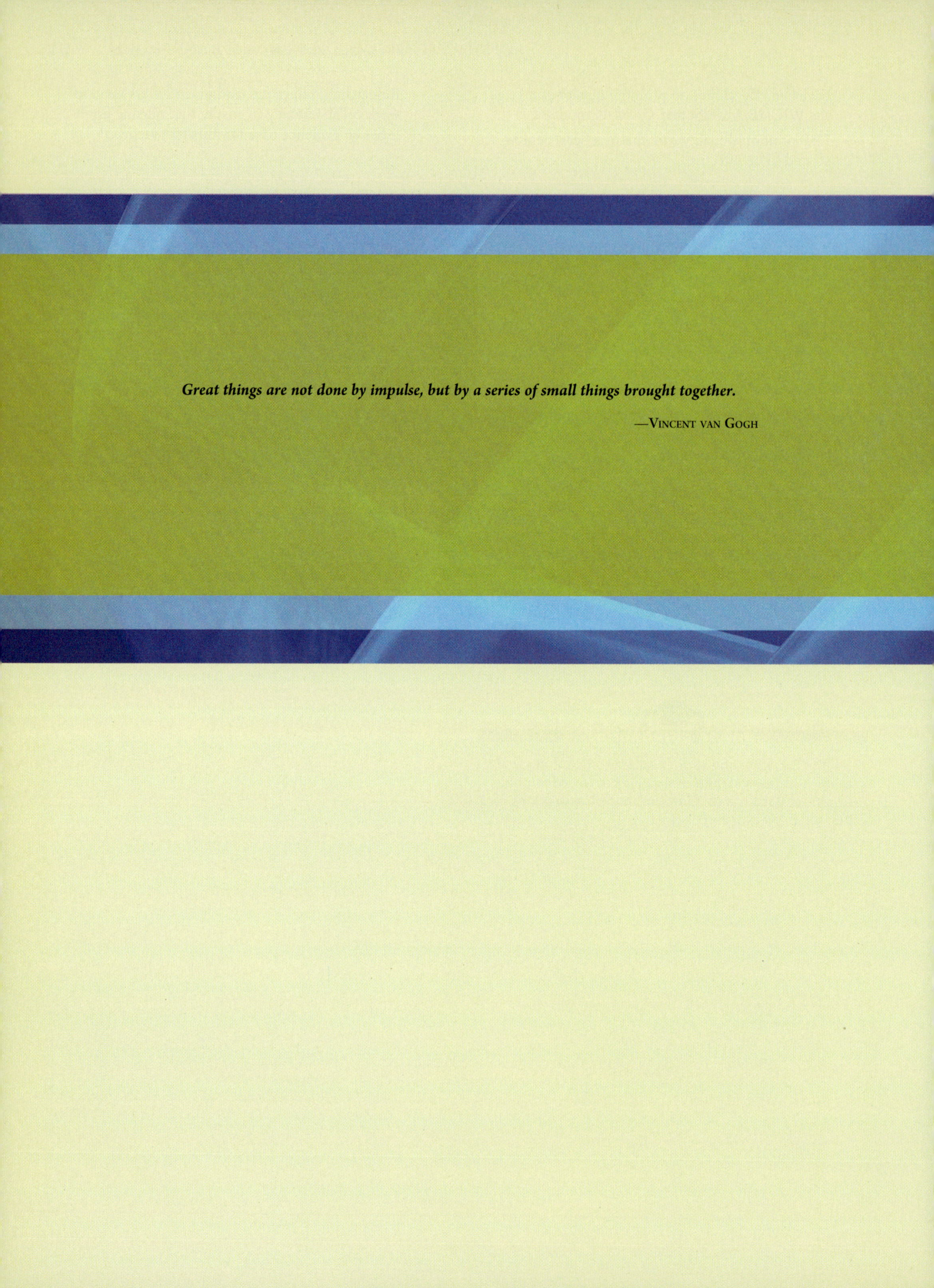

Great things are not done by impulse, but by a series of small things brought together.

—Vincent van Gogh

CHAPTER 4

Health Care Delivery, Quality, and the Continuum of Care

COMPETENCIES

1. Describe the current status of the U.S. health care delivery system.
2. Discuss the various health care settings through which health care services are delivered.
3. Identify the members of the health care team and respective roles.
4. Explain factors influencing health care delivery.
5. Explore the challenges that exist within the health care system.
6. Discuss nursing's role in meeting the challenges within the health care system.
7. Describe the emerging trends and issues for the health care delivery system.
8. Define the continuum of care concept.
9. Identify the levels of preventive care.
10. Discuss the phases of health care delivery that promote continuity of care.
11. Discuss methods for improving quality of health care delivery.
12. Explain the relationship between consumer satisfaction and quality.

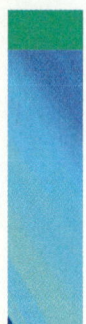

KEY TERMS

capitated rates	health care delivery system	process improvement
comorbidity	health maintenance organizations	quality
continuous quality improvement	managed care	quality assurance
cross-functional team	organizational culture	single-payer system
customer	performance improvement	single point of entry
exclusive provider organizations	preferred provider organizations	team
fee-for-service	primary care provider	total quality management
functional team	primary health care	

Nursing is a major component of the U.S. **health care delivery system**. Consequently, nurses must understand the changes occurring within this system as well as their role in shaping the changes. This chapter discusses the types of health care services available, various settings in which these services are provided, and the members of the health care team. The economics of health care and the challenges within the health care delivery system are also discussed. Nursing's role in meeting these challenges is described. In addition, this chapter discusses quality improvement in health care as well as continuity of care.

HEALTH CARE DELIVERY: ORGANIZATIONAL FRAMEWORKS

The U.S. health care delivery system is complex, involving myriad providers, consumers, and settings. Health care services in the United States are delivered by both the public (including official and voluntary) and private sectors. No single agency or group controls the entire health care system.

PUBLIC SECTOR

Public agencies are financed with tax monies; thus, these agencies are accountable to the public. The public sector includes official (or governmental) agencies, voluntary agencies, and nonprofit agencies. Figure 4-1 shows the hierarchy of the public sector of health care delivery.

At the local level, services provided include immunizations, maternal-child care, and activities directed at control of chronic diseases. Each state varies in the provision of public health services. Generally, a state department of health coordinates the activities of local health units.

At the national level, the U.S. Department of Health and Human Services (DHHS) is administratively responsible for health care services delivered to the public. The surgeon general is the chief officer of the U.S. Public Health Service (USPHS), the major agency that oversees the actual delivery of care services. Table 4-1 on page 55 lists the USPHS agencies and their purposes.

An important part of the public sector of the health care delivery system is voluntary agencies. These not-for-profit agencies exert significant legislative influence (e.g., the American Nurses Association [ANA] and the American Medical Association). Other voluntary agencies, such as the American Cancer Society and the American Heart Association, provide educational resources to the general public and to health care providers. Voluntary agencies are funded in a variety of ways, including individual contributions, corporate philanthropy, and membership dues.

Protecting public health is a shared responsibility among the federal, state, and local governments. Some local governments provide funding for indigent care through operating public hospitals and clinics. "Even as demands on the public health infrastructure have increased, support for public health has languished in recent decades". There is recognition of an increased need for local public health

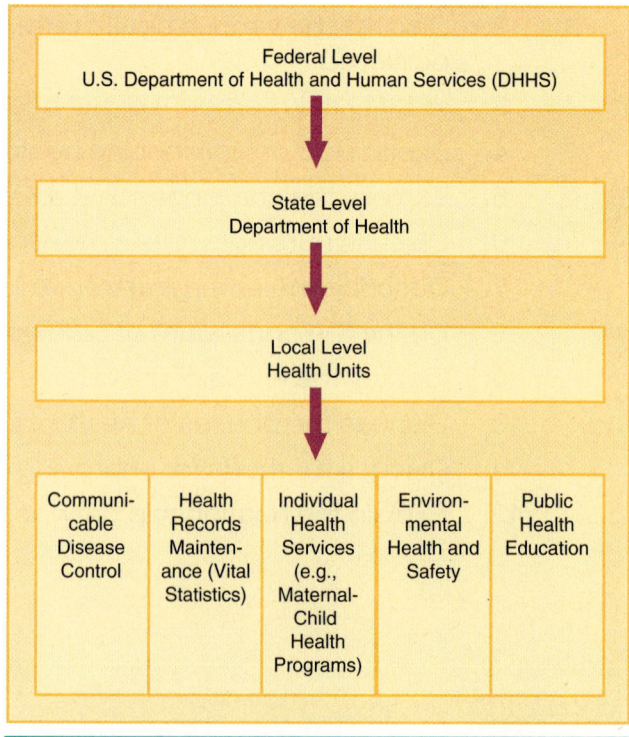

FIGURE 4-1 The Public Sector of Health Care Delivery DELMAR/CENGAGE LEARNING

TABLE 4-1 Agencies of the U.S. Public Health Service

AGENCY	PURPOSE
Health Resources and Services Administration (HRSA)	Provide health-related information Administer programs concerned with health care for the homeless, people with human immunodeficiency virus (HIV) and acquired immunodeficiency syndrome (AIDS), organ transplants, rural health care, and employee occupational health
Food and Drug Administration (FDA)	Protect the public from unsafe drugs, food, and cosmetics
Centers for Disease Control and Prevention (CDC)	Prevent the transmission of communicable diseases
National Institutes of Health (NIH)	Conduct research and education related to specific illnesses
Substance Abuse and Mental Health Services Administration (SAMHSA)	Improve quality and availability of substance abuse prevention, alcohol and drug addiction treatment, and mental health services
Agency for Toxic Substances and Disease Registry (ATSDR)	Maintain registry of certain diseases Provide information on toxic agents Conduct mortality and morbidity studies on defined population groups
Indian Health Service (IHS)	Provide health care services to Native Americans, including health promotion, disease prevention, alcoholism prevention, substance abuse prevention, suicide prevention, nutrition, and maternal-child health care
Agency for Healthcare Research and Quality (AHRQ)	Primary source of federal support for research related to quality and safety of health care delivery

Delmar/Cengage Learning

agencies to provide primary prevention services. Sanitation, immunization, and health surveillance are only some of the services provided at the local level. The threat of bioterrorism and natural disasters reinforces the need to have health resources available at the local level.

PRIVATE SECTOR

The private component of the health care system consists of all nongovernmental sources. It comprises the largest segment of the health care system because most health care facilities in the United States are run by private for-profit or nonprofit corporations. Also included in the private system are the health insurance industry, pharmaceutical companies, and suppliers of health care technology and equipment (Pulcini, Neary, & Mahoney, 2007). The variety of settings in which health care is delivered and the roles of nurses in these settings are directly influenced by social and economic factors.

HEALTH CARE TEAM

Health care services are delivered by a multidisciplinary team. Table 4-2 on page 56 provides a list of health care providers. Because nurses work with other care providers on an ongoing basis, it is necessary to understand the role of each provider. Nurses coordinate the care provided by the multidisciplinary team.

NURSE: ROLES AND FUNCTIONS

Nurses fulfill a variety of roles while assisting clients to meet their needs. Table 4-3 on page 57 defines the most common roles of nurses. Nurses work to promote, maintain, or restore health. A major aspect of nursing is to help individuals cope with the outcomes of illness or injury. Nurses are advocates and educators for individuals, families, and communities. Nursing roles are affected by changes in the health care environment. Nurses function in dependent, independent, and interdependent roles. The degree of autonomy nurses experience is related to client needs, expertise of the nurse, and practice setting.

ADVANCED PRACTICE NURSE: ROLES AND FUNCTIONS

The advanced practice of nursing has evolved as the profession has become more complex and specialized. Since the

TABLE 4-2 Health Care Providers

PROFESSIONAL	FUNCTION/ROLE
Nurse (RN)	Provides care to individuals who are unable to care for themselves; with a holistic approach, nurses assist clients to cope with illness or disability Addresses the needs of the client (individual, family, community) Emphasizes health promotion
Advanced practice registered nurse (APRN)	Diagnoses primary health care problems Prescribes therapeutic modalities Promotes continuity of care May specialize in a variety of areas (e.g., family practice, geriatrics, pediatrics)
Physician (MD)	Makes medical diagnoses and prescribes therapeutic modalities Performs medical procedures (e.g., surgery) May specialize in a variety of areas (e.g., gynecology/obstetrics, oncology, surgery)
Physician assistant (PA)	Provides medical services under the supervision of a physician
Pharmacist (RPh)	Prepares and dispenses drugs for therapeutic use Is often involved in client education
Dentist (DDS)	Diagnoses and treats conditions affecting mouth, teeth, and gums Performs preventive measures to promote dental health
Dietitian (RD)	Plans diets to meet special needs of clients Promotes health and prevents disease through education and counseling May supervise preparation of meals
Social worker (SW)	Assists clients with psychosocial problems (e.g., financial, marital) Conducts discharge planning Makes referrals for placement
Respiratory therapist (RT)	Administers pulmonary function tests Performs therapeutic measures to assist with respiration (e.g., oxygen administration, ventilators)
Physical therapist (PT)	Works with clients experiencing musculoskeletal problems Assesses person's strength and mobility Performs therapeutic measures (e.g., range of motion, massage, application of heat and cold) Teaches new skills (e.g., walking with crutches)
Occupational therapist (OT)	Works with clients with functional impairment to learn skills for activities of daily living
Chaplain	Assists in helping clients meet spiritual needs Provides individual counseling Provides support to families Conducts religious services
Unlicensed assistive personnel (UAP)	Assists in provision of client care activities under the direction of the RN May include certified nurses aide, personal care assistant, nursing assistant, orderly, and certified phlebotomist

Delmar/Cengage Learning

late 1960s, nurse practitioners (NPs), clinical nurse specialists (CNSs), certified nurse midwives (CNMs), and other advanced practice registered nurses (APRNs) have provided health care services to individuals, many of whom would have had inadequate or no access to services. APRNs possess advanced skills and in-depth knowledge in specific areas of practice. Even though there are differences in various advanced practice roles, all APRNs are experts who work with clients to prevent disease and to promote health (see Chapter 11).

TABLE 4-3 Nursing Roles

ROLE	DESCRIPTION
Caregiver	Traditional and most essential role Functions as nurturer Provides direct care Is supportive Demonstrates clinical proficiency Promotes comfort of client
Teacher	Provides information Serves as counselor Seeks to empower clients for self-care Encourages compliance with prescribed therapy Promotes healthy lifestyles Interprets information
Advocate	Protects the client Provides explanations in client's language Acts as change agent Supports client's decisions
Manager	Makes decisions Coordinates activities of others Allocates resources Evaluates care and personnel Serves as a leader Takes initiative
Expert	Advanced practice clinician Conducts research Teaches in schools of nursing Develops theory Contributes to professional literature Provides testimony at governmental hearings and in courts
Case manager	Tracks client's progress through the health care system Coordinates care to ensure continuity
Team member	Collaborates with others Possesses highly skilled communication methods Performs therapeutic measures to assist with respiration (e.g., oxygen administration, ventilators)

Delmar/Cengage Learning

APRNs must meet higher educational standards and higher clinical practice requirements than those of the basic nursing education and licensure required for all nurses. Many APRNs promote quality of health care by providing services to populations often underserved by other health care providers. They provide primary health care services by diagnosing and treating common acute illnesses and injuries. APRNs prescribe medications according to regulations that vary from state to state.

REIMBURSEMENT METHODS

Efforts to reform the health care system have been motivated primarily by health care costs. Control of costs has shifted from the health care providers to the insurers and, as a result, there are constraints on reimbursement. Historically, the predominant method of covering health care costs was the **fee-for-service** method, in which the recipient directly pays the provider for health care services when they are performed.

The U.S. health care system has a diverse financial base, comprising both private and public funding. As a result, administrative costs for health care reimbursement are higher in the United States than in countries with a **single-payer system**, a model in which the government is the only entity to reimburse health care costs (e.g., Canada). Despite the enormous expenditures of public funds, the United States does not provide adequate health care coverage for all citizens.

PRIVATE INSURANCE

A major source of financing health care services in the United States is private insurance. One of the largest sectors of the health care system is private insurance companies. Payment rates to health care providers vary among insurance companies. Insured individuals or their employers are paying substantial monthly premiums and deductibles for health care services. The cost of the premiums limits access for many Americans. Insurers will no longer pay for services that they deem unnecessary or, in many cases, have not been pre-approved by the insurer. The quality of care provided is being monitored by providers, third-party payers, regulatory bodies, legislators, and consumers.

MANAGED CARE

Managed care is a system of providing and monitoring care in which access, cost, and quality are controlled before or during delivery of services. The goal of managed care is the delivery of services in the most cost-efficient manner possible. Managed care seeks to control costs by monitoring delivery of services and restricting access to expensive procedures and providers. Managed care plans assume a significant portion of the risk of providing health care and, consequently, encourage both prudent use by consumers and prescription by providers.

The rationale for managed care is to give consumers preventive health services delivered by a **primary care provider** (PCP; a health care provider whom a client sees first for health care), which in turn results in less expensive interventions. PCPs are usually physicians or NPs.

The Health Maintenance Organization Act passed in 1973 provided federal grants and loans that were made available to **health maintenance organizations** (HMOs), prepaid health plans that provide primary health care services for a preset fee and focus on cost-effective treatment measures. The HMOs were mandated to comply with strict federal regulations as opposed to the less restrictive state requirements.

Managed care refers to an organizational structure. One type of managed care is represented by HMOs, which are both providers and insurers. Other variations are represented by **preferred provider organizations** (PPOs), a type of managed care model in which member choice is limited to providers within the system, and **exclusive provider organizations** (EPOs), organizations in which care must be delivered by providers in the plan for clients to receive reimbursement. The latter creates a network of providers (such as physicians and hospitals) and offers the incentive of consumer services with little or no copayment if these providers are used exclusively. Table 4-4 provides an overview of independent practice and managed care organizational structures.

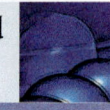

TABLE 4-4   Independent Practice and Managed Care Options

TYPE	DESCRIPTION
Independent practice	Fee-for-service Consumer choice of provider Disease-oriented philosophy
Health maintenance organizations (HMOs)	Fee is preset and prepaid Provide services to a group of enrolled persons Service provision is limited
Preferred provider organizations (PPOs)	Fees are preset and prepaid Networks of providers that give discounts to sponsoring organization Members are not mandated to select a specific primary care provider but must use a provider in the network
Exclusive provider organizations (EPOs)	Plan pays no benefit if member is treated outside the network Usually regulated by state insurance laws

Delmar/Cengage Learning

The impact of managed care is that caregivers and institutions must change from providing as many services as possible to providing fewer services so as to protect their financial interests.

Health Maintenance Organizations

HMOs often maintain primary health care sites and commonly employ health care professionals. They use **capitated rates** (a preset flat fee that is based on membership in, not services provided by, the HMO), assume the risk of clients who are heavy users, and exert control on the use of services. HMOs have been noted for their use of APRNs as PCPs, precertification programs to limit unnecessary hospitalization, and an emphasis on client education for health promotion and self-care.

Another common feature of HMOs is the practice of **single point of entry** (entry into the health care system is required through a point designated by the plan) through which primary care is delivered. **Primary health care** is the client's point of entry into the health care system and includes assessment, diagnosis, treatment, coordination of care, education, preventive services, and surveillance. It consists of the spectrum of services provided by a family practitioner (nurse or physician) in an ambulatory setting. PCPs serve as "gatekeepers" to the health care system in that they determine which, if any, referrals to specialists are needed by the client. To reduce costs, direct access to specialists is limited.

Preferred Provider Organizations

The most common type of managed care system is the PPO. A PPO is a contractual relationship between hospitals, providers, employers, and third-party payers to form a network in which providers deliver health services at a predetermined price. Currently, managed care is emerging as the preferred model for delivery of services.

GOVERNMENT PLANS

The federal government became a third-party payer for health care services with the advent of Medicare in 1965. The Centers for Medicare and Medicaid Services (CMS), formerly known as the Health Care Financing Administration, is a federal agency that regulates Medicare and Medicaid expenditures. Medicare was established to help retired older people pay for their health care expenses. Currently, three federal programs for reimbursing health care—Medicare, Medicaid, and the State Children's Health Insurance Program (SCHIP)—are administered by the CMS. Medicare is the federally funded program that provides health care coverage for older adults and people with disabilities. Medicaid is a program jointly administered between the federal and state governments to provide health care coverage for the economically disadvantaged.

The federal government created diagnosis-related groups (DRGs) to curtail spending for hospitalized Medicare recipients and to ensure that health care dollars would get to those who most need them. Through this system, an inclusive rate is established for each episode of hospitalization based on the client's age, principal diagnosis, and the presence or absence of surgery and comorbidity (existence of simultaneous disease processes within an individual). Hospitals are reimbursed only for services that are determined to be medically necessary by the CMS. An accelerating trend for the federal government is to give recipients of public monies the personal right to choose, through the use of vouchers, a managed care program in the private sector.

Another trend is that the CMS will no longer pay for certain incidents called "never events." The Medicare Modernization Act and Deficit Reduction Act of 2005 permit the CMS to reduce or refuse reimbursement to hospitals for certain medical events. The new rules went into effect in 2008. A never event is a serious, preventable adverse event that is a hospital-acquired condition (HAC). Examples of some of the HAC never events are surgical site infections, severe pressure ulcers, and falls. Other HAC events will experience reduced CMS reimbursement in the future.

Medicare

When Medicare was established in 1965, it was intended to protect individuals over the age of 65 from exorbitant costs of health care by providing public funds to cover the majority of health care services. Medicare does not pay for all health care expenses incurred by older adults. Some of the expenses not fully reimbursed include prescription drugs, preventive services (e.g., annual physical exams), dental care, and vision and hearing services. A major need of older adults not addressed by Medicare is reimbursement for long-term care and catastrophic illness. Also, Medicare does not provide adequate reimbursement to older people for the expense of medications. This imposes a great financial hardship since many older individuals take multiple expensive medications. In 1972, Medicare was modified to include individuals with permanent disabilities and those with end-stage renal disease.

Medicaid

Medicaid is a shared venture between the federal and state governments. Each state has latitude in determining who is "medically indigent" and thus eligible for public monies. Minimal services covered by Medicaid are defined by the federal government and include inpatient and outpatient hospital services, physician services, laboratory services (including x-rays), and rural health clinic services. States may elect to cover other services, such as dental, vision, and prescription drugs. Medicaid reimburses NPs and CNMs if state regulations have authorized the APRN to provide the services specified by the CMS.

State Children's Health Insurance Program

The Balanced Budget Act of 1997 established the SCHIP. This public health insurance program, administered at the state level, is like all other federal insurance plans in that it is funded from general taxes. Nurses play an essential advocacy role by helping parents of economically disadvantaged children to enroll in the SCHIP with their respective state health agencies.

In addition to Medicaid and SCHIP funds, states also administer the federally funded Title V Maternal-Child Block Grant Program. The objective of this program is to improve maternal, infant, and adolescent health. Also covered under this block grant are services for children at risk of chronic, disabling conditions.

States have a great deal of influence on health care reimbursement in that each state regulates insurance companies. Each state makes decisions about Medicaid financing and is, therefore, concerned about escalating health care costs. Several states offer some form of managed care to Medicaid participants in an attempt to control rising costs.

FACTORS INFLUENCING THE DELIVERY OF HEALTH CARE

Numerous social, political, and cultural factors influence the delivery of health care. Despite cost-containment efforts (such as DRGs established by the federal government and managed care by the insurers), the U.S. health care system still has problems with issues of cost, access, and quality. Other factors that influence health care delivery include regulatory mandates, the shortage of registered nurses, technological advances, increasing consumerism, and vulnerable population groups.

COST

Cost has been a driving force for change in the health care system as evidenced by the strength and numbers of managed care plans, increased use of outpatient treatment, and shortened hospital stays. The market force to maximize profits by minimizing costs is dominating the current changes in the health care system.

The United States spends more per person on health care than any other country. In 2007, the per capita health care expenses were $7,600 per person, with total health care spending representing 16% of the gross national product (National Coalition on Health Care [NCHC], 2008). Even though the United States has the most expensive health care system in the world, it ranks behind most other industrialized nations in the health of its citizens (Hunt, 2009). Every dollar that the government spends on health care is a dollar subtracted from other programs (e.g., education and housing) that affect citizens' well-being. Following are some of the factors that contribute to the escalation of health care costs:

- The aging population
- Technological advances
- A surplus of hospital beds
- Increased number of people with chronic illnesses

The cost of health care services is prohibitive to many people; thus, it is a major barrier to access to services. Another factor that contributes to the high cost of health care is the increase in health-related lawsuits that has resulted in the unnecessary use of services.

ACCESS

In addition to the issue of cost, access to health care services has a serious impact on the functioning of the health care system. As a result of the cost, health care for many people is crisis-oriented and fragmented. A large number of Americans are unable to gain access to health care services owing to low income or lack of insurance; therefore, their illnesses progress to an acute stage before intervention is sought. Services used by individuals during acute illnesses are typically those provided by emergency departments. Emergency room and acute care services are expensive when compared with early intervention and preventive measures. Poverty often adversely affects an individual's access to health care services. For example, limited transportation (lack of an automobile or funding for public transit) interferes with the ability to travel to health care facilities.

Approximately 47 million Americans are uninsured, which severely limits access to care (NCHC, 2008). Only a small portion of the medically indigent is covered by Medicare. In addition, many individuals are underinsured. These people are neither poor nor old, but middle-class unemployed Americans or those in jobs without adequate health care benefits.

In addition to poverty and unemployment, the following factors impede a person's ability to access available health care services:

- No provision for insurance by an employer due to prohibitive costs
- Inability to obtain individual insurance due to high costs
- Difficulty for people with certain medical problems (preexisting conditions) to obtain insurance
- Cultural barriers
- Shortages of health care providers in some geographic areas (especially rural or inner-city areas)
- Limited access to ancillary services (e.g., child care, transportation)

QUALITY

Many unnecessary diagnostic and medical procedures are performed in order to decrease the possibility of being sued for professional malpractice. This inappropriate use of resources can be traced to several causative factors, including:

- The litigious environment that creates the tendency toward defensive practice
- Resource consumption, which is highly influenced by the widely held American belief that more is better
- Lack of access to and continuity of services with subsequent misuse of acute care services

In an attempt to provide universal access to services in a cost-effective manner, quality does not have to be sacrificed. However, safety and quality are frequently compromised by inappropriate substitution of unlicensed personnel for registered nurses in direct care of clients. Sufficient numbers of registered nurses may decrease the occurrence of adverse events (Gordon, Buchanan, & Bretherton, 2008; Kane, Shamliyan, Mueller, Duval, & Wilt, 2007; Mark & Harless, 2007; Thungjaroenkul, Cummings, & Embleton, 2007).

Health care consumers and legislators, as well as the nursing profession, are concerned about the effects of fewer nurses in the workplace. Some states are instituting legislation that mandates the ratio of nursing staff to clients.

In an attempt to be cost-effective, some hospitals have decreased the number of registered nurses. Any movement toward reform must focus on providing quality nursing care to all consumers. According to Thungjaroenkul and colleagues (2007, p. 264), "Patient costs were reduced with greater RN staffing as RNs have higher knowledge and skill levels to provide more effective nursing care."

NURSING SUPPLY AND DEMAND

Currently an imbalance exists between the number of registered nurses and the demand for nursing services. The shortage of registered nurses in the United States could reach 500,000 by the year 2025 (Buerhaus, Staiger, & Aeurbach, 2009). Following is a list of some of the many factors that are increasing the gap between the demand for and supply of registered nurses:

- A declining number of nursing faculty
- Technological advances that result in treatment of more medical problems
- Increasing emphasis on preventive care
- Growing number of older adults who are more likely to need nursing care
- Declining numbers of enrollees in nursing schools

RESPONSES TO HEALTH CARE CHANGES

As the United States continues to look for ways to address the issue of health care reform, the implications for nursing will continue to increase. Some nurses feel threatened by impending changes, whereas others are excited about the possibility of transforming the health care system into something better. Advocating for clients, educating public policy makers, and continuing to provide direct quality care are only a few of the actions that nurses implement to ensure delivery of care in a safe, therapeutic manner.

NURSING AGENDA FOR HEALTH CARE REFORM

In response to the problems of high cost, limited access, and eroding quality that were affecting the U.S. health care system, the nursing community created a public policy agenda that is currently endorsed by more than 70 organizations. *Nursing's Agenda for Health Care Reform* (ANA, 2005) provides a valid framework for change in health care policy. A cornerstone of this policy statement is the delivery of health care services in environments that are easily accessible, familiar, and consumer-friendly. Another essential part of *Nursing's Agenda* is the empowerment of consumers for self-care. This goal has enormous implications for nurses as health educators and for the use of incentives for increasing personal accountability for one's own health status. Some elements of the ANA's Health Care Agenda 2005 are as follows:

- A nationally defined standard package of basic health care services available to all U.S. residents
- A phase-in of essential services that address vulnerable populations with limited access to health care
- Plans to decrease the costs of health care
- Activities that address long-term care needs with emphasis on consumer responsibility (ANA, 2005)

PUBLIC VERSUS PRIVATE PROGRAMS

The nursing profession supports an integration of public and private sector programs and resources for health care delivery. The competition between the two types of settings has encouraged quality and progress. Each setting provides benefits as well as drawbacks to health care recipients.

Public dollars are required to help the poor and those who do not receive health care benefits through the workplace. Actual services should be available through a variety of public and private sources. To safeguard the health care system from becoming a two-tiered process based on personal resources, both the poor and nonpoor and the privileged and nonprivileged need to be enrolled in the same programs: see Spotlight On: Caring and Compassion.

Finally, the basic required package of services must be defined in the same way in each state and required as the minimum for both public and private sector programs. The movement toward establishing national standards must be tempered with a respect for local needs and differences. In other words, set minimal national standards, but promote local planning and implementation. National standards are needed to promote equitable use of federal resources in the provision of health care services.

VULNERABLE POPULATIONS

Meeting the health care needs of underserved populations is especially challenging. Groups that may be unable to gain access to health care services include children, older adults, the homeless, and people living in poverty. Health is strongly related to socioeconomic status, with those in lower income brackets having poor health outcomes (Edelman & Mandle, 2006). See the accompanying Nursing Checklist for information about working with vulnerable individuals.

Our current health care system neglects the overall needs of children. Children are more likely than adults to be uninsured. As the federal and state governments continue to curb expenditures for health care, more children will be declared ineligible for Medicaid. Children who are covered by health insurance have a greater degree of well-being. Public health insurance provides significant benefits for children's access and use of health care services (Duderstadt, Hughes, Soobader, & Newacheck, 2006).

Many preschool children in the United States are not immunized. Preventive health care should be available to children of all ages, with an emphasis on early immunization. In addition, maternal-child health among some ethnic and racial minorities in certain geographic areas of the United States is poorer than that in developing countries. The ANA

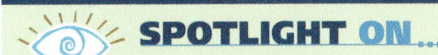

SPOTLIGHT ON...

Caring and Compassion
If you were to develop a core of basic health care services to which all Americans would have access, what would be included?

✓ NURSING CHECKLIST

Working with Members of Vulnerable Population Groups

- Establish an environment that is comfortable and nonthreatening
- Understand the verbal and nonverbal communication
- Learn about specific cultural practices that affect health care practices
- Collaborate with other care providers
- Make referrals to community agencies as necessary

and a coalition of allied nursing associations are working together in an attempt to immunize all children in the United States. The Centers for Disease Control and Prevention stated that in 2006, more than 77% of U.S. infants and toddlers received all the recommended immunizations. However, that number is below the 90% rate recommended by the Healthy People 2010 initiative.

Traditionally, rural areas have had few health care providers and facilities that were easily accessible. A large number of older people live in rural areas. Because people in rural areas tend to work for small businesses or are self-employed, many of them have no health insurance. Also, many hospitals in rural areas have been closed due to economic pressures.

Generally, adults in the United States who receive little assistance in health promotion maintain unhealthy lifestyles, which lead to the development of chronic illnesses. Older adults who have accumulated problems that could have been prevented are admitted to nursing homes, which are very costly (McCallion, 2007).

It is in the best interests of society to see that those who cannot afford the basic health services are not denied such services. The entire society's health is threatened when some sectors are denied basic care. As a group, nurses are concerned with the availability of health care services to everyone, regardless of their ability to pay (Hicks & Boles, 2008).

COMMUNITY NURSING ORGANIZATIONS

Community nursing organizations (CNOs) were established to help meet the needs of people in the community. The goal of CNOs is to provide quality health care services in a cost-effective manner. In CNOs, nurses are the PCPs. One

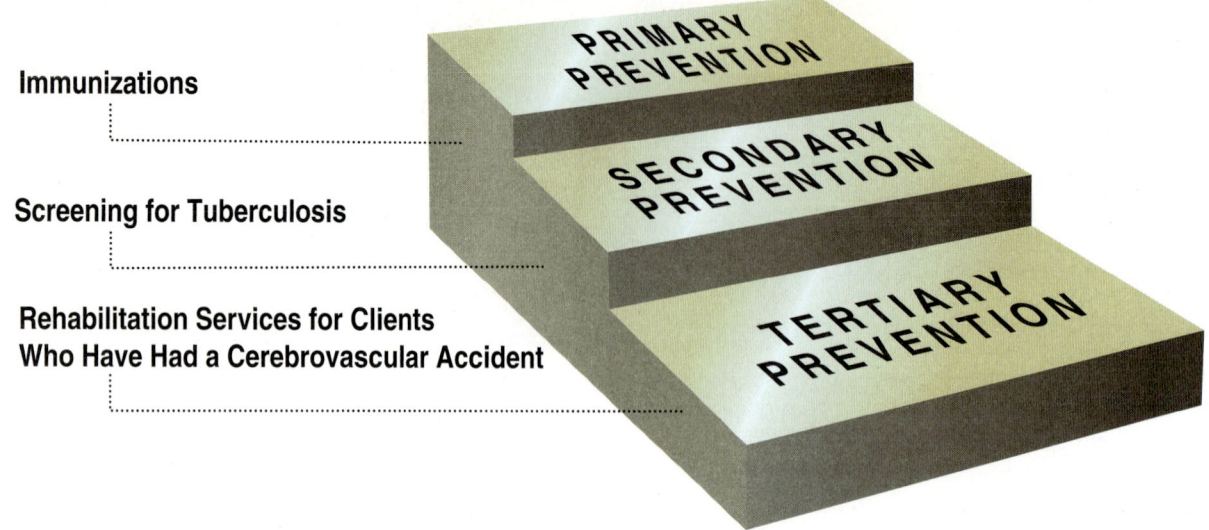

Immunizations

Screening for Tuberculosis

Rehabilitation Services for Clients
Who Have Had a Cerebrovascular Accident

FIGURE 4-2 Three Levels of Prevention and Examples DELMAR/CENGAGE LEARNING

example of a CNO is Columbia Advanced Practice Nurse Associates (CAPNA), which was established in 1998. CAPNA is affiliated with the Columbia University School of Nursing and provides primary care to the community at large.

CONTINUUM OF CARE

Acute care provided in hospitals constitutes only a small portion of health care services provided to the U.S. population. Clients need to have services provided over a broad spectrum of settings and time frames. Most large medical centers and hospitals provide a full range of services, including preadmission, outpatient, acute inpatient, long-term inpatient, hospitalization, and aftercare, which may consist of home health, hospice, subacute, or long-term care (e.g., nursing homes) Table 4-6 later in this chapter describes the settings in which health care services are provided.

LEVELS OF CARE

Basically, health care services can be categorized into three levels: primary, secondary, and tertiary (see Figure 4-2). The complexity of care varies according to the individual's need, provider's expertise, and delivery setting. Table 4-5 on page 63 provides an overview of the types of care.

Primary: Health Promotion and Illness Prevention

The major purposes of health care are to promote wellness and prevent illness or disability. Traditionally, the U.S. health care system has focused on disease prevention rather than health promotion. However, within the past decade, society has begun to engage in health-promoting behaviors. Illness prevention activities are directed at the individual, the family, and the community.

Secondary: Diagnosis and Treatment

Most health care services are the secondary type of health care interventions. Acute treatment centers (hospitals) are still the predominant site of delivery of health care services. There is a growing movement to have diagnostic and therapeutic services provided in locations that are more easily accessed by individuals.

Tertiary: Rehabilitation

Restoring an individual to the state that existed before the development of an illness is the purpose of rehabilitative (or restorative) care. In situations in which the person is unable to regain previous functional abilities, the goal of rehabilitation is to help the client reach the optimal level of self-care. Restorative care is holistic, in that the entire person is cared for—physiological, psychological, social, and spiritual dimensions.

HEALTH CARE SETTINGS

Health care services are delivered in a variety of settings; see Table 4-6 on page 63. Even though the majority of RNs currently are employed by hospitals, the fastest-growing employment opportunity for nurses in the near future is expected to be outpatient settings, i.e., clinics and home health care agencies (Bureau of Labor Statistics, 2007).

Technological advances have allowed many health care services to be delivered in outpatient settings. Such technology and increased medical specialization have resulted in improved health outcomes for many individuals. However, specialization has also led to a major problem, fragmentation of care.

COMMUNITY CONSIDERATIONS

Are there programs in your community in which nurses are delivering health services to vulnerable populations? What is the need for such services, taking into consideration populations such as children, older adults, the indigent, and the homeless?

TABLE 4-5 Types of Health Care Services

TYPE OF CARE	DESCRIPTION	EXAMPLES
Primary	• *Goal:* To decrease the risk to a client (individual, family, or community) for disease or dysfunction • *Explanation:* General health promotion Protection against specific illnesses	• Teaching • Lifestyle modification for health (e.g., smoking cessation, nutritional counseling) • Referrals • Immunization • Promotion of a safe environment (e.g., sanitation, protection from toxic agents)
Secondary	• *Goal:* Early intervention to alleviate disease and prevent further disability • *Explanation:* Early detection and intervention	• Screenings • Diagnosis • Acute care • Surgery
Tertiary	• *Goal:* To minimize effects of and permanent disability due to chronic or irreversible condition • *Explanation:* Restorative and rehabilitative activities to obtain optimal level of functioning	• Education and retraining • Provision of direct care • Environmental modifications (e.g., advising on necessity of wheelchair accessibility for a person who has experienced a cerebrovascular accident [stroke])

Delmar/Cengage Learning

FRAGMENTATION OF CARE

Health care often becomes fragmented when a person sees more than one health care provider and receives care at more than one facility. As a result of the fragmentation, clients may be misdiagnosed, receive unnecessary care, and be viewed as a "case" rather than a whole person. For example, a client who is being treated for hypertension by the PCP is referred to a gynecologist for an annual Pap smear, who then refers

TABLE 4-6 Health Care Settings

SETTING	SERVICES PROVIDED	NURSE'S ROLES/RESPONSIBILITIES
Hospitals	• Diagnosis and treatment of illnesses (acute and chronic) • Acute inpatient services • Emergency care • Ambulatory care services • Critical (intensive) care • Rehabilitative care • Surgical interventions • Diagnostic procedures	• Caregiver • Client educator • Provides ongoing assessment • Coordinates care and collaborates with other health care providers • Maintains client safety • Initiates discharge planning • Has a variety of areas in which to specialize: Cardiology Neurology Critical care Oncology Dialysis Orthopedics Emergency Pain management Geriatrics Psychiatry Infection control Rehabilitation Maternal-child Surgery

(continues)

TABLE 4-6 (Continued)

SETTING	SERVICES PROVIDED	NURSE'S ROLES/RESPONSIBILITIES
Extended care (long-term care) facilities (e.g., nursing homes, skilled nursing facilities)	• Intermediate and long-term care for people with chronic illnesses or those who are unable to care for themselves • Restorative care until client is ready for discharge to home	• Caregiver • Educator • Advocate • Provides care directed at meeting basic needs (e.g., nutrition, hydration, comfort, elimination) • Provides teaching and counseling • Plans and coordinates care • Administers medications, treatments, and other therapeutic modalities
Home health agencies	• Wide range of services, including acute and restorative	• Educator • Caregiver • Provides skilled nursing care • Coordinates health promotion activities (e.g., education)
Hospices	• Care of individuals with terminal illnesses • Improving the quality of end-of-life (EOL) care	• Caregiver • Counselor • Advocate • Plans and coordinates care • Promotes comfort measures • Provides pain control • Supports grieving families
Outpatient settings (clinics, ambulatory treatment centers)	• Treatment of illness (acute and chronic) • Diagnostic testing • Noncomplex surgical procedures	*Traditional Role:* • Checks vital signs • Assists with diagnostic tests • Prepares client for examination *Expanded Role:* • Provides teaching and counseling • Performs physical (or mental status) examination • In some settings, advanced practice registered nurses (APRNs) are the primary care providers
Schools	• School-based clinics are federally funded providers of physical and mental health services in elementary and secondary schools	• Caregiver • Educator • Advocate • Coordinates health promotion and disease prevention activities • Treats minor illnesses • Provides health education
Industrial clinics	• Maintain health and safety of workers	• Caregiver • Educator • Coordinates health promotion activities • Provides education for safety • Provides urgent care as needed • Maintains health records • Conducts ongoing screenings • Provides preventive services (e.g., tuberculosis testing)

(continues)

TABLE 4-6 (Continued)

SETTING	SERVICES PROVIDED	NURSE'S ROLES/RESPONSIBILITIES
Managed care organizations	• Reimbursement for health care services	• Caregiver • Educator • Case manager • Uses triage to determine the most appropriate intervention for clients
Community nursing centers	• Direct access to professional nursing services	• Caregiver • Treats client's responses to health problems • Promotes health and wellness
Rural primary care hospitals (RPCHs)	• Stabilize clients until they are physiologically able to be transferred to more skilled facilities	• Caregiver • Educator • Advocate • Performs assessments and provides emergency care

Delmar/Cengage Learning

the client to an oncologist for treatment of cervical cancer. The client is then treated by a hematologist, radiologist, and endocrinologist. Each specialty-care physician treats a certain problem instead of the entire person.

Fragmented care may also occur as the client progresses through various treatment settings. For example, the client may be seen in an outpatient clinic by one set of health care providers, then admitted to the hospital, and then discharged to home health care. Due to the variety of settings and care providers, the person's individuality may be overlooked. Many health care providers and organizations (such as HMOs) are implementing the concept of seamless service to overcome the delivery of fragmented services. Seamless service means that an organization provides preadmission, acute inpatient, and aftercare services to a client. Such a delivery system helps prevent a client from being lost in the system with resulting unmet needs.

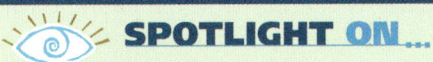

Professionalism
Before focusing on the problems within the current health care delivery system, stop and think!

The American health care system is first in technologic advances, biomedical research, and state-of-the-art clinical equipment and facilities. Yet even with these advantages, many consider that this system is in crisis. From your perspective, is the U.S. health care system in a position of strength or weakness? Explain why.

QUALITY MANAGEMENT IN HEALTH CARE

Quality of care, cost, and access are dominant themes in health care delivery. Health care services must be delivered in a manner that increases the occurrence of expected health outcomes. Nurses, as well as all other health care providers, are accountable for quality care. The challenge for nursing has never been greater as political, economic, and regulatory requirements increase and the demand for quality care intensifies.

DEFINING QUALITY

Health care has struggled for many years to define and measure quality. **Quality** is defined as meeting or exceeding requirements of the customer or client. A **customer** is anyone who uses the products, services, or processes of an organization. Quality is measured in terms of customer perspective with emphasis on the following:

- Accessibility and availability of service
- Timely and safe delivery of service
- Coordination and continuity of care between services
- Effectiveness of services (i.e., the delivery and outcome of care)

A health care organization must be concerned with *doing the right things* (efficacy, appropriateness) and *doing the right things well* (availability, timeliness, effectiveness, continuity, safety, efficiency, and respect and caring). **Performance improvement** consists of those activities and behaviors that each individual does to meet customers' expectations. It is doing the right thing well and continually striving to do better (Joint Commission, 2008).

Quality measurement consists of evaluating three inter-related components: structure, process, and outcome. Each of these components is interrelated. The ANA's *Nursing: Scope and Standards of Practice* (2004) uses these three components of care to guide nursing practice within the framework of the nursing process.

Quality management has its own array of terminology. Despite the similarities, there are differences in the concepts, as outlined here:

- **Quality assurance** (QA) is the traditional approach to quality management in which monitoring and evaluation focus on individual performance, deviation from standards, and problem solving.
- **Continuous quality improvement** (CQI) is the approach to quality management in which scientific, data-driven approaches are used to study work processes that lead to long-term system improvements. This concept has evolved into systems such as process improvement or performance improvement.
- **Total quality management** (TQM) is the method of management and system operation used to achieve CQI. TQM promotes an organizational culture that supports customer need, empowers employees to work as teams, emphasizes self-development, and requires a new leadership style in which employees are viewed as resources.

TQM is a system of operation, whereas CQI is the desired outcome of a quality management program. It is difficult to achieve performance improvement without a TQM culture. The goal of a quality management program is to focus on process improvement, which will ultimately improve the quality of care.

FACTORS INFLUENCING QUALITY IN HEALTH CARE

Today there are many consumers of health care in addition to clients and their families. One major consumer of health care is third-party payers, such as insurance companies, managed care organizations, and federal and state governments. The diversity of needs represented by these consumers requires improvement in health care delivery systems. The major factors that have influenced the development of the quality movement in health care are consumer demands, financial viability, professional accountability, regulatory requirements, progress in quality improvement techniques, and changes in health care delivery.

Consumer Demands

Health care consumers are sophisticated, knowledgeable, and selective. Clients no longer place blind trust in health care providers; they realize that variables in practice and results occur. Today's consumers negotiate services and compare health care costs among providers.

Financial Viability

Health care has entered an era of increased competitiveness for services, staff, and customers. There is a demand to reduce spending and contain costs. Budgetary constraints

continue to increase in both the private and public health sectors. Health care organizations must strive to reduce professional liability, increase reimbursement eligibility, and promote cost-effectiveness through increased efficiency.

Professional Accountability

Emphasis on clinician accountability and adherence to codes of ethical practice is increasing. Health care professionals must be dedicated to reducing practice variances in order to protect the public.

Regulatory Requirements

The CMS standards, Joint Commission standards, and numerous laws require quality improvement programs. The CMS is a subsidiary of the DHHS and is the federal agency responsible for administering the Medicare and Medicaid programs. The regulations established by these organizations for accreditation and reimbursement have facilitated the quality initiative in health care. Such externally mandated regulations have promoted the development of internal monitoring and evaluation systems within health care organizations.

Progress in Quality Improvement Techniques

During the past decade, health care providers have spent valuable resources on defining and measuring quality. As a result, evaluation methodologies have improved considerably. Information systems are available through which national and regional norms for comparative data can be obtained. Measurability methods have been upgraded and include a variety of process improvement models. **Process improvement** examines the flow of client care between departments to ensure that the processes work effectively and that acceptable levels of performance are achieved. Overall quality improvement methodologies enhance performance and work processes.

Changes in Health Care Delivery

Significant changes in health care delivery have occurred, and unprecedented change is anticipated in the future. Clients being admitted to hospitals today are more acutely ill yet are being discharged more quickly than in the past. Alternative care options such as home health care, in-home intravenous therapy, and intermediate care facilities have proliferated, resulting in an even greater need to coordinate a continuum of services.

Factors that have influenced the quality movement in health care have also protected those populations most vulnerable to inadequate health care (e.g., the uninsured, older adults, and low-income families). The quality movement has promoted access to care, standards of care, cost-effective service, and a continuum of care. Thus, the quality movement in health care has served as an advocate for consumers.

Legal Implications of Quality Improvement

Nurses, as well as other health care providers, must understand the roles that laws and regulations play in the quality movement. These aspects define professional practice. Laws define legal practice, while regulations define guidelines for delivery of care.

Legal considerations have an impact on quality management in several ways:

- Laws and regulations create the external structure for quality management.
- Failure to provide quality health care can result in lawsuits.
- Institutions can face liability for action taken against a practitioner if objective measures are not applied to performance and due process is not provided.

Quality management programs must protect against substandard care and ultimately reduce litigation. Organizations must have clearly defined processes for professional review. These responsibilities are based on federal regulations.

Federal Regulations

A number of federal agencies regulate health care standards, for example, the CMS, the Food and Drug Administration, and the Occupational Safety and Health Administration (OSHA). OSHA requires employers to protect employees from work-related injuries and illnesses (e.g., exposure to infectious materials). There are also federal laws that prohibit substandard care, promote health care provider peer review, and mandate the reporting of serious injury or death of clients resulting from unsafe use of medical devices.

Failure to adhere to the guidelines in these legislative acts can result in sanctions for violation of standards. Federal funding and payment for services can be denied for failure to provide quality care.

QUALITY AND HEALTH CARE ECONOMICS

Health care costs have skyrocketed in the past decades. The primary source of health insurance in the United States is employer coverage. Payers are becoming increasingly concerned about health care costs, and the issue of health care expenditures is being intensely debated.

Delivery of poor quality care has a negative financial impact on health care organizations. Management in some organizations argues that the quality improvement initiative is costly because of staff time involved in such activities. However, one must consider the cost of poor quality, which results in the following problems:

- Duplicated work between departments
- Loss of time due to inefficient task performance
- Loss of staff due to job dissatisfaction
- Recruitment and training of new employees
- Expenditure of energy and time in investigation of complaints and allegations
- Litigation and malpractice settlements
- Expenses related to overutilization of diagnostic tests to avoid malpractice

Originally, the perception of quality was that of doing more, that is, the performance of more tasks, which resulted in intensive intervention. Today, it is believed that efficiency can be improved without compromising quality.

Health care leaders must now look at the individual and collective effectiveness of organizational management. Organizations must also begin to examine the cumulative cost associated with a less-than-optimal ability to plan, delegate, communicate, and listen. The prevailing philosophy is to do more with less. Such an approach to health care management has resulted in downsizing, cross-training, and reduction of middle-management staff.

PRINCIPLES OF QUALITY IMPROVEMENT

Because CQI examines ways in which the entire organization can improve, the involvement of everyone, especially administration, is required. CQI is based on the following principles:

- Quality is a central theme to the organization. It is part of the organization's mission and the core of daily activities.
- Leadership is committed to and involved in creating an organizational culture (commonly held beliefs, values, norms, and expectations that drive the workforce) for quality improvement.
- All staff members are personally responsible for quality; therefore, decision making is done by the people doing the work.
- Education and training must be continual to improve skills and promote self-development.
- Processes and system operation, in addition to individual performance, are monitored.
- A scientific approach based on analysis of data is used.
- Accurate information is available and must be used in decision making. Individuals and institutions can no longer use opinion and intuition; they must manage by facts.

CUSTOMER SATISFACTION

Promoting customer satisfaction requires an organizational commitment from every employee to be sensitive to the needs, wants, and expectations of customers. This commitment requires putting the customer first. Customers include those internal and external to the organization, such as clients, suppliers, third-party payers, families, visitors, coworkers, and the community. Managers must meet employee needs and service delivery demands. The direct care provider must meet client needs, coworkers' needs, and organizational needs.

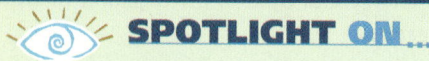

SPOTLIGHT ON...

Legal/Ethical

You are working in a skilled nursing facility. Regulations require that unlicensed personnel complete training and testing for certification as nursing assistants. You discover that there has been a recent turnover in staff and many newly employed nursing assistants are not yet certified.

What are the legal and ethical ramifications of this situation? What should you do?

Health care agencies do not have unlimited resources allocated solely to keeping customers happy. Therefore, the organization and each employee must understand the implications of customer dissatisfaction from a financial perspective. The loss of one admission is relatively insignificant to a multimillion dollar budget; however, multiple losses can have a substantial effect on a health care facility's financial well-being.

There is additional potential revenue loss from related ancillary services following hospitalization, such as home health care, laboratory procedures, pharmaceutical supplies, and office follow-up. A customer's dissatisfaction with one facet of service can be generalized to all related delivery systems.

Another effect of customer dissatisfaction is a tarnished community image. There is a multiplier (or ripple) effect in which one bad encounter can affect the attitude and opinion of many. An unhappy client may inform the immediate family, extended family, neighbors, friends, and coworkers. Seemingly simple acts, such as the following, can result in client dissatisfaction despite a positive health outcome:

- A cold food tray
- Failure to respond to a call light in a timely manner
- Waiting for tests
- Late treatment
- Unemptied bedpan
- Delayed pain medication
- Failure of health care provider to introduce himself or herself

Satisfaction is a subjective perception; therefore, health care providers must listen to the customer constantly to determine satisfaction and dissatisfaction. Then, improvements can be initiated.

ORGANIZATIONAL STRUCTURE FOR QUALITY MANAGEMENT

Because quality has become a central issue in health care delivery, nurses must consider the impact of organizational structure on the quality of care provided. Nurses are key in establishing a culture for excellence in most health care organizations.

Several factors within an organization affect quality management, including organizational culture, workforce diversity, empowerment, leadership, and teamwork. To improve the quality of care, the organization should be viewed as a system that is comprised of governance, management, clinical, and support devices. Many processes within the system involve more than one group. Therefore, a framework must be established to promote collaboration.

ORGANIZATIONAL CULTURE

Organizations have both formal and informal cultures. Incongruence between the formal operational style espoused by management and the style demonstrated by staff members may be evident. This can result in an ineffectual organization in which achieving continual improvement is difficult. Thus, the culture of an organization can affect the quality of care. A positive culture promotes trust, information sharing, collaboration, and risk taking, whereas a negative culture produces divisiveness, resistance, and a desire to maintain the status quo. In a negative culture, inertia develops and employees lack creativity and self-direction. Table 4-7 on page 69 compares characteristics of organizational culture within traditional and high-performance organizations.

Leadership

Organizational leadership contributes to the creation of the culture based on CQI beliefs and practice. Leadership must create a people-oriented culture. In today's fast-paced, high-tech, cost-driven health care environment, the human factor is frequently overlooked. Although staffing incurs the greatest expense and is a primary target for cost reduction, it is the people in the health care organization who are the greatest asset. Therefore, management must focus on ensuring a return on this important resource.

Teamwork

Improving quality requires team effort. Authoritarian, hierarchical, and traditional ways of management are no longer effective; therefore, health care organizations are turning to team-based strategies for organizing labor.

A **team** is a group of individuals who work together to achieve a common goal. The dynamics of team interaction are important. Teams must demonstrate commitment, cooperation, and communication. The way the team communicates and solves problems has a significant impact on outcome and delivery of service. For quality care to occur, work groups must function as teams.

To promote quality improvement, teams are used to study processes. There are two types of process improvement teams: functional and cross-functional. A **functional team** is a departmental or unit-specific group whose scope is limited to departmental or work area processes. A **cross-functional team** is an interdepartmental, multidisciplinary group that is assigned to study an organization-wide process

TABLE 4-7 Organizational Culture

DIMENSION	TRADITIONAL ORGANIZATION	HIGH-PERFORMANCE ORGANIZATION
Structure	• Authoritarian, hierarchical	• Team focused
Decision making	• Limited input, based on politics and alliances, dissonance	• By consensus, based on resources, commitment to action
Cooperation	• Territorial, departmentalized	• Organizational success emphasized • Widespread consideration
Conflict	• Open discussion of issues avoided	• Regarded as natural, even helpful • Focuses on issues, not person
Relationships	• Competitive, withholding, suspicious, partisan	• Trusting, respectful, supportive, collaborative
Information and communication	• Controlled at the top • Hoarded, withheld, flows mainly downward • Fiscal information secretive • Line staff uninformed, management unaware of staff opinion	• Full sharing, open, honest • Flows freely up, down, sideways • Fiscal information shared • Information considered credible
Listening	• Information from the lowest level does not reach the top • Management unresponsive	• Genuine listening at all levels • Feedback sought
Commitment and motivation	• Lack of strategic planning • Resistance to change • Individual interest considered over the group • Fear of punishment	• Commitment to vision, mission, and goals at all levels • Group achievement desired
Reward and compensation	• Based on subjective appraisal • Longevity considered over skills and positive reinforcement for negative performance	• Merit system based on ability • Unacceptable behavior results in termination
Atmosphere	• Intimidating, guarded, closed, political	• Open, nonthreatening, noncompetitive, participative
Labor-management relationship	• Adversarial • "We-they" mentality • Focus on grievance	• Collaborative problem solving with both parties committed to organizational welfare
Role of manager	• Expected to follow system • Conservative approach • Seniority system for promotion • Dictatorial style with emphasis on disciplinary action	• Managers considered important asset • Emphasis placed on recruitment, selection, development, training, and compensation of managers • Coaching skills essential
Attitude toward clients	• They need us; we know what is best	• Service attitude • Client is customer • Client's opinion is valued
Measurements of success	• Machines, equipment, materials • Quantitative output, volume	• Process improvement • Customer satisfaction

Data from Kilduff, M., & Krackhardt, D. (2008). *Interpersonal networks in organizations: Cognition, personality, dynamics and culture*. New York: Cambridge University Press; Michel, M., & Wortham, S. (2008). *Bullish on uncertainty: How organized cultures transform participants*. New York: Cambridge University Press.

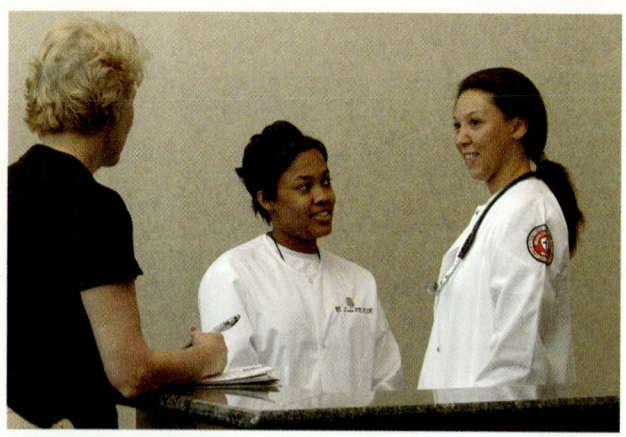

FIGURE 4-3 Members of a cross-functional health care team. How is the quality of health care improved by the involvement of more than one discipline? DELMAR/CENGAGE LEARNING

(see Figure 4-3). An effective team demonstrates mutual respect and trust, displays open communication, builds on skills of members, and seeks consensus.

The use of teams to restructure and improve work processes has many advantages, such as:

- Increased involvement and understanding
- More opportunities to share ideas
- Assistance in building relationships
- Involvement of staff in problem solving

The team approach is effective for coordinating and integrating interdepartmental work processes.

PROCESS IMPROVEMENT

For years, the focus of health care quality has been on performance improvement. No single individual's performance really stands alone. Each person's action in an organization is actually a performance step that is connected to the actions of others. This series of interconnected steps is known as a process; processes interconnect to form a system.

Tools for Measuring Quality

A variety of tools are used to collect and analyze data so that decisions can be made about organizational performance. Some mechanisms frequently used to obtain and measure data are:

- **Audit:** Reviewing client records for compliance to predetermined criteria that measure process and outcome of care
- **Peer review:** Evaluating care based on the judgment of a colleague with equal education and experience
- **Benchmarking:** Measuring service or practice against the competition
- **Clinical pathways:** Measuring the performance of care according to critical outcomes and key incidents that must occur within given time frames

In addition, comparative data can be obtained from the literature, practice guidelines, and external reference databases.

NURSING'S ROLE IN QUALITY MANAGEMENT

The primary purpose of nursing is to provide quality care to clients. Providing quality care means always seeking to improve the care delivered. Nurses function as clinicians, team members, and managers. Each of these roles has specific responsibilities for quality performance and requires certain skills to achieve the expected level of performance (see Table 4-8).

Whether functioning as a clinician, team member, or manager, nurses continually strive for excellence in everything they do. See the Uncovering the Evidence feature. By using a CQI approach, which examines structure and process instead of individual performance, nurses can move forward in the provision of quality care. Quality improvement identifies situations when nursing teams are more productive and functioning at a higher quality level.

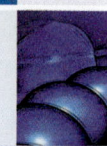

TABLE 4-8 Nursing Roles and Responsibilities: Quality Improvement	
ROLE	**RESPONSIBILITIES**
Clinician	• Maintain ethical standards of practice • Seek self-development via continuing education • Be self-directed • Serve as change agent • Practice efficient time management • Achieve customer satisfaction • Be committed to reducing cost and improving performance
Team member	• Be knowledgeable about group dynamics • Support colleagues • Promote mutual trust and respect • Build rapport with other disciplines • Practice active listening • Praise coworkers
Manager	• Develop leadership skills • Be knowledgeable about statistical analysis • Provide clear and direct communication • Delegate to and empower staff • Lead by example

Delmar/Cengage Learning

UNCOVERING THE

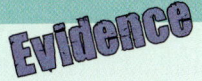

TITLE OF STUDY

"Quality Improvement: The Divergent Views of Managers and Clinicians"

AUTHORS

M. Price, L. Fitzgerald, and L. Kinsman

PURPOSE

Identify and explore nurse managers' and nurse clinicians' perceptions of quality improvement.

METHODS

This descriptive qualitative research study collected data via semistructured interviews. The data were analyzed using constant comparative analysis.

FINDINGS

The concept of quality improvement and how it applies to nursing practice varied between the two groups. Each group identified the importance of quality in delivery of care. However, managers and clinicians stated it was the other group that was responsible for decreased quality care delivery.

IMPLICATIONS

Nurse managers and clinicians provided divergent views of the deficiencies in the way quality improvement is implemented. In order to be successful, a quality improvement program must include the views of both managers and clinical nurses.

Price, M., Fitzgerald, L., & Kinsman, L. (2007). Quality improvement: The divergent views of managers and clinicians. *Journal of Nursing Management, 15*(1), 43–50.

TRENDS IN HEALTH CARE DELIVERY

As current trends continue, the delivery of health care services will continue to change. "Today the terms *change* and *chaos* are used interchangeably to describe the current state of the U.S. health care system. No one seems to have a clear vision of how health care services will be organized and delivered in the future" (Heinrich & Thompson, 2007, p. 208). Some factors that will continue to shape reform of the health care delivery system are:

- The aging of the U.S. population
- Increasing diversity in the U.S. population
- Increased number of single-parent families, with more children living in poverty
- Continued growth in outpatient settings with a greater demand for PCPs
- Advances in technology with a resultant ability to perform more services in outpatient settings (including the home)
- Emphasis on disease prevention and health promotion at the workplace
- Expectations of third-party payers and providers for clients to assume more personal responsibility for care

The states and private sector will lead the way through a process to a product suited to the American character. The nursing profession has reached a point in time where there are few questions about the direction or process of health care reform. "What is clear today is that economic incentives and concerns will continue to drive future health system changes, and that business and corporate Americans will increasingly have more of a say in how the future health care delivery system will be organized" (Heinrich & Thompson, 2007, pp. 211–212). The challenge is to improve the nation's delivery of health care services by positioning nursing to preserve its integrity and guarantee its preferred future. Nurses must continue to be in the forefront of change.

KEY CONCEPTS

- The three levels of health care services can be categorized as primary, secondary, and tertiary levels.
- Health care services are delivered by both the public (official, voluntary, and nonprofit agencies) and private (hospitals, extended care facilities, home health agencies, hospices, outpatient settings, schools, industrial clinics, managed care organizations, community nursing centers, and rural hospitals) sectors.
- The health care team is composed of nurses, APRNs, physicians, physician assistants, pharmacists, dentists, dietitians, social workers, therapists, and chaplains.

- Health care in the United States is financed through a combination of both private and public funding.
- Managed care organizations seek to control health care costs by monitoring the delivery of services and restricting access to costly procedures and providers.
- Managed care plans include HMOs, PPOs, and EPOs.
- The primary federal government insurance plans are Medicare, the program that provides health care coverage for older adults and people with disabilities, and Medicaid, the jointly administered program that provides health care services for the poor.

- Health care reform must address the three critical issues of cost, access, and quality of health care services to achieve equity for all Americans.

- *Nursing's Agenda for Health Care Reform,* written by the ANA and endorsed by over 70 professional organizations, outlines nursing's proposals for easing the current problems in health care delivery.

- The AHRQ aims to identify therapeutic standards for which the health care community can be held accountable.

- A primary goal of the nursing profession within the areas of public health, community health, and long-term care is to provide health care services that emphasize prevention and primary health care to clients in these settings and thus help reduce the cost and increase the quality of health care.

- The quality movement was initiated by consumer demands, financial viability, professional accountability, regulatory requirements, progress made in quality improvement techniques, and changes in health care delivery.

- Federal regulations establish guidelines for quality management.

- Continuous quality improvement focuses on studying work processes that promote system improvements.

- Total quality management is a method of organizational operation that establishes a work environment to achieve continuous improvement.

- A customer is anyone who uses the products, services, or processes within an organization. Clients, families, visitors, employees, suppliers, and the community are all considered customers within the health care system.

- Customer dissatisfaction can have significant financial implications for health care organizations.

- Quality management requires positive organizational culture, leadership, and teamwork.

- A variety of tools (e.g., audits, peer reviews, and benchmarking) are available through which data about variations in process improvement can be collected and analyzed.

- The nurse is responsible for quality improvement as a clinician, team member, and manager.

REVIEW QUESTIONS

1. A client asks the nurse, "Exactly what is an HMO?" The nurse's response should include which of the following information? Select all that apply.
   a. HMOs are groups of federally financed insurance companies.
   b. Many HMOs provide a continuum of care to individuals and families.
   c. HMOs were established to control the costs of health care delivery.
   d. An HMO provides unlimited services to its members.
   e. The HMO was developed as a type of fee-for-service reimbursement system.
   f. HMOs were intended to emphasize prevention rather than treatment of chronic conditions.

2. The largest insurer of health care services in the United States is the _____.

3. When working with a person from a vulnerable population, it is important for the nurse to do which of the following?
   a. Perform the nursing assessment as quickly as possible so the individual can return to the community.
   b. Learn about the person's specific cultural practices.
   c. Focus only on the client's verbal communication.
   d. Refer the client to another nurse who is from the same cultural group as the client.

4. The nurse who is working in a rehabilitation facility is providing which level of care?
   a. Primary
   b. Secondary
   c. Tertiary
   d. Palliative

5. Which of the following nursing actions will adversely affect customer satisfaction of hospitalized clients?
   a. Introducing self to client and family
   b. Assessing pain level
   c. Implementing a routine schedule for every client
   d. Documenting all care provided in a timely manner

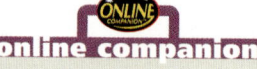

online companion

Visit the DeLaune and Ladner online companion resource at **www.delmar.cengage.com** for additional content and study aids. Click on Online Companions, then select the Nursing discipline.

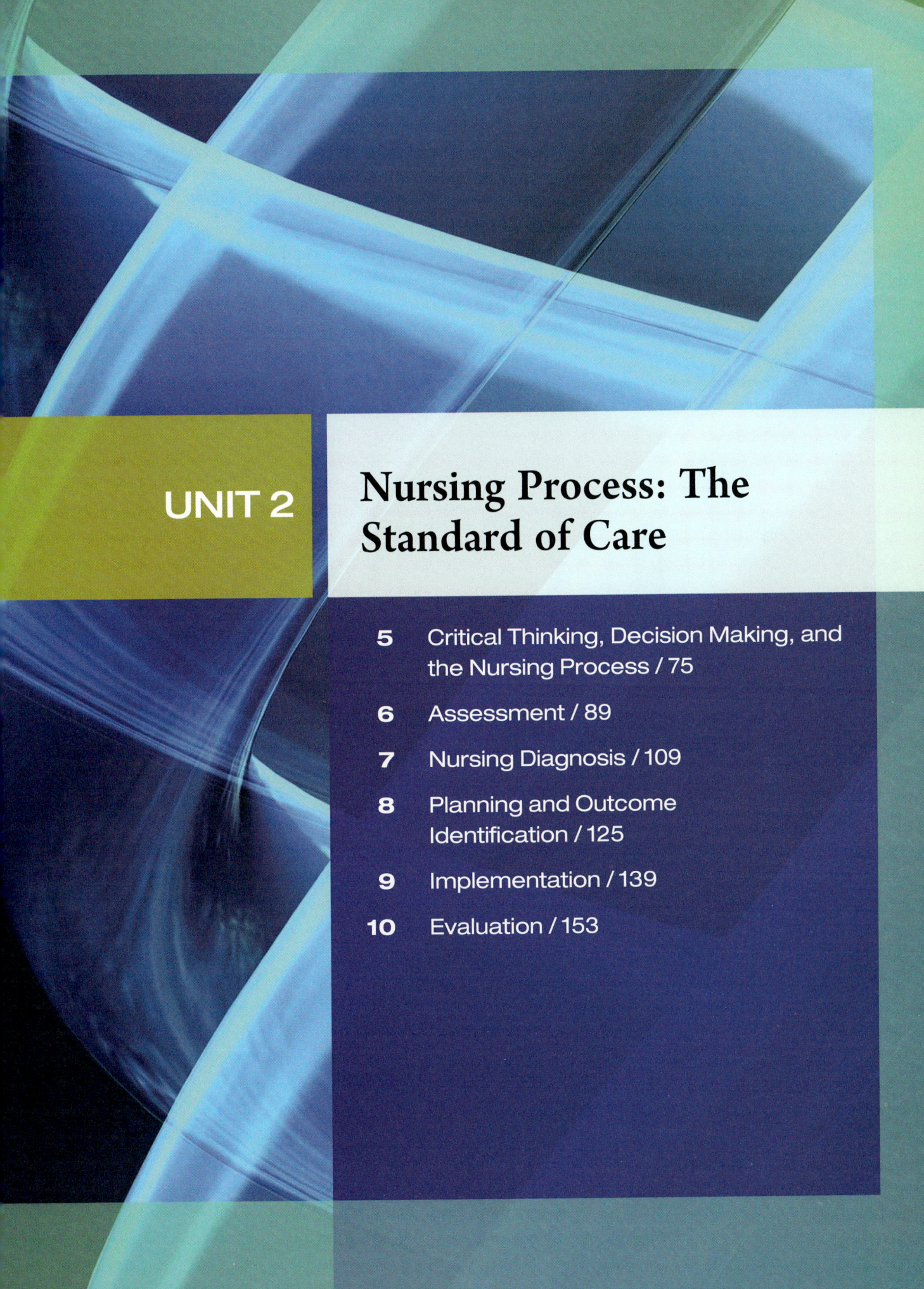

UNIT 2

Nursing Process: The Standard of Care

The principal goal of education is to create men and women ... who have minds which can be critical, can verify, and not accept everything they are offered.

—Jean Piaget

CHAPTER 5

Critical Thinking, Decision Making, and the Nursing Process

COMPETENCIES

1. Identify the components of critical thinking.
2. Describe the relationship between critical thinking, problem solving, and decision making.
3. Compare critical thinking and creative thinking.
4. Relate critical thinking to the nursing process.
5. Describe the assessment step of the nursing process.
6. Describe the process of nursing diagnoses.
7. List the tasks involved in the outcome identification and planning step of the nursing process.
8. Discuss the nursing implementation phase of the nursing process.
9. Discuss the evaluation process.

KEY TERMS

actual nursing diagnosis

analysis

assessment

collaborative problems

critical thinking

decision making

declarative knowledge

evaluation

expected outcomes

goal

groupthink

implementation

nursing diagnosis

nursing intervention

nursing process

objective data

operative knowledge

planning

possible nursing diagnosis

primary source

process

risk nursing diagnosis

secondary sources

subjective data

synthesis

wellness nursing diagnosis

Due to the constantly changing health care environment, critical thinking is a requisite skill in order for nurses to make complex decisions. Critical thinking is the process through which nurses analyze and make sense of situations in order to make sound clinical decisions. This chapter presents information about the relationship between problem solving, decision making, and the nursing process. Critical thinkers are people who know how to think. They possess intellectual autonomy, in that they refuse to accept conclusions without evaluating the evidence (facts and reasons) for themselves. Critical thinkers have the ability to think beyond the obvious and make connections between ideas. **Critical thinking** is the process that allows nurses to see the big picture (envision the overall perspective) instead of focusing only on details.

CRITICAL THINKING

There are many definitions of critical thinking, including Ennis's (1987) classic description, "reasonable reflective thinking that is focused on deciding what to believe or do" (p. 10). Critical thinking is a "skilled process that conceptualizes and applies information from observation, experience, reflection, inference, and communication" (Shin, Lee, Ha, & Kim, 2006, p. 182). Following is a brief summary of various definitions of critical thinking:

- The rational examination of ideas, assumptions, principles, conclusions, beliefs, and actions (Bandman & Bandman, 1995)
- Reasonable reflective thinking that focuses on decisions about actions and beliefs (Ennis, 1989)
- Purposeful, autonomous judgments that lead to interpretation, analysis, inference, evaluation, and explanation (Facione, 1990)
- Self-directed rational thinking that validates what we know and identifies what we do not know (Paul, 1992)
- A set of requisite abilities necessary for defining problems, recognizing assumptions, developing hypotheses, drawing conclusions, and validating inferences (Watson & Glaser, 1964)

Critical thinking is identified by the National League for Nursing (1997) as an essential nursing competency and an accreditation criterion; thus, nursing students and graduates must demonstrate competency in critical thinking skills.

COMPONENTS OF CRITICAL THINKING

Critical thinking has several components, including mental operations, knowledge, and attitudes.

Mental Operations

Mental operations include activities such as decision making and reasoning that are used to find or create meaning. Nurses engage in such activities whenever they search for solutions based on rationale and develop outcomes accordingly. The result of these mental operations is creative, appropriate problem solving. Critical thinking enables nurses to make sound clinical judgments by analyzing information and applying knowledge.

Knowledge

Critical thinking calls for a knowledge base that includes **declarative knowledge**, which is specific facts or information, and **operative knowledge**, which is an understanding of the nature of that knowledge. Nursing curricula assist the student in learning specific facts about nursing and the delivery of quality care. Students are also taught how to examine beliefs underlying facts in order to analyze and interpret those facts. In other words, students are not expected to merely repeat facts that have been memorized (learned by rote) but instead to understand the reasoning behind the knowledge. Finding meaning in what one is learning is the core of critical thinking.

In order to think critically, to solve problems, and to make decisions, nurses must develop a broad base of knowledge. Nurses' intuitive knowledge is essential for delivery of care. "Intuition is a rich source of nursing knowledge and … integral to the practice of nursing" (Billay, Myrick, Luhanga, & Yonge, 2007, p. 155). Nurses acquire a broad knowledge base that includes information from other disciplines such as physical science (anatomy, physiology, biology), psychology, and philosophy (logic). Nurses apply this knowledge to specific client situations through the use of critical thinking.

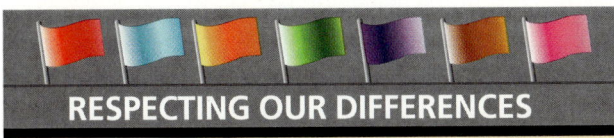

RESPECTING OUR DIFFERENCES

Cultural

You are working in the emergency department when a client is admitted for treatment of gunshot wounds. Consider how you would feel when caring for this client if you knew his injuries were:

Suffered during a robbery

Inflicted by his wife during a domestic disturbance

Caused by his homosexual lover in a fit of rage

Self-inflicted

The result of a gang-related revenge shooting

Experienced when he was selling drugs

Attitudes

Certain attitudes enhance a person's ability to think critically. One of the most important attitudes needed by a critical thinker is a sense of curiosity that allows the person to question assumptions upon which decisions are based. Analysis of basic assumptions allows the person to plan and act in a rational manner rather than out of habit or routine. Some attitudes demonstrated by critical thinkers are:

- Tolerance, open-mindedness, nonjudgmental mind-set
- Curiosity
- Persistence, intellectual courage
- Respect for others' perspectives
- Comfort dealing with ambiguity, uncertainty
- Intellectual humility (knowing that one does not have all the answers)
- Self-confidence (belief in own ability to think things through and make appropriate decisions)
- Flexibility
- Organization (Alfaro-LeFevre, 2008; Forehand, 2005)

The attitude of open-mindedness helps the nurse better care for clients whose lifestyle choices and values differ from those of the nurse; see the Respecting Our Differences box on reflective thinking and value systems. Critical thinkers question their assumptions and the effect of those assumptions on their actions.

DEVELOPMENT OF CRITICAL THINKING SKILLS

The development of critical thinking skills is a gradual process related to the individual's maturity, in that maturity enhances the ability to suspend judgment until the data have been collected. Perry (1970) developed a four-stage model describing cognitive development; see Table 5-1. It is important to note that every person does not function at the highest level of cognitive thinking. Also, the level of a person's cognitive function may vary according to the situation and professional experience. As people gain maturity and experience, their ability to think critically usually increases. The development of critical thinking is the aim of nursing educational programs. One longitudinal study (Standing, 2007) of newly graduated students showed that "as Registered Nurses they found having to 'think on your feet' without the 'comfort blanket' of student status both a stressful and formative learning experience" (p. 269). Thinking on one's feet mandates the use of the critical thinking process. The development of critical thinking occurs over time.

Following are some specific strategies that promote the development and application of critical thinking:

- Identify goals
- Determine what knowledge is required
- Assess the margin for error
- Determine the amount of time available for decision making
- Identify available resources
- Recognize factors (i.e., biases, fatigue) that may influence decision making (Alfaro-LeFevre, 2008)

Table 5-2 on page 78 lists skills necessary for critical thinking to occur.

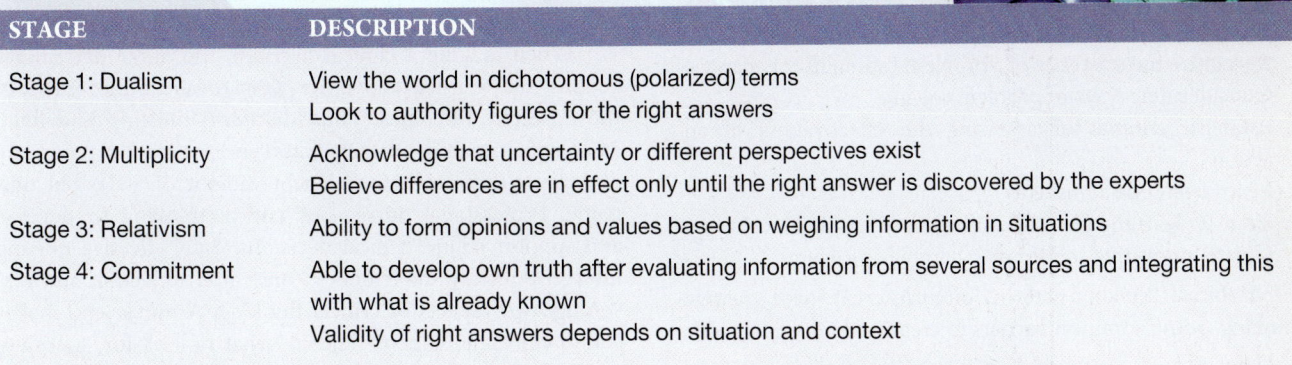

TABLE 5-1 **Stages of Cognitive Development**	
STAGE	**DESCRIPTION**
Stage 1: Dualism	View the world in dichotomous (polarized) terms Look to authority figures for the right answers
Stage 2: Multiplicity	Acknowledge that uncertainty or different perspectives exist Believe differences are in effect only until the right answer is discovered by the experts
Stage 3: Relativism	Ability to form opinions and values based on weighing information in situations
Stage 4: Commitment	Able to develop own truth after evaluating information from several sources and integrating this with what is already known Validity of right answers depends on situation and context

Data from Perry, W. G. (1970). *Forms of intellectual and ethical development in the college years*. New York: Holt, Rinehart, & Winston.

TABLE 5-2 Critical Thinking Skills

Interpretation	Categorize, decode sentences, clarify meanings
Analysis	Examine ideas, identify and analyze arguments
Influence	Query evidence, conjecture alternatives, draw conclusions
Explanation	State results, justify procedures, present arguments
Evaluation	Assess claims, assess arguments
Self-regulation	Self-examination, self-correction (if necessary)

Data from Pesut, D. J., & Herman, J. (1999). *Clinical reasoning: The art and science of critical and creative thinking.* Clifton Park, NY: Thomson Delmar Learning.

CRITICAL THINKING AND CREATIVITY

Critical thinkers are also creative thinkers. Critical and creative thinkers are those who question the status quo and search for innovative, yet practical, strategies for improvement. Those who think critically and creatively are the ones most likely to carry out research and apply the results of research studies. Creative nurses think in new ways when searching for solutions to problems. The process of creative problem solving is goal-directed thinking that leads to achievement by using new ideas or methods. The challenges presented by the current health care environment demand that nurses be creative thinkers. Critical thinking helps nurses make a smooth transition from the old to the new by facilitating analysis and planning.

Creative thinking is the foundation for individualizing client care, in that the nurse identifies the unique needs of each client and develops interventions specific to those needs. Without creative thinking, nursing care would become routine, that is, the same for every client.

There is a strong link between critical and creative thinking. In order to develop creative solutions to problems, the nurse needs to use critical intellect. Critical and creative thinkers engage in the following behaviors:

- Recognize the existence of a problem (stimulus for change)
- Consider new ways of problem solving
- Establish criteria for assessing the effectiveness of an action
- Learn from one's mistakes
- Transfer learning from one situation to another
- Create innovative solutions to complex problems

Habitual thinking patterns often interfere with creative thinking. Some common barriers to creative thinking include:

- Habit
- Comfort with the status quo
- Fear of making mistakes
- Tradition
- Use of meaningless routines and rituals
- Rigid mind-set

Groupthink, going along with the majority opinion while personally having another viewpoint, is also a major block to creativity. It takes intellectual courage to think something new and different from one's peers and then to act on those thoughts.

CRITICAL THINKING AND PROBLEM SOLVING

Critical thinking includes problem-solving and decision-making processes. With the problem-solving method, problems are identified, information is gathered, a specific problem is named, a plan for solving the problem is developed, the plan is put into action, and results of the plan are evaluated. However, this kind of problem solving is frequently based on incomplete data, and plans are sometimes based on guesses.

A formalized problem-solving approach, the nursing process, enables nurses to identify client needs and develop strategies for addressing those needs. It is a systematic and scientifically based process that requires the use of many cognitive and psychomotor skills. The following actions interfere with effective problem solving:

- Jumping too quickly to a conclusion before exploring all the aspects of a problem
- Failing to obtain critical facts, about either the problem or proposed change
- Selecting problems or changes that are too general, too complex, or poorly defined
- Failing to articulate a rational solution to the problem or proposed change
- Failing to implement and evaluate the proposal appropriately

Critical thinkers avoid such pitfalls by clearly defining the problem, analyzing the data, understanding the causes, and creating new ideas that will lead to problem resolution.

CRITICAL THINKING AND DECISION MAKING

With the rapid changes in health care and the influx of new technology, nurses must be able to use critical thinking. Decisions that provide optimal client care are the result of careful and deliberate use of critical thinking.

When making a clinical decision, the nurse determines actions that will help move the client toward achievement of the expected outcomes. Thus, **decision making** is defined as considering and selecting interventions from a repertoire of actions that facilitate the achievement of a desired outcome. Professional nurses use critical thinking to develop and support sound clinical decisions. Safe, effective nursing interventions are implemented only after reflection and reasoning, two aspects of critical thinking. A nurse who makes sound clinical judgments knows "what to look for, ... draws valid conclusions about what the signs mean, ... and knows what to do about it" (Chitty, 2007, p. 381).

Nurses exercise clinical judgment by making sound decisions; clinical judgment can be viewed as the application of critical thinking. Nursing judgments are formed after collecting assessment data, examining the relationships among those data in order to identify patterns, and taking appropriate action to address the problem(s).

Nurses make decisions every day. It is important that those decisions be the best decisions possible, that they be based on reliable information, and that they be made with as much critical thought as possible. Through a process of problem solving, one arrives at the point at which decisions can be made. The nursing process is the specific problem-solving method used by nurses to arrive at the point at which decisions about client care can be made.

THE NURSING PROCESS

The **nursing process** is the framework for providing professional, quality nursing care. It directs nursing activities for health promotion, health protection, and disease prevention and is used by nurses in every practice setting and specialty.

HISTORICAL PERSPECTIVE

Lydia Hall first referred to nursing as a "process" in a 1955 journal article, yet the term was not widely used until the late 1960s (Edelman & Mandle, 2006). Referring to the "nursing process" as a series of steps, Johnson (1959), Orlando (1961), and Wiedenbach (1963) further developed this description of nursing. Initially, the nursing process involved only three steps: assessment, planning, and evaluation. In their 1967 book *The Nursing Process,* Yura and Walsh identified four steps in the nursing process:

- Assessing
- Planning
- Implementing
- Evaluating

The *Standards of Practice,* first published in 1973 by the American Nurses Association (ANA), included eight standards. These standards identified each of the steps, including nursing diagnosis, that are now included in the nursing process.

Fry (1953) first used the term **nursing diagnosis**, but it was not until 1974, after the first meeting of the group now called the North American Nursing Diagnosis Association (NANDA), that nursing diagnosis was added as a separate and distinct step in the nursing process. Prior to this, nursing diagnosis had been included as a natural conclusion to the first step, assessment.

Following publication of the ANA standards, the nurse practice acts of many states were revised to include the steps of the nursing process specifically. The ANA made revisions to the standards in 1991 to include outcome identification as a specific part of the planning phase. Currently, the steps in the nursing process are:

- Assessment
- Diagnosis
- Outcome identification and planning
- Implementation
- Evaluation

The ANA (2004) practice standards address each step of the nursing process.

OVERVIEW OF THE NURSING PROCESS

A **process** is a series of steps or acts that leads to the accomplishment of some goal or purpose. The purpose of the nursing process is to provide care for clients that is individualized, holistic, effective, and efficient. The nursing process is not linear but involves overlapping steps that build on each other (see Figure 5-1). The steps are explained one after the other for ease of understanding. In actual practice, there may not be a definite beginning or end to each step. Work in one step may begin before work in the preceding step is completed.

The nursing process is dynamic and requires creativity for its application. The steps remain the same, but the application and results will be different in each client situation. The nursing process is designed to be used with clients throughout the life span and in any setting in which a nurse provides care. It is also a basic organizing system for the National Council Licensure Examination for Registered Nurses (NCLEX-RN).

ASSESSMENT

Assessment is the first step in the nursing process and includes collection, verification, organization, interpretation, and documentation of data. The completeness and correctness of the information obtained during assessment are directly related to the accuracy of the steps that follow. Assessment involves several steps:

- Collecting data from a variety of sources
- Validating the data
- Organizing data

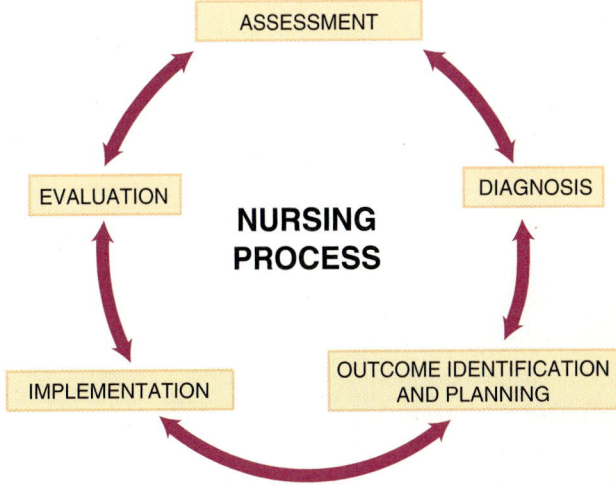

FIGURE 5-1 Components of the Nursing Process DELMAR/CENGAGE LEARNING

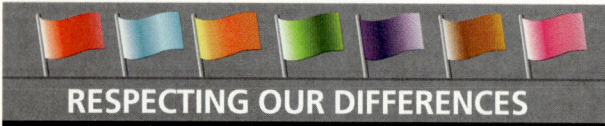

RESPECTING OUR DIFFERENCES

Cultural Influences

You are collecting data from a 35-year-old Asian American woman while her parents and older brother are in the room. Family is very important to this client, whose parents consistently interrupt her while she is answering your questions. If you ask the family to leave the room while you complete the interview, you risk offending the client and her family and creating barriers to your communication process. If you allow the family to remain in the room, the parents may influence the client's responses so that you are unable to perform an accurate assessment. How do you respect family dynamics while ensuring that the client receives the most appropriate care?

- Categorizing or identifying patterns in the data
- Making initial inferences or impressions
- Recording or reporting data

Data are collected from a variety of sources; however, the client should be considered the **primary source** of data (the major provider of information about self). As much information as possible should be gathered from the client, using both interview techniques and physical examination skills. Sources of data other than the client are considered **secondary sources** and include family members, other health care providers, and medical records. See the Respecting Our Differences feature about cultural influences.

Assessment provides information that will form the client database. Two types of information are collected through the assessment component: subjective and objective.

Subjective data are gathered by interacting with the client and include the client's feelings, perceptions, and concerns. The method of collecting subjective information is primarily the interview. Using therapeutic interviewing techniques, the nurse collects data that will be used to establish the client database. Examples of subjective information include such statements as:

- "I drink only coffee for breakfast."
- "I have had pains in my legs for three days now."

NURSING PROCESS HIGHLIGHT

Assessment

Think of all the ways you can use your senses when assessing clients. What type of information can you gather through vision, hearing, smell, and touch?

- "I go to sleep easily each night, but I wake up about two hours later and cannot go back to sleep until it is time to get up in the morning."

Objective data are observable and measurable and are obtained through physical examination and diagnostic tests. See the Nursing Process Highlight. The primary method of collecting objective information is the physical examination, which provides information about the function of body systems (see Figure 5-2). Examples of objective information include:

- T 98.6°F, P 100, R 12, BP 130/76
- Bowel sounds auscultated in all four quadrants
- Gait slow, shuffling, and unsteady

This objective information may add to or validate subjective information. Validation is a critical step in data collection to avoid omissions, prevent misunderstandings, and avoid incorrect inferences and conclusions.

Data that are collected must be organized in order to be useful to the health care professional collecting the data as well as others involved with the client's care. Clustering similar pieces of information assists the nurse in constructing a picture of the client's problems and strengths. There are a number of organizing frameworks for collection of data—for example, Gordon's functional health patterns. Many health care agencies use an admission assessment format, which assists the nurse in collecting data in specific categories of functioning.

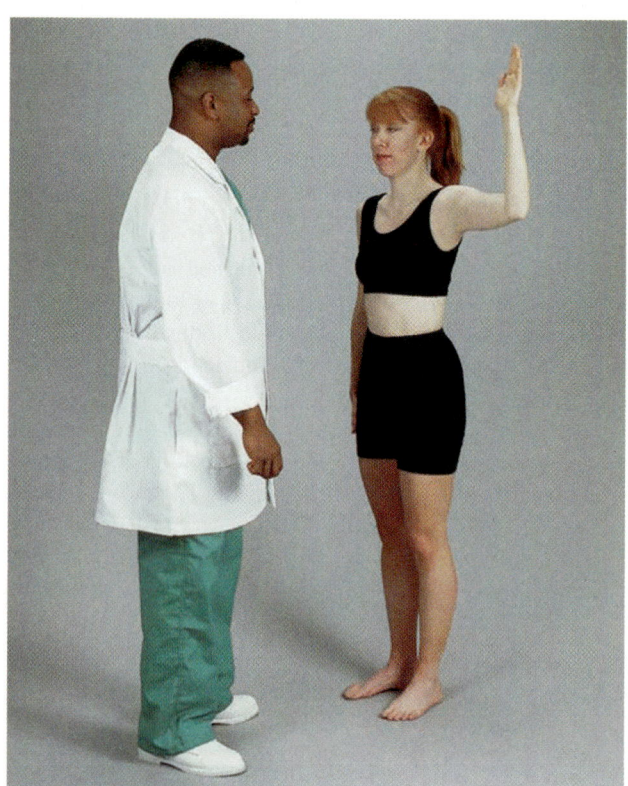

FIGURE 5-2 This nurse is gathering objective data through assessment of the client's ability to perform range-of-motion (**ROM**) activity DELMAR/CENGAGE LEARNING

Critical thinking is used in determining the significance of data collected. Once data are organized into categories, the data are clustered into groups of related pieces. Placing data into clusters helps the nurse to recognize patterns of response or behavior. When data are placed into clusters, the nurse can:

- Distinguish between relevant and irrelevant data
- Determine if and where there are gaps in the data
- Identify patterns of cause and effect

With this information, the nurse—through critical thinking—can begin to develop impressions or inferences about what the data mean.

Assessment data must be recorded and reported. The nurse makes a judgment about which data are to be reported immediately and which data need only to be recorded at that time. Data that reflect a significant deviation from the normal (e.g., rapid heart rate with irregular rhythm, severe difficulty in breathing, or high levels of anxiety) would need to be reported as well as recorded. Examples of data that need only to be recorded at the time include a report that prescribed medication has relieved a headache and a determination that an abdominal dressing is dry and intact.

Assessment does not end with the initial interview and physical examination. Assessment is dynamic and continues with each nurse-client interaction.

DIAGNOSIS

The second step in the nursing process involves further analysis (breaking the whole down into parts that can be examined) and synthesis (putting data together in a new way) of the data that have been collected. Formulation of the list of nursing diagnoses is the outcome of this process. A nursing diagnosis focuses on an individual, family, or community response to actual or potential health problems. The nursing diagnoses developed during this phase of the nursing process provide the basis for client care delivered through the remaining steps. Clients receive both medical and nursing diagnoses. Table 5-3 compares the two categories of diagnoses.

The nurse uses critical thinking and decision-making skills in developing nursing diagnoses. This process is facilitated by asking questions such as:

- Are there problems here?
- If so, what are the specific problems?
- What are some possible causes for the problems?
- Is there a situation involving risk factors?
- What are the risk factors?
- Is there a situation in which a problem can develop if preventive measures are not taken?
- Has the client indicated a desire for a higher level of wellness in a particular area of function?
- What are the client's strengths?
- What data are available to answer these questions?
- Are more data needed to answer the questions?
- If so, what are some possible sources of the data that are needed?

See the accompanying Nursing Process Highlight for a clinical example of applying critical thinking when determining nursing diagnoses.

Types of Nursing Diagnoses

Analysis of the collected data leads the nurse to make a diagnosis in one of the following categories:

- Actual problems
- Potential problems (including those where risk factors exist and there are possible problems)
- Wellness conditions
- Collaborative problems

See Table 5-4 on page 82 for examples of the various types of diagnoses.

An actual nursing diagnosis indicates that a problem exists and is composed of the diagnostic label, related factors, and signs and symptoms. An example of an actual diagnosis is impaired skin integrity related to prolonged pressure on bony prominence as manifested by (AMB) stage II pressure ulcer over coccyx, 3 cm in diameter.

A risk nursing diagnosis (potential problem) indicates that a problem does not yet exist, but special risk factors are present. A risk diagnosis is composed of the diagnostic label preceded by the phrase "risk for," with the specific risk factors listed. An example of a risk diagnosis is risk for impaired skin integrity related to inability to turn self from side to side in bed.

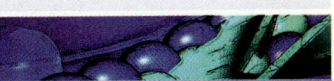

TABLE 5-3 Comparison of Medical Diagnoses and Nursing Diagnoses

MEDICAL DIAGNOSIS	NURSING DIAGNOSIS
Focuses on the illness, injury, or disease process	Focuses on the responses to actual or potential health problems or life processes
Remains constant until a cure is effected	Changes as the client's response or the health problem changes
Identifies conditions the physician is licensed and qualified to treat	Identifies situations in which the nurse is licensed and qualified to intervene

Delmar/Cengage Learning

TABLE 5-4 Types of Nursing Diagnoses

NURSING DIAGNOSIS	EXAMPLE
Actual diagnosis	*Deficient fluid volume* related to nausea and vomiting as manifested by dry skin and mucous membranes and decreased oral intake of fluids
Risk diagnosis	*Risk for infection* related to presence of invasive lines (intravenous line and indwelling bladder catheter)
Possible diagnosis	*Possible imbalanced nutrition:* less than body requirements related to insufficient oral intake
Wellness diagnosis	*Readiness for enhanced spiritual well-being*
Collaborative problem	*Potential complication* (PC): increased intracranial pressure

Delmar/Cengage Learning

A **possible nursing diagnosis** indicates a situation in which a problem could arise unless preventive action is taken. In addition, a possible diagnosis may state a "hunch" or intuition by the nurse that cannot be confirmed or elimi-nated until more data have been collected. A possible diagnosis is composed of the diagnostic label and related factors. An example of a possible diagnosis is *possible situational low self-esteem* related to recent retirement and relocation. The nurse may not yet have enough data to confirm this diagnosis or a more specific one. However, this diagnosis will alert other nurses to collect data that will either confirm this or another diagnosis, verify a risk diagnosis, or rule out the exis-tence of a problem.

A **wellness nursing diagnosis** indicates the client's expression of a desire to attain a higher level of wellness in some area of function. It is composed of the diagnostic label preceded by the phrase "readiness for enhanced." For example, a client who is neither overweight nor underweight tells the nurse that she knows she could improve her diet in some ways. She states that she eats only a small number of vegetables and fruits and thinks that the fat content of her diet is probably high. She expresses a desire to know more about how to improve her diet. The nurse would make a wellness diagnosis of *readiness for enhanced nutrition.*

Carpenito (2007) introduced the bifocal clinical practice model that includes nursing diagnoses and collaborative problems. **Collaborative problems** are defined as physio-logic complications monitored by nurses to assess changes in client status. Collaborative problems are managed through the use of interventions prescribed by other prescribing practitioners and nurses (Carpenito, 2007). Collaborative problems include those conditions in which the nurse seeks medical input for treatment of potential medical problems. Usually, collaborative problems involve alterations in organ or system function or structure (e.g., myocardial infarction, duodenal ulcer). Collaborative problems begin with the label *potential complication* (PC) followed by the situation—for example, *potential complication: hemorrhage.*

Analysis of the data also assists the nurse in identifying strengths of the client. For example, a client's supportive family would be identified as a strength. Client strengths will be reinforced and used as a basis for planning care for those areas in which functioning is less than optimal.

NURSING PROCESS HIGHLIGHT

Diagnosis

Example

Mr. Jona is a client on your unit. He is a 70-year-old widower, admitted 2 days ago with a broken left hip. While bowling with his church bowling league, Mr. Jona tripped, fell, fractured his hip, and sprained his right wrist. He has recently retired from an administrative position with a large company and moved to Florida from his home in Iowa. He has two children, who both live about 500 miles away. Mr. Jona lives alone in a one-bedroom apartment about 10 blocks from the hospital. In 2 days, Mr. Jona will be discharged and referred to the home health division for follow-up care.

Questions

1. Is he right-handed?
2. What tasks can he perform with his left hand?
3. Will there be anyone to stay with him when he gets home?
4. Who will shop for and prepare food?
5. Does he live in an upstairs apartment? If yes, is there an elevator?
6. Is there someone in his church who could help with errands and food?
7. Can his children stay with him for awhile?
8. Did you identify any other questions about Mr. Jona's situation?

After it is formulated, the list of diagnoses is presented to the client for confirmation if possible. If that is not possible, family members may be able to confirm the diagnoses. Finally, the list of nursing diagnoses is recorded in the client's record. Once this list is developed and recorded, the remainder of the client's plan of care can be completed. The list of nursing diagnoses is not static; rather, it is dynamic, changing as more data are collected, as client goals change, and as client responses to interventions are evaluated.

OUTCOME IDENTIFICATION AND PLANNING

Planning (the third step of the nursing process) involves developing a proposed course of action in regard to the client's health status. Once the nursing diagnoses have been established and client strengths have been identified, planning can begin. The planning phase involves several tasks:

- Prioritizing the list of nursing diagnoses
- Identifying and writing client-centered long- and short-term goals and outcomes
- Developing specific interventions
- Recording the plan of care

Once the list of nursing diagnoses has been developed from the data, decisions must be made about priority. Critical thinking enables the nurse to make decisions about which diagnoses are the most important and need attention first. A number of frameworks are used to prioritize nursing diagnoses; however, those diagnoses involving life-threatening situations are given the highest priority. For example, the following nursing diagnoses would be stated in this order of priority:

- *Ineffective airway clearance* related to excessive and thick secretions and pain secondary to surgery and inability to cough effectively; respirations: 25, shallow, wheezing
- *Risk for injury* (falls) related to unsteady gait
- *Imbalanced nutrition: less than body requirements* related to nausea and vomiting

Often, the words *goals* and *outcomes* are both used to describe expectations of what is to be achieved as a result of nursing actions. Goals and outcomes are measures for determining client progress.

Client-centered goals are established in collaboration with the client whenever possible. A **goal** is an aim, intent, or end. Goals are broad statements that describe the intended or desired change in the client's behavior. Goal statements refer to the diagnostic label (or problem statement) of the nursing diagnosis. If the client or significant others are unable to participate in goal development, the nurse assumes that responsibility until the client is able to participate. Client-centered goals assure that nursing care is individualized and focused on the client.

Expected outcomes are specific objectives related to the goals and are used to evaluate the nursing interventions. They must be measurable, have a time limit, and be realistic. Once goals and expected outcomes have been established,

nursing interventions are planned that enable the client to reach the goals.

Nursing Outcomes Classification (NOC) is a systematic process for organizing and evaluating expected results from nursing interventions. According to Moorhead, Johnson, Maas, and Swanson (2007), the NOC research has three aims:

- To identify and classify nursing-sensitive client outcomes
- To validate the classification system
- To use clinical data in order to measure the outcomes

Client outcomes are important in that they are the criteria for measuring the client's progress in response to nursing interventions. Because client outcomes are dynamic, the nurse uses critical thinking to reflect on status changes and to develop new interventions as necessary. There is a close relationship between nursing diagnoses and nursing outcomes; see Table 5-5.

A **nursing intervention** is the activity that the nurse will perform to promote accomplishment of the goals. Nursing interventions refer directly to the related factors in the actual nursing diagnoses and the risk factors in risk nursing diagnoses. If the nursing interventions can remove or reduce the related factors and the risk factors, the problem can be resolved or prevented. Nursing interventions also refer to the diagnostic label for possible diagnoses and focus on data needed to confirm or eliminate the diagnosis.

For each nursing diagnosis, there may be a number of nursing interventions. Nursing interventions are individualized and are stated in specific terms. Examples of nursing interventions are:

- Turn, cough, and deep breathe twice an hour beginning at 0800, 2/10.
- Teach "nipple care when breastfeeding" at 1000, 2/11.
- Weigh client at each visit.

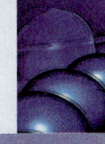

TABLE 5-5 NOC: Nursing Diagnoses and Nursing Outcomes, a Comparison

NANDA DIAGNOSIS	NOC OUTCOME
Constipation	Bowel continence
Diarrhea	Bowel elimination
Family Processes, Interrupted	Family functioning Family coping
Hopelessness	Hope
Deficient Knowledge	Knowledge: disease process Knowledge: medication

Delmar/Cengage Learning

Once the interventions have been determined for each diagnosis, the interventions are recorded on the client's plan of care. As is true with other steps in the nursing process, the list of interventions is not static. Interventions may change as the nurse interacts with the client, assesses responses to interventions, and evaluates those responses. Critical thinking is essential in every step of the nursing process, especially in developing client outcomes and relevant intervention strategies.

IMPLEMENTATION

The fourth step in the nursing process is implementation. **Implementation** involves the execution of the nursing plan of care derived during the planning phase. It consists of performing nursing activities that have been planned to meet client outcomes. Nurses may delegate some of the nursing interventions to other persons assigned to care for the client—for example, licensed practical nurses and unlicensed assistive personnel.

In 1996, the Iowa Intervention Project team developed the Nursing Interventions Classification (NIC), which is a system for organizing nursing actions using standardized language. Priority interventions are identified for selected nursing outcomes. These priority interventions "are the most obvious interventions to effect problem resolution, but this does not mean that they are the only interventions to be used. A variety of interventions should always be considered" (Wilkinson, 2006, p. xvii). Critical thinking enables the nurse to decide which interventions are most appropriate and therefore individualize client care.

Implementation involves many skills. The nurse must continue to assess the client's condition before, during, and after the interventions. Assessment prior to the intervention provides the nurse with baseline data. Assessment during and after the intervention allows the nurse to detect positive or negative client responses. If negative responses occur during the procedure, the nurse must take appropriate action. If positive responses occur, the nurse adds this information to the database for use in evaluating the efficacy of the intervention. See the Uncovering the Evidence box for an example.

The nurse must also possess psychomotor skills, interpersonal skills, and critical thinking skills in order to perform the nursing interventions that have been planned. The nurse uses psychomotor skills when performing procedures such as giving injections, changing dressings, and helping the client perform range-of-motion (ROM) exercises. Interpersonal skills are necessary as the nurse interacts with the client and the family to collect data, provide information in teaching sessions, and offer support in times of anxiety. Critical thinking skills enable the nurse to think through the situation, ask the appropriate questions, and make decisions about what needs to be done.

The implementation step also involves reporting and documentation. Data to be recorded include the client condition prior to the intervention, the specific intervention

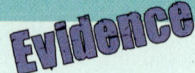

UNCOVERING THE Evidence

TITLE OF STUDY
"Nurses' Reported Thinking during Medication Administration"

AUTHORS
L. A. Eisenhauer, A. C. Hurley, and N. Dolan

PURPOSE
To document nurses' self-reported thinking processes during medication administration.

METHODS
Semistructured interviews and tape recordings were used to document the types of thinking processes used by nurses practicing in inpatient units.

FINDINGS
Content analysis led to identification of 10 types of thinking used by nurses. Situations requiring judgment about dosage, timing, or selection of specific medications gave the most definitive data about nurses' use of critical thinking and clinical judgment. A major theme identified was nurses' vigilance to ensure that appropriate medications were administered.

IMPLICATIONS
Nurses' thinking extended beyond mere considerations of policies, rules, and regulations. The thinking processes were based on professional knowledge and consideration of client data. Identification of thinking processes can help nurses explain the complex expertise required for safe medication administration.

Eisenhauer, L. A., Hurley, A. C., & Dolan, N. (2007). Nurses' reported thinking during medication administration. *Journal of Nursing Scholarship, 39*(1), 83–87.

performed, the client response to the intervention, and client outcomes. Critical thinking is essential for complete, accurate documentation to occur. Nurses must reflect on the care that was planned, consider the interventions performed, and evaluate the client's response to those interventions. Thorough documentation shows client progress in response to nursing interventions.

EVALUATION

Evaluation, the fifth step in the nursing process, involves determining whether client goals have been met, partially met, or not met. If the goal has been met, the nurse must

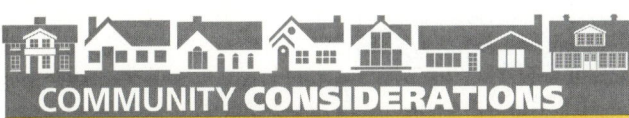

COMMUNITY CONSIDERATIONS

Priorities and Referrals

Mrs. Mendosa delivered a baby with congenital defects yesterday and is being discharged later today. You are responsible for her discharge planning, which includes the need for education about how to feed her infant. The baby is expected to be discharged in approximately 2 to 3 weeks. Think of the priority needs of Mrs. Mendosa. What follow-up care will be necessary for her and the infant? Which community agencies are available to provide support for both mother and child?

then decide whether nursing activities will cease or continue in order for the client's status to be maintained.

If the goal has been partially met or not been met, the nurse must reassess the situation. Data are collected to determine why the goal has not been achieved and what modifications to the plan of care are necessary. There are a number of possible reasons that goals are not met or are only partially met, including:

- The initial assessment data were incomplete.
- The goals and expected outcomes were unrealistic.
- The time frame was too optimistic.
- The goals and nursing interventions planned were not appropriate for the specific client.

Evaluation is an ongoing process. Nurses continually evaluate data in order to make informed decisions during other phases of the nursing process. Critical thinking promotes evaluation by helping nurses look at the overall picture in order to determine client status. Evaluation is an essential component of discharge planning that allows the nurse to work with clients and families in deciding whether further health care is needed and then providing necessary referrals; see the accompanying Community Considerations display.

CRITICAL THINKING APPLIED IN NURSING

Critical thinking is a skill that can be learned just as other skills are learned. The skill of critical thinking is important and useful in all aspects of a person's life. However, it is a vital tool for the nurse. Critical thinkers develop a questioning attitude and delve into situations in order to seek possible explanations for what is happening. See the Nursing

✓ NURSING CHECKLIST

Examples of Critical Thinking Questions for Use with the Nursing Process

- **ASSESSMENT**

Are the data complete? What other data do I need? What are some possible sources of those data? What assumptions or biases do I have in this situation? What is the client's point of view? Are there other points of view?

- **DIAGNOSIS**

What do these data mean? What else could be happening? Are there any gaps in the data? How are these data similar and how are they different? What assumptions or biases do I have in this situation? Have my assumptions affected my interpretation of the data? If so, in what way?

- **OUTCOME IDENTIFICATION AND PLANNING**

What are the goals for this client? What do I want to accomplish? How are my goals related to what the client wants to accomplish? What are the expected outcomes for this client? What interventions are to be used? Who is the best-qualified person to perform these interventions? How much involvement can the client and family or significant others have at this time? How much involvement does the client wish to have at this time?

- **IMPLEMENTATION**

What is the client's current status? What are the most critical steps in this intervention? How must I alter the intervention to best meet this client's needs and maintain principles of safety? What is the client's response during and after the intervention? Is there a need to alter the intervention in any way? If so, why and how?

- **EVALUATION**

Were the interventions successful in assisting the client to achieve the desired goals? How could things have been done differently? What data do I need to make new decisions? Where will I get the data? Were there assumptions, biases, or points of view that I missed that affected the outcomes? What can be done about these assumptions, biases, or points of view?

Checklist for examples of questions the nurse as a critical thinker might ask at each step in the nursing process. Table 5-6 on page 86 provides examples of how critical thinking is used in each phase of the nursing process.

TABLE 5-6 Application of Critical Thinking to the Nursing Process

ASSESSMENT	DIAGNOSIS	OUTCOME IDENTIFICATION AND PLANNING	IMPLEMENTATION	EVALUATION
• Gather pertinent data • Interpret data • Keep an open mind by questioning assumptions about data • Think about what information to collect • Determine the significance of data • Make conclusions based on the data	• Develop well-thought-out conclusions • Seek reasons and principles that justify nursing judgments • Test conclusions against criteria • Suspend judgment when data are insufficient • Differentiate essential and trivial data	• Explore alternative actions • Collaborate with others • Examine assumptions • Reframe problems in order to generate solutions • Generate ideas and possible solutions	• Communicate with others to solve complex problems • Accurately report data and clues • Base action on sound rationale	• Establish standards (criteria) based on logic rather than assumptions • Analyze course of action • Critique outcomes • Evaluate the soundness of conclusions

Delmar/Cengage Learning

KEY CONCEPTS

- Critical thinking, problem-solving, and decision-making skills are essential in nursing.
- Critical thinkers ask questions, evaluate evidence, identify assumptions, examine alternatives, and seek to understand various points of view.
- The nursing process is an organized method of planning and delivering nursing care.
- The nursing process is composed of five steps: assessment, diagnosis, outcome identification and planning, implementation, and evaluation.
- Assessment is the first step in the nursing process and involves collecting, validating, organizing, categorizing, and recording data.

- The second step in the nursing process involves further analysis and synthesis of the data and results in a list of nursing diagnoses.
- Planning, the third step in the nursing process, involves prioritizing nursing diagnoses, identifying and writing goals and client outcomes, developing nursing interventions, and recording the plan of care in the client's record.
- Implementation, the fourth step in the nursing process, involves performing or delegating nursing activities.
- Evaluation, the fifth step in the nursing process, involves deciding whether the client goals have been met, been partially met, or not been met.

REVIEW QUESTIONS

1. When reviewing a client's lab results, the nurse must have a knowledge base that includes which of the following types of knowledge in order to think critically?
   a. Affective
   b. Declarative
   c. Nonjudgmental
   d. Psychomotor

2. Which of the following phrases accurately describes the nursing process? Select all that apply.
   a. Applicable to every setting
   b. Can be implemented by unlicensed personnel
   c. Framework for licensure examination
   d. Is a linear process
   e. Organized care delivery framework
   f. Used with adults only

3. The nurse uses creative thinking in order to
   a. Express his or her own artistic tendencies
   b. Individualize care
   c. Liven up the work environment
   d. Please clients and families
4. Which of the following is an example of objective client data?
   a. 500 mL of amber-colored urine in collection bag
   b. Client complaint of nausea
   c. Client states pain is 9 on a scale of 1–10
   d. Self-report of insomnia
5. A client in the intensive care unit (ICU) has several health problems. Which of the following nursing diagnoses should be of priority concern to the nurse?
   a. Imbalanced nutrition: less than body requirements
   b. Impaired skin integrity
   c. Ineffective airway clearance
   d. Risk for injury (falls)
6. When referring to a client's medical record for information, the nurse is using which data source?
   a. Analytical
   b. Primary
   c. Secondary
   d. Tertiary

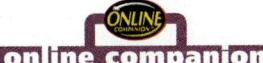

online companion

Visit the DeLaune and Ladner online companion resource at **www.delmar.cengage.com** for additional content and study aids. Click on Online Companions, then select the Nursing discipline.

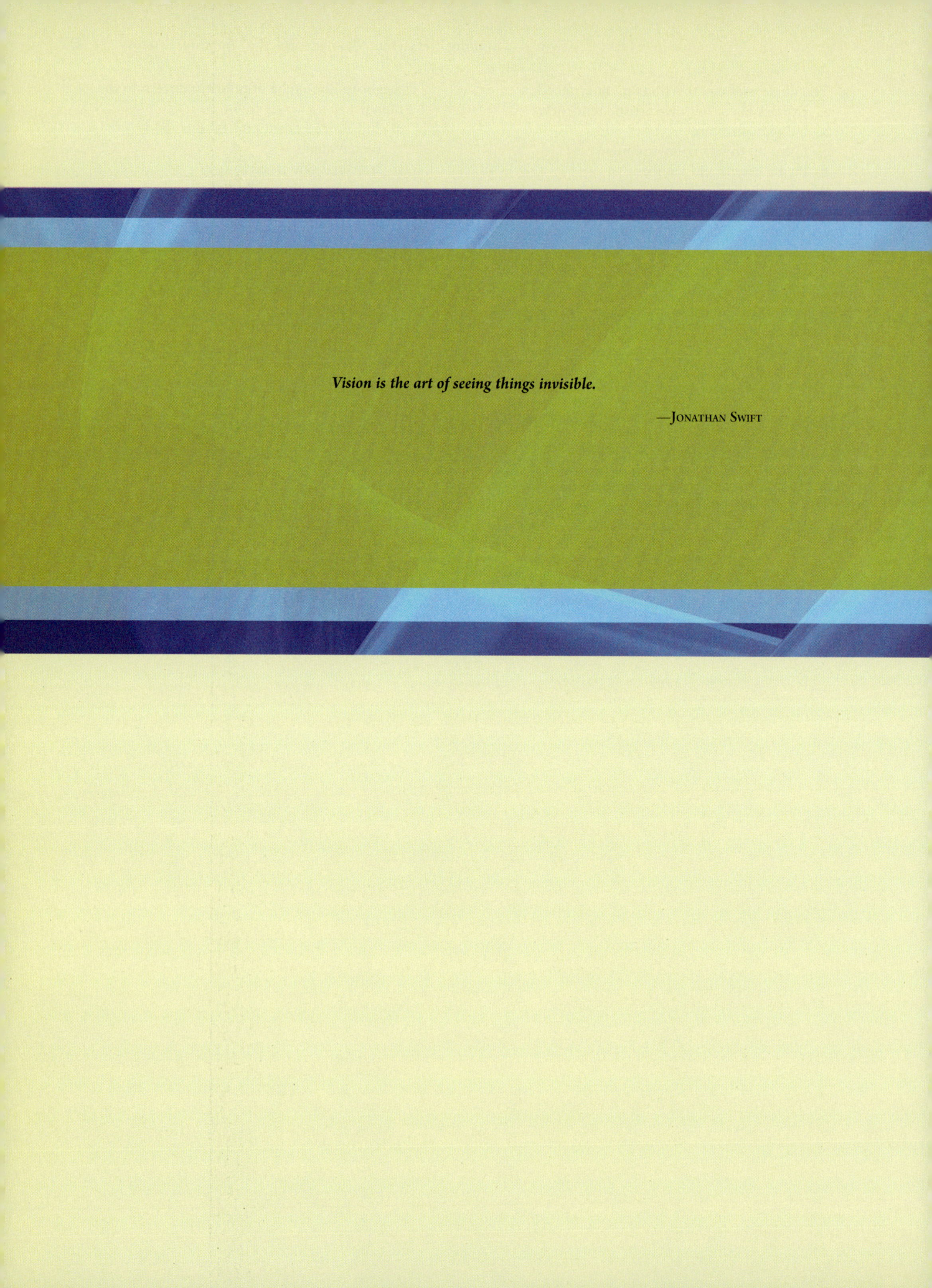

Vision is the art of seeing things invisible.

—Jonathan Swift

CHAPTER 6

Assessment

COMPETENCIES

1. Identify major purposes of data collection.
2. Describe three types of assessment.
3. Differentiate subjective and objective data.
4. Identify examples of nursing and nonnursing models used in collecting and organizing data.
5. Describe five methods involved in data collection.
6. Explain the stages of the assessment interview.
7. Outline the elements of the health history and their importance.
8. Describe the purposes of the physical assessment.
9. Discuss assessment techniques used in the physical examination.
10. Discuss the use of data clustering in organizing the information obtained about the client.
11. Identify four types of assessment formats.

KEY TERMS

assessment	data verification	ongoing assessment
assessment model	focused assessment	open-ended questions
auscultation	health history	palpation
closed questions	inspection	percussion
comprehensive assessment	interview	review of systems
data clustering	objective data	subjective data
data interpretation	observation	

Assessment is the first step in the nursing process and includes systematic collection, verification, organization, interpretation, and documentation of data for use by health care professionals. Effective planning of client care depends on a complete database and accurate interpretation of information. Incomplete or inadequate assessment may result in inaccurate conclusions and incorrect nursing interventions. Proper collection of assessment data guides the decision-making activities of professional nurses.

Assessment is the collection and analysis of data that are used in formulating nursing diagnoses, identifying outcomes and planning care, and developing nursing interventions. This chapter discusses the purpose of assessment, types of assessment, and the use of data in the assessment process.

PURPOSE OF ASSESSMENT

The purpose of assessment is to establish a database concerning a client's physical, psychosocial, and emotional health in order to identify health-promoting behaviors as well as actual and potential health problems. Through assessment, the nurse determines the client's functional abilities and the absence or presence of dysfunction. The client's normal routine for activities of daily living and lifestyle patterns are also assessed. Identification of the client's strengths provides the nurse and other members of the treatment team with information about the skills, abilities, and behaviors the client has available to promote the treatment and recovery process. Some examples of client strengths are family support, intelligence, spiritual beliefs, and coping skills (how previous problems have been solved). The assessment phase also offers an opportunity for the nurse to form a therapeutic interpersonal relationship with the client. During assessment, the client is provided an opportunity to discuss health care concerns and goals with the nurse. The essential elements of the assessment process are:

- Data collection
- Data verification
- Data organization
- Data interpretation
- Data documentation

Assessment, like all other phases of the nursing process, is client-centered.

TYPES OF ASSESSMENT

The type and scope of information needed for assessment are usually determined by the health care setting and needs of the client (see Figure 6-1). Three types of assessment are comprehensive, focused, and ongoing. Although a comprehensive assessment is most desirable in initially determining a client's need for nursing care, time limitations or special circumstances may dictate the need for abbreviated data collection, as represented by the focused assessment. The assessment database can then be expanded after the initial focused assessment, and data should be updated through the ongoing assessment process.

COMPREHENSIVE ASSESSMENT

A comprehensive assessment is usually performed upon admission to a health care agency and includes a complete health history to determine current needs of the client. This database provides a baseline against which changes in the client's health status can be measured and should include assessment of physical and psychosocial aspects of the client's health, the client's perception of health, the presence of health risk factors, and the client's coping patterns.

FOCUSED ASSESSMENT

A focused assessment is an assessment that is limited in scope in order to focus on a particular need or health care

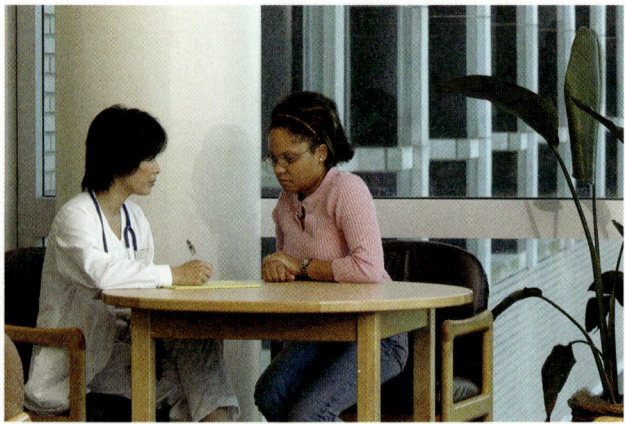

FIGURE 6-1 In this focused assessment, the nurse is collecting data about the client prior to elective surgery DELMAR/CENGAGE LEARNING

problem or potential health care risks. Focused assessments are not as detailed as comprehensive assessments and are often used in health care agencies in which short stays are anticipated (e.g., outpatient surgery centers and emergency departments), in specialty areas such as labor and delivery, and in mental health settings or for purposes of screening for specific problems or risk factors (e.g., well-child clinics). For example, the following is a list of sample questions used to assess a client experiencing labor:

- When did your contractions begin?
- How far apart are the contractions?
- Are they getting stronger?
- When did your water break?

ONGOING ASSESSMENT

Systematic follow-up is required when problems are identified during a comprehensive or focused assessment. An **ongoing assessment** is an assessment that includes systematic monitoring and observation related to specific problems. This type of assessment allows the nurse to broaden the database or to confirm the validity of the data obtained during the initial assessment. Ongoing assessment is particularly important when problems have been identified and a plan of care has been implemented to address these problems. Systematic monitoring and observation allow the nurse to determine client response to nursing interventions and to identify any emerging problems.

The nurse delivering care to a client at home uses ongoing assessment. Use of specific questions will be most helpful in eliciting specific information; see the accompanying Community Considerations box.

DATA COLLECTION

The nurse must possess strong critical thinking, interpersonal, and technical skills in order to elicit appropriate information and make relevant observations during the data collection process. This process often begins prior to initial contact between the nurse and the client, primarily through the nurse's review of biographical data and medical records. Upon meeting the client, the nurse continues data collection through interview, observation, and examination. A variety of sources and methods are used in compiling a comprehensive database.

TYPES OF DATA

Client data include information that clients communicate about perceptions of their own health status as well as specific observations made by the nurse. These two types of information are referred to as subjective and objective data. **Subjective data** are data from the client's point of view and include feelings, perceptions, and concerns. These data (also referred to as symptoms) are obtained through interviews with the client. They are called subjective because they rely on the feelings or opinions of the person experiencing them and cannot be readily observed by another.

Objective data are measurable data that are obtained through observation, standard assessment techniques performed during the physical examination, and laboratory and diagnostic testing. These data (also called signs) can be seen, heard, or felt by someone other than the person experiencing them. Assessments that are comprehensive and accurate include both subjective and objective data. See Table 6-1 on page 92 for examples of both types of data.

SOURCES OF DATA

A comprehensive database should consist of data from every possible source, including:

- Client
- Family and significant other
- Other health care professionals
- Medical records
- Interdisciplinary conferences, rounds, and consultations
- Results of diagnostic tests
- Relevant literature

The client should always be considered the primary source of information; however, other sources should not be overlooked. The client's family and significant others can also provide useful information, especially if the client is unable to verbalize information. In addition, other health care professionals who have cared for the client may contribute valuable information. Medical records, including the medical history and physical examination, should also be reviewed; results of laboratory and diagnostic tests and various health care professionals should also be consulted.

Pertinent literature should be investigated in order to pursue relevant information and plan appropriate nursing interventions. Written standards are valuable sources of data for comparison, for example, a standard table of infant growth to determine whether an infant's weight and height are within the normal growth range. Another valuable source of data is knowledge about the client's normal parameters of functioning. The nurse's knowledge based on experience is another important source of data.

COMMUNITY CONSIDERATIONS

Assessing Clients at Home

- What led up to your most recent hospitalization?
- What medications were prescribed for you during that time?
- What kind of diet were you on?
- What type of activities did you do while you were in the hospital?
- While in the hospital, what did you learn about … ?
- What adaptations for your comfort and care have you and your family made since your return home?

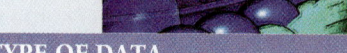

TABLE 6-1 Sample Application: Types of Data

DATA	TYPE OF DATA
Charlene Rhodes, age 47, has come to the clinic after "passing out" twice in the last 2 days. She tells the nurse that she becomes "lightheaded" after almost any type of activity. She has experienced some nausea since yesterday and vomited after eating breakfast this morning. She also tells the nurse that she is very nervous about these occurrences because she remembers her mother having similar symptoms when the mother suffered from a brain disorder. The nurse observes that the client's gait is unsteady and her skin is pale. The client also has large bruises on her right arm and the right side of her face, which she states occurred when she fell.	**Subjective** Report of fainting Complaint of dizziness Nausea Verbalization of anxiety Self-reported fall **Objective** Vomiting Unsteady gait Pale skin Bruises on right side of face and right arm

Delmar/Cengage Learning

METHODS OF DATA COLLECTION

The nurse collects information through the following methods: observation, interview, health history, symptom analysis, physical examination, and laboratory and diagnostic data. These approaches require systematic use of the assessment skills discussed in the following text.

Observation

The nurse uses the skill of observation to carefully and attentively note the general appearance and behavior of the client. These observations occur whenever there is contact with the client and include factors such as client mood, interactions with others, physical and emotional responses, and any safety considerations. Observation helps the nurse determine the client's status, both physical and mental. By carefully watching the client, the nurse can detect nonverbal cues that indicate a variety of feelings, including presence of pain, anxiety, and anger. Observational skills are essential in detecting the early warning signs of physical changes (e.g., pallor and sweating).

NURSING PROCESS HIGHLIGHT

Assessment

Sources of Data

Mrs. Palmer, age 76, was admitted to the hospital following a stroke. She is responsive but unable to speak or move extremities on the right side. Her daughter, who lives next door, is present at the bedside. What would be the best source of data in this situation?

Interview

An interview is a therapeutic interaction that has a specific purpose. The nurse interviews for a variety of reasons throughout the nurse-client relationship, including data collection, teaching, exploration of the client's feelings or concerns, and provision of support. Effective interviewing depends on the nurse's knowledge and ability to skillfully elicit information from the client using appropriate techniques of communication. Observation of nonverbal behavior during the interview is also essential to effective data collection.

INTERVIEW PREPARATION   The interview is more productive if the nurse has an opportunity to prepare for the interaction. Such preparation includes review of the client's medical records, conversations with other health care team members (e.g., personnel in emergency departments or long-term care facilities), and research of the presenting medical diagnosis. This information can be useful in obtaining the client's relevant history and formulating a current needs assessment.

INTERVIEW STAGES   Since the assessment interview often occurs at the beginning of a nurse-client relationship, it is helpful to begin the process with an orientation phase. During this period introductions are made, rapport is established, and roles are defined. The first few minutes of the nurse-client meeting may give an indication of the type of interviewing needed, so it is important that the nurse employ active listening skills. There are three phases to an interview: introduction, working, and closure.

Introduction Stage.   The introduction stage of the interview establishes the goals for the interaction. The primary goal of the assessment interview is the collection of data about the client. In this phase of the interview, the purpose and use of the data collection should be discussed. For example, the nurse might state, "I need to talk to you for a few minutes about your health so that we can better plan your care." Adequate time and privacy should be allowed for the interview so that the client feels free to share any information that may be relevant. The parameters of confidentiality must be clearly explained to the client; see Chapter 12 for more information on confidentiality. The nurse should also inform the client about the approximate duration of the interview.

The client is more likely to respond freely if the interview environment provides comfort and privacy and if rapport exists between the client and the nurse. The nurse should sit (if possible), establish eye contact with the client, and listen attentively. It is the nurse's responsibility to note nonverbal messages that may indicate that the client is uncomfortable, tired, or preoccupied with other matters. If any of these situations occur, it might be necessary to complete the interview at a later time. For example, if the client is guarding an incision and verbalizing discomfort or is extremely anxious about an impending procedure, only essential data are collected and the comprehensive interview is postponed until immediate needs have been met.

Working Stage. The working stage of the interview focuses on the details of data collection. The scope of the assessment interview depends on the type of assessment to be conducted (e.g., comprehensive or focused). The interview may be structured and formal (used in situations when a large amount of information needs to be obtained) or unstructured and informal (used in interactions that focus on a specific area of concern to the client). The nurse should be familiar with the specific assessment format used by the health care agency so that attention can be focused toward the client rather than the form itself.

The interview generally begins with questions about biographical and other nonthreatening information. The client's reason for seeking health care is also addressed early in the working phase. Information is usually gathered from the general to the specific, with details about intimate or potentially embarrassing topics reserved until later in the interview. The Nursing Checklist provides guidelines for interview preparation.

Techniques used during the interview will be determined by the setting and purpose of the interview. A comprehensive interview that seeks to identify problems and concerns is facilitated by open-ended questions, while an interview that focuses on specific details about a presenting problem will be facilitated by direct, closed questions. For example, an emergency setting would likely employ more direct, closed questions, while admission to a long-term care facility might require greater use of open-ended questions.

Closed questions are questions that can be answered briefly or with one-word responses. For example, the question "Have you been in the hospital before?" is a closed question that can easily be answered by a one-word response. Questions about the dates of and reasons for the hospitalizations are also closed questions that require brief answers.

Open-ended questions are questions that encourage the client to elaborate about a particular concern or problem. For example, the question "What led to your coming here today?" is open-ended and allows the client flexibility in response. Both closed and open-ended questions can be effective in collecting information; see the accompanying Nursing Process Highlight.

Closure Stage. Closure is established in the introduction phase when approximate time parameters are set. As the interview session is concluding, the nurse should indicate this fact by stating that almost all the information needed has been obtained or that the time for the interview is almost over. This action allows the client an opportunity to present any other relevant information, and it avoids surprises when the interview terminates. During the closure phase, the nurse summarizes what was covered or accomplished during the interview and requests validation of perceptions with the client. If the nurse or the client feels that additional time is needed for further exploration of specific points discussed during this session, plans can be made for future interviews.

Health History

A primary focus of the data collection interview is the health history. The **health history** is a review of the client's functional health patterns prior to the current contact with a health care agency. While the medical history concentrates on symptoms and the progression of disease, the nursing health history focuses on the client's functional health patterns, responses to changes in health status, and alterations in lifestyle. The health history is also used in developing the

---

✅ NURSING CHECKLIST

Preparing the Interview Environment

- Ensure adequate lighting.
- Maintain a comfortable room temperature.
- Select an environment that is as free of noise and distractions as possible.
- Maintain client privacy.
- Make sure that the interview is timed appropriately.
- Promote client comfort.

NURSING PROCESS HIGHLIGHT

Assessment

Interview Techniques: Questioning

Which questions—closed or open-ended—do you think will extract the most useful and complete information from the client? Under which circumstances would each type of question be best used?

plan of care and formulating nursing interventions. Following are elements of the health history:

- Demographic information
- Reason for seeking health care
- Client perception of health status
- Previous illnesses, hospitalizations, surgeries
- Client and family medical history
- Immunizations and exposure to communicable disease
- Allergies
- Current medications
- Developmental level
- Psychosocial history
- Sociocultural history
- Activities of daily living
- Review of systems

DEMOGRAPHIC INFORMATION Personal data include name, address, date of birth, gender, religion, race and ethnic origin, and occupation. This information may be useful in helping to foster understanding of a client's perspective.

REASON FOR SEEKING HEALTH CARE The client's reason for seeking health care should be described in the client's own words. For example, the statement "fell off four-foot ladder and landed on right shoulder; unable to move right arm" is the client's actual report of the event that precipitated the need for health care. The client's perspective is important because it explains what is significant about the event from the client's point of view. It is also important to determine the time of the onset of symptoms as well as a complete symptom analysis.

CLIENT PERCEPTION OF HEALTH STATUS Perception of health status refers to clients' opinions of their general health. It may be useful to ask clients to rate their health on a scale of 1 to 10 (with 10 being ideal and 1 being poor), together with the clients' rationales for their rating scores. For example, the nurse may record a statement such as the following to represent the client's perception of health: "Rates health a 7 on a scale of 1 (poor) to 10 (ideal) because he must take medication regularly in order to maintain mobility, but the medication sometimes upsets his stomach."

PREVIOUS ILLNESSES, HOSPITALIZATIONS, AND SURGERIES The history and timing of any previous experiences with illness, surgery, or hospitalization are helpful in order to assess recurrent conditions. It is also helpful to anticipate responses to illness, since prior experiences often have an impact on current responses.

CLIENT AND FAMILY MEDICAL HISTORY The nurse needs to determine any family history of acute and chronic illnesses that tend to be familial. Health history forms will frequently include checklists of various illnesses that can be used as the basis of the questions about this aspect. The client should be instructed that family history refers to blood relatives. It is also helpful to indicate *who* the relative is in relation to the client (e.g., mother, father, sister).

IMMUNIZATIONS AND EXPOSURE TO COMMUNICABLE DISEASE Any history of childhood or other communicable diseases should be noted. In addition, a record of current immunizations should be obtained. This is particularly important with children; however, records of immunizations for tetanus, influenza, and hepatitis B can also be important for adults. If the client has traveled out of the country, the time frame should be indicated in order to determine incubation periods for relevant diseases. The client should also be asked about potential exposure to communicable diseases, such as tuberculosis.

ALLERGIES Any drug, food, or environmental allergies should be noted in the health history. In addition to the name of the allergen, the type of reaction to the substance should be noted. For example, a client may report developing a rash or becoming short of breath. This reaction should be recorded. Clients may report an "allergy" to a medication because they developed nausea after ingesting it, which the nurse will recognize as a side effect that would not necessarily preclude administration of the drug in the future. A client's sensitivity to a drug can also change over time. Severe reactions may occur even though the client has successfully taken the drug or experienced only mild reactions to the drug in the past.

CURRENT MEDICATIONS All medications currently taken, both prescription and over the counter, are to be recorded by name, frequency, and dosage. Remind clients that this information should include medications such as birth control pills, laxatives, and nonprescription pain relief medications. Ask which, if any, herbal preparations the client uses. Patterns related to caffeine and alcohol intake and use of tobacco or recreational drugs should also be explored. Use of alternative or complementary treatment methods, including herbals, is often not shared by health care consumers. Some clients fear rejection or ridicule when divulging such information to health care providers. The nurse uses a sensitive, nonjudgmental approach when assessing the client's use of all healing practices.

DEVELOPMENTAL LEVEL Knowledge of developmental level is essential for considering appropriate norms of behavior and for appraising the achievement of relevant developmental tasks. Any recognized theory of growth and development can

▼ **SAFETY FIRST** ▼

ASSESSMENT FOR ALLERGIES
It is essential that the nurse explore possible allergies prior to administering any medications. Allergic reactions can be life threatening and can occur even with very low dosages of medications.

be applied in order to determine whether clients are functioning within the parameters expected for their age group. For example, if the nurse uses Erikson's stages of psychosocial development, evaluation of an adult client attaining the developmental task of generativity versus stagnation can be validated by a nurse's statement such as "client prefers to spend time with his family; very involved in children's school activities."

PSYCHOSOCIAL HISTORY Psychosocial history refers to assessment of dimensions such as self-concept and self-esteem as well as usual sources of stress and the client's ability to cope (see Chapter 23). Sources of support for clients in crisis (such as family, significant others, religion, or support groups) should be explored.

SOCIOCULTURAL HISTORY In exploring the client's sociocultural history, it is important to inquire about the home environment, family situation, and client's role in the family. For example, the client could be the parent of three children and the sole provider in a single-parent family. The responsibilities of the client are important data by which the nurse can determine the impact of changes in health status and thus plan the most beneficial care for the client.

ACTIVITIES OF DAILY LIVING The activities of daily living are a description of the client's lifestyle and capacity for self-care. This information is useful both as baseline information and as a source of insight into usual health behaviors. This database should include the following areas:

- *Nutrition:* Includes type of diet, foods eaten, and fluids consumed regularly; food preparation; the size of portions; and the number of meals per day. Food preferences and dislikes, as well as the client's need for assistance in food preparation or eating, should also be determined.
- *Elimination:* Includes both urinary and bowel elimination frequency and patterns. Any recent changes or problems in these patterns should be noted.
- *Rest and sleep:* Includes the usual number of hours of sleep, number of hours of sleep needed to feel rested, sleep aids used, and the time within the day or night when sleep usually occurs. Any bedtime rituals (especially with children) should also be noted.
- *Activity and exercise:* Includes types and patterns of exercise in a typical day or week. If assistance is needed with activities such as walking, standing, or meeting hygienic needs, this information should be noted.

REVIEW OF SYSTEMS The **review of systems** (ROS) is a brief account from the client of recent signs or symptoms associated with any of the body systems. This allows the client an opportunity to communicate any deviations from normal that have not been otherwise identified. The ROS relies on subjective information provided by the client rather than data from the physical examination. When a symptom is encountered, either while eliciting the health history or during the physical examination, the nurse should obtain as much information as possible about the symptom. Relevant data include:

- *Location:* The area of the body in which the symptom (such as pain) can either be pointed to or described in detail.
- *Character:* The quality of the feeling or sensation (e.g., sharp, dull, stabbing).
- *Intensity:* The severity or quantity of the feeling or sensation and its interference with functional abilities. The sensation can be rated on a scale of 1 (very little) to 10 (very intense).
- *Timing:* The onset, duration, frequency, and precipitating factors of the symptom.
- *Aggravating and alleviating factors:* The activities or actions that make the symptom worse or better.

Physical Examination

The purpose of the physical examination is to make direct observations of any deviations from normal and to validate subjective data gathered through the interview. Baseline measurements are obtained, and physical examination techniques are used to gather objective data.

BASELINE DATA Baseline data collection is the systematic organization of observations obtained during the physical examination. The baseline becomes the basis for comparison and evaluation to establish the status of a client at a given point in time. Measurement of height, weight, and vital signs (temperature, pulse, respirations, and blood pressure) is important for comparison with future measurements in order to judge the significance of any changes (progress or regression) over time.

ASSESSMENT TECHNIQUES The physical examination incorporates the use of visual, auditory, tactile, and olfactory senses and the use of systematic assessment techniques. The use of visual, auditory, and tactile senses will be described with each of the specific assessment techniques. In addition, olfaction (sense of smell) is helpful in detecting characteristic odors as well as those associated with altered health states. For example, presence of infection is sometimes first detected by a change in the characteristic odor of body fluids or drainage. The four assessment techniques used in physical examination are inspection, palpation, percussion, and auscultation.

Inspection. **Inspection** involves careful visual observation. The client is observed first from a general point of view and then with specific attention to detail. For example, the nurse first observes for patterns of skin lesions and then focuses on the specific characteristics of individual lesions. Instruments such as a penlight and otoscope are often used to enhance visualization. Effective inspection requires adequate lighting and exposure of the body parts being observed. Beginning nurses often feel self-conscious or embarrassed using the technique of inspection; however, most become comfortable with the technique over time. Nurses must also be sensitive to the client's feelings of embarrassment with the use of inspection and respond to this situation by discussing the technique with the client and using measures, such as draping for privacy, in order to increase the client's comfort level.

Palpation. **Palpation** uses the sense of touch to assess texture, temperature, moisture, organ location and size, vibrations and pulsations, edema, masses, and tenderness. Palpation requires a calm, gentle approach and is used systematically, with light palpation preceding deep palpation and palpation of tender areas performed last.

The technique of palpation uses the hands and fingers in different ways for assessment of:

- *Temperature:* Best detected using the dorsal (back) surface of the hand
- *Texture, pulses, and edema:* Best detected using fingertips
- *Vibration:* Best detected with the base of the fingers
- *Shape and consistency of organs or masses:* Best detected by grasping organ or mass between fingertips

▼ SAFETY FIRST ▼

PALPATION
Deep palpation is a technique requiring expertise and should not be employed by beginning nursing students without supervision.

Percussion. **Percussion** uses short, tapping strokes on the surface of the skin to create vibrations of underlying organs. It is used for assessing the density of structures or determining the location and the size of organs in the body. Structures with relatively more air (such as the lungs) produce louder, deeper, and longer sounds with percussion than more dense, solid structures (such as the liver), which produce softer, higher, and shorter sounds.

Auscultation. **Auscultation** involves listening to sounds in the body that are created by movement of air or fluid. Areas most often auscultated include the lungs, heart, abdomen, and blood vessels. Although direct auscultation is sometimes possible, a stethoscope is usually employed in order to amplify the sound.

Laboratory and Diagnostic Data

Results of laboratory and diagnostic tests can be useful objective data as these values often serve as defining characteristics for various altered health states; these can also be helpful in ruling out certain suspected problems. For example, diabetic clients who are poorly controlled on diet or medication will usually have an elevated blood glucose level. The pattern of these types of variations is useful in determining a plan of care. In addition, the effectiveness of nursing and medical interventions and progress toward health restoration are often monitored through laboratory and diagnostic test data.

DATA VERIFICATION

Data verification is the process through which data are validated as being complete and accurate. Once the nurse completes the initial data collection, the data are reviewed for inconsistencies or omissions. This process is particularly important if data sources are considered unreliable. For example, if a client is confused or unable to communicate, or if two sources provide conflicting data, it is necessary for the nurse to seek further information or clarification. Data verification is done by examining the congruence between subjective and objective data. For example, a client might exhibit nonverbal expressions of pain (e.g., guarding a part of the body, facial grimacing) but verbally deny feeling pain. The nurse would need to consider possible reasons for this discrepancy in findings and collect more information before formulating conclusions or planning care. Findings should also be compared with norms. Any grossly abnormal findings should be rechecked and confirmed. See the Uncovering the Evidence display.

UNCOVERING THE
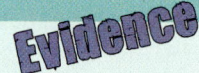

TITLE OF STUDY
"Passing the Audition—The Appraisal of Client Credibility and Assessment by Nurses at Triage"

AUTHORS
S. Edwards and D. Sines

PURPOSE
To build a grounded theory of the process of initial assessment at triage by nurses in emergency departments.

METHODS
A grounded theory and symbolic interactionist methodology were used in this study in which 38 recordings were made of live triage interactions between nurses and clients in an emergency department. The recording was stopped and the nurse was asked to describe his or her thoughts about each comment.

FINDINGS
The findings suggest that client manifestation of clinical problems was interpreted according to the nurse's perceptions of the problems. Triage is a process in which nurses judge clinical assessment data.

IMPLICATIONS
Nursing practice and research need to consider the client's input during triage decision making.

Edwards, B., & Sines, D. (2008). Passing the audition—The appraisal of client credibility and assessment by nurses at triage. *Journal of Clinical Nursing, 17*(18), 2444–2451.

DATA ORGANIZATION

After data collection is completed and information is validated, the nurse organizes, or clusters, the information together in order to identify areas of strengths and weaknesses. This process is known as **data clustering**. How data are organized depends on the assessment model used.

ASSESSMENT MODELS

An **assessment model** is a framework that provides a systematic method for organizing data. The use of a model helps to ensure comprehensive and organized data collection. A guiding framework also provides direction for decision making about nursing diagnoses. A number of nursing and nonnursing models are used to assist with organization of data. This section describes only a few of the many assessment models available to nurses.

Nursing Models

Nursing models have been developed to focus on a wide range of human responses to alterations in health status. These models typically include psychosocial, sociocultural, and behavioral data as well as biophysical data. Nursing models may offer the advantage of organizing information in a mode that more easily allows transition from data collection to nursing diagnoses.

FUNCTIONAL HEALTH PATTERNS Gordon's (2002) human functional health patterns model provides a systematic framework for data collection that focuses on 11 functional health patterns. Following is a list of the functional patterns that can be used in assessment of individuals, families, and communities:

- Health perception–health management pattern: Describes client's perceived pattern of health and well-being and how health is managed
- Nutritional-metabolic pattern: Describes pattern of food and fluid consumption relative to metabolic need and pattern indicators of local nutrient supply
- Elimination pattern: Describes patterns of excretory function (bowel, bladder, and skin)
- Activity-exercise pattern: Describes pattern of exercise, activity, leisure, and recreation
- Cognitive-perceptual pattern: Describes sensory-perceptual and cognitive pattern
- Sleep-rest pattern: Describes pattern of sleep, rest, and relaxation
- Self-perception–self-concept pattern: Describes self-concept pattern and perceptions of self
- Role-relationship pattern: Describes pattern of role engagements and relationships
- Sexuality-reproductive pattern: Describes patterns of satisfaction or dissatisfaction with sexuality; describes reproductive patterns
- Coping–stress-tolerance pattern: Describes coping pattern and its effectiveness in stress tolerance

- Value-belief pattern: Describes goals and value and belief patterns that underlie decision making (Gordon, 2002)

These functional health pattern areas allow gathering and clustering of information about a client's usual patterns and any recent changes in order to determine if the client's response is functional or dysfunctional. For example, if the activity-exercise pattern was assessed for a client who recently experienced a stroke, data collection would be focused on mobility and exercise patterns prior to the stroke, current muscle strength and joint mobility, and the effect of any changes on the client's lifestyle and functional ability.

HUMAN RESPONSE PATTERNS The North American Nursing Diagnosis Association (NANDA), in an effort to standardize terminology related to client problems, has developed a taxonomy of nursing diagnoses (NANDA, 2009). The first taxonomy was completed in 1973 and consisted of 31 diagnostic categories. This taxonomy has developed into over 100 diagnostic categories arranged in a hierarchical structure organized according to nine human response patterns (see Chapter 7). This framework suggests that a person's health status is evidenced by observable phenomena that can be classified into one of these response patterns. These human response patterns can then be used as a model for organizing data collection.

THEORY OF SELF-CARE The theory of self-care, developed by Orem (2001), is based on a client's ability to perform self-care activities. Self-care is a learned behavior and a deliberate action in response to a need. It includes activities that an individual performs to maintain health. A major focus of this theory is the appraisal of the client's ability to meet self-care needs and the identification of existing self-care deficits (see Chapter 2). Since this theory focuses on deficits in care, it primarily addresses illness states.

ROY ADAPTATION MODEL The Roy adaptation model is organized around adaptive behaviors (Andrews & Roy, 2008). The individual is considered a product of biological, psychological, and sociological influences and is in constant interaction with the environment. The ability of the person to cope with internal and external stressors determines the health status of the individual (see Chapter 2). Assessment is focused toward an individual's response to stimuli in the environment in the areas of physiological status, self-concept, role function, and interdependence.

Nonnursing Models

Nursing neither exists nor functions in a vacuum. Nurses use related health concepts from other disciplines, some of which are discussed in the following text.

BODY SYSTEMS MODEL Approaching data collection by examining body systems is sometimes referred to as the "medical model," since it is frequently used by physicians to investigate presence or absence of disease. This method organizes data collection according to the organ and tissue function in various body systems (e.g., cardiovascular, respiratory, gastrointestinal). Although nurses often use this method as well, the body systems model does not facilitate the formulation of nursing diagnoses. In addition, psychosocial aspects of the client's status are often neglected, with resultant fragmentation of care.

HIERARCHY OF NEEDS Maslow's hierarchy of needs model (1971) proposes that an individual's basic physiological needs must be met before progressing to higher-level needs. Maslow's framework can be used to prioritize client needs. Use of a hierarchy of needs model requires initial assessment of all physiological needs, followed by assessment of higher-level needs. Using Maslow's theory, a person's needs should be addressed in the following order:

- First: Physiologic needs—the basic survival needs, such as food, water, and oxygen
- Second: Safety and security needs—both physical (e.g., protection from bodily harm) and psychological (e.g., security and stability)
- Third: Need for love and belonging—humans have an innate need to be a part of a group and to feel accepted by others
- Fourth: Self-esteem needs—individuals need to feel they are valued and worthwhile
- Fifth: Self-actualization needs—the need to function at one's optimal level and to be personally fulfilled

DATA INTERPRETATION

Data clustering facilitates recognition of patterns and determination of further data that are needed. Data interpretation is necessary for identification of nursing diagnoses. Through data interpretation, the nurse examines all the information collected and seeks to make it meaningful in order to correctly determine pertinent client problems.

DATA DOCUMENTATION

Accurate and complete recording of assessment data are essential for communicating information to other health care team members. In addition, documentation is the basis for determining quality of care and should include appropriate data to support identified problems and diagnoses.

TYPES OF ASSESSMENT FORMATS

Health care agencies may choose from a variety of assessment forms for documentation depending on the type of agency, the population served by the facility, and the primary reasons for documentation. For example, clients seeking health care in a clinic or prescribing practitioner's office might be asked to complete a brief self-questionnaire, while a client admitted to an acute care facility for labor and delivery might be asked to provide only information directly related to pregnancy and child care needs. Four types of documentation

formats include open-ended, checklist, combination, and specialty. See Figure 6-2 on page 99 for an example of a form used in occupational nursing.

Open-Ended Formats

The open-ended format for documentation allows the nurse to write a narrative description of observations (see Figure 6-3 on page 100). This format is more time-consuming for the nurse but allows flexibility in recording findings.

Checklist Formats

Formats that include checklists facilitate documentation by summarizing findings in an abbreviated form (see Figure 6-4 on pages 101–104). They also provide more consistency in the recording of information and reduce the likelihood of omitting relevant information. However, checklists may discourage nurses from obtaining elaboration about observations from clients that require further explanation. For example, if a checklist indicates that mobility is impaired, further explanation is required in order to determine the extent of the impairment and thus plan the necessary interventions.

Combination Formats

Combination formats often allow the convenience of a checklist together with space to document a complete narrative description of any significant or abnormal findings (see Figure 6-5 on page 105). Some agencies provide cues on the form to alert personnel when further information is needed. This format provides for some consistency in recording data while allowing flexibility for documenting specific information.

Specialty Formats

Specialty areas such as outpatient surgery, labor and delivery, and psychiatric facilities may use abbreviated formats focused directly on assessment needs for the particular service provided. In addition, specialty assessment forms may be included together with comprehensive assessment forms for clients at particular risk for various conditions (e.g., falls, impaired skin integrity).

Documentation of assessment data is essential as a means of communication among health care team members to ensure accurate problem identification, determination of appropriate client outcomes, and continuity of care.

The Minimum Data Set

The Minimum Data Set (MDS) was developed by the Centers for Medicare and Medicaid Services (CMS) to promote the development of a comprehensive care plan for every resident of Medicare- or Medicaid-certified nursing homes. As such, the MDS is a standardized assessment instrument used in all long-term care facilities that are funded by CMS. The MDS is a comprehensive assessment tool designed to collect data about client needs.

Application: Assessment in the Industrial Clinic

The following is an example of an occupational health history used in industrial settings.

I.   Current Job:

    A. What is your current job title? _____

    B. How long have you had this job? _____

    C. What are specific tasks you perform on the job? _____

    _____

    _____

    D. Are you exposed to any of the following on your present job?

    ___Chemicals   ___Infectious agents   ___Stress

    ___Dust   ___Loud noise   ___Vapors, gases

    ___Extreme   ___Radiation   ___Vibrations
       temperature
       changes

    E. Do you think you have any work-related health problems?

       If so, describe: _____

    F. How would you describe your satisfaction with your job?

    ___Very satisfied ___Satisfied ___Somewhat satisfied ___Dissatisfied ___Very Dissatisfied

    G. Have there been any recent changes in your job or work hours?

    H. Do you use protective equipment or clothing on your job?

       If so, list items used: _____

II.   Past Work Experience:

Please provide the following information, starting with your first job:

Job Title	Dates Held	Brief Description of Job	Exposures	Injuries/Illnesses

FIGURE 6-2 Application: Assessment in the Industrial Clinic DELMAR/CENGAGE LEARNING

HEALTH HISTORY

Name_____ Date_____ Time_____

Demographic Data: Date of birth_____ Gender_____ Marital status_____

Reason for Seeking Health Care:_____

Perception of Health Status:_____

Previous Illness/Hospitalization/Surgeries:_____
_____

Client/Family Medical History:

Addiction (drugs/alcohol)_____   Diabetes_____   Mental disorders_____
Arthritis_____   Heart disease_____   Sickle cell anemia_____
Cancer_____   Hypertension_____   Stroke_____
Chronic lung disease_____   Kidney disease_____   Other_____

Immunizations/Exposure to Communicable Disease:_____
_____

Allergies:_____
_____

Home Medications:_____
_____

Developmental Level:_____
_____

Psychosocial History:

Alcohol use:_____
Tobacco use:_____
Drug use:_____
Caffeine intake:_____

Self-perception/Self-concept:_____
_____

Sociocultural History:

Family structure_____
Role in family_____
Cultural/ethnic group_____
Occupation/work role_____
Relationships with others_____

Activities of Daily Living:

Nutrition: Type of diet_____ Usual weight_____
Eating patterns_____
Types of snacks_____
Food likes/dislikes_____
Fluid intake: Type_____ Amount_____
Elimination (usual patterns): Urinary_____ Bowel_____
Sleep/Rest:
Usual sleep patterns_____
Relaxation techniques/patterns_____
Activity/Exercise:
Usual exercise patterns_____
Ability to perform self-care activities_____

Review of Systems:
Respiratory_____
Circulatory_____
Integumentary_____
Musculoskeletal_____
Neurosensory_____
Reproductive/Sexuality_____

Health Maintenance Activities:
Usual source of health care_____
Date of last exam (physical, dental, eye)_____
Other health maintenance activities_____

FIGURE 6-3 Sample Assessment Form: Open-Ended DELMAR/CENGAGE LEARNING

ADMISSION SUMMARY
FOR ADULT PATIENTS

ADMISSION   DATE:___/___/____   TIME:_____   Information from interview obtained from: ☐ Patient   ☐ Other:_____
Admitted from: ☐ Home   ☐ ER   ☐ MD Office   ☐ Other:_____
ARMBAND: ☐ Applied
PREVIOUS ADMISSION: ☐ No   ☐ Yes   If "yes," and less than 5 years ago, give date:_____
Reason for this admission according to patient/significant other:_____

Treatment in Progress:
IV Solution:_____   Site: _____

 Describe:

☐ Oxygen   _____

☐ Catheter   _____

☐ Drainage Tube   _____

☐ Feeding Tube   _____

☐ Other: _____

Height:_____   **Weight:**_____ kg.
Temperature:_____ oral/rectal/axillary
Pulse:_____ Radial/Apical
Quality of Pulse: ☐ Telemetry Channel
☐ Regular   ☐ Irregular   Verified
☐ Bounding   ☐ Thready   Rhythm:_____
Respiratory Rate:
 Quality of Respirations:
 ☐ Regular   ☐ Non-labored
 ☐ Labored   ☐ Shallow
Blood Pressure: ___ /___   O$_2$ Sat:_____

ALLERGIES: **Describe Reaction:**
Drugs: _____
_____
_____
_____
Latex:_____
Food:_____
Other: _____
_____

CURRENT MEDICATIONS
☐ See Medications listed in Physician Orders section of chart.
This list obtained from:
☐ Bottle Labels Available   ☐ Patient Interview
☐ Retail Pharmacy
Were medications brought to hospital?
☐ No   ☐ Yes
If "Yes," disposition: ☐ To Pharmacy
☐ Sent Home With: _____

Valuables Brought To Hospital: ☐ No   ☐ Yes   (If "yes," please complete applicable information below.)

	At Home	Kept by Pt.	Sent Home With:	Cashier	Comments:
Money	N/A				
Hearing Aid(s): ☐ Left ☐ Right					
Dentures: ☐ Upper ☐ Lower					
Denture Cup In Room ☐					
Eyeglasses					
Contacts					
Jewelry/Describe:					
Equipment/Describe:					
*Bio-Med Notified ☐ *Rehab Notified ☐					
Other/Describe:					

PERSONAL HABITS:
Do you use tobacco?   ☐ No   ☐ Yes (currently)   ☐ Yes (in the past)   If yes, what type?_____   How often?_____   How long in use?_____
How long have you been tobacco-free?_____
Do you use alcohol?   ☐ No   ☐ Yes (currently)   ☐ Yes (in the past)   If yes, what type?_____   How often?_____   How long in use?_____
How long have you been alcohol-free?_____
Do you take any drugs that are not prescribed?   ☐ No   ☐ Yes
If "Yes," please explain: _____

IS# 129.4 • 12/19/03

FIGURE 6-4 Sample Assessment Form: Checklist REPRINTED WITH PERMISSION FROM NORTH OAKS MEDICAL CENTER, HAMMOND, LA

DATE:___/___/_____

PAIN/COMFORT SCREENING

Location of Pain
(Mark area with an "X.")

Pain: ☐ No ☐ Yes

Pain Scale Reviewed: ☐ No ☐ Yes

New Pain: ☐ No ☐ Yes (less than 6 months)

Chronic Pain: ☐ No ☐ Yes (greater than 6 months)

If "yes," Location of Pain: _____

Origin of Pain:_____

Pain Intensity (on scale of 0 to 10): _____

Patient Unable to Evaluate? _____

Quality of Pain: ☐ Sharp   ☐ Stabbing   ☐ Dull
                 ☐ Burning ☐ Tingling   ☐ Constant
                 ☐ Intermittent ☐ Throbbing ☐ Tender
                 ☐ Cramping

Frequency (How often does your pain occur?):
   ☐ All of the Time   ☐ Following Activity   ☐ Daytime
   ☐ Late Afternoon   ☐ Bedtime

Onset: _____

Causative/Aggravating Factors:

☐ Body Position   ☐ Movement/Activity   ☐ Anxiety/Stress

Comfort Measures Used to Relieve Pain:

☐ Change in Body Position: _____

☐ Taking Medication (List.): _____

☐ Walking/Activity: _____

Were the measures effective? ☐ No ☐ Yes

Acceptable Level to Perform Daily Functions (Pain Goal):_____

PAIN EDUCATION: ☐ Verbal   ☐ Brochure

Comments: _____
_____
_____
_____
_____
_____
_____

Elimination:

Do you have trouble urinating? ☐ No ☐ Yes, Explain: _____

Are you a dialysis patient? ☐ No ☐ Yes

If "yes," and not urgent, notify Dialysis at ext. 2201.

If urgent, beep through PBX at ext.6305.

Do you have trouble with bowel movements? ☐ No   ☐ Yes

If "yes," explain: _____

Do you require laxatives?   ☐ No ☐ Yes

If "yes," what type and how often? _____

_____

Date of last B.M.:_____

* If greater than 3 days, must be addressed/documented. For patients on routine meds that cause constipation, address if no BM for 2 days.

FAMILY MEDICAL HISTORY	PATIENT		FAMILY	
	Yes	No	Yes	No
1. Hypertension				
2. Kidney Disease				
3. Anemia				
4. Cancer				
5. Heart Disease				
6. Ulcer				
7. Emphysema/COPD/Asthma				
8. Diabetes				
9. Arthritis				
10. Seizure Disorder				
11. Thyroid				
12. Glaucoma				
13. Sickle Cell Anemia				
14. Anesthesia Complications				
15. Other:				

Surgeries/Major Trauma (Explain): _____
_____
_____

Comments: _____
_____

Educational Assessment

Factors that may influence the patient's/significant other's ability and readiness to learn. (If any of the following are checked, explain in comments.):

☐ Cultural

☐ Motivation

☐ Cognitive Limitation

☐ Hearing/Vision/Speaking Impairment

☐ Language Barriers

☐ Religious Practices

☐ Psychosocial Factors

☐ None

Comments: _____

Patient able to read: ☐ No   ☐ Yes ☐ Print Only

How would you like your education provided?
            ☐ Explanation ☐ Audio ☐ Visual
            ☐ Demonstration ☐ Handout/Pamphlet

Reminder: Implement Patient Education Tool.

☐ Education channel 5

FIGURE 6-4 Continued

DATE:_____/_____/_____

QUALITY OF LIFE CONCERNS/NEEDS

Is patient within appropriate developmental stage as defined by age-specific policy/tool?   ☐ No   ☐ Yes

If "no," state specific delay and intervention necessary in addressing delay: _____

All areas identified will be addressed before discharge:

☐ **Nutrition:**

  Current diet:_____

  ☐ **Nausea/vomiting x 3 days or greater**

  ☐ **10 lbs +/- weight change in 6 months**

  ☐ **Dysphagia (Speech Therapy)**

  ☐ **Chewing problems**

☐ Lives Alone (if greater than 75 yrs. old)

☐ 3 or greater complex/chronic diagnosis

☐ Symptoms of depression (frequent crying spells, sleep disturbance, change in appetite, feelings of helplessness/hopelessness, fatigue, etc.)

☐ History of substance abuse

☐ Possible abuse or neglect

☐ Homeless/crime victim

☐ Suicide attempt/ideations

☐ Unable to perform ADL's, dress, bathe self and no support system in place

☐ Transient

☐ Fetal demise/miscarriage

☐ Infant under care of neonatologist

☐ Adoption arrangements made/requested

☐ Non-compliant with taking medication

  Explain:_____

☐ Other:_____

Are there any customs or religious beliefs that may affect your plan of care?   ☐ No   ☐ Yes

If "yes," explain: _____

_____

_____

_____

_____

_____

Pastoral follow-up requested by patient/family? ☐ No ☐ Yes

If "yes," did family request a specific pastor/priest? ☐ No ☐ Yes

If "yes," name of pastor/priest:_____

If "yes" to pastoral follow-up but no specific clergy member requested, was Volunteer Services notified? ☐ No ☐ Yes

VACCINATION STATUS
☐ Screening Tool Implemented

SAFETY
Yes

☐ Over 75 yrs. old _____

☐ History of falls _____

+ ☐ Visual impairment, not corrected _____

☐ Disability with physical impairment _____

+ ☐ Walker, crutches, cane, _____.

+ ☐ Confusion _____

☐ Agitation _____

☐ Impaired memory/judgment _____

☐ Hard of hearing _____

+ ☐ Altered level of consciousness _____

☐ Drugs that produce sedation _____

☐ Drugs that promote diuresis, affect GI mobility, alter thought processes, lower blood pressure

☐ • Weakness _____

+ ☐ • Paresis _____

☐ History of seizures or new onset seizures

☐ Seizure precautions initiated

Comments:_____

_____

NOTE: If patient meets 3 or more criteria above or one criteria designated by a cross (+), Fall Prevention should be instituted.

Yes

☐ Fall Prevention Instituted _____

☐ If "yes," is it entered into HBOC? _____

☐ Is a sign placed at bedside? _____

☐ Family/patient instructed on FPP? _____

FUNCTIONAL SCREENING
MAY REQUIRE REHAB

Ability to accomplish:

☐ Communication ability (Speech Therapy)

☐ Bed mobility skills (Physical Therapy/Occupational Therapy)

☐ Transfer skills (Physical Therapy/Occupational Therapy)

☐ Balance (Physical Therapy)

☐ Ambulation with or without assistive devices (Physical Therapy)

☐ Feeding skills (Speech Therapy/Occupational Therapy)

☐ Personal hygiene (Occupational Therapy)

☐ Bathing (Occupational Therapy)

☐ Dressing/fasteners (Occupational Therapy)

☐ Toileting (Occupational Therapy)

☐ Body position awareness (Physical Therapy/Occupational Therapy)

☐ Ability to understand or follow instructions (Speech Therapy/Occupational Therapy)

Deficit does not require rehab (e.g., old CVA).   ☐

FIGURE 6-4 Continued

DATE:___/___/_____

Explanation Given Regarding:
☐ Bed Mechanics ☐ Call Bell
☐ Telephone ☐ Activity Allowed

BRADEN SCALE

If Braden score is 17 - 23, pressure ulcer prevention precautions will be implemented.

If Braden score is 12 - 16, moderate pressure ulcer prevention precautions will be implemented.

If Braden score is 0 - 11, strict pressure ulcer prevention precautions will be implemented.

Clinical Condition Parameters

1. Sensory Perception: Response to Pressure-Related Discomfort

Completely Limited (unresponsive, quad, coma)	1
Very Limited (Responds only to painful stimuli, paraplegic, semicoma)	2
Slightly Limited (Responds with some sensory impairment CVA)	3
No Impairment (No limiting sensory deficit)	4

2. Moisture: Degree To Which Skin Is Exposed To Moisture

Constantly Moist (Always incontinent, 2 or more linen changes every 8 hours)	1
Moist (Often incontinent, linen change every 8 hours)	2
Occasionally Moist (Seldom incontinent, linen changes 2 every 24 hours)	3
Rarely Moist (Skin is dry, routine linen change)	4

3. Activity: Degree Of Physical Activity

Bed rest (Confined to bed)	1
Chairfast (Minimum weight bearing, ambulatory w/assist)	2
Walks Occasionally (Ambulatory short distance, sits mostly)	3
Walks Frequently (Ambulatory outside room, BID)	4

4. Mobility: Ability To Control, Change Body Position

Completely Immobile (Cannot move self)	1
Very Limited (Makes insignificant movements)	2
Slightly Limited (Makes slight changes independently)	3
No Limitations (Makes major, independent changes)	4

5. Nutrition: Usual Food Intake Pattern

Very Poor (NPO, IV greater than 5 days, less than 1/3 meals)	1
Problem Inadequate (Needs assistance, less than 1/2 meals)	2
Adequate (TPN, enteral needs met, greater than 1/2 meals)	3
Excellent (No supplement, eats most meals)	4

6. Friction and Shear: Ability To Maintain Body Position

Problem (Requires complete assist., slides down in bed/chair)	1
Potential Problem (Requires maximum assist., sometimes slides down in bed/chair)	2
No Apparent Problem (Moves independently, maintains good position in bed/chair)	3

Score_____

☐ Braden Score entered into HBOC ☐ Prevention Protocol Initiated

If all information not obtainable, please explain:
☐ Patient Non-verbal ☐ Patient Poor Historian ☐ No Family at Bedside
☐ Other: _____
_____
_____

SKIN ASSESSMENT

☐ No abnormalities noted.

☐ Abnormalities present. See "Skin Injury/Wound Assessment Flowsheet."

Note: Abnormalities include, but are not limited to, skin tears, surgical incisions (does not include healed scars), lacerations, decubitus ulcers, rashes, bruises and hematomas.

DISCHARGE INFORMATION
Who do you live with? _____
Number of children at home and ages: _____
Who will take care of you after discharge?
_____
Who will provide transportation upon discharge?
_____
Telephone #:_____
Where will you go at discharge?
☐ Home
☐ Home w/Home Health
Name of Current Home Health:
_____
☐ Nursing Home:
Name of Current Nursing Home:
_____
☐ Other: _____
Medical equipment used at home? ☐ No ☐ Yes
If "yes," please explain: _____
_____
Does patient use specialty bed? ☐ No ☐ Yes
If "yes," what type?
_____ _____
Name of Company: _____
Community Resources used:_____
_____
Anticipated needs at discharge:
☐ Equipment (explain):_____
☐ Supplies (explain):_____
☐ Transportation:_____
☐ Questionaire Reminder
☐ Other: _____

Signatures
Admit Nurse:_____
Date:_____ Time:_____
Reviewing RN: _____
Date:_____ Time:_____

FIGURE 6-4 Continued

ADMISSION ASSESSMENT

Date_____ Time_____

Admitted from: Home____ER____Other____

Allergies_____

Baseline Data: Ht____Wt____T____P____R____BP____

Mode of Transport: Stretcher____W/C____Amb____

Home Meds:
_____   _____
_____   _____
_____   _____

Mental Status			**Comment**
Alert/Oriented	Yes	No	_____
Confused	Yes	No	_____
Anxious	Yes	No	_____
Comatose	Yes	No	_____
Combative	Yes	No	_____

Other_____

Communication			**Comment**
Speaks English	Yes	No	_____
Aphasic	Yes	No	_____
Speech Impediment	Yes	No	_____

Sensory			**Comment**
Hearing Impaired	Yes	No	_____
Visually Impaired	Yes	No	_____
Amputation	Yes	No	_____
Hemiplegia	Yes	No	_____
Paraplegia	Yes	No	_____

Diet/Nutrition

Diet at Home_____

Likes/Dislikes_____

Appetite_____

Skin			**Location**
Warm/Dry	Yes	No	_____
Abrasions/Bruises	Yes	No	_____
Laceration/Scar	Yes	No	_____
Reddened Areas	Yes	No	_____
Decubitus Ulcers	Yes	No	_____
Burns	Yes	No	_____
Rash/Scaling	Yes	No	_____
Diaphoretic	Yes	No	_____

Other_____

Color: Pale   Normal   Cyanotic

Treatments in Progress:_____
_____
_____

Elimination			**Comment**
GI: Constipation	Yes	No	_____
Frequency	Yes	No	_____
Laxatives	Yes	No	_____

Other_____

GU: Frequency	Yes	No	_____
Burning	Yes	No	_____
Incontinent	Yes	No	_____

Other_____

Sleeping			**Comment**
Unable to fall asleep	Yes	No	_____
Awakens frequently	Yes	No	_____
Sleep meds	Yes	No	_____
Naps	Yes	No	_____

ADL   **Comment**

Assistance needed for:

Ambulation	Yes	No	_____
Eating	Yes	No	_____
Bathing	Yes	No	_____
Dressing	Yes	No	_____
Eliminating	Yes	No	_____
Turning	Yes	No	_____

Other_____

Denture	Yes	No	_____
Glasses	Yes	No	_____
Contact Lenses	Yes	No	_____

Personal Habits:

Tobacco use	Yes	No	_____ (quantity)
Alcohol use	Yes	No	_____ (quantity)

Chief Complaint:_____
_____
_____

Other Assessment Data:_____
_____
_____

FIGURE 6-5 Sample Assessment Form: Combination DELMAR/CENGAGE LEARNING

KEY CONCEPTS

- Assessment includes collection, verification, organization, interpretation, and documentation of data.

- The nurse uses the process of assessment to establish a database about the client, to form an interpersonal relationship with the client, and to provide the client with an opportunity to discuss health care concerns.

- Assessment can be comprehensive, focused, or ongoing, depending on the health care setting and needs of the client.

- The two types of data collected during the assessment process are subjective (data from the client's point of view) and objective (observable and measurable data that are obtained through both the physical examination and laboratory and diagnostic tests).

- Although a variety of sources should be used in data collection, the client is the primary source of information.

- Assessment models such as Gordon's functional health patterns, NANDA's human response patterns, Orem's theory of self-care model, Roy's adaptation model, the body systems model, and Maslow's hierarchy of needs model ensure comprehensive data collection and organization.

- Data are collected through the interview, health history, symptom analysis, physical examination, and laboratory and diagnostic tests.

- The three stages of assessment interview are the introduction, working, and closure phases.

- A comprehensive health history is useful in determining the client's functional health patterns, responses to changes in health status, and alterations in lifestyle.

- The elements of the health history are demographic information; reason for seeking health care; perception of health status; previous illnesses, hospitalizations, and surgeries; client and family medical history; immunizations and exposure to communicable disease; allergies; current medications; developmental level; psychosocial history; sociocultural history; activities of daily living; and review of systems.

- The purposes of the physical examination are to gather baseline data, confirm data obtained in the interview and health history, and evaluate progress toward established goals.

- The physical examination includes the techniques of inspection, palpation, percussion, and auscultation.

- Accurate and complete documentation of assessment findings is essential for communication to other health care team members.

- Data may be recorded on a variety of tools, such as open-ended, checklist, combination, and specialty formats.

REVIEW QUESTIONS

1. Which of the following nursing responses is an example of an open-ended statement?
   a. "Are you feeling better?"
   b. "Do you have any pain now?"
   c. "Tell me about your health."
   d. "Tell me how many children you have."

2. The process of assessment includes which of the following activities? Select all that apply.
   a. Collecting
   b. Documenting
   c. Interpreting
   d. Organizing
   e. Planning
   f. Verifying

3. A 72-year-old client comes to the emergency department for treatment of difficult, painful urination. What type of assessment is most appropriate for this client?
   a. Comprehensive
   b. Focused
   c. Ongoing

   d. Subjective

4. The nurse is performing an admission assessment. Which of the following are examples of objective data? Select all that apply.
   a. 10 cc of emesis in basin
   b. Cool, clammy skin
   c. Client says, "My feet are swollen."
   d. Complaint of nausea by client
   e. Oral temperature 103°F
   f. Rapid, thready pulse

5. When performing an assessment, which of the following would the nurse use as a primary source of data?
   a. All health care personnel
   b. Client
   c. Client family and/or friends
   d. Client medical records

6. Which of the following statements accurately describes the review of systems (ROS)?
   a. It is performed by the nurse at the earliest possible time.

b. It is the client's statement about perceived health status.

c. ROS should be performed only by advanced nurse practitioners.

d. The nurse does a head-to-toe physical examination of the client.

7. A newly admitted client states that she has a severe headache. What is the nurse's first action?

a. Administer pain medication as ordered in the client's medical record.

b. Check the client's vital signs.

c. Have the client sign consent forms for treatment and diagnostic procedures.

d. Orient the client to the unit and explain safety guidelines.

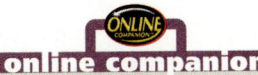

online companion

Visit the DeLaune and Ladner online companion resource at **www.delmar.cengage.com** for additional content and study aids. Click on Online Companions, then select the Nursing discipline.

We can have facts without thinking but we cannot have thinking without facts.

—JOHN DEWEY

CHAPTER 7

Nursing Diagnosis

COMPETENCIES

1. Describe nursing diagnosis as a critical step in clinical judgment.
2. Explain the purposes of nursing diagnoses.
3. List the types of nursing diagnoses and the components of each type.
4. Explore characteristics of the nursing diagnosis taxonomy.
5. Describe the process of developing a nursing diagnosis.
6. Identify common errors in developing a nursing diagnosis.
7. Discuss limitations of nursing diagnoses.
8. Explore barriers that can affect the use of a nursing diagnosis.
9. Describe strategies to overcome limitations of and barriers to using nursing diagnoses.
10. Describe how a nursing diagnosis enables the delivery of holistic, comprehensive nursing care.
11. Explain how a nursing diagnosis enhances accountability and empowerment in the nursing profession.

KEY TERMS

cluster	diagnostic label	related factors
cues	etiology	risk factors
defining characteristics	medical diagnosis	taxonomy of nursing diagnoses
definition	nursing diagnosis	
diagnosis	nursing informatics	

The **nursing diagnosis** is the second step in the nursing process and includes clinical judgments made about wellness states, illness states and syndromes, and the readiness to enhance current states of wellness experienced by individuals, families, and aggregate populations (communities). Diagnosing is based on a critical analysis of the assessment data. The purpose of a nursing diagnosis is to effectively communicate client needs among members of the health care team. Society tends to interpret nursing through the use of nursing language. When a nursing diagnosis is a part of the client's plan of care, the nurse is able to communicate the client's needs to other professionals involved in that care. These needs encompass physiologic, role function, self-concept, interdependence, and spiritual dimensions. To determine individualized therapeutic nursing interventions, the nurse must develop appropriate nursing diagnoses that are based on organized assessment data.

This chapter describes the nature of a nursing diagnosis, the purpose and types of nursing diagnoses, and the components of a nursing diagnostic statement. Development of nursing diagnoses and methods for avoiding diagnostic errors in the formulation of nursing diagnoses are also presented. Strategies for overcoming barriers to the use of nursing diagnoses are discussed.

WHAT IS A NURSING DIAGNOSIS?

Diagnosis is the science and art of identifying problems or conditions. Although this process has been linked primarily with physicians, it is also used by members of other professions, such as nurses, lawyers, social workers, mechanics, psychologists, and teachers. Though the term *nursing diagnosis* may convey multiple meanings, "in effect, nursing diagnosis defines nursing practice" (Ralph & Taylor, 2008, p. xxi).

Many definitions of nursing diagnosis have evolved over the past decades. The North American Nursing Diagnosis Association International (NANDA-I) defines nursing diagnosis as:

A clinical judgment about individual, family or community responses to actual and potential health problems or life processes. Nursing diagnoses provide the basis for selection of nursing interventions to achieve outcomes for which the nurse is accountable. (NANDA-I, 2009, p. 8)

Additional definitions of nursing diagnosis abound in the nursing literature. It is clear that although all definitions

are not exactly alike, there are similar attributes among them, such as a focus on client-centered problems; the promotion of nursing accountability; an awareness of the human response to health problems; the formation of clinical judgments about individuals, families, or communities; and the development of nursing interventions that a nurse is licensed to implement.

COMPARISON OF NURSING AND MEDICAL DIAGNOSES

It is important to differentiate a nursing diagnosis from a medical diagnosis (see Table 7-1). Clarification of this point is necessary to distinguish between the nursing and medical professions and the potential legal ramifications.

Delineation of "What is the nature of nursing?" versus "What is the nature of medicine?" is critical. In order to practice nursing, nurses need to know what it is that they do. Nursing diagnoses assist nurses in defining their scope of practice just as medical diagnoses assist physicians in defining their scope of practice. In addition, the use of diagnoses in nursing and medicine enables clarification of the legal boundaries for practice.

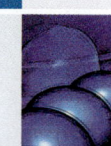

TABLE 7-1 Comparison of Selected Nursing and Medical Diagnoses	
NURSING (HUMAN RESPONSES)	**MEDICINE (DISEASE STATES)**
Ineffective breathing pattern	Chronic obstructive pulmonary disease
Activity intolerance	Cerebrovascular accident
Acute pain	Appendectomy
Disturbed body image	Amputation
Risk for imbalanced body temperature	Strep throat

Delmar/Cengage Learning

Medicine uses the term *medical diagnosis* and nursing uses the term *nursing diagnosis* to identify problems relating to a client's health status:

- **Medical diagnosis** is the terminology used for a clinical judgment by the physician that identifies or determines a specific disease, condition, or pathologic state.
- **Nursing diagnosis** is the terminology used for a clinical judgment by the professional nurse that identifies the client's or aggregate's actual, risk, wellness, or syndrome responses to a health state, problem, or condition.

There are both similarities and differences between medical and nursing diagnoses. The similarities include (1) using the diagnostic process, with "process" implying purpose, organization, and creativity (Bevis, 1978); (2) using cognitive, interpersonal, and psychomotor skills; (3) collecting and critically analyzing assessment data; (4) evaluating outcomes to ascertain continuation, resolution, or change of identified diagnosis; and (5) performing within legal dimensions and standards of the respective profession. An example of these similarities can be illustrated by considering a client who has a medical diagnosis of asthma. The physician and nurse would both collect assessment data on respiratory status. The physician would use this information to treat the disease of asthma and the nurse would use this information to focus on the client's response to the disease, which would result in a nursing diagnosis of *ineffective breathing pattern.*

Nursing diagnoses are different from medical diagnoses in (1) purpose, (2) goals, and (3) therapeutic interventions. The *purpose* of a nursing diagnosis is to focus on the human response or responses of the individual, family, or community to identified problems or conditions. Medical diagnoses center on the disease state or pathological condition. For example, if the medical diagnosis for a client is breast cancer, appropriate nursing diagnoses may include *fear, deficient knowledge* related to treatment measures, *grieving, disturbed body image, powerlessness,* and *ineffective coping.* In addition, the goals (aims, intent, or ends) that accompany these nursing diagnoses differ, as do the specific, individualized therapeutic nursing interventions (nursing actions to promote or restore health and enhance general well-being).

HISTORICAL PERSPECTIVE

The term *nursing diagnosis* has been in the literature since the early 1950s. Fry (1953) identified that nursing diagnosis is integral to the plan of nursing care and is an important tool for individualizing client care. However, these ideas were slow to gain momentum despite the interests of several nurse theorists and the focus on client-centered problems in the 1960s and the 1970s. In 1973, the First National Conference for the Classification of Nursing Diagnoses met to identify, develop, and classify nursing diagnoses. In 1982, at the fifth national conference, the organization was renamed the North American Nursing Diagnosis Association (NANDA).

Additional endorsement for nursing diagnosis came from the American Nurses Association (ANA) in 1973. Ongoing discussions occurred in the nursing literature, with increasing support evident by the 1980s for nursing diagnosis and the diagnostic process. The ANA continues to support nursing diagnosis as the second step of the nursing process. Key elements of the ANA standards for diagnosis state that diagnoses are:

- Based on data collected during assessment of client
- Validated with client, significant others, and health care providers
- Documented so that they can be used in further development of expected outcomes and plan of care (ANA, 2004)

Following the biennial conference in April 1994, the Taxonomy Committee identified the need to revise the structure of Taxonomy I. During the 14th biennial conference in April 2000, NANDA adopted Taxonomy II, which was designed to improve the flexibility of the nomenclature (NANDA-I, 2009). As NANDA's work continued to grow, countries outside the United States began to incorporate the nursing diagnosis taxonomy, translating it and contributing in turn to the organization. In 2002, at the 14th national conference, the organization was renamed NANDA-I to represent the many countries that participate in the work of the organization.

In 2003, the ANA (2004) revised nursing's social policy statement to include the essential features of professional nursing. Among these features is the processes of diagnosis through the use of critical thinking. NANDA-I officially began collaboration with the Center for Nursing Classification and Clinical Effectiveness (University of Iowa) to sponsor joint biennial conference meetings through the NNN (NANDA-NIC-NOC) Alliance to promote the development, dissemination, and utilization of standardized nursing languages.

RESEARCH

Since the inception of the first conference on nursing diagnoses in 1973, NANDA-I has supported research on the development of a nursing diagnosis classification system. The initial research conducted was identification studies, in which clinicians repeatedly observed a condition in order to label a nursing diagnosis.

PURPOSES OF NURSING DIAGNOSES

Nursing diagnosis is unique in that it focuses on a client's *response* to a health problem, rather than on the problem itself, and it provides the structure through which nursing care can be delivered. Although these characteristics have always been in existence within nursing, they were unidentified prior to the mid-twentieth century.

PROFESSIONALISM

One of the requisites of a profession is a unique body of knowledge. Clearer conceptualization of knowledge unique to nursing increases both professional accountability and autonomy (Carpenito-Moyet, 2007). Therefore, nursing diagnosis contributes to the professional status of the discipline. The diagnostic process includes data collection, interpretation, clustering of data (cues), and naming that cluster of cues. Nurses must be able to identify the phenomena of concern, determine appropriate outcomes, and then intervene to make those outcomes attainable.

COMMUNICATION

Nursing diagnosis also provides a means for effective communication. It is generally agreed among nurses, prescribing practitioners, and other health care professionals that there is a need for a common language within the health care sector. A mutual vocabulary that can be used for describing practice, research, and education benefits both the profession and the consumer. In addition, communication about nursing diagnoses is possible through computer-based searches.

HOLISTIC, INDIVIDUALIZED CARE

Holistic client care is facilitated with the use of nursing diagnosis. The list of NANDA-I–approved nursing diagnoses (NANDA-I, 2009) for clinical use provides assistance for the nurse in individualizing care and developing comprehensive therapeutic nursing interventions. See Table 7-2 for a listing of NANDA-I–approved diagnoses. "The interpretation of human responses is a complex nursing task that serves as the basis for selecting nursing interventions" (da Cruz, de Mattos Pimenta, & Lunney, 2006, p. 229). Quality care and continuity of care are enhanced with identified nursing diagnoses as part of the client's plan of nursing care. See the accompanying Community Considerations box, which illustrates the value of applying nursing diagnosis to a client receiving home health care.

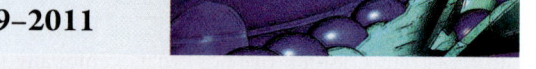

COMMUNITY CONSIDERATIONS

Home Health Care Setting

Individualizing care of the home health client is an important function of nursing diagnosis. For example, the following questions can be used as a guide in developing nursing interventions as a response to the nursing diagnosis of *compromised family coping* related to a caregiver appearing to be unable to assist a client with management of a health problem:

- Has the caregiver expressed concern or anxiety about performing certain functions for the client?
- Does the care performed by the caregiver for the client yield satisfactory results in terms of alleviation of symptoms?
- What changes have occurred within the family situation that have altered the dynamics between the client and caregiver?

NURSING DIAGNOSES AND NURSING INFORMATICS

Nursing informatics is a specialty within nursing that assists organizations, clients, and clinicians through its focus on the methods and tools needed for dealing with information within nursing practice (see Chapter 13). Standards of

TABLE 7-2 NANDA International Nursing Diagnoses 2009–2011

Activity Intolerance	Interrupted **B**reastfeeding
Ineffective **A**ctivity Planning	Ineffective **B**reathing Pattern
Risk for **A**ctivity Intolerance	Decreased **C**ardiac Output
Ineffective **A**irway Clearance	**C**aregiver Role Strain
Latex **A**llergy Response	Risk for **C**aregiver Role Strain
Risk for Latex **A**llergy Response	Readiness for Enhanced **C**hildbearing Process
Anxiety	Impaired **C**omfort
Death **A**nxiety	Readiness for Enhanced **C**omfort
Risk for **A**spiration	Impaired Verbal **C**ommunication
Risk for Impaired **A**ttachment	Readiness for Enhanced **C**ommunication
Autonomic Dysreflexia	Decisional **C**onflict (Specify)
Risk for **A**utonomic Dysreflexia	Parental Role **C**onflict
Risk-Prone Health **B**ehavior	Acute **C**onfusion
Risk for **B**leeding	Chronic **C**onfusion
Risk for Unstable **B**lood Glucose Level	Risk for Acute **C**onfusion
Disturbed **B**ody Image	**C**onstipation
Risk for Imbalanced **B**ody Temperature	Perceived **C**onstipation
Effective **B**reastfeeding	Risk for **C**onstipation
Ineffective **B**reastfeeding	**C**ontamination

(continues)

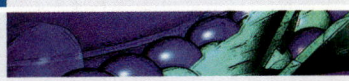

TABLE 7-2 (Continued)

Risk for **C**ontamination

Defensive **C**oping

Ineffective **C**oping

Readiness for Enhanced **C**oping

Ineffective Community **C**oping

Readiness for Enhanced Community **C**oping

Compromised Family **C**oping

Disabled Family **C**oping

Readiness for Enhanced Family **C**oping

Risk for Sudden Infant **D**eath Syndrome

Readiness for Enhanced **D**ecision Making

Ineffective **D**enial

Impaired **D**entition

Risk for Delayed **D**evelopment

Diarrhea

Risk for Compromised Human **D**ignity

Risk for **D**isuse Syndrome

Deficient **D**iversional Activity

Risk for **E**lectrolyte Imbalance

Impaired Urinary **E**limination

Readiness for Enhanced Urinary **E**limination

Disturbed **E**nergy Field

Impaired **E**nvironmental Interpretation Syndrome

Adult **F**ailure to Thrive

Risk for **F**alls

Dysfunctional **F**amily Processes

Interrupted **F**amily Processes

Readiness for Enhanced **F**amily Processes

Fatigue

Fear

Readiness for Enhanced **F**luid Balance

Deficient **F**luid Volume

Excess **F**luid Volume

Risk for Deficient **F**luid Volume

Risk for Imbalanced **F**luid Volume

Impaired **G**as Exchange

Grieving

Complicated **G**rieving

Risk for Complicated **G**rieving

Delayed **G**rowth and Development

Risk for Disproportionate **G**rowth

Ineffective **H**ealth Maintenance

Impaired **H**ome Maintenance

Readiness for Enhanced **H**ope

Hopelessness

Hyperthermia

Hypothermia

Disturbed Personal **I**dentity

Readiness for Enhanced **I**mmunization Status

Bowel **I**ncontinence

Functional Urinary **I**ncontinence

Overflow Urinary **I**ncontinence

Reflex Urinary **I**ncontinence

Stress Urinary **I**ncontinence

Urge Urinary **I**ncontinence

Risk for Urge Urinary **I**ncontinence

Disorganized **I**nfant Behavior

Risk for Disorganized **I**nfant Behavior

Readiness for Enhanced Organized **I**nfant Behavior

Ineffective **I**nfant Feeding Pattern

Risk for **I**nfection

Risk for **I**njury

Risk for Perioperative-Positioning **I**njury

Insomnia

Decreased **I**ntracranial Adaptive Capacity

Neonatal **J**aundice

Deficient **K**nowledge

Readiness for Enhanced **K**nowledge (Specify)

Sedentary **L**ifestyle

Risk for Impaired **L**iver Function

Risk for **L**oneliness

Risk for Disturbed **M**aternal/Fetal Dyad

Impaired **M**emory

Impaired Bed **M**obility

Impaired Physical **M**obility

Impaired Wheelchair **M**obility

Moral Distress

Dysfunctional Gastrointestinal **M**otility

Risk for Dysfunctional Gastrointestinal **M**otility

Nausea

Unilateral **N**eglect

Noncompliance

Imbalanced **N**utrition: Less than Body Requirements

Imbalanced **N**utrition: More than Body Requirements

Readiness for Enhanced **N**utrition

Risk for Imbalanced **N**utrition: More than Body Requirements

Impaired **O**ral Mucous Membrane

Acute **P**ain

Chronic **P**ain

Readiness for Enhanced **P**arenting

Impaired **P**arenting

Risk for Impaired **P**arenting

Ineffective Peripheral Tissue **P**erfusion

Risk for Decreased Cardiac Tissue **P**erfusion

Risk for Ineffective Cerebral Tissue **P**erfusion

Risk for Ineffective Gastrointestinal **P**erfusion

Risk for Ineffective Renal **P**erfusion

Risk for **P**eripheral Neurovascular Dysfunction

Risk for **P**oisoning

Post-Trauma Syndrome

Risk for **P**ost-Trauma Syndrome

Readiness for Enhanced **P**ower

Powerlessness

Risk for **P**owerlessness

Ineffective **P**rotection

(continues)

TABLE 7-2 (Continued)

Rape-Trauma Syndrome	Risk for **S**hock
Readiness for Enhanced **R**elationship	Impaired **S**kin Integrity
Impaired **R**eligiosity	Risk for Impaired **S**kin Integrity
Readiness for Enhanced **R**eligiosity	**S**leep Deprivation
Risk for Impaired **R**eligiosity	Disturbed **S**leep Pattern
Relocation Stress Syndrome	Readiness for Enhanced **S**leep
Risk for **R**elocation Stress Syndrome	Impaired **S**ocial Interaction
Impaired Individual **R**esilience	**S**ocial Isolation
Readiness for Enhanced **R**esilience	Chronic **S**orrow
Risk for Compromised **R**esilience	**S**piritual Distress
Urinary **R**etention	Risk for **S**piritual Distress
Ineffective **R**ole Performance	Readiness for Enhanced **S**piritual Well-Being
Bathing **S**elf-Care Deficit	**S**tress Overload
Dressing **S**elf-Care Deficit	Risk for **S**uffocation
Feeding **S**elf-Care Deficit	Risk for **S**uicide
Readiness for Enhanced **S**elf-Care	Delayed **S**urgical Recovery
Toileting **S**elf-Care Deficit	Impaired **S**wallowing
Readiness for Enhanced **S**elf-Concept	Ineffective Family **T**herapeutic Regimen Management
Chronic Low **S**elf-Esteem	Ineffective **T**hermoregulation
Situational Low **S**elf-Esteem	Impaired **T**issue Integrity
Risk for Situational Low **S**elf-Esteem	Ineffective Peripheral **T**issue Perfusion
Ineffective **S**elf-Health Management	Impaired **T**ransfer Ability
Readiness for Enhanced **S**elf-Health Management	Risk for **T**rauma
Self-Mutilation	Risk for Vascular **T**rauma
Risk for **S**elf-Mutilation	Impaired Spontaneous **V**entilation
Self-Neglect	Dysfunctional **V**entilatory Weaning Response
Disturbed **S**ensory Perception (Specify: Visual,	Risk for Other-Directed **V**iolence
Auditory, Kinesthetic, Gustatory, Tactile, Olfactory)	Risk for Self-Directed **V**iolence
Sexual Dysfunction	Impaired **W**alking
Ineffective **S**exuality Pattern	**W**andering

Nursing Diagnoses—*Definitions and classification 2009–2011* © 2009, 2007, 2005, 2003, 2001, 1998, 1994, NANDA International., Used by arrangement with Wiley-Blackwell Publishing, a company of John Wiley & Sons, Inc.

practice for nursing informatics, developed in 1995, address such topics as identifying, naming, organizing, grouping, collecting, processing, analyzing, storing, retrieving, communicating, transforming, and managing data or information (ANA, 2008). Certification is also available in nursing informatics. This specialty is absolutely critical to the implementation of NANDA and other nursing terminology systems within the clinical environment.

The advent of the electronic medical record has moved standardized nursing languages forward—perhaps faster than any other movement within health care. As more and more health care organizations computerize documentation, it becomes necessary for nursing to be able to efficiently and completely document both nursing care delivery and the clinical judgments (nursing diagnoses) that drive that care. The health care climate of recent years has been one of increasing mergers and partnerships between health care organizations that were formerly competitors. The task then is to be able to bring divergent computer systems together to meet the needs of the clients and the clinicians in these new alliances. Use of a standardized nursing language allows for ease in sharing and interpreting nursing care.

Nursing informatics has the ability to demonstrate nursing's value to clients and to improve client safety and quality of client care. Evidence-based nursing care, and the strong push toward measuring the quality of that care, has led organizations to harvest information out of all the data that are collected daily within their systems as a way of proving nursing's value. Point-of-care computing and clinical decision support are two of the many ways that informatics are improving the safety of client care, while at the same time making documentation of that care more efficient for nurses (see Chapter 13).

COMPONENTS OF A NURSING DIAGNOSIS

There are five components of a nursing diagnosis that should be understood by the student and practicing clinician alike. The **diagnostic label** (or concept) consists of one or more nouns (and may also include an adjective) that name the diagnosis and can be a word or a phrase that describes the pattern of related cues. The definition provides a clear description and differentiates one diagnosis from other similar diagnoses. The defining characteristics are observable manifestations of a specific diagnosis (NANDA-I, 2009). Risk factors are those elements that increase the chances of an individual, family, or community being susceptible to a disease state or life event that will have an impact on health. Finally, related factors can precede, be associated with, contribute to, or be related to nursing diagnoses in some type of patterned relationship (NANDA-I, 2009).

Several formats have been used to structure nursing diagnosis statements. Two formats that are frequently seen in the nursing literature are the two- and three-part statements. The two-part statement is NANDA-approved and is used by most nurses, in large part because of its brief and precise format. The three-part statement is preferred by those nurses desiring to strengthen the diagnostic statement by including specific manifestations, an attribute that is not possible through the use of the two-part format.

THE TWO-PART STATEMENT

The components of a nursing diagnosis typically consist of two parts. The first component is a problem statement or diagnostic label that describes the client's response to an actual, a possible, a risk for a health problem, or a wellness condition.

The second component of a two-part nursing diagnosis is the etiology. The etiology is the related contributing factor of the problem. The diagnostic label and etiology are linked by the term *related to* (RT). Examples of nursing diagnoses are *disturbed body image* RT loss of left lower extremity and *activity intolerance* RT decreased oxygen-carrying capacity of cells. Descriptive words or modifiers may be added to clarify specific nursing diagnoses. These modifiers, which limit or specify the meaning of a nursing diagnosis, are called judgments. NANDA-I (2009) recognizes the following: *anticipatory, compromised, decreased, defensive, deficient, delayed, disabled, disorganized, disproportionate, disturbed, dysfunctional, effective, enhanced, excessive, imbalanced, impaired, ineffective, interrupted, low, organized, perceived, readiness for,* and *situational.* These terms are placed before the problem statement.

The population for which a diagnosis is being used can also be named. The populations identified by NANDA-I (2009) include *individual, family, group,* and *community.* If a population is not specified within the diagnostic label, such as with *readiness for enhanced family processes,* it becomes the individual by default.

THE THREE-PART STATEMENT

The nursing diagnosis can also be expressed as a three-part statement. As in the two-part statement, the first two components are the diagnostic label and the etiology. The third component consists of defining characteristics (collected data that are also known as signs and symptoms, subjective and objective data, or clinical manifestations). In the three-part nursing diagnosis format, the third part is joined to the first two components with the connecting phrase "as evidenced by" (AEB). Defining characteristics list the relevant clinical manifestations, such as signs or symptoms for the identified client problem and the related etiology. Defining characteristics are identified for each NANDA-approved diagnosis. These characteristics continue to evolve as they are reviewed and updated. Defining characteristics may assist the nurse in identifying client goals, measurable client outcome criteria, and relevant nursing interventions.

Some nurses believe that the three-part statement strengthens the diagnostic process. However, other nurses prefer the two-part statement and refer to the defining characteristics as part of the original database. Table 7-3 depicts the components and relationship of the one-, two-, and three-part statements. Although the most commonly used format is the two-part statement, it is beneficial for the nurse to be knowledgeable about the use of the three-part statement for development of a nursing diagnosis. See Table 7-4 on page 116 for a comparison of selected NANDA-approved diagnoses in the two- and three-part statements.

CATEGORIES OF NURSING DIAGNOSES

Nursing diagnoses may be classified into four categories of health status: actual, risk, health promotion, and wellness. Health status indicates the place along the continuum from wellness to illness at which the nursing diagnosis is being made. The most common nursing diagnoses used are actual and risk diagnoses.

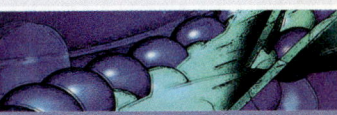

TABLE 7-3 Comparison of One-, Two-, and Three-Part Nursing Diagnosis Statements

ONE-PART STATEMENT	TWO-PART STATEMENT	THREE-PART STATEMENT
Part 1: Wellness condition or state to be enhanced (no related to, no etiology, and no defining characteristics)	Part 1: Problem related to Part 2: Etiology (no defining characteristics)	Part 1: Problem related to Part 2: Etiology Part 3: Defining characteristics

Delmar/Cengage Learning

TABLE 7-4 Examples of Nursing Diagnoses Expressed in Two- and Three-Part Statements

NURSING DIAGNOSIS	TWO-PART STATEMENT	THREE-PART STATEMENT
Feeding self-care deficit	*Feeding self-care deficit* RT decreased strength and endurance	*Feeding self-care deficit* RT decreased strength and endurance AEB inability to maintain fork in hand from plate to mouth
Ineffective airway clearance	*Ineffective airway clearance* RT fatigue	*Ineffective airway clearance* RT fatigue AEB dyspnea at rest
Anxiety	*Anxiety* RT change in role functioning	*Anxiety* RT change in role functioning AEB insomnia, poor eye contact, and quivering voice
Deficient knowledge	*Deficient knowledge* RT misinterpretation of information	*Deficient knowledge* RT misinterpretation of information AEB inaccurate return demonstration of self-injection
Spiritual distress	*Spiritual distress* RT separation from religious ties	*Spiritual distress* RT separation from religious ties AEB crying and withdrawal

Data from American Nurses Association. (2004). *Nursing: Scope and standards of practice.* Washington, DC: Author.

- *Actual diagnoses* are those problems that are already in existence. Examples of actual diagnoses include *excess fluid volume* RT intravenous infusion therapy overload and *anxiety* RT unknown results of breast biopsy.
- *Risk diagnoses* are identified when there is a recognized vulnerability for the client to exhibit a problem, but that response has not yet manifested itself. Examples of risk diagnoses include *risk for poisoning* RT increased mobility of infant and failure to have house childproofed and *risk for deficient fluid volume* RT excessive number of stools.
- *Health promotion diagnoses* identify behaviors that indicate a desire to increase well-being.
- *Wellness diagnoses* identify the client condition or state of being healthy that may be enhanced by deliberate health-promoting activities. These consist of a one-part statement (no "related to" phrase) that uses the label "readiness for enhanced" followed by the state to be enhanced. Examples of wellness diagnoses include *readiness for enhanced community coping* and *readiness for enhanced spiritual well-being.*

TAXONOMY OF NURSING DIAGNOSES

The **taxonomy of nursing diagnoses** classifies diagnostic labels based on which human responses the client is demonstrating in response to the actual or perceived stressor. Rather than consult the alphabetical listing of NANDA diagnoses, some nurses might find it more helpful to review the NANDA listing by pattern of human responses. This listing is called the NANDA Taxonomy II and organizes the NANDA-approved nursing diagnoses under the corresponding human

response category. NANDA Taxonomy II is composed of three levels: domains, classes, and diagnostic statements (nursing diagnoses). The 13 domains under which nursing diagnoses are placed are:

- Health promotion
- Nutrition
- Elimination/exchange
- Activity/rest
- Perception/cognition
- Self-perception
- Role relationship
- Sexuality
- Coping/stress tolerance
- Life principles
- Safety/protection
- Comfort
- Growth/development (NANDA-I, 2009, pp. 266–267)

CLINICAL JUDGMENT IN NURSING: DEVELOPING NURSING DIAGNOSES

Clinical judgment in nursing requires a firm foundation in the study of the humanities and life sciences in order to properly assess for cues related to diagnoses. The ability to cluster cues obtained during assessment, and the interpretation of assessment data to form hypotheses (potential nursing diagnoses), then drives additional assessment to validate or refute those hypotheses. The development of a nursing diagnosis is a systematic process in which certain activities

✓ NURSING CHECKLIST

DEVELOPING NURSING DIAGNOSES

- Collect data cues by comprehensive, accurate assessment activities.
- Validate data cues.
- Determine the meaning of data cues through application of critical thinking.
- Group data into clusters.
- Review the NANDA-approved list of diagnoses and related defining characteristics.
- Write the first part of the diagnostic statement.
- Identify and record the *related to* (RT) variables.
- Combine the last two steps into a two-part diagnostic statement.

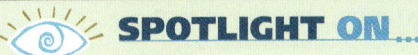

👁 SPOTLIGHT ON...

Professionalism

Identifying Data Cues

What are the relevant data cues that can be gathered from the following assessment data for Peter Zachary, age 44?

Subjective Data

"I am the father of two boys."

"I paint houses for a living."

"I go to church every Sunday."

"I always seem to be hungry, and I eat five or six times a day."

"I've gained twelve pounds this year."

Objective Data

Client is 5 feet 10 inches and weighs 204 pounds.

Protruding abdomen over belt and waist of pants.

Double chin.

Fleshy, loose upper arms.

Dimpling of buttocks.

One bowel movement every other day.

Vital signs: P 92; BP 130/80; R 17; T 98.9°F.

Red scaly patches on skin.

Nonproductive cough.

Birthmark right upper hip.

need to be executed; see the Nursing Checklist for steps in developing nursing diagnoses.

GENERATING CUES

In the assessment phase, the nurse collects data cues from the client. Cues are small amounts of data that are applied to the decision-making process. Nurses should be attentive to the cues gathered from the interview, health history, symptom analysis, physical examination, and laboratory and diagnostic data since they increase the index of suspicion and stimulate further observation of additional sets of cues. Examples of cues might be poor skin turgor, parched lips, dry skin, decreased urine output, and complaint of thirst. The expert nurse immediately processes these cues and together with the client determines a nursing diagnosis, plans client outcomes, and implements therapeutic nursing interventions. The novice nurse must proceed more cautiously and use additional time to process these data cues. See the accompanying Spotlight On display on identifying data cues.

VALIDATING CUES

After reviewing the data cues, the nurse validates that information and examines it carefully to determine if the information is accurate and complete (see Figure 7-1). This process involves verifying subjective and objective data. Verification can be done by interviewing the client again and reassessing data cues.

INTERPRETING CUES

Through interpretation of data cues and use of critical thinking strategies, the nurse assigns a meaning to the data cues. In order to interpret subjective and objective data cues, the nurse should ask the following questions that stimulate critical thinking:

- What is this information telling me?
- Is there a pattern?

- Can this information be put together?
- Is the information falling into a logical arrangement?
- Is the information forming natural groupings?

Interpreting data cues is one example of critical thinking that the nurse must do on a daily basis. Specifically, the synthesis of information that takes place when interpreting data

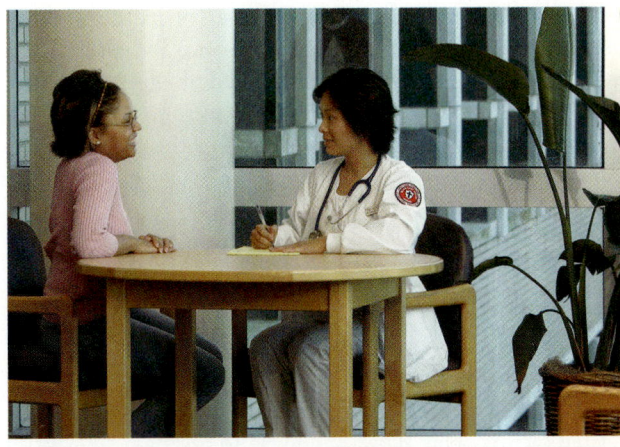

FIGURE 7-1 This nurse is validating the cues collected from this client during the assessment phase DELMAR/CENGAGE LEARNING

✓ NURSINGCHECKLIST

Critical Thinking

The following questions should be considered by the nurse in the development of a nursing diagnosis:

- Do I have enough data to formulate a nursing diagnosis?
- Are any data missing?
- Is there any information in my database that seems incomplete or uncertain?
- Should I talk to the client and family again?
- What data fit together or have something in common?
- What specific cues from the client made me form this conclusion?
- What elements of this situation, condition, or problem can be enhanced or resolved by therapeutic nursing interventions?
- What elements need to be referred to another discipline (e.g., medicine, social services, dietary)?

cues demonstrates how essential it is for the nurse to think critically. Interpreting cues is pivotal for correctly diagnosing actual or potential problems or wellness states. The accompanying Nursing Checklist provides questions that are helpful in developing appropriate diagnoses.

CLUSTERING CUES

Once the cues have been collected, validated, and interpreted, the data are then grouped into clusters. A cluster is a set of data cues in which relationships between and among cues are established to identify a specific health state or condition. Related pieces of information about the client are grouped together. Conclusions are drawn from the data cues. One piece of information by itself can be misleading. This idea is analogous to the assembly of a jigsaw puzzle. One puzzle piece by itself does not give an accurate idea of the picture. In the same way, one data cue (or piece of assessment data) does not have much relevance by itself. When more pieces of the puzzle are assembled or when more data assessment cues are put together, the nurse may have a beginning idea of what the puzzle picture or the client's health looks like.

USING NANDA-APPROVED NURSING DIAGNOSES

After the data have been organized into clusters, the nurse needs to consult the NANDA-approved diagnoses, carefully reviewing the definitions, defining characteristics, and risk or related factors. This allows the nurse to ascertain similarities and differences between the clusters and NANDA diagnoses. The clustered data are then matched with a particular

NANDA diagnosis. It is important that the nurse review the actual definitions and defining characteristics to ensure that the diagnosis being made is accurate; reliance on only the diagnostic statement can lead to inaccuracies in diagnosis.

WRITING THE NURSING DIAGNOSIS STATEMENT

The nursing diagnosis selected from NANDA-approved diagnoses becomes the diagnostic label, the first part of the diagnosis statement. Etiologies can be identified using the related factors listed with each nursing diagnosis. The appropriate etiology is selected and joined to the first part of the statement with the "related to" phrase. Because the NANDA list of nursing diagnoses is constantly evolving, there may be times when no etiology is provided. In such cases, the nurse should attempt to describe likely contributing factors to the client's condition. In a two-part statement, the nursing diagnosis for an overweight client would be *imbalanced nutrition: more than body requirements* RT excessive food intake. The three-part statement would be *imbalanced nutrition: more than body requirements* RT excessive food intake AEB weight gain, increased appetite, excess adipose tissue, and increased abdominal girth.

AVOIDING ERRORS IN DEVELOPMENT AND USE OF NURSING DIAGNOSES

Following is a discussion of common errors that may occur in the process of developing nursing diagnoses. Being aware of possible errors helps decrease the likelihood of their occurrence.

ASSESSMENT ERRORS

There is an underlying assumption that nurses have adequate assessment skills and are knowledgeable about what data need to be collected. However, this is not always the case. The novice nurse may have only rudimentary assessment skills and limited clinical experience. Experienced nurses are challenged to keep current and sometimes are ill equipped to collect appropriate assessment data. Errors may be made when writing a nursing diagnosis due to an incomplete database or inappropriately collected assessment data. When assessment data are missing, regardless of the cause, the end result is either an omission of nursing diagnoses, inaccurate diagnoses, or incorrect qualifying statements about the diagnoses.

Incomplete Assessment Data

Incomplete collection can occur when the nurse has neither had nor taken the time to appropriately address all subjective and objective data. For example, during admission of a new client to a health care facility, a nurse is interrupted during the data collection and fails to return to finish the admission process.

Restricted data collection occurs when a client is unable or unwilling to provide the necessary data. An example would be a newly admitted client with a cerebrovascular accident who has impaired speech and can provide only limited assessment data.

Validation Errors

Failure to validate occurs when the nurse does not confirm previously collected data. An example would be failure by the nurse to recheck an admission blood pressure that was elevated. A follow-up blood pressure may have revealed a transient elevation due to the stress of the admission process.

Misinterpreting Data

Misinterpretation can occur when the meaning attached to the data is incorrect. An example would be a client who comes to the ambulatory care clinic and presents with several signs and symptoms, including a reported 4-pound weight gain that month. Further investigation indicates this finding is not related to increased adipose tissue but, rather, is associated with fluid retention that accompanies an edematous state. See the accompanying Respecting Our Differences display.

DIAGNOSTIC ERRORS

Errors can also occur in the nursing diagnostic process during the clustering, interpretation, and statement of the diagnosis. Critical thinking skills and the use of standardized nursing language, such as NANDA diagnoses, help ensure accuracy in the diagnostic statement.

Inappropriate Data Clustering

Inappropriate data clustering may occur when the nurse lacks sufficient theoretical knowledge and clinical expertise in order to appropriately cluster data cues. An example would be the client who visits an industrial clinic with complaints of flulike symptoms, stomach cramps, and vomiting. The nurse attributes the vomiting to the influenza, but further analysis indicates that this client is actually manifesting symptoms of a toxic reaction to a prescribed drug that is causing the vomiting.

Incorrect Writing of the Nursing Diagnosis Statement

Incorrect writing of the statement can occur when the nurse does not follow the guidelines for formulating a two- or three-part statement. An example would be in the two-part statement *imbalanced nutrition: less than body requirements* RT renal disease. Renal disease is a medical diagnosis, and, according to the guidelines, the etiology must be a human response that the nurse is licensed and competent to treat. This diagnosis would be better stated as *imbalanced nutrition: less than body requirements* RT inadequate intake of an appropriate renal diet.

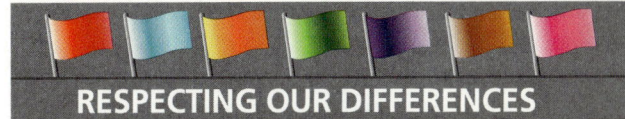

RESPECTING OUR DIFFERENCES

Errors in Data Interpretation

Your client, a 35-year-old married man with two children, has been discharged home following open-heart surgery. During your first two visits to assess the client's progress, you notice that the client seems reluctant to leave his bed and expresses minimal interest in topics other than the television programs he has been watching. When you inquire about his attempts to participate in leisure activities with his wife and children, he shrugs his shoulders and appears bored with the discussion. On the basis of this assessment, you formulate a nursing diagnosis of *deficient diversional activity* RT client's lack of engagement in recreational activities. If you were to determine on your third visit that the client has refrained from these kinds of activities because of his fear of reopening the incision, how would you reconcile the discrepancy between the assessment data gathered and the nursing diagnosis that was developed? Do you think that your values relating to this client's conduct may have played a role in the misinterpretation of the data and the resulting nursing diagnosis?

Values play an important role in interpretation of data, clustering of data, and ultimately the development of the diagnosis. Nurses must be cognizant of personal biases, being careful not to impose their value systems on clients. Personal prejudices should be avoided in the diagnostic statement. The Nursing Checklist provides selected questions that nurses

✓ NURSINGCHECKLIST

Avoiding Common Diagnostic Errors

When nurses are in the process of developing nursing diagnoses, the following questions should be considered:

- Am I saying the same thing twice?
- Am I using the medical diagnosis in my nursing diagnosis?
- Am I implying negligence or blaming anyone in my diagnosis?
- Have I stated the diagnosis with a client response or a client need?
- Am I making any value judgments about the client?

can ask themselves in order to avoid making mistakes when developing nursing diagnoses.

Nurses must also remember to focus on the client when developing a nursing diagnosis. The problem statement is client centered, not nurse centered. The nursing diagnosis directs nursing actions by providing the focus for evaluating outcomes.

LIMITATIONS OF NURSING DIAGNOSIS

A number of limitations and professional concerns are associated with nursing diagnosis. The primary concern is directed toward the lack of consensus among nurses regarding the NANDA-approved nursing diagnosis list. Criticisms about the list include disagreement over specific labels in the classification system and the perception that the list is confining, incomplete, illness and disease oriented, and confusing. Many nurses are not familiar with the NANDA list and do not know how to use it or feel "it doesn't have the diagnosis" they need. It should be noted that this list is not meant to be inclusive. Development and refinement of diagnoses continue to be a focus of NANDA conferences. In addition, nurses may disagree with or refuse to use diagnoses such as noncompliance or knowledge deficit (Carpenito-Moyet, 2007). In these instances, the nurse then has the choice and the right to not use these specific diagnoses.

Novice nurses need to know nursing diagnosis and nursing process in order to understand how the discipline of nursing intersects with the other health care providers. NANDA-I (2009) recognizes that health care continues to move toward an interdisciplinary, client-focused care environment that requires standardization of languages across disciplines. Many acute care facilities use an interdisciplinary care plan such as care maps or critical pathways to monitor client outcomes. All health care providers use the same care plan to document the client's response to specific interventions. Common "client problems" listed on a critical pathway are written as nursing diagnoses such as *risk for infection* or *risk for injury.*

Legal considerations concerning the use of nursing diagnoses also exist. Nurses are accountable for their actions and must document their interventions. If a nursing diagnosis is inappropriate or a nursing diagnosis list is incomplete and, as a result, the interventions are inappropriate or lacking, the nurse is liable for these errors in clinical judgment. These errors can be avoided by collecting comprehensive assessment data and by critically analyzing these data.

OVERCOMING BARRIERS AND LIMITATIONS TO NURSING DIAGNOSIS

NANDA's language is relatively new compared to medical language that has existed for several hundred years. Some nurses would rather wait until the NANDA listing is complete before they use it. However, it is unrealistic to think that a system such as NANDA should not be used until it is completed. Indeed, as nursing science continues to evolve, nursing diagnoses will be added, removed, or refined; there will never be a "completed" list of nursing or medical diagnoses for this very reason. The ever-changing health care scene dictates that nurses participate in evolving methods to communicate within the health care industry.

Another barrier to the use of nursing diagnoses is the numerous approaches for application that are found in the nursing literature. Due to these various methods, it may be difficult for nurses to choose one method with which they feel comfortable. Nurses may also be unable and unwilling to use nursing diagnoses because of incomplete knowledge about the process and disagreements about wording.

After identifying the existence of barriers to the use of nursing diagnoses, it is possible to design strategies to overcome them. One strategy is to develop a common nursing language that is globally used throughout the profession. Nursing diagnostic terminology serves this purpose. Familiarity with this language empowers the nurse to communicate more effectively with other nurses and health care team members. Effective communication, in turn, improves the accuracy in nursing diagnoses. Ultimately, the quality of care should improve, and the costs associated with that care should decrease. Due to the fact that many health care facilities are asking nurses to do more with fewer resources, nurses are challenged to learn more efficient ways of performing their duties. Nurses' time is spent more efficiently if less time is spent deciphering meanings of words.

The move toward electronic health records is making it more important than ever to have standardized nursing languages. As health care settings are required to communicate with other organizations to improve client management, it will be important to have standardized languages within those electronic systems so that different information systems are able to "talk to" one another by sending and receiving data that diverse systems can readily understand. The current method of "free text charting" will become a thing of the past, and standardized nursing languages representing nursing diagnoses, interventions, and outcomes will be critical to the success of these information systems. See the Nursing Process Highlight on page 121 in order to practice developing a diagnostic statement. The accompanying Uncovering the Evidence display on page 121 describes how education can improve the use and documentation of nursing diagnoses.

When a nurse encounters client situations that do not readily fit the nursing diagnosis language, every attempt should be made to describe the phenomena. The nurse may be on the threshold of documenting the need for a new, as-yet-undiscovered nursing diagnosis. Indeed, the work of NANDA is done by nurses working in client care areas, education, and research. Potential diagnoses are submitted to NANDA for approval based on research in the area of concern. Nurses are strongly encouraged to share their needs for nursing diagnosis language with NANDA so that the language will grow, become more inclusive, and become more usable for nurses in practice.

UNCOVERING THE

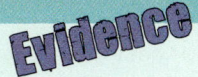

TITLE OF STUDY

"Improved Quality of Nursing Documentation: Results of a Nursing Diagnoses, Interventions, and Outcomes Implementation Study"

AUTHORS

M. Muller-Staub, I. Needham, M. Odenbreit, M. A. Lavin, and T. van Achterberg

PURPOSE

To evaluate the impact of the quality of nursing diagnoses, interventions, and outcomes in an acute care setting after implementation of an educational program.

METHODS

This experimental design study utilized pre- and post-tests on nurses who participated in two educational sessions about the use of nursing diagnoses, interventions, and outcomes. Nursing records were randomly selected for analysis before and after the implementation of the educational strategy.

FINDINGS

Significant improvements in the quality of documented nursing diagnoses, interventions, and outcomes were found following the implementation of the educational program.

IMPLICATIONS

Education can be a viable strategy for improving documentation of nursing diagnoses, interventions, and outcomes.

Muller-Staub, M., Needham, I., Odenbreit, M., Lavin, M. A., & van Achterberg, T. (2007). Improved quality of nursing documentation: Results of a nursing diagnoses, interventions, and outcomes implementation study. *International Journal of Nursing Terminologies & Classifications: The Official Journal of NANDA International, 18*(1), 1–2.

As nurses collaborate on the refinement of nursing diagnoses, it may be possible to agree on certain aspects of the language. The achievement of this goal will end the use of multiple approaches and will make choices less complicated. Enhanced communication among nurses in everyday settings and among professionals who convene nationally and internationally to exchange ideas about nursing diagnoses is essential.

Most nursing educational programs now offer standardized content related to nursing diagnoses. In addition, experienced nurses need opportunities to review principles of nursing diagnoses. See the Nursing Checklist for a list of strategies that are helpful for overcoming barriers to the use of nursing diagnoses.

✓ NURSING CHECKLIST

Strategies for Optimizing the Use of Nursing Diagnoses

Nurses should implement the following strategies when working with nursing diagnoses:

- Agree on a common language.
- Acknowledge and embrace the fluid nature of the language of nursing diagnosis.
- Discuss the purpose and value of nursing diagnosis with administrators and medical staff.
- Support colleagues when they use nursing diagnosis language.
- Adopt a positive attitude toward the principles and taxonomy of nursing diagnosis.
- Be willing to add to the existing body of knowledge by describing unusual nursing phenomena.
- Participate in conferences, workshops, and other educational activities that advance and promote nursing diagnosis.
- Continue communicating with other nurses about nursing diagnosis.

NURSING PROCESS HIGHLIGHT

Diagnosis

Example

Mr. Lowder is a 62-year-old male who was admitted last night through the emergency room because of difficulty breathing. He was also experiencing some difficulty voiding. His lower extremities are very swollen. History reveals he smokes one pack of cigarettes a day and has done this for the past 45 years. His vital signs are P 112; R 30; BP 172/96; T 101.1°F. He has an eighth-grade education, attends church every week, is estranged from his daughter, and says, "I hate hospitals because my mother died in one."

Questions

1. From the data cues in this case study, group data into clusters.
2. Look at the NANDA list of diagnoses and see which diagnoses "fit" best with your data clusters.
3. Write the first part of the NANDA diagnosis for each cluster.
4. Attempt to identify etiological (related to) factors for the list you started in Step 3.
5. Write two-part nursing diagnosis statements by combining Steps 3 and 4.
6. Identify whether the nursing diagnoses on your list are actual, possible, risk, or wellness-oriented nursing diagnosis statements.
7. Prioritize the nursing diagnoses.

KEY CONCEPTS

- Nursing diagnosis is the second step in the nursing process and is the clinical judgment about individual, family, or community (aggregate) responses to actual or risk problems, wellness states, or syndromes.

- Through the efforts of NANDA and the ANA, the identification and validation of nursing diagnosis as the second step of the nursing process has been substantiated and forms the basis for professional accountability.

- Nursing diagnosis contributes to a clearer understanding of knowledge unique to nursing, improves communication among nurses and other health care professionals, promotes individualized client care, and supports theory development and nursing research.

- Nursing diagnoses can be written as either two-part statements (diagnostic label and etiology) or three-part statements (diagnostic label, etiology, and defining characteristics).

- The NANDA nursing diagnosis taxonomy is composed of 13 domains: health promotion, elimination/exchange, perception/cognition, role relationship, coping/stress tolerance, safety/protection, growth/development, nutrition, activity/rest, self-perception, sexuality, life principles, and comfort.

- The process of developing a nursing diagnosis includes analysis of assessment cues, validation of cues, interpretation of cues, clustering of data, consulting NANDA's list of approved nursing diagnoses, and writing the nursing diagnosis statement.

- The nurse who is knowledgeable about the components of the nursing diagnosis process and is equipped to develop the diagnostic statement is able to make appropriate decisions regarding therapeutic nursing interventions.

- To avoid committing errors in the nursing diagnostic process, nurses should ensure that the data collection is complete, that the interpretation of the data is accurate and based upon the nursing and not the medical diagnosis, and that the client's response to a health problem is amenable to therapeutic nursing interventions.

- The barriers that have been identified as preventing the use of nursing diagnosis are the constraints on the time nurses can devote to client care, the continuing organization of health care according to medical diagnosis, the inapplicability of the list of nursing diagnoses to every client situation, the constantly evolving refinement of the nursing diagnosis language, and the availability of numerous approaches for formulation and application of nursing diagnoses.

- Although barriers to the use of nursing diagnosis may be present, they may be overcome by employing specific strategies such as agreeing on a common language, supporting colleagues' use of nursing diagnoses, adopting a nonjudgmental attitude, contributing to the development of nursing diagnosis language through submission of new diagnoses or revising existing diagnoses in the NANDA taxonomy, and continuing to communicate with other nurses at national and international levels.

REVIEW QUESTIONS

1. A nurse reads the following list of nursing diagnoses on a client's plan of care. Which of these statements is written correctly as a nursing diagnosis?
   a. Acute pain RT pain in right foot
   b. Impaired skin integrity RT infrequent repositioning by staff
   c. Impaired swallowing RT stasis of food in oral cavity after chewing
   d. Chronic confusion RT Alzheimer's disease

2. A client limps into the clinic with pain in the right foot. The physical examination shows that the client is 5 feet 6 inches tall, weighs 275 pounds, and has edema in the right lower extremity. Which of the following statements would be an accurate nursing diagnosis for this client?
   a. Acute pain RT pain in right foot
   b. Imbalanced nutrition: more than body requirements

   c. Impaired mobility RT pain
   d. Risk for injury RT obesity

3. A client who underwent hip replacement surgery has a nursing diagnosis of impaired physical mobility RT pain. Which of the following nursing interventions would be a priority for a client with this diagnosis?
   a. Elevating the client's foot
   b. Administering the prn analgesic medication as ordered
   c. Providing a walker for ambulation
   d. Teaching the client techniques for safely transferring from the bed to a wheelchair

4. An elderly client with thin, dry skin has a nursing diagnosis of impaired skin integrity. Which of the following nursing interventions should be implemented? Select all that apply.
   a. Repositioning the client every 2 hours

b. Keeping the bed linens dry
c. Reducing the client's fluid intake
d. Encouraging the client to consume a high-fiber diet
e. Making sure that the bed linens are wrinkle-free
f. Instructing the client to take deep breaths and cough

5. The nurse makes a nursing diagnosis of risk for impaired physical mobility RT pain. Which of the following is the risk factor for this client?
   a. Immobility
   b. Impaired skin integrity
   c. Malnutrition
   d. Pain

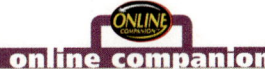

online companion

Visit the DeLaune and Ladner online companion resource at **www.delmar.cengage.com** for additional content and study aids. Click on Online Companions, then select the Nursing discipline.

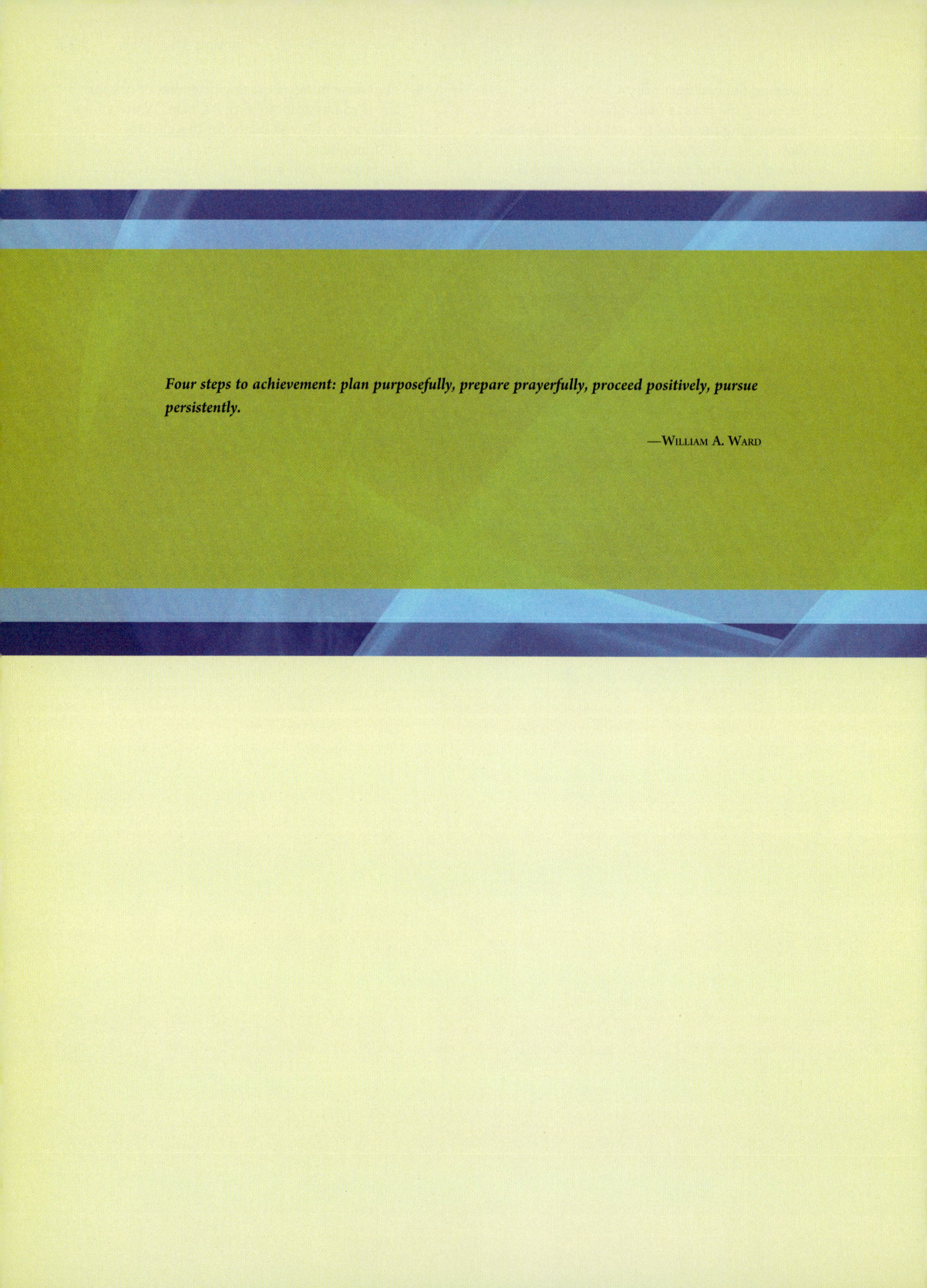

Four steps to achievement: plan purposefully, prepare prayerfully, proceed positively, pursue persistently.

—WILLIAM A. WARD

CHAPTER 8

Planning and Outcome Identification

COMPETENCIES

1. Explain the purposes of outcome identification and planning.
2. Describe four elements of the planning component.
3. Describe characteristics of goals and expected outcomes.
4. Discuss the five components in the construction of goals and expected outcomes.
5. Describe problems frequently encountered in planning nursing care.
6. Explain strategies to improve the planning of nursing care.
7. Differentiate dependent, independent, and interdependent nursing interventions.

KEY TERMS

collaboration	independent nursing	nursing order
consultation	interventions	ongoing planning
criteria	initial planning	planning
dependent nursing interventions	interdependent nursing	plan of care
discharge planning	interventions	rationale
expected outcome	long-term goal	short-term goal
goal	nursing intervention	

Planning, the third step of the nursing process, includes the formulation of guidelines used to establish the client's plan of care. Preceding this step is the collection of assessment data and the formulation of nursing diagnoses. After a nurse thoroughly assesses a client and determines the client's unique nursing diagnoses (or problems), a plan of action is developed with specific goals to resolve the nursing diagnoses or health problems. Following the planning component, the nursing process continues with implementation of nursing interventions and evaluation of the client's response to the plan of care.

This chapter explains the planning component of the nursing process. The planning concept is illustrated with theory and examples. Strategies for effective planning of quality nursing care are described together with problems frequently encountered in this stage of the nursing process. The role of critical thinking in planning and outcome identification is emphasized.

PURPOSES OF PLANNING AND OUTCOME IDENTIFICATION

The American Nurses Association (2004) identifies outcome identification and planning as essential principles for ensuring the delivery of competent nursing care and outlines these components in terms of their significance within the nursing process. Although the overall purpose of a client's plan of care should be to maintain or improve health at an optimal level, planning is a framework on which to base scientific nursing practice. Therefore, planning is done in order to provide quality nursing care. Planning also improves staff communication and provides continuity in the delivery of individualized, quality nursing care to all clients. The four critical elements of planning include:

- Establishing priorities
- Setting goals and developing expected outcomes (outcome identification)
- Planning nursing interventions (with collaboration and consultation as needed)
- Documenting

PROCESS OF PLANNING AND OUTCOME IDENTIFICATION

The five steps of the nursing process are at the very core of using scientific reasoning for the delivery of individualized, quality nursing care in any setting (Doenges, Moorhouse, & Geissler, 2006). The ability to make appropriate decisions based on a strong knowledge base and problem-solving strategies is an expected behavior of the professional nurse.

CRITICAL THINKING

Nurses must think critically in order to make intelligent decisions. By applying the critical thinking skills inherent in the nursing process to the client's identified nursing diagnoses, the nurse can focus on resolving the client's problems with greater proficiency.

Planning is sequential, dynamic, and future oriented. Planning includes establishing priorities, identifying goals and expected outcomes, developing nursing interventions, and documenting the client's plan of care. Appropriate guidelines are used to prioritize urgent needs. The client's nursing diagnoses are determined and then ranked by mutual agreement between the nurse and client or significant others. The planning component continues with thorough examination of this prioritized list of nursing diagnoses and determination of the client's goals and desired expected outcomes. After a clear picture is obtained regarding the diagnoses and goals, the nursing interventions can be planned to achieve the desired outcomes.

The planning of nursing care occurs in three phases: initial, ongoing, and discharge. Each type of planning contributes to the coordination of the client's comprehensive plan of care. **Initial planning** involves the development of the beginning of care by the nurse who performs the admission assessment and gathers the comprehensive admission assessment data. Because of progressively shorter lengths of hospitalization, initial planning is important in addressing each prioritized problem, identifying appropriate client goals, and correlating nursing care to hasten resolution of the client's problems. **Ongoing planning** entails continuous updating of the client's plan of care. Every nurse who cares for the client is involved in ongoing planning. As new information about the client is gathered and evaluated, revisions may be formulated and the initial plan of care becomes further individualized to the client. **Discharge planning** involves critical anticipation and planning for the client's needs after discharge. Discharge planning is a multidisciplinary team effort that focuses on providing a seamless transition across the continuum of care.

Establishing long-term goals is important in successful discharge planning. Goal setting assists in coordinating all health care team members to accomplish the same overall purpose, that is, client discharge. Coordination promotes continuity of care into settings such as restorative care or home health and requires the establishment of priority needs (see the accompanying Nursing Process Highlight display).

In the planning phase, the nurse uses organized (critical) thinking in order to make sound clinical decisions. To think critically is to examine an issue purposefully from a goal-directed perspective. Critical thinking is based on scientific principles and methodologies (Alfaro-LeFevre, 2008). Therefore, critical thinking is necessary for the development of objectives and in the formulation of a blueprint to achieve those objectives. The formulation of objectives is accomplished by using valid and reliable data previously gathered during the assessment phase of the nursing process.

ESTABLISHING PRIORITIES

When an individual client has more than one diagnosis, the nurse and client need to establish priorities to identify which nursing diagnosis will be addressed initially in the plan of care (Carpenito-Moyet, 2007). By communicating this decision-making process to other members of the health care team, the nurse encourages an orderly approach to the achievement of optimal health for each client.

The establishment of priorities is the first element of planning. When establishing priorities, the nurse examines the client's nursing diagnoses and ranks them in order of physiological or psychological importance. This method organizes a client's nursing diagnoses into a systematic framework for the planning of nursing care. The diagnoses should be mutually ranked by the nurse and client. Involving the client in shared decision-making power helps motivate the client and gives the client a feeling of control, which inspires successful achievement of each goal (Doenges et al., 2006).

Various guidelines are used in determining which nursing diagnosis will be addressed initially. The client's safety, basic needs, and desires, as well as anticipation of future diagnoses, must be considered. One of the most common methods of setting priorities is the consideration of Maslow's hierarchy of needs, which requires that a life-threatening diagnosis be given more urgency than a non–life-threatening diagnosis. Once the basic physiological needs (e.g., respiration, nutrition, hydration, elimination) are met to some degree, the nurse may consider needs on the next level of the hierarchy (e.g., safe environment, stable living condition) and progress up the hierarchy until all the client's nursing diagnoses have been prioritized.

A useful guide for the beginning nursing student would be to examine each nursing diagnosis, determine its level of need, and rank the need in order of priority. Table 8-1 illustrates this process.

Another consideration in the designation of priorities is client preferences. If at all possible, the client should be involved in the decision-making process of establishing priorities. The client must participate in the identification of priorities so that the nature of the problem as well as the client's values are reflected in the selected course of action. If the priorities are not mutually determined, the client's problems will likely remain unresolved. See the accompanying Nursing Process Highlight display on setting mutual priorities.

An additional point regarding the establishment of priorities is the anticipation of future diagnoses. Nursing diagnoses of low and moderate priorities often involve the prevention of anticipated potential or risk diagnoses. Although potential

NURSING PROCESS HIGHLIGHT

Planning

Prioritizing Nursing Diagnoses

Mr. Clyde Morrison, an elderly homeless client, was admitted to the hospital with a medical diagnosis of malnutrition. Identified nursing diagnoses include imbalanced nutrition, less than body requirements related to inability to procure appropriate food; constipation related to inadequate fluid intake; and disturbed body image related to feelings of inadequacy and inability to live up to identified standards. What should the priority ranking of this client's nursing diagnoses be?

TABLE 8-1 Ranking Nursing Diagnoses

NURSING DIAGNOSIS	MASLOW'S HIERARCHY OF NEEDS	RANK
Anxiety related to hospitalization	Safety and security	Moderate
Ineffective coping	Self-esteem	Low
Ineffective airway clearance related to excessive secretions	Physiological	High

Delmar/Cengage Learning

nursing diagnoses may not be a current threat to the client, their seriousness may require that the nurse consider the development of nursing interventions directed toward prevention of the problems. For example, a client in the postanesthesia care unit may have a high-priority nursing diagnosis of *ineffective breathing pattern* related to the anesthesia and sedative drugs. Despite the fact that the client currently has no problem in this area, this diagnosis is indeed the basis for the Postanesthesia Care Unit protocol of monitoring the client closely.

Establishing priorities does not mean that one diagnosis must be totally resolved before giving attention to another diagnosis. Nursing interventions for several diagnoses may be carried out simultaneously. However, at times, it is crucial that the nurse and client correctly identify the order of priority of the client's nursing diagnoses so that maximum effort can be directed toward resolution of the most urgent diagnosis; see Table 8-2.

ESTABLISHING GOALS AND EXPECTED OUTCOMES

After assessing the client, formulating nursing diagnoses, and establishing priorities, the nurse sets goals and identifies and establishes expected outcomes for each nursing diagnosis. The purposes of setting goals and expected outcomes are to provide guidelines for individualized nursing interventions and to establish evaluation criteria for measuring the effectiveness of the nursing care plan.

NURSING PROCESS HIGHLIGHT

Diagnosis

Setting Mutual Priorities

Mr. Jules Gordon has been admitted with third-degree burns of approximately 80% of his body. He is particularly concerned with the nursing diagnosis of *body image disturbance* related to scarring and disfigurement, whereas the nurse's major concern is with the nursing diagnosis of deficient fluid volume related to fluid shifts because it is far more life threatening. In this situation, the nurse's and client's priorities are not set mutually because they have separate primary goals. This situation may lead to conflict and interfere with goal accomplishment. What are some ways that this situation can be approached so that both nursing diagnoses may be resolved?

A **goal** is an aim, an intent, or an end. A goal is a broad or globally written statement describing the intended or desired change in the client's behavior, response, or outcome. An **expected outcome** is a detailed, specific statement that describes the methods through which the goal will be achieved. Expected outcomes are addressed through direct nursing care activities, such as client teaching.

Goals

Written goals need to be constructed clearly in order to improve the chances that goals will be achieved. When goals are clearly written, their establishment provides direction for the nursing plan of care and for determination of effectiveness in the evaluation of nursing interventions. A guideline is provided for the desired change in the client, and the client has a clear idea of the direction to be taken for achieving resolution of each nursing diagnosis. Goals establish appropriate evaluation criteria to measure the effectiveness of planned nursing interventions that are directed at resolving the client's individual nursing diagnoses.

Goals should be established to meet the immediate, as well as long-term prevention and rehabilitation, needs of the client. A **short-term goal** is a statement written in objective format demonstrating an expectation to be achieved in resolution of the nursing diagnosis in a short period of time, usually in a few hours or days. A **long-term goal** is a statement written in objective format demonstrating an expectation to be achieved in resolution of the nursing diagnosis over a longer period of time, usually over weeks or months (Alfaro-LeFevre, 2008). See Table 8-3 on page 129 for examples of short-term and long-term goals.

Another consideration is the accuracy in identifying the etiology of the problem. If the etiology of the problem is incorrectly identified, the client may meet the short-term

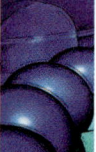

TABLE 8-2 Prioritizing Nursing Diagnoses with Accompanying Nursing Implications

PRIORITY	DIAGNOSIS	NURSING IMPLICATIONS
High	Ineffective breathing pattern	• Assess breath sounds. • Auscultate lungs. • Monitor vital signs. • Reposition client.
Moderate	Risk for impaired skin integrity	• Perform comprehensive skin assessment. • Keep skin clean and dry. • Provide turning schedule.
Low	Ineffective coping	• Assist to identify problem. • Encourage keeping daily journal. • Teach client strategies for expressing feelings.

Delmar/Cengage Learning

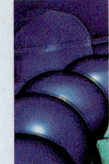

TABLE 8-3 Short- and Long-Term Goals

NURSING DIAGNOSIS: *CHRONIC PAIN* RELATED TO RHEUMATOID ARTHRITIS

Short-term: Focused on etiology	Verbalizes the presence of pain Identifies factors that influence the pain experience Self-administers pain medication as appropriate
Long-term: Focused on the problem	Verbalizes comfort

Delmar/Cengage Learning

TABLE 8-4 Relationship between Nursing Diagnoses and Goals and Expected Outcomes

NURSING DIAGNOSIS	GOALS	EXPECTED OUTCOMES
Sleep deprivation	Client will sleep uninterrupted for 6 hours.	Client will request back massage for relaxation. Client will set limits on family visitation.
Ineffective tissue perfusion: peripheral	Client will have palpable peripheral pulses within 1 week.	Client will identify three factors to improve peripheral circulation. Client's feet will be warm to touch.

Delmar/Cengage Learning

goal but the problem will not be resolved. Thus, it is important to correctly identify the etiology of the problem.

Expected Outcomes

After the goal is established, the expected outcomes can be identified based on the goal. Given the client's unique situation and resources, expected outcomes are constructed to be:

- Realistic
- Mutually desired by the client and nurse
- Attainable within a defined time period

These desired outcomes are the measurable steps toward achieving the previously established goals (Doenges et al., 2006). An expected outcome depicts measurable behavioral change or evidence of change in the client when the goal has been met. Several expected outcomes may be required for each goal. Expected outcomes are used in the evaluation process by providing a standard for comparison to determine if the client successfully accomplished the goal. Because nursing care is based on a holistic approach, expected outcomes may be written in the spiritual, emotional, physiological, developmental, and social dimensions.

When goals and outcomes are written clearly, the nurse can select nursing interventions to ensure that the client's baseline data are thoroughly assessed, individual client needs are identified, and appropriate approaches are used to address needs.

Usually, each nursing diagnosis has one global goal and several expected outcomes. In writing the goal statement, the nurse considers the nursing diagnosis for the formulation of a suitable client behavior that illustrates reduction or alleviation of the nursing diagnosis. These concepts are demonstrated in Table 8-4. In the construction of both goals and expected outcome objectives, essential components include the subject, task statement, criteria, conditions (if necessary), and time frame (Doenges et al., 2006).

See the Uncovering the Evidence on page 130 display for more on goal setting.

COMPONENTS OF GOALS AND EXPECTED OUTCOMES

There are five components of well-constructed goals and expected outcomes: subject, task statement, criteria, conditions, and time frame. An in-depth discussion of each component of an appropriately written goal follows. For clarity of each concept, examples are provided. The examples are designed with the intent of developing skills in goal construction.

Subject

The component to be considered initially in writing a goal is the subject. The subject identifies the person who will perform the desired behavior or meet the goal. In a client-centered plan of nursing care, the client is the person who needs to achieve a desired change in behavior. See the accompanying Nursing Process Highlight for an application of the subject component.

Task Statement

The next component in writing goals is the task statement or the action verb. This component describes what the client will do to achieve the expected change in behavior. The task statement enables the evaluator to determine achievement of the observable behavior. When the actual behavior is stated as a task statement that can be clearly and directly measured, the nurse can determine whether the client is demonstrating achievement of the goal.

Only one task statement should be used for each goal. It is clearer to write separate goals than to try to accurately

UNCOVERING THE

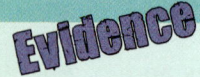

TITLE OF STUDY

"Healthcare Professional versus Patient Goal Setting in Intermittent Allergic Rhinitis"

AUTHORS

J. O'Conner, C. Seeto, B. Saini, S. Bosnic-Anticevich, I. Krass, C. Armour, and L. Smith

PURPOSE

To compare the effect of goal setting by a health care professional with client goal setting for the self-management of intermittent allergic rhinitis on severity of symptoms and quality of life.

METHODS

A 6-week parallel group study in which Group A participants designated relevant goals and strategies for responding to allergic rhinitis. Group B participants had their goals and strategies established by a health care professional. The main outcome measures were client-perceived symptom severity and quality of life.

FINDINGS

Both groups demonstrated significant improvements in quality of life and reduction of symptom severity. Group B symptom severity scores improved more. Group B set a greater number of goals that had more specific strategies for improvement.

IMPLICATIONS

Self-management goals established by a health care provider that are tailored to client symptoms lead to better outcomes than goals that are established solely by the client.

O'Conner, J., Seeto, C., Saini, B., Bosnic-Anticevich, B. S., Krass, I., Armour, C., et al. (2008). Healthcare professional versus patient goal setting in intermittent allergic rhinitis. *Patient Education and Counseling, 70*(1), 111–117.

NURSING PROCESS HIGHLIGHT

Planning

Subject of Goal

1. By Saturday, the client will ambulate the entire length of the hallway three times a day.
2. The client will demonstrate the technique for self-administration of insulin by Friday.
3. The client will take own radial pulse and obtain the same results as the nurse by Saturday.
4. By Friday, the client will plan a low-salt diet for 24 hours in accordance with the diet plan left by the dietitian.

Question

Who is to achieve the desired behavior in each of the preceding examples?

Because the plan of nursing care is based on the client, the subject is the client.

measure a combination of tasks. See the accompanying Nursing Process Highlight for examples of task statements.

Criteria

The next essential component is the criteria of a goal. **Criteria** are standards used to evaluate whether the behavior demonstrated indicates accomplishment of the goal. Criteria may be written in a variety of ways and may include:

- A time limit
- Amount of activity
- Characteristics of accurate performance
- Description of the performance to be followed

The nurse should specify the precise performance to be considered acceptable in accomplishment of the goal.

It is not always possible to specify a criterion with as much detail as one would like; however, the nurse should continue to communicate precise criteria as explicitly as possible. To provide better direction to the client, the nurse considers how well the client, family member, or significant other should perform the task. See the accompanying Nursing Process Highlight for examples of criteria.

Conditions

The next component to be included in writing effective goals is the conditions under which the client should perform or demonstrate mastery of the task. Although this component is optional in terms of writing goals, conditions may provide clarity and assist the client to demonstrate the expected behavior. The conditions may include the experiences that the client is expected to have before performing the task. See the accompanying Nursing Process Highlight for examples of conditions.

Time Frame

The last component to be included in writing goals appropriately is the time frame in which the client should perform or demonstrate mastery of the task. A written time frame serves as a parameter for evaluating goal achievement.

PROBLEMS FREQUENTLY ENCOUNTERED IN PLANNING

Planning care is a complex process. Nursing students, as beginners in the use of the nursing process, often fall into some common pitfalls when applying the process to practice.

NURSING PROCESS HIGHLIGHT

Planning

Task Statement

1. By Saturday, the client will ambulate the entire length of the hallway three times a day.
2. The client will demonstrate the technique for self-administration of insulin by Friday.
3. The client will take own radial pulse and obtain the same results as the nurse by Saturday.
4. By Friday, the client will plan a low-salt diet for 24 hours in accordance with the diet plan left by the dietitian.

Question

What is the action that the client is expected to do in each of the preceding examples?

The examples demonstrate exactly what the client is to perform ("will ambulate"; "will demonstrate"; "will take"; and "will plan").

NURSING PROCESS HIGHLIGHT

Planning

Criteria

1. By Saturday, the client will ambulate the entire length of the hallway three times a day.
2. The client will demonstrate the technique for self-administration of insulin with aseptic technique.
3. The client will take own radial pulse and obtain the same results as the nurse by Saturday.
4. By Friday, the client will plan a low-salt diet for 24 hours in accordance with the diet plan left by the dietitian.

Question

What are the standards that will be used to evaluate the client's achievement of the objective in each of the preceding examples?

The examples indicate the standards used to evaluate whether the behavior demonstrated by the client indicates that the goal has been reached. The first example includes a time limit and the amount of activity.

Example 2 demonstrates important characteristics of performance accuracy by stating "with aseptic technique."

Example 3 sets standards of performance accuracy and includes a time limit.

Example 4 includes a time limit and a sample plan to be followed.

NURSING PROCESS HIGHLIGHT

Planning

Conditions

1. By Saturday, the client will ambulate the entire length of the hallway three times a day with the use of a walker.
2. By Friday, the client will plan a low-salt diet for 24 hours in accordance with the diet plan left by the dietitian.

Question

What are the conditions under which the activity must be performed in each of the preceding examples?

Example 1 states the condition with which the activity must be performed ("with the use of a walker"). Example 2 cites the condition by which the activity must be performed ("in accordance with the diet plan left by the dietitian").

These pitfalls are described with the intent of providing a clear direction for the use of this process and proposing suggestions for avoiding common errors.

In regard to writing goals, errors frequently observed in this component involve improper format. Format errors include goals that are nurse centered instead of client centered, unrealistic, negative rather than positive, generically copied from a reference and not individualized to the client, unmeasurable, nonspecific, nonbehavioral, vague, wordy, and lacking a time frame.

Another challenge in the development of goals and expected outcomes is the establishment of appropriate time frames for accomplishment of the intended results. Although this component may be difficult at first to master, nursing students should practice writing goals that are realistic and include appropriate time frames using available literature and resources to gain expertise. It is preferable for a goal to include an excessively short, rather than an excessively long, time frame because the goal is brought to attention in the evaluation process more frequently. By inserting the time frame "daily" for specific goals, the expected outcome will be brought up frequently for evaluation. Through a process of building on continued professional growth and experience, students and novice nurses will become more adept and realistic in applying the nursing process to client situations.

Finally, novices as well as experienced nurses tend to make decisions for clients in a paternalistic fashion by deciding what is best for the client without input from the client. To correct this problem, the nurse must establish a trusting nurse-client relationship that promotes mutual understanding and caring. The nurse should encourage clients to make their own decisions regarding health care and respect those decisions.

PLANNING NURSING INTERVENTIONS

Once the goals have been mutually agreed on by the nurse and client, the nurse should use a decision-making process to select appropriate nursing interventions. A **nursing intervention** is an action performed by a nurse that helps the client to achieve the results specified in the goals and expected outcomes. These actions are based on scientific principles and knowledge from nursing, behavioral, and physical sciences. Usually, several nursing interventions are developed for each of the goals identified for the client (Ralph & Taylor, 2008). It is important to identify as many nursing interventions as possible so that if one proves to be unsuitable, others are readily available. The interventions are prioritized according to the order in which they will be implemented.

The delivery of quality, individualized nursing care is greatly enhanced by combining critical thinking and the scientific problem-solving approach. Through critical thinking, sound conclusions are reached in the selection of nursing interventions to prevent, reduce, or eliminate the nursing diagnoses or problems.

Several factors can assist the nurse in selecting nursing interventions. Just as the client's goals can be derived from the nursing diagnosis, the nursing interventions can be developed from the etiology of each nursing diagnosis. The effective nurse plans interventions that are directed toward the causative factors of the client's nursing diagnosis or problem. For example, for a client with angina who may have the nursing diagnosis of *pain* related to myocardial ischemia, an appropriate nursing intervention would be to help the client conserve energy (i.e., bed rest).

The nurse may use various guidelines in selecting appropriate nursing interventions. These guidelines include nurse practice acts, state boards of nursing regulations, and professional standards for nursing care. In addition to legal and professional guidelines, other factors affect the selection of appropriate nursing interventions. The Nursing Checklist provides a list of questions that are helpful in selecting interventions.

When determining which nursing interventions to use, the nurse should critically consider the consequences and the risks of each intervention. After considering these factors, the nurse selects interventions that are most likely to be effective with the minimum of risk. Table 8-5 applies the guidelines for selection of appropriate nursing interventions related to a specific nursing diagnosis.

After setting the goals and planning the appropriate nursing interventions, the nurse writes nursing orders to communicate the exact nursing interventions that are to be implemented for the client. A **nursing order** is a statement written by the nurse that is within the realm of nursing practice to plan and initiate. These statements specify direction and individualize the client's plan of care. For example, a prescribing practitioner's order to force fluids must be specified in the nursing order as the number of milliliters per hour or per shift (e.g., 100 mL/h on Day shift = 800 mL; Evening shift = 800 mL; Night shift = 400 mL).

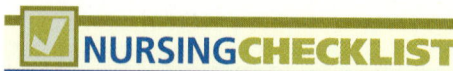

☑ NURSING CHECKLIST

SELECTING APPROPRIATE NURSING INTERVENTIONS

- Is the action realistic in terms of client ability?
- Can the intervention be performed safely and accurately by the nurse?
- Are the necessary resources available?
- Is the intervention compatible with the client's value system?
- Can the intervention be safely carried out with the other planned therapies?

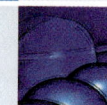

TABLE 8-5 Nursing Interventions: Selection Guidelines

Nursing diagnosis	Acute pain related to myocardial ischemia
Goal	Client will resume normal activities of daily living.
Expected outcome	Client will verbalize relief of pain.
Etiology	Myocardial ischemia
Nursing interventions	Assess pain characteristics such as location, quality, severity, duration, onset, relief.
	At first signs of pain, instruct client to relax and discontinue activity.
	Instruct client to take sublingual nitroglycerin as ordered.
	If pain continues after repeating doses every 5 minutes for a total of three pills, notify the prescribing practitioner.
	Administer oxygen as prescribed.
	Note time interval between episodes of pain.
	Maintain bed rest and quiet environment to decrease oxygen demands.
	Give analgesic medications as prescribed.
	Offer assurance and emotional support by explaining all treatments and procedures and by encouraging questions.

Delmar/Cengage Learning

Ensuring that nursing orders are well written requires several essential elements. These elements include the nursing order date, action verb, detailed description, time frame, and signature (Wilkinson, 2006). See Table 8-6 for a summary of the elements of a nursing order.

The type of nursing order written is determined by the client problem. The nurse is responsible for writing nursing orders that involve health promotion, observation, prevention, and treatment (Wilkinson, 2006). Table 8-7 gives examples of types of nursing orders.

Categories of Nursing Interventions

Nursing interventions are classified according to three categories: independent, interdependent, and dependent. **Independent nursing interventions** are nursing actions initiated by the nurse that do not require an order from another health care professional. These interventions are sanctioned by professional nurse practice acts derived from licensure laws. In many states, the nurse practice acts allow independent nursing interventions regarding activities of daily living, health education, health promotion, and counseling. An example of an independent nursing intervention is the nurse's action to elevate a client's edematous extremity.

Interdependent nursing interventions are those actions that are implemented in a collaborative manner by the nurse with other health care professionals. **Collaboration** is a partnership in which all parties are valued for their contribution. Collaboration is used to gather data, plan, implement, evaluate, and gain objectivity by examining another's viewpoint. Interdependent nursing interventions allow the client's nursing diagnoses to be resolved on the basis of recommendations by an interdisciplinary health care team. For example, a

TABLE 8-7 Types of Nursing Orders

TYPE	DESCRIPTION	EXAMPLE
Health promotion	Nursing orders that encourage behaviors leading to a higher level of wellness	Teach the importance of a daily exercise regimen.
Observation	Nursing orders that include observations regarding potential complications as well as observations of client's current responses	Auscultate lungs q4h.
Prevention	Nursing orders that direct nursing care in the reduction of risk factors or the prevention of complications	Turn, cough, and deep breathe q2h.
Treatment	Nursing orders that include teaching, referrals, or physical care necessary in the treatment of an existing problem	Refer client to occupational therapist for assistance with skills for activities of daily living.

Delmar/Cengage Learning

client care conference or a discharge planning committee uses an interdisciplinary approach that includes health care members such as a nursing supervisor, a home health care nurse, a dietitian, a social worker, and a physical therapist. The nurse assumes the responsibility of being both the primary coordinator of the client's plan of nursing care and the intermediary of interdepartmental collaboration (Doenges et al., 2006).

In addition to collaboration, the planning of interdependent nursing interventions may also include consultation. **Consultation** is a method of soliciting help from a specialist in order to resolve nursing diagnoses. The need for consultation arises when individual nurses identify a problem that cannot be solved using their own knowledge, skills, or resources. In the management of the client's plan of care, nurses may consult with other health care personnel such as clinical nurse specialists, nutritionists, physical therapists, and social workers. Nurses frequently consult to verify assessment data or to obtain clinical advice, for example, discussing the effects of chemotherapy on a client's self-esteem with an oncology clinical nurse specialist. Consultation can be informal or formal. An informal consultation may simply involve asking another practitioner for ideas regarding a nursing problem. Some agencies have a formal protocol for the consultation of a health professional and may require that certain

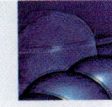

TABLE 8-6 Elements of Nursing Orders

Date	Date on which the order is written
	Is updated to reflect review and revision
Action verb	Directs nursing activities
	Example: explain, demonstrate, auscultate
Detailed description	Precise clarification of the action
	Explains what, where, when, by whom, and how
Time frame	Specifies frequency and duration that action is to be performed
Signature	Indicates person who writes the order
	Implies legal accountability

Delmar/Cengage Learning

forms be completed. Steps in formal consultation reflect a logical sequence and include:

- Identifying the problem
- Collecting all relevant data
- Selecting a suitable consultant
- Communicating unbiased data regarding the problem
- Discussing recommendations with the consultant
- Incorporating the recommendations into the client's plan of care

The consultation process often generates new approaches to the client's individualized plan of care. Acquiring supplementary knowledge may help in ensuring that the best conceivable plan of care is being developed. In addition, nurses who have sought the help of a consultant are presented with an opportunity to learn knowledge and/or skills that can be applied to future situations.

Dependent nursing interventions are those actions that require an order from another health care professional. An example of a dependent intervention is administration of a medication. Although this intervention requires specific nursing knowledge and responsibilities, in many states it is not within the realm of legal nursing practice to prescribe medications. The nurse may not order medications but, when administering them, the nurse is responsible for knowing the classification, the pharmacologic action, normal dosage, side effects, adverse effects, contraindications, and nursing implications of the drugs. Dependent nursing interventions must always be guided by appropriate knowledge and judgment. Many state nurse practice acts sanction advanced practice registered nurses to prescribe medications. In those states, prescriptive authority is an independent intervention for advanced practice nurses. Figure 8-1 illustrates the three categories of nursing interventions.

All nursing interventions require critical thinking in making appropriate nursing judgments. Alfaro-LeFevre (2008) states that the development of critical reasoning skills by nurses is a progressive process that requires a dedication to examine common health problems, participate in diverse clinical experiences, and prepare for delivery of care in clinical settings. Given the emphasis on critical thinking in the planning step of the nursing process, the nurse does not automatically carry out a prescribing practitioner's order without due

▼ SAFETY FIRST ▼

NURSING JUDGMENT
All nursing interventions must be guided by appropriate knowledge and judgment. An in-depth knowledge base is necessary to recognize an error and take corrective action.

consideration. All requested orders are given consideration for their appropriateness. See the Safety First display. The use of rationales helps the nurse practice decision making and substantiate judgments. The rationales should accompany the nursing intervention or nursing order statement on the written plan of nursing care. A **rationale** is an explanation based on theories and scientific principles of natural and behavioral sciences and the humanities.

EVALUATING CARE

Evaluating care involves determining the client's progress toward achievement of expected outcomes. Effective planning is essential if evaluation is to be effective. In other words, the planned outcomes are the yardsticks by which effectiveness of therapies is evaluated. If there is no stated expectation of care (i.e., client outcome), there is nothing against which to measure progress.

NURSING OUTCOMES CLASSIFICATION (NOC)

Recently, there has been increased emphasis by the nursing profession on evaluating outcomes. Nurse researchers (Moorhead, Johnson, Maas, & Swanson, 2007) at the University of Iowa have developed classifications of client outcomes, the Nursing Outcomes Classification (NOC). The NOC provides a standardized language that can be used to measure the effects of nursing practice on client outcomes. The NOC

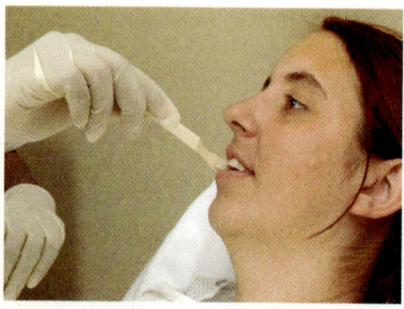
A.

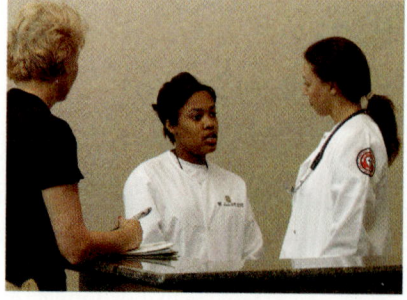
B.

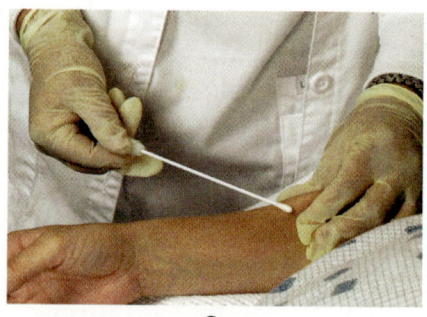
C.

FIGURE 8-1 Examples of types of nursing interventions: (A) Independent—assisting with hygiene needs; (B) Interdependent—multidisciplinary team meeting; (C) Dependent—performing a wound culture DELMAR/CENGAGE LEARNING

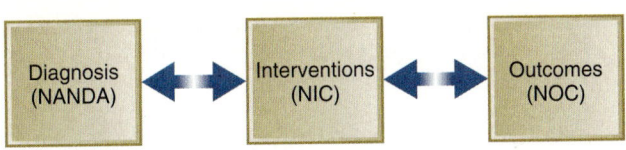

FIGURE 8-2 Relationship between Nursing Classification Systems DELMAR/CENGAGE LEARNING

outcomes, which are used in the United States and other countries, are constantly undergoing research to validate application to clinical practice. Figure 8-2 illustrates the relationship between the nursing classification systems. Just as the North American Nursing Diagnosis Association International (NANDA-I) and the Nursing Interventions Classifications (NIC) are continuing to develop standardized nursing language relative to diagnosis and intervention, the NOC is striving toward a similar goal of standardized language for classifying nursing outcomes. The NOC system can be used to enhance decision making in clinical practice and research.

Linking nursing interventions to improved client outcomes through scientific research is important. Nurse researchers who are observing, measuring, and studying client outcomes believe that outcomes indicate the quality or effectiveness of the nursing interventions provided. The use of classification systems in nursing promotes nurses' descriptions of their contributions and helps validate the value of nursing activities. The accompanying Community Considerations display lists some selected outcomes relevant to safety maintenance for an elderly client being cared for in the home. Strengthening the links between nursing interventions and client outcomes will benefit not only clients, but nursing as well. Having solid research evidence that documents the effectiveness of nursing care on client outcomes will influence political and financial decisions relative to nursing.

The NOC taxonomy focuses on function, physiology, psychosocial aspects, health knowledge and behavior, and perceived self-health and family health. The NOC system, which defines over 330 client outcomes that are sensitive to nursing interventions, allows nurses to evaluate client status over time.

PLAN OF CARE

The **plan of care** is a written guide that organizes data about a client's care into a formal statement that will be used to help the client achieve optimal health. Nursing care plans usually include components such as assessment, nursing diagnoses, goals and expected outcomes, nursing interventions, and evaluations. The nurse begins the nursing care plan on the day of admission and continually updates and individualizes the client's plan of care until discharge.

The plan of care directs the efforts of the entire health care team regarding each client. This plan promotes the health care team's delivery of holistic, individualized, and goal-oriented care to the client. Attention to a comprehensive assessment of the entire person allows for a holistic approach. Individualization is enhanced by continuous reviewing and

COMMUNITY CONSIDERATIONS

Nursing Outcomes Classification (NOC)

Knowledge of Personal Safety for a Home Health Client

- Description of fall prevention measures
- Description of risk reduction measures
- Description of home safety measures
- Description of emergency procedures
- Description of community safety risks

Adapted from Moorhead, S., Johnson, M., Maas, M., & Swanson, E. (2007). *Nursing outcomes classification (NOC)* (4th ed.). St. Louis, MO: Mosby.

updating of the plan of care. A carefully formulated written plan of care prioritizes problems and addresses short- and long-term needs of the client. The written plan of care authenticates activities of assessment by maintaining written records and providing evidence of nursing interventions, the client's response to nursing interventions, and changes in the client's condition.

Although plans of care differ in various institutions from handwritten to computerized forms, they all have the same basic elements in common. The plan of care is realistically designed and customized to each individual client's health status and is the final result of the planning component of the nursing process. The nursing plan of care documents health care needs, coordinates nursing care, promotes continuity of care, encourages communication within the health care team, and promotes quality nursing care.

TYPES OF CARE PLANS

There are several types of care plans. These different types include student-oriented, standardized, institutional, and computerized care plans.

Student-Oriented Care Plan

The student-oriented care plan promotes learning of problem-solving skills, the nursing process, verbal and written communication skills, and organizational skills. This comprehensive care plan focuses on teaching the process of planning care. Therefore, care plans developed by student nurses in educational settings are generally more detailed than the plans used by nurses in daily practice. Educational programs vary, but usually the student-oriented care plan begins with assessment and proceeds in a sequential manner, concluding with the plan for evaluation.

Standardized Care Plan

The standardized care plan is a preplanned, preprinted guide for the nursing care of client groups with common needs.

This type of care plan generally follows the nursing process format (i.e., problem, goals, nursing orders, and evaluation). The nurse may use standardized care plans when a client has predictable, commonly occurring problems. Individualization may be accomplished by the inclusion of additional handwritten notes on unusual problems or circumstances unique to the client.

Institutional Care Plan

Institutional nursing care plans are concise documents that become a part of the client's medical record after discharge. The Kardex nursing care plan is an example of this type of care plan. The institutional nursing care plan may simply include the problem, goal, and nursing action. In addition, the Kardex nursing care plan may be expanded to include assessment, nursing diagnosis, goal, implementation, and evaluation.

Computerized Care Plan

Computers are used for creating and storing nursing care plans and can generate both standardized and individualized nursing care plans. The nurse selects appropriate diagnoses from a menu of possible goals and nursing interventions. The nurse has the option of reading the client's plan of care from the computer screen or printing out an updated working copy.

STRATEGIES FOR EFFECTIVE CARE PLANNING

In planning quality nursing care for each client, the nurse assumes responsibility for the coordination of total nursing care. The nurse coordinates the participation of various health care team members to incorporate their recommendations into the delivery of quality nursing care. Critical thinking assists the nurse in establishing collaborative relationships with other members of the health care team and managing complex nursing systems; see the Spotlight On: Caring display that discusses coordination of care.

An important strategy for effective planning is clear communication of the client's plan of care to other health care personnel. The nurse must always communicate the plan of

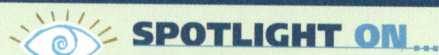

SPOTLIGHT ON...

Caring

Coordination of Care

Mr. Eduardo Rodriquez has been admitted with arthritis. His left knee is extremely edematous, and the prescribing practitioner has ordered heat application of 100°F to the left knee four times a day for 2 hours. In considering the appropriateness of this order, the nurse detects an error regarding the time frame because heat produces maximum vasodilation in 20 to 30 minutes to dissipate the edema; further application of heat may lead to a rebound phenomenon of tissue congestion and vessel constriction, as well as potential burns. At this point, the nurse needs to seek clarification of the order from the prescribing practitioner. What would be appropriate methods of handling this situation?

care in clear, precise terms, avoiding vague terminology such as *improved, adequate,* and *normal.*

Another strategy for effective planning is to establish a realistic nursing plan of care because this will avoid setting a goal that is too difficult or impossible to achieve. If a goal is too ambitious or is unattainable, the client and nurse may become discouraged or apathetic about the resolution of nursing diagnoses. In addition, goals should be measurable. Quantitative terms assist in the determination of measurement. Finally, the goals should be future oriented. Because a goal is an aim or a desired achievement, goals should be written in future tense format.

Once appropriate nursing diagnoses are individualized to the client, the plan of care has a stable framework on which an optimum level of wellness for the client can be based. Although some clients may not achieve complete resolution of all nursing diagnoses, the nursing plan of care that is individualized can improve health to the client's optimal level.

KEY CONCEPTS

- The outcome identification and planning component of the nursing process is a sequential, orderly method of using problem-solving skills and critical thinking to formulate a nursing plan of care to resolve nursing diagnoses.

- The planning component of the nursing process includes establishing priorities, setting goals, developing expected outcomes, selecting nursing interventions, and documenting the plan of care.

- The purposes of outcome identification and planning are to provide direction for nursing care, to improve staff communication, and to provide continuity of nursing care.

- The establishment of priorities may be guided by such factors as endangerment of well-being, Maslow's hierarchy of needs, client preferences, and anticipation of future diagnoses.

- Setting goals and expected outcomes provides guidelines for directing nursing interventions and establishes evaluation criteria by deciding on goals that illustrate a desired change in the client's behavior.
- Goals and expected outcome objectives include the components of subject, task statement, criteria, conditions, and time frame.
- Two common problems frequently encountered in planning goals are improper format and unrealistic, nonmeasurable qualities.
- In planning nursing care, the nurse uses an expansive scientific knowledge base and critical thinking to select independent, interdependent, and dependent nursing interventions guided by local and federal standards of care.
- The plan of care documents health care needs, coordinates nursing care, promotes continuity of care, encourages communication within the health care team, and promotes quality nursing care.
- Strategies for effective care planning include communication of the client's plan of care within the health care team, establishment of a realistic plan of care, and formulation of measurable and future-oriented goals.

REVIEW QUESTIONS

1. Which of the following best describes the plan of nursing care?
   a. Client assessment data, medical treatment regime and rationales, and diagnostic test results and significance
   b. Prescribing practitioner's orders, demographic data, and medication administration and rationales
   c. Collected documentation of all team members providing care for the client
   d. Assessment data, nursing diagnoses, goals and expected outcomes, and nursing interventions

2. What is the main purpose of the expected outcome?
   a. To describe the education plans to be taught to the client
   b. To describe the behavior the client is expected to achieve as a result of nursing interventions
   c. To provide a standard for evaluating the quality of health care delivered to the client during the hospital stay
   d. To make sure that the client's treatment does not extend beyond the time allowed under the diagnosis-related group system

3. Which of the following are the essential components of an expected outcome?
   a. Nursing diagnosis, interventions, and expected client behavior
   b. Target date, nursing action, measurement criteria, and desired client behavior
   c. Nursing action, client behavior, target date, and conditions under which the behavior occurs
   d. Client behavior, measurement criteria, conditions under which the behavior occurs, and target date

4. When planning care, which of the following should the nurse use as a guideline?
   a. Choose actions that a nurse can perform without leaving the unit or consulting with medical staff.
   b. Make intervention statements specific to ensure continuity of care.
   c. Write interventions in general terms to allow maximum flexibility and creativity in delivering nursing care.
   d. Make sure that nursing care activities receive priority over other aspects of the treatment regime.

5. Which of the following statements is correctly stated as a client expected outcome?
   a. Client will ambulate on fourth postoperative day.
   b. Client will ambulate safely.
   c. Client will be able to safely walk down the hallway.
   d. Client will safely walk unassisted to the end of the hallway within 4 days.

online companion

Visit the DeLaune and Ladner online companion resource at **www.delmar.cengage.com** for additional content and study aids. Click on Online Companions, then select the Nursing discipline.

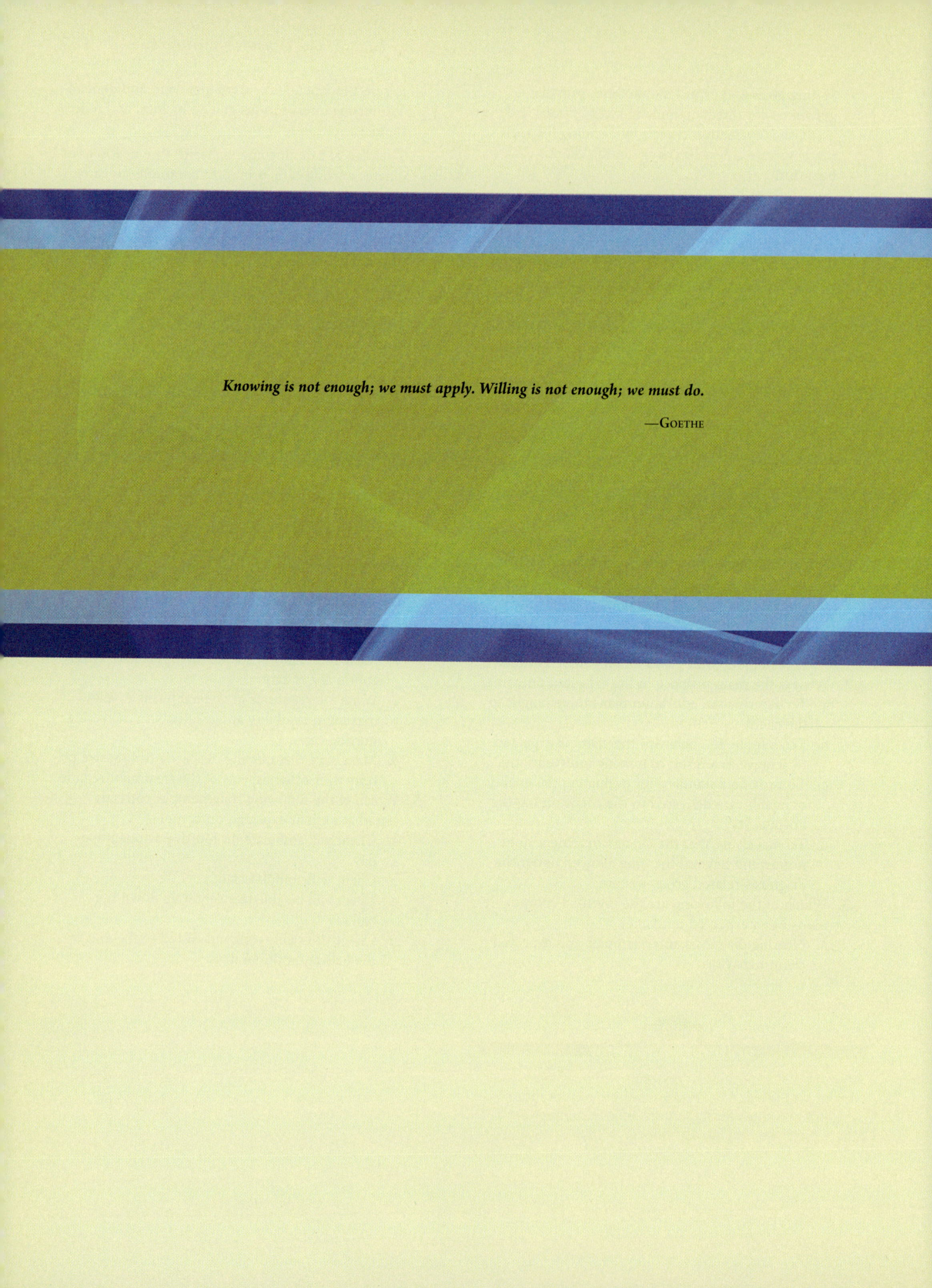

Knowing is not enough; we must apply. Willing is not enough; we must do.

—Goethe

CHAPTER 9

Implementation

COMPETENCIES

1. Describe the purposes of the implementation step of the nursing process.
2. Explore the types of skills required for effective implementation.
3. Discuss various implementation activities that nurses execute as directed by the nursing plan of care.
4. Explain the nurse's roles and responsibilities in the delegation of care to assistive personnel and their impact on implementation.
5. Identify the specific types of nursing interventions that are implemented by the nurse and the characteristics of each type.
6. Discuss the Nursing Interventions Classification (NIC) system.
7. Discuss the importance of documentation in the implementation process.

KEY TERMS

case management   modular nursing   rationale
delegation   nursing intervention   standing order
functional nursing   primary nursing   team nursing
implementation   protocol   total client care

Implementation, the fourth step in the nursing process, involves the execution of the nursing plan of care that was developed during the planning phase. It involves completion of nursing activities to accomplish predetermined goals and to make progress toward achievement of specific outcomes. The implementation phase of the nursing process, as with the other phases of the process, requires a broad base of clinical knowledge, careful planning, critical thinking and analysis, and judgment on the part of the nurse.

This chapter discusses the purposes of implementation, the specific skills associated with effectively implementing the nursing plan of care, and the activities involved in this process. Although identified as the fourth step of the nursing process, the implementation phase begins with assessment and continually interacts with the other steps of the process to reflect the changing needs of the client and the response of the nurse to those needs.

PURPOSES OF IMPLEMENTATION

Implementation is directed toward a fulfillment of client needs that results in health promotion, prevention of illness, illness management, or health restoration in a variety of settings including acute care, home health care, ambulatory clinics, or extended care facilities. Implementation also involves delegation of tasks and documentation of nursing interventions.

The American Nurses Association (2004) describes the standards applicable to implementation in terms of both a standard of care and standards of professional performance. Adherence to these standards requires that the nurse have a current knowledge base, be proficient with technical and communication skills, and use sound judgment in determining safe and efficient use of personnel and materials.

REQUIREMENTS FOR EFFECTIVE IMPLEMENTATION

The implementation phase of the nursing process requires cognitive (intellectual), psychomotor (technical), and interpersonal communication skills. These skills serve as vehicles with which effective nursing care can be delivered and are used either in conjunction with each other or individually as required by the client and the specific needs of the situation.

COGNITIVE SKILLS

Cognitive skills enable nurses to make appropriate observations, understand the rationale for the activities performed, and appreciate how differences among individuals influence nursing care. Critical thinking is an important element within the cognitive domain because it helps nurses to analyze data, organize observations, and apply prior knowledge and experiences to current client situations.

PSYCHOMOTOR SKILLS

Proficiency with psychomotor skills is necessary to safely and effectively perform nursing activities. Nurses must be able to handle medical equipment with a high degree of competency and to perform skills such as administering medications and assisting clients with mobility needs (e.g., positioning and ambulating).

INTERPERSONAL SKILLS

The use of interpersonal skills involves communication with clients and families as well as with other health care professionals. The nurse-client relationship is established through the use of therapeutic communication that helps ensure a beneficial outcome for the client's health status. Interaction between members of the health care team promotes collaboration and enhances holistic care of the client. Communication is also the mechanism by which nurses teach clients, families, and other community groups.

IMPLEMENTATION ACTIVITIES

Nurses perform a variety of activities that are designed to assist clients in meeting needs. Nursing implementation activities include:

- Ongoing assessment
- Establishment of priorities
- Allocation of resources
- Initiation of nursing interventions
- Documentation of interventions and client responses

These activities are interactive, and each is discussed in further detail.

ONGOING ASSESSMENT

The nursing plan of care is based on the initial assessment data collected by the nurse and the nursing diagnoses derived from those data. Because a client's condition can change rapidly, or new data may become available, ongoing assessment is necessary to validate the relevance of proposed interventions. Goals, expected outcomes, and interventions may need to be altered as new data are collected or progress toward outcome achievement is evaluated. Although a focused assessment should be completed during the initial interaction with the client, continuous observations during the implementation process allow for adaptations to be made to better individualize care. See the accompanying Nursing Process Highlight display.

It is not unusual for nursing diagnoses to change or to be resolved in a short period of time. For example, the nursing care plan for a preoperative client might include an intervention to teach her about the use of a patient-controlled analgesia (PCA) pump. As the use of this equipment is being demonstrated, the nurse observes that the client is unable to depress the button easily with the fingers of her right hand. The client informs the nurse that she forgot to mention that her joints swell occasionally and she has very little strength in her hand during these times. This information is essential for both developing a nursing diagnosis concerning the client's impaired physical mobility and determining appropriate teaching methods for use of the PCA pump.

Ongoing assessment demands attention to verbal and nonverbal cues from the client and requires knowledge of expected responses to specific interventions. If nurses observe that responses are different from those expected, this assessment data can lead to changes in expected outcomes and accompanying interventions.

Ongoing assessment is especially important in home health care or extended care settings when contact with skilled health care providers might occur less frequently and the length of time that the care is required varies (see the accompanying Community Considerations display). The nurse's assessment and clinical judgment often determine whether the client needs continued care or referral to other health care providers.

ESTABLISHMENT OF PRIORITIES

Following ongoing assessment and review of the problem list, priorities are determined for implementation of care. Priorities are based on:

- Which problems are deemed most important by the nurse, client, family, or significant others
- Activities previously scheduled by other departments (e.g., surgery, diagnostic testing)
- Available resources

The change-of-shift report can also be a valuable tool in determining priorities. A client's condition can change quickly and frequently—especially in acute care settings—requiring that the nurse exercise strong clinical judgment and maintain flexibility in organizing care. For example, the nursing care plan for a client who had hip replacement surgery might reflect a priority nursing diagnosis of *impaired physical mobility* with interventions focused toward learning to ambulate. When the nurse listens to the client's breath sounds on a particular morning, it is noted that breathing is more labored and crackles can be auscultated in the lung bases. This assessment is noted on the change-of-shift report, and the priorities of interventions change to focus on this new development.

Time management is important whether the nurse is caring for one client or a group of clients. It is helpful to

---

NURSING PROCESS HIGHLIGHT

Implementation

Relationship between Assessment and Implementation

Mrs. James, who has been diagnosed with diabetes, will be discharged from the hospital within a few days. The expected outcome in the nursing plan of care is that Mrs. James will correctly and accurately withdraw the prescribed amount of insulin and inject her own insulin. While implementing this teaching intervention, you observe that Mrs. James is unable to visualize the correct amount of insulin to withdraw in the syringe because of her impaired vision. How does the assessment of her response affect your interventions related to the teaching strategies that need to be implemented with the client?

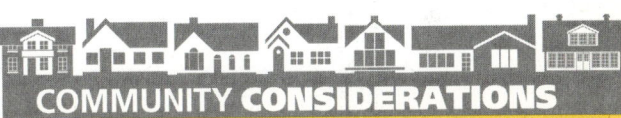

COMMUNITY CONSIDERATIONS

Care in the Home

An important element in the ongoing assessment of clients in the home is the appraisal for the risk of falls. The following questions can help the nurse determine the seriousness of this risk.

- Which medications are currently prescribed for the client, and what are their effects on the central nervous system?
- Are elimination problems such as incontinence being experienced?
- Has the mental status of the client recently changed in terms of orientation to time and place?
- Does the client's level of mobility require ambulatory assistance devices such as a cane, walker, or wheelchair?
- If the client has previously experienced a fall, what were the conditions under which it occurred?

make a list of tasks that need to be accomplished throughout the day and to create a worksheet outlining a target time for these activities. Those activities with specified times for completion should be scheduled first. For example, medications usually allow a narrow time frame for administration and must be scheduled at specific times on the worksheet. An example of a worksheet that outlines a plan for activities is shown in Table 9-1. The time allotted for activities depends on the complexity of the task and the amount of assistance required by the client. See Table 9-2 on page 143 for an example of a worksheet for a group of clients.

ALLOCATION OF RESOURCES

Before implementing the nursing plan of care, the nurse reviews proposed interventions to determine the level of knowledge and the types of skills required for safe and effective implementation. The assessment provides data for determining

TABLE 9-1	Sample Worksheet of Nursing Activities (One Client)	
TIME	**ACTIVITY**
6:45 AM	Listen to change-of-shift report.
7:00	Perform head-to-toe assessment of client, including vital signs.
7:10	Check routine medication times.
7:30	Chart assessment findings.
8:00	Serve breakfast. While client eats breakfast, review chart for new laboratory test data.
8:30	Record I and O after breakfast; remove breakfast tray.
8:40	Gather supplies for hygiene. Assist with AM care.
9:00	Administer medications.
9:15	Assist up to chair. Show films about diabetic skin care.
10:00	Document interventions and observations on chart.
10:15	Review care plan for any needed revisions.
10:30	Report status of client to charge nurse. Attend inservice on IV care.
11:45	Take and record vital signs.

Delmar/Cengage Learning

if an activity can be performed independently by the client, can be completed with assistance from family, or requires assistance of health care personnel.

Delegation of Tasks

Whereas some interventions are complex and require the knowledge and skills of a registered nurse, other interventions are relatively simple and can be delegated to assistive personnel. **Delegation** is the process of transferring a selected nursing task in a situation to an individual who is competent to perform that specific task. It must be remembered that although some activities can be assigned to other health care personnel, the registered nurse remains accountable for appropriate delegation and supervision of care provided by these individuals. See the accompanying Safety First display. See Chapters 11 and 12 for more information on delegation.

Types of Nursing Management Systems

Wise use of resources dictates that tasks be assigned to the most cost-effective level of personnel who can safely and proficiently perform the activity. The nursing management system often determines the numbers and types of personnel available. Changes in health care delivery in recent years have resulted in an increasing emphasis on cost containment and have subsequently created several unique management models. The redesign of the workplace in many health care agencies has included cross-training of employees, with nurses frequently assuming responsibilities formerly assigned to other health care providers. For example, nurses might draw blood for laboratory tests, perform electrocardiograms, or administer respiratory treatments, as care is focused around the client rather than the various departments in the agency. Nurses in community health settings have traditionally exercised a variety of roles in their practice. As health care delivery continues to evolve in this country, a variety of innovative approaches will emerge to better meet the needs of clients. The most common management systems currently used include functional nursing, team nursing, primary nursing, total client care, modular nursing, and case management.

FUNCTIONAL NURSING The **functional nursing** approach divides care into tasks to be completed and uses various levels of personnel depending on the complexity of the

▼ SAFETY FIRST ▼

LEGAL RESPONSIBILITY AND DELEGATION
The registered nurse is legally responsible for all nursing care given. Even though a task may be delegated, the nurse is accountable for safe performance of that task.

TABLE 9-2 Sample Worksheet of Nursing Activities (Group of Clients)

	7 AM	8 AM	9 AM	10 AM	11 AM	NOON
351 Hughes	V/S assess		Meds	Assist to chair	V/S Meds	Meds
352 Parsons	V/S assess	Feed	To PT	D/C plan	V/S	Telem. strip
353 Crowson	V/S assess	Ck. PTT results	Meds; Amb. in hall	Show video	BP sit/stand Meds	Telem. strip
354 Robinson	V/S assess	q2h I/O	Meds	q2h I/O		q2h I/O
355 Temple	Pre-op OR on call		Meds			
356 Anderson	V/S assess	NPO	Meds	V/S Gastro		Meds

Abbreviations: Amb., ambulate; BP, blood pressure; D/C, discharge; I/O, input/output; NPO, nothing by mouth; OR, operating room; PT, physical therapy; PTT, partial thromboplastin time; telem., telemetry; V/S, vital signs.

Delmar/Cengage Learning

assignment. Members of the staff perform their assigned tasks for each client. For example, one nurse may assess each client and document findings and another may give all medications and treatments. Another nurse may be assigned to complete client teaching or discharge planning (process that enables the client to resume self-care activities before leaving the health care environment). One nursing assistant might serve all trays and collect intake and output records for each client while another is responsible for giving baths or making beds.

The advantage of this system is that a large number of clients can be cared for by a relatively small number of personnel. In addition, it allows the use of less skilled (and less expensive) personnel for some tasks and allows personnel to be used in areas for which they have special knowledge or skill. However, this system can also result in fragmented and depersonalized care and may invite omissions in care because no *one* person is responsible for the total care of the client.

TEAM NURSING   The **team nursing** approach uses a variety of personnel (professional, technical, and unlicensed) in the delivery of nursing care. The registered nurse is the leader of the team and is responsible for supervision of the team members as well as planning and evaluating the results of caregiving activities. This management system uses professional nurses for skilled observations and interventions and provision of direct care to acutely ill clients, while licensed practical nurses care for less acutely ill clients and nursing assistants are responsible for serving trays, making beds, and assisting the nurses with other tasks. This management system is frequently used because it is cost-effective and provides more individualized care than the functional approach.

PRIMARY NURSING   In the **primary nursing** management system, the professional nurse assumes full responsibility for total client care for a small number of clients. Although care may be delegated to nurse associates for shifts when the primary nurse is not in attendance, the primary nurse maintains responsibility for total client care 24 hours a day (see Figure 9-1). The primary nurse sets health care goals with the client and plans care to meet those goals. The principal advantage of this approach is the continuity of care inherent

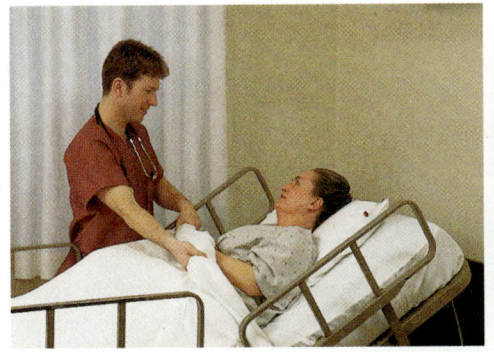
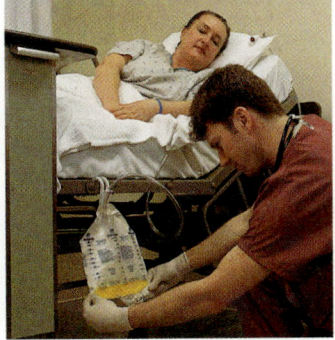
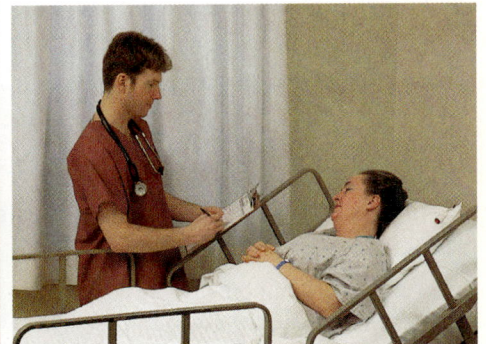

FIGURE 9-1 Delivery of care via the primary nursing management system. This primary nurse is responsible for meeting the total health care needs of this client. DELMAR/CENGAGE LEARNING

in the system. Primary nursing is most effective with a total staff of registered nurses, which makes this system expensive to maintain. Due to the expense and the current limited supply of registered nurses, the primary nursing model is rarely used except in critical care areas.

TOTAL CLIENT CARE AND MODULAR NURSING   Total client care and modular nursing are variations of primary nursing. Although these systems imply that one nurse is responsible for all the care administered to a client, responsibility for the client actually changes from shift to shift with the assigned caregiver. These systems use both registered nurses and licensed practical nurses; the registered nurses are assigned to more complex client situations. A unit manager or charge nurse typically coordinates activities on the unit. Modular nursing attempts to assign caregivers to a small segment or "module" of a nursing unit, ensuring that clients are cared for by the same personnel on a regular basis.

CASE MANAGEMENT   In the case management system, the nurse assumes responsibility for planning, implementing, coordinating, and evaluating care for a given client, regardless of the client's location at any given time. This approach is often used when care is complex and a number of health care team members are involved in providing care. Generally, a case management plan, or critical pathway, is developed based on the norm or typical course of the condition. The nurse evaluates the progress of the client in relation to what is expected, investigating and following up on any variance in the time required or the amount of improvement noted. Although the case load for the individual nurse might be smaller (thus making this approach expensive), continuity of care and collaboration are enhanced.

A case manager oversees client care across the continuum of practice settings to ensure comprehensive, less fragmented delivery of care. The goal of case management is to help the client maintain optimal health with the least amount of intervention from health care providers. Critical pathways and care maps are tools used by case managers to measure the client's progress according to predetermined time frames for achievement of expected objectives. The case manager seeks to improve the quality of health care by evaluating client outcomes, cost-effectiveness, and agency efficacy (Chitty & Black, 2007). See the accompanying Community Considerations display.

COMMUNITY CONSIDERATIONS

Factors Influencing a Case Manager's Decision for Home Care

- Assessment of home environment
- Learning needs of client and family
- Need for skilled nursing care
- Need for long-term care

NURSING INTERVENTIONS

After reviewing the client's current condition, verifying priorities, and examining resources, the nurse should be ready to initiate nursing interventions. A nursing intervention is an action performed by the nurse that helps the client to achieve the results specified by the goals and expected outcomes. All interventions must conform to professional standards of care. Nurses should understand the reason for any intervention, the expected effect, and any potential problems that may result. Understanding the reason for a nursing intervention is the hallmark of a professional nurse, in that the nurse is using logic and scientific reasoning as the basis of practice. It is important for novice nurses to identify the rationale (the fundamental principle) of all interventions in order to implement theory-based practice. Nursing interventions are a blend of science (rational acts) and art (intuitive actions).

Interventions are determined by and directed toward the cause of the problem, or factors contributing to the nursing diagnosis, and may vary for clients with similar nursing diagnoses depending on realistic expected outcomes for the individual. Prior to implementation, it is necessary to determine exactly:

- What is to be done
- How it is to be done
- When it should be done
- Who will do it
- How long it should be done

Consideration should be given to client preferences, the developmental level of the client, and availability of resources. In addition, the prescribing practitioner's orders often have an impact on nursing interventions by imposing restrictions on factors such as diet or activity.

Types of Nursing Interventions

Nursing interventions are written as orders in the care plan and may be nurse initiated, prescribing practitioner initiated, or derived from collaboration with other health care professionals. These interventions can also be categorized as independent, dependent, or interdependent, depending on the authority required for initiation of the activity; see Chapter 8 for more details.

Interventions can be implemented on the basis of standing orders or protocols. A standing order is a standardized intervention written, approved, and signed by a prescribing practitioner that is kept on file within health care agencies to be used in predictable situations or in circumstances requiring immediate attention. Nurses can implement standing orders in these situations after they have assessed the client and identified the primary or emerging problem. For example, nurses in an ambulatory clinic or home health care agency may have standing orders for administering certain medications or ordering laboratory tests when indicated, or a prescribing practitioner may establish standing orders on an inpatient unit that specify certain medications that can be administered for common complaints, such as headache.

Table 9-3 provides an example of standing orders used for client preparation for a barium enema.

A **protocol** is a series of standing orders or procedures that should be followed under certain specific conditions. They define what interventions are permissible and under what circumstances the nurse is to implement the measures. Health care agencies or individual prescribing practitioners frequently have standing orders or protocols for client preparation for diagnostic tests and for immediate interventions in life-threatening circumstances. These protocols prevent needless duplication of writing the same orders repeatedly for different clients and often save valuable time in critical situations.

Nursing Interventions Classification

In 1993, the Iowa Intervention Project developed a taxonomy of nursing interventions that includes both direct and indirect activities directed toward health promotion and illness management. This taxonomy, the Nursing Interventions Classification (NIC), is a standardized language system that describes nursing interventions performed in all practice settings. The NIC is a method for linking nursing interventions to diagnoses and client outcomes (Bulechek, Dochterman, & Butcher, 2007).

The format for each intervention is as follows: label name, definition, a list of activities that a nurse performs to carry out the intervention, and a list of background readings (Bulechek et al., 2007). See Table 9-4 on page 146. The NIC offers standardized language for research on nursing interventions and is a promising tool for determining reimbursement for nursing services in a variety of practice settings.

Nursing Intervention Activities

Implementing nursing interventions requires that consideration be given to client rights, nursing ethics, and the legal implications associated with providing care. Nursing interventions include:

- Assisting with activities of daily living (ADL)
- Delivering skilled therapeutic interventions
- Monitoring and surveillance of response to care
- Teaching
- Discharge planning
- Supervising and coordinating nursing personnel

Clients have the right to refuse any intervention. However, the nurse must explain the rationale for the intervention and possible consequences associated with refusing treatment. If the intervention refused was prescribed by another health care professional, that person should be informed of the refusal of care. Ethical standards require that clients be afforded privacy and confidentiality. Matters related to a client's condition and care should be discussed only with individuals directly involved with the client's care, and any discussion should be held in a location where information cannot be overheard by visitors or bystanders. From a legal standpoint, the nurse must ensure that the authority for prescribing any intervention has been satisfied and that applicable standards of care are maintained during implementation of all nursing interventions. See the accompanying Safety First display.

ACTIVITIES OF DAILY LIVING Clients frequently need assistance with ADL such as bathing, grooming, ambulating, eating, and eliminating. The goal for most clients is to return to self-care or to regain as much autonomy as possible. The nurse's role is to determine the extent of assistance needed and to provide support for ADL while at the same time fostering independence. Ongoing assessment is important for determining the appropriate balance between ensuring safety and promoting independence. For example, maintaining personal grooming is important for purposes of hygiene and comfort as well as for promoting self-esteem. The nurse must always provide privacy when assisting clients with personal hygiene. If these tasks are assigned to other personnel, adequate supervision is imperative to ensure compliance with these principles.

THERAPEUTIC INTERVENTIONS Therapeutic nursing interventions are those measures directed toward resolution of a

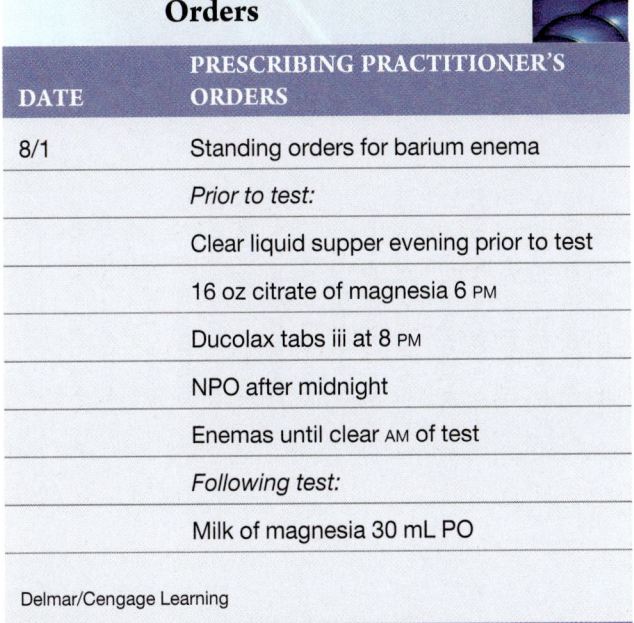

TABLE 9-3 Example of Standing Orders

DATE	PRESCRIBING PRACTITIONER'S ORDERS
8/1	Standing orders for barium enema
	Prior to test:
	Clear liquid supper evening prior to test
	16 oz citrate of magnesia 6 PM
	Ducolax tabs iii at 8 PM
	NPO after midnight
	Enemas until clear AM of test
	Following test:
	Milk of magnesia 30 mL PO

Delmar/Cengage Learning

▼ SAFETY FIRST ▼

MAINTAINING STANDARDS OF CARE
If nurses have never performed a specific procedure or feel unsure about their ability to safely perform the skill, they must always secure assistance before implementation.

TABLE 9-4 Nursing Interventions Classification (NIC) Taxonomy

	DOMAIN 1	DOMAIN 2	DOMAIN 3	DOMAIN 4	DOMAIN 5	DOMAIN 6
LEVEL 1: Domains	1. Physiological: Basic Care that supports physical functioning	2. Physiological: Complex Care that supports homeostatic regulation	3. Behavioral Care that supports psychosocial functioning and facilitates lifestyle changes	4. Safety Care that supports protection against harm	5. Family Care that supports the family unit	6. Health System Care that supports effective use of the health care delivery system
LEVEL 2: Classes	A *Activity and exercise management:* Interventions to organize or assist with physical activity and energy conservation and expenditure B *Elimination management:* Interventions to establish and maintain regular bowel and urinary elimination patterns and manage complications due to altered patterns C *Immobility management:* Interventions	G *Electrolyte and acid-base management:* Interventions to regulate electrolyte and acid-base balance and prevent complications H *Drug management:* Interventions to facilitate desired effects of pharmacologic agents I *Neurologic management:* Interventions to optimize neurologic functions J Interventions to provide care before,	O *Behavior therapy:* Interventions to reinforce or promote desirable behaviors or alter undesirable behaviors P *Cognitive therapy:* Interventions to reinforce or promote cognitive functioning or alter undesirable cognitive functioning Q *Communication enhancement:* Interventions to facilitate delivering and receiving verbal and	U *Crisis management:* Interventions to provide immediate short-term help in both psychological and physiological crises V *Risk management:* Interventions to initiate risk-education activities and continue monitoring risks over time	W *Childbearing care:* Interventions to assist in understanding and coping with the psychological and physiological changes during the childbearing period X *Lifespan care:* Interventions to facilitate family unit functioning and promote the health and welfare of family members throughout the life span	Y *Health system mediation:* Interventions to facilitate the interface between client/ family and the health care system a *Health system management:* Interventions to provide and enhance support services for the delivery of care b *Information management:* Interventions to facilitate communications among health care providers

(continues)

TABLE 9-4 (Continued)

DOMAIN 1	DOMAIN 2	DOMAIN 3	DOMAIN 4	DOMAIN 5	DOMAIN 6
to manage restricted body movement and the sequelae	during, and immediately after surgery	nonverbal messages			
D Nutrition support: Interventions to modify or maintain nutritional status	*K Respiratory management:* Interventions to promote airway patency and gas exchange	*R Coping assistance:* Interventions to assist another to build on own strengths, to adapt to a change in function, or to achieve a higher level of function			
E Physical comfort promotion: Interventions to promote comfort using physical techniques	*L Skin/wound management:* Interventions to maintain or restore tissue integrity	*S Client education:* Interventions to facilitate learning			
F Self-care facilitation: Interventions to provide or assist with routine activities of daily living	*M Thermoregulation:* Interventions to maintain body temperature within a normal range	*T Psychological comfort promotion:* Interventions to promote comfort using psychological techniques			
	N Tissue perfusion management: Interventions to optimize circulation of blood and fluids to the tissue				

Bulechek, G. M., Dochterman, J. M., & Butcher, H. K. (2007). *Nursing interventions classification (NIC)* (5th ed.). St. Louis, MO: Mosby. Reprinted with permission of Elsevier.

current problem and include activities such as administration of medications and treatments, performing skilled procedures, and providing physical and psychological comfort. Written orders must be verified before implementing interventions requiring prescriptive authority. Reassessment of the client is also needed to determine whether the intervention remains appropriate. In addition, a nurse must also understand the rationale, expected effects, and possible complications that could result from any intervention.

MONITORING AND SURVEILLANCE Observation of the client's response to treatment is an integral part of the implementation of any intervention. Monitoring and surveillance of the client's progress or lack of progress are essential in determining the effectiveness of the plan of care and detecting potential complications. Specific interventions require specific monitoring activities; however, typical monitoring activities include observations such as vital signs measurement, cardiac monitoring, and recording of intake and output. See the Uncovering the Evidence display.

TEACHING A major intervention in health promotion and illness management is educating clients in order to help them modify their behaviors in response to potential health risks and actual health alterations. As part of this teaching process, nurses must also discuss the rationales for the interventions in the nursing plan of care.

Numerous opportunities arise every day for informal teaching related to client care. For example, teaching clients about the medications they are taking and possible side effects should occur routinely as medications are administered. Similarly, as nurses perform assessment activities, the sharing of observations with the client can be informative in terms of what characteristics are desirable and what observations are sources of concern. This knowledge can be valuable to a client for self-monitoring.

Effective teaching requires insight into the client's knowledge base and readiness to learn. Realistic teaching goals and learning outcomes should be set on the basis of these factors. It is also desirable to include the family or significant others in teaching plans. A suitable learning environment should be created that is nonthreatening and allows active participation by the client.

Nurses should be careful to use terminology easily understood by the client. It is important that learning outcomes are validated to be sure that clients can safely and effectively care for themselves after discharge. See Chapter 21 for information about client education.

DISCHARGE PLANNING Preparation for discharge begins at the time of admission to a health care agency. As the average length of stay in acute care settings continues to decrease, early discharge planning becomes imperative. Expected outcomes dictate the type of planning required and the interventions necessary to attain the desired outcomes. Interventions directed toward discharge planning include activities such as teaching and consultation with other agencies (e.g., home health, rehabilitation facilities, nursing homes) concerning follow-up care. Teaching related to any changes in diet, medications, or lifestyle must be implemented; any barriers or problems in the home environment must be resolved before discharge from an acute or extended care facility. Some agencies employ personnel with the primary responsibility of teaching or discharge planning for groups of clients; however, the nurse who is caring for the individual client is also responsible for ensuring that all appropriate interventions have been implemented before discharge.

SUPERVISION AND COORDINATION OF PERSONNEL The management style and type of facility, as well as the needs of the client, determine the scope of interventions

---

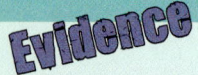

UNCOVERING THE Evidence

TITLE OF STUDY

"Patterns of Nursing Intervention Use across 6 Days of Acute Care Hospitalization for Three Older Patient Populations"

AUTHORS

L. L. Shever, M. Titler, J. Dochterman, Q. Fei, and D. M. Picone

PURPOSE

The purpose of this study was twofold: (1) to identify frequently used nursing interventions and (2) to describe patterns of interventions used for each of the three selected groups of clients.

METHODS

This secondary data analysis study used data from a medical center in which the Nursing Interventions Classification (NIC) was used to electronically document nursing care. Statistics were examined to determine the types, frequencies, and patterns of interventions used in providing care to older care recipients.

FINDINGS

Three interventions (surveillance, IV therapy, and diet staging) were used for all three groups of clients. There were some NIC treatment approaches that were unique to each client population.

IMPLICATIONS

The use of standardized nursing language (i.e., NIC) in electronic medical records enhances the collection and analysis of data. These data serve as guides for nurse managers in making decisions about staffing, resource allocation, and education.

Shever, L. L., Titler, M., Dochterman, J., Fei, Q., & Picone, D. M. (2007). Patterns of nursing intervention use across 6 days of acute care hospitalization for three older patient populations. *International Journal of Nursing Terminologies and Classifications*, 18(1), 18–29.

associated with supervision and coordination of client care. In a health care facility in which nurses are assigned clients within a total client care management system, responsibilities for supervision might be minimal, whereas facilities that use a variety of ancillary personnel for certain client activities might require a large percentage of time devoted to supervision of care. In home health care, for example, the primary role of the professional nurse might be supervision of personnel who provide assistance with ADL. Although a nurse might delegate certain tasks to other personnel, it is still the nurse's responsibility to ensure that the task was completed according to standards of care and to note the response of the client in order to evaluate progress toward expected outcomes.

Regardless of management style or type of facility, coordination of client activities among various health care providers remains the nurse's responsibility. For example, in acute care settings, the nurse needs to coordinate client activities around the schedule of diagnostic tests or physical therapy. Scheduling procedures, therapy, treatments, and medications for a number of clients often requires considerable organizational skills, creativity, and resourcefulness.

EVALUATING INTERVENTIONS

An important step to ensure the delivery of quality care is evaluation of nursing interventions. One approach to determining the efficacy of nursing interventions is by evaluating clients' achievement of expected outcomes. The NIC, previously described in this chapter, provides a systematic method for linking nursing activities to client outcomes. When treatment can be shown to directly improve client outcomes, both nursing and health care consumers benefit. Another taxonomy, the Nursing Outcomes Classification (NOC), has been specifically designed to measure client responses to nursing interventions.

DOCUMENTATION OF INTERVENTIONS

Communication concerning implementation of interventions must be provided through written documentation and should also be verbally conveyed when responsibility of the client's care is transferred to another nurse. The nurse is legally required to record all interventions and observations related to the client's response to treatment. This not only provides a legal record but also allows valuable communication with other health care team members for continuity of care and for evaluating progress toward expected outcomes. In addition, written documentation provides data necessary for reimbursement for services and tracking of indicators for quality improvement.

The recording of information can be in the form of either checklists, flow sheets, or narrative summaries. A complete description must be provided if there are any deviations from the norm or if any changes have occurred (see Chapter 13).

Verbal interaction among health care providers is also essential for communicating current information about clients. When delegating the tasks to unlicensed assistive personnel (UAP), the nurse must elicit feedback from the UAP about the activity performed and the client's response. In addition, assistive personnel should be alerted as to what additional data are meaningful, and these data should be conveyed to the nurse responsible for the client's care. For example, if a nursing assistant observes that a client hospitalized with a deep vein thrombosis of the left leg is having difficulty swallowing and has eaten very little, this information should be reported to the nurse. This is especially important if the behavior is a new occurrence and not a part of the established problem list, because the nurse might not otherwise seek this information.

Communication between nurses generally occurs at the change of shift, when the responsibility for care is transferred from one nurse to another. Nursing students must communicate relevant information to the nurse responsible for their clients when they leave the unit. Information that should be shared in the verbal report includes:

- Activities completed and those remaining to be completed
- Status of current relevant problems
- Any abnormalities or changes in client status
- Results of treatments (i.e., client response)
- Diagnostic tests scheduled or completed (and results)

All communication—whether written, verbal, or both—must be objective, descriptive, and complete. The communication includes observations rather than opinions and is stated or written so that an accurate picture of the client is conveyed. For example, if it is noted that a client is less alert today than yesterday, the *behavior* that led to that conclusion should be documented. This observation can be objectively and descriptively communicated by the statement "Does not respond unless firmly touched; quickly returns to sleep." This description results in a more complete picture of the client than simply stating, "Less alert today." Thorough and detailed communication of implementation activities is fundamental to ensuring that client care and progress toward goals can be adequately evaluated.

KEY CONCEPTS

- The implementation step of the nursing process is directed toward meeting client needs and results in health promotion, prevention of illness, illness management, or health restoration.
- Implementation involves delegation of nursing care activities to assistive personnel.

- Implementation requires application of cognitive, psychomotor, and intellectual skills to accomplish goals and make progress toward expected outcomes.
- Implementation activities include ongoing assessment, establishment of priorities, allocation of

resources, initiation of specific nursing interventions, and documentation of interventions and client responses.

- Ongoing assessment is necessary for determining effectiveness of interventions and for detecting new problems.

- Changing variables in clients and the environment demand clinical judgment and flexibility in organizing care.

- Time management skills are essential in implementing client care.

- The nurse maintains responsibility for care delegated to other health care personnel.

- The most common management systems currently used include functional nursing, team nursing, primary nursing, total client care, modular nursing, and case management.

- Interventions can be nurse initiated, prescribing practitioner initiated, or collaborative in origin and thus are considered dependent, independent, or interdependent.

- NIC is a system for sorting, labeling, and describing nursing interventions.

- Nursing interventions include assisting with ADL, skilled therapeutic interventions, monitoring and surveillance of client response to care, teaching, discharge planning, and supervision and coordination of nursing personnel.

- Communication concerning interventions should be provided verbally and in writing.

REVIEW QUESTIONS

1. Which of the following best describes the purpose of ongoing evaluation when implementing nursing activities?
   a. To be sure the activities performed are independent activities
   b. To determine client progress toward expected outcomes
   c. To ensure compliance with agency protocols
   d. To establish a nursing diagnosis

2. Establishing priority among several nursing interventions depends on which of the following? Select all that apply.
   a. Availability of resources
   b. Client perception
   c. Client's willingness to comply
   d. Education level of nurse
   e. Length of time necessary for the intervention
   f. Nurse determination of importance

3. Which of the following is an example of the functional nursing approach to care delivery?
   a. Team member has an assigned task to perform for the client.
   b. Full responsibility for total client care rests upon the registered nurse.
   c. The registered nurse coordinates care for the client across the entire care continuum.
   d. The registered nurse works with licensed practical/vocational nurses and unlicensed assistive personnel to deliver care.

4. Briefly answer the following question by filling in the blank:
   The nursing management system in which a group of care providers (RN, LPN, and UAP) coordinates activities to deliver care is defined as the _____ _____ nursing approach.

5. Which of the following should nurses do initially when performing a procedure they have never done before?
   a. Double-check the prescribing order.
   b. Seek help from another nurse who is proficient in performing the procedure.
   c. Inform the nursing supervisor that they are unwilling to do the procedure because it is a new skill for them.
   d. Try to remember all the steps of the procedure they learned in nursing school.

6. Which of the following statements made by a new nurse indicates a need for further guidance when giving a change-of-shift report?
   a. "The client had a good night."
   b. "The client is scheduled to have a CT scan this morning."
   c. "The client slept 5 uninterrupted hours after receiving Demerol."
   d. "We did not get all the blood glucose levels drawn this morning."

online companion

Visit the DeLaune and Ladner online companion resource at **www.delmar.cengage.com** for additional content and study aids. Click on Online Companions, then select the Nursing discipline.

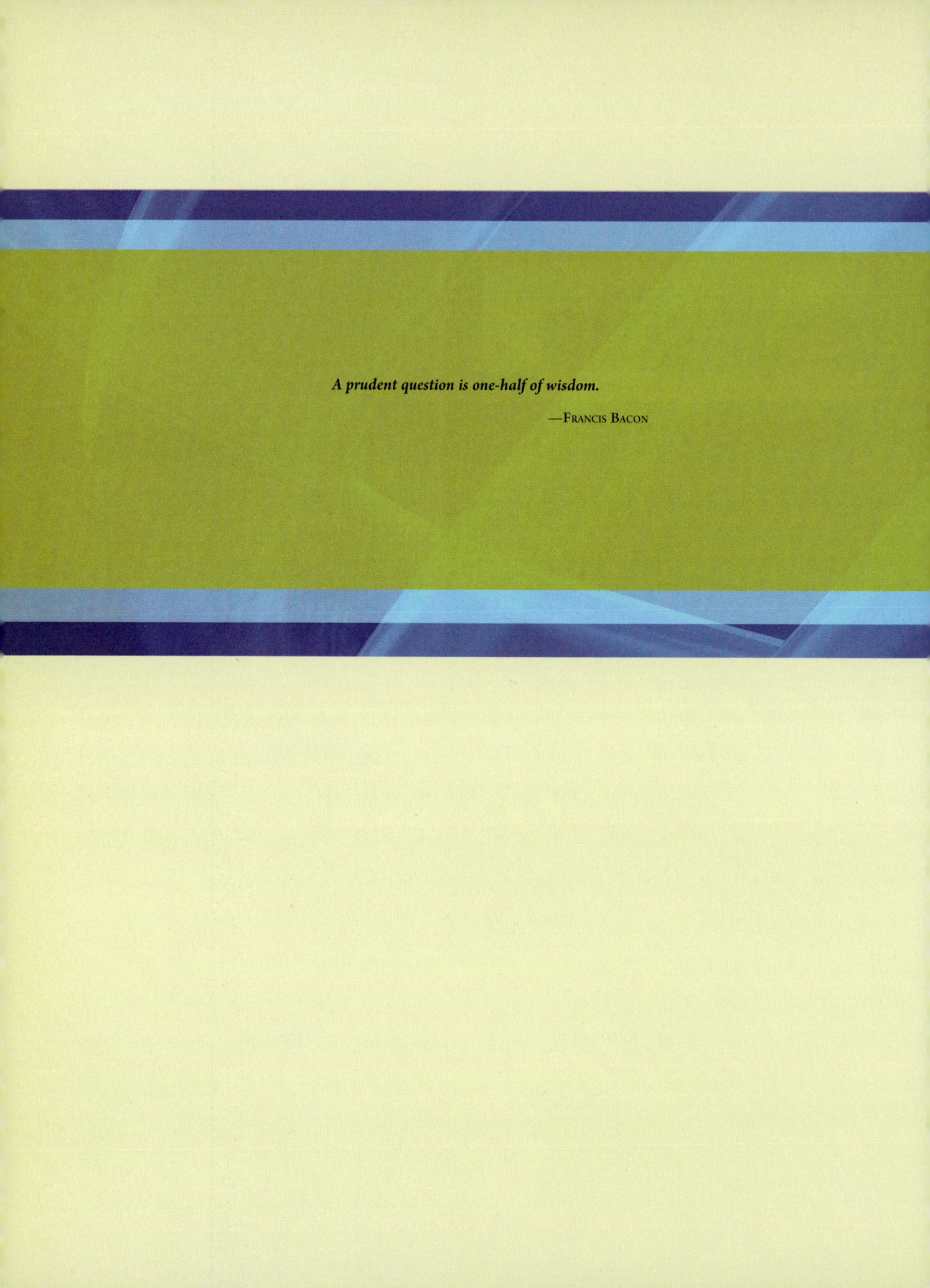

A prudent question is one-half of wisdom.

—FRANCIS BACON

CHAPTER 10

Evaluation

COMPETENCIES

1. Explain the purposes of evaluation in professional nursing practice.
2. Describe the components of comprehensive evaluation in nursing.
3. Describe the steps through which evaluation is conducted.
4. Describe the three types of evaluation.
5. Discuss the relationship between evaluation and accountability.
6. Explain the significance of multidisciplinary collaboration in evaluating client care.

KEY TERMS

evaluation	outcome evaluation	process evaluation
nursing audit	peer evaluation	structure evaluation

Evaluation is the fifth step in the nursing process and involves determining whether the client goals have been met, have been partially met, or have not been met. Even though it is the final phase of the nursing process, evaluation is an ongoing part of daily nursing activities. The major purpose of evaluation is to determine the effectiveness of those activities in helping clients achieve expected outcomes. Evaluation is not only a part of the nursing process but also an integral process in determining the quality of health care delivered. This chapter discusses the purposes, components, and methods of evaluation. The relationship between evaluation and quality of care is described.

EVALUATION OF CLIENT CARE

Evaluation is the measurement of the degree to which objectives are achieved. Therefore, evaluating the care provided to clients is an essential part of professional nursing. The American Nurses Association (2004) designates evaluation as a fundamental component of the nursing process. The purposes of evaluation include:

- To determine the client's progress or lack of progress toward achievement of expected outcomes
- To determine the effectiveness of nursing care in helping clients achieve the expected outcomes
- To determine the overall quality of care provided
- To promote nursing accountability

Evaluation is done primarily to determine whether a client is progressing—that is, experiencing an improvement in health status. Evaluation is not an end to the nursing process, but rather an ongoing mechanism that ensures quality interventions. Effective evaluation is done periodically, not just prior to termination of care. Evaluation is closely related to each of the other stages of the nursing process. The plan of care may be modified during any phase of the nursing process when the need to do so is determined through evaluation. Client goals and expected outcomes provide the criteria for evaluation of care. The Nursing Interventions Classification (NIC) and Nursing Outcomes Classification (NOC) taxonomies are methods useful in evaluating clients' achievement of outcomes and the efficacy of nursing interventions.

COMPONENTS OF EVALUATION

Evaluation is a fluid process that depends on all the other components of the nursing process. As shown in Figure 10-1, evaluation affects, and is affected by, assessment, diagnosis, outcome identification and planning, and implementation of

nursing care. Ongoing evaluation is essential if the nursing process is to be implemented appropriately. As Alfaro-LeFevre (2008) states:

> When we evaluate early, checking whether our information is accurate, complete, and up-to-date, we're able to make corrections *early*. We avoid making decisions based on outdated, inaccurate, or incomplete information. Early evaluation enhances our ability to act safely and effectively. It improves our *efficiency* by helping us stay focused on priorities and avoid wasting time continuing useless actions. (p. 20)

Specific criteria are to be used in the process of evaluation. The evaluation criteria must be planned, goal directed, objective, verifiable, and specific; that is, strengths, weaknesses, achievements, and deficits must be considered.

TECHNIQUES

Effective evaluation results primarily from the nurse's accurate use of communication and observation skills. Both verbal and nonverbal communication between the nurse and the client can yield important information about the accuracy of the goals, expected planned outcomes, and nursing interventions that have been executed for resolution of the client's problems. The nurse needs to be sensitive to clients' willingness or hesitation to discuss their responses to nursing actions and must use therapeutic communication techniques to collect all necessary data.

Effective nurses are aware of changes in the client's physiological condition, emotional status, and behavior. Because these changes are often subtle, they require astute observational skills on the part of the nurse. Observation occurs through use of the senses. In other words, what the nurse sees, hears, smells, and feels when touching the client all provide clues to the client's current health status.

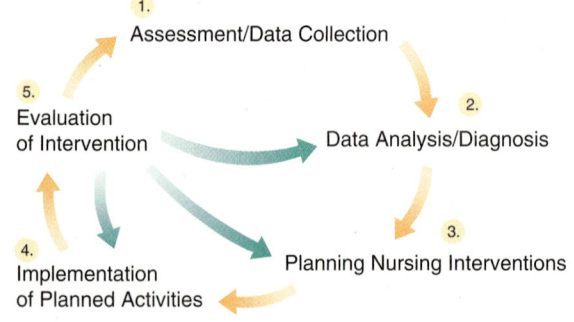

FIGURE 10-1 Relationship of Evaluation to Nursing Process
DELMAR/CENGAGE LEARNING

SOURCES OF DATA

Evaluation is a mutual process occurring among the nurse, client, family, and other health care providers. Both subjective and objective data are used in evaluating the client's status. Asking clients to describe how they feel results in subjective data. Objective data consist of observable facts, such as laboratory values and the client's behavior.

When a nurse communicates an assessment of a client's response to an actual or potential health problem, clients and families are empowered to discuss their concerns and questions. When feedback is given, the nurse must avoid being defensive because that attitude may cause clients or families to avoid being open and honest. As a result, clients may say only what they think the nurse wants to hear or they may refuse to participate in the evaluation process. The nurse's verbal and nonverbal communication establishes the atmosphere in which clients and families freely share their comments, both positive and negative.

GOALS AND EXPECTED OUTCOMES

The effectiveness of nursing interventions is evaluated by examination of goals and expected outcomes. Goals provide direction for the plan of care and serve as measurements for the client's progress, or lack of progress, toward resolution of a problem.

Realistic goals are necessary for effective evaluation. These goals must take into consideration the client's strengths, limitations, resources, and the time frame for achieving the objectives. Examples of client strengths are educational background, family support, and financial resources (e.g., money to purchase medications and foods that support the prescribed interventions). Examples of client limitations are delayed developmental level, poverty, and unwillingness to change (lack of motivation).

METHODS OF EVALUATION

The nurse who successfully evaluates nursing care uses a systematic approach that ensures thorough, comprehensive collection of data. Evaluation is an orderly process consisting of seven steps, which are explained here.

ESTABLISHING STANDARDS

Specific criteria are used to determine whether the demonstrated behavior indicates goal achievement. Standards are established before nursing action is implemented. Evaluation of criteria examines the presence of any changes, direction of change (positive or negative), and whether the changes were expected or unexpected.

COLLECTING DATA

Assessment skills are used to gather data pertinent to goals and expected outcomes. The nurse must be proficient in assessment skills in order for effective, comprehensive evaluation to occur. Evaluation data are collected to answer the following question: Were the treatment goals and expected outcomes achieved?

DETERMINING GOAL ACHIEVEMENT

Data are analyzed to determine whether client behaviors indicate goal achievement. This process is validated through analysis of the client's response to the specific nursing interventions that are developed in the plan of care. For example, these data can take the form of either physiological responses (such as the client's being able to cough productively in order to promote effective breathing patterns) or psychosocial responses (such as the client's being able to verbalize concerns about an impending surgical procedure in order to alleviate anxiety).

RELATING NURSING ACTIONS TO CLIENT STATUS

Nursing interventions are examined to determine their relevance to the client's needs and nursing diagnoses. Effective nursing actions are those that address pertinent client needs and help clients appropriately resolve actual or potential problems.

JUDGING THE VALUE OF NURSING INTERVENTIONS

Critical thinking skills are employed to determine whether nursing actions have contributed to the client's improved status. These skills enable the nurse to analyze the client's responses to the nursing interventions. Evaluating the benefits of nursing actions helps identify additional opportunities for changes in the plan of care.

REASSESSING THE CLIENT'S STATUS

The client's health status is reevaluated through use of assessment and observation skills. Evaluation focuses on the client's current health status and compares it with baseline data collected during the initial assessment. Omissions or incomplete data within the database are identified so that an accurate picture of the client's health status is obtained.

MODIFYING THE PLAN OF CARE

If the evaluation data indicate a lack of progress toward goal achievement, the plan of care is revised. These revisions are developed through the following process: reassessment of the client, formulation of more appropriate nursing diagnoses, development of new or revised goals and expected outcomes, and implementation of different nursing actions or repetition of specific actions to maximize their effectiveness (e.g., client teaching). See the Nursing Checklist for guidelines for evaluating effective application of the nursing process to client care.

☑ NURSING CHECKLIST

EVALUATING NURSING CARE

Following are guidelines useful in analyzing the application of the nursing process:

- Assessment is thorough and accurate.
- Nursing diagnoses are relevant.
- Client and family participate in goal setting.
- Goals are specific, measurable, and realistic.
- Nursing actions address client's problems.
- Client and family participate in evaluation.
- Evaluation is ongoing and results in a revised plan of care according to the client's status changes.
- Plan of care is revised according to the client's needs.
- Documentation reflects the client's status, including responses to nursing interventions.

Evaluation is performed by every nurse in all practice settings for each client. For example, the home health nurse evaluates the care provided regularly throughout the client's relationship with the agency. Evaluation of the home care client is carried out in order to determine whether the care was delivered in an effective and efficient manner, to modify the plan of care as needed, and to decide when the client is ready for discontinuation of home care services. The accompanying Community Considerations display provides an example of evaluation performed by the home health care nurse.

CRITICAL THINKING AND EVALUATION

Evaluation is a critical thinking activity. It is a deliberate mechanism used to analyze and make judgments. Evaluation

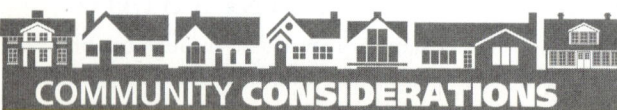

COMMUNITY CONSIDERATIONS

Evaluation in the Home Health Care Setting

When evaluating the effectiveness of care, the home health care nurse can use the following questions to examine client achievement of expected outcomes:

- Were the goals realistic in terms of client abilities and time frame?
- Were there external variables (e.g., housing problems, impaired family dynamics) that prevented goal achievement?
- Did the family have the resources (e.g., transportation) to assist in meeting the goals?
- Was the care coordinated with other providers to facilitate efficient delivery of care?

involves analysis and is much more complex than merely answering questions. Nurses need to remain objective when evaluating client care in order to modify care based on reason rather than emotion. Nurses use critical thinking throughout evaluative activities by comparing client responses to expected behaviors. They make conclusions about whether expected outcomes have been met. In order to make such conclusions, assessment data are needed to determine client progress toward achievement of objectives.

EVALUATION AND QUALITY OF CARE

Evaluation is performed at the individual and institutional levels. For example, individual evaluation focuses on the client's achievement of goals and also on the individual nurse's delivery of care. Quality and evaluation are closely related. This section examines the role of evaluation in ensuring the delivery of quality health care. Because it is the mechanism used by nurses in determining the need for improvement, evaluation assists in the provision of quality care. The aspects that need to be evaluated to determine the quality of health care are:

- Appropriateness (the care provided adhered to standards and resulted in achievement of goals)
- Clinical outcomes
- Client satisfaction
- Cost-effectiveness
- Access to care
- Availability of resources

Quality management involves constant, ongoing evaluation (monitoring of activities).

ELEMENTS IN EVALUATING THE QUALITY OF CARE

Organizational evaluation examines the agency's overall ability to deliver quality care. Evaluation can be classified according to what is being evaluated: the structure, the process, or the outcome. Figure 10-2 on page 157 illustrates the variables to be assessed in each type of evaluation.

Structure Evaluation

Structure evaluation is a determination of the health care agency's ability to provide the services offered to its client population. Structure evaluation examines the physical facilities, resources, equipment, staffing patterns, organizational patterns, and the agency's qualifications for staff. The majority of problems with providing effective health care stem from problems in the structural area. The purpose of structure evaluation is to identify any system errors that can be corrected.

Structure evaluation involves determining whether client care meets legal and professional standards. A frequently used method to evaluate whether the agency provides care within legal parameters is a review of policy and procedure

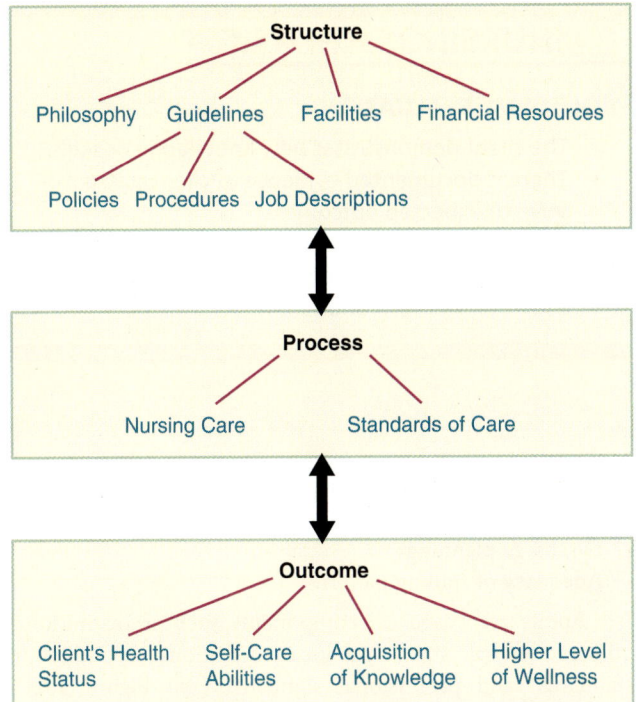

FIGURE 10-2 Elements within Each Type of Evaluation DELMAR/CENGAGE LEARNING

manuals to check for compliance with regulations. Table 10-1 describes ways to perform structure evaluation, which measures the adequacy of an agency to meet client needs.

Process Evaluation

Process evaluation is the measurement of nursing actions by examining each phase of the nursing process. This type of evaluation is done to determine whether nursing care was adequate, appropriate, effective, and efficient. Nursing interventions are judged to be effective when use of the action results in the desired outcome. See the Uncovering the Evidence display. Process evaluation determines the nurse's ability to establish an environment that promotes the client's health. See the Nursing Process Highlight for recommendations

for client evaluation. Note that these recommendations are applicable to all practice settings.

Outcome Evaluation

Outcome evaluation is the process of comparing the client's current status with the expected outcomes. This type of evaluation examines all direct care activities that affect the client's health status. Outcome evaluation focuses on changes in the client's health status. A basic question to ask when evaluating the outcome is "Has the expected change occurred?"

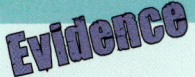

UNCOVERING THE Evidence

TITLE OF STUDY
"Evaluating the Effectiveness of Preoperative Interventions: The Appropriateness of Using the Children's Emotional Manifestation Scale"

AUTHOR
H. C. Li

PURPOSE
This study had two purposes: (1) to compare the effectiveness of two preoperative nursing interventions and (2) to examine the appropriateness of using the Children's Emotional Manifestation Scale for evaluating the efficacy of preoperative interventions.

METHODS
This was a randomized controlled trial in which children admitted for elective same-day surgery were assigned to one of two groups: the experimental group that received therapeutic play intervention and the control group that received routine preoperative information.

FINDINGS
Children receiving preoperative therapeutic play intervention reported significantly lower anxiety levels and fewer negative emotions and experienced lower heart rates and mean arterial blood pressures than children who received the routine preoperative preparation.

IMPLICATIONS
This study demonstrates the appropriateness of using the Children's Emotional Manifestation Scale to evaluate the effectiveness of preoperative nursing interventions. It also presents clear evidence that supports the efficacy of therapeutic play in preparing children for surgery.

Li, H. C. (2007). Evaluating the effectiveness of preoperative interventions: The appropriateness of using the Children's Emotional Manifestation Scale. *Journal of Clinical Nursing*, 16(10), 1919–1926.

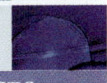

TABLE 10-1 Structure Evaluation

EVALUATION QUESTIONS	DATA SOURCES
• Are nursing policies readily available to staff? • Do orientation programs provide information necessary for job performance? • Do staffing patterns show ability to meet client needs?	• Orientation programs • Policy manuals • Procedure manuals • Staffing patterns

Delmar/Cengage Learning

NURSING PROCESS HIGHLIGHT

Evaluation

Client Evaluation

- Upon admission, each client is assessed by a registered nurse.
- Each client has an individualized plan of care.
- Nursing interventions are specified in the plan of care.
- Client responses to interventions are documented.

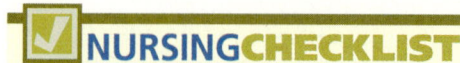

NURSINGCHECKLIST

OUTCOME EVALUATION

- The client demonstrates new knowledge or skills.
- There is documented evidence of client status relative to expected outcomes.
- There is documentation of client coping abilities.
- There is a discharge plan that specifies follow-up activities for client and family.

Another variable assessed during outcome evaluation is the client's self-care ability. Has the client demonstrated an improved ability to care for himself or herself? Does the client verbalize knowledge related to self-care needs? See the Nursing Checklist for suggested approaches to performing outcome evaluation. The accompanying Nursing Process Highlight shows the application of the North American Nursing Diagnosis Association (NANDA), NOC, and NIC systems with a client experiencing problems in feeding himself or herself.

NURSING AUDIT

A **nursing audit** is the process of collecting and analyzing data to evaluate the effectiveness of nursing interventions. A nursing audit can focus on implementation of the nursing process, client outcomes, or both in order to evaluate the quality of care provided. Nursing audits examine data related to:

- Safety measures
- Treatment interventions and client responses
- Preestablished outcomes used as basis for interventions
- Client teaching
- Discharge planning
- Adequacy of staffing patterns

Audits are based on components such as institutional policies; federal, state, and local regulations; accreditation standards; and professional standards (see Figure 10-3). Audits assist in identifying strengths and weaknesses that, in turn, provide direction for areas needing revision. Corrective

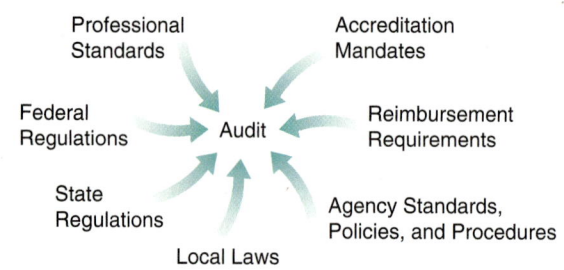

FIGURE 10-3 Influences Affecting Nursing Audit DELMAR/CENGAGE LEARNING

NURSING PROCESS HIGHLIGHT

Evaluation

Client with Feeding Self-Care Deficit

DIAGNOSIS (NANDA)	OUTCOMES (NOC)	INTERVENTION (NIC)
Self-care deficit: feeding	Be able to feed self independently	Assess energy level and activity tolerance
	Demonstrate adequate intake of food and fluids	Assess intake for nutritional adequacy
	Use adaptive devices to eat	Assess ability to use adaptive devices

From Bulechek, G. M., Dochterman, J. M., & Butcher, H. K. (2007). *Nursing interventions classifications (NIC)* (5th ed.). St. Louis, MO: Elsevier; Moorhead, S., Johnson, M., Mass, M., & Swanson, E. (2007). *Nursing outcomes classification (NOC)* (4th ed.). St. Louis, MO: Elsevier; North American Nursing Diagnosis Association. (2009). *Nursing diagnosis—Definitions and classification 2009–2011*. Philadelphia: John Wiley & Sons, Inc; Wilkinson, J. M. (2008). *Nursing diagnosis handbook* (9th ed.). Upper Saddle River, NJ: Prentice-Hall.

action plans are developed in accordance with the audit results.

PEER EVALUATION

Another method of evaluating quality of care is **peer evaluation** (also referred to as *peer review*), the process by which professionals provide to their peers critical performance appraisal and feedback that are geared toward corrective action. Peer evaluation, when performed appropriately, improves the quality of care by addressing specific behavior of the nurse being evaluated. It can be verbal or written depending on agency policy. Peer evaluation may be done formally or informally, with information being provided in a timely manner.

By evaluating itself, nursing is demonstrating an essential criterion by which professions are recognized. Peer evaluation promotes both professional and individual accountability. The quality of nursing care is strongly evident to coworkers and nurses who are expected to assess the work of their peers.

Such judgment may result in one of the following outcomes:

- Destructive: Complaints and attacks that undermine morale and cohesiveness
- Constructive: Positive feedback that improves the quality of care

Peer evaluation can be destructive if the parties involved begin to personalize the process, misunderstand the purpose, or deliver feedback in an unfeeling and nonobjective manner. Peer evaluation can be threatening when guidelines have not been established for the process and when the assessment focuses on emotions and personalities instead of on behaviors. Conversely, peer evaluation is constructive when the focus remains on quality improvement and encourages the continued growth and learning of all the parties involved. See the Spotlight On display.

EVALUATION AND ACCOUNTABILITY

Accountability means assuming responsibility for one's actions. Evaluation enhances nursing accountability by providing a mechanism for assisting the nurse to define, explain, and measure the results of nursing actions. Accountability is increased by ongoing evaluation; nurses are continually checking their own progress against predetermined standards.

Accountability is an integral part of professional nursing practice and is an important method through which commitment to quality client care can be demonstrated. Nurses are accountable for their judgments, decisions, and actions to:

- Clients, families, and significant others
- Colleagues
- Employers
- The general public (society)
- The nursing profession
- Themselves

Nurses demonstrate their commitment to accountability in a variety of ways, including maintaining expertise in skills and participating in continuing education programs. Other ways of demonstrating accountability are achieving and maintaining certification and participating in peer evaluation.

MULTIDISCIPLINARY COLLABORATION IN EVALUATION

Evaluating the quality of care provided is a responsibility shared among members of the health care team. In addition to those directly involved (the health care providers, clients, and families), others interested in the outcomes of evaluation include the community and third-party payers (both public and private reimbursement organizations).

An ongoing monitoring process is implemented to evaluate quality of care. Ideally, every discipline monitors its own quality efforts. No single discipline is responsible for all-inclusive evaluation of client care. However, in most health care agencies, nurses are actively involved in monitoring evaluation activities. Many agencies have nurses on staff who function either as quality management coordinators, utilization review evaluators, or both.

When health care providers from all the relevant disciplines are involved in evaluation, the result is decreased fragmentation of care. The team approach mandates active involvement of all care providers in the evaluation of quality care. Multidisciplinary evaluation helps promote a continuum of care for the client, from the preadmission phase to discharge planning and follow-up care.

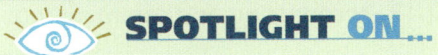 SPOTLIGHT ON...

Professionalism

Peer Evaluation and Friendship

Your coworker is also a close friend. You are assigned to perform a peer evaluation with her. Before the process begins, she asks you to be especially lenient when evaluating her performance. When collecting information about the quality of her work, you discover that she is often hurried and unorganized, a practice that results in her providing only mediocre care. You know that if the evaluation is not above average, your friend will likely experience disciplinary action from her supervisor. In view of your friendship, what do you do in this situation?

NURSING CARE PLAN

The Client Experiencing Self-Care Deficits and Risk for Injury

CASE PRESENTATION
Mr. Magee was admitted yesterday with right-sided weakness. His medical diagnosis is cerebral vascular accident (CVA). He is 68 years of age and resides alone in the house on his farm where he and his wife lived for 40 years. She died last year. He reports that he is right-handed and has difficulty holding a fork.

ASSESSMENT
- "I can't handle this milk carton with only one hand."
- "I do not like to use that walker. It gets in my way."
- Gait unsteady and shuffling
- Asymmetrical strength in arms and legs
- Unable to hold fork in right hand

NURSING DIAGNOSIS 1: *Feeding self-care deficit* related to weakness in right hand AEB inability to hold fork.
NOC: Client will be able to feed self independently.
NIC: Serve finger foods to promote independence.

EXPECTED OUTCOMES
The client will:

1. Attend a teaching session on feeding himself with his left hand at 1000 on 2/12.
2. Practice using adaptive spoon at 1400 on 2/12.
3. Use adaptive spoon for meals beginning with breakfast on 2/13.

INTERVENTIONS/RATIONALES
1. Present a teaching session "Feeding oneself with the nondominant hand" at 1000 on 2/12. For clients recovering from illness and/or injury, information about adapting to limitations fosters independence.
2. Provide the client with four foods of differing textures, adaptive spoons, and apron for a practice session at 1400 on 2/12. Providing practice time reinforces skills learned and fosters an improved confidence level in the learner.
3. Notify the dietary department to include a left-hand adaptive spoon with breakfast tray on 2/13. Using adaptive devices provides safety and promotes independence.
4. Encourage client to feed self independently at each meal, beginning 2/13. Recognizing and commending success promotes positive self-esteem.
5. Assist client with food preparation and feeding as needed at each meal, beginning 2/12. Assistance preserves strength, avoids tiring the client, promotes safety, and decreases frustration as the client strives for independence.

EVALUATION
1. Goal met. Mr. Magee attended teaching session on 2/12, asked questions, and participated in the practice session.
2. Goal partially met. Mr. Magee practiced using a spoon in his left hand to feed himself oatmeal, soup, ice cream, and canned peaches on 2/12. Successful self-feeding with all foods except soup. Continue practice, reevaluate 2/19.
3. Goal partially met. On 2/13, fed self 75% of each meal, using adaptive spoon. Continue. Reevaluate on 2/15.

NURSING DIAGNOSIS 2: *Risk for injury: falls* related to unsteady, shuffling gait.
NOC: Risk for fall will be decreased by environmental modifications.
NIC: Instruct client in fall prevention measures (e.g., handrails, grab bars, and shower mats).

(Continues)

NURSING CARE PLAN (Continued)

EXPECTED OUTCOMES

The client will:

1. Participate in physical therapy evaluation of mobility strengths and weaknesses on 2/11 at 1100.
2. Attend a muscle-strengthening class on 2/12 at 1600.
3. Perform all strengthening exercises prescribed BID at 1000 and 1600, beginning 2/13.

INTERVENTIONS/RATIONALES

1. Request physical therapy consultation for appropriate assistive devices, strengthening exercises, and gait training on 2/11. Collaboration with other health care providers provides the best care for the client.
2. Escort client to muscle-strengthening class on 2/12 at 1600. Provides safety and support as the client begins to learn new skills.
3. Assigned caregiver will record each exercise, number of repetitions, and client response BID. Documenting client progress toward the achievement of goals aids in outcome attainment and evaluation of care.

EVALUATION

1. Goal not met. Appointment not kept on 2/11. Dental emergency. Continue. Reevaluate 2/15.
2. Goal not met. Unable to evaluate on 2/12. Continue. Reevaluate on 2/15.
3. 2/15: Goal met. Client attended muscle-strengthening class and has performed exercises as prescribed two times each day.

KEY CONCEPTS

- Evaluation, the fifth step in the nursing process, involves determining whether client goals have been met, have been partially met, or have not been met.
- The purposes of evaluation are to determine the client's progress or lack of progress toward achievement of client objectives, to judge the efficiency of nursing actions in helping clients to achieve objectives, to determine the health care agency's overall ability to deliver care in an effective and efficient manner, and to promote nursing accountability.
- Evaluation is based primarily on the skills of communication and observation.
- Evaluation is a mutual, ongoing process occurring among the nurse, client, family, and other health care providers.
- The effectiveness of nursing interventions is evaluated by examination of goals and expected outcomes that provide direction for the plan of care and serve as standards by which the client's progress is measured.
- Evaluation is an orderly process consisting of seven steps: establishing standards, collecting data related to the goals and expected outcomes, determining goal achievement, relating nursing actions to client status, judging the value of nursing interventions in assisting clients to achieve goals and objectives, reassessing the client's status, and modifying the plan of care if necessary.
- There is a relationship between quality management and evaluation. Evaluation is necessary in the provision of quality care because it is the mechanism used by nurses in determining how to improve care.
- Structure evaluation judges a health care agency's ability to provide the services offered to its client population.
- Process evaluation measures nursing actions by examining each phase of the nursing process to determine the effectiveness of the actions in helping clients meet expected outcomes and goals.
- Outcome evaluation compares the client's current status with the expected outcomes and examines all direct care activities that affect the client's status.
- A nursing audit can focus on implementation of the nursing process, client outcomes, or both in order to evaluate the quality of care provided.
- Peer evaluation (peer review) is the process by which professionals provide to their peers performance appraisal feedback geared toward corrective action.

- Evaluation enhances professional nursing accountability by providing a mechanism for assisting the nurse to define, explain, and measure the results of nursing actions.

- Evaluating the quality of care is a shared responsibility among members of the health care team.

REVIEW QUESTIONS

1. Which of the following accurately describes the purposes of evaluation? Select all that apply.
   a. Determine client progress toward achievement of expected outcomes.
   b. Determine effectiveness of nursing care.
   c. Establish client expected outcomes.
   d. Establish priorities for nursing interventions.
   e. Promote nursing accountability.
   f. Write the plan of care, including specific measurable goals.

2. Which of the following client statements are indicators of client strengths? Select all that apply.
   a. "I don't think that I'll be able to stop smoking."
   b. "I dropped out of school in the eighth grade to go to work."
   c. "I have no relatives to bother me."
   d. "My company pays for my health insurance."
   e. "My family is willing to change their eating habits since I'm on a diet."
   f. "My wife and I are both employed as school teachers."

3. In which of the following situations is the nurse performing evaluation?
   a. Determining a client's baseline temperature
   b. Developing expected client outcomes

   c. Asking a client if pain is relieved after administration of analgesics
   d. Writing an individualized plan of care for a client

4. Which of the following statements best describes the evaluation of quality care?
   a. Carried out to determine whether the client feels better
   b. Determined after the project is completed
   c. Performed only by nursing
   d. Shared responsibility of multidisciplinary team

5. Which of the following mechanisms is based on honest confrontation and open communication?
   a. Establishing standards
   b. Outcome evaluation
   c. Peer review
   d. Structure evaluation

6. A nurse helps reposition a client who has difficulty breathing. Which of the following nursing actions, when performed after the intervention, demonstrates evaluation?
   a. Arranging pillows behind the client's back
   b. Changing the rate of flow for oxygen delivery
   c. Checking the client's respiratory status
   d. Instructing the client on the importance of mobility

online companion

Visit the DeLaune and Ladner online companion resource at **www.delmar.cengage.com** for additional content and study aids. Click on Online Companions, then select the Nursing discipline.

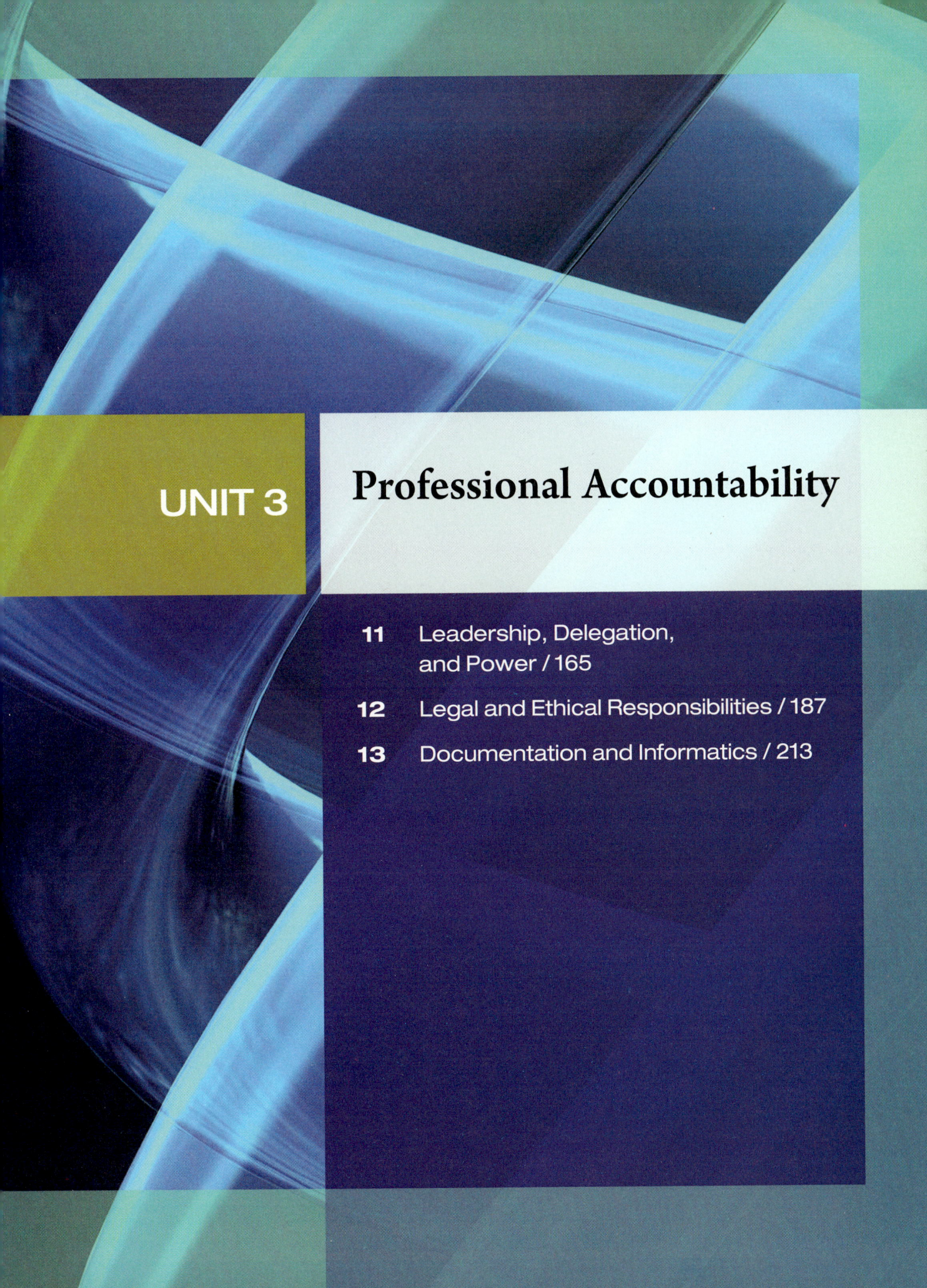

UNIT 3

Professional Accountability

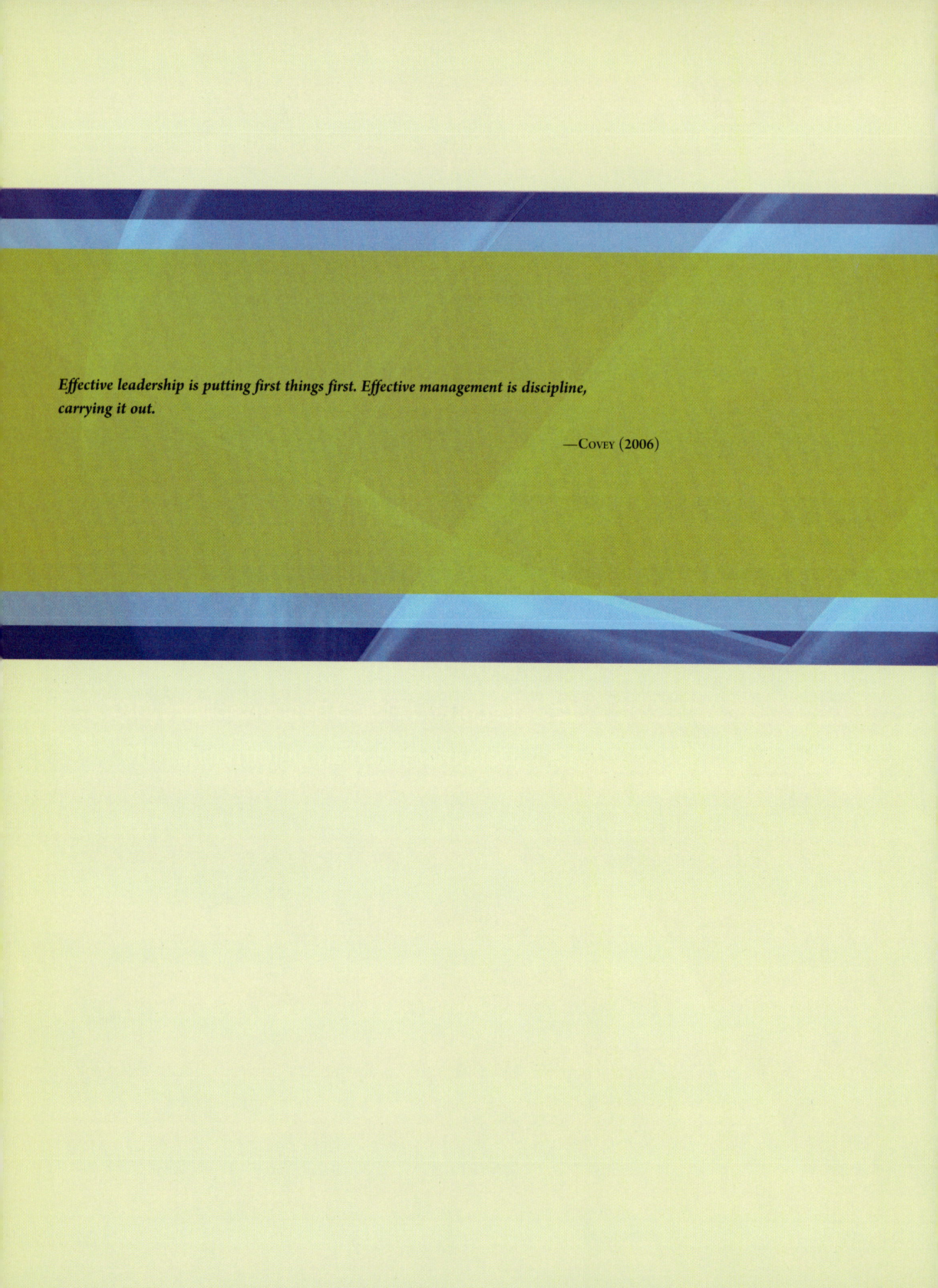

Effective leadership is putting first things first. Effective management is discipline, carrying it out.

—Covey (2006)

CHAPTER 11

Leadership, Delegation, and Power

COMPETENCIES

1. State criteria for professional nursing practice.
2. Describe the elements of professional accountability.
3. Explain the licensure process for professional nurses.
4. Discuss advanced practice nursing and professional accountability.
5. Discuss the characteristics of effective leaders.
6. Explain nursing responsibilities involved in delegation.
7. Describe the types of power and their sources.
8. State the actions through which nurses can increase political power.

KEY TERMS

accountability	leadership	politics
accreditation	legal regulation	power
advanced practice nursing	licensure	profession
autocratic leadership style	licensure by endorsement	professional regulation
certification	licensure by examination	professional standards
competency	management	scope of practice
delegation	mandatory licensure laws	situational leadership
democratic leadership style	networking	synergy
empowerment	nurse practice act	
laissez-faire leadership style	organization	

As nursing continues to evolve, many questions arise: Is nursing truly a profession? Are nurses really autonomous? Autonomy is related to accountability. As autonomy increases, so does the need to be accountable. To whom are nurses accountable?

This chapter addresses these issues and emphasizes the need to be involved in activities that advance the nursing profession. In addition, nursing leadership, power, and the politics of nursing are discussed in terms of their contributions to professional nursing practice.

PROFESSIONAL NURSING PRACTICE

Isabel Hampton Robb, the first president of the American Nurses Association (ANA), stated in the late nineteenth century that nursing lacked two elements of a profession—organization and legislation (ANA, 1976). Believing nurses were not capable of managing their own affairs, hospital authorities opposed any efforts of nurses to organize. Moreover, the lack of accepted standards for nursing education caused graduates of one nursing school to question the credentials of graduates of other nursing schools. The result of these negative responses to the autonomy of the nursing profession was the belief held by nurses that it was neither possible nor desirable to work collectively (ANA, 1976).

However, in the early twentieth century, nursing did organize. The primary goal was to establish legislation that would legitimize nursing practice and gain recognition of nursing as a profession. Even though nursing is often referred to as a profession, there is debate about whether nursing is a *true* profession when appraised against the criteria of a profession.

CRITERIA OF A PROFESSION

A **profession** is a group (vocational or occupational) that requires specialized education and intellectual knowledge. There has been much debate about whether nursing is a profession or an occupation. Registered nurses consider nursing to be a profession similar to other professions (e.g., accounting, engineering, pharmacy, law, and medicine). However, for nursing to be recognized as a profession by the society it serves, nursing must demonstrate on an ongoing basis that it meets the criteria of a profession (Table 11-1 on page 167). See the accompanying Spotlight On display.

Nursing has accomplished much in the way of establishing its body of knowledge, scope of practice, research base, and code of ethics. However, nursing continues to struggle with maintaining authority over its own practice. As political forces affect the health care delivery system, the challenge to maintain control over nursing practice will become even greater. If nursing is to maintain professional autonomy, it must have a strong political base that seeks to inform public policy makers about the role and scope of professional nursing.

A profession is only as good as its individual members. Every member of the profession must practice as a professional and contribute to nursing as a profession. Beginning nursing students should understand the significance of ascribing to professional attitudes and values and how their behavior can influence the public's view of the nursing profession.

As professionals, nurses are accountable for providing quality care. **Accountability** is the process in which individuals are answerable for their actions and have an obligation

SPOTLIGHT ON...

Professionalism

Indicators of Professionalism

Observe registered nurses in various practice settings. How do the nurses interact with one another? How do the nurses demonstrate professional commitment? Are they involved in professional activities, such as continuing education and professional association activities? How do these nurses contribute to the public's perception of the nursing profession?

TABLE 11-1 Comparison of Nursing to Criteria of a Profession

CRITERIA OF A PROFESSION	NURSING ACHIEVEMENTS
The work is intellectual and distinguished by a substantial body of knowledge.	• Professional nursing requires knowledge, judgment, and skills based on biological, sociological, psychological, and nursing sciences.
Provision of a unique service to society.	• Since the early twentieth century, the public has granted nursing the right and responsibility for self-regulation through state licensure laws. • Historically, the public has been concerned about having an adequate number of registered nurses to provide service.
An expanding body of knowledge.	• Nursing, by its nature, is expanding its knowledge base to meet the demands of health care delivery (i.e., increased technology, changing reimbursement systems, new practice settings). • Nurse theorists and nurse researchers contribute to the knowledge base.
Personal responsibility to the public for services provided.	• Professional registered nurses are held individually accountable to the public through such mechanisms as legal regulations and licensure.
A long period of education, including both theory and practice.	• Professional nursing is based on a broad knowledge base, requiring specialized knowledge, skills, and abilities. • Nursing education is both theory and practice based. • Nursing has successfully established its educational base away from the apprentice approach and moved into higher education.
Autonomy and the ability to develop policy about the discipline and control of the activity of one's members.	• Nurse practice acts generally grant authority for regulating the profession to an agency or board comprised of a majority of nurses. • Nurse administrators have achieved positions at levels comparable with other hospital administrators.
Members share a common identity, values, and attitudes.	• Registered nurses generally adhere to their dedication to care and identify their role as client advocates in the health care system. • Professional organizations share common values.
Career choice of its members is motivated by altruism and reflects a long-term commitment to the public.	• Historically, people entered the field of nursing to care for those in need; however, few individuals (predominantly female) anticipated long-term employment. Today, more men and minorities are entering nursing. Further, more registered nurses are employed full time in nursing than ever before and anticipate continuing this practice.
A code of ethics to which its members adhere.	• The ANA has a long-standing published code of ethics. Many of the values identified within this code have been incorporated into nurse practice acts, thus establishing them as legal requirements. • Violations of legal standards are grounds for disciplinary action against one's license. • Traditionally, registered nurses have ascribed to and supported the professional organization's responsibility to develop a code of ethics. • Registered nurses have demonstrated support of boards of nursing in enforcing professional practice and have participated by reporting violations.

Data from Chitty, K. K., & Black, B. P. (2007). *Professional nursing: Concepts and challenges* (5th ed.). St. Louis: Elsevier; Kelly, P. (2008). *Nursing leadership & management* (2nd ed.). Clifton Park, NY: Cengage Delmar.

(or duty) to act. Accountability is demonstrated by nurses in several ways. For example, the accountable nurse is one who demonstrates caring and compassion to clients and families. By providing client-centered holistic care, the nurse is meeting the expectations of society.

PROFESSIONAL ACCOUNTABILITY

Accountability is a term often used in nursing. How does a nurse demonstrate accountability? The nursing profession is accountable for establishing and maintaining standards that promote safe, effective care. Accountability involves responsibility—that is, being able and willing to respond. Nurses are accountable to many: themselves, clients and their families, the nursing profession, employers, and the general public for provision of safe, effective care established by the profession.

Accountability is one of the distinguishing characteristics of a profession. The professional nurse is accountable in several domains: professional, legal, and ethical. See Chapter 12 for complete discussion of legal and ethical accountability.

ELEMENTS OF PROFESSIONAL ACCOUNTABILITY

To appreciate one's accountability as a professional, it is important to first understand the social context of nursing. Professions arise from an identified public need for specialized knowledge and skills. The more specialized the knowledge and skills, the greater the risk to the public from an incompetent professional. Therefore, the public entrusts the profession to regulate itself on behalf of the public's best interests.

The public holds nursing accountable for safe nursing care and proper judgment in the provision of nursing services. The profession is held accountable by the public to

---

SPOTLIGHT ON...

Professionalism

Accountability

Think of the following actions as ways to demonstrate professional accountability:

- Assuming only those responsibilities that are within one's scope of practice
- Not assuming responsibility for activities in which competency has not yet been mastered
- Evaluating the outcomes of one's own actions
- Admitting mistakes rather than blaming others
- Documenting nursing interventions
- Select one day of your clinical experience and identify ways in which you demonstrated accountability.

---

ensure that only qualified individuals are granted the right to practice and that those who fail to uphold the professional standards are denied the future right to practice. See the accompanying Spotlight On display.

Professional accountability within nursing is fostered through the mechanisms by which nurses obtain the right to practice. These mechanisms include rights and responsibilities, organizational accountability, legislative regulations, individual accountability, and student accountability.

Rights and Responsibilities

The nurse has responsibility to the client to be competent, to render nursing services in accordance with standards of nursing practice, and to adhere to the profession's ethical code. The public trusts that an individual titled registered nurse will have appropriate knowledge and skills to render the services offered. This translates to accountability of nurses to accept assignments for which they are competent and to maintain the necessary knowledge and skills to perform such services.

When the registered nurse chooses a specific area of practice (e.g., emergency or home health nursing) additional knowledge, skills, and abilities will be required as the nurse evolves from novice to expert. The registered nurse is accountable for acquiring and maintaining these abilities. Furthermore, the nurse is accountable for adhering to the standards of care for that specialty. This process may be accomplished through various methods such as orientation, in-service education, peer review, continuing education, journal articles, professional association activities, and formalized advanced education. Although employers may provide some continuing education opportunities to the registered nurse, the ultimate accountability to gain and maintain competency rests with every nurse.

Organizational Accountability

Organization is the means by which members of a profession, such as nursing, join together to promote and protect the profession. **Professional regulation** is the process by which nursing ensures that its members act in the public interest by providing a unique service that society has entrusted to them (ANA, 2008). Professional regulation is the responsibility of professional organizations. The accompanying Spotlight On display on self-regulation lists ways in which the nursing profession regulates itself.

The basis of professional regulation in nursing is the scope of nursing practice. Professional standards evolve from the scope of nursing practice and provide the framework for the development of competency statements. **Professional standards** are authoritative statements developed by the profession by which the quality of practice, service, and education can be judged (ANA, 2004). Professional standards form the basis of educational outcomes and criteria for organized nursing services (ANA, 2008). In addition, professional standards provide the framework for accreditation and certification.

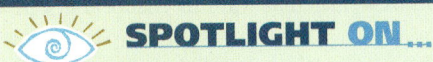

SPOTLIGHT ON...

Professionalism

Self-Regulation of the Nursing Profession

- Defining its practice base
- Providing for research and development of that practice base
- Establishing a system for nursing education
- Establishing the structures through which nursing services will be delivered
- Providing quality review mechanisms such as a code of ethics, standards of practice, structures for peer review, and a system of credentialing

Data from American Nurses Association (ANA). (2004). Nursing: Scope and standards of practice. Washington, DC: Author.

Standards of Nursing Practice

Professional nursing is responsible for determining standards of nursing practice. Every nurse is accountable for providing quality care by adhering to professional standards.

The ANA revised its standards of clinical nursing practice in 2004. As the professional organization representing all registered nurses, the ANA's focus was to develop a set of standards applicable to all nurses engaged in clinical practice. The ANA, as well as many specialty nursing associations, has developed standards of practice for specific areas of practice, for example, medical-surgical nursing, gerontology nursing, and perioperative nursing.

Nursing must be able to articulate the core of practice for which practitioners are accountable to the public regardless of clinical setting or specialty. The *Scope and Standards of Nursing Practice* (ANA, 2004) reflect both the caring and professional expectations of nursing (see Table 11-2).

In Canada, the Canadian Nurses Association (CNA) is the professional organization entrusted with the responsibility of developing professional standards. For nurses in Canada,

Accreditation

Accreditation is the process by which a nongovernmental agency appraises and grants status to institutions that meet predetermined criteria. The Joint Commission is one example of an accrediting body that promotes quality of health care by evaluating agencies' achievement of performance standards. Another type of accreditation is performed by the American Nurses Credentialing Center, which develops criteria for continuing nursing education agencies and evaluates those agencies in terms of meeting the criteria.

Accreditation and certification are mechanisms for promoting nursing accountability. The National League for Nursing (NLN) establishes educational standards and surveys educational programs to ensure that these standards are achieved by each accredited school of nursing. The ANA promotes the accountability of individual nurses through its certification process.

Certification

Certification is the process by which a nongovernmental agency certifies that an individual licensed to practice a profession has met predetermined standards specified for practice (ANA, 2008). Certification is an indicator that the nurse has obtained specialized knowledge and skills. Certification is one avenue for demonstrating and maintaining competence. It is a voluntary process through which nurses demonstrate their belief in the importance of ongoing education and excellence in clinical practice. Certification signifies a higher level of competence than is expected at the time of initial licensure.

The American Nurses Credentialing Center, a subsidiary of the ANA, develops and administers the certification examinations. It also requires a specified amount of continuing education in each specialty area for those nurses who choose to be certified.

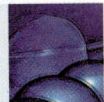

TABLE 11-2 Standards of Nursing Practice
STANDARDS OF CARE
I. Assessment: Collects data
II. Diagnosis: Analyzes data
III. Outcome Identification: Individualizes expected outcomes for client
IV. Planning: Develops plan of care
V. Implementation: Implements interventions in plan of care
VI. Evaluation: Determines client progress toward outcome achievement
STANDARDS OF PROFESSIONAL PERFORMANCE
I. Quality of Care: Evaluates quality and efficacy of nursing practice systematically
II. Performance Appraisal: Compares one's own nursing practice to professional standards of care
III. Education: Maintains current knowledge/skills
IV. Collegiality: Contributes to professional development of others
V. Ethics: Delivers care in an ethical manner
VI. Collaboration: Works with others to provide client care
VII. Research: Applies current research findings to practice
VIII. Resource Utilization: Considers safety, efficacy, and cost in care delivery

American Nurses Association. (2004). Nursing: Scope and standards of practice. Washington, DC: Author.

the guiding principles of practice are listed in the CNA ethical code (2008).

LEGISLATIVE ACCOUNTABILITY

For nurses to be recognized as professionals, nursing must have legislation that clearly defines the role and scope of nursing practice. Scope of practice refers to the legal boundaries of practice for health care providers as defined in state statutes. Legislation defines the legal rights granted to the profession by the public. It is essential to public well-being that nursing regulate its practice to ensure that only those individuals qualified to practice are allowed to do so.

Legal regulation is the process by which the state attests to the public that the individual licensed to practice is at least minimally competent to do so (ANA, 2008). The nurse practice act, the laws governing the practice of nursing, defines the legal scope of practice within a state or territory. Such laws generally authorize state boards of nursing to interpret the legal boundaries of safe nursing practice (ANA, 2008). Other laws may also have an impact on the scope of nursing practice, for example, licensure laws of other health care providers.

Although specific duties of boards of nursing vary among states or territories, the primary purpose is to protect the public from unqualified or incompetent practitioners. Boards of nursing are authorized to:

- Establish legal standards of practice
- Approve educational programs that prepare individuals for licensure
- Grant licensure to individuals who meet minimum qualifications
- Renew licensure for competent practitioners
- Discipline licensees as necessary to protect the public

Boards of nursing are authorized to adopt rules and regulations that establish legal standards for nursing education, practice, and licensure within the context of the nurse practice acts. Nurses are accountable for complying with the provisions of the nurse practice act and the related rules and regulations established by the board of nursing in their respective states. Regulating bodies for nursing have the legal authority to set practice standards for the protection of the general public. In the United States, boards of nursing in each state serve as the regulatory bodies, whereas in Canada the authority for governing nursing lies within the board in each province or territory. There is no national board of nursing in either the United States or Canada.

Licensure

Licensure is the method by which a state holds the nurse accountable for safe practice to citizens of that state. Licensure grants the nurse legal authority to perform certain acts, to use a specific title that reflects one's practice rights, and to offer one's services and receive compensation for those services in the state that issues the license. Licensure is granted based on evidence that the individual has attained the minimum degree of competency (the ability, qualities, and capacity to function in a particular way) to ensure that one is a safe practitioner.

Mandatory licensure laws prohibit any individual from practicing as a registered nurse without a current license. Licensure laws receive authority from the U.S. Constitution that defines the protection from harm as a constitutional right of every citizen. The Constitution entrusts the individual states with the inherent power to police human activities and to protect citizens in the human needs for safety, general welfare, and health. Laws enacted under the "police power" of the state are designed to protect society from ignorance, incapacity, deception, and fraud and must benefit the public primarily, *not* the members of the profession.

Licensure Process

There are two methods by which one may become initially licensed as a registered nurse in a particular state:

- Licensure by examination is the process by which an individual who has completed an approved nursing program seeks initial licensure by successfully passing a standardized competency examination.
- Licensure by endorsement is the process by which an individual who is duly licensed as a registered nurse under the laws of one state or country has those credentials accepted and approved by another state or country. Individuals are licensed to practice only in the state in which they initially took the licensing examination. Endorsement allows registered nurses to practice in states other than the one of initial licensure.

Nurse Licensure Compact

Nurses today are mobile and often travel to other states in which they practice temporarily. Also, electronic nursing means that nurses who are licensed in one state may be assessing, counseling, teaching, or otherwise caring for clients who are in another state. *Multistate licensure, interstate practice*, and *mutual recognition* are terms that refer to the practice of allowing a nurse to obtain one state licensure that grants privilege to practice across state lines. The Nurse Licensure Compact (NLC), which was first recognized by the National Council of State Boards of Nursing (NCSBN) in 1997, refers to a legal agreement between states to recognize the privilege of nurses to practice across state lines without having to apply for a license in each state (NCSBN, 2004). The nurse, however, is responsible for knowing and complying with the nursing licensure laws of each state in which the nurse practices. Each state must enact legislation that endorses the NLC and must adopt legal rules and regulations for implementing the compact. The NCSBN (2004) lists the following as some benefits of the NLC:

- Improved mobility for nurses
- Improved access to nursing care
- Clarification of the authority to practice for nurses working in interstate practice or telenursing
- Improved access to nurses during times of great need (i.e., a disaster)

The mutual recognition licensure system is based on states entering into an agreement, known as an interstate compact, to authorize practice by individuals licensed in one state to practice in the other state. The interstate compact defines such issues as jurisdiction, discipline, and information exchange between party states. Currently, 23 states are partners in NLC licensure (NCSBN, 2008).

The state boards of nursing have the authority and responsibility to determine that only qualified individuals are granted licensure. The boards of nursing may deny licensure based on information that indicates one to be "unfit" for such licensure. Examples of such activities are:

- A criminal history (especially a criminal act that affects one's ability to render safe nursing care)
- Chemical addiction
- Practicing without a current, proper license
- Aiding someone else who is unlicensed to pose as a nurse

State boards of nursing are required to report adverse actions taken against licensees to national data banks.

National Data Banks

Two national clearinghouses collect data about incompetent and fraudulent health care providers. The National Practitioner Data Bank was established by Congress and is administered by the U.S. Department of Health and Human Services. The Healthcare Integrity and Protection Data Bank is a national data collection program for information about adverse actions taken against health care providers. Both data banks are designed to improve the quality of health care by restricting the practice of health care providers who are incompetent. The need for creating such data banks was highlighted by incompetent and fraudulent practitioners who would move from one state to another to avoid restrictions on their professional practice.

The Data Banks' Proactive Disclosure Service Prototype (PDS) went online May 1, 2007. The PDS provides an opportunity for health care agencies (e.g., hospitals, HMOs) to continuously check up on their practitioners (U.S. Department of Health & Human Services, Health Resources & Services Administration, 2008). Types of adverse actions that must be reported to the data banks include:

- Health care–related civil judgments
- Health care–related criminal convictions
- Adverse actions taken by federal or state agencies responsible for licensing and certification
- Exclusions of prescribing practitioners, providers, and suppliers from participation in federal or state health care programs
- Actions taken by boards of nursing against licensees who violate state licensure laws

Licensure Examination

Each state is responsible for determining the licensing requirements for an individual to practice in that state.

Boards of nursing are entrusted to determine the appropriate examination to measure minimum competency for practice as a registered nurse. In the United States, through the NCSBN, the same examination is given nationally to qualified candidates. Known as the NCLEX-RN (National Council Licensure Examination for Registered Nurses), this examination has been adopted as the standard licensure examination by all 50 states and the U.S. territories.

A separate test (National Council Licensure Examination for Practical Nurses, NCLEX-PN) is administered to practical and vocational nurses. Use of a national licensure examination ensures uniformity in testing and facilitates endorsement of licensure in other states.

The examination is designed to distinguish qualified candidates from those who do not possess the necessary competencies for safe practice. The NCLEX-RN measures the competencies expected of a nursing graduate at the generalist level. The NCLEX-RN reflects the belief that nursing requires knowledge of:

- Safe and effective care environment
- Health promotion and maintenance
- Psychosocial integrity
- Physiological integrity (NCSBN, 2007)

The NCLEX-RN is not an examination for which one prepares in the last few weeks before graduation. Nursing students successfully complete this examination through careful study and achievement of nursing courses. Activities offered during the academic experience prepare students for registered nurse practice. Clinical experiences through which students learn the practice of nursing contribute to the ability to pass the licensure examination.

INDIVIDUAL ACCOUNTABILITY

Professional nurses must understand the method by which the board of nursing adopts rules and regulations in their state of licensure so that they can be active participants in the development of such regulations. Nurses can use a variety of ways to demonstrate individual accountability; two methods are continued competency and professional development.

Continued Competency

A registered nurse has the professional responsibility to attain and maintain competency. There has been much debate within the profession and consumer advocacy groups about the roles and responsibilities of health profession licensing boards to ensure that their members maintain minimum competency requirements for safe practice.

Once licensed, it is the responsibility of the registered nurse to maintain a current active license to practice in accordance with state requirements. Registered nurses must renew their licenses on an annual or biannual cycle before the expiration date and meet other requirements for license renewal as required by the individual state board of nursing.

The nursing profession has traditionally used three methods of ensuring accountability to the public—licensure examination, continuing education, and certification. These three methods are currently being scrutinized by the ANA in an attempt to ensure that nurses demonstrate competency. A variety of mechanisms are being considered as measures to improve accountability. Development of a professional portfolio is one avenue for demonstrating continued competence.

Professional Development

Active involvement in student organizations at the school, state, and national levels enables nursing students to develop critical professional skills and participate in events that may have an impact on their careers. Table 11-3 lists some professional organizations in which nurses can participate. In addition to these professional organizations, there are professional associations organized around specialty practice areas, including:

- American Academy of Nurse Practitioners
- American Association of Critical-Care Nurses
- American Association of Legal Nurse Consultants
- American Forensic Nurses
- American Holistic Nurses Association
- American Nursing Informatics Association
- American Psychiatric Nurses Association
- American Society of Pain Management Nurses
- Emergency Nurses Association
- Home Healthcare Nurses Association

Involvement with district and state nurses' associations is also encouraged. Nursing students can participate in these groups through continuing education, legislative activity, or political action. In addition, students have the opportunity of making contacts with registered nurses within these associations who will eventually be their colleagues. Such contacts are helpful when seeking guidance in employment opportunities and can develop into valuable mentoring relationships.

STUDENT ACCOUNTABILITY

Nursing students' accountability is directly related to their legal authority to practice. Nursing students function legally as an *exception* to the state licensure requirements *while enrolled in a nursing program* that is approved by the state board of nursing. Such exception is granted only when the student is engaged in learning activities structured within the program of studies. Performing nursing activities (other than those assigned to unlicensed individuals) outside the formalized clinical practicum of the nursing curriculum constitutes the illegal practice of nursing; see the accompanying Spotlight On display. Accountability for nursing care is shared by the student, faculty, educational institution in which the student is practicing, and clinical agency. The various responsibilities of each of these parties are determined by the respective state boards of nursing.

For nursing students, accountability for competency begins the first clinical day and continues throughout their careers. Therefore, students have the responsibility to:

- Be prepared for clinical practice
- Engage only in those skills for which they have gained competence
- Seek instruction as necessary

Students must not engage in client care activities without proper preparation, prior validation of competency by their instructor, and appropriate supervision (see Figure 11-1 on page 175). Nursing students have a responsibility to request clear information regarding the instructor's expectations and to seek direct supervision when uncertain of their own competency. See the accompanying Safety First display.

ADVANCED PRACTICE NURSING

Advanced practice nursing is the practice of nursing at a level requiring an expanded knowledge base and clinical expertise in a specialty area. Advanced practice registered nurses (APRNs) have an increased level of accountability to the public, the profession, and themselves. The autonomy that is experienced by nurses in advanced practice roles increases the sense of responsibility for personal decisions and actions. The general public also expects a higher level of ability and skills from APRNs just as it does from specialists in other professions. As APRNs assume leadership roles in

▼ SAFETY FIRST ▼

It is absolutely critical to client safety that nursing students verbalize any questions or concerns relative to their assignments before instituting care. Students must ask for directions if unsure of their abilities.

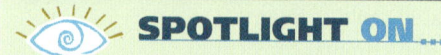

👁 SPOTLIGHT ON...

Legal

Student Accountability

You are working as a nursing assistant (unlicensed personnel) during your school break. What would be your appropriate response if asked to perform a nursing procedure such as medication administration? Would the fact that you have performed the procedure previously as a nursing student affect your response?

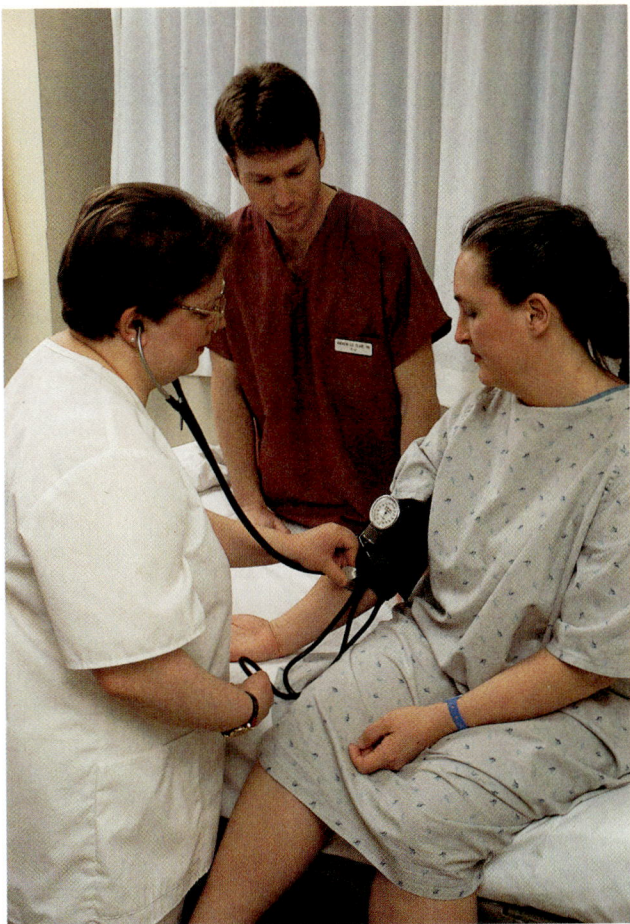

FIGURE 11-1 This nursing student is being taught to measure the client's blood pressure. If the instructor were temporarily called away from the bedside and the client asked the student about the measurement and its significance, what do you think the student should do? DELMAR/CENGAGE LEARNING

LEADERSHIP IN NURSING

Leadership is a method of modeling accountable behavior to others. Nursing has numerous leaders who demonstrate and encourage accountability. *Leadership* and *management* are terms often used interchangeably; however, some significant differences exist. **Management** is the accomplishment of tasks either by oneself or by directing others. **Leadership** is the interpersonal process that involves motivating and guiding others to achieve goals. Managers tend to be task oriented, whereas leaders focus on people. Every nurse, regardless of title or position, is a manager; each has the potential to be a leader.

MANAGERIAL FUNCTIONS

Essential functions that are performed by effective managers include:

- *Planning:* Determining objectives and identifying methods that lead to achievement of those objectives

- *Organizing:* Using resources (human and material) to achieve predetermined outcomes
- *Directing:* Guiding and motivating others to meet the expected objectives
- *Controlling:* Using performance standards as criteria for measuring success and taking corrective action, if necessary, to see that others comply with performance standards
- *Decision making:* Identifying a problem and deciding which alternatives can best achieve the objectives

These five functions are used daily by managers to accomplish the goal of providing quality care.

LEADERSHIP STYLES

Effective leaders accomplish goals by motivating and inspiring other people. In other words, they use the concept of **synergy** (the combined power of many) rather than attempting to achieve success alone.

The leader's behavior greatly determines the behavior of the group. There are basically three styles of leadership: autocratic, democratic, and laissez-faire (see Table 11-5 on page 177).

The **autocratic leadership style** is leader focused; that is, the leader maintains strong control, makes all decisions, and solves all problems. The leader dominates the group by issuing commands rather than making suggestions or seeking input.

The **democratic leadership style** (also called participative leadership) is based on the belief that every group member should have input into development of goals and problem solving. The democratic leader acts primarily as a facilitator and resource person. Concern for each member of the group as a unique individual is demonstrated by the leader.

In the **laissez-faire leadership style**, the leader assumes a passive, nondirective, and inactive approach. Leadership responsibilities are either assumed by the members of the group or completely abdicated. All decision making is left to the group, with the leader giving little, if any, guidance, support, or feedback. Almost any behavior by the group is permissible due to the leader's lack of limit setting and stated expectations. The tasks are unmet, and the relationship needs of group members are ignored.

No single style is superior to the other. Each leadership approach has its advantages and disadvantages (see Table 11-5). The effective leader will use **situational leadership**, which is a blending of styles based on current circumstances and events. The leader knows that behavior does not occur in a vacuum; thus, leadership styles are assumed according to the needs of the group and tasks to be achieved.

LEADERSHIP CHARACTERISTICS

There is debate about the development of effective leaders: Is leadership innate, or is it acquired through experience?

TABLE 11-4 Advanced Practice Registered Nursing (APRN) Roles

ADVANCED PRACTICE ROLE	EDUCATIONAL PREPARATION	MAJOR RESPONSIBILITIES
Clinical Nurse Specialist (CNS)	Graduate degree in a recognized nursing specialty	Authorized to provide direct nursing care to a select population
		Plans, guides, and directs care provided by other nursing personnel
Nurse Practitioner (NP)	Advanced preparation in a specific area of care	Authorized to provide primary care to individuals, families, and other groups in a variety of settings, including but not limited to homes, institutions, offices, industry, schools, and community agencies
		Conducts physical examinations
		Takes medical histories
		Orders and interprets laboratory and other diagnostic tests
		Diagnoses
		Treats minor illnesses (acute or chronic) or injuries
		Counsels and educates clients
Certified Nurse Midwife (CNM)	Advanced preparation in nursing and midwifery	Authorized to manage the care of women during all phases of pregnancy and newborns
Certified Registered Nurse Anesthetist (CRNA)	A registered nurse who is prepared in the science of anesthesiology	Authorized to select and administer anesthetics and ancillary services to clients

Delmar/Cengage Learning

The characteristics of effective leaders are discussed in the following sections.

Communication

Effective leadership relies on the individual's ability to communicate. Just as the effective nurse uses communication skills with clients, the effective manager uses communication as a tool for motivating others to be successful. Active listening is the major technique that managers use in order to understand others' needs and goals. Active listening is also the mechanism that allows the manager to instruct, to provide and receive feedback, and to keep the team moving forward. An effective nurse leader will:

- Listen actively to others
- Articulate thoughts in an intelligent, persuasive manner
- Differentiate aggressive, passive, and assertive behavior in order to communicate appropriately in a given situation

Aggressive behavior occurs when an individual meets one's needs regardless of the impact on others. *Passive behav-* ior is giving up one's rights and not having one's needs met. *Assertive behavior* occurs when an individual seeks to meet one's needs while respecting the rights of other people. Effective leaders communicate in an assertive manner; that is, they speak directly and honestly to others.

Credibility

A leader motivates others by demonstrating enthusiasm and exerting influence. To be influential, the leader must be credible. Credibility, the quality or power of inspiring beliefs, is based on competence. From competence comes confidence. Individuals who know what they are doing and perform well are those who can influence others.

Delegation

The nurse leader must be able to delegate effectively to coordinate the delivery of care. **Delegation** is the process of transferring a selected task in a situation to an individual who is competent to perform that specific task. Delegation is a

TABLE 11-5 Leadership Stages

STYLE	DESCRIPTION	LEADER BEHAVIORS	POTENTIAL IMPACT ON GROUP MEMBERS	ADVANTAGES	DISADVANTAGES
Autocratic	• Basic premise: Leader knows best. • Communication flows downward.	• Controlling • Directive • Makes all decisions and solves all problems • Issues commands	• Hostility • Rebellion	• Task oriented, high productivity • Facilitates a quick response • Often necessary in crisis situation	• Inhibits creativity and autonomy of members • Promotes mistrust and fear among followers • Members may become hostile or passive
Democratic ("participative leadership")	• Basic premise: Every member should have input. • Communication is open and mutual.	• Acts as a facilitator • Serves as resource person • Encourages members' active participation	• Improved productivity • More opportunity for personal growth • Increased cooperation and teamwork	• Promotes empowerment of team members • Facilitates communication • Increased creativity and autonomy	• Time-consuming • May be less efficient (in quantifiable terms) • Disagreements may happen as members express their viewpoints
Laissez-faire	• Basic premise: Leadership responsibilities are assumed by group. • Almost any behavior by the group is permissible due to the leader's lack of limit setting and stated expectations.	• Passive, nondirective approach • Provides little, if any, support, guidance, or feedback • Sets no limits	• Unmet tasks • Relationship needs of group members ignored • Apathy	• Promotes autonomy and creativity in some members	• May evoke passivity in team members • Aimless behavior often occurs • Chaos common • Inefficiency and low productivity

Delmar/Cengage Learning

multifaceted process involving communication, conflict resolution, feedback and evaluation, and knowledge of the person to whom a task is delegated (Hansten & Jackson, 2008).

Delegation is a helpful tool for nurse leaders in that it encourages team members to develop skills. Prior to delegating, the nurse manager must first assess the delegatee's ability to perform the specific task. Delegation is, therefore, a mechanism for encouraging staff members' growth as the effective manager will be available to teach and assist when necessary. The "five rights" of delegation must be followed to assure that the assignment is the *right task* delegated under the *right circumstances* to the *right person* with the *right directions and communication* and with the *right supervision and evaluation*

(NCSBN, 2006). The nurse uses professional judgment when determining which activities to delegate. Any activity that requires nursing judgment or independent nursing action cannot be legally delegated. See the Nursing Process Highlight.

In general, registered nurses are authorized by law to both provide nursing care to clients directly and supervise and instruct others to deliver this care. Further, the registered nurse is empowered to delegate selected tasks to either licensed or unlicensed nursing personnel (see Figure 11-2 on page 178). Decisions about delegation are guided by the needs of the client, the number and type of available personnel, and the nursing management system of the unit or agency.

NURSING PROCESS HIGHLIGHT

Planning

Delegation of the Nursing Process

Which steps of the nursing process may be legally and safely delegated?

Assessment: No. Input from other health care providers may be solicited (e.g., vital signs of client with noncomplex problem).
Diagnosis: No. Only registered nurses can establish nursing diagnoses.
Planning: No. Input is solicited from other members of the health care team.
Implementation: Yes. Certain tasks (e.g., hygiene, feeding, ambulating) can be delegated to other members of the care delivery team.
Evaluation: No. Input from others may be sought.

Data from American Nurses Association. (2005). *Principles for delegation.* Retrieved December 2, 2008, from http://www.safestaffingsaveslives.org// WhatisSafeStaffingPrinciples/PrinciplesforDelegationhtml.aspx.

The first consideration in determining the most appropriate nursing personnel to administer care is client safety. For example, administration of blood or blood products is not an act that can be legally delegated to licensed practical nurses or unlicensed assistive personnel in most states. Other activities, such as assisting clients with activities of daily living (ADL, those activities performed by a person usually on a daily basis), ordering supplies, or transcribing orders, can often be safely delegated to other personnel.

If delegation of a particular activity is legally allowed, the nurse should validate the knowledge and skill level of personnel before delegation. If uncertain about the level of competence of an individual to perform an activity, the nurse should not delegate the task.

The nurse practice act defines which aspects of care can be delegated and which must be performed by the registered nurse. Because nurse practice acts vary among the states and provinces, it is imperative that the nurse stay current with the rules and regulations promulgated by the respective state (or provincial) board of nursing regarding the delegation of nursing tasks. See Figure 11-3 on page 179 for elements to consider when delegating.

Even though a task may be delegated, the nurse who delegates maintains accountability for the overall nursing care of the client. Only the task, not the ultimate accountability, may be delegated to another. See the accompanying Spotlight On display.

Critical Thinking

Critical thinking is another characteristic of an effective leader. According to Alfaro-LeFevre (2008), "Critical thinking is the key to resolving problems. Nurses who don't think critically become *part* of the problem" (p. 13). The critical thinker has an open-minded, questioning attitude that facilitates problem solving (Figure 11-4 on page 179). This underlying curiosity leads the individual to search for answers based on rationales. The ineffective leader is one who falls into routine ways of thinking without even being aware of what is happening. See Chapter 5 for more information on critical thinking.

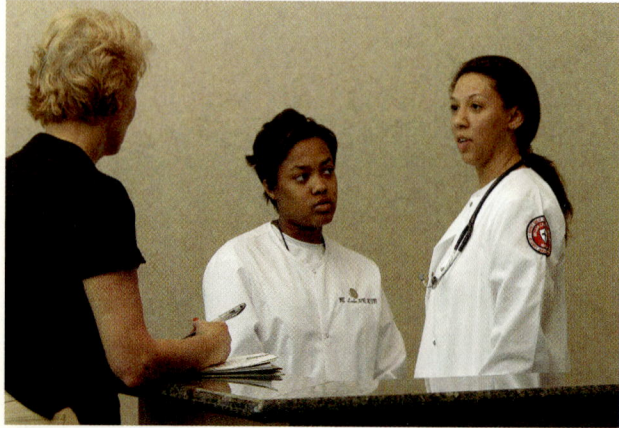

FIGURE 11-2 The registered nurse is responsible for delegating nursing tasks to other members of the health care team.
DELMAR/CENGAGE LEARNING

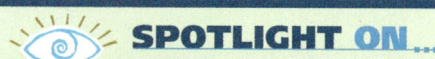 **SPOTLIGHT ON...**

Legal/Ethical

Delegation

Your employer, a large acute care hospital, has hired consultants to examine the cost of care expended in the facility and recommend a more cost-effective system. These consultants recommend decreasing the number of both registered nurses and licensed vocational nurses and increasing the responsibilities of unlicensed assistive personnel. As a registered nurse in charge of the care of medical-surgical clients, what questions would you ask regarding this proposal? In what ways do you think your responsibilities would increase because of this situation? Do you think your responsibilities would decrease significantly? What impact would this proposal have on the ethical delivery of care to clients, specifically the nurse's need to cause no harm and promote good? What are the legal implications of this recommendation?

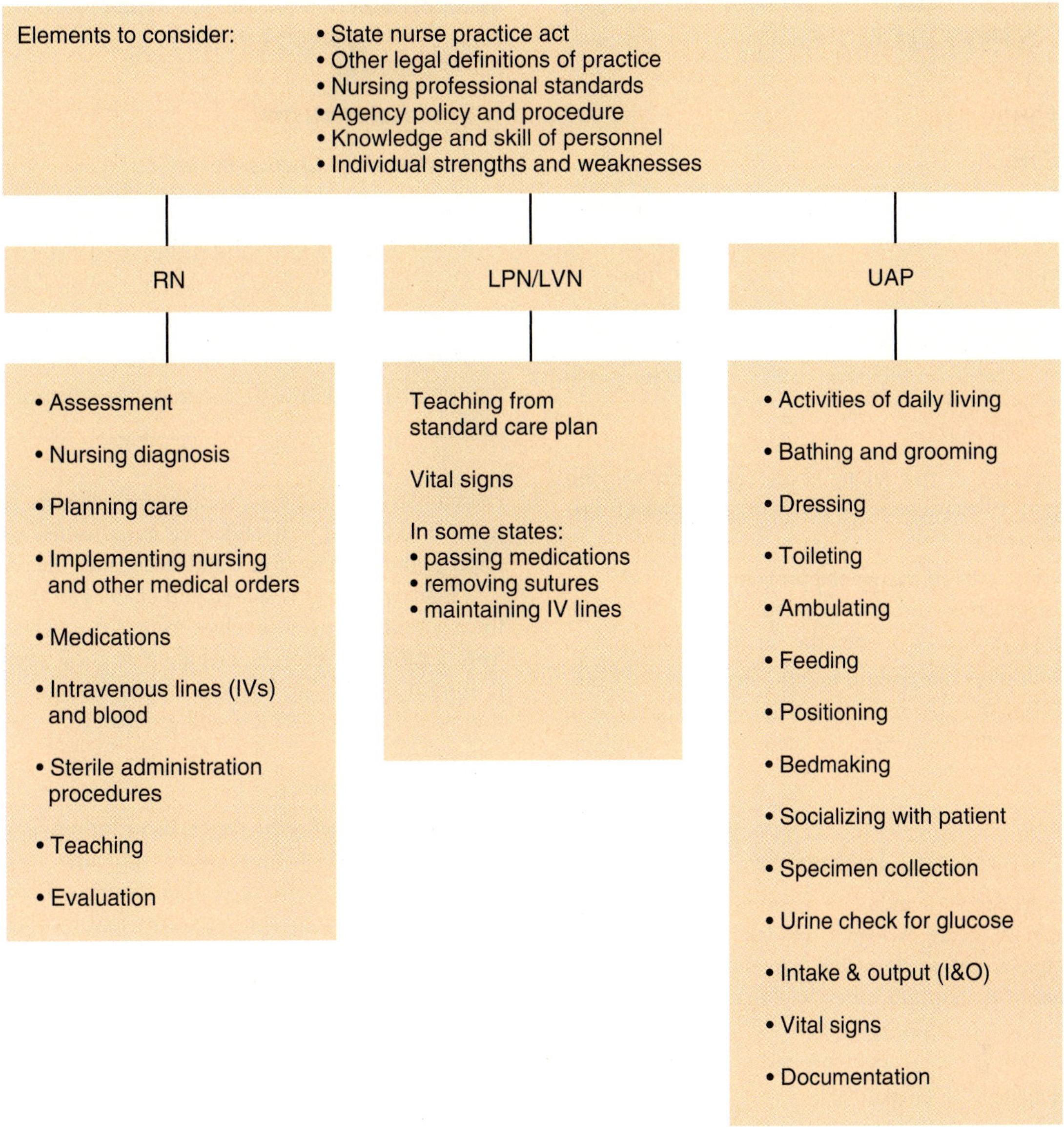

Elements to consider:
- State nurse practice act
- Other legal definitions of practice
- Nursing professional standards
- Agency policy and procedure
- Knowledge and skill of personnel
- Individual strengths and weaknesses

RN	LPN/LVN	UAP
• Assessment • Nursing diagnosis • Planning care • Implementing nursing and other medical orders • Medications • Intravenous lines (IVs) and blood • Sterile administration procedures • Teaching • Evaluation	Teaching from standard care plan Vital signs In some states: • passing medications • removing sutures • maintaining IV lines	• Activities of daily living • Bathing and grooming • Dressing • Toileting • Ambulating • Feeding • Positioning • Bedmaking • Socializing with patient • Specimen collection • Urine check for glucose • Intake & output (I&O) • Vital signs • Documentation

FIGURE 11-3 Considerations in Delegation POLIFKO-HARRIS, K. (2004). *CASE APPLICATIONS IN NURSING LEADERSHIP & MANAGEMENT.* CLIFTON PARK, NH: THOMSON DELMAR LEARNING.

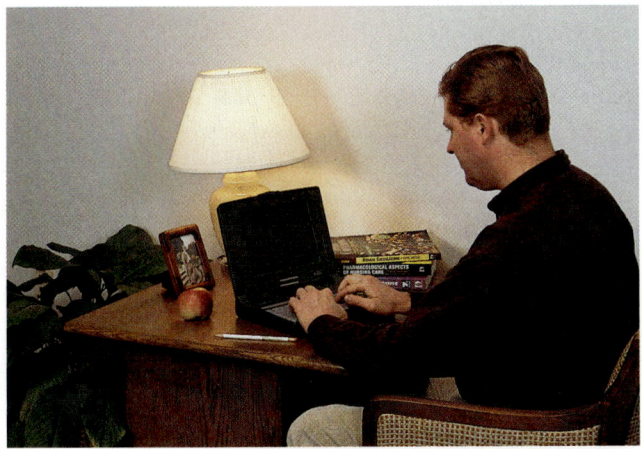

FIGURE 11-4 Critical thinking skills are integral to the analysis of problems and the development of leadership skills. How does critical thinking contribute to professional accountability? DELMAR/CENGAGE LEARNING

Initiating Action

In addition to thinking critically, a leader initiates action. Only by putting ideas into action does a person become a leader. A leader does not adopt a wait-and-see attitude with problems; instead, a leader initiates measures to solve problems. When taking action, the effective leader demonstrates flexibility. If one behavior is ineffective, the leader is not hesitant to try another approach. By initiating action, the proactive leader role-models successful behaviors and encourages others to strive for quality.

Risk Taking

Taking action to solve problems (i.e., to initiate change) involves taking a risk. People who take risks are those who are not satisfied with the status quo and strive continually for improvement. Effective risk takers are not reckless or haphazard; instead, their risk-taking activities are goal directed.

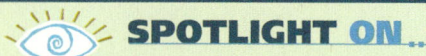

SPOTLIGHT ON...

Professionalism

Risk Taking

It is not always comfortable to assume the role of change initiator. However, whether you choose to act or not to act, you have made a choice. The question that must be answered is "Can I accept the consequences of my choice(s)?"

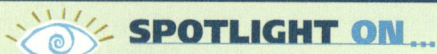

SPOTLIGHT ON...

Professionalism

Leadership Characteristics

How can you, in the preprofessional role, function as a leader? Think of all the situations in which you will attempt to motivate others to change, for example:

Encouraging clients and families

Interacting with team members

Collaborating with classmates and instructors

People engage in risk taking every day, often with no awareness of this behavior. Some common examples of risk-taking behaviors are:

- Volunteering to be in charge of a project
- Giving constructive criticism to others
- Expressing opinions even when they are unpopular

Effective leaders understand that the benefits of risk taking far outweigh the potential negative consequences and, therefore, act accordingly. See the accompanying Spotlight On display.

Persuasiveness and Influence

An effective leader uses influence to motivate and inspire others to achieve goals. A leader understands how to use power effectively, not to dominate but, rather, to motivate others. In order to motivate others, the leader must be able to inspire confidence. Ellis and Hartley (2007) have identified the following as behaviors of inspirational leaders:

- Being predictable and dependable
- Exercising good judgment
- Being knowledgeable and competent
- Demonstrating patience
- Recognizing efforts of others

Persuasiveness is a tool that managers can use to create enthusiasm for a project, encourage collaboration, and increase cohesiveness among team members. The persuasive leader is one who communicates effectively and demonstrates personal power. Persuasive people demonstrate enthusiasm for the task at hand and, therefore, are able to inspire others to work with them to accomplish goals. Because persuasive people exhibit enthusiasm, they are able to energize those around them. The accompanying Nursing Checklist provides some hints for increasing persuasiveness and influence. Also, see the accompanying Spotlight On display.

POWER

A leader is a powerful person. **Power** is the ability to do or act and results in the achievement of desired results. Power causes things to happen. Powerful people are able to modify behavior and influence others to change, even when others are resistant to change. Every person uses power to some degree to meet individual goals. Effective nurse leaders use power to improve the delivery of care and to enhance the profession.

Effective power is shared and enables all to work toward their potential. Power involves using force, which is derived from a variety of sources, including physical strength, ability to reward and punish, financial incentives, legal actions, position within an organization, and expertise.

Types of Power

The type of power used depends on various power sources or bases. Table 11-6 on page 181 provides an overview of types of power according to their sources. Personal power can be developed by building trust and gaining the confidence of coworkers. Another way to develop power is to focus on solving problems rather than complaining about them. Creating outcomes is powerful!

Principles of Power

Nurse leaders must recognize certain guiding principles when obtaining and using power. Effective nurse leaders understand that power is an expendable resource, so they are careful to renew their sources of power in order to maintain an adequate power base. Power requires the leader to be committed to organizational goals; a leader who loses sight of the objectives also loses the power to influence others. The leader who uses power effectively will use only as much power as necessary to achieve the expected goal.

✓ NURSING CHECKLIST

WAYS TO INCREASE PERSUASIVENESS AND INFLUENCE

- Role-model expected behaviors.
- Use effective problem-solving skills.
- Communicate expectations clearly.
- Give praise for accomplishments.
- Maintain one's own competency.
- Encourage others to participate in decision making.

TABLE 11-6 Types and Sources of Power

TYPE	SOURCE	EXAMPLE
Coercive power	Ability to punish	A head nurse assigns a staff nurse who has been "insolent" to an undesirable shift.
Expert power	An excellent knowledge base and skill level; the person has expertise in an area not held by those who are to be influenced by the leader	The instructor exerts power with students.
Informational power ("positional")	Based on the types and amount of information that an individual can access	A staff nurse has just learned through her experience a new way to teach a client. She tells her coworkers about the approach. Knowledge is shared and power increases.
Legitimate power	Based on one's position within a hierarchy	The nurse executive has legitimate power over a staff nurse within the same agency or institution.
Personal power	Derives from a high degree of self-confidence that is based on positive self-esteem	A nurse with a take-charge attitude is powerful during a crisis.
Referent power	Charisma; others wanting to associate with one	A unit manager is powerful because he is popular with both his superiors and subordinates.
Reward power	Ability to provide incentives	A nurse manager can decide when to schedule vacation time for staff nurses.

Delmar/Cengage Learning

Developing a Power Base

Power can be a positive element in nursing. For example, a nurse manager can use personal power to promote cohesiveness and teamwork with subordinates. The power of a work group can be harnessed by a leader who is skilled in communication and time management techniques. Power is a force used by nursing leaders to accomplish goals. However, many nurses do not want to be labeled as powerful because of a perceived negative connotation of the word. In the past, many nurses have tended to abdicate their power by negating their own contributions and expertise. Power is abdicated by:

- Focusing on the negative
- Failing to seize power and use it
- The way one dresses
- Body language (hesitant voice tone, slouched posture)
- Always playing it safe rather than taking risks

Expanded practice roles have increased nursing's power. For example, NPs are empowered legally through licensure to use advanced knowledge and skills. Expansion of the scope of nursing practice results in greater accountability to one's self, the profession, and the public. Competence of APRNs increases their power to exert a positive influence on the health care delivery system.

In addition to advanced practice nursing, another way for nurses to achieve power is affiliation. There are a variety of ways to build affiliations, including mentorship and networking.

MENTORING

A mentor is an experienced person who serves as a guide to a novice. Mentors help novices develop skills. When seeking out a mentor, it is wise for nursing students or graduate nurses to look for a person who communicates directly and focuses on the positive. In selecting a mentor, the novice nurse should choose a person who can provide criticism in a supportive, constructive manner through teaching and role modeling (Zerwekh & Claborn, 2008).

NETWORKING

Networking, the process of building connections with others, is essential for the success of nurses because it is a way to increase power. Networking helps nurses to become

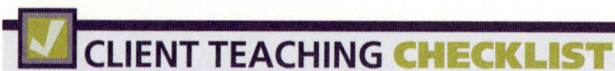

☑ NURSING CHECKLIST

NETWORKING STRATEGIES

- Seek opportunities to help others develop.
- Role-model successful behaviors.
- Share "secrets" for success.
- Encourage others to take professional risks.
- Provide support.
- Teach those who are less experienced.
- Express pride in others' achievements.
- Respect colleagues' judgment and work.
- Consult with colleagues and respect their input.
- Introduce others to contacts.
- Acknowledge all help received from contacts.
- Make frequent contact with network members.

☑ CLIENT TEACHING CHECKLIST

CLIENT EMPOWERMENT

- Determine client's learning needs, focusing on the client's perception of importance.
- Speak in terms easily understood by the client and family.
- Demonstrate the skill and ask client to perform a repeat demonstration.
- Provide feedback immediately to reinforce the learning.
- Ask clients to state in their own words what has been learned about the topic.

more influential because it encourages sharing of information and creates a synergistic effect for all those involved. Establishing and maintaining connections with others can be accomplished in a variety of ways (including mentoring and preceptorship), some of which are shown on the accompanying Nursing Checklist.

EMPOWERMENT

Empowerment, the process of enabling others to do for themselves, is an interpersonal process. Empowerment occurs when individuals are able to influence what happens to them.

Many elements are necessary for creating an atmosphere conducive to empowerment. Open communication built on trusting relationships is of utmost importance; the environment must be supportive and caring. Nurses who work in a nurturing environment are more likely to be empowered than those working in settings that do not attend to employee needs. Another element for establishing empowerment is mutual goal setting and decision making; personal power increases as these become shared responsibilities. Nurses who are empowered are the ones who are motivated to become active problem solvers. They become more confident and competent as a result of empowerment.

Empowerment of Clients

Client teaching is a major tool used by nurses to empower clients. By teaching clients how to better meet their needs, nurses are promoting client independence and power. For clients to be truly empowered (i.e., enabled to care for themselves), many health care providers need to shift their thinking away from the paternalistic belief that is based on the need for control. Paternalism is the process of treating adults like children by telling them what to do. Some health care providers still use a paternalistic approach to clients (e.g., telling a client to do something "for your own good"). Nurses who empower others treat clients as partners in

health care. An example of client empowerment is a nurse teaching a client how to self-administer insulin injections. The accompanying Client Teaching Checklist offers suggestions for empowering clients.

Another mechanism for nurses to empower clients is advocacy. Acting as client advocates, nurses can work through the political and legislative processes to bring about positive changes for vulnerable populations. For example, nurses exert influence with policy makers regarding health care needs of the elderly, children, those who are economically impoverished, and homeless individuals.

Empowerment of Nurses

Empowerment is not something that is given to nurses. It is encouraged by enlightened leaders who value the work of their colleagues. Nurses will continue to create environments that promote the process of empowerment. Some ways to promote nurse empowerment include:

- Sharing power and resources (including knowledge) with others
- Admitting when a mistake is made (demonstrates trustworthiness and honesty)
- Avoiding power struggles
- Using persuasion
- Using accurate information in decision making

An example of nurse empowerment is self-governance (the process of having nurses work together to develop their own schedule for unit staffing coverage).

POLITICS OF NURSING

Politics is often used to refer to governmental and legislative issues. However, politics is a much broader concept in that it refers to how things are done within an organization. **Politics** is the way in which people try to influence decision making, especially decisions about the use of resources. See the

UNCOVERING THE
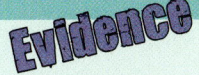

TITLE OF STUDY

"Nursing Leadership: Championing Quality and Patient Safety in the Boardroom"

AUTHORS

M. F. Mastal, M. Joshi, and K. Schulke

PURPOSE

Identify the extent to which hospital boards of trustees, CEOs, and CNOs (chief nursing officers) are engaged in quality and safety at the leadership and governance level.

METHODS

A total of 73 telephone interviews were conducted with hospital board chairs, CEOs, and CNOs from a convenience sample of 36 hospitals in the United States. The telephone interviews were followed up by a focus group consisting of nurse executives.

FINDINGS

There were significant differences in the perceptions of CNOs versus those of board chairs and CEOs. CNOs reported greater increases in understanding quality and client safety than did board chairs. Board chairs and CEOs have limited comprehension of inherent nursing quality issues, including client safety.

IMPLICATIONS

Nurse executives have a critical role in championing client safety and quality improvement issues among the power brokers of health care.

Mastal, M. R., Joshi, M., & Schulke, K. (2007). Nursing leadership: Championing quality and patient safety in the boardroom. *Nursing Economics, 25(6),* 323–330.

Uncovering the Evidence display. Organizational politics determine the following:

- Who has the power

✓ NURSING**CHECKLIST**

BUILDING POLITICAL POWER WITHIN AN ORGANIZATION

- Call attention to oneself by volunteering to serve on committees.
- Know what the organization values, both the written and the unwritten rules of expected conduct.
- Prepare oneself by earning the credentials needed for the particular position that is being sought.
- Communicate ideas, both verbally and in writing.
- Develop an extensive network by getting to know people who work in other areas of the organization.
- Become involved in professional associations.
- Seek out a mentor (membership in professional organizations facilitates this goal).
- Project a positive image, not only in dress and posture, but also in one's behavior.

- Who controls the resources
- Who is rewarded
- Who makes the decisions

Every nurse is affected by organizational politics. It is up to the individual nurse to decide whether to join the political "game" or whether to let others make decisions.

Nurses who are able to advance their careers have determined where the opportunities lie and have taken advantage of these opportunities. Some specific ways that nurses can increase their political power within an organization are listed in the Nursing Checklist.

Nurses need to be involved not only in organizational politics but also in politics that affect society at large. Because nurses provide essential services, they possess much potential power. However, nurses need better organization to fully actualize that potential. When that potential is realized, nursing will become even more powerful and, therefore, better able to influence the delivery of health care.

KEY CONCEPTS

- The criteria for professional nursing practice include intellectual work, provision of a unique service, an expanding body of knowledge, personal responsibility to the public, an extended period of education that includes theory and practice, autonomy, a common identity shared by members, a sense of altruism and commitment to the public, and a code of ethics upheld by its members.

- Accountability is a process that requires individuals to be answerable for their actions. Being accountable means having an obligation (or duty) to act.

- As a profession, nursing is accountable for establishing and maintaining standards that promote safe, effective care.

- Professional accountability within nursing is fostered through mechanisms by which nurses obtain the right to practice and is the basis for understanding the responsibility nurses have to the public.

- Professional standards provide the framework for the development of competency statements.

- Nurse practice acts, which vary from state to state, clearly define the role and scope of nursing practice.

- Licensure gives an individual the right to offer one's services and receive compensation as a registered nurse.

- An individual can be granted the right to practice nursing within a state or territory by licensure through examination or licensure through endorsement.

- The registered nurse has the professional responsibility to attain and maintain competency.

- Nursing students have the responsibility to be prepared for clinical practice, to perform those skills for which competency has been achieved, and to seek instruction as necessary.

- Advanced practice nursing requires specialized knowledge and clinical proficiency. Advanced practice nursing roles include clinical nurse specialist,

nurse practitioner, certified nurse midwife, and certified registered nurse anesthetist.

- Leadership involves motivating and guiding others to achieve goals.

- Managerial functions can be categorized into five major areas: planning, organizing, directing, controlling, and decision making.

- Characteristics of effective leaders include communication, credibility, delegation, critical thinking ability, initiating action, risk taking, and persuasiveness and influence.

- Types of power (rewarding, coercive, referent, expert, legitimate, personal, and informational) are derived from sources such as ability to provide incentives, ability to punish, charisma, expertise, position within an organization, self-confidence, and information.

- Through empowerment, both nurses and clients can achieve their professional and personal goals.

- Nurses influence the delivery of health care services through participation in organizational politics.

REVIEW QUESTIONS

1. Which of the following is the primary legal guide for professional nursing practice?
   a. Agency-specific job description
   b. American Nurses Association *Ethical Code for Nurses*
   c. Federal nurse practice act
   d. State nurse practice acts

2. Which of the following is an ineffective leader behavior?
   a. Clarifying a misunderstanding
   b. Confronting a supervisor
   c. Yelling at a coworker
   d. Yielding on an unimportant issue

3. A nurse manager understands that the autocratic leadership style is most appropriate:
   a. during crisis situations.
   b. when a manager prefers a "telling" style.
   c. when followers cannot agree on a course of action.
   d. when problems are routine.

4. A nurse is licensed through a multistate compact to practice in Tennessee, Kentucky, and North Carolina. The nurse, who was originally licensed to practice in Tennessee, is providing diabetic education to a client residing in North Carolina. Which of the following correctly describes this situation?
   a. Only the Tennessee State Board of Nursing has regulatory authority over this nurse's actions.

   b. The client must go to Tennessee in order to be treated by this nurse legally.
   c. The nurse is guilty of professional malpractice due to practicing without a license.
   d. The nurse's practice must be in compliance with rules and regulations of the North Carolina State Board of Nursing.

5. Which of the following statements correctly describes a state's nurse practice act?
   a. Legislative act that defines nursing practice and sets standards for the profession in that state
   b. Means of regulating health care institutions under a voluntary standard of accreditation
   c. Professional credential that is granted by a professional nursing organization to demonstrate excellence in practice
   d. Reference to a nurse's legal responsibilities for harm caused to a client by inappropriate nursing action

6. The nurse manager calls a meeting of the nursing staff to discuss cost-cutting strategies. Staff members are encouraged to share their ideas and comments. The manager is demonstrating the importance of using which type of leadership style?
   a. Autocratic
   b. Democratic
   c. Laissez-faire
   d. Social trait

7. In planning care for a group of clients, which assignment planned by the registered nurse would be most appropriate?
   a. Asking a nursing assistant to explain to the client how to empty a urine collection bag
   b. Assigning the nursing assistant to orient a new graduate practical nurse to the unit
   c. Delegating the administration of all medications to the practical nurse
   d. Delegating the administration of an intermittent tube feeding to the practical nurse

8. When the nurse is preparing to assign duties to the unit staff, which element must be present to ensure effective delegation?
   a. A solid information base
   b. Adequate supplies and equipment
   c. Experienced staff members
   d. Informed clients and families

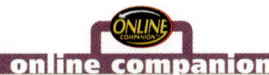

online companion

Visit the DeLaune and Ladner online companion resource at **www.delmar.cengage.com** for additional content and study aids. Click on Online Companions, then select the Nursing discipline.

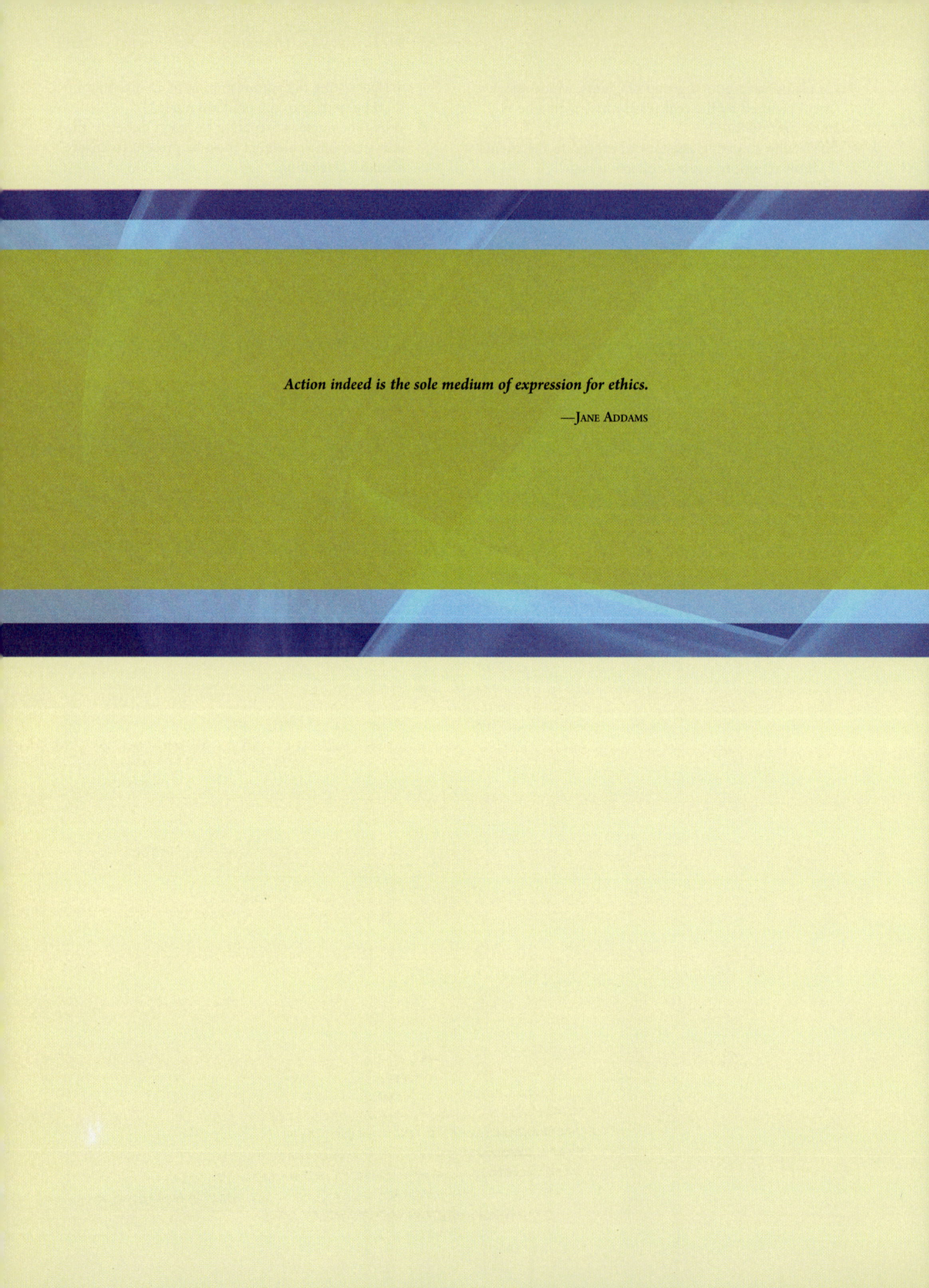

Action indeed is the sole medium of expression for ethics.

—JANE ADDAMS

CHAPTER 12

Legal and Ethical Responsibilities

COMPETENCIES

1. Explain the relationship between ethics and law.
2. Identify the sources of public law and their implications for nursing practice.
3. Describe the sources of civil law and their impact on the nursing profession.
4. Explain the actions that constitute unintentional and intentional torts.
5. List the legal responsibilities of nurses in delivering client care.
6. Discuss actions that nurses can implement to avoid potential liability.
7. Explain the role of the nurse in the informed consent process.
8. Define the three types of advance directives.
9. Describe the legal and ethical considerations for nurses involved in client care situations involving abortion, pronouncement of death, do not resuscitate orders, euthanasia, care of the deceased, wills, organ donation, autopsies, and refusal of treatment.
10. Discuss the ethical theories of teleology and deontology.
11. Describe the major ethical principles that affect health care.
12. Explain the link between ethics and values.
13. Identify the rights of the client as established by the American Hospital Association.
14. Discuss the roles of the nurse as client advocate and whistle-blower in the delivery of ethical nursing care.
15. Apply the steps identified in the ethical decision-making framework to selected dilemmas.

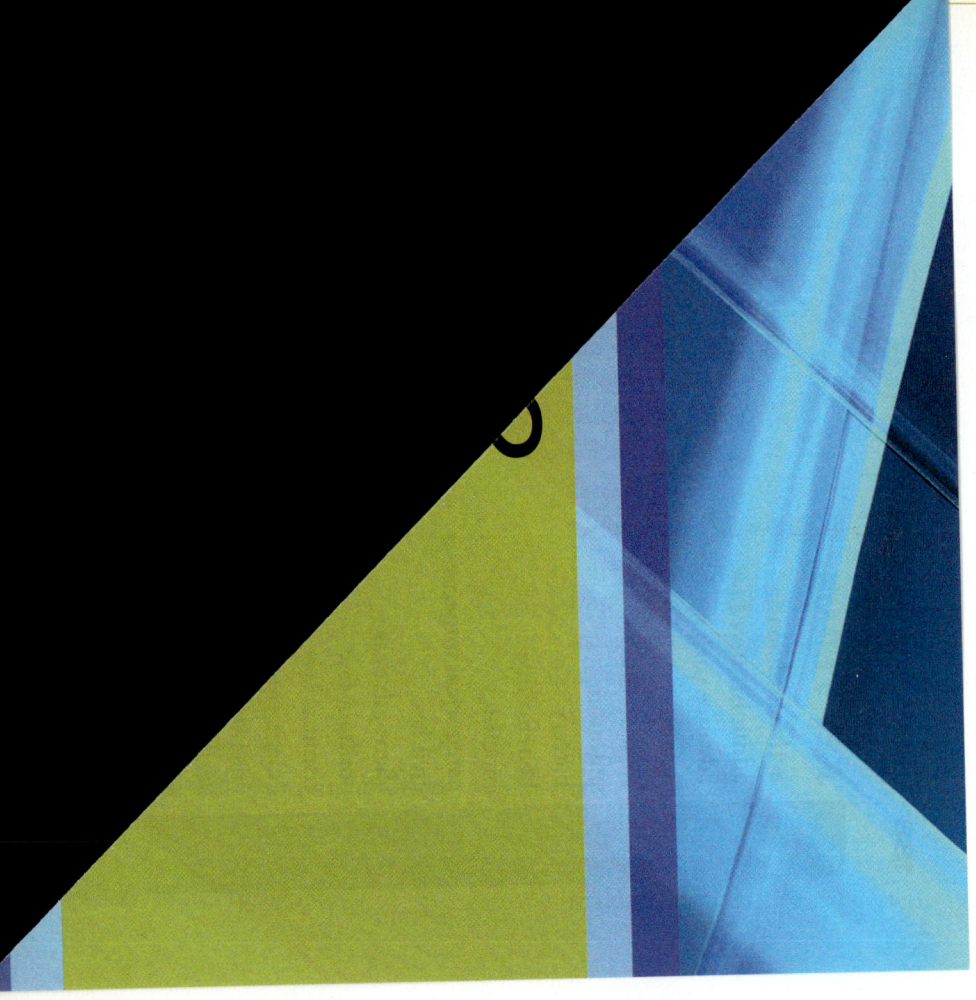

material principle of justice
misdemeanor
morality
negligence
nonmaleficence
passive euthanasia
paternalism
plaintiff
public law
statutory law
teleology
testimony
tort
tort law
unprofessional conduct
utility
values
values clarification
veracity
whistle-blowing

Law, like nursing, is responsive to changing needs, roles, and relationships in society. As the nursing profession has continued to evolve, the scope of applicable law has enlarged considerably. This chapter discusses laws affecting nursing practice and the legal responsibilities of nurses. In addition to legal standards, nurses must also practice according to ethical guidelines. Therefore, this chapter also explores the concept of ethics, ethical theories and principles, ethical codes, and the application of ethical decision-making guidelines in nursing practice.

LEGAL FOUNDATIONS OF NURSING

The word **law** is derived from an Anglo-Saxon term meaning *that which is laid down or fixed*. The two types of law are **public law**, which deals with an individual's relationship to the state, and **civil law**, which deals with relations between individuals.

SOURCES OF LAW

The three sources of public law at the federal and state levels are constitutional, administrative, and criminal. The three sources of civil law at the federal and state levels are contracts, torts, and protective and reporting laws.

Public Law

As shown in Table 12-1 page 189, public law governs the legal aspects of constitutional, administrative, and criminal law. The law of the United States is set forth in the Constitution. Laws enacted by legislative bodies are referred to as **statutory law**. State boards and professional practice acts, such as nurse practice acts, are created and governed under statutory laws.

Administrative law (regulatory law) is developed by groups who are appointed to governmental administrative agencies and who are entrusted with enforcing the statutory laws passed by the legislature. Under administrative law, state boards of nursing are given the power to further delineate the rules and regulations governing nursing as set forth in nurse practice acts. In these administrative rules, boards identify specific processes such as:

- Licensure
- Grounds for disciplinary proceedings
- Establishment of fees for the services
- Penalties rendered by the board

The most common example of public law is **criminal law**, which refers to acts or offenses against the welfare or safety of the public. In criminal law there are two types of crimes, felonies and misdemeanors. A **felony** is a crime of a serious nature, usually punishable by imprisonment in a state penitentiary at hard labor or by death, or a crime in violation of federal statute in which punishment is more than 1 year

TABLE 12-1 Types of Public Law

| CONSTITUTIONAL LAW | | ADMINISTRATIVE LAW | | CRIMINAL LAW | |
FEDERAL	STATE	FEDERAL	STATE	FEDERAL	STATE
• U.S. Constitution • Civil Rights Act	• State constitutions	• Food, Drug, and Cosmetic Act • Social Security Act • National Labor Relations Act	• Practice acts (e.g., nurse, medical, pharmacy) • Workers' compensation laws • State Labor Relations Act • Employment Security Act	• Controlled Substances Act • Kidnapping	• Criminal codes (define murder, manslaughter, criminal negligence, rape, fraud, illegal possession of drugs, theft, assault, and battery)

Data from Aiken, T. D. (2008). *Legal and ethical issues in health occupations* (2nd ed.). St. Louis, MO: Elsevier.

incarceration. A **misdemeanor** is an offense that is less serious than a felony and may be punished by a fine or sentence to a local prison for less than 1 year.

Civil Law

Civil law deals with crimes against a person or persons in such legal matters as contracts, torts, and protective/reporting law (see Table 12-2). Malpractice, also referred to as professional liability, is a violation of civil law (Aiken, 2008).

CONTRACT LAW.   **Contract law** is the enforcement of agreements among private individuals. A legal contract has three essential elements:

1. Promise(s) between two or more legally competent individuals stating what each individual must do or not do
2. Mutual understanding of the terms and obligations that the contract imposes on each individual
3. Compensation for lawful actions performed

Contracts are recognized at the state level as shown in Table 12-2.

TABLE 12-2 Types of Civil Law

| CONTRACT LAW | | TORTS | | PROTECTIVE AND REPORTING LAWS | |
FEDERAL	STATE	FEDERAL	STATE	FEDERAL	STATE
• None	• Employment contracts • Business contracts with clients • Contracts with allied groups • Uniform Commercial Code	• Federal Torts Claims Act	• State torts claims acts (to allow claims against the state) • Negligence (common law claim) • Malpractice statutes (professional liability) • Assault • Battery • False imprisonment • Invasion of privacy • Libel • Fraud	• Child Abuse Prevention and Treatment Act • Privacy Act of 1974	• Age of consent statutes (medical treatment, drugs, sexually transmitted disease) • Privileged communication statutes • Abortion statutes • Good Samaritan acts • Abuse statutes (child, elderly, domestic violence) • Involuntary hospitalization statutes • Living will legislation

Data from Aiken, T. D. (2008). *Legal and ethical issues in health occupations* (2nd ed.). St. Louis, MO: Elsevier.

The terms of a contract may be agreed on orally or in writing; however, a written contract (**formal contract**) cannot be changed legally by an oral agreement. With an **expressed contract**, the conditions and terms of the contract are usually given in writing by the concerned parties. An **implied contract** recognizes a relationship between parties for services.

In accord with U.S. and Canadian contract law, the nurse, as an employee, is legally required to:

1. Adhere to the employer's policies and standards unless they are in conflict with federal or state law
2. Fulfill the terms of contracted service with the employer
3. Respect the rights and responsibilities of other health care providers, especially in areas that promote the continuity of client care

Accompanying these legal responsibilities are the nurse's rights to:

1. Expect adequate and qualified assistance in providing care
2. Receive reasonable and prudent conduct from the client
3. Expect from the employer compensation for services and provision of a safe environment with the necessary resources to perform the services
4. Be treated with prudent, reasonable behaviors by other health care providers

TORT LAW. **Tort law** is the enforcement of duties and rights among individuals independent of contractual agreements. **Tort** is an act that harms a person. Tort liability can be classified as unintentional (negligence and malpractice) and intentional (assault and battery, false imprisonment, invasion of privacy, defamation, and fraud). Intentional torts must prove that the defendant intended to commit the act. Examples of tort law are listed in Table 12-2.

THE JUDICIAL PROCESS

Courts interpret a state's laws as they apply to everyday events. Once a court in the same jurisdiction, such as a state or city, interprets a law in a certain manner, other courts tend to follow the same interpretation. This is referred to as setting a precedent.

Additionally, lower courts in the same jurisdiction must adhere to the interpretations of higher courts in the same region. Thus, all of a state's lower courts must adhere to the interpretations and procedures specified by that state's supreme or highest court, and all courts in the United States must follow the rules established by the U.S. Supreme Court. This body of judge-made law is referred to as **jurisprudence**. A well-known and controversial example of jurisprudence is the constitutional right to an abortion recognized by the Supreme Court.

LEGAL LIABILITY IN NURSING

When the nurse fails to meet the legal expectations of care, the client can initiate action if harm or injury is incurred by the client.

Negligence and Malpractice

Liability is an obligation one has incurred or might incur through any act or failure to act. The term **malpractice** refers to a professional person's wrongful conduct, improper discharge of professional duties, or failure to meet the standards of acceptable care that results in harm to another person (Zerwekh & Claborn, 2008). **Negligence** (breach of duty) is the failure of an individual to provide care that a reasonable person would ordinarily use in a similar circumstance. In other words, action that is contrary to the conduct of a reasonable person and results in harm is considered to be negligent behavior. When a nurse commits a negligent act that results in injury, it is known as malpractice.

Proof of liability depends on four elements:

1. **Duty** is an obligation created either by law or contract or by any voluntary action. It is the first element that must be proved for malpractice.
2. Breach of duty occurs when a nurse fails to act in accord with the standard of care. An act of commission or omission of the nurse may constitute a breach of the standard of care.
3. Injury (physical, financial, or emotional harm) must be demonstrated by the person making the claim to prove negligence.
4. Causation is the breach of duty that must be proved to have legally caused the injury. A cause-and-effect relationship must be clearly established.

To succeed in a malpractice suit, the **plaintiff** (the party who initiates a lawsuit that seeks damages or other relief) must first show that the **defendant** (the person being sued) owed him or her a duty. The plaintiff must then show that the defendant did not meet the duty and that this breach of duty caused harm, requiring compensation. Once the plaintiff files charges, the defendant must either refute the charges by demonstrating that if a duty was owed, the duty was fulfilled or that if a duty was breached, the breach was not the cause of the plaintiff's complaint of injury.

A person typically has no difficulty showing that a nurse owed a duty. All that needs to be demonstrated is that the nurse was working on the day of the injury and was responsible for the person's care as verified by the staffing schedules and assignment sheets. It is more difficult to prove that the duty owed was breached.

Courts usually apply the *reasonable person standard*, which asks, "What would a reasonable nurse do in a similar situation?" To answer this question, courts look to the institution's policies and procedures to determine how client care is to be performed in that facility. When determining a breach of a duty, the actions of the nurse are also compared against the professional standards of nursing care. This is done by using published nursing standards developed by specialty nursing groups or by having another nurse testify as an expert witness. An **expert witness** is a person called upon by parties in a malpractice suit who is a member of the same profession as the party being sued and who is qualified to testify about the expected behaviors performed by members of the profession in a similar situation.

When a nurse is called to testify in a malpractice lawsuit, either as the defendant or as an expert witness, the **testimony** (written or verbal evidence given by a qualified expert in an area) must be based on facts. The jury and the court must form an opinion on their own; they are interested in the facts, not the witness's opinions, on the matter in dispute.

Nurses are expected to administer client care based on both institutional policy and procedure and the professional standards of care. The nurse defendant would use the same methods to prove that a breach of duty did not occur: showing that the facility's policies and procedures were followed and that the actions followed professional nursing standards. An expert witness is often asked to describe the relevant standards of care that will demonstrate that the client had the right to receive a *duty owed* from the nurse.

It is not sufficient to imply that the nurse breached a duty. The claimant must also show that this breach caused harm. A person cannot be compensated for a breach that caused no harm. Frequently, complaints against nurses are in one of the following categories: client falls, medication errors, failure to monitor a client in restraints, improper technique in giving treatment, failure to follow hospital procedures, and failure to supervise nonlicensed employees.

Informed Consent

Laws regarding informed consent protect the client's right to self-determination. A client is able to make an informed decision about consenting to or refusing a treatment regime only if adequate information has been presented.

The law requires that clients, or their representatives, be given sufficient information regarding various treatment modalities so that the consent is an informed process. A consent is a voluntary act by which a person agrees to allow someone else to do something. **Informed consent** means that the client understands the reason for the proposed intervention, and its benefits and risks, and agrees to the treatment by signing a consent form (see Figure 12-1). Consent forms must be obtained for all **invasive** (accessing body tissues, organs, or cavities through some type of instrumentation) procedures.

The client must be mentally competent to give consent for medical procedures. Obtaining the informed consent requires client teaching by the health care provider since clients must understand procedures and consequences of treatment and nontreatment.

The health care provider may not coerce the client to sign the consent. The client has the right to refuse the information, waive the informed consent, and undergo treatment. The client's refusal must be documented in the client's medical record. The signing of an informed consent can also be waived for urgent medical and surgical intervention as long as institutional policy so indicates. Obtaining the client's informed consent is the responsibility of the health care provider who is to perform the therapeutic activity; see the

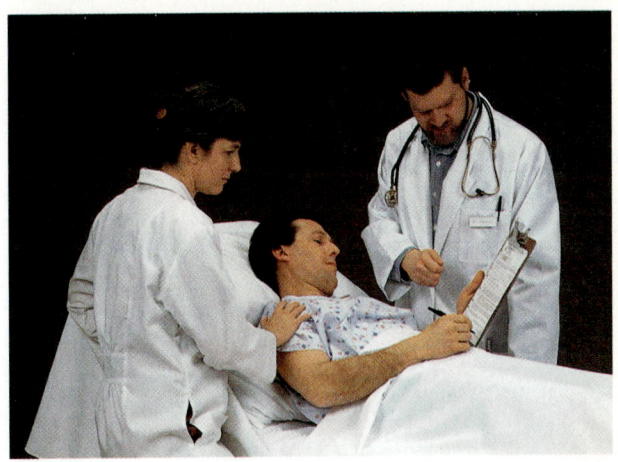

FIGURE 12-1 This nurse is witnessing the signing of a consent form after the prescribing practitioner has fully informed the client about the proposed treatment. How does the nurse's compliance with the policy of informed consent decrease the nurse's liability in terms of this client's care? DELMAR/CENGAGE LEARNING

Safety First display. When nurses sign a consent form as a witness, in actuality they are validating that they have seen the client sign the consent form. See Figure 12-2 on page 192 for an example of a consent to treatment form.

Parental or guardian consent should be obtained before treatment is initiated on a minor. There are three exceptions to this ruling: an emergency; situations where the consent of the minor is sufficient, such as treatment of a sexually transmitted disease; and situations where a court order or other legal authorization has been obtained. If a client is a minor and the parents or legal guardian deny the lifesaving treatment, the court may overrule the decision. Under the laws of most states and Canadian provinces, an emancipated minor (one who is married, pregnant, a parent, or financially independent) can give a valid consent to treatment.

Assault and Battery

Assault is a stated intent to touch a person in an offensive, insulting, or physically intimidating manner. **Battery** is the touching of another person without the person's consent. The legal issues arising from assault and battery are usually based on whether the client consented to the touching that occurred.

▼ **SAFETY FIRST** ▼

It is the legal responsibility of the health care provider performing the procedure to obtain the client's informed consent.

TULANE MEDICAL CENTER
Hospital and Clinic
1415 Tulane Avenue
New Orleans, Louisiana   70112

Consent for medical procedure and acknowledgement
of receipt of information

Date_____

In keeping with the Louisiana State Law, you are being asked to sign a confirmation that we have discussed your contemplated operation or medical procedure. We have already discussed with you the common problems or risks. We wish to inform you as completely as possible. Please read the form carefully. Ask about anything that you do not understand and we will be pleased to explain it.

1.] I hereby authorize and direct Dr._____ , with associates or assistants of his choice, to perform

upon_____ , the following surgical, diagnostic, or medical procedure

_____

_____

including any necessary or advisable anesthesia.

2.] In general terms, the nature and purpose of this operation or medical procedure is:

_____

_____

3.] This procedure has been explained to me. Alternate methods have also been explained to me, as have the advantages and disadvantages. I am advised that though good results are expected, the possibility and nature of complications cannot be accurately anticipated and that, therefore, there can be no guarantee as expressed or implied either as to the result of surgery or as to cure. The possible risks include death, brain damage, quadriplegia, paraplegia, loss of organ, loss of an arm or leg, or disfiguring scars.

4.] I authorize the administration of a blood transfusion and such additional transfusion as may be deemed advisable in judgement of the attending physician, or his associates or assistants.
It has been fully explained that blood transfusions are not always successful in producing a desirable result and that there is a possibility of ill effects, such as the transmission of infectious hepatitis or other diseases or blood impairments. Also, it has been explained that emergencies may arise when it may not be possible to make adequate cross-matching tests, and that immediate need may make it necessary to use existing stocks of blood which may not include compatible blood types.

5.] I further authorize the doctors to perform any other procedure that in their judgement is advisable for my well being. I hereby authorize and direct the above named physician and associates or assistants to provide such additional services as they may deem reasonable and necessary including, but not limited to, the administration of any anesthetic agent, or the services of the X-ray department or laboratories, and I hereby consent thereto.

6.] I hereby state that I have read and understand this consent, all questions about the procedure or procedures have been answered in a satisfactory manner, and that all blanks were filled in prior to my signature.

Witness_____   Signature_____
                                                      (patient or person authorized to consent)

Witness_____   Relationship_____
   (required only for telephone consent or consents signed with an X)

I certify that all blanks in this form were filled in prior to signature and that I explained them to the patient or his representative before requesting the patient or his representative to sign it.

Signature_____
                         (above named physician to sign)

†

**CONSENT FOR MEDICAL PROCEDURE AND ACKNOWLEDGEMENT
OF RECEIPT OF INFORMATION**

Order by priority when consenting to medical/surgical procedure (except for care and treatment of mentally ill)

1. Any competent adult, age 18 or older, for himself.
2. Any parent, whether an adult or minor, for his minor child.
3. Any married person, whether an adult or minor, for his/her spouse if spouse is unable to consent.
4. Any person temporarily standing in place of a parent whether formally served or not for the minor under his care and any guardian for his ward.
5. Any female regardless of age or marital status, for herself when given in connection with pregnancy or childbirth.
6. In the absence of a parent, any adult, for his minor brother or sister.
7. In the absence of a parent, any grandparent for his minor grandchild.

FIGURE 12-2 **Example of a Consent Form** COURTESY OF TULANE UNIVERSITY HOSPITAL AND CLINIC, NEW ORLEANS, LA

Because assault and battery both deal with *acts of touching,* the client's cultural values, beliefs, and practices must be respected by the nurse. If the nurse fails to recognize cultural differences, undesired outcomes may occur in the nurse-client relationship.

False Imprisonment

False imprisonment occurs when clients are led to believe they cannot leave a place. The most common example of this tort is telling a client not to leave the hospital until the bill is paid (Zerwekh & Claborn, 2008). Another example of false imprisonment is the misuse of physical or chemical restraints; see the Safety First display.

RESTRAINTS AND SECLUSION. The Omnibus Budget Reconciliation Act (OBRA) of 1987 outlines the rights of the client and the responsibilities of health care providers regarding the use of both physical and chemical restraints. The nurse is to use safety measures, such as keeping the client's bed in a low position and frequently assessing the client, in an effort to avoid the use of restraints. Chemical restraints, primarily psychotropic medications (e.g., sedatives, hypnotics, antianxiety agents, and neuroleptics), are used to control hyperactive behavior of agitated clients.

If a competent client refuses to follow orders and the nurse uses restraints, the nurse can be charged with false imprisonment, assault and battery, or both. In an emergency situation when a client becomes violent and is in imminent danger of harming himself or herself or others, the nurse may apply restraints and then immediately obtain an order from the prescribing practitioner. The law mandates that the use of restraints or seclusion must have a prescribing practitioner order. The nurse is legally accountable for the client in restraints or seclusion. Care of clients in restraints requires documentation according to specific agency policies.

Privacy and Confidentiality

An essential component of nursing practice is protecting the client's confidentiality and privacy. The American Nurses Association (ANA) *Guide to the Code of Ethics for Nurses* (2008a) identifies privacy and confidentiality as key elements in maintaining the integrity of the nursing profession. Nurses are accountable for respecting the client's right to privacy. State laws that respect privilege doctrine guarantee that no one will reveal confidential information without the client's

permission. Nurses must obtain the client's permission before disclosing any information regarding the client, going through the client's personal belongings, performing procedures, and photographing the client.

The Canadian Nurses Association (CNA) has developed its own code of ethics. The CNA's *Code of Ethics for Nursing* (2008) has involved nurses in all provinces and territories in Canada. Within the CNA's *Code of Ethics,* the value that applies to confidentiality states that the nurse is responsible to hold confidential all information about a client learned in health care settings. The nurse-client relationship is based on trust. Any violation of the client's privacy or breach of confidentiality may interfere with trust.

Nurses must ensure that clients understand their privacy rights, including withholding information, such as their diagnoses, from the family. For example, clients with sexually transmitted diseases or who are positive for the human immunodeficiency virus (HIV) may choose to withhold this information from their family.

Privacy involves more than protecting confidential communication. Nursing care should be delivered with a caring attitude that provides for privacy, such as keeping the door to the client's room closed, knocking before entering the client's room, closing the curtains around the bed before exposing the client, and draping the client appropriately for procedures.

A rapidly increasing problem that threatens privacy and confidentiality is access to electronic data. The technological proliferation of cellular phones, facsimile machines, and electronic health records (EHRs) may jeopardize the privacy of information. In 2004, a presidential executive order called for the adoption of EHRs by 2014 (Westra, Delaney, Konicek, & Kennan, 2008). As the use of EHRs expands, there will be more issues about protecting the privacy of shared health information.

In 1996, Congress enacted the Health Insurance Portability and Accountability Act (HIPAA) to ensure the privacy of individual health care information. HIPAA rules require written confirmation that clients have been informed about their privacy rights (U.S. Department of Health and Human Services, 2002). As a result of the HIPAA, the following changes have been implemented in health care settings:

- Posting a client's name near the room door is prohibited.
- Charts containing clients' names cannot be within public view.
- Calling out clients' names (e.g., in clinic waiting rooms) is prohibited.
- Medical records must be stored in secure areas.
- Clients' health care information must be discussed in private areas.

Defamation

Defamation occurs when information is communicated to a third party that causes damage to someone else's reputation either in writing (libel) or verbally (slander). The most common examples of this tort are giving out inaccurate or inappropriate information from the medical record; discussing

---

▼ SAFETY FIRST ▼

Restraints are legal only if they are necessary to protect the client or others from harm. The rationale for use of restraints must be documented in the client's health care record.

clients, families, or visitors in public areas; and speaking negatively about coworkers (Zerwekh & Claborn, 2008).

Fraud

Fraud results from a deliberate deception intended to produce unlawful gain. Fraudulent billing practices include overcharging for services and billing for services that were not provided. Other examples of fraud in health care include obtaining and using false credentials and falsifying medical records. Nursing activities to deter fraud include the following:

- Documenting facts accurately
- Reporting illegal activities
- Educating peers and the public as to what constitutes fraud

Unprofessional Conduct

Conduct of a health care provider that could adversely affect the health and welfare of the public constitutes unprofessional conduct. The following actions or omissions constitute unprofessional conduct:

- Breach in client confidentiality
- Failure to use sufficient knowledge, skills, or nursing judgment when practicing nursing
- Physically or verbally abusing a client
- Assuming duties without sufficient preparation
- Knowingly delegating nursing tasks to unlicensed personnel that places the client at risk for injury
- Failure to accurately maintain a record for each client or falsifying a client's record
- Leaving a nursing assignment without properly notifying appropriate personnel

Use of Controlled Substances

The improper use of controlled substances may lead to criminal penalties under laws governing the distribution and use of controlled substances (narcotics, depressants, stimulants, and hallucinogens). Agencies that distribute controlled substances must follow federal and state regulations regarding the security and access to these drugs. Title II of the Comprehensive Drug Abuse Prevention and Control Act of 1970 (Controlled Substances Act) requires accurate documentation of narcotic administration.

THE IMPAIRED NURSE. If a nurse suspects a coworker is abusing chemicals, the nurse has a duty to report the individual to nursing administration in a confidential manner with the goal of treatment being the priority issue. Nursing administration should then notify the board of nursing regarding the nurse's behavior.

Nurses must safeguard the client and the public by reporting the incompetent, unethical, or illegal practice of any person. Some boards of nursing will discipline a nurse for failing to report a fellow nurse who is abusing drugs. An impaired nurse is habitually intemperate or is addicted to

the use of alcohol or habit-forming drugs. Some indicators of substance abuse in nurses are:

- Social isolation (e.g., requesting to work the night shift)
- Changes in personal appearance and mood
- Excessive work-related tardiness, absences, and accidents
- Excuses for being unavailable while on duty
- Resistance to change
- Defensive when questioned about client complaints and discrepancies in the narcotic control sheet
- Failure to meet schedules and deadlines
- Inaccurate and sloppy documentation

With the formation of the Task Force on Addiction and Psychological Disturbance by the ANA in 1981, many states have initiated programs to identify, treat, and assist impaired nurses. Intervention programs allow the nurse to seek and comply with a treatment regimen as an alternative to disciplinary action, such as suspension of nursing license.

Safety

The promotion of physical safety is one of the most important responsibilities of the nurse. There are four areas regarding client safety in which nurses are at legal risk: (1) failure to monitor client status, (2) medication errors, (3) falls, and (4) use of restraints.

Failure to monitor means that the nurse must be aware of the client's condition at all times. This calls for frequent assessment of all clients and adherence to policy guidelines regarding assessment of clients with special needs, such as those who are immobile, critically ill, or unconscious.

A major safety issue in health care is the prevention of medication errors. Medication errors not only jeopardize client safety but are also expensive. "Besides harming patients, they can lead to expensive follow-up care, litigation, and monetary awards for damages" (Austin, 2008, p. 36). Some of the most common types of medication errors are improper dosing, administration of the wrong drug, and omitting to administer a medication. Nurses play a major role in the prevention of adverse drug events by careful drug administration and client assessment. See Chapter 30 for information on safe administration of medication.

Another major area for potential liability is client falls. Elderly clients are especially at risk for fall-related injuries. The most important measures for preventing lawsuits related to falls are assessing for fall potential and taking action to prevent falls (Aiken, 2008).

Another potential problem is the use of medical equipment. Whenever nurses are confronted with unfamiliar medical equipment, they are expected to seek out information and training on use of the machinery. Nurses must always use equipment according to the manufacturer's instructions. Nurses must also report malfunctioning or broken equipment according to the employing agency's policies. Austin suggests, "Never try guessing how to use equipment" (2008, p. 39).

Understaffing

Understaffing refers to the failure of a facility to provide a sufficient number of professional staff to meet client needs.

Health care providers must have written staffing guidelines for each client population and setting to comply with the standards of the Joint Commission. Usually staffing policies are in place to direct the decision making regarding increasing or downsizing staff numbers.

Reassignment.   Questions are often raised by nurses in hospitals regarding the liabilities of "floating" (reassignment to work on an unfamiliar unit). This is an acceptable, legal practice used by hospitals to solve their understaffing problems. Legally, a nurse cannot refuse to float unless a union contract guarantees that nurses work only in a specified area or the nurse can prove the lack of knowledge for the performance of assigned tasks.

When reassignment occurs, nurses should set priorities and identify potential areas of harm to the client. The nurse is legally mandated to be competent before performing procedures; inexperience is no legal excuse for errors. Nurses who are required to float should receive orientation prior to reassignment.

Executing Prescribed Orders

Medical practice acts of states and provinces usually define medicine as any act of diagnosis, prescription, surgery, or treatment of illness. This definition allows for the initiation of written or verbal prescribing practitioner orders. In accord with nurse practice acts, nurses are obligated to follow the orders of a licensed prescribing practitioner *unless the orders would result in client harm.*

The nurse has a legal responsibility to the client to ensure that the order is clear and appropriate to the client's treatment. When the nurse questions an order, the prescribing practitioner should be contacted to provide clarification. If, after prescribing practitioner clarification, the nurse still questions the order, the nurse should institute agency policy (e.g., notify the supervisor). Following the agency's policy in this matter protects the nurse from employer disciplinary action. See the Safety First display.

LEGAL RESPONSIBILITIES AND ROLES

Nurses are legally responsible to practice nursing as defined by nurse practice acts and professional standards of care. There are several roles performed by nurses related specifically to legal accountability.

▼ SAFETY FIRST ▼

The nurse remains liable for incorrectly administering a medication even if it is ordered incorrectly by the prescribing practitioner. Sound nursing judgment is required for every medication that is administered.

Provider of Care

The nurse is legally responsible to ensure that the client receives competent, safe, and holistic care. Nurses are expected to:

- Render care based on their education, experience, and circumstances (standard of "reasonable, prudent person")
- Discuss with the client the associated risks and outcomes inherent in the plan of care
- Supervise and evaluate aspects of care that have been delegated to licensed and unlicensed caregivers
- Document the care the client receives and other significant events affecting the client
- Maintain clinical competency

The nurse is also responsible for the client's physical safety as discussed in this chapter's section on safety.

Expert Witness

To qualify as an expert witness, the nurse's education and experience are presented to the court to prove the nurse is knowledgeable about current standards and practice. The credentials of an expert witness have to match or exceed a defendant's qualifications. During the trial, the plaintiff's and the defendant's attorneys have the right to use the testimony of the expert witness for their respective cases.

Forensic Specialist

Another role for nurses is that of forensic nurse. The ANA's *Scope and Standards of Forensic Nursing Practice* (2008b) describes some of the responsibilities of forensic nurses as treating incarcerated clients, investigating trauma cases, and serving as expert witnesses in court. As violence continues to escalate in the United States, there will be an increased demand for forensic nurses.

Client Educator

Safe nursing care requires that the client has a thorough understanding of the treatment plan. Although the prescribing practitioner has specific responsibilities regarding client education, the nurse must also provide client teaching and document the degree of learning. See Chapter 21 for a complete discussion of the nurse's responsibilities for client education.

Reporting Responsibilities

Nurses should know which situations have to be reported because reporting statutes vary among the states and provinces; refer to Table 12-2 for protective and reporting laws. Criminal acts of rape and sexual assault must also be reported in most states and provinces.

LEGAL RESPONSIBILITIES OF STUDENTS

Nursing students must act as reasonably prudent persons, equivalent with education and experience, when performing nursing duties. When employed as caregivers, nursing students must perform only tasks that they are competent to perform; see the Spotlight On display.

LEGAL SAFEGUARDS FOR NURSING PRACTICE

There is a common set of actions a nurse can take to protect against ligation. Although each client encountered presents a unique situation that can place the nurse at legal risk, certain general nursing care activities decrease this risk (see the Nursing Checklist). Implementing the guidelines in the checklist should help protect nurses from lawsuits as well as provide defense in the event of a suit.

Institutional Policies

All health care facilities have policies for delivering safe, effective care. Nursing students and registered nurses are obligated to know the policies and follow the procedures and protocols that flow from policy. Although policies are not laws, courts generally rule against nurses who violate policies.

Professional Liability Insurance

Nurses should purchase their own liability insurance for protection against malpractice lawsuits. When securing liability insurance, the nurse should validate the company's reputation. Most professional nursing organizations offer group liability insurance.

Nurses may erroneously assume that they are protected by their employer's professional liability policies. Usually when a nurse is sued, the employer is also sued for the nurse's actions or inaction. Even though this is the norm, nurses are encouraged to have their own malpractice insurance. Having one's own insurance also provides the nurse protection as an individual and allows the nurse to have an attorney who has only the nurse's interests in mind.

As Willson (2007, p. 11) states:

In Canada, most nurses are covered by their employer's liability insurance and therefore have representation by a lawyer appointed by the employer's insurer. This means that the lawyer acting on behalf of the hospital is also acting on behalf of you as an employee. An exception to this is if your alleged

conduct fell outside the scope of your employment or if it was criminal in intent, in which case you may not be eligible for legal representation through your employer.

NURSING CHECKLIST

Actions to Decrease the Risk of Liability

- Communicate with clients by keeping them informed and listening to what they say.
- Acknowledge unfortunate incidents and express concern about these events without either taking the blame, blaming others, or reacting defensively.
- Chart and time observations immediately while facts are still fresh in mind.
- Take appropriate actions to meet the client's nursing needs.
- Follow the facility's policies and procedures for administering care and reporting incidents.
- Acknowledge and document the reason for any omission or deviation from agency policy, procedure, or standard.
- Maintain clinical competency and acknowledge one's own limitations. Nurses who do not know how to do something should ask for help.
- Promptly report any concern regarding the quality of care, including the lack of resources with which to provide care, to a nursing administration representative.
- Implement appropriate standards of care.
- Time and document changes in conditions requiring notification of the prescribing practitioner and include the prescribing practitioner's response.
- Delegate client care based on the documented skills of licensed and unlicensed personnel.
- Treat all clients and their families with kindness and respect.

Risk Management Programs

Risk management is a method of identifying, evaluating, and decreasing the agency's risk of financial loss. Most health care facilities are required to have formal risk management programs in place by agencies such as the Department of Health and Human Services, accrediting bodies, and liability insurance carriers. These programs are based on systematic reporting of incidents or unusual occurrences (e.g., client falls).

INCIDENT REPORTS. In accord with the agency's policies, nurses are required to file incident reports when a situation arises that could or did cause client harm. When filing an incident report, the nurse should state only the *facts* surrounding the incident. The nurse's opinions or conclusions about the incident are not to be documented. Also, the

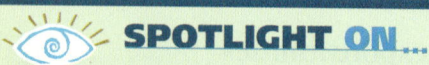

SPOTLIGHT ON...

Legal

Legal Implications for Nursing Students

When agency policy conflicts with the nurse practice act, what should you do? Remember that the state legislature empowers the board of nursing to define and monitor practice. If, as a nursing student, you willfully violate the state board's ruling, what future implication(s) could this have on your ability to apply for licensure?

client's medical record should not contain any reference to the filing of an incident report. See Chapter 13 for more information on incident reports.

LEGISLATION AFFECTING NURSING PRACTICE

There are legal, as well as ethical, implications inherent in nursing practice that require nurses to know and comply with the specific existing health care laws and regulations in their state of licensure. Following is a discussion of some laws that impact nursing.

Patient Self-Determination Act

The Patient Self-Determination Act (PSDA) of 1990 requires that on admission to any health care service, clients are to be given the opportunity to determine what type of life-prolonging or lifesaving actions they want performed. The PSDA applies to all health care settings, including hospitals, home health agencies, and long-term care centers. Often, the nurse is the person designated to educate the client on care options. Ideally, health care decisions would be made before an emergency arises. Ellis and Hartley (2007, p. 297) state:

> One suggestion has been that these matters first be discussed in the health care provider's office, before admission. When this is possible, it allows for more time to consider alternatives and consult significant others. The final decision is then made away from the pressure of the health care environment.

The three types of documents that comply with the PSDA include the following:

1. A **living will** is a document prepared by a competent adult that provides direction regarding medical care in the event that the person becomes unable to make decisions personally.
2. **Durable power of attorney** (health care proxy) is an authorization that enables any competent individual to name someone to exercise decision-making authority, under specific circumstances, on the individual's behalf.
3. An **advance care medical directive** is a document in which an individual, in consultation with the prescribing practitioner, relatives, or other personal advisors, provides precise instructions for the type of care the client wants or does not want in a number of scenarios.

The living will is the most widely available instrument for recording future health care–related decisions. Figure 12-3 on page 198 presents a sample document of a living will. All states provide for a general durable power of attorney.

Roe v. Wade

The 1973 Supreme Court decision of *Roe v. Wade* increased the safety and availability of abortions in the United States.

Health care agencies and practitioners in various states may be required to report abortions performed as well as other information about the client, the procedure, and any resulting complications. Some states require the reporting of abortions only for minors.

Nurses may need to explore their own feelings or beliefs about abortion before assisting with these procedures. The nurse should also be aware of the client's feelings before the abortion so that appropriate referral can be made for postprocedure care if necessary.

The Americans with Disabilities Act

Passed by the U.S. Congress in 1990, the Americans with Disabilities Act (ADA) prohibits discrimination on the basis of disability in employment, public services, and public accommodations. The ADA defines a person with a disability as having a physical or mental impairment that substantially limits one or more of the major life activities. See the Respecting Our Differences display.

Good Samaritan Acts

Good Samaritan acts are laws that provide protection to health care providers by ensuring immunity from civil liability when assistance is provided at the scene of an emergency when the caregiver does not intentionally or recklessly cause client injury. The caregiver will be evaluated by how a reasonable and prudent caregiver would have responded in a similar situation. Good Samaritan acts are examples of common and statutory laws as determined by the individual states. Although all 50 states and the District of Columbia have Good Samaritan acts, some of the Canadian provinces (e.g., Ontario and Quebec) do not have such acts.

Good Samaritan acts vary in coverage from state to state, and it is the responsibility of caregivers to know the law for their own jurisdictions. Keep in mind that some states cover only nurses licensed in that state and that these acts are amended periodically by legislation. Good Samaritan acts do not provide immunity to the nurse who is providing care as an employee (Zerwekh & Claborn, 2008). See the accompanying Spotlight on page 198 On display.

RESPECTING OUR DIFFERENCES

Hearing Impaired Coworker

How would you feel about a nurse coworker who is hearing impaired and cannot hear heart, lung, and bowel sounds? What are your responsibilities in such a situation?

Declaration

Declaration made this _____ day of _____(month, year).

I, _____, being of sound mind, willfully and voluntarily make known my desire that my dying shall not be artificially prolonged under the circumstances set forth below and do hereby declare:

If at any time I should either have a terminal and irreversible incurable injury, disease, or illness or be in continual profound comatose state with no reasonable chance of recovery, certified by two physicians who have personally examined me, one of whom shall be my attending physician, and the physicians have determined that my death will occur whether or not life-sustaining procedures are utilized and where the application of life-sustaining procedures would serve only to prolong artificially the dying process, I direct that such procedures be withheld or withdrawn and that I be permitted to die naturally with only the administration of medication or the performance of any medical procedure deemed necessary to provide me with comfort care.

In the absence of my ability to give directions regarding the use of such life-sustaining procedures, it is my intention that this declaration shall be honored by my family and physician(s) as the final expression of my legal right to refuse medical or surgical treatment and accept the consequences from such refusal.

I understand the full import of this declaration and I am emotionally and mentally competent to make this declaration.

Signed:_____

City, Parish, and State of Residence_____

The declarant has been personally known to me and I believe him or her to be of sound mind.

Witness:_____

Witness:_____

FIGURE 12-3 **Sample of a Living Will** COURTESY OF LOUISIANA HOSPITAL ASSOCIATION, BATON ROUGE, LA

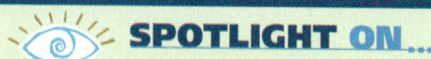

SPOTLIGHT ON...

Legal

Good Samaritan Acts

If, as a nurse, you charge or accept a fee for the services rendered during an emergency situation, will you still be protected by a Good Samaritan act? What are the legal implications for accepting compensation for your professional services?

Health Care Quality Improvement Act

The Health Care Quality Improvement Act was enacted in 1986 to identify unsafe health care providers and restrict their unsafe practice. The major goal of this legislation was to deter incompetent practitioners from moving to a new state without having to report on problematic care delivery in previous states. This legislation established the National Practitioner Data Bank to serve as a clearinghouse for information on unsafe practitioners and to provide immunity to those who report incompetent peers.

Occupational Safety & Health Administration

In 1970, the Occupational Safety & Health Administration (OSHA) was established to ensure safe work environments for Americans. The intent of the act was to decrease work-related injuries. The act was expanded in 1991 to develop standards for safety of those who may experience work-related exposure to bloodborne contaminants. OSHA also provides guidelines for health care workers' potential exposure to drugs and chemicals, biological agents (e.g., influenza virus), radioactivity, and threats to respiratory health. Ergonomic hazards from lifting and repetitive movements are also addressed by OSHA (2008). Employers are fined if they violate OSHA rules and regulations.

LEGAL ISSUES RELATED TO DEATH AND DYING

Nurses encounter numerous legal and ethical challenges when caring for clients who are dying. The following section discusses do not resuscitate orders, wills, pronouncement of death, care of the deceased, autopsies, and organ donation.

Do Not Resuscitate Orders

Cardiac arrest requires the initiation of cardiopulmonary resuscitation (CPR) by competent persons. In health care settings, caregivers (often nurses) perform CPR and other lifesaving measures according to agency policy unless the primary prescribing practitioner has written a *do not resuscitate (DNR)* order in the client's medical record. The prescribing practitioner's DNR order provides an exception to the universal standing order to resuscitate.

Health care agencies are required to have policies in place that provide a mechanism for reaching a DNR decision as well as for resolving conflicts in decision making. The principles of informed consent must be respected by the prescribing practitioner who writes a DNR order. When the client is either comatose or near death, there should be knowledgeable concurrence by the prescribing practitioner and the client's family or guardian about actions to prolong the client's life. It is the responsibility of the nurse to know and follow the client's wishes relative to resuscitation and the application of life-support systems. This information must be documented in the client's medical record.

Wills

The United States and Canada have laws regarding the legal requirements for written and oral wills. Nurses are usually required to notify the prescribing practitioner and nurse supervisor before acting as a witness and signing a will. Nurses should refrain from assisting the client with the wording of the will, as this should be done with legal advice from an attorney. When serving as a witness, a nurse is verifying that it is indeed the client who is actually signing the documents.

Pronouncement of Death

Medicine has yet to agree on one acceptable definition of death. The various definitions are as follows: the absence of awareness of external stimuli, lack of movement or spontaneous breathing, absent reflexes, a flat brain wave repeated twice in 24 hours, and the Uniform Definition of Brain Death, which requires irreversible cessation of all functioning of the brain (Zerwekh & Claborn, 2008). See the accompanying Spotlight On display.

State regulatory boards have initiated laws to protect the public when dealing with issues of death. It is usually within the scope of practice of medicine to pronounce a client dead. However, some boards of nursing allow the nurse, in certain circumstances and with thorough documentation, to make a determination and pronouncement of death. Because state laws vary concerning this issue, it is important for registered nurses to know the laws in their own state or province of licensure.

Care of the Deceased

When a client dies, the nurse is obligated to treat the deceased with respect and dignity. The nurse should prepare the body for removal to the morgue in accordance with agency policies. The nurse is responsible for properly identifying the body. Wrongful identification of the body could result in severe distress for the family of the deceased as well as negative legal ramifications for both the health care agency and the nurse.

Autopsies

An autopsy is performed to determine the cause of death. Autopsy results are used in cases of suspicious death or the presence of communicable disease. The cause of death also has implications regarding payment from insurance policies and workers' compensation.

Some states require consent for an autopsy in writing, whereas other states accept telegrams or documented telephone conversations. Regardless of how consent is obtained, the prescribing practitioner must document that consent was obtained and identify in the client's record who authorized the autopsy. In some states, consent for an autopsy is not required in unwitnessed deaths because this situation requires a mandatory autopsy. The nurse is responsible for ensuring that all documentation is in place before releasing a body for autopsy.

Organ Donation

All 50 states have adopted the Uniform Anatomical Gift Act for cadaver organ donation. In the United States and Canada, any person aged 18 or older may become an organ donor by

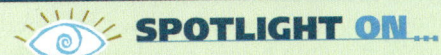

SPOTLIGHT ON...

Legal

What Constitutes Death?

Considering the various definitions of death, is it absolutely clear when the moment of death occurs? Based on these definitions, when can the life-supporting machines be turned off? Although the right of the client to refuse treatment, which may lead to death, has been established, can you identify clinical circumstances where the client might be deprived of the right to die?

written consent. In the absence of appropriate documentation, a family member or legal guardian may authorize donation of the organs. Nurses and other caregivers are expected to approach families for organ donation in the absence of documentation of the client's wishes. Consent for an organ donation requires the collaborative efforts of the nurse with prescribing practitioners, social workers, and clergy to ensure timely removal of the organs.

ETHICAL FOUNDATIONS OF NURSING

Every day, nurses encounter situations in which they must make decisions based on the determination of right and wrong. How do they make such decisions? Which values determine the rightness of an action?

The delivery of ethical health care is becoming an increasingly difficult and confusing issue in contemporary society. Nurses are committed to maintaining clients' rights related to health care. This desire to maintain clients' rights, however, often conflicts with professional duties and institutional policies. It is essential to balance these two perspectives so that the primary objective, delivery of quality care, is achieved. See the Uncovering the Evidence display.

It is also necessary to realize that there are no absolute right answers. Dealing with the gray areas (ambiguities) causes discomfort for some nurses. Unlike mathematics and other empirical sciences, there are no apparent absolute rules governing ethics. Scientists can say for certain that two plus two always equals four—regardless of the time factors, circumstances, feelings, or beliefs of those involved in the calculations. Ethical guidelines are less clear and more open to interpretation. In other words, ethical decisions may vary according to each individual and each situation. Because clients and nurses are humans, no two situations can ever be exactly alike.

CONCEPT OF ETHICS

Ethics is the branch of philosophy that examines the differences between right and wrong. Simply put, ethics is the study of the rightness of conduct. Ethics deals with one's responsibilities (duties and obligations) as defined by logical argument. Ethics looks at human behavior—what people do under what type of circumstances. But ethics is not merely a philosophical discussion; ethical persons put their beliefs into action.

Often the term *morals* is mistakenly used when ethics is meant. **Morality** is behavior in accordance with custom or tradition and usually reflects personal or religious beliefs. An example of a moral belief is a person's desire to maintain his or her right to die. Ethics is the free, rational, and publicly stated assessment of alternative actions in relation to theories, principles, and rules. Ethics is rooted in the legal system and reflects the political values of our society. An example of an ethical belief is the practice of parents' teaching their children the importance of telling the truth.

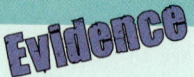

UNCOVERING THE Evidence

TITLE OF STUDY
"Ethical Dilemmas among Nurses as They Transition to Hospital Case Management: Implications for Organizational Ethics, Part II"

AUTHOR
L. T. O'Donnell

PURPOSE
To describe the ethical concerns experienced by clinical nurses as they moved into their new role of hospital case management.

METHODS
An interpretive phenomenological approach was used to identify themes in ethical concerns and relate them to the role of hospital nurse case management. Interviews were conducted to explore participants' resolution of ethical dilemmas.

FINDINGS
As nurses are promoted to the expanded role of case manager, they face situations that require ethical decision making and clinical judgment.

IMPLICATIONS
(1) Nurse case managers are confronted daily with ethical dilemmas. (2) There is a need for continued education of the case manager role.

O'Donnell, L. T. (2007). Ethical dilemmas among nurses as they transition to hospital case management: Implications for organizational ethics, Part II. *Professional Case Management, 12*(4), 219–231.

Relationship between Legal and Ethical Concepts

There is a connection between acts that are legal and acts that are ethical. Sometimes, it is difficult to separate legalities from ethics. Some legal acts are considered to be unethical and vice versa. According to Burkhardt and Nathaniel (2007), the following contribute to the occasional discrepancies between law and ethics:

- Ethical opinions reflect individual differences.
- Human behavior and motivation are too complex to be accurately reflected in law.
- The legal system judges action rather than intention.
- Laws change according to social and political influences.

Professional nursing actions are both legal and ethical. See the accompanying Spotlight On display on page 201.

Bioethics

The application of general ethical principles to health care is referred to as **bioethics**. Ethics affects every area of health care, including direct care of clients, allocation of finances, and utilization of staff. Ethics does not provide easy answers but can help provide structure by raising questions that ultimately lead to answers.

Ethics is exerting an ever-increasing influence on health care today. Several factors contribute to an increased need to provide health care in an ethical manner. Some of these factors are:

1. An increasingly technological society. The nature of advanced technology creates situations that involve complicated issues that never had to be considered before. As a result of technological advances:
   - Many newborns are surviving at earlier gestational ages, and many of them have serious health problems.
   - People are living much longer than ever before.
   - Organ transplants and the use of bionic body parts are becoming more common.
2. The changing fabric of our society. Family structure is moving from extended families to nuclear families, single-parent families, and nonrelated individuals living together as families.
3. Clients are becoming more knowledgeable about their health and health-related interventions. As consumer demand for information increases, health care providers must adapt quickly. The result is a focus on a consumer-driven system.

Nurses face situations in which they must make decisions that transcend technical and professional concerns. These situations may or may not involve life-or-death issues. Such situations raise complex problems that cannot be answered completely with technical knowledge and professional expertise. Technological advances have created unprecedented choices, not only for society at large, but specifically for clients and nurses.

There is emphasis on ethical issues involving life-or-death situations. However, nurses daily encounter challenges about what *ought* to be done, even in the most ordinary circumstances. The accompanying Spotlight On display lists

ethical dilemmas that frequently occur in nursing practice. The way in which nurses relate to clients, families, and other health care providers is the true demonstration of ethical behavior.

ETHICAL THEORIES

Ethical theories were debated by ancient philosophers such as Plato and Aristotle, and the debate continues today. No theory in and of itself can provide the "correct" answer to any single ethical conflict. However, ethical theories can be used as a way to analyze ethical problems.

Teleology

Teleology is the ethical theory stating that the value of a situation is determined by its consequences. Thus, the outcome of an action—not the action itself—is the criterion for determining the goodness of that action. This theory (also called the consequentialist theory) was advocated by the philosopher John Stuart Mill. The principle of **utility** is a basic concept of teleology; utility states that an act must result in the greatest amount of good for the greatest number of people involved in a situation. "Good" refers to positive benefit. Any act can be ethical if it delivers "good" results. Every alternative is assessed for its potential outcomes, both positive and negative. The selected action is the one that results in the most benefits and the least amount of harm for all those involved.

Deontology

Deontology is the ethical theory that considers the intrinsic significance of the act itself as the criterion for determination of good. That is, in determining the ethics of a situation, a person must consider the motives of the actor, not the consequences of the act.

This theory (also called formalism) was postulated by the philosopher Immanuel Kant. Kant established the concept of the categorical imperative, which states that one should act only if the action is based on a principle that is universal (everyone would act in the same way in a similar situation). The **categorical imperative** also mandates that a person

---

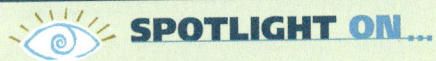

SPOTLIGHT ON...

Legal/Ethical

Legal and Ethical Concepts

Which of the following behaviors are ethical and illegal? Legal and unethical? Illegal and unethical? Legal and ethical?

> Working in a clinic that performs abortions
>
> Honoring a terminally ill client's request to have "no heroic" actions taken
>
> Discontinuing a comatose client's life support at the request of the family
>
> Diverting medications from a client for your own use

SPOTLIGHT ON...

Ethics

Frequently Occurring Ethical Dilemmas

> Informed consent
> Refusal of treatment
> Use of scarce resources
> Cost-containment initiatives that negatively affect client well-being
> Incompetent health care providers

should never be treated as a means to an end. Adherence to this concept may pose an ethical concern to health care researchers, who sometimes may risk the well-being of a person participating in an experimental procedure for the sake of finding a drug that will save many from suffering.

ETHICAL PRINCIPLES

Ethical principles are tenets that direct or govern actions. They are widely accepted and generally are based on the humane aspects of society. Ethical decisions are principled; that is, they reflect what is best for the client and society. Table 12-3 summarizes the major ethical principles. Each principle is discussed in detail in the following paragraphs.

By applying ethical principles, nurses become more systematic in solving ethical conflicts. Ethical principles can be used as guidelines in analyzing dilemmas; they can also serve as a justification (rationale) for the resolution of ethical problems. Remember that these principles are not absolute; there can be exceptions to each principle in any given situation.

Autonomy

The principle of autonomy refers to the individual's right to choose and the ability to act on that choice. The individuality of each person is respected when autonomy is maintained. This respect for personal liberty is a dominant value of mainstream American society.

Nurses must respect clients' right to decide and protect those clients who are unable to decide for themselves. The ethical principle of autonomy reflects the belief that every competent person has the right to determine his or her own course of action. The right to free choice rests on the client's competency to decide.

Informed consent is based on clients' right to decide for themselves. Upholding autonomy means that the nurse accepts the client's choices, even when those choices are not in the client's best interests. Following are examples of clients' autonomous behavior that can impair recovery or treatment:

- Smoking after a diagnosis of emphysema or lung cancer
- Refusing to take medication

- Continuing to drink alcohol when one has cirrhosis
- Refusing to receive a blood transfusion because of religious beliefs

The PSDA of 1990 was legislated to ensure that clients have the right to make their own health care decisions. Based on the principle of autonomy, this act requires that every person admitted to a health care facility be informed of the right to self-determination.

Nonmaleficence

Nonmaleficence is the duty to cause no harm to others. Harm can take many forms: physiological, psychological, social, or spiritual. Nonmaleficence refers to both actual harm and the risk of harm. The principle of nonmaleficence helps guide decisions about treatment approaches; the relevant question is "Will this treatment modality cause more harm or more good to the client?" Determining whether technology is harmful to the client is not always a clear-cut decision. Factors to consider include the following:

- The treatment must offer a reasonable prospect of benefit.
- It must not involve excessive expense, pain, or other inconvenience.

Nonmaleficence requires that the nurse act thoughtfully and carefully, weighing the potential risks and benefits of research or treatment. Sometimes it is easier to weigh the risk than to measure the benefit. It is possible to violate this principle without acting maliciously and without ever being aware of the harm.

Nonmaleficence is considered a fundamental duty of health care providers. Both nursing's Nightingale Pledge and medicine's Hippocratic Oath state that providers are to cause no harm to clients. Some clinical examples of nonmaleficence are:

- Preventing medication errors (including drug interactions)
- Being aware of potential risks of treatment modalities
- Removing hazards (e.g., obstructions that might cause a fall)

See the accompanying Spotlight On display on page 203.

When upholding the principle of nonmaleficence, the nurse practices according to professional and legal standards

TABLE 12-3 Overview of Ethical Principles

PRINCIPLE	EXPLANATION
Autonomy	Respect for an individual's right to self-determination; respect for individual liberty
Nonmaleficence	Obligation to do or cause no harm to another
Beneficence	Duty to do good to others and to maintain a balance between benefits and harms
Justice	Equitable distribution of potential benefits and risks
Veracity	Obligation to tell the truth
Fidelity	Duty to do what one has promised

Delmar/Cengage Learning

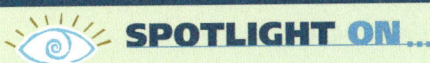

SPOTLIGHT ON...

Ethics

Nonmaleficence

Weighing the potential benefit and harm of treatment approaches is value laden. At what point does pain, inconvenience, or expense become excessive? Who determines excessiveness? Is the result of a therapy that will prolong the client's life a benefit or a burden? Who determines what is an acceptable and what is an unacceptable quality of life?

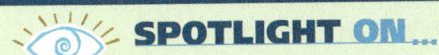

SPOTLIGHT ON...

Ethics

Paternalism

Listen to the messages communicated to clients by health care professionals. What comments can you think of that would be considered paternalistic? Would you consider the following comments to be paternalistic? Why or why not?

- "Just follow the doctor's orders and everything will be OK."
- "We know what's best for you; trust us."
- "This is for your own good."

of care. The question most frequently asked in court of a nurse is "Did you cause any harm?"

Beneficence

Beneficence is the ethical principle that means the duty to promote good and to prevent harm. There are two elements of beneficence:

1. Providing benefit
2. Balancing benefits and harms

One undesirable outcome of beneficence is **paternalism**, an occurrence in which health care providers decide what is "best" for clients and then attempt to coerce (or "encourage") them to act against their own choices. Paternalistic health care providers treat competent adults as if they are children who need protection.

Paternalism is usually not considered an ethical approach. However, in some situations paternalism may be advisable. For example, when prevention of harm overrides the loss of individual freedom and when an individual's ability to choose is limited by incompetency, paternalism may be justified. See the accompanying Spotlight On display.

Justice

The principle of **justice** is based on the concept of fairness. The major health-related issues of justice involve fair treatment of individuals and allocation of resource distribution. Justice considers action from the point of view of the least fortunate in society. As a result of equal and similar treatment of people, benefits and burdens are distributed equally.

The ethical principle of justice requires that all people be treated equally unless there is a justification for unequal treatment. The **material principle of justice** is the rationale for determining when unequal allocation of scarce resources is appropriate. This concept specifies that resources should be allocated:

- Equally
- According to need
- According to individual effort
- According to the individual's merit (ability)
- According to the individual's contribution to society

An application of the material principle of justice is the Department of Veteran Affairs (VA). Individuals who gave to their country by serving in the military are eligible to receive health care through the VA in ambulatory, acute care, and psychiatric facilities.

According to the ANA (2008a), three types of actions are considered to be unjust:

- Discrimination or arbitrary unequal treatment in enforcing policies and rules
- Exploiting (taking unfair advantage of) another
- Making unfair (false or derogatory) remarks about others

In health care institutions, the principle of justice is being strenuously tested on the issue of allocation of one important resource: nursing personnel. Many institutions and agencies are downsizing their professional staff as a cost-containment measure. As a result, some health care facilities are so poorly staffed or have such a high ratio of underqualified personnel providing care that quality care is being sacrificed.

The principles of justice and beneficence often conflict. For example, should federal funds be spent on a costly transplant that will benefit only one Medicaid recipient, or should the funds be spent on less expensive measures that would prevent disease in many (e.g., immunizations)?

Veracity

Veracity means truthfulness, neither lying nor deceiving others. Deception can take many forms: intentional lying, nondisclosure of information, or partial disclosure of information. Veracity often is difficult to achieve. It may not be difficult to tell the truth, but it is not always easy to decide how much truth to tell. See the accompanying Spotlight On display on page 204.

Fidelity

The concept of **fidelity**, which is the ethical foundation of nurse-client relationships, means faithfulness and keeping promises. Clients have an ethical right to expect nurses to act in their best interests. As nurses function in the role of

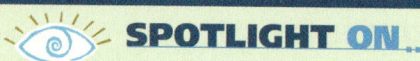

SPOTLIGHT ON...

Ethics

Veracity

Is honesty always the best policy?

Is withholding information the same as lying?

Can you ethically justify withholding information?

Can you ethically justify telling white lies?

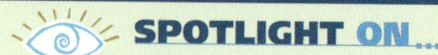

SPOTLIGHT ON...

Legal/Ethical

Client Advocate

A 15-year-old girl visits a family planning clinic because she suspects she is pregnant. Her suspicion is confirmed after an examination. She informs the nurse practitioner that she wants an abortion, and she refuses to tell her parents about the situation. In considering this dilemma, keep in mind that the client is a minor. What are the ethical obligations of the nurse practitioner? Do the ethical obligations coincide or conflict with the legal responsibilities? How would you resolve this conflict?

client advocate (a person who speaks up for or acts on behalf of the client), they are upholding the principle of fidelity. Fidelity is demonstrated when nurses:

- Represent the client's viewpoint to other members of the health care team
- Avoid letting their own personal values influence their advocacy for clients
- Support the client's decision even when it conflicts with the nurse's preferences or choices

See the accompanying Spotlight On display.

VALUES AND ETHICS

The close relationship between ethics and values both illuminates and complicates the nurse's approach toward balancing the principles of health care delivery with those of the client. Nurses need to examine their own value systems in order to determine the best approach in managing the care of clients whose values differ. In order to practice ethically, nurses must understand the impact of their own values. **Values** influence the development of beliefs and attitudes and thus affect behaviors indirectly. Almost nothing in life is value free, even though individuals often fail to consider the impact of values on decisions and resultant behaviors. Values are similar to breathing; one does not think about them until there is a problem.

Nurses often care for clients whose value systems conflict with theirs. Determining what is meaningful to the client is based on an understanding of the client's value system. The nurse's values can become problematic when they conflict with the values of clients.

Values Clarification

Through values clarification, a nurse can increase self-awareness and become better able to care for people with different values. **Values clarification** is the process of analyzing one's own values to better understand what is truly important. In their classic work *Values and Teaching*, Raths, Harmin, and Simon (1978, p. 47) formulated a theory of values clarification and proposed a three-step process of valuing, as follows:

1. *Choosing:* Beliefs are selected freely (that is, without coercion) from among alternatives. The choosing step involves analysis of the consequences of various alternatives.

2. *Prizing:* The beliefs that are selected are cherished (prized).
3. *Acting:* The selected beliefs are demonstrated consistently through behavior.

Nurses must understand that values are individual rather than universal; therefore, nurses should not impose their own values on clients. The provision of ethical nursing care is directly related to one's values. For example, the nurse who strongly values the sanctity of life may experience an ethical conflict when caring for a terminally ill client who refuses treatment that may extend life for a short period of time.

ETHICAL CODES

One hallmark of a profession is the determination of ethical behavior for its members. Several nursing organizations have developed codes as guidelines for ethical conduct. The International Council of Nurses (ICN) first developed its ethical code in 1953 and revised it in 2006. The *ICN Code for Nurses* (ICN, 2006) emphasizes nursing's respect for human rights, including the right to life, the right to dignity, and the right to be treated with respect. The ICN code promotes an environment that respects the values, customs, and spiritual beliefs of the individual.

The ANA (2008a) code for ethical conduct spells out the nurse's obligations to clients and society at large. Some of those obligations include maintaining clients' privacy and safety, improving the standards of nursing care, and assuming responsibility for one's nursing actions. The ethical code, which provides broad principles for determining and evaluating nursing care, is not legally binding for registered nurses. In most states, however, the board of nursing has authority to reprimand nurses for unprofessional conduct that results from violation of the ethical code.

The CNA developed a code of ethics in 1980 and revised it in 2008 (CNA, 2008). The CNA code serves as a guide for professional nurses to assist in working through ethical dilemmas encountered in all practice settings.

CLIENTS' RIGHTS

The concept of rights is often misused, overused, and abused. Society tends to take rights for granted; rights and obligations are culturally defined. The dominant American society has an ethnocentric perspective in believing that its rights and values are shared globally.

Clients have certain rights including, but not limited to, the right to

- Make decisions regarding their care
- Be actively involved in the treatment process
- Be treated with dignity and respect

These rights apply to all clients regardless of the setting for delivery of care. For example, during the initial assessment, the home health nurse discusses these rights with the client. When clients are admitted to short-term acute care agencies or extended care facilities, they are also entitled to certain rights. In 1972, the American Hospital Association (AHA) established A Patient's Bill of Rights, which includes the rights and responsibilities of clients receiving care in hospitals. This document was revised and renamed in 2003 (see Box on next page). The *Patient Care Partnership* (AHA, 2003) increases health care providers' awareness of the need to treat clients in an ethical manner and encourages all health care providers to protect the rights of clients.

ETHICAL DILEMMAS

An **ethical dilemma** occurs when there is a conflict between two or more ethical principles. Ethical dilemmas are situations of conflicting requirements for which there is no right or wrong option. The most beneficial decision depends on the circumstances. Ethical analysis is not an exact science. When an ethical dilemma occurs, the nurse must make a choice between two alternatives that are equally unsatisfactory. In some cases, even after a dilemma seems to have been resolved, questions remain. This ambiguity makes it emotionally painful for the persons involved. The emotional discomfort is often a result of the nurse's trying to second-guess the decision and may lead to such self-messages as "If only I had done this" or "Maybe I should have...." See the accompanying Spotlight On display.

Euthanasia

Most people hope to experience a peaceful gentle death when their "time comes." The word **euthanasia** comes from the Greek word *euthanatos*, which literally means "good, or gentle, death." In current times, euthanasia refers to mercy killing (deliberate ending of life as a humane action). See the accompanying Spotlight On display.

Active euthanasia refers to taking deliberate action that will hasten the client's death. In contrast, **passive euthanasia** means cooperating with the client's dying process. Passive euthanasia is the omission of an action that would prolong life.

Assisted suicide is a form of active euthanasia in which health care professionals provide clients with the means to end their own lives. Recently, physician–assisted suicide has been

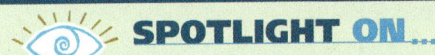

SPOTLIGHT ON...

Ethics

Ethical Conflicts

As a nurse, you will often be caught in a dilemma involving what you ought to do (on the basis of one ethical principle) and what you ought not to do (on the basis of another principle). For example, should you tell a client who has been diagnosed as having breast cancer the complete truth about the diagnosis, or should you soft-pedal the bad news because it might result in loss of hope? The dilemma is a conflict between the principles of veracity and nonmaleficence. Also, the principle of autonomy is involved. Not telling violates autonomy by denying the client the right to make an informed choice.

the topic of much controversy. In 1997, the U.S. Supreme Court decided that there was no constitutionally protected right to physician–assisted suicide for clients who are terminally ill.

Nurses have differing opinions regarding assisted suicide. Some view it as a violation of the ethical principles upon which the practice of nursing is based: autonomy, nonmaleficence, beneficence, justice, veracity, and fidelity. Other nurses view assisted suicide as a humane act. Regardless of a nurse's personal viewpoint, assisted suicide is still illegal except in Oregon, the only state that has designated assisted suicide as a legal action. Other nurses may see assisted suicide as an ethical dilemma; they agree that it violates some ethical principles but question whether it violates others. For example, does assisted suicide violate the principle of autonomy? From one standpoint, it is *refusal* to assist a suicide that violates a client's autonomy. In its *Position Statement: Active Euthanasia,* the ANA (1994) states that participation in active euthanasia violates nursing's ethical code.

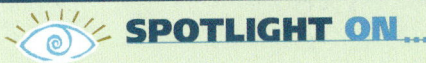

SPOTLIGHT ON...

Ethics

Ethical Debate: Euthanasia

What does the phrase "good death" mean to you? For some people, it means:

Dying with dignity

Being pain-free

Dying in the company of loved ones and friends

To others, dying a good death means:

Being at home

Determining when death will occur (maintaining control)

AMERICAN HOSPITAL ASSOCIATION PATIENT CARE PARTNERSHIP

THE PATIENT CARE PARTNERSHIP: UNDERSTANDING EXPECTATIONS, RIGHTS AND RESPONSIBILITIES

When you need hospital care, your doctor and the nurses and other professionals at our hospital are committed to working with you and your family to meet your health care needs. Our dedicated doctors and staff serve the community in all its ethnic, religious and economic diversity. Our goal is for you and your family to have the same care and attention we would want for our families and ourselves.

The sections explain some of the basics about how you can expect to be treated during your hospital stay. They also cover what we will need from you to care for you better. If you have questions at any time, please ask them. Unasked or unanswered questions can add to the stress of being in the hospital. Your comfort and confidence in your care are very important to us.

WHAT TO EXPECT DURING YOUR HOSPITAL STAY

High-quality hospital care. Our first priority is to provide you the care you need, when you need it, with skill, compassion, and respect. Tell your caregivers if you have concerns about your care or if you have pain. You have the right to know the identity of doctors, nurses and others involved in your care, and you have the right to know when they are students, residents or other trainees.

A clean and safe environment. Our hospital works hard to keep you safe. We use special policies and procedures to avoid mistakes in your care and keep you free from abuse or neglect. If anything unexpected and significant happens during your hospital stay, you will be told what happened, and any resulting changes in your care will be discussed with you.

Involvement in your care. You and your doctor often make decisions about your care before you go to the hospital. Other times, especially in emergencies, those decisions are made during your hospital stay. When decision-making takes place, it should include:

- *Discussing your medical condition and information about medically appropriate treatment choices.* To make informed decisions with your doctor, you need to understand:
  — The benefits and risks of each treatment.
  — Whether your treatment is experimental or part of a research study.
  — What you can reasonably expect from your treatment and any long-term effects it might have on your quality of life.
  — What you and your family will need to do after you leave the hospital.
  — The financial consequences of using uncovered services or out-of-network providers. Please tell your caregivers if you need more information about treatment choices.
- *Discussing your treatment plan.* When you enter the hospital, you sign a general consent to treatment. In some cases, such as surgery or experimental treatment, you may be asked to confirm in writing that you understand what is planned and agree to it. This process protects your right to consent to or refuse a treatment. Your doctor will explain the medical consequences of refusing recommended treatment. It also protects your right to decide if you want to participate in a research study.
- *Getting information from you.* Your caregivers need complete and correct information about your health and coverage so that they can make good decisions about your care. That includes:
  — Past illnesses, surgeries or hospital stays.
  — Past allergic reactions.
  — Any medicines or dietary supplements (such as vitamins and herbs) that you are taking.
  — Any network or admission requirements under your health plan.
- *Understanding your health care goals and values.* You may have health care goals and values or spiritual beliefs that are important to your well-being. They will be taken into account as much as possible throughout your hospital stay. Make sure your doctor, your family and your care team know your wishes.
- *Understanding who should make decisions when you cannot.* If you have signed a health care power of attorney stating who should speak for you if you become unable to make health care decisions for yourself, or a "living will" or "advance directive" that states your wishes about end-of-life care; give copies to your doctor, your family and your care team. If you or your family need help making difficult decisions, counselors, chaplains and others are available to help.

(Continues)

(Continued)

Protection of your privacy. We respect the confidentiality of your relationship with your doctor and other caregivers, and the sensitive information about your health and health care that are part of that relationship. State and federal laws and hospital operating policies protect the privacy of your medical information. You will receive a Notice of Privacy Practices that describes the ways that we use, disclose and safeguard patient information and that explains how you can obtain a copy of information from our records about your care.

Preparing you and your family for when you leave the hospital. Your doctor works with hospital staff and professionals in your community. You and your family also play an important role in your care. The success of your treatment often depends on your efforts to follow medication, diet and therapy plans. Your family may need to help care for you at home.

You can expect us to help you identify sources of follow-up care and to let you know if our hospital has a financial interest in any referrals. As long as you agree that we can share information about your care with them, we will coordinate our activities with your caregivers outside the hospital. You can also expect to receive information and, where possible, training about the self-care you will need when you go home.

Help with your bill and filing insurance claims. Our staff will file claims for you with health care insurers or other programs such as Medicare and Medicaid. They also will help your doctor with needed documentation. Hospital bills and insurance coverage are often confusing. If you have questions about your bill, contact our business office. If you need help understanding your insurance coverage or health plan, start with your insurance company or health benefits manager. If you do not have health coverage, we will try to help you and your family find financial help or make other arrangements. We need your help with collecting needed information and other requirements to obtain coverage or assistance.

While you are here, you will receive more detailed notices about some of the rights you have as a hospital patient and how to exercise them. We are always interested in improving. If you have questions, comments, or concerns, please contact_____.

Reprinted with permission of the American Hospital Association, copyright 2003. All rights reserved.

Refusal of Treatment

The client's right to refuse treatment is based on the principle of autonomy. In fairness, the client can refuse only after the treatment methods and their consequences have been explained. A client's right to refuse treatment and the right to die challenge the values of most health care providers.

Consider the use of ventilators. Medical technology makes it possible for clients to continue breathing as long as they are connected to a machine; without the machine, these clients would die. But what are the costs—emotional, physical, psychological, and fiscal? And what is the quality of a life prolonged by technology?

Use of Scarce Resources

With the current emphasis on containing health care costs, the use of expensive services is being examined closely. The use of specialists, organ transplants, and distribution of services is being influenced by social and political forces. For example, the length of stay in a hospital and the number of office visits allowable for individual clients are already predetermined by many third-party payers. In addition to economics, the availability of goods (such as organs) is contributing to a scarcity of resources. In many situations, clients experience extended waiting periods before receiving a donated organ. The allocation of scarce resources is emerging as a major ethical dilemma in today's health care environment.

As a result of technological advances and the aging of the population, there is an increased demand for health care services. There is a critical need for decisions regarding the fair and equitable use of health care services in the United States. See the accompanying Spotlight On display.

ETHICAL ROLES AND RESPONSIBILITIES OF PROFESSIONAL NURSES

As professionals, nurses are accountable for protecting the rights and interests of the client. Consequently, sound nursing practice involves making ethical decisions. Ethics affects

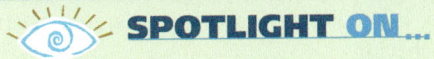

SPOTLIGHT ON...

Ethics

Allocation of Scarce Resources

The following two people are in desperate need of a liver transplant:

A 62-year-old alcoholic who is destitute and has no family

A 24-year-old mother of three young children

One liver is available. In your opinion, who should get the liver? What influenced your decision?

nurses in every health care setting, and each practice setting presents the nurse with its own set of ethical concerns. For example, consider home health nursing. With the increased acuity level of clients cared for in the home setting, home health nurses face ever-increasing ethical challenges of continuing to provide quality care under federally mandated cost-containment initiatives.

Whatever the setting, nurses need to balance their ethical responsibilities to each client with their professional obligations. Often there is an inherent conflict. The Nursing Checklist provides guidelines for promoting ethical care.

Ethics Committees

The provision of ethical health care requires self-examination of the care provider and the opportunity for dialogue with other health care providers. Many health care agencies now recognize the need for a systematic approach for discussing ethical concerns. Formation of multidisciplinary committees, referred to as institutional ethics committees, is one approach for facilitating dialogue regarding ethical dilemmas. In addition to serving as a forum where ethical issues are discussed, ethics committees can lead to the establishment of policies and procedures for prevention and resolution of dilemmas.

Client Advocacy

When acting as a client advocate, the nurse's first step is to develop a meaningful relationship with the client. The primary ethical responsibility is to protect clients' rights to make their own decisions. The nurse who functions as a client advocate is adhering to the ANA code of ethics. Specific examples of advocacy behaviors include empowerment of clients through education, providing support, actively listening to clients' concerns, and acting as a liaison between clients and other health care providers.

Whistle-Blowing

The term **whistle-blowing** refers to calling attention to unethical, illegal, or incompetent actions of others. This behavior is based on the ethical principles of veracity and nonmaleficence. Even though nurses are expected to "blow the whistle" on incompetent health care providers, many are reluctant to do so. Why? Because there are inherent risks in whistle-blowing behavior.

Federal law and state laws (to varying degrees) provide protection to whistle-blowers. The federal government encourages whistle-blowers to report Medicare and Medicaid fraud (Centers for Medicare and Medicaid Services, 2003). Unfortunately, however, the inclination to protect one's coworkers and fear of reprisal may deter a nurse from fulfilling the ethical obligation to report substandard behaviors. See the accompanying Spotlight On display on page 209.

ETHICAL DECISION MAKING

Nurses must understand the rationale for their decisions. **Ethical reasoning** is the process of thinking through what one ought to do in an orderly, systematic manner to provide justification of actions based on principles. Ethical decisions cannot be based entirely on intuition or emotions. Ethical decision making is used in situations in which the right decision is not clear or in which there are conflicts of rights and duties. A framework for resolving ethical dilemmas follows.

Framework for Ethical Decision Making

Once an ethical dilemma is identified, the nurse must determine the relevant parts of the conflict in order to resolve it. When making an ethical decision, the nurse must consider the following relevant parts:

- Which theories are involved?
- Which principles are involved?
- Who will be affected?
- What will be the consequences of the alternatives (ethical options)?

To resolve ethical dilemmas, the nurse must be able to make decisions in a systematic fashion. Figure 12-4 illustrates a method for making ethical judgments that uses steps similar to those of the nursing process.

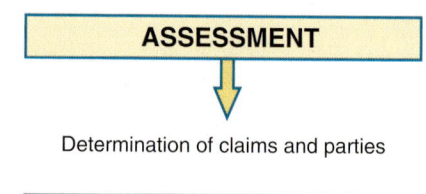

ASSESSMENT

Determination of claims and parties

ANALYSIS AND DIAGNOSIS

Problem identification: Statement of the ethical dilemma

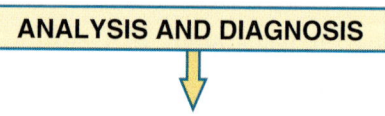

PLANNING

Consideration of priorities of claims;
Generation of alternatives for resolving the dilemma;
Consideration of the consequences of alternatives

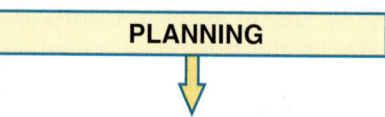

IMPLEMENTATION

Carrying out selected actions

EVALUATION

Assessing the outcome of actions;
"Were the actions ethical?"
"What were the consequences?"

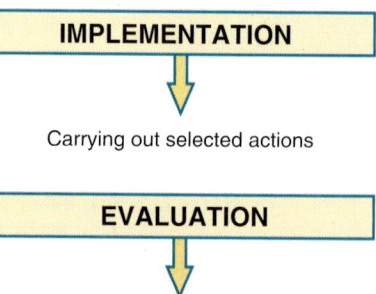

FIGURE 12-4 **Ethical Decision-Making Model** DELMAR/CENGAGE LEARNING

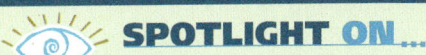

NURSINGCHECKLIST

Providing Ethical Care

- Initiate dialogue concerning the client's wishes. Do more listening than talking. (For example, the following is a question you might ask to help determine the client's wishes: "If your heart stopped, would you want us to try to start it again?")
- Assess the client's understanding of the illness and available treatment options.
- Allow time for the client to explore values and to communicate.
- Facilitate communication of the client's desires to family and other health care providers.

SPOTLIGHT ON...

Ethics

Whistle-Blowing

A coworker often takes Tylenol from a client's medication drawer. When you confront her about the behavior, she states: "It's only Tylenol. Besides, the client's not taking it anymore anyway." Should you blow the whistle? Why or why not? Would your response be different if your coworker were taking narcotics from the client?

The first step of ethical analysis is to gather relevant data in order to identify the problem. Determine what type of ethical problem exists: Do principles conflict with principles? Do actions conflict with actions? Do actions conflict with principles?

Next, consider all the people involved. What are their rights, responsibilities, duties, and decision-making abilities? Who is the most appropriate person to make the decision? It is important to identify several possible alternatives and predict the outcome of each. Then, and only then, select a course of action that ends in resolution of the problem. The final step of ethical decision making is evaluation of the resolution process.

KEY CONCEPTS

- Laws define and limit relationships among individuals and the government.
- The three sources of public law at the federal and state levels are constitutional law, administrative law, and criminal law.
- Administrative law empowers state boards of nursing to protect the public by regulating the scope of nursing practice.
- The three sources of civil law at the federal and state levels are contract law, tort law, and protective and reporting laws.
- A nurse employed by a health care facility is legally responsible for the terms of an implied contract.
- The two types of tort law at the state level are unintentional torts, which include negligence and malpractice, and intentional torts, which include assault and battery, false imprisonment, invasion of privacy, defamation, and fraud.
- Protective and reporting laws, such as the ADA and Good Samaritan acts, protect a designated group of individuals.
- The legal responsibilities of the nurse, defined in practice acts and standards of care, include elements such as providing services to clients and acting as expert witnesses in malpractice suits.

- Incident reports are filed by the nurse when a situation arises that might or did cause client harm.
- To prevent incurring liability due to the policy of floating, nurses should set priorities, identify potential areas of harm to the client, and receive orientation and cross-training before reassignment.
- Legal instruments such as informed consent and advance directives uphold the right of all people to control decisions relating to their own health care.
- Nurses may witness the signing of a consent form by a client as permitted by institutional policies; however, if the nurse discovers circumstances that render a signed consent form invalid, the nurse should notify the prescribing practitioner and, if necessary, the nurse manager.
- In terms of specific client care issues such as abortion, pronouncement of death, DNR orders, euthanasia, care of the deceased, wills, organ donation, and autopsies, nurses must know and comply with the existing laws and regulations that pertain to these areas in their individual states and provinces of licensure.
- Ethics is the study of the rightness of conduct.
- Ethics examines human behavior—what people do under what circumstances.

- Morality is not the same as ethics. Morality is behavior in accordance with custom or tradition and usually reflects personal or religious beliefs.

- There is a connection between acts that are legal and acts that are ethical. Professional nursing actions are both legal and ethical.

- Teleology is an ethical theory that states that the moral nature of a situation is determined by its consequences.

- Deontology is an ethical theory that considers the intrinsic moral significance of the act itself as the criterion for determination of good.

- Ethical decisions are based on the principles of autonomy, nonmaleficence, beneficence, justice, veracity, and fidelity.

- Nurses need to explore their own values in order to acknowledge the sometimes different value systems of clients.

- Values clarification is a process through which nurses can gain knowledge of their values and apply that understanding to the care of clients.

- Ethical codes that have been developed by nursing organizations such as the ICN, the ANA, and the CNA establish guidelines for the ethical conduct of nurses.

- The AHA's *Patient Care Partnership* is designed to guarantee ethical care of clients in terms of health care decision making.

- Nurses must apply the process of ethical reasoning to resolve ethical dilemmas in which conflict exists between principles and duties.

- The framework for ethical decision making consists of five steps: assessment, analysis and diagnosis, planning, implementation, and evaluation.

- The roles of client advocate and whistle-blower enable nurses to protect their clients' rights and ensure the ethical and competent actions of their peers within the nursing profession.

REVIEW QUESTIONS

1. Which of the following is based on the teleological theory of ethics?
   a. Dialysis for clients with end-stage renal disease (ESRD)
   b. Immunizations for all preschool children
   c. Parenting classes in outpatient prenatal clinics
   d. Protection of health care workers

2. A nurse tells a client, "You must take the medication. If you don't swallow it, I'll have to give you an injection." Which of the following best describes this nurse's illegal act?
   a. Assault
   b. Battery
   c. False imprisonment
   d. HIPAA violation

3. Which of the following statements best describes professional liability insurance for a registered nurse?
   a. Advanced practice registered nurses are the only nurses who need to purchase professional liability insurance.
   b. Each nurse should purchase professional liability insurance.
   c. Nurses are protected by their employer's insurance.
   d. Nurses will be represented by the employer's attorney.

4. A nurse is preparing a client for a surgical procedure. Which of the following should the nurse do if there is no surgical consent form signed by the client?

   a. Explain the procedure and its risks to the client and have the client sign the consent form.
   b. Notify the surgeon of the client's need for informed consent.
   c. Send the client to surgery with a notation that the consent form is unsigned.
   d. Tell the client that the form must be signed prior to surgery.

5. A nurse who usually works on a medical-surgical unit with adult clients is reassigned ("floated") to the pediatric unit. Which of the following accurately describes the nurse's legal obligations?
   a. File a grievance against the hospital for changing the assignment.
   b. Participate in orientation to the new unit.
   c. Refuse to work in another specialty area.
   d. Work on the newly assigned unit and follow the actions of the other nurses there.

6. A nurse thinks that too much medication has been ordered for a client due to the client's weight. Which of the following actions should the nurse take?
   a. Administer a smaller dose of medication to the client.
   b. Ask the nursing supervisor what should be done.
   c. Contact the prescriber and clarify the order.
   d. Give the medication as ordered by the prescriber.

7. Which of the following nursing actions is based on the ethical principle of autonomy?

a. Removing a throw rug from the client's bedside
b. Respecting a client's refusal of treatment
c. Telling a client the truth about a negative diagnosis
d. Using a paternalistic approach when answering client questions

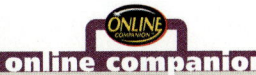

online companion

Visit the DeLaune and Ladner online companion resource at **www.delmar.cengage.com** for additional content and study aids. Click on Online Companions, then select the Nursing discipline.

8. The allocation of scarce resources involves which of the following ethical principles?
   a. Autonomy
   b. Beneficence
   c. Fidelity
   d. Justice

Much more precise might be our observation even than this and much more correct our conclusions.

—Nightingale (in Skretkowicz, 1992)

CHAPTER 13

Documentation and Informatics

COMPETENCIES

1. Describe the role of information in nursing.
2. Discuss the use of information technology in promoting client safety.
3. Explain the purposes of documentation in health care.
4. Identify the HIPAA requirements related to security and privacy.
5. Discuss the principles of effective documentation.
6. Describe various methods of documentation.
7. Describe various types of documentation records.
8. Explain how to verify verbal orders.
9. Identify the entry-level informatics competencies for a nurse.
10. Describe the ways that computers and informatics support evidence-based practice and the research process.

KEY TERMS

advance directive	focus charting	problem, intervention, evaluation
case management	incident reports	(PIE)
charting by exception (CBE)	informatics	problem-oriented medical record
communication	information literacy	(POMR)
computer literacy	information technology	SOAP
critical pathway	informed consent	source-oriented (SO) charting
documentation	Kardex	variations
durable power of attorney	narrative charting	
E-prescribing	nursing informatics	

Throughout the development of modern nursing, a variety of documentation systems have emerged in response to changes inherent in health care delivery. Changes in consumer and legal expectations, federal and state regulations, accreditation standards, and research findings direct provider accountability for the documentation of services. Systems of recording and reporting data pertinent to the care of clients have evolved primarily in response to the demand for health care practitioners to be held accountable to societal norms, professional standards of practice, legal and regulatory standards, and institutional policies and standards.

As with all facets of health care, advanced technology has affected the expectations for documentation. Benchmarking activities in quality improvement and cost containment have also increased the demands on prescribing practitioners to create efficient documentation systems. Efficiency is measured in terms of time, thoroughness, and the quality of the observations being recorded. The documentation systems in use today reflect the specific needs and preferences of the numerous health care agencies.

Since client safety is the major standard that directs nursing care, the ability to communicate information clearly, accurately, and promptly is vital to providing the safest care possible. In the changing world of health care and economics, the profession of nursing, like all other disciplines, is being challenged to decrease waste and reduce cost. Within the infrastructure of nursing informatics is an emerging system that fosters improvement in efficiency, safety, and quality client care.

INFORMATICS

In order to understand one method of documentation, computerized documentation, nurses need to be familiar with informatics. **Informatics** is a science of turning data into information. According to Hebda and Czar (2009), the broad definition of **nursing informatics** (NI) is the use of information and computer technology to support all aspects of nursing practice, including direct delivery of care, administration, education, and research.

The American Nurses Association (ANA) first defined the role of the informatics nurse specialist in 1992. The ANA revised its definition in 1994, 2001, and 2007 to define the evolving scope of practice:

Nursing informatics is a specialty that integrates nursing science, computer science, and information science to manage and communicate data, information, knowledge and wisdom into nursing practice. Nursing informatics facilitates the integration of data, information, knowledge and wisdom to support patients, nurses, and other providers in their decision making in all roles and settings. This support is accomplished through the use of information structures, information processes, and information technology. (ANA 2007, p. 1)

Computer literacy refers to a familiarity with the use of personal computers, including the use of software tools such as word processing, spreadsheets, databases, presentation graphics, and e-mail (Hebda & Czar, 2009). **Information literacy** is the ability to recognize when information is needed as well as the skills to find, evaluate, and use needed information effectively (Association of College and Research Libraries, 2008). **Information technology** (IT) refers to the management and processing of information with the assistance of computers (Hebda & Czar, 2009). This technology has allowed organizations to develop management information systems such as a hospital information system (HIS) that focus on the types of data needed to manage client activities. An information system refers to the use of computer hardware and software to process data into information to solve a problem.

There are two basic types of HISs: clinical information systems (CISs) and administrative information systems. CISs are large computerized database management systems with subsystems such as order entry, admission, result retrieval admissions (e.g., laboratory, pharmacy, and radiology), and documentation that support and enhance health care. Administrative information systems manage financial and demographic information and provide reporting capabilities to support client care.

CLINICAL INFORMATION SYSTEMS

The main purpose of CISs is to allow health care providers and researchers to gain quick and safe access to information, order appropriate medications and treatments, and implement cost-effective, evidence-based care without duplicating services. For example, the nurse documents client allergies in the initial assessment; these data are then accessible to all health care providers, such as the prescribing practitioner and the pharmacist. The tools or subsystems of this clinical system include electronic health records, clinical decision support systems, and bedside medication administration using positive client identification, computerized prescribing practitioner order entry, client surveillance, and clinical data warehouses (Hebda & Czar, 2009).

Computerized physician (provider or prescriber) order entry (CPOE) is the process by which the prescribing practitioner directly enters orders for client care into an HIS. Information is drawn from several systems, such as pharmacy and laboratory systems, with drug databases to warn the prescriber of potential problems with dosages, drug interactions, allergies, and contraindications.

E-prescribing refers to the electronic transmission of drug prescriptions to a pharmacy from a hospital-based inpatient ordering system (CPOE), personal digital assistants, wireless computers, or other handheld devices. This system reduces error regarding illegible handwriting; it also incorporates lists of client allergies and other medications the client is taking.

Positive client identification is accomplished through the use of barcodes or radio frequency identification (RFID). Barcodes are the dominant technology in use to reduce identification errors. In 2004 the Food and Drug Administration required barcodes on most prescription and some over-the-counter medications to decrease medication errors. The barcode system requires scanning of the nurse's identification, the client's identification bracelet, and all prescription medications during the medication administration process. Once scanned into the computer, the information is processed and confirms the right client, drug, and dosage. RFID technology produces data when stimulated by radio frequency energy; it is a costly system and is not as widely used as barcoding.

Decision-support software (DSS) refers to a computer application that analyzes data, such as laboratory values or standards of care, and presents it in a fashion that facilitates decision making. For example, DSS guides the triage nurse through a series of observations, questions, interventions, and safety alerts when a client presents with a specific complaint.

ELECTRONIC HEALTH RECORD

Client safety, accessibility to health information, and economics are the driving forces of the government, professional organizations, and accrediting bodies toward the development and implementation of the electronic health record (EHR). The Bush administration called for the adoption of the EHR by 2014 to help transform health care in the United States. The traditional paper medical record is episode oriented, with a separate record for each client visit to a health care agency (Hebda & Czar, 2009). Critical information, such as client allergies, may be lost from one episode of care to the next, jeopardizing client safety.

The EHR is a longitudinal electronic record of client health information generated by one or more encounters in any health care setting (Healthcare Information and Management Systems Society [HIMSS], 2008). Because the EHR system stores the complete record of every clinical encounter, health care providers can access clinical data to identify quality issues, link interventions with positive outcomes, and make evidence-based decisions. The EHR also provides interactive client access and allows the client to append information.

The HIMSS (2008) developed a definitional model for EHR with these attributes:

- Provides secure, reliable, real-time access to client health record information where and when it is needed to support care
- Records and manages episodic and longitudinal EHR information
- Functions as clinicians' primary information resource during the provision of client care
- Assists with the work of planning and delivery of evidence-based care to individuals and groups of clients
- Captures data used for continuous quality improvement, utilization review, risk management, resource planning, and performance management
- Captures the client health-related information needed for medical records and reimbursement
- Provides longitudinal, appropriately masked information to support clinical research, public health reporting, and population health initiatives
- Supports clinical trials and evidence-based research

The development of the EHR relies on an operational electronic medical record and a national health information network. The Department of Health and Human Services formed the EHR collaborative with professional organizations in 2003 to facilitate rapid input from the health care community to support the adoption of standards for the EHR. Hebda and Czar (2009) cite the benefits of the EHR for nursing: It facilitates comparison of data from different health care encounters, maintains an ongoing record of a client's education and learning in all encounters, eliminates the need for repetitive demographic data, ensures administration and documentation of medications and treatments, facilitates research, automates critical and clinical pathways, and allows recognition of nursing work in measurable units when used with a common unified structure for nursing language. During the last decade, the use of EHRs has become more widespread, from large academic medical centers to community-based acute care and outpatient facilities (Kossman & Scheidenhelm, 2008).

NURSING INFORMATION SYSTEMS

A nursing information system is a subsystem of CISs, supports the use and documentation of nursing processes and interventions, and provides tools for managing the delivery of nursing care. The system should provide access to the information nurses need: client medical records, test results, progress notes, hospital policy and procedures, and tools for online literature searches such as the Cumulative Index of Nursing and Allied Health Literature (CINAHL), Medline, and automated drug information.

Nursing information systems have two basic approaches to nursing care and documentation: the nursing process and critical pathways or protocols. The traditional nursing process approach uses established formats such as admission and postoperative assessments, problem lists, care plans, discharge planning instructions, and intervention lists. A more organized version incorporates standardized nursing languages such as the North American Nursing Diagnoses Association (NANDA), Nursing Interventions Classification (NIC), and Nursing Outcomes Classification (NOC).

The nursing process approach uses traditional paper forms for automated documentation. The documentation of nursing and admission assessment and discharge instructions relies on a menu-driven approach to obtain essential information. A menu list with related commands directs the nurse through assessment, such as a client's past medical history, advance directives, psychosocial history, and review of systems. Once the assessment data are entered into a computer, a program will offer menu lists for the nurse to select appropriate nursing diagnoses and interventions for an individualized care plan and discharge instructions. The program will generate printed copies of discharge instructions, medication information, and follow-up appointments for nurses to review with clients on discharge.

The nursing process approach also includes system formats for the following:

- Generating a nursing work list that directs routine scheduled activities related to client care
- Documenting discrete data or activities such as vital signs, weight, and intake and output measurements
- Documenting routine client care activities such as bathing, positioning, blood glucose measurement, dietary intake, and/or wound care in a flow sheet format
- Documenting nursing care in progress notes using one of the following charting formats: narrative, charting by exception, or flow sheet
- Documenting medication administration

These systems require acceptance of the nursing process by each nurse and sufficient technical equipment to provide for nurse documentation.

The second design is based on evidenced-based clinical protocols or critical pathways, often used in a multidisciplinary manner, with many types of care providers accessing the system for information and to document care. This system allows for the selection of one or more appropriate critical pathways for a client. Standard prescribing practitioner order sets can be included with each critical pathway and may be automatically processed by the system. The system identifies variances of the anticipated outcomes when charted and provides aggregate variance data for analysis by the care provider.

Hakes and Whittington (2008) measured nurse documentation time before and after the implementation of an electronic medical record and found that there was no difference in documentation time between the preelectronic medical

record and the postelectronic medical record. Although there are an insufficient number of studies that show the impact of computerized record systems on nursing practice and client outcomes, there is an increase of computers in health care settings. Anecdotal reports and descriptive studies suggest that computerized documentation enhances the systematic approach to client care through standardized protocols, teaching documents, data management, and communication.

DOCUMENTATION AS COMMUNICATION

Communication is a dynamic, continuous, and multidimensional process for sharing information as determined by standards or policies. Reporting and recording are the major communication techniques used by health care providers to direct client-based decision making and continuity of care. The medical record serves as a legal document for recording all client activities assessed and initiated by health care practitoners.

DOCUMENTATION DEFINED

Documentation is defined as written (paper and pen or electronic) evidence of:

1. The interactions between and among health professionals, clients, their families, and health care organizations
2. The administration of tests, procedures, treatments, and client education
3. The results or client response to these diagnostic tests and interventions

Documentation provides written records that reflect client care provided on the basis of assessment data and the client's response to interventions.

Nurses rely on documentation tools, including computerized systems, that support the implementation of the nursing process. These tools are the charting records and systems that facilitate a logical sequencing of events. All the tools used by nurses to record their nursing care should form a system. Systematic documentation is critical because it presents the care administered by nurses in a logical fashion, as follows:

1. Assessment data (obtained by interviewing, observing, and inspecting) identify the client's specific alterations and provide the foundation of the nursing care plan.
2. The risk factors and the identified alteration in the functional health pattern direct the formulation of a nursing diagnosis.
3. Identifying the nursing diagnosis promotes the development of the client's short-term goals, long-term goals, and expected outcomes and also triggers the nursing interventions. These activities occur during the planning and implementation phases of the nursing process.

4. The plan of care identifies the nursing interventions necessary to resolve the nursing diagnosis.

5. Implementation is evidenced by actions the nurse performed to assist the client in achieving the expected outcomes.

The effectiveness of the nursing interventions in achieving the client's expected outcomes becomes the criterion for evaluation that determines the need for subsequent reassessment and revision of the plan of care.

The system becomes a vehicle for expressing each phase of the nursing process. Nurses rely on systems that provide thorough, accurate charting reflective of the nurse's decision-making ability and the client's plan of care. The nurse's critical thinking skills, judgments, and evaluation must be clearly communicated through proper documentation.

PURPOSES OF HEALTH CARE DOCUMENTATION

Professional responsibility, accountability, and client safety are the primary reasons why practitioners document. Other reasons to document include communication, education, research, meeting legal and practice standards, and reimbursement. Documentation provides written evidence of the nurse's accountability to the client, the institution, the profession, and society. See the accompanying Nursing Checklist display.

Communication

Recording is a method of communication that validates the care provided to the client. It should clearly communicate all important information regarding the client. Thorough documentation provides:

- Accurate data needed to plan the client's care in order to ensure the continuity of care
- A method of communication among the health care team members responsible for the client's care
- Written evidence of what was done for the client, the client's response, and any revisions made in the plan of care
- Compliance with professional practice standards (e.g., the ANA)
- Compliance with accreditation criteria (e.g., the Joint Commission)
- Compliance with the Health Insurance Portability and Accountability Act (HIPAA)
- A resource for review, audit, reimbursement, education, and research
- A written legal record to protect the client, institution, and practitioner

The client's medical record contains documents for record keeping. The type of document that constitutes the medical record is determined by the health care institution. References will be made to the various types of medical record documents throughout this chapter; refer to Table 13-1 on page 218 for an explanation of these documents. These medical record documents are either on paper or contained within a computerized system.

Education

The documentation contained within the client's medical record can be used for the purpose of education. Health care students use the medical record as a tool to learn about disease processes, complications, medical and nursing diagnoses, and interventions. The results of physical examination and laboratory and diagnostic testing provide valuable information regarding specific diagnoses and interventions.

Nursing students can enhance their critical thinking skills by examining the records in chronological order, analyzing the results, and following the health care team's plan of care (e.g., how it was developed, implemented, and evaluated). Students and all health care professionals need to be aware of confidentiality issues before reading any client's chart; these are discussed later in the chapter.

Clinical rounds and case conferences, which rely heavily on information contained in the medical record, have also proved to be effective teaching tools. These learning experiences usually involve several disciplines that contribute to the review and discussion of client outcomes.

Student nurses need to learn the "flow" of documenting clinical data according to institutional policy in a legible, descriptive, and time-sequenced fashion. A good way to learn this flow is to review the client's condition as presented in the chart before hearing the report. The data obtained from chart review should direct the assessment of signs and symptoms on rounds.

Research

Researchers rely heavily on clients' medical records as a clinical data source to determine if clients meet the research criteria of a study. Researchers use computers to expedite collection and

---

✓ NURSINGCHECKLIST

REVIEWING A CHART

- Can the assessment data that triggered the nursing diagnosis be identified?
- When the defining characteristics of a specific nursing diagnosis are compared to the client's presenting signs and symptoms, is there supporting evidence?
- Were critical questions asked during the client interview?
- Did the nurse use the data obtained from both the interview and physical assessment in establishing the diagnoses?
- Can any assumptions that might have misled the nurse's judgment be identified?
- Are the nursing data correlated with the results of the physical examination and findings from diagnostic tests?
- Are the expected outcomes realistic?

TABLE 13-1 Medical Record Documents

DOCUMENT	INFORMATION
Face sheet	Biographical data: name, date of birth, address, phone number, Social Security number, marital status, employment, race, gender, religion, closest relative; insurance coverage; allergies; attending prescribing practitioner; admitting medical diagnosis; assigned diagnosis-related group; statement of whether the client has an advance directive.
Consent form	*Admit:* Gives the institution and prescribing practitioner the right to treat. *Surgery:* Explains the reason for the operation in lay terms, the risks for complications, and the client's level of understanding. *Blood transfusion:* Permission to administer blood or blood products.
Medical history and physical examination	Results of the client's initial history and physical assessment as performed by the health care provider.
Prescriber order sheet	Medical orders to admit and the treatment plan.
Progress notes	Evaluation of the client's response to treatment; may contain the progress recording of interdisciplinary practitioners (e.g., dietary or social services).
Consultation sheet	Initiated by the prescribing practitioner to request the evaluation or services of other practitioners.
Diagnostic results	The results from laboratory and diagnostic tests (e.g., x-ray, hematology).
Nursing admit assessment	Recording of data obtained from the interview and physical assessment conducted by the RN.
Nursing plan of care	Contains the treatment plan (e.g., nursing diagnosis or a problem list, initiation of standards of care, or protocols).
Graphic sheet	Data recording regarding vital signs and weight.
Flow sheet	Contains all routine interventions that can be noted with a check mark or other simple code; allows for a quick comparison of measurement.
Nurses' progress notes	Additional data that do not duplicate information on the flow sheet (e.g., client's achievement of expected outcome or revision of the plan of care).
Medication administration record (MAR)	Contains all medication information for routine and prn drugs: date, time, dose, route, site (for injections).
Client education record	Recording of nurses' teaching of clients, families, and other caregivers and the learners' responses.
Health care team record	Treatment and progress record for nonmedical and nonnursing practitioners, when the prescribing practitioner's progress notes are not used by other practitioners (e.g., respiratory, physical therapy, dietary).
Clinical pathway	A multidisciplinary form for each day of anticipated hospitalization that identifies the interventions and achievement of client outcomes; the practitioner's initial implementation and variances from the norm are explained in the progress notes.
Discharge plan and summary	A multidisciplinary form used before discharge from a health care facility containing a brief summary of care rendered and discharge instructions (e.g., food-drug interactions, referrals, follow-up appointments).
Advance directive or living will	Federal law requires that health care providers discuss with clients the use of advance directives (e.g., the living will and the durable power of attorney). Most states recognize the living will as a legal document. If the client has advance directives, they are reviewed at the time of admission and placed in the medical record.

Delmar/Cengage Learning

analysis of data. Mobile devices such as notebook computers at the study site can transmit data to another computer for compilation and analysis. Documentation also can validate the need for research. For example, if documentation demonstrates an increased infection rate with intravenous catheters, researchers can identify and study the nursing intervention variables that may be associated with the increased infection rate.

Legal and Practice Standards

The client's medical record is a legal document, and in the case of a lawsuit, the record serves as the description of exactly what happened to a client. The legal issues of documentation require:

- Legible and neat writing for paper records
- Proper use of spelling and grammar
- Use of authorized abbreviations
- Factual and time-sequenced descriptive notations

These elements of effective documentation are discussed later in this chapter.

Nurses are responsible for the care the client receives and can be held liable if appropriate interventions are not implemented in a timely manner when information is available that would dictate otherwise. The nurse is responsible for documenting on the chart when a "prescribing practitioner was notified" along with what significant information was orally communicated. If the nurse does not get a response from the prescribing practitioner that recognizes the urgency of the information, the nurse must document the prescribing practitioner's response and notify the supervisor of the situation.

DeMilliano (2009) and the Nurses Service Organization, which is a medical malpractice, professional liability, and risk management company, identified common charting errors that can result in malpractice:

- Failing to record pertinent health or drug information
- Failing to record nursing actions
- Failing to record that medications have been given
- Recording on the wrong chart
- Failing to record drug reactions or changes in the client's condition
- Transcribing orders improperly or transcribing improper orders
- Writing illegible or incomplete records
- Failing to document a discontinued medication

In addition to these omissions, nurses should chart only their own actions; never chart for someone else unless the caregiver has left the unit and calls with additional information that needs to be documented. Follow agency policy when documenting a late entry, as discussed later in this chapter.

HEALTH INSURANCE PORTABILITY AND ACCOUNTABILITY ACT (HIPAA)

The HIPAA of 1996 was the first federal legislation to protect automated client records. This act called for the establishment of electronic record systems and privacy rules to legally protect personal health information (PHI). PHI is any information contained in automated records that is transmitted or maintained in any form or medium, including verbal discussions, electronic communications regarding clients, and written communications (Hebda & Czar, 2009). Examples of PHI include name, address, birth date, Social Security number, allergies, claims data, laboratory results and other diagnostic history, prescription history, past visits to a prescribing practitioner, emergency rooms and other health care encounters, vaccination records, and prior in- and outpatient procedures.

The HIPAA privacy rule mandates how an organization must address administrative and technical procedures to protect privacy (Hebda & Czar, 2009). Examples of administrative procedures include information access controls; formal mechanisms for processing records; security incident procedures, training, and management processes; and termination procedures. Technical measures require audit controls, authorization controls, data authentication, communication and network controls, encryption, and other types of authentication such as event reporting and message integrity.

In 2003 HIPAA published the security rule that mandates safeguards for the physical storage, maintenance, transmission, and access to PHI to ensure its confidentiality, data integrity, and availability when required for treatment (Hebda & Czar, 2009). The HIPAA law provides for penalties of noncompliance with either the privacy rule or the security rule.

HIPAA allows for student access but demands individual accountability for viewing PHI (Milo & Carlton, 2008). Using IT and learning to perform clinical documentation is an important facet in the education of student nurses and needs to be integrated into all clinical courses (Milo & Carlton, 2008; Thede, 2008).

Hospital and nursing information systems must ensure rapid access to accurate and complete client information to legitimate users, while safeguarding client privacy and confidentiality (Hebda & Czar, 2009). HIPAA requires health care organizations to demonstrate measures that protect client information and comply with accreditation criteria.

In IT language, privacy refers to the client's right to determine what information is collected, how it is used, and the ability to access collected information to review its security and accuracy. HIPAA requires that all clients be given clear written explanations of how facilities and providers may use and disclose client health data. Nurses are held legally accountable by the ANA *Code of Ethics* and state practice laws to protect client privacy.

Confidentiality is necessary for the accurate assessment, diagnosis, and treatment of health problems, and it refers to a situation in which a relationship has been established and private information is shared. The ethical duty of confidentiality requires that information shared during the course of a professional relationship is kept secure and secret from others. Appropriate security mechanisms must address the storage and transmission of private information; ensure that the equipment used for storage and transmission is secure; and prevent the interception of e-mail, instant messages, faxes, and other correspondence containing private information. Fax numbers should be confirmed prior to sending confidential information. All printed information, such as faxes and e-mails, that contains confidential information must be destroyed. Most agencies have shredders or locked receptacles for shredding and later incineration of client record information.

Information privacy requires informed consent for the release of specific information. Information security is the protection of information against threats to its integrity, inadvertent disclosure, or availability. Consent is when an individual authorizes health care providers to release information based on an informed understanding of how this information will be used. As with all consents, the individual must be made aware of any risks that may exist to privacy as well as the security measures taken to protect privacy.

Security mechanisms use a combination of two basic protection measures: logical and physical restrictions such as firewalls and the installation of antivirus and spyware detection software. Automatic sign-off is an example of logical restriction; this mechanism logs off a user from the system after a specific period of inactivity on the computer.

Identification management deals with identifying individuals in a system and controlling access to resources within that system by associating user right and restriction with the established identity. Identity must be authenticated to determine whether someone is who he or she professes to be. Some examples of authentication are passwords, digital certificates, and public or private keys used for encryption and biometric measures.

Access codes and passwords are collections of alphanumeric characters that users type into the computer. The password is usually required after the entry and acceptance of the access code, often called the *user name*. The password should not be known to anyone but the user. A strong password should contain letters, numbers, and symbols to ensure a high level of security. The user should log off when leaving the computer unattended.

A firewall is a barrier between systems to protect those systems from unauthorized access. A firewall screens traffic, allowing only approved transactions to pass through them, and restricts access to other systems or sensitive areas such as client information, payroll, or personal data (Hebda & Czar, 2009).

Antivirus software refers to a set of computer programs that can locate and eradicate viruses and other malicious programs from scanned memory sticks, storage devices, individual computers, and networks. These systems require updating to combat the constant creation of new viruses. Users can install and activate antivirus software to automatically run a virus check on a personal computer or server on a scheduled basis in addition to performing random checks. Network computers automatically perform a virus scan of new files and update antivirus files; administrators can also set privileges to prohibit unauthorized file downloads.

Another security concern is spyware. Spyware is a self-installing data collection mechanism that is installed without the user's permission. This may happen when the user is browsing the Web or downloading software. Spyware often includes cookies that track Web use as well as applications that capture credit card, bank, and PIN numbers or other PHI stored on that computer for illicit purposes by an authorized person (Hebda & Czar, 2009). Indicators of a computer spyware infection are the presence of pop-up ads, keys that do not work, random error messaging, and poor system performance. Spyware detection software should be installed on computers because of this security threat.

COMPONENTS OF A POLICY TO PROTECT AND SECURE PHI IN COMPUTERIZED RECORDS

- Computer access is governed by user passwords that should not be shared with anyone.
- Once the user is logged into the computer, the computer screen should not be left unattended or accessible for public viewing.
- All unnecessary computer-generated paper must be shredded.
- Users must know how to correct an entry error.
- Users must know how to chart client-sensitive material, such as a diagnosis of AIDS.
- A firewall protects the server from unauthorized access.

Most health care agencies allow student and graduate health professionals access to client records for the purpose of education and research. Client records are used to support learning such as conferences, rounds, and nursing care plans. Students must comply with ethical codes and legal and agency regulations such as HIPAA to hold all client information in confidence. The student is responsible for protecting the client's privacy by not using a name or any statements in the notations that would identify the client (Hebda & Czar, 2009). Health care agencies, in compliance with HIPAA mandates, specifically the Security Rule of 2005, have policies and procedures to ensure the privacy and confidentiality of PHI stored in computers; see Box above for a sample policy that protects the privacy and security of computerized records.

SPOTLIGHT ON...

Legal/Ethical

Is this just a cliché: "If it wasn't charted, it wasn't done"? Since the purpose of the medical record is to document the care administered to the client, how can a practitioner convince a jury that care was administered if it is not documented in the medical record? Consider the following. A nurse, by habit, always administers an intramuscular injection in the ventrogluteal site, although both the ventrogluteal and dorsogluteal sites are within the accepted guidelines of care. The nurse, however, fails to chart the site on the medication administration record (MAR). The client files a suit for sciatic nerve damage. Knowing that there is an identified greater risk factor for sciatic nerve injury with the dorsogluteal site, do you think it would be difficult to defend care given in this case?

▼ **SAFETY FIRST** ▼

THE IMPORTANCE OF COMMUNICATION
Important information obtained from an assessment that warrants immediate intervention should not only be documented in the medical record but also communicated orally to the other practitioners. The element of time must direct decision making when critical information is obtained.

▼ **SAFETY FIRST** ▼

CONSENT FROM SEDATED CLIENTS
Sedated clients should never be requested or allowed to sign an informed consent; they may not be capable of understanding the nature of and risks associated with the procedure, so the consent will be invalid, and the nurse and institution will be at legal risk. Wait instead for the client to be competent and free of sedation, or have a legally acceptable family member brought into the decision.

INFORMED CONSENT **Informed consent** means that the client understands the reason for and the risks of the proposed intervention and agrees to the treatment by signing a consent form. Legally, the client must be mentally competent, and the prescribing practitioner who is to perform the procedure is responsible for obtaining the client's informed consent (refer to Chapter 12). Failure to provide educational opportunities for a client to participate in decision making could open the door to litigation.

In order to assist the prescribing practitioner with proper documentation of teaching, many facilities have preprinted informed consent documents that explain procedures in lay terms and identify the risk factors and possible complications. These documents are usually duplicate copies: The original goes in the medical record, and the copy is given to the client. This procedure provides the client with a written copy of the information that can be reviewed at a later time in a more relaxed environment.

Nurses are responsible for ensuring that the client understands the procedure or intervention and has signed the informed consent. The best way to assess client knowledge of an intervention is to ask clients to explain, in their own words, what is going to be done and the common risks and possible complications. If the informed consent has not been signed or if the nurse assesses a lack of understanding on the client's part, the prescribing practitioner should be notified and the client should not be allowed to undergo the procedure. If the intervention is a surgical procedure, the nurse should notify the operating room at the time the surgeon is notified.

Although most informed consents deal with medical interventions, nurses are sometimes responsible for implementing the interventions: For example, administering blood or blood products requires informed consent. It is also the responsibility of the nurse to obtain oral consent for certain nursing interventions, such as initiating intravenous therapy or inserting a nasogastric tube or urinary catheter. Remember that consents require client education with an explanation of outcomes and documentation of the client's understanding of the procedure.

Once the client has been educated by the prescribing practitioner and nurse about the intervention, the informed consent needs to be signed by the client and witnessed. Witnessing the signing of the consent confirms that the person who signs the consent is in fact the client and *is competent,*

alert, and aware of all actions at that point in time. Refer to Chapter 12 for further discussion of informed consent.

ADVANCE DIRECTIVES An **advance directive** is a statement made by clients that defines care they deem acceptable if they become incapacitated. It effectively allows clients, while competent, to participate in end-of-life decisions and to choose the types of life-sustaining procedures they will permit if they become unable to make their own decisions at a later time. A **durable power of attorney** allows the client to appoint a person to make health-related decisions when the client is incapable of making them. The Patient Self-Determination Act of 1990 requires health care facilities (hospitals, skilled-nursing facilities, and home health agencies) to inform adult clients of their rights regarding advance directives and to document in the medical record whether the client has such a directive. The implementation of advance directives is discussed in Chapter 12.

AMERICAN NURSES ASSOCIATION STANDARDS OF CARE Standards of documentation are established by professional organizations. The ANA's Standards of Clinical Nursing Practice serve as guidelines for determining safe, quality nursing care and practice. The nursing process gives structure to the standards of care, with specific measurement criteria for each phase in the process. For each of the six standards (assessment, diagnosis, outcome identification, planning, implementation, and evaluation), there is a measurement criterion that states "are documented." ANA standards make explicit the role of data collection and documentation in nursing practice. They specify that data collection be systematic and continuous and that data be accessible, communicated, and recorded (ANA, 1997).

STATE NURSE PRACTICE ACTS In an attempt to recognize and control the practice of nursing, nurse practice acts, on a state-by-state basis, have established guidelines to ensure safe practice and to demonstrate accountability to society. The standards of care, as set forth in the practice acts, are based on the phases of the nursing process and require evidence of compliance by documentation. Nurses should be familiar with the practice acts and rules of the state in which they work.

THE JOINT COMMISSION The Joint Commission surveys health care facilities to measure compliance with its standards for safe health care provision. Although facilities voluntarily submit to this accreditation process, reimbursement eligibility for Medicare, Medicaid, and private funding is dependent upon Joint Commission accreditation.

The Joint Commission recommends the use of an HIS and requires that reports be submitted using computerized formats. The Joint Commission's National Patient Safety Goal for 2008 requires organizations to develop technology that will assist with the process of positive client identification. National initiatives are focused on reducing identification errors for procedures and nursing interventions such as medication administration, bedside glucose checks, and the administration of intravenous fluids and blood transfusion.

In 1994 the Joint Commission issued information management standards for health care organizations. The standards addressed these areas:

- Measures to protect information confidentiality, security, and integrity
- Uniform definitions and methods for data capture as a means to facilitate data comparison within and among health care agencies
- Education on the information management principles and training for system use
- Accurate and timely transmission of information
- Integration of clinical systems such as pharmacy, nursing, laboratory, and radiology and nonclinical systems such as medical records and admissions
- Client-specific data and information related to outcomes that facilitate care, provide financial and legal records, aid research, and support decision making
- Aggregate data and information records that support operations and research and improve performance and care
- Knowledge-based information capable of providing literature in print or electronic form
- Data that facilitate comparison of one institution with other agencies

The Joint Commission revised these standards in 2006 to provide for business continuity and disaster recovery planning, data and information retention, decision support, and specific documentation areas and formats (Hebda & Czar, 2009).

The Joint Commission no longer requires that health care organizations have traditional nursing care plans, but documentation of an individualized plan of care must be evident for each client. The Joint Commission's standards require:

- The involvement of the client or family in the development of the plan, which must be documented in the medical record
- Interdisciplinary planning and implementation of all aspects of care

The use of interdisciplinary tools has proven to be an effective approach to documenting client and family education for agencies not yet using critical pathways (discussed later in the chapter) or care mapping.

During the accreditation survey, the reviewer looks for evidence of an organized and systematic method of monitoring and evaluating client care that is reflected through documentation in the medical record. Documenting the steps of the nursing process ensures compliance with the Joint Commission's plan of care requirements.

Reimbursement

Peer review organizations (PROs), consisting of prescribing practitioners and nurses, are required by the federal government to monitor and evaluate the quality and appropriateness of care given. Medical record documentation is the mechanism for the PRO review, which evaluates the intensity of services and the severity of illness on the basis of a comparison of sample medical records from different facilities against specific screening criteria.

The federal enactment of the diagnosis-related group (DRG) classification system changed the health care provider reimbursement process from a cost-per-case formula to a prospective payment system (PPS). With PPS, the medical record must provide documentation that supports the DRG and the appropriateness of care. Nursing documentation must also show evidence of client and family education and discharge planning.

From a hospital's perspective, when information in the medical record demonstrates compliance with Medicare and Medicaid standards, the reimbursement is maximized. If nurses fail to document the equipment or procedures used daily (e.g., feeding pump; daily weight, intake and output; intravenous therapy; drug additives), reimbursement to the facility can be denied.

Another federal law, the Comprehensive Omnibus Budget Reconciliation Act (COBRA), allows employees to temporarily carry their employer-provided health insurance benefits for 90 days after termination, reduction in the work hours, or retirement. The law requires that for any COBRA client receiving care in an emergency room, the client's condition must be stabilized before the client can be transferred to another facility. If the client's condition is not stable, then the institution cannot initiate a transfer.

Facilities in violation of COBRA laws are fined and stand to lose their eligibility to Medicare and Medicaid funding. Compliance with this law is evaluated through medical record review. The documentation concerning client transfers must include:

- Chronology of the event
- Measures taken or treatment implemented
- Client's response to treatment
- Results of measures taken to prevent the client's condition from deteriorating

SPOTLIGHT ON...

Legal/Ethical

Why would an emergency room want to transfer a COBRA client who has insurance? Do you think these clients are considered high risk? Suppose a pregnant client in the seventh month of gestation comes to the emergency room in labor. The client is assessed by the prescribing practitioner and nurse. Labor is in progress, but delivery is not imminent, and the client's blood pressure is 210/124. Treatment is initiated; however, the blood pressure remains high (190/110). Can this client be transferred? If not, why not? Why would this health care provider want to stabilize and transfer the client before delivery?

PRINCIPLES OF EFFECTIVE DOCUMENTATION

Documentation requirements will differ depending on the health care facility (hospital, nursing home, home health agency) and the setting within the facility (e.g., emergency room, perioperative, medical-surgical unit) and with specific client populations (e.g., obstetrics, pediatrics, geriatrics). Regardless of what client care is administered, the documentation of that care must reflect the nursing process. General documentation guidelines for paper records and computerized charting are listed in the accompanying display.

Nursing notes must be logical, focused, and relevant to care and must represent each phase in the nursing process. Nursing documentation based on the nursing process facilitates effective care because client needs can be traced from assessment, through the identification of the problems, to the care plan, implementation, and evaluation. A brief reminder of the elements of the nursing process follows:

- *Assessment:* Summarize, without duplication, assessment data that are related to an actual or potential health care need. With reassessment, highlight any new findings or any changes in the client's condition (e.g., increased pain). The accompanying display outlines some assessment-specific documentation guidelines.
- *Diagnosis:* Identify the client's problem or need using NANDA terminology.
- *Outcome identification and planning:* Discuss with the client and communicate to members of the multidisciplinary team the expected outcomes or goals of client care.
- *Implementation:* After the intervention has been performed, document observations, treatments, teaching, and related clinical judgments. Client teaching should include learning needs, teaching plan content, methods of teaching, who was taught, and the learners' responses.

GENERAL DOCUMENTATION GUIDELINES

- Ensure that you have the correct client record or chart and that the client's name and identifying information are on every page of the record.
- Document as soon as the client encounter is concluded to ensure accurate recall of data (follow institutional guidelines on frequency of charting).
- Date and time each entry.
- Sign each entry with your full legal name and with your professional credentials, or per your institutional policy.
- Do not leave space between entries.
- If an error is made while documenting, use a single line to cross out the error, then date, time, and sign the correction (check institutional policy); avoid erasing, crossing out, or using correction fluid.
- Never change another person's entry, even if it is incorrect.
- Use quotation marks to indicate direct client responses (e.g., "I feel lousy").
- Document in chronological order (if chronological order is not used, state why).
- Write legibly.
- Use a permanent-ink pen (black is usually preferable because of its ability to photocopy well).
- Document in a complete but concise manner by using phrases and abbreviations as appropriate.
- Document all telephone calls that you make or receive that are related to a client's case.
- Keep computer passwords confidential.
- Once logged on to the computer, do not leave the computer screen unattended or accessible to public viewing.

- *Evaluation:* Evaluate and document the effectiveness of the interventions in terms of the expected outcomes: progress toward goals; client response to tests, treatments, and nursing interventions; client and family response to teaching and significant events; and questions, statements, or complaints voiced by the client or family.
- *Revisions of planned care:* Document the reasons for the revisions with the supporting evidence and client and family agreement.

Charting in accordance with the nursing process ensures thorough documentation in compliance with the ANA's standards of care, practice acts, and reimbursement and accreditation criteria.

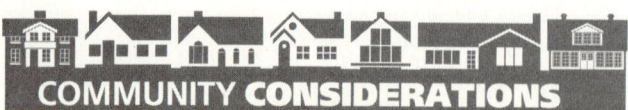

COMMUNITY CONSIDERATIONS

Home Health Care

Home health agencies also keep documents: prescribing practitioner orders, history and physical forms, home care team records, and nursing records (initial assessment form, plan of care, problem list for daily progress notes, client teaching activities, and discharge summary). Home health care providers are required to comply with state and federal regulations that affect health care, documentation, and reimbursement.

ELEMENTS OF EFFECTIVE DOCUMENTATION

Effective documentation requires:

- Use of a common vocabulary
- Legibility and neatness
- Use of only authorized abbreviations and symbols
- Factual and time-sequenced organization
- Accurately including any errors that occurred

The following discussion of effective charting refers to all nursing documents, such as flow sheets, progress notes, and so on. Add to the nursing documents when:

- A change occurs in the client's condition
- Measuring the client's response to an intervention or expected outcome
- The client or family voices a complaint

Use of Common Vocabulary

The use of a common vocabulary in nursing is considered critical by many nurse leaders in order for nurses to define the practice of nursing. A common vocabulary allows nurses to provide continuity of care as well as researchers to collect and compare data among large groups of clients, facilitating the development of evidence-based practice (EBP). When nurses use multiple terms for describing nursing assessment, diagnoses, interventions, and client outcomes, it is difficult to conduct comparisons of nursing care.

With the formulation of nursing diagnoses by the NANDA as well as the NIC and NOC, nursing is moving toward a coordinated set of clinical languages. This system should provide nursing care with decision support and a standardized language to describe nursing activities.

In the early 2000s, nursing leaders in the United States began meeting with international groups to determine acceptable nursing terminologies to be computable and semantically interoperable with one another. In 2003 the international summit members adopted the first model of standards, and by 2008 the group shifted from developing standards to reviewing, revising, and implementing standards

ASSESSMENT-SPECIFIC DOCUMENTATION GUIDELINES

- Record all data that contribute directly to the assessment (e.g., positive assessment findings and pertinent negatives).
- Document any parts of the assessment that are omitted or refused by the client.
- Avoid using judgmental language such as "good," "poor," "bad," "normal," "abnormal," "decreased," "appears to be," and "seems."
- Avoid evaluative statements (e.g., "client is uncooperative," "client is lazy"); cite instead specific statements or actions that you observe (e.g., "client said 'I hate this place' and kicked trash can").
- State time intervals precisely (e.g., "every 4 hours," "b.i.d.," instead of "seldom," "occasionally").
- Do not make relative statements about findings (e.g., "mass the size of an egg"); use specific measurements (e.g., "mass 3 cm × 5 cm").
- Draw pictures when appropriate (e.g., location of scar, masses, skin lesion, decubitus, deep tendon reflex).
- Refer to findings using anatomical landmarks (e.g., left upper quadrant [of abdomen], left lower lobe [of lung], midclavicular line).
- Use the face of the clock to describe findings that are in a circular pattern (e.g., breast, tympanic membrane, rectum, vagina).
- Document any change in the client's condition during a visit or from previous visits.
- Describe what you observed, not what you did.

(Ozbolt & Saba, 2008). By 2008 the basic groundwork was laid with the data and terminology tools for computability and semantic interoperability.

Legibility

Whatever is charted must be easily readable, without any chance of error. If your handwriting is not readable, print. If you make a mistake, do not erase or obliterate it; draw one line through the erroneous entry and state the reason for the error, then sign and date the correction.

Abbreviations and Symbols

Facilities usually have a list of acceptable abbreviations and symbols, approved by the Medical Records Committee, to be used when documenting information in the client's record. The National Coordinating Council for Medication Error Reporting and Prevention and the Joint Commission have both issued dangerous abbreviations to be avoided by all health care providers. These dangerous abbreviations (e.g., "U," "IU," and the use of "zero" with a decimal point) are not to be used in any clinical documentation; see the accompanying display and Chapter 30 on dangerous abbreviations and use of the decimal point. The use of trailing zeros is banned because the overlooked decimal point can lead to a tenfold overdose. However, the "zero" before a decimal point should always be used when prescribing and recording.

Always refer to the facility's approved listing (see Symbols and Abbreviations on the inside back cover of this book). Avoid abbreviations that can be misunderstood; see Chapter 30 for a list of dangerous abbreviations. For example, when qd (every day) is not written legibly, it may be read as q.i.d. (four times a day).

Organization

Start every entry with the date and time. Chart in a chronological order—assessment data, observation, intervention, and evaluation. Comply with the time frame indicated in the facility's guidelines for documentation (e.g., the frequency of charting observations for a client with restraints or the time frame within which the admit assessment must be completed).

Chart in a timely fashion to avoid the omission of pertinent data; it is not a good practice to wait until the end of the shift to chart on all the clients. Chart medications immediately after administration to avoid errors. Sign your name after each entry.

When the nurse forgets to document significant data, it is appropriate and advisable to include these data at a later date. There are several reasons why a late entry might have to be made:

- The chart was not available (e.g., the chart was with the client in a special procedures lab).
- Entries had to be added after notes were completed.
- Information was documented on the wrong record.

As with other aspects of documentation, follow the facility's policy for charting a late entry. Common practice is to enter the date and time and label "Late entry" to indicate that it is out of sequence. Then record the date and time it should have been made in the body of the entry.

Accuracy

Accurate and objective data are crucial if the documentation is to be useful either clinically or for research. Use factual, descriptive terms to chart exactly what was observed or done. See the accompanying display for incorrect and correct examples.

Use correct spelling and grammar, and write complete sentences. Differentiate who does what; for example, "Dr. Smith inserted a triple-lumen, 20-gauge catheter into the right subclavian vein." Read the notes recorded by nurses on previous shifts and make further comments on their findings to maintain the continuity of care.

Documenting a Medication Error

Facilities require nurses to report medication errors on incident reports (discussed later in this chapter and Chapter 12).

This information should also appear on the MAR with a notation in the nurses' progress notes. Remember, the purpose of the medical record is to report any care or treatment the client receives.

When a medication error occurs, the following should be charted:

1. Chart the medication on the MAR to prevent other caregivers from giving the client additional doses of the drug, similar drugs, or drugs that may be contraindicated.
2. Document the error in the nurses' notes as follows: name and dosage of the medication, time it was given, client's response to the medication, name of the prescribing practitioner who was notified of the error, time of the notification, nursing interventions or medical treatment to counteract the error, and client's response to treatment.

Confidentiality

Nurses are bound by ethical codes and laws to treat all client information in a confidential and professional manner; this includes the client's record. The written documentation contained in the client's chart is a legal record of care, and it should be available only to members of that client's health care team. The client's significant others, insurance companies, and other parties not directly involved in the care provided by the health care team may not have access to clients' records; it is the nurse's responsibility to protect the privacy and confidentiality of client interactions, assessments, and care. Even clients themselves must submit a written request to have their information released, and then they must specify exactly what information is to be released and to whom. In many institutions, particularly teaching hospitals, client records may be used for educational or research purposes. Members of these educational and research teams are held to the same standards of privacy protection and may not

DANGEROUS ABBREVIATIONS AND USE OF THE DECIMAL POINT

Incorrect	Correct
25 U of regular insulin	25 units of regular insulin
.9 mg	0.9 mg

FACTUAL DESCRIPTIVE TERMS

Incorrect	Correct
"Wound appears the same."	"Wound is 2.5 cm by 1.0 cm."
"Large amount of drainage."	"Foul-smelling, yellowish drainage completely saturated two 4 × 4s."

legitimately use client information for any purposes other than education or research or in any manner that would identify specific clients in any way.

METHODS OF DOCUMENTATION

Documentation must reflect the complexity of care, and it must embody accuracy, completeness, and evidence of professional practice with efficient and cost-effective systems. The clinical standards (structure, outcome, process, and evaluation) are used to develop a system that complies with legal, accreditation, and professional practice requirements of documentation.

Many methods are used for documentation, including:

- Narrative charting
- Source-oriented (SO) charting
- Problem-oriented charting
- PIE charting
- Focus charting
- Charting by exception (CBE)
- Computerized documentation
- Case management with critical paths

NARRATIVE CHARTING

Narrative charting, the traditional method of nursing documentation, is a story format that describes the client's status, interventions and treatments, and the client's response to treatments. Before the advent of flow sheets, this was the only method for documenting care.

Narrative documentation is easy to use in emergency situations, in which a simple, chronological order is needed. However, in this type of documentation it is often difficult to avoid being subjective, and there is normally a lack of analysis and critical decision making on the part of the nurse. Narrative charting is now being replaced by other formats because:

- The flow of care is disorganized. It is difficult to show a relationship between data and critical thinking skills. Each nurse writes with a unique style, making continuity of care difficult to identify.
- It fails to reflect the nursing process. The focus is on tasks without emphasis on assessment data or progress toward achievement of outcomes.
- It is time-consuming. The paragraphs are free-flowing, so it takes more time to record accurate data and for others to read it.
- The information is difficult to retrieve. The same problems may not be addressed from shift to shift, so it is difficult to track the client's progress. Auditors often disallow charges for equipment and supplies because consistent usage cannot be identified.

In a nursing information system, narrative charting is accomplished using free text entry or menu selections.

SOURCE-ORIENTED CHARTING

Source-oriented (SO) charting is described as a narrative recording by each member (source) of the health care team

on separate records. Because each discipline has a separate record, care is often fragmented and communication between disciplines becomes time-consuming. SO charting has similar advantages and disadvantages to narrative charting since nurses use an unstructured approach to documenting in the progress notes.

PROBLEM-ORIENTED CHARTING

The problem-oriented medical record (POMR) was introduced in 1969 by Lawrence Weed, a physician at Case Western Reserve University. The focus of POMR documentation is on the client's problem, with a structured, logical format to narrative charting called SOAP:

- S: subjective data (what the client or family states)
- O: objective data (what is observed/inspected)
- A: assessment (conclusion reached on the basis of data formulated as client problems or nursing diagnoses)
- P: plan (actions to be taken to relieve client's problem)

SOAPIE and SOAPIER refer to formats that add:

- I: intervention (measures to achieve an expected outcome)
- E: evaluation (effectiveness of interventions)
- R: revision (changes from the original plan of care)

See the accompanying display for a sample of SOAPIE charting. As you chart according to these systems, think about which piece of information corresponds with each letter in the SOAP, SOAPIE, or SOAPIER entry.

The POMR system was modified by nonmedical caregivers and is referred to as the problem-oriented record (POR). The system is used by hospitals, nursing homes, and home care agencies.

There are four critical components of POMR/POR:

- Database: Assessment data, representative of all disciplines (history, physical, nursing admit assessment, laboratory findings, educational and discharge needs), which become the basis for a problem list evaluation of the client's condition.
- Problem list: Derived from the database: a listing of the client's problems as identified, with each problem numbered and labeled as acute, chronic, active, or inactive. Nurses use NANDA terminology in writing client problems as nursing diagnoses; the list is revised as new problems arise and others are resolved.
- Initial plan: Based on problem identification; the starting point for care plan development with client participation in setting goals, expected outcomes, and learning needs.
- Progress notes: Charting based on the SOAP, SOAPIE, or SOAPIER format.

The POR system uses flow sheets to record routine care and a discharge summary that addresses each problem on the list and notes whether it was resolved. SOAP entries are usually made every 24 hours on any unresolved problem or whenever the client's condition changes.

SOAPIE CHARTING—PROBLEM 2 KETOACIDOSIS

Date/Time	**S:** Client states, "I feel sick all over." Client claims difficulty in breathing, abdominal pain, and nausea.
	O: Lungs clear, R 28/min, labored. Abdomen distended, bowel sounds underactive all four quadrants, 5+ abdominal pain.
	A: Alteration in nutrition and comfort R/T ketoacidosis. Blood sugar 458 mg/dL. Ketones strongly positive, pH < 7.3.
	P: Maintain IV infusion of 0.9% NS with regular insulin as ordered. NPO. Oral hygiene hrly. Maintain accurate I & O. Assess for rales, hypotension, cardiac dysrhythmias. Monitor blood glucose & electrolytes. (Signature)
Date/Time	**I:** Called Dr. Smith, blood sugar 458 mg/dL, IV bolus regular insulin given as ordered, 1000 mL 0.9% NS infusing @ 1 L/H central line 1 via infusion pump. 50 units regular insulin in 500 mL NS infusing @ 50 mL/H central line 2 via infusion pump. EKG taken, placed on telemetry. (Signature)
Date/Time	**E:** Lungs clear, R 24/min, nonlabored, NSR, 3+ abdominal pain. Urinary output 750 mL/hr. Blood glucose 360 mg/dL. (Signature)

FOCUS CHARTING

Focus charting is a method of identifying and organizing the narrative documentation of client concerns to include data, action, and response. This method is not limited to client "problems" but allows for the identification of all "concerns" such as a significant event (e.g., results of a diagnostic test). Focus charting was created in 1981 at Eitel Hospital in Minneapolis, when the results from a SOAP audit revealed weaknesses in writing care plans and charting the client's response to care. Focus charting uses a columnar format within the progress notes to distinguish the entry from other recordings in the narrative notes, as shown in the accompanying display on focus charting on page 230.

CHARTING BY EXCEPTION

Charting by exception (CBE) is a charting method that requires the nurse to document only deviations from preestablished norms. CBE was instituted in 1983 by St. Luke Medical Center in Milwaukee to overcome the recurring problem of lengthy, repetitive notes and to enable the identification of trends in client status. The CBE system has three key components:

1. Flow sheets: Highlight significant findings and define assessment parameters and findings.
2. Reference documentation: Is related to the standards of nursing practice. (All standards are met unless otherwise documented.)
3. Bedside accessibility: Is related to the documentation forms. CBE requires the nurse to document significant findings and exceptions to predefined norms.

PIE CHARTING

After SOAP charting gained in popularity, the **problem, intervention, evaluation (PIE)** system was instituted at Craven Regional Medical Center in 1984 to streamline documentation. Whereas SOAP was developed on a medical model, PIE charting has a nursing origin. PIE is an acronym for problem, intervention, and evaluation of nursing care. The key components of this system are assessment flow sheets and nurses' progress notes with an integrated plan of care that eliminates the need for a separate care plan. Each client problem is labeled and numbered for easy reference. When interventions are implemented to manage the client's problem, the problem number is identified; see the accompanying display on PIE charting. This system eliminates the traditional care plan by incorporating an ongoing plan of care into the daily documentation.

PIE CHARTING—IMBALANCED NUTRITION R/T KETOACIDOSIS

• Date/Time	**P4:** Imbalanced nutrition R/T ketoacidosis. Blood glucose 458 mg/dL, ketones strongly positive, pH 7.2. **I4:** Called Dr. Smith, blood sugar 458 mg/dL. IV bolus regular insulin given as ordered. 1000 mL 0.9% NS infusing @ 1 L/H central line 1 via infusion pump. 50 units regular insulin infusing @ 50 mL/H central line 2 via infusion pump. EKG taken, placed on telemetry.
• Date/Time	**E4:** Lungs clear, R 24/min, nonlabored. 3+ abdominal pain. Urinary output 750 mL/H (0730–0830). Blood sugar 360 mg/dL. (Signature)

COMPUTERIZED DOCUMENTATION

Computerized clinical records systems allow nurses to use computers to store client data. These systems allow nurses to record client assessment, medication administration (see Figure 13-1), client teaching, progress notes, care plan updating, client acuity, and charges into either a bedside computer terminal or a small, portable handheld terminal. Figure 13-2 on page 229 provides an example of a computer-generated vital sign graphic record that allows nurses to see at a glance trends in the client's vital signs.

To document nursing interventions and client responses, the nurse chooses from standardized lists of terms or enters narrative information into the computer. Automated documentation should provide all normal standards and allow the nurse to document any exception by menu selection or free text entry. Flow sheet charting should provide for routine aspects of care to be documented in tabular form; a pointing device such as a mouse is used to make menu selections or text entries. The automated MAR is one form of flow sheet charting.

CASE MANAGEMENT PROCESS

Case management is defined as a methodology for organizing client care through an episode of illness so that specific clinical and financial outcomes are achieved within an allotted time frame. The outcome of this process is a DRG-specific case management plan that contains daily assessment documentation, care plan, outcome-oriented multidisciplinary interventions, teaching, and discharge planning.

At admission, the nurse case manager and the admitting practitioner individualize the case management plan (called a

---

12/26/05
1033

MEDICATION ADMINISTRATION RECORD

Tulane University

DIAGNOSIS: WOUND INFECTION
WT: 195lb 0.0oz (88.450kg) HT: 5ft7.0in (170.1cm) BSA: 2.07m2
AGE: 44   SEX: F   Serum Cr: Est. CREATININE CL: LAB RESULTS N/A
ADMIT: 12/20/05
NOTES:

UNIT #   D.5EA
ACCT#

ALLERGIES:

ADMINISTRATION PERIOD: 0000 12/25/05 TO 2359 12/25/05	START/STOP	0000 - 0659	0700 - 1459	1500 - 2359

ASPIRIN (ASPIRIN)
81 MG (1 TAB.EC)   ORAL   ONCE DAILY
    AVOID ALCOHOL: TAKE WITH MEALS
    03603139
		12/20/05	1125 RPB	

ANCEF 1GM PLASTIC BAG 50 ML		12/23/05 12/23/05 12/23/05 12/23/05 12/23/05		*1910 RPB OF 50.00 MLS 2327 RLD 50.00 MLS SITE: CL

100 MLS/HR   INTRAVEN.   Q8H
    ADMINISTER OVER 30 MIN
    03607985				

DILTIAZEM HCL (CARDIZEM CD)
240 MG (1 UDCAP.SA) ORAL   ONCE DAILY
    AVOID GRAPEFRUIT JUICE. AVOID ALCOHOL.
    03603135
		12/20/05	1125 RPB	

ENOXAPARIN (LOVENOX) **40 MG-0.4 ML (1 SYR)** SUBCUTANEOUS ONCE DAILY 03603649		12/21/05	1125 RPB SITE: RA	

* Meds not given REASON CODES OF - OFF FLOOR	USER NAME AND TYPE	INIT	USER NAME AND TYPE	INIT
		RPB VLM		RLD
INJECTION SITES CL - CENTRAL LINE RA - RIGHT ARM				

FIGURE 13-1 Electronic Medication Administration Record REPRINTED WITH PERMISSION BY TULANE UNIVERSITY HOSPITAL & CLINIC, NEW ORLEANS, LA

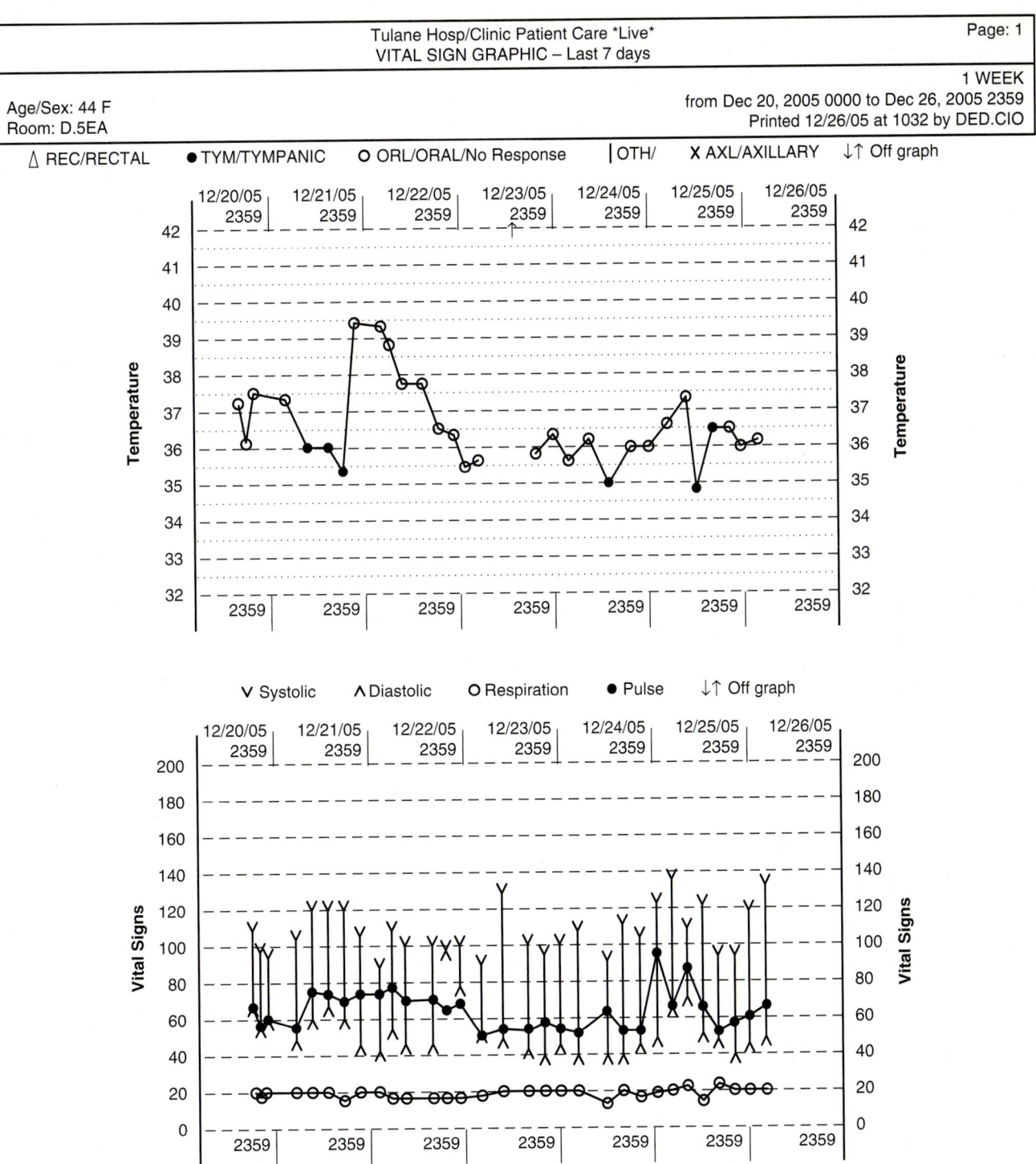

FIGURE 13-2 A computer-generated vital sign graphic record is capable of trending results over time. REPRINTED WITH PERMISSION BY TULANE UNIVERSITY HOSPITAL & CLINIC, NEW ORLEANS, LA

critical pathway) to meet the client's specific needs. A **critical pathway** (or critical path) is an abbreviated summary of key elements from the case management plan. The pathway is used by all health care providers as a monitoring and documentation tool to ensure that interventions are performed on time and that client outcomes are achieved on time. See Chapters 32 and 36 for sample critical pathways.

Variations, sometimes referred to as a variance, are goals not met or interventions not performed within the time

frame. The nurse documents on the back of the critical pathway the unexpected event (e.g., hospital-acquired decubiti), actions taken in response to the event, and appropriate discharge planning.

The advantages of case management are that it makes efficient use of time and increases the quality of care, with the expected outcomes identified on the plan. It also promotes collaboration, communication, and teamwork, which work to the advantage of the client and the facility, with

---

FOCUS CHARTING—IMBALANCED NUTRITION R/T KETOACIDOSIS

Date/Time	
	D: Client experiencing labored breathing, 5+ abdominal pain, and nausea. Blood sugar 458 mg/dL; ketones strongly positive; pH 7.2, T 99.8, R 28, P 110, BP 100/56.
	A: Auscultation reveals lungs clear and underactive bowel sounds in all 4 quadrants. Abdomen distended. Dr. Smith notified of blood glucose, ketones, and pH. IV bolus of regular insulin given as ordered. IVs infusing as ordered through central lines with infusion pumps. Stat EKG done, telemetry, NPO, oral hygiene admin, measuring I & O. (Signature)
Date/Time	**R:** Within 1 H (0730–0830) blood glucose 360 mg/dL, R 24, nonlabored. Urinary output 750 mL/H. Client identified abdominal pain, 3+. (Signature)

---

discharge occurring in a timely manner. Case management also has several limitations; mainly, it is useful for clients with only one or two diagnoses. When clients have more than two diagnoses or variations, documentation becomes complicated because of limited space. This situation requires additional documentation forms to complement the pathway, such as intervention flow sheets and nurses' notes.

FORMS FOR RECORDING DATA

Several types of forms are used in record keeping: Kardex, flow sheets, nurses' progress notes, and discharge summaries. All these forms are designed to facilitate record keeping, reduce duplicate activity, and ensure quick and easy access to information.

KARDEX

A **Kardex** (client profile and client summary sheets) is a summary worksheet reference of basic client care information that traditionally is not part of the medical record. The Kardex, a concise client data source, is used as a reference throughout the shift and during change-of-shift reports. Kardexes come in various sizes, shapes, and types (and they may also be computer generated). The Kardex is designed to complement the care delivery setting. For example, a home health Kardex would contain information related to family contacts, prescribing practitioners, other services, and emergency referrals. The Kardex usually contains the following information:

- Client data: Name, age, marital status, religious preference
- Medical diagnoses: Listed by priority
- Nursing diagnoses: Listed by priority
- Medical orders: Diet, medications, IV therapy, treatments, diagnostic tests and procedures (inclusive of dates and results), and consultations
- Activities permitted: Functional limitations, assistance needed in activities of daily living, and safety precautions

FLOW SHEETS

Flow sheets have vertical or horizontal columns for recording dates and times to show assessment and interventions, making it easy to track changes in the client's condition. Client teaching, use of special equipment, and IV therapy are other aspects of the flow sheet. Because the flow sheets have small spaces for recording, these forms usually contain legends that identify the approved abbreviations to chart data (see Figures 13-3 on page 231 and, on page 233, 13-4). It is important to fill out flow sheets completely because blank spaces imply that an intervention was not completed, attempted, or recognized.

The information on the flow sheet can be formatted to meet the specific needs of client populations (special needs, activity, and measurement and intervention). For example, recording assessment data may be different in pediatric clinics and pediatric hospital units than in facilities for adults. Flow sheets in critical care settings are more comprehensive than are those on a medical-surgical unit. Flow sheets can also complement other types of records of specific interventions (e.g., MAR, IV therapy).

Flow sheets are used as supplements to most documentation systems because they decrease the redundancy of charting in the nurses' progress notes. But they do not replace the progress notes. Nurses still need to document observations, client responses and teaching, detailed interventions, and other significant data in the progress notes.

NURSES' PROGRESS NOTES

The nurses' progress notes are used to document the client's condition, problems, and complaints; interventions; response to interventions; and achievement of outcomes. Progress notes include the following forms: nurses' notes, MARs, personal care flow sheets, teaching records, intake and output forms, vital sign records, and specialty forms (e.g., diabetic flow sheet and neurologic assessment form). The progress notes can be completely narrative or incorporated into a standardized flow sheet to complement SOAP(IE), PIE, focus charting, and other documentation systems.

DISCHARGE SUMMARY

Discharge summaries highlight the client's illness and course of care. When a narrative discharge summary is entered into the progress notes, it includes:

- The client's status at admission and discharge
- A brief summary of the client's care
- Intervention and education outcomes

TULANE UNIVERSITY MEDICAL CENTER

Tulane Hospital for Children

Date:_____ PEDIATRIC FLOW SHEET

7A - 7P PHYSICAL ASSESSMENT

	ASSESSMENT TIME	07	08	09	10	11	12	13	14	15	16	17	18	19	20	21	22	23	24	01	02	03	04	05	06
RESPIRATORY	Quality																								
	Cough																								
	Sputum																								
	Breath Sounds																								
	Suction (Y / N)																								
	Cough, Deep Breathe (Y / N)																								
	Other:																								
CARDIOVASCULAR	Heart Sounds																								
	Edema																								
	Capillary refill Sec.																								
	Nail bed color																								
	Peripheral pulses: Radial																								
	Pedal																								
	Other:																								
NEUROLOGICAL	LOC																								
	Pupils																								
	Fontanel (<2YRS.)																								
	Other:																								
ELIMINATION	Bowel sounds																								
	Abdomen																								
	Stool Color																								
	Urine Color																								
	Other:																								
SKIN INTEGRITY	Oral mucosa																								
	Turgor																								
	Skin discoloration																								
	Break in skin integrity (Y / N)																								
	IV site																								
	IV tubing change (Y / N)																								
COMFORT/PAIN	Discomfort/Pain (Y / N)																								
	Rating																								
MOBILITY	Range of motion																								
	Upper extremity strength																								
	Lower extremity strength																								
	OOB/ambulate (Y / N)																								
	Turn/Position																								
	Other:																								
SAFETY	Attendant																								
	Safety check (Y / N)																								
	Initials																								

FIGURE 13-3 Assessment and Intervention Flow Sheet REPRINTED WITH PERMISSION BY TULANE UNIVERSITY HOSPITAL & CLINIC, NEW ORLEANS, LA

TULANE UNIVERSITY MEDICAL CENTER

Date: _____ PEDIATRIC FLOW SHEET

NURSE'S NOTES

NURSE'S NOTES (Continued)

LEGEND

Resp. Quality
RG-regular
G-grunting
R-retracting
P-periodic
A-apneic
S-shallow
L-labored
F-nasal flaring

Heart Sounds
RG-regular
M-murmur
I-irregular

Pupils
R-reactive
NR-non-reactive

Urine Color
C-clear
Y-yellow
L-cloudy
B-bloody

ROM
F-full
A-active
P-passive
C-contracted
L-limited

Cough
NP- non
    productive
PC-productive
    cough

Edema
N-none
D-dependent
G-generalized
O-periorbital
P-pitting
T/P-tibial/pedal

Fontanel
S-soft
FL-flat
Sn-sunken
B-bulging
F-full
T-tense

Oral Mucosa
P-pink
W-pale
D-dusky
C-cyanotic
M-moist
DR-dry

Strength
N-normal
P-paretic
D-decerebrate
DC-decorticate
F-flaccid
W-weak

Sputum
C-clear
T-tenacious
P-purulent
G-green
Y-yellow
B-bloody
W-white

Nail bed Color
P-pink
W-pale
C-cyanotic
D-dusky

Bowel Sounds
P-present
A-absent
⇓-decreased
⇑-hyperactive

Turgor
G-good
F-fair
P-poor
T-tenting

Turn/Position
Sf-self
L-left
R-right
P-prone
S-supine

Breath Sounds
C-Clear
A-Absent
W-Wheezes
CS-Coarse
CR-Crackles
D-Decreased

Pulses
3+-bounding
2+-normal
1+-weak
0 -absent

Abdomen
S-soft
F-flat
D-distended
H-hard

Skin Discoloration
N-none
W-pale
D-dusky
C-cyanotic
J-jaundice
M-mottled

Attendant
A-absent
P-present

O₂ Route
RA-Room air
M-Mask
N-Nasal Cannula
T-Tent
Tr-Trach Tube

LOC
A-awake/alert
L-lethargic
F-flaccid
S-sedated
R-respond to pain
C-coma

Stool
N-Soft/formed
W-watery
S-seedy
F-frothy
B-bloody
T-tarry
H-hard

I.V. Site
N-Dry & intact
I-Infiltrated
P-Phlebotic
E-Edematous

FIGURE 13-3 (Continued)

**Tulane University
Hospital and Clinics**

	ID #:	Gender: unknown
	Hospital Admit Date: 12/23/2005 1751	Bed: D.SIC D.3376
	Age:	Attending MD:
	Allergies:	

SICU FLOWSHEET   **Condition Report**

Statistics		12/26 0700	12/26 0800	12/26 0900	12/26 1000	12/26 1100	12/26 1200	12/26 1300	12/26 1400	12/26 1500	12/26 1600	12/26 1700	12/26 1800
SICU Admit Date		*12/23/>	--------->	--------->	--------->	--------->	--------->	--------->	--------->	--------->	--------->	--------->	--------->
Art Insert Date		12/23/05	--------->	--------->	--------->	--------->	--------->	--------->	--------->	--------->	--------->	--------->	--------->
TLC Insert Date		12/23/05	--------->	--------->	--------->	--------->	--------->	--------->	--------->	--------->	--------->	--------->	--------->
ETT Insert Date		12/23/05	--------->	--------->	--------->	--------->	--------->	--------->	--------->	--------->	--------->	--------->	--------->
Vent Start Date		12/23/05	--------->	--------->	--------->	--------->	--------->	--------->	--------->	--------->	--------->	--------->	--------->
Weight Pre–op	kg	77	--------->	--------->	--------->	--------->	--------->	--------->	--------->	--------->	--------->	--------->	--------->
Weight–Yesterday	kg		77.2	--------->	--------->	--------->	--------->	--------->	--------->	--------->	--------->	--------->	--------->
Weight Today	kg	77.2	--------->	--------->	--------->	--------->	--------->	--------->	--------->	--------->	--------->	--------->	--------->
Intake–Last 24 hrs	cc	2627	--------->	--------->	--------->	--------->	--------->	--------->	--------->	--------->	--------->	--------->	--------->
Output–Last 24 hrs	cc	1450	--------->	--------->	--------->	--------->	--------->	--------->	--------->	--------->	--------->	--------->	--------->

Vital Signs													
Heart Rate	bpm	93,	81,	75,	78								
NIBP Systolic	mmHg	127	124	124	124								
NIBP diastolic	mmHg	64	67	63	67								
Temperature	degC		36.3										
Temp Site:			Tympanic										

Hemodynamics													
CVP	mmHg	12,	11,	13,	242								
CVP	mmHg	12,	11,	13,	242								

Chemistry													
Accu_Chek			101										

Respiratory Status													
Resp. Rate	bpm	17,	13,	16,	21								
SpO2	%	86,	98,	96,	98								
O2 Device		Room Air	Room Air		Room Air								

Intake–Oral													
NG Fluid	cc		60		30								

Intake–IV													
NS Flush	cc	3	3	3	3								
TPN	cc	83	83	83	83								
Piggyback					* 100								

Piggyback
12/26/2005 1000   100   1000 Zosyn 2.25gm IVPB infusing via distal port of R SC TLC.
Watkins RN   ENTERED AT: 12/26/2005 1008

# Unreviewed	> Partial Display	! Exceeds Warning Range
? Invalid	* Comment Attached	!! Critical
, Hidden Data	^ Revised	

Flowsheet printed at: 12/26/2005 1008

Signature: _____

From: 12/26/2005 0700
Until: 12/26/2005 1859

Page: 1 of 1

FIGURE 13-4 Surgical Intensive Care Unit (SICU) Flow Sheet REPRINTED WITH PERMISSION BY TULANE UNIVERSITY HOSPITAL & CLINIC, NEW ORLEANS, LA

- Resolved problems and continuing care needs for unresolved problems, inclusive of referrals
- Client instructions regarding medications, diet, food-drug interactions, activity, treatments, follow-up instructions, and other special needs

Many facilities have a documentation form that itemizes discharge and client instructions. The form has a duplicate copy for the client; the original goes in the medical record. Figure 13-5 on page 234 shows the common elements of this tool.

Tulane
UNIVERSITY
Medical Center

COORDINATION OF DISCHARGE CARE

DISCHARGE ASSESSMENT

DESCRIPTION			COMMENT	DESCRIPTION			COMMENT	DESCRIPTION				COMMENT
LOC	NL	AB		respiration quality	NL	AB		Foley removed/voided	N	Y	NA	
pupils	NL	AB		lung auscultation	NL	AB		bladder habit problems	N	Y		
range of motion	NL	AB		heart sounds	NL	AB		sleep problems	N	Y	UTO	
extremity strength	NL	AB		telemetry removed	N	Y	NA	IV removed and intact	N	Y	NA	
appetite	NL	AB	UTO	peripheral pulses	NL	AB		break in skin integrity	N			
swallowing difficulty	N	Y	UTO	bowel sounds	NL	AB		discomfort/pain	N	Y	UTO	
feeds self	N	Y		bowel habit problems	N	Y	Date Last BM					

Signature _____ RN _____ Date _____ Time _____

DISCHARGE MEDICATIONS

☐ None	Medication	Dosage	Route	Schedule	Special Instructions ▼ medication instruction sheets given interaction sheet given ▼		RX given food/drug
					☐		☐
					☐		☐
					☐		☐
					☐		☐
					☐		☐
					☐		☐
					☐		☐
					☐		☐
					☐		☐

HOME ROUTINE

Activity: ☐ As tolerated ☐ Restrictions_____
Diet: ☐ Regular ☐ Modified
Special Instructions: (document discharge sheet given to patient)

_____
_____
_____
_____
_____
_____
_____

Social Services:

_____
(SIGNATURE)

Physical Therapy ☐ Exercise Program ☐ Equipment
☐ Gait Instruction
(SIGNATURE)
Occupational Therapy:

_____
(SIGNATURE)
Nutrition Care:

_____
(SIGNATURE)
Other Services:

_____
(SIGNATURE)

FOLLOW-UP CARE

Your MD is: _____ To Contact Call: _____ In An Emergency Call: _____

☐ No Appointment ☐ Appointment(s) made:

Name	clinic/floor	date/time	phone #
Name	clinic/floor	date/time	phone #

Appointment(s) not made:

Call _____ phone # ext. _____ for an appointment in _____ days/weeks with _____ MD
Call _____ phone # ext. _____ for an appointment in _____ days/weeks with _____ MD

I understand the above instructions.

_____ Patient or Guardian's Signature _____ Date Time of Discharge _____ Nurse's Signature & Title _____

FIGURE 13-5 Common Elements of an Interdisciplinary Discharge Tool REPRINTED WITH PERMISSION BY TULANE UNIVERSITY HOSPITAL & CLINIC, NEW ORLEANS, LA

REPORTING

Reporting is the verbal communication of data regarding the client's health status, needs, treatments, outcomes, and responses. When a report is given, it needs to summarize the current critical information that facilitates clinical decision making and continuity of care. As with recording, reporting is based on the nursing process, standards of care, and legal and ethical principles. The nursing process provides structure for an organized report, a challenge inherent in verbal communications. In order to verbally communicate an efficient and well-organized report, the nurse must consider:

- What needs to be said
- Why it needs to be said
- How to say it
- What the expected outcomes are

Considering these aspects of reporting before the communication will provide for a concise, organized report.

Another critical element in reporting is listening (see Chapter 15). Reports require participation from everyone present. When receiving a report, the nurse focuses behaviors to enhance listening skills: The nurse eliminates distractions, puts thoughts and concerns aside, concentrates on what is being said, and does not anticipate what the presenter will say next. The reporting process is an integral component of developing effective interpersonal and intrapersonal relationships that promote continuity of client care. Regardless of the type of communication, planned presentation of client data is a key to accurate, concise, effective reporting. Summary reports, walking rounds, telephone reports and orders, and incident reports are all types of reporting.

SUMMARY REPORTS

Summary reports summarize pertinent client information that focuses on the client's needs as identified by the nursing process for the new caregiver. Summary reports commonly occur at the change of shift and when the client is transferred to another area.

A summary, or end-of-shift, report should be presented as follows:

- Background data obtained from client interactions and assessment of the functional health patterns
- Primary medical and nursing diagnoses and priority problems

- Identification of client risk problems
- Recent changes in condition or in treatments (e.g., new medications, elevated temperature)
- Effective interventions or treatments of priority problems, inclusive of laboratory and diagnostic results (e.g., client's response to pain medication)
- Progress toward expected outcomes: priority problems, teaching or discharge planning
- Adjustments in the plan of care
- Client or family complaints

This format will provide structure and organization to the data that are both logical and time sequenced since the format follows the nursing process. The new caregiver needs to receive an accurate, concise report about what has happened during the previous shift in order to provide continuity of care. Client and family complaints should be addressed last for each client because these situations usually generate questions and discussion.

TELEPHONE REPORTS AND ORDERS

Telephone communications are another way nurses report transfers, communicate referrals, obtain client data, solve problems, and inform the prescribing practitioner and the client's family members regarding a change in the client's condition. Nurses are expected to demonstrate phone courtesy and professionalism when initiating and receiving telephone reports and orders.

When initiating a phone call, organize the information to be reported or received. For example:

1. Make sure all lab results are back; if they are not, identify in advance which ones are missing and phone the lab or check the computer to determine if other results are available. Write down which tests have been performed and the results. Spell the client's name and provide the client's medical record number to avoid error in getting the results on the wrong client.

2. Review your notes and have your assessment data readily available, especially any significant client data related to the call. If you have not assessed the client, do an assessment before telephoning the practitioner; otherwise, the practitioner might ask you questions that you will not be able to answer.

3. Let the charge nurse or someone else at the nurses' station know that you are placing the call so that you will not be interrupted while on the phone.

When you place the call, state the reason you are calling: For example, "I am calling Dr. Smith regarding the blood sugar results for Mrs. White." Be brief and listen carefully. Repeat the test results and any orders the prescribing practitioner gives over the phone.

Record accurately in the medical record the date and time the phone call was placed, the client data you reported on the phone, the name of the person you spoke with, and whether an order was obtained. Do not chart "prescribing practitioner notified, no orders obtained." Rather, chart "Dr. Smith notified by phone, blood sugar 260 mg (drawn by the

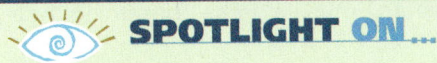

SPOTLIGHT ON...

Professionalism
Can nurses give a detailed enough shift report by telephone? If you give a report by telephone, can you then skip the face-to-face update with the oncoming nurse? Does the telephone shift report really save time, or does it double the time of giving a report?

lab at 1300), orders received and recorded on the prescribing practitioner order sheet." Charting telephone orders and documentation in the nurses' progress notes should be done as soon as possible after the phone call to prevent an entry by another caregiver before you chart the telephone report. The Joint Commission (2008) revised communication goals regarding orders and critical test results delivered verbally, whether in person or by telephone, require the receiver of the information to write it down or enter it into the computer, and then read it back. This new requirement is applicable to all spoken orders, not just medication orders. The only exception to writing down the verbal order prior to repeating the order is during surgery or a code when the spoken order can be just repeated.

A telephone order should be documented as follows on the prescribing practitioner's order sheet: Date and time the entry; record the order as given by the prescribing practitioner; then sign the order beginning with *t.o.* (telephone order), write the prescribing practitioner's name, and sign your name. If another nurse witnesses the phone order, that nurse's signature should go after yours.

The prescribing practitioner needs to countersign the order within a time frame as specified by the facility's policy. Fax machines have decreased the need for lengthy or complicated telephone orders, both saving time and avoiding error. To confirm the prescribing practitioner's identity as the initiator of the fax orders, telephone the prescribing practitioner. The prescribing practitioner needs to countersign the fax orders according to agency policy.

INCIDENT REPORTS

Incident reports, or occurrence reports, are used to document any unusual occurrence or accident in the delivery of client care, such as falls or medication errors. The *Code for Nurses* (ANA, 1985) states that nurses are expected "to protect the client when safety is affected." Ethical practice requires that nurses file an incident report to protect the client, not to punish the caregiver.

The filing of incident reports is not only an internal device for the facility but also a requirement by federal, national, and state accrediting agencies. Nurses are often advised not to document the filing of an incident report in the nurses' notes for legal reasons, but as previously discussed, documenting medication errors requires an incident report and documentation in the nurses' notes to ensure that the client receives safe care.

The incident report serves two functions:

1. It informs the facility's administration of the incident, so risk management personnel can consider changes that might prevent similar occurrences in the future.
2. It alerts the facility's insurance company to a potential claim and the need for further investigation.

Litigation can be avoided if the facility takes prompt action by investigating an occurrence. The incident report is not part of the medical record, but it may be used later in litigation.

Each person with firsthand knowledge of the occurrence should fill out and sign a separate report. Although the incident report format varies from one facility to another, key elements must be addressed when filing a report:

- Record the date, exact time, and place you discovered the occurrence.
- Identify the person(s) involved in the occurrence, including witnesses.
- Document accurately and objectively the exact occurrences that you witnessed or first saw after the incident:

NURSING PROCESS HIGHLIGHT

Implementation

Documentation of Client Fall

Assessment

- Check for bruises, lacerations, or abrasions.
- Check blood pressure, pulse, respirations.
- Perform a neurologic assessment (slurred speech, weakness, mental status).
- Check for incontinency (urinary or fecal).
- Note any pain or deformity in the extremities (arm, lumbar spine, hip, or leg).

Interview the Client

- Were there any symptoms prior to the fall (lightheadedness, impaired vision, dizziness, weakness, palpitations, shortness of breath, chest pain)?
- What were your actions prior to the fall (movements, muscle jerks, breathing pattern)?
- How did the fall occur (getting out of bed, while walking in the room)?
- Did anyone witness the fall?

Be sure to chart what you observe ("Client prone on floor"), not what you conclude ("Client fell out of bed"). Document all data in the nurses' progress notes and on the incident report.

▼ SAFETY FIRST ▼

DOCUMENTATION ERRORS

Charting procedures or medications before they are completed constitutes a documentation error; the error can cause a client to miss a dose of medication or a treatment and can confuse, misrepresent, or mask a client's real condition. Likewise, errors are committed when nurses fail to document observations of the client such as deterioration, pain, or agitation or particular signs of complications related to the illness or therapies.

For example, record, "Found the client sitting on the floor. Client stated that …" rather than "Client fell."

- Record the exact details, in time sequence, of what happened, and the consequences for the persons involved.
- Record your actions to provide care and results of your assessment for injuries and client complaints.
- Notify the supervisor on duty and record the time and name of the prescribing practitioner notified; if telephone orders were received from the prescribing practitioner, document as previously discussed and implement the orders.
- Do not record your opinions, judgments, conclusions, or assumptions about what occurred; point blame; or suggest how to prevent occurrence of a similar incident.
- Forward the incident report to the designated person as defined in the facility's policy.

As an additional safeguard, the nurse can write a brief, accurate description of the incident and keep it at home. In the description, include the details of the incident and the names of the people who were involved, especially if they can substantiate the information. Lawsuits may take several years from the time of an incident until the case goes to court; personal notes will help with accurate recall of the incident. Use the same elements described earlier in filing an incident report because your personal notes may be read by the plaintiff's attorney.

Special attention should be given to documenting falls; client falls are the main reason nurses are sued. (See Chapter 29 for information on how to prevent client falls and their legal ramifications.) The Nursing Process Highlight identifies the required nursing documentation when a client falls.

COMPUTERS IN NURSING

Documentation is not the only reason registered nurses must have a basic level of computer literacy. Nurses are involved in many activities that require computer technology: administrative nursing functions such as staffing and quality assurance, educating nurses and clients, communicating with health care providers and clients, and accessing EBP and conducting research.

THE PROFESSIONAL NURSE AS AN INFORMATION CONSUMER AND PRODUCER

"Healthcare delivery systems are knowledge-intensive settings with nurses as the largest group of knowledge workers within those systems" (Hebda & Czar, 2009, p. 7). According to the Institute of Medicine (2007), there is a failure on the part of the present health care delivery system to consistently translate new knowledge into practice and apply new technologies safely, appropriately, and expediently. When nurses learn and use IT such as research-driven evidence-based care or online drug databases, this new knowledge can have a positive outcome on client care. IT tools can assist nurses in

expanding decision-making skills and client monitoring. Hebda and Czar (2009, pp. 9–10) provide these examples:

- Data gatherer: The nurse collects clinical data such as vital signs.
- Information user: The nurse interprets and structures clinical data, such as a client's pain, into information that can be used to assist clinical decision making and client monitoring.
- Knowledge user: The nurse takes individual client data and compares them with existing nursing knowledge.
- Knowledge builder: The nurse aggregates clinical data and shows patterns across clients that serve to create new knowledge or can be interpreted within the context of existing nursing knowledge.

Data collected and documented by nurses using automated systems can benefit other health care professionals such as aggregate critical pathways and laboratory and pharmacy information systems. The interface of these systems eliminates redundant data collection such as client allergies, current medications, demographic data, and diagnoses.

INFORMATICS COMPETENCIES FOR NURSES

The 1998 Pew Health Professions Commission recommended 21 competencies for health care professionals in the twenty-first century (see Chapter 1). One of the Pew competencies addresses the need to use communication and IT effectively and appropriately. The American Association of Colleges in Nursing (AACN) endorsed a new set of competency standards that will enhance the ability of baccalaureate-prepared nurses to provide safe, high-quality client care. Of the 9 essential competencies identified by AACN, 1 addresses the need for professional nursing practice to be grounded in the analysis and application of evidence for practice. Informatics competencies are deemed necessary to facilitate the delivery of safer, more efficient care; to add to the knowledge base for the profession; and to transition toward EBP. "The federal mandate that all Americans have an electronic medical record by 2014 makes informatics competencies necessary for all healthcare professionals" (Hebda & Czar, 2009, p. 15).

The competencies for the beginning nurse focus primarily on the ability to retrieve and enter data in an electronic format that supports client care, analyze and interpret information in planning care, use informatics applications designed for nursing practice, and implement polices relevant to information. The ANA (2007) has identified the following informatics competencies for the beginning nurse:

- The ability to demonstrate basic computer literacy, inclusive of basic desktop applications and electronic communications
- The ability to use IT to support clinical and administrative processes such as information literacy to support EBP
- The ability to access data and perform documentation with computerized records
- The ability to support safety initiatives through the use of IT
- The ability to define the role of informatics in nursing

The ANA has also identified competencies for the experienced nurse and the informatics nurse.

NI competencies are also available on the TIGER (Technology Informatics Guiding Educational Reform) Web site and the Quality and Safety Education for Nurses (QSEN) site. The TIGER competencies are organized into four domains: basic computer, information literacy, information management and informatics, and attitude and awareness. The QSEN site was developed as part of a Robert Wood Johnson–funded project designed to facilitate reform in nursing education in the areas of quality and safety.

As communications and technology continue to evolve, competencies will need to be frequently reviewed and updated in contexts such as education, practice, and administration (Hebda & Czar, 2009). Educators must ensure that students have the knowledge, skills, and attitudes to fully engage in the technology of nursing practice. Nurses in practice must develop an attitude of continuous learning while nurse administrators must strive to assess and evaluate staff competencies, offer continuing education in core competencies, and continuously advocate for improvement in IT (Androwick, Kraft, & Haas, 2008).

APPLICATIONS OF NURSING INFORMATICS

"Nursing is a function of healthcare, which is, increasingly, a business that reflects and responds to the society in which it operates" (Simpson, 2008, p. 253). IT has to be part of health care change to support the work of health care professionals and consumers. Hebda and Czar (2009, pp. 35–36) cite the following examples of how informatics and computers support various areas of nursing and consumer health. Nursing education:

- Online course registration and scheduling and completion of mandatory education requirements
- Course delivery and support for Web-based education
- Computerized student tracking, testing, grade management, and communications with students
- Access to remote library and Internet resources
- Capability for podcasts, Webcasts, teleconferencing, and presentation of prepared slides and handouts

Nurse educators are challenged to transform curricula and teaching methods to integrate information resources into the cognitive, psychomotor, and organizational processes of professional practice (see Uncovering the Evidence). Nursing practice:

- Staff reminders of planned nursing interventions and documentation prompts to ensure comprehensive charting
- Computer-generated nursing care plans, critical pathways, and client documentation such as discharge instructions and medication information
- Monitoring devices for vital signs and other measurements directly into the client's record
- Automatic billing for supplies or procedures with documentation

- Access to computer-archived client data from previous encounters
- Online drug information

Nursing research:

- Computerized literature searching
- Standardized language related to nursing terms
- Internet access for obtaining data collection tools and conducting research
- Collaboration with other researchers

IT applications regarding consumer health may include communications with health care providers through e-mail and instant messaging, online scheduling of tests or procedures, support groups, and remote monitoring and other teleheath services. Information access has fostered consumerism that will make all of health care more accountable (Simpson, 2008).

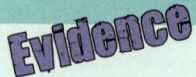

UNCOVERING THE Evidence

TITLE OF STUDY

"One Strategy to Reduce Medication Errors: The Effect of an Online Continuing Education Module on Nurses' Use of the Lexi-Comp Feature of the Pyxis MedStation 2000"

AUTHOR

M. Straight

PURPOSE

To evaluate the impact of an online self-learning module on nurse knowledge and use of the Lexi-Comp feature of the Pyxis MedStation Rx 2000 system, a point-of-care medication delivery system.

METHODS

Data were collected among nurse-users at a community-based health care organization (N = 41). Pre- and posttraining surveys were used to evaluate training effects.

FINDINGS

Posttraining, completion of the tutorial and knowledge and use of the Lexi-Comp feature increased by 23% and 53%, respectively. One month posttraining, a drop in medication error on administration was observed.

IMPLICATIONS

These findings suggest that evaluative and instructional tools improve integration of technology and clinical practice and improve client outcomes in medication error reduction.

Straight, M. (2008). One strategy to reduce medication errors: The effect of an online continuing education module on nurses' use of the Lexi-Comp feature of the Pyxis MedStation 2000. *CIN: Computers, Informatics, Nursing, 26*(1), 23–30.

TELEHEALTH SERVICES

Consult with colleagues
Assess and monitor clients
View diagnostic images
Review slides and laboratory reports
Decrease health care costs
Provide health education
Improve the coordination of care
Improve the equity of access to services
Improve the quality of client care

Hebda, T., & Czar, P. (2009). *Handbook of informatics for nurses & healthcare professionals*. Upper Saddle River, NJ: Pearson Prentice Hall.

Nursing administration has a set of applications to assist with staff scheduling and online bidding for unfilled shifts, electronic mail, cost analysis and budget trends, quality assurance and outcomes analysis, and client tracking and placement of case management (Hebda & Czar, 2009). One of the greatest challenges to chief nurse executives is to select and implement IT enabling tools that allow nurses to learn continuously while never losing sight of nursing's caring mission (Simpson, 2008).

TELEHEALTH

One of the goals of Healthy People 2010 includes eliminating health disparities among populations and improving quality of life and life expectancy. Telehealth is seen as a venue for improving health care access in vulnerable populations through the use of electronic devices in the clients' homes that monitor and assess for early complications (Prinz, Cramer, & Englund, 2008).

Telehealth refers to the use of telecommunication technologies and computers to exchange health care information and to provide services to clients at another location such as health promotion, disease prevention, diagnosis, consultation, education, and therapy. Telehealth nursing refers to the utilization of the nursing process via telecommunications devices with individual clients or defined client populations (Prinz et al., 2008). Telehealth devices allow the nurse to monitor pulse oximetry, heart rate, blood pressure, and weight. Some of the tools used to support these services are voice only (regular telephone), video images (digital pictures), data exchange (keyboard and mouse operations), and virtual contact (videoconferencing); see the Box on the following page regarding some of the professional services provided by telehealth.

EVIDENCE-BASED PRACTICE AND RESEARCH

Client safety is the dominant principle on which all nursing care is based; nursing has an ethical obligation to the client to use all the resources at its disposal to ensure client safety (Straight, 2008). Although technologies such as electronic medical records and barcoding allow nurses to make treatment decisions and ensure proper medications are being administered, none of the technologies address the need for instant access to human knowledge and expertise through timely communications. In health care, the ability to communicate information clearly, accurately, and promptly is vital to providing the best possible care for clients and ensuring that no critical matters involving a client's well-being are overlooked or left unattended (Kuruzovich, Angst, Faraj, & Agarwal, 2008).

EBP is an approach to providing care that integrates nursing experience and intuition with valid and current clinical research to achieve best client outcomes (Salmond, 2007). Although there is agreement that EBP is imperative for ensuring quality, cost-effective, safe care and more predictable outcomes for health care consumers, the initial expectations have not been fully realized, and there is little evidence showing how use in practice brings the intended value. There are issues with standardized nursing terminologies—the NANDA, NOC, and NIC versus the languages recognized by the ANA's Committee on Nursing Practice Information Infrastructure—for incorporation into the EHR. Nurses and administrators need education to appreciate the importance and power of standardized language so that nursing records can be integrated with other records to support communication and retrieval of critical information.

EBP requires the application of current research. To apply research to practice, the nurse must be knowledgeable about the research process; specifically, the nurse must be able to perform a research synthesis (systematic review). A research synthesis is a review of a clearly formulated question that uses systematic and explicit methods to identify, select, and critically appraise relevant research and to collect and analyze data from the studies (Newhouse, 2008). Stevens (2008) recommends the steps outlined in the *Cochrane Handbook* for conducting a systematic review: Evidence should be reviewed by two people, the approach should be explicit, evidence should be rated and graded, and both reviewers should produce recommendations for practice. The Cochrane Collaboration and *Worldviews on Evidence-Based Nursing* are reliable sources for systematic reviews in nursing. EBP is possible only as a result of IT's ability to collect, aggregate, and present client and practice data whenever and wherever nurses need it in the provision of care (Simpson, 2008).

CRITERIA FOR EVALUATING VALIDITY OF INFORMATION

Professional accountability requires all health care providers to critically evaluate the quality of online information and assist consumers to judge all retrieved materials. According to Hebda and Czar (2009), the following criteria should be used to evaluate online resources:

1. Credentials of the source: Large professional associations such as hospitals, universities, government, and official health organizations tend to have the most reliable Web sites.

2. Ability to validate information: When facts and studies are cited, the original source should be retrieved for review, allowing the user to draw conclusions.

3. Accuracy: Internet content should identify contact persons or cite references that may be checked to allow evaluation of posted information.

4. Comprehensiveness of information: If the site is comprehensive, it should have all relevant information on that site; for example, if the site deals with medications, it should discuss indications, contraindications, protocols, and dosage.

5. Date of issue or revision: All valid Web sites should indicate when material was written, revised, or reviewed so that the user can determine if the information is current or outdated.

6. Bias or sponsorship: The content should be well organized, with hyperlinks to current Web pages, and load easily.

7. Intended purpose and audience: Terminology and reading level should be appropriate for the intended audience.

8. Disclaimers: Sites that allow for individual opinions should contain a statement to that effect to help users distinguish between fact and opinion.

9. Site of accreditation: To ensure the quality of information found on health-related Web sites, some sites display a "seal" that indicates that the site has voluntarily met a set of predetermined standards for the quality of information posted.

10. Privacy policies: Sites that collect personal information need to identify how that information may be used so the user can determine whether to disclose the information.

Material found on the Internet and Web should be credited to the authors, just like any other media; failure to cite sources is copyright infringement.

KEY CONCEPTS

- Informatics is the application of computer and statistical techniques to the management of information.

- Nursing informatics is the use of information and computer technology as a tool to process information to support all areas of nursing.

- A health care information system consists of clinical and administrative systems.

- A nursing information system using the nursing process approach should support the use and documentation of nursing processes and provide tools for managing nursing care activities.

- Critical pathways or protocol approaches to nursing information systems provide a multidisciplinary format for planning and documenting client care.

- Documentation provides a system of written records that reflect client care provided on the basis of assessment data and the client's response to interventions.

- The medical record can be used by health care students as a teaching tool and is a main source of data for clinical research.

- Nurses are responsible for assessing and documenting that the client has an understanding of the treatment prior to the intervention.

- Competent adult clients have the right, through an advance directive, to make decisions regarding life-sustaining interventions when they become incapacitated or terminally ill.

- Standards of care, as set forth by state boards of nursing and the ANA, require nurses to use the nursing process in their documentation.

- Accreditation and reimbursement agencies require accurate and thorough documentation of the nursing care rendered and the client's response to interventions.

- Effective documentation requires clear, concise, accurate recording of all client care and other significant events in an organized and chronological fashion, representative of each phase of the nursing process.

- Client safety requires appropriate reporting and recording of medication errors and other occurrences in compliance with the facility's policy, as well as the avoidance of dangerous abbreviations and inappropriate use of the decimal point.

- Narrative charting requires an organized presentation of the client's problems and response to interventions in chronological order.

- Problem-oriented charting provides structure when documenting the client's problems and responses in the nurses' progress notes.

- Computerized documentation saves time, increases legibility and accuracy, provides standardized nursing terminology, enhances the nursing process and decision-making skills, and supports continuity of care.

- Technology advances are providing systems that promote client safety such as the electronic administration system.

- Managed care incorporates client participation in planning the care while focusing on the quality of care provided in a timely fashion.

- Critical pathways document the key interventions of managed-care plans.

- Flow sheets are used to document assessment findings, activity, measurements, treatments, and equipment.
- The discharge summary is used to highlight the client's illness, course of care, and aftercare instructions.
- Incident reports are used to document any unusual occurrence in the delivery of client care.
- The competencies for the beginning nurse focus mainly on developing and using skills that rely on

the ability to retrieve and enter data in an electronic format that is relevant to client care.
- An example of the application of NI is computer-generated client documentation that includes discharge instructions and medication information.
- As technology advances, it ensures that telehealth can emerge as a viable solution to providing accessible, quality health care.
- Nurses need to use critical thinking skills to evaluate information found on the Internet.

REVIEW QUESTIONS

1. Which best describes the client's medical record?
   a. It serves as a legal document for recording all client activities assessed and initiated by prescribing practitioners.
   b. It provides a written record for nurses to document all phases of the nursing process.
   c. It is a systematic documentation of critical elements of care performed by nurses.
   d. It contains the client's medical record that can be used for educational purposes.

2. A client tells the nurse, "I have a headache and feel nauseous." This is an example of what type of data?
   a. Assessment
   b. Historical
   c. Subjective
   d. Objective

3. Which of the following charting entries is written in the most accurate way?
   a. Client up, out of bed, walked to the bathroom with assistance, tolerated well.
   b. Client up, out of bed, walked 40 feet to the bathroom and back to bed, tolerated well.
   c. Client up, out of bed, walked 40 feet to the bathroom and back to bed with assistance from the nurse.
   d. Client up, out of bed, walked 40 feet to the bathroom and back to bed with assistance from the nurse, heart rate 84 and regular before exercise, 92 and regular after exercise.

4. The case manager nurse should be assigned to provide services to which of the following clients?
   a. A mother experiencing her first pregnancy
   b. A client with newly diagnosed diabetes mellitus
   c. A client with a broken arm following a bicycle accident

   d. A group of teenagers who are members of SADD (Students against Drunk Driving)

5. The nurse has to document the assessment findings of a surgical incision with staples and retention sutures; however, the pop-up screen on the computer provides for only staples. How should the nurse document the findings regarding the retention sutures?
   a. Document the assessment of the staples on the computer screen, and click to go to the next screen with no mention of the retention sutures.
   b. Document the retention sutures assessment on the paper chart.
   c. Document assessment of the retention sutures as free text in summary notes attached to the appropriate nursing documentation computer page.
   d. Call the surgeon, give an oral report of the assessment findings, and document the phone call in the computerized nursing progress notes.

6. Which of the following actions by the nurse would make her or him more vulnerable to legal action?
   a. Documenting all pertinent client information
   b. Following agency documentation policies
   c. Discussing a client's case with a peer in the elevator
   d. Assisting a client to find appropriate Web sites

7. The major concern in implementing an electronic health record is:
   a. Cost
   b. Utilization
   c. Privacy
   d. Accuracy

online companion

Visit the DeLaune and Ladner online companion resource at **www.delmar.cengage.com** for additional content and study aids. Click on Online Companions, then select the Nursing discipline.

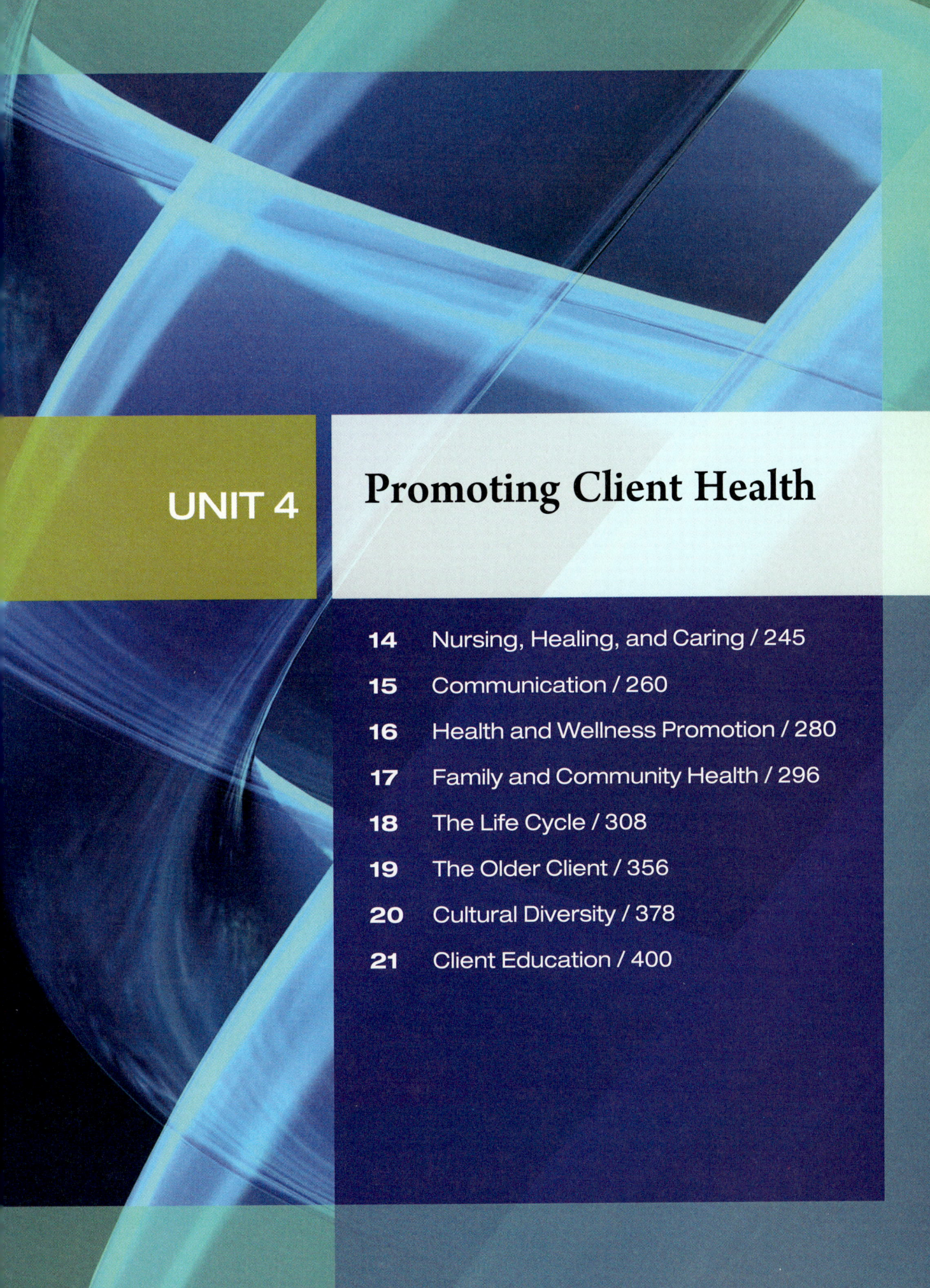

Above all, nursing is caring.

—Diers (1986)

CHAPTER 14

Nursing, Healing, and Caring

COMPETENCIES

1. Describe the influence of caring and compassion on the practice of professional nursing.
2. Explore the value of nursing care in today's technologically advanced health care system.
3. Compare selected perspectives on the relationship between caring and nursing.
4. Explain the primary nursing functions in each phase of the nurse-client relationship.
5. Discuss the impact of communication on the delivery of compassionate care.
6. Describe the characteristics of a therapeutic relationship.
7. Explain nursing roles that are important in demonstrating care and compassion.

KEY TERMS

active listening

attending behaviors

catharsis

client advocate

depersonalization

empathy

empowerment

healing

nurse-client relationship

orientation (or introductory)
   phase

paraverbal communication

presence

rapport

role

termination (or concluding)
   phase

therapeutic

therapeutic relationship

therapeutic use of self

transcultural nursing

working (or exploitative) phase

This chapter presents information about caring—*the fundamental value in nursing*. The relationship between caring and nursing is explored and nursing's impact on healing is examined. The nurse-client relationship is discussed, and the stages of this relationship are described with attendant nursing goals and the behaviors usually exhibited by clients in each stage.

NURSING'S THERAPEUTIC VALUE

Nursing is both an art and a science that leads to therapeutic outcomes in clients. The term **therapeutic** refers to activities that are beneficial to the client. When therapeutic interventions are performed in a caring compassionate manner, an environment that promotes healing is established.

DEFINITION OF NURSING

According to the American Nurses Association (2004), nursing is defined as "the protection, promotion, and optimization of health and abilities, prevention of illness and injury, alleviation of suffering through the diagnosis and treatment of human response, and advocacy in the care of individuals, families, communities, and populations" (p. 7). This definition places nursing's focus on the individual experiencing a health problem rather than on the problem (or disease) itself—that is, on caring for clients as they deal with health issues fundamental to the practice of professional nursing.

The Canadian Nurses Association (1986), similarly, describes nursing as a caring relationship that helps the client achieve and maintain an optimal level of health.

NURSING: A BLEND OF ART AND SCIENCE

Nursing creates therapeutic change through the application of scientific principles. As the science of nursing has rapidly progressed over the past decade, nurse theorists have formulated various frameworks by which to organize nursing's unique body of knowledge. While continuing to expand its theoretical base, nursing must remain firmly rooted in its essence—caring. In other words, nursing does not rely on

science alone. The application of knowledge and skills enables the nurse to value the uniqueness of each client (Warelow, Edward, & Vinek, 2008).

Caring is a universal value that directs nursing practice. Leininger and McFarland (2002, p. 21) define caring in the nurse-client relationship as "the direct (or indirect) nurturant and skillful activities, processes, and decisions related to assisting people to achieve or maintain health." Even though clients cannot always be cured, caring is ongoing within the nurse-client relationship.

A prerequisite for the nursing art is the nurse's commitment to helping the client; this trait is also referred to as intentionality. Intention occurs when we consciously focus on someone in order to learn something about and to help that person (Dossey, Keegan, & Guzzetta, 2008). Caring is more than an intuitive process; it can be learned both intellectually and interpersonally. One learns caring by interacting with others who demonstrate caring. When nurses exhibit caring behaviors, they are serving as role models—to students, colleagues, clients, and families.

PURPOSES OF NURSING

A **therapeutic relationship** is one that benefits the client's health status. The therapeutic relationship is based on the belief that a person has a natural drive toward optimal health. Caring—being willing and able to nurture others—is an attribute of the effective nurse. Curing rids the client of the disease or disability; caring nurtures the person even if the disorder is incurable. When it is understood that complete, or perhaps even partial, recovery is not possible, nursing goals focus on facilitating comfort by alleviating pain and promoting as much client autonomy as possible.

Nursing promotes healthy lifestyle behaviors, prevents the development of illness and injury, and restores individuals to their optimal level of functioning. Another purpose of nursing is to improve client satisfaction with the delivery of health care services.

Consumer satisfaction greatly influences where services are provided. Nurses who demonstrate caring behaviors enhance the quality of care provided; thus, clients are more satisfied with care delivered in a caring, compassionate manner.

NURSING AND HEALING

Nursing is a humanistic discipline that provides care from a holistic framework. Seeing and responding to the client as a whole person instead of a disease, disorder, or case lead to complete care of the total person. Healing is the process of recovery from illness, accident, or disability. This return to an optimum level of functioning may occur rapidly or gradually. Healing encompasses the physical, emotional, and spiritual domains of individuals. Nursing and caring are essential components in the healing process. See Chapter 31 for further discussion of nurses as healers.

THEORETICAL PERSPECTIVES OF CARING

There are numerous theoretical concepts relative to caring in nursing. Some major ideas related to caring have been postulated in Watson's theory of human caring, Leininger and McFarland's theory of transcultural caring, and Benner's novice to expert model; see Table 14-1.

The theory of human caring evolved from Watson's beliefs, values, and assumptions about caring. In Watson's view (2007), care and love comprise the primal, universal psychic energy and are the basis for our humanity.

Watson's theory is composed of 10 carative factors, which are classified as nursing actions or caring processes. Watson's carative factors are:

1. Formation of a humanistic-altruistic system of values
2. Nurturing of faith-hope
3. Cultivation of sensitivity to one's self and to others
4. Developing a helping-trusting, human caring relationship
5. Promotion and acceptance of the expression of positive and negative feelings
6. Use of creative problem-solving method processes
7. Promotion of transpersonal teaching and learning
8. Provision for a supportive, protective, or corrective mental, physical, sociocultural, and spiritual environment
9. Assistance with gratification of human needs
10. Allowance for existential-phenomenological forces (Watson, 2007)

The first 3 carative factors serve as the philosophical foundation for the science of caring. The remaining 7 provide more specific direction for nursing actions.

Transcultural nursing focuses on the study and analysis of different cultures and subcultures with respect to cultural care, health beliefs, and health practices, with the goal of providing health care within the context of the client's culture (Leininger & McFarland, 2002). A basic assumption of transcultural nursing is that when health care providers see problems from the client's cultural viewpoint, they are more open to understanding, appreciating, and working effectively with those clients. Other assumptions of transcultural nursing theory are:

- Every culture has some kind of system for health care that is based on values and behaviors.
- Cultures have certain methods for providing health care. These methods of care are often unknown by nurses from other cultures (Leininger & McFarland, 2002).

TABLE 14-1 Perspectives of Caring in Nursing

THEORIST	THEORY	MAJOR CONCEPTS
Watson	Theory of human caring	- Caring is central to nursing practice. - Emphasis is on the dignity and worth of individuals. - Each person's response to illness is unique. - Caring is demonstrated interpersonally. - Caring involves a commitment to care and is based on knowledge.
Leininger and McFarland	Transcultural care theory	- Caring is the essence of nursing. - Caring is universal, occurring in all cultures. - Caring behaviors are determined by and occur within a cultural context.
Benner	Novice to expert	- Caring is central to all helping professions. - Caring is the foundation of being. - People and interpersonal concerns are important. - Caring is communicated through actions. - Problem solving is a major component of caring. - Advocacy is caring.

Data from Benner, P. (2001). *From novice to expert: Excellence and power in clinical nursing practice* (comm. ed.). Upper Saddle River, NJ: Prentice-Hall; Leininger, M., & McFarland, M. R. (2002). *Transcultural nursing: Concepts, theories, research, and practice* (3rd ed.). New York: McGraw-Hill; Watson, J. (2007). *Nursing: Human science and human care* (rev. ed.). Boston: Jones & Bartlett; Watson, J. (2008). *The philosophy and science of caring* (rev. ed.). Denver: University Press of Colorado.

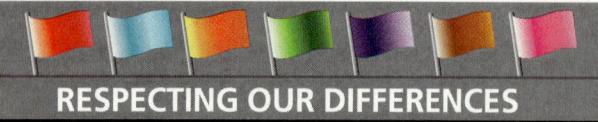

RESPECTING OUR DIFFERENCES

Caring Behaviors That Occur in Different Cultures

Attention	Presence
Comfort	Protection
Compassion	Restoration
Empathy	Support
Instruction	Surveillance
Love	Tenderness
Nurturance	Touch
Personalized help	Trust

Data modified from Leininger, M., & McFarland, M. R. (2002). *Transcultural nursing: Concepts, theories, research, and practice* (3rd ed.). New York: McGraw-Hill.

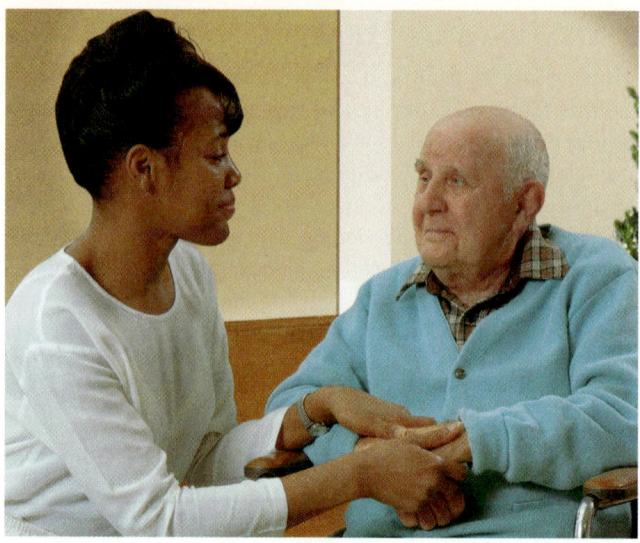

FIGURE 14-1 Clasping the client's hand is one way to communicate caring through touch. DELMAR/CENGAGE LEARNING

Leininger and McFarland identify several behaviors as caring and state that these behaviors occur in various cultures; see the accompanying display on caring behaviors.

Benner (2001, p. 49) describes the caring nurse as one who has "courage to be with the patient, offering whatever comfort the situation allows." Caring occurs within the context of a relationship that consists of several steps. First, hope is mobilized for both the client and nurse. Second, the relationship focuses on discovering the meaning of the illness, pain, or emotion. Finally, the client is aided in using social and spiritual support (Benner, 2001).

Caring—being willing and able to nurture others—is a hallmark of the effective nurse. It occurs when a nurse acts in a genuine, authentic manner with the client. Caring is a process and an art that requires commitment and knowledge; it is a combination of behaviors and attitudes. The way in which nursing actions are implemented expresses caring. Specific behaviors that indicate caring are provision of information, relief of pain, spending time with clients and families, and promoting client autonomy. Treating each client in a dignified, courteous manner is the true expression of caring.

Touch is an effective method for communicating a sense of caring (see Figure 14-1). Touch is a powerful nonverbal medium for communication that can be used to soothe, comfort, and establish rapport. It can communicate a sense of caring—as it does when a nurse holds a person's hand during

SAFETY FIRST

Avoid touching clients who are suspicious, hostile, or very confused as the nurse's intent may be misinterpreted.

a painful procedure—or it can be perceived as intrusive or hostile. Touch, no matter how well intended, may sometimes be misinterpreted by a client; see the Safety First display.

CARE IN THE HIGH-TECHNOLOGY ENVIRONMENT

Caring is the soul of nursing. Nurses demonstrate caring in various ways, such as anticipating client requests and providing information. Clients feel supported and more comfortable in the presence of a nurse who, through caring, helps alleviate fears and anxieties. Although technological advances have resulted in many possibilities in health care, the major risk of reliance on technology is that clients may be perceived as objects. The focus of attention becomes the disease, instead of the individual experiencing the illness. The compassionate nurse treats each client with respect and dignity.

Depersonalization is the process in which individuals are treated as objects instead of people. Some examples of dehumanizing actions are checking on the equipment and not the person, failing to respond to the client, and communicating a lack of interest in what the client says. When the machinery becomes the focus of the nurse's activities, depersonalization of the client is likely to occur. Critical care nursing, with its multiple technological activities, presents a challenge to the development of a therapeutic nurse-client relationship (O'Connell, 2008). Spending time with the client is one way to counteract depersonalization; see Figure 14-2.

Nursing care counteracts depersonalization by emphasizing a client's individuality. It is through caring that the nurse humanizes the client. The reason people are admitted to acute care facilities is to receive nursing care. Caring is what clients want and need most from nurses. While receiving care, people want to be treated with compassion. The nontechnical element of care makes clients feel cared for as individuals; the use of high-touch activities communicates

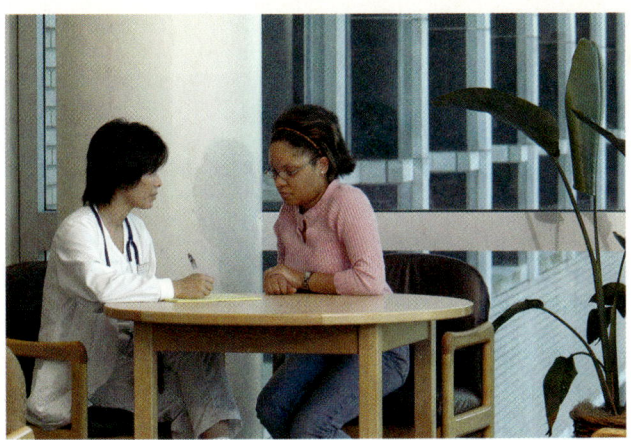

FIGURE 14-2 Nursing is caring. It is showing concern for and interest in the client. Identify behaviors of the nurse that demonstrate caring. DELMAR/CENGAGE LEARNING

UNCOVERING THE

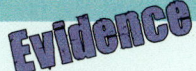

TITLE OF STUDY

"The Challenges of Caring in a Technological Environment: Critical Care Nurses' Experiences"

AUTHOR

M. McGrath

PURPOSE

To examine the behaviors and feelings of experienced critical care nurses in a technological setting.

METHODS

Data, which were collected from unstructured interviews with 10 critical care nurses, were analyzed according to the Walters data analysis system.

FINDINGS

The use of technology may create an "alien environment" by increasing distance between the nurse and client. However, this study demonstrates that experienced critical care nurses can use technology to increase the bond between nurses and clients and families.

IMPLICATIONS

Experienced critical care nurses can transcend the barrier created by technology. However, nursing education should place more emphasis on the use of technology in order to help novice nurses bridge the chasm sometimes created by technology.

McGrath, M. (2008). The challenges of caring in a technological environment: Critical care nurses' experiences. *Journal of Clinical Nursing, 17*(8), 1096–1104.

caring. As society continues to place a high value on technology, caring is often undervalued. Nurses make a crucial contribution by valuing both care *and* technology.

Although the concept of caring is being de-emphasized in today's health care environment because of exploding technology and cost-containment strategies, nursing must persevere in delivering compassionate care to clients. The challenge of nursing is to create moments of caring through human-to-human interaction in the face of the fast-paced world of health care. "Caring professionals need to balance state-of-the-art technology with integrated and comprehensive care" (Almerud, Alapack, Fridlund, & Ekebergh, 2008, p. 136).

NURSE-CLIENT RELATIONSHIP

Caring is communicated interpersonally; thus, the vehicle for communicating a caring intent is the nurse-client relationship. The **nurse-client relationship** is the one-to-one interactive process between client and nurse that is directed at improving the client's health status or assisting in problem solving. The primary goal of the relationship is the client's achievement of therapeutic outcomes. The nurse-client relationship is a planned process that focuses on meeting the needs of the client. There are many differences between the therapeutic nurse-client relationship and a social relationship; see Table 14-2 on page 250.

The interactive process between client and nurse greatly influences the client's progress in healing. Peplau (1952), the first nurse theorist to define nursing as an interpersonal process, viewed the nurse-client relationship as the basis of nursing. Interpersonal skills are the foundation for establishing the therapeutic relationship. Only through interacting does the nurse have the ability to adequately assess the client's needs, teach methods for best meeting those needs, empower the client to achieve goals, and evaluate the outcome of nursing interventions.

PHASES OF THERAPEUTIC RELATIONSHIP

The three phases of the nurse-client relationship are orientation, working, and termination. These phases overlap and influence each other. Each phase is characterized by specific client behaviors and nursing goals. Figure 14-3 on page 250 illustrates the phases of the interactive relationship.

Orientation Phase

The **orientation (or introductory) phase** is the first stage of the therapeutic relationship, in which the nurse and client become acquainted with each other, establish trust, and determine the expectations of the other. Usually, the only knowledge the client and nurse have of each other is preconceived ideas. The nurse gets to know the client as an individual by giving up biases and judgmental thoughts. The orientation stage is especially important because it is the time in which the foundation for the relationship is established.

TABLE 14-2 Comparison of Social and Therapeutic Relationships

SOCIAL	THERAPEUTIC
• Is spontaneous, just happens. • Is mutually beneficial. • Often has no planned agenda. • Is based on mutual interests. • Each participant expects to be liked by the other. • Problems are shared. • Communication is spontaneous.	• Is planned and goal directed. • Seeks to meet clients' needs. • Is based on theory. • Privileged information is available to health care provider. • Clients are emotionally vulnerable. • Clients must be accepted as they are. • Communication is planned. • Has clear-cut boundaries.

Delmar/Cengage Learning

CLIENT BEHAVIORS The usual response of the client in the orientation stage is anxiety, which can result from several factors including:

• Fear of the unknown
• Pain or distress
• Unfamiliar environment
• Undergoing unfamiliar, often painful, procedures
• Loss of freedom and control

As a result of the client's insecurity, anxiety escalates. Because anxiety is communicated interpersonally, the nurse should project a calm, relaxed attitude during every interaction with the client to decrease anxiety.

Another behavior frequently exhibited by the client during the orientation stage is testing. The client attempts to determine the degree of the nurse's trustworthiness. Through behavior, the client is asking:

• Is the nurse truly willing to help?
• Is the nurse competent to help?
• Is the nurse reliable and trustworthy?

The nurse answers such questions through consistent, reliable behavior that promotes the development of trust.

NURSE BEHAVIORS The most important nursing actions during the orientation phase are assessment and creating a climate conducive to rapport. The nurse must determine the client's needs, knowledge base, strengths and limitations, coping mechanisms, and support system. Often clients do not express their needs directly; behavior is the only clue to their needs. The nurse's goal is to determine the real meaning of the behavior and to assess the client's perception of the most crucial needs and problems.

To reduce a client's anxiety and promote trust, the nurse provides some specific information. Information the client should receive during the orientation phase includes:

• Nurse's name
• Nurse's role
• Reasons the nurse must ask questions
• Confidentiality and its parameters

See the Spotlight On display, which addresses confidentiality.

Working Phase

The **working (or exploitative) phase** is the second stage of the therapeutic relationship, in which problems are identified,

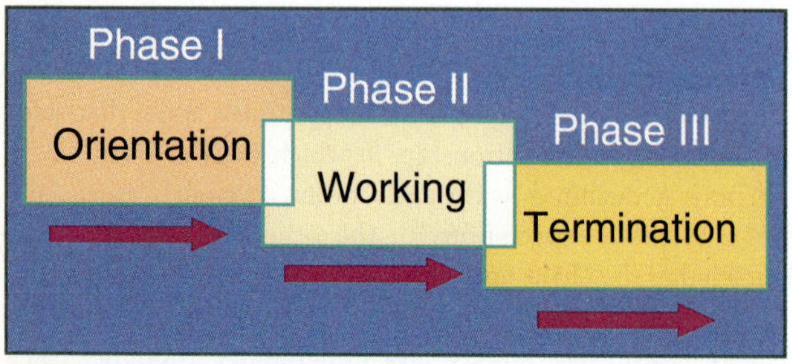

FIGURE 14-3 Phases of the Nurse-Client Relationship DELMAR/CENGAGE LEARNING

SPOTLIGHT ON...

Legal/Ethical

Confidentiality in the Therapeutic Relationship

Nurses have ethical and legal responsibilities to protect client confidentiality. Consider what you would do in each of the following situations:

You are assisting Ms. Adams with her AM care when she says, "Isn't it just terrible about Mr. Denton across the hall? I heard his tests came back negative. What are his chances of making it?"

Your neighbor asks you if a mutual friend is being treated for AIDS.

In a crowded elevator at work, you overhear two coworkers discussing a client's condition.

goals are established, and problem-solving methods are selected. Attainable goals play an important part in the client's perception of control (Reb, 2007). Actions are chosen after carefully considering both the consequences of actions and the client's values. It is necessary to consider the client's value system when determining problem-solving methods. Client participation increases when consideration of values is incorporated into care planning. It is important that nurses consider clients' feelings of personal control and intervene to increase perceptions of control, especially for clients treated in inpatient facilities (Williams, Dawson, & Kristjanson, 2008).

CLIENT BEHAVIORS The client engages with the nurse in active problem solving to achieve mutually developed outcomes. Behaviors that indicate the client is in the working phase are:

- Asking questions about his or her own problems
- Seeking clarification from the nurse
- Being attentive to instructions
- Asking for more information about his or her own role in recovery

NURSE BEHAVIORS The nurse seeks to maximize the client's success in problem solving. Nursing goals to be achieved during the working phase are to:

- Reevaluate goals and related activities as new information arises
- Support realistic problem-solving activities of the client

Termination Phase

The **termination (or concluding) phase**, the third and final stage of the therapeutic relationship, focuses on the evaluation of goal achievement and effectiveness of treatment. It is important that the client has been prepared for the final stage of the relationship by encouraging discussion of feelings.

CLIENT BEHAVIORS Some clients welcome this final phase, whereas other clients who have become overly dependent on their nurse will be more resistant to saying goodbye. Planning for termination is actually initiated during the beginning of the relationship. A relationship that ends abruptly is likely to place the client at risk for difficulties such as increased:

- Anxiety levels
- Frustration
- Suspiciousness
- Unwillingness to engage in future relationships with health care providers

NURSE BEHAVIORS Evaluation is the primary goal for the client and nurse in the third stage of the nurse-client relationship. Questions to be answered include:

- Were the goals meaningful?
- Were the goals realistic?
- Were the client and family actively involved?

See the Nursing Checklist, which can be used to evaluate skills in establishing a therapeutic nurse-client relationship.

THERAPEUTIC USE OF SELF

The interpersonal process between nurse and client is a therapeutic process because interventions are planned and implemented to benefit the client. The nurse's most effective tool for helping the client is the **therapeutic use of self**, a process in which nurses deliberately plan their actions and approach the relationship with a specific goal in mind before interacting with the client. The nurse's most effective tool for demonstrating caring is not some technologically sophisticated machine but rather one's self. Figure 14-4 illustrates therapeutic use of self. Therapeutic use of self provides an opportunity for the nurse and client to make a person-to-person connection. The term **presence** refers to the process of "just being with" another. Presence requires the nurse to demonstrate patience in a caring manner.

Therapeutic use of self involves verbal and nonverbal communication. Just as important as what one says is *how* one says it. With a deliberate, planned approach, the nurse communicates a sense of caring and willingness to help: The nurse is committed to helping clients find ways to help themselves. The nurse's true expression of humanistic concern for a client is shown by taking the time to simply be with the client.

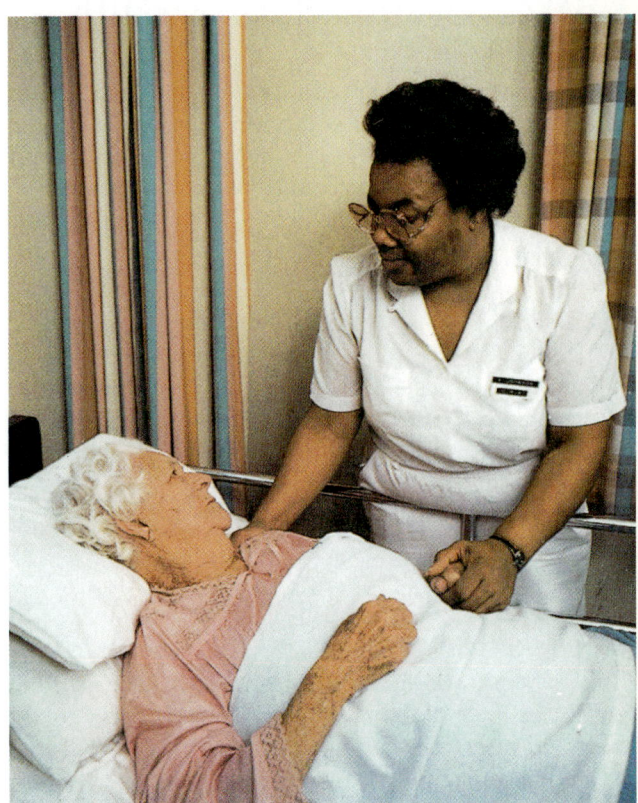

FIGURE 14-4 In this situation, what factors indicate that rapport has been established between nurse and client? DELMAR/CENGAGE LEARNING

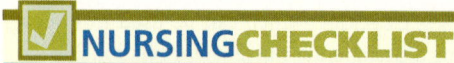

NURSINGCHECKLIST

ESTABLISHING THERAPEUTIC RELATIONSHIPS

- Introduce self on initial contact
- Explain own role
- Develop groundwork for trust
- Establish therapeutic boundaries
- Determine client's perception of problem(s)
- Understand client's expectations of care
- Communicate at client's level of comprehension
- Involve client in evaluating treatment

CARING AND COMMUNICATION

Communication is the mechanism for demonstrating compassion and caring. Therapeutic communication is deliberately planned by the nurse to result in positive client outcomes.

Therapeutic communication:

- Is purposeful and goal-directed
- Has well-defined boundaries
- Is client-focused
- Is nonjudgmental
- Uses well-planned, selected techniques

There are numerous techniques that are helpful in promoting therapeutic communication; see Chapter 15 for an explanation of these techniques.

CHARACTERISTICS OF THERAPEUTIC RELATIONSHIPS

Compassionate delivery of care is based on the establishment of a therapeutic relationship between client and nurse. In order to establish therapeutic relationships, the nurse must possess certain interpersonal skills. Some characteristics of therapeutic nurses are:

- Warmth
- Hope
- Rapport
- Trust
- Empathy
- Acceptance
- Humor
- Compassion
- Self-awareness
- Flexibility
- Risk taking
- Active listening
- Nonjudgmental approach

Catharsis, which refers to the relief experienced from verbalizing one's problems, is often referred to as "getting things off one's chest." It is a universal experience that is therapeutic for individuals experiencing stress.

Nurses use interpersonal skills to help clients express their feelings and meet their needs. A discussion of each characteristic follows.

Warmth

Warmth is the demonstration of positive behaviors toward the client. Respect, genuine interest, caring—all are expressions of warmth. The nurse who demonstrates warmth is approachable and available rather than aloof. Warmth means projecting an interested attitude without overwhelming the client. The nurse demonstrating warmth responds to the client as one human being to another. The therapeutic nurse is approachable and available yet maintains objective boundaries.

Hope

Hope means anticipating the future by helping clients look realistically at their potential. Hope is strengthened by relationships with others; social isolation reinforces a sense of despair. Many clients, especially those with great losses, experience distress, despair, and hopelessness. The reemergence of hope may be a gradual process. Hope is not to be confused with false reassurance, which is countertherapeutic; see the accompanying Spotlight On display.

Providing opportunities for clients to socialize and making resources available are two ways in which nurses can help instill hope in clients. Hope is necessary for coping with severe stressors, such as illness. Nurses must determine the client's source of hope, which may include the following:

- Relationships with others
- Positive emotions
- Anticipating the future
- Availability of resources

The instillation of hope helps clients meet their spiritual needs. Since spirituality is closely related to hope, nurses can also assess clients' spiritual needs to determine which interventions are most appropriate; see Chapter 24.

SPOTLIGHT ON...

Caring and Compassion

Hope Versus False Reassurance

Consider the following example of false reassurance. Mrs. Ngyuen is awaiting results of diagnostic testing that will confirm or deny the suspected diagnosis of cancer. She says to her nurse, "I think it's taking a long time to get the results. Something must be wrong." The nurse replies, "Oh, don't worry, everything's going to be just fine!"

What do you suppose motivated the nurse's response?

What will be the impact of the nurse's behavior on Mrs. Ngyuen?

Rapport

Rapport is a bond between two people that is based on mutual trust. This connection does not just happen spontaneously; it is planned by the nurse who purposefully implements behaviors that promote trust. When seeking to establish trust, the nurse recognizes the client as a unique individual and reinforces that individuality. In other words, actions that humanize the client are therapeutic. To establish rapport, the nurse's actions show that the client is considered important. Actions are implemented to boost the level of the client's self-esteem. Nonverbal interventions are of utmost importance in helping establish rapport.

Interacting with family and significant others is also helpful in establishing rapport with the client (see Figure 14-5). Recognizing the importance of the family's influence on the healing process allows the nurse to bond with those who will encourage and support the client. "The nurse must know when to move aside and allow family members a greater role in the care of the patient and when to relieve the family member" (Benner, 2001, p. 66).

Trust

Trust must be present for help to be given and received. A therapeutic relationship is firmly rooted in trust. The nurse sets the tone of the relationship by creating an atmosphere in which the client feels free to express feelings. How does the nurse promote a trusting relationship? Three major activities will facilitate the development of trust: *consistency, respect,* and *honesty.* Table 14-3 lists actions that facilitate the development of trust. The basis of trust is a caring relationship that is essential for most nursing interventions. Being consistently trustworthy is an expression of the nurse's personal integrity and builds the foundation for a therapeutic relationship.

Empathy

Empathy—understanding another person's perception of the situation—is a key element in the therapeutic relationship. The phrase "Walk a mile in my shoes" describes empathy

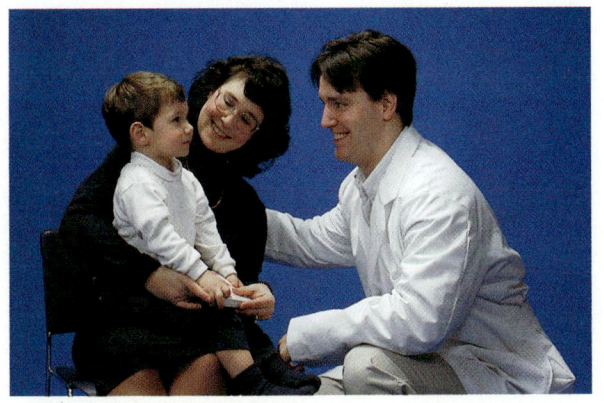

FIGURE 14-5 Through interaction with the client's family, how can the nurse help the client obtain optimal health? DELMAR/
CENGAGE LEARNING

TABLE 14-3 Trust: Essential Behaviors		
CONSISTENCY	**RESPECT**	**HONESTY**
• Follow through on plans.	• Call client by name.	• Ask client about personal preferences.
• Adhere to schedule.	• Provide clear explanations.	• Keep any promises.
• Seek out client for extra time to interact.	• Recognize own strengths and limitations.	• Maintain confidentiality.
• Be straightforward; no hidden motives.	• Listen to client.	• Be flexible in responding to requests.

Delmar/Cengage Learning

well. The empathic nurse understands that the client's perception of the situation is real to the client. By perceiving clients' understanding of their own needs, the nurse is better able to assist clients in determining which actions are most appropriate. Empathy enables the nurse to assist the client to become a fully participating partner in treatment rather than a passive recipient of care.

Through empathy, the nurse validates the experiences of the client. The challenge for the nurse is to see the world from the client's perspective with as much understanding as possible. This involves understanding the client's perspective and communicating that understanding to the client. According to Kirk (2007), empathy is built on intentionality. Empathy is not the same as sympathy. Sympathy is rarely therapeutic; in fact, a barrier occurs when the nurse sympathizes and becomes paralyzed by the expression of pity. For example, empathic listening allows the nurse to encourage clients to find meaning in their experiences and move on to problem solving.

Acceptance

Accepting the client as a person worthy of dignity and respect is basic to providing nursing care. Acceptance means compassionately working with clients, even those who demonstrate negative behaviors. It is extremely important for the nurse to show acceptance of the client while setting limits on unhealthy or undesirable behavior. The accepting nurse conveys the message that the client does not have to put on a front. The client knows it is safe to be genuine because of the nurse's acceptance; see the accompanying Spotlight On display.

Active Listening

Active listening (listening that focuses on the speaker) is the basic skill for interpersonal effectiveness. Active listening is facilitated by **attending behaviors**, a set of nonverbal listening skills that conveys interest in what the other person is

SPOTLIGHT ON...

Caring and Compassion

Acceptance of Clients

Think of some client behaviors that you may not approve of, such as smoking, using alcohol, refusing to comply with treatment, or aborting a fetus. Even when clients engage in behavior that nurses think is wrong, bad, or immoral, those clients still have a legal and ethical right to quality nursing care. How will you respond when caring for someone whose behavior opposes your basic values?

saying. These behaviors allow the nurse to show caring, concern, and acceptance. Behaviors such as sitting down, facing the client, maintaining eye contact, and head nodding are indicators of active listening. Active listening requires the nurse to turn down inner dialogue because total attention must be focused on what the client is saying.

Also, it is important for the nurse to avoid looking rushed or distracted. The primary message that is communicated through active listening is the nurse's concern and intent to assist in problem solving. Active listening is required in *every* nurse-client relationship.

The active listener is cognizant of all three elements of communication: the *verbal, paraverbal,* and *nonverbal.* The verbal message is *what* is said. **Paraverbal communication** is the way in which a person speaks, including voice tone, pitch, and inflection, and the nonverbal message is body language. The active listener pays attention to all three aspects in order to hear the true intent of the communicator.

Active listening means that the nurse focuses on the feelings behind the words, *not* just the words themselves. It is important for the nurse to note any incongruities between the client's verbal and nonverbal messages. For example, if the client says, "Oh, I'm just fine!" and is slumped over with head hanging down, there is an incongruity—the behavior and the words do not match.

The client's expression of feelings demonstrates trust in the nurse. This expression of trust must be recognized and respected. By listening carefully to the client, the nurse is able to learn what the client perceives as the most crucial problem. *Listening is the first step in personalizing care for each client.* Listening can improve client outcomes by letting clients know their input is essential and increasing their sense of control. "For clients, being able to control one's own life is a source of power" (Oudshoorn, Ward-Griffin, & McWilliam, 2007, p. 1443). Some outcomes of active listening are:

- Establishment of rapport
- Expression of genuine concern
- Communication of intent to assist in problem solving
- Promotion of comfort level
- Decreased level of anxiety

- Client empowerment for self-care
- Facilitation of learning

Humor

Humor is another characteristic of therapeutic nurses. The use of humor as a therapeutic intervention is not a new concept for nurses. Nightingale (1969) recognized the influence of the mind on the body and acknowledged humor as an important nursing intervention.

As shown in Figure 14-6, humor can assist in establishing a relationship because it helps break the ice, decreases fear, and promotes trust. Humor is a medium for sharing; thus, it can be used to strengthen the therapeutic relationship. Humor also stimulates creative thinking, which is helpful for both clients and nurses in problem solving.

Humor is influenced by one's cultural background, so it is imperative that the nurse be sensitive to the client's interpretation and use of humor. A humor assessment can be conducted by noting:

- What makes the client smile or laugh
- The use of jokes by clients
- Type of humor expressed by the client

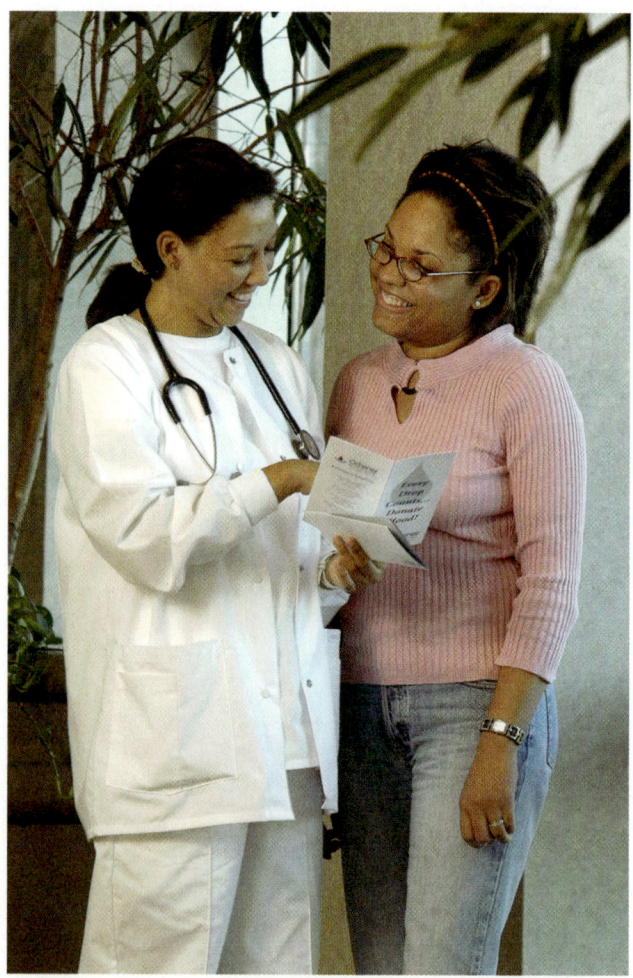

FIGURE 14-6 Note the exchange of laughter between client and nurse. What are some therapeutic outcomes facilitated by the nurse's deliberate use of humor? DELMAR/CENGAGE LEARNING

Humor is a powerful tool for coping. Humor helps individuals to alleviate stress and to express anger in a socially acceptable manner.

Nurses use humor to defuse the negative effects of stress. Although humor can relieve tension and stabilize high-stress situations, it must be used with caution since it can be destructive if used carelessly. For example, when using humor as a therapeutic intervention, the nurse must differentiate between *laughing at* and *laughing with* another.

Compassion

Compassion is truly caring about what happens to another person. Kindness and genuine concern are demonstrated through compassionate acts. Some behaviors that communicate the nurse's compassion include:

- Acting on the belief that everyone is equally deserving of care
- Treating individuals with dignity
- Respecting a client's privacy—which includes simple acts such as keeping the client covered and knocking on the door before entering the room

Other examples of compassion are a nurse caring for the homeless in a shelter or holding the hand of a person with acquired immunodeficiency syndrome (AIDS).

Self-Awareness

Being aware of one's feelings is the first step in developing therapeutic behavior. Knowledge of one's assets is necessary in that effective nurses are able to identify their own skills and abilities. Conversely, only after identifying deficits in knowledge and skills can the nurse initiate necessary improvements. This process of analyzing one's strengths and limitations is an ongoing part of learning. The therapeutic nurse knows learning is a lifelong process that contributes to growth—personally and professionally. Self-awareness allows the nurse to remain objective, that is, separate enough to distinguish one's own feelings and needs from those of the client.

Nonjudgmental Approach

Nonjudgmental behavior must be used if nursing interventions are to be therapeutic. Nonjudgmental means acting without biases, preconceptions, or stereotypes. Nonjudgmental nurses do not evaluate the client's moral values nor tell the client what to do; these nurses accept people as they are. Nonjudgmental nurses do not stereotype people nor expect others to behave in certain ways because they belong to a certain group.

Judgment influences perceptions because people tend to see what they expect to see. Judgmental behavior interferes with the therapeutic value of nursing interventions. It is nontherapeutic for nurses to allow biased views that stem from personal values to influence their actions. The initial assessment of clients is often influenced by preconceived ideas. See the Respecting Our Differences display.

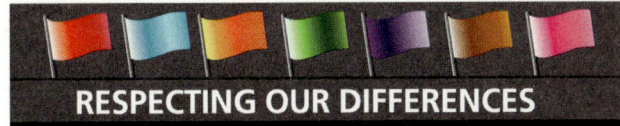

RESPECTING OUR DIFFERENCES

Getting to know people with diverse cultural backgrounds expands the knowledge base and helps one become more tolerant and open-minded.

Becoming nonjudgmental is an ongoing process consisting of the following steps:

- The first step is the most difficult—recognizing that one's thoughts are biased and prejudicial.
- Second, in order to change, nurses must accept their own feelings.
- The third step consists of identifying the source of the negative feelings—not to blame but to gain an understanding of the origins.

Flexibility

Flexibility is another trait necessary for creating a therapeutic relationship. A flexible nurse is one who is ready for the unexpected—knowing that every day is filled with unplanned events and situations. The flexible nurse is able to adapt by taking things in stride and making necessary adjustments. Some of the unexpected events require immediate actions. The flexible nurse is able to establish priorities by determining which needs are urgent and which can be tended to later. Staying calm during a crisis is characteristic of the flexible nurse.

Risk Taker

A risk taker is a person who takes steps to find innovative solutions in problem solving. To become effective risk takers, nurses must give themselves permission to try something new, to step outside their comfort zones, and to not be bound by tradition or fear. The result of risk taking is creative solutions to problems. Successful risk takers give themselves credit for trying something new regardless of the outcome. Smart risk takers learn from those risk-taking ventures that are less than successful. They do not allow themselves to become complacent, that is, content to stay at a comfortable plateau.

THERAPEUTIC VALUE OF THE NURSING PROCESS

The nursing process provides a framework for the delivery of compassionate care. It gives direction by organizing the nurse's actions: assessing, diagnosing, planning, implementing, and evaluating.

The nursing process itself is therapeutic because it focuses on the client's response to illness, disease, or disability rather than just on the problem. By focusing on the caring aspects, the nursing process helps nursing define its practice. Professional accountability is reinforced by the use of this process, which is client centered. When functioning within the parameters of the nursing process, the nurse assumes a variety of roles, including:

- Caregiver
- Counselor
- Teacher
- Client advocate
- Change agent
- Team member
- Resource person

NURSING ROLES

A role is a set of expected behaviors associated with an individual's status or position. A role includes behaviors, rights, and responsibilities. Nurses function in a variety of roles every day. Often roles overlap, which may lead to a conflict in expectations or responsibilities. A discussion of some predominant nursing roles follows.

Caregiver

The caregiver is the role most commonly associated with nursing by the general public. In the role of caregiver, the nurse provides direct care when clients are unable to meet their own needs. Specific activities characteristic of the caregiver role include feeding, bathing, and administering medications. When individuals are ill, they are more likely to be dependent upon others for assistance in meeting their basic needs, referred to as activities of daily living (ADL). Such dependency may result in the person experiencing a perceived loss of control and feelings of helplessness. Effective nurses understand the importance of helping clients maintain control as much as possible. To promote healing, nurses must help clients regain or maintain a sense of control. "Many patients feel alienated from their recovery and treatment; frequently it is the nurse who assists the patient in regaining a sense of participation and control" (Benner, 2001, p. 61).

Counselor

When acting as a counselor, the nurse assists clients with problem identification and resolution. The counselor facilitates client action by helping clients to make their own decisions. Counseling is done to help clients increase their coping skills. Effective counseling is holistic, in that it addresses the individual's emotional, psychological, spiritual, and cognitive dimensions. The counselor role is most often fulfilled by the nurse who intervenes with clients experiencing chronic conditions and those who are grieving.

Teacher

Teaching is an intrinsic part of nursing. The nurse views *each* interaction as an opportunity for education; both client and nurse can learn something from every encounter with each

other (see Figure 14-7). Client education focuses on client empowerment, that is, enabling clients to do as much as possible for themselves. Compassionate nurses provide information that is easily understood by clients and that will assist them in problem solving.

Client Advocate

A client advocate is a person who speaks up for or acts on behalf of the client. Advocacy empowers clients to be partners in the therapeutic process rather than passive recipients of care. The relationship that encourages client empowerment is one of mutual participation by client and nurse. Clients and families are actively involved in establishing goals.

Frequently, clients and families do not communicate their concerns to prescribing practitioners but will do so to the nurse with whom a bond has been established. Nurses function as client advocates by listening and communicating the expressed concerns to other health care providers and including those concerns in care planning.

Change Agent

Nurses who function in the role of change agent recognize that change is a complex process. The change agent is proactive (takes the initiative to make things happen) rather than reactive (responding to things after they have happened). Change should not be done in a random manner. It should be planned carefully and implemented in a deliberate way to facilitate the client's progress.

The compassionate nurse understands that the decision to change rests with the client. For example, consider the client who is instructed to lose weight in order to lower cholesterol levels. The nurse provides the necessary information but knows that the client has ultimate control in determining whether to make the necessary lifestyle modifications recommended by the health care providers. In other words, caring nurses do not attempt to force people to change.

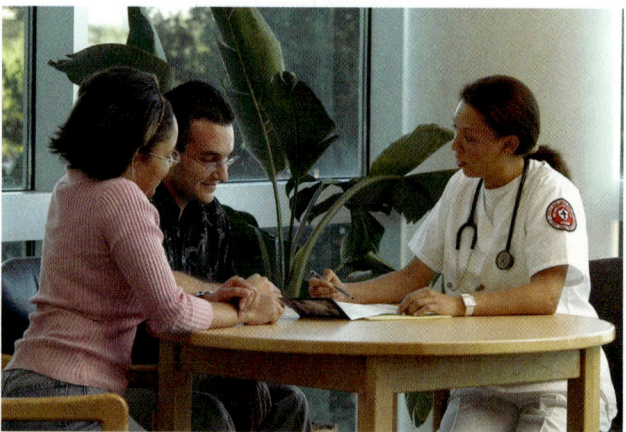

FIGURE 14-7 In this situation, the nurse is providing prenatal instructions to the clients. DELMAR/CENGAGE LEARNING

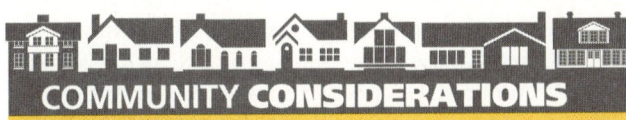

COMMUNITY CONSIDERATIONS

Referrals

The nurse must have a broad understanding of community resources in order to connect clients with support services that are accessible. For example, an emergency room nurse may need to refer a woman to a battered women's shelter. Or a nurse who works in an obstetric clinic may need to refer a client to a local health unit in order to receive information about the supplemental nutrition program for women, infants, and children (WIC).

Team Member

A vital role of the nurse is that of team member. The nurse does not function in isolation but rather works with other members of the health care team. Collaboration requires the nurse to use effective interpersonal skills and promotes continuity of care. See Chapter 15 for a discussion on promoting healthy relationships with clients and colleagues.

Resource Person

The nurse functions as a resource person by providing skilled intervention and information. Identifying resources and making referrals as needed also fall under the auspices of this role (see Community Considerations accompanying display). Nurses must consider clients' strengths as well as availability of resources, including physical, intellectual, economic, social, and environmental factors.

KEY CONCEPTS

- Caring is the fundamental value in nursing.
- Today's high-tech environment requires that nurses provide humanistic caring.
- The therapeutic nurse-client relationship is the one-to-one interactive process between client and nurse that is directed at improving the client's health status or assisting in problem solving.
- Therapeutic relationships differ from social relationships in that they are deliberately planned, focus on client problems, and communicate acceptance of the client.
- Nursing is an interpersonal process between someone who needs help in meeting needs and someone who is competent to assist in meeting those needs.
- The three interwoven phases of the nurse-client relationship are orientation, working, and termination.

- Therapeutic use of self is a process in which nurses deliberately plan their actions and approach the relationship with a specific goal in mind before interacting with the client.
- Several interpersonal characteristics and skills can be developed to increase the therapeutic value of a nurse's interventions. These include warmth, hope, rapport, trust, empathy, acceptance, active listening, humor, compassion, awareness, nonjudgmental attitude, flexibility, and risk taking.
- The nursing process is the framework for providing compassionate care.
- Nurses function in a variety of roles when working with clients. The roles overlap and have specific responsibilities.

REVIEW QUESTIONS

1. The nurse is assigned a new client. Which of the following nursing actions will facilitate the development of a therapeutic relationship? Select all that apply.
   a. Clarifying client's expectations for care
   b. Determining the nurse's perception of problems
   c. Discussing the nurse's problems
   d. Establishing boundaries
   e. Explaining the guidelines for confidentiality
   f. Setting the groundwork for trust
2. Which of the following client behaviors is indicative of the working phase of the nurse-client relationship?
   a. Asking questions about treatment methods
   b. Changing the topic frequently

   c. Demonstrating elevated anxiety
   d. Testing the nurse's reliability
3. When planning care for a client, the nurse will decide to use touch if the client demonstrates:
   a. Confusion
   b. Cooperativeness
   c. Hostility
   d. Suspiciousness
4. A nurse manager observes a newly hired staff nurse providing care to a client. Which of the following staff nurse behaviors indicates that depersonalization has occurred?
   a. Calling the client by name
   b. Checking the client's vital signs without speaking

   c. Knocking on the client's door before entering the room

   d. Talking to the client

5. The nurse is talking with a client scheduled for surgery the next day. The client expresses much anxiety about the procedure. Which of the following nursing responses is an example of empathy?

   a. "Everyone feels like this before surgery."

   b. "I'm sure everything will work out fine."

   c. "Things always look worse before they get better."

   d. "You sound very anxious about the surgery."

6. Which of the following nursing actions demonstrates that the nurse is acting as a client advocate?

   a. Administering medications according to the prescribing practitioner's orders

   b. Discussing the client's concerns at a treatment team meeting

   c. Insisting that the client make all health care decisions without family input

   d. Urging the client to consent to a treatment procedure that the client is refusing

7. During the nurse-client interaction, when the nurse tries to gain an understanding of the client's viewpoint, the nurse is exhibiting the use of _____.

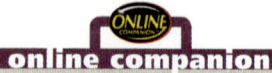

online companion

Visit the DeLaune and Ladner online companion resource at **www.delmar.cengage.com** for additional content and study aids. Click on Online Companions, then select the Nursing discipline.

I learn a great deal by merely observing you, and letting you talk as long as you please, and taking note of what you do not say.

—T. S. Eliot

CHAPTER 15

Communication

COMPETENCIES

1. Explain the process of communication.
2. Describe the modes of communication.
3. Discuss the types of communication.
4. Discuss the principles of therapeutic communication.
5. Explore the barriers to effective therapeutic communication.
6. Utilize approaches that facilitate therapeutic communication between nurses and clients.
7. Describe the benefits of communicating with other health care professionals.

must be aware of the different levels ... tion is conducted between nurses and clients and among members of the health care team.

This chapter discusses the communication process, modes of communication, types of communication, and barriers to therapeutic interaction. Knowledge of these aspects of communication helps the nurse establish a therapeutic relationship with the client and deliver quality nursing care.

THE COMMUNICATION PROCESS

Communication, the process of transmitting thoughts, feelings, facts, and other information, includes verbal and nonverbal behavior. Kneisl (2009) describes communication as every aspect of behavior and, therefore, more than simply transmitting or imparting facts. Meaning must be assigned to those facts for communication to occur. All people engage in the dynamic process of communication. In fact, people cannot *not* communicate.

In nursing, communication is the vehicle for establishing a therapeutic relationship with a client. There would be a void if the nurse did not relate to clients—if there were no fondness, no closeness, no bonding. In fact, communication *is* the relationship between nurse and client (Kneisl, 2009). The quality of the relationship between nurse and client is directly associated with the quality of their communication.

COMPONENTS OF THE COMMUNICATION PROCESS

The five major components of the communication process are sender, message, channel, receiver, and feedback. See Figure 15-1, which provides a framework for understanding the process of communication.

The Sender

The communication process begins when a person, known as the **sender**, generates a message. Messages stem from a person's need to relate to others, to create meanings, and to understand various situations. Messages are generated by external stimuli, such as what the sender sees, hears, touches, tastes, or smells. However, the sender also perceives internal stimuli that generate messages. Examples of internal stimuli that affect communication include hunger, fatigue, or the mental activities of fantasizing and thinking (i.e., self-talk). The source (or encoder) is the stimulus, such as the idea, event, or situation. **Encoding** involves the use of language and other specific signs and symbols for sending messages.

The Message

The **message** is a stimulus produced by a sender and responded to by a receiver. Messages may be verbal, nonverbal, written materials, and artistic. Verbal and nonverbal

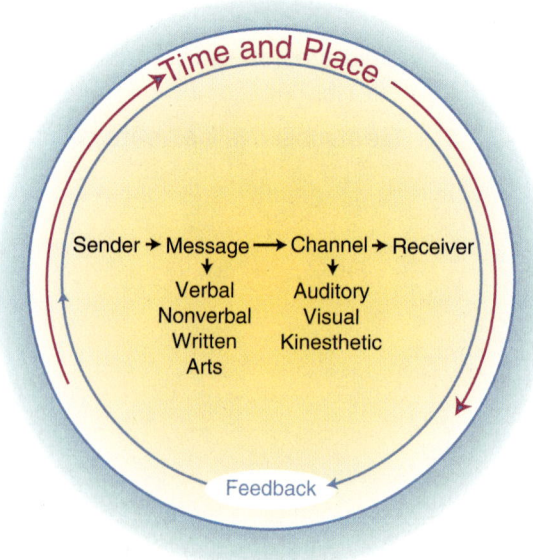

FIGURE 15-1 A Communication Model DELMAR/CENGAGE LEARNING

transmissions of messages are discussed at length later in this chapter.

The Channel

The channel is the medium through which a message is transmitted. There are three major communication channels: visual, auditory, and kinesthetic. The visual channel consists of sight and observation. The auditory channel consists of spoken words and cues. The kinesthetic channel refers to experiencing sensations. See Table 15-1. Each person has a dominant channel that influences communication. See the Respecting Our Differences display.

The Receiver

The receiver is the person who intercepts the sender's message. Receiving is influenced by complex physiological, psychological, and cognitive processes.

The physiological component involves the process of hearing. An intact, healthy auditory system, including those areas of the brain involved in the hearing process, enables the receiver to hear messages. Good eyesight allows for the reception of messages via the visual channel. Likewise, homeostasis in those bodily structures where touch is applied allows for reception of tactile stimuli.

The psychological process refers to mental mechanisms that affect human behavior. This component may enhance or impede the receiving process. For example, anxiety may restrict the perceptual field, causing the client to hear, see, or feel less accurately. However, during mild and moderate levels of anxiety, the perceptual field broadens, causing the client to be more alert, with increased perception.

The cognitive aspect is the "thinking" part of receiving and involves interpretation of stimuli, thus converting them into meaning. The receiver assigns meaning through his or her own method of perceiving and "self-talk," or communication with oneself. Engaging in too much self-talk may cause

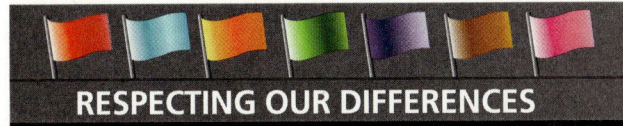

RESPECTING OUR DIFFERENCES

Your Dominant Channel

Culture influences the way a person processes information. To determine which channel—visual, auditory, or kinesthetic—is your dominant mode, ask yourself these questions. How do I learn best: by seeing, hearing, or doing? When people speak, what do I pay most attention to: their appearance, their words, or their actions?

the receiver to do a poor job of listening. Controlling this self-talk requires continuous focusing and validating of the sender's message. Through cognitive processing, the receiver decodes messages, interprets them, and then provides feedback to the sender.

Feedback

Feedback is the information the sender receives about the receiver's reaction to the message. The function of feedback is to provide the sender with information about the receiver's perception of a situation. Having this information, the sender can then adjust the delivery of the message to communicate more effectively.

Communication is reciprocal in that both the sender and receiver must be involved; the sender must transmit the message, and the receiver must provide feedback for a communication transaction to be complete. Characteristics of effective feedback include:

- Specific rather than general
- Descriptive

TABLE 15-1 Communication Channels

CHANNEL	MODE OF TRANSMISSION	CONGRUENT WORDS
Visual	Sight	• "I see what you mean."
	Observation	• "It looks perfectly clear that . . ."
Auditory	Hearing	• "I hear you." • "Tell me what you mean."
	Listening	• "Sounds like you're saying . . ." • "Tell me what you mean."
Kinesthetic	Procedural touch	• "How does that feel?"
	Caring touch	• "That is so touching."

Delmar/Cengage Learning

- Supportive and nonthreatening
- Timely delivery (as soon as possible after the behavior or the message)
- Clear and unambiguous
- Direct and honest

FACTORS INFLUENCING COMMUNICATION

In addition to channels, there are many other variables that influence communication. The primary influential factors are discussed in the following text.

Perception

Perception is a person's sensing and understanding of the world. Perception of an event or situation is unique in that it varies from person to person. Perceptions help a person determine the meaning of the words and the content of the messages being communicated. It is important for listeners to confirm what they think they have heard because interpre-

tation of the message depends upon the hearer's perception of the message.

Cultural Context

Because behavior is learned, nonverbal communication varies from culture to culture. For example, the messages communicated by touch and eye contact depend to a great extent on one's cultural context. See the accompanying Respecting Our Differences display on page 265 and Chapter 20 for a complete discussion of cultural variations related to communication.

Space and Distance

Proxemics is the study of the distance between people and objects. Each person has an invisible boundary, buffer zone, or personal space. Table 15-2 describes the types of personal space. Culturally defined boundaries alert a person as to how close another can comfortably approach. Invasion of personal space produces discomfort, anxiety, and the fight-or-flight response; see Chapter 23. The nurse respects the client's personal space in several ways, such as not touching or moving the client's possessions unless necessary.

TABLE 15-2 Types of Personal Space

TYPE	DESCRIPTION	NURSING IMPLICATIONS

Intimate distance (0 to 18 inches around the person's body)	• Reserved for people with whom one has a relationship
	• Vision is affected in that it is restricted to one portion of the other's body; may be distorted
	• Tone of voice may seem louder
	• Body smells noticeable
	• Increased sensation of body heat
		• Nurses often must intrude on this space to provide care
		• Explain intention to client
		• Respect client's space as much as possible
		• May be used for comforting and protecting
		• Therapeutic examples:
		  —Rocking a toddler
		  —Administering a massage
		  —Checking vital signs (temperature, pulse, respiratory rate, and blood pressure)

Personal distance (zone extends 1.5 to 4 feet around person's body)	• Usually maintained with friends
	• Vision is clear since more of the other person is visible
	• Tone of voice is moderate
	• Sensations of body smells and heat are lessened
		• Better able to read nonverbal communication at this distance
		• Therapeutic examples:
		  —Conversation between client and nurse usually occurs in this zone
		  —One-to-one teaching
		  —Counseling

Social or public distance (zone extends from 4 feet and beyond)	• Generally used when conducting impersonal business
	• Communication is more formal and less intense
	• Sensory involvement is less intense
	• Increased eye contact
		• Therapeutic examples:
		  —Making rounds
		  —Leading a group
		  —Teaching a class

Data from Kneisl, C. R. (2009). Therapeutic communication. In C. R. Kneisl & E. Trigoboff, *Contemporary psychiatric mental health nursing* (2nd ed.). Upper Saddle River, NJ: Prentice-Hall; Spector, R. E. (2008). *Cultural diversity in health and illness* (7th ed.). Upper Saddle River, NJ: Pearson.

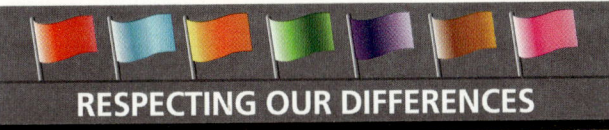

RESPECTING OUR DIFFERENCES

When talking with clients from diverse cultures, it is especially important to attend to nonverbal messages. Eye contact, voice volume and tone, facial expression, and gestures can be used to enhance communication with individuals of every cultural background. When communicating with people who do not understand English, what do you do to promote effective communication?

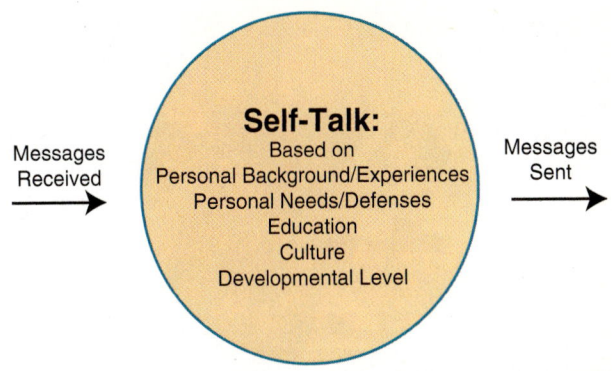

FIGURE 15-2 Intrapersonal Communication DELMAR/CENGAGE LEARNING

Time

The study of the effects of time on the communication process is referred to as **chronemics**. The entire communication process is influenced by time. For example, the same message received at 3:00 AM will be perceived and responded to differently at 3:00 PM. The amount of time spent in communicating depends on the client's needs. Some clients will require more of the nurse's time than others. The client who is seriously ill or nontrusting may respond better to brief, frequent contact than to prolonged, infrequent contact. If the nurse is hurried during the interaction with the client, a nonverbal message of impatience may be transmitted. Keeping clients waiting conveys a message that they are unimportant. On the other hand, the nurse who is prompt and who allows time for the client to talk communicates nonverbally, "You are important to me" and "I value you as a person."

LEVELS OF COMMUNICATION

Communication occurs at different levels, with each level influencing the others. The following text discusses the intrapersonal, the interpersonal, and group levels of communication.

Intrapersonal Level

Intrapersonal communication consists of the messages one sends to oneself, including self-talk, or communication with oneself. A person receiving internal or external messages organizes, interprets, and assigns meaning to the messages. Figure 15-2 illustrates the process of self-talk. The result of this process is the individual's unique way of perceiving. The message of the speaker may differ from that heard by the receiver because of the intrapersonal communication of each. Also, self-talk can interfere with attention to others and cause much to be missed during interpersonal exchanges.

Interpersonal Level

Interpersonal communication is the process that occurs between two people either in face-to-face encounters, over the telephone, or through other communication media. Interpersonal communication builds on the intrapersonal level in that each person communicating must communicate with the

self in order to communicate with others. An important outcome of interpersonal communication is the development of an interpersonal relationship (see Figure 15-3). Interpersonal skills are essential competencies for nurses.

Group Level

Group communication occurs when three or more people meet in face-to-face encounters or through another communication medium, such as a conference call or webinar. This level of communication is complex because of the number of people communicating intrapersonally and interpersonally and the combinations of the people involved.

The study of the events that take place during group interaction is called **group dynamics**. The dynamics of any group influence the productivity of the group. Nurses deal with groups as they interact with families of clients, treatment teams, therapy groups, and committees within their health care settings (see Figure 15-4 on page 266). Table 15-3 on page 266 highlights some of the differences between one-to-one and small group interactions.

In dealing with groups, the nurse should be aware of the various nonverbal messages derived from the spatial arrangement of group members. For example, the leader tends to sit at the end or head of the table. Timid or uninterested

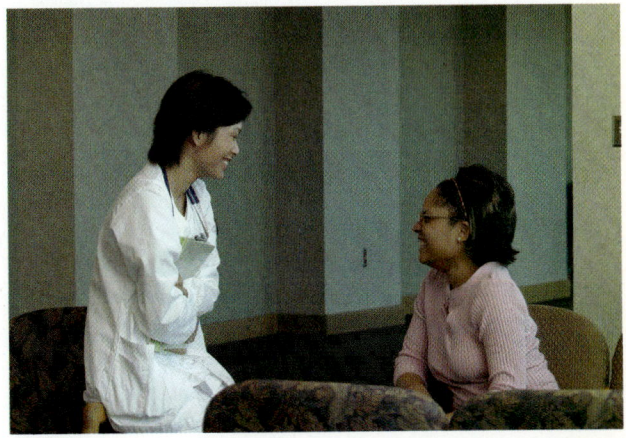

FIGURE 15-3 A Nurse Communicating with a Client on the Interpersonal Level DELMAR/CENGAGE LEARNING

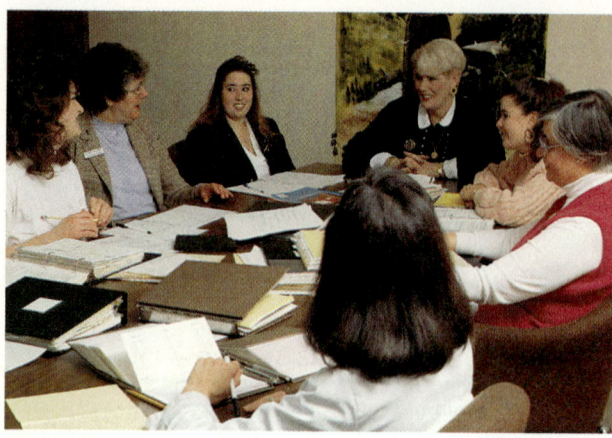

FIGURE 15-4 Team Conference: What factors could improve communication in this situation? DELMAR/CENGAGE LEARNING

Since groups are interventions to improve a client's health status, it is important for nurses to refer clients to groups when necessary. Following are three mechanisms used by nurses to connect clients with health-promoting groups:

1. Communication—The nurse actively listens to the client to determine needs.
2. Critical thinking—The nurse uses cognitive processes to decide which groups are congruent with the client's needs.
3. Collaboration—The nurse works with multidisciplinary team members (i.e., social workers, physicians, clergy) to start the referral process.

MODES OF COMMUNICATION

Communication occurs in a variety of ways: through words, actions, or a combination of words and actions. When there is congruence ("a match") between one's words and actions, communication is enhanced.

VERBAL MESSAGES

Verbal messages are messages communicated through words and language, either spoken or written. Verbal messages are accompanied by **paraverbal (or paralinguistic) cues**: tone and pitch of voice; speed, inflection, and volume; and grunts and other nonlanguage vocalizations. Paraverbal cues embellish a verbal message, thus adding to its meaning. Paraverbal communication often influences the listener more than the actual words do. Even when the words themselves are not understood, the power of the paraverbal cues can lead to understanding. For example, when a person speaking a foreign language is angry, the paraverbal cues of yelling,

participants tend to sit at the back of the room. Seat clients in a circle rather than in rows to promote interaction and cohesion. The study of proxemics in small group situations is called **small group ecology** and provides a potent source of nonverbal messages about participants.

A group is formed around a common purpose or goal; this common goal is the factor that leads to **cohesiveness** (bonding among group members). Several types of groups exist; see Table 15-4 on page 267 for a listing of groups in which nurses usually participate. Nurses' participation in groups depends upon educational level. According to the American Nurses Association (2004), nurse generalists (those prepared at the baccalaureate level or below) may lead and colead all types of groups except psychotherapy groups. Only nurse specialists (those with graduate degrees) are to lead psychotherapeutic groups.

TABLE 15-3 Differences between One-to-One and Group Communication

ONE-TO-ONE INTERACTIONS	GROUP INTERACTIONS
• One sender and one receiver, each with his or her own unique perceptions.	• Numerous senders and receivers, each with unique perceptions.
• Influenced by dynamics of creating, maintaining, and terminating a therapeutic nurse-client relationship.	• Influenced by group dynamics.
• Requires understanding of nurse-client relationship theory, communication theory, and an overall theoretical approach (e.g., Rogers, Peplau, Reusch).	• Requires understanding of underlying modalities as well as a theoretical framework to guide both interventions and interpretations (e.g., psychoanalytic, behavioral, or interpersonal model).
• Problem identification and problem solving are done by the client, with input from the nurse.	• Problem identification and problem solving are done by the group, with assistance from the leader.
• The nurse is the major support for the client during the interaction.	• The group is the major support for the client during the interaction.
• The logical outcome of one-to-one communication is the development of the nurse-client relationship.	• The logical outcomes are group cohesiveness and group productivity.

Delmar/Cengage Learning

TABLE 15-4 Types of Groups

TYPE	DESCRIPTION	EXAMPLES
Task group	• Focuses on achievement of a specific goal • Emphasizes problem solving and decision making	• Diabetes education group • Committee to study staffing issues • Student Nurses Association
Therapeutic group	• Increases members' coping abilities • Offers support • Provides education and information	• Stress management class • Bereavement and grieving group • Exercise group (i.e., mall-walkers club)
Therapy group	• Helps members learn about and change problematic behaviors • Focuses on emotional and behavioral disorders	• Cognitive-behavioral group • Psychotherapy group
Self-help group	• Focuses on a common experience of all members • Often led by nonprofessionals	• Weight Watchers • Reach for Recovery (a group for women who have had mastectomies) • Alcoholics Anonymous

Delmar/Cengage Learning

shouting, grunting, or hissing through clenched teeth convey the message across language barriers.

NONVERBAL MESSAGES

Nonverbal messages are messages communicated without words, that is, through body language. Much of the communication between people is nonverbal. Unspoken messages often carry more weight than verbal and paraverbal ones, and they can be more reliable. Nurses must pay attention to nonverbal communication in order to determine the meaning of changes in client behavior. See the accompanying Spotlight On display. Major nonverbal aspects of communication are discussed in the following text.

The nurse must never assume the meaning of a person's body language. Nonverbal messages can have several interpretations. Consider a client who crosses his or her arms when listening to the nurse. What does the client's nonverbal communication mean? It could be a signal that the client is shutting out the nurse's words, is trying to get warm, or is repositioning for comfort. It is essential that the nurse validate the intended meaning of the message with the client.

Facial Expression

The face is the greatest conveyor of nonverbal messages. Facial expressions give clues that support, contradict, or disguise the verbal message. Many types of feelings and reactions are reflected in a person's face. Facial expressions serve as clues to emotionally charged topics and often communicate the client's needs.

The eyes often belie facial expressions because there is little voluntary control over the eyes. For example, a frightened client might say, "I am fine," and voluntarily control the muscles of the face to portray inner calm. However, the pupils of the eyes dilate widely in fear, thus alerting the receiver to the real message. Eyes, together with the use of the eyebrows and eyelashes, give numerous signals to others. They show interest, concern, sadness, dishonesty, or honesty. The eyes may also indicate shock, shyness, pleasure, displeasure, excitement, and flirtation. They exemplify all feelings: anger, happiness, sadness, and fear.

The lips also communicate several messages, such as:

• Warmth and friendliness when they smile
• Malevolence when they snarl

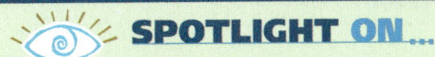 **SPOTLIGHT ON...**

Professionalism

Elements of Communication

Nonverbal behavior is a more accurate indicator of the individual's intended message than words. Why do you think the adage "Actions speak louder than words" is true? A client yells, "I am NOT angry!" while pounding his fist on the bedside table. Which message—the verbal or the nonverbal—do you heed? Why?

- Anger when they pout
- Fear when they quiver

People who do not wish to share their feelings might clamp their jaws shut or purse their lips. Anxious people often chew their bottom lips. The nurse can use such clues to understand the client's messages.

Posture

Much about an individual may be learned by observing and interpreting posture. Posture indicates anxiety, relaxation, and negative or positive self-image. Leaning forward usually indicates interest; leaning backward may communicate aversion or rejection. Standing straight and tall with chest forward generally shows confidence, whereas individuals who are depressed, tired, or bored often slump.

Gestures

Gestures refer to the movement of body parts. Shrugging the shoulders, waving the hands, tapping the feet—all add a distinct dimension to verbal communication. The nurse communicates openness and a willingness to listen by facing the client in a relaxed position, with hands resting palms up on the lap. Crossed arms pulled closely against the body may indicate nonacceptance and a lack of desire to hear the client.

Touch

Touch is a powerful nonverbal medium for communication. It can be used to soothe, comfort, and establish rapport. Touch can communicate a sense of caring—as it does when a nurse holds a person's hand during a painful procedure—or it can be perceived as intrusive or hostile. Touch should be used cautiously with clients who are:

- *Confused:* They may misinterpret the intent of the touch.
- *Aggressive:* They may see the touch as a threat and lash out.
- *Suspicious:* They may think the touch is harmful.
- *Victims of abuse:* They may be frightened by touch.

The nurse must understand various cultural perceptions of touch in order to prevent problems. See the Respecting Our Differences display, and see Chapter 20 for discussion of the cultural significance of touch.

Physical Appearance and Artifacts

Physical appearance and **artifacts** (specific types of nonverbal messages that include items in the client's environment, grooming, or use of clothing and jewelry) convey nonverbal messages that enhance or detract from the spoken words. For example, uniforms often send nonverbal messages that stifle interpersonal exchange by setting up a boundary of superiority. For this reason, nursing uniforms are not worn in certain areas, such as pediatrics, psychiatry, and some home health settings. If worn, a uniform that is clean and pressed, along with shoes that are polished, can help inspire confidence in the caregiver.

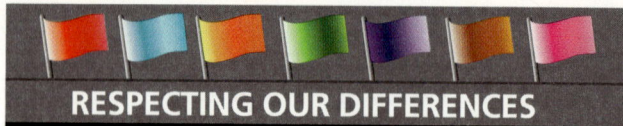

RESPECTING OUR DIFFERENCES

Interpreting Nonverbal Behavior

Never assume that a nonverbal behavior has the same meaning for everyone. Interpretation of various nonverbal aspects of communication varies among people because of developmental, cultural, and experiential factors.

METACOMMUNICATION

Metacommunication is the relationship aspect of communication. It refers to the message about the message. For example, a person who is silent is still sending out messages through nonverbal communication. Metacommunication refers to all the factors that influence how messages are received. It involves focusing on the communication process rather than only on the content. The "reading between the lines" that occurs in metacommunication allows the receiver to better understand the sender's true message (Edelman & Mandle, 2006).

TYPES OF COMMUNICATION

There are several types of communication: social, therapeutic, and formal. Formal communication, which consists of written messages and the arts, may include lectures, reports, charting in the client's record, and public speaking. Usually, with formal communication, there is one sender transmitting messages to several others.

INTERDISCIPLINARY COMMUNICATION

The health care team consists of the client and all medical personnel involved in providing care. All members of the team perform important, though different, roles in the health care delivery system. See Chapter 4 for a complete discussion of the roles of health care team members. It is important that all health care team members communicate with each other regarding assessment, intervention outcomes, and client status. The interdependent nature of teams requires thoughtful and effective communication. Breakdown of communication between different team members can interfere with the client's treatment.

THERAPEUTIC COMMUNICATION

Therapeutic communication is the use of communication for the purpose of creating a beneficial outcome for the client. Therapeutic communication:

- Is purposeful and goal-directed
- Has well-defined boundaries
- Is client-focused

- Is nonjudgmental
- Uses well-planned, selected techniques

Ruesch (1961), who originated the term *therapeutic communication,* stated that the purpose is to improve the client's ability to function. Furthermore, therapeutic communication facilitates the establishment of the nurse-client relationship and fulfills the purposes of nursing (Kneisl, 2009). Therapeutic communication forms a connection between client and nurse. Technological advances cannot replace the need for communication between client and nurse. The "high-tech" environment demands the presence of "high-touch" nursing care. Table 15-5 on page 270 presents the essential elements of therapeutic communication: empathy, trust, honesty, validation, caring, and use of active listening.

Principles of Therapeutic Interaction

Regardless of the type of interaction, principles and guidelines of therapeutic communication are used to direct the nurse when relating with clients. A discussion of basic principles for guiding therapeutic communication follows.

Plan to interview at an appropriate time. The time frame within which an interaction occurs influences the outcome. For example, it is unwise to plan to talk with a client during visiting hours, during change of shift, or when the client is distracted by environmental stimuli (e.g., the homebound client is watching a favorite television show). In such situations, the nurse may be rushed or the client may be preoccupied. Neither situation would be conducive to effective interaction.

Ensure privacy. Clients are entitled to confidentiality. It is both a legal mandate and an ethical obligation that nurses respect the client's confidence; this includes spoken words and medical records. No one wants to discuss private matters when or where other people are listening. Privacy can be arranged by screening the client's bed, closing the door to the room, or finding a quiet secluded place in which to talk. See the accompanying Community Considerations display.

Establish guidelines for the therapeutic interaction. During the initial contact with the client, the nurse should share certain information such as the nurse's name and affiliation, purpose of the interaction, the expected length of the contact with the client, and the assurance of confidentiality. The client needs to have this basic information, and it serves as an introduction to the development of the therapeutic nurse-client relationship.

COMMUNITY CONSIDERATIONS

Ensuring Privacy in the Home Setting

In the home setting, it may be necessary to ask family members or visitors for time and space to promote confidentiality. Federal laws protect the confidentiality of every client in every health care setting, including those treated in community settings.

✓ NURSING CHECKLIST

Meeting the Client's Comfort Needs

- Regulate the temperature of the environment.
- Sit in comfortable chairs or help position client comfortably on bed or stretcher.
- Provide adequate room ventilation.
- Implement measures to decrease pain.
- Institute actions to protect privacy.

Provide for comfort during the interaction. Discomfort can be distracting. Pain interferes with a person's ability to concentrate; thus, communication becomes impaired. See the Nursing Checklist, which provides guidelines for promoting a client's comfort in order to improve communication.

Accept the client exactly as is. Being judgmental blocks communication. Nurses who put aside personal prejudices, curiosities, feelings, and values are more receptive to the feelings and behaviors of the client, regardless of content stated by the client. Nonjudgmental nurses are less encumbered by their own personal needs.

Encourage spontaneity. The nurse gathers more data when the client is talking freely. Also, the client experiences relief and freedom from worries by talking without inhibition.

Focus on the leads and cues presented by the client. Asking questions just for the sake of talking or for the satisfaction of one's own curiosity does not contribute to effective interviewing. Therapeutic interaction involves discussing the client's problems, needs, or concerns. Therefore, allow the client to initiate the topic to be discussed; then, use techniques to focus on that topic. Pay attention to the verbal, paraverbal, and nonverbal cues and signals of the client, and focus on them when they occur.

Encourage the expression of feelings. Simply allowing the client to talk is not interviewing. Therapeutic interaction occurs when the client is permitted to voice feelings about troublesome events or interpersonal situations. Doing so requires the nurse to identify those areas that are emotionally charged and to focus on them.

Be aware of one's own feelings during the interaction. The nurse's feelings influence the interaction. For example, the nurse who becomes anxious may change the subject or make comments that finalize the session. The nurse must make a conscious effort to prevent personal feelings from getting in the way of the client's progress. Identifying one's own feelings and behavior and recognizing the way they affect the client lead to better communications.

THERAPEUTIC APPROACHES WITH CLIENTS

In addition to using the interviewing principles discussed previously, there are numerous techniques that help promote therapeutic communication. It is important to use the communication techniques as tools for building relationships with clients. See Table 15-6 on page 271 for an analysis of these techniques.

TABLE 15-5 The Elements of Therapeutic Communication

DEFINITION	BEHAVIORS OF THE NURSE	OUTCOMES
Empathy: An emotional linkage between two or more people through which feelings are communicated; involves trying to imagine what it must be like to be in another person's situation	*Verbal comments:* • "This must make you feel sad." *Nonverbal actions:* • Nodding the head to indicate understanding	• Promotes understanding of the client's feelings and condition • Provides the client with cues that the nurse is following and understanding what is being said
Trust: The client's belief that the nurse will behave predictably and competently while responding to the client's needs	• Ensuring confidentiality • Being consistent • Doing exactly what you say you will do for the client • Being consistently open and honest	• Establishes the foundation of the therapeutic relationship • Provides the basis for progress during future encounters • Makes the client feel comfortable with the nurse, rather than guarded or afraid
Honesty: The ability to be truthful, frank, and sincere	• Providing realistic reassurance • Avoiding false reassurance • Developing insight into the way your feelings and reactions affect the client • Accepting yourself	• Promotes the development of trust • Enables the nurse to gain personal insight and modify behavior as needed
Validation: Listening to the client and responding congruently in order to be sure that the nurse and client have the same understanding of a problem or issue	*Verbal comments:* • "So you are saying that . . ." • "Tell me what you understand about what I just said."	• Clarifies communication • Helps the client to feel accepted, respected, and understood
Caring: The level of emotional involvement between the nurse and the client	*Nonverbal actions:* • Spending quality time with the client • Paying attention to the client's needs • Using tactile messages, such as a pat on the back, to show support	• Helps the client feel accepted • Provides the client with the knowledge that the nurse is willing to help
Active listening: Hearing and interpreting language, noticing nonverbal and paraverbal enhancements, and identifying underlying feelings	• Taking time to listen • Giving the client your undivided attention • Making eye contact • Responding to verbal and nonverbal leads, cues, and signals from the client • Suspending judgment • Noticing discrepancies between facts and feelings • Noticing things omitted such as topics that the client should be discussing but avoids • Using communication principles and techniques to be a sounding board	• Promotes understanding of the client • Allows the client to express himself or herself more freely • Helps the client gain a better understanding of the problem(s) • Promotes problem solving by the client • Enhances the client's self-esteem

Data from Antai-Otong, D., & Wasserman, F. (2007). Therapeutic communication. In D. Antai-Otong & P. Hawkins (Eds.), *Psychiatric nursing: Biological and behavioral concepts* (2nd ed.). Clifton Park, NY: Delmar Learning; Kneisl, C. R. (2009). Therapeutic communication. In C. R. Kneisl & E. Trigoboff (Eds.), *Contemporary psychiatric mental health nursing* (2nd ed.). Upper Saddle River, NJ: Pearson.

TABLE 15-6 Therapeutic Communication Techniques

TYPE	DESCRIPTION	EXAMPLES
TECHNIQUES THAT ALLOW THE CLIENT TO SET THE PACE		
Offering self	• Nurse is available, physically and emotionally • Indicates nurse's willingness and intent to help • Nurse's presence is reassuring; may prompt client to continue • Indicates nurse's attention and interest	• "I'll sit with you awhile." • "Go on." • "Uh-huh." • Head nodding
Broad openings	• Encourage client to choose topic for discussion • Demonstrate respect for client's thoughts • Emphasize importance of client's needs	• "What do you want to talk about?" • "Can you tell me more about that?" • "How have things been going?"
Silence	• Gives client time to reflect • Encourages client to express self • Indicates interest in what client has to say • Increases nurse's understanding of client's message • Helps to structure and pace the interaction • Conveys respect and acceptance	• Sit quietly and observe client's behavior • Use appropriate eye contact • Employ attending behaviors • Control own discomfort during quiet periods or conversation lulls
TECHNIQUES THAT ENCOURAGE SPONTANEITY		
Open-ended comments	• Unfinished sentences that prompt client to continue • Questions that require more than a one-word answer • Allow client to decide what content is relevant	• "Tell me about your pain" instead of "Are you in pain?" • "Tell me about your family" rather than "How many children do you have?"
Reflection	• Focuses on content of client's message and feelings • Repeating client's words in order to prompt further expression • Lets client know the nurse is actively listening • Communicates nurse's interest	*Client:* "Do you think I should tell the doctor I stopped taking my medication?" *Nurse:* "What do you think about that?" *Client:* "I probably should. But the medicine makes me so tearful and agitated." *Nurse:* "You sound a bit agitated now."
Restating	Repeating or paraphrasing client's main idea Indicates nurse is listening to client Encourages further dialogue Gives client an opportunity to explain or elaborate	*Client:* "I told the doctor that I had problems with this medicine, but he just didn't listen to me!" *Nurse:* "Sounds like you're angry at him." *Client:* "I don't sleep well anymore." *Nurse:* "You're having problems sleeping?"
TECHNIQUES THAT FOCUS ON THE CLIENT BY RESPONDING TO VERBAL, PARAVERBAL, AND NONVERBAL CUES		
Exploring	• Attempts to develop in more detail a specific area of concern to client • Identifies patterns or themes	• "Tell me more about how you feel when you do not take your medication." • "Could you tell me about one of those times when you felt so upset?"
Recognition	• Nurse points out observed cues to client	• "I notice that you became embarrassed when . . ." • "I see that you have some pictures of the new baby."

(Continues)

TABLE 15-6 (Continued)

TECHNIQUES THAT FOCUS ON THE CLIENT BY RESPONDING TO VERBAL, PARAVERBAL, AND NONVERBAL CUES		
Focusing	• Questions or statements that help client develop or expand an idea • Directs conversation toward key topics	• "You mentioned that you are having a problem with . . ." • "You say you feel nauseous a lot."
Directing	• Comments that elicit specific information from the client • Is used to collect assessment data, not to satisfy nurse's curiosity	*Client:* "They told me I needed to see a specialist." *Nurse:* "What made them say that to you?" or "When were you told this?" or "How do you feel about seeing another doctor?"

TECHNIQUES THAT ENCOURAGE EXPRESSION OF FEELINGS		
Verbalizing the implied	• An attempt to detect the true meaning of verbal messages	*Client:* "How much is this x-ray going to cost?" *Nurse:* "You're worried about your medical bills?"
Making observations	• Nurse calls attention to behavior indicative of feelings	• "You seem sad today." • "You're limping as if your leg hurts."
Clarifying	• Makes the meaning of client's message clear • Prevents nurse from making assumptions about client's message	*Client:* "Whenever I talk to my doctor, I feel upset." *Nurse:* "Tell me what you mean by upset." *Client:* "They said I could be discharged tomorrow." *Nurse:* "Who told you this?"

TECHNIQUES THAT ENCOURAGE THE CLIENT TO MAKE SOME CHANGES		
Confronting	• Nurse's verbal response to incongruence between client's words and actions • Encourages client to recognize potential areas for change	*Client:* "I am so angry at her" (stated while smiling). *Nurse:* "You say you're angry, yet you're smiling." *Client:* "I never know which of my symptoms to pay attention to. I think maybe I'm just a hypochondriac." *Nurse:* "You say you're not sure which symptoms are important, yet you knew when to come to the clinic for help."
Limit setting	• Stating expectations for appropriate behavior • Establishing behavioral parameters	*Nurse:* "It seems that you are feeling unsure of how to behave right now." *Client:* "What do you mean?" *Nurse:* "Well, you're asking me a lot of personal questions. The reason you're here is because you have some health problems. How can I help you tell me more clearly what brought you here to the clinic?"

Data from Antai-Otong, D., & Wasserman, F. (2007). Therapeutic communication. In D. Antai-Otong & P. Hawkins (Eds.), *Psychiatric nursing: Biological and behavioral concepts* (2nd ed.). Clifton Park, NY: Delmar Learning; Kneisl, C. R. (2009). Therapeutic communication. In C. R. Kneisl & E. Trigoboff, *Contemporary psychiatric mental health nursing* (2nd ed.). Upper Saddle River, NJ: Pearson; Stuart, G. W., & Laraia, M. T. (2004). Therapeutic nurse-patient relationship. In G. W. Stuart & M. T. Laraia (Eds.), *Principles and practice of psychiatric nursing* (8th ed.). St. Louis, MO: Elsevier.

BARRIERS TO THERAPEUTIC INTERACTION

Communication barriers present real challenges to the nurse, but need not stop communication. Rather, barriers pose hurdles that the nurse is able to scale by using creative and different approaches with the client. The nurse develops strategies for overcoming barriers by use of critical thinking skills. Common communication barriers are discussed in the text that follows.

LANGUAGE DIFFERENCES

When English is the clients' second language, they may have problems navigating through the health care system. An inability to communicate effectively with health care providers adversely affects clients' responses to interventions. The impact of this barrier can be lessened by learning the client's language (or parts of it), or by using interpreters, pictures and symbols, and foreign language dictionaries. Other ways of ameliorating language problems are discussed later in this chapter.

Communication problems can also occur even when everyone speaks the same language. For example, complex sentence structure and the different meanings of words may lead to communication difficulties. The use of value-laden terms also blocks the exchange of information, ideas, and feelings.

CULTURAL DIFFERENCES

Various cultures and subcultures use language differently. People's communication patterns reflect their culture. In some cultures, expression of thoughts and feelings is spontaneous and exuberant, whereas people of other cultural groups may be reserved and stoic in their verbalizations. Some of the communication variables that are culture specific include eye contact, proximity to others, direct versus indirect questioning, and the role of social small talk. See Chapter 20 for a discussion of the influence of culture on communication.

GENDER

Sending, receiving, and interpreting messages can vary between men and women. The effect and use of nonverbal cues are often gender dependent. For example, women tend to be better decoders of nonverbal cues, and men prefer more personal distance between themselves and others than do women (Boggs, 2006). See the Respecting Our Differences display on gender roles and expectations.

HEALTH STATUS

One's health status affects communication. For example, the client who is oriented will communicate more reliably than a client who is delirious, confused, or disoriented. Communi-

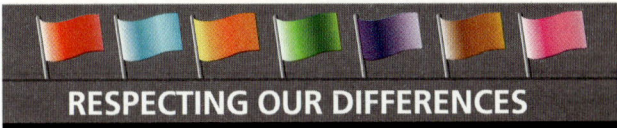

RESPECTING OUR DIFFERENCES

Gender Roles and Expectations

Traditional sex-role beliefs support the idea that women bear the primary responsibility for family well-being. How might the gender-biased expectations of both nurse and client affect the messages communicated? What are your gender-biased expectations of women as either clients or care providers? What approaches could you take to make your communication more gender conscious?

cation is affected by sensory perceptual alterations, such as loss of vision or hearing.

DEVELOPMENTAL LEVEL

Failure to communicate at the client's developmental level can be a roadblock. For example, communicating with children requires the use of different words and approaches than those used with adults because a child cannot think in abstract concepts. Relating at the client's developmental level is necessary for understanding. A discussion of communicating with children is presented later in this chapter.

KNOWLEDGE DIFFERENCES

All people need to be understood. Nurses consistently assess the knowledge levels of clients in order to determine the best way to correct knowledge deficits. When assessing knowledge level, the nurse should:

- Take note of the client's vocabulary
- Observe the numbers and kinds of facts verbalized by the client
- Determine the client's educational background

With this information, the nurse is able to assess the teaching needs of the client and determine the most appropriate method of instruction.

EMOTIONAL DISTANCE

Satisfying encounters are described by words such as *rapport* and *empathy,* and they occur when both parties are willing to be "present" as persons. Emotional distance, on the other hand, involves treating the client as a curiosity, a problem, or a disease, thus preventing satisfying interaction and possibly causing hostility. For instance, a client who is on strict isolation for an infectious disease, or someone who is confused and disoriented, is at risk for experiencing emotional isolation. By maintaining rapport with clients regardless of their status, nurses are able to decrease emotional distance.

EMOTIONS

When the nurse or the client is anxious, communication may change, stop, or take a nonproductive course. Nurses should be aware of their own feelings and try to control them in order to ensure progress in the interview. It is important that the nurse present a calm manner in order to ease the client's apprehension and, thus, improve the quality of communication.

DAYDREAMING

People can hear words faster than they can speak. Therefore, the listener's mind may wander, and the point of a message may be missed. Mind-wandering can also happen because the listener is bored or preoccupied with worrisome thoughts. Nurses can keep themselves from daydreaming by constantly attending to what the client has to say, by staying alert, and by controlling their own thoughts.

USE OF HEALTH CARE JARGON

The use of health care jargon can provoke anxiety in the client. Nurses and other health care providers have a language unique to their subculture. Nurses who use health care jargon with clients are likely contributing to blocked communication. Terms or phrases such as "CBC," "prn," "intake," "BP," and "take your vitals" are often misinterpreted by clients and families. It is important that nurses use language that is easily understood and explain medical terminology so that it is clear to clients and families.

COMMUNICATION BLOCKS

Certain responses (e.g., giving advice and agreeing) that would be acceptable during social conversation are not useful during therapeutic interaction. Unhelpful techniques are those that halt the progress of the interview and may result in the client's experiencing feelings of inadequacy, intimidation, or confusion. Table 15-7 on page 275 describes several communication roadblocks that are to be avoided. Nurses must constantly be aware of potential barriers to effective communication between themselves, their clients, and members of the health care team, and they must develop strategies to maximize their therapeutic interactions with clients.

COMMUNICATION, CRITICAL THINKING, AND NURSING PROCESS

Critical thinking is an important part of effective communication. Critical thinking involves analysis to determine why a certain conclusion has been reached. In other words, nurses

carefully formulate questions and propose answers by thinking critically. Interpersonal skills (as evidenced by effective communication) and critical thinking are competencies upon which nursing practice is based; see the accompanying Nursing Process Highlight for examples of the use of communication throughout the nursing process.

ASSESSMENT

Therapeutic communication is the vehicle for establishing a partnership between client and nurse. Peplau (1960) stated, "To encourage the patient to participate in identifying and assessing his problem is to engage him as an active partner—an enterprise of great concern to him" (p. 47). When performing the admission assessment, the nurse seeks to understand the client's entire message by focusing on both verbal and nonverbal communication. For example, note what a client is doing when stating, "I have a terrible headache." What nonverbal cues support the words?

NURSING PROCESS HIGHLIGHT

Relationship between Communication and Nursing Process

Assessment
- Asking questions to elicit key information
- Observing nonverbal behavior
- Reading medical records

Diagnosis
- Posing questions to help analyze and cluster data into meaningful patterns
- Talking with client and family or significant others to determine perception of needs and problems

Planning/Outcome Identification
- Talking with clients to mutually determine areas of concern and to formulate goals and objectives
- Staff meetings with coworkers to develop plans of care
- Writing and reading plans of care

Implementation

Determination of most appropriate intervention or method of responding; calls for input from client, significant others, and health care team members

Evaluation

Critiquing the client's response to interventions; requires direct communication with client and significant others

TABLE 15-7 Communication Roadblocks

ROADBLOCK	DEFINITION	EXAMPLES
Reassuring	Comments that indicate to the client that concerns or fears are unwarranted	• "Everything will be fine." • "You will feel better soon."
Agreeing	Comments that indicate that the nurse's views are those of the client	• "I agree." • "I think you are right."
Approving	Comments that indicate that the client's views, actions, needs, or wishes are "good" rather than "bad"	• "That's good." • "I think you did the right thing."
Defending	Comments that are aimed at protecting the nurse, someone else, or something from verbal attack	• "I did not say that." • "Doctor Jones is a good physician." • "I am sure your father meant nothing by that comment."
Using closed questions	Questions or comments that can be answered by the client with one word	• "Are you tired?" • "Could we talk now?" • "Did you sleep well?"
Using stereotyped comments	"Pat" answers or clichés that indicate that the client's concerns are unimportant or insignificant	• "C'est la vie." • "That's the way the ball bounces." • "It will all come out in the wash."
Changing focus	Switching to a topic that is more comfortable to discuss	*Client:* "I wish I were dead." *Nurse:* "Did your wife visit today?"
Judging	Comments or actions by the nurse that indicate pleasure or displeasure with what the client says	• A stern look • Rolling the eyes • "I like that." • "I do not like that."
Blaming	Accusing the client of misconduct; undermining the client's need to be loved and accepted	• "You should know better than to talk like that." • "If you had not moved, I would have been able to complete this venipuncture."
Belittling the client's feelings	Indicating to the client that feelings expressed are unwarranted or unimportant	• "Don't feel that way." • "Be a big boy and stop crying."
Advising	Giving the client opinion or direction about solving a problem	• "If I were you, I would talk to your husband about this." • "I think you should do something for yourself for a change."
Rejecting	Indicating to the client that certain topics are not open to discussion	• "Let's not talk about that right now."
Disapproving	Indicating displeasure about comments or behaviors or placing a value on them	• "That's bad."
Probing	Pressuring the client to discuss something before he or she is ready	• "Why do you feel this way?" • "Why did you come to the hospital?" • "Why are you angry with your son?"

Data from Antai-Otong, D., & Wasserman, F. (2007). Therapeutic communication. In D. Antai-Otong & P. Hawkins (Eds.), *Psychiatric nursing: Biological and behavioral concepts* (2nd ed.). Clifton Park, NY: Delmar Learning; Kneisl, C. R. (2009). Therapeutic communication. In C. R. Kneisl & E. Trigoboff, *Contemporary psychiatric mental health nursing* (2nd ed.). Upper Saddle River, NJ: Pearson; Stuart, G. W., & Laraia, M. T. (2004). Therapeutic nurse-patient relationship. In G. W. Stuart & M. T. Laraia (Eds.), *Principles and practice of psychiatric nursing* (8th ed.). St. Louis, MO: Elsevier.

TABLE 15-8 Classification of Aphasias

Broca's aphasia	Slow hesitant speech
	Difficulty selecting and organizing words
	Naming, word, and phrase repetition
	Writing impaired
	Slight comprehension defects
Wernicke's aphasia	Auditory comprehension impaired
	Impaired speech content
	Client unaware of deficits
Anomic aphasia	Unable to name objects or places
	Comprehension and repetition of words and phrases intact
Conduction aphasia	Difficulty repeating words; substitutes incorrect sounds for another
Global aphasia	Severe impairment of oral and written comprehension
	Impaired naming and repetition of words
	Impaired writing ability

Delmar/Cengage Learning

NURSING PROCESS HIGHLIGHT

Diagnosis

Nursing Diagnosis: Impaired Verbal Communication
Definition: State in which a person experiences a decreased, delayed, or absent ability to process, receive, or transmit meaning

Defining Characteristics

- Disorientation
- Inability or unwillingness to speak
- Difficulty speaking
- Difficulty expressing thoughts verbally
- Partial or total visual defect
- Stuttering or slurring of words
- Willful refusal to speak
- Unable to speak dominant language

Related Factors

- Cultural differences
- Decreased cerebral blood flow
- Physical barrier (e.g., tracheostomy)
- Anatomical defect (e.g., cleft palate)
- Developmental differences

Data from North American Nursing Diagnosis Association International. (2009). *Nursing diagnoses—Definitions and classification 2009–2011*. Philadelphia: John Wiley & Sons, Inc.

Or is there an incongruity between the words and behavior? Assessing the client's communication ability involves collecting data relevant to the presence of physical and psychological barriers. Assessment of the client's ability to communicate must be ongoing. The presence of aphasia (impairment or absence of language function) should not be misinterpreted as confusion. Table 15-8 describes the types of aphasia.

NURSING DIAGNOSIS

Accurate diagnosis of client problems can be achieved by establishing a therapeutic relationship with the client. By paying meticulous attention to the client's communication, nurses are able to determine pertinent needs and, thus, develop accurate diagnostic judgments. Through effective communication, the nurse develops an atmosphere in which the client feels safe to express all relevant concerns.

The North American Nursing Diagnosis Association International (2009) defines communication as the ability to receive and transmit a system of symbols. Whenever a client is unable to send, receive, or interpret messages accurately, the diagnosis *Impaired verbal communication* is applicable; see the Nursing Process Highlight.

Other diagnoses that may be relevant for the person experiencing communication difficulties include the following:

- Social isolation related to impaired verbal communication
- Anxiety related to impaired verbal communication

✓ NURSING CHECKLIST

Overcoming Language Barriers

- Speak slowly and distinctly in a normal tone of voice.
- Use gestures or pictures to emphasize meaning of words.
- Avoid cliches, medical jargon, or value-laden terms.
- Avoid defensive or challenging body language.
- Provide reading material written in the appropriate language.
- Use an interpreter who is fluent in health care terminology.
- Speak to the client rather than to the interpreter.
- Use the same interpreter for every interaction if feasible.

TABLE 15-9 Communicating with Vulnerable Populations

Clients who are hearing impaired	Determine if the client reads lips. If so, face the client and reduce background noise to a minimum.
	If client is using a hearing aid, check to see that it is in working order.
	Always face the client.
	Speak at a normal pace in a normal tone of voice.
	Focus on nonverbal cues from the client.
	Use gestures and facial expressions to reinforce verbal messages.
	Provide pen and paper to facilitate communication if client is literate.
Clients who are visually impaired	When speaking to visually impaired clients, always face them as if they were sighted.
	Follow the cues of the clients in order to allow as much independence as possible.
	Look directly at the client.
	Speak in a normal tone of voice; it is demeaning to yell.
	Ask for permission before touching the client.
	Orient the client to the immediate environment.
Clients who are aphasic	Assess the client's usual method of communication; adapt the interaction to accommodate the client's abilities.
	Use a written interview format, letter boards, or yes/no cards.
	Allow additional time for client's responses.
	Do not answer for the client.
	Use closed (one-word response) questions when possible.
	Repeat or rephrase the comment if client does not understand.
	Speak directly to the client, not to the intermediary.
	To reinforce verbal messages, use facial expressions, gestures, and voice tone.
Unconscious clients	Assume the client can hear.
	Talk to the client in a normal tone of voice.
	Engage in normal conversational topics as with any client.
	Speak to the client before touching.
	Use touch to communicate a sense of presence.
Confused clients	Maintain appropriate eye contact.
	Keep background noises to a minimum.
	Use simple, concrete words and sentences.
	Use pictures and symbols.
	Use closed rather than open-ended questions.
	Give the client time to respond.
Angry clients	Use caution when communicating with a client who has a history of violent behavior or poor impulse control.

(Continues)

TABLE 15-9 (Continued)

Do not turn your back on the client. Arrange the setting so that the client is not between you and the door to the room.
Focus on the client's body language.
Be alert for physical indicators of impending aggression: narrowed eyes, clenched jaw, clenched fist, or a loud tone of voice.
Model the expected behavior by lowering your tone of voice.
Stay within the client's line of vision.
Do not use touch.

Delmar/Cengage Learning

UNCOVERING THE

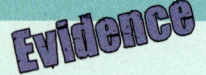

TITLE OF STUDY

"Impact of Patient Communication Problems on the Risk of Preventable Adverse Events in Acute Care Settings"

AUTHORS

G. Bartlett, R. Blais, R. Tamblyn, R. J. Clermont, and B. MacGibbon

PURPOSE

To assess whether communication problems are associated with an increased risk of preventable adverse events.

METHODS

A total of 2,355 medical records were randomly selected and reviewed to assess the cause of adverse events. Reviewers abstracted client characteristics, including communication problems, in order to examine the cause of adverse events that occurred in general hospitals.

FINDINGS

Clients with preventable adverse events were significantly more likely than those without such events to have communication problems.

IMPLICATIONS

Clients with communication problems appeared to be at higher risk for preventable adverse events. Interventions to reduce the risk for these clients need to be developed.

Bartlett, G., Blais, R., Tamblyn, R., Clermont, R. J., & MacGibbon, B. (2008). Impact of patient communication problems on the risk of preventable adverse events in acute care settings. *Canadian Medical Association Journal, 178*(12), 1573–1574.

PLANNING AND OUTCOME IDENTIFICATION

After identifying communication problems, the nurse and client work together to develop goals and outcomes. The nurse then formulates nursing interventions to promote goal achievement. A major goal for every client is to develop an ability to communicate effectively, whether by verbalization or alternate means. See the Nursing Checklist on page 276 for guidelines in dealing with language barriers.

IMPLEMENTATION

Communication is the major tool by which nurses deliver safe, effective care. Research evidence indicates that effective communication increases client safety (Bartlett, Blais, Tamblyn, Clermont, & MacGibbon, 2008). Therefore, it is crucial that nurses communicate effectively with all clients. See the Uncovering the Evidence display.

It is extremely challenging for nurses to communicate with clients experiencing communication disorders. Technological advances have led to the development of telecommunication relay services (TRS), which often can be used with clients experiencing communication disorders. See Table 15-9 on page 277 for a description of methods for communicating with clients who have special needs. Also see Chapter 21 for specific guidelines on communicating with children, adolescents, and elderly clients.

EVALUATION

Evaluation of communication effectiveness involves both nurse and client. Communication is a major tool for evaluating a client's achievement of expected outcomes. For example, the nurse observes nonverbal behavior, talks with the client, and listens actively to the client's comments. The nurse uses critical thinking to analyze the client's responses as well as his or her own use of communication skills.

KEY CONCEPTS

- Communication is a vital aspect of all phases of nursing practice.

- The five components of the communication process are the sender, message, channel, receiver, and feedback.

- Factors such as perception, cultural context, space and distance, and time influence communication.

- The three levels of communication are intrapersonal, interpersonal, and group.

- Using language or other symbols, the sender produces verbal, paraverbal, and nonverbal messages that are delivered through a channel (visual, auditory, or kinesthetic) to a receiver.

- Interdisciplinary communication is a type of interaction by which members of the health care team collaborate on a client's care.

- Therapeutic communication is the use of communication for the purpose of creating a beneficial outcome for the client.

- Elements of effective therapeutic communication include empathy, trust, honesty, validation, caring, and active listening.

- The nurse needs to observe specific principles and techniques in order to initiate and maintain therapeutic communication with clients.

- Barriers such as language differences, sociocultural differences, gender, health status, developmental level, knowledge differences, emotional distance, emotions, and daydreaming can pose challenges for nurses in communication with clients.

- Communication barriers can be overcome if creativity, innovation, awareness, sensitivity, and critical thinking skills are used by the nurse.

REVIEW QUESTIONS

1. A client who is crying states, "I just don't understand why they won't let me get up." Which of the following nursing responses demonstrates the use of clarification?
   a. "I'm sure they are just doing what they think is best for you."
   b. "Maybe you just misunderstood them."
   c. "Tell me who they are."
   d. "Well, of course, you can get up. I'll help you."

2. A nurse is conducting a medication education class. Which of the following client behaviors indicates that a client's dominant sensory channel is visual?
   a. Asking the nurse to explain in more detail about the medications
   b. Asking the nurse to repeat the information
   c. Demonstrating self-administration of an injection
   d. Reading the handout distributed by the nurse

3. A nurse manager is meeting with a staff nurse to provide feedback on inferior performance of a specific task. Which of the following actions by the manager demonstrates the effective use of feedback? Select all that apply.
   a. Avoiding discussion of the poor performance in order to boost the staff nurse's self-confidence
   b. Discussing the staff nurse's performance in a staff meeting
   c. Scheduling the feedback session immediately following the poor performance

   d. Stating exactly what needs to be done to show improvement
   e. Using words that clearly describe the unsatisfactory performance
   f. Waiting to discuss the staff nurse's actions at the annual performance evaluation

4. Which of the following communication techniques encourages the client to be spontaneous during an interaction?
   a. Confronting
   b. Making observations
   c. Open-ended comments
   d. Focusing

5. Which of the following nursing comments demonstrates the use of reassuring?
   a. "I think you should talk with your friend about that."
   b. "That's the way the cookie crumbles."
   c. "You shouldn't feel like that."
   d. "You will feel better soon."

6. A client who is scheduled for surgery tomorrow tells the nurse that he is afraid. Which of the following nursing responses is therapeutic for this client?
   a. "Are you saying you've changed your mind about having the surgery?"
   b. "I'm sure you will be fine."
   c. "Tell me more about that."
   d. "You have nothing to worry about. Your surgeon is the best!"

online companion

Visit the DeLaune and Ladner online companion resource at **www.delmar.cengage.com** for additional content and study aids. Click on Online Companions, then select the Nursing discipline.

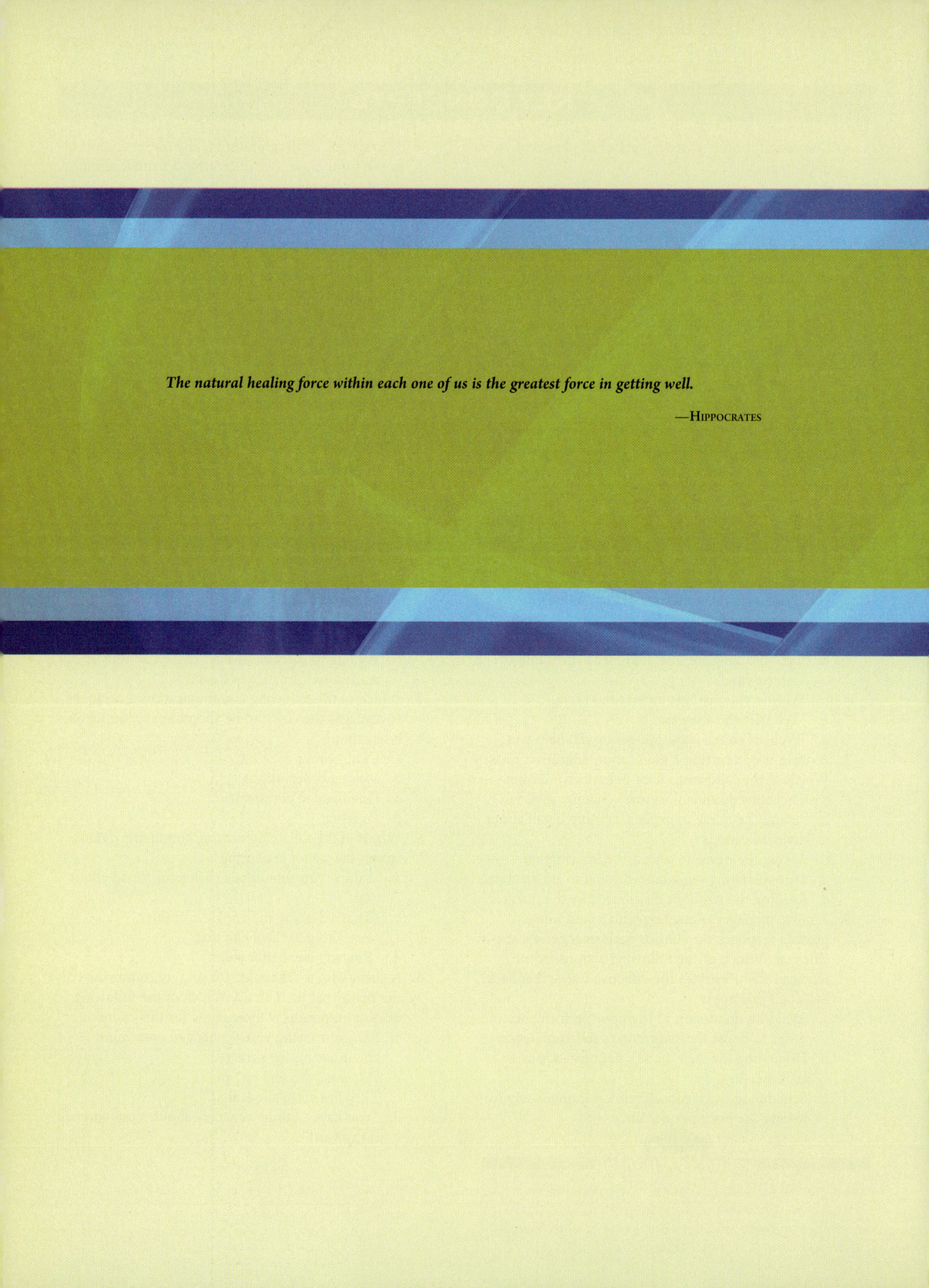

The natural healing force within each one of us is the greatest force in getting well.

—Hippocrates

CHAPTER 16

Health and Wellness Promotion

COMPETENCIES

1. Differentiate health, illness, and wellness.
2. Identify assumptions of selected theoretical models of health.
3. Relate the achievement of basic needs to health status.
4. Explain the relationship of variables such as lifestyle, locus of control, self-efficacy, health care attitudes, and self-concept to health behaviors.
5. Discuss the impact of holism on health and health care delivery.
6. Discuss nursing's role in health promotion.
7. Discuss the nurse's role in promoting the sexual health of clients.

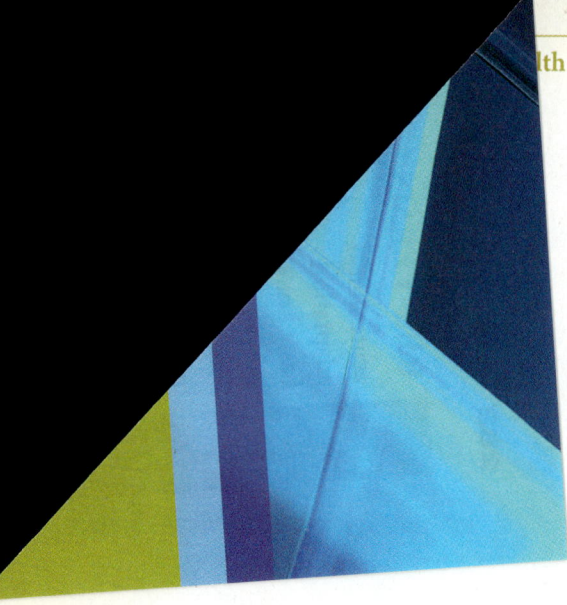

health promotion	self-concept
health-seeking behaviors	self-efficacy
heterosexuality	self-esteem
high-level wellness	sex roles
homeostasis	sexuality
homosexuality	sexual orientation
illness	spirituality
locus of control	transsexuality
need	wellness
psychoneuroimmunology	

Health and illness can be defined in many ways. Health is a concept that includes physical and mental status, emotional well-being, and spiritual well-being. Historically, Western cultures have defined health as the absence of illness. It is easier to measure illness than it is to measure health because definite parameters can be used to determine whether an individual has symptoms indicative of disease processes. What criteria are used for determining one's health? Is health merely the absence of disease, or is health more comprehensive?

In addition to examining these questions, this chapter describes health promotion activities with an emphasis on nursing's role. There is a discussion of holism, basic human needs, and the physiological, psychological, sociocultural, intellectual, spiritual, and sexual dimensions of the individual.

HEALTH, ILLNESS, AND WELLNESS

Health, the process through which a person seeks to maintain an equilibrium that promotes stability and comfort, is a dynamic process that varies according to a person's perception of well-being. The traditional definition of health as the absence of illness is a narrow concept. Illness is the inability of an individual's adaptive responses to maintain physical and emotional balance with subsequent impairment of functional abilities. Wellness is the condition in which an individual functions at optimal levels. An in-depth discussion of wellness appears later in this chapter.

Health is a global term because it refers to every aspect of a person's life, including:

- Physical status
- Emotional well-being
- Social relationships
- Intellectual functioning
- Spiritual condition
- Sexuality

MODELS OF HEALTH

There are several theoretical models of health (see Table 16-1 on page 283). These models help clarify the link between the states of well-being and illness and clients' responses to these processes.

Dossey and Guzzetta (2008) describe health as a maintenance of harmony and balance among body, mind, and spirit. Balance refers to homeostasis, which is an equilibrium among psychological, physiological, sociocultural, intellectual, and spiritual needs. The process by which a person adjusts to achieve homeostasis is called adaptation. When people describe their health status, three basic areas are considered:

- Presence or absence of symptoms (physical and emotional)
- How they feel (emotionally and physically)
- What they are able to do (ability to function)

Health can be studied both in individuals and in groups (e.g., families and communities). Health status is influenced by:

- Beliefs and attitudes
- Cultural factors
- Lifestyle behaviors

An individual, within the context of the family unit, gives meaning to health and makes adjustments necessitated by the illness. A family's adaptation to changes in health status is strongly influenced by each member's personal resources and support systems (i.e., social, spiritual).

Cultural Influences on Health

Health-related concepts evolve within the context of one's culture; that is, culture affects how an individual views health and illness. Cultural background influences health-related behaviors and expectations of treatment when illness occurs. For example, how an individual cares for himself or herself is directly related to cultural norms. See Chapter 20 for a complete discussion of cultural beliefs and behaviors affecting health.

TABLE 16-1 Theoretical Perspectives of Health

MODEL	THEORIST	ASSUMPTIONS
Clinical model	Traditional perspective	Health is the absence of illness. Individuals who are not "sick" (i.e., experiencing a disease) are healthy.
Health-belief model	Rosenstock	Expectations direct behaviors that lead to fulfillment of the expectations. Group values exert influence on beliefs about health. Beliefs may change as a person grows and develops.
High-level wellness model	Dunn	Health is influenced by the interaction between the individual, family, and community. Health is viewed as an attempt to achieve one's fullest potential.
Social learning theory	Bandura, Rosenstock	Beliefs strongly influence actions. Behavior is influenced by expectations and reinforcements (or incentives).
Host-agent-environment model ("ecologic" model)	Leavell and Clark	Health depends on the interaction of host, agent, and environment. Balance among these elements results in health. Illness occurs when there is an imbalance in one of the three elements. Model is used most often in predicting risk of illness.
Health promotion model	Pender	Model focuses on activities that improve wellness and prevent disabilities. People use health-promoting activities when they: • Value health • Perceive health as being within their control • Can identify benefits in self-care activities • Have a positive perception of their own health status

Data from Bandura, A. (1977). *A social learning theory*. Englewood Cliffs, NJ: Prentice-Hall; Becker, M. H. (1974). The health belief model and sick role behavior. *Health Education Monogram*, 2, 409–419; Dunn, H. (1961). *High-level wellness*. Arlington, VA: R. W. Beatty; Edelman, C., & Mandle, C. L. (2006). *Health promotion throughout the life span* (6th ed.). St Louis, MO: Mosby Elsevier; Leavell, H., & Clark, A. E. (1965). *Preventive medicine for doctors in the community*. New York: McGraw-Hill; Pender, N. J. (1987). *Health promotion in nursing practice*. East Norwalk, CT: Appleton & Lange; Rosenstock, I. (1974). Historical origin of the health belief model. In M. H. Becker (Ed.), *The health belief model and personal health behavior*. Thorofare, NJ: Charles B. Slack.

Family Influences on Health

Because health is defined uniquely by each client's culture, the nurse must assess the family's health definitions and beliefs. Generally, families are the first to identify signals of impending illness. Also, families help determine the following:

• Whether to seek treatment
• What type of treatment is appropriate
• Who should provide the treatment or care
• Where the treatment or care should be provided

See the accompanying Community Considerations display.

Families are often the major caregivers for individuals experiencing illness. Extended families and communities have traditionally acted as a buffer against excessive stress and illness. Lack of social support from family or significant others often results in psychological and spiritual isolation, which negatively affects a person's physiological state. Thus, it is

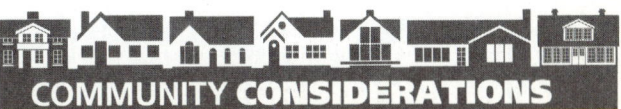

COMMUNITY CONSIDERATIONS

Rewarding Healthy and Unhealthy Behaviors

In general, Western society does not reward health-promoting behaviors. For example, children get attention when they are sick, not when they are well. This attention takes the form of goodies, treats, and relief from responsibilities such as homework and chores. This attention reinforces the value of being sick to children. Another example of our society's rewarding illness occurs in the workplace. Most employees are entitled to sick days, but time off is not given for "well days." What message is communicated by such behaviors?

important to help clients identify, strengthen, and use their social support systems. Sometimes, families need guidance in order to optimize healthy behaviors. Nursing assessment must include the client's and family's perspectives of the most pressing problem. See the Community Considerations display for a listing of nursing actions that promote family collaboration.

ILLNESS PERSPECTIVES

Illness means different things to different people and is more than just the existence of physical signs and symptoms. Illness is the result of a disease (either physiological or psychological) or injury that affects functioning and occurs when there is an inability to meet one's needs.

There are two major classifications of illness: acute and chronic. An **acute illness** is a disruption in functional ability usually characterized by a rapid onset, intense manifestations, and a relatively short duration. Acute illnesses are usually reversible. A **chronic illness** is a disruption in functional ability usually characterized by a gradual, insidious onset with lifelong changes that are usually irreversible. Chronic illnesses last a long time, frequently throughout the individual's life. An example of an acute illness is influenza; arthritis is an example of a chronic illness. It is possible for a person to have both a chronic illness and an acute illness at the same time, for example, the person with diabetes (chronic) who also develops pneumonia (acute).

Chronic illness affects individuals across the life span. Approximately 20% of American children are affected by disabilities, such as learning or behavioral problems (Cagle, 2006, p. 583). Adolescents experiencing chronic illnesses need two major nursing interventions: support and education.

Even though many elderly individuals have multiple chronic conditions, it is important to remember that chronicity is *not* an experience unique to the elderly. However, as life expectancy continues to increase, an increasing number of people are living with chronic illness. The implications for nursing are far reaching. Some of the goals of caring for people with chronic illnesses include:

- Coping with lifestyle changes and the subsequent modification of self-care activities
- Coping with long-term discomfort or pain
- Establishing or maintaining a sense of personal control
- Maintaining a positive self-esteem (Edelman & Mandle, 2006)

WELLNESS PERSPECTIVES

Wellness further describes health status by putting health on a continuum from one's optimal level (wellness) to a maladaptive state (illness); see Figure 16-1. Wellness is a dynamic process that is ever changing. The well person usually has some degree of illness, and the ill person usually has some degree of wellness. This concept of a health continuum negates the idea that wellness and illness are opposite because they may occur simultaneously in the same person in varying degrees. The classic description of wellness was developed by Dunn in the early 1960s. According to Dunn (1961), **high-level wellness** means functioning to one's maximum health potential while remaining in balance with the environment.

HEALTH BEHAVIORS

To understand how people influence their health status, it is important to know about health behaviors. **Behavior** is defined as the observable response of an individual to external stimuli. An important concept to remember when caring for clients is that *all behavior has meaning*. In other words, behavior is the individual's attempt to achieve satisfaction of needs. Nurses must sometimes act as detectives to determine the need(s) underlying client behavior. Thorough assessment is the key for nurses in determining the meaning of client behavior. **Health-seeking behaviors** are those activities directed toward attaining and maintaining a state of well-being.

COMMUNITY **CONSIDERATIONS**

Actions to Promote Collaboration with Families

- Listen as family members express feelings.
- Assess the extent to which family members wish to be involved in the treatment process.
- Involve family members to the extent they desire.
- Encourage participation in problem-solving activities.
- Participate in family support groups.
- Answer questions asked by client and family.
- Allow time for everyone to talk.
- Discuss aftercare plans to promote continuity of care.

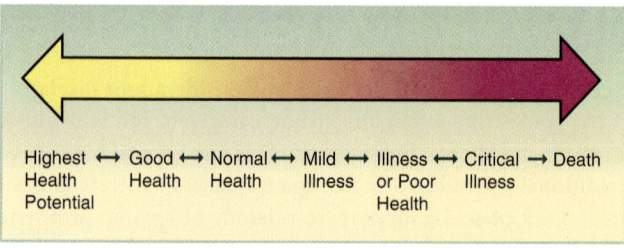

Highest ↔ Good ↔ Normal ↔ Mild ↔ Illness ↔ Critical → Death
Health   Health   Health   Illness   or Poor   Illness
Potential   Health

FIGURE 16-1 **Health Continuum** DELMAR/CENGAGE LEARNING

VARIABLES INFLUENCING HEALTH BEHAVIORS

There are several variables that influence health including:

- Lifestyle
- Perceived locus of control
- Perceived ease or difficulty in accomplishing a task (self-efficacy)
- Health care attitudes
- Self-concept

Lifestyle

Individuals determine their health status through their actions (see Figure 16-2). Lifestyle consists of a person's usual daily activities and routines that are acceptable practices in the person's life. Such routines and habits influence health status. For example, smoking and a sedentary lifestyle negatively affect health status. Lifestyles are developed within one's family and one's cultural environment. The family is the primary influence on a child's development of health-promoting (or health-defeating) behaviors.

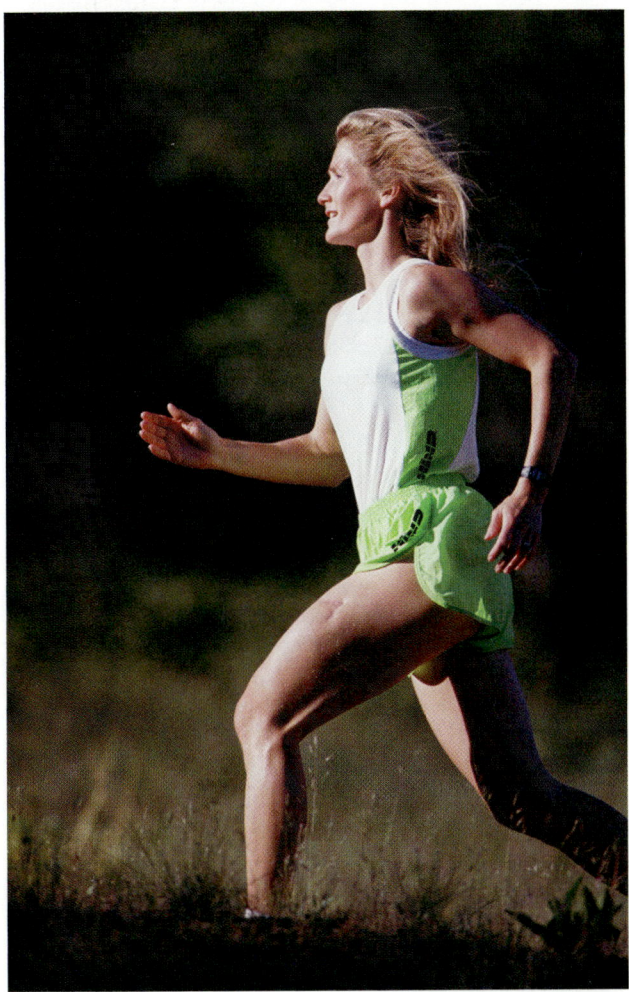

FIGURE 16-2 Through exercise, this woman is demonstrating a lifestyle choice that will enhance her health status. How does this type of behavior promote wellness? DELMAR/CENGAGE LEARNING

When lifestyle modifications are necessary to improve health, many individuals have difficulty implementing the suggested changes. Individuals are less likely to comply with recommended lifestyle changes if there is a perception of increased inconvenience and cost. Also, the required degree of change in lifestyle may affect compliance.

Locus of Control

Locus of control refers to individuals' sense of being able to influence events and situations affecting their lives. A person with an external locus of control feels like a victim with little, if any, control over life events. However, people with an internal locus of control feel able to influence significant events and occurrences affecting them; that is, they see themselves as responsible for their own lives. Thus, those with an internal locus of control are more willing to make lifestyle changes that lead to wellness.

Self-Efficacy

Bandura (1977) used the term self-efficacy to describe an individual's perception of one's own ability to perform a certain task. Self-efficacy has a powerful impact on initiating behavior change.

Self-efficacy is a form of self-confidence that leads to successful behavior performance. As described by Bandura (1986), self-efficacy encompasses two types of expectations:

1. *Outcome expectations:* Beliefs about whether behavior will produce desirable results
2. *Efficacy expectations:* Beliefs the person has about his or her own ability to perform the behavior

Health implies moving toward self-care, in other words, becoming and remaining independent. Self-responsibility, as it relates to health-promoting activities, is a fairly new concept to many Americans. For years, individuals have looked to prescribing practitioners to "fix things" and "make it better." Only when individuals enter into active partnerships with their primary health care provider (nurse, physician, or other healer) will self-responsibility for health become a reality. See the Uncovering the Evidence display on page 286.

When clients are able to make informed decisions about their health behaviors and feel that they are successful in these areas, they are more likely to attempt behavior change. Thus, an essential component of nursing care is to provide opportunities for clients to achieve this level of self-motivation. For example, when teaching a client how to self-administer injections, the nurse breaks the task down into small manageable objectives and asks the client to do a return demonstration. The client receives immediate feedback, which encourages further success.

Health Care Attitudes

Beliefs are powerful shapers of behavior. Health behaviors are based on beliefs. Attitudes about health and personal vulnerability (which are initially learned in the family unit)

UNCOVERING THE

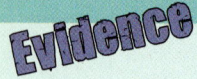

TITLE OF STUDY

"Incorporating Self-Efficacy and Interpersonal Support in an Intervention to Increase Physical Activity in Older Women"

AUTHORS

C. Costanzo and S. N. Walker

PURPOSE

The purpose of this study was twofold: (1) to compare the efficacy of five sessions versus one session of behavioral counseling in a 12-week intervention to increase self-efficacy and family and friend support for activity and (2) to examine self-efficacy and support as mediators of activity among 45 urban older women.

METHODS

This was a randomized, controlled trial in which outcomes were examined with repeated-measures analysis of variance and path analysis.

FINDINGS

No significant change was observed in self-efficacy in the five-session group; however, a significant decrease was observed in the one-session group. Family and friend support increased significantly in the five-session group. The intervention effect on activity was mediated through change in self-efficacy and family support.

IMPLICATIONS

Self-efficacy can be increased and/or maintained through repeated counseling sessions and family support.

Costanzo, C., & Walker, S. N. (2008). Incorporating self-efficacy and interpersonal support in an intervention to increase physical activity in older women. *Women & Health, 47*(4), 91–108.

Self-Concept

Self-concept is an individual's perception of self. It includes **self-esteem** (an individual's perception of self-worth) and **body image** (perception of one's physical self). The relationship between self-concept and health is strong.

Self-concept influences individuals' health behaviors in that people who think highly of themselves will tend to take care of themselves. On the other hand, a person with a negative self-concept may engage in reckless or self-destructive behaviors that endanger health. People with a low self-concept frequently ignore their own needs because they are perceived to be less important than the needs of other people.

Self-concept is dynamic and may change according to health status. Not only does self-concept influence health, but changes in health status may also influence self-concept. For example, consider the person who has lost a limb due to amputation. This person's self-concept might be altered as a result of the physical change. See Chapter 22 for further discussion of self-efficacy.

HEALTH PROMOTION

Prior to the 1990s, most health-related research focused on behaviors that prevent illness. Currently, however, the trend among health care professionals is to emphasize behaviors that promote wellness. Health promotion refers to any activity that improves the quality of health and well-being of individuals, families, and communities. The aim of health promotion is to empower people to make choices regarding lifestyles and activities (Maville & Huerta, 2007).

The U.S. Department of Health and Human Services (DHHS) (2005), in its Healthy People initiative, focuses on the individual's responsibility in promoting health. Individuals are viewed as having the ability to influence their own health and also that of the country. There are several approaches to health maintenance:

- Health promotion
- Health protection
- Disease prevention (U.S. DHHS, 2005)

COMMUNITY CONSIDERATIONS

The Media and Health Beliefs

The media are extremely powerful in shaping attitudes and beliefs. Here are some examples of how various media discourage health-promoting behaviors:

Advertising foods with high sugar, salt, and fat content

Promoting alcohol use

Encouraging use of tobacco products

What other examples can you identify? Recently, there seems to be an emerging trend to advertise healthier lifestyles. What examples come to mind?

greatly influence behavior. Socialization (which occurs within the family) influences the development of beliefs about health care. Societal values also affect the development of beliefs about health care; see the accompanying Community Considerations display. These beliefs determine the person's willingness to participate in health care. For example, if the person believes in the use of herbs or folk healers, these practices could either enhance or interfere with traditional treatment approaches.

Nurses must be sensitive to the fact that all clients do not share the same beliefs about health care issues. Using a nonjudgmental attitude helps the nurse to be more accepting of clients with diverse beliefs and behaviors.

In 1979, the U.S. DHHS mobilized public health agencies to work toward developing healthier Americans. This initiative, Healthy People, is now in its fourth decade and is called Healthy People 2020. The program, coordinated by the Office of Disease Prevention and Health Promotion under the U.S. DHHS, focuses on allowing equal access of all Americans to preventive health care services. Most states use the Healthy People framework to guide the development and implementation of local health policies and programs. Healthy People 2020 recognizes the need to focus on improving the quality of life as well as reducing disparities in the type of health care services received by Americans.

The Healthy People initiative is implemented through the efforts of health care agencies, both public and private. The leading health indicators, which are used to measure the nation's health, reflect the major health concerns of the nation; they include the following:

- Physical activity
- Overweight and obesity
- Tobacco use
- Substance abuse
- Responsible sexual behavior
- Mental health
- Injury and violence
- Environmental quality
- Immunization
- Access to health care (U.S. DHHS, 2005)

HEALTH PROMOTION ACTIVITIES

Health promotion is a process undertaken to increase the levels of wellness in individuals, families, and communities. It involves activities and programs provided by nurses and other health care providers to foster lifestyle behaviors conducive to optimum health status. Major goals of health promotion activities include the following:

- Respect and support clients' right to make decisions
- Identify and use client strengths and assets
- Empower clients to promote their own health or healing

Nurses identify high-risk individuals and determine and strengthen their social support, thus encouraging disease prevention. Clients who are attempting to adopt health-promoting behaviors (actions that increase well-being or quality of life) must receive support and reinforcement for their attempts. As beginning health care providers, nursing students are encouraged to develop their own health-promoting behaviors in order to be better role models for clients. See the accompanying Spotlight On display.

Individuals are becoming more aware of the relationship between daily behavior and health status. Types of health promotion programs can include smoking cessation, nutrition, and exercise. Changing health behaviors means focusing on the whole person within the context of the environment.

Health promotion activities are holistic in that they target physical and emotional health concerns. Some

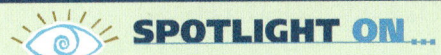

SPOTLIGHT ON...

Caring

Nurses as Healthy Role Models

Nurses have an opportunity to model healthy behaviors. Think about the messages many nurses communicate through certain behaviors such as smoking, overwork, and inadequate use of stress management techniques.

Do you think nurses have an obligation to demonstrate healthy behaviors? Explain the rationale for your answer.

What type of health-promoting behaviors do you demonstrate?

nursing activities that promote and protect mental health include:

- Teaching conflict resolution skills
- Providing support to grieving families
- Monitoring for abuse of children, partners, and elders
- Teaching stress management techniques

HEALTH PROTECTION ACTIVITIES

Health protection includes a variety of activities. Prevention of accidental injury in the home, at school, and in the workplace is an example. Programs that focus on occupational safety and health are designed to protect employees' health. Governmental efforts to ensure the safety of food and drug products are another example of health protection. Environmental strategies, such as water purification, sewage disposal, and air quality control, are used to protect the health of individuals and communities.

DISEASE PREVENTION ACTIVITIES

Disease prevention occurs on a continuum, from averting the development of disease to limiting its course once developed. The purpose of *primary prevention* is to decrease the person's vulnerability to disease. Primary preventive measures include parenting education, attention to personal hygiene, and avoidance of toxins. The goal of *secondary prevention* is early detection of disease to initiate early intervention. Examples of secondary preventive activities are screening for particular diseases and preventing the spread of communicable disease. When a disease (such as a chronic condition) already exists, *tertiary prevention* is used to minimize its effects and to prevent further disability.

Nurses who work in rehabilitation settings, including the home, are engaged in tertiary prevention. The focus is on restorative care, that is, therapeutic interventions directed at helping clients reach and maintain their optimal level of functioning.

NURSE'S ROLE IN HEALTH PROMOTION

Nurses play a major role in promoting health and wellness. Health promotion enables the individual to develop behavior patterns that promote a healthy lifestyle and reduce the risk of disease. When behaviors that once worked for the individual are no longer effective, the client must give up the old behaviors in order to be able to adopt new, healthier ones. The challenge for nurses is to find ways to motivate clients and families to develop health-promoting behaviors. Client teaching is a major intervention for promoting health (see Figure 16-3). An essential component of teaching is encouraging clients to make necessary lifestyle changes to promote health.

Motivation is a key component of achieving and maintaining health. Nurses can better help clients engage in healthy behaviors by considering the client's beliefs and experiences when planning care. How do nurses encourage the development of healthy behaviors in clients? Merely providing information is not the key. The key is to inspire clients to want to change. Price (2006) refers to this process as getting the attention of the client. Many factors help clients feel motivated to change health behaviors:

- Perception of self as able to succeed (self-efficacy)
- Belief that health status will improve
- Response to attempts to change in the form of feeling healthier and receiving confirmation of these changes from others

HEALTH PROMOTION AND VULNERABLE POPULATIONS

Risk factors that threaten the health of individuals include poverty and chronic disease (Go, 2006). The health of certain population groups is threatened; especially vulnerable groups include:

- Children
- Older adults

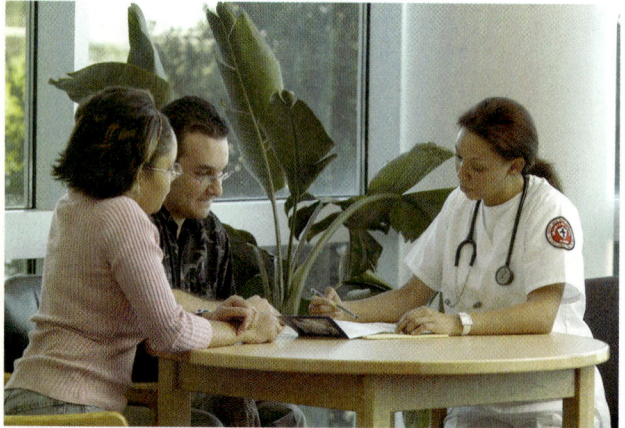

FIGURE 16-3 To promote the health of this expectant couple and their baby, the nurse is providing information about nutritional intake during pregnancy. What incentives can the nurse offer in this situation that would encourage these clients to practice health-promoting behaviors? DELMAR/CENGAGE LEARNING

RESPECTING OUR DIFFERENCES

Inexpensive Health-Promoting Behaviors

Several behaviors, such as walking and breastfeeding, are relatively inexpensive and promote health.

Think of some other examples of inexpensive behaviors that nurses can encourage people of all socioeconomic groups to incorporate into their lifestyles.

- Those who are economically disadvantaged
- Those who are immunocompromised
- The homeless

One primary variable affecting health promotion is socioeconomic status. Middle- and upper-income families are more likely to demonstrate healthy behaviors as they have the financial means to purchase nutritional foods, buy exercise equipment, and pay for recreation. The monies of lower socioeconomic families are typically used in meeting basic needs such as food, shelter, and acute medical care. Health-promoting options must be affordable and readily available to people of all economic levels; see the accompanying Respecting Our Differences display. Political involvement is one avenue for nursing to advance the health status of all. Nurses must be actively involved in shaping health care policy in order to influence the establishment of resources for underserved, disenfranchised groups.

Another variable affecting health is age. Elderly individuals tend to describe themselves as well when they are physically active, relatively free from pain, and able to maintain meaningful social ties. Maintaining independence and quality of life are of great importance for most elders. Nurses must promote self-care activities with elders to facilitate wellness.

THE INDIVIDUAL AS A HOLISTIC BEING

Due to the interwoven nature of the body and mind, it is impossible to separate physiological needs from psychosocial ones. **Psychoneuroimmunology** (the study of the complex relationship between the cognitive, affective, and physical aspects of individuals) is based on recognition of the concept that mind, body, and spirit are one. For example, a person who is physically ill also experiences psychosocial disruptions. On the other hand, when a person is anxious or depressed, physical manifestations occur.

The practice of body-mind medicine is not new and is rooted in the origins of healing, as shown in the following examples:

- Hippocrates taught physicians to establish trust with their patients.

- Hippocrates taught physicians to observe the emotional states of patients.
- Socrates suggested that curing the soul leads to healing.
- The fundamental principle of traditional Chinese medicine is to honor the spirit.
- Florence Nightingale understood the connection between the physical and spiritual aspects of clients.

Holism guides the total care of the individual as a *complete being* rather than fragmented care focused on parts of the person. Only when nurses treat clients as individuals and not as "cases" to be "cured" do nurses respond in a holistic, caring way. A major role for nurses is to put the *caring* back into the process of healing.

NEEDS AND HEALTH

Since human beings are not merely physiological creatures, basic needs occur in the emotional, sociocultural, intellectual, and spiritual realms as well as the physiological realm. The entire person (body, mind, and spirit) is influenced by satisfaction of needs. A variety of needs emerge, are met, and reemerge in each area of a person's life.

A **need** is anything that is absolutely *essential* for one's existence. **Basic human needs** (also known as universal needs) are those that are necessary for every person's survival. Table 16-2 provides an overview of basic needs.

Maslow (1970) classified human needs on a tier, with the most basic needs as the foundation of the hierarchy (see Figure 16-4). These basic needs must be met before the individual can satisfy higher-level needs. For example, an individual who is starving must be fed before achieving the need for acceptance. An individual with a deficient self-esteem and who is hemorrhaging must have the biologic needs met first. The satisfaction of basic needs enhances wellness. Con-

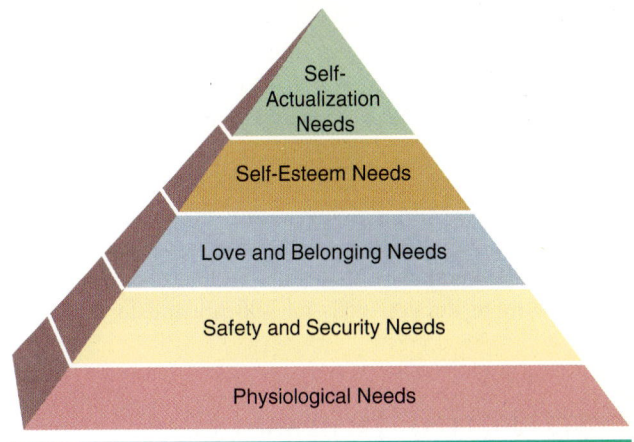

FIGURE 16-4 Maslow's Hierarchy of Needs ADAPTATION BASED ON MASLOW'S HIERARCHY OF NEEDS

versely, an impairment in the satisfaction of basic needs can result in a client's altered health status.

The following section describes basic needs related to the physiological, psychological, sociocultural, intellectual, spiritual, and sexual dimensions. There is extensive discussion of the nursing process as it relates to spirituality and sexuality to demonstrate how the process can be applied to all dimensions of an individual's being. See Chapter 24 for further further discussion of spiritual needs.

PHYSIOLOGICAL DIMENSION

Providing physiological care focuses on achievement of the basic needs such as oxygenation, circulation, sleep and comfort, nutrition, and elimination. Refer to Chapters 32, 34, 35, and 39 for a thorough discussion of the nurse's role in helping to meet these basic physiological needs.

PSYCHOLOGICAL DIMENSION

Individuals have psychological needs for security, a sense of belonging, and self-esteem. Nursing actions that promote a sense of emotional comfort include the following:

- Treating the client as a unique individual
- Protecting confidentiality and privacy
- Using touch and personal space in a therapeutic manner
- Recognizing and respecting cultural differences
- Decreasing anxiety through stress management techniques

Goals for clients experiencing unmet psychological needs usually revolve around the following issues:

- Improve self-esteem
- Establish trusting relationships
- Develop social skills
- Cope with losses

SOCIOCULTURAL DIMENSION

As social creatures, all people rely on others to some extent. It is difficult for some people to ask for help or to accept

TABLE 16-2 Basic Human Needs	
NEED	**EXAMPLE**
Physiological	Oxygen, water, food, temperature (shelter and clothing), elimination, sleep, activity, and sex
Psychological	Self-esteem, feelings of security, happiness, sadness
Sociocultural	Feelings of belonging, relationships
Intellectual	Thinking, learning
Spiritual	Being connected to others, having a sense of purpose

Delmar/Cengage Learning

assistance when it is offered. Nurses need to assess the client's degree of dependence. Often, the nurse becomes involved in a balancing act in an effort to maintain equilibrium between the client's needs for dependence and independence.

Empowerment is a process of enabling others to do for themselves. It consists of encouraging the client to be an active participant in treatment rather than a passive recipient of care. Nurses empower clients by teaching them and their families how to develop skills for self-care and for healthier living.

INTELLECTUAL DIMENSION

The intellectual dimension consists of cognitive functions such as judgment, orientation, memory, and the ability to take in and process information. See Chapter 38 for information on cognition and perception.

Piaget conducted landmark studies on children to determine how children think at various developmental stages. See Chapter 18 for a complete discussion of cognitive development throughout the life cycle.

Intellectual functioning can be impaired by multiple factors, including infection, exposure to toxins, substance abuse, trauma, and psychological problems. It is important for nurses to determine the client's intellectual abilities in order to communicate effectively. Using words that are easily comprehended by the client and implementing teaching strategies appropriate to developmental level promote client learning.

SPIRITUAL DIMENSION

Spirituality is multidimensional in that it refers to one's relationship with one's self, a sense of connection with others, and a relationship with a higher power or divine source. Spirituality assists a person in determining the sense of meaning or purpose in one's life. It is an integral component of one's being. Spirituality is somewhat difficult to define as it is determined at an individual level.

Spirituality is *not* the same as religion, which refers to a set of beliefs and practices associated with a particular church, synagogue, mosque, or other formal organized group. Spirituality is a personal, individualized set of beliefs and practices that are not church related.

Health status can have an impact on spiritual beliefs and vice versa. For example, when they are seriously ill, many people turn to religion for support. On the other hand, serious illness may cause some people to question their beliefs; see Chapter 24.

PROMOTING SEXUAL HEALTH

Sexuality is a complex set of human characteristics that refers not just to genital sex but to all the aspects of being male or female, including feelings, attitudes, beliefs, and behavior. Sexuality is a pervasive aspect of the total self from birth to death and is an important aspect of health for people of all ages. Sexuality includes a person's attitudes toward relationships with people of the same sex, toward relationships with those of the opposite sex, and about touching and being touched. The ways in which people dress, talk, and relate to others are indicators of their sexuality.

Sex roles are culturally determined patterns associated with being male and female. These patterns are developed as a result of cultural expectations, customs, norms, habits, and traditions. For example, the differences between the sexes are evident in the ways infants are treated during their first days of life. Infant boys and infant girls are talked to, cuddled, and, many times, dressed differently. In many cultures, the role of the man is to be strong and protective, whereas the woman is expected to be passive and nurturing. Sex roles change as societal norms change and may be accepted or rejected by individuals. "In North American culture, gender roles are more strictly enforced for males than for females, and males are socially punished for female behavior" (Fontaine, 2009, p. 406).

DEVELOPMENT OF SEXUALITY

Physiological sexual development begins with conception. Chromosomes from each parent transport programming information to the embryo. During the first 6 weeks of fetal development, there is no anatomic difference between males and females. At approximately 7 to 8 weeks, if there is a high level of testosterone, testes develop. Ovaries form in fetuses with lower levels of testosterone (Guyton & Hall, 2005).

Human sexual feelings develop throughout the life span. Feelings, attitudes, and behavior related to sexuality are learned in the family of origin and reflect the cultural context. See the Respecting Our Differences display.

GENDER IDENTITY

Gender identity is a person's sense of identity as a male or female. It is how the person expresses sexuality in behaviors with others of the same and opposite sex. This perspective on one's sexuality is not inborn but rather evolves throughout the life span (Fontaine, 2009).

Sexual orientation describes an individual's preference for ways of expressing sexual feelings. Like all human behavior, sexual behavior is complex. Sexual orientation is a dynamic lifelong process of growth. The prevailing sexual orientation in current Western society is heterosexuality (sexual activity between a man and a woman). There are

RESPECTING OUR DIFFERENCES

There are no universally accepted sexual values. For example, a sexual practice that is considered normal in one culture may be prohibited in another culture.

many other types of sexual orientation, including **homosexuality** (sexual activity between two members of the same sex), **bisexuality** (having an equal or almost equal preference for partners of either sex), and **transsexuality** (the belief that one is psychologically of the sex opposite his or her anatomic gender). In many cultural groups, homosexuals, bisexuals, and transsexuals are discriminated against due to their alternative lifestyles. Nurses must respect all individuals, regardless of sexual orientation.

SEXUAL NEEDS

Sexual integrity is an integral part of a person's well-being. Even though there are no universal values about sexuality, individuals do experience some common sexual needs, including:

- Tenderness
- Intimacy
- Sensuality
- Attachment
- Caring
- Procreation

HUMAN SEXUAL RESPONSE

The human sexual response is a combination of physiological responses and emotional responses (thoughts and feelings). Masters and Johnson (1966) were the first to describe the physiological phases that occur during the sexual response. These four phases are experienced by both men and women:

- **Excitement:** Begins with sexual stimulation; characterized by vasocongestion of the genitals (results in vaginal lubrication and penile erection)
- **Plateau:** Characterized by maintenance of sexual arousal and the building of excitement leading to orgasm
- **Orgasm:** A highly pleasurable reflex characterized by muscle spasms and male ejaculation
- **Resolution:** Characterized by a gradual return to the pre-excitement phase

SEXUALITY AND HEALTH

Nurses often encounter clients whose sexuality is threatened. Illness, disability, surgery, medications, and hospitalization may impair a person's sexual integrity. Chronic illnesses may also negatively affect sexuality. Other conditions that may contribute to the development of sexual problems appear in the accompanying box, which lists risk factors for sexual dysfunction.

Medications, especially those used to treat hypertension, diabetes, and depression, can also interfere with normal sexual activity. In such cases, the medication should be changed if possible. Also, clients and their sexual partners need to be informed about the cause of the problems. Chronic pain may also interfere with clients' sexual functioning. Clients who experience chronic pain need to be taught methods for increasing their comfort level (e.g., relaxation techniques). Clients

RISK FACTORS FOR SEXUAL DYSFUNCTION

Anemia	Hypertension
Anxiety	Multiple sclerosis
Cardiovascular disease	Previous traumatic
Cigarette smoking	sexual experience
Concern about sexual	Prostate surgery
performance	Renal failure
Depression	Spinal cord injuries
Diabetes	Substance abuse
Hormonal imbalances	Thyroid abnormalities
Hyperlipidemia	Vascular bypass surgery

who are hospitalized may experience sexual dysfunction for a variety of reasons. For example, being in unfamiliar surroundings, separation from significant others, and loss of privacy all may interfere with sexual function. Nurses who are sensitive create an atmosphere that communicates consideration of the client's need for confidentiality and a nonjudgmental manner. See the accompanying Spotlight On display on page 292.

NURSING PROCESS AND SEXUALITY

Sexuality is a significant part of health, whether the client is sexually active or not. Talking and listening to clients promotes intimacy. Some nurses, as well as clients, are embarrassed to talk about sexuality. It is imperative to deal with one's own feelings in order to decrease the client's discomfort. Nurses must not express shock or disapproval regarding a client's sexual practices. It is not necessary to change beliefs and attitudes, but it may be necessary to suspend them in order to spare the client any judgment, directly or indirectly. A question as simple as "what sexual concerns do you have?" may be used to introduce the topic of sexuality in a nonthreatening manner. Questions about sexual orientation must be asked in a nonjudgmental, matter-of-fact manner.

Assessment

Discussion about sexuality must be sensitive to cultural and religious differences. The sensitive nurse will establish an atmosphere that encourages clients to freely discuss their concerns. Some actions that are conducive to such discussion include the following:

- Ensure privacy and maintain confidentiality.
- Use simple, direct language.
- Provide explanations in terms understood by the client.
- Allow time for the client's questions.
- Demonstrate respect by adopting a nonjudgmental attitude.
- Use open-ended questions to elicit more information.

Sexual assessment may produce feelings of fear, anxiety, indignity, and loss of control in many people. These feelings

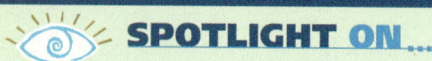

SPOTLIGHT ON...

Values

Client's Sexual Activity

You walk into an adult client's room and find her engaged in sexual intercourse with a visitor. You know that the visitor is not the married client's husband. What should you do?

can be alleviated by the sensitivity of the nurse throughout the assessment process.

Before beginning the genitalia examination, consider the client's cultural background and the beliefs that may affect the examination. For example, some cultures forbid assessment of a female by a male caregiver. The accompanying Nursing Checklist describes some guidelines useful in preparing for the sexual assessment.

Diagnosis

The North American Nursing Diagnosis Association International (2009) has established two diagnoses related to sexuality; see Table 16-3.

Planning and Outcome Identification

It is impossible to provide holistic client care without considering the client as a person with sexual needs. In order to plan accurate delivery of nursing care, it is necessary to ask all clients, regardless of age, about their sexual history. Some nurses do not discuss sexual concerns with adolescents due to their own values about adolescents, sexual behavior, and engaging in sexual behavior prior to marriage. In such instances, the nurses are countertherapeutic to clients. Many nurses reflect the societal belief that older adult clients are asexual. Acting on such a belief ignores clients' needs.

Planning takes into consideration the age-specific variations regarding the need for information on sexuality; see Table 16-4 on page 293. Planning of care also calls for consideration of the client's history of possible sexual abuse. No client, regardless of age, should be excluded from evaluation for sexual abuse. See the Safety First display on page 293 for signs of sexual abuse.

TABLE 16-3 Diagnoses Related to Sexuality

DIAGNOSIS	DEFINITION	DEFINING CHARACTERISTICS	RELATED FACTORS
Sexual dysfunction	Change in sexual function that is viewed as unsatisfying, unrewarding, inadequate	• Values conflicts • Changed interest in self and others • Verbalization of a sexual problem • Alterations in achieving perceived sex role • Actual or perceived limitations as a result of disease or treatment	• Misinformation or lack of knowledge • Abusive relationships • Physical abuse • Inability to achieve desired satisfaction • Altered body structure or function • Lack of privacy
Ineffective sexuality pattern	Expressions of concern regarding own sexuality	• Verbalized difficulties, limitations, or changes in sexual behaviors or activities	• Lack of significant other • Conflict with sexual orientation • Fear of acquiring a sexually transmitted disease • Fear of pregnancy • Ineffective or absent role models • Lack of privacy • Lack of knowledge

Data from North American Nursing Diagnosis Association International. (2009). *Nursing diagnoses—Definitions and classification 2009–2011.* Philadelphia: John Wiley & Sons, Inc.

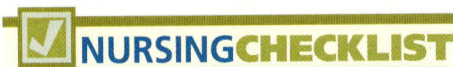

NURSING CHECKLIST

PREPARING FOR THE SEXUAL ASSESSMENT

- Review the client's medical history.
- Greet the client and explain the assessment techniques that you will be using.
- Assess the client's anxiety level, and provide reassurance that this is normal.
- Ensure that the room temperature is warm and comfortable.
- Use a quiet room that will be free from interruptions; it may be necessary to post a "do not disturb" sign on the door of the client's room or the examination room.
- Have the client void prior to the examination.

▼ SAFETY FIRST ▼

INDICATORS OF SEXUAL ABUSE

- Bruises, lacerations, scars in genital area
- Presence of sexually transmitted diseases
- Extreme anxiety or guarding during the physical examination
- Suspiciousness or reluctance in answering questions
- Lack of eye contact

TABLE 16-4 Sexual Information: Age-Specific Needs

Children	• Parenting skills to decrease possibility of child abuse • Children need to learn to differentiate "good" touching and "bad" touching • Teach children how to say "no" when they are uncomfortable with any touch • The importance of reporting any sexual advances to parents, teachers, or other adults
Adolescents	• Education about physiological changes (i.e., signs of onset of puberty; growth and development concepts) • Information on psychosocial responses to physiological changes (i.e., body image changes) • Sexual abuse prevention (including date rape) • Safe sex education (contraception, STD prevention) • Information on sexual preference or orientation
Young adults	• Safe sex education (contraception, STD prevention) • Establishment and maintenance of intimate relationships • Pregnancy and childbirth • Parenting skills
Middle-aged adults	• Effects of aging on sexuality (e.g., menopause, erectile dysfunction) • STD prevention • Contraception
Older adults	• Effects of aging on sexuality • STD prevention • Ways other than intercourse to express sexuality and to meet intimacy needs • Specific information for older women: (1) If vaginal secretions are decreased, use a water-soluble lubricant. (2) Extended foreplay may help in achieving orgasm. (3) Provide a reminder that there is no pregnancy risk. • Specific information for older men: (1) Avoid factors that interfere with circulation (i.e., smoking, alcohol abuse, sedentary lifestyle). (2) Encourage dietary changes to reduce fat and cholesterol. (3) Stress management. (4) Compliance with medications prescribed for diabetes and cardiovascular disorders. (5) Need for a relaxed atmosphere and patience.

Most states have laws mandating nurses to report suspected incidences of abuse. It is important to also know the employing agency's policies about reporting abuse and suspected abusive situations. It is critical that the nurse plan to establish an environment that communicates a sense of safety to clients who may have experienced abuse, neglect, or exploitation. See Chapter 19 for more information about elder abuse.

Implementation

When addressing sexual concerns of clients, there are two major nursing interventions that must be employed: communication and education. These nursing activities should be implemented in order to help promote clients' sexual health.

Communication skills are necessary to ensure optimal exchange of essential information regarding sexual concerns. Reminding the client that the information discussed is confidential helps reinforce a trusting relationship. Self-awareness can help improve communication and, therefore, overall effectiveness when working with sexual issues, particularly issues that can be value laden such as sexually transmitted diseases (STDs). It is helpful for nurses to assess their attitudes toward sexual practices and STDs. Other nursing actions useful in working with clients with STDs include maintenance of a nonjudgmental approach, avoiding imposing one's own values on the client, and not talking down to the client. See the Spotlight On display.

Education is an integral part of treating clients with sexual problems. The nurse must teach prevention of STDs. It is also important to discuss the effects of aging on the sexual response to allay clients' anxieties and to correct any misperceptions.

Another essential education topic related to sexuality focuses on preventive measures: breast self-examination (BSE)

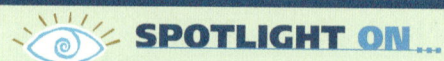

SPOTLIGHT ON...

Compassion and Values

Clients With Recurrent Sexually Transmitted Diseases

Ask yourself how you feel about clients who seek treatment for recurrent STDs. Will your personal feelings influence the quality of nursing care you provide? How would you feel if such a client showed no interest in learning about ways to avoid contracting STDs?

and testicular self-examination (TSE). See Chapter 27 for details on performing BSE and TSE.

Evaluation

To determine the client's achievement of expected outcomes, nurses use observation and communication. Client and partner verbalizations help in evaluating outcome achievement. The nurse observes the client and partner for expressions of intimacy. During the evaluation process, it is important that the nurse remain open-minded and nonjudgmental when working with clients who may have sex alone, with one partner of the opposite gender, with one partner of the same gender, or with several partners of either gender. Personal values can interfere with, or encourage, the client's achievement of expected outcomes and, thus, discourage or promote the client's sexual wholeness.

Because sexuality is such an integral part of individuals and their health status, it is addressed throughout the remainder of this text when relevant.

KEY CONCEPTS

- Health is a process through which the person seeks to maintain an equilibrium that promotes stability and comfort and varies depending on context and situation.

- Illness is the inability of an individual's adaptive responses to maintain physical and emotional balance and results in an impairment in functional ability.

- Wellness is the condition in which an individual functions at optimal levels and is a dynamic process that occurs in varying degrees.

- The various theoretical models of health, such as the clinical, health-belief, high-level wellness, social learning, host-agent-environment, and health promotion models, help nurses to understand the relationship between the experience of health and illness and clients' behaviors in response to this process.

- The two major classifications of illness are acute and chronic. Acute illness is usually characterized by rapid onset, short duration, and intense symptoms. Chronic illness is usually characterized by a gradual insidious onset, lifelong duration, and irreversible changes.

- Lifestyle, locus of control, self-efficacy, health care attitudes, and self-concept are examples of variables that influence health-promoting behaviors.

- The three approaches to health maintenance (health promotion, health protection, and disease prevention) are centered on the individual's responsibility in promoting one's own health.

- Nurses play a key role in helping clients to adopt healthy lifestyles and use approaches such as role modeling and formal teaching to motivate client change.

- Nurses must focus their efforts on improving the health status of vulnerable populations.
- The satisfaction of basic human needs, such as physiological, psychological, sociocultural, intellectual, and spiritual needs, is necessary for every person's survival.
- An impairment in meeting basic needs results in an altered health status.

- A holistic viewpoint helps nurses to recognize the body-mind connection and see the client as a whole person rather than fragmented parts.
- Spirituality is the aspect of a person that seeks a sense of meaning and purpose in life and that also can provide support in times of stress.
- Sexuality affects an individual's relationships with others, male and female, and evolves throughout a person's life.

REVIEW QUESTIONS

1. Which of the following client statements indicates self-efficacy?
   a. "Every problem has a solution."
   b. "I've been on so many diets before, why should this one work?"
   c. "I've solved problems before, so I can probably do so again."
   d. "There's no point in trying to change."

2. Which of the following statements accurately describes Pender's health promotion model? Select all that apply.
   a. A person is more likely to perform health-promoting behaviors when he or she can identify the benefits of the behavior.
   b. Group values exert much influence on an individual's behaviors.
   c. Health is viewed as an attempt to achieve one's fullest potential.
   d. Individuals who perceive health as being within their control are more likely to perform healthy behaviors.
   e. People engage in self-promoting behaviors when they value health.
   f. People who are ill are more motivated than healthy ones to develop health-promoting behaviors.

3. Which of the following nursing statements encourages a client to rely on an internal locus of control?
   a. "I think that an exercise program is just what you need."

   b. "We'll have to see what the prescribing practitioner recommends for you."
   c. "What has worked for you in the past?"
   d. "You should start losing weight as soon as possible."

4. Listed below are nursing activities implemented to promote a client's health. Rank them in terms of priority according to Maslow's hierarchy of needs. Rank in order of 1 = to be done first, 2 = to be done second, and so forth.
   _____ Administering analgesic medication for a headache
   _____ Identifying client strengths in order to boost self-esteem
   _____ Lowering the client's bed and placing the call light within reach
   _____ Referring the client to a support group that consists of peers with similar health problems

5. A nurse is preparing to talk to a client about healthy lifestyle changes. Which of the following actions must the nurse do initially with the client?
   a. Assess the client's motivation for change
   b. Assess the client's pain level
   c. Determine the client's current knowledge level
   d. Distribute teaching materials that are written at the client's level of comprehension

online companion

Visit the DeLaune and Ladner online companion resource at **www.delmar.cengage.com** for additional content and study aids. Click on Online Companions, then select the Nursing discipline.

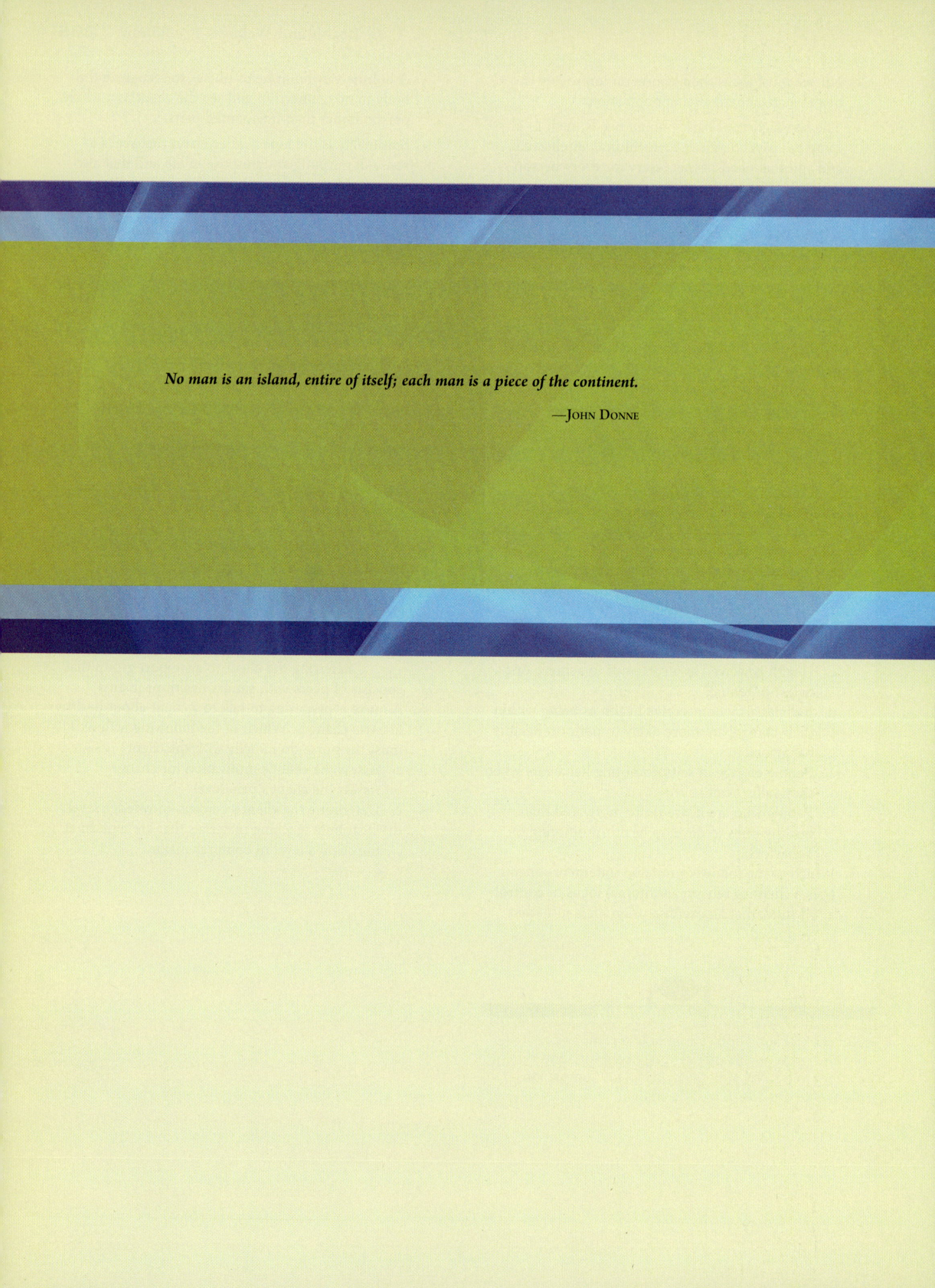

No man is an island, entire of itself; each man is a piece of the continent.

—JOHN DONNE

CHAPTER 17

Family and Community Health

COMPETENCIES

1. Discuss family structure, types, roles, and functions.
2. Describe characteristics of healthy families.
3. Discuss theoretical perspectives of family development.
4. Discuss domestic violence as a threat to family integrity.
5. Identify health-related community needs.
6. Differentiate community health nursing and public health nursing.
7. Discuss nursing's role in promoting community health.
8. Describe nursing's role in disaster preparedness.

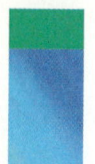

KEY TERMS

aggregates	enmeshment	family roles
community	epidemiology	family structure
community health nursing	family	
disaster	family functions	

Individuals do not exist in a vacuum, but instead interact with and are products of families and communities. Families and communities benefit from nursing care, as do individuals. This chapter describes the health-related needs of families and communities and the nursing responses that address those needs.

FAMILY HEALTH

A family is a dynamic system of people living together who are united by significant emotional bonds. The family is the basic unit of society in that it provides the foundation for a person's view of the world and social interactions.

Due to sociocultural changes, the American family is undergoing transformation. For example, increasing divorce rates, cohabiting adults, and adoption by unmarried individuals have led to a proliferation of single-parent families. The traditional concept of family is being challenged by many living arrangements in current society; for example, many individuals who are unrelated through biological or legal bonds and live together often are considered to be a family. It is necessary for the nurse to ask clients who they consider to be their family members in order to include significant others in the provision of health care. The family performs a variety of functions, including the transmission of cultural values from one generation to the next. The family also teaches socially acceptable behaviors and provides a sense of belonging to its members. Early family interactions help children learn important skills such as problem solving and communication.

FAMILY STRUCTURE

Family structure is the form that a family takes in order to maintain function. Family structures vary depending on cultural context. There is no "typical" family structure even though the nuclear family is often portrayed as such by the media; see Figure 17-1. Types of families include, but are not limited to, the following:

- Nuclear family—composed of husband, wife, and children (naturally conceived, adopted, or both)
- Blended family—combination of two divorced families through remarriage; may include stepchildren, half-siblings, or combinations
- Extended family—usually members of a nuclear family and other blood-related people (such as grandparents, aunts, uncles, and cousins)

Table 17-1 on page 299 further describes various forms of families.

The structure of a family affects its health status. An extended family has several members living in one household;

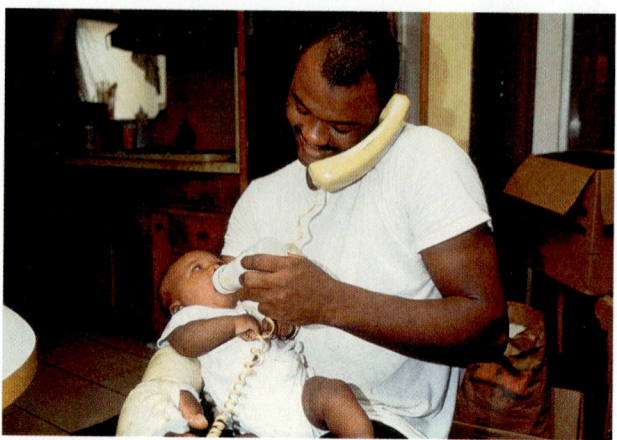

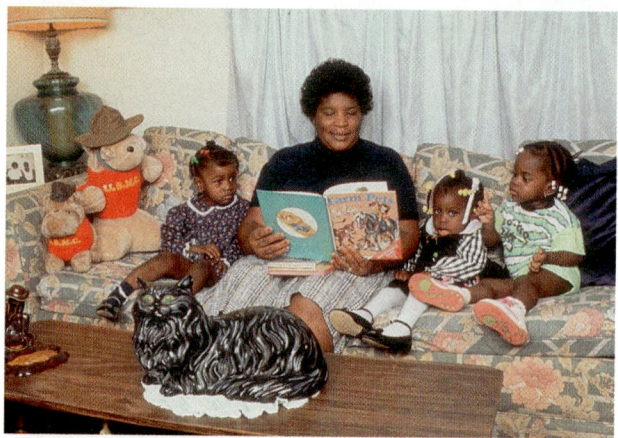

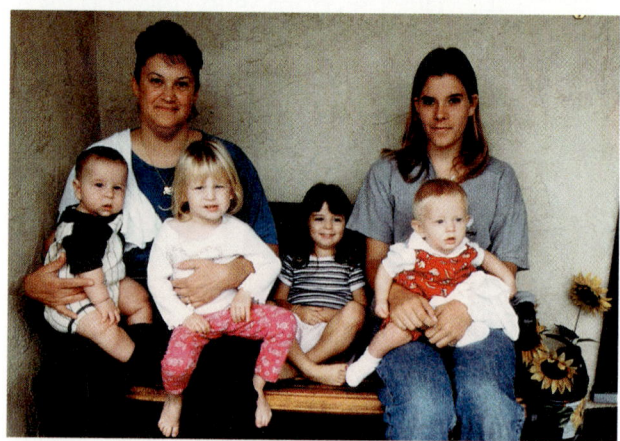

FIGURE 17-1 There are diverse family structures and types, as shown in these photographs DELMAR/CENGAGE LEARNING

therefore, people are available to help care for the sick. A person living in a nuclear family often experiences self-reliance. A client who has a nuclear family "often has different needs from

TABLE 17-1 Various Family Forms

FAMILY STRUCTURE	EXAMPLES
Legally married	• Traditional nuclear • Blended • Coparenting
Dual-career	• Both adults in same household are employed • Commuter marriages
Adoptive	• Adults (either married or single) and one or more children
Foster	• Adults (either married or single) who care for children on a temporary basis
Voluntarily childless	• Married adults who have decided not to procreate
Unmarried	• Adults who never married • Cohabitation, with or without children • Same-sex relationship
Formerly married	• Widowed • Divorced (includes custodial parent, joint custody parents, and noncustodial parents)
Multiadult household	• Communes
Extended family	• Grandparents, parents, and children • Adult children who move back home with parents • Siblings living together, with or without parents or children

Delmar/Cengage Learning

the client with numerous extended family members living in the same household or nearby" (Hunt, 2009, p. 10).

FAMILY ROLES AND FUNCTIONS

Family roles are the behaviors expected of family members. These roles are learned and transmitted within the family unit and help the family to fulfill its functions. Roles also provide the foundation for the children's future interactions as adults. **Family functions** are the roles that allow family members to adapt in order to develop as individuals and as members of the family unit. Family roles include, but are not limited to, the following:

• Nurturance and support
• Allocation of resources
• Development of life skills
• Division of labor
• Socialization of members (Antai-Otong, 2007)

CHARACTERISTICS OF HEALTHY FAMILIES

The family unit exerts much influence on the health of its individual members. For example, the family that places a high value on proper nutrition will encourage children to develop dietary practices that will promote health throughout the life cycle. Each family is a dynamic system whose members form a unit that interacts with the community. Differentiating healthy and unhealthy families is often difficult. Some traits of a healthy family are as follows:

• Supporting members
• Teaching respect for others
• Helping with problem solving
• Communicating

Healthy families are often described as functional, in that they are able to cope with stressors and deal with crises as they arise. Eggenberger and Nelms (2007) state that "being a family unit is what gives most families the ability to endure the emotional upheaval and suffering that come with the critical illness experience" (p. 1628). See the accompanying Uncovering the Evidence display on page 300. *Dysfunctional* families, on the other hand, often lack problem-solving skills and deteriorate in adaptive abilities when confronted with stressors. Table 17-2 on page 301 compares healthy and unhealthy families. Healthy families typically have family rituals, or traditions, that promote bonding between family members; see the accompanying Spotlight On display.

UNCOVERING THE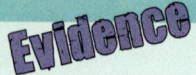

TITLE OF STUDY

"Being Family: The Family Experience When an Adult Member Is Hospitalized with a Critical Illness"

AUTHORS

S. K. Eggenberger and T. P. Nelms

PURPOSE

To understand the family experience when an adult family member is hospitalized for treatment of a critical illness.

METHODS

Semistructured interviews were conducted with 11 families of critically ill, hospitalized adults. The family experience was examined according to Van Manen's concepts of lived space, lived relation, lived body, and lived time.

FINDINGS

Most families are able to cope with the stressors of a critical illness and hospitalization as a result of a strong sense of being a family. Family bonds increase the strength of family members during a crisis.

IMPLICATIONS

Nurses can exert a powerful influence on families by acting on a commitment to be with the family. Family caring is increased by the presence of caring nurses.

Eggenberger, S. K., & Nelms, T. P. (2007). Being family: The family experience when an adult member is hospitalized with a critical illness. *Journal of Clinical Nursing, 16*(9), 1618–1628.

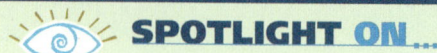

SPOTLIGHT ON…

Family Rituals

Apply the following questions to your own family:

What are some traditions valued by your family (e.g., special holiday celebrations)?

Are there rituals performed by your family (e.g., having a special meal or going to a special place on vacation)?

How have these traditions and rituals strengthened your sense of family?

A newer perspective of the family development cycle was proposed by Carter and McGoldrick in 1989, with several revisions over time. Carter and McGoldrick's (2004) model describes six stages of the family life cycle that are more reflective of adult needs in current society. Table 17-3 on page 302 compares the models developed by Duvall and by Carter and McGoldrick.

THREATS TO FAMILY INTEGRITY

A healthy family supports and protects its members from harm. However, several variables, such as violence and poverty, can interfere with the family's health and integrity. One major threat is domestic violence, which is becoming an increasing problem for many family units.

Domestic Violence

Domestic violence, which occurs in all socioeconomic groups, is an ever-increasing social problem; see the accompanying Spotlight On display. Approximately 10% of children in the United States live in homes with reported violence (Moore, Probst, Tompkins, Cuffe, & Martin, 2007). In addition to its impact on specific victims, domestic violence has negative effects on communities. Several studies document the harmful effects of family violence that may include acute trauma, death, unwanted pregnancy, depression, suicide, posttraumatic stress disorder, and substance abuse (Binder et al., 2008; Bradley et al., 2008; Moore et al., 2007; Widom, DuMont, & Czaja, 2007). Victims of violence within families are primarily children, older adults, and female spouses or intimate partners. Children are affected by family violence even if they are not the direct victims; witnessing domestic violence can have adverse effects on a child's emotional well-being. Domestic violence becomes a repetitive cycle in that people who were abused as children learn that violence is normal behavior; thus, they will use violence in an attempt to solve problems.

CHILD ABUSE   According to the Administration for Children and Families, U.S. Department of Health and Human Services (2008), 950,000 children were victims of abuse or

FAMILY DEVELOPMENT THEORIES

The developmental approach to viewing families is similar to the developmental approach to viewing individuals. That is, the family unit has a developmental process with expected tasks that are to be achieved at each developmental stage. The family that achieves specific developmental tasks is considered to be a healthy family. The way in which a family achieves the tasks of one developmental stage greatly influences the family's ability to handle subsequent developmental issues.

The classic work of Duvall and Miller (1985) is often used as the basis for assessing a family's developmental progress. However, Duvall's theory is somewhat limited in that it assumes that the family unit consists of a married couple that becomes involved in child-rearing activities. From Duvall's perspective, the nuclear family is the standard by which all others are assessed. Duvall's model describes eight stages of the family life cycle.

TABLE 17-2 Comparison of Healthy and Unhealthy Families

CHARACTERISTIC	FUNCTIONAL (HEALTHY) FAMILY UNIT	DYSFUNCTIONAL (UNHEALTHY) FAMILY UNIT
Communication	• Clear, direct, and truthful	• Ambiguous, indirect, dishonest
Problem-solving ability	• Focused and appropriate	• Fails to solve problems, with resultant family crisis
Affective responsiveness	• Members are encouraged to express feelings • Feelings are respected	• Emotions are repressed • Members become guarded, suspicious, and untrusting
Affective involvement	• Family members care about each other	• Family members are focused on protecting self
Behavioral control	• Rules are flexible • Feedback is timely and constructive	• Rigid rules, usually in an autocratic hierarchy • Feedback is negative
Boundaries	• Provide safety and security • Encourage growth of individual members	• Are blurred, rigid, and inconsistent • Lead to **enmeshment** (overinvolvement or lack of separateness of family members)
Role allocation	• Roles are flexible according to family needs and situations	• Roles are rigid (e.g., ''That's woman's work'')

Delmar/Cengage Learning

neglect in 2006. This number most likely does not reflect the total number of children abused because underreporting is common. Young children are more vulnerable to abuse than are older ones; see Figure 17-2.

Many factors are related to child abuse and neglect. These factors include stress, financial problems, inadequate parenting skills, parental substance abuse, parental impulsivity, social isolation, and parents themselves being abused as children. Child abuse results in physical pain and emotional damage that may last a lifetime.

OLDER ADULT ABUSE Maltreatment of older adults takes many forms, including physical, sexual, and psychological abuse and financial exploitation. In the majority of cases, the perpetrator of abuse of older adults is a family member, usually an adult child or spouse. Factors associated with abuse of older adults include increasing age, nonwhite race, low income status, functional impairment, and impaired cognitive ability. Older adults who have chronic illnesses are also at increased risk. Social isolation is a serious problem that affects many elderly, especially those with chronic illnesses (Holley, 2007). Lack of transportation, lack of employment, and strained relationships with caregivers may lead to inadequate care, including maltreatment. See Chapter 19 for more discussion on maltreatment of older individuals.

SPOUSE AND PARTNER ABUSE The vast majority of assaults by partners are directed at women. Women are also at greater risk than men for being killed during intimate partner violence (Hunt, 2009, p. 299). The greatest cause of injury to women in the United States is violence (Fontaine, 2009). Some of the risk factors for intimate partner abuse include young age, low income status, pregnancy, mental health problems, substance abuse by victims or perpetrators, separated or divorced status, and history of childhood sexual or physical abuse.

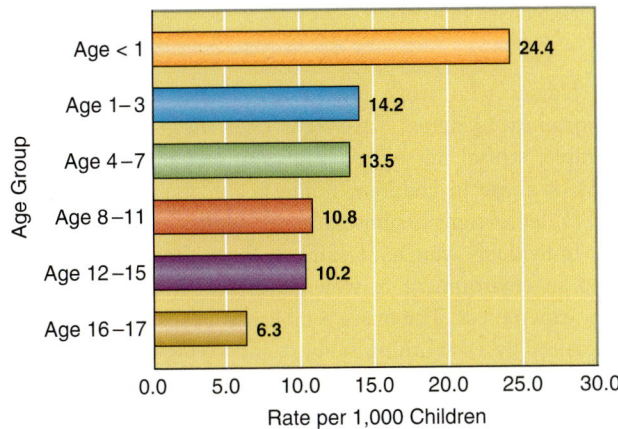

FIGURE 17-2 Child Victimization Rates by Age Group, 2006
DATA FROM ADMINISTRATION FOR CHILDREN AND FAMILIES, U.S. DEPARTMENT OF HEALTH AND HUMAN SERVICES. RETRIEVED FROM HTTP://WWW.ACF.HHS.GOV/PROGRAMS/CB/PUBS/CM06.PDF.

TABLE 17-3 Family Developmental Stages

DUVALL	CARTER AND MCGOLDRICK	DEVELOPMENTAL TASKS
No formal stage identified	1. The unattached young adult	• Successfully separate from parents as a young adult • Develop financial independence • Accept emotional responsibility for self
1. Marriage: the beginning family	2. The newly married couple	• Develop and commit to a new family unit (establishment of couple identity) • Adjust to parenthood
2. Childbearing families	3. Families with young children	• Establish and maintain a household • Incorporate new members into the family unit
3. Families with preschool children		• Nurture children • Adjust to separation by parents and children
4. Families with school-aged children		• Socialize and educate children • Adapt as a family to school influences
5. Families with teenagers	4. Families with adolescents	• Balance adolescents' freedom and responsibility • Develop flexibility to respond to increased independence of children • Extend caring activities to previous generation (aging parents, grandparents)
6. Families launching young adults	5. Launching children	• Let go of young adult children • Accept exits from and entrances into family unit • Renegotiate marital relationship
7. Middle-aged parents (empty nest up to retirement)		• Reinvest in couple identity • Accept changes in generational roles (i.e., grandparenting)
8. Retirement to death of both spouses	6. Families in later life	• Review life and integrate it • Accept the reality of death

Adapted from Carter, B., & McGoldrick, M. (2004). *The expanded life cycle: Individual, family, and societal perspectives* (3rd ed.). Boston: Allyn & Bacon; Duvall, E. M., & Miller, B. C. (1985). *Marriage and family development* (6th ed.). New York: ; Hitchcock, J. E. (2006). Frameworks for assessing families. In J. E. Hitchcock, P. E. Schubert, & S. A. Thomas (Eds.), *Community health nursing: Caring in action* (2nd ed.). Ventura, CA: CRAM101.

NURSING RESPONSE TO FAMILY VIOLENCE The best treatment of family violence is prevention; see Table 17-4 on page 303. Prevention is based on assessment and education; therefore, nurses in every practice setting and specialty must be vigilant for signs of violence. Nurses who work in schools, emergency departments, outpatient clinics, and women's health and geriatric settings should be especially vigilant for signs of abuse. When abuse is suspected, the nurse should document the findings and report them to the appropriate protective services agencies. Documentation should include verbatim statements of the victim, photographs, and description of the injuries. Telephone numbers of local shelters and crisis lines should be given to the client. Clients who have been abused also need to be referred to mental health professionals for counseling.

Nurses who work in the community have a unique opportunity to detect early signs of domestic violence. For example, school nurses are often the first people to detect signs of abuse in children; home health nurses may be the first to detect signs of abuse of older adults.

Individuals who have suffered abuse, regardless of age, need an environment in which they feel safe to talk about their experiences. The nurse establishes a sense of psychological safety by establishing rapport and laying the foundation for trust. In order to do this, the nurse must be nonjudgmental when talking with both the abused person and the suspected perpetrator. Self-awareness helps the nurse increase sensitivity when listening to clients discussing emotional issues such as abuse and neglect.

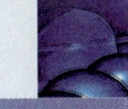

TABLE 17-4 Levels of Prevention of Child Abuse

LEVEL OF PREVENTION	EXAMPLES
Primary	• Parenting classes that provide information about childhood growth and development • Identification of at-risk households • Telephone "hot lines" for parents who are feeling out of control
Secondary	• Behavior management programs for at-risk families, such as those referred to child protective services • Assessment of signs of abuse
Tertiary	• Removal of children from homes with abusive parents • Family therapy for abusive parents

Data from Kaakien, J. R., Hanson, S. M., & Birenbaum, L. K. (2007). Family development and family nursing assessment. In M. Stanhope & J. Lancaster (Eds.), *Community and public health nursing* (7th ed.). St. Louis, MO: Mosby.

SPOTLIGHT ON...

Prevalence of Violence

Do you believe that family violence is prevalent in your community? Read your local newspaper for 1 week. Observe the number of stories that are printed about domestic violence. Consider what public initiatives could be taken to reduce the incidence of domestic violence in your community.

Poverty

Food insecurity means having limited access to nutrients; obviously, there is a link between poverty and food insecurity. As defined by the Economic Research Service of the U.S. Department of Agriculture (2006), food insecurity occurs when a member of a household has an altered eating pattern as a result of lack of money for food. There are higher rates of health problems in families affected by food insecurity. "Mental health problems in mothers and children are more common when mothers are food insecure, a stressor that can potentially be addressed by social policy" (Whitaker, Phillips, & Orzol, 2006, p. 868). Nurses have an opportunity to improve the health status of families through advocacy and education of legislators who develop social policies.

COMMUNITY CONSIDERATIONS

Detecting Abuse

Home health and public health nurses have a unique opportunity to detect indicators of abuse (in children, elders, and intimate partners). Assessing the home and community environment can provide cues to abuse and, thus, trigger early intervention.

COMMUNITY HEALTH

Every community (a group of people united by some common element or shared interest) is different and, therefore, has its own specific needs. However, all communities need to be safe and promote the health of their constituents. The safety and health of any community may be threatened by epidemics or disasters, either natural or man-made. "The measure of a healthy community, then, is not the complete absence of problems, but rather how well the community prepares for and responds to them" (Dreher, Shapiro, & Asselin, 2006, p. 120). Community health is achieved through meeting the collective needs of the community and society by identifying problems and supporting community participation in the process. One way to measure the health of a community is to assess its progress in achievement of the Leading Health Indicators established by the U. S. public health department's Healthy People initiative; see Chapter 16 for further discussion. Community-based nursing focuses on individuals, families, and aggregates (subgroups) living and working within a community. An aggregate is a particular population of people with a common identifying variable; there are no relationships among members of an aggregate other than similar factors. Examples of aggregates include teenage pregnant girls, persons who smoke cigarettes, and people with tuberculosis.

When working with an individual or family, the community health nurse considers them within the context of the entire community. The specialty area of community health nursing is divided into public health and home health care nursing. The major goal of community health nursing is the preservation and improvement of the health of populations and communities worldwide. In order to accomplish this goal, community health nurses practice in neighborhoods and homes in rural and urban areas. Settings in which community health nurses commonly practice include:

• Primary care offices
• Schools
• Workplaces
• Public health units

The services provided by community health nurses range from examining infants in a clinic setting to providing case management services to frail older adults in the home. Community health nurses also identify vulnerable populations, such as the homeless, those living in poverty, those exposed to communicable diseases, and those living in violence-prone neighborhoods, in order to plan specific strategies to address the special needs.

Community health nurses conduct epidemiological investigations and participate in health policy analysis and decision making. Epidemiology is the study of the distribution and determinants of health-related states or events in populations. For example, "invasive methicillin-resistant *Staphylococcus aureus* (MRSA) infection affects certain populations disproportionately. It is a major public health problem ..." (Klevens et al., 2007, p. 1763). One study (Hota et al., 2007) states that the risk for development of community-associated methicillin-resistant *Staphylococcus aureus* (CA-MRSA) is increased in people who are incarcerated or who live in public housing complexes. Community health nurses target these at-risk populations for surveillance and preventive education. Community nursing uses a holistic approach that requires both disease prevention and health promotion activities, including education and advocacy. Nurses who work in the community make a commitment to improving the health of the entire community.

The nursing process can be applied to individuals, families, and aggregates. Use of the nursing process enables nurses to:

- Determine needs and health concerns that could lead to potential health risks
- Formulate a plan of care incorporating health promotion activities such as teaching and counseling
- Evaluate plans of care to determine whether they are promoting client well-being

PUBLIC HEALTH NURSING

Public health nursing, a specialization within community-based nursing, has never before been so essential to the health of U.S. citizens. The emergence of new infectious diseases (such as SARS, H1N1 virus, and *Clostridium difficile* infections) and bioterrorism threats increase the demand for services from a health care system at a time when the nursing workforce is becoming more scarce.

The public health perspective focuses on prevention as opposed to illness. In order to promote community health, public health nurses perform the following functions:

- Prevention of epidemics and spread of disease
- Protection against environmental hazards
- Prevention of injuries
- Promotion of health behaviors
- Response to disasters

Some public health initiatives have led to improvements in blood pressure control, automobile safety restraints, and cessation of tobacco use by many. See Table 17-5 for a listing of some of the factors affecting the public's health, with specific nursing interventions.

DISASTER PREPAREDNESS

A disaster is any event (human-made or natural) that causes destruction that cannot be relieved without assistance. See the Community Considerations display on page 305 for examples.

The disaster plan for any community must include preparation for both physical and emotional reactions to the disaster. Nurses have always been actively involved in disaster preparedness and response. Nurses play a vital role in disaster response and usually work in extremely challenging

TABLE 17-5 Nursing Responses to Factors Affecting Public Health

VARIABLE	EXAMPLES	NURSING RESPONSES
Behavioral	• Dietary practices • Lifestyle (active or sedentary) • Tobacco usage	• Education • Screening • Counseling
Environmental	• Living conditions • Air quality • Water quality	• Education of clients and policy makers • Advocacy • Political action
Social	• Workplace safety	• Health screenings • Health promotion programs
Educational	• Basic knowledge about disease causation and prevention	• Public education announcements • Educational programs about disease prevention and health promotion

Delmar/Cengage Learning

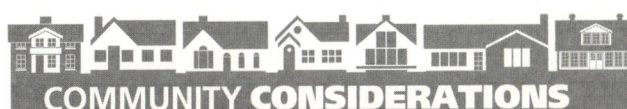

COMMUNITY CONSIDERATIONS

Types of Disasters

Natural Disasters

- Blizzards
- Droughts
- Earthquakes
- Floods
- Forest fires (i.e., ignited by lightning)
- Hurricanes
- Tornadoes

Human-Made Disasters

- Bombings
- Fires (arson)
- Toxic spills
- Transportation accidents
- Wars

SPOTLIGHT ON...

Nursing Process in a Disaster

Imagine yourself as part of the disaster response team following the devastation of two hurricanes. Consider the potential human responses of the hurricane victims as you study these questions.

What is being done to meet the public's needs?
What are the potential human responses to the disaster?
What is being done to help the internal environment of the individuals affected?
What is being done to help the community cope and rebuild?
Consider how your answers might vary if these questions were applied to victims of a terrorist act.

circumstances to deliver necessary care. For example, the nurse may need to provide care in the absence of electricity, water, adequate number of care providers, or other essential resources. In 2008, the American Nurses Association (ANA) developed guidelines for adapting standards of care during disasters and other emergencies. According to the ANA (2008, p. 10):

Decision-making during extreme conditions, however, shifts ethical standards to a utilitarian framework in which the clinical goal is the greatest good for the greatest number of individuals. As a result, not everyone may receive the optimal services that might be available at other times or places.

Nurses are expected to meet the following standards, which have been identified by the ANA as the most critical standards for provision of care during an extreme emergency:

- Maximize safety of care provider and client
- Maintain respiration and circulation
- Maintain or establish infection control interventions (ANA, 2008, p. 16)

The accompanying Spotlight On display lists questions to consider when applying the nursing process in a disaster.

KEY CONCEPTS

- A family is a dynamic system of people living together who are united by significant emotional bonds.

- The family is the basic unit of society in that it provides the foundation for a person's view of the world and social interactions.

- The nurse must ask clients who they consider to be their family members in order to include significant others in the provision of health care.

- Family structure is the form that a family takes in order to maintain function. Family structures vary depending on cultural context.

- Family roles are the behaviors expected of family members. These roles are learned and transmitted within the family unit and help the family to fulfill its functions.

- Family functions are the roles that allow family members to adapt in order to develop as individuals and as members of the family unit.

- A healthy family is characterized by these traits: communicates and listens, supports its members, teaches respect for others, develops trust, plays and shares a sense of humor, has a strong sense of family (as evidenced by rituals and traditions), and seeks help with problems as necessary.

- Healthy families are often described as functional, in that they are able to cope with stressors and deal with crises as they arise.

- Dysfunctional families lack problem-solving skills and deteriorate in adaptive abilities when confronted with stressors.

- The family unit has a developmental process with expected tasks that are to be achieved at each developmental stage.
- Domestic violence, which occurs in all socioeconomic groups, is an ever-increasing social problem.
- Domestic violence becomes a repetitive cycle in that people who were abused as children learn that violence is normal behavior; thus, they may use violence in an attempt to solve problems.
- In the majority of cases, the perpetrator of abuse of older adults is a family member.
- The vast majority of assaults by partners are directed at women.
- The best treatment of family violence is prevention.
- Community-based nursing focuses on individuals, families, and aggregates living and working within a community.
- The major goal of community health nursing is the preservation and improvement of the health of populations and communities worldwide.

- Community health nurses practice in neighborhoods and homes in rural and urban areas. Settings in which community health nurses commonly practice include primary care offices, schools, workplaces, and public health units.
- Public health nursing is a specialization within community-based nursing practice.
- New infectious diseases and bioterrorism threats are increasing the demand for public health services.
- The public health perspective focuses on prevention as opposed to illness.
- Public health nurses perform the following functions: prevention of epidemics and spread of disease; protection against environmental hazards; prevention of injuries; promotion of health behaviors; and response to disasters.
- A disaster is any event (human-made or natural) that causes destruction that cannot be relieved without assistance.
- Nurses have always been actively involved in disaster preparedness and response.

REVIEW QUESTIONS

1. A school nurse is teaching a class on domestic violence to high school students. Which of the following student statements indicates a need for further teaching?
   a. "Abusers are often excessively jealous and possessive."
   b. "If you are educated and have money, abuse does not happen."
   c. "The abuser will often apologize and promise to stop."
   d. "Violence often begins in a dating relationship."
2. The community health nurse is teaching a parenting skills class to new parents. Which of the following parent statements indicates that the teaching has been effective? Select all that apply.
   a. "In order to be considered a family, those living together must be related by blood."
   b. "My family is typical because we have a husband, wife, and soon-to-be two children."
   c. "My husband has a child by another marriage, so when our child is born we will be a blended family."
   d. "Our family's beliefs may affect the health of our children."
   e. "There are many different types of families."

3. Which of the following is a trait of a functional (healthy) family?
   a. Ambiguous communication
   b. Enmeshment
   c. Hierarchy of rules
   d. Timely feedback
4. Approximately _____% of children in the United States live in homes with reported violence. (Fill in the blank.)
5. Two priority actions of the community nurse that address family violence are:
   a. Assessment
   b. Diagnosing
   c. Education
   d. Interdisciplinary communication
   e. Planning
   f. Political advocacy
6. Which of the following is an example of tertiary prevention activities for the nurse to perform with abused children?
   a. Assessing for signs of child abuse
   b. Identifying at-risk households
   c. Performing family therapy for abusive parents
   d. Teaching parenting classes on developmental milestones

7. According to the American Nurses Association, which of the following standards of care must be implemented during response to a disaster? Select all that apply.
   a. Airway, breathing, and circulation maintenance
   b. Confidentiality
   c. Documentation of care
   d. Elective procedures
   e. Infection control practices
   f. Safety for both nurse and client(s)

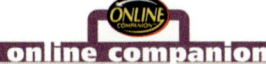

online companion

Visit the DeLaune and Ladner online companion resource at **www.delmar.cengage.com** for additional content and study aids. Click on Online Companions, then select the Nursing discipline.

The strongest principle of growth lies in human choice.

—George Eliot (in Herrmann, 1990)

CHAPTER 18

The Life Cycle

COMPETENCIES

1. Discuss basic principles of growth and development.
2. Explain factors that influence growth and development.
3. Discuss the major theories related to physiological, psychosocial, cognitive, moral, and spiritual development.
4. Identify critical milestones for each developmental stage.
5. Describe specific nursing interventions that are relevant to each developmental stage.

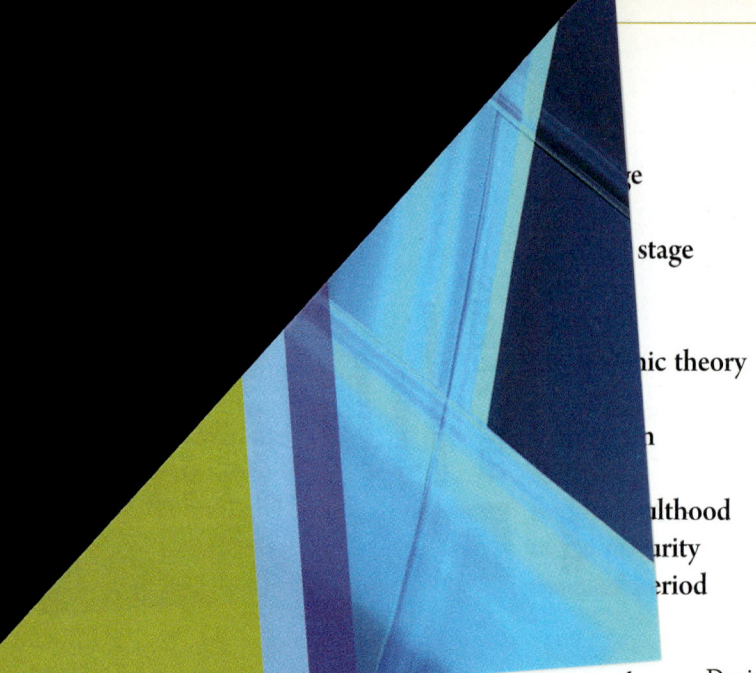

changing. Physical growth, psychosocial development, emotional maturation, cognitive development, moral development, and spiritual growth occur throughout life. Progression through each developmental stage influences health status. A thorough understanding of developmental concepts is essential for the delivery of quality nursing practice. This chapter discusses the changes occurring in each stage of the life cycle.

FUNDAMENTAL CONCEPTS OF GROWTH AND DEVELOPMENT

Development occurs continuously through the life span. Adults continue to have transition periods during which growth and development occur. Individuals experience changes in all dimensions of life, from conception to death.

Growth is the quantitative (measurable) changes in physical size of the body and its parts, such as increases in cells, tissues, structures, and systems. Examples of growth are physical changes in height, weight, bone density, and dental structure. Even though growth is not a steady process through the life cycle, growth patterns can be predicted. Variations in growth, such as rapid increases contrasted with slower rates of physical change, occur with each individual. Rapid growth is most common in the prenatal, infant, and adolescent stages. **Development** refers to behavioral changes in functional abilities and skills. Thus, developmental changes are qualitative, that is, not easily measured. **Maturation** is the process of becoming fully grown and developed and involves physiological and behavioral aspects of an individual. Maturation depends on biological growth, functional changes, and **learning** (assimilation of information with a resultant change in behavior). During each developmental stage of the life cycle, certain goals (**developmental tasks**) must be achieved. These developmental tasks set the stage for future learning and adaption.

The **critical period** is the time of the most rapid growth or development in a particular stage of the life cycle.

During these critical periods, an individual is most vulnerable to stressors of any type.

Growth, development, maturation, and learning are interdependent processes. For learning to occur, the individual must be mature enough to grasp the concepts and make required behavioral changes. Cognitive maturation precedes learning. Physical growth is also a prerequisite for many types of learning; for example, a child must have the physical ability to control the anal sphincter before toilet training skills are learned.

PRINCIPLES OF GROWTH AND DEVELOPMENT

All persons have individual talents and abilities that contribute to their development as unique entities. *There are no absolute rules in predicting the exact rate of development for an individual.* However, some general principles relate to the growth and development of all humans (see Table 18-1 on page 311).

The sequence of development is predictable even though the emergence of specific skills varies with each person. For example, not all infants roll over at the same age, but most roll over before they crawl.

FACTORS INFLUENCING GROWTH AND DEVELOPMENT

Multiple factors such as heredity, life experiences, health status, and cultural expectations influence a person's growth and development. The interaction of these factors greatly influences how an individual responds to everyday situations. The choices a person makes regarding health behaviors are also greatly determined by these factors.

Heredity

A complex series of processes transmits genetic information from parents to children. The genetic composition of an individual determines physical characteristics such as skin

TABLE 18-1 Principles of Growth and Development

PRINCIPLE	EXAMPLE/DESCRIPTION
Development occurs in cephalocaudal (head-to-toe) direction.	An infant raises the head before sitting up.
Development occurs in a proximodistal manner.	The infant is able to move the arms before picking up objects with the hands and the fingers. Functions closer to the midline (proximal) of the body develop before functions farther away from the body's midline (distal).
Development occurs in an orderly manner from simple to complex and from the general to the specific.	An infant crawls before walking. A child holds a crayon with the entire hand before being able to grasp it between thumb and finger. Gross motor control is achieved before fine motor coordination.
The pattern of growth and development is continuous, orderly, and predictable. However, growth and development do not proceed at a consistent rate.	Periods of rapid growth (similar to growth spurts of adolescence) alternate with periods of slower growth (as seen in middle adulthood).
All individuals go through the same developmental processes.	Individual differences occur, but the process is consistent.
Every person proceeds through stages of growth and development at an individual rate.	A child who grows more slowly may be shorter than other children of the same age.
Every stage of development has specific characteristics.	An infant is dependent on others for physical and emotional survival. Adolescence is characterized by a search for identity.
Each stage of development has certain tasks to be achieved or acquired during that specific time. Tasks of one developmental stage become the foundation for tasks in subsequent stages.	An infant must master the psychological task of developing trust in order to mature as an adolescent who can establish a separate identity.
Some stages of growth and development are more critical than others.	The first trimester of pregnancy is a critical time for fetal development. During this critical phase, the developing human is most vulnerable to damage from toxins (e.g., drugs, chemicals, viruses).

Delmar/Cengage Learning

color, hair texture, facial features, body structure, as well as a predisposition to certain diseases (e.g., Tay-Sachs, sickle cell anemia). Heredity is a genetic blueprint from which an individual grows and develops; it determines to a great extent the rate of physical and mental development. See the accompanying Respecting Our Differences display.

Life Experiences

A person's experiences can also influence the rate of growth and development. For example, compare physical growth rates of a child whose family can afford food, shelter, and health care with those of a child whose family has little, if any, resources. The child whose family is economically disadvantaged has a higher risk of experiencing physical and mental delays in growth and development.

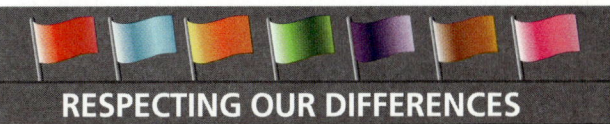

RESPECTING OUR DIFFERENCES

Nature or Nurture?

What determines a person's behavior—heredity or environment? This "nature versus nurture" issue remains a controversy today. What do you think is most important in determining a person's behavior: an individual's genetic predisposition or the response of other people and socialization? This question has no simple answers. As you continue to develop in your professional role, keep an open mind regarding the factors influencing behavior.

Another example of the influence of life experiences is an older adult who is enjoying retirement and has both an adequate income and an active support system. If this individual had an impairment in any of these variables, psychological development would likely be affected in a negative way.

Health Status

Individuals experiencing wellness are progressing normally along the life cycle. However, illness or disability can interfere with the achievement of developmental milestones. Individuals with chronic conditions will often experience a delay in meeting developmental milestones.

Cultural Expectations

Society expects people to master certain skills in each developmental period. The age at which an individual masters a particular task is determined in part by culture. For example, the time for mastery of toilet training is greatly influenced by cultural norms. The following are examples of how societal expectations hinder one's growth and development:

- A child who grows up in an economically deprived home may receive inadequate food, shelter, emotional nurturing, and intellectual stimulation with resultant impairments in physical, psychosocial, and cognitive development.
- A woman may not be expected to fully use her intellectual abilities; thus, she has altered cognitive development.
- A man may be discouraged from showing tenderness and nurturing behaviors; such discouragement results in dysfunctional psychosocial development.

See the accompanying Spotlight On display.

THEORETICAL PERSPECTIVES OF HUMAN DEVELOPMENT

Nurses must have a thorough understanding of human growth and development in order to provide individualized care. It is necessary to remember that chronological age and developmental age are not synonymous. An overview of the major developmental theories is presented in the following text. These theories are discussed more fully in the specific sections about each developmental period.

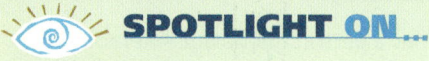

SPOTLIGHT ON...

Values

Stereotyping

Consider how people are stereotyped today. Society labels certain characteristics as "masculine" or "feminine." How do you think these gender stereotypes influence a child's development?

PHYSIOLOGICAL DIMENSION

Physiological growth (physical size and functioning) of an individual is influenced primarily by interaction of genetic predisposition, the central nervous system (CNS), the endocrine system, and maturation. The role of heredity in human development is complex and not yet fully understood. Genetics is the foundation for achievement of specific tasks. Factors such as the psychosocial environment and health status influence individuals' ability to achieve their genetic potential.

PSYCHOSOCIAL DIMENSION

The psychosocial dimension of growth and development consists of subjective feelings and interpersonal relationships. A favorable **self-concept** (view of one's self, including body image, self-esteem, and ideal self) is likely the most important key to a person's success and happiness. Following are characteristics of an individual with a positive self-concept:

- Self-confidence
- Willingness to take risks
- Ability to receive criticism without defensiveness
- Ability to adapt effectively to stressors
- Innovative problem-solving skills

People with a healthy self-concept believe in themselves; as a result, they set goals that can be achieved. Goal achievement reinforces the positive belief about one's self. See Chapter 22 for a complete discussion about self-concept.

A person with a positive self-concept is likely to engage in health-promoting activities. For example, a person who values him- or herself is more likely to change unhealthy habits (such as smoking and sedentary lifestyle) in order to improve health status. There are many different psychosocial theories that explain the development of self-concept. This chapter presents the intrapsychic and interpersonal models of personality development.

Intrapsychic Theory

Intrapsychic theory (also called psychodynamic) focuses on an individual's unconscious processes. Feelings, needs, conflicts, and drives are considered to be motivators of behavior, learning, and development. Sigmund Freud and Erik Erikson are two major intrapsychic theorists.

Freud's theories, developed in the early 1930s, continue to influence current concepts related to human development. A basic belief of the Freudian model is that *all behavior has some meaning.*

According to Freud (1961), in order to mature, a person must successfully travel through five stages of development (see Table 18-2 on page 313). In each stage, there is a task to be mastered; if the task is not achieved, the individual is halted (develops a fixation) at this stage. A **fixation** is characterized as either inadequate mastery or failure to achieve a developmental task. A fixation in earlier stages inhibits healthy progression through subsequent stages.

Erikson (1968) expanded Freud's concept of developmental stages by theorizing that psychosocial development

TABLE 18-2 Freud's Stages of Psychosexual Development

STAGE	AGE	DESCRIPTION
Oral	Birth–18 months	Management of anxiety by using mouth and tongue
Anal	18 months–3 years	Control of muscles, especially those controlling urination and defecation
Phallic ("Oedipal")	3–6 years	Awareness of sex and genitalia
Latency	6–12 years	Exhibition of latent sexual development and energy
Genital	12 years–adulthood	Reemergence of sexual interests and development of relationships with potential sexual partners

Data from Freud, S. (1961). *Civilization and its discontents.* New York: Norton.

is a lifelong process that does not stop at the end of adolescence. Just as physical growth patterns can be predicted, certain psychosocial tasks must be mastered in each developmental stage. Erikson's model proposes that psychosocial development is a series of conflicts that can have favorable or unfavorable outcomes. These conflicts occur in eight developmental stages of life that are described in Table 18-3.

Havighurst (1972) theorized that there are six developmental stages of life, each with essential tasks to be achieved. Mastery of a task in one developmental stage is essential for mastery of tasks in subsequent stages. When a task in one stage is mastered, it is learned for life, independent of subsequent neurological change (which may occur with disease or injury). Table 18-4 on page 314 presents Havighurst's developmental stages and associated tasks.

TABLE 18-3 Erikson's Stages of Psychosocial Development

STAGE	AGE	TASK TO BE ACHIEVED	IMPLICATIONS
Trust vs. mistrust	Birth–18 months	Develop a sense of trust in others	Consistent, affectionate care promotes successful mastery.
			Inadequate, inconsistent care produces an unfavorable outcome at this stage.
Autonomy vs. shame and doubt	18 months–3 years	Learn self-control	The child needs support, praise, and encouragement to use newly acquired skills of independence.
			Shaming or insulting the child will lead to unnecessary dependence.
Initiative vs. guilt	3–6 years	Initiate spontaneous activities	Give clear explanations for events, and encourage creative activities.
			Threatening punishment or labeling behavior as "bad" leads to development of guilt and fears of doing wrong.
Industry vs. inferiority	6–12 years	Develop necessary social skills	To build confidence, recognize the child's accomplishments.
			Unrealistic expectation or excessively harsh criticism leads to a sense of inadequacy.

(Continues)

TABLE 18-3 (Continued)

STAGE	AGE	TASK TO BE ACHIEVED	IMPLICATIONS
Identity vs. role diffusion	12–20 years	Integrate childhood experiences into a personal identity	Help the adolescent make decisions.
			Encourage active participation in home events.
			Assist with planning for the future.
Intimacy vs. Isolation	18–25 years	Develop commitments to others and to a life work (career)	Teach the young adult to establish realistic goals.
			Avoid ridiculing romances or job choices.
Generativity vs. stagnation	21–45 years	Establish a family and become productive	Provide emotional support.
			Recognize individual accomplishments and provide appropriate praise.
Integrity vs. despair	45+ years	View one's life as meaningful and fulfilling	Explore positive aspects of one's life. Review contributions made by the individual.

Data from Erikson, E. (1968). *Childhood and society*. New York: Norton; Varcarolis, E., & Halter, M. J. (2008). *Essentials of mental health psychiatric nursing: A communication approach to evidence-based care*. St. Louis, MO: Elsevier.

TABLE 18-4 Havighurst's Developmental Stages and Tasks

DEVELOPMENTAL STAGE	DEVELOPMENTAL TASKS
Infancy and early childhood	• Eat solid foods • Walk • Talk • Control elimination of wastes • Relate emotionally to others • Distinguish right from wrong • Learn sex differences and sexual modesty • Achieve psychological stability • Form simple concepts of social and physical reality
Middle childhood	• Learn physical skills required for games • Build healthy attitudes toward oneself • Learn to socialize with peers • Learn appropriate masculine or feminine role • Gain basic reading, writing, and mathematical skills • Develop concepts necessary for everyday living • Formulate a conscience based on a value system • Achieve personal independence • Develop attitudes toward social groups and institutions

(Continues)

TABLE 18-4 (Continued)

DEVELOPMENTAL STAGE	DEVELOPMENTAL TASKS
Adolescence	• Establish more mature relationships with same-age individuals of both sexes • Achieve a masculine or feminine social role • Accept own body • Establish emotional independence from parents • Achieve assurance of economic independence • Prepare for an occupation • Prepare for marriage and establishment of a family • Acquire skills necessary to fulfill civic responsibilities • Develop a set of values that guides behavior
Early adulthood	• Select a partner • Learn to live with a partner • Start a family • Manage a home • Establish self in a career or occupation • Assume civic responsibility • Become a part of a social group
Middle adulthood	• Fulfill civic and social responsibilities • Maintain an economic standard of living • Assist adolescent children to become responsible, happy adults • Relate to one's partner • Adjust to physiological changes • Adjust to aging parents
Later maturity	• Adjust to physiological changes and alterations in health status • Adjust to retirement and altered income • Adjust to death of spouse • Develop affiliation with one's age group • Meet civic and social responsibilities • Establish satisfactory living arrangements

Data from Havighurst, R. J. (1972). *Developmental tasks and education*. New York: Longman.

Levinson (1978) studied men to determine developmental phases of young and middle adulthood. As a result of Levinson's research, five "seasons" or "eras" (phases) were identified; see Table 18-5 on page 316. The midlife transition, which begins at approximately age 40, includes examining and structuring one's life to one's own satisfaction (Edelman & Mandle, 2006).

Interpersonal Theory

Harry Stack Sullivan (1953) theorized that relationships with others influence how one's personality develops. Approval and disapproval from significant others shape the formation of one's personality. To form satisfying relationships with others, an individual must complete six stages of development, which are shown in Table 18-6 on page 316.

COGNITIVE DIMENSION

The cognitive dimension is characterized by the intellectual process of knowing (which includes perception, memory, and judgment) and develops as an individual progresses through the life span. Intelligence is an adaptive process used by individuals to adapt by changing the environment to meet their needs and by altering their responses to environmental stressors. The ability to change behavior in response to the demands of an ever-changing environment is characteristic of intelligent beings. Four factors are catalysts to intellectual development:

1. Maturation of the endocrine and nervous systems
2. Action-centered experience that leads to discovery ("learning by doing")
3. Social interaction, with opportunities for receiving feedback
4. A self-regulating mechanism that responds to environmental stimuli (Murray, Zentner, & Yakimo, 2008)

Piaget (1963) studied the differences between children's thinking patterns at different ages and how intelligence is used to solve problems and answer questions. He theorized that children learn to think by playing.

TABLE 18-5 Levinson's Seasons of Adulthood

SEASON (PHASE)	AGE	CHARACTERISTICS
Early adult transition	18–20 years	Seeks independence by separating from family
Entrance into the adult world	21–27 years	Experiments with different careers and lifestyles
Transition	28–32 years	Makes lifestyle adjustments
Settling down	33–39 years	Experiences greater stability
Pay-off years	45–65 years	Is self-directed and engages in self-evaluation

Data from Levinson, D. (1978). *The seasons of a man's life*. New York: Knopf.

Piaget and Inhelder (1969) categorized intellectual development into four phases: sensorimotor, preoperational, concrete operations, and formal operations. Table 18-7 on page 317 provides a description of each phase. Each phase is characterized by the ways in which the child interprets and uses the environment. Approximate ages are indicated for each phase, but there is great variation among individuals.

The individual learns by interacting with the environment through three processes: assimilation, accommodation, and adaptation. **Assimilation** is the process of taking in new experiences or information. **Accommodation** allows for readjustment of the cognitive structure (mindset) to take in the new information; thus, understanding is increased. **Adaptation** refers to the changes that occur as a result of assimilation and accommodation (Murray et al., 2008).

MORAL DIMENSION

The moral dimension consists of a person's value system that helps in differentiating right and wrong. **Moral maturity**, the ability to independently decide for oneself what is "right," is closely related to emotional and cognitive development. Kohlberg (1977) established a framework for understanding how individuals determine a moral code to guide their behavior. Kohlberg's model states that a person's ability to make moral judgments and behave in a morally correct manner develops over a period of time.

Kohlberg defines six stages of moral development. Each stage is built on the previous stage and becomes the foundation for successive stages. Moral development progresses in relationship to cognitive development. Individuals who are able to think at higher levels have the necessary reasoning skills on which to base moral decisions. Table 18-8 on page 318 provides an overview of Kohlberg's stages of moral development. Kohlberg (1977) stated that individuals move through the six stages in a sequential fashion; however, not everyone reaches Stages 5 and 6 in their development of personal morality.

Gilligan's theory of moral development is based on research that focused on women. Women tend to describe moral issues in the context of human relationships and seek to avoid hurting others (Gilligan, 1982). Women's moral judgment revolves around three basic issues: a concern with survival, a focus on goodness, and an understanding of others' need for care (Gilligan & Attanucci, 1988). Table 18-9 on page 318 provides an overview of Gilligan's theory.

TABLE 18-6 Sullivan's Interpersonal Model of Personality Development

STAGE	AGE	DESCRIPTION
Infancy	Birth–18 months	Infant learns to rely on caregivers to meet needs and desires.
Childhood	18 months–6 years	Child begins learning to delay immediate gratification of needs and desires.
Juvenile	6–9 years	Child forms fulfilling peer relationships.
Preadolescence	9–12 years	Child relates successfully to same-sex peers.
Early adolescence	12–14 years	Adolescent learns to be independent and forms relationships with members of opposite sex.
Late adolescence	14–21 years	Person establishes an intimate, long-lasting relationship with someone of the opposite sex.

Data from Sullivan, H. S. (1953). *Interpersonal theory of psychiatry*. New York: Norton.

TABLE 18-7 Piaget's Phases of Cognitive Development

PHASE	AGE	DESCRIPTION
Sensorimotor	**Birth–2 years**	**Sensory organs and muscles become more functional.**
Stage 1: Use of reflexes	Birth–1 month	Movements are primarily reflexive.
Stage 2: Primary circular reaction	1–4 months	Perceptions center around one's body. Objects are perceived as extensions of the self.
Stage 3: Secondary circular reaction	4–8 months	Becomes aware of external environment. Initiates acts to change the environment.
Stage 4: Coordination of secondary schemata	8–12 months	Differentiates goals and goal-directed activities.
Stage 5: Tertiary circular reaction	12–18 months	Experiments with methods to reach goals. Develops rituals that become significant.
Stage 6: Invention of new means	18–24 months	Uses mental imagery to understand the environment. Uses fantasy ("make-believe").
Preoperational	**2–7 years**	**Emerging ability to think.**
Preconceptual stage	2–4 years	Thinking tends to be egocentric. Exhibits use of symbolism.
Intuitive stage	4–7 years	Unable to break down a whole into separate parts. Able to classify objects according to one trait.
Concrete Operations	**7–11 years**	**Learns to reason about events in the here and now.**
Formal Operations	**11+ years**	**Able to see relationships and to reason in the abstract.**

Data from Piaget, J. (1963). *The origins of intelligence in children*. New York: Norton.

SPIRITUAL DIMENSION

The spiritual dimension is characterized by a sense of personal meaning. Spirituality refers to relationships with one's self, with others, and with a higher power or divine source. Spirituality does not refer to a specific religious affiliation; rather, it can be defined as the core of a person. Development of spirituality is an ongoing, lifelong process. See the accompanying Spotlight On display.

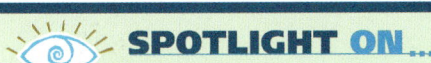

SPOTLIGHT ON...

Caring

Spiritual Awareness

The term *spirit* is derived from the Latin word meaning breath, air, and wind. Thus, spirit refers to whatever gives life to a person. What animates you? What is the core of your spirituality (life force)? The answers to these questions are truly individual. Remember that each client has a personalized definition of spiritual self, even though some clients seem to be unaware of their spiritual nature.

Fowler's (1981) theory of spiritual development, which was influenced by the works of Erikson, Piaget, and Kohlberg, is composed of a prestage and six distinct stages of faith development. Even though individuals will vary in the age at which they experience each stage, the sequence of stages remains the same. Table 18-10 on page 319 describes Fowler's theory.

HOLISTIC FRAMEWORK FOR NURSING

Providing care to the whole person is a basic concept of professional nurses. Knowledge of growth and development concepts is essential because nursing interventions must be appropriate to each client's developmental stage. Nursing's holistic perspective recognizes the progression of individual development across the life span. Developmental progress, or lack of progress, in one aspect affects all other dimensions of life. Figure 18-1 on page 319 illustrates the holistic nature of individuals.

Growth and development theories are useful to nurses as assessment parameters because alterations in expected patterns are indicators for early intervention. Following are situations in which knowledge of developmental milestones

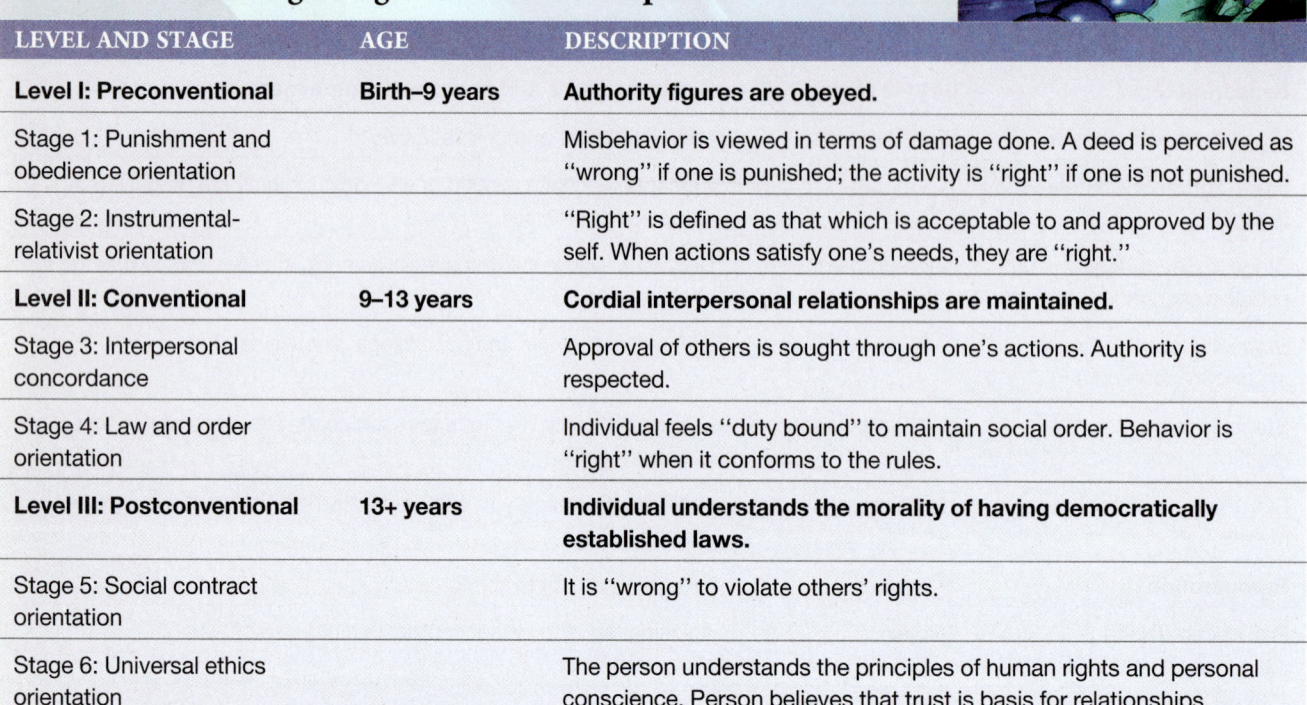

TABLE 18-8 Kohlberg's Stages of Moral Development

LEVEL AND STAGE	AGE	DESCRIPTION
Level I: Preconventional	**Birth–9 years**	**Authority figures are obeyed.**
Stage 1: Punishment and obedience orientation		Misbehavior is viewed in terms of damage done. A deed is perceived as "wrong" if one is punished; the activity is "right" if one is not punished.
Stage 2: Instrumental-relativist orientation		"Right" is defined as that which is acceptable to and approved by the self. When actions satisfy one's needs, they are "right."
Level II: Conventional	**9–13 years**	**Cordial interpersonal relationships are maintained.**
Stage 3: Interpersonal concordance		Approval of others is sought through one's actions. Authority is respected.
Stage 4: Law and order orientation		Individual feels "duty bound" to maintain social order. Behavior is "right" when it conforms to the rules.
Level III: Postconventional	**13+ years**	**Individual understands the morality of having democratically established laws.**
Stage 5: Social contract orientation		It is "wrong" to violate others' rights.
Stage 6: Universal ethics orientation		The person understands the principles of human rights and personal conscience. Person believes that trust is basis for relationships.

Data from Kohlberg, L. (1977). *Recent research in moral development*. New York: Holt, Rinehart, & Winston.

TABLE 18-9 Gilligan's Theory of Moral Development

LEVEL	CHARACTERISTICS
I. Orientation of individual survival transition	• Concentrates on what is best for self • Is selfish • Is dependent on others
Transition 1: From selfishness to responsibility	• Recognizes connections to others • Makes responsible choices in terms of self and others
II. Goodness as self-sacrifice	• Puts needs of others ahead of own • Feels responsible for others • Is dependent • May use guilt to manipulate others when attempting to "help"
Transition 2: From goodness to truth	• Makes decisions based on intentions and consequences, not on others' responses • Considers needs of self and others • Wants to help others while being responsible to self • Increases social participation
III. Morality of nonviolence	• Sees self and others as morally equal • Assumes responsibilities for own decisions • Holds basic tenet to hurt no one, including self • Experiences conflict between selfishness and selflessness • Is not dependent on others' perceptions for self-judgment but rather on consequences and intentions of actions

Data from Gilligan, C., & Attanucci, D. (1988). Two moral orientations: Gender differences and similarities. *Merrill-Palmer Quarterly*, 34(3), 332-333; Gilligan, C. (1982). *In a different voice: Psychologic theory and women's development*. Cambridge, MA: Harvard University Press.

TABLE 18-10 Fowler's Stages of Faith

STAGE	AGE	CHARACTERISTICS
Prestage: Undifferentiated faith	Infant	• Trust, hope, and love compete with environmental inconsistencies or threats of abandonment
Stage 1: Intuitive-projective faith	Toddler, preschooler	• Imitates parental behaviors and attitudes about religion and spirituality • Has no real understanding of spiritual concepts
Stage 2: Mythical-literal faith	School-aged child	• Accepts existence of a deity • Religious and moral beliefs are symbolized by stories • Appreciates others' viewpoints • Accepts concept of reciprocal fairness
Stage 3: Synthetic-conventional faith	Adolescent	• Questions values and religious beliefs in an attempt to form own identity
Stage 4: Individuative-reflective faith	Late adolescent and young adult	• Assumes responsibility for own attitudes and beliefs
Stage 5: Conjunctive faith	Adult	• Integrates other perspectives about faith into own definition of truth
Stage 6: Universalizing faith	Adult	• Makes concepts of love and justice tangible

Data from Fowler, J. W. (1981). *Stages of faith: The psychology of human development and the quest for meaning.* New York: Harper & Row.

is essential for prompt identification of problems and comprehensive intervention:

• The infant who does not sit, crawl, or walk at expected times

• The adolescent girl who has not experienced menarche at the expected time

• The adult who has failed to develop adequate problem-solving skills

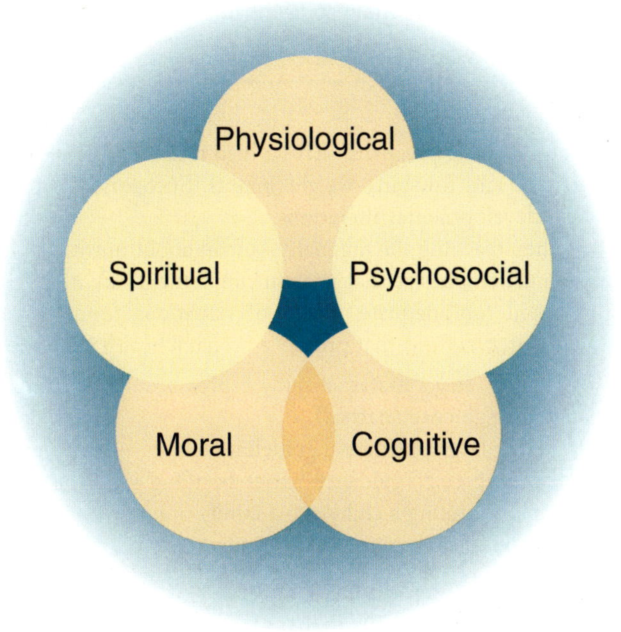

STAGES OF THE LIFE CYCLE

For purposes of this discussion, 11 developmental stages are presented: prenatal period, neonate, infant, toddler, preschooler, school-age child, preadolescent, adolescent, young adult, middle adult, and older adult. For each stage, the manifestations of growth and development in the physiological, psychosocial, cognitive, moral, and spiritual dimensions are discussed with the relevant nursing implications.

Nurses can intervene to promote health and wellness during each stage of the life cycle. The Centers for Disease Control and Prevention (2007a) has developed health protection goals that are specific to each developmental stage; see Table 18-11 on page 320.

PRENATAL PERIOD

The **prenatal period**, the developmental stage beginning with conception and ending with birth, is a critical time in a human being's development and consists of three developmental phases: the germinal, embryonic, and fetal stages. The **germinal stage** begins with conception and lasts approximately 10 to 14 days. This stage is characterized by

FIGURE 18-1 Holistic Nature of Human Beings DELMAR/CENGAGE LEARNING

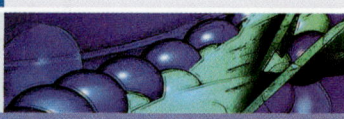

TABLE 18-11   Centers for Disease Control and Prevention's Health Protection Goals: Healthy People in Every Stage of Life

DEVELOPMENTAL STAGE	GOAL	DESCRIPTION
Infants and toddlers (ages 0–3)	Start strong	Increase the number of infants and toddlers who have a strong start for healthy and safe lives.
Children (ages 4–11)	Grow safe and strong	Increase the number of children who grow up healthy, safe, and ready to learn.
Adolescents (ages 12–19)	Achieve healthy independence	Increase the number of adolescents who are prepared to be healthy, safe, independent, and productive members of society.
Adults (ages 20–49)	Live a healthy, productive, and satisfying life	Increase the number of adults who are healthy and able to participate fully in life activities and enter their later years with optimum health.
Older adults and seniors (ages 50+)	Live better, longer	Increase the number of older adults who live longer, high-quality, productive, and independent lives.

Centers for Disease Control and Prevention. (2007a). *Health protection goals*. Atlanta, GA: Author. Retrieved November 20, 2008, from http://www.cdc.gov/osi/goals/people/index.html. (Courtesy of U.S. Centers for Disease Control and Prevention.)

rapid cell division and implantation of the fertilized egg in the uterine wall. In this very early stage, the central nervous system (CNS) is already beginning to form.

The **embryonic stage**, the first 2 to 8 weeks after fertilization of an egg by a sperm, is characterized by rapid cellular differentiation, growth, and development of the body systems. This critical period is when the embryo is most vulnerable to noxious stimuli, which may lead to a spontaneous abortion (miscarriage) (Murray et al., 2008).

The **fetal stage**, the intrauterine developmental period from 8 weeks to birth, is characterized by rapid growth and differentiation of body systems and parts. Table 18-12 on page 321 provides an overview of fetal development.

Nursing Implications

Pregnant women need to have physical examinations and screenings during the entire pregnancy. Early prenatal care is essential for a positive pregnancy outcome. See the accompanying Spotlight On display.

Learning that one is pregnant is accompanied by several emotions: happiness, fear, sadness, excitement, and anxiety. Emotions lead to alterations in biochemicals; therefore, the mother's emotional state can bring about biochemical changes in the fetus. By teaching pregnant women how to relax, the nurse can promote a supportive environment for the developing embryo and fetus.

WELLNESS PROMOTION   The uterus is the primary environment affecting prenatal growth and development. Ideally, this environment nurtures positive growth of the embryo and fetus.

An ample supply of nutrients must be provided by the gestating woman. Women who consume insufficient amounts

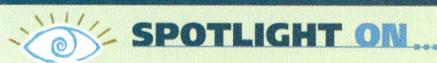

SPOTLIGHT ON...

Ethical

Nutrition and the Economically Disadvantaged

Do you think it is the responsibility of the federal government to ensure that pregnant women have adequate diets? What would happen if government-sponsored nutritional programs for pregnant women were abolished?

of protein during pregnancy have a high risk of giving birth to premature and low-birth-weight infants. Such infants are at risk for developmental alterations.

When teaching the pregnant woman about nutrition, the nurse must emphasize that vitamin supplements are *not* to be substituted for adequate intake of nutritious food. Other nursing interventions that promote prenatal health include:

- Screening (e.g., maternal blood pressure measurement and urine glucose analysis)
- Teaching (e.g., nutritional guidelines)
- Counseling (e.g., guidance about bonding with the child and incorporating a child into a family unit)
- Promoting the use of complementary and alternative modalities (e.g., imagery) to reduce stress
- Working with economically disadvantaged clients to obtain prenatal care

SAFETY CONSIDERATIONS   The fetus is especially vulnerable to substances consumed by the mother. In addition to

TABLE 18-12 Embryo and Fetus: Growth and Development

AGE	CHARACTERISTICS
Weeks 1–3	• Rapid cell differentiation • Heart starts to pulsate • CNS formation • Presence of all organs
Week 4	• Beginnings of respiratory system • Basic structures for eyes and ears • Limb buds distinguishable
Week 5	• Embryo has a C-shaped body with a tail and large head • Each body system present in at least a rudimentary form • Umbilical cord developed • Brain vesicles developed • Nerve tissues more fully developed
Week 6	• Establishment of circulatory pathway (including heart with septa) • Limbs distinguishable as arms and legs • Intestine elongating • Lungs formed, with bronchi beginning to branch out • Liver begins production of blood cells
Week 9	• Fingers, toes, eyelids, nose, and jaw evident
Week 12	• Body growth speeds up while growth of head slows
Week 16	• Ossification of skeleton begins • Fingers and toes separated
Week 20	• Fetal movement felt by mother • Wake and sleep cycles evident • Formation of small amounts of body fat
Week 24	• Circulation of blood in vessels is visible • Accelerated weight gain • Ovaries or testes developed • Kidney tubules branch out • Brain grows rapidly
Week 28	• Eyes open and close • Thick hair on head • Lanugo (thick coating of body hair) is present • Rhythmic breathing patterns begin to be established
Week 32	• Maturation of respiratory system and temperature-regulating mechanism • Fat deposited in arms and legs • Fingernails and toenails present
Week 36	• Protrusion of mammary glands in both sexes • Lack of melanin leads to white skin in all fetuses at this stage
Week 40	• Completion of fetal development • Fetus is ready for extrauterine environment • Optimal time for birth

Data from Guyton, A. C., & Hall, J. (2005). *Textbook of medical physiology* (11th ed.). Philadelphia: Elsevier; Hockenberry, M. J., Wilson, D., & Jackson, C. (2006). *Wong's nursing care of infants and children* (8th ed.). St. Louis, MO: Elsevier.

▼ **SAFETY FIRST** ▼

TOBACCO AND ALCOHOL USE DURING PREGNANCY

Total abstinence from cigarette smoking is advised during pregnancy. Because there has been no determination of "safe" amounts of alcohol consumption, caution all pregnant women to avoid drinking alcohol.

providing the fetus with wholesome nutrients, maternal blood can also transport toxins.

Cigarettes contain several toxic substances, such as nicotine, that cross the placental barrier and interfere with the transport of oxygen to the fetus. Such toxins often result in increased risk of premature birth, retarded growth, learning difficulties, and fetal death.

Use of alcohol during pregnancy can result in **fetal alcohol syndrome** (FAS), a condition in which fetal development is impaired and is manifested in the infant by characteristic physical attributes and intellectual problems. Typically, FAS infants are small, have facial abnormalities (such as thin upper lips and short, upturned noses), and may have some degree of brain damage. Alcohol consumption is most dangerous during the first 3 months of pregnancy when the embryo's brain and other vital organs are developing. The effects of alcohol on the fetus are permanent. FAS is considered to be the leading cause of mental retardation among infants, and the incidence continues to increase (Hockenberry, Wilson, & Jackson, 2006).

In addition to nicotine and alcohol, there are many other teratogenic substances. A **teratogenic substance** is any substance that can cross the placental barrier and impair normal growth and development. See the accompanying Safety First display.

Client education consists of teaching pregnant women to check labels of *all* medicines for information about potential effects on the fetus; this includes over-the-counter (OTC) medications and herbal remedies. The Food and Drug Administration requires that all manufactured drugs list their potential for causing birth defects. The use of illegal drugs by pregnant women presents a very serious threat to the unborn. Substance abuse prevention programs can be effective in preventing or reducing this risk.

NEONATAL PERIOD

The **neonatal period**, the first 28 days of life following birth, is a time of major adjustment to extrauterine life. The energies of the neonate (newborn) are focused on achieving equilibrium through stabilization of major body systems. Table 18-13 on page 323 describes neonatal development.

The neonate's activities, which are reflexive in nature, consist primarily of sucking, crying, eliminating, and sleeping (see Figure 18-2 on page 324). The neonate blinks in response to bright lights and demonstrates the startle reflex in response to loud noises. Neonatal reflexes play a major role in

▼ **SAFETY FIRST** ▼

NEONATAL REFLEXES

A complete assessment of neonatal reflexes should be performed immediately after birth. Early detection of problems is essential in order to perform life-saving interventions.

the ability to survive. Table 18-14 on page 325 lists the reflexive activities of the neonate.

During the first month of life, the neonate progresses developmentally from a mass of reflexes to behavior that is more goal directed (purposeful). In addition to the major physiological adjustments necessitated by extrauterine life, the neonate also undergoes psychological adaptation.

The major psychological task of neonates is to adjust to the parental figures. **Bonding**, the formation of attachment between parent and child, begins at birth when the neonate and parent make initial eye contact. The quality of parent-neonate bonding lays the foundation for trust that is necessary for the development of future interpersonal relationships. Figure 18-3 on page 325 shows bonding between neonate and parent.

Nursing Implications

A complete and thorough assessment of the neonate, which is performed immediately after delivery, includes evaluation of the neonate's reflexes. In addition to focusing on the reflexes, the assessment also evaluates respiratory and cardiac functioning. Table 18-15 on page 325 shows the Apgar assessment tool that is performed by the nurse at 1 minute and again at 5 minutes after birth.

In the first few hours after birth, encourage the parents to cuddle the newborn. Explain the neonate's interactive abilities. Encourage mutual eye contact between neonate and parents by showing parents how to hold the child facing them.

WELLNESS PROMOTION   Teaching is one of the most important nursing activities for promoting neonatal wellness. First-time parents need information about basic newborn needs (to be held, rocked, and talked to), nutrition, infection control (especially handwashing and hygienic diaper changing practices), care of the umbilicus, and incorporating the newborn into the family unit.

Knowledge of growth and development milestones is necessary for parents to provide appropriate neonatal stimulation and have realistic expectations.

Other nursing interventions that promote neonatal wellness are the following:

- Continually assessing the neonate's physiological status
- Providing a warm environment (Neonates breathe more easily when they are warm.)
- Monitoring nutritional status (It is normal for neonates to lose up to 10% of birth weight during the first week of life.)
- Providing a clean environment to protect neonates from infection and teaching parents that neonates need a clean environment, not a sterile one

TABLE 18-13 Neonate: Growth and Development

DIMENSION	CHARACTERISTICS	NURSING IMPLICATIONS
Physiological	Circulatory function shifts from the umbilical cord to heart.	Accurately assess neonate's cardiovascular status.
	Gas exchange (oxygen and carbon dioxide) is transferred from placenta to lungs. Respiratory reflexes are activated seconds after birth.	Immediately after birth, hold the neonate with head lower than body to allow for drainage of fluids that may block respiratory passages.
		If spontaneous respirations do not occur, resuscitate immediately.
	Weak neck and shoulder muscles.	Carefully support the neonate's head.
	Immature temperature-regulating mechanism.	To conserve heat: • Dry neonate immediately after birth and place in a warmed bassinet. • Place a stockinette cap on neonate's head.
	Incomplete ossification (process of cartilage changing to bone).	Protect the anterior fontanelle on neonate's skull.
	Poor visual acuity; visual focus is generally rigid.	Instruct parents to be directly in front of the neonate (about 9–12 inches away from child's face) when communicating.
Motor	Reflexes direct the majority of movement.	
	The full-term neonate has some limited ability to hold the head erect. Able to lift head slightly when lying prone.	Support neck and head when lifting.
Psychosocial	Crying is the neonate's method of communication. There is a reason for the cry.	Teach parents about the dynamics of crying to avoid having the neonate labeled as "fussy" or the parents developing the misconception that they are inadequate caregivers.
		Encourage parents to learn to discriminate crying patterns.
	The bonding process begins shortly after birth.	Teach parents the importance of interacting with the neonate during every contact (feeding, bathing, changing, cuddling).
Cognitive	Neonates learn through sensory experiences. Learning is enhanced by an environment that provides stimuli without bombarding the neonate. Learning occurs by repeated exposure to stimuli.	To promote learning, encourage parents to provide frequent sensory stimuli (touching, talking, looking the neonate in the eyes).

Data from Estes, M. E. Z. (2010). *Health assessment and physical examination* (4th ed.). Clifton Park, NY: Delmar/Cengage Learning; Murray, R. B., Zentner, J. P., & Yakimo, R. (2008). *Nursing assessment and health promotion through the lifespan* (8th ed.). Upper Saddle River, NJ: Prentice-Hall; Hockenberry, M. J., Wilson, D., & Jackson C. (2006). *Wong's nursing care of infants and children* (8th ed.). St. Louis, MO: Elsevier.

- Conducting screening tests (e.g., the blood test for phenylketonuria (PKU), a genetic disorder that, if untreated, can lead to impaired intellectual functioning)
- Promoting early parent-neonate interaction

Selection of a feeding method for the neonate is a major decision for parents. Breastfeeding is the most natural option. However, commercially prepared formula is sometimes used due to the neonate's special needs or parental choice. For a comparison of feeding methods, see the discussion about infant nutrition.

SAFETY CONSIDERATIONS Safety is of primary concern when caring for neonates because they are totally dependent on others to meet their needs. Accidents are the primary cause of neonatal mortality (Murray et al., 2008). One of the most important neonatal accident prevention methods is to teach

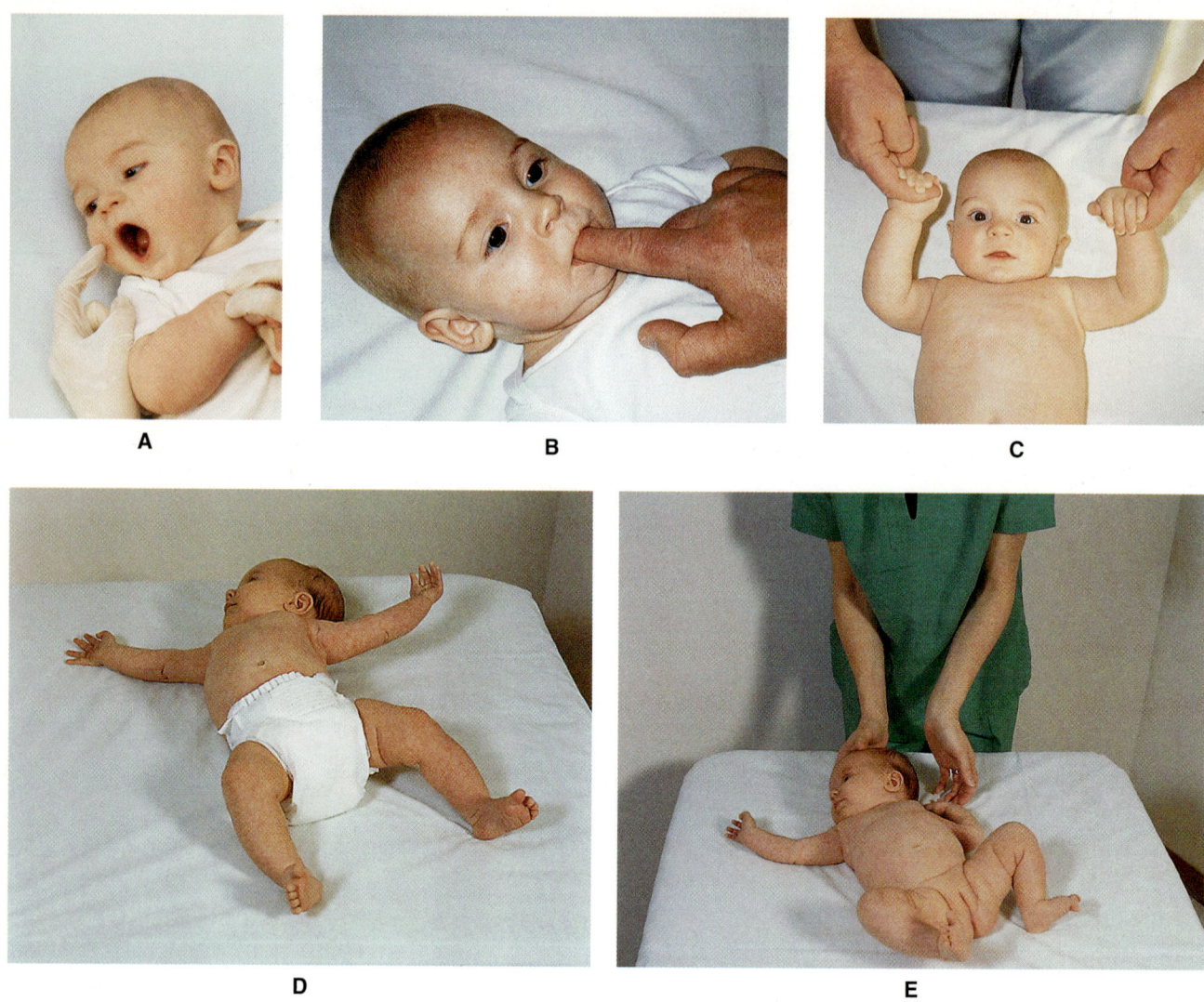

FIGURE 18-2 **Selected Neonatal Reflexes: A,** rooting; **B,** sucking; **C,** grasp; **D,** Moro; **E,** tonic neck. DELMAR/CENGAGE LEARNING

parents about the proper use of infant car seats. Under current federal law, neonates and infants must be secured in an approved infant car seat *every* time the child travels in a car.

In addition to accidents, infections pose a serious health risk to the neonate. Newborns should not be in contact with anyone experiencing an infectious disease. The skin is the body's major defense against invasion by disease-producing microorganisms; therefore, it is essential that the neonate's skin integrity be maintained. Parents must be taught the importance of skin cleanliness. Diaper rash is a common skin problem for newborns and infants because of the ammonia from urine in wet diapers. The ammonia burns and irritates the skin, resulting in localized irritation, blisters, or fissures. In addition to prompt changing of wet diapers, bathing and use of protective creams are useful in preventing skin breakdown.

INFANCY

Infancy, the developmental stage from the first month to the first year of life, is a time of continued adaptation. During

this stage, the infant experiences rapid physiologic growth and psychosocial development (see Figure 18-4 on page 326). Table 18-16 on page 327 provides an overview of infant development in the physical, motor, psychosocial, cognitive, moral, and spiritual dimensions.

Nursing Implications

The nurse caring for an infant must focus on safety, prevention of infection, and teaching parents about incorporating the child into the family. Nursing care involves the provision of support, reassurance, and information to the parents.

WELLNESS PROMOTION Nurses promote infant wellness by teaching growth and development concepts to parents and other caregivers. Knowledge of the type of behavior to expect at certain times during infancy serves as both guidance and reassurance for parents. Three specific areas in which parents need guidance from the nurse in caring for their infants are nutrition, protection from infection, and promotion of sleep.

TABLE 18-14 Major Neonatal Reflexes

REFLEX	DESCRIPTION
Rooting	Turning the mouth and nose in the direction of any facial touch
Sucking	Using the tongue and mouth to take in liquid or food
Swallowing	Movement of throat muscles to push food from mouth to esophagus
Grasp	Firm contraction of hand muscles around an object
Babinski	When foot stroked, toes fan upward and outward
Moro	When startled, arms and legs swing quickly out, then immediately back, and neonate curls up into a ball
Smiling	Turning lips upward; neonate looks "happy"
Blinking	Rapid closing and opening of eyelids
Sneezing	A violent, spasmodic, sudden expiration of breath
Coughing	Explosively expelling air from the lungs
Crying	Making a loud, wailing sound
Tonic neck	When head is turned to side, arm and leg on same side are extended in a fencing posture
Extrusion	Tongue pushes outward when touched by an object at the tip
Head turning	Moving face to one side or the other when airway is blocked by a surface, such as a bed or pillow

Delmar/Cengage Learning

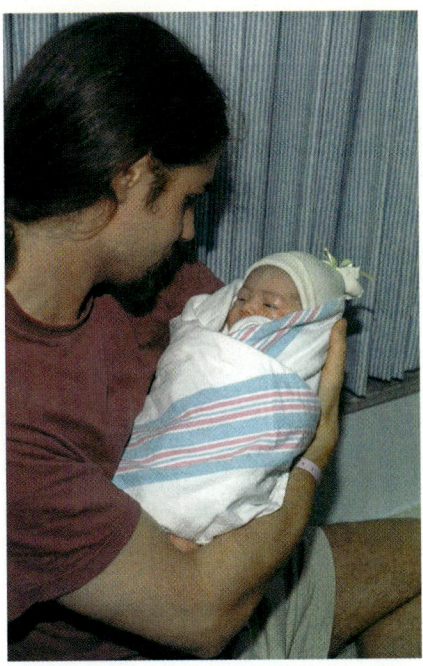

FIGURE 18-3 Bonding between a parent and neonate. Consider the factors that may have an impact on the early attachment between this father and daughter. DELMAR/CENGAGE LEARNING

A major factor influencing health maintenance of the infant is the provision of adequate nutrients delivered in a loving, consistent manner. Caregivers should be taught that the nutrients must be germ free and provide the recommended amounts of carbohydrates, protein, calcium, iron, and vitamins. It is recommended that infants be breastfed for the first 6 to 12 months (Murray et al., 2008). Breast milk has several benefits over commercially prepared formulas, including that it:

- Boosts immune functioning (e.g., contains immunoglobulins, lymphocytes, and other bacteria growth retardants)
- Is more easily digested because of smaller curds than those in cow's milk and formula
- Promotes absorption of fat and calcium
- Is readily available and economical

TABLE 18-15 Apgar Assessment Tool

SIGN	VALUE 0	1	2
Heart rate	Absent	Less than 100 beats per minute	Over 100 beats per minute
Respiratory effort	Absent	Slow and irregular	Crying
Muscle tone	Flaccid	Some flexion of extremities	Active movement
Reflex irritability	No response	Weak cry or grimace	Vigorous cry
Color	Blue or pale	Pink body, cyanotic extremities	Entire body is pink

Delmar/Cengage Learning

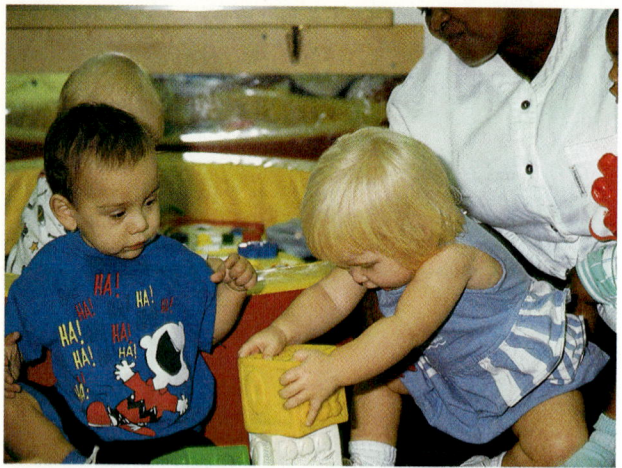

FIGURE 18-4 These children are exploring their world and are demonstrating mastery of both the physiological and cognitive dimensions of their development. DELMAR/CENGAGE LEARNING

The act of breastfeeding promotes maternal-infant bonding (Hockenberry et al., 2006). There are some cultural sanctions against breastfeeding, and some cultures view bottle-feeding as a status symbol.

Normal growth and development can occur without breastfeeding. "There is no doubt that human breastmilk is the perfect formulation for growth, development and the establishment of an infant's immunity. Sometimes, breastfeeding is not an option so if a mother chooses to partially or totally feed her baby with formula there is no reason for her to feel guilty" (Mainstone, 2008, p. 612). Special formulas are available for infants who are hypersensitive to protein, who have PKU, and who experience fat malabsorption. Whole cow's milk is not recommended for infants under 1 year of age. Human milk and commercially prepared formula are more easily digested. Soy-based formulas have been developed for the infant with lactose deficiency or who is allergic to regular formula. Infants who are formula fed generally have greater deposits of subcutaneous fat (Murray et al., 2008). The Nursing Checklist on page 329 provides teaching strategies for parents of bottle-fed infants. See the accompanying Safety First and the Uncovering the Evidence displays. It is important that the nurse provide accurate information about the types of feeding available and support the parents' decision about the method chosen.

Solid foods are usually introduced at 3 to 4 months of age. Rice cereal is the first solid food of choice because it has the fewest allergic responses (Murray et al., 2008).

Infants are especially vulnerable to developing infections because the immune system is not fully matured. Immunizations are of utmost importance in preventing infections.

▼ SAFETY FIRST ▼

BOTTLE FEEDING
Never prop a bottle in the baby's mouth because choking may result.

Nurses should confirm that infants receive all necessary immunizations. Figure 18-5 on page 328 provides a recommended schedule for childhood immunization.

Parents often need information about normal sleep patterns of infants and how the patterns change with maturation. Activities that promote sleep include:

- Providing a quiet room for the infant
- Scheduling feedings and other care activities during periods of wakefulness instead of drowsy times
- Developing sensitivity to the unique sleep and rest periods established by the infant

UNCOVERING THE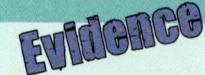

TITLE OF STUDY
"Complex Pediatric Feeding Disorders: Using Teleconferencing Technology to Improve Access to a Treatment Program"

AUTHORS
B. Clawson, M. Selden, M. Lacks, A. V. Deaton, B. Hall, and R. Bach

PURPOSE
The overall goal of this study was to provide treatment options to children in order to help them eat effectively, thereby improving their overall health status. The study was done to determine the efficacy of teleconferencing in improving children's access to treatment for feeding disorders.

METHODS
This pilot study included children with complex feeding disorders referred from locations from 300 to 3,500 miles from the treatment center. Fifteen teleconferencing visits were carefully planned, implemented, and evaluated. Follow-up to the teleconferencing sessions was accomplished by phone, letter, and a questionnaire.

FINDINGS
Of the initial consultations, 50% resulted in recommendations that allowed the children to be treated in their communities. The reduced cost of care for teleconferencing was an advantage for families of children with feeding disorders.

IMPLICATIONS
The availability of teleconferencing as an option for screening and follow-up care enables children with complex feeding disorders to be treated effectively within their communities.

Clawson, B., Selden, M., Lacks, M., Deaton, A. V., Hall, B., & Bach, R. (2008). Complex pediatric feeding disorders: Using teleconferencing technology to improve access to a treatment program. *Pediatric Nursing, 34*(3), 213–216.

TABLE 18-16 Infant: Growth and Development

DIMENSION	CHARACTERISTICS	NURSING IMPLICATIONS
Physiological	• Physical growth is rapid. Birth weight usually triples by end of first year. Height increases by approximately 50%. • Progressive maturation of all body systems. • Body temperature stabilizes. • Heart rate slows (approximately 80–130 beats per minute). • Blood pressure rises. • At approximately 4–6 months, eruption of teeth begins. • Rapid growth of brain (reaches about half the adult size).	• Inform parents of the developmental norms. • Encourage parents to have "well-baby checkups" as recommended.
	• Posterior fontanel closes at approximately 2 months. • Eyes begin to focus.	• Protect infant's skull.

Motor	• Physical maturation allows for development of motor skills.
	• Primitive reflexes are replaced by movement that is more voluntary and goal directed.
	• Motor skills develop rapidly:
	    6 months: rolls over voluntarily
	    6–7 months: crawls
	    8 months: sits alone
	• Grasping objects is reflexive for first 2–3 months and gradually becomes voluntary.
		• Teach parents anticipated ages for motor skill development.

Psychosocial	• *Freud:* Oral stage • *Erikson:* Trust vs. mistrust • A sense of self begins to develop. • Responds to caregiver's voice. • Anxiety separation occurs at approximately 6 months.	• Seeks immediate gratification of needs. Receives pleasure and comfort through mouth, lips, and tongue. • Encourage parents to feed in a prompt, consistent manner (feed on demand rather than a fixed schedule). • Other activities that promote trust are providing warmth, diapering, and comforting.
	• *Havighurst:* Learns to eat solid food, crawl, walk, and talk.	• Teach parents approximate ages that developmental milestones are expected to occur.
Cognitive	• *Piaget:* Sensorimotor stage • Infant learns by interacting with the environment.	• Encourage parents to provide a variety of sensory stimuli: visual, sensory, auditory, and tactile (e.g., colorful mobiles; musical toys; soft plush animals; rubbing, patting, stroking the infant's skin).
	• Language development includes babbling, repetition, and imitation.	• Caregivers need to talk to infant often. Encourage caregivers to name objects that are the focus of infant's attention.
Moral	• *Kohlberg:* Preconventional stage	• Teach parents that now is the time to start teaching (by role modeling) the difference between "right" and "wrong."
Spiritual	• *Fowler:* Stage of undifferentiated faith	• Encourage caregivers to model the values they want the infant to learn.

Data from Murray, R. B., Zentner, J. P., & Yakimo, R. (2008). *Nursing assessment and health promotion through the lifespan* (8th ed.). Upper Saddle River, NJ: Pearson; Hockenberry, M. J., Wilson, D., & Jackson, C. (2006). *Wong's nursing care of infants and children* (8th ed.). St. Louis, MO: Elsevier.

Recommended Immunization Schedule for Persons Aged 0 Through 6 Years—United States • 2009
For those who fall behind or start late, see the catch-up schedule

Vaccine ▼ Age ▶	Birth	1 month	2 months	4 months	6 months	12 months	15 months	18 months	19–23 months	2–3 years	4–6 years
Hepatitis B[1]	HepB	HepB	HepB	see footnote 1	HepB	HepB	HepB	HepB			
Rotavirus[2]			RV	RV	RV[2]						
Diphtheria, Tetanus, Pertussis[3]			DTaP	DTaP	DTaP	see footnote 3	DTaP	DTaP			DTaP
Haemophilus influenzae type b[4]			Hib	Hib	Hib[4]	Hib	Hib				
Pneumococcal[5]			PCV	PCV	PCV	PCV	PCV			PPSV	
Inactivated Poliovirus			IPV	IPV	IPV	IPV	IPV	IPV			IPV
Influenza[6]					Influenza (Yearly)						
Measles, Mumps, Rubella[7]						MMR	MMR	see footnote 7			MMR
Varicella[8]						Varicella	Varicella	see footnote 8			Varicella
Hepatitis A[9]						HepA (2 doses)				HepA Series	
Meningococcal[10]										MCV	

▨ (yellow)	Range of recommended ages
▨ (purple)	Certain high-risk groups

FIGURE 18-5A Recommended Immunization Schedule for Persons Aged 0–6 Years—United States, 2009 COURTESY OF U.S. CENTERS FOR DISEASE CONTROL AND PREVENTION

Recommended Immunization Schedule for Persons Aged 7 Through 18 Years—United States • 2009
For those who fall behind or start late, see the schedule below and the catch-up schedule

Vaccine ▼ Age ▶	7–10 years	11–12 years	13–18 years
Tetanus, Diphtheria, Pertussis[1]	see footnote 1	Tdap	Tdap
Human Papillomavirus[2]	see footnote 2	HPV (3 doses)	HPV Series
Meningococcal[3]	MCV	MCV	MCV
Influenza[4]	Influenza (Yearly)		
Pneumococcal[5]	PPSV		
Hepatitis A[6]	HepA Series		
Hepatitis B[7]	HepB Series		
Inactivated Poliovirus[8]	IPV Series		
Measles, Mumps, Rubella[9]	MMR Series		
Varicella[10]	Varicella Series		

▨ (yellow)	Range of recommended ages
▨ (green)	Catch-up immunization
▨ (purple)	Certain high-risk groups

FIGURE 18-5B Recommended Immunization Schedule for Person Aged 7–18 Years—United States, 2009 COURTESY OF U.S. CENTERS FOR DISEASE CONTROL AND PREVENTION

- Providing comfort and security measures (e.g., rocking, singing)
- Establishing routine times for sleep

SAFETY CONSIDERATIONS The majority of infant injuries and deaths are related to motor vehicle accidents. Therefore, the consistent, proper use of infant car seats is one of the most effective measures parents can take to ensure their infant's safety.

▼ SAFETY FIRST ▼

AIDING THE CHOKING INFANT
Never use the Heimlich maneuver on an infant who is choking. Instead, use alternating back blows and chest compressions to dislodge the object.

✓ **NURSING**CHECKLIST

Bottle Feeding

- The baby should be in a semireclining position cradled close to the mother's body with the mother in a comfortable position.
- Use care if heating bottles. Do not warm bottles in the microwave because the hot liquid can cause esophageal and oropharyngeal burns.
- Avoid using the bottle as a pacifier because this action may result in tooth decay and set the stage for future obesity.

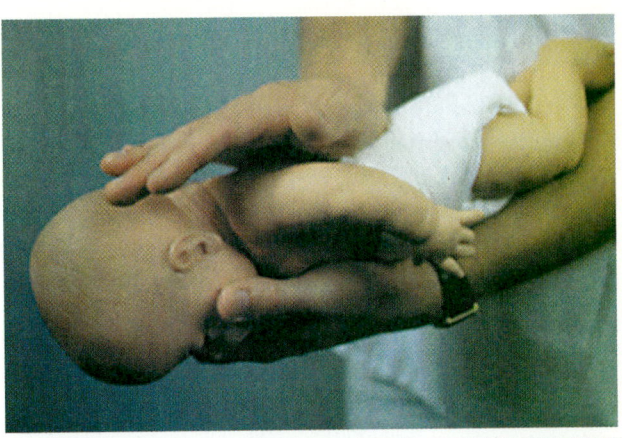

FIGURE 18-6 Intervention for a choking infant. Emergency care for an infant who is choking consists of a series of five blows to the back between the shoulder blades, followed by five thrusts midline on the chest approximately 1 inch below the nipple line. DELMAR/CENGAGE LEARNING

During this oral phase of development, infants tend to test out their environment and seek pleasure through the mouth. Aspiration accidents are common with infants who choke on objects such as buttons, coins, and food. The Heimlich maneuver is *not* used with infants because it may force the foreign object further down the trachea. Figure 18-6 illustrates the proper technique to use with an infant who is choking. See the accompanying Safety First display on page 328 and Client Teaching Checklist below for guidelines that the nurse can share with parents to prevent infant accidents.

TODDLER

The toddler period begins at 12 to 18 months of age, when a child starts to walk alone, and ends at approximately age 3. The family is very important to the toddler in that the family promotes language development and teaches toileting skills. During this stage, the child becomes more independent. Frequently, when attempts to demonstrate autonomy are prevented, the child will have a temper tantrum; thus, this stage is often referred to as "the terrible twos." Parents must understand that the toddler's frequent use of the word "no" is an expression of developing autonomy.

Nurses can greatly influence the quality of parent-child interaction by teaching parents about developmental concepts. This information helps parents form realistic expectations of the toddler's behavior. Setting firm limits in a consistent manner helps the toddler learn while providing parameters for safe and socially acceptable behavior. Table 18-17 on page 330 describes the toddler's growth and development in the physiological, motor, psychosocial, cognitive, moral, and spiritual dimensions.

Nursing Implications

Nurses who work with toddlers must be sensitive to the fact that children of this age are likely to be anxious and fearful in the presence of strangers. The establishment of rapport with the child will help alleviate this stranger anxiety. Play is an effective tool for building rapport with toddlers.

When toddlers are hospitalized (for an extended time or only a day), fear and anxiety can make the experience a negative one. The major stressor resulting from hospitalization is the toddler's separation from parents. An unfamiliar environment also results in stress for the toddler. Nurses can help reduce stress in the hospitalized toddler by teaching both the child and parents about procedures. Parents can alleviate the toddler's stress by holding the child and talking in a calm manner when in the presence of the health care provider (see Figure 18-7 on page 331).

✓ CLIENT TEACHING **CHECKLIST**

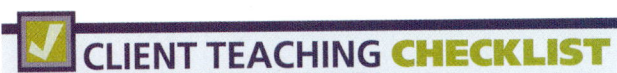

PREVENTING ACCIDENTS IN INFANTS

- To avoid vehicular accidents: Use infant seats, and keep the infant out of the paths of automobiles and other vehicles. Many infants can crawl very quickly.
- To prevent burns: Keep infant away from open heaters, furnaces, fireplaces, hot stoves, and matches.
- To protect from falls: Keep crib rails up at all times, never leave the infant lying unattended on furniture, and use protective gates and barriers to block stairways.
- To prevent drowning: Never leave the infant unattended near water (bathtubs, buckets, swimming pools).
- To prevent electrocution: As the infant begins to crawl, use plastic safety plugs to cover all electrical outlets and keep electrical cords out of infant's reach.
- To prevent choking: Closely monitor the infant who is exploring the environment.

TABLE 18-17 Toddler: Growth and Development

DIMENSION	CHARACTERISTICS	NURSING IMPLICATIONS
Physiological	• Overall rate of growth slows. By 24 months, the toddler usually weighs four times more than at birth. • Rapid growth of brain.	• Instruct parents on need for vitamin D, calcium, and phosphorus.
	• Bones in extremities grow in length.	• Recognize that "growing pains" are normal.
	• Physiological readiness for bowel and bladder training develops.	• Instruct parents of timing for toilet training and need for consistency and patience.
Motor	• Walks and runs. • Becomes more coordinated.	• Assess home environment for safety as toddler becomes more mobile.
Psychosocial	• *Freud:* Anal stage (receives pleasure from contraction and relaxation of sphincter muscles)	• Instruct parents to avoid overemphasis on toilet training.
	• *Erikson:* Autonomy vs. shame and doubt	• Teach parents to encourage toddler's attempts at independence (e.g., trying to feed and dress self).
	• *Havighurst:* Developmental tasks include: —Beginning to learn sex differences —Learning to talk	• Explain that sexual curiosity is normal. • Encourage parents to talk to child frequently.
	• Engages in parallel play (playing near other children but not necessarily interacting with them).	• Provide opportunities for child to socialize with peers.
	• A reemergence of separation anxiety often occurs. • By age 3, most toddlers are able to tolerate being left with strangers.	• Reassure child that parents will return.
Cognitive	• *Piaget:* Preoperational stage • Concrete thought processes. • Short attention span.	
	• Can follow simple directions.	• Instruct parents to give only one direction at a time.
	• Is able to anticipate future events.	• Use a calendar to show today's date and the number of days until a significant event.
	• Comprehends self as a separate entity.	• Teach caregivers importance of calling child by name.
	• Language: At approximately 1 year, can make two-syllable sounds (e.g., ma-ma, da-da). • At approximately 2 years, can form short sentences. • Has a vocabulary of approximately 900 words.	• Talk to child frequently, avoiding use of "baby talk."
Moral	• *Kohlberg:* Preconventional stage • Learns to distinguish right from wrong.	• Parents need to be consistent in setting limits. • Understand the significance of modeling desired behavior to child. • Spiritual
Spiritual	• *Fowler:* Intuitive-projective stage of faith	• Instruct parents to provide simple answers to questions related to religion. • Instruct on importance of incorporating religious rituals and ceremonies into daily life.

Data from Murray, R. B., Zentner, J. P., & Yakimo, R. (2008). *Nursing assessment and health promotion through the lifespan* (8th ed.). UpperSaddle River, NJ: Pearson; Hockenberry, M. J., Wilson, D., & Jackson, C. (2006). *Wong's nursing care of infants and children* (8th ed.). St. Louis, MO: Elsevier.

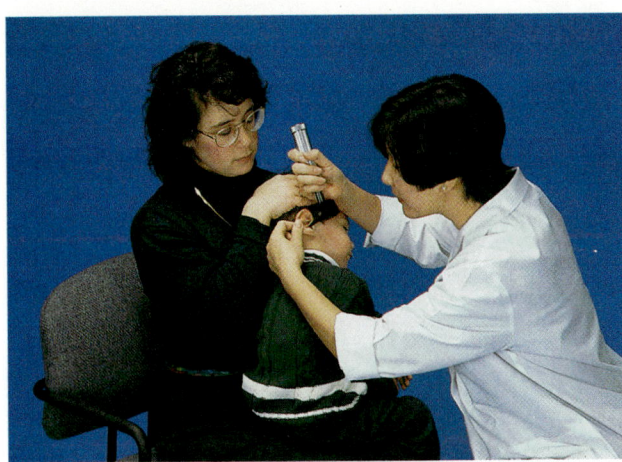

FIGURE 18-7 By participating in this health examination, this mother is helping her son overcome his anxiety. DELMAR/CENGAGE LEARNING

Some specific nursing approaches to use with toddlers are the following:

- Explain what is being done in a calm tone of voice.
- Use play to alleviate anxiety (e.g., have the child examine a teddy bear or doll).
- Give short, simple directions.
- After a painful procedure, comfort the child (cuddling, rocking).
- Encourage parents' active participation in the care.

WELLNESS PROMOTION Teaching is done with both toddlers and their parents. Play can be used to establish an effective relationship with the child. Play is a valuable process for toddlers in that it is the primary mechanism for socialization and learning. To facilitate learning, approach toddlers at eye level and use terminology that they can understand.

Respiratory infections are common health threats to the toddler. Parasitic diseases are also fairly common. Toddlers need to have regular health examinations, and immunizations remain an essential part of health care. Encourage parents to be involved during the examination and immunizations. Teaching parents preventive measures becomes the focus of wellness promotion.

Nutritional needs change during the toddler period as the rate of growth slows. The need for calories decreases from the requirements for infants. The required amount of protein is also lower than that of the infant; however, toddlers still need more protein than do older children. The toddler needs fewer fluids than the infant (Hockenberry et al., 2006). Because most toddlers become selective ("picky") about the foods they enjoy, it is sometimes difficult to provide increased intake of calcium and iron due to the toddler's food habits. The toddler should consume an average of 2 to 3 cups of milk a day to ensure adequate calcium intake. The toddler who drinks more than a quart of milk per day is at increased risk of developing anemia because the high milk consumption limits the amount of other nutrients taken in (Hockenberry et al., 2006).

Nurses can play a key role in the toddler's nutritional counseling. The following points should be shared with parents about dietary practices:

- Avoid using food as a reward because this may encourage overeating.
- Do not serve large helpings because the child may be overwhelmed and refuse to eat.
- Expect sporadic eating patterns (e.g., toddler eats a lot one day and very little the next; enjoys one food for several days and then suddenly will refuse it).
- Avoid power struggles related to meals. Trying to force a child to eat is counterproductive to establishing healthy eating habits.
- Establish a mealtime routine and follow it (rituals are comforting to toddlers).
- Provide nutritional snacks to meet dietary requirements.

SAFETY CONSIDERATIONS Accidents, especially those involving automobiles, are the most frequent cause of disability and death in toddlers (Edelman & Mandle, 2006; Murray et al., 2008). The information on the use of car seats for neonates and infants is applicable to toddlers.

Another common type of accident occurring with toddlers involves toys. Parents need to be taught to inspect toys for age appropriateness, sharp objects, small parts that can be swallowed, and flammable or toxic materials (e.g., lead-based paint). As children gain new skills, parents should be taught to reassess the safety of toys and of the home environment.

Toddlers, with their increased mobility and curiosity, are especially prone to accidental poisonings. Parents should be informed of the need for careful observation of the toddler and childproofing the home.

PRESCHOOLER

The developmental stage from the ages of 3 to 6 is called the **preschool stage**. During this stage, physical growth slows and psychosocial and cognitive development are accelerated. Table 18-18 on page 332 describes preschool development in detail.

During this period of childhood, curiosity becomes pronounced and the child is better able to communicate. When teaching the parents, let them know that the child's frequent use of the word "why" is necessary for normal cognitive and psychosocial development.

The child's world begins to expand outside the immediate home environment. Play is the mechanism used by the preschooler to learn about and develop relationships.

Nursing Implications

Play is a tool that can be used by nurses with preschoolers to help reduce fear and anxiety. Through the use of play, preschoolers learn about the environment, incorporate socially defined expectations for behavior, and reduce tension (see Figure 18-8 on page 333).

WELLNESS PROMOTION When working with a preschooler, it is important for the nurse to communicate at the

TABLE 18-18 Preschooler: Growth and Development

DIMENSION	CHARACTERISTICS	NURSING IMPLICATIONS
Physiological	• Physical growth slows; average weight at age 5 is 45 pounds. • Size of head is approximate adult size.	
	• Has a full set of deciduous teeth; these "baby teeth" start to fall out and be replaced by permanent teeth.	• Can eat larger meals and a variety of foods.
Motor	• Development of fine motor skills (e.g., ability to skip, throw a ball overhand, use scissors, tie shoelaces).	• Provide a safe environment for play and exploration. • Praise attempted independent activities.
Psychosocial	• *Freud:* Phallic stage • Oedipal conflict leads to development of superego (conscience)	
	• *Erikson:* Initiative vs. guilt	• Inform parents that preschoolers learn self-control through interacting with others.
	• *Havighurst:* Developmental tasks include: —Learning sex differences and modesty —Increasing language development and basic ability to formulate concepts —Developing reading readiness —Distinguishing right from wrong	• Inform parents to provide sex education information at the child's comprehension level. • Encourage parents to read to child.
Cognitive	• *Piaget:* Preoperational stage • Improved ability to use reason and logic and increased curiosity result in frequent use of questioning. • Play becomes more reality based. • As a result of increased ability to communicate, there is greater socialization with peers.	• Parents need to know that children of this age learn through frequent use of the word "why."
Moral	• *Kohlberg:* Preconventional stage • A conscience begins to develop. • Child fears wrongdoing. • Child seeks parental approval.	• Teach child basic values, ideally by role modeling. • Provide consistent praise and acceptance of child.
Spiritual	• *Fowler:* Intuitive-projective stage of faith • Not yet able to understand spiritual concepts. • Imitates parental behaviors.	• Remind parents that teaching by example is the best approach for a child this age.

Data from Murray, R. B., Zentner, J. P., & Yakimo, R. (2008). *Nursing assessment and health promotion through the lifespan* (8th ed.). Upper Saddle River, NJ: Pearson; Hockenberry, M. J., Wilson, D., & Jackson, C. (2006). *Wong's nursing care of infants and children* (8th ed.). St. Louis, MO: Elsevier.

child's level of comprehension without talking down to the child. Include the child in activities and decisions as much as possible. The preschool years are the optimum time for the child to begin showing interest in health. The astute nurse capitalizes on this by making health education fun in order to promote the development of lifelong health-promoting lifestyles.

A major wellness intervention for preschoolers is immunization. Teach parents about and encourage them to adhere to the recommended schedules. Each state in the United States has immunization requirements as prerequisites for school admission. The nurse should encourage parents to have children immunized and to keep the immunization records current.

SAFETY CONSIDERATIONS Accidents are the leading cause of death in young children. Eagerness to explore the environment and cognitive immaturity lead to the

increases and vocabulary expands greatly to accommodate the expression of needs, thoughts, and feelings.

As the school-age child's cognitive abilities expand, creativity is expressed in a variety of unique ways. Involvement in academics, sports, and social activities stimulates the development of creativity and provides outlets for its expression.

Nursing Implications

The most common health problems of school-age children are accidents and minor illnesses such as upper respiratory infections. Health promotion teaching is a major role of the nurse caring for school-age children.

WELLNESS PROMOTION Lifestyles begin to be established during childhood; nurses can intervene to promote the development of healthy lifestyles with children in schools. Schools are an area in which health promotion behaviors can be taught in a cost-effective manner. Nurses can promote wellness in the school-age child by teaching parents to:

- Encourage healthy lifestyles (nonsedentary activities, nutritious meals)
- Provide nutritious meals
- Have children immunized
- Teach children appropriate hygienic measures
- Schedule regular checkups with the primary health care provider
- Schedule dental checkups and encourage daily brushing and flossing
- Establish sleep patterns alternating with periods of activity
- Report any symptoms of illness immediately to the health care provider
- Teach safety precautions

SAFETY CONSIDERATIONS Many accidents experienced by school-age children occur during play. Injuries related to the use of skates, skateboards, in-line skates, bicycles, and scooters are common. Children should be taught safety rules for use of such toys (e.g., use of protective equipment; Figure 18-9 on page 335). Parents must frequently remind children of the danger of playing near traffic. Children in this developmental stage must also be taught to use caution with strangers because of the possibility of abductions.

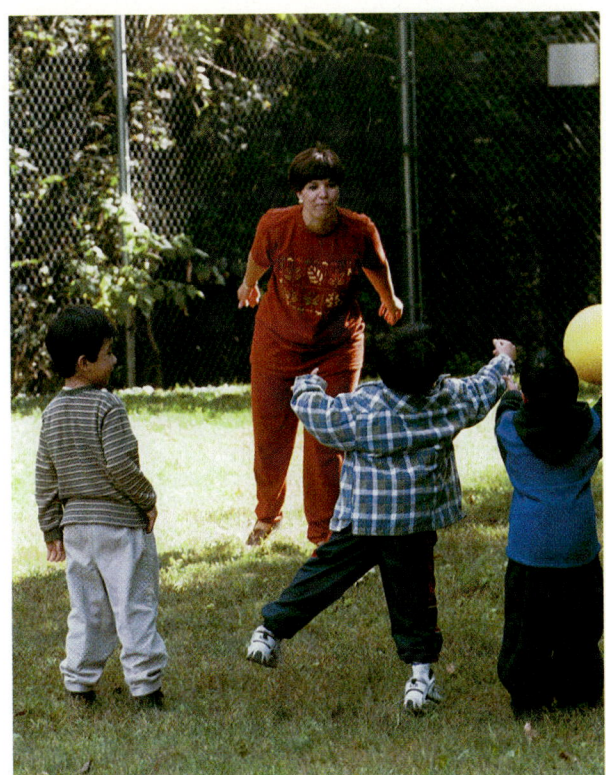

FIGURE 18-8 Play is an important tool for socializing among preschoolers. Describe a few health care activities that nurses can incorporate through play that would correspond to a preschooler's level of development. DELMAR/CENGAGE LEARNING

preschooler's risk for accidents. Children in this stage often act impulsively and cannot be expected to remember and follow all safety rules. Parents must understand the importance of teaching young children the meaning of "no" to prevent accidents. Common accidents that affect preschoolers are automobile accidents, burns, falls, drowning, animal bites, and ingestion of poisonous substances.

It is important for the nurse to emphasize education about protection from potential hazards. The safety practices that are developed by the preschooler will tend to be lifelong. Adults can best teach preschoolers about accident prevention through role modeling. For example, parents who buckle their seat belts every time they get into a car are not only protecting themselves but are also teaching their children an important accident preventive measure.

SCHOOL-AGE CHILD

During the **school-age period** (developmental stage from the ages of 6 to 12 years), physical changes occur at a slow, even, continuous pace. Table 18-19 on page 334 gives an overview of growth and development of the school-age child.

The school-age child's world expands greatly. Participation in school activities, team sports, and play contributes to an enlarging social network. For children in school, play time becomes more structured and less spontaneous. Communication

PREADOLESCENT

Preadolescence, the developmental stage from the ages of 10 to 12 years, is marked by rapid physiological changes with accompanying psychological and social implications. The child is beginning to experience hormonal changes that will result in the onset of **puberty** (appearance of secondary sex characteristics). Girls generally experience preadolescence at a younger age than boys—approximately age 9 to 10 for girls and age 10 to 11 for boys (Edelman &

TABLE 18-19 School-Age Child: Growth and Development

DIMENSION	CHARACTERISTICS	NURSING IMPLICATIONS
Physiological	• Physical growth is steady (approximately 3–6 pounds and 2–3 inches per year). • Due to changes in amount and distribution of fat, body has an overall slimmer shape. • Maturation of CNS is nearly completed.	• Emphasize with parents the need for a balanced diet to sustain growth requirements.
	• By age 12, all permanent teeth are present (except second and third molars).	• Teach parents need for dental hygiene (daily brushing and flossing) and regularly scheduled visits to dentist. • Instruct to change toothbrushes every 3 months.
Motor	• Continued development of motor control.	• Encourage participation in physical activities.
	• Becomes less dependent on parents for activities of daily living.	• Provide praise for independent activities.
Psychosocial	• *Freud:* Latency stage • Same-gender companions preferred. • *Erikson:* Industry vs. inferiority	• To develop a sense of confidence, encourage child to: —Participate in both group and individual activities —Become involved in a variety of activities
	• Develops initiative and high level of self-esteem as shown in school and sports. • Exhibits less dependency on family. • *Havighurst:* Developmental tasks include ability to perform more complex motor functions (e.g., ride a bicycle, catch a ball)	• Encourage parents to praise child's efforts.
Cognitive	• *Piaget:* Concrete operations stage	
	• Ability to cooperate with others and begins to be able to see the other's point of view, which leads to more meaningful communication. • Reasoning ability moves from intuitive toward logical and rational.	• Encourage child to engage in group activities.
	• Ability to think in the abstract is not fully developed. • Develops the concept of time: —Knows difference between past and present —Begins to learn to tell time —Understands the process of aging better • Able to order, categorize, and classify groups of objects as evidenced in increased interest in collections (coins, stamps, rocks). • Sees relationships between objects.	• Communicate at child's level of comprehension.
Moral	• *Kohlberg:* Conventional stage • Can understand what society deems as unacceptable behavior but cannot always choose between right and wrong without assistance.	• Provide consistent limits. • Role-model appropriate behavior. • Provide praise for appropriate behavior.
Spiritual	• *Fowler:* Mythical-literal stage of faith • Accepts existence of a deity. • Beliefs are symbolized through stories.	• Encourage parents to discuss their beliefs. • Storytelling and use of parables can reinforce understanding of spiritual concepts.

Data from Edelman, C. L., & Mandle, C. L. (2006). *Health promotion throughout the lifespan* (6th ed.). St. Louis, MO: Mosby; Murray, R. B., Zentner, J. P., & Yakimo, R. (2008). *Nursing assessment and health promotion through the lifespan* (8th ed.). Upper Saddle River, NJ: Pearson.

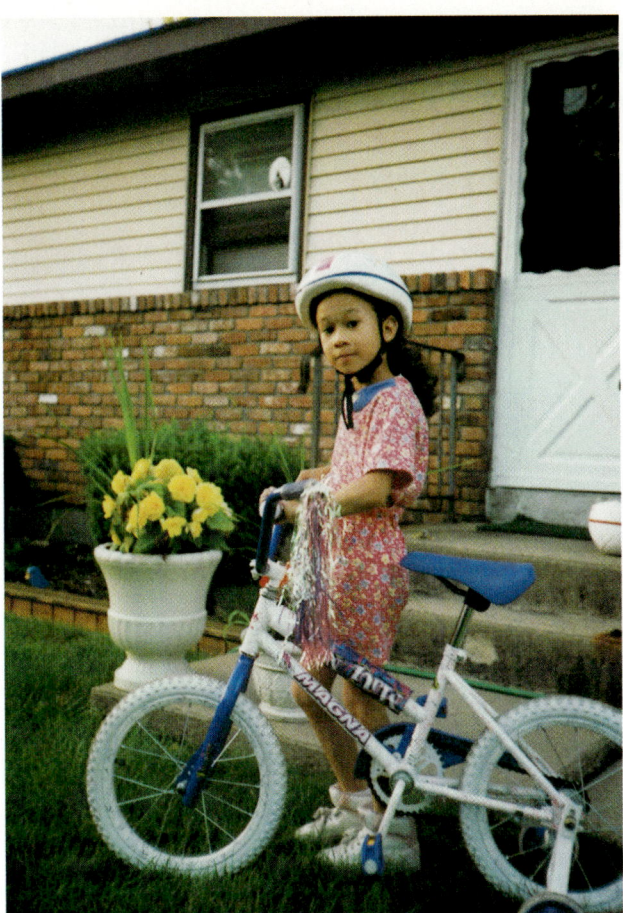

FIGURE 18-9 The use of equipment, such as safety helmets, helps to protect school-age children from injury. DELMAR/CENGAGE LEARNING

Mandle, 2006). Table 18-20 on page 336 provides an overview of preadolescent development.

In girls, breast development begins between the ages of 10 and 11. Further breast development is stimulated by the release of estrogen that occurs during puberty. Premature adrenarche refers to early onset of secretion of adrenal androgens, which results in the isolated development of pubic hair before the age of 8 years in girls and 9 years in boys. Premature adrenarche may result in the development of polycystic ovary syndrome and/or syndrome X (Leung & Robson, 2008). Nurses must inform parents of the need for observation and reporting of indicators of adrenarche. The pattern of female breast development is described in Table 18-21 on page 338. Other aspects of female sexual development are described in Table 18-22 on page 339.

Approximately 2 years after the appearance of breast buds, **menarche** (onset of the first menstrual period) occurs. The first menstrual periods are usually irregular and scant, and they may or may not be accompanied by ovulation. The average age of menarche in the United States is 12.8 years, which has gradually declined over the past century. This is probably due to improved general health status, particularly nutrition and sanitation (Hockenberry et al., 2008).

The menstrual cycle is a complex blend of physiological and psychological changes that occur approximately every month. After approximately the first 6 to 12 months, a girl's cycle will become established in a regular pattern. Some girls may have received inadequate or incorrect information regarding the onset of menstruation. Client teaching should include information about the physiological changes, emotional changes, and hygienic practices. Teaching should emphasize that the cyclical hormone-induced changes are normal.

In preadolescent boys, the first signs of puberty are:

- Testicular enlargement
- Penile enlargement
- The scrotum becomes thinner and redder
- Pubic hair growth

Table 18-23 on page 340 illustrates the physiological changes in boys during sexual development of male genitalia.

Nursing Implications

Sensitivity is essential for the nurse working with the preadolescent. To increase one's sensitivity, the nurse uses a nonjudgmental approach and attends to the child's body language. It is imperative that the nurse establish a trusting relationship with the preadolescent in order to encourage the child to ask questions about any health-related concerns.

WELLNESS PROMOTION   The preadolescent needs information about nutrition, rest and activity, and physiological changes that are occurring. The child must learn about the growth spurt, sexual changes, and psychosocial changes. By preparing the preadolescent for upcoming changes, the nurse is promoting physical and emotional health.

SAFETY CONSIDERATIONS   The preadolescent is at risk for injury from sports and play activities. Another major health risk posed to many preadolescents is violence, both in and away from the home. Education is a major preventive approach to violence; it is the tool for helping break the intergenerational cycle of child abuse.

Other topics for promoting preadolescent safety are substance abuse prevention, sex education, and development of healthy lifestyles.

ADOLESCENT

Adolescence, the developmental stage from the ages of 13 to 20 years, begins with the onset of puberty. During adolescence, the individual undergoes the major transition from child to adult. Numerous physiological changes and rapid physical growth occur during this stage. The rapid changes that occur during adolescence are not only physical. Many psychosocial adjustments must be made by the adolescent. Establishing a sense of personal identity uses a great amount of the adolescent's psychic energy. Questions such as "Who am I?" and "What is *really* important?" are common for adolescents to consider. See Table 18-20 for an overview of adolescent development.

TABLE 18-20 Preadolescent and Adolescent: Growth and Development

DIMENSION	CHARACTERISTICS	NURSING IMPLICATIONS
Physiological *Physiological changes*	• Accelerated physical growth with changes in body proportion. Extremities grow first, then trunk and hips.	• Teach the child and parents about expected growth spurts.
	• Growth in skull and facial bones results in changes in physical appearance.	• Provide reassurance that it is not uncommon for facial appearance to change in only a few months.
Reproductive and sexual changes	• Hypothalamus stimulates secretion of pituitary gonadotropins, leading to reproductive maturity. • Development of both primary and secondary sex characteristics. • Beginning of puberty is evidenced in girls by: —Breast development —Pubic and axillary hair growth —Menarche (onset of menses) —Increases in height • Beginning of puberty is evidenced in boys by: —Genital development —Growth of facial, pubic, and axillary hair —Nocturnal ejaculations —Height increases —Voice changes	• Provide support and information about emerging sexual changes. • Remember that the physiological changes are accompanied by psychological and social alterations.
Musculoskeletal changes	• Ossification of bones. • Increased muscle mass and strength.	• Encourage physical activities and intake of adequate amounts of calcium.
Cardiovascular changes	• Heart increases in size and strength. • Heart rate decreases to adult norms. • Increased blood volume and blood pressure.	
Respiratory changes	• Rate decreases to an average of 15–20 respirations per minute. • Increased respiratory volume and vital capacity.	
	• Growth of larynx, laryngeal cartilage, and vocal cords and deepening of voice pitch.	• Instruct about anticipated changes.
Gastrointestinal and genitourinary changes	• Spleen, liver, kidneys, and digestive tract enlarge but experience no functional changes.	
Dental changes	• Eruption of last four molars.	• Emphasize importance of continued dental hygiene.
Integumentary changes	• Skin becomes thicker and tougher. • Activation of sebaceous glands leads to possibility of acne. • Appearance of pubic hair.	• Teach proper skin care: —Wash two to three times daily with soap and water. —Avoid vigorous scrubbing. —Females should avoid cosmetics with a fat or grease base.

(Continues)

TABLE 18-20 (Continued)

DIMENSION	CHARACTERISTICS	NURSING IMPLICATIONS
		—Use sunscreen and avoid prolonged exposure to sunlight. —Provide support to children experiencing acne.
Motor	• Able to be completely independent with self-care activities.	
Psychosocial	• *Freud:* Genital stage • *Erikson:* Identity vs. role diffusion • Major task: Develop a sense of identity. • Develops a new body image. • Establishes intimacy with members of opposite gender. • Peer group is the primary mechanism of support. • Rebels against adult authority. • *Havighurst:* Achieves personal independence and establishes more mature relationships with others.	• Offer support. • Continue to provide sex education. • Inform parents that rebellion is a normal developmental experience. • Encourage attempts to achieve independence while providing assistance and support as needed.
Cognitive	• *Piaget:* Formal operations stage • Logical, organized, consistent approach to thinking. • Thinks in terms of cause and effect. • **Note:** Not all adolescents achieve this level of cognitive development. Some are capable of flights from reality. • Tends to be extremely idealistic. • Egocentric (self-centered) thinking is common with views of themselves as omnipotent. • Sees self as exceptional, special, and unique, and possesses a belief that one is immune to problems.	• Teach parents expected developmental changes in thinking patterns. • A false sense of immunity (''It can't happen to me'' attitude) has an impact on health behaviors. • Teach safety issues to children: —Safe sex practices —Avoid driving and use of alcohol or other drugs
Moral	• *Kohlberg:* Postconventional stage • Tends to support the morality of law and order to determine right from wrong. • Begins to question status quo and discards and chooses different values. • Moral maturity varies in context of the situation and the relationship. • Peer pressure may override the adolescent's own moral reasoning.	• Teach parents that questioning of values is normal. • Teach child assertiveness skills to use in communicating with peers.
Spiritual	• *Fowler:* Synthetic-conventional stage of faith • Questions values and beliefs.	• Inform parents that curiosity about other religious beliefs is normal.

Data from Edelman, C. L., & Mandle, C. L. (2006). *Health promotion throughout the lifespan* (6th ed.). St. Louis, MO: Mosby; Varcarolis, E., & Halter, J. (2008). *Essentials of psychiatric mental health nursing: A communication approach to evidence-based practice.* St. Louis, MO: Elsevier.

TABLE 18-21 Sexual Maturity Rating for Female Breast Development

DEVELOPMENTAL STAGE

1. Preadolescent state (before age 10)
- Nipple is small, slightly raised.

2. Breast bud stage (after age 10)
- Nipple and breast form a small mound.
- Areola enlarges.
- Height spurt begins.

3. Adolescent stage (10–14 years)
- Nipple is flush with breast shape.
- Breast and areola enlarge.
- Menses begin.
- Height spurt peaks.

4. Late adolescent stage (15–19 years)
- Nipple and areola form a secondary mound over the breast.
- Height spurt ends.

5. Adult stage.
- Nipple protrudes.
- Areola is flush with the breast shape.

Data from Estes, M. E. Z. (2010). *Health assessment and physical examination* (4th ed.). Clifton Park, NY: Delmar/Cengage Learning.

Most adolescents are greatly concerned about their appearance. This emphasis on physical attractiveness sometimes results in eating disorders, such as **anorexia nervosa**, a self-imposed starvation that results in a 15% loss of body weight. Approximately 1% to 2% of female adolescents are affected by anorexia; the rate in males is much lower—about 5% to 10% of the anorectic population is male (Kneisl & Trigoboff, 2009). Other types of eating disorders common in adolescents are **bulimia** (episodic binge eating followed by purging) and **obesity** (weight that is 20% or more above the

TABLE 18-22 Sexual Maturity Rating for Female Genitalia

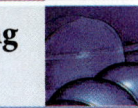

DEVELOPMENTAL STAGE

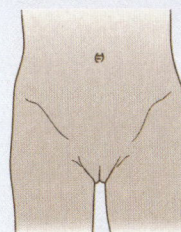

Stage 1 (before age 11)
No pubic hair, only body hair (vellus hair).

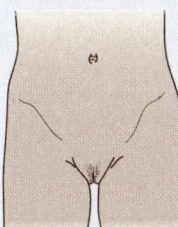

Stage 2 (11–12 years)
Sparse growth of long, slightly dark, fine pubic hair, slightly curly and located along the labia.

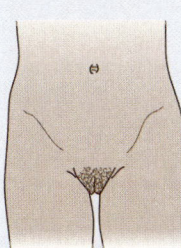

Stage 3 (12–13 years)
Pubic hair becomes darker, curlier, and spreads over the symphysis.

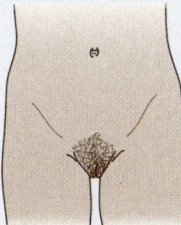

Stage 4 (13–15 years)
Texture and curl of pubic hair are similar to those of an adult but not spread to thighs.

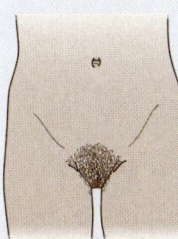

Stage 5 (adult stage)
Adult appearance in quality and quantity of pubic hair. Growth is spread to inner aspect of thighs and abdomen.

Data from Estes, M. E. Z. (2010). *Health assessment and physical examination* (4th ed.). Clifton Park, NY: Delmar/Cengage Learning.

Nursing Implications

Nurses support adolescents by providing information about the numerous bodily changes. Adolescents should be encouraged to share their health concerns with parents. However, the nurse must honor the adolescent's choice to withhold sensitive information from parents. The use of a nonjudgmental attitude is essential to the establishment of rapport when working with adolescents. Adolescents should be treated in a respectful, dignified manner. Avoid using a condescending attitude when communicating with them. The accompanying Nursing Checklist discusses therapeutic approaches that can be used when working with adolescent clients.

WELLNESS PROMOTION The nurse promotes the adolescent's wellness primarily through teaching. Areas to be emphasized in health education of adolescents include hygiene, nutrition, sex education, developmental changes, and substance abuse prevention.

Adolescents need education about the physical changes they are undergoing. Health teaching is often done by school nurses, and the establishment of nurse-managed clinics in schools is one avenue for promoting wellness among adolescents.

SAFETY CONSIDERATIONS Unhealthy behaviors contribute to the three major causes of adolescent death: accidents, homicide, and suicide. The following developmental factors increase the adolescent's risk for accidents:

- Impulsive behavior
- Sense of being invulnerable to accidents (a feeling that "It can never happen to me!")
- Testing limits
- Rebelling against adult advice

As a result, many adolescents engage in unhealthy behaviors such as smoking, consuming alcohol and other drugs, reckless driving, violence, and unprotected sexual activity. See the accompanying Respecting Our Differences display on page 341.

Many health problems in adolescents are related to sexual behaviors, including acquired immunodeficiency syndrome (AIDS), sexually transmitted diseases (STDs), and unplanned pregnancy. The effect of teen pregnancy on families and communities is great. Many pregnant teens become trapped in a cycle of school failure (or dropout), limited employment opportunities, and poverty. Adolescents who

✓ CLIENT TEACHING CHECKLIST

Preventing Eating Disorders

- Promote an increased sense of self-esteem.
- Emphasize the importance of a healthy lifestyle rather than physical appearance.
- Avoid pressuring children to seek perfection or to strive for unrealistic goals.
- Recognize the indicators of eating disorders.

ideal body weight). See the accompanying Client Teaching Checklist for essential information about eating disorders to share with clients and families.

TABLE 18-23 Sexual Maturity Rating for Male Genitalia

	PUBIC HAIR	PENIS	SCROTUM
	Developmental Stage 1 No pubic hair, only fine body hair (vellus hair).	Preadolescent; childhood size and proportion	Preadolescent; childhood size and proportion
	Developmental Stage 2 Sparse growth of long, slightly dark, straight hair.	Slight or no growth	Growth in testes and scrotum; scrotum reddens and changes texture
	Developmental Stage 3 Becomes darker, coarser, and slightly curled and spreads over symphysis.	Growth, especially in length	Further growth
	Developmental Stage 4 Texture and curl of pubic hair are similar to an adult's but hair does not spread to thighs.	Further growth in length; diameter increases; development of glans	Further growth; scrotum darkens
	Developmental Stage 5 Adult appearance in quality and quantity of pubic hair; growth is spread to medial surface of thighs.	Adult size and shape	Adult size and shape

Data from Estes, M. E. Z. (2010). *Health assessment and physical examination* (4th ed.). Clifton Park, NY: Delmar/Cengage Learning.

become pregnant experience developmental difficulties in that they must make adult decisions. Infants born to adolescent mothers are likely to experience health-related problems such as prematurity and low birth weight. The pregnant adolescent needs expert prenatal care, a supportive environment, and information. Client teaching must emphasize the prevention of STDs because the pregnancy itself is evidence of high-risk (unprotected) sexual activity.

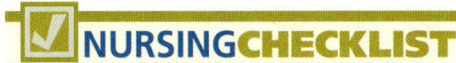

NURSING**CHECKLIST**

Therapeutic Approaches with the Adolescent Client

- Treat the adolescent as an active participant in health care to form a collaborative partnership.
- Answer all questions honestly.
- Be especially sensitive to nonverbal clues. Adolescents are often too embarrassed to initiate discussion of their health-related concerns.
- Remember that the peer group is of major importance to adolescents, and use group settings whenever possible to provide health education.
- Demonstrate acceptance of the adolescent, especially if limits need to be established to intervene with unhealthy or inappropriate behaviors.
- Questioning adult authority is a normal part of adolescent rebelliousness. Do not personalize testing behaviors. Nurses who personalize client behavior become defensive and lose their interpersonal effectiveness with adolescents.

STDs present a serious health threat for adolescents. Diseases such as genital herpes virus, human papillomavirus (which causes genital warts), chlamydia, syphilis, and gonorrhea are spread through sexual contact. The human immunodeficiency virus (HIV), which causes AIDS, is also transmitted through unprotected sexual activity. Table 18-24 on page 342 describes the most common STDs. Nurses must educate adolescents about methods for preventing the spread of STDs. Preventive education should include the following topics:

- Methods of transmission
- Incubation period
- Clinical manifestations
- Treatment methods
- Consequences of lack of or inadequate treatment
- Notification of sexual partner(s)

Nurses who teach adolescent clients about safe sex practices need to be especially sensitive to cultural influences on sexual activity. See the accompanying Spotlight On display.

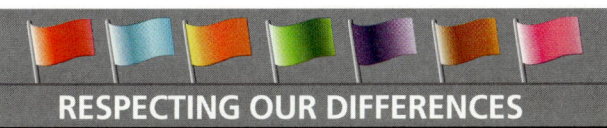

RESPECTING OUR DIFFERENCES

Adolescent Behaviors

Think of the type of behaviors adolescents often demonstrate to prove that they are "grown up." Which of these behaviors have a negative impact on health? Which have a positive impact?

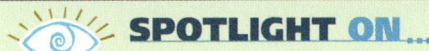

SPOTLIGHT ON...

Values

Values Clarification

As a nurse, you will often encounter clients whose value systems conflict with your own beliefs. How will you provide care to sexually active adolescents if you think their behavior is immoral or "wrong"? Is it ethical for you to try to change the adolescent's values to be congruent with yours? Should you change your values to be congruent with those of the client?

Laws concerning the dissemination of information about STDs vary among states and provinces. However, most have legislation that requires nurses to report the names of clients with certain STDs to the state or provincial health department. The nurse must know the requirements for his or her state or province.

Another major health problem during adolescence is the high risk of suicide. Often, suicide is perceived by the adolescent as the only alternative to an overwhelming situation. Low self-esteem, lack of maturity, and impulsive behaviors may increase the risk of suicidal behavior. The rate of suicide is higher among adolescent males than females.

When assessing for suicidal potential, the nurse should always directly question the adolescent about any plans for harming or killing him- or herself. Signs indicative of suicide risk in adolescents include:

- Writing suicide notes
- Talking about suicide
- Substance abuse
- Preoccupation with death
- Giving away treasured objects
- Sudden changes in behavior
- Verbal cues (e.g., "You won't have to worry about me much longer")

When teaching suicide prevention, inform people to *immediately* contact a health care professional if someone is exhibiting any of the indicators of suicide risk. Many communities have a special telephone suicide-cope-line available. See the accompanying Safety First display.

▼ SAFETY FIRST ▼

SUICIDE PREVENTION
Never leave the suicidal adolescent alone. Close observation is a strong deterrent to suicide.

TABLE 18-24 Sexually Transmitted Diseases: An Overview

DISEASE	CHARACTERISTICS	NURSING IMPLICATIONS
Acquired immunodeficiency syndrome (AIDS)	• Incurable and often fatal disease • In addition to sexual activity, other modes of transmission are: —Direct exposure to infected blood or blood products —Intrauterine transmission from infected woman to fetus	• Know that the incubation period can range up to 15 years from time of initial exposure. • The only "cure" is prevention. • Teach safe sex methods (use of latex condoms). • Provide information about the disease. • Treatment is primarily supportive. • Provide physical care and psychological support. • Always follow standard precautions guidelines.
Chancroid	• A small, irregular-shaped papule (on the penis, labia, or vaginal opening) that develops into a painful ulcer that drains pus or blood • Dysuria (painful urination) • Painful regional lymph nodes (inguinal tenderness)	• Partner(s) having sex within 10 days before onset of client's symptoms need to be assessed. • Client should be reassessed within 7 days after treatment begins. • Instruct in proper use of condoms. • Medication education.
Chlamydia	*Males:* • Painful urination • Urethral discharge *Females:* • Usually none • May experience purulent discharge • **Note:** If untreated, pelvic inflammatory disease (PID) can develop.	• Instruct client to notify sexual partner(s) of past 2 months of their need for treatment. • Instruct clients to avoid sexual activity or to use condoms until both client and partner(s) are symptom free. • Medication education.
Genital herpes: herpes simplex virus 2 (HSV-2)	• Vesicles on penis, vagina, labia, perineum, or anus • Can progress to painful ulceration • Lesions may last up to 6 weeks • Recurrence is common • **Note:** May be asymptomatic	• Refer sexual partner(s) for examination. • Teach that virus can be transmitted even when the person is asymptomatic. • Instruct in use of condoms. • Teach females of need for annual Pap smear. • Medication education.
Gonorrhea	*Males:* • Urethritis (inflammation of the urethra) • Purulent discharge • Urinary frequency • Epididymitis (inflammation of the epididymis) *Females:* • Is often asymptomatic • May lead to PID or salpingitis (inflammation of the fallopian tube) • Can occlude the fallopian tubes, with resultant sterility	• Instruct client to return for further treatment if symptoms persist. • Sexual partner(s) within past 60 days need to be assessed. • Instruct to avoid sexual activity until symptoms subside in both client and partner(s). • Medication education.

(Continues)

TABLE 18-24 (Continued)

DISEASE	CHARACTERISTICS	NURSING IMPLICATIONS
Hepatitis B virus (HBV)	• Varies greatly from asymptomatic state to severe hepatitis to cancer	• Partner(s) should receive medical prophy-laxis within 14 days after exposure. • For client and partner(s): Recommend three-dose immunization series when this episode has abated.
Human papillomavirus (genital warts)	• Fleshy, cauliflower-like growth on genitalia	• Inform and treat sexual partner(s). • Medication education.
Syphilis	• Disease consists of four stages with distinct manifestations:	
	Primary: • A painless papule on penis, vagina, or cervix • Serologic blood test usually negative • Highly infectious during this stage	• Interview client to identify sexual contacts. • Protect confidentiality of all involved. • All those exposed to the disease should be given penicillin.
	Secondary: • Rash, especially prevalent on palms and soles • Low-grade fever • Sore throat • Headache	• Educate client and sexual contacts about the disease. • Medication education.
	Early Latency: • Infectious lesions may occur, otherwise asymptomatic. • Reactive serologic tests	• Counsel and educate client.
	Late Latency: • Lesions may be present in central nervous and cardiovascular systems. • Noninfectious except to fetus of pregnant woman	• Counsel and educate client.
Trichomoniasis	• Petechial lesions • Profuse urethral or vaginal discharge that is foul smelling, yellow, and foamy	• Treat sexual partners simultaneously with metronidazole (Flagyl). • Medication education.

Data from Hale, P. J. (2006). HIV, hepatitis, and sexually transmitted diseases. In M. Stanhope & J. Lancaster (Eds.), *Foundations of community health nursing* (2nd ed.). St. Louis, MO: Mosby; Ignatavicius, D. D., & Workman, M. L. (2009). *Medical-surgical nursing: Critical thinking for collaborative care* (6th ed.). St. Louis, MO: Elsevier.

Another significant health problem for many adolescents is substance abuse. Using alcohol or other drugs is a common maladaptive attempt to cope with the stressors of adolescence. Some indicators of substance abuse in adolescents are:

- Decline in academic performance
- Mood swings
- Changes in personality (e.g., confusion, euphoria, belliger-ence, withdrawal)
- Fatigue
- Drowsiness
- Behaviors indicative of depression (e.g., appetite changes, insomnia, weight loss, apathy)

Nurses can play a key role in substance abuse prevention with adolescents. A comprehensive substance abuse preven-tion educational program includes:

- Hazards of drug use
- Misuse of legal substances, such as tobacco and alcohol
- Self-esteem-boosting methods

- Assertive communication skills (how to say "no" to peers)
- Adaptive coping mechanisms for dealing with stress

By providing such information, nurses can help adolescents make responsible, informed decisions before experimentation with drugs begins.

YOUNG ADULT

Physical growth stabilizes during **young adulthood**, the developmental stage from the age of 21 to approximately 40 years. Young adults experience physical and emotional changes at a slower rate than adolescents. Table 18-25 on page 345 describes the development of young adults. Young adulthood is a time of transition from an adolescent to a person capable of assuming adult responsibilities and making adult decisions.

Pregnancy, a time of transition and lifestyle adjustment, is experienced by many young women. Table 18-26 on page 346 lists a few of the changes commonly experienced during pregnancy. Throughout pregnancy, women experience changes in self-concept and may need reassurance that such changes are normal.

Nursing Implications

Usually, young adulthood is the healthiest time in a person's life. Consequently, concern for health is low among people in this age group, and wellness is often taken for granted. Preventive measures for young adults focus on three primary areas:

1. Avoidance of accident, injury, and violence
2. Development of health-promoting behaviors (e.g., lifestyle modification)
3. Maintenance of current recommended immunizations (see Figure 18-10 on page 346)

The nurse plays an important role in each of these areas of health promotion by teaching and counseling. Other topics that are developmentally appropriate for the nurse to address are vocational counseling and establishing relationships.

WELLNESS PROMOTION Decision making by young adults affects their health status. Since young adults tend to take excessive risks, they are at greater risk for death from accident, suicide, or homicide (Edelman & Mandle, 2006). For example, driving recklessly, driving while intoxicated, engaging in unprotected sex, and participating in gang activities illustrate the lack of a sense of fear that is demonstrated by many young adults.

STD is a leading cause of infection with resultant reproductive dysfunction in young adults. The information presented about STDs in the discussion of safety considerations for adolescents is also applicable to young adults. Nurses should teach women how to perform a monthly breast self-examination (BSE). Men need to learn how to perform a testicular self-examination (TSE); see Chapter 27.

SAFETY CONSIDERATIONS Because vehicular accidents are a major cause of health problems for young adults, providing information about driving safety is a must. Another activity that poses a health risk for many young adults is sunbathing. Exposure to direct sunlight with the resultant radiation or use of tanning salons is directly linked to skin cancer. Nurses can be influential in decreasing the occurrence of skin cancer through teaching and by role modeling safe behaviors.

MIDDLE-AGED ADULT

Middle adulthood, the developmental stage from the ages of 40 to 65 years, is characterized by productivity and responsibility. For most middle-aged adults, the majority of activity revolves around work and parenting, and success and achievement are measured in terms of career accomplishments and family life.

Physiological changes that affect many of the body systems occur during middle adulthood. Table 18-27 on page 348 lists the major changes experienced by the middle-aged person.

The primary developmental task of the middle-aged adult revolves around the conflict of generativity (a sense that one is making a contribution to society) versus stagnation (a sense of nonmeaning in one's life). When an individual successfully resolves this developmental conflict, acceptance of age-related changes occurs. Achievement of the developmental task is indicated by the following:

- Demonstrating creativity
- Guiding the next generation
- Establishing lasting relationships
- Evaluating goals in terms of achievement

The evaluation of goals often leads to a midlife crisis, especially if individuals feel they have accomplished little or failed to live up to earlier self-expectations.

Nursing Implications

A large proportion of the U.S. population consists of middle-aged adults (Edelman & Mandle, 2006). Individuals of the baby-boom generation have entered their midlife stage and will require more nursing care to maintain wellness and cope with illness.

Nurses have the opportunity to help middle-aged clients improve their health status (and thus quality of life) by identification of risk factors and early intervention. The major risk factors for adults in the middle years can be modified because they are primarily environmental and behavioral. Assisting the middle-aged client to change unhealthy behaviors can be done through one-to-one intervention or in group settings.

WELLNESS PROMOTION As health educators, nurses can encourage middle-aged adults to assume more responsibility for their own health (see Figure 18-11 on page 347). Self-care education topics appropriate for the middle-aged adult include:

- Acceptance of aging
- Nutrition

TABLE 18-25 Young Adult: Growth and Development

DIMENSION	CHARACTERISTICS	NURSING IMPLICATIONS
Physiological *Physiological changes*	• Physical growth stabilizes. • Time of optimum physical functioning. • Maturation of body systems complete.	• The person is at physical peak and therefore less likely to be concerned with own health. • Teach importance of health promotion behaviors. • Encourage development of healthy lifestyles.
Cardiovascular changes	• Men are more likely to have increased cholesterol levels than women.	
Gastrointestinal changes	• After age 30, decreased digestive juices.	
Dental changes	• By mid-20s, dental maturity is achieved with emergence of last four molars ("wisdom teeth").	
Musculoskeletal changes	• At approximately age 25, skeletal growth is complete.	
Reproductive and sexual changes	• System is completely matured. • *Women:* Ages 20–30 are optimal years for reproduction. • *Men:* Beginning at about age 24, male hormones slowly decrease; does not affect ability to reproduce.	
Psychosocial	• *Erikson:* Intimacy vs. isolation —Engages in productive work. —Develops intimate relationships. • *Havighurst:* —Becomes part of a social group. —Selects a partner. —Assumes civic responsibility.	• Emphasize need for social support as the person assumes new roles. • Teach time management skills. • Provide sex education information, including prevention of STDs.
Cognitive	• *Piaget:* Formal operations stage —Problem-solving abilities are realistic. • Demonstrates less egocentricism. • Many young adults are engaged in formal educational activities.	• Encourage the development and use of appropriate judgment.
Moral	• *Kohlberg:* Postconventional stage —Defines right and wrong in terms of personal beliefs and principles. • *Gilligan:* Women consider morality to be based on caring for others and avoiding harm.	• Assess the person's value system and respect beliefs.
Spiritual	• *Fowler:* Individuative-reflective faith • Assumes responsibility for own beliefs.	• Encourage client to use spiritual support system.

Data from Edelman, C. L., & Mandle, C. L. (2006). *Health promotion throughout the lifespan* (6th ed.). St. Louis, MO: Mosby; Ignatavicius, D. D. & Workman, M. L. (2009). *Medical-surgical nursing: Critical thinking for collaborative care* (6th ed.). St. Louis, MO: Elsevier.

TABLE 18-26 Changes Experienced during Pregnancy

	PHYSIOLOGICAL	PSYCHOLOGICAL
First trimester	• Fatigue • Nausea and vomiting • Urinary frequency • Constipation • Breast tenderness and enlargement	• Emotional detachment as thoughts begin to focus on developing child • Labile (rapidly changing) mood • Ambivalence about the pregnancy • Increased dependency on others
Second trimester	• Perception of fetal movement • Fetal heart tones can be detected with fetoscope • Increased libido	• Doubts and fears about ability to care for an infant • Bond with mate either strengthened or threatened • Excited by fetal movement • Initial attachment with fetus strengthened
Third trimester	• Backache • Stretch marks on abdomen or breasts • Urinary frequency • Heartburn • Shortness of breath • Varicose veins on legs	• Feeling less attractive • Increased irritability • Insomnia • Anticipation of birth • Plans for incorporating child into family unit

Data from Edelman, C. L., & Mandle, C. L. (2006). *Health promotion throughout the lifespan* (6th ed.). St. Louis, MO: Mosby; Ignatavicius, D. D., & Workman, M. L. (2009). *Medical-surgical nursing: Critical thinking for collaborative care* (6th ed.). St. Louis, MO: Elsevier.

Recommended Adult Immunization Schedule
UNITED STATES · 2009
Note: These recommendations *must* be read with the footnotes that follow containing number of doses, intervals between doses, and other important information.

VACCINE ▼ AGE GROUP▶	19–26 years	27–49 years	50–59 years	60–64 years	≥65 years
Tetanus, diphtheria, pertussis (Td/Tdap)[1,*]	Substitute 1-time dose of Tdap for Td booster; then boost with Td every 10 yrs				Td booster every 10 yrs
Human papillomavirus (HPV)[2,*]	3 doses (females)				
Varicella[3,*]	2 doses				
Zoster[4]				1 dose	
Measles, mumps, rubella (MMR)[5,*]	1 or 2 doses		1 dose		
Influenza[6,*]	1 dose annually				
Pneumococcal (polysaccharide)[7,8]	1 or 2 doses				1 dose
Hepatitis A[9,*]	2 doses				
Hepatitis B[10,*]	3 doses				
Meningococcal[11,*]	1 or more doses				

*Covered by the Vaccine Injury Compensation Program.

☐ (yellow) For all persons in this category who meet the age requirements and who lack evidence of immunity (e.g., lack documentation of vaccination or have no evidence of prior infection)

☐ (purple) Recommended if some other risk factor is present (e.g., on the basis of medical, occupational, lifestyle, or other indications)

☐ (white) No recommendation

FIGURE 18-10(A) Recommended Adult Immunization Schedule, by vaccine and age group. COURTESY OF THE U.S. CENTERS FOR DISEASE CONTROL AND PREVENTION BY VACCINE AND AGE GROUP

Vaccines that might be indicated for adults based on medical and other indications

VACCINE ▼	INDICATION ► Pregnancy	Immuno-compromising conditions (excluding human immunodeficiency virus [HIV])[13]	HIV infection[3,12,13] CD4+ T lymphocyte count <200 cells/µL	HIV infection[3,12,13] CD4+ T lymphocyte count ≥200 cells/µL	Diabetes, heart disease, chronic lung disease, chronic alcoholism	Asplenia[12] (including elective splenectomy and terminal complement component deficiencies)	Chronic liver disease	Kidney failure, end-stage renal disease, receipt of hemodialysis	Health-care personnel
Tetanus, diphtheria, pertussis (Td/Tdap)[1,*]	Td	Substitute 1-time dose of Tdap for Td booster; then boost with Td every 10 yrs							
Human papillomavirus (HPV)[2,*]		3 doses for females through age 26 yrs							
Varicella[3,*]	Contraindicated		2 doses						
Zoster[4]	Contraindicated		1 dose						
Measles, mumps, rubella (MMR)[5,*]	Contraindicated		1 or 2 doses						
Influenza[6,*]	1 dose TIV annually								1 dose TIV or LAIV annually
Pneumococcal (polysaccharide)[7,8]	1 or 2 doses								
Hepatitis A[9,*]	2 doses								
Hepatitis B[10,*]	3 doses								
Meningococcal[11,*]	1 or more doses								

*Covered by the Vaccine Injury Compensation Program.

For all persons in this category who meet the age requirements and who lack evidence of immunity (e.g., lack documentation of vaccination or have no evidence of prior infection)

Recommended if some other risk factor is present (e.g., on the basis of medical, occupational, lifestyle, or other indications)

No recommendation

FIGURE 18-10(B) Vaccines that might be indicated for adults based on medical and other indications COURTESY OF THE U.S. CENTERS FOR DISEASE CONTROL AND PREVENTION

- Exercise and weight control
- Substance abuse prevention
- Stress management
- Recommendations for health screening (cholesterol screening, prostate examination, mammogram, Papanicolaou [Pap] test).

SAFETY CONSIDERATIONS Automobile accidents, especially those involving the use of alcohol, are a serious health problem for middle-aged adults. Another significant problem is occupational health hazards, such as exposure to environmental toxins. Middle adulthood is also the time when a lifelong accumulation of unhealthy lifestyle practices, such as smoking, sedentary habits, inadequate nutrition, and overuse of alcohol, begins to exert adverse effects.

Most middle-aged individuals have increased leisure time. Consequently, there is an increased risk for recreational accidents (e.g., boating accidents, sports-related injuries, jogging mishaps).

OLDER ADULT

Older adulthood is the developmental stage occurring from age 65 and beyond. Chapter 19 provides an in-depth discussion of the elderly adult. Therefore, this section only highlights the concepts of growth and development as they relate

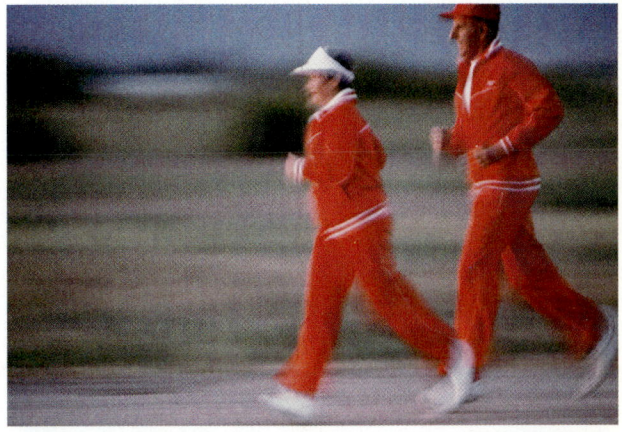

FIGURE 18-11 Through activities such as running, these middle-aged adults have taken responsibility for their health and are learning to cope with the physiological changes that occur during this stage. DELMAR/CENGAGE LEARNING

to the older adult. Table 18-28 on page 351 provides an overview of growth and development in the older adult.

Older adults have several psychosocial tasks to accomplish, such as:

- Developing a sense of satisfaction with the life that one has lived (to find meaning in one's life)

TABLE 18-27   Middle Adult: Growth and Development

DIMENSION	CHARACTERISTICS	NURSING IMPLICATIONS

Physiological *Cardiovascular changes*	• Decreased functional aerobic capacity results in decreased cardiac output.
	• Blood vessels become thicker and lose elasticity.
		• Decreased capacity for physical activity. Instruct client about necessity of remaining physically active.
		• Predisposition for hypertension (high blood pressure), coronary artery disease, and cerebral vascular accidents (''strokes'').
		• Teach client about lifestyle modifications related to cardiovascular health:
		  —Smoking cessation
		  —Avoiding secondary tobacco smoke
		  —Nutrition (low fat, low cholesterol)
		  —Engaging in physical activity

Neurological changes	• Cellular changes (regulation, repair, and atrophy) occur gradually.
	• A gradual loss in efficiency of nerve conduction to impaired sensation of heat and cold.
		• Explain age-related changes.
		• Provide support and reassurance.
		• Teach safety precautions regarding:
		  —Exposure to sunlight
		  —Sensitivity to heat stroke
		  —Sensitivity to frostbite

Gastrointestinal changes	• Slower gastrointestinal motility results in constipation.	• Teach client about:
		  —Nutrition (high-fiber foods; adequate amounts of fluid)
		  —Maintaining physical activity

Genitourinary changes	• Nephron units diminish in number and size; diminished blood supply to kidneys. • Decreased glomerular filtration rate leads to decrease in urinary output with resultant dehydration.	• Teach normal age-related changes. • Teach signs indicative of dehydration. • Inform client of need to maintain adequate fluid intake.
Integumentary changes	• Decreased moisture and turgor of skin and loss of subcutaneous fat lead to development of wrinkles. • Hair thins and turns gray.	• Instruct client about effects of sun and cigarette smoking on the skin. • Assess client for body image alterations. • Use nonjudgmental listening. • Provide support.

Musculoskeletal changes	• Decreased bone mass and density.
	• Slight loss of height may occur (1–4 inches).
	• Thinning of intervertebral disks.
	• Generalized decrease in muscle tone; ''flabby'' appearance and less agility.
		• Instruct client about:
		  —Need for calcium intake
		  —Importance of decreasing caffeine and alcohol consumption
		  —Effects of sedentary versus active lifestyle on osteoporosis
		• Increased risk of injury. Instruct client of need for proper posture (especially sitting), exercise, and adequate fluid intake.
		• Instruct client on need for adequate physical activity.

Endocrine changes	• Decreased metabolism results in reduced production of enzymes and increased hydrochloric acid.
	• Lead to acid indigestion and belching.
		• Instruct client to:
		  —Avoid foods that are spicy or fried
		  —Avoid eating within 2 hours before bedtime

(Continues)

TABLE 18-27 (Continued)

DIMENSION	CHARACTERISTICS	NURSING IMPLICATIONS
Reproductive and sexual changes	*Women:* • Cessation of estrogen and progesterone production during menopause. • Regression of secondary sex characteristics (decreased breast size, loss of pubic hair). • Decreased vaginal secretions. • Note: With no pregnancy risk, some post-menopausal women enjoy sexual activity more. *Men:* • Decreased levels of testosterone. • Reduced amount of viable sperm. • Decline in sexual energy; takes longer to achieve an erection; erection is sustained longer. • Adaptation to developing chronic diseases and sexual problems may diminish self-esteem.	• Teach clients about age-related sexual and reproductive changes. • Encourage responsible sexual behavior. • Teach about prevention of sexually transmitted diseases.
Psychosocial	*Erikson:* Generativity vs. stagnation • Adults who have achieved generativity feel good about their lives and are comfortable with themselves. • Become more involved in altruistic acts (e.g., community activities). • Usually experience changing family roles (e.g., grandparent, caregiver for aging parents). *Havighurst:* • Fulfill social and civic responsibilities. • Assist children to become independent. • Adult children leaving home may lead to happiness or depression ("empty nest syndrome"). • Maintain relationship with one's partner.	• Provide support as the client deals with aging. • Encourage to become involved in community activities, volunteer work. • Teach leisure skills. • Instruct in the need to care for self while caring for others.
Cognitive	*Piaget:* • Will use all stages, depending on the task (e.g., can move between formal operations, concrete operations, and problem solving as needed). • Able to reflect on the past and anticipate the future. • Reaction time diminishes during late middle age. • Memory is unimpaired. • Learning ability remains intact if person is motivated and material is meaningful.	• Encourage middle-aged clients who are anticipating returning to school or engaging in other intellectually stimulating activities.

(Continues)

TABLE 18-27 (Continued)

DIMENSION	CHARACTERISTICS	NURSING IMPLICATIONS
Moral	*Kohlberg:* Postconventional stage *Gilligan:* • Women tend to judge morality of issues according to a sense of fairness and avoiding hurt to others. • Establishes moral beliefs that are independent of what others think.	• Use nonjudgmental approach when client discusses values. • Respect personal differences by individualizing care.
Spiritual	*Fowler:* Conjunctive faith • Is able to appreciate others' belief systems. • Becomes less dogmatic with own beliefs. • Religion is usually a source of comfort.	• Encourage use of spiritual support. • Refer to clergy if desired by client.

Data from Edelman, C. L., & Mandle, C. L. (2006). *Health promotion throughout the lifespan* (6th ed.). St. Louis, MO: Mosby; Ignatavicius, D. D., & Workman, M. L. (2009). *Medical-surgical nursing: Critical thinking for collaborative care* (6th ed.). St. Louis, MO: Elsevier.

• Establishing meaningful roles
• Adjusting to infirmities (if any exist)
• Coping with losses and changes
• Preparing for death

Nursing Implications

Professional nursing care is important in assisting aging people to develop a sense of well-being. Nurses who work with older adults must be especially sensitive to their own feelings, attitudes, and beliefs about aging and be aware of the effect of these responses on their care.

When assessing the older adult for health-related needs, the nurse needs to learn about the client's background, family history, work history, hobbies, and achievements (see Figure 18-12). Clients should be encouraged to talk about their life experiences. When planning care, it is important to build on the client's lifelong interests. By recognizing each client's unique experiences and assets, the nurse is more likely to individualize care.

When clients express dissatisfaction and regrets about the past, the nurse should listen in a nonjudgmental manner and avoid trying to convince them that things are really better than they remember or perceive. It is important, however, to help clients put disappointments into perspective by balancing them with accomplishments and achievements. Nurses should encourage families to engage in a positive life review with older adult clients. Most nursing interventions for older adults center around introspection and reflection on their lives. Life review (or reminiscence therapy) promotes a positive self-concept in older people (Kneisl & Trigoboff, 2009).

COMMUNITY CONSIDERATIONS

Resources for Senior Citizens

Many communities have senior citizens' centers to promote socialization. What types of resources are available in your community that help improve functional abilities of older citizens?

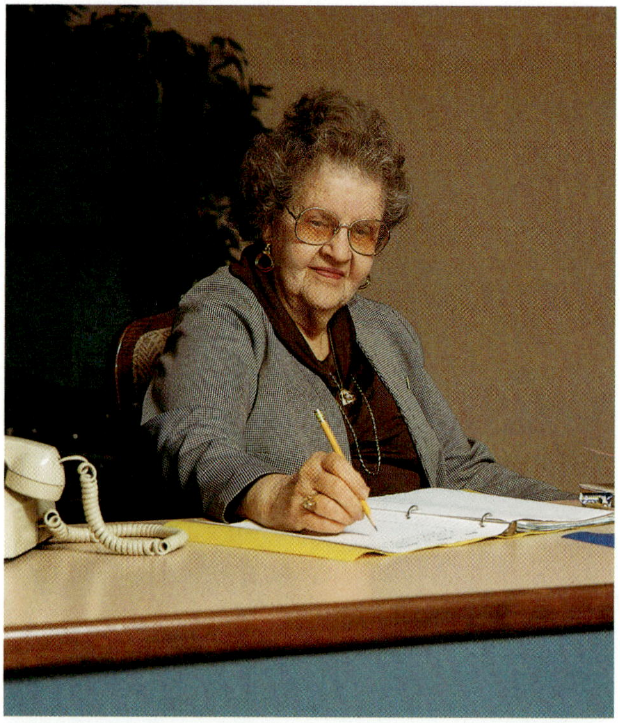

FIGURE 18-12 This older adult is able to maintain her independence and self-esteem through volunteer work. Describe the importance of incorporating information such as the ability and desire to make a contribution to society into an older adult's nursing care. DELMAR/CENGAGE LEARNING

TABLE 18-28 Older Adult: Growth and Development

DIMENSION	CHARACTERISTICS	NURSING IMPLICATIONS
Physiological *Cardiovascular changes*	• Reduced elasticity of heart muscle and arteries. Less efficient functioning of cardiovascular system; increased systolic blood pressure. • Increased fat deposits on heart lead to reduced oxygen supply. • Thickening of aortic and mitral valves leads to incomplete closure; murmurs may occur. • Arterial diameter decreases as a result of arteriosclerosis. • Orthostatic hypotension may occur as the inelastic vessels are unable to constrict rapidly in response to postural changes. • Thickening of venous walls leads to decreased elasticity. • Development of varicose veins is common.	• Decreased capacity for physical activity. Instruct client about the importance of remaining physically active and to balance activity with adequate rest and sleep. • Teach client lifestyle modifications that promote cardiovascular health: —Avoid smoking and other use of tobacco. —Avoid secondary tobacco smoke. —Maintain proper diet (low fat, low cholesterol). —Avoid sedentary lifestyle.
Neurological changes	• Decreased number of neurons. • Fewer neurotransmitters. • Slower transmission of nerve impulses. • Decreased sensory threshold. • The vestibulocochlear nerve (associated with balance and equilibrium) has decreased number of fibers.	• A generalized slower response to environmental changes leads to increased risk for falls, burns, and other injuries. • Teach safety measures. • Teach fall preventive measures.
	Vision • Pupils decrease in size and are less responsive to light. • Cataracts or glaucoma often occurs. • Fewer tears are produced by the lacrimal glands, so the cornea is likely to become irritated. • Decreased ability to see colors; pastels fade; monotones, blacks, and whites are difficult to see.	• Be aware of client's increased sensitivity to glare; allow time for eyes to accommodate changes in lighting. • The use of eye drops or artificial tears is helpful. • Brighter colors compensate for decline in color discrimination.
	Hearing • Ear canal may become blocked with cerumen (wax), which diminishes transmission of sound. • Tympanic membrane is thinner and may become sclerotic. • Diminished ability to hear high-frequency sounds.	• Teach proper hygiene for cleaning ears. • Caution client to avoid inserting objects into ear during cleaning. • Lower tone of voice and rate of speech; instruct family members to do likewise.
	Taste and smell • General decline in taste perception. • Diminished salivation often occurs with aging. • Olfactory nerve cells decrease in number.	• Many elders prefer more highly seasoned foods, salt, and sugar; teach healthy diet plans. Increased loss of appetite often occurs; make food visually appealing and know the client's food preferences. • Be alert for safety hazards associated with decreased sense of smell (inability to detect smoke, leaking gas, or spoiled food).
Respiratory changes	• Decreased elasticity and muscle tone. • Fewer functioning alveoli.	• Instruct client how to deep breathe and cough effectively.

(Continues)

TABLE 18-28 (Continued)

DIMENSION	CHARACTERISTICS	NURSING IMPLICATIONS
	• Calcification of chest wall and rib cage. • Decreased number of cilia results in ineffective clearing of respiratory system. • Lungs tend to remain hyperinflated on exhalation, which causes decreased vital capacity.	• Encourage a balance between exercise/activity and rest/sleep.
Musculoskeletal changes	• Loss of calcium from bones. • Bone loss is a greater problem in women since it is accelerated by menopause. • A gradual decrease in height results from bone loss. • Less flexibility; muscle stiffness due to decreased number of elastic fibers in muscle tissues. • General posture is flexion. • Center of gravity shifts, with resultant changes in movement and balance.	• Instruct women of all ages about importance of calcium consumption. • Encourage the elderly to engage in physical activity, especially walking. • Teach safety measures, including fall preventive measures. • Encourage exercise to promote flexibility. • Perform passive range-of-motion exercises for those who need it.
Gastrointestinal changes	*Mouth* • Atrophy of oral mucosa. • Connective tissue loses elasticity. • Decreased number of nerve cells. • Saliva production is decreased and becomes more alkaline. • Ability to chew food is impaired by loss of teeth, gum recession, and degeneration of jaw bone.	• Decreased absorption of nutrients as a result of changes. • Instruct on importance of adequate nutrition, especially fluids and bulky foods. • Keep client well hydrated; instruct client to drink at least 8 glasses of fluid daily. • Provide foods that are easily chewed.
	Gastrointestinal tract • Peristalsis slows; decreased emptying of esophagus and stomach; slowed intestinal motility. • Shrinkage of gastric mucosa leads to decreased amounts of hydrochloric acid. • Reduction of pancreatic enzymes. • Delayed time for emptying gallbladder; bile is thicker. • Elimination is often impaired.	• Encourage client to remain physically active. • Teach importance of having a regular time for toileting. • Avoid spicy and fried foods. • Avoid eating within 2 hours of bedtime.
Endocrine changes	• Metabolism slows. • Alteration in pancreatic activity.	• Inform client of need for fewer calories.

Reproductive and sexual changes	• Decreased amounts of growth hormone, estrogen, and testosterone blood levels.
	  Men:
	    • Enlargement of prostate gland.
	    • Decreased reserves of testosterone.
	    • Testes softer and smaller.
	    • Sperm production decreased or inhibited.
	    • Ejaculations less forceful.
	  Women:
	    • Breast tissue loses elasticity (starts to sag).
		• Provide information about the normal changes associated with aging.
		• Use nonjudgmental approach when client discusses sexual issues.
		• Teach about effects of aging on reproduction and sexuality.
		• Teach STD preventive measures.

(Continues)

TABLE 18-28 (Continued)

DIMENSION	CHARACTERISTICS	NURSING IMPLICATIONS
	• Decreased size of uterus and fallopian tubes. • Vaginal walls thin. • Vaginal secretions decrease. • Vulva and external genitalia shrink (due to loss of subcutaneous body fat).	
Integumentary changes	• Decreased activity of sebaceous glands leads to drying. • Decreased turgor. • Thinning of epidural layer. • Decreased number of sweat glands (can result in heat exhaustion). • Loss of subcutaneous fat increases susceptibility to cold. • Wrinkles become more pronounced. • Hair turns gray and thins.	• When bathing: —Avoid excessive use of soap, hot water, and brisk rubbing. —Pat, do not rub, skin dry. —Use tepid water. • Use lotion for itching and dryness. • Avoid prolonged pressure on bony prominences. • Protect from temperature extremes. • Assess for body image alterations. • For those with body image alterations: —Assist with grooming as necessary. —Use photographs to help adjust to changing appearance. —Use touch to help clarify body boundaries.
Psychosocial	*Erikson:* Integrity vs. despair • Accepts one's life as it is. • Feels a sense of worth when helping others. *Havighurst:* • Adjusts to retirement and changed financial status. • Adjusts to decline in physical strength. • Fulfills civic responsibilities. • Meets social obligations. • Adjusts to death of significant others. • Develops affiliation with peers and age group (sees self as "old"). • Retirement from employment affects finances, social activities, leisure time, and role identity (may be positive or negative impact). • Potential for social isolation as significant others and peers die.	• Ask the older person for advice. • Identify and use the older adult's strengths. • Encourage the use of reminiscence (life review). • Encourage to express feelings concerning aging. • Promote socialization with peers.
Cognitive	*Piaget:* Formal operations stage • There is no decline in IQ associated with aging. • Reaction time is usually slowed.	• Allow client time to respond to questions or instructions.
	Memory • Short-term: decreased capacity for recall. • Long-term: remains unchanged.	• Be alert for the possibility of medication-induced confusion with resultant impact on memory.
Moral	• *Kohlberg:* Postconventional stage • Makes moral decisions according to own principles and beliefs.	• Support decision making. • Respect client values even when different from own.

(Continues)

TABLE 18-28 (Continued)

DIMENSION	CHARACTERISTICS	NURSING IMPLICATIONS
Spiritual	*Fowler:* • Universalizing stage of faith. • Is generally satisfied with one's spiritual beliefs. • Tends to act on beliefs.	• Listen carefully to determine spiritual needs. • Acknowledge losses and encourage appropriate grieving.

Data from Ebersole, P., Hess, P., Luggen, A. S., Touhy, T., & Jett, K. (2007). *Toward healthy aging: Human needs and nursing response* (7th ed.). St. Louis, MO: Elsevier; Edelman, C. L., & Mandle, C. L. (2006). *Health promotion throughout the lifespan* (6th ed.). St. Louis, MO: Mosby; Ignatavicius, D. D., & Workman, M. L. (2009). *Medical-surgical nursing: Critical thinking for collaborative care* (6th ed.). St. Louis, MO: Elsevier; Murray, R. B., Zentner, J. P., & Yakimo, R. (2008). *Nursing assessment and health promotion through the lifespan* (8th ed.). Upper Saddle River, NJ: Prentice-Hall.

WELLNESS PROMOTION Health promotion activities should be implemented with older adults in order to maintain functional independence. Health promotion activities are aimed at maximizing the person's abilities and strengths. Specific topics that are developmentally appropriate for older clients are use of leisure time, increased socialization, engaging in regular physical activity, maintaining a positive mental attitude, and developing and maintaining healthy lifestyles.

SAFETY CONSIDERATIONS Falls pose a major health threat to older adults. See Chapter 29 for information related to fall prevention and other specific safety promotion practices for older individuals. See Chapter 19 for information on other safety measures for older adults.

KEY CONCEPTS

- Growth is the quantitative changes in physical size of the body and its parts.
- Development refers to behavioral changes in functional abilities and skills.
- Maturation is the process of becoming fully grown and developed and involves both physiological and behavioral aspects of an individual.
- During each developmental stage, certain developmental tasks must be achieved for normal development to occur.
- Growth and development of an individual are influenced by a combination of factors, including heredity, life experiences, health status, and cultural expectations.
- According to Freud, certain developmental tasks must be achieved at each developmental stage; failure to achieve or a delay in achieving the developmental task results in a fixation at a previous stage.
- Erikson stated that psychosocial development is a series of conflicts that occur during eight stages of life.
- Sullivan stated that personality development is strongly influenced by interpersonal relationships.
- Piaget's theory states that there are four stages of cognitive development: sensorimotor, preoperational, concrete operations, and formal operations. Each stage is characterized by the ways in which the person interprets and uses the environment.
- Kohlberg's theory describes six stages of moral development through which individuals determine a moral code to guide their behavior.
- Gilligan states that women's moral judgment revolves around three issues: a concern with survival, a focus on goodness, and an understanding of others' need for care.
- Fowler's theory states that there are six distinct stages of faith development and, even though individuals will vary in the age at which they experience each stage, the sequence of stages remains the same.
- Providing care to the whole person is a basic concept of professional nurses, and knowledge of growth and development concepts guides holistic care of clients.
- The stages of the life cycle are the prenatal, neonate, infant, toddler, preschooler, school-age child, preadolescent, adolescent, young adult, middle adult, and older adult.
- Nurses have important roles in promoting the health and safety of individuals at each stage of the life cycle.

REVIEW QUESTIONS

1. During a clinic visit, a mother of a 4-month-old child tells the nurse, "My baby is not sitting up yet. Does this mean there's a problem?" Which of the following is the most therapeutic nursing response?
   a. "Be sure to tell the doctor so he can order some tests for your baby."
   b. "Every child develops at his or her own pace."
   c. "Most babies start to sit alone at about 8 months of age."
   d. "Oh, don't worry, your baby's fine."

2. Which of the following are developmentally appropriate for older adults? Select all that apply.
   a. Acceptance of life as it is
   b. Decreased reaction time
   c. Expanded circle of friends
   d. False sense of immunity
   e. Questioning one's values and beliefs
   f. Sense of generativity

3. When teaching accident prevention to high school students, which of the following topics is most important for the nurse to include?
   a. Fall prevention
   b. Fire prevention
   c. Motor vehicle safety
   d. Transmission of STDs

4. Which of the following statements made by a woman in the first trimester of pregnancy indicates a need for further prenatal teaching?
   a. "Every morning I feel so sick to my stomach, like I'm going to vomit."
   b. "I feel tired most of the time."
   c. "I take prenatal vitamins every day."
   d. "It's OK for me to drink wine as long as I do so in moderation."

5. Which of the following statements made by a 50-year-old person indicates achievement of developmental tasks?
   a. "At this stage of my life, everyone should take care of me."
   b. "I'm busy with my family and job."
   c. "I'm not sure which direction my life is going."
   d. "I've had a full, happy life and am ready to die when my time is up."

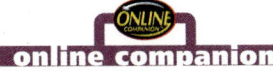

online companion

Visit the DeLaune and Ladner online companion resource at **www.delmar.cengage.com** for additional content and study aids. Click on Online Companions, then select the Nursing discipline.

The setting sun is as beautiful as the rising sun.

—Japanese proverb

CHAPTER 19

The Older Client

COMPETENCIES

1. Discuss theories of aging.
2. Refute common myths about aging.
3. Describe the impact of physical changes associated with aging on functional ability.
4. Explain ways in which the older adult adapts to the physiological changes associated with aging.
5. Discuss the psychosocial impact that retirement, changes in social relationships, changes in living arrangements, and loss may have on the older client.
6. Define polypharmacy and its significance for nurses caring for older clients.
7. Identify physical and psychological signs of abuse in older adults.
8. Outline safety considerations for the older adult living at home.
9. Discuss the use of the nursing process with older adult clients.

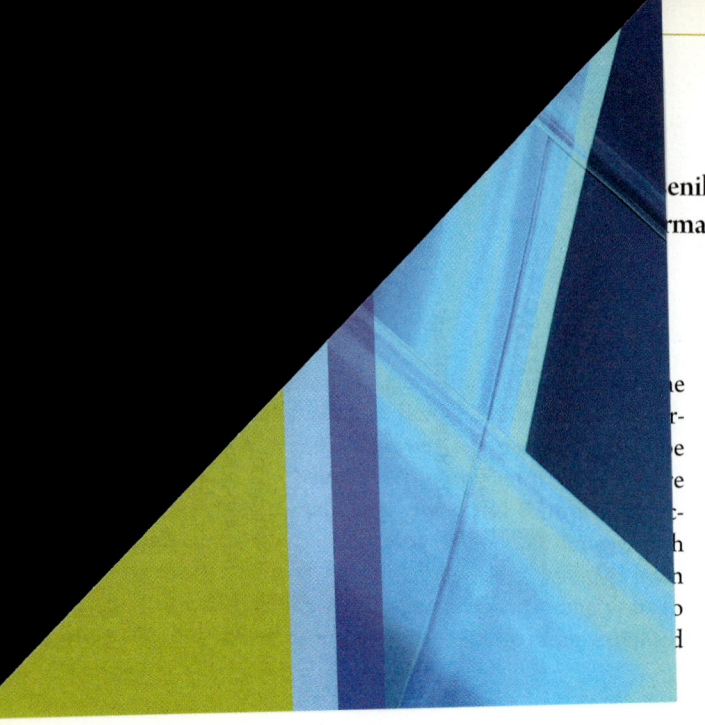

enilis
rmacy

presbycusis
restorative nursing care

baby boomers (individuals born between 1946 and 1964) start turning age 65 in 2011. The number of older people will subsequently increase rapidly during the period of 2010–2030 (Federal Interagency Forum on Aging Related Statistics, 2007); see Figure 19-1 on page 359.

The rapidly expanding population will have an enormous impact on health care as the graying of America's baby boomers increases the demand for nurses and other health care providers. It will be essential that nurses are sensitive to and understanding of the needs, requirements, and capabilities of the older adult.

DEFINING OLD AGE

It is difficult to define *old age* in an era when factors such as medical breakthroughs and advanced health care techniques have extended the average lifetime. The most obvious measure of age is a person's **chronological age**, or the exact age of a person from birth. But a person's chronological age does not dictate the state of health, attitude toward daily life, or beliefs about living. There are enormous differences among individuals. People in their 70s may look and act more as if they were 50, whereas some people in their 30s think and act in ways that reinforce negative stereotypes of the older generation. For these reasons, age is difficult to define.

When does old age begin? For many centuries, people in their 50s were considered old. Today, Americans in their 50s generally consider themselves still young and, if asked at what age old age begins, are likely to respond "80" (see Table 19-1). The U.S. population is rapidly aging, as the

THEORIES OF AGING

Aging is a complex process of biological, psychosocial, cultural, and experiential changes. No one theory completely embraces and explains all the many facets of aging. Following is a discussion of several biological and psychosocial theories that offer a frame of reference for providing nursing care to older adults.

Biological Theories

There are several biological theories that address the physical changes of aging. The *stress theory* suggests that irreversible structural and chemical changes occur in the body as a result of stress throughout the life span and that individuals must learn to adapt to these changes. The *cross-linkage theory* describes the deterioration of tissues and organs as the cause of loss of flexibility and functional mobility that occurs with aging. The *somatic mutation theory* states that changes in DNA that are not repaired lead to replication of mutated cells, which brings about decreased cellular functioning and loss of organ efficiency. The *programmed aging theory* states that life span is determined by heredity and that an internal genetic clock is responsible for the rate at which an individual develops, ages, and eventually dies.

Psychosocial Theories

Psychosocial theories on aging present the position that many factors in addition to genetics contribute to the aging process. The *disengagement theory* posits that as individuals age, they inevitably withdraw from society and society withdraws from them in a process of separation. The *continuity theory* suggests that an individual's values and personality develop over a lifetime and that goals and individual characteristics will remain constant throughout life. An individual thus learns to adapt to changes and will tend to repeat those reactions and behaviors that led to success in the past. The *activity theory* proposes that an individual's satisfaction

TABLE 19-1	Chronological Classification of Age Groups	
AGE	CLASSIFICATION
65–74	Young-old
75–84	Old
85–94	Old-old
95 and older	Elite-old, chronologically gifted

Data from Mauk, K. L. (2006). Introduction to gerontological nursing. In K. L. Mauk (Ed.), *Gerontological nursing: Competencies for care*. Boston: Jones & Bartlett.

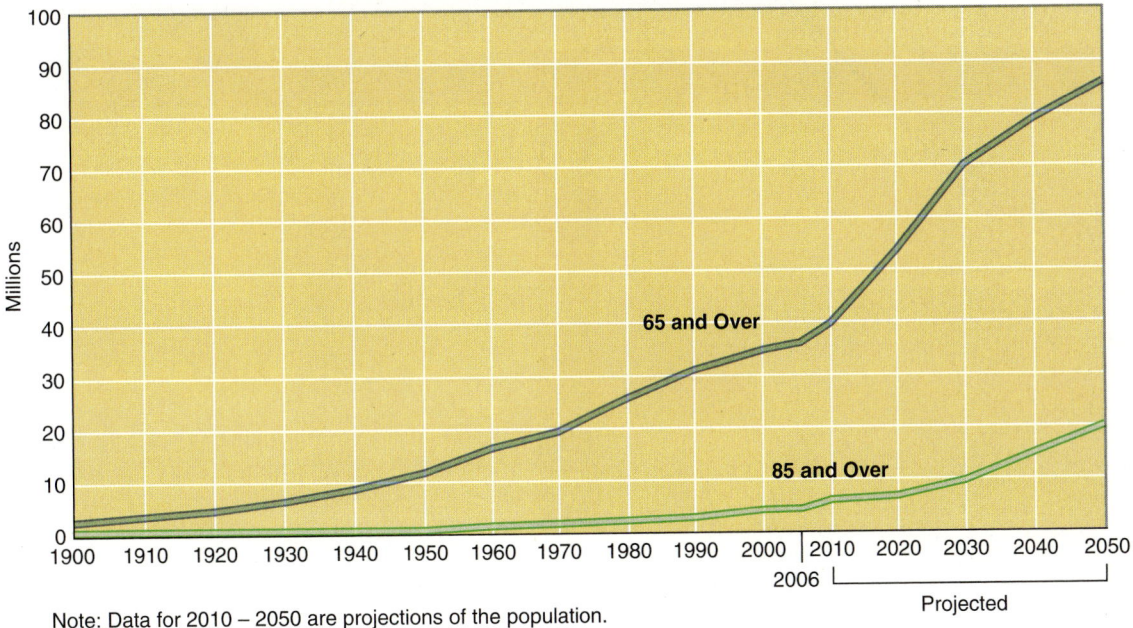

Number of People Age 65 and Over, by Age Group, Selected
Years 1900–2006 and Projected 2010–2050

Note: Data for 2010 – 2050 are projections of the population.
Reference population: These data refer to the resident population.
U.S. Census Bureau, Decennial Census, Population Estimates and Projections.

FIGURE 19-1 **Number of People Age 65 and Older** FEDERAL INTERAGENCY FORUM ON AGING RELATED STATISTICS. (2007). *OLDER AMERICANS 2008.* RETRIEVED NOVEMBER 22, 2008, FROM HTTP://WWW.AGINGSTATS.GOV/AGINGSTATSDOTNET/MAIN_SITE/DATA/2008_DOCUMENTS/POPULATION.PDF.

with life depends on involvement in new interests, hobbies, roles, and relationships. Volunteering is one way that many retirees stay connected to the community. In addition to providing social connection, volunteer activities provide a daily routine, a way to make a contribution, and a sense of being needed.

MYTHS AND STEREOTYPES OF AGING

In the youth-obsessed society of the United States, old age has a negative connotation. In many cultures, older adults are accorded a position of respect, and young people feel a moral and familial responsibility to care for parents and older

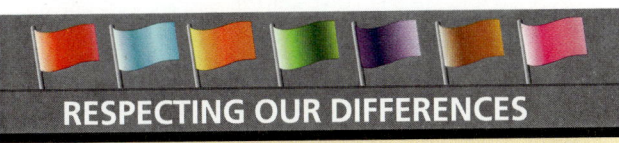

RESPECTING OUR DIFFERENCES

Personal Views on Aging

Consider your own beliefs about aging. Do you feel that one of these theories best represents the older adult population? Would you classify your opinion of older adults as basically positive or basically negative? On what information have you based your views?

relatives. In American culture, misconceptions about older adults abound; see Table 19-2, on page 360, for common myths about older adults. There are many reasons these myths develop and persist. For example, many young people today have little personal contact with older family members such as grandparents; also, health care providers usually see only older people who are acutely or chronically ill, and are hospitalized or live in a long-term care setting.

Older adults are often stereotyped as being ill, bald, hard of hearing, forgetful, rigid, grumpy, or boring, simply on the basis of their age and regardless of their competencies and individual characteristics. Many younger Americans also believe that all older people live in nursing homes and fail to consider the independence of the older generation and their contributions to society. These types of attitudes are known as **ageism** (the process of stereotyping and discriminating against people because they are old).

To many, aging is synonymous with death; these individuals have a negative view of the aging process, which usually results from fear, lack of exposure to older individuals, and a lack of understanding of how varied experiences can enhance the overall quality of life. Surprisingly, many older adults have negative attitudes toward other older adults; these often result from fear of stereotypes and social stigmas, or a sense of anxiety over "guilt by association." Nurses need to be aware of these myths and stereotypes and to separate them from the realities of the aging process in order to provide sensitive and appropriate care to older clients.

TABLE 19-2 Refuting Common Myths about Older Adults

MYTH	FACT
Most older Americans are economically disadvantaged.	In 2006, approximately 9% of Americans over age 65 lived below the poverty threshold. This is a great improvement as compared to 1951 when the percentage of elders living in poverty was 35%.
The majority of older individuals are ill.	During 2004–2006, 74% of people age 65 and older rated their health as good or better.
Most older people live in extended care facilities.	In 2005, 5% of people age 65–84 and 17% of those aged 85 or older lived in long-term facilities.
Older individuals are uninterested in or unable to engage in sexual activity.	Most people ages 57–85 think of sexuality as an important part of life. The frequency of sexual activity declines slightly during the 50s, 60s, and 70s.

Data from Centers for Medicare and Medicaid Services. (2008). Alternatives to nursing home care. Retrieved November 22, 2008, from http://www.cms.hhs.gov; Federal Interagency Forum on Aging Related Statistics. (2007). *Older Americans 2008.* Retrieved November 22, 2008, from http://agingstats.gov/agingstatsdotnet/main_site/data/2008_documents/population.pdf; Lindau, S. T., Schumm, L. P., Laumann, E. O., Levinson, W., O'Muircheartaigh, C. A., & Waite, L. J. (2007). A study of sexuality and health among older adults in the U.S. *New England Journal of Medicine, 357*(8), 762–774; U.S. Census Bureau. (2008). *Current population survey, annual social and economic supplement, 1960–2007.* Retrieved November 22, 2008, from http://www.census.gov.

QUALITY OF LIFE AMONG OLDER ADULTS

Quality of life is gaining more emphasis in today's aging society. The increasing life span has both positive and negative outcomes. One of the greatest fears associated with advancing age is poor health. Most people want to live a long life, as long as it is a long healthy life. Older adults do have more chronic health problems than the general population.

Currently, the trend is for people to live longer and healthier lives. Many Americans over 65 live in relative financial comfort, able to continue working or start enjoying their retirement years. Good nutrition, proper exercise, continued work, travel, recreation, hobbies, and companionship are just a few of the healthy lifestyle choices many older people now have the means to afford.

A positive outlook and adaptive ability contribute to the high quality of life enjoyed by many older adults today. Although many people over 65 have some kind of chronic health problem, most have found ways to keep these ailments from interfering with their enjoyment of life. Most older people accept a certain amount of declining health as a normal, expected part of aging, but do not allow health issues to interfere with the vigorous pursuit of enjoyment; see Figure 19-2.

CHANGES ASSOCIATED WITH AGING

Change is an ongoing part of life. People who have a difficult time accepting change, and therefore adapt poorly to it, will experience problems. Changes of aging can be viewed as developmental, physiological, or psychosocial in nature.

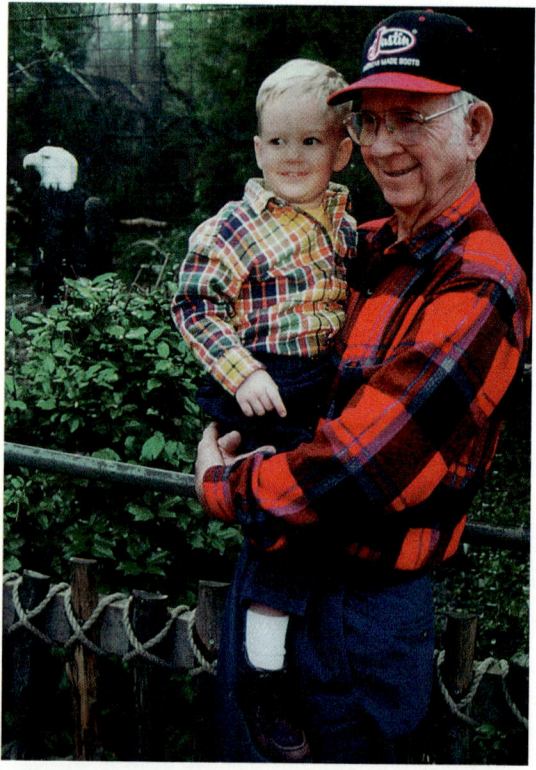

FIGURE 19-2 Older adults often assume new roles, such as grandparent, as they mature, and can gain immense pleasure in spending time with family and sharing wisdom and ideas with the younger generation. DELMAR/CENGAGE LEARNING

DEVELOPMENTAL CHANGES

At every stage of life, including old age, new developmental challenges constantly arise. Like developmental challenges faced earlier in life, these occasions are opportunities for success or failure. Older people may experience feelings of satisfaction or success over completing certain developmental tasks associated with aging, such as:

- Gaining insight or wisdom, even if physical powers are in decline
- Developing improved social skills, with more same-sex friendships
- Becoming more open-minded and tolerant
- Finding an active and pleasurable sexual dimension
- Seeing children transform into responsible, successful adults
- Becoming a grandparent
- Holding civic and community positions of responsibility
- Achieving mastery of one's occupation or skills
- Developing new skills, hobbies, and avocations
- Renewing and deepening one's relationship with one's spouse
- Gaining new knowledge and experiences
- Adjusting to physical changes associated with aging
- Coping with aging spouses and friends

On the other hand, any person would be challenged to find successful ways to cope with other developmental events of aging, such as:

- Adjusting to the death of a spouse or partner
- Adapting to major declines in health or physical ability
- Adjusting to the loss of social role, prestige, occupation, income, or sense of usefulness
- Accepting loss of independent living
- Adjusting to loneliness or loss without boredom or depression

It is important for the nurse to assess the nature of any developmental challenges a client may be experiencing because a client's adaptation to changes can have a profound effect on health status.

PHYSIOLOGICAL CHANGES

From the moment of birth, the human body begins the aging process. Each person ages differently as the rate of age-related changes varies from one individual to the next. However, some generalized physiological changes occur with the aging process, including:

- Decreased rate of cell mitosis
- Deterioration of specialized nondividing cells (i.e., neurons)
- Decreased elasticity and increased rigidity of connective tissue
- Decreased functional capacity

Some of the physical changes of aging, such as graying of hair and decreased visual acuity, are readily apparent. Other changes are more subtle and may go undetected until a problem occurs.

The rate of aging is influenced by:

- Genetic composition
- Lifestyle (dietary and exercise patterns)
- Presence of chronic illnesses
- Previous experience (e.g., adaptive responses to stressors)

Neurological Changes

Aging brings about several changes in the nervous system that alter sensory and perceptual responses. Murray, Zentner, and Yakimo (2008) identify some of the age-related neurological changes as:

- Fewer neurons
- Transmission of nerve impulses slowed
- The number of neurotransmitters (chemical messengers of the central nervous system) decreased
- Sensory threshold decreased (affects pain and tactile sensations)

As a result of these changes, reaction time is usually slowed. The generalized slower response to environmental changes leads to increased risk for falls, burns, and other injuries.

It is important that the nurse allow older clients time to respond to questions and instructions. Teaching safety measures is a preventive aspect of nursing that must not be overlooked when dealing with older clients.

Sensory and Perceptual Changes

Sensory changes are progressive and may cause some limitations in later years. The resultant changes may impair the individual's ability to enjoy life to the fullest as well as present related health problems.

VISION The aging process causes some visual changes. For example, pupils decrease in size and are less responsive to light. Usually a loss of visual acuity occurs because of degenerative changes related to aging. By the age of approximately 42, the lens cortex becomes thicker, impairing its ability to change shape and focus. This condition, presbyopia, causes farsightedness and is corrected by the use of bifocals.

Cataracts, glaucoma, and age-related macular degeneration are the most common pathological visual problems experienced by older adults. Cataracts (or opacity of the lens) can be surgically corrected. If untreated, glaucoma can result in blindness; thus, annual screening is recommended for all individuals over age 40. Age-related macular degeneration is the loss of central vision; magnification must be used to compensate for the changes. Diabetes, hypertension, and other systemic diseases will exacerbate macular degeneration. As a result of aging, fewer tears are produced by the lacrimal glands, so the cornea is likely to become irritated. Most older adults normally experience a decreased ability to see colors; pastels fade, and monotones, blacks, and whites are difficult to see.

The nurse caring for older clients must be aware of the client's increased sensitivity to glare and allow time for the eyes to accommodate changes in lighting. The use of eye-drops or artificial tears may also be beneficial. Brighter colors compensate for the decline in color discrimination.

HEARING Generally, hearing is diminished with age. There is a drying and wrinkling of the auricle with a noticeable increase of hair in the auditory canal. Cerumen becomes drier and can cause impaction, which blocks transmission of sounds. The hearing loss associated with old age is called presbycusis. In the middle ear, bony joints show some degeneration. However, the major changes occur in the inner ear, where degeneration of the vestibular system and simultaneous atrophy of the cochlea and the organ of Corti produce deficits in equilibrium and hearing.

Nurses need to be very patient in their approach to the older client. With anticipated changes in sensory perception, it is important that nurses face their clients, speak slowly and clearly, and protect them from injury. It is important when teaching clients that nurses ask for feedback and evaluate client comprehension.

TASTE AND SMELL With aging, taste perception declines and salivation is diminished. Many older clients prefer highly seasoned foods, with additional salt and sugar to compensate for a decreased sensation of taste. Increased loss of appetite often occurs and may be medication-related in some individuals. It may be helpful for older adults to eat small portions frequently throughout the day. The nurse seeks to make food visually appealing and know the client's food preferences. It is important to teach clients about healthy eating patterns.

Olfactory nerve cells decrease in number. The nurse should instruct family members and other caregivers to be alert for safety hazards associated with decreased sense of smell, such as the inability to detect smoke, leaking gas, or spoiled food.

Cardiovascular Changes

As a result of aging, functioning of the cardiovascular system becomes less efficient. Reduced elasticity of the heart muscle and arteries causes a subsequent increase in systolic blood pressure. Increased fat deposits in the blood vessels lead to a reduced supply of oxygen. The arterial diameter decreases as a result of arteriosclerosis. Thickening of venous walls leads to decreased elasticity. Thickening of aortic and mitral valves leads to incomplete closure; heart murmurs may occur in some older people. The development of varicose veins is common. As a result of decreased cardiac output, many older people experience a decreased capacity for physical activity. A diminished cardiac output is problematic when the older person becomes physically, mentally, or emotionally impaired (Ebersole, Hess, Luggen, Touhy, & Jett, 2007).

The nurse should instruct the client about the importance of remaining physically active and the need to balance activity with adequate rest and sleep. Older clients also need information on lifestyle modifications that promote cardiovascular health. Such instruction would include the following:

- Avoid smoking and use of other forms of tobacco.
- Avoid secondary tobacco smoke.
- Eat a healthy diet (low fat, low cholesterol).
- Avoid a sedentary lifestyle, which can result in impaired cardiac output with resultant fatigue.

Respiratory Changes

Most older adults experience a decreased functional respiratory reserve capacity, with a generalized decreased elasticity and tone of muscles, including the muscles necessary for respiration. Physical changes in the lungs include fewer functioning alveoli and a decreased number of cilia. Therefore, ineffective clearing of the respiratory system occurs. Calcification of the chest wall and rib cage causes the lungs to remain hyperinflated on exhalation, thereby decreasing vital capacity.

To deal with respiratory changes, the nurse teaches the client how to breathe deeply and cough effectively. The client needs to establish a balance between exercise and activity to conserve respiratory effort while at the same time improving vital capacity. Because physical exercise increases lung capacity, nurses should encourage older clients to walk.

Gastrointestinal Changes

Aging brings about several alterations in gastrointestinal functioning. The major changes are described in the following sections.

MOUTH Many older people lose their teeth for a variety of reasons, including years of inadequate dental hygiene and extended use of medication (e.g., anticonvulsant drugs). Other physiological changes include atrophy of oral mucosa, loss of elasticity in connective tissue, and a decreased number of nerve cells that control chewing, swallowing, and taste. Saliva production is decreased, and saliva becomes more alkaline. The older person's ability to chew food is often impaired by loss of teeth, gum recession, and degeneration of the mandible. The nurse should instruct the client and caregivers to have available foods that are easily chewed and swallowed.

GASTROINTESTINAL TRACT There is a decrease in peristaltic action with a relaxation of the lower esophageal sphincter. This causes a decreased emptying of the esophagus and stomach. Shrinkage of gastric mucosa leads to changes in the levels of hydrochloric acid, with subsequent heartburn. Older adults often have an inability to tolerate large amounts of foods containing fat.

Elimination is often impaired in older clients; as a result, there is decreased absorption of nutrients. Intestinal motility is slowed, and some loss of sphincter control may be noted. Nurses should instruct older clients about the importance of adequate nutrition, especially fluids and high-fiber foods. Keep clients well hydrated by instructing them to drink at least 8 glasses of fluid daily. Other methods to prevent constipation are physical activity and adhering to a regular time for toileting.

Genitourinary Changes

Major changes in the structure and function of the urinary system are associated with aging. The kidneys, bladder, and ureters are all affected by the aging process.

The loss of some muscle tone in the bladder and urethra can result in incomplete emptying of the bladder. Residual urine can lead to bladder infection. Decreased bladder capacity may cause subsequent nocturia and polyuria.

Renal function is the major determinant of an individual's fluid and electrolyte balance. In older adults, renal function is often affected by diminished blood flow to the kidneys as a result of arteriosclerosis, hypertension, and other cardiovascular disorders. The glomerular filtration rate slows, and there are fewer functioning nephrons.

The risk of renal failure increases with age, as does fluid retention. Dehydration is a very real threat for many older adults. The aging body loses some of its functional ability to adapt to changes in total body water, which is essential for metabolism. The composition of body water declines to about 40% of an older adult's total body weight.

Nursing measures address the underlying problems that result in a fluid and electrolyte imbalance. For example, if clients are dehydrated, they should be instructed to drink 2000 mL (10 glasses) of liquid a day. Note that the fluid intake should be limited to 2 hours before bedtime to decrease the likelihood of nocturia.

Endocrine Changes

During the aging process, the following changes occur in the endocrine system:

- Slowing of metabolism
- Alteration in pancreatic activity
- Decreased blood levels of growth hormone, estrogen, and testosterone

As a person ages, the number of hormonal receptors in the adrenal and thyroid glands decreases. Thus, the person's ability to respond effectively to stress is diminished. Aging is associated with altered functioning of the pancreas; there is an increased level of insulin and circulating glucose.

The major changes of aging that affect men are enlargement of the prostate gland (benign hypertrophy) and decreased reserves of testosterone. The age-related changes for women include a loss of elasticity in breast tissue with resultant sagging of the breasts, decreased size of the uterus and fallopian tubes, and decreased motility in fallopian tubes.

The nurse must provide information about the normal changes associated with aging. It is also necessary to listen in a nonjudgmental manner when clients discuss their concerns about the physical changes.

Reproductive and Sexual Changes

To promote discussion of sexuality, it is important for the nurse to adopt an understanding and accepting attitude.

Sensitivity to verbal and nonverbal cues will also promote the client's expression of concerns. The nurse must not assume that the older client is heterosexual, sexually inactive, or uninterested in sex (Figure 19-3). It is important to recognize older clients as sexual beings and to provide privacy to promote intimacy. See the accompanying Respecting Our Differences display, on page 364, for a listing of age-related changes in sexual responses in older adults.

Older adults who are sexually active may need education about sexually transmitted diseases (STDs), including AIDS. This is one learning need that is frequently overlooked in health promotion for older people.

When caring for clients of either gender, the nurse should teach about the effects of aging on reproduction and sexuality. It is important that nurses use a nonjudgmental approach when clients discuss sexual issues.

CHANGES IN MEN As men age, the testes become softer and smaller as a result of decreased concentration of testosterone in the bloodstream. The production of sperm is inhibited or decreased, and ejaculations are less forceful. Sexual dysfunction increases in prevalence with aging; however, it is not an inevitable result of the aging process. Several factors contribute to the possible development of erectile dysfunction (ED), also referred to as impotence. Some factors that contribute to ED in older men are anemia, diabetes, hypertension, and medications.

CHANGES IN WOMEN Older women experience a decline in serum levels of estrogen. As a result, the vaginal walls thin and vaginal secretions decrease. The vulva and external genitalia shrink because of loss of subcutaneous body fat. Postmenopausal changes, such as vaginal dryness, may cause the woman to experience pain during intercourse. The nurse needs to explain that using water-soluble lubricants helps relieve the pain and discomfort that may occur during intercourse.

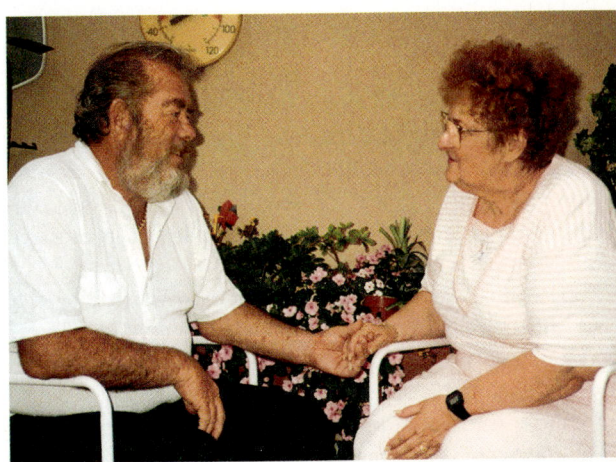

FIGURE 19-3 Older adults need companionship, as intimacy and sexuality remain important throughout the entire life span.
DELMAR/CENGAGE LEARNING

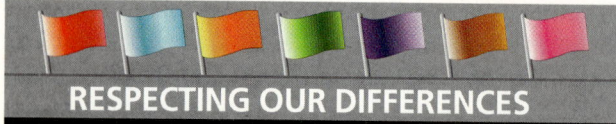

RESPECTING OUR DIFFERENCES

Age-Related Changes in Sexual Responses

Women

- Nipple erections during sexual excitement may last several hours postorgasm.
- Orgasms are usually unchanged, except that vaginal contractions may be of shorter duration.
- Vaginal lubrication is decreased.
- Urinary frequency and urgency occur after intercourse.
- Clitoral response to stimulation is the same as in youth.
- Skin is less flushed due to superficial vasocongestive skin response.

Men

- It takes longer to achieve an erection.
- More direct physical stimulation is required for erection.
- Erection is more readily lost after interruption.
- There is an increased ability to prolong time before ejaculation.
- Ejaculation may be less forceful or may not occur.
- Orgasm is similar to that experienced in youth.
- Less flushing of skin occurs.

Data from Dowdall, S. M., Taplay, K., Flores-Vela, A., & Maville, J. A. (2007). Promoting health in the older adult. In J. A. Maville & C. G. Huerta (Eds.), *Health promotion in nursing* (2nd ed.). Clifton Park, NY: Delmar Cengage Learning; Kautz, D. D. (2006). Appreciating diversity and enhancing intimacy. In K. L. Mauk (Ed.), *Gerontological nursing: Competencies for cure.* Boston: Jones & Bartlett.

Musculoskeletal Changes

Many people experience a decrease in height as they age. Long bones take on a disproportionate size, and many older people assume a stooped posture. These postural changes occur primarily as a result of calcium loss from bone, creating osteoporosis and kyphosis. These conditions are more common in women than in men and are implicated in estrogen loss that occurs with aging.

Ligaments, tendons, and joints are also affected by age. They show results of collagen loss and become thicker, more rigid, less flexible, and predisposed to tears. Cartilage wears down around the joints, making flexion painful. Walking and a consistent exercise pattern can promote function and prevent the disabling effects of many of these changes (Ebersole et al., 2007).

The nurse should instruct women about the importance of calcium consumption. Foods with a high calcium content include dairy products and green leafy vegetables. Encourage

exercise, especially walking, to promote flexibility and perform passive range-of-motion exercises for those who need it. It is essential to teach safety measures, including fall prevention measures, to both clients and caregivers.

Integumentary Changes

Older adults frequently experience dry, wrinkled, flaccid skin. This is an expected condition that occurs with aging because the skin loses many of the properties that help make it appear youthful. It takes approximately 20 days for epidermal cells to be replaced in a young person, whereas in the older adult, this process takes about 30 days. Therefore, it takes longer for an older client's wounds to heal. Because of collagen loss, the skin of an older person loses its ability to stretch, and thus tears more easily. Loss of subcutaneous fat, moisture content of the skin, and elastic fibers causes the older person's skin to wrinkle, dry, and sag, leading to the development of elongated ears, jowls, and double chin. If the client has had years of sun exposure, skin drying is accelerated. For the aging smoker, dehydration of the skin is further exacerbated.

The development of **lentigo senilis** (brown pigmented areas on the face, hands, and arms of older people) can cause older adults concern over their appearance. Sometimes called liver spots or age spots, these colorations are benign. Some cosmetic agents may lighten or almost eliminate these spots.

Skin appendages (hair and nails) also undergo changes associated with aging. Hair loses its original color as the production of melanin decreases, turning it gray and, eventually, white. Hair also tends to thin, both on the head and elsewhere on the body. Nails thicken and become more brittle. Care of the toenails often becomes a problem for many older people because they may not have the flexibility to reach their feet easily. Referrals to a podiatrist may be necessary for an older person to receive adequate care of the toenails.

As a person ages, the number of sweat glands decreases; this decrease can result in heat exhaustion. The decreased amount of subcutaneous fat may lead to increased susceptibility to cold.

The accompanying Client Teaching Checklist on page 365 provides guidelines for dealing with integumentary changes. Some older clients will have body image changes as a result of these visible signs of aging. The nurse must assess for body image alterations. If the client has an altered body image, it may be appropriate to:

- Assist with grooming as necessary.
- Use photographs of client to help adjust to changing appearance.
- Use touch to help clarify body boundaries.

Alterations in Mental Status

Alterations in mental status that occur with aging can be mild and have little impact on a client's functioning, or they can be severe and require the older adult to have assistance in managing psychosocial and physical needs. The nurse must understand the types of cognitive deficits and their impact on the client's health status.

✔ CLIENT TEACHING CHECKLIST

Responding to the Older Adult's Integumentary Alterations

- Instruct client to avoid excessive use of soap, hot water, and brisk rubbing when bathing.
- Teach client to pat skin dry instead of briskly rubbing.
- Inform client of the need to use tepid bathwater.
- Use lotion for itching and dryness.
- Use a humidifier to help reduce dryness.
- Avoid prolonged pressure on bony prominences.
- Protect the skin from temperature extremes.
- Protect skin from sun exposure (wear protective clothing, hats, and sunglasses, and use sunblock with a high sun protection factor [SPF]).
- Soak nails in water before trimming.
- Dress appropriately for weather and climate.

Acute confusion is a state of diminished awareness and attention, usually with a short duration (hours to weeks). The level of confusion often varies according to the time of day, worsening at night; this may cause sleep pattern disturbances. The individual is usually unaware of the setting, time of day, or day of the week and needs frequent reorientation to reality. Acute confusion occurs as a result of many conditions, many of which are reversible with appropriate treatment. Dehydration, infection, trauma, and medications may result in acute states of confusion.

Some individuals with dementia experience chronic confusion, usually of a long duration (months to years). Individuals with dementia may exhibit personality changes, difficulty with sequential speech and thoughts, and a lack of orientation to reality. Alzheimer's disease is a type of dementia that causes numerous deficits, including diminished intellectual abilities, confusion, and impaired judgment.

Depression is an altered state of mood that lasts at least 6 weeks. Individuals suffering from depression typically are alert and oriented to their environment but are characterized by exaggerated sadness, apathy, and preoccupation with negative thoughts. Table 19-3, on page 366, offers guidelines for differentiating acute confusion, dementia, delirium, and depression in older adults. Many people believe that it is normal for older adults to become sad and withdrawn. This is a false assumption that leads to lack of diagnosis and treatment of a serious health problem. Late-life depression can be successfully treated if it is not dismissed as an inevitable part of the aging process.

PSYCHOSOCIAL CHANGES

The multitude of physical changes that occur with aging are accompanied by numerous psychosocial changes. Major life events such as retirement, changes in social relationships and roles, changes in living arrangements, and dealing with loss are usually experienced during the later years of life and can affect an individual's health status and outlook on life.

Retirement

An individual's view of retirement is a product of many factors, including overall life attitude, support of significant others, financial status, and personal expectations. For individuals who, during their adult years, defined themselves and their success according to their work contributions, retirement is likely to produce feelings of uneasiness and anxiety. An individual who views retirement as the end of the productive years will dread the change in life pattern and social status and may fear being a burden to others, both socially and financially.

Many adults, though, look forward to retirement as their reward for years of hard work and contributions and fill their days with activities, travel, hobbies, and interests that time constraints had prohibited them from pursuing during their earlier years (see Figure 19-4). These individuals typically led more balanced lives during their working years, viewing their value as a combination of many factors including work, family, and community involvement; they adjust more easily to the loss of employment status by balancing this change with other positive aspects of their lives. The transition to retirement involves two major challenges: adjustment to the loss of the work role and the social ties of work (van Solinge & Henkens, 2008). Individuals who have planned for retirement and made arrangements (financial, housing, social) ahead of time tend to adjust more readily to this change in work status.

Social Relationships and Roles

Relationships and roles change over time as an individual grows and develops. For the older adult, these changes may

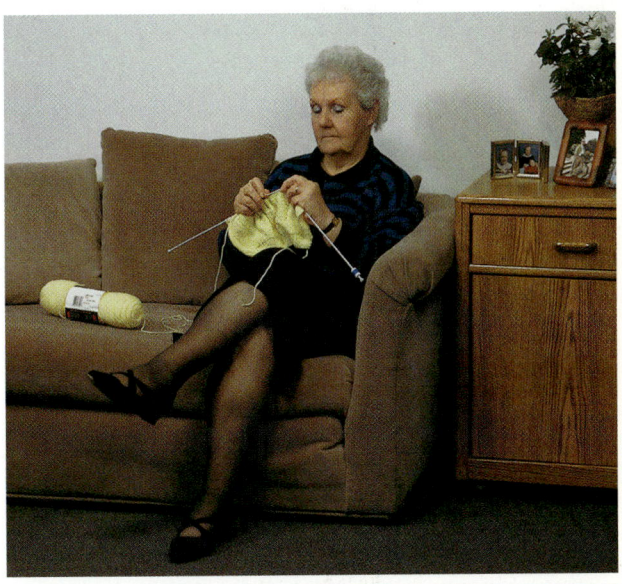

FIGURE 19-4 Retirement often means having time to develop new hobbies or interests. DELMAR/CENGAGE LEARNING

TABLE 19-3 Distinguishing Acute Confusion, Delirium, Dementia, and Depression

PARAMETER	ACUTE CONFUSION	DELIRIUM	DEMENTIA	DEPRESSION
Definition	Inability to think with usual clarity, speed, and coherence	Perceptual disorder characterized by heightened awareness, hallucinations, vivid dreams, and intense emotional outbursts	Deterioration of all cognitive functions with little or no disturbance of consciousness or perception	Altered emotional state characterized by feelings of intense sadness, helplessness, and hopelessness
Onset	Variable	Sudden	Gradual	Variable
Duration	Reversible	Reversible	Irreversible	Reversible
Pathophysiology	• Metabolic disorders • Toxic substances • Cerebrovascular accident (CVA) • Trauma • Febrile states • Medications	• Drug intoxications • Withdrawal from alcohol and other drugs • Encephalitis • Trauma • Febrile states • Hypoxia • Fluid and electrolyte imbalance	• Alzheimer's disease • Metabolic disorders • CVA • Head injury	• Neurochemical abnormalities • Significant loss • Chronic disease • CVA • Medications
Attention	Impaired: dulled	Impaired: heightened or dulled	Impaired	Intact
Memory	• Short term: impaired • Long term: may be impaired	• Short term: impaired • Long term: intact	• Short term: impaired first • Long term: intact until disease progresses to later stages	• Variable, depending on the ability to concentrate
Judgment	• Impaired	• Grossly impaired • Impulsive • Volatile	• Impaired	• Impaired
Insight	Impaired	Impaired	Impaired	Impaired
Spatial perception	May be impaired	Intact	Impaired	Intact
Thought process and content	Impaired, incoherent	Impaired, hallucinations	Impaired	Intact

Delmar/Cengage Learning

take on even more meaning because activities and involvement in other areas of life may change or diminish. One study (Radina, Lynch, Stalp, & Manning, 2008) suggests that belonging to groups, such as social clubs, provides connections and prevents social isolation. Club membership offers older people the opportunity to obtain instrumental and social support. Changes in relationships and roles typically occur in conjunction with major life events, such as marriage, divorce, birth, death, relocation, and change in employment status. For instance, the older adult who has been a husband for 40 years will find his life and his roles greatly changed when

he becomes a widower. The birth of his children's children will bring him new status as a grandparent, and his retirement will remove him from the full-time workforce and present opportunities for the development of new relationships.

A key to successful aging is staying connected to others. One way in which many older adults maintain connections is by volunteering. Several studies (Ayalon, 2008; Hao, 2008; Piliavin & Siegl, 2008; Windsor, Anstey, & Rodgers, 2008) suggest a strong relationship between volunteerism and well-being in older individuals. Volunteering is one way for older adults to add a sense of purpose and to establish social connections.

Another type of relationship that many older adults experience is grandparenthood. This relationship may be a source of pride and happiness, or it can become a negative stressor. For many older Americans, grandparenting has become a full-time responsibility, as they are the sole caretakers of grandchildren. Over 4.5 million families in the United States are maintained by grandparents (American Association of Retired Persons Foundation, 2007). Some grandparents who assume the role of rearing grandchildren experience anger about the extra responsibilities (Belsky, 2007). However, not all grandparents are overwhelmed by the role of childrearing for a second generation; many find it rewarding.

Following are some of the factors that have contributed to the increasing numbers of grandparents who are raising their grandchildren on a full-time basis:

- Divorce
- Unemployment
- Teen pregnancy
- Death of a grandchild's parent
- Abuse or neglect of the child
- Substance abuse

Nurses should be knowledgeable about potential areas of stress imposed by the additional responsibilities of the grandparenthood role. Also, knowledge of community resources is essential for appropriate referral. Some grandparents may also need information about current childhood problems that were not as prevalent when they were parenting their own offspring (e.g., cyberporn, school violence).

Living Arrangements

Advancing age often brings with it changes in living arrangements. Older people have many living options depending on income, health status, activity level, functional ability, level of independence, and family or other support systems; see Figure 19-5. A change in living arrangements is a significant event for any individual, but for older adults, this change may mean leaving family, friends, neighbors, and routines that have been a part of life for decades. Most older adults prefer to remain in their homes or dwellings, in a familiar environment and with familiar routines. In some cases, older adults may move in with their adult children and their families or have the adult children move in with them. The degree of physical, psychological, and financial independence of the older adult, and the status of the relationship with the children, will likely determine the success of this arrangement.

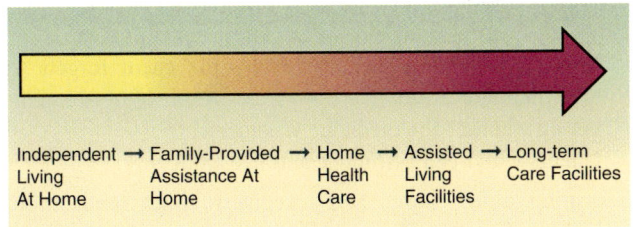

FIGURE 19-5 Continuum of Living Arrangements for Older Adults DELMAR/CENGAGE LEARNING

Older adults needing assistance to remain in their homes may take advantage of home care services, which provide assistance in the tasks of daily living, or day care services, which provide limited health and rehabilitation intervention. Assisted living facilities (ALFs) are a new option to help ease the transition between living independently at home and residing in a nursing home. Other options include foster care, group living arrangements, and hospice. When health needs necessitate extensive or full-time supervision and care, a long-term care facility (such as a nursing home) may be the best living option. Nursing homes offer a variety of services to support the medical, personal, and psychosocial needs of the aging client.

"Personal autonomy—the ability to make freely self-directed choices in one's life—is considered critical to an older person's quality of life" (Matsui & Capezuti, 2008, p. 141). Older adults who are able to participate in the decisions regarding their living arrangements generally adapt better to such changes than those who are unable to participate or are not involved in their care decisions. Nurses can enhance an older client's autonomy by encouraging independence, providing information, and working with the client's support system.

Coping with Loss

Loss is an inevitable part of life, and the longer a person lives, the more losses will be experienced. Losing a lifetime partner is one of the most stressful loss experiences an individual can face, and many older people will face loss through death of a spouse at some point in their lives. As the years pass, deaths of children and friends may leave older adults grieving and feeling as if everyone they have known and loved is gone. Feelings of isolation and hopelessness may arise; these can be compounded if the individual suffers multiple losses within a short period of time.

Individuals who feel isolated and abandoned often feel angry and hopeless. Helping older adults stay connected with others in the community is an effective intervention for those who are experiencing loss and resultant depression. Some avenues for helping older adults develop a social support system are churches, senior citizen centers, neighborhood and apartment associations, and community support groups. Often, loss will lead older clients to reflect on their lives and their relationships and to review their successes and shortcomings.

Nursing actions that promote a sense of hope in older adults include making time to involve the client in the discussion and asking about daily plans. It is imperative that nurses avoid expressing pity toward lonely older clients, as pity decreases hope and exacerbates the sense of loss. See the accompanying Spotlight On display on page 368.

MEDICATIONS AND THE OLDER ADULT

Many older adults take multiple medications for both acute and chronic conditions. As a result, nurses need to focus on

SPOTLIGHT ON...

Understanding the Meaning of Loss

Consider the perspective of an older client who has experienced the loss of loved ones, such as a spouse of 50 years or a child. How many losses of this magnitude have you experienced? Do you feel you will be able to relate to and show empathy to an older adult whose life experiences may differ dramatically from your own? What steps can you take to ensure that you treat these clients with dignity, respect, and compassion?

TABLE 19-4 Factors Affecting Pharmacokinetics in Older Clients

FACTOR	AGING-RELATED CHANGES
Absorption	• Increased gastric pH • Decreased gastrointestinal motility and gastrointestinal blood flow
Distribution	Decreased total body water, lean body mass, serum albumin, and body fat
Hepatic metabolism	Decreased liver size, liver blood flow, and enzyme activity
Renal clearance	Decreased renal blood flow, glomerular filtration, and tubular secretion
Excretion	Decreased creatinine clearance, increased half-life

Data from Cowely, J., Diebold, C., Gross, J. C., & Hardin-Fanning, F. (2006). Management of common problems. In K. L. Mauk (Ed.), *Gerontological nursing: Competencies for care.* Boston: Jones & Bartlett.

two major issues, response to medication and compliance, both of which are discussed in the following sections.

RESPONSES TO MEDICATION

The physiological changes of aging can complicate drug therapy in the older adult. For example, the normal effects of aging alter the body's metabolism and excretion of drugs. Therefore, older adults are more sensitive to both the toxic and therapeutic effects of medications. Another factor affecting the older person's drug use is **polypharmacy** (the concurrent use of several medications). Older adults take more medicine than those who are young, and as a result, they are at greater risk for adverse drug reactions (ADRs). The presence of multiple diseases and the use of several medications place the older person at risk. In addition to increased risk of an ADR, other problems associated with polypharmacy are:

- Medication errors
- Inappropriate prescribing
- Excessive drug costs
- Noncompliance

The symptoms of many ADRs are subtle and often are confused with the changes of aging or chronic illnesses. For example, confusion, constipation, fatigue, and dizziness are nonspecific symptoms of many conditions, including ADRs. The effectiveness of drug therapy in the older individual depends on the properties of the particular drug and the impact of age-related changes (Table 19-4).

The older client's response to drugs is highly individualized. Therefore, the nurse must accurately monitor the client for therapeutic effectiveness and signs of ADRs. See the accompanying Safety First display.

MEDICATION COMPLIANCE

In addition to assessing the client's responses to medications, the nurse also must assess the client's knowledge of medications being used. Knowledge about the medication, its intended effects, possible side effects, and how to alleviate the side effects can increase the client's compliance with the

▼ SAFETY FIRST ▼

MONITORING DRUG USE
Watch for nonspecific side effects, such as appetite disturbance, altered behavior, and falls. Many side effects of medication use are subtle and, therefore, not detected.

medication regimen. Factors that may negatively affect medication compliance are as follows:

- Complicated dosing schedules and regimens
- Multiple dosing throughout the day
- Polypharmacy
- Cost of drugs
- Limited mobility and range of motion (e.g., the client with arthritis who is unable to open childproof containers)
- Impaired memory (e.g., omission—the client forgets to take the medication; overdosing as a result of not remembering whether the medicine was taken)
- Clients who need assistance and live alone

Educating older clients and caregivers about medication, self-administration, and ways to increase compliance is a major nursing intervention. See the accompanying Nursing Checklist on page 369.

✔ NURSING CHECKLIST

Improving Medication Compliance

- Provide easily understood information about the medications.
- Schedule administration of the medication around certain activities of daily living as a reminder to the client.
- Provide the client with a name and telephone number of a person to contact when questions arise.
- Assess how the medications are stored and arranged in the client's home. Make sure the medication is accessible.
- Perform a complete drug history to determine all medications being taken. Instruct the client or caregiver to provide this information to the prescribing practitioner.
- Encourage client and caregiver to discuss any concerns regarding the medication.

SIGNS OF PHYSICAL MISTREATMENT

- Contusions
- Abrasions
- Sprains
- Burns
- Bruising
- Human bite marks
- Sexual molestation
- Untreated but previously treated conditions
- Misuse of medications
- Depression
- Erratic hair loss from hair pulling
- Lacerations
- Fractures
- Dislocations
- Oversedation
- Over- or undermedication
- Welts
- Scratches
- Decubiti
- Dehydration
- Malnutrition
- Freezing
- Poor hygiene
- Head and face injuries (especially orbital fracture, black eyes, broken teeth)

Data from Fontaine, K. L. (2009). Persons at risk for violence. In C. R. Kneisl & E. Trigoboff (Eds.), *Contemporary psychiatric-mental health nursing* (2nd ed.). Upper Saddle River, NJ: Pearson Prentice Hall; Wallace, M. (2006). Older adult. In C. L. Edelman & C. L. Mandle (Eds.), *Health promotion throughout the lifespan* (6th ed.). St. Louis, MO: Elsevier.

MISTREATMENT OF THE OLDER ADULT

Mistreatment of the older adult (elder abuse) is a serious and ever-increasing problem and disturbing trend. Approximately 1 out of 20 older adults is abused each year in the United States (Dowdall et al., 2007). There are many forms of abuse, including:

- *Physical abuse*—willful infliction of injury
- *Neglect*—withholding goods or services (such as food, attention) to the detriment of the older person's physical or mental health
- *Psychological abuse*—withholding affection or imposing social isolation
- *Exploitation*—dishonest or inappropriate use of the older person's property, money, or other resources

Nurses in the home, clinic, hospital emergency department, and long-term care settings are often the first to identify signs of mistreatment in older people; see the accompanying display on signs of physical mistreatment. Abused older adults may either cling to or act in a very guarded manner toward the abuser. Another indicator of possible abuse is vague explanations offered for the cause of the injuries. Psychosocial indicators of abuse may be anger and rage, depression, anxiety, and conflictual interactions between the older adult and the abuser.

When assessing for mistreatment, the nurse must be nonjudgmental and avoid any signs of disapproval that may evoke further feelings of anger or shame in the older client. A private setting should be used for interviewing to promote disclosure; if the older victim thinks the perpetrator is able to hear the interview, the victim may withhold information or refuse to talk. It is essential that the interview findings be documented in an accurate and unbiased manner.

Nursing interventions for the abused older client are primary, secondary, and tertiary. Primary intervention strategies emphasize prevention. Secondary nursing interventions consist of early identification and prompt treatment to minimize the long-term effects of the abuse. Tertiary interventions occur after the abuse and promote recovery and rehabilitation. Tertiary interventions are restorative in nature.

If the nurse suspects abuse or neglect, this concern should first be addressed with the client. Many abused older adults may not admit to abuse because of embarrassment and fear of reprisal. Most states and many local governments have an Adult Protective Services program. Nurses are responsible for knowing the local statues on mandatory reporting of abuse, as these laws may vary.

NURSING PROCESS AND THE OLDER ADULT

An ever-increasing number of nurses will provide care to older clients. Client education is a major nursing intervention that helps people change their behavior in order to take advantage of increased longevity. Some areas in which older adults need to develop health-promoting behaviors are nutrition, exercise, and the use of health screenings. Increasing numbers of gerontological nurses are needed to provide quality of care. Professional standards for gerontological nurses were developed by the American Nurses Association in 1995 and revised in 2001. These standards are addressed in the next section.

ASSESSMENT

The data-gathering phase of assessment begins with the first encounter with the older adult client. Overall appearance, dress, gait, presentation, and general behavior can be noted during the first meeting with a client. Assessment of the older client can be a time-consuming yet rewarding process when the nurse works thoughtfully and sensitively with the client in order to discover strengths, resources, and limitations.

When interviewing the older client in the home, it is important to also include the client's caregivers in the assessment. The home care nurse assesses:

- Family interactions
- Caregiver motivation to participate in the rehabilitation process
- The motivational impact of the caregivers on the older person to accept some control over his or her own care
- Feelings of caregivers toward their role (i.e., level of satisfaction or burnout)

Health History

Older adults are not only individuals of age and vintage, but also individuals with a long history that deserves telling. The nurse's role in conducting a health history with the older client is to draw out facts and interpretations from the client that will shed light on current health status and health concerns. Eliciting these data requires time and patience on the part of both nurse and client, but it can be a rewarding and interesting process. To gather pertinent health data, the nurse may interview the client and the client's support members to determine the client's past coping strategies, strengths, and health habits. A holistic approach will include discussion of physical, emotional, psychological, spiritual, and sociocultural aspects that contribute to the client's overall health. The nurse respects the client's dignity and independence during the interview process by facing the client, speaking directly to the client in a clear manner, and reacting appropriately to client concerns and needs.

Physical Examination

The nurse must be knowledgeable about the normal changes of aging in order to conduct an accurate physical examination of the older client. The physical changes must be noted; the impact these changes have on the client's quality of life and activities of daily living (ADL) must also be determined. The assessment tools may need to be adjusted to the older person's abilities and limitations. For instance, the physical examination may need to be performed in more than one session to prevent client fatigue. Client positioning may need to be adjusted according to client comfort. The client may need assistance with disrobing or position changes, and the

nurse must always be alert to protect the client from potential injury, such as falls.

NURSING DIAGNOSIS

Nursing diagnoses developed from assessment of older clients will be as varied as the clients themselves. Nurses must keep in mind that older clients may present with many needs, both physical and psychosocial, and that the nursing diagnoses will need to be prioritized. Client status may change frequently, so reevaluation of nursing diagnoses on a regular basis is warranted. Selected nursing diagnoses (North American Nursing Diagnosis Association International, 2009) that are frequently seen in older clients include:

- Physical
  - *Impaired physical mobility* related to intolerance to activity or decreased strength and endurance; pain or discomfort; perceptual/cognitive impairment; neuromuscular impairment; musculoskeletal impairment; depression or severe anxiety
  - *Activity intolerance* related to bed rest or immobility; generalized weakness; sedentary lifestyle
  - *Dressing/grooming self-care deficit* related to intolerance to activity; decreased strength and endurance; physical, perceptual, or cognitive impairment
- Psychosocial
  - *Impaired social interaction* related to absence of supportive significant others; alterations in physical appearance; alterations in mental status; inadequate personal resources
  - *Risk for loneliness:* risk factors include affectional deprivation; physical isolation; social isolation
  - *Ineffective role performance* related to change in self-perception of role; change in physical capacity to resume role; change in usual patterns of responsibility
  - *Impaired home maintenance* related to disease or injury; insufficient finances; impaired cognitive or emotional functioning; inadequate support systems
  - *Acute confusion* related to age; dementia; alcohol abuse; drug abuse; delirium

OUTCOME IDENTIFICATION AND PLANNING

Outcomes must be developed and individualized for each client. Outcomes identified in the plan of care must be developed in partnership with the older client and the client's support system. Outcomes should be realistic for the client's current status and desired goals and should be targeted to maintaining a certain level of health or restoring the client to a former state of health. See the accompanying Client Teaching Checklist, on page 371, for a discussion of a teaching plan for an older client.

IMPLEMENTATION

Nursing interventions for the older client will typically focus on the areas of maintaining physical health, supporting

☑ CLIENT TEACHING CHECKLIST

Teaching Plans for Older Adults

When developing a teaching plan:

- Plan for a quiet, private environment that is conducive to learning.
- Assess the client's readiness to learn as well as previous knowledge.
- Treat the client as a partner whose input is valuable in the planning and outcome identification process.
- Assess sensory status, especially sight and hearing, and adjust actions according to client needs.
- Use language that is clear and easy to understand.
- Encourage clients to ask questions and verbalize their understanding of what is being taught. For instance, state, "I want you to feel free to ask questions; all your questions are important."
- Plan to include the family and significant others in the teaching session, not as a substitute for the client, but for support and reinforcement.
- Plan for active learning experiences (e.g., use examples, simulations, games, and audiovisuals when appropriate).
- Pace the learning. Do not give too much information at one time, and progress at the individual's learning pace. Stop if you see that the client is distracted or fatigued.
- Plan to summarize and reinforce what has been taught.

☑ NURSING CHECKLIST

Communicating with Older Clients

- Get the client's attention before you speak.
- Minimize environmental stimuli.
- Sit directly facing the client and maintain eye contact.
- Speak slowly and clearly.
- Use short, simple sentences.
- Give the client time to respond.
- Speak loudly enough for the client to hear you, but avoid yelling.

- Promotes ability to attain perspective and find meaning (Trigoboff, 2009)

See the accompanying Spotlight On display.

Maintain Physical Health

During the assessment phase, the nurse will identify which physical changes are the result of normal aging and which have underlying pathology. Clients will need to be educated as to what these changes mean, what impact they may have on daily activities, and what strategies can be used to meet needs. It is critical to emphasize clients' assets and abilities, instead of focusing on limitations, in order to maintain a healthy self-concept and to show clients how much independence they still maintain.

Specific interventions related to the physical changes of aging will depend on the nature of the alterations. For instance, skin changes such as dryness, wrinkling, or flaccidity can be partially overcome through the use of oils, moisturizers, and a humidifier. If deteriorating eyesight is a problem, nurses should instruct the client to avoid reading when fatigued, to use large-print materials, and to ensure that the reading environment is well lit with an overhead light and desk lamp that do not create glare. If cardiovascular changes result in fatigue and shortness of breath on exertion, nurses should help clients learn the signs indicating their activity tolerance level and to adjust activity accordingly (e.g., plan for

psychosocial well-being, promoting safety, and providing restorative care. Three major interventions used effectively with older adults are education, communication, and life review. See Chapter 21 for specific guidelines for teaching older clients. The Nursing Checklist provides information on communicating effectively with older adults.

Life review (reminiscence therapy) is a structured intervention in which the nurse guides the client through remembrance of life, stage by stage. This intervention is especially therapeutic for clients who feel alienated and depressed, as it helps people develop a sense of meaning and promotes achievement of the sense of integrity identified by Erikson (1968). Some of the therapeutic outcomes of reminiscence are that it:

- Provides an outlet for catharsis ("getting things off one's chest")
- Assists in resolving conflicts
- Maximizes long-term memory when short-term memory is impaired
- Maintains identity and self-esteem

👁 SPOTLIGHT ON...

Compassion

As the nurse manager of a nursing home, you want to establish a program to encourage clients to engage in life review. You decide to conduct a weekly class for interested residents who want to share their life experiences. How would you prepare for the class? What agenda would you establish? How would you evaluate the effectiveness of the class?

frequent rest periods, sit or lie down when fatigued, avoid carrying heavy parcels when ambulating).

Support Psychosocial Well-Being

An older client's psychosocial health is as important as physical well-being. The use of touch and therapeutic communication helps the client overcome feelings of isolation and enhances a positive self-concept. Encouraging the older adult to be active in social groups, leisure activities, and hobbies supports a higher level of self-esteem and pleasure with life and helps the client to focus on positive traits and abilities.

The client's significant others can have a major impact on maintaining the client's psychosocial functioning. They can assist the client in maintaining a relatively independent lifestyle and may be able to help the client sustain ADL outside of an institutional environment. For clients without support systems, teaching how to cope with alterations in mental status (e.g., using calendars to orient to reality, reading the daily paper to keep aware of current events) and how to work within those parameters can help clients maintain a sense of independence and dignity.

Promote a Safe Environment

Many environmental factors may negatively affect an older person's safety, including:

- Decreased visual acuity
- Poor vision in dimly lit areas
- Less foot and toe lift when walking
- Altered center of gravity
- Slower reflexes
- Impaired muscle control
- Orthostatic hypotension (blood pressure related to posture)
- Urinary frequency (Ebersole et al., 2007)

Ongoing assessment includes observing the client's immediate environment for safety. This is especially critical for clients who will be remaining in a home situation where they, not the health care staff, are responsible for maintaining a safe environment. Significant others should be included in the efforts to create a safe environment for the older client (see Figure 19-6).

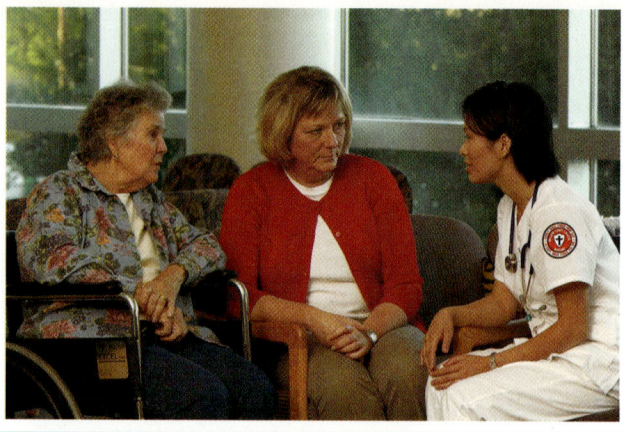

FIGURE 19-6 Educating the older client and family is an essential nursing function that is facilitated by the use of clear step-by-step instructions. DELMAR/CENGAGE LEARNING

Falls are a major safety issue with many older adults. See Chapter 29 for additional information on safety and preventing falls.

In order to promote a safe home environment for the older client, the nurse may suggest the following environmental actions:

- Provide adequate nonglare lighting.
- Place night-lights in bedroom, bathroom, and hall.
- Install slip-proof mats in tub and shower.
- Place a chair in tub and shower.
- Install grab bars in tub and shower, and next to toilet.
- Have handrails next to stairs and in long hallways.
- Use sturdy chairs with armrests.

Over the past 20 years, the older population has had an increased crime victimization rate. According to the U.S. Department of Justice (2008), property crime is the major type of attack on people over age 65. Older people are often easy targets for car theft, robbery, and burglary. Nurses can educate older clients on protecting themselves from crime by reminding them to lock doors and windows at home, install an alarm system, have income checks deposited directly into the bank, and be alert for false claims of "miracle cures" to health problems.

NURSING CARE PLAN

An Older Adult Who Is Confused

CASE PRESENTATION

Winston Evans, an 82-year-old man, is a retired grocer who was widowed 6 years ago. Until last year, Mr. Evans lived alone in a small home, was involved with his family, went to church regularly, and enjoyed socializing with peers at the community senior center. He now lives in his daughter's home. His daughter brings him to the clinic today, stating, "We can't go on like this! Last night he walked out of the house and was missing for hours. The policeman brought him home while we were looking for him." This is Mr. Evans's

(Continues)

NURSING CARE PLAN (Continued)

fourth episode of wandering within the past 3 months. The daughter also states that Mr. Evans is unable to take care of himself. "I have to feed and bathe him every day." Mr. Evans is unable to state the date, day of week, month, or year. He also does not know where he is, even though he has been treated by the nurse practitioner (NP) for several years at the clinic. He cannot remember the names of any family members except his daughter. He is observed by the NP to be restless, and his speech is rambling and confused. Mr. Evans tells the NP, "Get away from me. No one's gonna hurt me." His medical diagnosis is severe arthritis, glaucoma, and congestive heart failure. He weighs 115 pounds (a weight loss of 24 pounds over the past 4 months). He "picks at his food," is constipated, sleeps most of the day, and is usually loud and restless at night. During the assessment, Mr. Evans is agitated and cries out several times, "Help me, help me!"

ASSESSMENT
- Disoriented
- Forgetful
- Restless
- Paranoid
- Wandering behavior
- Insomnia
- Decreased appetite
- Constipation

NURSING DIAGNOSIS 1: *Risk for injury* related to confused mental status
NOC: Risk control
NIC: Environmental management

EXPECTED OUTCOME
Mr. Evans will be free from injury to himself or others.

INTERVENTIONS/RATIONALES
1. Approach in a calm, nonthreatening manner. To decrease anxiety level, which impairs mental status.
2. Determine the presence of personal or environmental risk factors. Identification of safety hazards is the first step in minimizing such hazards.
3. Orient Mr. Evans regularly to his environment. To decrease client's frustration level and better understand client needs.
4. Closely supervise Mr. Evans at night to assess safety. To determine which risk factors are present and what safety measures should be implemented.
5. Set limits on self-destructive behavior. To promote safety of client and others.
6. Monitor judgment, decision-making ability, and impulse control. Impaired judgment and impulsivity increase the likelihood of unsafe behaviors.
7. Minimize specific hazards in the home (e.g., remove stove knobs, store cleaning products and medications in a locked area, clear floor and hallway of obstacles). To make the home environment safer.
8. Keep night-lights on at night. To decrease the potential for falls.
9. Provide an ID bracelet for Mr. Evans to wear at home, and participate in local police registry if available. To increase possibility of client's quick return to home if he wanders away.
10. Instruct family to install an alarm system on all exit doors. To minimize the possibility of wandering.

EVALUATION
Goal met. Mr. Evans remains free from physical injury and does not injure anyone else. He has not wandered off alone in the past week.

(Continues)

NURSING CARE PLAN (Continued)

NURSING DIAGNOSIS 2: *Sleep deprivation* related to altered mental status
NOC: Sleep
NIC: Environmental management

EXPECTED OUTCOME
Mr. Evans will experience at least 4 hours of uninterrupted sleep at night.

INTERVENTIONS/RATIONALES
1. Monitor and keep a record of sleep patterns. To determine a baseline for future evaluation of progress or lack of progress.
2. Minimize daytime napping. Older adults need less sleep, so daytime napping only subtracts from amount of sleep occurring at night.
3. Schedule exercise 2 hours prior to scheduled bedtime. To provide relaxation.
4. Teach simple relaxation techniques. Keeping instructions simple helps the client who is confused to better absorb the information. Relaxation techniques can be used to promote sleep.
5. Limit caffeine intake. Caffeine exerts an energizing effect and thus can interfere with sleep.
6. Ensure quiet environment with a soft night-light. To promote relaxation and a sense of comfort.
7. Provide comfort measures and teach such measures to family. The use of back rubs and rearranging linens can promote comfort and relaxation.

EVALUATION
Goal partially met. Family reports that Mr. Evans is sleeping every night in approximately 3-hour intervals.

NURSING DIAGNOSIS 3: *Bathing/hygiene self-care deficit* related to cognitive impairment
NOC: Self-care: Activities of daily living (ADL)
NIC: Self-care: Assistance: Bathing/hygiene

EXPECTED OUTCOME
Mr. Evans will perform ADL with optimal independence.

INTERVENTIONS/RATIONALES
1. Monitor ability to perform ADL. To determine the client's level of functional ability and the amount of assistance that is needed.
2. Encourage client to perform the skills that are present. To prevent functional disuse and to promote independence and self-esteem.
3. If necessary, give step-by-step directions in clear simple terms with only one step at a time. Breaking a task down into small segments increases the likelihood of successful completion.
4. Instruct family to purchase clothing (or modify existing wardrobe) with Velcro fasteners instead of buttons and zippers. Decreases amount of effort client must expend to dress himself appropriately without assistance.

EVALUATION
Goal partially met. Mr. Evans is able to dress himself if the clothes are laid out by someone else. He follows step-by-step directions but is unable to initiate or complete the task alone.

From Carpenito, J. L. (2007). *Handbook of nursing diagnosis* (12th ed.). Philadelphia: Lippincott, Williams & Wilkins; Doenges, M. E., Moorhouse, M. F., & Geissler, A. C. (2006). *Nursing care plans: Guidelines for individualizing patient care* (7th ed.). Philadelphia: F. A. Davis; North American Nursing Diagnosis Association International. (2009). *Nursing diagnoses: Definitions and classification, 2009–2011*. Philadelphia: Author.

Restorative Care

Restorative nursing care (also referred to as rehabilitative care) seeks to assist the client in regaining maximal functional ability. Restorative care is provided to clients who have residual impairment from disease or injury in order to increase the client's independence. Nurses providing restorative care understand that sometimes the impairment in functional ability will remain. In such cases, the goal is to help the client function at the maximal level possible. Nurses constantly balance the client's need for dependence with the need for independence. In other words, nurses provide care as needed while encouraging the client to do for himself or herself as much as possible. Restorative care is provided in home health, assisted living, and long-term care facilities (e.g., nursing homes).

See the Nursing Checklist for interventions most useful in providing restorative care. Nurses need to be especially alert in monitoring follow-up care for seniors living in poverty. "Low-income seniors frequently have more multiple chronic medical conditions for which they often fail to receive the recommended standard of care" (Counsell et al., 2007, p. 2673); see the Uncovering the Evidence display.

EVALUATION

Evaluation is a major determinant of the need for continuing care of older clients. The nurse must decide whether the original assessment is still pertinent and if its

---

UNCOVERING THE
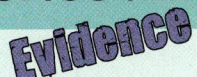

TITLE OF STUDY
"Geriatric Care Management for Low-Income Seniors: A Randomized Controlled Trial"

AUTHORS
S. R. Counsell, C. M. Callahan, D. O. Clark, W. Tu, A. B. Buttar, T. E. Stump, and G. D. Ricketts

PURPOSE
To test the effectiveness of a geriatric care management model on improving the quality of primary care for low-income older adults.

METHODS
This controlled clinical trial was conducted on 952 adults 65 years or older with an annual income below poverty level. One group of study participants received 2 years of home-based management care provided by a nurse practitioner (NP) and social worker. The control group received no home-based management care from the NP and social worker.

FINDINGS
Data analysis reveals significant improvements for the clients who received the intervention. The improvements occurred in four areas: general health, vitality, social functioning, and mental health.

IMPLICATIONS
Home-based geriatric care leads to improved quality of care and better quality of life for elderly low-income persons.

Counsell, S. R., Callahan, C. M., Clark, D. O., Tu, W., Buttar, A. B., Stump, T. E., et al. (2007). Geriatric care management for low-income seniors: A randomized controlled trial. *Journal of the American Medical Association, 298*(22), 2673–2674.

✓ NURSINGCHECKLIST

Guidelines for Providing Restorative Care

- Encourage independence.
- Use a positive, reassuring approach.
- Be alert to limitations and client-expressed need for help.
- Encourage client decision making.
- Communicate with words easily understood by clients. Ask clients to repeat directions in order to assess their comprehension.
- Provide positive reinforcement often.
- Use repetition through words and actions (i.e., demonstration).
- Provide rest periods as needed.
- Ensure client safety by safeguarding against injury at all times.

---

accompanying diagnoses have been resolved. New diagnoses need to be established on the basis of client progress and changing needs. New goals must be developed in order to foster maximum health status based on the client's abilities and capabilities to provide continuity of care. The nurse should consider the ongoing needs of the client and offer resources or make referrals to ensure that the health and well-being of the client will continue to be monitored and enhanced.

KEY CONCEPTS

- Persons in the late adulthood years are often classified as "young-old" (those between 65 and 75); "middle-old" (those between 75 and 85); and "old" (those 85 and older).

- Biological theories of aging state that the physical changes of aging are universal and inevitable.

- Psychosocial theories of aging consider factors other than genetics when describing the aging process.

- Numerous myths about aging can be viewed as ageism, which is stereotyping and discrimination based on age.

- Advances in medicine and technology have greatly improved life expectancy as well as the quality of life for the older adult.

- Developmental tasks of the older adult include enhancing skills, gaining and sharing wisdom, renewing relationships, expanding knowledge, and adjusting to losses and change.

- The multiple physical changes associated with aging can have a profound impact on an older adult's functional ability and performance of ADL.

- Retirement, changes in social relationships, changes in living arrangements, and loss may affect an older client's self-esteem and lead to feelings of isolation.

- Individuals who have had a positive outlook on the aging process over the years tend to adapt better to life changes than do individuals who fear or do not understand the aging process.

- Physical assessment of the older client will need to be tailored to the client's functional level and activity tolerance.

- Including significant others in planning and implementing care for older clients enhances achievement of outcomes.

- Restorative nursing care (also referred to as rehabilitative care) seeks to assist the client in regaining maximal functional ability.

- Restorative care is provided to clients who have residual impairment as a result of disease or injury; it aims to increase the client's ability to perform self-care independently.

- Safety is a primary concern when caring for older clients; this can be addressed through comprehensive assessment and through client and family teaching.

REVIEW QUESTIONS

1. The nurse is administering medications to an older client. Which of the following is most important for the nurse to assess in order to prevent drug toxicity?
   a. Central nervous system function
   b. Genitourinary system function
   c. Renal function
   d. Thyroid function

2. A female client says to the nurse, "I just don't think I can go on. It's too much for me to raise my grandchildren." Which of the following nursing responses is most therapeutic?
   a. "How could your daughter abandon her children?"
   b. "I think your grandchildren are very lucky to have you care for them."
   c. "Many people your age are raising grandchildren, and they do just fine."
   d. "You sound overwhelmed. Let's look at some options for you."

3. A resident of a nursing home says to the nurse, "Most of the other people here are much older than I am, and a lot of them are sicker than I am. Is that what I have to look forward to?" Which of the following is the most therapeutic nursing response?
   a. "Every resident is here for a different reason."
   b. "Everyone ages at his or her own rate."

   c. "They are not that much older than you."
   d. "You just need to concentrate on yourself and not worry about others."

4. Which of the following nursing interventions is appropriate for an older female client in order to promote bone health?
   a. Encourage to avoid physical activity
   b. Instruct to eat dairy products
   c. Remind of need to be more sedentary
   d. Teach the importance of consuming antioxidants

5. A nurse is discussing a client's complaint of pain in the lower back and legs. A nursing assistant replies, "What do you expect? The client is 90 years old." Which of the following is the best response by the nurse to the assistant?
   a. "Pain is not an expected result of aging."
   b. "The client is probably exaggerating."
   c. "The client is probably just seeking attention."
   d. "Yes, everyone's pain level increases as they get older."

6. Which of the following age-related physiological changes may lead to the development of hypertension (high blood pressure)? Select all that apply.
   a. Calcification of the chest wall
   b. Decreased elasticity of blood vessels
   c. Decreased percentage of body fat

    d. Increased cardiac output
    e. Development of heart murmurs
    f. Decreased arterial diameter

7. Which of the following statements about older adults is true?
    a. Most older adults live in poverty.
    b. Older adults have sexual needs.
    c. The majority of older adults see themselves as ill.
    d. The majority of older adults reside in extended care facilities.

8. Which of the following nursing actions should be implemented for a client experiencing age-related visual changes?
    a. Instruct on the need to avoid use of artificial tears
    b. Suggest the use of eyedrops
    c. Use monotone colors to avoid sensory overload
    d. Use pastel colors to reduce eyestrain

9. A nursing assistant is helping an older client bathe. Which of the following statements by the nursing assistant indicate the need for further teaching? Select all that apply.
    a. "Be sure to use hot water when you're able to get into the bathtub."
    b. "Here's some lotion for your feet."
    c. "I must add water to your room humidifier."
    d. "I need to rub your back well with the towel to make sure it's dry."
    e. "You need to use a lot of soap."
    f. "You should not use any kind of cream or lotion."

10. Which of the following foods is not helpful in promoting musculoskeletal health of older adults?
    a. Cheese
    b. Red meat
    c. Spinach
    d. Yogurt

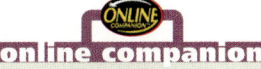

online companion

Visit the DeLaune and Ladner online companion resource at **www.delmar.cengage.com** for additional content and study aids. Click on Online Companions, then select the Nursing discipline.

There is a richness to diversity that is lacking in a homogeneous environment. We need to embrace and cultivate that richness.

—Fralic (1995)

CHAPTER 20

Cultural Diversity

COMPETENCIES

1. Discuss the concepts of culture, ethnicity, race, ethnocentrism, and stereotyping.
2. Describe dominant values in the United States.
3. Discuss the six organizing phenomena of culture.
4. Discuss the impact of culture on health beliefs and health behaviors.
5. Recognize the impact of cultural values on utilization of health care services.
6. Describe the process of transcultural nursing.
7. Explain the process for maintaining sensitivity to cultural diversity.
8. Discuss nursing strategies that ensure delivery of culturally competent care.

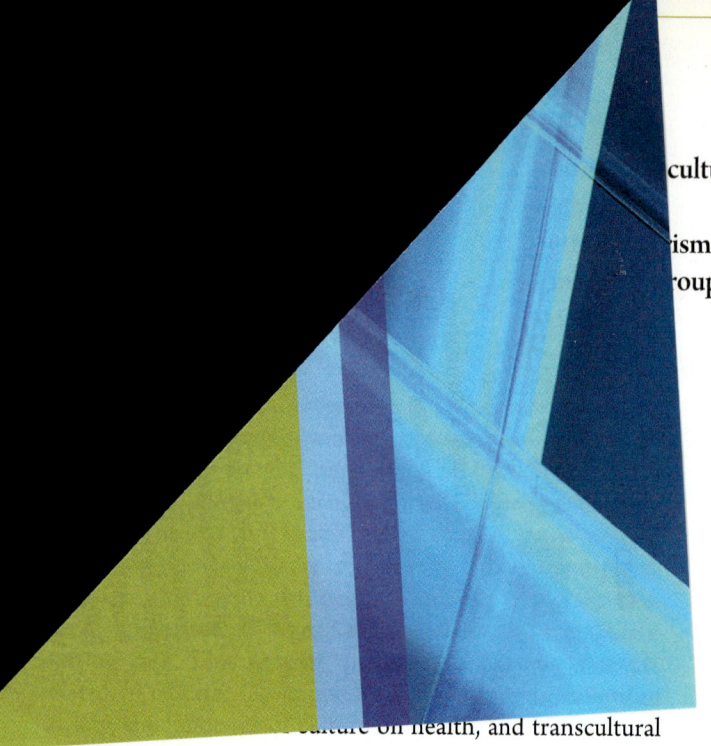

culture

~~~ism

~~~oup

race
racism
stereotyping
transcultural nursing

... culture on health, and transcultural nursing.

demonstration, and discussion (see Figure 20-1). Differences exist among cultural groups and among individuals within a single culture. Despite these variances, all cultures exhibit the characteristics shown in Table 20-1.

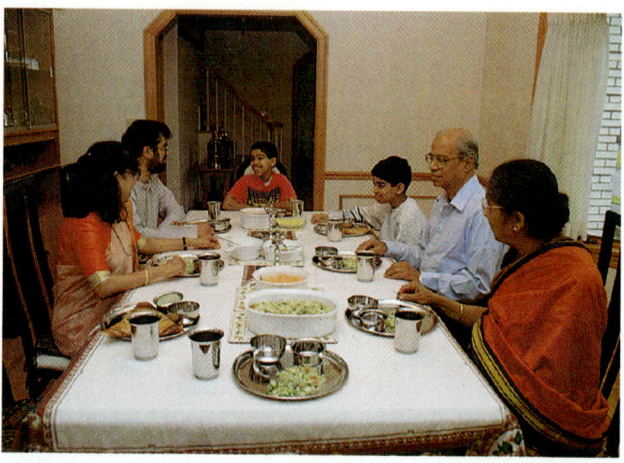

FIGURE 20-1 Cultural expectations and traditions are shared through formal and informal activities such as meal times. DELMAR/ CENGAGE LEARNING

CONCEPTS OF CULTURE

Each individual is culturally unique. Behavior, self-perception, and judgment of others all depend on one's cultural perspective. This section discusses the concepts of culture, race, ethnicity, and stereotyping and provides an overview of the dominant cultural values in the United States. To provide holistic care, the nurse needs a thorough understanding of the following concepts.

CULTURE

Culture refers to knowledge, beliefs, behaviors, ideas, attitudes, values, habits, customs, languages, symbols, rituals, ceremonies, and practices that are unique to a particular group of people. This structure of knowledge, behaviors, and values provides a group with a "blueprint" or a road map for ways to think and act.

Culture is not static, nor is it uniform among all members within cultural groups. Culture represents adaptive dynamic processes learned through life experiences. People have culturally predetermined values and beliefs that may change as new information is gained. There is much diversity among cultural groups. Cultural messages are transmitted in a variety of ways such as through families, schools, and churches. The various media are also powerful transmitters and shapers of culture.

People learn about culture through traditions. When people state "That's how we've always done it," they are describing cultural traditions. Cultural beliefs, values, customs, and behaviors are transmitted from one generation to another. Grandparents, other elders, and parents teach children cultural expectations and norms through role modeling,

TABLE 20-1 Characteristics of Culture	
CHARACTERISTIC	**EXPLANATION**
Learned and taught	Culture is transmitted from one generation to another. Cultural concepts are learned through socialization.
Shared	Sharing common practices provides a group with part of its cultural identity.
Social in nature	Culture develops in groups. Cultural practices are communicated within groups.
Dynamic and adaptive	Cultural change occurs slowly in response to group needs. Adaptation allows a culture to survive.

Delmar/Cengage Learning

ETHNICITY AND RACE

Ethnicity is a cultural group's perception of themselves (group identity). This self-perception influences how the group's members are perceived by others. Ethnicity is a sense of belongingness and a common social heritage that is communicated from one generation to the next. Members of an ethnic group demonstrate their shared sense of identity in common customs and traits.

Race refers to a grouping of people based on biological similarities. Members of a racial group have similar physical characteristics such as blood group, facial features, and color of skin, hair, and eyes. There is often overlap between racial and ethnic groups because the cultural and biological commonalities support one another (Spector, 2008). The similarities of people in racial and ethnic groups reinforce a sense of commonality and cohesiveness.

LABELING AND STEREOTYPING

Problems arise when differences across and within cultural groups are misunderstood. Misperception, confusion, and ignorance often accompany people's expectations of others. There are numerous ways in which people are different and, thus, classified by others. See the accompanying Respecting Our Differences display.

Members of some cultural groups have historically and globally experienced oppression in the forms of racism, sexism, and classism. The basic underlying premise of these biases is that one way is assumed to be better or "right" and every other way is inferior. **Ethnocentrism** is the belief that one's own culture is superior to all others. Ethnocentrism results in **oppression**, which occurs when the rules, modes, and ideals of one group are imposed on another group. Oppression is based on cultural biases, which stem from values, beliefs, tradition, and cultural expectations. **Racism**, a form of oppression, is defined as discrimination directed toward individuals who are misperceived to be inferior due to biological differences.

Stereotyping is an expectation that all people within the same racial, ethnic, or cultural group act alike and share the same beliefs and attitudes. Stereotyping results in labeling people based on the values of cultural preconceptions; therefore, an individual's unique identity is often ignored.

DOMINANT VALUES IN THE UNITED STATES

Cultural differences refer to values, practices, and rituals that vary from those of the dominant culture. The dominant culture of the United States is white middle-class Protestants of European ancestry. A **dominant culture** is the group whose values prevail within a society. The European value orientation has had an important influence on U.S. culture, as illustrated by the following dominant beliefs:

- Achievement and success
- Individualism, independence, and self-reliance
- Activity, work, and ownership
- Efficiency, practicality, and reliance on technology

RESPECTING OUR DIFFERENCES

Ways in Which People Differ

- Age
- Gender
- Educational level
- Language
- Occupation
- Residence (rural, urban, suburban)
- Socioeconomic status
- Religion
- Functional abilities
- Cognitive abilities
- Racial composition
- Nationality
- Family structure and ties

- Material comfort
- Competition and achievement
- Youth and beauty

See the accompanying Respecting Our Differences display.

Frequently, these dominant values (which may be blatant or subtle) conflict with the values of minority groups. A **minority group** can be composed of an ethnic, racial, or religious group that constitutes less than a numerical majority of the population. Minority groups are labeled and treated differently from others in the society. Minority groups are usually considered to be less powerful than the dominant group (Spector, 2008).

People assume the characteristics of the dominant culture through **acculturation** (process of learning the norms, beliefs, and behavioral expectations of a group). Acculturation is encouraged through schools and the media. **Cultural assimilation** occurs when individuals from a minority group are absorbed by the dominant culture and take on the characteristics of the dominant culture. "Through assimilation, a person develops a new cultural identity" (Spector, 2008, p. 82).

RESPECTING OUR DIFFERENCES

Comparison of Personal Values with Dominant U.S. Values

Consider the dominant U.S. values, and compare them with your personal beliefs. For example, how do you measure success? Are you results oriented? How important are independence and self-reliance to you? Do you value material comfort? If so, what are you willing to do to gain it? How do you feel about older adults? How do you feel about people who have a physical appearance that is different from yours?

MULTICULTURALISM IN THE UNITED STATES

Cultural diversity is ever increasing in the United States. The numbers of immigrants and refugees entering the United States from non-European countries have added to this multicultural composition within the American universal culture. It is estimated that by the year 2050, one of every four persons in the United States will be of Hispanic ethnicity (Weidel, Provencio-Vasquez, Watson, & Gonzales-Guarda, 2008). "The percentage of Americans who identify themselves as Hispanic or Asian continues to increase" (National Center for Health Statistics, 2007, p. 20); see Figure 20-2.

VALUE OF DIVERSITY

Cultural diversity refers to the differences among people that result from ethnic, racial, and cultural variables. The United States has a vast potential of human resources that, with divergent viewpoints and behaviors, enriches the sociopolitical climate. New ideas, varying perspectives, diverse problem-solving approaches, and increased tolerance are all outcomes of a diverse population. In addition to these advantages, there are also some disadvantages to living and working within such a culturally diverse environment. For example, the amount and types of variances can lead to ethnocentrism and discrimination.

Cultural diversity presents special challenges for nurses who must provide care that is congruent with a person's expectations. Nurses caring for clients who are different from themselves must remember to determine the client's perception and significance (meaning) of the event (illness). The nurse honors each individual's differences while understanding that culture influences how clients are viewed and treated within health care settings.

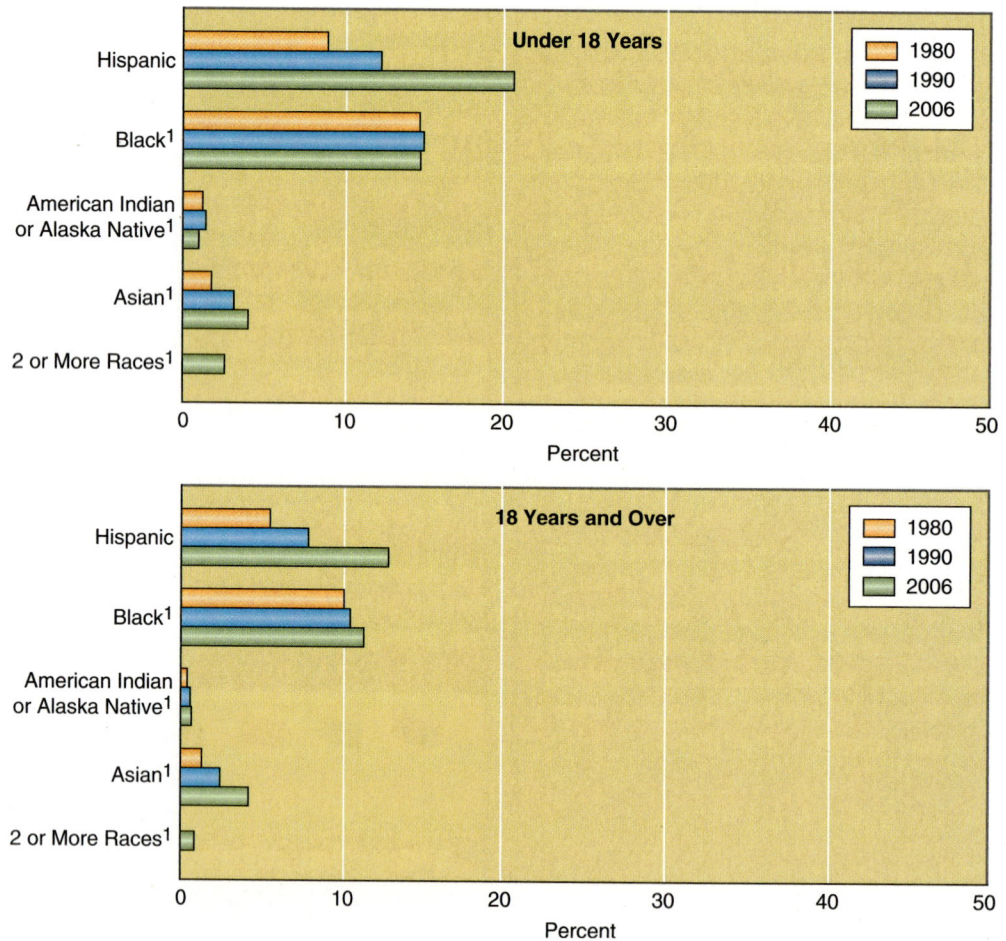

[1]Not Hispanic.

Notes: Persons of Hispanic origin may be of any race. Race data for 2006 are not directly comparable with data for 1980 and 1990. Individuals could report only one race in 1980 and 1990, and more than one race in 2006. Persons who selected only one race in 2006 are included in single-race categories; persons who selected more than one race in 2006 are shown as having 2 or more races and are not included in single-race categories. In 1980 and 1990, the Asian category included Asian and Native Hawaiian or Other Pacific Islander; in 2006, this category includes only Asian.

Adapted from U.S. Census Bureau.

FIGURE 20-2 **Population in Selected Race and Hispanic Origin Groups, by Age: United States, 1980–2006** NATIONAL CENTER FOR HEALTH STATISTICS. (2007). *HEALTH, UNITED STATES, 2007: WITH CHARTBOOK ON TRENDS IN THE HEALTH OF AMERICANS.* HYATTSVILLE, MD: AUTHOR. RETRIEVED DECEMBER 19, 2008, FROM HTTP://WWW.CDC.GOV/NCHS/DATA/HUS/HUS07.PDF.

ORGANIZING PHENOMENA OF CULTURE

Cultural factors determine the worth of behaviors, whether behaviors are acceptable, and whether behaviors are incorporated into daily living. When these behavioral concepts are applied to health, they influence the individual's expectation of health care. The nurse must be sensitive to the client's cultural context in order to provide care that meets individual needs. Each cultural group has the following basic organizational factors:

- Communication
- Space
- Orientation to time
- Social organization
- Environmental control
- Biological variations

Following is a discussion of the six organizing factors that must be considered when delivering culturally competent care. Table 20-2, on page 384, presents specific examples of cultural variances in these six phenomena.

COMMUNICATION

Communication is the vehicle for transmitting and preserving culture. To share complete and accurate information, nurses must be aware of the cultural variances related to communication. Culturally appropriate nurses attend to both verbal and nonverbal messages and are aware that messages can be easily misinterpreted due to cultural variances.

Nurses provide information to clients by using two types of communication: verbal and nonverbal. Verbal communication consists of words, both spoken and written. When cultural variances exist, communication problems may occur; see the Safety First display. The nurse must validate the meaning of and interpret words to ensure that clients receive the intended message. For example, a communication barrier exists when different languages are spoken by the client and nurse. In such cases, the use of an interpreter facilitates communication. Even when client and nurse speak the same language, communication problems may occur because words have different meanings according to the cultural context.

Nonverbal communication consists of body language (e.g., facial expressions, posture, gestures), the use of silence, and paralinguistic cues (e.g., voice tone, pitch, rate). An example of how nonverbal communication can be culturally misunderstood is the presence or absence of eye contact. For example, in Native American and Asian American cultures, eye contact is considered intrusive and disrespectful. However, in the dominant U.S. cultural group, eye contact between individuals indicates trustworthiness.

SPACE

An individual's personal space includes one's body, the surrounding environment, and objects and people within that environment; see Chapter 15. Culture determines the amount of social distance tolerated by a person. People of British and German heritages usually require more personal space than do people of Hispanic and French backgrounds (Spector, 2008).

Nurses must be aware of the client's degree of comfort with closeness, since diverse groups have varying norms for the use of touch. Touch may be perceived as invasive by clients from some cultures. Who can touch a person, when a person can be touched, and what forms of touch are appropriate are culturally determined. For example, members of the dominant U.S. culture often greet each other with handshakes while it is commonly accepted in European cultures to greet others with a kiss on the cheek.

ORIENTATION TO TIME

Time orientation (being focused on the past, the present, or the future) varies according to cultural group. European Americans are future oriented as evidenced by their development of plans, such as retirement savings. Many Native Americans have a different concept of time in that they tend to live in the present moment (Spector, 2008); see the Respecting Our Differences display. For many Native Americans, watching the clock and timeliness or tardiness have little importance. Time is considered a circular, rather than a linear, process. The nurse's nonverbal behavior can be changed to build interpersonal rapport by spending time, sitting down with clients, and demonstrating presence.

▼ **SAFETY FIRST** ▼

ASSUMPTIONS AND COMMUNICATION
When the nurse assumes that the client understands the intended message and fails to confirm client understanding, cultural blindness can hamper the communication process. Thus, client safety can be severely compromised.

RESPECTING OUR DIFFERENCES

Time Orientation

In the mainstream American culture, time is a valuable commodity (i.e., "Time is money!"). When caring for clients of diverse cultures, be sensitive to the fact that they may view time differently. Avoid jumping to conclusions that the client who is late for an appointment is lazy or inconsiderate.

TABLE 20-2 **Application of Cultural Phenomena to Nursing Care**

CULTURAL GROUP	COMMUNICATION	SPACE	TIME ORIENTATION	SOCIAL ORGANIZATION	ENVIRONMENTAL CONTROL	BIOLOGICAL VARIATIONS	NURSING IMPLICATIONS
African American	*Language(s):* • English *Silence:* • Head nodding does not mean agreement. *Eye contact:* • Direct eye contact is often viewed as being rude. *Other:* • Nonverbal communication is very important. • It is intrusive to ask personal questions of someone one has just met.	*Social distance:* • Close, personal space *Touch:* • Touching another's hair is sometimes viewed as offensive	• Present over future • Flexible concept of time	*Family:* • Large, extended family networks are important. *Gender roles:* • Strong matriarch *Religion:* • Protestant (Baptist) • Strong church affiliation with community *Other:* • Social organizations are strong within communities.	*Definition of health:* • Harmony with nature • No separation of body, mind, and spirit *Causative factors of illness:* • Disharmonious state that may be caused by demons or spirits • Can be prevented by nutritious meals, rest, and cleanliness	*Dietary practices and preferences:* • Foods are slow cooked in added fat. • Some pregnant African Americans engage in pica (ingestion of nonfood items, such as laundry starch). *Increased susceptibility:* • Lactose intolerance • Keloid formation • Sickle cell anemia • Hypertension • Cancer (especially stomach and esophageal) • Coronary heart disease	• Encourage involvement of extended family. • Know that a folk healer (or herbalist) may be consulted before individual seeks other treatment. • Clarify meaning and intent of client's words. • Validate the meaning of client's nonverbal behavior.
Asian American	*Language(s):* • Chinese (especially Mandarin) • Japanese • Korean • Vietnamese • English *Silence:* • Is valued *Eye contact:* • Considered to be rude	*Social distance:* • Avoid physical closeness. *Touch:* • Usually do not touch others during conversation. • Is unacceptable with members of opposite sex	• Present oriented	*Family:* • Highly value immediate and extended family • Honor elders and ancestors • Family unit is very structured and hierarchical. • Family loyalty and honor are valued.	*Definition of health:* • A state of physical and spiritual harmony with nature • A balance between positive and negative energy forces (yin and yang) • A healthy body is viewed as a gift from ancestors.	*Dietary practices and preferences:* • Soy sauce • Raw fish • Rice *Increased susceptibility:* • Lactose intolerance • Hypertension • Cancer (stomach and liver)	• Expect that a traditional healer will probably be consulted first. • Clarify responses to questions. • Avoid excessive touch. • Limit eye contact.

(Continued)

TABLE 20-2 (Continued)

CULTURAL GROUP	COMMUNICATION	SPACE	TIME ORIENTATION	SOCIAL ORGANIZATION	ENVIRONMENTAL CONTROL	BIOLOGICAL VARIATIONS	NURSING IMPLICATIONS
	Other: • Criticism or disagreement is not expressed verbally. • The word "no" is avoided to show respect for others. • An upturned palm is offensive.	*Touch:* • Touching someone on the head is disrespectful because the head is considered to be sacred.		*Gender roles:* • Men have the power and authority. • Women are expected to be obedient. *Religion:* • Taoism • Buddhism • Islam • Christianity *Other:* • Education is viewed as important.	*Causative factors of illness:* • Yin and yang imbalance • Contributing factors include: – Prolonged sitting or lying – Overexertion		• Avoid gesturing with your hands. • Touch the client's head only when necessary and explain before doing so. • Avoid rigidly scheduling care procedures; be flexible with time use.
European American	*Language(s):* • National languages • English *Silence:* • Can be used to show respect or disdain for another, depending on the situation *Eye contact:* • Indicates trust worthiness	*Social distance:* • Tend to avoid close physical contact • Aloof *Touch:* • Handshakes for formal greetings	Future over present	*Family:* • Nuclear family is basic unit. • Extended family is important. *Gender roles:* • The male is the dominant figure. *Religion:* • Judeo-Christian *Other:* • Community social organizations are important.	*Definition of health:* • Usually viewed as absence of disease or illness *Causative factors of illness:* • Often viewed as punishment for sins • Tend to be stoical when expressing complaints	*Dietary practices and preferences:* • Carbohydrates (potatoes) • Red meat *Increased susceptibility:* • Heart disease • Thalassemia • Breast cancer • Diabetes	• Focus on client's body language. • Respect client's personal space. • Help client decrease fatalistic viewpoint of illness. • Know that home remedies may be the first method of treatment used.

(Continues)

TABLE 20-2 (Continued)

CULTURAL GROUP	COMMUNICATION	SPACE	TIME ORIENTATION	SOCIAL ORGANIZATION	ENVIRONMENTAL CONTROL	BIOLOGICAL VARIATIONS	NURSING IMPLICATIONS
Hispanic American	*Language(s):* • Spanish or Portuguese with many dialects *Silence:* • Tend to be verbally expressive *Eye contact:* • Eye behavior is significant. The "evil eye" can be given to a child if a person looks at and admires a child without touching the child. • Avoidance of eye contact indicates respect and attentiveness. *Other:* • Direct confrontation is disrespectful. • Dramatic body language (gestures, facial expressions) is used to express emotions or pain. • Confidentiality is important.	*Social distance:* • Comfortable with close proximity to others *Touch:* • Very tactile (use of embraces, handshakes) • Values physical presence of others *Other:* • Politeness is essential. • Modesty is necessary.	• Present oriented • Concept of time is flexible.	*Family:* • Nuclear family is basic unit. • Extended family is highly regarded. • Needs of family take precedence over needs of individual. *Gender roles:* • Man is the decision maker and breadwinner. • Woman is the caretaker and homemaker. *Religion:* • Catholicism	*Definition of health:* • May be a reward from God or the result of good luck • Results from a state of balance between "hot" and "cold" forces and "wet" and "dry" forces *Causative factors of illness:* • God's punishment for sins • *Susto* (fright) • *Mal ojo* (evil eye) • *Envidia* (envy)	*Dietary practices and preferences:* • Beans • Fried foods • Spicy foods *Increased susceptibility:* • Lactose intolerance • Diabetes • Parasites	• Offer to call priest or other clergy because of significance of religious practices related to illness (e.g., sacrament of anointing the sick person). • Protect privacy. Maintain confidentiality. • Communicate with male head of family. • Always touch a child you are admiring or examining. • Avoid rigidly scheduling care procedures; be flexible with use of time. • Pay particular attention to dietary preferences.

(Continues)

TABLE 20-2 (Continued)

CULTURAL GROUP	COMMUNICATION	SPACE	TIME ORIENTATION	SOCIAL ORGANIZATION	ENVIRONMENTAL CONTROL	BIOLOGICAL VARIATIONS	NURSING IMPLICATIONS
	• Expression of negative feelings is impolite.						
Native American (Referred to as Native American in the United States and as Aboriginals in Canada)	*Language(s):* • English • Tribal languages *Silence:* • Indicates respect for the speaker *Eye contact:* • Is avoided because it is a sign of disrespect *Other:* • Body language is important mode of communication. • Speak in low tone of voice. • Expect others to be attentive.	*Social distance:* • Personal space is very important. • Space has no boundaries. *Touch:* • Will lightly touch another person's hand during greetings • Massages given to newborns to promote bonding between infant and mother • Touching a dead body is prohibited.	• Usually present oriented	*Family:* • Basic unit is extended family, often including people from several households. • Family is highly valued. • In some tribes, grandparents are viewed as family leaders. • Elders are honored. *Gender roles:* • The father does all the work outside the home. • The mother assumes responsibility for domestic duties. *Religion:* • Sacred myths and legends provide spiritual guidance.	*Definition of health:* • Health is a state of harmony between the person, the family, and the environment. *Causative factors of illness:* • Supernatural forces • Disequilibrium between person and environment • Everything that happens is the result of something else (past or future events).	*Dietary practices and preferences:* • Vary greatly according to tribal customs and geographical location. • Navajos prefer meat and blue cornmeal and tend to avoid the consumption of milk. *Increased susceptibility:* • Tuberculosis • Diabetes • Heart disease • Arthritis • American Eskimos are susceptible to glaucoma.	• Elicit input from extended family members. • Actively accommodate extended family visitors in hospital and clinic settings. • Closely monitor own use of body language. • Encourage client to personalize space in which health care is delivered (e.g., bring personal items, objects to hospital room). • Clarify messages. • Understand that the client may be attentive even when eye contact is absent.

(Continues)

TABLE 20-2 (Continued)

CULTURAL GROUP	COMMUNICATION	SPACE	TIME ORIENTATION	SOCIAL ORGANIZATION	ENVIRONMENTAL CONTROL	BIOLOGICAL VARIATIONS	NURSING IMPLICATIONS
				• Religion and healing practices are blended with each other. *Other:* • Community social organizations are important. • Children are taught to respect traditions.		• Because there are over 400 tribes in North America (including Eskimos and Aleuts), expect diversity according to specific tribe.	

Data from Berry-Caban, C. S., & Crespo, H. (2008). Cultural competency as a skill for health care providers. *Hispanic Health Care International, 6*(3), 115–121; Spector, R. E. (2008). *Cultural diversity in health and illness* (7th ed.). Upper Saddle River, NJ: Prentice-Hall; Stanhope, M., & Lancaster, J. (2006). *Foundations of community health nursing* (2nd ed.). St. Louis, MO: Mosby.

SOCIAL ORGANIZATION

Social organization refers to the ways in which groups determine rules of acceptable behavior and roles of individual members. Examples of social organizations include family and other kinship ties, religious groups, and ethnic groups.

Family

General systems theory (GST) considers the family to be a system that seeks to maintain balance. From the GST perspective, the family functions as a unit. Thus, if an event affects one family member, all the other members will be affected in one way or another. Nurses must know which family members will be involved in making health care decisions. Including the family according to their cultural expectations is a hallmark of quality nursing care. Various types of family structures are described in Table 20-3. Family patterns usually are of one of three types: linear, collateral, or individualist. See Table 20-4 for an explanation of these types of family patterns.

In many cultures, the family assumes greater importance than the individual (see Figure 20-3 on page 390). For example, in most Native American tribes, the extended family is the basic family structure. The extended family is also extremely important in Hispanic American cultural groups. In some Hispanic groups, the family may include third and fourth cousins as well as close friends who are not related by ties of kinship.

GENDER

Gender roles vary according to cultural context. For example, in families with a patriarchal structure (the man is the head

TABLE 20-3 Types of Family Structures	
TYPE	**DEFINITION**
Nuclear	Parents and children
Extended	Parents, children, and other relatives (e.g., grandparents, cousins)
Attenuated	Single parent with children
Incipient	Married couple with no children
Blended	Married couple and their children from previous unions; may indicate stepparents, stepsiblings, half siblings

Delmar/Cengage Learning

of the household and chief authority figure), the husband and father is the dominant person. Such expectations are the cultural norm for Latino, Hispanic, and traditional Muslim families. The husband and father is the one who makes decisions regarding health care for all family members. Also, in such cultures, the wife is responsible for child care and household maintenance, whereas the father's role is to protect and support the family members (Munoz & Luckmann, 2005).

TABLE 20-4 Family Patterns		
KINSHIP PATTERN	**EXPLANATION**	**MOST COMMON CULTURAL CONTEXT**
Linear	• Goals focus on needs of extended and hereditary family. • Patriarchal structure is present. • Enculturation of children is an important function. • Elders are respected.	• Asian • Middle Eastern • Upper-class Euro-American
Collateral	• Individual members' goals are less important than those of the family. • Nuclear family is present. • Men are "head of household," yet women contribute to decision making (especially about child care). • Children are highly valued. • Socialization revolves around family groups.	• Hispanic • Native American
Individualist	• Individuals' goals take precedence over those of family. • Emphasis is on individual accountability and self-responsibility. • There is less respect for authority figures. • Elders are not as honored. • Family responsibilities are shared between men and women.	• Middle-class Euro-American • Single-parent family • Gay family

Delmar/Cengage Learning

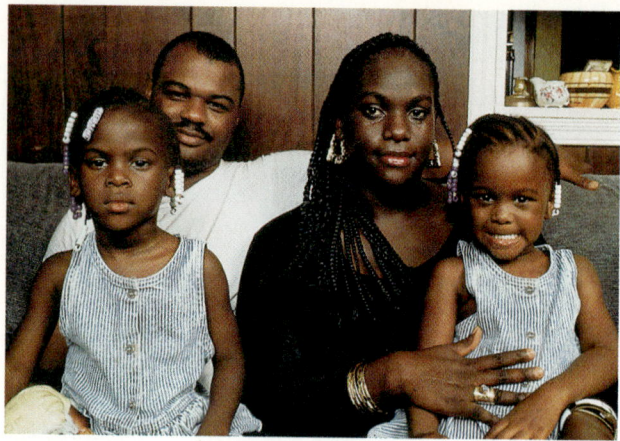

FIGURE 20-3 Within this family, decisions about health care are made on a very personal level among the parents and children. DELMAR/CENGAGE LEARNING

LIFESTYLE

In addition to an increased heterogeneity of population groups in the United States, lifestyles are also becoming more diverse. Some examples of alternative lifestyles are homosexual couples and communal groups. Nurses must demonstrate respect for clients' lifestyles even when they differ from those of the nurse. Some specific ways in which nurses can respect clients with differing lifestyles are:

- Use self-awareness to determine the impact of own beliefs and values.
- Be aware of own tendency to be ethnocentric.
- Be sensitive to client's needs, especially those expressed nonverbally.

Often the nurse and client are of different cultural backgrounds; see Figure 20-4. The nurse must be culturally sensitive in order to promote the development of a therapeutic nurse-client relationship.

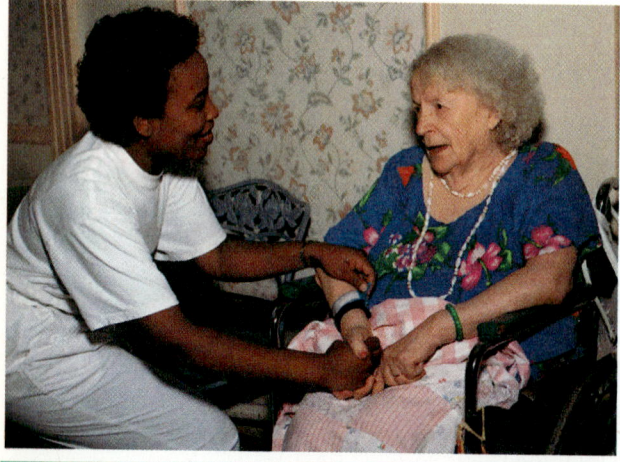

FIGURE 20-4 Provision of culturally sensitive care depends on establishing a therapeutic nurse-client relationship. DELMAR/CENGAGE LEARNING

RELIGION

Religious beliefs influence a person's response to major life events such as birth, illness, and death. Religious practices are a source of comfort during stressful life events and provide support for many people during the healing process. Table 24-3 presents an overview of the practices of selected major world religions that relate to issues such as diet, birth, death, and health care. Crises such as illness and treatment modalities are often the catalyst for increased spiritual needs.

CULTURAL DISPARITIES IN HEALTH AND HEALTH CARE DELIVERY

Language and other cultural differences often result in barriers to necessary health care including:

- Appointment procedures
- Transportation
- Written directions

Language and culture strongly affect access and response to health care services (Berry-Caban & Crespo, 2008). It has been noted that in the United States, "many measures of disease and disability differ significantly by race and ethnicity" (National Center for Health Statistics, 2007, p. 20). There are disparities in the health of Americans. "Racial and ethnic minorities often receive lower-quality health care than white patients ..." (Smith et al., 2007, p. 654). One of the major objectives established by the U.S. Office of Public Health in its *Healthy People* objectives is the elimination of disparities in health status by providing equitable services for people of all groups (U.S. Department of Human Services, n.d.).

VULNERABLE POPULATIONS

As a result of societal changes, more people are at risk for health problems. Groups that are especially susceptible to health-related problems include the poor, the homeless, migrant workers, abused individuals, older adults, pregnant adolescents, and people with sexually transmitted diseases (STDs) such as acquired immunodeficiency syndrome (AIDS).

The United States is currently facing many economic, social, and political challenges related to the delivery of health care services to vulnerable population groups (Edelman & Mandle, 2006). As a result, many vulnerable populations are underserved because of the high demand for services, lack of services, and limited availability and access to services.

The Indigent

Poverty affects health status and accessibility to health care services. Living in poverty means being unable to meet the financial demands of basic living expenses, such as food, shelter, and clothing. Socioeconomic status is determined by family income, educational level, and occupation. In 2007, the average poverty threshold for a family of four was $21,203 (U.S. Census Bureau, 2008). The poor population has more complex health problems including a higher incidence of chronic illness; see the accompanying Spotlight On display.

Increasing numbers of federally mandated health care initiatives are being implemented to address the historic racial and class disparities in health care. Entitlement programs imply that the government is legally mandated to provide services to the programs' eligible populations. Entitlement programs such as Medicare, Medicaid, and Women, Infants, and Children (WIC) were developed, in part, because of social and political pressures. WIC, a special supplemental food program for women, infants, and children, is a U.S. Public Health–sponsored program that targets low-income pregnant and breastfeeding mothers and their children age 5 years or younger. WIC links health care services, food supplements, and health education into a combined service package for eligible members. Medicaid is a program designed to provide access to health care for medically needy infants, children, and adults. Medicare is an entitlement program that finances health care services for individuals over the age of 65; see Chapter 4.

Poverty interferes with a child's ability to be housed, clothed, and fed adequately and can deprive the child of a safe (physical and psychological) environment. Children with access to health care have the possibility of getting necessary health care services. Children with health insurance (public or private) are much more likely than children without insurance to have a regular and accessible source of health care. In 2008, over 9 million children in the United States were uninsured (National Conference of State Legislatures, 2008). Basic health care services, such as routine screenings and immunizations, establish the foundation of healthy lives for children. However, the lack of insurance prevents receipt of such services by children who live in poverty.

The Homeless

Millions of people are homeless in the United States. Societal factors that contribute to homelessness are:

- Lack of affordable housing
- Increasingly stringent criteria for public assistance
- Decreased availability of social services
- Inadequate or lack of employment
- A history of psychosocial trauma
- Deinstitutionalization of clients from mental health facilities without adequate community support (such as halfway houses and group homes)

One reason that homelessness is such a major problem is that there are multiple causative factors that cross lines of age, gender, and socioeconomic status (Edelman & Mandle, 2006). See the accompanying Community Considerations display.

Many homeless people are on the streets because they have some form of mental illness or are addicted to alcohol or other drugs. Those who are homeless are at greater risk for illness and injuries (Edelman & Mandle, 2006), including STDs, and substance abuse. Access to basic health care services is limited because the homeless lack health insurance coverage. Those few facilities that do provide services to the homeless are not always accessible due to lack of transportation. See Table 20-5, on page 392, on common health problems of homeless people.

ENVIRONMENTAL CONTROL

Environmental control refers to the relationships between people and nature and to a person's perceived ability to control activities of nature, such as factors causing illness. Environmental factors that affect health status include air quality, water pollution, soil contamination, noise pollution, and sanitation. See Table 20-6, on page 392, for other examples of environmental health problems and see the Uncovering the Evidence display, on page 394, that discusses a social-environmental problem.

FOLK MEDICINE

The use of a folk medicine system (also referred to as alternative medicine) can present challenges to nurses caring for clients from diverse cultures. In order to work effectively with clients who use folk remedies, the nurse needs to have knowledge of cultural beliefs about illness. See Chapter 31

SPOTLIGHT ON...

Values

Socioeconomic Status and Health Care

Think about the following questions regarding poverty and health:

When you see a child who is hungry, what do you feel?

When an adult approaches you on the street asking for money, what do you do?

What do you think causes a person to be economically impoverished? Is poverty a result of socioeconomic, political conditions; the individual's lack of initiative; or other factors?

How do you feel about a person who cannot afford adequate health care services?

COMMUNITY CONSIDERATIONS

Is Basic Shelter a Guarantee?

Every person in this country has a basic right to shelter. Do you agree or disagree with this statement? Consider the ethical ramifications of this statement. In light of the current political and social climate, what do you think the homeless population can expect from government and society?

TABLE 20-5 Common Health Problems Experienced by Homeless People

PROBLEM	IMPACT OF HOMELESSNESS
Diabetes	• Lack of regularly scheduled nutritious meals • Inadequate rest • Insufficient exercise
AIDS	• Higher rate of sexual assault • Intravenous drug use • Lack of treatment or inadequate follow-up
Respiratory diseases (e.g., tuberculosis, pneumonia)	• Crowded living conditions • Inadequate nutrition • Limited or no access to treatment facilities
Cardiovascular diseases	• Impaired peripheral circulation as a result of extended time walking on the streets or sleeping in upright, seated position • Food served in many shelters has a high sodium content • Consumption of alcohol and tobacco products
Parasitic infestations	• Shared personal items (clothing, bedding, hairbrushes) • Close physical contact (as in shelters) • Lack of facilities for baths, showers • Inability to treat all those in contact with the affected person

Stanhope, M., & Lancaster, J. (2006). *Foundations of community health nursing* (2nd ed.). St. Louis, MO: Mosby.

TABLE 20-6 Environmental Health Problems

ENVIRONMENTAL AREA	POTENTIAL PROBLEMS
Air quality	• Gaseous pollutants • Spraying of herbicides and pesticides • Disappearing ozone layer
Food quality	• Bacterial contamination • Altered food chain as result of ecosystem destruction • Food additives • Genetic engineering/alteration
Living patterns	• Exposure to secondhand smoke • Noise exposure • Substance abuse • Urban crowding • Violence/unsafe neighborhoods
Radiation threats	• Nuclear facility emissions • Radioactive hazardous wastes • Radon gas • X-ray exposure

Adapted from Hall, J. M., Robinson, C. H., & Broyles, T. J. (2007). Environmental health. In M. A. Nies & M. McEwen (Eds.), *Community/public health nursing: Promoting health of populations* (4th ed., p. 237). Philadelphia: Saunders Elsevier.

for a complete discussion of complementary and alternative treatment methods.

Folk healers are knowledgeable about cultural norms and are usually familiar to the one seeking care (Edelman & Mandle, 2006). Table 20-7 on page 393 presents the various healers within different cultures and describes common folk healing practices within these cultures. Nurses must be able to relate care and treatment to the client's cultural context to incorporate informal caregivers, healers, and other members of the clients' support system as allies in treatment.

BIOLOGICAL VARIATIONS

Biological variations that distinguish one cultural group from another include enzymatic differences and susceptibility to disease (Spector, 2008). Enzymatic differences account for diverse responses of some groups to dietary therapy and drugs (see Table 20-8 on page 394). "Cultural variations and differences may affect the breakdown, distribution, and action of pharmacologic agents for ethnically and culturally diverse persons" (Warren, 2008, p. 293). Nutritional variations include food preferences that may contribute to health problems (see Table 20-9 on page 395).

TRANSCULTURAL NURSING

Acknowledgment and acceptance of cultural differences and understanding of culturally specific responses to illness are prerequisites for providing safe and effective care. The conceptual framework for understanding cultural diversity and providing culturally competent care is based on Leininger's transcultural nursing theory. **Transcultural nursing**, according to Leininger (2005), focuses on the study and analysis of different cultures and subcultures with respect to cultural

TABLE 20-7 Folk Medicine: Healers and Practices

CULTURAL GROUP	TRADITIONAL HEALERS	HEALING PRACTICES
African American	• Elderly women healers • "Community Mother" or "Granny" • "Root doctor" • Voodoo healer ("Mambo" or "oungan") • Spiritualist	• Herbs, roots • Poultices • Oils • Religious healing through rituals (e.g., laying on of hands) • Talismans are worn around the wrist or neck, or carried in a pouch to ward off disease
Asian American	• Herbalist • Physician	• Use of hot and cold foods • Herbs (e.g., ginseng root, which is used as a restorative potion) • Soups • Cupping, pinching, and rubbing • Meditation • Acupuncture (puncturing the skin at specified areas with metal needles) • Acupressure (applying pressure with the fingertips to specified areas of the body) • Application of tiger balm (a salve) to relieve muscular pains • Energy to restore balance between yin and yang
European American	• Nurse • Physician	• Exercise • Medication (prescribed and over the counter) • Modified diets • Amulets • Religious healing rituals
Hispanic American	• *Curandero* • *Espiritualista* • *Yerbero* (herbalist) • *Brujo* (healer who uses witchcraft) • *Sobadora* • *Santiguadora*	• Hot and cold foods to treat some conditions • Herbal teas, such as Manzanilla, used to treat gastrointestinal problems, insomnia, and menstrual cramps • Prayers and religious medals • Massage • *Azabache*, a black stone worn as a necklace or bracelet to ward off the "evil eye" • Some Haitian mothers practice the "three baths" ritual: They bathe for the first 3 postpartum days in water boiled with special leaves
Native American	• Shaman • Medicine man or woman	• Use of plants and herbs • Medicine bundle or bag filled with herbs that have been blessed by a medicine man or woman during a healing ceremony • Sweet grass (herbs) burned to purify the ill person • *Estafiate* (dried leaves) boiled to produce a tea for treating stomach disorders • The Blessingway ceremony (a healing ritual conducted by the medicine man or woman) • In some Navajo tribes, the medicine man or woman uses sand painting as a diagnostic method

Data adapted from Degazon, C. (2006). Cultural diversity and community health nursing practice. In M. Stanhope & J. Lancaster (Eds.), *Foundations of community health nursing* (2nd ed.). St. Louis, MO: Mosby; Edelman, C. L., & Mandle, C. L. (2006). *Health promotion throughout the lifespan* (6th ed.). St. Louis, MO: Mosby; Spector, R. E. (2008). *Cultural diversity in health and illness* (7th ed.). Upper Saddle River, NJ: Prentice-Hall.

UNCOVERING THE
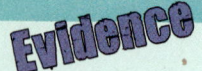

TITLE OF STUDY

"Is Immigrant Status Relevant in School Violence Research? An Analysis with Latino Students"

AUTHOR

A. A. Peguero

PURPOSE

To investigate the effect of immigrant status and English proficiency on the experiences of Latino students with school violence–related outcomes.

METHODS

This investigative study is based on data from the Education Longitudinal Study of 2002. The study examined 1,457 nationally representative public school Latino students' experiences with school violence–related outcomes.

FINDINGS

Data analysis reveals that third-generation immigrant students were more likely than first- and second-generation students to be victimized while at school. First-generation immigrant students were the most likely to feel unsafe at school. Nonnative English-speaking students were more likely to report being a victim of school violence in comparison to native English speakers.

IMPLICATIONS

There is a great need for further study of school and community characteristics of immigration and assimilation and their impact on children's lives. Children's exposure to violence must be investigated more thoroughly in school and community settings.

Peguero, A. A. (2008). Is immigrant status relevant in school violence research? An analysis with Latino students. *Journal of School Health*, *78*(7), 397–404.

TABLE 20-8 Effects of Biological Variations on Selected Drugs

CULTURAL GROUP	EFFECT OF BIOLOGICAL VARIANCE ON DRUGS
African American	• Isoniazid (drug used to treat tuberculosis) is rapidly metabolized, thus becoming inactive quickly; occurs in approximately 60% of population. • An enzyme deficiency interferes with metabolism of primaquine (used to treat malaria); occurs in approximately 35% of population. • Antihypertensive drugs (e.g., propranolol) need to be administered in higher doses to produce same effects as in European Americans.
Asian American	• Isoniazid (drug used to treat tuberculosis) is rapidly metabolized, thus becoming inactive quickly; occurs in approximately 85%–90% of population. • Rapid metabolism of alcohol results in excessive facial flushing and other vasomotor symptoms. • Chinese men need only about half as much propranolol (antihypertensive drug) as European American men. • Asian people need smaller doses of alprazolam (antianxiety drug) to achieve same blood levels as their European American counterparts; the drug is also metabolized more slowly (remains in the bloodstream longer) in Asian men.
European American	• Due to liver enzyme differences, caffeine is metabolized and excreted faster than by people of other cultural groups.
Native American	• Isoniazid (drug used to treat tuberculosis) is rapidly metabolized, thus becoming inactive quickly; occurs in approximately 60%–90% of population. • Rapid metabolism of alcohol results in excessive facial flushing and other vasomotor symptoms.

Data adapted from Spector, R. E. (2008). *Cultural diversity in health and illness* (7th ed.). Upper Saddle River, NJ: Prentice-Hall.

care, health beliefs, and health practices with the goal of providing health care within the context of the client's culture.

A basic assumption of transcultural nursing is that health care providers who see problems from the client's cultural viewpoint are more open to understanding, appreciating, and working effectively with these clients (Figure 20-5 on page 396). Other assumptions of transcultural nursing theory are:

- Every culture has some type of system for health care that is based on values and behaviors.
- Cultures have certain methods for providing health care. These methods of care are often unknown to nurses from other cultures (Leininger, 2005).

Due to rapid globalization, every nurse must have an understanding of human conditions in diverse societies. Nurses do not need to travel to foreign countries to engage in international nursing. Nurses encounter cultural diversity

TABLE 20-9 Food Preferences and Related Effects on Health

CULTURAL GROUP	FOOD PREFERENCES	NUTRITIONAL EXCESS	RELATED HEALTH PROBLEM
African American	• Pork • Greens • Rice • Fried foods	• Calories • Cholesterol • Carbohydrates • Sodium	• Obesity • Cardiovascular illnesses (hypertension, coronary heart disease) • Diabetes
Asian American	• Raw fish • Rice • Soy sauce	• Calories • Cholesterol • Carbohydrates • Sodium	• Coronary heart disease • Liver disease • Stomach cancer • Ulcers
Hispanic American	• Beans • Fried foods • Chili • Carbonated beverages	• Calories • Cholesterol • Carbohydrates • Sodium	• Obesity • Coronary heart disease • Diabetes
Native American	• Blue cornmeal • Fish • Game • Fruits and berries	• Calories • Carbohydrates	• Malnutrition • Diabetes

Data adapted from Spector, R. E. (2008). *Cultural diversity in health and illness* (7th ed.). Upper Saddle River, NJ: Prentice-Hall.

everywhere—from inner-city hospitals to suburban clinics, from technologically sophisticated institutions to homes in rural, inner-city, and suburban areas.

CULTURAL COMPETENCE

Community, social and kinship ties, religion, language, food, and cultural perceptions of illness are all areas that need to be considered by the nurse when working with clients. Diversity challenges nurses to bridge gaps with clients by providing culturally relevant care. An understanding of the client's cultural context permits nurses to become familiar with the client as a person instead of focusing only on the illness or problem.

Cultural competence is the process through which the nurse provides care that is appropriate to the client's cultural context. Culturally competent nurses are those who demonstrate understanding of the client's values related to health and illness. Also, nurses who provide care in a culturally sensitive manner are flexible in their approaches and thinking.

CULTURAL COMPETENCE AND NURSING PROCESS

Cultural sensitivity is required in every phase of the nursing process. The nurse's role in providing culturally competent care includes performing a cultural assessment, formulating nursing diagnoses, identifying expected client outcomes, planning care to assist clients in achieving the expected

outcomes, intervening to address the client's nursing diagnoses, and evaluating the plan of care. The College of Nurses of Ontario (2008) identifies four elements of providing culturally sensitive care: self-reflection, facilitating client choice, gaining cultural knowledge, and effective communication. These four elements permeate the nursing process.

ASSESSMENT

Caring for a client from a different culture can be challenging to the nurse. With every client, take time, listen carefully, and convey warmth, openness, and honesty when collecting information. Using the client's strengths and respecting the client's values are essential components of effective nursing care. To begin providing culturally competent care, the nurse should use questions to gather information about the client's cultural background. Factors pertinent to cultural assessment are listed in the Nursing Process Highlight on page 396. Cultural assessment can either be incorporated into a general nursing assessment or performed separately.

NURSING DIAGNOSIS

Diagnoses approved by the North American Nursing Diagnosis Association (NANDA, 2009) are used extensively by nurses. However, one stated disadvantage to NANDA diagnostic statements is that sometimes the diagnoses are worded in ways that result in cultural bias (Munoz & Luckmann, 2005). The accompanying Nursing Process Highlight, on page 396, lists some diagnoses that may be culturally biased.

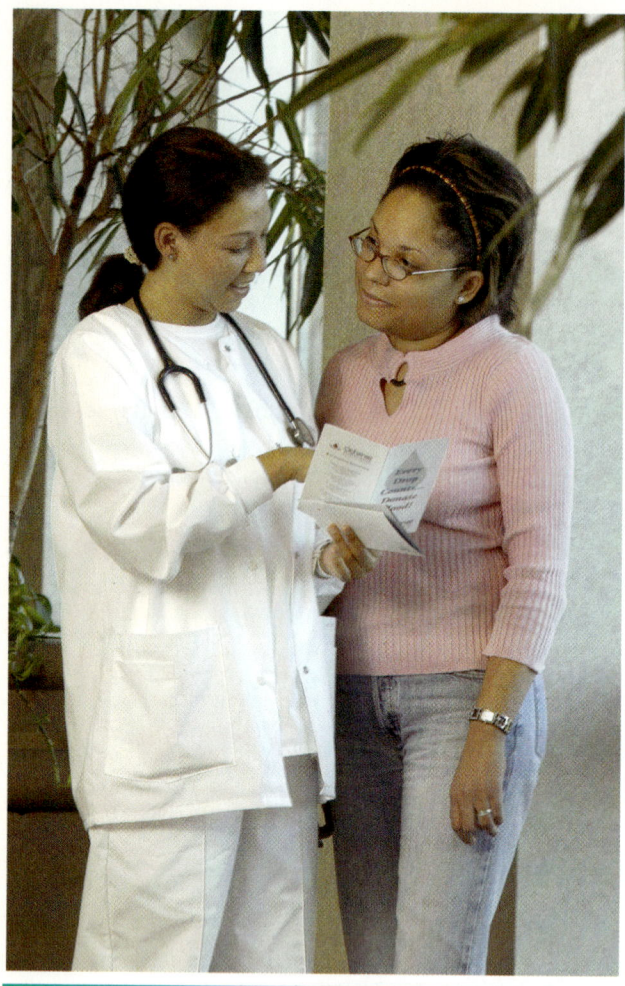

FIGURE 20-5 The relationship between this nurse and client is based on a mutual acceptance of each other's cultural viewpoints. In your interactions with clients, what factors or cultural phenomena would you explore to ensure acknowledgment of the client's cultural beliefs and values? DELMAR/CENGAGE LEARNING

Consider the following examples of ways in which these diagnoses may be used in a culturally inappropriate manner:

- Applying the diagnosis *Impaired verbal communication* to clients who speak a language different from the nurse

NURSING PROCESS HIGHLIGHT

Assessment

Cultural Assessment Factors

- Client's ethnic heritage
- Family role and function
- Religious practices
- Food preferences
- Native language
- Social networks
- Educational experiences (formal and informal)
- Health care beliefs
- Family patterns of health care

NURSING PROCESS HIGHLIGHT

Diagnosis

Nursing Diagnoses That May Be Culturally Biased

- Noncompliance
- Impaired verbal communication
- Impaired social interaction
- Deficient knowledge
- Disturbed thought processes
- Powerlessness

- Using the diagnosis *Noncompliance* with clients who reject a prescribed treatment method in order to adhere to their culturally sanctioned folk healing methods

PLANNING AND OUTCOME IDENTIFICATION

Cultural groups are not homogeneous; there are individual variations in personality, behavior, and expectations. It is important not to consider one member of a particular group to be like all the others of that same group.

In order to develop effective plans of care, nurses need to understand cultural definitions of health and illness. It is also necessary to consider how the client's beliefs may affect the plan of care. Cultural beliefs greatly influence perceptions about health and, therefore, may create barriers to adhering to prescribed treatment plans.

IMPLEMENTATION

Caring for culturally diverse clients requires three major nursing interventions: self-awareness, use of a nonjudgmental approach, and client education. Each of these aspects are discussed in the following sections. The accompanying Community Considerations display, on page 397, offers guidelines for providing culturally sensitive care for clients at home.

Self-Awareness

In an increasingly diverse society, the nurse must be aware of the potential for bias or misunderstanding and see the influence of the nurse's cultural background on the delivery of care. Self-awareness can be used to help nurses recognize their own stereotypes, biases, and prejudgments about clients who are culturally different. Further experience, introspection, and study empower nurses to appreciate their own cultural perspectives as well as the strengths of other cultures.

Nonjudgmental Approach

A nonjudgmental attitude is essential in the provision of culturally sensitive care. When caring in a manner sensitive to the client's cultural background, the nurse enables the client to offer open, honest feedback; to disagree; and to discuss

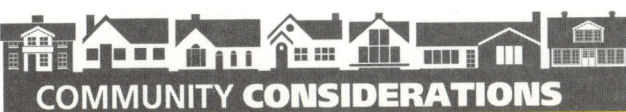

COMMUNITY CONSIDERATIONS

Providing Culturally Sensitive Nursing Care in the Home

- The setting for care is controlled by the client and family, not by the health care provider.
- The nurse is often viewed as a guest by the client and family. Social chatter may be necessary to facilitate rapport.
- The nurse must be nonjudgmental about the condition of the home (e.g., presence of clutter and disarray).
- Show respect and consideration for the client. For example:
  - Wipe your feet before entering the home.
  - Ask permission to use sink or bathroom to wash your hands.
  - Ask permission before moving client's belongings, and replace items after you have finished the task.
- Take advantage of the home environment to assess cultural values and norms. Cultural clues may include:
  - Orderliness and decor of the home
  - Assignment of family roles and tasks
  - Types of interactions among family members
  - Value placed on privacy
  - Value placed on possessions

✓ CLIENT TEACHING CHECKLIST

Culturally Sensitive Teaching Guidelines

When caring for clients from diverse cultures, the nurse should consider the following guidelines for client teaching.

- Assess and incorporate family history of health care:
  - Fluency in English
  - Extent of family support or disintegration of family
  - Community resources
  - Level of education
  - Change of social status as a result of coming to this country
- Affirm client strengths and potential for growth.
- Recognize informal caregivers (family members and significant others) as an integral part of treatment.
- Evaluate the client's current knowledge base by asking the client to state what he or she knows about the specific topic.
- To ascertain the client's perception of need, ask the client/family what they need/want to learn.
- Observe the interaction between the client and family to determine family roles and authority figures. Include the dominant family member in your teaching.
- Use language easily understood by the client.
- Clarify your verbal and nonverbal messages with the client.
- Have the client repeat the information taught. If feasible, have the client do a return demonstration of material taught.

real or perceived problems. A health care partnership is the outcome of such an approach.

Client Education

Educating clients is an integral part of nursing practice. Education not only must be relevant to the client's needs but also must be provided in a culturally sensitive manner. See the Client Teaching Checklist for culturally sensitive teaching guidelines.

EVALUATION

The final phase of the nursing process, evaluation, is extremely important in determining the client's achievement of expected outcomes and the efficacy of nursing interventions in delivery of culturally sensitive care.

Provision of culturally competent care requires that the nurse view the client as an actively participating partner of the health care team. It is important to demonstrate caring behaviors rather than just tolerating cultural variations in client behavior. Awareness of cultural similarities and variations allows nurses to accept and appreciate the impact of culture on health care. Evaluation of client response provides valuable data about the efficacy of nursing care.

KEY CONCEPTS

- Every aspect of a person's life is influenced by culture.
- Behavior affecting health is culturally determined.
- Culture is a dynamic structure of behaviors, ideas, attitudes, values, habits, beliefs, customs, languages, rituals, ceremonies, and practices that are unique to a particular group of people. This structure of knowledge, behaviors, and values provides a group with a blueprint for behavior.
- Cultural norms are transmitted from one generation to another.

- Ethnicity is described as a sense of belongingness that is shared by other members of the same group. Ethnic groups are usually composed of people with the same racial composition.

- Race refers to a grouping of people based on biological similarities. Members of a racial group have similar physical characteristics, such as blood type, facial features, and color of skin, hair, and eyes.

- Members of some racial and ethnic groups have experienced oppression in the forms of racism, sexism, ageism, and classism.

- The dominant values of the United States include achievement and success; individualism, independence, and self-reliance; activity, work, and ownership; efficiency, practicality, and reliance on technology; material comfort; competition and achievement; and youth and beauty.

- There is great value in cultural diversity, including a broader perspective of others, enhanced problem-solving ability and creativity, and improved productivity in the workplace.

- The six organizing phenomena of culture are communication, space, orientation to time, social organization, environmental control, and biological variations.

- Transcultural nursing is based on the belief that nurses who view problems from clients' cultural viewpoints are more open to understanding and working effectively with clients from other cultures.

- Understanding and accepting cultural differences and responses to illness are prerequisites for providing quality nursing care.

- The provision of culturally sensitive care is achieved through the use of approaches such as nonjudgmental attitudes and self-awareness and tools such as cultural assessment guides and client education strategies.

REVIEW QUESTIONS

1. A nurse tells a client who recently emigrated from Asia, "You will have to follow the rules here in order to get better." Which of the following is illustrated by the nurse's statement?
   a. Cultural competence
   b. Cultural sensitivity
   c. Ethnocentricism
   d. Transcultural nursing

2. Which of the following are examples of culturally competent nursing care? Select all that apply.
   a. Asking who makes health care decisions for the client
   b. Contacting a rabbi to see a Jewish client before consulting with the client
   c. Determining client food preferences
   d. Explaining how the client must comply with the hospital regulations
   e. Including family members in client teaching
   f. Insisting that family members leave when answering client questions

3. Which of the following nursing actions is culturally inappropriate for an Asian American client?
   a. Avoiding physical closeness when feasible
   b. Limiting eye contact with the client
   c. Patting the client's child on the head
   d. Using very few hand gestures when talking with the client

4. Which of the following actions would be appropriate for the nurse when caring for a client of Hispanic culture?
   a. Avoid touching a child you are admiring.
   b. Communicate with the female head of household.
   c. Expect the client to adhere to an exact time schedule.
   d. Touch the client frequently during communication.

5. When performing an admission assessment on a Native American client, the nurse should understand which of the following?
   a. Absence of eye contact indicates attentiveness.
   b. Interactions should include the client and members of the immediate (nuclear) family.
   c. Limit visitors to only two or three at a time.
   d. The client should be encouraged to touch the deceased.

6. When assessing a homeless client in an outpatient clinic, the nurse must look for indicators of which of the following?
   a. Breast cancer
   b. Cataracts
   c. Hearing deficits
   d. Parasitic infestations

online companion

Visit the DeLaune and Ladner online companion resource at **www.delmar.cengage.com** for additional content and study aids. Click on Online Companions, then select the Nursing discipline.

All men by nature desire knowledge.

—ARISTOTLE

CHAPTER 21

Client Education

COMPETENCIES

1. Explain the importance of client education in today's health care climate.
2. Relate principles of adult education to client teaching.
3. Identify common barriers to learning.
4. Explain how learning varies throughout the life cycle.
5. Discuss the nurse's professional responsibilities related to teaching.
6. Relate the teaching-learning process to the nursing process.
7. Describe teaching strategies that make learning meaningful to clients.

Client education, a quality nursing care, is a fiscally responsible intervention that encourages health care consumers to engage in self-care and to develop healthy lifestyle practices. This chapter offers an overview of the teaching-learning process, including learning barriers and teaching responsibilities of nurses.

THE TEACHING-LEARNING PROCESS

The teaching-learning process is a planned interaction for promoting behavioral change that is not a result of maturation or coincidence. Teaching is an active process in which one individual shares information with others to provide them with the information to make behavioral changes. Teaching refers to all the activities used by a teacher to assist the learner to absorb new information; it consists of activities that promote change. Teaching is a goal-directed process that provides the opportunity for learning.

Learning is the process of assimilating information with a resultant change in behavior. Nurses and clients have shared responsibilities in the teaching-learning process. Knowledge is power. By sharing knowledge with clients, the nurse empowers clients to achieve their maximum level of wellness. The teaching-learning process will be familiar to nurses in that it mirrors the steps of the nursing process: assessment, identification of learning needs (nursing diagnosis), planning, implementation of teaching strategies, and evaluation of learner progress and teaching efficacy.

PURPOSES OF CLIENT TEACHING

According to Edelman and Mandle (2006), the goal of health education is to help individuals achieve optimum states of health through their own actions. Teaching, one of the most important nursing functions, addresses clients' need for information. Often, a knowledge deficit about the course of illness and self-care practices hinders a client's recovering from illness or engaging in health-promoting behaviors. The nurse's charge is to help bridge the gap between what a client knows and what a client needs to know in order to achieve optimum health. (See Table 21-1.)

Client teaching is done for a variety of reasons, including:

- Promotion of wellness
- Prevention of disease and injury
- Restoration of health
- Facilitation of coping abilities

Client education focuses on the client's ability to practice healthy behaviors. The client's ability to care for himself or herself is enhanced by effective education.

In order to be more effective teachers, nurses need a basic understanding of learning theories. There are many schools of thought (theories) about how people learn. Table 21-2, on page 403, provides an overview of major learning theories.

TABLE 21-1 Client Education Topics

Health promotion	• Parenting Skills • Nutrition • Exercise • Family planning
Health restoration	• Medication information • Community resources • Information about treatment modalities
Illness and injury prevention	• Immunizations • Health screenings • Smoking cessation • Breast self-examination • Safety measures (e.g., car seat, restraining devices)
Facilitating coping	• Safe use of medical equipment • Dietary modifications • Information about the disease process • Counseling related to anger, grief, self-esteem • Stress management

Delmar/Cengage Learning

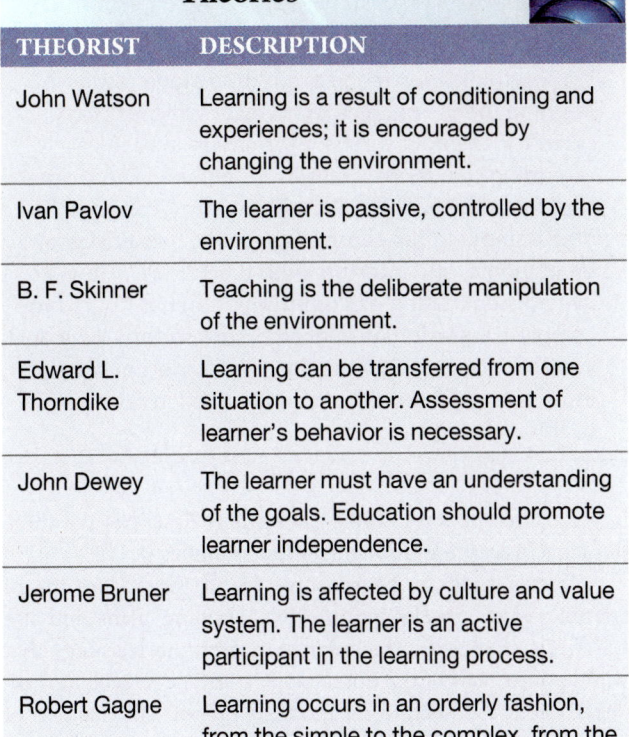

TABLE 21-2 Overview of Learning Theories

THEORIST	DESCRIPTION
John Watson	Learning is a result of conditioning and experiences; it is encouraged by changing the environment.
Ivan Pavlov	The learner is passive, controlled by the environment.
B. F. Skinner	Teaching is the deliberate manipulation of the environment.
Edward L. Thorndike	Learning can be transferred from one situation to another. Assessment of learner's behavior is necessary.
John Dewey	The learner must have an understanding of the goals. Education should promote learner independence.
Jerome Bruner	Learning is affected by culture and value system. The learner is an active participant in the learning process.
Robert Gagne	Learning occurs in an orderly fashion, from the simple to the complex, from the concrete to the abstract.
Albert Bandura	Behavior is regulated by internal mechanisms, such as self-efficacy

Delmar/Cengage Learning

Each nurse needs to develop an individual **philosophy** (statement of beliefs that is the foundation for behavior) of learning. When formulating a philosophy about teaching-learning, nurses need to consider the common beliefs about learning listed in the accompanying Spotlight On display.

FACILITATORS OF LEARNING

Certain fundamental principles of education can be used by nurses to facilitate client learning. Knowles (1984) stated four basic assumptions about adult learners, which are applicable to client education:

- *Assumption:* An individual's personality develops in an orderly fashion from dependence to independence. *Nursing application:* Plan teaching-learning activities that promote client participation, thus encouraging independence; this increases client control and self-care through empowerment.
- *Assumption:* Learning readiness is affected by developmental stage and sociocultural factors. *Nursing application:* Conduct a thorough psychosocial assessment before planning the teaching-learning activities.
- *Assumption:* An individual's previous learning experiences can be used as a foundation for further learning. *Nursing application:* Perform a complete assessment to determine

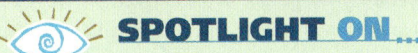

SPOTLIGHT ON...

Professionalism

Your Beliefs about Learning

Consider the information in Table 21-2. Which statements mirror your own philosophy about learning? Which statements are most congruent with a nursing philosophy that views clients not as recipients of care but as partners in the caring and healing process?

what the client already knows and build on that knowledge base.
- *Assumption:* Immediacy reinforces learning. *Nursing application:* Provide opportunities for immediate application of knowledge and skills. Incorporate feedback as a continuous part of each nurse-client interaction.

Table 21-3 describes key learning principles.

TABLE 21-3 Principles of Learning

PRINCIPLE	EXPLANATION
Relevance	The material should be: • Meaningful to client • Easily understood by client • Related to previously learned information
Motivation	Client should: • Want to learn • Perceive value of information
Readiness	Client should be able and willing to learn.
Maturation	Client should be developmentally able to learn and have requisite cognitive and psychomotor abilities.
Reinforcement	Feedback to learner should be: • Positive • Immediate
Participation	Active involvement promotes learning.
Organization	The material should: • Incorporate previously learned information • Be presented in sequence of simple to complex
Repetition	Retention of material is reinforced by practice, repetition, and presentation of same material in a variety of ways.

Delmar/Cengage Learning

Learning plateaus, or peaks in effectiveness of teaching and depth of learning, will occur in relation to the client's motivation, interest, and perception of relevance of the material. Frequent reinforcement of learning through immediate feedback and continual reassessment of effectiveness will enhance the value of the learning process. Making the information acquisition process as user-friendly as possible will also increase satisfaction and success. This can be done by organizing content from the simple to the complex and from the familiar to the new, making learning as creative and interesting as possible, and adopting a flexible approach to allow the learning process to be dynamic.

BARRIERS TO LEARNING

Receiving information does not, in and of itself, guarantee that learning will occur. Several barriers can impede the learning process. In a nursing situation, learning barriers can be classified as either internal (psychological or physiological) or external (environmental or sociocultural). Examples of these barriers are shown in Table 21-4. See the accompanying Spotlight On display.

The nurse must assess for the presence of barriers in order to facilitate the learning process. Specific assessment information is presented later in this chapter.

DOMAINS OF LEARNING

Bloom, in his classic work (1977), identified three areas or domains in which learning occurs: the cognitive domain (intellectual understanding), the affective domain (emotions and attitudes), and the psychomotor domain (motor skills). Each domain responds to and processes information

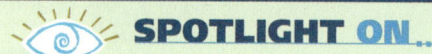

SPOTLIGHT ON...

Caring

Barriers to Learning

Do you think knowledge acquisition alone results in learning (behavior change)? Why or why not? Consider, for example, all the information available regarding the harmful effects of smoking. Every cigarette package has a similar statement: "Warning: Cigarette smoking can cause lung cancer, heart disease, emphysema, and interfere with pregnancy." However, dissemination of this information has not led to complete cessation of smoking in our society. Why do you think this is so? What learning barriers may be interfering with smokers' taking action in response to this warning?

in very different ways. Table 21-5 briefly describes the three domains of learning through clinical examples.

Nurses need to be sensitive to all three domains of learning when developing effective teaching plans and use teaching strategies (techniques to promote learning) that will tap into each of the domains. For instance, teaching a diabetic client the need to measure the proper daily balance of insulin against glucose levels is within the cognitive domain. Helping this client learn to self-administer insulin falls within the psychomotor domain. Helping the client learn to view

TABLE 21-4 Barriers to Learning

External Barriers

Environmental
- Interruptions
- Lack of privacy
- Multiple stimuli

Sociocultural
- Language
- Value system
- Educational background

Internal Barriers

Psychological
- Anxiety
- Fear
- Anger
- Depression
- Inability to comprehend

Physiological
- Pain
- Fatigue
- Sensory deprivation
- Oxygen deprivation

Delmar/Cengage Learning

TABLE 21-5 Domains of Learning

DOMAIN	DEFINITION	CLINICAL EXAMPLE
Cognitive	Learning that involves the acquisition of facts and data. Used in problem solving and decision making.	Client states the name and purpose of prescribed medications.
Affective	Learning that involves changing attitudes, emotions, beliefs. Used in making judgments.	Client accepts that he or she has a chronic illness.
Psychomotor	Learning that involves gaining motor skills. Used in physical application of knowledge.	Client gives himself or herself an injection.

Delmar/Cengage Learning

diabetes as only one part of an entire individual is an example of affective learning.

PROFESSIONAL RESPONSIBILITIES RELATED TO TEACHING

Through teaching, the nurse empowers clients in their self-care abilities. Teaching is the tool for providing information to clients about specific disease processes, treatment methods, and health-promoting behaviors.

LEGAL ASPECTS

The American Nurses Association (2003), in its *Social Policy Statement*, identifies health teaching as an essential function of nursing. Each state has its own definition of nursing practice; in most states, teaching is a required function of nurses. For example, as stated by the Louisiana State Board of Nursing (2004, p. 9), "The practice of a registered nurse includes such activities as health instruction, and health counseling."

Client teaching is also mandated by several accrediting bodies, such as the Joint Commission. The American Hospital Association (2003) calls for the client's understanding of health status and treatment approaches. Informed consent for treatment procedures can be given only by clients who are well informed. The nurse assesses the client's level of understanding about treatment methods and corrects any knowledge deficits. The nurse is often an interpreter to the client—explaining in easily understood terms, clarifying, and referring messages between the client and other health care providers.

Teaching supports behavior change that leads to positive adaptation. Thus, teaching involves decreasing the fear of change. Reducing anxiety and anticipatory stress is an important component of teaching.

Client teaching is an essential function of every professional nurse regardless of the practice setting. Table 21-6 outlines learning needs as they relate to the three phases of nursing care: primary, secondary, and tertiary. Clients who are hospitalized need information regarding their condition, the hospital environment, and expectations regarding treatment.

DOCUMENTATION

The reasonable, prudent standard calls for nurses to document client education. See Chapter 12 for a discussion of this standard. From a legal perspective, if the nurse teaches the client and fails to document it, then the educational activities never occurred. Documentation of teaching promotes continuity of care and facilitates accurate communication to other health care providers.

Many different approaches can be used to document client teaching. Figure 21-1, on page 406, provides one example of documentation for client teaching in an inpatient setting. Because client education is a standard and essential component of nursing practice, teaching interventions and the client's response must be documented. Elements for documenting client education in all practice settings include:

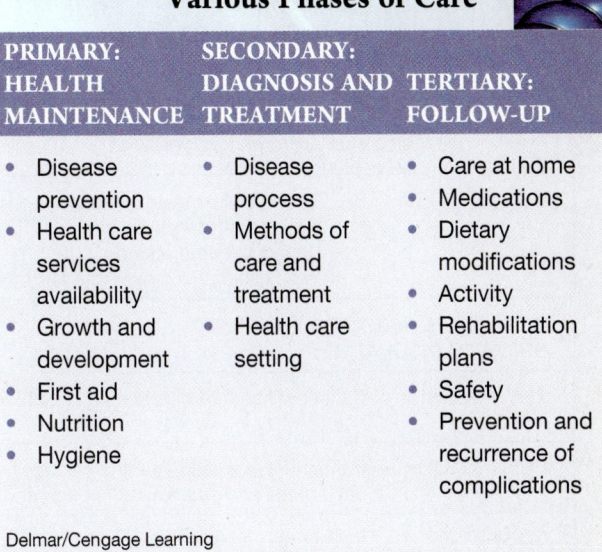

TABLE 21-6 Learning Needs in Various Phases of Care

PRIMARY: HEALTH MAINTENANCE	SECONDARY: DIAGNOSIS AND TREATMENT	TERTIARY: FOLLOW-UP
• Disease prevention • Health care services availability • Growth and development • First aid • Nutrition • Hygiene	• Disease process • Methods of care and treatment • Health care setting	• Care at home • Medications • Dietary modifications • Activity • Rehabilitation plans • Safety • Prevention and recurrence of complications

Delmar/Cengage Learning

- Content taught
- Teaching methods used
- Who was taught (e.g., client, which family member, other caretaker)
- Client and family response to teaching activities

LEARNING THROUGHOUT THE LIFE CYCLE

One basic assumption underlies teaching effectiveness—all people are capable of learning. This ability to learn varies from person to person and from situation to situation. Most clients—because of anxiety, pain, or other stressors related to illness—have only limited adaptive resources. They may not have much energy or interest to invest in learning.

Learning needs and learning abilities change throughout life. The client's chronological age and developmental stage greatly influence the ability to learn. The principles of learning discussed earlier in this chapter have relevance to learners of all ages. However, teaching approaches must be modified according to the client's developmental stage and level of understanding. Specific information about teaching children, adolescents, and older adults is provided in the following sections. Table 21-7, on page 407, lists teaching strategies for different age groups.

CHILDREN

Readiness for learning (evidence of willingness to learn) varies during childhood according to maturational level. Responding to knowledge deficits of young children requires the nurse to work closely with the child's caretaker. Including the family or significant others in teaching is essential when caring for young children.

Young children learn primarily through play, which can be incorporated into teaching activities (Figure 21-2 on page 408).

Tulane
UNIVERSITY
Medical Center

PATIENT TEACHING PROTOCOL

LEVEL: Interdependent

TITLE: Teaching the Patient with Diagnosis of Gastrointestinal (GI) Bleed

COMMENT KEY   S = Successfully meets outcome
N = Needs further instruction
U = Unable to comprehend
⋆ = See Nursing Progress Note for Patient/Family Education

OUTCOME STANDARDS TO BE MET PRIOR TO DISCHARGE:	DATE / INITIALS		
	INITIATED	MET	NOT MET
PHYSIOLOGIC: Patient will be free of evidence of GI bleed.			
PSYCHOLOGIC: Patient will express fears and concerns with diagnosis of GI bleed and procedures to be performed.			
COGNITIVE: Patient will verbalize understanding of information presented.			

PATIENT LEARNING OUTCOMES (PLO)	Information to be Presented/ Patient Learning Activities	Date Time	PLO #	Initials		Comment (See Key)
				Nurse	Pt.	

1. Patient will verbalize understanding and compliance with diagnostic procedures and treatment measures.	1. Discuss with patient and offer literature for various tests/procedures ordered:
	– Colonoscopy
	  Barium Enema
	  EGD
	  Gastrointestinal Series (upper GI)
	  Sigmoidoscopy
	– Nasogastric Tube if applicable
	– NPO, clear liquids
	– Collection of Stool specimens for blood
	– Intake and output recorded
	– IV fluids if ordered
	– Medications					

2. Patient will verbalize those signs/symptoms to report to nurse/M.D.	2. Discuss with patient those signs and symptoms to be reported: – Severe abdominal pain – Abdominal swelling – Cramping – Increased nausea/vomiting, diarrhea or bleeding – Increased weakness					
3. Patient will verbalize fears, concerns and anxieties regarding diagnosis, procedures, and prognosis.	3. Encourage patient to ventilate fears, feelings, and concerns during hospital stay and provide emotional support prn.					

TABLE 21-7 Teaching across the Life Span

	TEACHING STRATEGY	NURSING IMPLICATIONS
Infants	• Be consistent in actions. • Use brightly colored toys and objects. • Role-play nurturing behavior for parent to model.	• Teach the primary caregivers. • Emphasize the need for consistency in approach. Learning needs: Safety, growth and development concepts, infant care, nutrition, sleep patterns, skin integrity (diaper rash)
Toddlers	• Play with appropriate medical equipment and supplies (e.g., bandages, surgical caps). • Use child's comfort toy. • Positive simple commands • Picture books • Coloring books • Puppets, dolls • Audiotapes	• Involve parents to decrease child's anxiety level. • Use words easily understood by the child without being condescending. • Assess for signs of sensory overload (toddlers tire quickly); avoid trying to teach when the child is overwhelmed or irritable. Learning needs: Safety, immunizations, nutrition, dental hygiene
Preschoolers	• Provide immediate reinforcers (rewards) for positive behavior (e.g., smiley-face stickers). • Encourage play. • Books and coloring books • Music: singing, audiotapes	• Preschoolers often use words without fully understanding their meanings. • Feelings are expressed through actions instead of words. Learning needs: Immunizations, safety, nutrition, dental hygiene, parenting skills
School-aged children	• Toys • Computer games • Books • Demonstration • Role-play	• Able to follow simple directions • Understand the use of symbols • Often seek approval by doing the "right" thing • Assess child's reading ability. Learning needs: Safety, hygiene, nutrition, socialization with peers
Adolescents	• Printed material (at appropriate literacy level) • Role-play • Demonstration	• Peer approval is important; group sessions may be useful unless the material to be taught is too threatening. • Maintain privacy. • Assess for and correct any misinformation. • A sense of invulnerability leads to an "it can't happen to me" attitude. • Emphasize immediate benefit of learning information. Learning needs: Physiologic changes, sexuality (including contraception), substance abuse prevention, self-esteem, automobile safety, prevention of sports injuries
Young adults	• Printed materials appropriate to literacy level • Discussion • Demonstration • Role-play	• Content must be perceived as relevant to young adults. • Recognize strong need for independence; provide choices. • Encourage input into decision making. Learning needs: Nutrition, exercise, stress management, time management, sexuality issues (e.g., contraception); some may need parenting skill classes.

(Continues)

TABLE 21-7 (Continued)

	TEACHING STRATEGY	NURSING IMPLICATIONS
Middle-aged adults	• Printed materials geared to level of comprehension • Discussion • Demonstration • Role-play	• Increased awareness of personal vulnerability • Generally, a recognition of the need for lifestyle changes • Assess reading skills. Learning needs: Nutrition, exercise, stress management, warning signs of illness
Older adults	• Assess for reading skills • Frequent repetition • Demonstration • Discussion • Assess for sensory perceptual changes and match with corresponding materials.	• May need large-print materials • Often a strong desire for independence; offer choices. • Chronic illness (e.g., arthritis) may impair mobility and dexterity. • Aging does not lead to an overall decreased intelligence. Learning needs: Loss and grief, disease-specific information, stress management, socialization skills, elimination patterns, dental hygiene

Data from Edelman, C. L., & Mandle, C. L. (2006). *Health promotion throughout the life span* (6th ed.). St. Louis, MO: Elsevier Mosby; Hunt, R. (2009). *Introduction to community-based nursing* (4th ed.). Philadelphia: Lippincott, Williams & Wilkins.

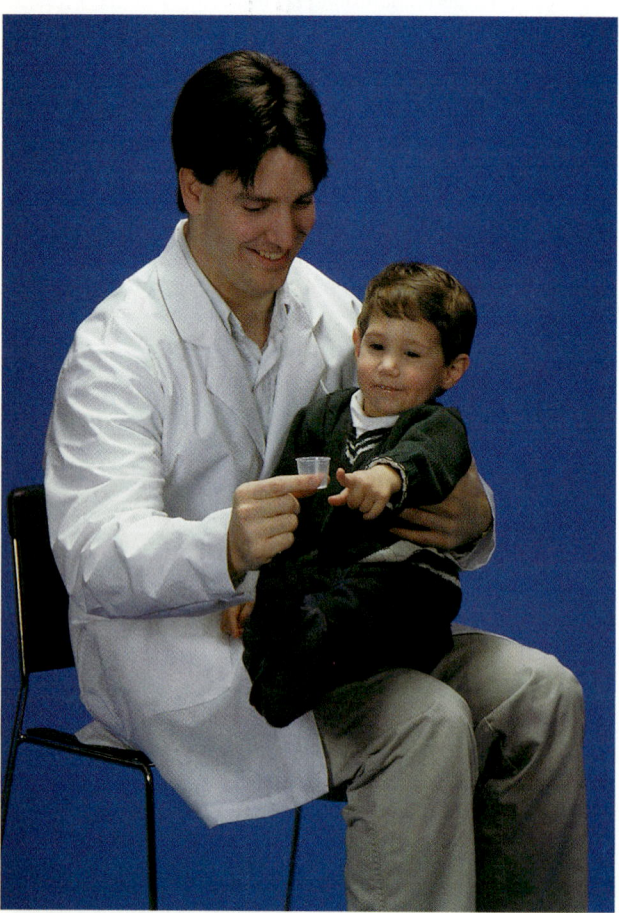

FIGURE 21-2 The use of play and games helps children learn and decreases their anxiety about the health care setting. DELMAR/ CENGAGE LEARNING

For example, puppets, toys, and coloring books can be effective teaching tools for the young child.

Older children can also benefit from the use of art materials and medical supplies (e.g., medicine cups, putting bandages on dolls). While the child is involved in play, the nurse is alleviating anxiety by teaching the child what to expect

✓ NURSING CHECKLIST

GUIDELINES FOR TEACHING CHILDREN

- Make sure the client is comfortable.
- Encourage caregiver participation.
- Assess developmental level. Do not equate age with developmental level.
- Assess client's learning readiness and motivation.
- Assess client's psychological status.
- Determine self-care abilities of client and caregiver.
- Use play, imitation, and role-play to make learning fun and meaningful.
- Use different visual stimuli such as books, chalkboards, and videos to convey information and check understanding.
- Use terms that are easily understood by the client and caregiver.
- Provide frequent repetition and reinforcement.
- Develop realistic goals that are consistent with developmental abilities.
- Verify client's understanding of information presented.

regarding treatment procedures. The accompanying Nursing Checklist provides guidelines for teaching children.

ADOLESCENTS

As children approach adolescence, they are better able to conceptualize relationships between things. Usually, reading skills and comprehension ability have advanced, and the adolescent can understand more complex information. One of the strongest influences on an adolescent is peer support; therefore, group sessions are often useful in teaching (see Figure 21-3). Nurses also teach by acting as role models and relating to adolescents on their level. See the accompanying Respecting Our Differences display. Listening allows the nurse to hear the adolescent's feedback relative to learning needs. It is also important when teaching adolescents to focus on the present and to be aware of their need to maintain control. The nurse must assist the adolescent as needed while at the same time encouraging as much independence as possible. Show respect for adolescents by recognizing that they still have to gain the knowledge and experience of adulthood while struggling to break away from the grasp of childhood. The accompanying Nursing Checklist provides additional guidelines for teaching adolescents.

OLDER ADULTS

Aging is accompanied by many physiological changes. As a result of these changes, some older adults have perceptual impairments such as impaired vision and hearing. The nurse must assess for perceptual changes and adjust teaching materials accordingly. For example, provide large-print written material and make sure the client can hear all the nurse's instructions and directions. The accompanying Nursing Checklist on page 410 provides guidelines for teaching older adults.

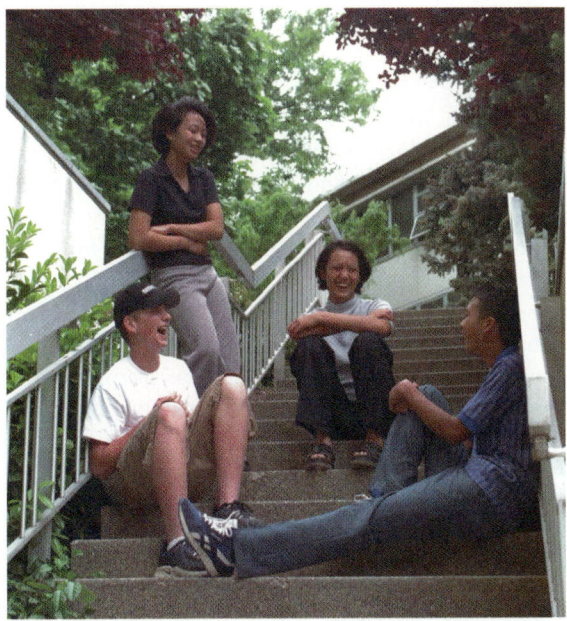

FIGURE 21-3 Adolescents are greatly influenced by peer pressure. How can this concept be used when teaching adolescent clients? DELMAR/CENGAGE LEARNING

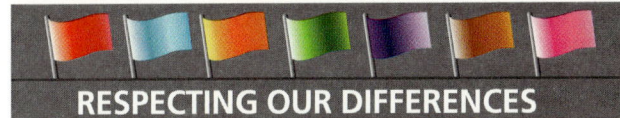

RESPECTING OUR DIFFERENCES

Do As I Say

The adage "Do as I say and not as I do" goes against all wisdom. Individuals learn from examples set by role models. Adolescents are especially sensitive to discrepancies between an adult's words and actions. How does this apply to you as a beginning practitioner of nursing? What messages are communicated by your health behaviors?

TEACHING-LEARNING AND THE NURSING PROCESS

The teaching-learning process and the nursing process are similar. Both are dynamic and consist of the same phases: assessment, diagnosis, planning, implementation, and evaluation. Figure 21-4, on page 410, compares the nursing process and the teaching-learning process. See Chapter 5 for more information about the nursing process.

ASSESSMENT

Primary and secondary data sources are used by nurses for assessment of learning needs. See Chapter 6 for a discussion of these sources. Communicating with the client and family or significant others is the foundation of assessment related to learning. Several factors need to be considered during assessment, including:

- Learning styles
- Learning needs
- Potential learning needs

✓ NURSINGCHECKLIST

GUIDELINES FOR TEACHING ADOLESCENTS

- Boost adolescents' confidence by asking for their input and opinions on health care matters.
- Encourage adolescents to explore their own feelings about self-concept and independence.
- Be sensitive to peer pressure.
- Help adolescents identify their positive qualities and build on those.
- Use language that is clear yet appropriate to the health care setting.
- Gear teaching to the adolescent's developmental level.
- Engage adolescents in problem-solving activities to encourage independent and informed decision making.

TEACHING-LEARNING PROCESS

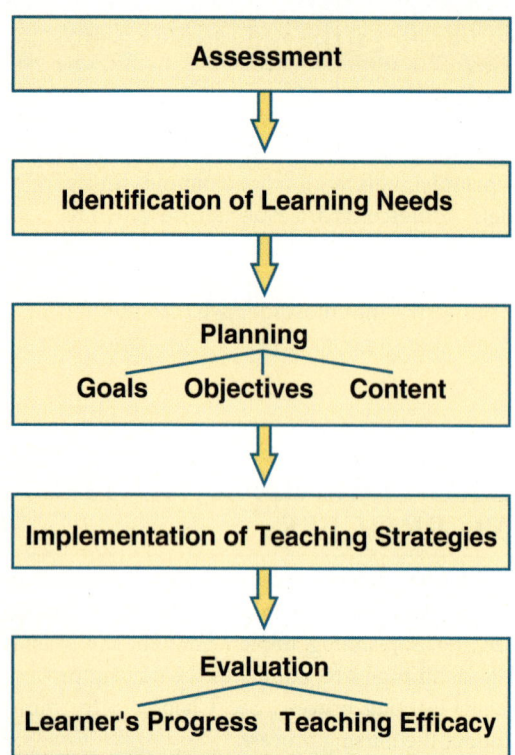

NURSING PROCESS

FIGURE 21-4 Teaching-Learning Process and Nursing Process: A Comparison DELMAR/CENGAGE LEARNING

✔ NURSINGCHECKLIST

GUIDELINES FOR TEACHING OLDER ADULTS

- Offer positive reinforcement for every attempt by the older learner to participate.
- Use silence as a reflective tool to allow older learners additional time to process information.
- Encourage reflection, particularly when sensitive issues are being discussed.
- Stimulate both visual and auditory senses in the presentation of the material to increase the probability that content matter will be retained.
- Use a variety of teaching methods, such as role-playing, games, examples, open discussion, charts, and reading material.
- Use true/false, multiple-choice, or open-ended questions to evaluate progress.
- Ask specific questions designed to elicit a response from participants. Avoid general inquiries such as "Do you have any questions?"
- Utilize the older learner's experience and expertise.

Data from Ebersole, P., Hess, P., Luggen, A. S., Touhy, T., & Jett, K. (2007). *Toward healthy aging: Human needs and nursing response* (7th ed.). St. Louis, MO: Elsevier.

- Ability to learn
- Readiness to learn
- Client strengths
- Previous experience and knowledge base

Learning Styles

Each individual has a unique way of processing information. The manner in which an individual incorporates new data is called **learning style**. Some people learn information by seeing it (**visual learners**), others by listening to words (**auditory learners**), and others by doing (**kinesthetic learners**). The nurse should use a variety of techniques (e.g., lecture, discussion, small group work, role-play, return demonstration, imitation, problem solving, games, question-and-answer sessions) to match different learning styles of clients. A good way to discover learning style is to ask the client, "What helps you to learn?" or "What kinds of things do you enjoy doing?"

Learning Needs

Everyone who receives health care services has some need for information. Client teaching may be indicated when a client:

- Has a need for new skills
- Expresses a need for information to make decisions

- Desires to make modifications in lifestyle
- Is in an unfamiliar environment

Comprehensive assessment is a mutual process between client and nurse. A crucial step in teaching is to determine the client's learning needs—what the client needs to know and what the client already knows. The nurse must evaluate the client's knowledge about the content that is to be taught. This previous knowledge can then be used as a foundation for new concepts. If the client is misinformed, the nurse develops a remediation plan. Determination of the client's learning needs is accomplished in a variety of ways, including:

- Questioning the client directly
- Observing client behaviors
- Interacting with the client's family or significant others

It is imperative that the nurse first address the client's immediate need for knowledge. This is facilitated by assessing the client's perception of learning needs and prioritizing those needs with client input. See the accompanying Nursing Process Highlight for needs assessment guidelines.

Potential Learning Needs

The nurse also assesses for potential learning needs. These potential needs influence anticipatory planning to avert a relapse in recovery and to maintain wellness. Some examples of anticipatory learning needs include:

- A female client is pregnant for the first time. *Potential learning need:* Infant care
- A male client has just been diagnosed with diabetes that is currently controlled by dietary modifications. He has been told that he may have to take insulin daily in the future. *Potential learning need:* Self-administration of insulin

NURSING PROCESS HIGHLIGHT

Assessment

Needs Assessment

Listen to what the client's words and actions are communicating.

- Does the client express uncertainty or anxiety over an upcoming procedure?
- Is the client able to tell you about medications, purposes, and side effects?
- Can the client describe necessary lifestyle modifications?
- Does the client perform self-care activities correctly?
- Is the client able to demonstrate necessary treatment procedures (e.g., colostomy irrigations, injections, blood glucose monitoring)?

Ability to Learn

The nurse assesses the client for characteristics that will hinder or facilitate learning. One such characteristic is the client's developmental stage. For example, do not automatically assume that an adult client has mastered the developmental tasks of childhood. Age is not synonymous with developmental level; observation of behavior provides the clearest clue to developmental level.

The client's maturity level greatly influences the ability to learn information. Every developmental stage is characterized by unique skills and abilities that affect the response to various teaching tools. Developmental stage greatly determines the type of data to be taught, the method(s) to be used, the language that is used, and the location for teaching. In addition to developmental stage, assessment should include evaluation of the client's cognitive skills, problem-solving abilities, and attention span.

Readiness to Learn

Another characteristic to be assessed is the client's learning readiness. Table 21-8 shows some factors that influence readiness.

Readiness is closely related to growth and development; for example, does the client have the requisite cognitive and psychomotor skills for learning a particular task? Can the client comprehend the information? Learning readiness is present when the client asks questions. Another indicator that the client is ready to learn is client participation in learning activities, such as actively participating in return demonstration of a dressing change. Some behaviors that indicate lack

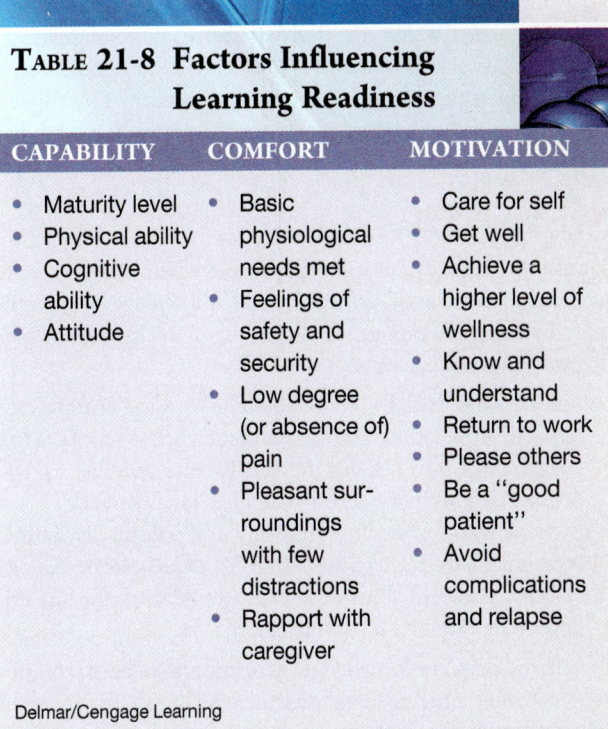

TABLE 21-8 Factors Influencing Learning Readiness

CAPABILITY	COMFORT	MOTIVATION
• Maturity level	• Basic physiological needs met	• Care for self
• Physical ability		• Get well
• Cognitive ability	• Feelings of safety and security	• Achieve a higher level of wellness
• Attitude	• Low degree (or absence of) pain	• Know and understand
	• Pleasant surroundings with few distractions	• Return to work
		• Please others
	• Rapport with caregiver	• Be a "good patient"
		• Avoid complications and relapse

Delmar/Cengage Learning

of client readiness are anxiety, avoidance, denial, lack of participation in discussion or demonstration, and lack of participation in self-care activities.

Closely related to readiness is client motivation. Individuals must believe that they need to learn the information before learning occurs. Does the client perceive relevance (meaningfulness) in the current information to be taught? If an individual sees the information as being personally valuable, the information is more likely to be learned. However, if the client does not think that the content is relevant, learning is less likely to occur. Relevance is determined individually; the nurse must assess the personal meaning of learning content for each client.

Bandura (1977) described the concept of **self-efficacy** (a belief that one will succeed in attempts to change behavior) as having a profound influence on motivation; see Chapter 16. If clients feel they will not achieve the goals, they will lack motivation to try. To maximize motivation, keep the teaching-learning goals realistic. Break the content down into small steps that are achievable and provide feedback on the progress.

Client Strengths

Identifying the client's strengths and limitations provides a foundation for realistic expectations. An understanding of the client's strengths and weaknesses allows the nurse to plan successful teaching-learning experiences. Determination of client strengths assists the nurse in selecting appropriate teaching methods.

Previous Experience and Knowledge Base

The client has a knowledge base acquired through life experiences. Previous knowledge affects the client's attitudes about learning and perception of the importance of information to be learned and is related to the client's type of educational experiences.

Culture plays an important role in knowledge acquisition. Attitudes (which are derived from a cultural context) toward what is appropriate to learn and who should teach may require alterations in the nurse's approach. The nurse's sensitivity to cultural values affects every aspect of the teaching-learning process.

NURSING DIAGNOSIS

Several nursing diagnoses are applicable when barriers to the learning process exist. When lack of knowledge is the primary barrier to learning, the diagnosis of *Deficient knowledge* is applicable. For example:

- A client who does not understand how to use crutches for assisted ambulation may have the diagnosis of *Deficient knowledge: Crutchwalking* related to inexperience as evidenced by multiple questions and hesitancy to walk.
- A client who has had a colostomy and will be discharged soon may have a diagnosis of *Deficient knowledge: Follow-up care* related to colostomy care and maintenance as evidenced by requests for information.

An inadequate knowledge base may also be a component of other nursing diagnoses in which risk or impaired behavior exists. For instance, *Risk for infection* may relate to a client's compromised health status; this risk can be modified or reduced through certain physical and environmental changes and also through proper client education. A client presenting with a diagnosis of a *Bathing/hygiene self-care deficit* may need assistance in acquiring the physical supplies to remedy the deficit as well as instruction in techniques.

PLANNING AND OUTCOME IDENTIFICATION

Informal teaching can occur in any setting at any time; formal teaching is planned and goal directed. Teaching is a goal-directed, purposeful process, which means that teaching-learning activities must be planned. Learning does not just happen by chance—it is planned. Planning, an ongoing phase of the teaching process, involves consideration of the following:

- What to teach
- How to teach
- Who will teach and who will be taught
- When teaching will occur
- Where teaching will be done

Content

Determination of *what* to teach is done through comprehensive assessment. The content to be taught depends greatly on the client's knowledge base, readiness to learn, and current health status. Examples of teaching topics are disease processes, medications, self-care activities, and health promoting behaviors.

Methods

Deciding *how* to teach involves matching teaching strategies with client's learning needs, readiness, and ability. The nurse who is an effective teacher uses methods that capture the client's interest. A variety of teaching methods (e.g., discussion, demonstration, written materials) can be used to match the client's learning styles.

Individuals

Planning also means deciding *who* will teach the client. Effective client education is the result of a multidisciplinary effort. However, the nurse is the coordinator of the health care team's teaching activities. Responsibility for planning a comprehensive teaching approach, from admission to postdischarge, remains with the nurse. Continuity of care is greatly affected by the teaching plan.

The "who" part of planning also means determining who should be taught. In addition to the individual client, the nurse must determine who else in the family needs to be taught about the illness and recovery process. An enormous wealth of health educational materials is available to families.

Timing

The decision of *when* to teach should be carefully planned. The nurse recognizes that *every* interaction with the client is an opportunity for informal teaching. Whenever a client asks a question, there is an opportunity for teaching. These windows of teaching opportunities must never be closed. Nothing destroys a client's motivation for learning more quickly than hearing such comments as "Ask your doctor that" or "We'll talk about that later, right now take your medicine." The best time for teaching is when the client is comfortable—physically and psychologically.

In addition to capitalizing on informal teaching time, the nurse must plan time during which formal teaching can be done. Teaching must match the pace of the client's progress. Some clients learn more quickly than others; some need much repetition. Timing of the teaching session is crucial. The more information presented, the more a client is likely to forget. Therefore, teaching sessions should be kept brief in order to avoid overwhelming the client. Throughout the teaching session, use repetition and frequently ask the client questions to help pace the delivery of information.

Location

The location for teaching activities must also be well planned. *Where* teaching occurs affects the quality of learning. Some factors to be considered in determining the location of teaching include provision for privacy and availability of equipment. Selection of teaching methods is often determined by the location. For example, videos can often be used effectively in inpatient settings; however, the same information may need to be presented with flipcharts or brochures in the home setting. The nurse needs to determine whether environmental factors (e.g., loud noises, uncomfortable room temperature) are present that may interfere with learning.

Goal Setting

An important part of planning in the teaching-learning process is goal setting. The client and family or significant others must be involved in setting goals since mutually determined learning goals promote learning. Specific learning goals should include these elements:

- Measurable behavioral change
- Time frame
- Methods and intervals for evaluation

Teaching-learning goals must be realistic, that is, based on the abilities of both learner and teacher.

Establishing teaching-learning goals involves setting priorities. One way to prioritize goals is to teach the "need-to-know" information (that which is necessary for survival) before moving on to the "nice-to-know" content. For example, a client who is in her first trimester of pregnancy *must* know guidelines for diet and exercise ("need-to-know" goal); learning about infant care can occur later in the pregnancy ("nice-to-know" goal).

Teaching Vulnerable Populations

When planning to teach individuals with special needs, it is important that the usual teaching strategies be modified according to the client's individual needs. This section describes education of individuals who experience developmental delays, chronic illness, low literacy skills, and sensory impairments.

DEVELOPMENTAL DELAYS Individuals with limited cognitive abilities have a medical diagnosis of mental retardation if the IQ level is 70 or less (American Psychiatric Association, 2000). The client's learning depends upon the degree of cognitive impairment, so teaching strategies must be selected accordingly. For example, a client who has mild mental retardation (IQ level of 50–70) may be able to learn by discussion of simple concepts that are stated in easily understood terms. Note that it is important to use concrete language and frequent repetition with clients in this category; the use of simple games is often effective. On the other hand, a client who is profoundly mentally retarded (IQ level below 25) may be unable to learn in the traditional sense. Frequent communication and repetition are required when working with a client with this degree of mental impairment. See the Respecting Our Differences display.

CHRONIC ILLNESS Clients who experience chronic illness (e.g., arthritis, hypertension, diabetes, asthma) have many learning needs, both actual and potential. Some chronic disorders, such as arthritis, may impair mobility and thus interfere with learning psychomotor skills as a result of decreased flexibility and dexterity of the fingers. Other chronic illnesses, such as diabetes, require ongoing assessment of the client level of understanding about self-care (e.g., diet, exercise, and lifestyle changes). Essential hypertension, another chronic disease process, often leads to client noncompliance with the prescribed treatment regimen. Ongoing education related to antihypertensive medication helps improve compliance.

LOW LITERACY SKILLS Health literacy involves reading, comprehension, basic mathematical abilities, and the ability to make health care decisions (Schaefer, 2008). Low health literacy levels are linked to poor health status. It is imperative that nurses assess the reading and comprehension abilities of clients before using printed educational materials. The majority of health care teaching involves the use of printed materials. However, approximately one-third of the U.S. population has limited health literacy (Weld, Padden, Ramsey, &

RESPECTING OUR DIFFERENCES

When working with clients with low IQ levels, you will demonstrate respect by making expectations clear. The use of repetition is necessary to help clients with developmental delays to learn. What other techniques will you use to teach clients who are cognitively impaired?

Bibb, 2008). It is a common mistake to equate the highest educational level achieved with reading level. When teaching clients with low literacy skills, it is helpful for nurses to use simple, noncomplex terms and give examples. Other therapeutic approaches are to avoid the use of medical terminology and provide clear definitions and explanations. See the accompanying Respecting Our Differences display.

SENSORY IMPAIRMENTS Many clients have sensory impairments as a result of illness, injury, or the aging process (see Figure 21-5). Effective nurses modify their teaching approaches in order to accommodate such impairments. A common mistake many people make when talking with someone who has a sensory impairment is to talk loudly. Screaming and yelling do not help the person who has auditory or visual impairments. See the accompanying Nursing Checklist for guidelines in working with clients who have visual, auditory, or memory impairments.

IMPLEMENTATION

There are several characteristics of nurses that influence the outcome of the teaching-learning process. Nursing self-awareness, an all-important first step in teaching, focuses on the concepts discussed in the following sections. The Client Teaching Checklist on page 415 provides some implementation guidelines for making teaching more meaningful to clients.

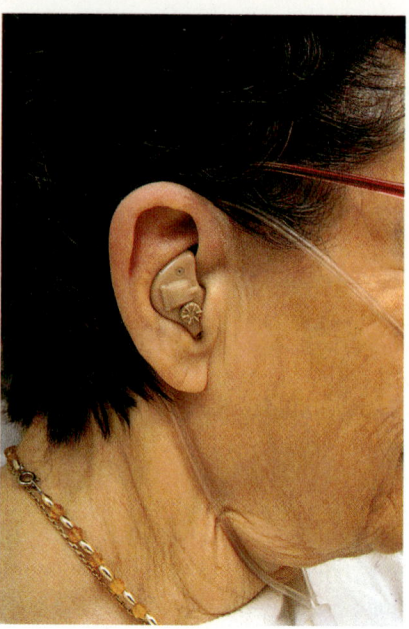

FIGURE 21-5 If a hearing aid is used, make sure it is functional before client teaching begins. For example, is the hearing aid turned on? Are the batteries working? DELMAR/CENGAGE LEARNING

Knowledge Base

It is impossible for nurses to teach if they lack the knowledge or skills that are to be taught. Staying current in knowledge and proficient in skills is the first step to maintaining efficacy and credibility as a teacher. It is impossible for one individual to be an expert in every area of nursing. Therefore, knowing when to refer the client to others for teaching can augment learning.

Interpersonal Skills

Effective teaching is based on the nurse's ability to establish rapport with the client. The nurse who is empathic to the client shows sensitivity to the client's needs and preferences. An atmosphere in which the client feels free to ask questions

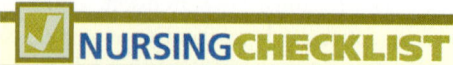

NURSINGCHECKLIST

GUIDELINES FOR TEACHING CLIENTS WITH SENSORY IMPAIRMENTS

For memory-impaired clients:

- Use repetition.
- Use a variety of cues (verbal, written, pictures, and symbols).

For visually impaired clients:

- Provide large-print materials.
- Provide prescription eyeglasses and magnifying glasses.
- Provide adequate lighting while reducing glare.

For hearing-impaired clients:

- Face the client directly when you speak.
- Use short sentences and words that are easily understood.
- Use signals to reinforce verbal information—point, gesture, demonstrate.
- Eliminate distracting noises or activities from the environment as much as possible.

Data from Ebersole, P., Hess, P., Luggen, A. S., Touhy, T., & Jett, K. (2007). *Toward healthy aging: Human needs and nursing response* (7th ed.). St. Louis: Elsevier; Mauk, K. L. (2010). Teaching older adults. In K. L. Mauk (Ed.), *Gerontological nursing: Competencies for care*. Boston: Jones & Bartlett.

RESPECTING OUR DIFFERENCES

Checking Literacy

"Lscean uyro sdhna. Seu yver dloc rweat."

The preceding statement is what many of your clients will see when you give them printed educational materials. Be sure to assess clients' ability to comprehend written materials, and avoid making assumptions about your clients' literacy level. Check for comprehension through return explanation of the written material.

promotes learning. Activities that help establish an environment conducive to learning include:

- Showing genuine interest in the client.
- Including the client in *every* step of the teaching-learning process.
- Using a nonjudgmental approach.
- Communicating at the client's level of understanding.

The effective nurse will deliberately plan to communicate a sense of empathy and caring. See the accompanying Spotlight On display.

Teaching Clients at Home

Clients who are recovering at home and their families have significant learning needs. A primary role of the home health nurse is to teach clients how to care for themselves at home; this often involves teaching family members how to provide care (Figure 21-6). Home-based clients need information regarding their illness, accident, or injury. They also need to learn how to achieve and maintain a maximum state of wellness. Accurate teaching plans for the home-based client and family are established by assessing multiple factors, some of which are listed in Table 21-9 on page 416. See the accompanying Community Considerations display.

EVALUATION

Evaluation of teaching-learning is a twofold process:

1. Determining what the client has learned
2. Assessing teaching effectiveness of the nurse

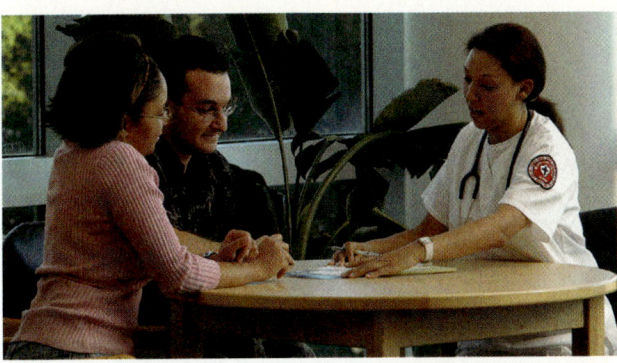

FIGURE 21-6 Preparing clients to reenter their home environment often means including family members in the teaching process. DELMAR/CENGAGE LEARNING

The evaluation process is ongoing and may lead to changes in the teaching plan and strategies used by the nurse.

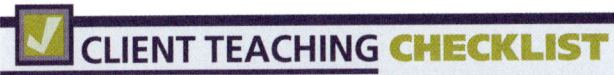

COMMUNITY **CONSIDERATIONS**

Client Teaching in the Home Setting

Preparing the client and family for home care begins not at the time of hospital discharge but rather with hospital admission. Effective teaching is the key to thorough follow-up care in the home. Discharge planning considers the current learning needs of clients and caregivers as well as potential needs after discharge. Thus, teaching includes consideration of community resources and possible referral.

✔ CLIENT TEACHING **CHECKLIST**

GUIDELINES FOR EFFECTIVE CLIENT TEACHING

- Assess client's knowledge and needs.
- Focus on client's perceived needs.
- Relate material to prior knowledge.
- Encourage client's active participation.
- Provide opportunity for immediate application of knowledge or skill.
- Expect learning plateaus to occur.
- Reinforce learning frequently.
- Provide immediate feedback to facilitate learning.
- Ensure a comfortable environment.
- Organize content from the simple to the complex, building on what the client already knows.
- Use a variety of teaching methods.
- Emphasize verbal instructions with writing and pictures.
- Stay flexible in your approach.
- Be creative!

👁 SPOTLIGHT ON...

Professionalism

Medical Jargon and Teaching

Consider the language used by most nurses—think of the terms nurses take for granted. When you ask a client to "void," does the client understand what is meant? Think of the following frequently used terms, which can easily be misunderstood by clients and families: ambulate, defecate, dangle, NPO, vital signs, contraindicated.

Listen to the language you use when communicating with clients. How can you communicate without using professional jargon?

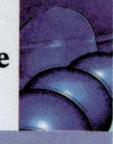

TABLE 21-9 Factors Affecting Learning Needs of Home Health Clients

TYPE	EXAMPLE
Environmental	• Accessibility of home to client with physical disability • Need for availability of equipment and supplies • Space to accommodate special needs of client • Need for information about environmental cleanliness as it relates to health • Need for assistance with self-care activities
Economic	• Ability to purchase medications, equipment, and supplies • Available financial assistance
Support system	• Persons available to assist with caregiving • Caregiver's deficient knowledge regarding necessary care
Community resources	• Resources in the immediate area • Awareness of and access to support services • Available respite to the family

Delmar/Cengage Learning

Evaluation of Learning

Evaluation, a continuous process, consists of determining what the client has learned. Is there a behavior change? Is the behavior change related to learning activities? Is further change necessary? Will continued behavior change promote health? The following strategies can be used to evaluate client learning:

- Verbal questioning
- Observation
- Return demonstration
- Written follow-up (e.g., questionnaires)

The accompanying Nursing Process Highlight provides guidelines for evaluation of learning.

Evaluation of Teaching

A major purpose of evaluation is to assess the effectiveness of the teaching activities and decide which modifications, if any, are necessary. When learning objectives are not met,

---

NURSING PROCESS HIGHLIGHT

Evaluation

Evaluation of Learning

- Did the client meet mutually established goals and objectives?
- Can the client demonstrate skills?
- Have the client's attitudes changed?
- Can the client cope better with illness-imposed limitations?
- Does the family understand health problems and know how to help?

UNCOVERING THE

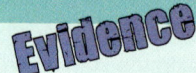

TITLE OF STUDY

"Discharge Knowledge and Concerns of Patients Going Home with a Wound"

AUTHORS

B. Pieper, M. Sieggreen, C. K. Nordstrom, B. Freeland, P. Kulwicki, M. Frattaroli, D. Sidor, M. T. Palleschi, J. Burns, and D. Bednarsk

PURPOSE

To examine clients' wound care knowledge prior to discharge from an acute care hospital.

METHODS

This is a comparative descriptive study of 67 persons, ages 20 to 83 years, who were all scheduled for discharge from a large urban acute care hospital; 58 clients had acute wounds, and 9 had chronic wounds. A questionnaire was completed by each participant.

FINDINGS

Data reveal that the participants' greatest concerns about going home were activity restrictions, wound pain, and watching for complications, including infection. Participants had appropriate knowledge about handwashing, nutrition, going out of the home, and cigarette smoking. They had incorrect information about drying out wounds and leaving them open to promote healing.

IMPLICATIONS

Client concerns about discharge can be used to help plan discharge teaching. Teaching literature could include ways to avoid misinformation about wound care. Discharge teaching needs to begin early so that clients have adequate time to learn and ask questions.

Pieper, B., Sieggreen, M., Nordstrom, C. K., Freeland, B., Kulwicki, P., Frattaroli, M., et al. (2007). Discharge knowledge and concerns of patients going home with a wound. *Journal of Wound and Ostomy Continence Nursing, 34*(3), 245–253.

NURSING CARE PLAN

The Client with Ineffective Breastfeeding

CASE PRESENTATION
Mrs. Gozalo is a 32-year-old attorney who presents to the clinic requesting help in breastfeeding her 3-day-old daughter. She states that her first few attempts at breastfeeding in the hospital were marginally successful and that her baby was given formula by the staff prior to her discharge. Since being home, she has given the baby bottled formula when she cannot get the baby to latch on and suck successfully; these unsuccessful attempts at breastfeeding have made her question whether the effort to breastfeed is worthwhile. She says her husband has suggested using only bottle feedings, and she is frustrated and confused but wants to be successful at breastfeeding, which she describes as ''the right thing to do.''

ASSESSMENT
- Verbalizations of desire to be successful at breastfeeding
- Lack of understanding of correct latch-on procedure

NURSING DIAGNOSIS: *Ineffective breastfeeding* related to unsatisfactory breastfeeding process as evidenced by infant's receiving supplemental feedings with artificial nipple, interruption in breastfeeding, maternal anxiety, and deficient knowledge

NOC: Knowledge: Breastfeeding

NIC: Teaching: Individual

EXPECTED OUTCOMES
The client will:

1. Explain and demonstrate correct latch-on and breastfeeding procedure (cognitive and psychomotor domains)
2. Express confidence that breastfeeding will be successful (affective domain)
3. Demonstrate desire to continue efforts at breastfeeding (affective domain)

INTERVENTIONS/RATIONALES
1. Ask client, or determine through the interview process, what teaching strategies (lecture, literary, visuals) are most likely to be effective for her, and tailor teaching accordingly. Matching teaching strategies to learning styles and needs increases the chance of successful education.
2. Explain briefly the mechanics of the breastfeeding process, such as milk letdown, signs of breastfeeding readiness, and signs of infant hunger and satisfaction. Knowledge of the process of correct breastfeeding will help bring client expectations in line with reality.
3. Demonstrate correct infant holds and maternal postures. Proper position of both the child and mother facilitates breastfeeding.
4. Teach client effective techniques for latch-on, such as supporting the breast to correctly position it in the baby's mouth and tickling the baby's lips or cheeks to stimulate rooting. Use of correct techniques greatly enhances the likelihood of latch-on.
5. Show client video or literature demonstrating successful breastfeeding. Seeing other women breastfeed successfully helps promote confidence and maintain desire to learn correct process.
6. Encourage client to have her husband participate in the breastfeeding process by bringing the baby to her when she cries, stroking the baby's head while she is nursing, and burping the baby after each feeding. Partner support and involvement in the breastfeeding process will boost client's confidence and strengthen desire to continue breastfeeding process.

EVALUATION
Client verbalizes confidence and comfort level with attempts at breastfeeding. Client achieves correct latch-on with minimal difficulty. Client states the signs of successful breastfeeding and states that she will look for such signs as the breasts feeling less full and the infant sucking strongly and seeming content at each feeding.

reassessment is the basis for planning modification of teaching-learning activities. Several activities can be used to evaluate teaching effectiveness, including the following:

- Feedback from the learner
- Feedback from colleagues
- Situational feedback
- Self-evaluation

Evaluation is facilitated through the use of goals that are measurable and specific. Use of the accompanying Nursing Checklist facilitates evaluation of teacher effectiveness. See the Uncovering the Evidence display on page 416.

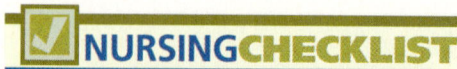

NURSINGCHECKLIST

EVALUATION OF TEACHER EFFECTIVENESS

- Was content presented clearly and at the client's level of comprehension?
- Did the nurse use a variety of teaching aids?
- Were the teaching aids appropriate for the client and the content?
- Was client participation encouraged?
- Was the nurse supportive?
- Did the nurse communicate an interest in the client and in the material?
- Did the nurse give frequent feedback and allow for immediate return demonstration?
- Were learning objectives stated in behavioral terms (i.e., easy to evaluate)?

KEY CONCEPTS

- Client education is done to help individuals achieve and maintain optimum states of health.
- The teaching-learning process is a planned interaction that promotes behavioral change that is not a result of maturation or coincidence.
- Teaching supports behavioral change that leads to positive adaptation.
- Learning is the process of assimilating information with a resultant change in behavior.
- Learning occurs in three domains: the cognitive (intellectual), the affective (emotional), and the psychomotor (motor skills).

- Learning readiness is affected by developmental and sociocultural factors and is a lifelong process that occurs in every developmental stage.
- Elements for documenting client education include the content taught, teaching methods used, who was taught, and response of the learners.
- The teaching-learning process and the nursing process are interdependent dynamic processes.
- Evaluation of the teaching-learning process involves two aspects: (1) determination of what the client has learned and (2) efficacy of the teacher.

REVIEW QUESTIONS

1. Which of the following methods can be used by the nurse to determine the client's dominant channel for learning new information? Select all that apply.
   a. Administering the client a written questionnaire on learning styles
   b. Asking clients how they learn best
   c. Asking family members what types of activities are enjoyed by the client
   d. Observing a client's behaviors
   e. Using a variety of teaching strategies

2. A client with hearing loss is being started on a new medication. Which of the following nursing actions is most appropriate for this client?
   a. Avoid the use of gestures.
   b. Face the client directly when speaking.
   c. Raise voice pitch and tone.
   d. Speak loudly.

3. The nurse is teaching a client how to self-administer insulin. Which of the following statements indicates the client's readiness to learn?
   a. "Are you sure this won't hurt a lot?"
   b. "I always watched my mother give herself injections."
   c. "I don't think I can ever get used to sticking myself."
   d. "I need to learn how to do this so I can take care of myself."

4. A nurse is planning to teach an adolescent client about skin care, focusing on hygiene. Which of the following teaching strategies would best promote client learning?
   a. Have the client initiate questions, then provide answers.
   b. Include the client in a group session on hygiene.

   c. Provide one-on-one instruction.

   d. Show a video that demonstrates the relationship between cleanliness and healthy skin.

5. Which of the following activities addresses the client's psychomotor learning needs?

   a. Asking a client to describe his feelings about self-administering injections

   b. Encouraging the client to accept a recent diagnosis of a chronic illness

   c. Helping the client read instructions on a prescription label

   d. Showing a client how to self-administer an injection

6. Which of the following nursing statements is most helpful for teaching a postoperative client how to safely ambulate?

   a. "If you don't get out of bed, you could develop pneumonia."

   b. "Walking will help you recover more quickly."

   c. "You must ambulate in order to avoid complications."

   d. "You need to dangle your feet before getting up to ambulate."

7. Which of the following is a priority nursing action for client education?

   a. Assessing client learning needs

   b. Selecting teaching methods

   c. Self-awareness

   d. Using clear, simple terms when teaching

8. The nurse is teaching a client who has an IQ of 68. Which of the following nursing actions is appropriate for meeting this client's learning needs?

   a. Ask multiple questions to capture the client's interest.

   b. Avoid repeating the information.

   c. Incorporate simple games into learning sessions.

   d. Use abstract terms when communicating.

9. Which of the following factors will most likely interfere with the client's ability to learn?

   a. Curiosity

   b. Decreased self-efficacy

   c. Headache

   d. Knowledge deficit

10. A client says, "I don't understand why my prescribing practitioner wants me to get out of bed so much." Which of the following nursing responses would encourage teaching-learning to occur?

   a. "I don't know what the prescribing practitioner was trying to say."

   b. "I will come back to talk with you after I finish giving medications to the other clients."

   c. "You need to ask your prescribing practitioner about that."

   d. "You sound confused about the need to walk."

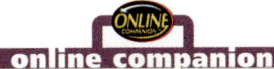

online companion

Visit the DeLaune and Ladner online companion resource at **www.delmar.cengage.com** for additional content and study aids. Click on Online Companions, then select the Nursing discipline.

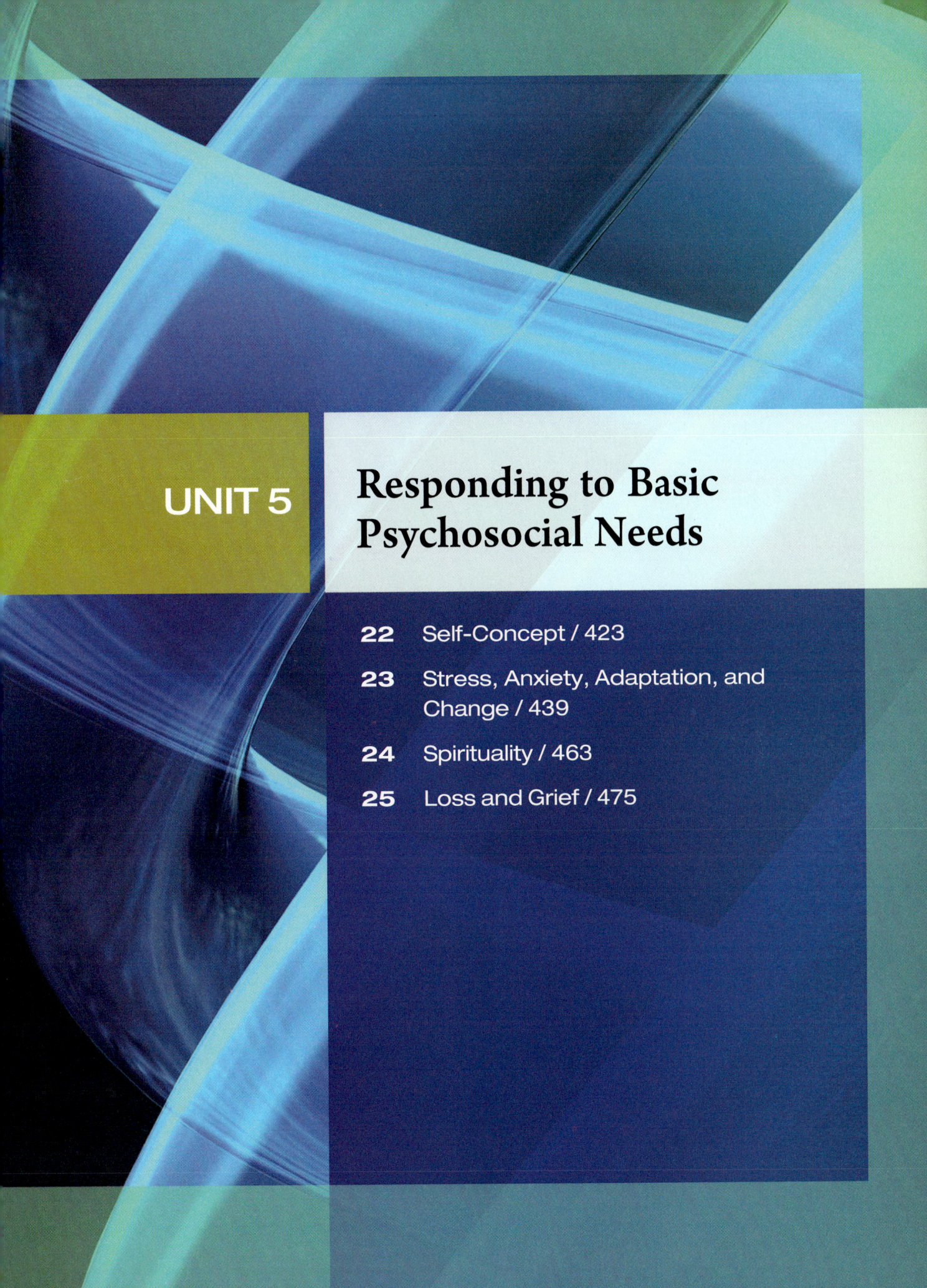

UNIT 5

Responding to Basic Psychosocial Needs

So much is a man worth as he esteems himself.

—Milton, 1532 (in McWilliams & McWilliams, 1991)

CHAPTER 22

Self-Concept

COMPETENCIES

1. Describe the four components of self-concept.
2. Explain the development of self-concept throughout the life span.
3. Discuss factors affecting self-concept.
4. Describe behaviors indicative of altered self-concept.
5. Discuss application of the nursing process with clients experiencing self-concept alterations.

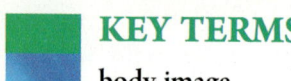

KEY TERMS

body image	role	self-concept
identity	role conflict	self-esteem

Self-concept (an individual's perception of self) affects every aspect of life, including relationships, functional abilities, and health status. No two people have an identical self-concept as self-concept is what helps make each individual unique. Everyone has both positive and negative self-assessments in the physical, emotional, intellectual, and functional dimensions, which change over time and according to the context of the situation. Because self-concept is an individual's frame of reference for perceiving and interacting with the world, it exerts a powerful influence on one's life. Though neither visible nor tangible, a positive self-concept is one of the greatest strengths a person can possess.

One's view of self affects the ability to function. A person who sees himself or herself as a competent individual will behave competently and vice versa. Individuals with a positive self-concept approach new experiences and tasks with confidence; they expect to be accepted by others and to succeed. Conversely, the person with a negative self-concept tends to shy away from others and to avoid challenges. Self-concept greatly influences health status. For example, a person with a positive self-concept is more likely to care for one's self—physically, emotionally, and spiritually. The relationship of the components of self-concept and mental health are discussed in Table 22-1.

COMPONENTS OF SELF-CONCEPT

Self-concept is composed of four components: identity, body image, self-esteem, and role performance (see Figure 22-1). By considering these four elements of self-concept, nurses can respond more effectively to clients.

IDENTITY

A sense of personal **identity** is what sets one person apart as a unique individual. A well-formulated identity provides the answer to the question "Who am I?" Identity includes a person's name, gender, ethnic identity, family status, occupation, and various roles.

During childhood, a person begins to develop identity, which is constantly reinforced and modified throughout life. First, parents or caretakers provide a child with elements of an emerging identity. Children may be told they are good or naughty, shy or outgoing, creative or dull, powerless or powerful. Children believe what they are told by others, and these beliefs influence their developing identities. During adolescence, conflict often arises as the teenager struggles to become independent and establish a unique identity. Eventually, people learn to observe themselves objectively, as their social environment expands. Feedback from others may support and strengthen an aspect of identity already implanted, or it may contradict an aspect and be a catalyst for change.

BODY IMAGE

Body image is an attitude about one's physical attributes and characteristics, appearance, and performance. Body

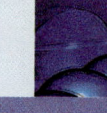

TABLE 22-1	**Self-Concept and Mental Health**

COMPONENT OF SELF-CONCEPT	RELATIONSHIP TO MENTAL HEALTH
Strong sense of identity	• The person experiences self as a unique, valuable individual.
Accurate and positive body image	• A healthy awareness of one's body is based on reality testing.
Positive self-esteem	• A person with a high degree of self-esteem respects self and treats self with dignity.
Satisfying role performance	• The person with healthy role performance relates well with others and receives gratification from fulfilling role expectations.

Delmar/Cengage Learning

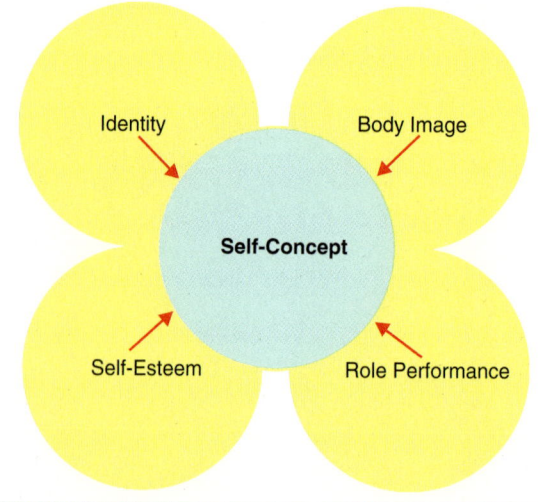

FIGURE 22-1 The Interrelationship of Components of Self-Concept DELMAR/CENGAGE LEARNING

image is dynamic because any change in body structure or function, including the normal changes of growth and development, can affect body image. Adolescence is an example of the interplay between an individual's physical changes and a developing sense of body image. Many teenagers have harmless body image distortions. It is not at all uncommon for adolescents to feel self-conscious because they think their noses are too big, or their hips too wide, or their blemishes too prominent. Usually, these are normal concerns. Adolescents generally find that their perceptions continue to evolve as their physical development progresses, resulting in a healthy body image.

SELF-ESTEEM

Self-esteem is an individual's generalized sense of worth and value, or how a person regards himself or herself. Self-esteem refers to an individual's self-evaluation, whereas self-concept is a broader term encompassing an individual's overall self-description.

The level of self-esteem at any given moment can be influenced by many factors. Individuals make decisions on what life factors (e.g., physical attributes, skills, social accomplishments) they deem important and calculate their self-esteem on the basis of their achievement of the factors they value most highly. These values are based on the individual's familial and cultural backgrounds and influenced by societal standards. Self-esteem varies over time, depending on the situation (e.g., new job), the environment (e.g., cocktail party with strangers), and an individual's level of development and overall self-confidence.

ROLE PERFORMANCE

Role refers to a set of expected behaviors that are determined by familial, cultural, and social norms. Individuals fulfill several roles simultaneously—parent, sibling, friend, spouse, student nurse. Each role has a set of expected behaviors, that is, a belief about how a person in that role should behave. See the accompanying Respecting Our Differences display on the sick role.

The nurse may assume several different roles (defined by Peplau, 1959), such as counselor, teacher, leader, or surrogate parent. As the relationship progresses, the client feels free to express feelings to the nurse because the nurse has assumed the roles of listener and counselor. As counselor, the nurse responds to the client's feelings or behavior, helping the client to gain insight, self-care, and a health-affirming outlook. As teacher, the nurse may provide information to the client or correct misconceptions.

Stressors Affecting Role

Roles have accompanying responsibilities. Whenever a person is unable to fulfill role responsibilities, self-concept is impaired. When an individual has too many roles to fulfill simultaneously, overload can occur. The person becomes overwhelmed by multiple demands of several roles. The individual feels unable to cope since coping skills are greatly taxed.

In addition to overload, another common problematic role experience is role conflict, which occurs when the expectations of one role compete with the expectations of other roles. The person may feel unable to establish priorities among competing role expectations. See the accompanying Spotlight On display and Table 22-2, on page 426, which describe the various types of role conflict.

DEVELOPMENT OF SELF-CONCEPT

Self-concept evolves throughout life and depends to an extent on an individual's developmental level. Self-concept changes during each developmental stage. According to Stuart and Laraia (2008), the ongoing process of self-concept development is facilitated by the following:

- Interpersonal and cultural experiences
- Self-perceived competence
- Self-actualization (living up to one's potential)

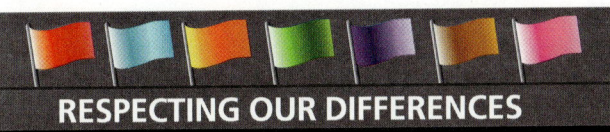

RESPECTING OUR DIFFERENCES

Sick Role

It is difficult enough for a healthy person to manage multiple roles, conflicts, and stresses. But what happens when illness forces an individual to assume the "sick role"? What are the social expectations of a sick person, and what effect does this new and often unexpected role have on all the other roles of the individual?

SPOTLIGHT ON...

Professionalism

Personal Roles

Consider the various roles you currently fulfill. What are some of the potential conflicts inherent in your multiple roles? For example, your role of student may at times conflict with your role of friend or parent (e.g., you need to be in class at the same time you need to attend a parent-teacher conference or be available to your friend who is undergoing a crisis). Or your need to study for an examination (student role) is superseded by your need to work (role of wage earner).

TABLE 22-2 Types of Role Conflict

TYPE	DESCRIPTION	EXAMPLE
Interrole conflict	Expectations of one role oppose expectations of another role.	A woman's job requires travel at the same time her child's dance recital is scheduled.
Interpersonal role conflict	Incompatible role expectations are held by one or more people.	A husband and wife disagree on parental expectations (e.g., disciplinary methods).
Role overload	Excessive demands of numerous roles have conflicting priorities.	A nurse must decide which urgent task to do first.
Person-role conflict	The individual's values are violated by demands of a role.	A nurse who believes in always telling the truth is directed by the supervisor to withhold a diagnosis from a client.

Delmar/Cengage Learning

Self-concept is developed primarily in response to social interactions and experiences. Sullivan (1953) stated that self-concept is developed according to perceptions mirrored by others to the individual. A person's concept of self depends, to an extent, on what one thinks that others think about oneself. As individuals mature, they can accept or reject the appraisals of others and change their behavior in ways that lead to a more positive self-concept.

CHILDHOOD

Self-concept is not innate; rather, it develops throughout the life cycle as a result of social interactions. An infant whose basic needs are met in a warm, consistent manner develops positive feelings about self. Formation of self-concept occurs in the following manner: (1) During infancy, the child develops a self-perception of being separate from the environment (including parents); (2) as the child ages, perspectives (especially of the parents) are internalized; and (3) society's norms (e.g., expectations of appropriate behavior) are then internalized by the child.

A child's sense of self is shaped by family experiences and interactions with parents and other relations. Children learn about their individual worth and their ability to be competent in the family unit, and their sense of self changes as they move through each developmental stage. Infants learn to trust based on the degree to which their needs are met, and they begin to develop a sense of self as distinct from the primary caretaker and their surroundings. As new skills are mastered, toddlers begin to develop a sense of autonomy and self-image, yet they still remain very self-centered. Pre-schoolers have increasing initiative and self-awareness as their expanding language and motor skills broaden their horizons, and they begin to have an awareness of emotions and values that are held by their families. When children reach school age, they will incorporate experiences and values of their new contacts and environments into their image of self and may start to have an understanding of their strengths as well as their shortcomings (see Figure 22-2).

Positive experiences, role models, and family environment are all crucial to the healthy self-concept of the growing child. The impact of early parent-child experiences on the shaping of a child's self-concept was emphasized by Sullivan (1953), whose interpersonal theory of psychiatry has greatly influenced nursing. The child develops a sense of self according to the type of feedback received from significant others (parental figures). Positive feedback reinforces the development of a "Good-Me" sense of self. A negative self-concept ("Bad-Me") is reinforced by feedback that is consistently negative and anxiety provoking (Sullivan, 1953).

ADOLESCENCE

The numerous changes in physical, emotional, and psychosocial status that characterize the adolescent years bring about rapid changes in self-concept. Impressions about self from childhood may be internalized or challenged. The primary benchmark for arriving at an overall perception of self can

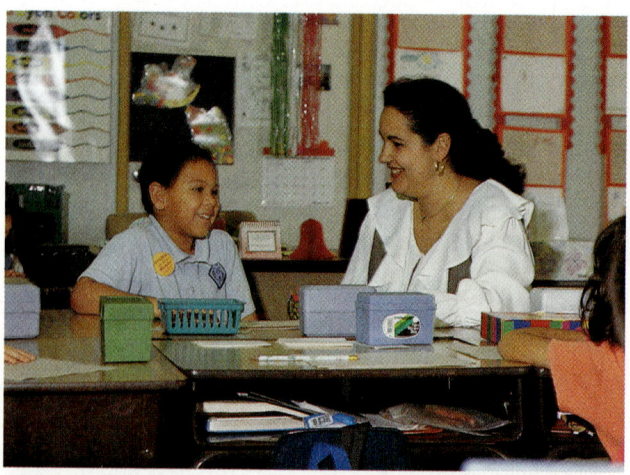

FIGURE 22-2 For a school-aged child, praise from teachers and a feeling of accomplishment in school can boost self-esteem. DELMAR/CENGAGE LEARNING

▼ SAFETY FIRST ▼

ADOLESCENTS AND SELF-CONCEPT
Due to the emphasis on body image, teens are at particular risk for feelings of disturbed body image, which may lead to serious health concerns such as anorexia nervosa and bulimia nervosa.

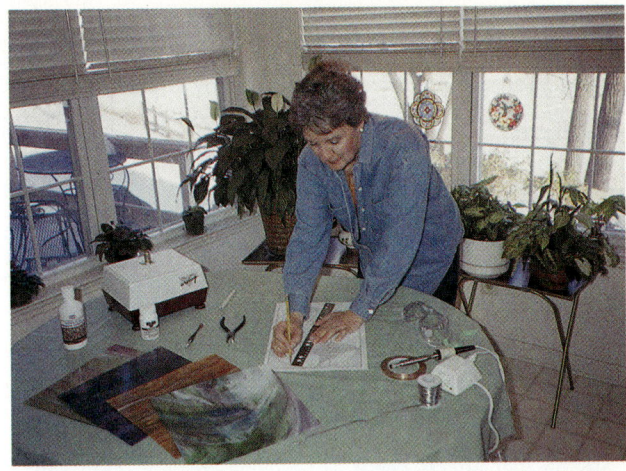

FIGURE 22-3 The mature adult's self-concept can be enhanced by learning new skills and enjoying new activities. DELMAR/CENGAGE LEARNING

change from family values to those held by peers or embodied in desired role models. Teens typically invest tremendous energies in physical appearance and social status and often fail to see their positive traits if they feel deficient in these areas. Adolescents often cannot separate their opinion of their own body image from their overall self-concept. For example, the teen who views herself as fat, when in fact she is emaciated, is likely to have a disturbed self-concept based on her distorted body image, regardless of what other positive qualities she may possess. The nurse needs to learn to distinguish between what might be a normal body image distortion ("I wish I were 3 inches taller") and one that can have serious, even fatal, consequences ("Weighing 100 pounds is the most important thing in the world for me"). Determining a teen's self-concept will help the nurse differentiate perceptions that are normal reactions to the changes of adolescence and those that are potentially harmful.

ADULTHOOD

Self-concept continues to develop and change as an individual progresses through the adult years. Periods of relative stability in self-image may be interspersed with realizations of physical changes in body size, proportion, characteristics, and energy levels, all of which will influence perception of self. Involvement in family, work, and community obligations and activities contributes significantly to an individual's self-concept, as roles and responsibilities change and new roles are introduced. Healthy adjustment to these changes results in a positive self-concept (see Figure 22-3).

As the years pass, the older adult's perception of self continues to develop. Learning to adapt to the numerous physical changes that normally occur with aging (e.g., diminished eyesight and hearing, lower stamina levels, loss and change in color of hair) can be a true challenge for many individuals; see Figure 22-4. Accompanying these changes is often the desire to look back on one's life and evaluate its overall success. Such reminiscence is usually a critical factor in an older adult's self-concept.

FACTORS AFFECTING SELF-CONCEPT

There is a universal need for positive self-concept, which includes a high degree of self-esteem and self-acceptance.

Any type of threat (real or imagined, actual or anticipated) may challenge one's self-concept.

ALTERED HEALTH STATUS

Illness evokes anxiety in most people; in turn, anxiety can result in illness. Every client will have some element of anxiety

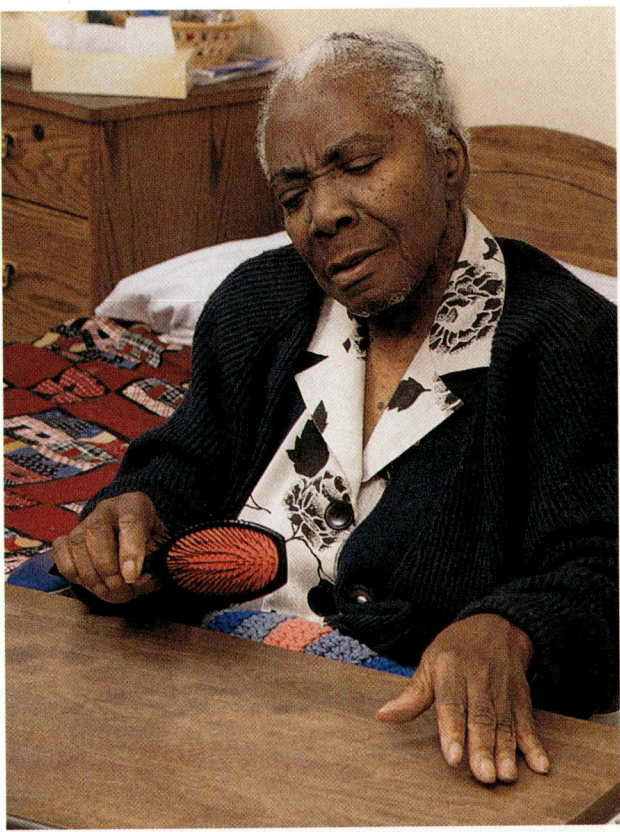

FIGURE 22-4 Older adults need to adjust their self-concept, especially body image, in accordance with physical changes that affect appearance. DELMAR/CENGAGE LEARNING

that influences behavioral and emotional responses. Most ill people are somewhat uneasy, especially if they are being treated in an unfamiliar environment or by a new health care provider. When anxiety level is heightened, recovery is compromised. Nurses, as professionals who focus on the human response to illness, must be aware of client anxiety level in order to promote effective adaptation. Table 22-3 shows common stressors frequently experienced during illness.

By their very nature, some illnesses may impair self-concept. For example, there is a social stigma against mental illness; the reactions of other people to the mentally ill person affect the client's self-perceptions. Many people fear cancer and isolate those affected with the disease. A diagnosis of acquired immunodeficiency syndrome (AIDS) may also carry a stigma that affects client self-esteem. Society often shuns those with AIDS, which may make them feel embarrassed or ashamed about their illness. To improve the client's quality of life, the nurse caring for individuals with any of these disorders must intervene to promote positive self-concept.

Compromised health status that requires surgery can also lead to several psychological alterations, including an impaired body image. Altered body image may result from loss of a body part or function after surgical procedures. Some procedures (e.g., mastectomy, amputation, colostomy) may leave the individual feeling mutilated or flawed. Bodily changes as a result of surgery have different meanings to different individuals. For example, consider a mastectomy. The woman whose feminine identity is symbolized by a voluptuous shape will likely be adversely affected by the surgery. Other common sequelae of surgery—decreased independence, loss of control, and disruption of routine—can also negatively affect self-concept. Self-esteem deficits related to surgery often include interference with role performance and impaired sexuality.

DEVELOPMENTAL TRANSITIONS

Developmental processes may affect self-concept by introducing changes or challenges to an individual's identity, body image, self-esteem, and role expectations. For example, pregnancy is a process with resultant changes in all these factors of self-concept; see Figure 22-5. In the early part of pregnancy, the woman incorporates the baby into her self-image. As the pregnancy progresses, the woman's body image adjusts to accommodate the idea that the baby is a separate individual (Edelman & Mandle, 2006). After delivery, the woman who has positive self-esteem will accept and love the

TABLE 22-3 Stressors Associated with Illness	
THREAT	**EXAMPLE**
Threats to physical safety	Undergoing painful procedures (the thought of receiving an injection evokes anxiety in many)
	Fear of pain
	Fear of death
Threat to psychological integrity	One's image of self is threatened or challenged by new situations (such as moving to a nursing home)
Inability to exert control	Having little or no input into important decisions; clients often feel as if they have no input into decision making regarding their treatment plan
	Loss of control may have a negative impact on self-concept and self-esteem, which in turn evokes anxiety
Unmet biological needs	Hunger
	Thirst
	Urge to eliminate and lack of bathroom or privacy for toileting
	Physical pain, discomfort

Delmar/Cengage Learning

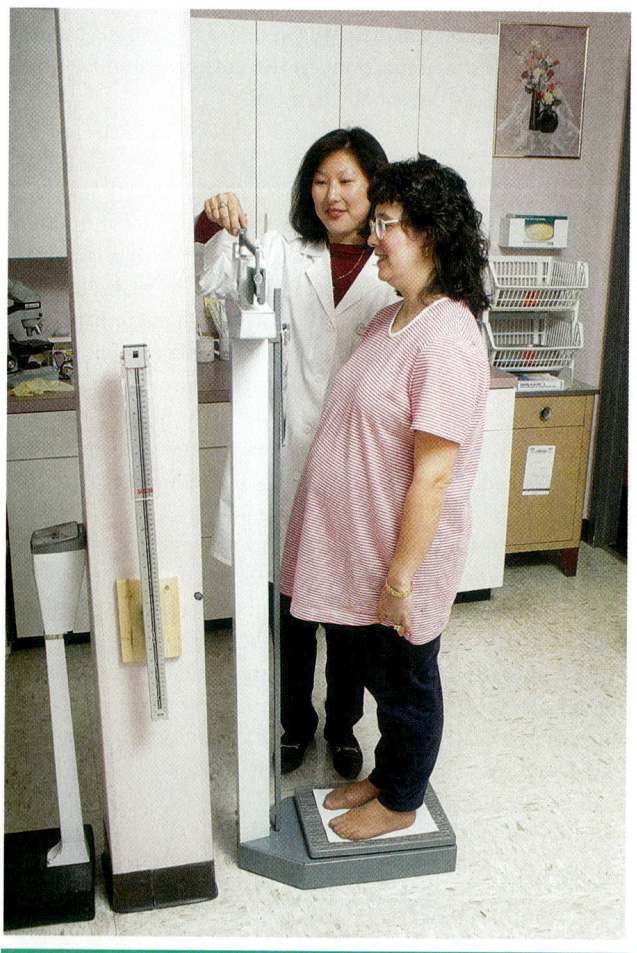

FIGURE 22-5 Body image changes with developmental events such as pregnancy. What do this client's nonverbal cues indicate about her self-concept? DELMAR/CENGAGE LEARNING

baby. One who feels unlovable or unattractive may make disparaging remarks about the infant (Edelman & Mandle, 2006) and have difficulty bonding appropriately and adjusting to the life changes a new baby introduces. The role of parent needs to be incorporated into a revised self-concept, and identity and self-esteem must be adjusted on the basis of new expectations.

Another example of a developmental issue that can affect the self-concept of an individual is menopause. The nurse must understand the meaning of this transitional period to the client and know that it varies with each individual. This normal developmental transition may have a negative psychological impact on some women. Some people view the female climacteric (menopausal phase) as an indication of loss of femininity with resultant decrease in value as a person. Other women view menopause as a sign of freedom from the risk of childbearing. Some common misconceptions about menopause are:

- Menopause is a disease.
- The menopausal woman has decreased sex drive.
- Menopause means the end of femininity.
- A woman who has experienced menopause is "old."
- The physical symptoms of menopause are unbearable.

EXPERIENCE

Self-concept is also influenced by an individual's experiences. Individuals who have experienced several failures begin to view themselves as failures. Their behavior often becomes self-fulfilling in that they perform at an unsuccessful level because they feel that is all they are capable of achieving. A negative self-concept is the result of repeated failures. On the other hand, people who achieve a task begin to see themselves in a positive manner, thus establishing the foundation for a positive self-concept.

NURSING PROCESS AND SELF-CONCEPT

Nursing care is individualized for each client as determined by specific needs. Therefore, client self-concept greatly influences application of the nursing process. Each phase of the nursing process must consider the client's perception of self.

ASSESSMENT

When assessing a client's self-concept, the nurse must consider both the client's developmental level and chronological age. Clients need to be addressed at a level that reflects their current condition as well as their cognitive competence. For example, very young clients and those with low literacy skills may not be able to read; thus, the use of pictures or diagrams may be helpful.

It is necessary to determine the client's perception of self-concept and the factors affecting it. For example, an adjustment to and recovery from an appendectomy may

be uneventful for one person and difficult for another. The person who sees the surgery as a means to recovery will be healthier than the one who feels mutilated by scarring.

Behavior, thoughts, and emotions are affected by self-concept. It is important to attend to the client's verbal and nonverbal cues. Self-concept is reflected in a person's behavior and conversation. Individuals who feel they are unable to accomplish goals will experience changes in eating, sleeping, and activity patterns (Edelman & Mandle, 2006).

The accompanying Nursing Process Highlight offers some questions useful in assessing body image and self-esteem. Table 22-4, on page 430, lists some indicators of high and low levels of self-esteem. To provide quality care, the nurse must determine the client's strengths. Doing so enables assessment of characteristics that can be used for coping and problem solving. The client's strengths are a foundation on which to build therapeutic interventions. Some areas to assess include the client's ability to:

- Develop and maintain appropriate relationships
- Care for himself or herself in order to meet basic needs
- Adapt to stressors in a positive manner

The nurse should encourage clients to make a list of all the positive things they have done and then review the list. Also, the nurse can help clients identify how they have handled problems in the past: "When you were in a similar situation, what did you do? Was it helpful? Are you able to try that now? If not, what else can you do?"

The nurse should ask clients to describe their appearance and abilities. This information is an indicator of awareness of strengths as well as limitations; it is also important to assess clients' personal meaning of these assets and liabilities.

NURSING PROCESS HIGHLIGHT

Assessment

Questions for Assessing Body Image and Self-Esteem

Body Image

- What do you like best about your body?
- What do you like least about your body?
- If you could change how you look, what would you change?

Self-Esteem

- What do you like best about yourself?
- What do you like least about yourself?
- How do you describe yourself to others?
- How would others describe you?
- What are your strengths and weaknesses?

TABLE 22-4 Indicators of High and Low Self-Esteem

	HIGH SELF-ESTEEM	LOW SELF-ESTEEM
Communication	• Assertive • Direct and honest	• Passive or aggressive • Indirect, dishonest
Posture	• Erect • Moves briskly	• Stooped • Slow movement and activity
General appearance	• Well groomed	• Unkempt and dirty
Eye contact	• Frequent and appropriate to context of situation	• Avoidance or intrusive staring
Speech	• Well modulated • Speech flows smoothly	• Monotone • Mumbling • Hesitant
Self-care	• Attends to own needs	• Denies or minimizes own needs • Neglects own needs by always caring for others first
Self-talk	• Praises self	• Puts self down • Highly self-critical
Behavior	• Appropriate to situation and context of interpersonal relationship	• Socially inappropriate • Violates social norms • Counterproductive
Measure of worth	• Values self	• Has feelings of worthlessness
Decision making	• Makes decisions appropriately for context of situation	• Indecisive • Hesitant
Locus of control	• Internal	• External
Autonomy	• Self-directed	• Overly dependent on others
Emotions	• Able to experience a wide range of emotions • Varies appropriately according to situation	• Wide range of emotions inappropriately expressed • Hostile • Dependent

Delmar/Cengage Learning

DIAGNOSIS

Individuals experiencing self-concept disturbances usually have feelings of anxiety, hostility, guilt, and shame. Self-concept alterations affect every aspect of a person's life: emotions, relationships, and functional ability.

The nurse must conduct a thorough assessment to determine the nature and extent of problems in order to formulate accurate nursing diagnoses. Because of the extensive impact of self-concept problems, several diagnoses may be established by the nurse. The accompanying Nursing Process Highlight, on page 431, lists some primary nursing diagnoses associated with self-concept disturbances as defined by the North American Nursing Diagnosis Association (2009).

OUTCOME IDENTIFICATION AND PLANNING

For clients with an altered self-concept, a major nursing goal is to promote the client's sense of well-being and to facilitate growth. This involves teaching coping skills and the effective use of personal resources.

Together the nurse and client develop specific goals because mutually established goals encourage the client to assume an active role in recovery. Realistic planning involves examination of options. What is available to use in helping a client regain responsibility for self-care? Realistic goals should be stated in terms of specific behavior that is

NURSING PROCESS HIGHLIGHT

Diagnosis

Nursing Diagnoses Related to Self-Concept

- Disturbed body image
- Impaired parenting
- Disturbed personal identity
- Ineffective role performance
- Chronic low self-esteem
- Situational low self-esteem
- Anxiety
- Social isolation
- Hopelessness
- Powerlessness

From North American Nursing Diagnosis Association. (2009–2011). *Nursing Diagnoses—Definitions and Classification 2009–2011* © 2009, 2007, 2005, 2004, 2001, 1998, 1996, 1994 NANDA International. Used by arrangement with Wiley-Blackwell Publishing, a company of John Wiley & Sons, Inc.

measurable and should have an appropriate time frame for evaluation of outcome achievement.

IMPLEMENTATION

Regardless of the setting in which they practice, nurses will inevitably encounter clients who are experiencing alterations in self-concept. Whether a client is experiencing an optimal level of health or an alteration in health, a high degree of self-esteem is necessary for a positive outcome. The nurse needs to find ways to support positive self-esteem. A high degree of self-esteem can be associated with several different dimensions of the person, such as success in relationships, intelligence, or being a member who is held in high regard by an ethnic or cultural group. In attempting to support the client's high self-esteem, the nurse should learn sources of self-esteem for the client and seek to reinforce them. "Respect is the act of esteeming another. Demonstrated by word and deed, it is fostered by attending to the whole person by involving the patient and family in decision making ..." (Rushton, 2007, p. 155).

Initiate Therapeutic Interaction

Self-concept, or lack of it, affects the nurse-client relationship. The nurse is a role model of an individual who has self-respect and also respects others. By using a nonjudgmental approach, the nurse encourages clients to feel more positive about themselves.

The use of open-ended statements facilitates honest communication. Active listening is essential in working with clients experiencing self-concept alterations. By thoughtfully applying therapeutic communication skills, the nurse facilitates the development of trust and rapport.

Support Healthy Defense Mechanisms

Use of defense mechanisms is a common reaction to anxiety or a perceived threat. See Chapter 23 for a discussion of defense mechanisms. When caring for a client with altered or threatened self-concept, it is wise to first identify the client's strengths and successful coping mechanisms before formulating and implementing a plan of care. It is important to avoid taking away a client's defensive processes until another method of coping with anxiety has been developed. For example, breaking through a client's denial too soon can result in overwhelming anxiety. On the other hand, encouraging the use of denial beyond its time of therapeutic value will result in reality distortion.

Ensure Satisfaction of Needs

The relationship between satisfaction of basic needs and psychological comfort is undeniable. When needs are unmet, anxiety increases. Nursing interventions must be focused on helping clients fulfill basic needs.

PHYSICAL NEEDS Self-concept stems in part from the client's perception of personal appearance, competencies, and limitations. It includes the client's self-perception as well as others' perceptions. By assisting the client to maintain personal appearance, the nurse is also helping the client improve self-esteem. Being unable to meet one's basic needs usually results in self-concept impairment. Self-esteem is generally decreased as a person becomes more dependent on others.

Providing for the client's well-being and comfort is the foundation of quality nursing care. When clients are treated in a caring, competent manner and their physical needs are met, self-concept is positively influenced.

PSYCHOSOCIAL NEEDS Uncertainty escalates anxiety. All clients in every health care setting need clear statements of expected behavior. Explain procedures, telling the client what is expected and what is going to occur. The following nursing actions promote the client's psychological safety:

- Respect a client's privacy. Loss of privacy triggers anxiety in most individuals. During treatment in any setting, personal probing questions must be asked; procedures often violate physical space and can be offensive; elimination activities often occur in the presence of others. Be sure to protect privacy as much as possible.
- Treat each client as an individual worthy of dignity. This means being sensitive to the feelings of others.
- Encourage the client to be as independent as possible while providing assistance as needed.

Promote Positive Self-Esteem across the Life Span

The nurse understands that self-esteem is affected by developmental level. Thus, nursing interventions are planned and implemented differently according to a client's placement in the life span.

CHILDHOOD The child's self-concept develops over time and is greatly influenced by interactions and experiences with others. The child who feels successful and competent with tasks has a more positive self-concept than does the child who fails to achieve task mastery.

Some of the changes occurring with physical growth and maturation may be anxiety provoking for the child; for instance, anxiety may result when the child loses baby teeth or experiences menstruation for the first time. The onset of physical changes of puberty can be frightening or unsettling to the child. The nurse is most effective by providing education and support. The accompanying Client Teaching Checklist provides information essential in helping parents promote positive self-concept development in children.

ADOLESCENCE An adolescent's sense of self is greatly influenced by others, especially peers. Acceptance and a sense of belonging to a peer group influence the adolescent's sense of worth and well-being; see Figure 22-6. Feelings about one's self intensify during puberty. Adolescents may become very self-conscious because they often think everyone else is watching them.

As adolescents' bodies change, they must keep revising their body images. A severe or deep-rooted distortion of body image may be a manifestation of a mental illness, such as anorexia nervosa or bulimia nervosa, which occur primarily during adolescence. The nurse needs to help the adolescent redirect energies, focus on positive traits, and view himself or herself as a compilation of many factors, not just one (e.g., weight). See the Uncovering the Evidence display.

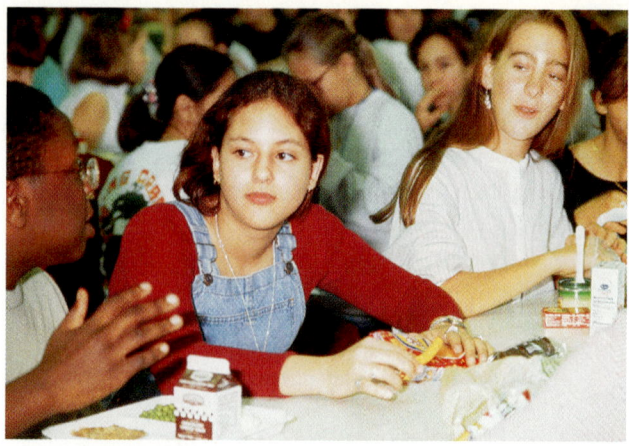

FIGURE 22-6 Peers exert much influence on the adolescent's changing self-concept. DELMAR/CENGAGE LEARNING

UNCOVERING THE

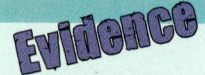
Evidence

TITLE OF STUDY
"Ecological Strategies to Promote Healthy Body Image among Children"

AUTHORS
R. R. Evans, J. Roy, B. F. Geiger, K. A. Werner, and D. Burnett

PURPOSE
To examine approaches that may be used to promote development of healthy body images in children.

METHODS
This study systematically applied the ecological model to components of coordinated school health, including attitudes and behaviors about eating; exercise and physical appearance modeled by parents, teachers, and peers; opportunities to learn new habits; and social praise for healthy choices. Strategies for each component were developed in the areas of health education, exercise science, and dietetics.

FINDINGS
For each strategy, applicable health and physical education standards and resources were provided to assist educators in supporting healthy body images among students.

IMPLICATIONS
Educators and school nurses may effectively use a coordinated approach to guide multiple activities aimed at increasing healthy habits and the development of healthy body images of children.

Evans, R. R., Roy, J., Geiger, B. F., Werner, K. A., & Burnett, D. (2008). Ecological strategies to promote healthy body image among children. *Journal of School Health, 78*(7), 359–367.

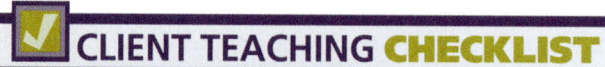

✔ CLIENT TEACHING **CHECKLIST**

Actions of Parents to Promote Positive Self-Concept in Children

- Encourage expression of feelings.
- Promote mutual respect and trust by establishing and maintaining open lines of communication
- Demonstrate a willingness to talk about any subject.
- Listen carefully to children, and use words they understand.
- Use examples and anecdotes to promote learning.
- Teach by example. Role-model problem solving and coping skills.
- Encourage children's talents and accept their limitations. Be realistic in your expectations, and avoid comparing one child to another.
- Celebrate children's accomplishments.
- Demonstrate confidence in their abilities.
- Provide children with unconditional love.

ADULTHOOD As adults continue to mature, self-concept changes in response to new self-perceptions and roles. Young adults make a transition to independent living without parental assistance. The degree of ease or discomfort in making such a transition affects the young adult's self-concept by demonstrating a sense of competency.

The self-concept of an older person is the culmination of a variety of factors, including life experiences and interactions with others. Some life experiences that shape the older adult's self-concept are adjusting to role loss and dealing with the loss of significant others. Spending time with significant others may increase the older client's self-esteem by making him or her feel valued; see Figure 22-7.

Throughout life, the individual has developed coping resources. Because self-concept is intertwined with competency, it is important for nurses to allow older clients the time to complete tasks that are meaningful to them. Some of the many factors that may negatively affect the older adult's self-esteem are shown in the accompanying Respecting Our Differences display. When caring for older clients, it is important to plan activities that promote a healthy self-concept.

EVALUATION

A client's behavior and attitudes will reflect the degree of progress toward restoring an altered self-concept. The nurse must reconsider the alignment of the client's targeted self-concept with the plan of care to assess if the two are still congruent. Input from family members or significant others can be useful in seeing the client in a larger context of differing roles and expectations and may also highlight some of the similarities and differences between the client's perceived self-image and the impressions of those closest to him or her.

Another crucial factor in evaluating the success of attaining goals is the consideration of time. Because self-concept is based on personal attitudes, feelings, and impressions, it

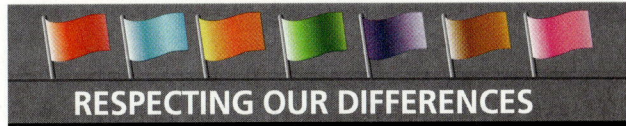

RESPECTING OUR DIFFERENCES

Factors Contributing to Self-Concept Alterations in the Older Client

- Changes in environment
- Ageism (social stigma against older adults)
- Loss of significant others (including pets)
- Social isolation
- Illness, acute or chronic
- Financial change

✓ NURSINGCHECKLIST

Promoting Self-Concept in the Older Client

- Increase socialization.
- Encourage involvement and participation in care.
- For clients in the home setting, urge family members to allow client to be involved with household tasks and routines as much as possible.
- Elicit client feedback.
- Use touch to decrease feelings of isolation and to promote feelings of security and acceptance.
- Modesty is often important to the older client; therefore, maintain and promote privacy. For example, perform physical examinations or procedures without completely exposing the client.
- Do not remove all personal belongings because these are often invested with symbolic meaning (e.g., let the older woman keep her purse at her bedside).
- Demonstrate patience; allow clients time to complete sentences and to finish one task before moving on to the next.
- Involve family or significant others as much as possible in the provision of care.
- Encourage the client to reminisce, especially focusing on individual strengths and accomplishments.

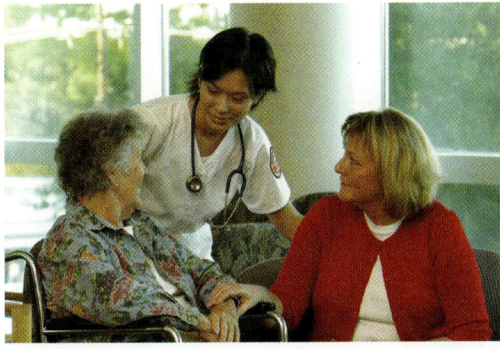

FIGURE 22-7 Identify some factors that may contribute positively to this older client's self-esteem. DELMAR/CENGAGE LEARNING

often requires months or even years to change. Nurses, clients, and families all need to learn to be patient and to work together to improve or restore a client's self-concept.

NURSING CARE PLAN

The Client with Ineffective Role Performance

CASE PRESENTATION

Todd Lloyd is a 31-year-old civil engineer who has just left his job of 10 years to care full-time for his new-born daughter, Sarah. He and his wife decided that after their child was born, she would return to work full-time outside the home, and he would be the primary caregiver for their daughter during the day. Mr. Lloyd presents at the clinic stating, "I am very eager and excited about being a full-time dad, but I'm also a little nervous because I really don't know what to expect."

ASSESSMENT

- Lack of knowledge about new parenting role
- Concern over changes in responsibilities

NURSING DIAGNOSIS

Ineffective role performance related to change in roles and usual patterns of responsibility, as evidenced by verbalization of concern over lack of knowledge about new role

NOC: Parenting Performance

NIC: Parent Education: Infant Care

EXPECTED OUTCOMES

The client will:

1. Explain specific concerns about new roles.
2. Demonstrate role competence.
3. Verbalize satisfaction with role performance.

INTERVENTIONS/RATIONALES

1. Encourage the client to express his feelings about his new role. Opens the door to communication and problem solving.
2. Outline with client what aspects of his role(s) will be changing and what will be the same. Helps client identify the ways in which his role is changing, so he can face the changes from a realistic frame of mind. Also highlights similarities, not just differences, between his past and present roles, thus helping client feel less overwhelmed.
3. Assist the client in identifying concerns he has regarding the change in roles. Helps the client determine his specific concerns so they can be addressed.
4. Encourage client to discuss concerns with wife and to seek help together. Support of spouse will be critical to client's success in overcoming concerns about changing roles.
5. Help client gain confidence and competence with new role by demonstrating new role behaviors, offering literature and resources, and providing referral to parenting courses or counselors. Assures client that resources are available to help him meet his needs and helps lessen his anxiety and his feeling of being overwhelmed.
6. Have client return demonstrate new behaviors and offer encouragement and additional teaching. Allows client to try out new behaviors in a "safe" environment and provides a means for immediate feedback.
7. Ask client for feedback on the new behaviors and information acquired. Provides chance for client to evaluate progress in new role, which will increase client's confidence.

EVALUATION

Mr. Lloyd is able to identify specific concerns about his new role as parent and has demonstrated a growing competence in some of the behaviors that will support this new role. He read the literature and has ordered a videotape designed for new parents. He is also planning to subscribe to a newsletter entitled "The Full-Time Father." Mr. Lloyd agrees that his wife's input would be very valuable to his gaining comfort and confidence in his new role, and he agrees to visit the clinic again with her in a week.

KEY CONCEPTS

- Self-concept (an individual's perception of self) affects every aspect of a person's life.

- People who see themselves as competent individuals will behave competently and vice versa.

- Self-concept consists of four interrelated components: identity, body image, self-esteem, and role performance.

- A well-formulated identity provides the answer to the question "Who am I?" and may consist of a person's name, family status, occupation, and various roles.

- Body image refers to a person's mental picture of and attitudes about his or her body. It includes physical attributes and characteristics, appearance, and performance.

- Self-esteem is the individual's generalized sense of worth and value.

- Role refers to a set of expected behaviors that are determined by social norms.

- The development of self-concept begins at birth and depends, to a degree, on interactions with others as the child grows and matures.

- The person's developmental level affects self-concept; with maturity comes a stronger self-concept.

- Illness evokes anxiety in most people, and anxiety can exacerbate illness. Any threat to self-concept arouses anxiety. When anxiety level is heightened, recovery is compromised.

- Surgery can result in body image disturbances. Altered body image results from loss of a body part or function and distortion of body image.

- Assessment of self-concept must consider both developmental level and chronological age.

- Identification of client strengths enables the nurse to determine the presence of factors the client can use for coping and problem solving.

REVIEW QUESTIONS

1. Which of the following are indicators that a person has a high degree of self-esteem? Select all that apply.
   a. Appropriate decision-making skills
   b. Assertive communication
   c. Disheveled clothing
   d. Erect posture
   e. Intrusive staring
   f. Mumbling, hesitant speech

2. A student nurse is teaching a group of clients how to improve self-esteem. Which of the following client statements indicates that further teaching is needed?
   a. "I will do something, like take a walk, the next time I feel down."
   b. "If I just wait long enough, I'll start to feel better."
   c. "When I feel bad, I should think of something positive."
   d. "When I feel good about myself, I have good self-esteem."

3. When working with a client who has anorexia nervosa, which of the following nursing diagnoses is most applicable?
   a. Anxiety
   b. Chronic low self-esteem
   c. Disturbed body image
   d. Social isolation

4. A student nurse has clinical scheduled at the same time as his child's parent-teacher conference. Which of the following is the student nurse experiencing?

   a. Body image disturbance
   b. Person-role conflict
   c. Role conflict
   d. Role overload

5. Which of the following are client strengths that may be used in health promotion?
   a. Ability to perform self-care
   b. History of multiple job changes
   c. Relying on others for assistance with activities of daily living
   d. Role overload

6. The nurse is planning a parenting class on building self-esteem in children. Which of the following topics is important for the nurse to include when teaching parenting skills classes? Select all that apply.
   a. Accept the child's limitations and strengths.
   b. Compare younger siblings to older ones to encourage the development of competition.
   c. Provide conditional love to children.
   d. Role-model expected behaviors.
   e. Talk to children in adult terms so they will develop language skills quickly.
   f. Use abstract terms when talking to young children.

7. Which of the following client statements indicates a high degree of self-esteem?
   a. "I am so tired of failing."
   b. "I've solved problems before so feel like I can do so now."

c. "There's no use in trying because nothing will change."

d. "Why bother! Everything I do turns out wrong anyway."

8. Which of the following factors is most influential on the development of an adolescent's body image?

a. Life experiences

b. Parental feedback

c. Peer approval

d. The need for modesty

9. Which of the following actions can be implemented by the nurse to improve the self-concept of older clients?

a. Decrease socialization in order to lower anxiety level.

b. Encourage the client to talk about current events, instead of those in the past.

c. Remove personal items to keep the health care environment free of clutter.

d. Use touch to promote feelings of acceptance.

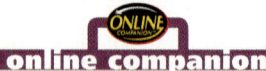

online companion

Visit the DeLaune and Ladner online companion resource at **www.delmar.cengage.com** for additional content and study aids. Click on Online Companions, then select the Nursing discipline.

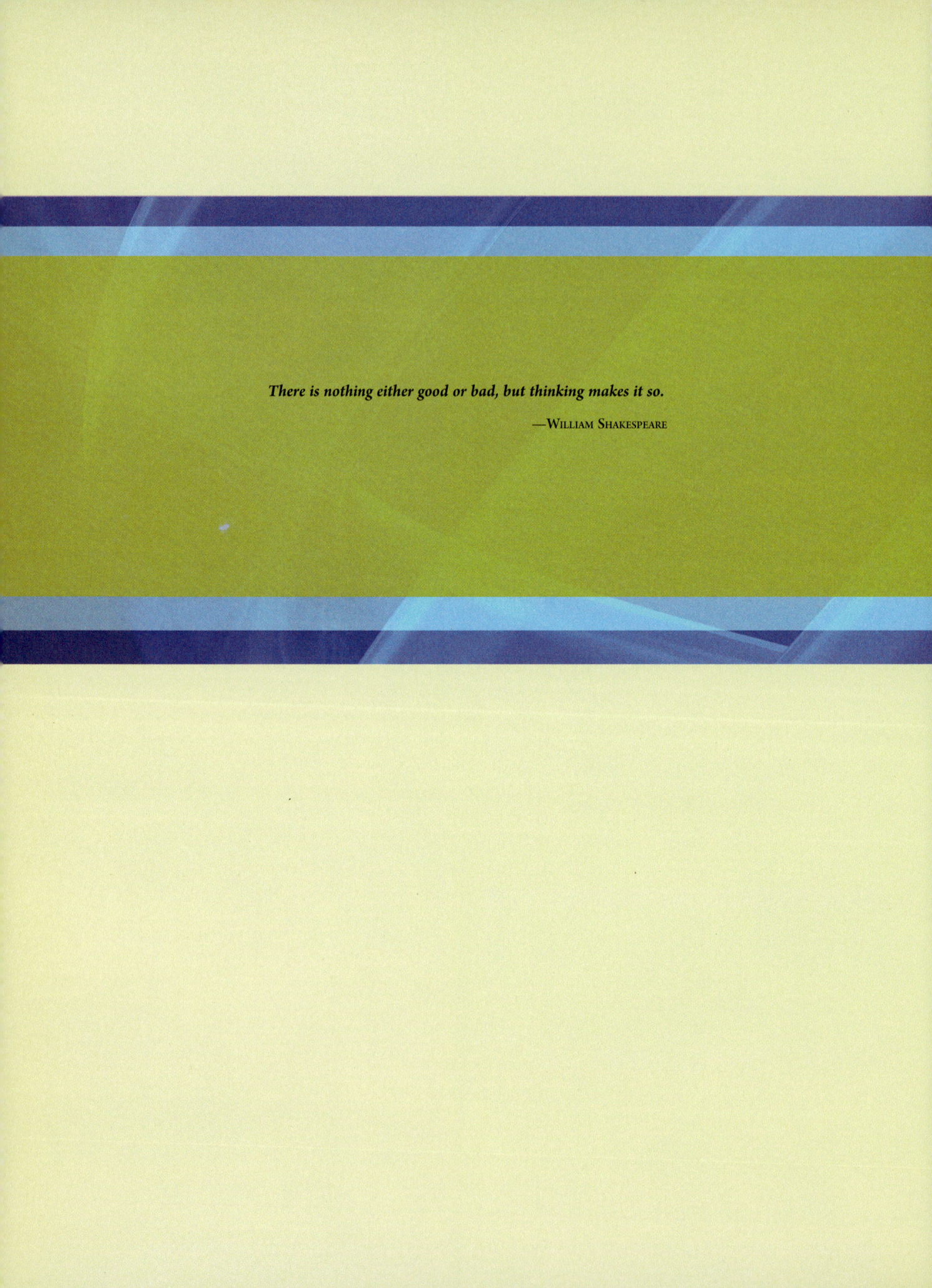

There is nothing either good or bad, but thinking makes it so.

—WILLIAM SHAKESPEARE

CHAPTER 23

Stress, Anxiety, Adaptation, and Change

COMPETENCIES

1. Discuss stress, anxiety, and adaptation as they affect health.
2. Identify factors contributing to the stress response.
3. Describe the general adaptation syndrome (GAS).
4. Explain stressors inherent in the change process.
5. Discuss the role of the nurse as a change agent.
6. Explain nursing interventions that promote positive adaptation to stress.
7. Develop an individualized stress management plan for use as a nurse.

Stress, a universal experience, can be the catalyst for positive change or it can be the source of discomfort and pain. Nurses help clients learn to cope with the stress imposed by illness, injury, disability, or treatment approaches. How does stress affect nurses? Caring for clients who are experiencing high levels of anxiety can be stress-provoking for nurses. Successful stress management is necessary for wellness of both clients and nurses. This chapter discusses the major concepts related to stress, anxiety, and adaptation and presents strategies for coping with stress and change.

STRESS, ANXIETY, AND ADAPTATION

Stress is the body's physiological reaction to any stimulus that evokes a change. Any situation, event, or agent that threatens a person's security is a **stressor**. A stressor is a stimulus that evokes the need to adapt and can be internal or external. For example, a headache is an internal stressor, whereas a difficult assignment is an external stressor. A stressor can be physical (e.g., a laceration), physiological (e.g., hypertension), or psychosocial (e.g., graduation from school). Even pleasant events can be stressful in that they evoke the need to adapt. Stressors in themselves are neutral; in other words, a stressor is neither good nor bad. The individual's perception of the stressor greatly determines whether the outcome is positive or negative.

Anxiety, a pervasive feeling of dread or apprehension, is a subjective response that occurs when a person experiences a threat to well-being. There is a close relationship between stress and anxiety. Stress is the person's physiological response to a stimulus, whereas anxiety is the psychological response to a threat. Anxiety can be both an activator of stress and a response to stress. It is usually activated by stress and may, in and of itself, lead to more stress.

Adaptation is an ongoing process by which individuals adjust to stressors in order to achieve **homeostasis** (equilibrium between physiological, psychological, sociocultural, intellectual, and spiritual needs). Adaptation is a holistic response that involves all dimensions of an individual.

Individuals, as holistic beings, seek to maintain a *steady state* (another term for homeostasis) in all dimensions of life: physiological, psychological, cognitive, social, and spiritual. Wellness is an adaptive state; that is, the well person is one who is coping effectively with stressors to maintain a high level of well-being. The nurse's goal is to identify and support the client's positive adaptive responses.

SOURCES OF STRESS

Individuals experience stress from multiple sources, primarily their bodies, their thoughts, and the environment. A situation or event that evokes stress in one person may not affect another. Examples of factors contributing to stress are shown in Table 23-1 on page 441.

RESPONSES TO STRESS

Every individual has unique responses to stress. A person's response to stress is influenced by several variables: mental attitude, lifestyle, perception, and heredity.

PHYSIOLOGICAL RESPONSE

The stress response, which can be adaptive or maladaptive, is the nonspecific response of the body to any demand (Selye, 1974). When the response is adaptive, the individual achieves and is able to maintain homeostasis. If the stress response is maladaptive, health status is altered.

General Adaptation Syndrome

Selye (1976) introduced the concept of the **general adaptation syndrome** (GAS), the physiological response to stress. The GAS is the same whether the stressor is actual or imagined, present or potential. In other words, the physiological reactions of the body are essentially the same regardless of the source of the stress. For example, the mind can imagine a stressor, and the physiological response (GAS) will be the same as if the body had actually experienced the stressor.

TABLE 23-1 Common Stressors

TYPE OF STRESSOR	EXAMPLES
Physiological	• Maturation (moving from one developmental stage to another) • Trauma • Illness • Poor nutrition • Sleep disturbances • Hunger • Discomfort • Pain
Psychological	• Worry • Fear • Anger • Happiness
Cognitive	• Thoughts • Perceptions • Interpretation of events
Environmental	• Temperature (weather) • Air pollution • Noise pollution • Crowding • Time pressures
Sociocultural	• Job loss or promotion • Changes in interpersonal relationships • Interpersonal conflict • Living conditions

Delmar/Cengage Learning

See the accompanying Respecting Our Differences display. According to Selye, all stress reactions involve similar physiological reactions. The three stages of the GAS are described in Figure 23-1.

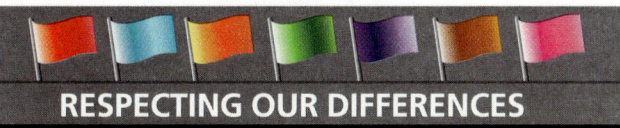

RESPECTING OUR DIFFERENCES

Anticipatory Stress

Each person worries about different stressors. Consider what happens when you worry about a situation. Your thoughts are stressors that trigger the GAS. While you are reviewing these "movies of the mind," your body responds as if you were actually experiencing the events in the present moment.

Stage One: ALARM
When stressors are threatening or perceived to be threatening, the body activates physiological changes that ready it for fight or flight.

⬇

Stage Two: RESISTANCE
The fight-or-flight response occurs. Long-term coping with stressors depletes adaptive energy, resulting in exhaustion.

⬇

Stage Three: EXHAUSTION
When the body has used up its adaptive energy and can no longer cope with stressors, it breaks down in disease, collapse, or death.

FIGURE 23-1 Stages of the General Adaptation Syndrome (**GAS**) DELMAR/CENGAGE LEARNING

FIGHT-OR-FLIGHT RESPONSE During the resistance stage of the GAS, an individual attempts to defend against the stressor through the **fight-or-flight response**. The body becomes physiologically ready to defend itself by either fighting or running away from the danger (stressor). Hormones, such as adrenaline and norepinephrine, are secreted, causing various biological changes. Arousal of the autonomic nervous system (ANS) characterizes the fight-or-flight phenomenon (see Figure 23-2 on page 442). The endocrine system is also involved in maintaining physiological homeostasis.

Local Adaptation Syndrome

The **local adaptation syndrome** (LAS) is the physiological response to a stressor (e.g., trauma, illness) affecting a specific part of the body. For example, if a person experiences a puncture wound on the foot, the LAS is activated, resulting in localized inflammation. The classic symptoms of inflammation (redness, warmth, and edema) occur at the injured site. The LAS is usually a temporary process that is resolved when the traumatic area is restored to its steady state. However, if the inflammation is not resolved with the LAS, the individual will then experience the GAS as the entire body becomes affected.

MANIFESTATIONS OF STRESS

The manifestations of stress are numerous and affect every dimension of a person. Common manifestations of stress are described in Table 23-2 on page 442.

OUTCOMES OF STRESS

Stress is an experience that provides the individual with two possibilities: (1) an opportunity for personal growth or (2) the risk of disorganization and distress. When stressors are

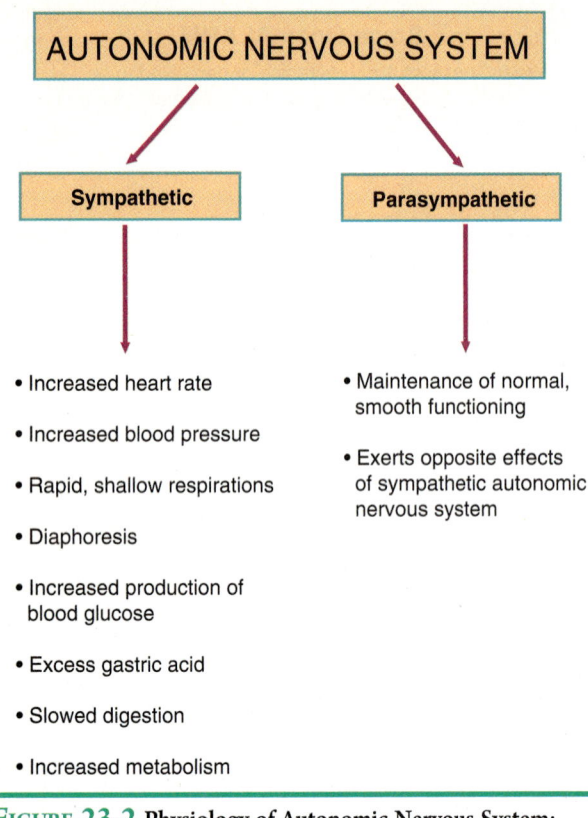

FIGURE 23-2 Physiology of Autonomic Nervous System: Arousal and Homeostasis ADAPTED FROM DELAUNE, S. C. (2009). ANXIETY AND DISSOCIATIVE DISORDERS. IN C. R. KNEISL & E. TRIGOBOFF (EDS.), *CONTEMPORARY PSYCHIATRIC-MENTAL HEALTH NURSING* (2ND ED.). UPPER SADDLE RIVER, NJ: PRENTICE-HALL.

responded to appropriately, adaptation is successful and the body returns to its normal steady state.

When stress is not resolved within a short period of time, however, problems may occur. Individuals who experience chronic periods of stress are the ones who have the greatest risk of becoming ill. Selye (1976) refers to the effects of chronic stress as "dis-ease," which occurs in the third stage of the GAS, exhaustion. The person becomes dis-eased when coping mechanisms are ineffective. The inability to adapt to continued demands of stress can have harmful results such as illness. The process of coping ineffectively with stressors is referred to as **maladaptation**.

The term **eustress** is used to describe a type of stress that results in positive outcomes. Consider, for example, students who have an examination scheduled the following week. The stress over the impending test motivates them to study early. As a result, they pass the examination.

When stressors evoke an ineffective response, **distress** is experienced. For example, consider students who have an examination scheduled for the next day. They had plenty of time to study, but because they delayed studying until the last minute, they take the examination unprepared. As a result of studying all night, they are not alert, do not know the material, and fail the examination; they are experiencing distress. In general, when people say *stress* they are referring to distress, the negative outcomes of an ineffectual stress response. See the Respecting Our Differences display on page 443.

TABLE 23-2 Manifestations of Stress

TYPE OF STRESSOR	EXAMPLES
Physiological	• Cardiovascular and respiratory effects 　—Increased pulse 　—Increased blood pressure 　—Rapid, shallow breathing • Neurological effects 　—Dizziness 　—Headaches 　—Dilated pupils • Gastrointestinal effects 　—Nausea 　—Altered appetite 　—Diarrhea or constipation • Genitourinary effects 　—Polyuria • Musculoskeletal effects 　—Tension 　—Twitching • Endocrine effects 　—Increased levels of blood glucose and cortisol
Psychological	• Irritability • Increased sensitivity (feelings are easily hurt) • Sadness, depression • Feeling "on edge"
Cognitive	• Impaired memory • Confusion • Impaired judgment and decision making • Delayed response time • Altered perceptions • Inability to concentrate
Behavioral	• Pacing • Sweaty palms • Rapid speech • Insomnia • Withdrawal • Exaggerated startle reflex
Spiritual	• Alienation • Social isolation • Feeling of emptiness

Delmar/Cengage Learning

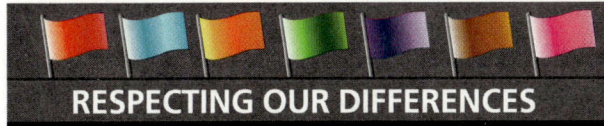

RESPECTING OUR DIFFERENCES

Everyone Responds to Stress Differently

Personal Stressors: Eustressful

Think about some of the stressors in your life. Identify those that are eustressful, that is, stimulating and positive.

Personal Stressors: Distressful

Think of the last time you felt "stressed out" and anxious. How did your body respond? What did you feel? What were you thinking? How did you respond behaviorally?

Crisis

When stressors exceed the person's ability to cope, a crisis develops. A **crisis** (an acute state of disorganization) occurs when the individual's usual coping mechanisms are no longer effective. Crisis is characterized by extreme anxiety, inability to function, and disorganized behavior. A crisis is time limited; that is, no one can remain in acute disequilibrium for a long period of time because of the degree of discomfort that is experienced. See the Safety First display on page 444. The treatment method of crisis intervention is discussed later in this chapter.

A crisis can be a negative experience, but it also has the potential to be an opportunity for growth and learning. The outcome of crisis is unique according to each individual's perception and coping abilities. Nurses are challenged to help clients discover the opportunity in their crises to adapt in a positive, healthy manner.

Not every person will experience a crisis as a result of stressful events. Each crisis is unique according to the individual and circumstances. However, there are some characteristics common to all crises, including the following:

- A crisis is experienced as a sudden event.
- A crisis has an identifiable precipitating event.
- The situation is perceived as overwhelming or life threatening.
- The situation cannot be resolved with usual coping skills.
- Intervention is required for equilibrium to be achieved.

A crisis is *not* a mental illness even though it is not uncommon for a person experiencing the acute discomfort and anxiety to fear "I'm losing my mind." There are three types of crises; see Table 23-3.

BALANCING FACTORS   There are three factors that influence a person's resolution of a crisis (Stuart & Laraia, 2008); see Figure 23-3. During a crisis, one (or sometimes more) of these factors is out of balance. When the factors return to a balanced state, the individual is better able to resolve the

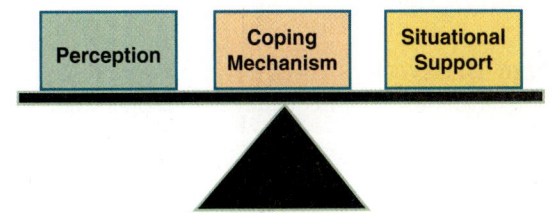

FIGURE 23-3 Balancing Factors of a Crisis ADAPTED FROM AGUILERA, D. C. (1997). *CRISIS INTERVENTION: THEORY AND METHODOLOGY* (8TH ED.). ST. LOUIS, MO: MOSBY

TABLE 23-3 Types of Crises		
TYPE	**DEFINITION**	**EXAMPLES**
Developmental or maturational	• Occur as a person ages and moves from one developmental stage to another • Are universal	• An adolescent attempting to gain independence from parents • A middle-aged woman experiencing menopause
Situational	• Can occur at any time and are not predictable • Are not experienced by everyone • Occur when there is change in role or function	• Illness • Loss (death, divorce) • Graduation • Job promotion • Retirement
Adventitious	• Are unpredictable events that rarely occur	• Being in an airplane crash • Losing one's home in a tornado • Being a victim of a school shooting • Winning a $10 million lottery

Delmar/Cengage Learning

▼ **SAFETY FIRST** ▼

Because of the time-limited nature of a crisis, a client experiencing a crisis needs immediate intervention in order to reach a successful resolution.

crisis effectively. Nursing interventions focus on reestablishing equilibrium among these factors.

Anxiety

Anxiety is the most common emotional (affective) response to stress. Individuals feel anxious whenever they are threatened, whether the threat is perceived or actual. Anxiety occurs on a continuum; some degree of anxiety is necessary as it serves as a motivator for adaptation. High levels of anxiety, however, can overwhelm the person and impair the ability to think and function. As the severity of anxiety increases, the person becomes less able to function effectively; see Table 23-4 on page 445.

COPING BEHAVIORS There are many ways to cope with stress. The following are frequently used coping strategies:

- Talking
- Crying
- Laughing
- Exercising

These strategies can result in successful adaptation. However, they become ineffective if they are the only coping methods used by the individual.

DEFENSE MECHANISMS Just as the body has physiological mechanisms (e.g., the immune system, the inflammatory response) to defend against infection and disease, the mind has psychological protective mechanisms. Defense mechanisms are unconscious operations that protect the mind from anxiety (see Table 23-5 on page 446). Defense mechanisms are employed to achieve and maintain psychological homeostasis. Illness and the resultant treatment evoke anxiety in everyone; thus, all clients use defense mechanisms (also called mental mechanisms).

Defense mechanisms are universal. Their use does not indicate psychosocial imbalance or mental illness; however, defense mechanisms are pathological when they become a stereotyped pattern, that is, the only way that an individual responds to a threat. Defense mechanisms are also considered to be pathological when they limit the individual's ability to function.

Defense mechanisms operate at the unconscious level of awareness and are involuntary and automatic; that is, the individual does not consciously decide to use a defense mechanism. Suppression is a conscious mechanism whereby a

person decides to avoid dealing with a stressor at the present time. See the Nursing Process Highlight.

The nurse who is unfamiliar with defense mechanisms is likely to be judgmental about clients who do not respond according to the nurse's expectations. If, for example, the nurse tries to break through a client's denial too quickly by presenting reality, the client will likely be overwhelmed by anxiety and will panic. See the Safety First display.

STRESS AND ILLNESS

Everyone experiences stress and accompanying anxiety; this anxiety is increased during illness and the recovery process. Illness and stress are interwoven to such a degree it is difficult to determine which precedes the other. When a person's adaptive attempts are unsuccessful, illness occurs; a person who is ill has fewer adaptive resources available to cope with stressors. Even though some stressors may not directly cause illness, stress is a significant component in the onset and progression of many diseases. Table 23-6, on page 447, lists some disorders commonly associated with stress.

A major outcome of prolonged periods of stress is impairment of the immune system. As the body continues to

NURSING PROCESS HIGHLIGHT

Planning

Clinical Example: Suppression

Mrs. James, a 34-year-old mother of two small children, has just been informed by her prescribing practitioner that she has cervical cancer. She is also told that her prognosis is dire; she has about 3 months left to live. Mrs. James asks questions and appears to be very calm. Later, the nurse asks Mrs. James if she wants to talk. Mrs. James replies, "I can't deal with this right now. I'll wait until my family is here and then I'll talk to you." How does suppression affect Mrs. James's plan of care?

▼ **SAFETY FIRST** ▼

TO PREVENT PANIC
To prevent panic, never attempt to take away a defense mechanism until the client has learned another method of coping. Denying a client the use of a defense mechanism will cause more anxiety.

TABLE 23-4 Levels of Anxiety

ANXIETY LEVEL	CHARACTERISTICS OF ANXIOUS PERSON	NURSING IMPLICATIONS
Mild	• Increased degree of alertness • Increased vigilance	• Optimal time for client teaching because of heightened awareness and increased perceptual field
Moderate	• Subjective distress • Decreased perception and attention	• Help the client to determine a cause-and-effect relationship between stressor and anxiety
Severe	• Increased subjective distress • Selective attention • Distorted perception	• Encourage verbalization • Engage in motor activity • Give specific directions
Panic	• Major perceptual distortion • Immobilization; inability to function • Impaired communication	• Provide limits and structure • Maintain client safety (both physical and psychological)

Data from Peplau, H. E. (1952). *Interpersonal relations in nursing*. New York: Putnam; and Sullivan, H. S. (1953). *The interpersonal theory of psychiatry*. New York: Norton.

fight off the threat (actual or perceived), steroid production is increased. Increased steroid production is helpful on a short-term basis because steroids speed up the healing process. However, increased steroid production over a period of time will impair the immune system. Thus, the body is less able to protect itself from disease.

IMPACT OF ILLNESS AND TREATMENT

Everyone entering the health care system experiences a change in their usual routine. For example, hospitalization, surgery, receipt of home health care, and admission to a long-term care facility are major disruptions in one's routine. Such changes evoke the stress response. See the Community Considerations display.

Being in an unfamiliar environment, losing control over one's schedule, and being dependent on others for care are all issues with which clients must cope. Each of these issues is a stressor that requires adaptation in order to maintain a steady state. Most clients do not have the energy to cope with the numerous changes simultaneously. Some cues that a person may be reacting adversely to assumption of the client role include:

- Increased stress response
- Higher levels of anxiety
- Increased or impaired use of coping mechanisms
- Inability to function
- Disorganized behavior

The greater the threat (or perceived threat), the greater the level of the client's anxiety. The nurse must be sensitive to stress and anxiety stemming from the multiple changes imposed by illness on the client, family, and significant others. The nurse's sensitivity to the client's stress reduces the risk of depersonalizing the client. See the Respecting Our Differences display.

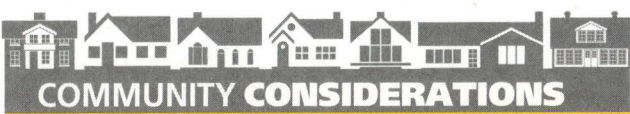

COMMUNITY CONSIDERATIONS

Client Role Stressors

Individuals do not have to be hospitalized to experience stressors associated with the client role. Consider, for example, the person having "minor" surgery at an outpatient center, the employee being treated at an industrial clinic for a work-related injury, or the adolescent being treated by the school nurse. Even clients who are treated by home health agencies experience stressors associated with having a health care provider enter their personal environment.

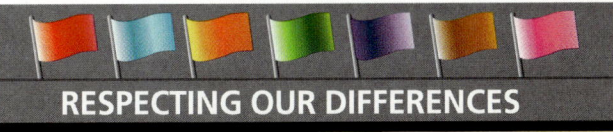

RESPECTING OUR DIFFERENCES

Stressors Associated with Illness

Think of some major changes that people experience when they are ill. Can you identify at least three changes? What can you do to significantly reduce threats (real or perceived) in acute care settings? In long-term care settings? In outpatient settings?

TABLE 23-5 Common Defense Mechanisms

MECHANISM	DESCRIPTION	EXAMPLE
Denial	Negation of reality of threatening situations, despite factual evidence	The client refuses to admit to anger, even though the situation warrants it and the client's voice indicates anger.
Projection	Attribution of one's own thoughts, feelings, or impulses to others	"I'm not attracted to him. My best friend is."
Repression	Unconscious blocking from awareness material that is threatening or painful	"I never got angry at my father; our family lived in harmony and love" (when such descriptions of the family life would not fit with anyone else's interpretation of the events).
Rationalization	Intellectual explaining away of threatening circumstances	"The test had too many trick questions; I really knew all the material, but our instructor was out to get me."
Introjection	Incorporating, without examination or thought, the qualities or attitudes of others	An adolescent takes on all the values and styles of an admired teacher.
Displacement	Transfer of feelings or reactions evoked by one topic or event to another that is less threatening	A husband who is angry at his wife yells at the family dog rather than dealing directly with his anger.
Reaction formation	Expression of a feeling that is the opposite of one's authentic feeling or of feelings that would be appropriate in the situation	A client brings gifts to the nurse with whom he is really angry.
Regression	Retreat to a previous developmental level	A child starts to suck his thumb (after 2 years of not thumb sucking) when admitted to the hospital.
Suppression	Conscious attempt to keep threatening material out of consciousness	A student nurse decides not to think about a family problem at the moment so he can study for an upcoming examination.
Sublimation	Channeling of socially unacceptable impulses into socially acceptable activities	A young man deals with aggression by playing football.
Symbolization	Use of an object, idea, or act to express emotion that is not expressed directly	The client leaves the nurse a flower rather than directly saying she cares about the nurse.

Delmar/Cengage Learning

Depersonalization describes the process in which an individual is treated as an object instead of as a person. Literally, it involves taking away clients' unique aspects by treating them as nonhuman. Nurses who demonstrate caring and compassion avoid depersonalizing clients. In order to prevent depersonalization, nursing interventions focus on helping the client reduce feelings of unfamiliarity and loss of control. The accompanying Nursing Checklist, on page 447, suggests some actions for promoting client control.

STRESS AND CHANGE

Change, a dynamic process in which an individual's behavior is altered in response to a stressor, is an inherent part of life. It is the process that causes individuals to adapt. Whether it is planned or unplanned, change is both inevitable and constant. Change, whether constructive or destructive, is stressful to individuals because it activates the GAS. Some characteristics of change are that it:

- Is an inevitable part of life.
- May be eustressful or distressful.

TABLE 23-6 Stress-Related Disorders: A Partial List

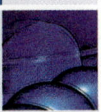

Respiratory disorders	• Chronic bronchitis • Asthma
Cardiovascular disorders	• Hypertension • Cardiac arrhythmias • Migraine headaches
Endocrine disorders	• Thyroid problems • Amenorrhea, anovulation • Diabetes • Excessive weight gain or weight loss
Musculoskeletal disorders	• Chronic back pain • Arthritis
Genitourinary disorders	• Enuresis • Urinary frequency
Sexual and reproductive disorders	• Decreased libido • Impotence (erectile dysfunction, or ED) • Menstrual irregularities
Gastrointestinal disorders	• Irritable bowel syndrome • Chronic constipation • Ulcers • Gastritis
Integumentary disorders	• Eczema • Hives • Psoriasis

Delmar/Cengage Learning

- Can be self-initiated or externally imposed.
- Can occur abruptly or have a gradual onset with insidious progression.
- Requires energy to effect as well as to resist.

The pace of change is rapidly increasing in health care agencies, which have been changing and continue to change in response to consumer demands. Some changes that have evolved from consumer demands and needs include:

- Sports medicine clinics
- Substance abuse treatment programs
- Day treatment programs for geriatric and psychiatric clients
- Weight control programs
- Exercise programs
- Emergency department fast-track programs

TYPES OF CHANGE

Change is either planned or unplanned. Unplanned change is the change that "just happens"; it is unpredictable and may

✔ NURSINGCHECKLIST

Actions to Promote Client Control

- Communicate clearly. Use terms easily understood by clients and families. Avoid using medical jargon with clients.
- Answer questions thoroughly. Validate client's and family's level of understanding.
- Teach the use of relaxation techniques, such as progressive muscle relaxation (a stress management technique involving the tensing and relaxing of muscles) and guided imagery (a relaxation technique in which the individual uses the imagination to experience a pleasant, soothing image).
- Instruct clients on the use of cognitive reframing (a technique in which individuals change their negative perception of a situation or event to a more positive, less-threatening perspective).
- Provide support and reassurance. The nurse's presence ("being with" the client) can alleviate anxiety levels. The most therapeutic tool in alleviating client anxiety is the nurse's therapeutic use of self.
- Break down the information shared with clients. Too much information at once can make the client feel overwhelmed and less likely to listen. When clients have adequate information, they can make informed decisions and maintain some degree of control over their lives.

be imposed by others or by uncontrollable natural events (e.g., losing one's home in a flood). On the other hand, planned change results from a deliberate effort to improve a situation. In addition to planned and unplanned change, there are other types of change (see Table 23-7 on page 448).

THEORIES OF CHANGE

Nurses must be able to initiate and cope with change. Proficiency in critical thinking and problem-solving skills is necessary to initiate positive change. Two major theories of change are discussed in the following text.

Lewin's Theory

A classic theory of change was developed by Lewin (1951), who stated that the change process occurs in three stages: unfreezing, moving, and refreezing (see Figure 23-4 on page 448). In the unfreezing stage, the person recognizes a need for change and becomes motivated to move in a new direction. Stage 2, changing, is the actual implementation of the change. In the third stage, refreezing, new changes are incorporated into behavior and these new behaviors stabilize. Because the change process is dynamic, these stages are not rigid. The process of change may quickly move through all stages, or it may become stuck in one stage.

TABLE 23-7 Types of Change

TYPE OF CHANGE	DESCRIPTION
Developmental	• Physical and emotional changes that occur at different stages of the life cycle • Generally predictable • Usually occur gradually
Reactive	• Adaptive responses to external stimuli • Efforts to cope with change imposed by others
Covert	• Occur without person's conscious awareness
Overt	• Person is aware of the change • Usually not under individual's direct control

Delmar/Cengage Learning

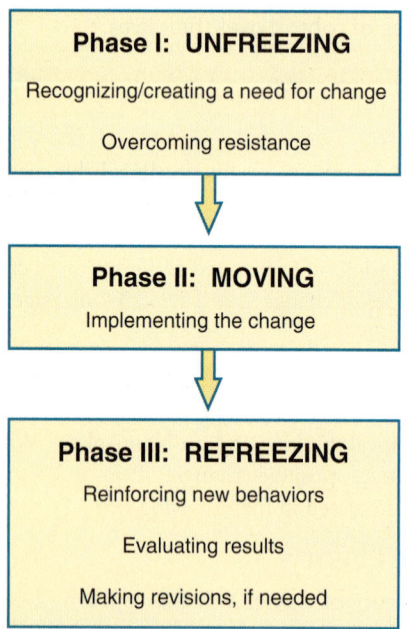

FIGURE 23-4 Lewin's Theory of Change DATA FROM LEWIN, K. (1951). *FIELD THEORY IN SOCIAL SCIENCE.* NEW YORK: HARPER.

Lippitt's Theory

Lippitt, Watson, and Westley (1958) proposed a theory of change that consists of seven phases:

1. Diagnose the problem (need for change).

2. Assess the change target's motivation and capacity for change.
3. Assess the change agent's motivation and capacity for change.
4. Establish objectives for change.
5. Determine the role of the change agent.
6. After change has occurred, maintain it.
7. Terminate the role of the change agent.

RESISTANCE TO CHANGE

Many people tend to resist change because of the energy required to adapt. Conversely, energy is also required to resist change, or to maintain the status quo. Individuals differ in their ability to tolerate (or even thrive on) change.

There are many reasons people tend to resist change (see Table 23-8 on page 449). There are no absolute guarantees that the change activity will lead to positive outcomes; this uncertainty about outcomes is a major barrier to change.

CHANGING PARADIGMS

Changing involves questioning and frequently results in the development of a new **paradigm** (a pattern, model, or mind-set that strongly influences one's decisions and behaviors). One's paradigm greatly colors one's behaviors. By changing paradigms, an individual can determine what is positive in the old system and use it to create a newer, better system (Alfaro-LeFevre, 2008).

It is risky to initiate change, to challenge one's own paradigms and those of others. One of the first signs of the need for change is questioning. The nurse who wonders "Why?" or "Why not?" or "What if?" is the nurse who will likely take risks to initiate change activity. The risk taker who is effective is neither reckless nor overly cautious. Successful risk takers consider possible outcomes before initiating action. See the Spotlight On display.

Overcoming Barriers to Change

Because change is inevitable, learning how to deal with it is crucial for nurses. Resistance occurs when the individual rejects proposed new ideas without critically thinking about the proposal.

SPOTLIGHT ON...

Professionalism

Nurses as Risk Takers

Do you think nurses are encouraged to be risk takers? What empowers you to take risks as a student? What barriers to risk taking can you identify in academic and health care settings?

TABLE 23-8 Reasons People Resist Change

Conformity	Often referred to as "groupthink"; complying with the group's expectations; going along with others to avoid conflict.
Dissimilar beliefs and values	Differences in attitudes and expectations regarding health and illness behaviors; differences between client and nurse that can impede positive change.
Fear	Fear of failure and fear of the unknown especially block change.
Habits	Routine, "set" behaviors are often hard to change.
Satisfaction with status quo	Seeing only advantages to the present system can blind one to the possible need for change. Satisfaction with the way things are now reinforces resistance to change.
Secondary gains (outcomes other than alleviation of anxiety)	Benefits or payoffs of the sick role (e.g., gaining attention and sympathy, avoiding responsibilities, getting financial compensation or reward) often are so desirable that the client has little incentive to change.
Threats to satisfying basic needs	Change may be perceived as a threat to self-esteem, security, or survival.
Unrealistic goals	Set up the individual for failure in change efforts.

Delmar/Cengage Learning

Overcoming this barrier doesn't mean embracing every new idea uncritically. It means being willing to suspend judgment long enough to make an informed decision on whether the change is worthwhile. (Alfaro-LeFevre, 2008, p. 32)

Coping with change of any type calls for flexibility, adaptability, and resilience.

NURSE AS CHANGE AGENT

Initiating change is an expectation for professional nurses. Nurses experience stress daily as a result of changes within their immediate work environment as well as changes in the entire health care delivery system. Uncertainty about the future of health care is very distressful to some nurses. Others see opportunity for positive change in the future.

In bringing about change to promote positive adaptation, the nurse serves as a **change agent** (a person who intentionally initiates and creates change). True change agents constantly seek ways to make improvements. They use critical thinking skills to develop creative, innovative solutions. Critical thinking is also required to determine the outcomes of change. Evaluating the effects of change is key to bringing about positive change.

To be most effective, change should be planned and directed by people who are **proactive** (initiating change rather than responding to change imposed by others). Proactive individuals assume responsibility for their own lives. On the other hand, a reactive person responds only to externally imposed change. Proactive nurses are change agents who affect the entire health care system as well as individual clients.

Change agents keep the change process moving toward a positive outcome. As an advocate for change, the nurse empowers the client to initiate change in order to adapt more successfully; client education is a powerful tool for initiating change. Teaching a client about a disease process, a treatment modality, or a lifestyle alteration provides the client with an opportunity to change. In fact, learning results in behavioral changes.

ASSESSMENT

When caring for an anxious client, the nurse must first determine the client's perception of the situation. This determination is done by directly asking for the client's input and carefully listening to the client's response. Because the nurse's nonverbal behavior can affect the client's anxiety level, nurses must be aware of their own body language. Anxiety is a subjective experience; thus, it cannot be directly observed. Therefore, the nurse must look for the signs indicative of anxiety (previously discussed in Table 23-2).

A thorough assessment of stress and anxiety levels includes eliciting client input to evaluate the following factors:

- Patterns of stressors
- Typical responses to stressful situations
- Cause-and-effect relationships between stressors and thoughts, feelings, and behaviors
- Past history of successful coping mechanisms

Assessing the client's coping abilities can be done in various ways. For example, use open-ended questions to determine previously used coping mechanisms. Some sample questions are:

- "What is the problem?"
- "What have you tried before?"
- "How well did it work?"
- "Who is available to help you?"

Identification of the client's coping abilities assists in establishing appropriate nursing diagnoses and developing an effective plan of care. Assessment, which relies heavily on the nurse's observation and listening skills, provides the data necessary for formulating nursing diagnoses.

NURSING DIAGNOSIS

There are several nursing diagnoses that may apply to clients experiencing anxiety. See Table 23-9, on page 451, for selected diagnoses and their defining characteristics and related factors. In addition to the four diagnoses listed in Table 23-9, the following North American Nursing Diagnosis Association International (2009) diagnoses may also be appropriate for anxious clients.

- *Impaired adjustment*
- *Ineffective role performance*
- *Disturbed thought processes*
- *Ineffective coping*
- *Fear*
- *Posttrauma syndrome*
- *Impaired social interaction*
- *Spiritual distress*

OUTCOME IDENTIFICATION AND PLANNING

Client involvement in planning care is essential because helping clients learn to cope successfully is part of the empowerment process. Planning means exploring with the client self-responsibility issues. Here are some issues to consider when planning care for an anxious client. The client:

- Identifies situations that increase stress and anxiety levels.
- Verbalizes a plan to decrease effects of common stressors.
- Differentiates positive and negative stressors in his or her life.
- Classifies stressors into categories of those that can be eliminated, can be controlled, or cannot be controlled directly by himself or herself.
- Demonstrates the accurate use of selected stress management exercises (e.g., progressive muscle relaxation, guided imagery, thought stopping).
- Verbalizes a plan for stress management, including necessary lifestyle modifications.

IMPLEMENTATION

Teaching, a major nursing intervention for managing stress, is inherent in holistic nursing practice. Stress management approaches can be taught to clients of every age and developmental stage in all health care settings: acute care (inpatient and outpatient), long-term care, and the home.

Teaching clients to reduce their own levels of stress is a major step in promoting self-care; client education provides clients with options. Clients who have a thorough understanding of their options can make informed decisions about necessary lifestyle changes (see Figure 23-5). Following is a

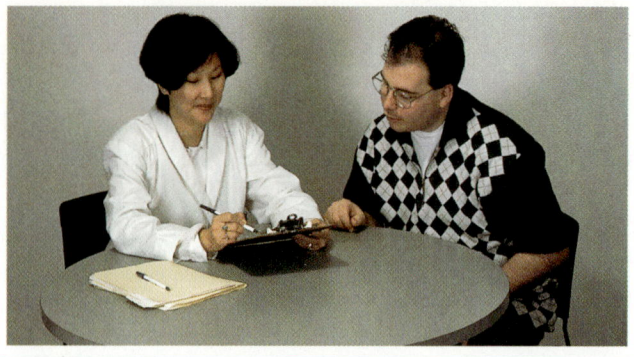

FIGURE 23-5 By discussing options for care with this client, the nurse is providing him with the information he needs to plan effective lifestyle changes. What methods can the nurse use to assess whether the client fully understands the information?
DELMAR/CENGAGE LEARNING

discussion of some of the many interventions that can be used with anxious clients.

MEETING BASIC NEEDS

There is a close relationship between basic physiological needs and stress. Anything that interferes with the satisfaction of basic needs evokes the stress response and attendant anxiety. Clients who are cold, hungry, or in pain have higher anxiety levels than those who are comfortable. When anxiety levels increase, so does the perception of pain. Nurses who empower clients to meet basic needs are building the foundation for a less stressful, more caring treatment process. By reducing anxiety, the nurse is improving the client's healing potential.

ENVIRONMENTAL STRATEGIES

Because an individual's immediate environment can influence stress levels, it is important for the nurse to decrease environmental stimuli that may contribute to anxiety. Some specific ways to limit environmental stimuli are:

- Close the door to the client's room.
- Turn off the television.
- Lower the tone of the telephone ringer or take the phone off the hook if feasible.
- Turn off the lights or close the blinds.
- Limit the number of visitors (unless isolation increases the client's anxiety).
- Decrease environmental clutter.
- Personalize the environment.

VERBALIZATION

Encouraging clients to express their feelings is especially valuable in stress reduction. Freud (1959) used the term **catharsis** to describe the process of talking out one's feelings. People instinctively know the value of "getting things off their chest" through verbalization. Verbalization promotes

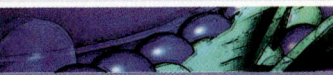

TABLE 23-9 Nursing Diagnosis: Clients Experiencing Anxiety

NURSING DIAGNOSIS: DEFINITION	DEFINING CHARACTERISTICS	RELATED FACTORS

Anxiety: Feelings of apprehension and arousal of the autonomic nervous system in response to a threat (which may be specific or vague)	Note: Manifestations will vary according to the level of anxiety.
	• Physiological
	  —Changes in vital signs (increased pulse, respirations, blood pressure)
	  —Diaphoresis (increased sweating)
	  —Restlessness, tremors
	  —Frequent urination
	• Emotional
	  —Verbalization of feelings of helplessness, losing control, nervousness, fear
	  —Inability to relax
	  —Increased irritability
	  —Withdrawal or angry outbursts
	• Cognitive
	  —Forgetfulness
	  —Impaired ability to concentrate
	  —Indecisiveness
		• Any threat, real or perceived
		• Unmet needs (biological, safety and security, belonging, self-esteem)
		• A loss (e.g., of a relationship as a result of death or divorce, a job, functional ability)
		• Loss of control (over one's situation or events)
		• Conflict (interpersonal or intrapersonal)
		• Environmental changes

Ineffective coping: The inability to manage stressors because problem-solving behaviors are no longer effective	• Unmet basic needs • Inability to solve problems • Altered patterns of communication • Inappropriate use of defense mechanisms • Verbalization of inability to ask for help • Destructive behavior toward self or others	• Low self-esteem • Alterations in body integrity (e.g., disfigurement secondary to trauma or surgery, loss of body part) • Disruption of emotional ties • Inadequate support system • Separation from home and family • Sensory overload
Ineffective denial: Occurrence in which the person minimizes or negates symptoms to the point of being injurious to his or her health status	• Refusal of health care treatment • Delay in seeking treatment • Resistance to treatment program • Failure to perceive danger of presence of symptoms • Relinquishing of self-responsibility (frequent verbalizations of "I can't") • Blaming other people or circumstances ("It's not my fault") • Inability or unwillingness to admit impact of illness or trauma on self	• Presence of chronic or terminal disease • Loss (e.g., of job, significant other, income) • Personal vulnerability • Fear • Difficulty handling new situations • Learned response • Cultural factors • Personal and family value system
Powerlessness: Situation in which the person perceives a lack of control over situations or events	• Verbalization of dissatisfaction over inability to control the situation • Passive, "giving-up" behavior or aggressive, hostile behavior • Difficulty in expressing self directly • Anxiety • Resignation • Depression	• Illness (both acute and chronic) • Hospitalization or institutionalization • Expressed feelings of insecurity and resentment • Multiple life changes or losses

Data from Carpenito, L. J. (2007). *Handbook of nursing diagnosis* (12th ed.). Philadelphia: Lippincott, Williams & Wilkins; Doenges, M. E., Moorhouse, M. F., & Murr, A. C. (2006). *Nursing care plans: Guidelines for individualizing client care* (7th ed.). Philadelphia: F. A. Davis; North American Nursing Diagnosis Association International. (2009). *Nursing Diagnoses—Definitions and Classification 2009–2011* © 2009, 2007, 2005, 2003, 2001, 1998, 1996, 1994, NANDA International. Used by arrangement with Wiley-Blackwell Publishing, a company of John Wiley & Sons, Inc.

relaxation primarily in two ways. First, when a feeling is described, it becomes *real*. Once the problem is identified, the person can begin to deal effectively with it. Also, the actual activity of talking uses energy and, therefore, reduces anxiety.

INVOLVEMENT OF FAMILY AND SIGNIFICANT OTHERS

The client's developmental stage influences the type of intervention for stress management. Children and adolescents have varying coping skills; children of all ages rely on their parents to some degree for security and support. It is important to include the entire family in the care of the client whenever possible (see Figure 23-6). Such an approach is useful in decreasing the stress levels of everyone involved because families provide essential support for clients.

Family members who are extremely anxious often have a negative impact on the client's health status. Therefore, nurses often need to help family members relax; one way to accomplish this is by providing explanations and information. Thus, it is often necessary for nurses to teach stress management techniques to the client's family.

STRESS MANAGEMENT

There are a variety of stress management techniques that can easily be taught to clients and significant others. Many of these techniques are considered to be complementary (integrative) modalities as they are used in conjunction with traditional medical treatment methods (i.e., medication, radiation therapy). Some of the most frequently used approaches for managing stress are discussed in the following text.

Exercise

Physical exercise is a powerful way to reduce anxiety and can be used by clients of all ages and with varying physical

abilities; see Figure 23-7. Client teaching should emphasize the need for incorporating exercise into one's lifestyle (see the accompanying display, on page 453, on establishing an exercise program). In other words, if exercise is to reduce anxiety, it must be done on an ongoing and regular basis. The physiological benefits of regular exercise are shown in Table 23-10 on page 453.

Lack of physical exercise contributes to obesity, which leads to many health problems. Approximately 34% of adults in the United States are obese; for children and adolescents, the obesity rate is 17% (Centers for Disease Control and Prevention, 2008). People who are overweight or obese are at higher risk for developing hypertension and diabetes than are people of normal weight. Sedentary people are at greater risk for developing conditions associated with obesity.

In addition to the physical benefits, individuals who exercise regularly also experience psychological benefits, such as the following:

- Enhanced feelings of well-being
- Improved concentration and memory
- Reduced depression
- Reduced insomnia
- Reduced dependence on external stimulants or relaxants
- Increased self-esteem
- Sense of self-control over anxiety

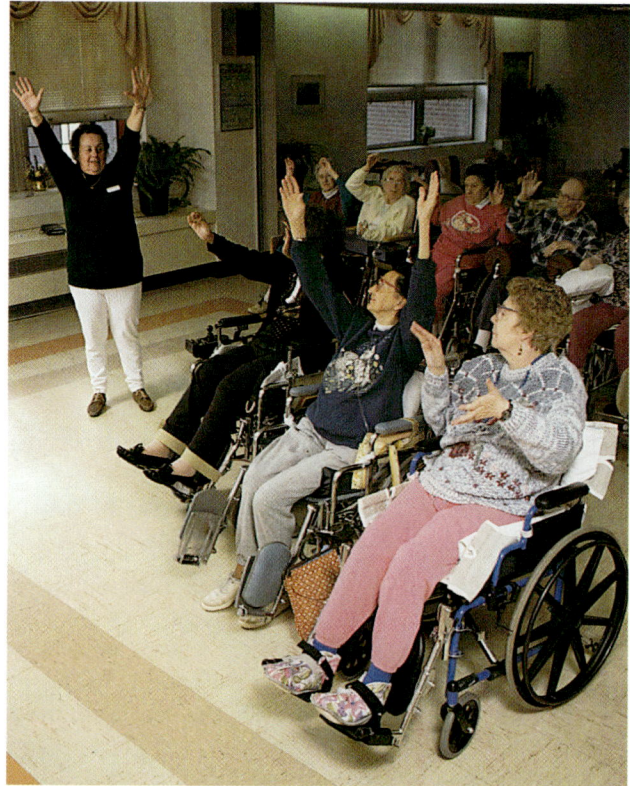

FIGURE 23-7 Exercise provides physiological and psychological benefits to individuals of all ages with varying degrees of functional abilities. Notice that the individuals in this figure are also experiencing socialization during the physical activity. DELMAR/CENGAGE LEARNING

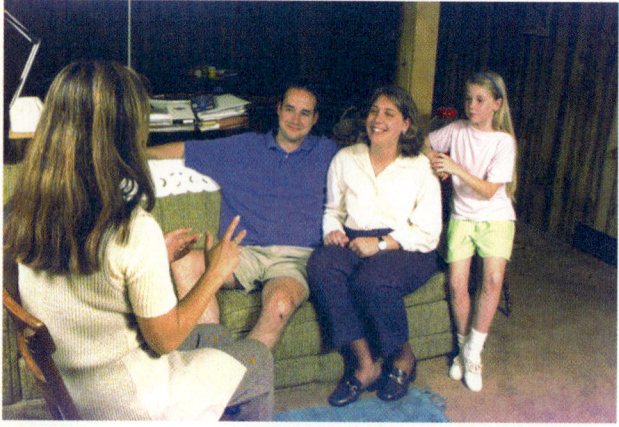

FIGURE 23-6 Nurses can encourage the interaction of clients with family members and significant others in various health care settings. This involvement is helpful in easing the client's anxiety and can also serve as a method through which family members are kept informed about the client's care. DELMAR/CENGAGE LEARNING

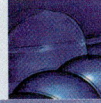

TABLE 23-10 Physiological Benefits of Exercise

EFFECT OF EXERCISE	BENEFIT
Promotes metabolism of adrenalin and thyroxine	• Decreased amounts of these substances in the bloodstream minimize autonomic arousal and hypervigilance.
Reduces musculoskeletal tension	• Reduction of the tension in muscles reduces feelings of being tense and "uptight."
Improves circulation, resulting in better oxygenation of bloodstream and brain	• Increased alertness and concentration enhance problem-solving ability.
Stimulates endorphin production	• Endorphins (a group of opiate-like substances produced naturally by the brain) raise the body's pain threshold, produce sedation and euphoria, and promote a sense of well-being.
Decreases cholesterol levels	• Reduces risk of atherosclerosis.
Decreases blood pressure	• Reduces risk of myocardial infarction (heart attack) and cerebral infarction (stroke).
Increases acidity of blood (lowered pH)	• Improves digestion. • Improves energy level. • Improves utilization of food for energy (promotes metabolism).
Improves elimination (through lungs, skin, bowels)	• Reduces buildup of toxins in the body.

Data from Keegan, L. (2008). Nutrition, exercise, and movement. In B. M Dossey & L. Keegan (Eds.), *Holistic nursing: A handbook for practice* (5th ed.). Boston: Jones & Bartlett; Rentfro, A. R. (2006). Health promotion and the individual. In C. L., Edelman & C. L., Mandle (Eds.), *Health promotion throughout the lifespan* (6th ed.). St. Louis, MO: Mosby.

Relaxation Techniques

There are several approaches that help individuals relax. See Chapter 31 for a discussion of complementary and alternative modalities (e.g., aromatherapy, herbals, music, humor) that promote relaxation. A discussion of some specific relaxation techniques that are easily learned and can be effective for a variety of stressors follows.

GUIDELINES FOR ESTABLISHING AN EXERCISE PROGRAM

- Explore the availability of different exercise programs.
- Consult with a health care provider about the safety of a specific exercise program.
- Set realistic goals.
- Plan a routine, and allow for a warm-up and cool-down period using stretch exercises.
- Engage in activity that increases heart rate for a period of time and is followed by a cool-down period.

PROGRESSIVE MUSCLE RELAXATION Progressive muscle relaxation (PMR) is a method of inducing relaxation by tensing and releasing various muscle groups. For example, the individual tightens the hands into a fist, holds the tension for a few seconds, then slowly relaxes the fingers and hands, paying particular attention to the different sensations of tension and relaxation (see Figure 23-8). This tense-release action is applied to all muscle groups of the body. PMR is especially helpful in promoting sleep. PMR is a technique that can successfully be taught to clients for use in any health care setting, including the home (see the Client Teaching Checklist on page 454).

GUIDED IMAGERY Another technique for helping clients manage stress successfully is guided imagery, a process in which the person uses all the senses to experience the sensation of relaxation. During guided imagery, the client is

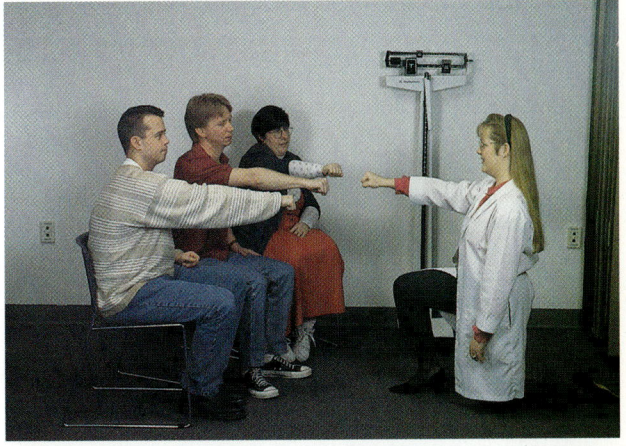

FIGURE 23-8 This nurse is demonstrating the technique of progressive muscle relaxation in a client education program. **How does instruction in this method enhance the self-responsibility that clients need to develop in order to manage their stress?** DELMAR/CENGAGE LEARNING

✓ CLIENT TEACHING CHECKLIST

Progressive Muscle Relaxation

After explaining the purpose and process of progressive muscle relaxation (PMR), instruct the client to:

1. Assume a comfortable position in a quiet environment.
2. Close eyes and keep them closed until the exercise is completed.
3. Inhale deeply to a count of 4.
4. Hold breath for a count of 4.
5. Exhale to a count of 4.
6. Continue to breathe slowly and deeply.
7. Tense both feet until muscle tension is felt. Caution the client to tighten the muscles only until the muscles are tensed, not to the point of pain. Hold a gentle state of tension in both feet for a count of 3.
   NOTE: If muscle cramps occur, stop the procedure and gently massage the affected area. Then begin the cycle of slight muscle tension and relaxation again.
8. Slowly release the tension from the feet.
9. Fully experience the difference between tension and relaxation.
10. Repeat Steps 3–6.

Repeat the above sequence with all the muscle groups to experience relaxation throughout your body. To be effective, this procedure requires approximately 20 to 30 minutes. Like all other relaxation exercises, PMR is most effective with repetition.

THOUGHT STOPPING: A COGNITIVE REFRAMING TECHNIQUE

- Listen to self-talk (thoughts).
- Recognize when the self-talk is negative.
- When a negative thought is detected, do something physical to stop the train of thought. For example, clap your hands or snap a rubber band on your wrist. Tell yourself, "Stop!"
- Replace the negative thought with one that is both positive and realistic.

Like all other relaxation exercises, thought stopping becomes more effective with repetition.

directed to concentrate on a pleasant scene or image in order to become more relaxed. In many situations, music is a helpful adjunct to guided imagery (see Figure 23-9). The Client Teaching Checklist, on page 455, describes the steps involved in using this technique. See Chapter 31 for further discussion of guided imagery. Note that imagery is not recommended for individuals experiencing emotional instability.

COGNITIVE REFRAMING AND THOUGHT STOPPING

Cognitive reframing is a technique based on a theory proposed by Aaron Beck (1976), who stated that a person's emotional response is determined by the meaning attached to an event. For example, if an event is perceived to be threatening, the client is likely to feel anxious. If the interpretation of the event can be modified, the client will be less anxious. Reframing is a technique used to alter one's perceptions and interpretations by changing one's thoughts. The accompanying display describes the thought-stopping process, a cognitive behavioral technique.

CRISIS INTERVENTION

Some clients will be in an acute crisis state and require **crisis intervention**, a specific technique that helps clients regain equilibrium. This approach views clients as having the ability to control their own lives. The five steps of crisis intervention are illustrated in Figure 23-10 on page 455.

The client is an active participant in the process of resolving the crisis in order to restore equilibrium. If the client is unable to participate in problem solving (e.g., because of delayed developmental stage or altered mental status), then crisis intervention should not be attempted. However, the family can be approached with the crisis intervention method.

Sometimes clients need more assistance than the nurse is able to provide. Recognition of such situations calls for prompt consultation with and, sometimes, referral to other health care providers, such as:

- Psychiatric clinical nurse specialists
- Nurse psychotherapists
- Psychologists
- Social workers
- Psychiatrists
- Clergy and other counselors

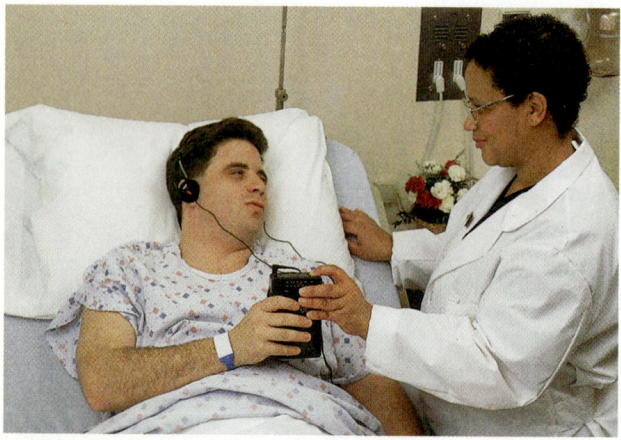

FIGURE 23-9 To help relieve this client's stress, the nurse is encouraging the client to listen to music. In your opinion, are there any situations in which this type of intervention may be inappropriate? DELMAR/CENGAGE LEARNING

✓ CLIENT TEACHING CHECKLIST

Guided Imagery

After explaining the purpose and process of guided imagery, instruct the client to:

- Assume a comfortable position in a quiet environment.
- Close eyes and keep them closed until the exercise is completed.
- Inhale deeply to a count of 4.
- Hold breath for a count of 4.
- Exhale to a count of 4.
- Continue to breathe slowly and deeply.
- Think of a favorite place and prepare to take an imaginary journey there. Select a place in which you are relaxed and at peace.
- Picture in your mind's eye your favorite place. Look around you. See all the colors, the light and shadows. Look at all the pleasant sights.
- Listen to all the sounds. Pay attention to what you hear.
- Feel all the physical sensations . . . the temperature . . . the textures . . . the movement of the air.
- As you take in a deep breath, smell the aromas of your favorite place.
- Taste the foods and drinks you usually consume in your favorite place. Savor each taste fully.
- Focus all your attention totally on your favorite place.
- Inhale deeply to a count of 4.
- Hold breath for a count of 4.
- Exhale to a count of 4.
- Resume your usual breathing pattern.
- Slowly open your eyes and stretch, if desired.

This procedure works best when all five senses are used. Like all other relaxation exercises, guided imagery becomes more effective with repetition. This technique (like all imagery exercises) is not recommended for individuals with emotional instability.

Identification of the Problem

It is necessary to be as specific as possible when naming the underlying issue(s). Being specific promotes clarity in planning.

Identification of Alternatives

Client and nurse need to list all the possible options for resolving the crisis. The greater the number of alternatives identified, the greater the likelihood of successful resolution.

Selection of an Alternative

The potential outcomes of each option are examined and one alternative is chosen.

Implementation

The selected alternative is carried out.

Evaluation

The overall effectiveness of the plan is evaluated in terms of process and outcome.

FIGURE 23-10 Steps of Crisis Intervention DELMAR/CENGAGE LEARNING

Process Highlight for some questions that the nurse may consider in evaluating the effectiveness of interventions to reduce anxiety.

NURSING PROCESS HIGHLIGHT

Evaluation

Evaluating Client Response to Relaxation Techniques

Consider these questions when evaluating the effectiveness of anxiety-reducing interventions:

- Does the client exhibit decreased fidgeting and pacing?
- Is the client's tone of voice calm?
- Is the client's problem-solving ability unimpaired?
- Is the ability to concentrate intact?
- Are the vital signs within normal limits (client's baseline)?

EVALUATION

Evaluating the effectiveness of clients' coping abilities is an ongoing comprehensive process that must include client input. It is imperative that the nurse evaluate client outcomes as well as the process of delivering nursing care.

In addition to eliciting verbal input from the client and significant others, nurses also collect evaluation data by observation of client behavior. See the accompanying Nursing

PERSONAL STRESS MANAGEMENT APPROACHES FOR THE NURSE

There are many stressors inherent in nursing. Therefore, nurses must learn effective coping skills. Two major reasons nurses must cope successfully with stress are to maintain their own wellness and to model health-promoting behaviors to others. In order to help clients learn to manage stress, nurses must first be able to manage their own stress. "Before nurses can care for clients, they must first learn to value and care for themselves" (Fontaine, 2004, p. 18).

Caring for one's self includes the following activities:

- Taking time out for oneself
- Using effective communication skills with coworkers, family, and significant others
- Managing conflict effectively (intrapersonal and interpersonal)

See the accompanying Spotlight On display on page 457.

Here are some complementary and alternative methods that nurses can use to promote self-care:

- Imagery
- PMR
- Prayer
- Humor
- Music
- Communion with nature
- Journaling
- Meditation

NURSING BURNOUT

High stress levels among nurses are associated with **burnout**, a state of physical and emotional exhaustion that occurs when caregivers deplete their adaptive energy. Nurses who have experienced such an overwhelming degree of stress tend to treat clients in depersonalizing ways. Such nurses also lack feelings of personal accomplishment. Burnout exacts a high price not only on individual nurses themselves but also on the profession. Highly qualified professionals leave nursing and, as a result, the quality of care declines. "Creating a healthy work environment for nursing practice is crucial to maintain an adequate nursing workforce; the stressful nature of the profession often leads to burnout, disability, and high absenteeism, and ultimately contributes to the shortage of nursing" (Shirley, 2006, p. 256).

Several work-related factors can contribute to the development of nursing burnout:

- Cost-containment measures
- Nursing shortages
- Innate job-related stress (for example, the stress evoked by caring for dying people)
- Workload
- Interpersonal conflict in the work environment
- Rapid restructuring of health care organizations (e.g., mergers, partnerships)

In order to avoid developing the classic symptoms of burnout—absenteeism, poor morale, and illness—nurses need to nurture themselves. Burnout prevention and recovery depend on stress management.

There are many strategies that nurses can use to help manage professional and personal stress (see Table 23-11). The following Nursing Checklist, on page 457, provides some other strategies that are also helpful in managing professional stress. See the Uncovering the Evidence display on page 457. Guidelines that are helpful in changing from a negative to a positive outlook include these points:

- Expect to be successful.
- Remember the power of self-fulfilling prophecies and deliberately focus on the positive.

TABLE 23-11 Strategies for Coping with Professional Stress

STRATEGY	EXPLANATION
Use time management methods.	Encourages recognition of your own needs as priorities.
Focus on accomplishments instead of uncompleted tasks.	Being focused on unfinished business increases anxiety; paying attention to successes boosts self-esteem.
Practice slow, focused breathing.	Alleviates muscle tension by increasing the amount of oxygenated blood. Consciously thinking about breathing serves as a diversionary tactic.
Do not assume personal responsibility for others' behaviors or problems.	Encourages avoidance of assuming a rescuer role.
Know your own limits.	Clarifies expectations, strengths, and limitations. Learn to differentiate what's really important. Know when a problem is beyond your control.
Whenever possible, distance yourself from stressors that have a negative impact.	Avoids exposure to needless stress and subsequent draining of adaptive resources.
Identify and change the stressors that you can directly influence.	Increases your sense of personal power; avoids needless expenditure of energy.
Vary tasks between physical and mental activities.	Helps restore a sense of balance; conserves energy by reducing fatigue.

Delmar/Cengage Learning

✓ NURSING **CHECKLIST**

Managing Professional Stress

- Develop and maintain active support systems, both at work and away from work. Having friends who are not health care providers helps maintain a sense of balance and separateness between personal and professional domains.
- Develop decision-making skills. For example, break large tasks down into small, realistic, achievable objectives. This strategy avoids your becoming overwhelmed by the seemingly impossible task before you.
- Avoid consumption of noxious substances. Practice a substance-free lifestyle to manage stress well. Do not depend on these unhealthy behaviors as avenues to relaxation: smoking, overeating, drinking alcohol and caffeine.
- Nourish your body with a healthy diet and adequate amounts of sleep and rest balanced with activity and exercise. Care for yourself as you would for clients.
- Maintain a sense of humor while you work. Humor helps a person maintain a positive outlook; therefore, it can be used to reframe situations to reduce distress (see Figure 23-11).

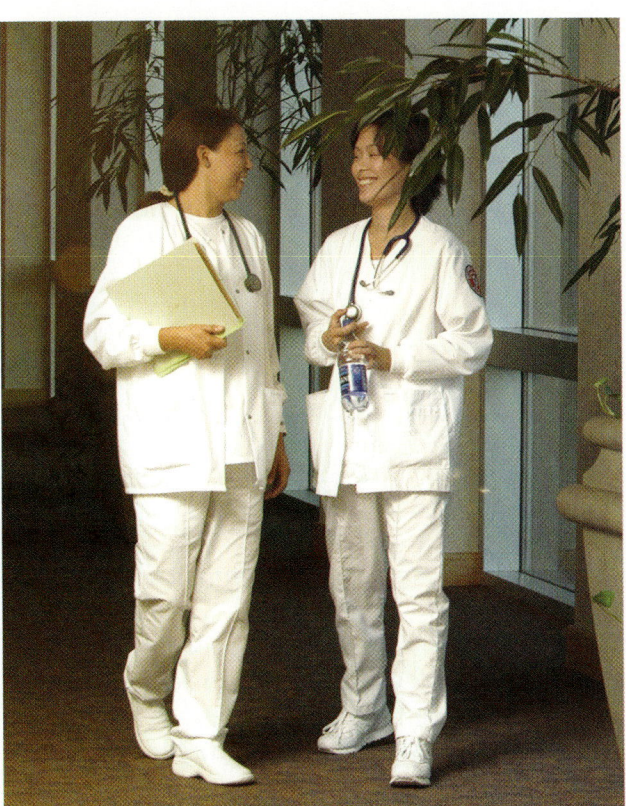

FIGURE 23-11 Humor helps nurses manage the stress created by the nature and intensity of their work. What can you do to help your fellow nursing students cope with the anxiety that is inherent in this stage of your academic experience? DELMAR/CENGAGE LEARNING

UNCOVERING THE

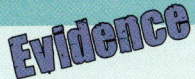

TITLE OF STUDY

"Relationships among the Nurse Work Environment, Self-Nurturance and Life Satisfaction"

AUTHORS

M. A. Nemcek and G. D. James

PURPOSES

(1) To determine the relationship among self-nurturance, perceived Magnet features, and life satisfaction and (2) to evaluate the predictive effects of self-nurturance and Magnet features on life satisfaction.

METHODS

This descriptive, correlational study is based on a survey of a convenience sample of 310 registered nurses (RNs).

FINDINGS

Self-nurturing RNs were more satisfied with life and perceived that more Magnet features were present in the workplace.

IMPLICATIONS

Higher levels of perceived Magnet features and frequent self-nurturance choices have a positive effect on RNs' life satisfaction. Increased life satisfaction reduces job dissatisfaction and improves retention rates.

Nemcek, M. A., & James, G. D. (2007). Relationships among the nurse work environment, self-nurturance and life satisfaction. *Journal of Advanced Nursing, 59*(3), 240–247.

- Let go of the need to be perfect.
- Listen to your self-talk.
- Encourage the use of appropriate humor in the workplace.

Nurses who cultivate the hardiness factor will likely be resilient to stress. Kobasa (1979) originated the concept of

👁 SPOTLIGHT ON...

Caring

Self-Nurturers

Society often labels people who take care of themselves as selfish. Do you agree? Why or why not? Consider how taking care of yourself can help you be a better care provider to others. What are some specific things you can do now to take better care of yourself?

hardiness in the late 1970s. Hardiness consists of a set of attitudes, beliefs, and behaviors that result in individuals being more resilient (or hardy) to the negative effects of stress. There are three components to stress hardiness:

- *Commitment.* Becoming involved in what one is doing
- *Challenge.* Perceiving change as an opportunity for growth rather than an obstacle or threat
- *Control.* Believing that one is influential in directing what happens to oneself rather than feeling helpless and victimized

According to studies (Kobasa, 1979; Kobasa, Maddi, & Kahn, 1982), individuals who have higher degrees of hardiness are healthier than are individuals with low degrees of hardiness. Such people develop fewer illnesses when they experience multiple stressors.

Many nurses need to relearn the value of play and to know when to stop working. Nursing students, who spend many hours a week working and studying, may need to schedule some time for play as it is a method to manage stress and, thereby, to become a more effective care provider.

NURSING CARE PLAN

The Client Experiencing Anxiety

CASE PRESENTATION
Kathryn Markham is a 38-year-old female who is seeking treatment in the emergency department of a metropolitan hospital. She is tearful, pacing, and wringing her hands. She is complaining of severe chest pain, a pounding headache, and back pain. She is sweating profusely and exhibits fine hand tremors. Her blood pressure and pulse are elevated, and her respirations are rapid and shallow. She says that she hasn't slept well since her husband left her 3 months ago. She states that "I'm afraid I'm losing my mind! My heart is racing and I can't sit still. Help me! I feel like I'm going to die."

ASSESSMENT
- Autonomic hyperactivity (rapid pulse, elevated blood pressure)
- Verbalized feelings of apprehension and uneasiness
- Restlessness

NURSING DIAGNOSIS
Anxiety related to feelings of powerlessness and lifestyle change
NOC: Anxiety self-control
NIC: Coping enhancement

EXPECTED OUTCOMES
The client will:

1. Identify effective coping mechanisms.
2. Report that anxiety is reduced to a manageable level.
3. Demonstrate relaxation skills.

INTERVENTIONS/RATIONALES
1. Establish a trusting relationship. The client may perceive the nurse or emergency department as a threat, and thus anxiety will increase.
2. Have the client identify and describe physical and emotional feelings. The first step in coping with anxiety is to recognize the anxiety and become aware of feelings in order to link emotions with maladaptive coping responses.
3. Help the client to relate cause-and-effect relationships between stressors and anxiety. Increases the client's sense of control and power over the situation.
4. Encourage the client to use coping mechanisms that have previously been successful. Increases confidence in own abilities to cope.

(Continues)

NURSING CARE PLAN (Continued)

5. Teach the client relaxation techniques (such as imagery and meditation). The relaxation response is the opposite of the stress response and, therefore, counters the physiological effects of the stress response. The relaxation response leads to lowered blood pressure, decreased heart rate, and deeper and slower respirations.
6. Administer antianxiety medication as indicated. Antianxiety agents provide relief from the immobilizing effects of anxiety. **NOTE:** This is a collaborative dependent nursing action.

EVALUATION
The client is visibly relaxed. Vital signs are within normal limits. The client verbalizes that she is calmer and no longer afraid.

KEY CONCEPTS

- Stress is an individual's physiological response to stimuli.
- Individuals who experience prolonged periods of stress are at risk for developing stress-related diseases.
- Anxiety is the psychological response to a threat to the health and well-being of an individual and activates the stress response.
- An individual seeks equilibrium through the process of adaptation. When adaptation is effective, homeostasis (the body's self-regulation of physiological processes) is maintained.
- Many factors, such as physiological, psychological, cognitive, or environmental changes, contribute to stress.
- The general adaptation syndrome (GAS), the physiological response to stress, consists of three stages: alarm, resistance, and exhaustion. The GAS is the same whether the stressor is actual or imagined, present or potential.
- Illness and hospitalization are major stressors for individuals and their families. To alleviate the stress of hospitalization, nursing interventions should reduce the client's feelings of unfamiliarity and loss of control.
- Change can be perceived as stressful because of a fear of failure, a threat to security, a potential for loss

of self-esteem, and the need to develop new paradigms.
- Nurses act as change agents by consciously empowering the client through education to initiate change.
- Nursing interventions that promote positive adaptation to stress are the empowerment of clients to meet basic needs; the minimization of environmental stimuli; the encouragement of verbalization of feelings; the inclusion of significant others into client care; and the use of various relaxation techniques, such as progressive muscle relaxation (PMR) and guided imagery.
- Stress management techniques can be used by both clients and nurses to facilitate effective coping.
- The thought-stopping technique, a cognitive approach to stress management, involves removing or reducing anxiety by changing negative thoughts to positive and realistic thoughts.
- Burnout occurs when the nurse is overwhelmed by stress. As a result, the nurse experiences physical, emotional, and behavioral dysfunction, including decreased productivity.
- Elements of a stress management plan for professional nurses consist of maintaining support systems, developing time management and decision-making skills, identifying and changing stressors that can be managed, and knowing personal limits.

REVIEW QUESTIONS

1. When assessing a client for anxiety, which of the following indicators would the nurse look for? Select all that apply.
   a. Decreased blood pressure
   b. Dry skin
   c. Increased pulse rate
   d. Increased respiratory rate
   e. Rapid, shallow breathing
   f. Shortness of breath verbalized by client

2. A medical-surgical unit has just reorganized its scheduling system. Members of the nursing staff have become comfortable with the new system and state they are pleased with the new self-scheduling method. According to Lewin's theory, the nursing staff is best defined as being in which phase of change?
   a. Moving
   b. Refreezing
   c. Status quo
   d. Unfreezing

3. Which of the following statements accurately describes a crisis situation?
   a. A crisis can be successfully resolved without intervention from others.
   b. Crisis has a slow, insidious onset.
   c. Prompt intervention is necessary to prevent an extended period of crisis.
   d. The client perceives the event as overwhelming.

4. Which of the following is an example of suppression used by a nursing student?
   a. Arguing with a roommate instead of expressing concerns to the instructor
   b. Deciding to go to bed early the night before the exam instead of cramming
   c. Stating that poor performance was a result of poorly written test questions
   d. Stating that the instructor was "out to get me"

5. Which of the following is an example of a situational crisis?
   a. Being a victim of a school shooting
   b. Hospitalization following an automobile accident
   c. Losing one's home due to a hurricane
   d. Sadness experienced by a woman during menopause

6. A nurse is planning to teach a client about safe medication usage. Which of the following activities should the nurse do first?
   a. Administer medication to help the client relax.
   b. Assess the client's anxiety level.
   c. Determine the client's need for information.
   d. Develop a specific teaching plan.

7. A unit nurse manager wants to implement a new system for making staff assignments. When planning the change process, which of the following should the nurse expect?
   a. Change efforts should be stopped if the staff members verbalize negative comments.
   b. Staff morale could be permanently damaged by the change.
   c. Staff may resist the change.
   d. Staff will quickly embrace the change.

8. A mother brings her 4-year-old son to the clinic for an annual checkup. The mother tells the nurse that the child began sucking his thumb 2 months ago when his little brother was born. The nurse recognizes the child's behavior as an example of which of the following defense mechanisms?
   a. Denial
   b. Reaction formation
   c. Regression
   d. Symbolization

9. Which of the following environmental strategies can be performed by the nurse to reduce client anxiety?
   a. Assign the client to a room across from the nurses' station.
   b. Keep the door to the client's room open.
   c. Keep the room brightly lit.
   d. Remove clutter from the room.

10. A nurse has been teaching a client the thought-stopping technique for stress reduction. Which of the following client statements indicates a need for further teaching?
    a. "I need to pay attention to what I'm thinking."
    b. "I should tense and relax my muscles whenever I feel anxious."
    c. "I will try to replace my negative thoughts with positive ones."
    d. "This technique needs to be repeated several times a day."

online companion

Visit the DeLaune and Ladner online companion resource at **www.delmar.cengage.com** for additional content and study aids. Click on Online Companions, then select the Nursing discipline.

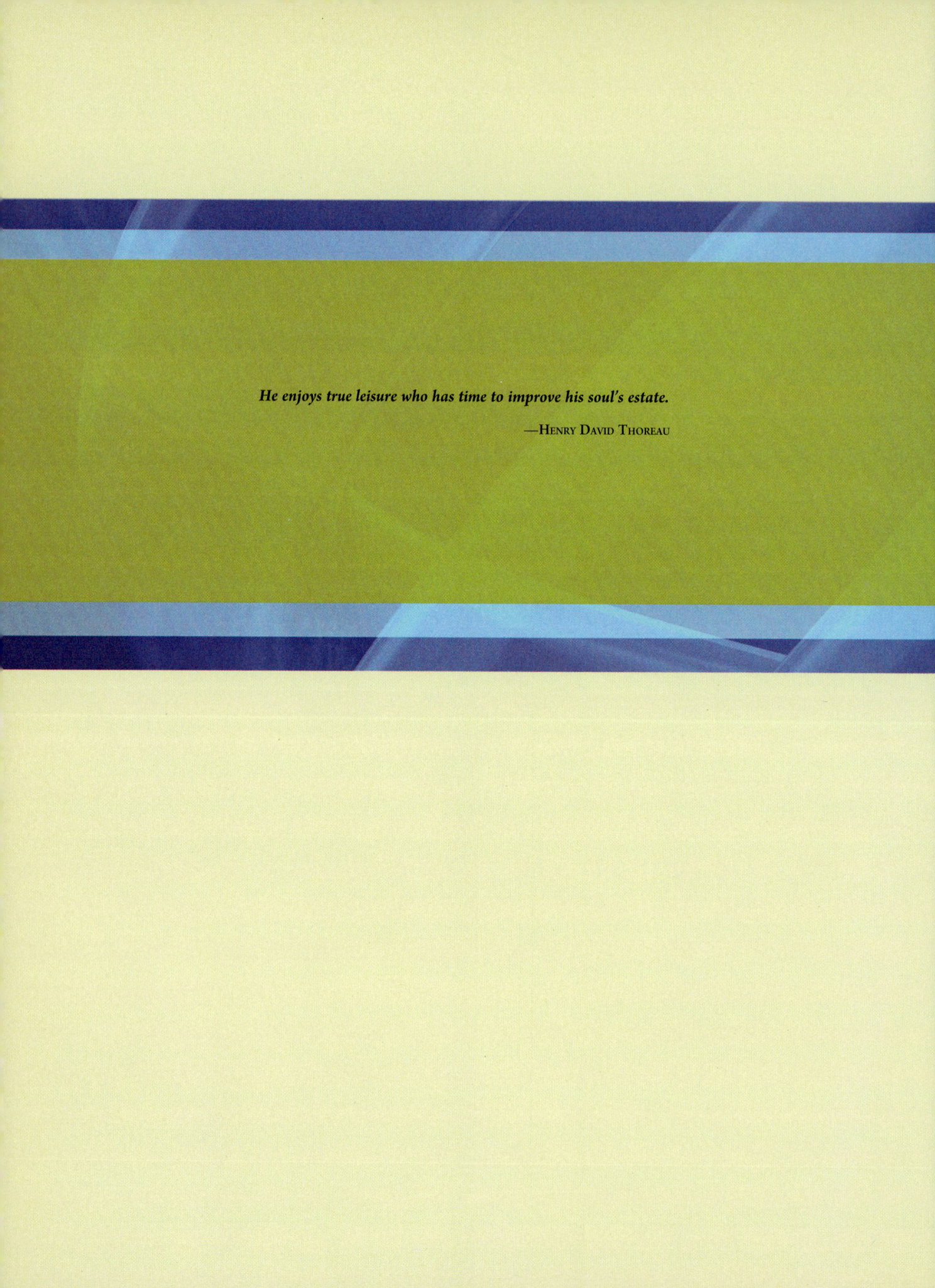

He enjoys true leisure who has time to improve his soul's estate.

—Henry David Thoreau

CHAPTER 24

Spirituality

COMPETENCIES

1. Describe the characteristics of spirituality.
2. Describe the connection between health and spiritual well-being.
3. Describe ways in which nurses help clients regain a sense of balance and harmony.
4. Discuss application of the nursing process as it relates to client spirituality.

KEY TERMS

faith	religion	spiritual well-being
hope	spiritual distress	spirituality
mindfulness		

Throughout history, people have dealt with pain, illness, and healing in spiritual ways. Ancient Babylonians and Egyptians performed elaborate healing rituals in temples; the ancient Greeks used dream-inducing methods to treat various disorders. In many primitive cultures, the roles of physician, psychiatrist, and priest were combined into one.

Nurses are entrusted with the holistic care of clients, that is, caring for the soul and spirit as well as for the body. The holistic framework challenges nurses to assess and respond to the physical, mental, emotional, and spiritual dimensions of each client.

SPIRITUALITY DEFINED

Spirituality is multidimensional in that it refers to one's relationship with one's self, a sense of connection with others, and a relationship with a higher power or divine source. Spirituality assists people in determining the sense of meaning or purpose in their lives. It is an integral component, or core, of one's being.

The classic work of Frankl, *Man's Search for Meaning* (1985), emphasized that the need for meaning is the primary motivating force in a person's life. By asking questions such as "what does this mean?" and "why me?" a person seeks to find meaning. According to Frankl, people find meaningfulness by what they take from the world, what they give to the world, and the attitude they choose for themselves in response to suffering. See the Respecting Our Differences display.

RESPECTING OUR DIFFERENCES

Spiritual Questions

Questions are powerful tools in shaping our thoughts, feelings, and behaviors. Allow yourself some silence in which to ponder your answers to the following questions:

What are the questions that I live with?

In what ways do I ask these questions?

How do I seek responses to these questions?

What makes life meaningful to me?

What sense do I make of pain and suffering?

Where do I see beauty in the world?

Be open to whatever arises within as you consider these questions. Know that your answers to these questions are strongly influenced by your cultural heritage.

The challenge that nurses face today is emphasizing the importance of spirituality in a health care system affected by advancing technology, ongoing organizational change, and limited resources. According to Pipe and colleagues,

Hospitalized patients may be at risk for experiencing a sense of fear and anxiety. Today's shorter hospital stays make it more challenging for the patient and health care team to form a meaningful relationship. This transpersonal connection may be even more important as the health care environment becomes more complex and efficiency focused. (2008, p. 248)

In order for nurses to meet this challenge, they must first begin their own healing journeys, caring for the soul and spirit as well as the body. Promoting **spiritual well-being** (a sense of connectedness between self, others, nature, and a higher power that can be accessed through prayer or other means) is a goal of holistic nursing. "Gaining an understanding of patients' expectations regarding spiritual care is essential to entering into a truly holistic, caring relationship with patients" (Davis, 2006, p. 1).

Healing, **faith** (a belief in and relationship with a higher power), spirituality, religiosity, and **hope** (a factor that enables one to cope with distressing events) are interrelated. When individuals deal with a life-threatening illness, serious medical condition, or loss, they often rely on spiritual support.

Spirituality is *not* the same as **religion**, which refers to a set of beliefs and practices associated with a particular church, synagogue, mosque, or other formal organized group. Spirituality is a personal, individualized set of beliefs and practices that are not affiliated with an institution or sect. See Table 24-1 for a comparison of religion and spirituality. Table 24-2 on page 465 describes the characteristics of spirituality.

Factors that affect spirituality include cultural context, family, developmental stage, and health status. Families influence a person's development of spiritual beliefs. Nurses

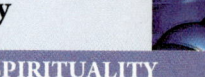

TABLE 24-1	Comparison of Religion and Spirituality	
RELIGION	**SPIRITUALITY**
A subset of spirituality	Universal
Denominational	Ecumenical
Behavioral rituals	Spontaneous
Cognitive	Affective
Public	Private

Delmar/Cengage Learning

TABLE 24-2 Characteristics of Spirituality

CHARACTERISTIC	DESCRIPTION
Relationship with self	Knowledge of who one is and one's capabilities
Relationship with others	Caring for others when they need help
	Sharing of self
Harmony with nature	Knowledge of plants and animals
	Preserving nature
	Communing with nature (being outdoors)
Relationship with a higher power	Meditation
	Prayer
	Participating in religious services
	Performing religious rituals

Data from Burkhardt, M. A., & Nagai-Jacobson, M. G. (2008). Transcultural and spiritual issues. In M. A. Burkhardt & A. K. Nathaniel (Eds.), *Ethics & issues in contemporary nursing* (3rd ed.). Clifton Park, NY: Delmar/Cengage Learning.

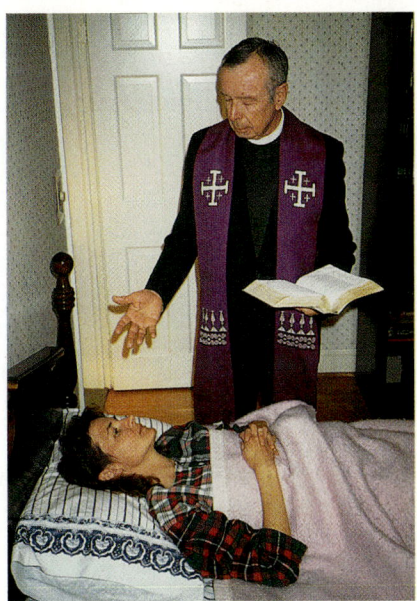

FIGURE 24-1 Rituals such as prayer may be an integral part of some individuals' expressions of spirituality. DELMAR CENGAGE LEARNING

Koenig, 2007; Newlin, Melkus, Tappen, Chyun, & Koenig, 2008; Reyes-Ortiz et al., 2008), religiousness and spirituality predicted fewer physical symptoms and better cognitive function in people experiencing medical and mental disorders.

NURSING PROCESS AND SPIRITUALITY

Spiritual care is an essential component of holistic care. The International Council of Nursing (2006) ethical code calls for nurses to promote an environment that respects the client's spiritual beliefs. Spiritual care, in addition to being an ethical duty of nurses, is now a requirement of some accreditation organizations. The right of clients to receive care that respects spiritual values was added to the Joint Commission's accreditation standards in 1998. In response to these criteria, some hospitals have revised policies to reflect the staff's duty to minister to persons of diverse cultural and religious backgrounds.

ASSESSMENT

Assessment primarily consists of observation and communication, which is based on a therapeutic nurse-client relationship. Some clients may be hesitant or embarrassed to discuss their spiritual beliefs. The nurse's presence communicates to the client that it is appropriate for clients to discuss all their concerns and issues. Presence helps establish the nurse-client relationship that is built on trust. As clients develop trust in the nurse, they are more likely to discuss sensitive issues. The use of open-ended questions and indirect questions encourages discussion of spiritual concerns. Hoffert,

understand the importance of families in providing spiritual support and encourage the provision of that support. Spirituality evolves throughout one's life. See Chapter 18 for a discussion of the development of spirituality related to Fowler's stages of faith.

Health status can also have an impact on spiritual beliefs and vice versa. For example, when they are seriously ill, many people turn to religion for support. On the other hand, serious illness may cause some people to question their beliefs. In some cases, a person's belief system may interfere with the prescribed medical treatment regimen. For example, a person's religious or spiritual beliefs may require fasting. Acceptance or rejection of prescribed therapies may be rooted in spiritual beliefs (see Figure 24-1). Table 24-3 on page 466 presents an overview of the practices of selected major world religions that can relate to issues such as diet, birth, death, and health care.

Individuals with spiritually satisfying lives are those people who have a source of inner strength. Spiritual beliefs can enhance self-esteem and help protect individuals from stress. Such beliefs help people adjust to stressful events such as illness, injury, and loss. There are several health-related benefits of engaging in spiritual practices, some of which include reduced stress levels, decreased blood pressure, lower cholesterol levels, and improved sleep patterns. According to several studies (Dew, Daniel, Goldston, & Koenig, 2008;

TABLE 24-3 World Religions and Health Implications

BELIEFS AFFECTING DIETARY PRACTICES	BELIEFS ABOUT BIRTH	BELIEFS ABOUT DEATH	BELIEFS AFFECTING HEALTH CARE	COMMENTS
Baptist				
• Alcohol prohibited	• No infant baptism	• Believe in heaven and hell • Prayer and counseling from clergy with client and family	• See physician as an instrument for God's intervention • Oppose abortion • Some believe in healing power of "laying on of hands"	• Those who believe in predestination (i.e., see illness as "God's will") often respond passively to treatment approaches
Buddhism				
• Alcohol and drug use discouraged • Some sects are vegetarian	• No infant baptism • Infant presentation	• Chanting of last rite at bedside immediately following death	• See illness as a result of negative karma • View cleanliness as very important • Often hesitant to receive treatment (such as surgery) on holy days	• When a death occurs, contact the priest
Christian Science				
• No restrictions or requirements	• No baptism	• No last rites • Organ donation usually opposed	• View illness as a mental concept that can be changed by prayer • Reject drugs or other therapies	• Will accept legally mandated immunizations • Many will refuse all treatment (including emergency care) until they have consulted with a reader
Church of Jesus Christ of Latter-Day Saints (Mormon)				
• Alcohol, coffee, and tea prohibited • Limited consumption of meat • First Sunday of the month is time for fasting	• No baptism at birth • Infant is blessed by clergy in church as soon as possible after birth	• No last rites • Many want church elders with them when dying • Cremation discouraged	• Medical therapy not prohibited • Many believe in divine healing with "laying on of hands" by church elders • Believe healing can occur by anointing with oil	• While hospitalized, may request sacrament on Sunday
Hinduism				
• Beef and veal prohibited • Many are vegetarian; limited consumption of meat • Fasting occurs on specific days of the week, according to which god the person worships	• No ritual	• Last rites are carefully prescribed • Priest pours water into mouth of the dead and ties a thread around the wrist to indicate a blessing	• Illness viewed as result of sins committed in previous life	• Will accept most medical interventions

(Continues)

TABLE 24-3 (Continued)

BELIEFS AFFECTING DIETARY PRACTICES	BELIEFS ABOUT BIRTH	BELIEFS ABOUT DEATH	BELIEFS AFFECTING HEALTH CARE	COMMENTS
• Children are not allowed to participate in fasting • Fasting rituals vary from complete abstinence to consumption of only one meal per day • Fasting may occur over a 1-month period or be observed only on holy days		• Family is particular about who touches the dead body • Cremation preferred		
Islam				
• Pork prohibited • Any meat product not ritually slaughtered prohibited • Avoidance of alcohol and drugs • During Ramadan (ninth month of Muhammadan year), fasting occurs during daytime	• No baptism	• Family must be with dying person • Dying person must confess sins and ask forgiveness • Family washes body • Only family and friends may touch the body • Usually oppose autopsy	• Faith healing unacceptable • Ritual washing after prayer (which occurs five times a day)	• May have fatalistic view that interferes with compliance to treatment plan
Jehovah's Witnesses				
• Prohibition of any food to which blood has been added • Can consume animal flesh that has been drained of blood	• No infant baptism	• No last rites • Autopsy only as required by law	• Opposed to blood transfusions	• No restrictions on giving blood sample • May have to obtain court order for treatment consent of child
Judaism				

• Dietary kosher laws must be adhered to by Orthodox believers
• Only the following meats are allowed:
  —Animals that are vegetable eaters
  —Animals with split hooves
  —Animals that are ritually not slaughtered
  —Fish that have scales and fins
	• No infant baptism
	• Male infants ritually circumcised on eighth day
		• Body is ritually cleansed
		• Burial should occur as soon as possible
		• Autopsy prohibited
		• No organ donation or transplantation unless approved by rabbi
			• Needs imposed by illness supersede dietary laws
			• During Sabbath (sundown Friday to sundown Saturday), may refuse surgical procedures
				• Body parts that are surgically removed should be made available to family for burial
				• If irreversible brain damage occurs, often opposed to prolongation of life

(Continues)

TABLE 24-3 (Continued)

BELIEFS AFFECTING DIETARY PRACTICES	BELIEFS ABOUT BIRTH	BELIEFS ABOUT DEATH	BELIEFS AFFECTING HEALTH CARE	COMMENTS
• Any combination of meat and milk prohibited • During Yom Kippur, 24-hour fasting • Pregnant women and those who are seriously ill are exempt from fasting • During Passover week, only unleavened bread eaten				
Methodist				
• No restrictions or requirements		• No last rites	• Before surgery, communion may be requested	• Donation of body or body parts to science is encouraged
Pentecostal (Assembly of God)				
• Abstention from alcohol • Avoid consumption of anything to which blood has been added • Some avoid pork	• No infant baptism	• No last rites	• Prayer is viewed as the tool for deliverance from illness • Illness is considered to be God's punishment or an intrusion of Satan	• May speak in tongues
Roman Catholicism				
• Optional fasting during Lenten season • During Lent, no meat on Fridays • Children and ill people exempt from fasting	• Infant baptism mandatory • May be performed by anyone if child is gravely ill	• Mandatory rite for anointing the sick • Last rites performed by priest • Autopsy acceptable • Organ donation and transplantation acceptable	• Life is viewed as sacred; abortion and contraceptive use are prohibited by church doctrine	• For many, religious articles and objects are important
Russian Orthodoxy				
• Abstention from meat and dairy products on Wednesday, Friday, and during Lent • During Lent, all animal products (including dairy) are forbidden	• Baptism performed only by priest	• Arms and fingers of the deceased are crossed • Opposed to autopsy and embalming • Cremation prohibited	• Major themes include fear, sin, and punishment • Believe in divine healing but will accept medical treatment	• Do not remove cross necklace unless absolutely necessary; replace as soon as possible

(Continues)

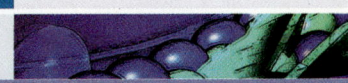

TABLE 24-3 (Continued)

BELIEFS AFFECTING DIETARY PRACTICES	BELIEFS ABOUT BIRTH	BELIEFS ABOUT DEATH	BELIEFS AFFECTING HEALTH CARE	COMMENTS
• Fasting during Advent • Exceptions from fasting during illness and pregnancy				
Seventh Day Adventists; Church of God				
• No alcohol • Coffee and tea prohibited • Some groups prohibit meat	• No infant baptism	• No last rites	• Practice anointing with oil and use of prayer for those who are ill • Some believe in divine healing • Some groups oppose hypnosis as a therapeutic modality • When ill, may want baptism or communion	• Literal acceptance of the Bible • For many, Saturday is the Sabbath

Data from Carpenito-Moyet, L. J. (2007). *Nursing diagnosis: Application to clinical practice* (12th ed.). Philadelphia: Lippincott, Williams & Wilkins; Giger, J. N., & Davidhizar, R. E. (2007). *Transcultural nursing: Assessment and intervention* (5th ed.). St. Louis, MO: Mosby Elsevier; Hockenberry, M. L., Wilson, D., & Jackson, C. (2006). *Wong's nursing care of infants and children* (8th ed.). St. Louis, MO: Elsevier Science.

Henshaw, and Mvududu (2007) suggest the use of these questions: "What gives you strength?" and "Who do you turn to in tough times?" (p. 68). See Table 24-4 on page 470, which provides a tool for assessing clients' spirituality.

DIAGNOSIS

Nurses must differentiate spiritual well-being from **spiritual distress** in a client. Spiritual distress is the client's perception that the client's belief system, or the client's place within it, is threatened. Following are some ways in which spiritual distress is manifested:

- Expressed anger toward God (e.g., "It's not fair! Why is God doing this to me?")
- Inner conflict about one's beliefs (e.g., "I'm not even sure what the right thing to do is anymore. Things used to be so clear.")
- Questions about the meaning of life, illness, death (e.g., "I wonder what I'm supposed to learn from all this.")
- Crying and sighing
- Withdrawn behaviors

- Verbal requests for spiritual assistance (e.g., "Keep me in your prayers.")

Spirituality helps individuals to find meaning in suffering. Receiving a diagnosis of a terminal condition such as cancer or acquired immunodeficiency syndrome (AIDS) often triggers a spiritual crisis. The North American Nursing Diagnosis Association International (NANDA) has established three diagnoses related to spirituality; see Table 24-5 on page 471.

PLANNING AND OUTCOME IDENTIFICATION

Planning of nursing care is directed at helping clients meet their needs, including spiritual needs.

In order to be healthy and respond appropriately to daily stress, an individual must experience a balance among mind, body, and spirit. The spiritual dimension provides the beliefs that affect the mind-body response to stress. Spiritual beliefs provide one with one's own uniqueness and

TABLE 24-4 Spiritual Assessment Tool

DIMENSION	QUESTIONS
Meaning and purpose	• What gives your life meaning? • Do you have a sense of purpose in your life? • How hopeful are you about getting better?
Inner strengths	• What brings you peace and joy? • What do you like about yourself? • What are your life goals? • What do you believe in?
Interconnectedness	• Who are the important people in your life? • Do you belong to any groups? • Can you ask others for help when you need it? • Do you participate in any religious activities? • Do you believe in God or a higher power?

Data from Dossey, B. M., & Keegan, L. (2008). *Holistic nursing: A handbook for practice* (5th ed.). Boston: Jones & Bartlett.

creativity, allowing one to listen to the inner voice and respond accordingly. Just as the mind and body must be fed, the spirit must be nourished. Spiritual nourishment may be in the form of prayer, reading, meditation, visualization, massage, music, art, or quiet time alone or in the presence of a loved one. **Mindfulness**, a form of meditation in which one focuses only on the present moment, is one way to heighten an appreciation of spiritual aspects in one's life. It is very difficult for many people to experience mindfulness because they are too busy, have too many things on their minds, or are worrying about the past or anticipating the future. Deliberately slowing down one's thinking helps one to experience an awareness of the present moment. See the accompanying Spotlight On display on page 472.

IMPLEMENTATION

Addressing the spiritual needs of clients often evokes anxiety in nurses. "Nurses who have reviewed their personal beliefs are likely to be more comfortable discussing the spiritual needs of a patient" (Loustalot, 2008, p. 22). However, it is imperative that nurses use self-awareness to prevent their own feelings from interfering with the fulfillment of clients' needs. The Nursing Checklist on page 472 provides guidelines for working with clients who need spiritual intervention.

Nurses are the professionals who are there to "just listen" and communicate compassion and support. Being there and listening to clients is a demonstration of nursing presence, which communicates caring and compassion. Essential nursing interventions directed at spiritual needs include helping clients to find meaning in their current situations and assisting clients to use their sources of strength.

Instillation of hope helps clients meet their spiritual needs. Hope is necessary for coping with severe stressors, such as illness. "People are partly enabled to endure suffering by maintaining hope in one or both of two ways: i) trusting in a higher being and ii) finding meaning through relationships with a higher being and/or with other people" (Vivat, 2008, p. 859). Spirituality provides a feeling that one is not alone. Nurses must determine the personal meaning of clients' experiences to help bolster spiritual support. The nurse should determine the client's source of hope, which may include the following:

- Relationships with others
- Positive emotions
- Anticipating the future
- Availability of resources

It has been proposed that religious and spiritual interventions could provide support for individuals experiencing chronic diseases, such as cancer and cardiovascular disease (Griffin, Salman, Lee, Seo, & Fitzpatrick, 2008).

Interventions for clients experiencing spiritual distress relate to (1) nursing priorities for assessing contributing factors, (2) assisting people to deal with feelings and the situation, and (3) promoting wellness. Examples of specific interventions include:

- Noting expressions of inability to find meaning in life
- Listening to expressions of anger or alienation from God
- Determining religious or spiritual orientation and influence of beliefs
- Asking how the nurse can be of the most help
- Providing a quiet setting
- Developing a therapeutic relationship that supports free expression of feelings and concerns
- Assisting client in developing goals for dealing with illness and other distressing situations
- Assisting client in identifying spiritual resources and other supports (Burkhardt & Nagai-Jacobson, 2008)

The nurse who takes time to be with clients in a caring way communicates a strength that can promote healing. The nurse's caring manner can act as a catalyst to promote self-healing by restoring a spiritual sense of balance and harmony. Use of meditative techniques helps clients to mentally

TABLE 24-5 Diagnosis Related to Spiritual Needs

DIAGNOSIS	DEFINITION	RELATED FACTORS
Spiritual distress	Impaired ability to experience and integrate meaning and purpose in life through a person's connectedness with self, others, art, music, literature, nature, or a power greater than oneself	• Self-alienation • Loneliness or social alienation • Anxiety • Sociocultural deprivation • Death and dying of self or others • Pain • Life change • Chronic illness of self or others
Readiness for enhanced spiritual well-being	Ability to experience and integrate meaning and purpose in life through connectedness with self, others, art, music, literature, nature, or a power greater than oneself	Not identified by NANDA
Risk for spiritual distress	At risk for an impaired ability to experience and integrate meaning and purpose in life through a person's connectedness with self, other persons, art, music, literature, nature, and/or a power greater than oneself	Risk factors: • Energy-consuming anxiety • Low self-esteem • Mental illness • Physical illness • Poor relationships • Blocks to self-love • Physical or psychological stress • Substance abuse • Loss of loved one • Natural disasters • Situational losses • Maturational losses • Inability to forgive

Data from North American Nursing Diagnosis Association International (NANDA). (2009). *Nursing Diagnoses—Definitions and Classification 2009–2011* © 2009, 2007, 2005, 2003, 2001, 1998, 1996, 1994 NANDA International. Used by arrangement with Wiley-Blackwell Publishing, a company of John Wiley & Sons, Inc.

relax, relieve tension, and honor their own intuition. Fostering trust through the demonstration of respect and empathy encourages the client to express feelings and spiritual beliefs. See the Uncovering the Evidence display.

Collaboration

The Joint Commission has criteria regarding spiritual care delivery that health care providers must meet. Clients should be asked if they would like to see their spiritual leader or advisor, with the understanding that not all clients will want to meet with a clergy member. Nurses need to know and use various resources available for providing spiritual support to clients. Many inpatient facilities have pastoral care departments that conduct formal services, visit and pray with clients, and conduct support groups (e.g., bereavement). Family members are the major spiritual support for some clients. Nurses can also identify colleagues who have more experience in dealing with spiritual concerns and use those individuals as resources.

EVALUATION

Evaluation focuses on client achievement of expected outcomes or objectives and on the efficacy of nursing care provided. Estes (2010) identifies the following as indicators that the client's spiritual distress has lessened:

- Acceptance of spiritual support from the source with which the client feels most comfortable
- Decrease in restlessness, insomnia, and crying
- Decrease in statements of worthlessness and hopelessness
- Verbalization of satisfaction with spiritual beliefs and the comfort provided by them

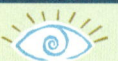 **SPOTLIGHT ON**...

Caring

Spiritual Nourishment

In what ways do you nurture your spiritual self? Think of your favorite "soul food" ingredients, for example, talking with a loved one, experiencing solitude, or enjoying nature.

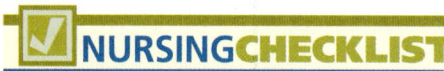 **NURSINGCHECKLIST**

Providing Spiritual Care

- Listen actively. Avoid using cliches, and take the client's concerns seriously.
- Demonstrate an interested, empathetic response to the client's comments.
- Respect the client's beliefs. For example, allow the client to pray without interruption.
- Provide privacy for the client to perform religious practices or rituals. For example, if the client's religious practice involves chanting, find a location where this can be done.
- Make referrals to clergy when appropriate. Ask the client's permission first to avoid imposing the nurse's own values on the client.

UNCOVERING THE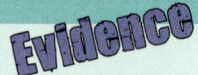

TITLE OF STUDY
"A Prospective Descriptive Study Exploring Hope, Spiritual Well-Being, and Quality of Life in Hospitalized Patients"

AUTHORS
T. B. Pipe, A. Kelly, G. LeBrun, D. Schmidt, P. Aterton, and C. Robinson

PURPOSE
To explore the relationships among hope, spiritual well-being, and quality of life in hospitalized clients across the time points spanning admission, discharge, and 6 weeks after discharge.

METHODS
A prescriptive, longitudinal, descriptive design was used. Selected data elements were collected from reviews of the participants' medical records. Participants responded on three occasions to interviews using standardized surveys that measured hope, spiritual well-being, and quality of life. Open-ended questions were also included pertaining to aspects of care that participants found most meaningful.

FINDINGS
Hope, spiritual well-being, and quality of life were correlated significantly and positively with each other at all three time intervals.

IMPLICATIONS
Clients often rely on nurses to provide psychosocial and spiritual care and comfort. Much of nursing is grounded in the transpersonal relationship that emphasizes caring. Psychosocial needs were associated with length of stay, reinforcing the need to identify these needs early. Findings suggest that nursing care can impact quality of life and length of stay.

Pipe, T. B., Kelly, A., LeBrun, G., Schmidt, D., Atherton, P., & Robinson, C. (2008). A prospective descriptive study exploring hope, spiritual well-being, and quality of life in hospitalized patients. *MEDSURG Nursing, 17*(4), 247–257.

KEY CONCEPTS

- Nurses are entrusted with the holistic care of clients, that is, caring for the soul and spirit as well as for the body.
- Spiritual care is a component of holistic care.
- Spirituality helps one determine a sense of meaning or purpose in one's life.

- Spirituality is not the same as religion, which refers to a set of beliefs and practices associated with a formal organized group.
- Factors affecting spirituality include cultural context, family, developmental stage, and health status.
- Spirituality develops across the life span.

- Nurses must emphasize the importance of spirituality in a health care system affected by advancing technology, ongoing organizational change, and limited resources.
- During assessment, nurses must differentiate spiritual well-being and spiritual distress in a client.
- There are three primary nursing diagnoses related to spirituality: spiritual distress, risk for spiritual distress, and readiness for enhanced spiritual well-being.
- When planning for client care, the nurse seeks to help the client maintain a balance among mind, body, and spirit.

- When implementing spiritually based care, the nurse must listen actively, demonstrate empathy, respect client beliefs, provide privacy, and make referrals to clergy as appropriate.
- Indicators that the client's spiritual distress has lessened are acceptance of spiritual support from others; decreased restlessness, insomnia, and crying; decreased statements of worthlessness and hopelessness; and verbalization of satisfaction with spiritual beliefs and the comfort provided by them.

REVIEW QUESTIONS

1. Parents of which of the following religious groups are most likely to request infant baptism for their very ill infant? Select all that apply.
   a. Baptist
   b. Buddhism
   c. Christian Science
   d. Hinduism
   e. Roman Catholic
   f. Russian Orthodoxy

2. Which of the following examples illustrates nursing sensitivity to a client's spiritual needs?
   a. Delivering a dinner tray to a Hindu client that has the following foods: green salad, cheeseburger, gelatin, and milk
   b. Insisting that a Jehovah's Witness client be given a blood transfusion
   c. Placing a do not disturb sign on the door of an Islamic client who is praying
   d. Scheduling an elective procedure for a Jewish client on Saturday

3. When should a nurse perform a spiritual assessment on a hospitalized client?
   a. At time of discharge
   b. Just prior to discharge or transfer to another facility
   c. On admission
   d. When client is admitted and throughout hospitalization

4. Which of the following is the initial nursing action when providing spiritual care to a client?
   a. Assessment of client needs
   b. Calling the clergy to minister to the client
   c. Praying with the client
   d. Self-awareness

5. A client has recently been informed of a terminal diagnosis. The client says, "I wonder why God is doing this to me. It's not fair!" Which of the following nursing diagnoses is appropriate for this client?
   a. Energy field disturbance
   b. Readiness for enhanced spiritual well-being
   c. Risk for spiritual distress
   d. Spiritual distress

6. The practice of focusing only on the present moment is known as:
   a. Collaboration
   b. Mindfulness
   c. Mysticism
   d. Spiritual distress

7. A client who is dying says, "You know I wonder what will happen to me after I die?" Which of the following nursing responses demonstrates provision of spiritual care?
   a. "I hate to interrupt your prayer but it's time for your pain medication."
   b. "I have asked my pastor to add your name to the prayer list."
   c. "Oh, don't talk like that. You'll feel better soon."
   d. "You sound anxious. Let's talk about it."

online companion

Visit the DeLaune and Ladner online companion resource at **www.delmar.cengage.com** for additional content and study aids. Click on Online Companions, then select the Nursing discipline.

Everyone can master grief but he that has it.

—Shakespeare

CHAPTER 25

Loss and Grief

COMPETENCIES

1. Discuss theoretical perspectives of loss, grief, and dying.
2. Describe various losses that affect individuals across the life span.
3. Describe characteristics of an individual experiencing grief.
4. Differentiate adaptive grief and pathological grief.
5. Explain the relationship between loss and grief.
6. Discuss the holistic needs of the dying person and family.
7. Discuss use of the nursing process with a grieving individual.
8. Describe end-of-life (EOL) care, including hospice.
9. Discuss nursing responsibilities when a client dies.
10. Describe ways in which nurses can cope with their own grief.

KEY TERMS

algor mortis	grief	mourning
anticipatory grief	grief work	palliative care
autopsy	hospice	rigor mortis
bereavement	liver mortis	situational loss
complicated grief	loss	uncomplicated grief
dysfunctional grief	maturational loss	

In contemporary society, individuals constantly experience loss. Frequent episodes of terrorism, natural disasters, and personal crises result in the universal experience of loss. Throughout the life cycle, people are faced with loss, without which growth would not continue. Many people consider loss only in terms of death and dying; however, loss of every type occurs daily. Nurses must be aware of the potential for loss in today's world, as well as the processes by which individuals adapt.

Every day nurses encounter clients who are responding to grief associated with losses. Thus, nurses must have an understanding of the major concepts related to loss and grieving. Grief is a response to losses of all types. Nurses also care for dying clients. This chapter provides information on meeting the special needs of terminally ill clients and their families.

LOSS

Loss is any situation (either actual, potential, or perceived) in which a valued object is changed or is no longer accessible to the individual. Because change is a major constant in life, everyone experiences losses. Loss can be actual (e.g., a spouse is lost through divorce) or anticipated (a person is diagnosed with a terminal illness and has only a short time to live). A loss can be tangible or intangible. For example, when a person is fired from a job, the tangible loss is income, whereas the loss of self-esteem is intangible.

Losses occur as a result of moving from one developmental stage to another. An example of such a maturational loss is the adolescent who loses the younger child's freedom from responsibility. Other examples of losses associated with growth and development are discussed later in this chapter. A situational loss occurs in response to external events, usually beyond the individual's control (such as the death of a significant other).

LOSS AS CRISIS

Loss precipitates anxiety and a feeling of vulnerability—which may lead to crisis. When a significant other dies, one's sense of safety and security is disrupted. Grieving is a mechanism for crisis resolution. When an individual feels overwhelmed by stress and the usual coping mechanisms are no longer effective, crisis occurs. Crisis intervention may be necessary to help the person grieve successfully. See Chapter 23 for a discussion of crisis and crisis intervention.

TYPES OF LOSS

Loss occurs when a valued object is changed or is no longer available. Not everyone responds to loss in the same way because the significance of the lost object or person is determined by individual perceptions. There are many types of loss, including:

- *Actual loss:* Death of a loved one, theft of one's property
- *Perceived loss:* Occurs when a sense of loss is felt by an individual but is not tangible to others
- *Physical loss:* Loss of an extremity in an accident, scarring from burns, permanent injury
- *Psychological loss:* Such as a woman feeling inadequate after menopause and resultant infertility

There are four major categories of loss: loss of external objects, loss of familiar environment, loss of aspects of self, and loss of significant other.

Loss of an External Object

When an object that a person highly values is damaged, changes, or disappears, loss occurs. The significance of the lost object to the individual determines the type and amount of grieving that occurs. The valued object may be a person, pet, prized possession, or one's home. The loss of a pet, especially for those who live alone, can be devastating.

Loss of Familiar Environment

The loss of a familiar environment occurs when a person moves to another home or a different community, changes schools, or starts a new job. Also, a client who is hospitalized or institutionalized experiences loss when faced with new surroundings. This type of loss evokes anxiety caused by fear of the unknown.

Loss of Aspect of Self

Loss of an aspect of self can be physiological or psychological. A psychological aspect of self that may be lost is ambition, a sense of humor, or enjoyment of life. An example of physiological loss is loss of physical function as a result of illness or injury. Loss also occurs when there is disfigurement or disappearance of a body part, such as having an amputation or mastectomy. Loss of an aspect of self can result from illness, trauma, or treatment methodologies (e.g., surgery).

Loss of Significant Other

The loss of a loved one is a significant loss. Such a loss can be the result of separation, divorce, running away, moving to a different area, or death. Responses to loss are highly individualized, as each person perceives the meaning of loss differently. For example, the death of a spouse is generally perceived differently by men and women (see Figure 25-1).

GRIEF

Grief is a series of intense physical and psychological responses that occur following a loss. It is a normal, natural, necessary, and adaptive response to a loss. Loss leads to the adaptive process of **mourning**, the period of time during which the grief is expressed and resolution and integration of the loss occur. **Bereavement** is the period of grief following the death of a loved one.

THEORIES OF THE GRIEVING PROCESS

There is no one comprehensive theory to explain the grief process, which may consist of a series of phases. Several theories have allowed us to delineate predictable symptoms and states in response to loss. When reviewing the following theories, remember that everyone does not experience each phase in the order described. The theories of Lindemann, Engle, Bowlby, and Worden are discussed in the following sections.

Lindemann

In 1944, after the Coconut Grove fire in Boston, in which over 400 people died, Lindemann studied survivors of the disaster and their families. Lindemann coined the phrase **grief work**, which is still used today to describe the process experienced by the bereaved. During grief work, the person experiences freedom from attachment to the deceased, becomes reoriented to the environment in which the deceased is no longer present, and establishes new relationships (Lindemann, 1944). Lindemann's classic work is the foundation for current crisis and grief resolution theories. See Table 25-1, which provides a description of Lindemann's concepts.

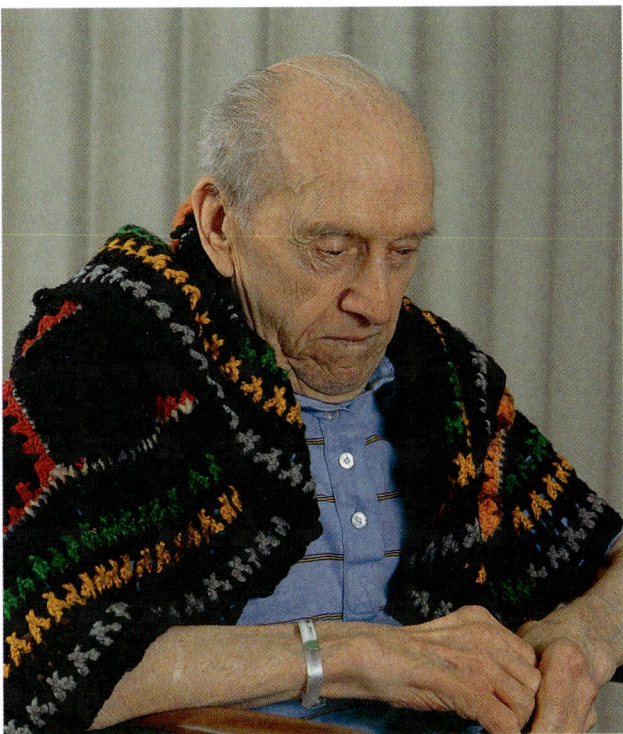

FIGURE 25-1 Losing a spouse or partner who has been a part of their lives for many years is common for older adults. How can nurses support these individuals during the grieving process? DELMAR/CENGAGE LEARNING

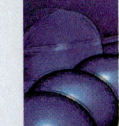

TABLE 25-1 Lindemann's Theory: Reactions to Normal Grief

STAGE	DESCRIPTION
Somatic distress	Episodic waves of discomfort in duration of 10–60 minutes Multiple somatic complaints Emotional pain
Preoccupation with image of the deceased	A sense of unreality Emotional detachment from others Overwhelming preoccupation with visualizing the deceased
Guilt	Bereaved consider the death to be a result of their own negligence or lack of attentiveness Look for evidence of how they could have contributed to the death
Hostile reactions	Relationships with others become impaired owing to the bereaved's desire to be left alone, irritability, anger
Loss of patterns of conduct	Inability to sit still (generalized restlessness) Continually searching for something to do

Data from Lindemann, E. (1944). Symptomatology and management of acute grief. *American Journal of Psychiatry, 101*, 141–148.

Engle

Grief is a typical reaction to loss of a valued object. There are three stages of mourning, and progression through each stage is necessary for healing. The grieving process, which may take several years to complete, cannot be accelerated. The goal of the grieving process is for the mourner to accept the loss and let go of the deceased. See Table 25-2, which provides an overview of Engle's theory of grief.

Bowlby

Bowlby stated that grief results when an individual experiences a disruption in attachment to a love object. His theory proposes that grief occurs when attachment bonds are severed. There are four phases that occur during grieving:

- Numbing
- Yearning and searching
- Disorganization and despair
- Reorganization (Bowlby, 1982)

Worden

Worden (1982) has identified four tasks that an individual must perform in order to successfully deal with a loss:

- Accept the fact that the loss is real.
- Experience the emotional pain of grief.
- Adjust to an environment without the deceased.
- Reinvest the emotional energy once directed at the deceased into another relationship.

Worden categorized the behavioral responses that grieving individuals experience; see Table 25-3 on page 479.

TYPES OF GRIEF

Grief is a universal, normal response to loss. Grief drains people, both emotionally and physically. Because grief consumes so much emotional energy, relationships may be impaired and health status may become altered. There are different types of grief including uncomplicated ("normal"), dysfunctional, and anticipatory.

Uncomplicated Grief

Many individuals use the term *normal grief*. Engle (1961) proposed use of the term **uncomplicated grief** to describe a grief reaction that normally follows a significant loss. Uncomplicated grief runs a fairly predictable course that ends with the relinquishing of the lost object and resumption of the previous life. Even though the bereaved person's life is changed forever, the person is able to regain the ability to function.

Some common responses experienced by grieving individuals are shown in Table 25-4 on page 479. Not every mourner will experience all the reactions, but the reactions most often experienced in response to a recent loss are listed.

Many grieving people experience feelings of anger or blame; these feelings may be directed toward those perceived to have caused or contributed to the death. Often the anger associated with grief is directed at one's self, that is, expressed as guilt or depression. Some survivors have a strong need to assign blame. If someone else can be blamed, then the survivors can rid themselves of any responsibility. Those who are experiencing grief must be provided an opportunity to express feelings—both positive and negative—in order to alleviate guilt.

Nurses play an important role in assisting mourners to develop and understand the normal grieving process and the complex feelings exhibited when grief becomes more complicated. Nurses with a sound knowledge base of both normal grief and dysfunctional grief will be better prepared to assist the survivors than nurses who believe that all grief is the same.

TABLE 25-2 Engle's Theory of Grief: Three Stages of Mourning

STAGE	CHARACTERISTICS
Stage I: Shock and disbelief Can last from minutes to days	Disorientation Perceived helplessness Denial gives protection until person is able to face reality
Stage II: Developing awareness May last from 6 to 12 months	Emotional pain occurs with increased reality of loss Recognition that one is powerless to change the situation Feelings of helplessness Anger and hostility may be directed at others Guilt Sadness Isolation Loneliness
Stage III: Restitution and resolution Marks the beginning of the healing process and may take up to several years	Emergence of bodily symptoms May idealize the deceased Mourner starts to come to terms with the loss Establishment of new social patterns and relationships

Data from Engle, G. L. (1961). Is grief a disease? *Psychosomatic Medicine, 23*, 18–22; Engle, G. L. (1964). Grief and grieving. *American Journal of Nursing, 64*(9), 93–98.

TABLE 25-3 Manifestations of Normal Grief (Worden)

EMOTIONS	PHYSICAL SETTINGS	BEHAVIORS	THOUGHT PROCESSES
• Sadness • Anxiety • Guilt • Relief • Emancipation • Self-blame • Fatigue • Numbness • Shock • Helplessness • Yearning • Loneliness	• Increased sensitivity to noise • Constricted feeling in throat and chest • Shortness of breath • Hollow feeling in stomach • Dry mouth • Muscular weakness • Lethargy	• Disrupted sleep patterns • Dreaming about the deceased • Forgetfulness • Crying • Avoiding reminders of the deceased • Treasuring objects belonging to the deceased • Social withdrawal	• Disbelief • Preoccupation • Confusion • Sense of presence of the deceased • Hallucinations (e.g., as seeing or hearing the deceased)

Delmar/Cengage Learning

TABLE 25-4 Reactions Commonly Experienced during Grief

PHYSICAL REACTIONS	PSYCHOSOCIAL REACTIONS	COGNITIVE REACTIONS	BEHAVIORAL REACTIONS
• Loss of appetite • Weight loss • Insomnia • Fatigue • Decreased libido • Decreased immune functioning (increased susceptibility to illness) • Multiple somatic complaints (e.g., headache, backache) • Restlessness	• Profound sadness • Helplessness • Hopelessness • Denial • Anger • Hostility • Guilt • Nightmares • Ennui (overwhelming sense of emptiness) • Preoccupation with lost object • Loneliness	• Inability to concentrate • Forgetfulness • Impaired judgment • Decreased problem-solving ability • Impaired decision-making ability	• Impulsivity • Indecisiveness • Social withdrawal • Distancing • Crying

Delmar/Cengage Learning

Dysfunctional Grief

Persons experiencing **dysfunctional grief** do not progress through the stages of overwhelming emotions associated with grief, or they may fail to demonstrate any behaviors commonly associated with grief. The person experiencing pathologic grief continues to have strong emotional reactions, does not return to a normal sleep pattern or work routine, usually remains isolated, and has altered eating habits. The bereaved may have the need to endlessly tell and retell the story of loss but without subsequent healing. Visits to the grave site or mausoleum may be made often or not at all.

Dysfunctional grief is a demonstration of a persistent pattern of intense grief that does not result in reconciliation of feelings. A person experiencing chronic grief continues to focus on the deceased, may overvalue objects that belonged to the deceased, and may engage in depressive brooding. The pathologically grieving person is unable to reestablish a routine. Several factors predispose a person to experience dysfunctional grieving, including:

- Uncertain, sudden, or overcomplicated circumstance surrounding the loss
- A loss that is socially unspeakable or socially negated (e.g., suicide)
- A relationship with the deceased characterized by ambivalence or excessive dependency (Worden, 1991)

Anticipatory Grief

Anticipatory grief is the occurrence of grief work before an expected loss. Anticipatory grief may be experienced by the terminally ill person as well as family. This phenomenon promotes adaptive grieving by freeing up the mourner's emotional energy. Although anticipatory grieving may be helpful in adjusting to the loss, it may also result in some disadvantages. For example, for the dying client, anticipatory grieving may lead to family members' distancing themselves and not being available to provide support. Also, if the family members have separated themselves emotionally from the dying client, they may seem cold and distant and thus may not meet society's expectations of mourning behavior. This response can prevent the mourners from receiving their own much-needed support from others.

FACTORS AFFECTING GRIEF

The experience of grief is individual and is influenced by various factors. Factors that influence grief include the person's developmental level, religious and cultural beliefs, relationship to the lost object, and the cause of death.

Developmental Considerations

Certain kinds of loss at key developmental points may have a profound effect on a person's ability to work through grief and may result in inadequate achievement of the developmental task. Depending on a client's developmental level, the grief response to a loss will be experienced differently. For example, a pregnant woman will, to some degree, experience loss after delivery, even delivery of a normal healthy infant. See Table 25-5 for other examples of developmental losses that may precipitate grieving.

TABLE 25-5 Losses Associated with Developmental Stage

DEVELOPMENTAL STAGE	RELATED LOSS
Infants	Intrauterine environment (warmth and protection)
	Comfort of sucking breast or bottle
Toddlers and preschoolers	Spontaneity of bodily function as a result of toilet training
	Immediate gratification of needs as child gains independence
	Familiar environment as child attends day care or nursery school
School-aged children	Periodic loss of body function caused by normal childhood illnesses and injuries
	Friends and significant others (teachers, coaches) as they progress through school
Adolescents	Familiar body with onset of puberty
	Childhood freedoms in response to social expectation to act mature
	First love (as adolescent "crushes" end) functions
	Familiar environment when leaving home for work or education
Young adults	Friends through leaving school, moving, changing jobs
	Financial support from parents when leaving home
	Freedom when assuming more adult responsibilities
	Sexual partner
Middle adults	Spouse, through separation, divorce, or death
	Children as they leave home
	Friends through job changes, moving, or death
	Parents through death
	"Youth" (as related to physical appearance, libido, and physical stamina)
	Women experience loss of fertility through menopause

(Continues)

TABLE 25-5 (Continued)

DEVELOPMENTAL STAGE	RELATED LOSS
Older adults	Spouse and friends through death
	Sensory perceptual acuity
	Job, as a result of retirement
	Body image changes related to decline in some physiological functions
	Independence

Delmar/Cengage Learning

CHILDHOOD   Children vary in their ability to comprehend the meaning of death. It is important to understand how a child's concept of death evolves because it varies with developmental level (see Table 25-6).

Well-meaning adults often try to protect children from the realities of death by excluding them from mourning rituals. However, children need to be included in family activities as appropriate to their developmental level. Children who are grieving need explanations about death that are honest and in language that they can easily understand. See Table 25-7, on page 482, for suggestions on talking to children about death.

ADOLESCENCE   Most adolescents value physical attractiveness and athletic abilities. Grief may occur when the adolescent suffers the loss of a body part or function. Because of the strong influence of peer groups, adolescents seek approval from their friends and fear being rejected if a loss

TABLE 25-6 Perception of Death by Children and Adolescents

DEVELOPMENTAL STAGE	PERCEPTION	POTENTIAL DEVELOPMENTAL DISRUPTIONS
Infancy and toddler	• Is not aware of death • Is aware of disruptions in normal routine • Can react to family's expressions of grief	• If the mother or surrogate dies during the first 2 years of life, the child may have significant, long-lasting psychosocial problems
Preschool	• Views death as a temporary separation • Able to react to the gravity of death in accordance with the reactions of parents or other adults	• May have significant psychosocial problems if either parent is lost at this stage, especially between ages 4 and 6 (owing to magical thinking, in which children may believe death is their fault)
School-age	• Appreciates that death is final and inevitable • Fantasizes about and tends to personify death ("the bogeyman")	• May have nightmares • May engage in death-avoidance behaviors (e.g., hiding under the covers, leaving the lights on, closing closet doors) • May experience intense guilt and a sense of responsibility for the death
Preadolescent and adolescent	• Recognizes that death is final • Understands that death is inevitable • Preadolescents: tend to worry about dying • Adolescents: tend to deny that death could happen to them	• Loss of a parent may interfere with mastery of the young adulthood task of forming intimate relationships with members of opposite sex

Delmar/Cengage Learning

TABLE 25-7 Communicating with Children about Death

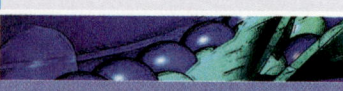

THERAPEUTIC	NONTHERAPEUTIC
• Use simple, concrete language. • Involve the child in mourning rituals (e.g., take to funeral home and cemetery); explain what is going to happen. • Encourage the child to express feelings. • Reassure children that they will not be abandoned. • Answer all questions truthfully.	• Use of euphemisms (e.g., ''he's gone to sleep'' or ''she went away'') • Overexplanations • Minimizing child's experience • Judgmental statements

Delmar/Cengage Learning

affects their acceptance by others (e.g., grief after a disfiguring accident is usually intense in adolescents). Even though they have an intellectual understanding of death, adolescents feel they are immune to death and therefore do not accept the possibility of their own mortality. This perception is caused by the sense of invulnerability that normally occurs during adolescence.

EARLY ADULTHOOD In the young adult, grief is usually precipitated by loss of role or status. For example, unemployment or breakup of a relationship causes significant grief for the young adult. The concept of death in this age group is primarily a reflection of cultural values and spiritual beliefs.

MIDDLE ADULTHOOD During middle adulthood the potential for experiencing loss increases. The death of parents begins to occur. As an individual ages, it can be especially threatening for peers to die because their death forces acknowledgment of one's own vulnerability to death. Other losses frequently experienced during middle age are those associated with changes in employment and relationships (e.g., divorce), children leaving home, and decreasing functional abilities.

OLDER ADULTHOOD During late adulthood, most individuals recognize the inevitability of death. Most older adults experience numerous losses as they age. Losses commonly experienced by older adults include loss of (Bowlby, 1961):

- Loved ones and friends
- Occupational role as a result of retirement
- Material possessions
- Dreams and hopes

In the United States, women live longer than men and are, therefore, more likely to experience the loss of a spouse. According to the U.S. Census Bureau (2008), in 2007 the population of those age 75 years or older is 4.7% male and 7.5% female. Regardless of gender, the bereaved may need to develop new skills in order to adapt. For example, a man who was married for 50 years may have to learn meal preparation after his wife dies.

Religious and Cultural Beliefs

Religious and cultural beliefs can have a significant effect on an individual's grief. Every culture has certain religious beliefs about the significance of death as well as rituals for care of the dying; see Table 25-8. See Chapters 20 and 24 for

TABLE 25-8 Religious Traditions Related to Death

RELIGION	BELIEFS AND RITUALS
Buddhism	May prefer quality of life rather than quantity
	Last-rite chanting at bedside
	Cremation usually preferred
Catholicism	Believe life should be prolonged by ordinary, not extraordinary, means
	Sacrament of the sick
	Organ donation and autopsy acceptable
	Practice of ''waking'' (keeping watch) over the dead is common
	Usually burial instead of cremation

(Continues)

Table 25-8 (Continued)

RELIGION	BELIEFS AND RITUALS
Christian Science	Opposed to euthanasia
	No organ transplantation
	Disposal of body to be decided by the family
Greek Orthodox	May isolate dying person and withhold truth about prognosis
	Dying at home is important
	Widow wears dark mourning clothes for rest of life
Hinduism	Believe in reincarnation
	Autopsy and organ donation are acceptable
	Religious chanting before and after death
	Cremation is preferred
	Non-Hindus should not touch the body
	Thread is tied around wrist of the deceased to signify a blessing
Islam	Euthanasia forbidden
	Organ donation acceptable
	Autopsy only if legally or medically necessary
	Deceased body is washed only by Muslim of same gender
	Body usually remains at home, wrapped in white cloth
	Burial within 24 hours of death
Jehovah's Witness	Euthanasia prohibited
	Autopsy only for legal purposes
	Organ donation forbidden
Judaism	Euthanasia forbidden
	No autopsy or organ donation
	Relatives remain with dying person
	Do not mandate life support
	Body is ritually washed
	Eyes must be closed at death
	Burial is done within 24 hours or as soon as possible
	Recognize a 7-day period of mourning
Protestantism	May be some restrictions on prolonging life
	Uphold individual decisions regarding autopsy, organ donation, and burial or cremation

Data from Spector, R. E. (2008). *Cultural diversity in health and illness* (9th ed.). Upper Saddle River, NJ: Prentice-Hall.

discussion of the impact of religious and cultural beliefs. Beliefs about an afterlife and faith in a higher power, redemption of the soul, and reincarnation are important aspects that often assist one in grief work.

Relationship with the Lost Object

It is usually more difficult to cope with the loss of an ambivalent relationship, as such relationships are characterized by many "if only" and "I should have" thoughts. Unfinished business and regrets about the deceased make coping with the loss more problematic. When individuals in conflicted relationships have time to work on issues prior to the death, grieving is usually facilitated.

In general, the more intimate the relationship with the deceased, the more intense the grief experienced by the bereaved. The death of a child poses a particular risk for dysfunctional grieving. The death of a parent or a sibling can pose a major challenge for children. The child's feelings may often go unrecognized by adults who fail to understand the child's need to mourn.

Individuals experiencing parental grief usually have intense reactions and responses. It is expected that children outlive their parents. When a child dies, the parent not only loses the child but also experiences losses of the parental role. Bowlby (1961) describes parents who talk about losing a part of themselves as a result of their child's death. The uniqueness of parental grief for a deceased child may be the loss of the perceived potential for the child who has died. It is the loss of the hopes of the parents for the child, for "the things that could have been." Table 25-9, on page 485, provides a listing of characteristics of parents whose children have died.

Cause of Death

The intensity of the grief response changes according to the cause of death, be it unexpected, traumatic, or a suicide.

UNEXPECTED DEATH The loss occurring with an unexpected death poses particular difficulty for the bereaved in achieving closure. Unanticipated death, such as a death resulting from a natural disaster or other tragedy (e.g., airplane crash), leaves survivors shocked and bereaved. Often, the inability to say goodbye compounds the trauma of the death and may be a factor contributing to altered grieving.

TRAUMATIC DEATH   **Complicated grief** is associated with traumatic death such as death by homicide or suicide. Although traumatic death does not necessarily predispose the survivor to complications in mourning, survivors suffer emotions of greater intensity than those associated with normal grief.

When loved ones die violently, the grievers may suffer from traumatic imagery, that is, reliving the terror of the incident or imagining the feelings of horror felt by the victim. Traumatic imagery is a common occurrence with traumatic death. Such thoughts, coupled with intense grief, can lead to

posttraumatic stress disorder (PTSD). Nurses must be aware of the possibility of PTSD and be alert for the presence of symptoms, which may include:

- Sleep disturbances, such as recurrent, terror-filled nightmares
- Psychological distress
- Chronic anxiety

Unless complicated grief is recognized and the survivors are encouraged to express the intense feelings, they will not be able to progress through the normal, adaptive grieving process.

SUICIDE The loss of a loved one to suicide is frequently compounded by feelings of blame in the survivors. They feel guilty for failing to recognize clues that may have enabled the victim to receive help. These feelings of guilt and self-blame can be transformed into anger at the victim for inflicting such pain, at themselves, and at caregivers. Feelings of shame for having a suicide in the family may also be present.

NURSING CARE OF THE GRIEVING PERSON

Resolution of a loss is a painful process and must be done by clients in their own way. Grief changes people by affecting self-esteem, triggering the development of new ways of coping, and precipitating a change in lifestyle without the deceased.

Nurses can play an active role in assisting people to grieve. Encourage clients to do their grief work, that is, to experience their feelings to the fullest in order to work through them. Provide support and explain to the bereaved that it will take time to grieve the loss and to gain some closure to the relationship.

Assessment

A thorough assessment of the grieving client and family begins with a determination of the personal meaning of the loss. Another key assessment area is deciding where the person is in terms of the grieving process. The nurse understands that the stages of grieving are not necessarily mastered sequentially, but that instead individuals may vacillate in progression through the stages of grief. Levin (1998) recommends that assessment be done to differentiate the signs of healthy grieving from at-risk behavior.

Diagnosis

The North American Nursing Diagnosis Association International (NANDA, 2009) defines *Complicated grieving* as "a disorder that occurs after the death of a significant other, in which the experience of distress accompanying bereavement fails to follow normative expectations and manifests in functional impairments" (p. 98); see the Nursing Process Highlight on page 486.

TABLE 25-9 Characteristics of Parents Whose Children Die

DEATH	CHARACTERISTICS
Spontaneous abortion (miscarriage) and stillbirth	Parents may have feelings of intense sadness, anger, or guilt.
	The death is often unacknowledged by others, especially if the loss occurs in early weeks of pregnancy.
	The death may be considered a personal failure.
	Parents may dwell on details, designating blame to themselves or others.
	Grief from previous losses may be relived.
	Anticipatory grief may occur if the infant's condition is known early.
	Ambivalence experienced in early pregnancy may increase grief.
	Hopes for the future must be modified or changed.
	Despair may peak when the parents must leave the hospital without the baby.
Neonatal death	Feelings are similar to stillbirth.
	Parents have had time to form a bond with the infant, intensifying the grief.
	Grief may be intense for both parents.
Sudden infant death syndrome (SIDS)	Death is unexplainable and unexpected.
	Pain is increased by lack of knowledge and misinformation.
	Parental bonding is complete.
	Death is silent, with no signs of distress.
	Guilt is often present.
	Police may investigate, adding to the guilt.
	Grief is acute due to lack of time to prepare.
	Parents may be preoccupied with the details of the death.
Abortion	Shame, secrecy, and guilt may accompany grief.
	Highly ambivalent feelings may be present.
	Little support or comfort is offered by others.
	Feelings of relief are expected, but despair and depression may surface.
	No guilt may be felt, especially if the woman did not want a child.

Delmar/Cengage Learning

Outcome Identification and Planning

It is important to clarify the expected outcomes when planning care for the grieving client. Following are some expected outcome criteria for the person experiencing grief:

- Verbalize feelings of grief
- Share grief with significant others
- Accept the loss
- Renew activities and relationships

Some of these expected outcomes will take a long period of time to achieve, and some must be achieved before others are mastered. For example, to accept the loss, the person must begin to share grief with others by verbalizing feelings. Two expected outcomes for mourners are discussed in the sections that follow.

ACCEPTANCE OF THE LOSS Only by going through grief work are individuals able to reach some acceptance and,

NURSING PROCESS HIGHLIGHT

Diagnosis

Complicated Grieving

Defining Characteristics (partial listing):

- Decreased functioning in life roles
- Decreased sense of well-being
- Depression
- Fatigue
- Preoccupation with thoughts of the deceased
- Searching for the deceased

Related Factors (partial listing):

- Death of a significant other
- Emotional instability
- Lack of social support

Data from North American Nursing Diagnosis Association International. (2009). *Nursing Diagnoses—Definitions and Classification* 2009–2011 © 2009, 2007, 2005, 2003, 2001, 1998, 1996, 1994 NANDA International. Used by arrangement with Wiley-Blackwell Pubishing, a company of John Wiley & Sons, Inc.

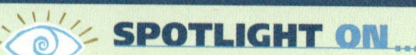

SPOTLIGHT ON...

Compassion

Allowing Time to Grieve

Your coworker, who is also your friend, has just lost a loved one whose funeral was today. Tomorrow your friend must return to work because his 3-day bereavement leave is over. He is dealing with many intense emotions as well as a lack of energy. Society dictates that he return to work. How do you deal with his lack of productivity at work? How do you provide support to him?

ultimately, resolution of feelings about the loss. Often, people try to find some meaning in their situations. This search involves introspection in which spiritual support is of therapeutic value.

RENEWAL OF ACTIVITIES AND RELATIONSHIPS The very core of grief work revolves around acceptance of the fact that the needs met by key people in one's life can be met in other ways and by other people. The deceased cannot be replaced; however, enough healing must occur so that new relationships can be initiated.

How long does the process of adaptive grieving take? Grief work takes time. There are no definite time frames in which grief should occur. The length of time for grief to be resolved is as individual as the person experiencing it and its intensity. Each person grieves in his or her own way and at his or her own pace. See the accompanying Spotlight On display.

Implementation

Therapeutic nursing care is based on an understanding of the significance of the loss to the client. To understand the client's perspective, the nurse must spend time listening. As the client expresses feelings, the nurse must demonstrate acceptance, even if the client is not responding according to the nurse's expectations or belief system. The nurse's nonjudgmental, accepting attitude is essential while listening to the bereaved. The nurse communicates an understanding of the client's anger—and avoids personalizing and using defensive behaviors.

Grieving people need reassurance, counseling, and support; see Figure 25-2. One mechanism of providing support on a long-term basis is support groups. Thus, the nurse needs to be aware of the availability of such groups within the community in order to make appropriate referrals. When bereaved people join support groups, they will be with others who have experienced similar situations. This sharing decreases the feelings of loneliness and social isolation that are so common in grief. The accompanying Nursing Checklist, on page 487, provides guidelines for nurses working with grieving clients.

Evaluation

People follow their own time schedule for grief work. In general, it takes months or years for resolution of grief. It is important to teach grieving individuals that resolution of the loss is generally a process of lifelong adjustment. Therefore, nurses usually do not have an opportunity to be with the bereaved family when grief work is completed. However, the nurse has a unique opportunity to lay the foundation for adaptive grieving by encouraging the bereaved to share their

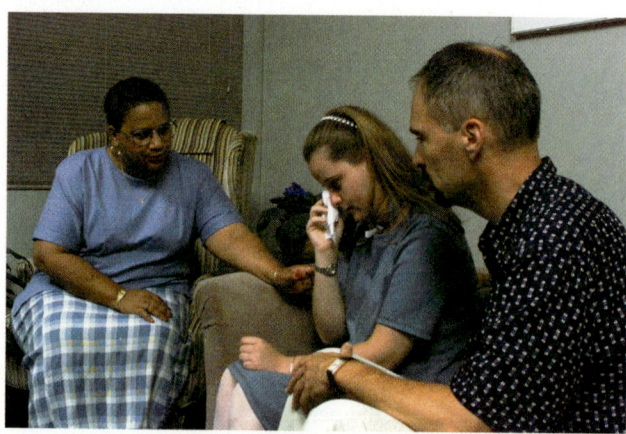

FIGURE 25-2 Note the nurse's nonverbal expression of support for this couple's grief over the loss of their child. What specific actions can the nurse implement to provide support? DELMAR/ CENGAGE LEARNING

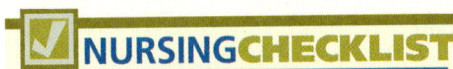

NURSINGCHECKLIST

CARING FOR GRIEVING CLIENTS

- Approach the client with a nonjudgmental attitude.
- Understand that each person's expression of grief is individualized.
- Encourage clients to express feelings at their own pace.
- Demonstrate compassion.
- Employ empathy, not sympathy.

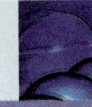

TABLE 25-10 Kübler-Ross's Stages of Dying and Death

STAGE	EXAMPLE
First stage: **Denial**	*Verbal:* "This can't be happening to me!"
	Behavioral: Client is diagnosed with terminal lung cancer; client continues to smoke two packs of cigarettes daily.
Second stage: **Anger**	*Verbal:* "Why me?"
	Behavioral: Client strikes out at caregivers.
Third stage: **Bargaining**	*Verbal:* Client prays, "Please, God, just let me live long enough to see my grandchild graduate."
	Behavioral: Client tries to "make deals" with caregivers.
Fourth stage: **Depression**	*Verbal:* "Go away. I just want to lie here in bed. What's the use?"
	Behavioral: Client withdraws and isolates self.
Fifth stage: **Acceptance**	*Verbal:* "I feel ready. At least, I'm more at peace now."
	Behavioral: Client gets financial or legal affairs in order. Client says good-bye to significant others.

Data from Kübler-Ross, E. (1969). *On death and dying.* New York: Macmillan.

feelings and continue to verbalize their experience with significant others. Goals mutually established with client and family are the foundation for evaluation.

DEATH

In today's social climate, death is viewed as something to be avoided at all costs; medicine, with its technological advances, pursues immortality. Death is considered to be an unusual occurrence by many Americans. "People in our country deny death, believing that medical science can cure any patient. Death is often seen as a failure of the health care system rather than a natural aspect of life" (American Association of Colleges of Nursing [AACN], 2008, p. 1). Scientific advances do not change the fact that death is a part of every human existence.

STAGES OF DEATH AND DYING

In her classic works, Elizabeth Kübler-Ross (1969, 1974) identified five possible stages of dying experienced by clients and their families (Table 25-10). Every person does not move sequentially through each stage. These stages are experienced in varying degrees and for varying lengths of time. The client may express anger and, a few minutes later, express acceptance of the inevitable, then express anger again. The value in Kübler-Ross's work is that it helps increase sensitivity to the needs of the dying client.

Denial

In the first stage of dying, the initial shock can be overwhelming. Denial, which is an immediate response to loss experienced by most people, is a useful tool for coping. It is an essential and protective mechanism that may last for only a few minutes or may manifest itself for months.

Anger

The initial stage of denial is followed by anger. The client's security is being threatened by the unknown. All the normal daily routines have become disrupted. The client has no control over the situation and thus becomes angry in response

to this powerlessness. The anger may be directed at himself or herself, God, and others. Often the nurse is the recipient of the anger when the client lashes out; see Figure 25-3 on page 488.

Bargaining

The anticipation of the loss through death brings about bargaining through which the client attempts to postpone or reverse the inevitable. The client promises to do something (e.g., be a better person, change lifestyle) in exchange for a longer life.

Depression

When the realization comes that the loss can no longer be delayed, the client moves to the stage of depression. This depression is different from dysfunctional depression in that it helps the client detach from life in order to be able to accept death.

Acceptance

The final stage of acceptance may not be reached by every dying client. Verbalization of emotions facilitates acceptance.

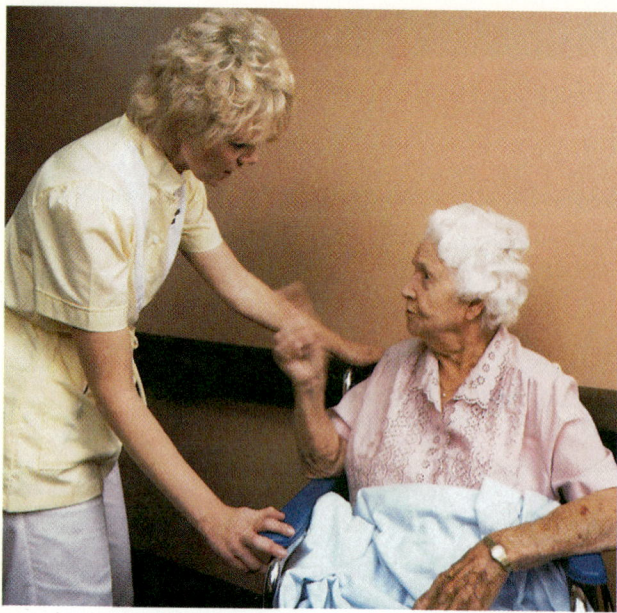

FIGURE 25-3 **Anger is a common response of grieving individuals. What is the nurse's priority action in the situation with this angry client?** DELMAR/CENGAGE LEARNING

With acceptance comes growing awareness of peace and contentment. The feeling that all that could be done has been done is often expressed during this stage. Reinforcement of the client's feelings and a sense of personal worth are important during this stage.

ETHICAL IMPLICATIONS

Death is associated with ethical dilemmas that occur almost daily in health care settings. Many health care agencies have ethics committees to develop and implement policies that deal with end-of-life issues. See Chapter 12 for a discussion of the ethical implications of euthanasia, assisted suicide, and refusal of treatment. One of the most difficult dilemmas is determining the difference between killing and allowing someone to die by withholding life-sustaining treatment methods.

The American Nurses Association (ANA) differentiates relieving pain and mercy killing (euthanasia or assisted suicide). Pain relief is a central value in nursing, whereas euthanasia is unethical. "Nurses, individually and collectively, have an obligation to provide comprehensive and compassionate end-of-life care, which includes the promotion of comfort and the relief of pain, and, at times, supporting the patient in foregoing life-sustaining treatments" (ANA, 1997).

ASSESSMENT

Nursing interventions are based on a thorough assessment of the client's holistic needs. Pertinent information to be determined when assessing a terminally ill client includes:

- Client's awareness of the terminal nature of illness
- Availability of support systems
- Physical condition
- Emotional status
- Presence of advance directives for health care decisions
- History of previous positive coping skills
- Unfinished business expressed by client or family

DIAGNOSIS

One NANDA-approved nursing diagnosis that is applicable for many dying clients is *Powerlessness,* that is, the "perception that one's own action will not significantly affect an outcome; a perceived lack of control over a current situation or immediate happening" (NANDA, 2009, p. 168). Another response that is often experienced by the dying is described by the diagnosis *Hopelessness,* a "subjective state in which an individual sees limited or no alternatives or personal choices available and is unable to mobilize energy on own behalf" (NANDA, 2009, p. 107). See Table 25-11, on page 489, for description of these two diagnoses.

OUTCOME IDENTIFICATION AND PLANNING

The dying client must be treated as a unique individual worthy of respect rather than as a diagnosis or a case to be cured. Essential elements to consider when planning care of the dying person include:

- Schedule time to be available to client.
- Offer to contact clergy.
- Balance the client's need for independence and need for assistance.
- Respect the client's confidentiality.
- Answer all questions and provide factual information to client and family.

Nursing care promotes the optimal quality of life, which means treating the client and family in a respectful manner and providing a safe environment for the expression of feelings. Sensitive nursing care recognizes and respects the cultural, ethnic, spiritual, and religious beliefs of clients and families. Planning focuses on meeting the holistic needs of the client and family.

IMPLEMENTATION

The nurse's first priority is to communicate a caring attitude to the client. Establishment of rapport facilitates the client's verbalization of feelings. The nurse establishes a safe environment in which the client does not feel chided or chastised for experiencing those feelings. Nonverbal communication can be used very effectively with dying individuals.

End-of-Life (EOL) Care

No one expects to die. It is something that happens to someone else and to someone else's loved ones. Dying was once considered to be a normal part of the life cycle, whereas today it is often considered to be a medical problem that

TABLE 25-11 Nursing Diagnoses for Powerlessness and Hopelessness

DIAGNOSIS	DEFINING CHARACTERISTICS	RELATED FACTORS
Powerlessness	**Major** • Expressions of dissatisfaction about inability to change the situation **Minor** • Reluctance or refusal to be involved in decision making • Anxiety • Apathy • Depression • Resignation	• Diagnosis of terminal illness • Chronic pain • Deficient knowledge • Lack of explanation from care providers • Social isolation • Being in a threatening situation
Hopelessness	**Major** • Expressions of overwhelming apathy in response to a situation in which there is no perceived solution (may say something like ''What's the use? I can't make things change.'') • Lack of energy • Expression of a feeling of incompetence • Passive, giving-up behavior • Decreased affect • Rigid thinking patterns **Minor** • Loss of appetite • Weight loss • Irritability • Muscular tension • Social withdrawal • Depression • Suicidal thoughts	• Diagnosis of terminal illness • Chronic pain • Deterioration of health status • Altered body image • Prolonged discomfort • Inability to care for self

Data from Carpenito, L. J. (2007). *Handbook of nursing diagnosis* (12th ed.). Philadelphia: Lippincott, Williams & Wilkins; North American Nursing Diagnosis Association International. (2009). *Nursing Diagnoses—Definitions and Classification* 2009–2011© 2009, 2007, 2005, 2003, 2001, 1998, 1996, 1994 NANDA International. Used by arrangement with Wiley-Blackwell Publishing, a company of John Wiley & Sons, Inc.

should be handled by health care providers. Technological advances in medicine have caused care of those who are dying to become depersonalized and mechanical.

In an attempt to humanize care of the dying, proponents of improved EOL care are looking to nurses. The highly technological health care environment calls for application of high-touch intervention with the dying. In other words, appropriate care of the dying is administered by compassionate nurses who are both technically competent and able to demonstrate caring. The United States is facing the realities of an aging population, recognition of the limits and inappropriate use of technological resources, and concerns about the capabilities of health care providers. Additionally, the increase in demand for assisted suicide and apprehensions of

the public about suffering and expenses associated with dying that may be prolonged unnecessarily by technology contribute to a renewed interest in humane EOL care (AACN, 2008).

Proficient nursing care during the final stage of life requires a unique knowledge base and skills. In 1999, the AACN developed a list of competencies necessary to provide quality EOL care. These competencies are revised as necessary by the AACN (2004); see the accompanying display, on page 490, on competencies necessary for nurses to provide quality EOL care. These competencies follow the position of the International Council of Nurses (1997) that nurses have the primary responsibility for a person's experiencing a peaceful death. See the Uncovering the Evidence display on page 490.

COMPETENCIES NECESSARY FOR NURSES TO PROVIDE HIGH-QUALITY CARE TO CLIENTS AND FAMILIES DURING THE TRANSITION TO THE END OF LIFE: AACN

1. Recognize changes (social, demographic, economic) necessitating improved end-of-life (EOL) care.
2. Promote provision of comfort care to the dying.
3. Communicate with client, family, and colleagues about EOL issues.
4. Recognize one's own attitudes, feelings, values, and expectations about death; acknowledge diversity (individual, cultural, and spiritual) in beliefs and customs.
5. Demonstrate respect for the client's view and wishes during EOL care.
6. Collaborate with interdisciplinary team members during EOL care.
7. Use scientifically based standardized tools to assess symptoms experienced by client at the end of life.
8. Use assessment data to plan and intervene using traditional and complementary approaches.
9. Evaluate the impact of traditional, complementary, and technological therapies on client-centered outcomes.
10. Assess and treat multiple dimensions (physical, psychological, social, and spiritual needs) to improve quality at the end of life.
11. Assist client, family, colleagues, and one's self in coping with suffering, grief, loss, and bereavement in EOL care.
12. Apply legal and ethical principles in the analysis of complex EOL issues.
13. Identify barriers and facilitators to clients' and caregivers' effective use of resources.
14. Demonstrate skill at implementing a plan for improved EOL care.
15. Apply knowledge gained from palliative care research to EOL education and care.

Adapted from American Association of Colleges of Nursing. (2004). *Peaceful death: Recommended competencies and curricular guidelines for end-of-life nursing care.* Retrieved January 2, 2009, from http://www.aacn.nche.edu.

UNCOVERING THE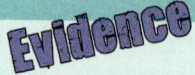

TITLE OF STUDY
"Practice of Expert Critical Care Nurses in Situations of Prognostic Conflict at the End of Life"

AUTHORS
C. M. Robichaux and A. P. Clark

PURPOSE
To (1) explore the practice of expert critical care nurses in end-of-life (EOL) conflicts and (2) describe actions taken when the nurses thought continued aggressive medical interventions were unwarranted.

METHODS
A qualitative design was used with analysis of interview data. Data were collected from interviews with 21 nurses who were nominated as experts by their coworkers.

FINDINGS
Three recurrent themes emerged from data analysis: (1) protecting or advocating for clients, (2) presenting a realistic picture (to clients and families), and (3) experiencing frustration and resignation.

IMPLICATIONS
The transition from curative to EOL care in the critical care setting is often accompanied by ambiguity and frustration. Expert nurses demonstrated the ability and willingness to actively protect and speak up for their clients even in situations in which the nurses' actions did not directly influence the outcomes.

Robichaux, C. M., & Clark, A. P. (2006). Practice of expert critical care nurses in situations of prognostic conflict at the end of life. *American Journal of Critical Care, 15*(5), 480–490.

and mobility. Table 25-12, on page 491, provides information on meeting the client's physiological needs.

Promoting Comfort

The primary activities directed at promoting physical comfort include pain relief, keeping the client clean and dry, and providing a safe, nonthreatening environment. The nurse who demonstrates a respectful, caring attitude promotes the client's psychological comfort by establishing rapport. Use of **palliative care** (a focus on alleviating symptoms rather than finding a cure) is rapidly increasing in the United States. Palliative care is not confined to EOL situations; it can be provided at any time during the course of illness and disability (Center to Advance Palliative Care, 2009). The goal of palliative care is to promote comfort in all dimensions—physiological, psychosocial, and spiritual.

Physiological Needs

According to Maslow's hierarchy of needs, physiological needs must be met prior to others because they are essential for existence. Areas that are often problematic for the terminally ill client are nutrition, respiration, elimination, comfort,

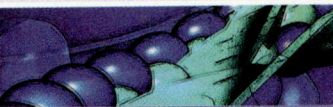

TABLE 25-12 Meeting the Physiological Needs of the Terminally Ill Client

AREA OF NEED	DISCUSSION	NURSING IMPLICATIONS
Nutrition	Presence of nausea and vomiting decreases appetite.	• Identify the cultural, social, and ethnic practices that influence eating patterns.
	Psychological factors (e.g., depression) may interfere with appetite.	• Use specific measures that promote food intake and retention, such as favorite foods, easy-to-swallow foods, and eating small amounts frequently.
	Some treatment modalities (e.g., chemotherapy, radiation) affect appetite and impair immune functioning.	• Give antiemetic drugs as needed. • Recommend that client avoid fried foods, alcoholic drinks, and gas-producing vegetables (corn, cauliflower, beans, broccoli). • Instruct client to avoid raw meat and raw eggs.
Energy	Weakness and exhaustion may occur as a result of metabolic demands.	• Schedule care activities to ensure uninterrupted times for rest.
	Fatigue and weakness may impair self-care abilities.	• Encourage client to conserve energy (do strenuous tasks for the client).
Hygiene	Diaphoresis and incontinence often occur in final stages of illness.	• Provide bed bath as necessary. • Perform oral care. • Change linens frequently to keep client dry (promotes skin integrity).

Delmar/Cengage Learning

Clients may experience many fears related to death. They may fear helplessness, dependence on others, loss of abilities, mutilation, or uncontrollable pain. The fear of a painful death is almost universal. Many, though certainly not all, dying clients experience pain. Comfort should be maximized by management of pain and other discomforting factors. The Nursing Checklist provides a list of interventions to promote comfort. See Chapter 35 for further discussion of pain management.

Hospice Care

Hospice, a type of care for the terminally ill, is founded on the concept of allowing individuals to die with dignity and be surrounded by those who love them. Hospice care is one of the fastest-growing segments of the health care industry. Clients enter hospice care when aggressive medical treatment is no longer an option or when the client refuses further aggressive medical treatment. Clients are usually referred to hospice when life expectancy is approximately 6 months or less (Hospice Foundation of America, 2008). Hospice, which provides an environment that emphasizes caring instead of curing, initiated the concept of palliative care.

Managing the care of a dying person requires many skills. Because of the complexity of care required by the

✔ NURSINGCHECKLIST

MEETING THE COMFORT NEEDS OF THE TERMINALLY ILL CLIENT

- Encourage client to verbalize presence of pain.
- Discuss pain relief options with client and family.
- Administer medication on a regular schedule instead of prn basis to ensure maximum pain relief.
- Assist client and family to identify the stressors that influence pain.
- Teach noninvasive pain relief measures:
  - Relaxation techniques such as deep breathing, imagery
  - Use of heat and cold
  - Massage
  - Topical ointments, such as soothing salves, deep-heating rubs, herbal-scented lotions
  - Aromatherapy

hospice client, an interdisciplinary team is essential for delivering quality, compassionate care. The interdisciplinary team consists of nurses, physicians, social workers, psychologists, clergy, ancillary personnel, and volunteers.

Home Care

A dying person is often not given the opportunity to be surrounded by family and friends. Many Americans die in hospitals or nursing homes. Home care is an alternative for the dying client, if the family members are physically and emotionally able to provide care. Hospices provide therapeutic interventions to bereaved family members. Ideally, health care providers should share the responsibility of home care of the dying with the family through respite time and frequent visits.

Psychosocial Needs

Death presents a threat not only to one's physical existence but also to psychological integrity. See Table 25-13 for a discussion of ways to meet the psychosocial needs of the dying client.

Spiritual Needs

In times of crisis, such as death, spirituality may be a source of comfort and support for the client and family. Spiritual and religious beliefs often determine the appropriate course of action. Nurses respect clients' reliance on spiritual support by listening and contacting clergy and spiritual guides if requested.

Nurses play a major role in promoting the dying client's spiritual comfort. Dying is a personal and, frequently, lonely

TABLE 25-13 Meeting the Psychosocial Needs of the Terminally Ill Client

PROBLEM	DISCUSSION	NURSING IMPLICATIONS
Anxiety	• A combination of factors contribute to anxiety of the dying client and family: —Client's fear of death (and loss of the known world) —Caregiver's fear of loss of the loved one —Client's sense of abandonment by the family, friends, and health care providers • Loss of independence and social isolation increase anxiety.	• Spend as much time as possible with the dying client. • Encourage verbalization of feelings. • Listen in nonjudgmental manner. • Answer all questions in an honest, factual manner. • Provide explanation of all procedures. • Encourage family and friends to spend time with client.
Decreased independence	• Independence is threatened by powerlessness. • Independence is promoted by having control over one's life.	• Seek client's opinion on treatment issues. • Involve client in developing plan of care. • Encourage continued interaction of client with family and friends. • Assist the client to develop goals that are realistic within the limitations of the illness (realistic hope). • Avoid always focusing only on limitations. • Allow client and family to ventilate feelings about not being able to change the course of events. • Help the client to identify those things over which he or she does have power.
Social interaction	• Loneliness is increased when others detach themselves in order to disengage from the dying person's pain. • Health care providers tend to avoid interacting with the dying. • Sensory deprivation (dimly lit rooms and out-of-the-way rooms) can increase feelings of abandonment.	• Encourage family to remain with the dying person. • Stay with the dying person as much as possible. • Provide support through your presence and active listening. • Be available to discuss the client's situation. • Use touch to communicate caring. • Provide meaningful sensory stimuli.

process. The nurse can serve as a sounding board for the client who expresses values and beliefs related to death. The following are therapeutic nursing interventions that address the spiritual needs of the dying:

- Communicating empathy
- Playing music
- Using touch
- Praying with the client
- Contacting the clergy if requested by the client
- Reading religious literature aloud at the client's request

Family Support

Family members need to be involved in the care of their dying loved one. Unrealistic guilt is increased by feelings of powerlessness; thus, it is important to involve family members in the caregiving. Families facing the impending death of a loved one require much support from nurses and other caregivers. The nurse's presence, just being there with the family, is extremely important.

Learning Needs of Client and Family

Bereaved families need much support and information; thus, the nurse must teach family members what they need to know. For instance, families must be assisted with acquiring the tools that will help them help their loved one. An example may be for the family to understand that the dying person needs to conserve energy. One simple action on the part of the family to assist with energy conservation would be to schedule activities after a rest period or early in the morning when the client is strongest. This is not an earth-shattering revelation, but simple interventions can be overlooked during this highly charged emotional time.

Client and family knowledge deficits can be related to:

- Insufficient information about physical condition
- Insufficient information about the treatment regimen
- Inability to anticipate medical crises
- Inexperience with personal threat of death
- Unfamiliarity with protocol to follow for emergency care when not in the hospital

The accompanying Client Teaching Checklist provides guidelines for educating families of dying people.

CARE AFTER DEATH

Caring for the deceased body and meeting the needs of the grieving family are nursing responsibilities. This section discusses care of the body and responding to the needs of families of the deceased.

CARE OF THE BODY

The body of the deceased needs to be treated in a way that respects the sanctity of the human body. Nursing care includes maintaining privacy and preventing damage to the body.

✓ CLIENT TEACHING CHECKLIST

GUIDELINES FOR TEACHING A FAMILY CAREGIVER

- Discuss the nature and extent of the disease process.
- Use adult education principles.
- Reinforce material frequently.
- Clearly explain the purpose of palliative care while maintaining a sense of realistic hope.
- Inform client and family of available community resources; reassure them that they are not alone.
- Teach steps for caregiver to follow if an emergency arises at home.
- Provide written instructions for caregiver to follow. These should include important telephone numbers and persons to be contacted.
- Inform about the purpose of hospice.

Physiological Changes

Several physiological changes occur after death. The body temperature decreases with a resultant lack of skin elasticity (**algor mortis**). Therefore, the nurse must use caution when removing tape from the body to avoid skin breakdown. Another physiological change, **liver mortis**, is the bluish purple discoloration that is a by-product of red blood cell destruction. This discoloration occurs in dependent areas of the body; therefore, the nurse should elevate the head to prevent discoloration from the pooling of blood. Approximately 2 to 4 hours after death, **rigor mortis** occurs; this is stiffening of the body caused by contraction of skeletal and smooth muscles. To prevent disfiguring effects of rigor mortis, as soon as possible after death the nurse should close the eyelids, insert dentures (if applicable), close the mouth, and position the body in a natural position.

In preparing the body for family viewing, the nurse seeks to make the body look comfortable and natural. This means removing all tubes and positioning the body as previously described. After the family has viewed the body, the nurse places identification tags on the body's toe and wrist. The body is then placed in a plastic or fabric shroud, and the shroud is tagged. Then the body is transported to the morgue according to the agency's policy. The nurse is also responsible for returning the deceased's possessions to the family. Jewelry, eyeglasses, clothing, and all other personal items are returned to the family.

LEGAL ASPECTS

In most states, the physician is legally responsible for determining the cause of death and signing the death certificate. The nurse may, in certain situations, be the person responsible for certifying the death. It is important for nurses to know their legal responsibilities, which are defined by their state or provincial board of nursing.

Autopsy

An **autopsy** (postmortem examination to determine the cause of death) is mandated in situations in which an unusual death has occurred. For example, an unexpected death and a violent death are circumstances that would necessitate an autopsy. As with all other aspects of postmortem care, the nurse must be sensitive to the family's cultural beliefs. For example, some religious groups (e.g., Judaism) prohibit autopsy. Other religious sects (e.g., Islam and Jehovah's Witness) allow autopsy only when legally mandated.

Organ Donation

The donation of organs for transplantation is a matter that requires compassion and sensitivity from the caregivers. It is essential that families of the deceased know the importance of and process for organ donation. There is an inadequate supply of organs and tissues to meet the demand for transplants. The following organs and tissues are used for transplantation:

- Kidneys
- Heart
- Lungs
- Liver
- Pancreas
- Skin
- Corneas
- Bones (long bones and middle ear bones)

At the time the family gives consent for donation, the nurse notifies the donor team that an organ is available for transplant. Time is of the essence because the organ or tissue must be harvested and transplanted quickly to maintain viability. Health care agencies are required to have policies

---

NURSING CARE PLAN

Terminally Ill Client with Lung Cancer

CASE PRESENTATION

Mr. Charles Jefferson is a 57-year-old man who is terminally ill with lung cancer. He has a wife, three adult children who are married, and two grandchildren. He was employed until 2 months ago, when radiation therapy, chemotherapy, and cancer (which has metastasized to his bones and other vital organs) rendered him too weak to pursue regular daily activities. He is a religious man who is considered by all to be the "heart" of his family. He has always been generous, and his friends are many. He is currently bedridden. His cognitive abilities and sense of humor remain intact. His current problems include pain, nausea, constipation, difficulty urinating, and dry skin. He has lost 60 pounds. He has not yet received his Social Security disability income or pension money. Tomorrow he is being discharged from the hospital; he states he is going home to die.

ASSESSMENT

- 60-pound weight loss
- Constipation
- Urinary difficulty
- Dry skin

NURSING DIAGNOSIS 1: *Imbalanced nutrition:* Less than body requirements
NOC: Mr. Jefferson will report adequate energy levels.
NIC: Provide a variety of high-calorie, nutritious foods from which to select.

EXPECTED OUTCOMES

1. Mr. Jefferson will identify factors that affect the consumption and retention of food and fluids.
2. Mr. Jefferson will maintain his current body weight.

INTERVENTIONS/RATIONALES

1. Ask client to state his food preferences. Including the client in problem solving increases the likelihood of compliance. Knowing the client's food preferences helps in planning a diet that is more likely to be appealing.

(Continues)

NURSING CARE PLAN (Continued)

2. Discuss findings about dietary preferences with the family. Providing information to family members is essential because they are the ones preparing meals at home.
3. Weigh the client at the same time of day while he is wearing similar clothing. Provides an accurate reflection of weight stability and fluctuations.

EVALUATION

Goal partially met. Mr. Jefferson stated his food likes and dislikes to the home health nurse. He has lost 2 more pounds because, he states, "I'm just not hungry anymore."

NURSING DIAGNOSIS 2: *Acute pain* related to metastasis of cancer
NOC: Mr. Jefferson will use analgesic and nonanalgesic relief measures appropriately.
NIC: Correct any misconceptions about narcotic or opioid analgesics, and teach the use of nonpharmacologic techniques.

EXPECTED OUTCOME

1. Mr. Jefferson will verbalize pain relief.

INTERVENTIONS/RATIONALES

1. Communicate your understanding of his pain. Validation of client's experience reduces anxiety.
2. Provide frequent opportunities to rest. Pain is exacerbated by fatigue.
3. Provide pain medication at a level that it is effective. For a terminally ill client, pain relief is the primary goal of care.
4. Teach the client and family noninvasive pain relief measures (massage, deep breathing, imagery). Knowledge of noninvasive methods helps the client and family feel in control. Such methods complement the effectiveness of medication in pain relief.

EVALUATION

Goal partially met. Mr. Jefferson reports being pain-free for up to 2 hours at a time.

related to the referral of potential donors to organ procurement agencies.

CARE OF THE FAMILY

At the time of death, the nurse provides invaluable support to the family of the deceased. Informing the family of the type and circumstances surrounding the death is extremely important. The nurse provides information about viewing the body, asks the family about donating organs, and offers to contact support people (e.g., other relatives, clergy). Sometimes, the nurse needs to help the family with decision making regarding a funeral home, transportation, and removal of the deceased's belongings. Demonstrating compassion is essential in providing information and support to families.

NURSE'S SELF-CARE

Working with dying clients can evoke both a personal and a professional threat in the nurse. Because many nurses are confronted with death and loss daily, grief is a common experience for nurses. Frequent exposure to death can interfere in the nurse's effectiveness because of subsequent anxiety and denial.

Whether working in a hospice, hospital, long-term care facility, or home, nurses are at particular risk for experiencing negative effects from caring for the dying. Often nurses do not want to confront their grief and will use some of the common defenses against grieving, such as keeping busy, taking care of others, being strong, and suffering in silence. Nurses need to stop pretending that they do not experience grief and subsequent suffering by talking about the intense emotions associated with caregiving.

To cope with their own grief, nurses need support, education, and assistance in coping with the death of clients. Staff education should focus on decreasing staff anxiety about working with grieving clients and families, how to seek support, and how to provide support to coworkers; see the accompanying Spotlight On display on page 496.

Often, the nurses' fears and doubts about death cause anxiety related to feelings about their own mortality. Even though such feelings are normal, caring for the dying client and the family can be emotionally draining. Therefore, nurses must remember to care for themselves.

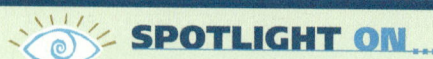

SPOTLIGHT ON...

Caring

Nurses and the Vulnerability of Grieving

Nurses need to feel as free to ask for help in dealing with feelings about a dying client as they would in asking for assistance in lifting and repositioning a client in bed. Asking for help means taking a risk to be vulnerable; some nurses fear appearing emotionally vulnerable or overwhelmed. How can nurses support each other in dealing with the grief of caring for dying people?

KEY CONCEPTS

- Loss is a universal response experienced by an individual when someone (or something) of value is no longer available.

- Grief is a psychological response to loss characterized by deep mental anguish and sorrow. Grieving people experience various stages of grief.

- The difference between normal and pathologic grief is the inability of the individual with pathologic grief to adapt to life without the loved one.

- There are five psychological stages involved in the dying process: denial, anger, bargaining, depression, and acceptance.

- Complicated grief is associated with traumatic death such as homicide or suicide.

- Hospice care offers terminally ill clients an alternative to hospitalization when aggressive medical treatment is no longer an option.

- After death, the nurse focuses on supporting the family and caring for the deceased body.

- Nurses must care for themselves in order to provide quality, compassionate care to the dying person.

REVIEW QUESTIONS

1. Which of the following nursing actions is therapeutic for dying clients?
   a. Apply nursing presence.
   b. Avoid the use of touch.
   c. Discuss only issues over which the client has control.
   d. Limit family visits in order to conserve client energy.

2. Which of the following postmortem activities by the nurse helps decrease the effects of rigor mortis?
   a. Close the body's eyelids and mouth.
   b. Lower the head of the bed.
   c. Place the body in high-Fowler's position.
   d. Remove tape carefully from skin.

3. A client who has just learned that she is terminally ill with breast cancer says, "Not me. This can't be happening to me!" Which stage of death and dying as described by Kübler-Ross is this client exhibiting?
   a. Anger
   b. Bargaining

   c. Denial
   d. Depression

4. A client is admitted to the hospital and is in the terminal stage of cancer. The nurse enters the client's room to administer some medicine and finds the client crying. Which of the following is the most therapeutic nursing action?
   a. Administer the client's medication and leave so the client can cry in private.
   b. Call the family to come to the hospital to stay with the client.
   c. Sit down and hold the client's hand.
   d. Tell the client that you will call the client's minister.

5. A terminally ill client has been referred to hospice care. Which of the following information should a nurse give this client and family?
   a. "Hospice uses minimal pain medication in order to improve the quality of life."

b. "Hospice will make you accept the impending death."

c. "The focus of hospice is to make you more comfortable."

d. "The major purpose of hospice is to support the family after their loss."

6. A recently widowed client describes how she is having difficulty sleeping. She states that last night she woke up because she heard the voice of her husband calling her name. Which nursing response is most therapeutic?

a. Inform the prescribing practitioner that the client needs a prescription for sleeping pills.

b. Reassure the client that these behaviors are a normal part of grieving.

c. Refer the client to a mental health clinic for immediate assessment.

d. Tell the client that she will feel better soon.

7. The nurse is providing postmortem care for a client. Which of the following interventions would be appropriate prior to allowing the family to visit?

a. Call the prescribing practitioner to verify the time of death before allowing the family to see the body.

b. Keep the sheet over the client's face until the family is comfortably seated in the room.

c. Prepare the body to look as clean and natural as possible.

d. Wear sterile gloves to pack the anal canal with gauze.

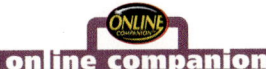

online companion

Visit the DeLaune and Ladner online companion resource at **www.delmar.cengage.com** for additional content and study aids. Click on Online Companions, then select the Nursing discipline.

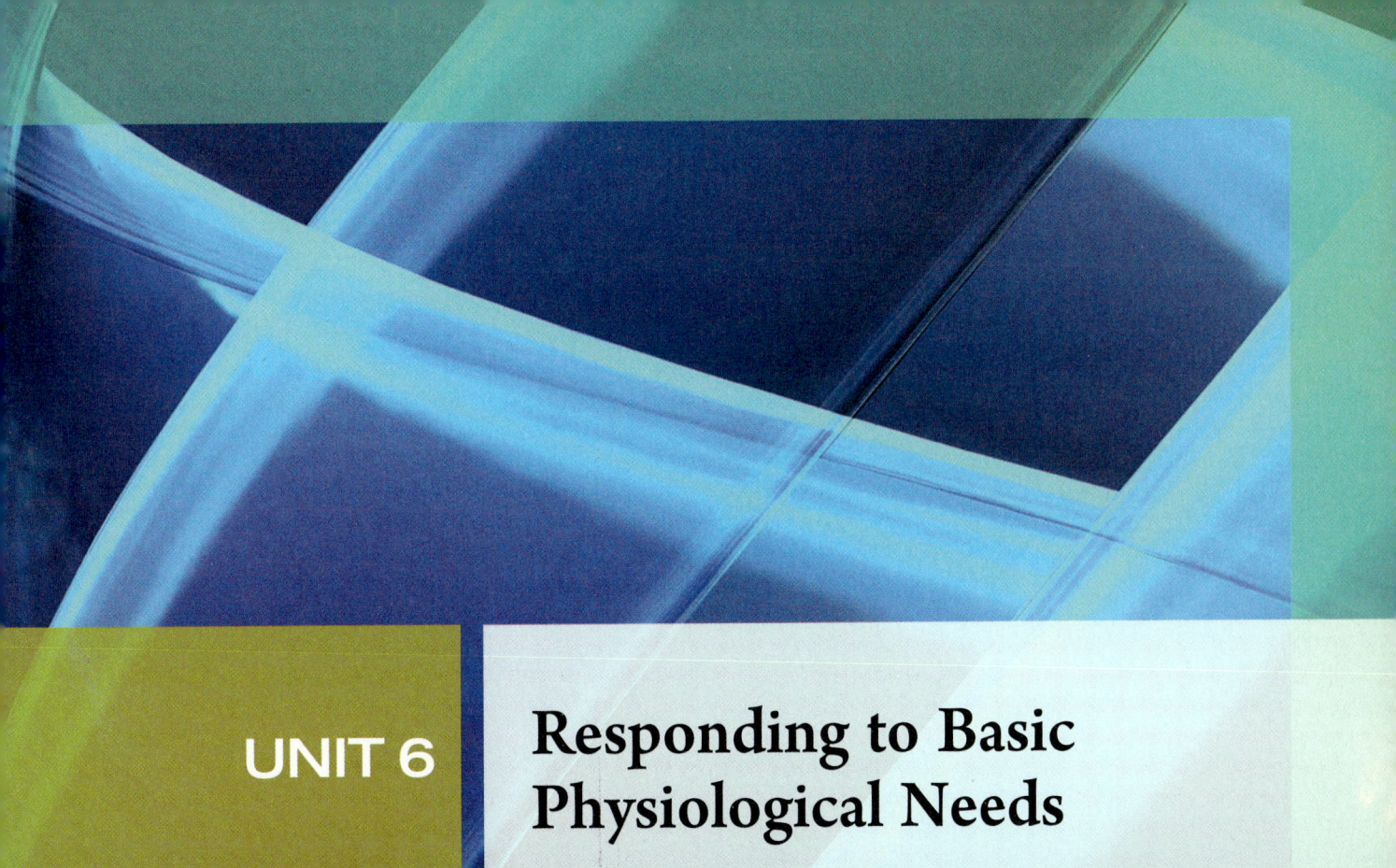

UNIT 6

Responding to Basic Physiological Needs

Nurses [need] to have technical skills and a strong knowledge base, [yet] it is especially important to be fully present with patients, and listen to the story they have to tell …

—Dossey (in Gray, 1995)

CHAPTER 26

Vital Signs

COMPETENCIES

1. Describe the physiological mechanisms governing temperature, pulse, respiration, and blood pressure.
2. Identify the normal age-related variations for vital sign measurements.
3. Select the appropriate equipment used to take vital signs and perform a physical examination.
4. Describe the correct positioning of the client for performing a physical examination.
5. Identify the sites for measuring vital signs.
6. Assess temperature, pulse, respiration, and blood pressure.

KEY TERMS

apnea monitor
atherosclerosis
auscultatory gap
basal metabolic rate (BMR)
baseline values
blood pressure
bradycardia
bradypnea
cachexia
cardiac output
conduction
convection
costal (thoracic) breathing
cyanosis
degrees
diaphragmatic (abdominal)
   breathing
diastole
dyspnea
dysrhythmia

eupnea
evaporation
expiration
external respiration
hemodynamic regulation
hypertension
hyperventilation
hypotension
hypoventilation
insensible heat loss
inspiration
internal respiration
neurogenic fever
orthostatic hypotension
osteoporosis
oximeter
piloerection
pleura
pulse
pulse deficit

pulse pressure
pulse quality
pulse rate
pulse rhythm
pulse volume
pyrexia
pyrogens
radiation
respiration
stroke volume
systole
tachycardia
tachypnea
thermoregulation
vasoconstriction
vasodilation
vital capacity
vital signs

Assessing and monitoring a client's clinical condition is the main reason nursing care is required. Nursing decisions are based on assessment data. One of the most frequent data collection interventions a nurse performs is taking **vital signs**, meaning the measurement of a client's temperature (T), pulse (P), respiration (R), and blood pressure (BP). These measurements indicate the physiological functioning of the circulatory, respiratory, neural, and endocrine systems. The data obtained from these measurements are used by the nurse, in conjunction with a client's physical assessment and health history, to determine a client's clinical care.

The body's physiological responses in terms of temperature, pulse, respiration, and blood pressure, how these responses are measured, and special nursing considerations, as appropriate, will be presented in this chapter. The latest research released by the National High Blood Pressure Education Program (*The Seventh Report of the Joint National Committee on Prevention, Detection, Evaluation, and Treatment of High Blood Pressure* [JNC 7]; National Institutes of Health [NIH], 2003) is presented in the section on hypertension. This report is referred to throughout the chapter as the JNC 7. The eighth report of the JNC is scheduled for release in 2009.

VITAL SIGNS

Vital signs are fundamental to assessment to establish baseline values of the client's cardiorespiratory integrity. **Baseline values** establish the norm against which subsequent measurements can

be compared. Variations from normal findings may indicate potential problems regarding the client's health status. Nurses should confirm "normal" measurements with clients because the perception of what is normal may vary among clients.

Vital signs are taken whenever the client is admitted to a health care facility or service, for example, home health care, clinic, or other ambulatory setting, and on a routine basis in the hospital. The frequency of vital sign measurements for the hospitalized client is determined by the client's health status, the prescribing practitioner's orders, and the established standards of care for the particular clinical setting or service. Whenever a change is suspected in the client's status, the nurse should measure the vital signs, regardless of the setting.

The sequence for recording vital signs measurement in the nurses' notes is T-P-R and BP. Agencies usually have special graphic forms to record vital signs findings. These forms facilitate data comparison at a glance because the data are plotted on a graph.

PHYSIOLOGICAL FUNCTION

Healthy people have the ability to meet their own needs; however, during illness, people need assistance (in proportion to the degree of dysfunction) in meeting their basic needs. The assessment of physiological functioning provides specific data regarding the client's current condition. Data analysis allows the nurse to plan nursing care that is responsive to the preventive and restorative needs of the client. See Chapters 5 through 10 for a complete discussion of the steps of the nursing process.

Thermoregulation

Thermoregulation is the body's physiological function of heat regulation to maintain a constant internal body temperature. The heat of the body is measured in units called **degrees**. The "core" internal temperature of 98.6° Fahrenheit (F) (37° centigrade [C]) does not vary more than 1.4°F (0.77°C) and is higher than the skin and external temperatures. In contrast, the skin temperature rises and falls in accordance with changes in environmental temperature.

HEAT PRODUCTION Heat is produced in the body's cells through food metabolism that results in the release of energy. The body converts energy supplied by metabolized nutrients to energy forms that can be used directly by the body. One form of this energy is thermal energy for regulation of body temperature. Energy is measured in terms of heat. A kilocalorie is an energy value (heat measure) of a given food; 1 kilocalorie equals 1,000 calories (the amount of heat required to raise the temperature of 1 kilogram of water 1°C). This type of heat liberation is usually expressed as the metabolic rate and measured as the **basal metabolic rate**, or **BMR** (the rate of energy use in the body needed to maintain essential activities). See Chapter 34 for a complete discussion of calories, kilocalories, and metabolic rate.

Factors that affect the metabolic rate of heat liberation, such as age and exercise, are discussed later in this chapter. The thyroid hormones thyroxine and triiodothyronine increase basal metabolism by breaking down glucose and fat. Muscular activity also produces heat from the breakdown of carbohydrates and fats and through shivering.

Body temperature is controlled by balancing metabolic heat production with heat loss. Most heat production comes from the deep tissue organs (brain, liver, and heart) and the skeletal muscles. The skin, subcutaneous tissues, and fat of the subcutaneous tissues serve as heat insulators for the body. Sweat glands in the dermis are innervated by sympathetic nerves of the autonomic nervous system and are controlled by the anterior hypothalamus to regulate sweating.

When body heat rises, the hypothalamus transmits impulses to reduce body heat by triggering perspiration, **vasodilation** (the widening of blood vessels), and the inhibition of heat production. The opposite physiological functioning occurs in response to a decrease in body heat. In this situation the hypothalamus transmits impulses to stimulate heat production through **vasoconstriction** (the narrowing of blood vessels), muscle shivering, and **piloerection** (hairs standing on end).

HEAT LOSS Most body heat is lost from the skin's surface to the environment by the processes of radiation, conduction, convection, and evaporation (see Table 26-1 on page 504). **Insensible heat loss** is the heat that is lost through the continuous, unnoticed water loss that occurs with vaporization, accounting for 10% of basal heat production. Evaporation accounts for the greatest heat loss when body heat increases.

BEHAVIORAL CONTROL OF BODY TEMPERATURE In addition to the heat production and heat loss mechanisms described earlier, the body has another potent mechanism for temperature control, known as behavioral control. In response to the body's signaling conditions of being either overheated or too cold, the person makes appropriate environmental adjustments to reestablish comfort. Guyton and Hall (2007) recognize this mechanism as the most effective one for body heat control in severely cold environments.

Respiration

Respiration is the act of breathing. Respiration is defined by physiological functioning as:

- **External respiration**—the exchange of oxygen and carbon dioxide between the alveoli of the lungs and the pulmonary blood system
- **Internal respiration**—the interchange of oxygen and carbon dioxide between the circulating blood and cells throughout the body
- **Inspiration** (inhalation)—the intake of air into the lungs
- **Expiration** (exhalation)—the movement of gases from the lungs to the atmosphere
- **Vital capacity**—the amount of air exhaled from the lungs after a minimal full inspiration

These five major physiological pulmonary functions provide oxygen to the tissues and remove carbon dioxide:

1. Ventilation—the inflow and outflow of air between the atmosphere and the lung alveoli
2. Circulation—the quantity of blood flowing through the lungs is approximately 4 to 6 L/min
3. Diffusion—the exchange of oxygen and carbon dioxide between the alveoli and the blood
4. Transport—the carrying of oxygen and carbon dioxide in the blood and body fluids to and from the cells
5. Regulation—the neurogenic system that adjusts the rate of alveolar ventilation to meet the demands of the body. The arterial blood oxygen pressure (P_{O_2}) and arterial blood carbon dioxide pressure (P_{CO_2}) may be altered during times of strenuous exercise and other types of respiratory stress. See Chapter 32 for a complete discussion about oxygenation.

The mechanics of pulmonary ventilation depend on abdominal recti and internal intercostal muscles that cause lung expansion and contraction. Normal breathing is accomplished by:

1. The downward and upward movement of the diaphragm to lengthen or shorten the chest cavity
2. The elevation and depression of the ribs to increase and decrease the anteroposterior diameter of the chest cavity

Children and men normally breathe with their diaphragm muscles; adult women generally breathe with their upper chest muscles.

Hemodynamic Regulation

Hemodynamic regulation is the physiological function of blood circulating to maintain an appropriate environment in

TABLE 26-1 Methods of Heat Loss

METHOD	CHARACTERISTICS	EXAMPLE
Radiation: Loss of heat in the form of infrared rays	All objects that are not at absolute zero radiate heat rays from the surface of one object to the surface of another object that is not in physical contact with the first object.	If the temperature of the body is greater than the surroundings, heat is lost from the body to the environment. A nude person in a room with normal temperature will lose about 60% of total loss by radiation.
Conduction: Loss of heat to an object in contact with the body	Heat is lost to other objects that are cooler than the skin. As much as 15% of the body's total heat loss is transferred to the air. Once the temperature of the air adjacent to the skin equals the skin temperature, there is no further loss of body heat.	Bathing a client in cool or tepid water will lower the client's temperature.
Convection: Movement of heat away from the body's surface	Convection accompanies conduction when the warmed air or water is replaced with cooler elements.	The use of fans enhances convected heat loss by air. Water adjacent to the skin can absorb far greater quantities of heat than can air. Clothing entraps air next to the skin, decreasing heat loss from the body by conduction and convection.
Evaporation: Continuous insensible water loss from the skin and lungs when water is converted from a liquid to a gas	It takes approximately 0.58 calories of heat for a gram of water to evaporate.	Insensible water loss is continuous. Insensible loss occurs regardless of body temperature; thus, it is not a major regulator of temperature.

Delmar/Cengage Learning

tissue fluids. Circulation transports nutrients to the tissues, removes waste products, and carries hormones from one part of the body to another. When the body's circulatory needs change, the heart rate either accelerates or decelerates. This is a compensatory mechanism under the control of the cardiac centers that are located in the medulla of the brain stem. The sensory receptors in the tissues transmit impulses to the cardiac centers, which in turn trigger a change in the heart rate through the sympathetic and parasympathetic nervous systems that innervate the heart. When the physiological needs of the tissues are met, the heart rate returns to normal.

Systemic circulation supplies blood to all the tissues of the body except the lungs (which is accomplished through pulmonary circulation). Approximately 84% of the entire blood volume is in the systemic circulation, with the heart containing 7% and the pulmonary vessels containing 9%. The circulatory system is composed of:

- Arteries—large vessels that transport systemic blood under high pressure to the tissues
- Arterioles—the smallest branches of the arterial system that act as control valves to release blood into the capillaries
- Capillaries—thin-walled vessels permeable to small molecular substances that exchange fluids, nutrients, electrolytes,

hormones, and other substances between the blood and interstitial fluid
- Venules—vessels that collect blood from the capillaries and gradually coalesce into progressively larger veins
- Veins—vessels that transport systemic blood from the tissues back to the heart and serve as a reservoir for extra blood

The normal physiological function of the cells requires continuous blood flow and appropriate volume and distribution of blood to the cells that need nutrients. This is accomplished through the heart's contraction and ejection of blood into the aorta and the distensibility of the arterial system. The combination of arterial distensibility and resistance reduces the pressure pulsations, allowing continuous blood flow to the tissues. The dynamics of distensibility and resistance maintain a constant blood flow; otherwise, blood would flow to the tissues only during **systole** (phase in which the ventricles contract to eject blood) with an absence of blood flow during **diastole** (phase in which ventricles are relaxed and no blood is being ejected).

The cardiac cycle has two phases: systole and diastole. At the onset of systole there is an increase in ventricular pressure that causes the mitral and tricuspid valves to close. The closing of these valves produces the first heart sound (S_1).

Ventricular pressure continues to increase until it exceeds the pressure in the pulmonary artery and the aorta, causing the aortic and pulmonic valves to open and allowing the ventricles to eject blood into these arteries. Ventricular emptying and relaxation cause a decrease in ventricular pressure and closure of the aortic and pulmonic valves. Closure of these valves produces the second heart sound (S_2). During diastole the pressure in the ventricles is less than that in the atria, causing the mitral and tricuspid valves to open and allowing blood to flow from the atria into the ventricles until the end of diastole, when the atria contract to send the rest of the blood into the ventricles. Ventricular filling causes an increase in pressure that closes the mitral and tricuspid valves (the beginning of systole) and starts another cardiac cycle.

Stroke volume is the measurement of blood that enters the aorta with each ventricular contraction. With each ventricular contraction, the heart ejects 60 to 70 mL of blood into the aorta. **Cardiac output** is the volume of blood pumped by the heart in 1 minute and is measured by multiplying the heart rate by the ventricle's stroke volume. For example, a client with a heart rate of 80 beats per minute times a stroke volume of 60 mL of blood would have a cardiac output of 4,800 mL. **Pulse pressure** is a measurement of the ratio of stroke volume to compliance (total distensibility) of the arterial system.

PULSE   The **pulse** is the bounding of blood flow in an artery that is palpable at various points on the body. The pulse is caused by the stroke volume ejection and distension of the walls of the aorta, which creates a pulse wave as it travels rapidly toward the distal ends of the arteries. As the pulse wave reaches a superficial peripheral artery and travels over an underlying bone or muscle, the pulse can be palpated by applying gentle pressure over a pulse point (a specific area where the peripheral pulses can be palpated). Figure 26-1 shows the location of pulse points throughout the body.

BLOOD PRESSURE   Both the blood pressure and pulse are measurements that determine the volume of ejected blood into the arterial system with each ventricular contraction. **Blood pressure** is the measurement of pressure pulsations exerted against the blood vessel walls during systole and diastole. It is measured in terms of millimeters of mercury (mm Hg). In a healthy young adult, the pressure at the height of each pulse (the systolic pressure) is less than 120 mm Hg, and the pressure at the lowest point of each pulse (diastolic pressure) is less than 80 mm Hg. The pulse pressure is the difference between these pressures, which is 40 mm Hg. If 1 mm Hg caused a vessel originally containing 10 mL of blood to increase its volume by 1 mL, the distensibility would be 0.1/mm Hg, or 10%/mm Hg (Guyton & Hall, 2007).

The body has four hemodynamic regulators for blood pressure control:

1. Blood volume—the volume of blood in the circulatory system. Blood pressure is proportional to the blood volume. Hemorrhage causes a loss in blood volume that, in turn, lowers the blood pressure. Rapid infusion

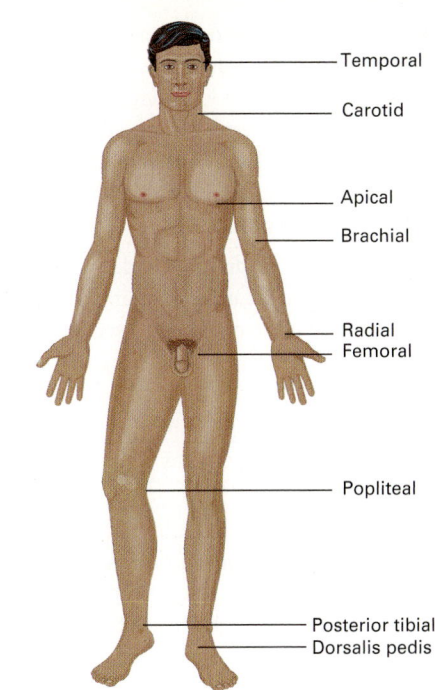

FIGURE 26-1 Pulse Points DELMAR/CENGAGE LEARNING

of intravenous fluids causes an increase in volume and a subsequent rise in pressure.
2. Cardiac output—the major factor that influences systolic pressure.
3. Peripheral vascular resistance—the size and distensibility of the arteries, which is the most important determinant of diastolic pressure. Arterial resistance (decreased distensibility) is encountered when the left ventricle pumps blood from the heart under pressure during the systolic phase. The arteries contain smooth muscles that allow them to contract, which decreases their compliance (tone) and causes resistance. The varying degrees of tone allow some of the arterioles to remain constricted while others dilate to protect the body's circulatory system from accommodating a greater blood capacity than the actual blood volume. If all of the arterioles were to dilate at one time, there would not be enough blood to fill them.
4. Viscosity—the thickness of the blood based on the ratio of proteins and cells to the liquid portion of blood. The greater the viscosity, the harder the heart must work to pump blood, with a resultant increase in blood pressure.

These regulators work in unison to create a constant blood pressure. For instance, when the blood volume decreases, the body compensates with an increased heart rate and vasoconstriction that increases peripheral resistance to maintain normal pressure and functions of the vital organs.

Blood pressure is a result of the cardiac output and peripheral vascular resistance. Normal arteries expand during systole and contract during diastole, creating two distinct pressure phases:

• Systolic blood pressure is a measurement of the maximal pressure exerted against arterial walls during systole (when myocardial fibers contract and tighten to eject blood from the ventricles), primarily a reflection of cardiac output.

- Diastolic blood pressure is a measurement of pressure remaining in the arterial system during diastole (period of relaxation that reflects the pressure remaining in the blood vessels after the heart has pumped), primarily a reflection of peripheral vascular resistance.

Serial blood pressure readings provide significant clinical data relative to the client's cardiovascular and fluid volume status. See Chapter 33 for a complete discussion of maintenance of fluid volume.

FACTORS INFLUENCING VITAL SIGNS

Several factors can cause changes in one or more of the vital signs: age, gender, heredity, race, lifestyle, environment, medications, pain, and other factors such as exercise and metabolism, anxiety and stress, postural changes, diurnal variations, and hormones.

AGE

The normal values and variations in vital sign measurement are usually based on age. Tables 26-2, 26-3, and 26-4 present age-related changes in temperature, pulse, and respiration. In newborns, thermoregulation and the respiratory center are immature. The newborn's temperature fluctuates with the environment. Clothing must be adequate to maintain body heat. For example, the newborn's head should be covered because up to 30% of body heat can be lost through the head. The newborn's respiratory rate is from 30 to 50 breaths per minute, with a slightly irregular rhythm. Temperature regulation becomes stable when children reach puberty.

TABLE 26-3 **Normal Age-Related Variations in Resting Pulse**

AGE	NORMAL RANGE	AVERAGE RATE/MINUTE
Newborn	100–170	140
1 year	80–170	120
3 years	80–130	110
6 years	75–120	100
10 years	70–110	90
14 years	60–110	90
Adult	60–100	80

Delmar/Cengage Learning

TABLE 26-4 **Normal Age-Related Variations in Resting Respiration**

AGE	NORMAL RANGE	AVERAGE RATE/MINUTE
Newborn	30–50	40
1 year	20–40	30
3 years	20–30	25
6 years	16–22	19
14 years	14–20	17
Adult	12–20	18

Delmar/Cengage Learning

In the elderly, the efficiency of thermoregulation is reduced by the physiological changes of aging, including loss of subcutaneous fat, decreased sweat gland activity, reduced metabolism, and poor vasomotor control. Financial status and environmental conditions experienced by the elderly may also affect diet, activity, and ability to control the external temperature.

The normal aging process causes changes in the elderly person's respiratory functions. Major physiological alterations include:

- Ventilation—Bony changes in the thorax and vertebrae and the decline in respiratory and abdominal musculature reduce the ability of the lungs to distend.
- Circulation and diffusion—The increase in dead air space in the respiratory tree decreases the quantity of blood flowing through the lungs and gaseous exchange.
- Transport—**Atherosclerosis** (plaques in the inner walls of arteries) and **dysrhythmia** (irregular heartbeat) reduce the amount of blood flow available to tissues.

TABLE 26-2 **Normal Age-Related Variations in Body Temperature**

AGE		NORMAL RANGE CELSIUS	FAHRENHEIT
Newborn	Axillary	35.5–39.5°C	96.0–99.5°F
1 year	Oral	37.7°C	99.7°F
3 years	Oral	37.2°C	99.0°F
5 years	Oral	37.0°C	98.6°F
Adult	Oral	37.0°C	98.6°F
	Axillary	36.4°C	97.6°F
	Rectal	37.6°C	99.6°F
70+ years	Oral	36.0°C	96.8°F

Delmar/Cengage Learning

- Regulation—The inability of lung function to perform maximal breathing for extended periods of time reduces the rate of alveolar ventilation to meet the demands of the body.

See Chapter 19 for a complete discussion of the physiological changes that occur in the older client.

Blood pressure varies throughout life (see Table 26-5). From early childhood throughout adolescence, the blood pressure varies according to body size. An adult's blood pressure continues to increase with age. The JNC 7 (NIH, 2003) states that men over age 45 and women over age 55 are at higher risk for developing high blood pressure (hypertension). In some women, blood pressure can increase if they use birth control pills, become pregnant, or take hormone therapy during menopause.

GENDER

Women usually experience greater temperature fluctuations than men because of hormonal changes. Temperature variations occur during the menstrual cycle mainly in response to the progesterone level. As the progesterone level increases during ovulation, temperature gradually rises. During menopause, the instability of the vasomotor controls may cause periods (30 seconds to 5 minutes) of intense body heat and sweating. Males in general have higher blood pressure than do females of the same age.

HEREDITY

Although many studies have been conducted to relate hereditary factors to specific cardiovascular disease occurrence, the results are often inconclusive regarding the influence of hereditary versus environmental factors. For example, studies have been conducted to relate elevated blood cholesterol levels to a single gene. Giger and Davidhizar (2008) describe studies of Jews and non-Jews and compare Ashkenazi Jews with Oriental Jews based on the theory that elevated blood cholesterol levels may be caused by a single gene. These studies indicate a higher occurrence of elevated blood cholesterol levels among Jews than among non-Jews and that Ashkenazi Jews may have a higher frequency of the gene than Oriental Jews. The conclusion of this research indicates a need for further studies to be done to determine the frequency of heart disease among Jews as well as the interplay between heredity and environment (Giger & Davidhizar, 2008). Genetic and environmental factors also are believed to be contributing factors to hypertension in African Americans. A family history of hypertension increases one's chances of developing hypertension (NIH, 2003).

RACE

Some ethnic groups are more susceptible than others to hemodynamic alterations. African Americans have a higher prevalence and greater severity of hypertension than do other minorities and whites. Hypertension-related deaths are higher in this population.

LIFESTYLE

Lifestyle factors, such as cigarette smoking, cause chronic changes in the lungs as manifested by impaired ventilation. Stimulants such as caffeinated beverages and tobacco elevate the heart rate. Eating too much salt and not enough potassium and consuming alcohol also can raise blood pressure (NIH, 2003). The effects of exercise and stress are discussed later.

ENVIRONMENT

Environmental factors such as temperature and noise level can alter the heart rate. Acid rain and industrialized areas are often associated with a high occurrence of respiratory conditions, such as infections and chronic lung diseases.

Primary prevention is a major role of occupational (industrial) health nurses. A health screening examination relies heavily on vital sign measurements and physical examination findings. The occupational health nurse should perform health screening examinations that focus on the short-term results of certain environmental conditions (diseases) and monitor for the development of chronic trends; see the accompanying Respecting Our Differences display, on page 508, on health screening criteria.

MEDICATIONS

Some medications can directly or indirectly alter the pulse, respiration, or blood pressure. Digitalis preparations (cardiac glycosides) decrease the pulse rate. Narcotic analgesics (pain medications) can depress the rate and depth of respirations and lower the blood pressure.

Always ask clients what medications they are currently taking, and be aware of the side effects of any medications administered. Certain drugs may either increase or decrease pulse rate and blood pressure. If the drug alters the client's pulse, respiration, or blood pressure, provide appropriate

TABLE 26-5	Normal Age-Related Variations in Blood Pressure
AGE	**BLOOD PRESSURE (MM HG)**
Newborn	Up to 70/45
5 years	Up to 115/75*
6 to 12 years	Up to 125/80*
13 to 15 years	Up to 126/78*
16 to 18 years	Up to 132/82*
Over 18 years	<120/80

*These blood pressure measurements are general guidelines and may not be accurate if a child is particularly tall or short for his or her age. < means "less than."

The Heart Center Online. Retrieved September 8, 2008, from http://www.heartcenteronline.com.

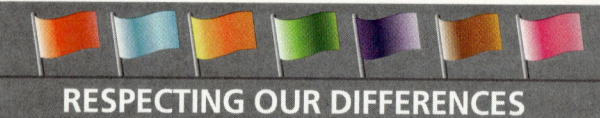

RESPECTING OUR DIFFERENCES

The performance of a health screening examination is justified when the disease being screened for has:

- A significant effect on the longevity or the quality of life
- A sufficiently high prevalence rate to justify the cost of the screening program
- Been shown to have better therapeutic results if detected in the early stage and worse results with delayed detection and treatment
- A significant asymptomatic period allowing an opportunity for detection and treatment that will reduce the rate of morbidity and mortality
- An acceptable method of treatment

Data from Edelman, C. L., & Mandle, C. L. (2006). *Health promotion throughout the life span* (6th ed., p. 231). St. Louis, MO: Elsevier Health Sciences.

client teaching so that the client is able to compensate for the variations in these functions.

PAIN

Each person reacts to pain in varying degrees. With acute pain, sympathetic stimulation increases the heart rate, which increases the cardiac output and vasoconstriction, causing increased peripheral vascular resistance. These changes result in increased pulse and respiratory rates, depth of respirations, and blood pressure. Chronic pain causes parasympathetic stimulation and decreases the pulse rate. See Chapter 35 for a complete discussion about pain and measures to promote comfort.

OTHER FACTORS

Table 26-6 discusses the effects of exercise and metabolism, anxiety and stress, postural changes, and diurnal (daily) variations (also called circadian) on vital sign measurements. Routine exercise increases metabolism and heat production and strengthens the cardiac muscles. The normal, untrained person can increase cardiac output fourfold with exercise, and the trained athlete can increase cardiac output about sixfold (Guyton & Hall, 2007).

Anxiety and stress stimulate the sympathetic nervous system to:

- Increase the production of epinephrine and norepinephrine, with a resultant increase in metabolic activity and heat production
- Increase the heart rate, which, in turn, increases the cardiac output and causes vasoconstriction with a subsequent increase in peripheral vascular resistance

Sympathetic stimulation causes an increase in the pulse rate and blood pressure. See Chapter 23 for a complete discussion about stress, anxiety, adaptation, and change.

TABLE 26-6 Factors Influencing Vital Signs

FACTOR	TEMPERATURE	PULSE	RESPIRATION	BLOOD PRESSURE
Exercise and metabolism	Increases	Short-term: increases • Long-term: lowers the resting rate and return time to the resting rate postexercise	Rate and depth increase	Increases
Anxiety and stress	Increases	Increases	Increases	Increases
Postural changes	No change	Increases with sitting or standing; decreases when lying down	Decreases with stooped or slumped positions due to decreased chest expansion	Decreases with sitting or standing
Diurnal variations (circadian rhythm)	Lowest level: 0400–0600 h Highest level: 2000–2400 h	Decreases during sleep	None	Lowest level: early morning Highest level: late afternoon or early evening

Postural changes occur in response to stimulation of the baroreceptors (spray-type nerve endings of the autonomic nervous system) that are located in the walls of the arteries. The baroreceptor reflex is the primary mechanism for maintaining a relatively constant arterial pressure. When a person stands up after lying down, the arterial pressure in the head and upper part of the body immediately tends to fall. This falling pressure elicits an immediate baroreceptor reflex, resulting in strong sympathetic discharges throughout the body. This response minimizes the decrease in pressure in the head and upper body (Guyton & Hall, 2007). The person's blood pressure decreases when going from a lying to a sitting or standing position. However, the pulse is lower in a lying position and increases in a sitting or standing position.

Each person has a different temperature pattern, with a normal variance ranging from 0.5°C to 1°C (0.9°F–1.8°F) for a 24-hour period. Table 26-6 identifies when the lowest temperature and pulse variances occur.

The skin temperature rises and falls with a change in environmental temperature. Infants and older adults are most susceptible to environmental changes because their temperature-regulating mechanisms are less effective. Warm environments decrease conduction and increase body temperature, which, in turn, increases the metabolic rate, resulting in an increased pulse rate. Improper clothing in cold climates may lead to a decrease in body temperature through radiation and conductive heat loss that results in shivering to raise body temperature.

Other factors can contribute to vital signs being above or below the established normal limits. A review of the client's health history data will reveal pertinent information regarding the factors that influence vital signs.

MEASURING VITAL SIGNS

Measuring a client's vital signs is a routine yet important nursing function that all nurses must master and execute skillfully.

EQUIPMENT

The measurement of the client's vital signs requires the appropriate instruments. All pieces of equipment should be maintained to function accurately. Table 26-7 on page 510, describes the common types of equipment used to assess vital signs.

Equipment should be gathered before entering the client's room. However, certain pieces of equipment, such as the sphygmomanometer, may be permanently installed in the examination and inpatient rooms. The nurse should observe what equipment is in the client's room during the first visit. The necessary equipment for clients who are maintained on isolation precautions should be kept inside the room because items should not be taken in and out of isolation rooms.

MEASUREMENT OF HEIGHT AND WEIGHT

Measuring height and weight is as important as assessing the client's vital signs. Routine measurement provides data related to growth and development in infants and children and signals the possible onset of alterations that may indicate illness in all age groups. The client's height and weight are routinely taken upon admission to acute care facilities and during visits to prescribing practitioners' offices, clinics, and other health care settings.

Height

Measurement of height is expressed in inches (in.), feet (ft), centimeters (cm), or meters (m). See the accompanying display on conversion equivalents for height measurements from one system to another.

A scale for measuring height, calibrated in either inches or centimeters, is usually attached to a standing weight scale. This type of scale is used for measuring the height of children and adults. The nurse should ask the client to stand erect on the scale's platform. The metal rod attached to the back of the scale should be extended to gently rest on top of the client's head, and the measurement should be read at eye level.

When measuring an infant's length, the nurse should place the infant on a firm surface. Extend the knees, with the feet at right angles to the table. Measure the distance from the vertex (top) of the head to the soles of the feet with a measuring tape. The procedure usually requires two nurses, one to hold the infant still and the other to measure the length. If the nurse needs to perform the measurement without assistance, an object should be placed at the infant's head, the infant's knees should be extended, and a second object should be placed at the infant's feet. Lift the infant and measure the distance between the two objects.

Height increases gradually from birth to the prepubertal growth spurt. Girls usually reach their adult height between the ages of 16 and 17 years, whereas boys usually continue to grow until the ages of 18 to 20 years. The older adult usually decreases in height as a result of a gradual loss of muscle mass and changes in the vertebrae that occur in conditions such as **osteoporosis** (a process in which reabsorption exceeds accretion of bone).

Weight

Measurement of weight is expressed in ounces (oz), pounds (lb), grams (g), or kilograms (kg); see the accompanying display, on page 512, on conversion equivalents. Weight

---

CONVERSION EQUIVALENTS FOR HEIGHT MEASUREMENT

1 in. = 2.5 cm   1 cm = 0.4 in.
1 ft = 30.5 cm or 0.3 m   1 m = 39.4 in. or 3.28 ft

TABLE 26-7 Equipment Used for Vital Signs Measurement

INSTRUMENT		DESCRIPTION
Thermometer		
Electronic	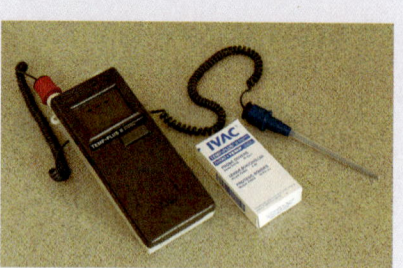	Battery-powered display unit with a sensitive probe (blue for oral and red for rectal) covered with a disposable plastic sheath for individual use.
Disposable (chemical), single-use	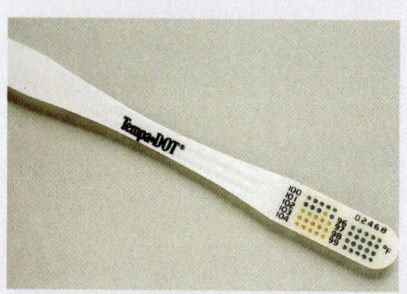	Thin strips of plastic with chemically impregnated dots that change color to reflect temperature.
Tympanic	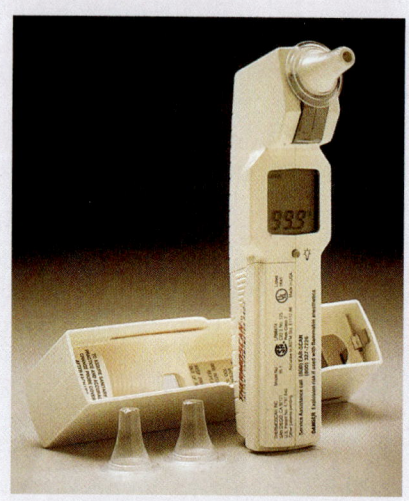	Battery-powered display unit with disposable speculums and infrared-sensing electronics. (Photograph courtesy of The Gillette Company)
Stethoscope		
Acoustic	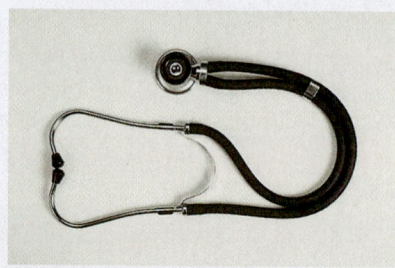	Closed cylinder that prevents dissipation of sound waves and amplifies the sound through a diaphragm. Flat-disc diaphragm transmits high-pitched sounds, and the bell-shaped diaphragm transmits low-pitched sounds.

(continues)

TABLE 26-7 (Continued)

INSTRUMENT		DESCRIPTION
Ultrasound (Doppler)	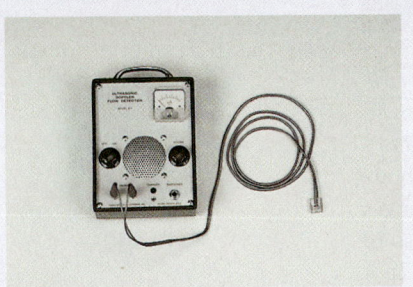	Battery-operated headset with earpieces attached to a volume-controlled audio unit and ultrasound transducer that detects movement of red blood cells through a vessel.
Sphygmomanometer		
Mercury manometer	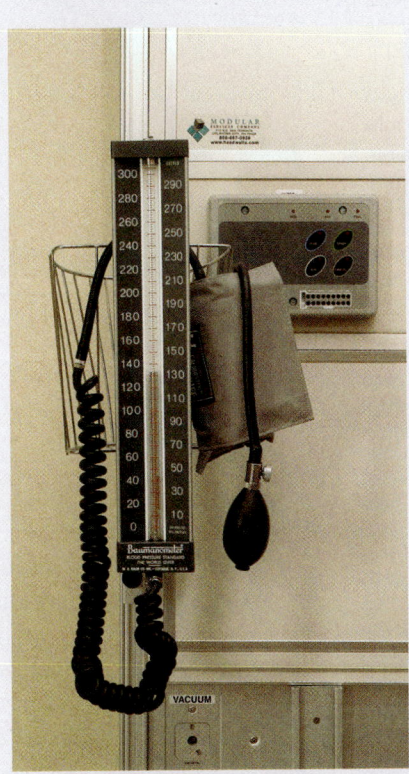	Wall unit that contains a mercury-filled glass column, calibrated in millimeters; the mercury rises and falls in response to pressure created when the cuff is inflated.
Aneroid manometer	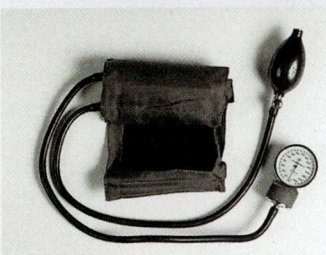	Portable unit with a glass-enclosed gauge containing a needle to register millimeter calibration and a metal bellows within the gauge that expands and collapses in response to pressure variations from the inflated cuff.

Delmar/Cengage Learning

CONVERSION EQUIVALENTS FOR WEIGHT MEASUREMENT

1 lb = 0.45 kg   1 kg = 2.2 lb
1 oz = 28.4 g   1 g = 0.35 oz

increases gradually from birth until the prepubertal growth spurt. Height and weight changes occur in the adolescent's torso. The resulting redistribution of body fat gives the body an adult appearance. (See Table 26-8 for the normal ranges of body height and weight according to age.) The loss of muscle mass and changes in dietary habits usually cause weight loss in older adults.

When a client has an order for "daily weight," the weight should be obtained at the same time of the day on the same scale, with the client wearing the same type of clothing. Standing scales are used for clients who can bear their own weight (see Figure 26-2). When standing on a scale, the client should wear some type of light foot covering, such as disposable operating room slippers, to prevent the transmission of infection and to enhance comfort. The Nursing Checklist describes the procedure for calibrating a scale and measuring the weight for children and adults (see Figure 26-3 on page 513).

Several types of scales, such as stretcher, chair, and bed scales, are available for clients who are unable to bear weight or who are confined to bed. Figure 26-4 on page 513, shows a scale that is equipped with a mechanical lift. A sheet should be placed between the client's skin and the surfaces of the belts.

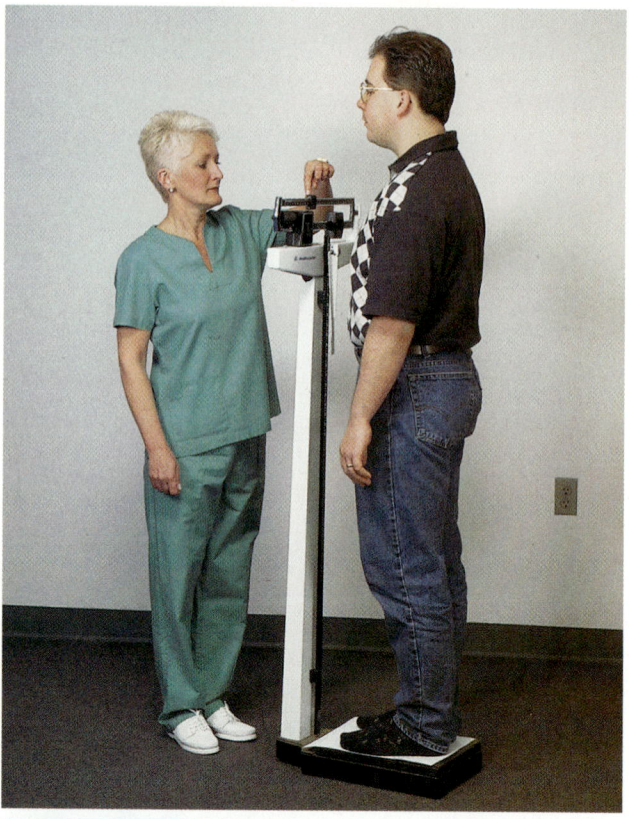

FIGURE 26-2 Weighing a Client on a Standing Scale DELMAR/CENGAGE LEARNING

TABLE 26-8 Normal Age-Related Variations in Height and Weight

AGE	HEIGHT	WEIGHT
Newborn	50 cm (20 in.)	3.38 kg (7.5 lb)
1–6 mos	63 cm (25 in.)	2 × birth weight
6–12 mos	71 cm (28 in.)	3 × birth weight
Toddler	75–83 cm (30–33 in.)	15 kg (33 lb)
Preschooler	100 cm (40 in.)	18.2–20.5 kg (40–45 lb)
School-age	115–140 cm (46–56 in.)	35.5–38.6 kg (75–85 lb)
Growth Spurt		
Girls 8–14 yrs	120–160cm (48–64 in.)	40.9–63.6 kg (90–140 lb)
Boys 10–16 yrs	125–170 cm (50–68 in.)	40.9–68.2 kg (90–150 lb)

Delmar/Cengage Learning

✓ NURSING CHECKLIST

Calibrating the Scale and Measuring Weight of Children and Adults

- Calibrate the standing scale by setting both weight indicators to zero. The balance beam will be at the top (Figure 26-3A). When calibrated, the balance beam will be at the midway point.
- Digital display scales should read zero. If they do not, follow the manufacturer's instructions to recalibrate the scale.
- Assist the client to a standing position. Have the client empty his or her bladder before the weight measurement.
- Make sure the scale is sitting evenly on the floor, and assist the client onto the scale. Instruct the client to remain still. Avoid touching him or her.
- Slowly move the standing scale's weight indicators on the balance beam until the tip of the beam registers in the middle of the mark (Figure 26-3B). Digital scales will automatically display the weight.
- Read and record the weight.
- Assist the client back to the former position.

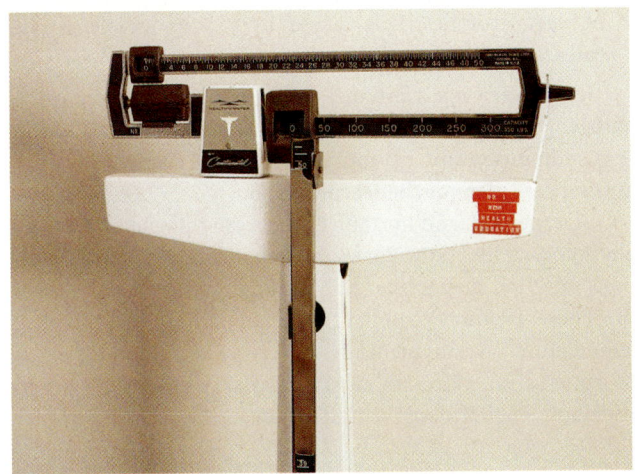

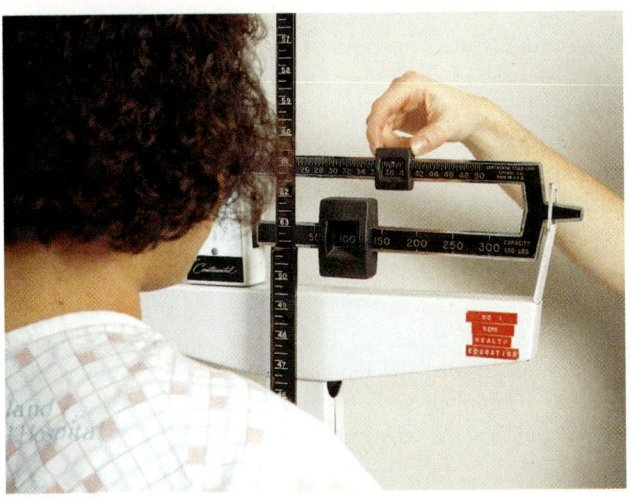

A

B

FIGURE 26-3 **Calibrating the Scale and Weighing the Client.**
A. Set both weight indicators to zero. **B.** With the client standing
on the scale, move the weight indicators on the balance beam until
the tip of the beam registers in the middle of the mark. DELMAR/CENGAGE
LEARNING

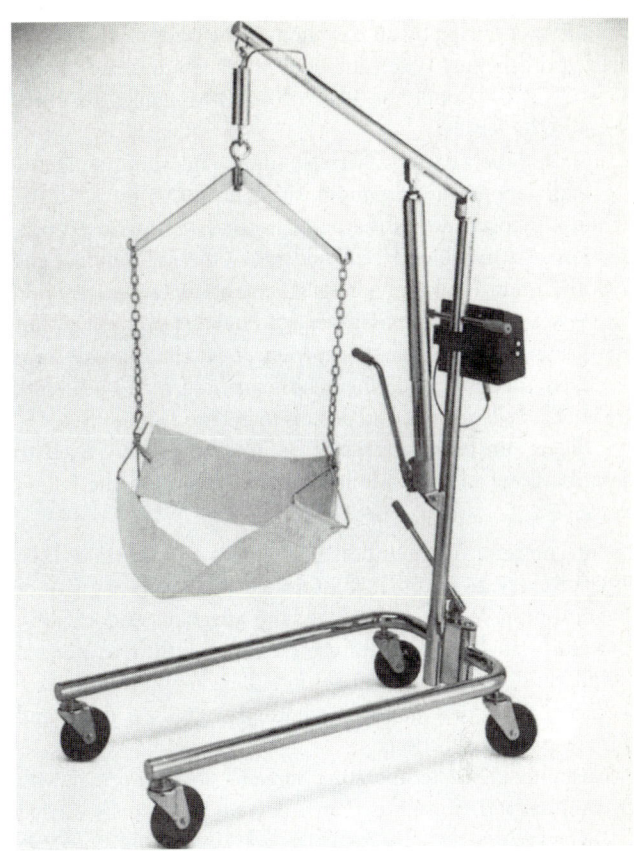

FIGURE 26-4 Scales equipped with mechanical lifts are used
for clients who are either unable to bear their weight on sta
nding scales or who are confined to bed. PHOTO COURTESY OF HEALTH O METER

DOCUMENTATION   The height and weight measurements
are recorded on the appropriate form, such as the admit
assessment form. Daily weights are usually recorded on the
vital signs record. If the weight is taken at a different time or
on a different scale, the variation should be recorded.

Infants can be weighed on platform or cradle scales.
Before weighing the infant, the nurse should make sure the
room is warm. The infant's clothing and diaper should then
be removed, and the nurse should place a light blanket on
the scale's surface. The nurse should face the infant, keeping
one hand over the top of the infant to prevent accidental
injury while adjusting the scale with the other hand. The
reading should be noted as quickly as possible, and the nurse
should return the infant to the crib and dress her or him.

Nursing Considerations

Accurate recordings of weight are imperative because they are
used in drug dosage calculations and in evaluating the effectiveness of drug, fluid, and nutritional therapy. Weights above
the normal range may indicate obesity or fluid retention.
Weights below the normal range may indicate malnutrition,
delayed growth and development, or cachexia (weight loss
marked by weakness and emaciation that usually occurs with a
chronic illness such as tuberculosis or cancer). Height is compared with weight to evaluate growth of infants and children.

THE NURSING PROCESS AND VITAL SIGNS

Monitoring vital signs is a critical nursing intervention that
provides data necessary to evaluate the client's condition and
prevent complications. The nursing process, in order to be an
effective tool of assessment and accountability, must have a
system of measurement based on nursing vocabularies and taxonomies (Moorhead, Johnson, & Maas, 2008). The ongoing
work of the North American Nursing Diagnosis Association
(NANDA) International, Nursing Outcomes Classification
(NOC), and Nursing Interventions Classification (NIC) is to
create vocabularies and taxonomies that define nursing; see
Unit 2 for a complete discussion of the nursing process.

NURSING PROCESS AND THERMOREGULATION

When heat production exceeds heat loss and body temperature rises above the normal range, pyrexia occurs. This

condition is caused by an elevation of the body's set point in the hypothalamus. When the body's temperature rises above 37.4°C (101°F) orally or 38°C (100.4°F) rectally, the client is said to be febrile.

Pyrogens (bacteria, viruses, fungi, and some antigens) are endogenous or exogenous substances that cause fever. When a pyrogen enters the body, it causes an increased production of white blood cells and raises the set point of the hypothalamus. It takes the body several hours to generate and conserve sufficient heat to achieve the new set point. It is during this time that the person experiences the clinical symptoms of chills and shivering. When the temperature and set point are equal, chills subside and fever is manifested clinically.

There are four patterns of occurrence that are used to describe fever and provide information regarding the fever's cause:

- Intermittent: The temperature returns to normal at least once every 24 hours; it is associated with gram-negative or gram-positive sepsis, abscesses, and infectious endocarditis.
- Remittent: The temperature does not return to normal but varies only a few degrees in either direction; it is associated with viral upper respiratory tract, *Legionella*, and *Mycoplasma* infections.
- Sustained: The temperature remains above normal with minimal variations, less than 1 degree; it is usually caused by drugs.
- Recurrent (relapsing): This pattern is characterized by one or more episodes of fever, each as long as several days, with one or more days of normal temperature between episodes; it is caused by various infectious diseases, including fungal.

The fever cycle continues until the body overcomes the pyrogen either naturally or through clinical intervention (e.g., administration of antibiotics). See Chapter 29 for a nursing care plan for the febrile client.

Age, gender, and hormonal levels can influence "normal" physiological function. For example, an older adult with a serious infection may trigger only a modest fever or no fever at all. These factors account for the differences in individual temperature measurements relative to fever. When a person is exposed to extreme environmental conditions, several alterations in thermoregulation can occur (see Table 26-9).

Assessment

Body temperature is measured by using one of the instruments described in Table 26-7. Frequent monitoring is required for clients who have or who are at risk for infection, for example, postoperative clients or those with a suppressed white blood cell count. Accuracy of temperature measurement is essential in the clinical management of clients because it guides nursing and medical decision making and interventions.

TEMPERATURE SCALES The nurse should consistently measure and record the temperature using either the centigrade or Fahrenheit scale as defined in specific health care agency policies. A centigrade-calibrated scale ranges from

TABLE 26-9 Alterations in Thermoregulation

ALTERATION	DEFINITION	CHARACTERISTICS
Heat exhaustion	An increase in body temperature (38°C–40°C, 100.4°F–104.0°F) in response to environmental conditions that, in turn, causes diaphoresis (profuse perspiration)	Loss of excessive amounts of water and sodium from perspiring leads to thirst, nausea, vomiting, weakness, and disorientation.
Heat stroke	A critical increase in body temperature (41°C–44°C, 100.6°F–112.0°F) resulting from exposure to high environmental temperatures	Dry, hot skin is the most important sign. The person becomes confused or delirious and experiences thirst, abdominal distress, muscle cramps, and visual disturbances. Loss of consciousness occurs if untreated.
Hypothermia	A body temperature of 35°C (95°F) or lower resulting from cold weather exposure or artificial induction	Decrease in metabolism leads to impaired mental functioning and depressed pulse, respiration, and blood pressure; can result in cardiac arrest if untreated.
Frostbite	Freezing of the body's surface areas (earlobes, fingers, and toes) in extremely low temperatures	Circulatory impairment may be followed by gangrene.

Delmar/Cengage Learning

34°C to 42°C, and a Fahrenheit-calibrated scale ranges from 94°F to 108°F. Conversions from one scale to another are based on the formula that 0°C is equal to 32°F (see the accompanying display on centigrade and Fahrenheit conversion formulas).

SITES Although the prescribing practitioner may order a specific site to measure the temperature, nursing judgment usually determines the best site based on the client's age and physical and mental condition. Traditional sites for measuring the body's internal (core) temperature are oral (OT), rectal (RT), and axillary (AT), using either glass or electronic thermometers.

Advances in clinical thermometry provide other devices and sites, such as thermistors for pulmonary artery temperature (PAT) and infrared thermometers for ear canal temperature (ET). ET is the most common site used for temperature measurements in adults because it is a safe and an efficient method; however, it is less sensitive in detecting fever in infants and young children. ET should not be used in infected or draining ears or if adjacent lesions or incisions exist. The most reliable measure of core temperature is PAT. Since PAT requires placement of a thermodilution pulmonary artery catheter, it is impractical for routine care.

Oral and rectal temperature measurements are higher than axillary because the measuring device is in contact with the mucous membrane. Rectal measurements are higher than oral because of the seal created by the anal sphincter, which decreases contact with environmental air. With the availability of electronic measuring devices, a glass thermometer should never be used for oral readings because of the possibility of the client biting and breaking the thermometer.

The axilla is commonly used as a site for infants and children with disabilities because it is the safest, even though the least accurate, method. Axillary or rectal sites are used for clients who are uncooperative or comatose, or who have a nasogastric or feeding tube in place. Rectal temperature measurement is contraindicated in clients with cardiovascular alterations because the thermometer may stimulate the vagus nerve and cause an irregular cardiac rhythm. It is also contraindicated in leukemia and rectal surgery clients because the insertion of the thermometer may traumatize the mucosa or incision line, causing bleeding.

Temporal artery (TA) thermometers measure temperature using a scanning infrared thermometer that compares arterial temperature in the temporal artery of the forehead to the temperature in the room and calculates the heat balance to approximate the core temperature of the blood in the pulmonary artery. Place the TA probe in the middle of the forehead. With the red button depressed, slide the probe slowly from the midline across the forehead to the hairline. Lift the probe from the forehead, touch it on the neck just behind the earlobe, and release the button. The probe is touched behind the earlobe if the client has perspiration; this allows the thermometer to compensate for evaporative cooling (Exergen Corporation, 2008).

ASSESSING BODY TEMPERATURE Assess the client for the most appropriate site and gather the necessary equipment; refer to Table 26-7 for the devices that are used to measure temperature. The mercury-in-glass thermometer was once the standard device for measuring temperature; however, federal regulation prohibits the use of mercury-containing medical devices because of potential health and environmental hazards. Mercury is a reproductive toxin and a potent neurotoxin affecting both the brain and central nervous system. Basically two types of thermometers are used in health care facilities: electronic and disposable. A third type, the glass gallium-indium-tin (galinstan), is available commercially for in-home use. Nurses must understand the limitations of each device and must receive training on proper thermometry technique.

When checking the client's oral temperature, the nurse should confirm that the client has consumed neither hot or cold food or beverages or smoked for 15 to 30 minutes before the measurement. Mouth breathing and tachypnea may also cause an inaccurate oral reading. Herpes viruses are extremely contagious and require implementation of Standard Precautions of the Centers for Disease Control and Prevention. Clients with herpetic lesions should have their own glass thermometer to prevent transmission to others.

When using a glass thermometer stored in a disinfectant solution, the nurse should rinse it under cold water to remove the solution. Hot water should not be used on the thermometer because it will cause the mercury to expand and could break the thermometer. Procedure 26-1 describes the actions involved in measuring body temperature according to site.

Nursing Diagnosis

The nurse examines the assessment data and clusters the defining characteristics to form a nursing diagnosis for clients with altered body temperature; see the accompanying display, on page 516, on body temperature alterations. A diagnosis identifies a client's state that is altered or has the potential to be altered or improved; nursing diagnoses describe problems, actual or potential, that the nurse seeks to resolve through interventions. For example, a decrease in body temperature below the normal range, pallor, shivering, cyanotic nail beds, and blood pressure and pulse above the normal range are the defining characteristics for the diagnosis

---

CENTIGRADE AND FAHRENHEIT CONVERSION FORMULAS

- Centigrade to Fahrenheit conversion: multiply the centigrade reading by 9/5 and add 32:

  $$°F = (°C \times 9/5) + 32$$

- Fahrenheit to centigrade conversion: deduct 32 from the Fahrenheit reading and multiply by 5/9: $°C = (°F − 32) \times 5/9$

▼ SAFETY FIRST ▼

Children left in vehicles in sweltering summer temperatures are at high risk for hyperthermia. The temperature inside the car can climb 20°F within 10 minutes, even with the windows rolled down.

hypothermia. Once the diagnosis is made, the nurse must determine the related factor(s): exposure to a cold environment and evaporation from the skin in a cold environment; medications causing vasodilation; or decreased metabolism. In hypothermia, a related factor of exposure to a cold environment will result in different interventions than a related factor of medications causing vasodilation. Once the nursing diagnosis is formulated, *hypothermia* related to exposure to a cold environment, the nurse then establishes nursing goals and client outcomes to measure the effectiveness of interventions.

Planning and Outcome Identification

During the planning phase, the nurse synthesizes assessment findings and integrates all client data to formulate nursing goals, interventions, and outcomes for clients with body temperature alterations. Care plan development must involve the client and/or the family, must be based on professional standards of care, and must utilize research findings or best practices.

When a client has a fever, nursing care includes treating the cause as prescribed and providing supportive care. Controversy exists regarding whether or not to treat the fever itself since fever acts as a protective mechanism. In order for bacteria to multiply, bacteria need large amounts of iron and zinc, but during fever, the liver and spleen do not release these elements (Beard & Day, 2008). Since fever increases

NURSING DIAGNOSES: BODY TEMPERATURE ALTERATIONS

- *Risk for imbalanced body temperature*—at risk for failure to maintain body temperature within normal range
- *Hyperthermia*—body temperature elevated above normal range
- *Hypothermia*—body temperature below normal range
- *Ineffective thermoregulation*—temperature fluctuation between hypothermia and hyperthermia

Source: Data from North American Nursing Diagnosis Association International. (2007). *Nursing diagnoses: Definitions and classification 2007-2008* (pp. 21, 108, 109, and 225). Philadelphia: Author.

metabolism, this action helps the body to heal itself. One study suggests that aggressively treating fever may lead to higher mortality rates in certain clients (Schulman, 2005).

Implementation

Once the client's plan of care is defined, the nurse implements those interventions that will assist the client in achieving the specific outcomes. Vital signs measurements are often delegated by the professional nurse to other health care providers. Since professional nurses may delegate certain nursing interventions to other nursing personnel, either licensed or unlicensed, certified or uncertified, it is imperative that nurses document the competency of those individuals performing the nursing interventions. Delegation is a legal action, as defined in nurse practice acts by the various state boards of nursing. Although an intervention may be delegated to other nursing personnel, such as a licensed practical nurse or unlicensed ancillary personnel, the registered nurse is held responsible and accountable for the outcome. (See Chapter 11 for a complete discussion regarding delegation.)

The nurse teaches the client health-seeking behaviors to promote a balance between heat production and heat loss, such as client activity and clothing and environmental temperature. Health education and self-modification assistance for a client who exercises should address the need to wear light-fitting, light-colored clothing; to be exposed gradually to a hot climate; to exercise only in well-ventilated areas; to avoid strenuous exercise in hot, humid weather; and to drink fluids such as water before, during, and after exercise.

The nurse should place the client experiencing heat exhaustion in a cool environment. The goal of nursing care is to stop diaphoresis by administering fluid and electrolytes as prescribed by a prescribing practitioner. See Chapter 33 for a complete discussion of fluid and electrolyte therapy.

Victims of heat stroke do not perspire because of severe electrolyte loss and impaired hypothalamic function, as discussed in Table 26-9. Heat stroke victims are usually discovered outdoors, with emergency measures instituted to lower the temperature during transport to an emergency center. Nursing's primary role relative to heat stroke is prevention. The nurse is usually involved in teaching preventive measures, such as drinking liquids before, during, and after exercise; avoiding strenuous exercise in humid, hot weather; and wearing light-colored, loose-fitting clothing and covering the head when working outdoors in hot climates.

Hypothermia and frostbite victims found injured in cold weather or who were immersed in cold water are

COMMUNITY CONSIDERATIONS

Homeless

Clients most at risk for hypothermia are homeless persons who lack adequate heating, shelter, diet, or clothing.

▼ **SAFETY FIRST** ▼

ORAL LESIONS
Assess for oral lesion, especially herpetic lesions, because herpes viruses are highly contagious and require the implementation of Standard Precautions; clients with herpetic lesions should have their own disposable thermometer to prevent transmission to others.

treated while in transit to an emergency center with heating blankets and instillation of warm fluids into the stomach. Nursing's role is to teach preventive measures to groups at risk, such as the homeless, and to parents or guardians of mentally challenged or handicapped clients who live in cold environments.

Many clients with traumatic brain injury such as a skull fracture may develop **neurogenic fever**, described as a long-term elevation of body temperature thought to result from a disruption of the normal body temperature set point. Neurogenic fever is caused by damage to the hypothalamus from central nervous system trauma, intracerebral bleeding, or an increase in intracranial pressure. Neurogenic fever increases the metabolic demands on the body and can increase swelling of the brain, further increasing the risk of neurological damage. Nurses should monitor traumatic brain injury clients with unexplained temperature elevation to facilitate early diagnosis and treatment of neurogenic fever.

DOCUMENTATION Record the temperature measurement and the site on the designated medical record form. Temperature measurements are usually plotted on a graph to identify alteration patterns, such as sharp elevations and declines in temperature (a condition known as spiking).

Evaluation

Nursing interventions are evaluated by comparing the client's actual response to the nursing-sensitive client outcome, such as body temperature that is maintained within the normal range. If the client is not able to achieve the outcome, with body temperature increased to 38.8°C (101.8°F), then the plan of care may require revisions. After any nursing intervention, the nurse measures the client's temperature at a time that is appropriate to assess the client's response to the intervention. The nurse also uses other evaluative measures such as palpation of the skin and assessment of pulse and respiration when evaluating the client's response to nursing interventions. Based on the client's ability to respond effectively to nursing interventions, the body temperature and other vital signs will return to normal ranges, and the client will report a feeling of comfort.

PULSE

Pulse assessment is the measurement of a pressure pulsation created when the heart contracts and ejects blood into the aorta. Assessment of pulse characteristics provides clinical data regarding the heart's pumping action and the adequacy of peripheral artery blood flow.

Sites

There are multiple pulse points. The most accessible peripheral pulses are the radial and carotid sites. Because the body shunts blood to the brain whenever a cardiac emergency such as hemorrhage occurs, the carotid site should always be used to assess the pulse in these situations.

Variances exist among health care agencies regarding which pulse sites to assess. The common sites for each type of assessment are:

- Complete physical assessment—apical and all bilateral peripheral pulses
- Initial assessment—apical and bilateral peripheral radial and dorsalis pedis pulses
- Routine vital signs assessment—apical and radial pulses in adults and apical and temporal pulses in infants and children.

Disorders that alter the client's cardiovascular status require different pulse point assessments (Table 26-10 on page 518). Whenever circulation is compromised, the corresponding pulse point should be assessed.

Assessing Pulse Rate

The nurse should begin the assessment by speaking with the client about the normal pulse rate. The client's medical record should be reviewed for baseline data, if available, and any medications that could affect the heart rate should be noted. Because physical activity increases the heart rate, ensure that the client rests 5 to 10 minutes before the pulse is assessed.

Clinical data regarding the efficacy of blood circulation to an extremity are obtained by assessing the characteristics (quality, rate, rhythm, and volume) of the peripheral pulses. These attributes are described in the section entitled Pulse Characteristics. Palpate a peripheral pulse by placing the first two fingers on the pulse point with moderate pressure. A firm pressure will obliterate the pulse; if the pressure is too light, the pulse cannot be felt.

A Doppler ultrasound stethoscope (DUS) is used on superficial pulse points to detect and magnify heart sounds and pulse waves when the peripheral pulse cannot be palpated. The DUS, which has an earpiece similar to that of a stethoscope, is connected by a cord to a volume-control audio unit with an ultrasound transducer. See Chapter 32 for a complete discussion about other devices to monitor the heart rate.

Normal radial and apical pulses are identical in rate. The stethoscope is used to auscultate the heart's rate and rhythm. The stethoscope should be placed on the fifth intercostal space at the midclavicular line, as described in Procdeure 26-2. Count the rate for a full minute, noting the regularity (rhythm).

When an irregular peripheral pulse is present, the nurse needs to assess for a **pulse deficit** (condition in which the apical pulse rate is greater than the radial pulse rate). A pulse deficit results from the ejection of a volume of blood that is too small to initiate a peripheral pulse wave. When a discrepancy exists between the apical and radial pulses, the deficit is assessed by simultaneously measuring the apical and radial pulses for a

TABLE 26-10 Pulse Point Assessment

PULSE POINT	ASSESSMENT CRITERIA
Temporal: over temporal bone, superior and lateral to eye	Accessible; used routinely for infants and when radial is inaccessible
Carotid: bilateral, under lower jaw in neck along medial edge of sternocleidomastoid muscle	Accessible; used routinely for infants and during shock or cardiac arrest when other peripheral pulses are too weak to palpate; also used to assess cranial circulation
Apical: left midclavicular line at fourth to fifth intercostal space	Used to auscultate heart sounds and assess apical-radial deficit
Brachial: inner aspect between groove of biceps and triceps muscles at antecubital fossa	Used in cardiac arrest for infants, to assess lower arm circulation, and to auscultate blood pressure
Radial: inner aspect of forearm on thumb side of wrist	Accessible; used routinely in adults to assess character of peripheral pulse
Ulnar: outer aspect of forearm on finger side of wrist	Used to assess circulation to ulnar side of hand and to perform the Allen's test
Femoral: in groin, below inguinal ligament (midpoint between symphysis pubis and anterosuperior iliac spine)	Used to assess circulation to legs and during cardiac arrest
Popliteal: behind knee, at center in popliteal fossa	Used to assess circulation to legs and to auscultate leg blood pressure
Posterior tibial: inner aspect of ankle between Achilles tendon and tibia (below medial malleolus)	Used to assess circulation to feet
Dorsalis pedis: over instep, midpoint between extension tendons of great and second toe	Used to assess circulation to feet

Delmar/Cengage Learning

minute. This procedure is usually performed by two nurses; however, it can be performed by one nurse if necessary.

PULSE CHARACTERISTICS A normal pulse has defined characteristics: quality, rate, rhythm, and volume (strength or amplitude). **Pulse quality** refers to the "feel" of the pulse, its rhythm and forcefulness.

Pulse rate is an indirect measurement of cardiac output obtained by counting the number of apical or peripheral pulse waves over a pulse point. A normal pulse rate for adults is between 60 and 100 beats per minute. **Bradycardia** is a heart rate less than 60 beats per minute in an adult. **Tachycardia** is a heart rate in excess of 100 beats per minute in an adult.

▼ SAFETY FIRST ▼

CAROTID PULSE ASSESSMENT
When assessing a carotid pulse, apply light pressure to only one carotid artery to avoid disruption of cerebral blood flow.

Pulse rhythm is the regularity of the heartbeat. It describes how evenly the heart is beating: regular (the beats are evenly spaced) or irregular (the beats are not evenly spaced). Dysrhythmia (arrhythmia) is an irregular rhythm caused by an early, late, or missed heartbeat.

Pulse volume is a measurement of the strength or amplitude of force exerted by the ejected blood against the arterial wall with each contraction. It is described as normal (full, easily palpable), weak (thready and usually rapid), or strong (bounding). To facilitate data comparison of this measurement, a standard pulse volume scale should be used in documenting findings (see Table 26-11 on page 519). Procedure 26-2 describes the actions involved in assessing the pulse rate.

Nursing Considerations

An irregular pulse rate, if not previously documented in the medical record, should be reported immediately. The following equipment is used to identify the type of dysrhythmia causing the irregular heartbeat:

- Electrocardiogram (ECG or EKG) provides an electrical representation of the heart's activity. The primary pacemaker of the heart is the sinoatrial (SA) node. If another

TABLE 26-11 Pulse Volume Scale

SCALE	DESCRIPTION OF PULSE
0	Absent pulse
1+	Weak and thready pulse
2+	Normal pulse
3+	Bounding pulse

Delmar/Cengage Learning

site within the heart initiates the electrical activity, the ECG tracing will identify the area serving as the pacemaker.

- A Holter monitor is a portable device worn for a 24-hour interval to identify the dysrhythmia pattern.
- Cardiac telemetry transmits the heart's electrical activity to a site for continuous monitoring.

See Chapter 32 for additional information regarding these cardiac monitoring devices.

Clients on certain cardiac medications, such as cardiovascular agents and cardiac glycosides, need to monitor their pulse rate. Clients receiving cardiovascular agents (verapamil hydrochloride) and cardiac glycosides (digoxin) may experience an irregular pulse or pulse rate change that should be reported to their prescribing practitioner. In addition, clients who follow an exercise regimen should assess their pulse rate to measure their heart's response to the exercise. Routine or regular exercise lowers the resting and activity pulses. When teaching clients how to monitor their own heart rate, nurses should show them the procedure in assessing the radial or carotid pulse points.

DOCUMENTATION All pulse measurements are documented by recording in the client's medical record on the appropriate forms (e.g., the vital signs flow sheet). The nurse should report and document an irregular pulse.

RESPIRATIONS

Respiratory assessment is the measurement of the breathing pattern. Assessment of respirations provides clinical data regarding the pH of arterial blood.

Sites

Normal breathing is slightly observable, effortless, quiet, automatic, and regular. It can be assessed by observing chest wall expansion and bilateral symmetrical movement of the thorax. Another method the nurse can use to assess breathing is to place the back of the hand next to the client's nose and mouth to feel the expired air.

Assessing Respirations

When assessing respirations, ascertain the rate, depth, and rhythm of ventilatory movement. The nurse should assess the rate by counting the number of breaths taken per minute.

Note the depth and rhythm of ventilatory movements by observing the normal thoracic and abdominal movements and symmetry in chest wall movement. Normal respirations are characterized by a rate ranging from 12 to 20 breaths per minute. Procedure 26-3 describes the actions involved in assessing respirations.

One inspiration and expiration cycle is counted as one breath. The nurse should observe the rise and fall of the chest wall and count the rate by placing the hand lightly on the chest to feel its rise and fall. Count the number of respirations as explained in Procedure 26-3.

MOVEMENT OF THE DIAPHRAGM When the chest wall moves, so do the lungs because the lungs are attached to the inner wall of the thoracic cavity by the outer layer of the **pleura** (lining of the chest cavity). The movement of the chest wall should be even and regular, without noise and effort. On inspiration, the chest changes shape and expands as the rib cage is raised and the diaphragm is lowered. Before inspiration, the pressure inside the chest cavity is negative (-4.5 to -9.0 mm Hg below atmospheric pressure). Air flows along the concentration gradient from a higher atmospheric pressure to the lower intrathoracic pressure.

The opposite action occurs with expiration. The muscles relax, causing the rib cage to lower and the diaphragm to rise, compressing the chest. Intrathoracic pressure decreases to -3 to -6 mm Hg to allow the air to escape into the atmosphere.

CHARACTERISTICS OF NORMAL AND ABNORMAL BREATH SOUNDS Different respiratory wave patterns are characterized by their rate, rhythm, and depth. See Chapter 32 for a complete discussion of wave patterns. **Eupnea** refers to easy respirations with a normal rate of breaths per minute that is age specific. **Bradypnea** is a respiratory rate of 10 or fewer breaths per minute. **Hypoventilation** is characterized by shallow respirations. **Tachypnea** is a respiratory rate greater than 24 breaths per minute. **Hyperventilation** is characterized by deep, rapid respirations.

The nurse can also observe alterations in the movement of the chest wall: **costal (thoracic) breathing** occurs when the external intercostal muscles and the other accessory muscles are used to move the chest upward and outward; **diaphragmatic (abdominal) breathing** occurs when the diaphragm contracts and relaxes as observed by movement of the abdomen. **Dyspnea** refers to difficulty in breathing as observed by labored or forced respirations through the use of accessory muscles in the chest and neck to breathe. Dyspneic clients are acutely aware of their respirations and complain of shortness of breath.

Nursing Considerations

Respiratory alterations may cause changes in skin color as observed by a bluish appearance in the nail beds, lips, and skin. The bluish color (**cyanosis**) results from reduced oxygen levels in the arterial blood. Changes in the level of consciousness may also occur with decreased oxygen levels. Dyspneic clients will assume a forward-leaning position to increase the expansion capacity of the lungs.

▼ SAFETY FIRST ▼

POSITIONING FOR DYSPNEIC CLIENTS

Dyspneic clients should never be placed flat in bed; maintain them in a semi-Fowler's or Fowler's position. To facilitate maximal lung expansion, place the client in a forward-leaning position over a padded, raised overbed table with arms and head resting on the table.

CONTRAINDICATIONS FOR BRACHIAL ARTERY BLOOD PRESSURE MEASUREMENT

When the client has any of the following, *do not* measure blood pressure on the involved side:

- Venous access devices, such as an intravenous infusion or arteriovenous fistula for renal dialysis
- Surgery involving the breast, axilla, shoulder, arm, or hand
- Injury or disease to the shoulder, arm, or hand, such as trauma, burns, or application of a cast or bandage

---

Clients with respiratory alterations require additional nursing assessment. Noninvasive oxygen assessment can be performed with an oximeter (a machine that measures the oxygen saturation of the blood through a probe clipped to the fingernail or earlobe) or an apnea monitor (a machine with chest leads that monitors the movement of the chest). Both noninvasive machines have alarm features that are set to specific parameters. For example, if the client's respirations fall below 6 breaths per minute, the apnea monitor alarm will sound. The apnea monitor is used in the home environment for apneic clients; when the alarm sounds, it wakes the person and causes him or her to breathe.

DOCUMENTATION   Document the assessment findings for the respiratory rate, depth, rhythm, and character on the appropriate form (e.g., the vital signs flow sheet). Report a respiratory rate outside of the normal age range, an irregular rhythm, an inadequate depth, or any abnormal characteristics such as dyspnea.

BLOOD PRESSURE

Blood pressure measurement is performed during a physical examination, at initial assessment, and as part of a routine vital signs assessment. Depending on the client's condition, the blood pressure is measured by either a direct or an indirect technique. The direct method requires an invasive procedure in which an intravenous catheter with an electronic sensor is inserted into an artery and the artery-transmitted pressure on an electronic display unit is read. The indirect method requires use of the sphygmomanometer and stethoscope for auscultation and palpation as needed.

Sites

The most common site for indirect blood pressure measurement is the client's arm over the brachial artery. When the client's condition prevents auscultation of the brachial artery, the nurse should assess the blood pressure in the forearm or leg sites (see the accompanying display on contraindications for brachial artery blood pressure measurement).

When pressure measurements in the upper extremities are not accessible, the popliteal artery, located behind the knee, becomes the site of choice. The nurse can also assess the blood pressure in other sites, such as the radial artery in the forearm and the posterior tibial or dorsalis pedis artery in the lower leg. Because it is difficult to auscultate sounds over the radial, tibial, and dorsalis pedis arteries, these sites are usually palpated to obtain a systolic reading.

Assessing Blood Pressure

Selecting the proper equipment and following procedural technique are basic to ensuring an accurate reading. Psychomotor skills, acquired with practice, are needed to manipulate the blood pressure equipment. Procedure 26-4 describes the actions involved in assessing blood pressure.

As shown in Table 26-7, a sphygmomanometer is a device used to measure indirect blood pressure. A sphygmomanometer consists of a mercury or an aneroid manometer and a cuff that contains an inflatable rubber bladder connected to two pieces of rubber tubing. One piece of tubing connects the bladder to the manometer or gauge, and the second tubing is attached to a pressure bulb with a release valve to inflate and deflate the cuff. When pressure is applied to the bulb, air enters the bladder and inflates the cuff.

The sphygmomanometer wears with usage. If there is a defect in any part of the system, the blood pressure reading will be inaccurate. The aneroid gauge needle or mercury in the manometer column should be at a zero reading when the cuff is deflated and should rise evenly when pressure is applied to the bulb. The valve should turn freely, and all tubing should be intact, with secured connections to prevent air from leaking out of the system.

An accurate reading also requires the correct width of the blood pressure cuff as determined by the circumference of the client's extremity. The bladder cuff must encircle the width and length of the site. The bladder width should be approximately 40% of the circumference or 20% wider than the diameter of the midpoint of the extremity. To measure the width of the bladder, the nurse should place the cuff lengthwise on the client's extremity and extend the width to cover 40% of the extremity's circumference (see Figure 26-5). The length of the sphygmomanometer bladder should be twice the width. Table 26-12, recommends bladder sizes based on different arm circumferences. A falsely elevated reading will result if the bladder is too narrow, and a falsely low reading will result if it is too wide.

Electronic sphygmomanometers are used by clients for self-measurements. A stethoscope is not required because the device electronically inflates and deflates the cuff while simultaneously reading and displaying the systolic and diastolic pressures. The electronic device is useful for clients who must monitor their own pressure at home. However, it must be recalibrated routinely to ensure an accurate reading.

AUSCULTATION A stethoscope is used to auscultate the blood pressure (hear the sounds created by blood flowing through the artery). As discussed in Procedure 26-4, the blood pressure cuff is inflated 30 mm Hg higher than the palpated pressure so that the inflated pressure causes the artery to collapse; blood flow ceases, and sound is absent on auscultation. As the pressure is released from the bladder, blood begins to flow through the artery and creates the first sound, which is the systolic pressure.

The Korotkoff's sounds, described in Table 26-13 and Procedure 26-4, are named after the Russian surgeon who first identified the five distinct phases of sound heard with a stethoscope during auscultation. Korotkoff's sounds are correlated to the pressure dynamics of measurement.

Bilateral readings should be done with the initial blood pressure assessment. A pressure variance of 5 to 10 mm Hg normally exists between arms. The arm with the higher reading should be used for routine measurements.

When measuring a popliteal blood pressure, the nurse should select a cuff wide and long enough to fit the girth of the thigh. Although the American Heart Association does not specify cuff sizes for thigh BP readings, the association emphasizes that the cuff should be wider and longer than an arm cuff to allow for the greater girth. Place the client in a supine position with the legs in a nondependent position for at least 10 minutes. (A prone position is also acceptable.) Apply the

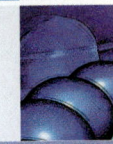

TABLE 26-12 Guidelines for Sphygmomanometer Selection

MIDPOINT* ARM CIRCUMFERENCE**	BLADDER CUFF WIDTH**	BLADDER LENGTH**
5–7.5 (newborn)	3	5
7.5–13 (infant)	5	8
13–20 (child)	8	13
24–32 (average adult)	13	24
32–42 (large adult)	17	32

*Distance between the acromion and olecranon processes.
**Measurement in centimeters (cm).

Delmar/Cengage Learning

bladder cuff to the client's thigh with the center of the bladder over the popliteal artery. Wrap the cuff snugly, and place it far enough above the popliteal fossa to allow for auscultation of arterial sounds. Help the client slightly flex the knee and abduct the hip. This position will facilitate palpation of the pulse and placement of the stethoscope. Place the diaphragm of the stethoscope over the area where the pulse was palpated, and follow the same procedure as presented for brachial artery auscultation (see Procedure 26-4). When the BP cuff is removed, inspect the area, and note abnormalities such as bruising, hematoma, or skin tear. Document in the medical record the systolic and diastolic BP, the site, and the size of the BP cuff. In the thigh, systolic readings may be 10 to 40 mm Hg higher than in the arm, but diastolic readings are generally the same.

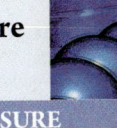

TABLE 26-13 Korotkoff's Sounds Correlated to Pressure Dynamics

PHASE	PRESSURE DYNAMICS
I. Clear, soft tapping that increases to a thud or loud tap (systolic sound).	1. Ventilation
II. Tapping changes to a soft, swishing sound.	2. Circulation
III. Clear tapping sound returns.	3. Diffusion
IV. Muffled, blowing sound (diastolic sound in children or physically active adults).	4. Transport
V. Disappearance of muffled, blowing sound (second diastolic sound).	5. Regulation

Delmar/Cengage Learning

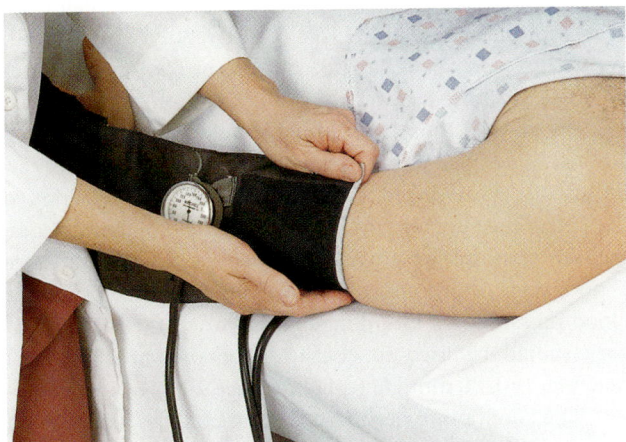

FIGURE 26-5 Measure width of arm by holding cuff against client's upper arm. DELMAR/CENGAGE LEARNING

UNCOVERING THE

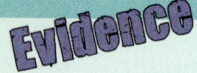

TITLE OF STUDY

"A Comparison of Blood Pressure Measurement over a Sleeved Arm versus a Bare Arm"

AUTHORS

G. Ma, N. Sabin, and M. Dawes

PURPOSE

To determine whether the measurement of blood pressure over a sleeved arm varies from that taken on a bare arm.

METHOD

Between September 2004 and November 2006, 376 clients (ages 18 to 85 years) were recruited from a family medicine clinic. All clients had their blood pressures recorded using the same automatic oscillometric device, with the cuff placed over their bare arms for the first reading. Each client was than randomly assigned to either the bare-arm group, for which the second blood pressure reading was also taken on a bare arm, or the sleeved-arm group, for which the second reading was taken with the cuff placed over the sleeved arm.

FINDINGS

No clinically important differences were found between the bare-arm group and the sleeved-arm group in age, sex, or body mass index.

IMPLICATIONS

There was no significant difference in blood pressure recorded over a sleeve or on a bare arm. The decision to measure blood pressure on a bare arm or over a sleeved arm should be left to the judgment of the health care professional taking the blood pressure.

Ma, G., Sabin, N., & Dawes, M. (2008). A comparison of blood pressure measurement over a sleeved arm versus a bare arm. *Canadian Medical Association Journal*, 178(5), 585–589.

PALPATION When the client's hemodynamic regulation is compromised to the degree that Korotkoff's sounds cannot be heard, such as with myocardial infarction or shock, the blood pressure has to be monitored by palpation or direct measurement. To palpate the systolic blood pressure, apply the cuff over the brachial artery, inflate the cuff, place the fingers over the radial artery, slowly release the pressure, and note the reading on the manometer when the first pulse (systole) is felt. With palpation, it is difficult to assess the diastolic pressure. Direct measurement is obtained with the insertion of an intravenous catheter.

HYPOTENSION Hypotension refers to a systolic blood pressure less than 90 mm Hg or 20 to 30 mm Hg below the client's normal systolic pressure. Hypotension is caused by a disruption in hemodynamic regulation, such as:

- Decreased blood volume (e.g., hemorrhage)

- Decreased cardiac output (e.g., myocardial infarction [heart attack])
- Decreased peripheral vascular resistance (vascular dilation; e.g., shock)

A hypotensive client manifests symptoms relative to the degree of hypotension regardless of the cause.

One of the initial compensatory responses to a falling blood pressure is an increased pulse rate. For example, if a blood vessel cauterized during surgery begins to bleed internally, at the point at which the circulating blood volume is compromised the heart will automatically beat faster to compensate for the decreased circulating volume. If the falling pressure is untreated, the body's compensatory mechanisms will fail and the client will exhibit the symptoms of shock: cool, clammy skin; fast, thready pulse; a gradual decrease in urinary output; and disruption to cerebral blood flow that causes confusion, progressing to coma.

Orthostatic hypotension (postural hypotension) refers to a sudden drop of 25 mm Hg in systolic pressure and 10 mm Hg in diastolic pressure when the client moves from a lying to a sitting or a sitting to a standing position. Orthostatic hypotension usually occurs with aging and is a common antiadrenergic side effect of several medications, such as chlorpromazine hydrochloride. When measuring orthostatic blood pressure:

1. Place the client in a supine position for 5 minutes to allow for equilibration of the blood pressure, and measure the pulse and blood pressure.
2. Assist the client to a standing position, and wait 1 minute to obtain a full evaluation of the initial orthostasis, then recheck the pulse and blood pressure.
3. Reassess the vital signs after 2 minutes to allow for an evaluation of the client's mechanisms to compensate for the presence of any orthostasis.

Clients with orthostatic hypotension should be advised to rise slowly from a supine position and to sit down immediately if they feel faint.

HYPERTENSION Hypertension increases the risk for cardiovascular disease, the leading cause of death in the United States. Until May 2003, people with blood pressure measurements below 140/90 mm Hg were considered normal; however, with the release of the JNC 7 (NIH, 2003), people with systolic pressures of 120 to 139 mm Hg or diastolic pressures of 80 to 89 mm Hg were classified as prehypertensive, at higher risk than those with lower blood pressures. They are advised to adopt healthy lifestyles to decrease the risk of cardiovascular disease (see Table 26-14 on page 523). Prior to the JNC 7, **hypertension** was classified into three stages; the new classification provides for prehypertension and stage 1 and stage 2 hypertension. When systolic and diastolic blood pressures fall into different categories, the higher category should be used to classify blood pressure level. For example, 160/80 mm Hg would be stage 2 hypertension.

The adoption of health-promoting lifestyles is critical for the prevention and management of hypertension. According to the JNC 7 (NIH, 2003), the following major lifestyle changes have been shown to lower blood pressure:

- Maintain normal body weight.

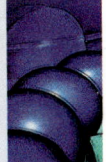

TABLE 26-14 Categories for Blood Pressure Levels in Adults (Ages 18 Years and Older*)

CATEGORY	BLOOD PRESSURE LEVEL (MM HG)		
	SYSTOLIC		DIASTOLIC
Normal	<120	and	<80
Prehypertension	120–139	or	80–89
High Blood Pressure			
Stage 1 hypertension	140–159	or	90–99
Stage 2 hypertension	>160	or	>100

*For adults 18 and older who are not on medicine for high blood pressure, do not have a short-term serious illness, or do not have another condition such as diabetes or kidney disease.

Source: National High Blood Pressure Education Program, National Institutes of Health. (2003). *The Seventh Report of the Joint National Committee on prevention, detection, evaluation, and treatment of high blood pressure.* Retrieved September 8, 2008, from http://www.nhlbi.nih.gov/guidelines/hypertension/jnc7full.pdf.

- Adopt the Dietary Approaches to Stop Hypertension (DASH) eating plan, which includes a diet rich in fruits, vegetables, and low-fat dairy products with a reduced content of saturated and total fat.
- Reduce dietary sodium intake to 2.4 g sodium or 6 g sodium chloride.
- Engage in regular aerobic physical activity, such as brisk walking at least 30 minutes a day, most days of the week.
- Limit alcohol consumption: men, two drinks a day, women, one drink a day.

By making the dietary changes just discussed, a 1,600-mg-sodium DASH eating plan has an effect similar to single-drug therapy; a combination of two (or more) lifestyle modifications can achieve greater results (NIH, 2003).

▼ SAFETY FIRST ▼

LUER CONNECTORS

Some automatic blood pressure monitoring devices are designed with male and female Luer connectors, the same type of connectors used on intravenous tubing. Normally the BP device cycles at preset intervals, inflating the cuff with more than 500 mL of air at pressures up to 300 mm Hg; if no resistance is met with an inflated cuff, two additional cycles occur. If the BP Luer is inadvertently connected to an intravenous line when the device cycles, more than 1,500 mL of air can enter the client's vascular system.

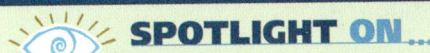

SPOTLIGHT ON...

Professionalism

Vital Signs Measurement

What happens when we do anything routinely? Do we recognize the significance of a routine action? Vital signs are taken routinely. The nurse should be able to identify possible negative consequences of this routine nursing action.

The majority of clients will require medications to achieve their goal blood pressure reading of less than 140/90 mm Hg. According to the JNC 7 (NIH, 2003), stage 1 hypertension should be treated with a thiazide-type diuretic, and stage 2 hypertension will require two or more antihypertensive medications.

Another strategy addressed in the new guidelines is to build trusting provider-client relationships that will motivate clients to achieve good health. Clients' attitudes are influenced by their cultural backgrounds, beliefs, and previous experiences with the health care system; thus, the plan of therapy must be client centered.

Nursing Considerations

Before checking a blood pressure, review the client's chart for brachial artery contraindications, and make sure that the client has not exercised or eaten for the past 30 minutes. Clients who have recently eaten, ambulated, or experienced an emotional upset will have a falsely high blood pressure reading. When the vital signs are taken correctly in sequence (T-P-R and BP), the client should be calm from sitting or lying quietly.

Faulty techniques that constrict blood flow will produce a falsely high pressure reading:

- A cuff too narrow for the extremity
- A cuff that does not fit snugly around the extremity
- A cuff that is deflated too slowly

Other false high readings occur when the mercury column in the manometer is not positioned flat on a firm surface or is read above eye level or the extremity is below the heart's apex level.

False low readings occur when the extremity is above the heart's apex level, the cuff is too wide for the extremity, or the mercury column in the manometer is read below eye level. If the nurse fails to recognize the **auscultatory gap**, the temporary disappearance of sounds at the end of Korotkoff's sounds phase I and beginning of phase II, the systolic pressure is read at a falsely low pressure.

DOCUMENTATION The nurse should record the blood pressure measurement on the appropriate form. If the brachial artery is not used for the measurement, indicate the site when recording the results. If the pressure was obtained by palpation, record "80 systolic by palpation."

Monitoring blood pressure changes in relation to T-P-R measurements is one of the major responsibilities of the registered nurse. One element of critical thinking is having concrete, objective clinical data, as provided by vital signs measurements, to direct decision making.

<table>
<tr><td>
PROCEDURE 26-1
</td><td>
Measuring Body Temperature
</td></tr>
</table>

EQUIPMENT

- Thermometer (one of the following)
  — Electronic thermometer with disposable protective sheathing
  — Tympanic membrane thermometer with probe cover
  — Disposable, single-use chemical strip thermometer
- Lubricant for rectal thermometer
- Two pairs of nonsterile gloves
- Tissues

ACTION	RATIONALE
1. Review medical record for baseline data factors that influence vital signs.	1. Establishes parameters for client's normal measurements, provides direction in device selection, and helps determine site to use for measurement. Vital signs are measured in the order of temperature, pulse, and respiration (TPR) and blood pressure (BP), usually without interruptions, to provide the nurse with an objective clinical database to direct decision making.
2. Explain to the client that vital signs will be assessed. Encourage the client to remain still; refrain from drinking, eating, and smoking; and avoid mouth breathing, if possible.	2. Encourages participation, allays anxiety, and ensures accurate measurements. Cold or hot liquids and smoking alter circulation and body temperature. Mouth breathing can alter temperature.
3. Assess client's toileting needs, and proceed as appropriate.	3. Prevents interruptions during measurements, communicates caring, and promotes client's comfort.
4. Gather equipment.	4. Facilitates organized assessment and measurement.
5. Provide for privacy.	5. Decreases embarrassment.
6. Perform hand hygiene/wash hands, and apply gloves when appropriate.	6. Reduces transmission of microorganisms. Hands are washed before and after every contact with a client. Gloves are worn to avoid contact with bodily secretions and to reduce transmission of microorganisms.

ORAL TEMPERATURE—ELECTRONIC THERMOMETER

7. Repeat Actions 1 to 6.	7. See Rationales 1 to 6.
8. Place disposable protective sheath over probe (see Figure 26-6 on page 525).	8. Reduces transmission of microorganisms.
9. Grasp top of the probe's stem. Avoid placing pressure on the ejection button.	9. Pressure on the ejection button releases the sheath from the probe.
10. Place tip of thermometer under the client's tongue and along the gumline to the posterior sublingual pocket lateral to center of the lower jaw (see Figure 26-7 on page 525).	10. Sublingual pocket contains superficial blood vessels.

(Continues)

PROCEDURE 26-1
Measuring Body Temperature (Continued)

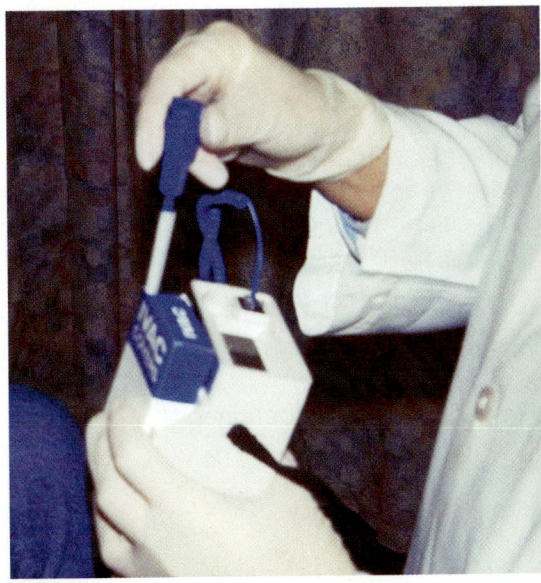

FIGURE 26-6 Place disposable sheath over probe. DELMAR/CENGAGE LEARNING

11. Instruct client to keep mouth closed around thermometer.

12. Thermometer will signal (beep) when a constant temperature registers (see Figure 26-8).
13. Read measurement on digital display of electronic thermometer. Push ejection button to discard disposable sheath into receptacle, and return to storage well.
14. Inform client of temperature reading.
15. Remove gloves and perform hand hygiene.
16. Record reading according to institution policies.

17. Return electronic thermometer unit to charging base.

18. Wash hands/hand hygiene.

11. Maintains thermometer in proper place and decreases amount of time required for an accurate reading.
12. Signal indicates final temperature reading.
13. Reduces transmission of microorganisms. Ensures that the electronic system is ready for next use.
14. Promotes client's participation in care.
15. Reduces transmission of microorganisms.
16. Accurate documentation by site allows for comparison of data.
17. Ensures charging base is plugged into electrical outlet and ready for next use.
18. Reduces transmission of microorganisms.

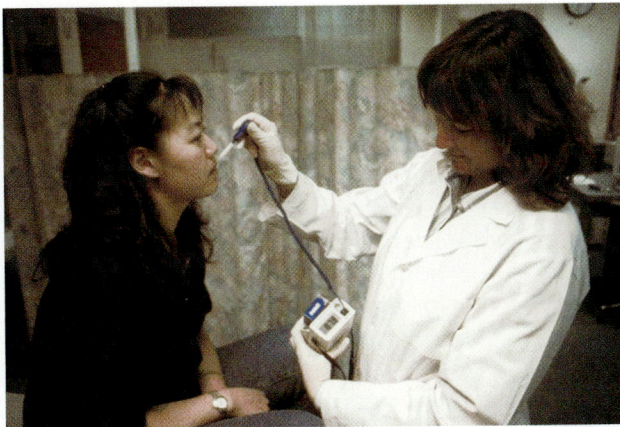

FIGURE 26-7 Place probe tip in the posterior sublingual pocket. DELMAR/CENGAGE LEARNING

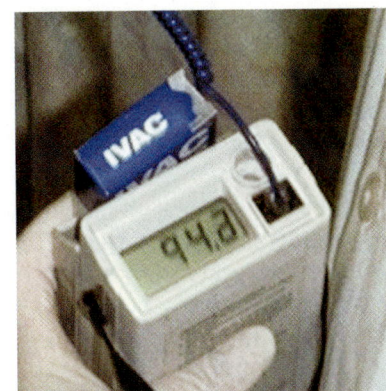

FIGURE 26-8 Listen for audible beep signal when temperature registers. DELMAR/CENGAGE LEARNING

(Continues)

PROCEDURE 26-1
Measuring Body Temperature (Continued)

TYMPANIC TEMPERATURE: INFRARED THERMOMETER

19. Repeat Actions 1 to 6.
20. Position client in Sims' or sitting position.
21. Remove probe from container, and attach probe cover to tympanic thermometer unit (see Figure 26-9).
22. Turn client's head to one side. For an adult, pull pinna upward and back; for a child, pull down and back. Gently insert probe with firm pressure into ear canal (see Figure 26-10).

23. Remove probe after the reading is displayed on digital unit (usually 2 seconds).
24. Remove probe cover and replace in storage container.
25. Return tympanic thermometer to storage unit.

26. Record reading according to institution policy.

27. Wash hands/hand hygiene.

19. See Rationales 1 to 6.
20. Promotes access to ear.
21. Prevents contamination.

22. Provides access to ear canal. Gentle insertion prevents trauma to external canal. Firm pressure is needed to ensure probe will record an accurate temperature.
23. Reading is displayed within seconds.

24. Prevents damage to the reusable probe.
25. Recharges batteries of unit for future use.
26. Promotes accurate documentation for data comparison.
27. Reduces transmission of microorganisms.

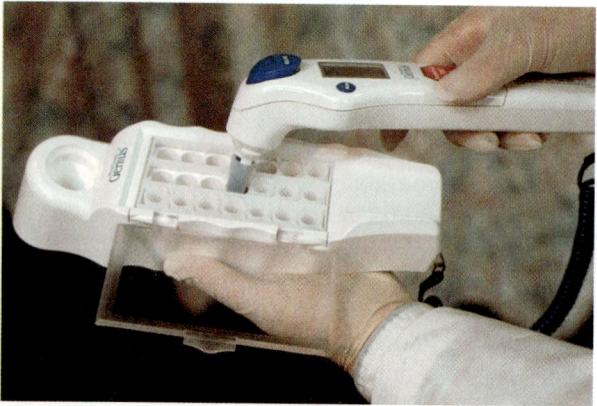

FIGURE 26-9 Attach disposable probe cover to unit.
DELMAR/CENGAGE LEARNING

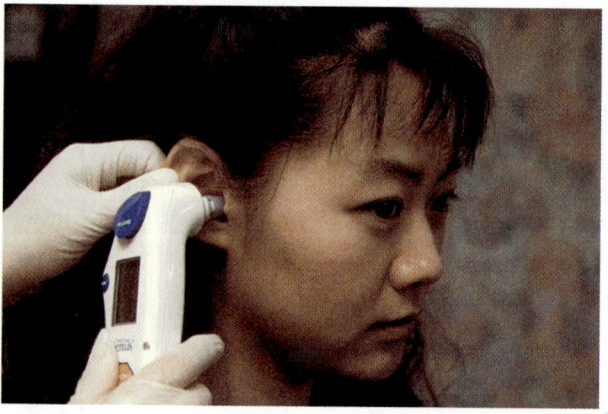

FIGURE 26-10 Insert temperature probe into ear canal.
DELMAR/CENGAGE LEARNING

ORAL GLASS THERMOMETER

28. Repeat Actions 1 to 6.
29. Hold end (tip will be blue) of glass thermometer by fingertips (see Figure 26-11 on page 527), rinse under cool water, and wipe dry with a tissue from bulb's end toward fingertips.

30. Read mercury level while gently rotating thermometer at eye level. It should read 35.5°C (96°F). If the mercury is above desired level, grasp tip of thermometer securely, stand away from solid objects, and sharply flick wrist downward.
31. Place thermometer into oral sublingual pocket as shown in Figure 26-7; leave thermometer in place 3 minutes.

28. See Rationales 1 to 6.
29. A blue tip usually denotes an oral thermometer. Rinsing removes disinfectant, and cool water prevents expansion of the mercury. Holding the thermometer at the opposite end reduces contamination of the bulb.
30. Thermometer must be below normal body temperature. Briskly shaking lowers mercury level in glass tube.

31. Ensures contact with large blood vessel under the tongue.

(Continues)

PROCEDURE 26-1
Measuring Body Temperature (Continued)

Remove thermometer, and wipe off secretions with a clean tissue, moving toward the bulb. With the thermometer at eye level, read finding. Shake thermometer down, cleanse with soapy water, rinse with cool water, and store thermometer in storage container.

Thermometer must stay in place long enough to obtain an accurate reading. Mucus on the thermometer may interfere with disinfectant solution's effectiveness. Wipe from area of least contamination to area of most contamination. Ensures accurate reading.

32. Wash hands/hand hygiene.
33. Record temperature, indicate the method, and discard the thermometer.
34. Repeat Actions 1 to 6.
35. Position the client in a sitting or lying position with the head of the bed elevated from 45 degrees to 60 degrees for measurement of all vital signs except those designated otherwise.

32. Reduces transmission of microorganisms.
33. Nursing documentation, practice clean technique.
34. See Rationales 1 to 6.
35. Promotes comfort, and improves site access for all measurements. Activity and movement can elevate heart and respiratory rates.

RECTAL TEMPERATURE—ELECTRONIC THERMOMETER

36. Repeat Actions 1 to 9.
37. Place client in the Sims' position with upper knee flexed. Adjust sheet to expose only anal area.

38. Place tissues in easy reach. Apply gloves.

39. Lubricate tip of rectal probe (a rectal probe usually has a red cap; see Figure 26-11).
40. With dominant hand, grasp top of the probe's stem. With other hand, separate buttocks to expose anus (see Figure 26-12 on page 528).

41. Instruct the client to take a deep breath. Insert the probe gently into anus: infant, 1.2 cm (0.5 inches); adult, 3.5 cm (1.5 inches). If resistance is felt, do not force insertion.
42. Repeat Actions 12 to 18.

36. See Rationales 1 to 6.
37. Proper positioning ensures visualization of anus. Flexing knee relaxes muscles for ease of insertion.
38. Tissue is needed to wipe anus after device is removed.
39. Promotes ease of insertion of thermometer or probe.
40. Aids in visualization of anus.

41. Relaxes anal sphincter. Gentle insertion decreases discomfort to client and prevents trauma to mucous membranes.

42. See Rationales 12 to 18.

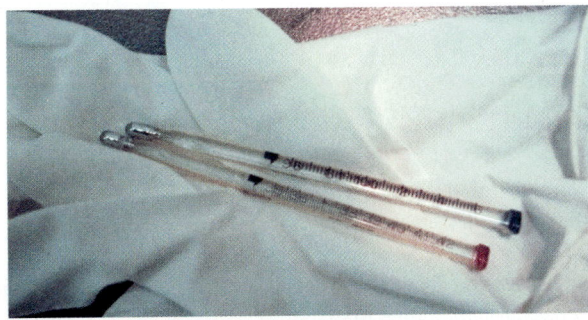

FIGURE 26-11 Oral (blue tip) and rectal (red tip) glass thermometers. ALTMAN, G. B. (2004). DELMAR'S FUNDAMENTAL & ADVANCED NURSING SKILLS. CLIFTON PARK, NY: DELMAR/CENGAGE LEARNING.

(Continues)

PROCEDURE 26-1
Measuring Body Temperature (Continued)

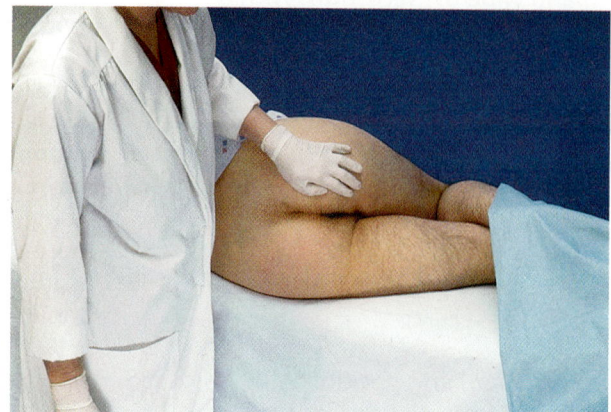

FIGURE 26-12 Preparation for the insertion of a rectal thermometer. DELMAR/CENGAGE LEARNING

AXILLARY TEMPERATURE

43. Repeat Actions 1 to 10.
44. Remove client's arm and shoulder from one sleeve of gown. Avoid exposing chest.
45. Make sure axillary skin is dry; if necessary, pat dry.

46. Place probe into center of axilla. Fold the client's upper arm straight down, and place arm across the client's chest.
47. Repeat Actions 12 to 18.

43. See Rationales 1 to 10.
44. Exposes axillary area.
45. Removes moisture and prevents a false low reading.
46. Puts device into contact with axillary blood supply. Maintains the device in proper position.
47. See Rationales 12 to 18.

DISPOSABLE (CHEMICAL STRIP) THERMOMETER

48. Repeat Actions 1 to 6.
49. Apply tape to appropriate skin area, usually forehead.

50. Observe tape for color changes.

51. Record reading and indicate method.

52. Wash hands/hand hygiene.

48. See Rationales 1 to 6.
49. Tape must be in direct contact with the client's skin.
50. Color indicates temperature reading (refer to the manufacturer's instructions).
51. Promotes accurate documentation for data comparison.
52. Reduces transmission of microorganisms.

delegation tip

The skill of temperature measurement is often delegated to ancillary personnel; however, the nurse retains responsibility for knowledge of the client's temperature and appropriate actions. The expectation is that ancillary personnel will have documented instruction and competency validation of their ability to:

- *Select the correct route for measurement of the temperature*
- *Correctly position the client for measurement*
- *Correctly perform the measurement according to established guidelines and record on the appropriate flow sheet (clinical record)*
- *Recognize and report abnormal findings to the nurse*

nursing tips

After giving antipyretic medication to a client, a temperature measurement should be taken 30 minutes after the intervention and then every 2 to 4 hours. Nursing intervention policy may vary across institutions.

PROCEDURE 26-2   Assessing Pulse Rate

EQUIPMENT

- Watch with a second hand
- Stethoscope
- Alcohol swab
- Gloves

ACTION	RATIONALE
TAKING A RADIAL (WRIST) PULSE	
1. Wash hands/hand hygiene.	1. Reduces transmission of microorganisms.
2. Inform client of the site(s) where pulse will be measured.	2. Encourages participation and allays anxiety.
3. Flex client's elbow and place lower part of arm across chest.	3. Maintains wrist in full extension and exposes artery for palpation. Placing client's hand over chest will facilitate later respiratory assessment without undue attention to the nurse's action. (It is difficult for any person to maintain a normal breathing pattern when someone is observing and measuring.)
4. Support client's wrist by grasping outer aspect with thumb.	4. Stabilizes wrist and allows for pressure to be exerted.
5. Place index and middle fingers on inner aspect of client's wrist over the radial artery, and apply light but firm pressure until pulse is palpated (see Figure 26-13).	5. Fingertips are sensitive, facilitating palpation of pulsating pulse. The nurse may feel his or her own pulse if palpating with thumb. Applying light pressure prevents occlusion of blood flow and pulsation.
6. Identify pulse rhythm.	6. Palpate pulse until rhythm is determined. Describe as regular or irregular.
7. Determine pulse volume.	7. Quality of pulse strength is an indication of stroke volume. Describe as normal, weak, strong, or bounding.
8. Count pulse rate by using second hand on watch (see Figure 26-14).	8. An irregular rhythm requires a full minute of assessment to identify the

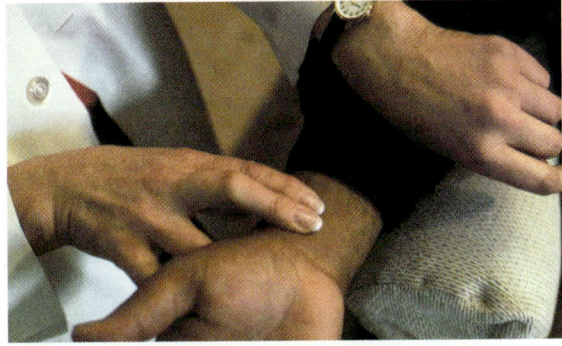

FIGURE 26-13 Place index and middle fingers over radial artery. DELMAR/CENGAGE LEARNING

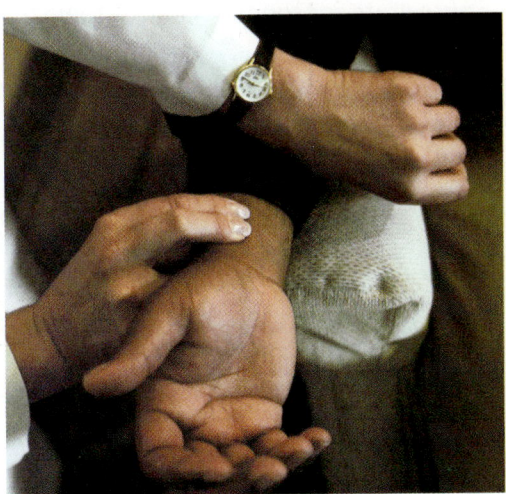

FIGURE 26-14 Count pulse rate for 30 seconds. Multiply by 2. DELMAR/CENGAGE LEARNING

(Continues)

PROCEDURE 26-2
Assessing Pulse Rate (Continued)

ACTION	RATIONALE
• For a regular rhythm, count number of beats for 30 seconds and multiply by 2. • For an irregular rhythm, count number of beats for a full minute, noting number of irregular beats.	number of inefficient cardiac contractions that fail to transmit a pulsation, referred to as a "skipped" or irregular beat.

TAKING AN APICAL PULSE

9. Wash hands/hand hygiene.
10. Raise client's gown to expose sternum and left side of chest.
11. Cleanse earpiece and diaphragm of stethoscope with an alcohol swab.

12. Put stethoscope around neck.

13. Locate apex of heart:
   • With client lying on left side, locate suprasternal notch.
   • Palpate second intercostal space to left of sternum.
   • Place index finger in intercostal space, counting downward until fifth intercostal space is located.
   • Move index finger along fourth intercostal space left of the sternal border and to the fifth intercostal space left of the mid-clavicular line to palpate the point of maximal impulse (PMI) (see Figure 26-15).
   • Keep index finger of nondominant hand on the PMI.
14. Inform client that his or her heart will be listened to. Instruct client to remain silent.
15. With dominant hand, put earpiece of the stethoscope in ears and grasp diaphragm of the stethoscope in the palm of the hand for 5 to 10 seconds.

16. Place diaphragm of stethoscope over the PMI and auscultate for sounds S_1 and S_2 to hear lub-dub sound (see Figure 26-16).

9. Reduces transmission of microorganisms.
10. Allows access to client's chest for proper placement of stethoscope.
11. Decreases transmission of microorganisms from one prescribing practitioner to another (earpiece) and from one client to another (diaphragm).
12. Ensures stethoscope is nearby for frequent use.
13. Identification of landmarks facilitates correct placement of the stethoscope at the fifth intercostal space in order to hear PMI.
   • Ensures correct placement of stethoscope.

14. Elicits client support. Stethoscope amplifies noise.
15. Dominant hand facilitates psychomotor dexterity for placement of earpiece with one hand. Heat warms metal or plastic diaphragm and prevents startling client.

16. Movement of blood through the heart valves creates S_1 and S_2 sounds. Listen for a regular rhythm

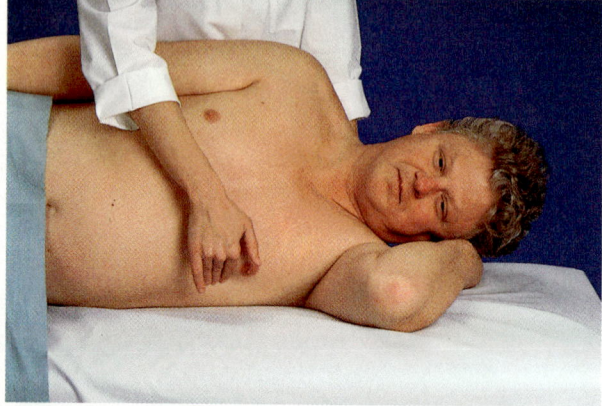

FIGURE 26-15 Palpating the apical pulse. DELMAR/CENGAGE LEARNING

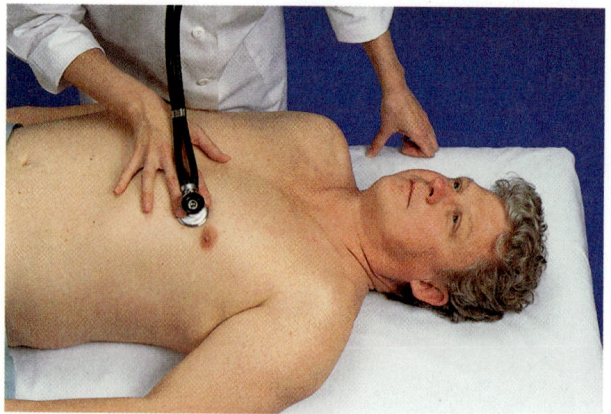

FIGURE 26-16 Place diaphragm of stethoscope over the PMI to hear the heart rate. DELMAR/CENGAGE LEARNING

(Continues)

PROCEDURE 26-2
Assessing Pulse Rate (Continued)

ACTION	RATIONALE
	(heartbeats are evenly spaced) before counting.
17. Note regularity of rhythm.	17. Establishment of a rhythmic pattern determines length of time to count the heartbeats to ensure accurate measurement.

18. Start to count while looking at second hand of watch. Count lub-dub sound as one beat:
  • For a regular rhythm, count rate for 30 seconds and multiply by 2.
  • For an irregular rhythm, count rate for a full minute, noting number of irregular beats.
	18. Ensures sufficient time to count irregular beats.

19. Share findings with client.	19. Promotes client participation in care.
20. Record by site the rate, rhythm, and, if applicable, number of irregular beats.	20. Record rate and characteristics at bedside to ensure accurate documentation.
21. Wash hands/hand hygiene.	21. Reduces transmission of microorganisms.

delegation tip

The radial pulse assessment is often delegated to trained ancillary personnel; however, the nurse is responsible for knowing the results. Assessment of the apical pulse may be delegated to specially prepared staff. The assessment of peripheral circulation is delegated after proper training in the monitoring of peripheral sites for the presence of abnormal color, motion, or sensation in the extremity. The absence of pulses must be immediately reported for further assessment by the nurse, and the nurse is responsible for reviewing the data collected in a timely manner and revalidating the results, if indicated. The institution's policy should clearly indicate the training and validation requirements before the nurse delegates the monitoring of apical pulses and peripheral vascular assessments on stable clients. These tasks should not be delegated if the client is unstable.

nursing tips

If taking an apical pulse, have the client breathe normally through the nose; breathing through the nose decreases breath sounds and makes the heart sounds easier to hear.

PROCEDURE 26-3
Assessing Respiration

EQUIPMENT

- Watch with a second hand
- Stethoscope, if needed

ACTION	RATIONALE
1. Wash hands/hand hygiene.	1. Reduces transmission of microorganisms.
2. Be sure chest movement is visible. Client may need to remove heavy clothing.	2. Facilitates observation of chest wall and abdominal movements.

(Continues)

PROCEDURE 26-3
Assessing Respiration (Continued)

ACTION	RATIONALE
3. Observe one complete respiratory cycle. If it is easier, place the client's hand across the abdomen and your hand over the client's wrist.	3. Helps determine what constitutes a breath. Helps determine what to count. Hand rises and falls with inspiration and expiration.
4. Start counting with first inspiration while looking at the second hand of a watch (see Figure 26-17). • Infants and children: Count a full minute. • Adults: Count for 30 seconds and multiply by 2. If an irregular rate or rhythm is present, count for a full minute.	4. Respiratory rate is one complete cycle (inspiration and expiration). • Infants and children usually have an irregular rate.
5. Observe character of respirations: • Depth of respirations by degree of chest wall movement (shallow, normal, or deep) • Rhythm of cycle (regular or interrupted)	5. Reveals volume of air movement into and out of the lungs.
6. Replace client's gown if needed.	6. Prevents embarrassment and chilling.
7. Record rate and character of respirations.	7. Record rate and characteristics at bedside to ensure accurate documentation.
8. Wash hands/hand hygiene.	8. Reduces transmission of microorganisms.

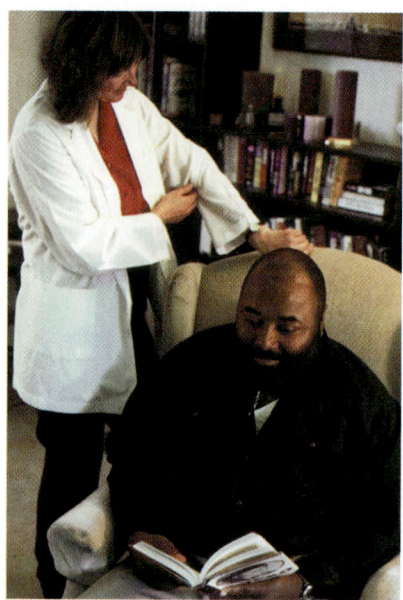

FIGURE 26-17 Count inspirations for a full 30 seconds. Multiply by 2. DELMAR/CENGAGE LEARNING

delegation tip

The skill of respiratory rate measurement is often delegated to properly trained ancillary personnel; however, the nurse is responsible for this information and appropriate action. Respiration counts over 30 (adult) or 60 (child) should immediately be reported to the nurse for further assessment.

nursing tips

Fear, pain, and anger can easily raise the respiratory rate. If these emotions are present, consider assessing the rate again at a later time when the client appears calmer.

PROCEDURE 26-4 — Assessing Blood Pressure

EQUIPMENT

- Stethoscope
- Gloves, if required
- Alcohol swabs
- Sphygmomanometer/bladder with mercury column or aneroid dial

ACTION	RATIONALE
AUSCULTATION METHOD USING BRACHIAL ARTERY	
1. Wash hands/hand hygiene.	1. Reduces transmission of microorganisms.
2. Determine which extremity is most appropriate for reading. Do not take a pressure reading on an injured or a painful extremity or one in which an intravenous line is running.	2. Cuff inflation can temporarily interrupt blood flow and compromise circulation in an extremity already impaired or a vein receiving intravenous fluid.
3. Select a cuff size appropriate for the client. Estimate by inspection or measure with a tape the circumference of the bare upper arm at the midpoint between the shoulder (acromion) and the elbow (olecranon process) (see Figure 26-18).	3. The bladder inside the cuff should encircle 80% of the arm in adults and 100% of the arm of children less than 13 years old. If in doubt, use a larger cuff to ensure equalization of pressure on the artery and accurate measurement.
4. Have the client's bare arm resting on a support so the midpoint of the upper arm is at the level of the heart. Extend the elbow with palm turned upward.	4. Blood pressure increases when the arm is below the level of the heart and decreases when the arm is above the level of the heart.
5. Make sure the bladder cuff is fully deflated and the pump valve moves freely. Place the manometer so the center of the mercury column or aneroid dial is at eye level and easily visible to the observer.	5. Equipment must be visible and must function properly to obtain an accurate reading.
6. Palpate the brachial artery, in the antecubital space, and place the cuff so that the midline of the bladder is over the arterial pulsation. Next, wrap and secure the cuff snugly around the client's bare upper arm. The lower edge of the cuff should be 1 inch (2 cm) above the antecubital fossa (bend of the elbow), where the head of the stethoscope is to be placed (see Figures 26-19 and 26-20 on page 534).	6. Ensures even pressure distribution over the brachial artery. Rolling up the sleeve may form a tourniquet around the upper arm. Always use a bare arm.

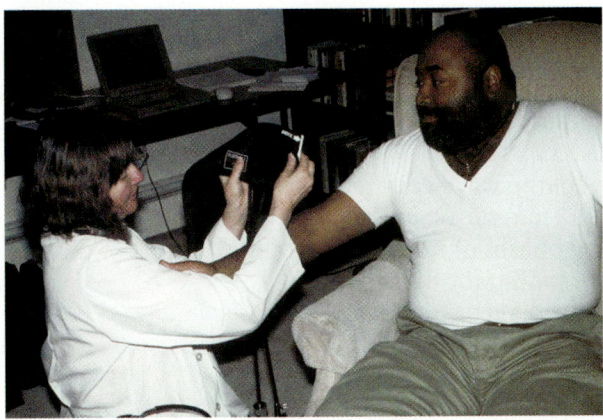

FIGURE 26-18 Select proper cuff size. An obese client may need a larger-size cuff to obtain an accurate reading. DELMAR/CENGAGE LEARNING

(Continues)

PROCEDURE 26-4
Assessing Blood Pressure (Continued)

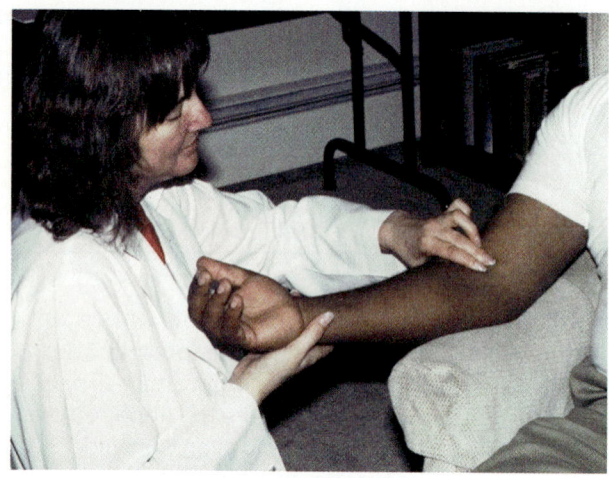

FIGURE 26-19 Palpate the brachial artery to determine placement of the stethoscope. DELMAR/CENGAGE LEARNING

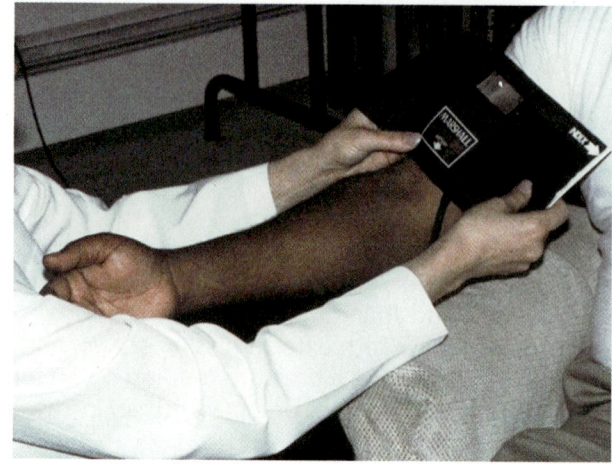

FIGURE 26-20 Center the blood pressure cuff over the brachial artery. DELMAR/CENGAGE LEARNING

ACTION	RATIONALE
7. Inflate the cuff rapidly to 70 mm Hg and increase by 10-mm increments while palpating the radial pulse. Note the level of pressure at which the pulse disappears and subsequently reappears during deflation.	7. The palpatory method provides the necessary preliminary approximation of systolic blood pressure to ensure an accurate reading. When frequent measurements are required, such as every 15 minutes, the palpatory method is generally not incorporated with each pressure check.
8. Insert the earpieces of the stethoscope into the ear canals with a forward tilt to fit snugly.	8. The bell, the low-frequency position of the stethoscope, enhances sound transmission from chestpiece to ears.
9. Relocate the brachial artery with nondominant hand, and place the bell of the stethoscope over the brachial artery pulsation. The bell should be held firmly in place, ensuring that the head is in direct contact with the skin and not touching the cuff (see Figure 26-21 on page 535).	9. Sound is heard best directly over the artery. Wedging the head of the stethoscope under the edge of the cuff results in considerable extraneous noise and may cause an inaccurate reading.
10. With dominant hand, turn the valve clockwise to close. Compress the pump to inflate the cuff rapidly and steadily until the manometer registers 20 to 30 mm Hg above the level previously determined by the palpation (see Figure 26-22 on page 535).	10. Prevents air leaks during inflation. Ensures the cuff is inflated to a pressure greater than the client's systolic pressure.

11. Partially unscrew (open) the valve counterclockwise to deflate the bladder at 2 mm/sec while listening for the appearance of the five phases of Korotkoff's sounds. Note the manometer reading for these sounds.
   I. A faint, clear, tapping sound that increases in intensity
   II. Swishing sound
   III. Intense sound
	11. Maintains constant release of pressure to ensure hearing first systolic sound. Identify manometer readings for each of the five phases.
	  • For children less than 13 years old, use phase IV sounds as the diastolic level. Even though five phases of Korotkoff's

(Continues)

PROCEDURE 26-4
Assessing Blood Pressure (Continued)

ACTION	RATIONALE
IV. Abrupt, distinctive, muffled sound V. Sound disappears (See Table 26-13 for more information about Korotkoff's sounds.)	sounds have been identified, most clients have only two clearly distinct sounds (phase I and V), identified as the systolic and diastolic sounds.
12. After the last Korotkoff's sound is heard, deflate the cuff slowly for at least another 10 mm Hg to ensure that no other sounds are audible; then, deflate rapidly and completely (see Figure 26-23).	12. Prevents arterial occlusion and client discomfort from numbness or tingling.

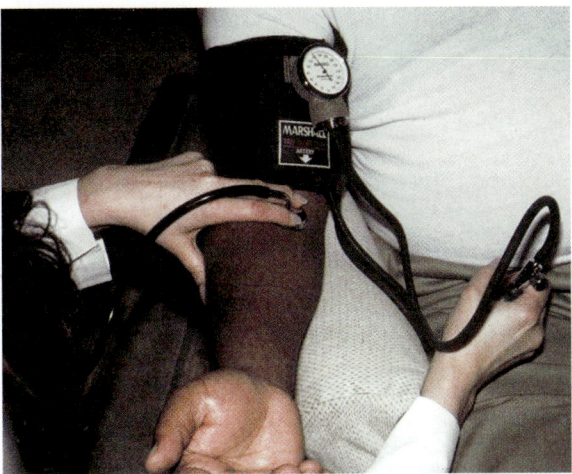

FIGURE 26-21 The stethoscope chestpiece should not touch the blood pressure cuff. DELMAR/CENGAGE LEARNING

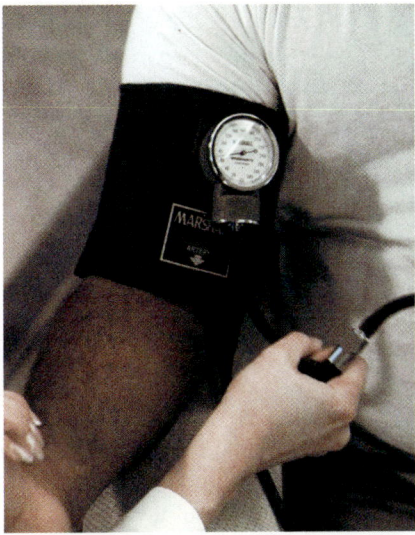

FIGURE 26-22 Compress the pump to inflate the blood pressure cuff. DELMAR/CENGAGE LEARNING

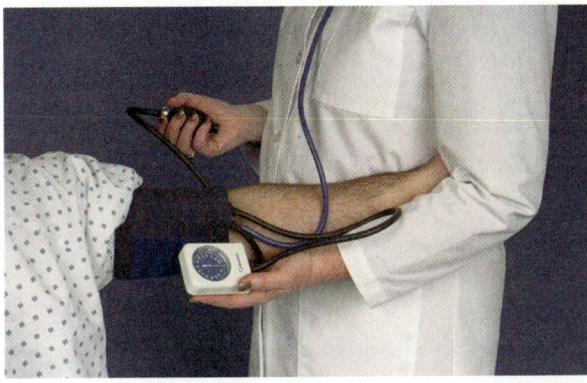

FIGURE 26-23 Deflate the cuff completely and wait at least 2 minutes before taking a second reading. DELMAR/CENGAGE LEARNING

(Continues)

PROCEDURE 26-4
Assessing Blood Pressure (Continued)

ACTION	RATIONALE
13. Allow the client to rest for at least 30 seconds and remove cuff. Take two or more additional readings and average them. (The American Heart Association recommends that the repeated measurements should be done after 30-minute intervals in the same or opposite arm; the Joint National Commission recommends a 2-minute interval between repeated measurements.)	13. Releases trapped blood in the vessels. Ensures accurate measurement.
14. Inform the client of the reading.	14. Promotes client's participation in health care.
15. The systolic (phase I) and diastolic (phase V) pressure should be immediately recorded, rounded off (upward) to the nearest 2 mm Hg.	15. Ensures accuracy. In children and when sounds are heard nearly to the level of 0 mm Hg, the phase IV pressure should also be recorded.
16. If appropriate, lower bed, raise side rails, and place call light within easy reach.	16. Promotes client's safety.
17. Put all equipment within proper place.	17. Fosters maintenance of equipment.
18. Wash hands/hand hygiene.	18. Reduces transmission of microorganisms.

delegation tip

The measurement of blood pressure is often delegated to ancillary personnel who have been properly educated to use both manual and electronic equipment; however, the nurse is responsible for carefully monitoring this information for significant changes and taking appropriate action. The measurement of blood pressure would be reserved for a client in stable physical condition and measured at sites without intravenous solutions infusing, dialysis shunt or fistula, painful extremity, or recent mastectomy.

nursing tips

A blood pressure cuff that is too small for the client's arm will often come unfastened as it is inflated.

KEY CONCEPTS

- Baseline values establish the norm; variations from normal may indicate possible problems with the client's health status.

- The assessment of physiological functioning provides specific data regarding the client's current condition.

- Thermoregulation is the body's physiological function of heat regulation to maintain a constant internal body temperature.

- Hemodynamic regulation is the body's physiological function of blood circulation to maintain an appropriate environment in all the tissue fluids.

- The pulse is caused by the stroke volume ejection and distension of the walls of the aorta, which creates a pulse wave as it travels rapidly toward the distal ends of the arteries.

- Blood pressure is the measurement of pressure pulsations exerted against the blood vessel walls during cardiac systole and diastole. It is measured in terms of millimeters of mercury (mm Hg).

- Several factors cause changes in one or more of the vital signs: age, sex, exercise and metabolism, anxiety and stress, postural and diurnal variations, hormones, pain, medications, and alterations in physiological functions.

- The normal values and variations in vital signs measurement are usually based on age.

- All pieces of equipment used to measure the vital signs and to perform a physical assessment should be maintained to function accurately.

- Clinical data regarding the efficacy of blood circulation to an extremity are obtained by assessing all of the characteristics (rate, quality, rhythm, and volume) of the peripheral pulses.

- When assessing ventilation, ascertain the rate, depth, and rhythm of ventilatory movement.

- Before checking a blood pressure, review the client's chart for brachial artery contraindications, and make sure the client has not exercised or eaten for the past 30 minutes.

REVIEW QUESTIONS

1. The measurement of blood that enters the aorta with each ventricular contraction is called the
   _____.
   a. Pulse
   b. Stroke volume
   c. Cardiac output
   d. Pulse pressure

2. A 69-year-old woman is admitted with dizziness, confusion, and dyspnea. Which vital sign should not be delegated to trained ancillary personnel?
   a. Temperature
   b. Pulse
   c. Respiratory rate
   d. Blood pressure

3. Prioritize your nursing interventions based on the vital signs.
   a. Temperature 102.4°F (39.1°C), oral, electronic thermometer
   b. Heart rate 130 beats/min, apical
   c. Respiratory rate 25 breaths/min
   d. BP 145/80

4. A client is admitted with a head injury and may develop neurogenic fever. Which nursing diagnosis would be most appropriate for this client?
   a. *Risk for imbalanced body temperature*
   b. *Hyperthermia*
   c. *Hypothermia*
   d. *Ineffective thermoregulation*

5. According to the JNC's seventh report, a BP reading of 144/96 would be considered _____.
   a. Normal
   b. Prehypertension
   c. Stage 1 hypertension
   d. Stage 2 hypertension

6. Developing a trusting provider-client relationship encourages the client to _____.
   a. Talk about his or her feelings and needs
   b. Take his or her medicines
   c. Live a productive life
   d. Maintain a positive attitude toward his or her illness

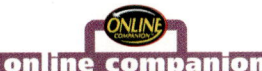

online companion

Visit the DeLaune and Ladner online companion resource at **www.delmar.cengage.com** for additional content and study aids. Click on Online Companions, then select the Nursing discipline.

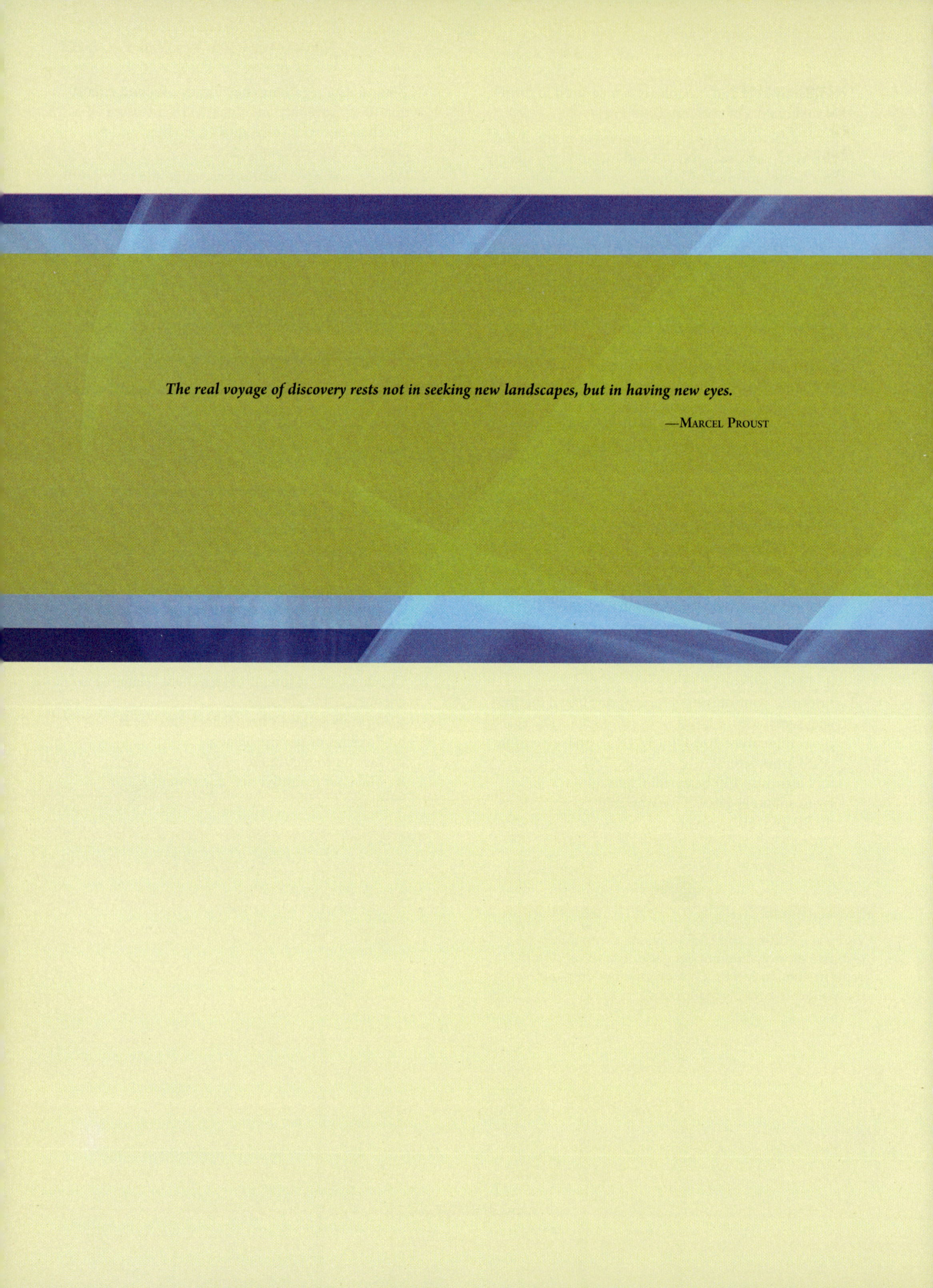

The real voyage of discovery rests not in seeking new landscapes, but in having new eyes.

—Marcel Proust

CHAPTER 27

Physical Assessment

COMPETENCIES

1. Describe the correct positioning of the client for performing a physical examination.
2. Explain techniques used in conducting a physical examination.
3. Describe the significance of assessment findings obtained from a physical examination.
4. Discuss documentation of data obtained from a physical examination.

KEY TERMS

adventitious breath sounds
aneurysm
angina
aphasia
arthritis
ascites
atrophy
bronchial sounds
bronchovesicular sounds
bruits
crackles
crepitus
cystocele
dermatome map
dullness

extinction
Glasgow Coma Scale
goniometer
graphesthesia
heaves
hypertonicity
hypertrophy
hypotonicity
integumentary system
ischemia
murmur
myocardial infarction
nystagmus
osteoarthritis
pleural friction rub

regurgitation
rhonchi
Snellen chart
stenosis
stereognosis
striae
stridor
supernumery nipples
tactile fremitus
thrills
tympany
vesicular sounds
wheezes

The physical examination is performed in all health care settings on clients of every age in order to gather comprehensive, pertinent assessment data. The physical examination provides a complete picture of the client's physiological functioning. When combined with a health and psychosocial assessment, it forms a database to use in decision making. See Chapter 6 for a discussion of psychosocial assessment and health history. The nurse uses information from the assessment, health history, and physical examination to develop a client profile. Health history ascertains the client's chief complaint and directs the focus of physical examination.

PURPOSES OF PHYSICAL EXAMINATION

The physical examination provides the database from which all interventions are planned. The complete assessment data are used to:

- Ascertain the client's level of health and physiological function
- Identify factors placing the client at risk for problems
- Determine areas of preventive nursing
- Confirm alterations, disease, or inability to perform the activities of daily living
- Identify the need for additional testing or examination
- Evaluate the outcomes of treatment and therapy

The physical examination is done in a sequential, head-to-toe fashion to ensure a thorough assessment of the client. This method not only prevents the nurse from forgetting to examine an area, it also decreases the number of times the nurse and the client have to change positions.

After gaining proficiency in performing the physical examination, nurses should be able to integrate assessment into daily care activities. For example, while weighing the client, observe posture, motor activity, and gait. This chapter provides in-depth information with detailed descriptions for conducting a complete physical examination. Keep in mind that none of these skills should override the nurse's use of observation and inspection; see the Uncovering the Evidence display on page 542.

PREPARATION FOR PHYSICAL EXAMINATION

Many clients become anxious about being physically exposed and/or experiencing pain during the examination. Because the client will experience some anxieties, it is important for the nurse to keep the client informed while performing the examination. The nurse needs to be organized and demonstrate respect for the client's apprehension during the examination.

It is important that the nurse appear calm, organized, and competent. A review of the agency's physical examination form before meeting with the client ensures that the nurse can fully explain the actions that will be performed and prevents omission of any area required to be assessed.

Environment

The client and the environment require special consideration. The nurse needs to determine that the environment will accommodate any special needs of the client. Adjust the environment to allow for placement of the equipment on a surface that is clean and free from movement. Remove from the floor any items that would place the client at risk for falling.

The room needs to be quiet, warm, without drafts, and adequately lit. Depending on the setting, make the necessary adjustments to ensure privacy. Inform other personnel about the time of the examination to avoid interruptions, which are frustrating to both client and nurse.

Equipment

The nurse should review the protocol relative to a physical examination and secure the forms required for documenting the assessment findings. Wash hands and gather the necessary equipment. Table 27-1 discusses the equipment needed to conduct a physical examination. Several other items that are frequently used in the physical examination include:

- Aromatic substances (e.g., vanilla) to test the 1st cranial (olfactory) nerve

- Cotton balls to assess sensory response to light touch
- Toothpick to assess sensory response to slight pain
- Drapes to cover the client
- Gloves to reduce the transmission of microorganisms
- Calibrated tape measure for assessing circumference, length, and width
- Tongue depressor to inspect mouth and to stimulate gag reflex for assessing 9th and 10th (glossopharyngeal and vagus) cranial nerves

TABLE 27-1 Equipment and Supplies Used for a Physical Examination

INSTRUMENT		DESCRIPTION AND USAGE
Laryngeal mirror		Metal instrument with mirror to inspect pharynx and oral cavity
Lubricant		Facilitates insertion of instruments into body cavities
Ophthalmoscope		Lighted instrument attached to a battery tube to visualize the eye's interior
Otoscope		Special ear speculum that attaches to an ophthalmoscope to visualize external and middle ear (eardrum)
Penlight		Flashlight to test pupillary reaction to light and assess third, fourth, and sixth (oculomotor, trochlear, and abducens) cranial nerves
Percussion hammer		Instrument with rubber head to test reflexes
Tuning fork		Metal fork that vibrates when tapped and is used to perform Rinne test to assess eighth (acoustic) cranial nerve

Delmar/Cengage Learning

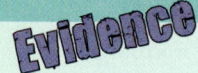

UNCOVERING THE Evidence

TITLE OF STUDY

"A Survey of Physical Assessment Techniques Performed by RNs: Lessons for Nursing Education"

AUTHOR

Jean F. Giddens

PURPOSE

To identify physical examination skills performed by nurses in the clinical setting to better understand the competencies needed by nursing school graduates.

METHODS

This is a descriptive study that involved the administration and analysis of a survey of registered nurse participants. The participants, who were randomly selected, were direct care providers in both inpatient and outpatient settings. The survey consisted of a list of 126 physical examination techniques; participants indicated the average frequency they performed each of the techniques. Eighty percent of the surveys were returned. Simple descriptive statistical applications were used to analyze the data.

FINDINGS

Thirty core techniques were identified by the sample. The majority of these techniques involve inspection and general observation. One-third of the techniques are associated with cardiovascular and respiratory assessment.

IMPLICATIONS

The findings suggest that this sample of registered nurses incorporates a small set of physical examination skills into practice on a regular basis. The majority of these skills involve inspection. The implication for nurse educators is to help students develop greater skills in observing and recognizing cues indicative of changes in client status; in order to do this, it is suggested that less time be spent in great detail on physical examination techniques that are not actually used in clinical practice.

Giddens, J. F. (2007). A survey of physical assessment techniques performed by RNs: Lessons for nursing education. *Journal of Nursing Education, 46*(2), 83–87.

Positioning and Draping

The nurse should position the client to ensure accessibility to the body part being assessed. Table 27-2 on page 543 presents the positions used in conducting a physical examination; contraindications for each position are also described.

The primary purpose of draping the client is to prevent unnecessary exposure during the examination. Feelings of embarrassment elicit tension and restlessness and may decrease the client's ability to cooperate. The drapes also prevent the client from being chilled.

The drape may be paper or cloth, for example—a bath blanket, sheet, or towel. The client's gown can be rearranged to expose or cover different body parts. When the client is in a sitting, supine, Sims', or prone position, use a gown or towel to cover the upper chest and a bath blanket or sheet to cover the rest of the body.

Draping a client in the lithotomy position requires a sheet and boots. The nurse should apply the boots, if available, to cover each of the client's feet and legs. Fold and place the sheet in a diamond-shaped arrangement over the body: top diamond under chin with opposite corner pointing toward the toes and lateral corners pointing toward the sides of the table. Ask the client to flex the knees, and with the lateral corners of the sheet, wrap it in a spiral fashion around the legs and feet. The bottom corner covers the perineum and is folded back over the abdomen to expose the perineum when the examination begins.

GENERAL SURVEY

Assessment begins at the initial contact with the client. Proper terminology and agency-approved abbreviations should be used when recording assessment data.

Assess the following areas during a general survey:

- Signs of distress: labored breathing, pallor or cyanosis, protection of a painful part, sweating or cold moist palms, anxious face
- Client's state of health, stature, and sexual development
- Weight, height, and vital signs
- Posture, motor activity, and gait; dress, grooming, and personal hygiene; and any odors of body and breath
- Client's facial expressions; behaviors; and manner, affect, and reaction to persons and things in environment
- Quality of speech and level of consciousness (See Chapter 38.)

When performing the general survey, it is important to remember the client's cultural context; see the Respecting Our Differences display on page 544. Document general survey data in an organized fashion to portray a clinical picture of the client. Certain clients, such as those who are older, disabled, or abused, will require special consideration during the physical examination.

Sexual History

Prior to performing a physical examination of the genitalia, the nurse should refer to the information obtained from the client's sexual history. Illness and medical interventions can interfere with sexual functioning; for example, antihypertensive medication can cause men to experience ejaculation or erection difficulties. Sexual responsiveness can be altered in both men and women who are taking narcotics, sedatives, antidepressants, and antispasmodic medications. Prolonged therapies, such as chemotherapy or radiation, may cause physiologic changes that affect sexual desire and function; refer to the Nursing Process Highlight on page 544 for elements of a sexual history. "While not every nurse can be a sexual counselor, listening to concerns of

TABLE 27-2 Positioning for a Physical Examination

POSITION	BODY PART ASSESSED	KEY POINTS AND CONTRAINDICATIONS
Sitting	Head, neck, back, posterior thorax and lungs, anterior thorax and lungs, breast, axillae, heart, and extremities	Client can expand lungs; nurse can inspect symmetry. Institute risk precautions (e.g., falls) for older adults and debilitated clients.
Supine	Head, neck, anterior thorax and lungs, breast, axillae, heart, abdomen, and extremities	Client relaxed; decreases abdominal muscle tension; nurse can palpate all peripheral pulses. Contraindicated in clients with cardiopulmonary alterations.
Sims'	Rectum and vagina	Relaxes rectal muscles. Painful for clients with joint deformities.
Prone	Posterior thorax and lungs, hip	Assessment of hip extension. Contraindicated in clients with cardiopulmonary alterations.
Knee-chest	Rectum	Maximal rectal exposure. Contraindicated in clients with respiratory alterations.
Lithotomy	Female genitalia, rectum, and genital tract	Maximal genitalia exposure; embarrassing and uncomfortable for client. Contraindicated in clients with joint disorders.

Delmar/Cengage Learning

patient and family, presenting factual information in a non-threatening manner, managing noncomplex disease and treatment related symptoms, and providing appropriate referrals can be easily incorporated into routine care" (Krebs, 2007, p. 529).

Older Adults

When nurses assess older clients, it is important to know the normal changes that result from aging. See Chapter 19 for a

NURSING PROCESS HIGHLIGHT

Assessment

Sexual History

- Age at which sexual activity began
- History of sexual activity with women, men, or both
- Number of current sexual partners
- Satisfaction in current relationship
- Concerns regarding sexuality or sexual identity
- History of sexually transmitted diseases (STDs)
- Desire for parenting, at present or in the future
- Current or past contraceptive methods
- History of childhood or adult sexual trauma, rape, or domestic abuse

Data from Krebs, L. U. (2007). Sexual assessment: Research and clinical. *Nursing Clinics of North America, 42*(4), 525–529.

complete discussion about caring for older clients. Aging may reduce the body's resistance to illness and tolerance of stress and increase the time needed to recuperate from illness. Make sure the client understands and can follow instructions, and allow extra time if the client has difficulty changing positions.

Disabled Clients

Determine the client's ability to participate before conducting the examination. When assessing disabled clients, nurses should adapt their interactions to the client's ability; for example, a hearing-impaired client should be given a written questionnaire. An intellectually impaired client might require simple, direct sentences and questions or use of pictures. To allay the disabled client's fears and anxiety, allow a family member to remain with the client during the examination. The nurse should ascertain and encourage the client's level of independence.

RESPECTING OUR DIFFERENCES

Cultural Values and Assessment

Cleanliness is highly valued by mainstream American society. However, in some cultures, a daily bath is not perceived as necessary or desirable. Some cultures do not define natural body odors as offensive. It is important to consider the client in the context of cultural beliefs before labeling a client. Think of the terms "dirty," "unkempt," or "foul smelling." These value-laden terms can cloud the assessment process and subsequently the care provided to the client.

Abused Clients

Nurses need to be observant for signs of abuse, especially in children and older adults. The symptoms may be psychological as well as physical, for example, not wanting to be touched, unable to maintain eye contact, or unwillingness to talk about bruises, burns, or other injuries. Abuse-related bruises or lacerations usually appear on breasts, buttocks, thighs, or genitalia. The nurse should also inspect for healed scarring or burns. The nurse needs to know state laws and agency policies for reporting possible abuse. See the accompanying Spotlight On display.

Clients who have been sexually abused require special care. Registered nurses with specialized education and clinical training may serve as a sexual assault nurse examiner (SANE). The SANE nurse is responsible for collecting forensic evidence, documenting the forensic examination, providing appropriate counseling and referral, and coordinating communication with other involved agencies. Many SANE programs provide follow-up with the victim and postexamination services.

ASSESSMENT TECHNIQUES

Chapter 6 describes the assessment techniques of inspection, palpation, percussion, and auscultation; this section demonstrates how these techniques are used in performing a physical examination. The specific techniques used to assess each body system are identified and explained within the context of the assessment. See the assessment tables throughout this chapter to reinforce appropriate techniques for assessment of each body system.

The nurse should use the senses of sight, hearing, smell, and touch when gathering information during the physical examination. The nurse uses the sense of sight by visually inspecting the client's body parts and assessing the client's normal behaviors. For example, the skin is inspected for color, tone, texture, and presence of scars, lesions, abrasions, and rashes. Throughout the examination the nurse should visually observe the client's movement, motor dexterity, contour and symmetry of the body, and abnormalities.

The nurse uses the sense of touch when performing palpation. The skin is thinner on the backs of the hands and more sensitive to temperature changes. The back of the hand can be used to assess skin temperature over an inflamed joint or a leg with impaired circulation. The fingerpads are also sensitive and are used to palpate the size, position, and consistency of various body parts, such as lymph nodes and breast tissue. Figure 27-1 on page 545 demonstrates how to perform light palpation.

SPOTLIGHT ON...

Legal

Caring for Abused Clients

What would you do if a child in the emergency room in which you were practicing showed signs of abuse? How would you conduct the physical examination?

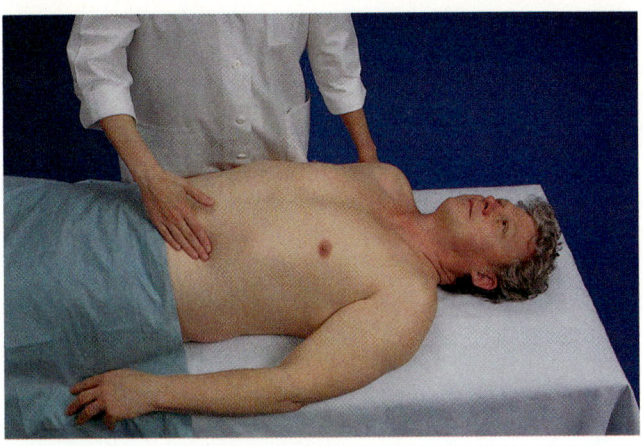

FIGURE 27-1 Light Palpation DELMAR/CENGAGE LEARNING

Learning the technique of percussion is challenging; it can be practiced on any surface to improve accuracy. See Figure 27-2, and practice percussion as follows:

1. Hyperextend the middle (pleximeter) finger of the nondominant hand and press its distal phalanx and joint firmly on the surface to be percussed (see Figure 27-2A). Only the distal phalanx and joint should be touching the surface. Having other parts of the hand in contact with the surface will dampen the vibrations.
2. Position the forearm of the dominant hand close to the surface, with the hand cocked upward (see Figure 27-2B) and the middle finger partially flexed, relaxed, and poised to strike.
3. With a quick, sharp, but relaxed *wrist* motion, strike the pleximeter finger with the tip of the right plexor finger of the dominant hand (see Figure 27-2C). Only the wrist joint is flexed, not the finger or elbow.
4. Quickly withdraw the plexor finger to avoid damping the vibration.
5. Strike one or two blows in one location, then move on, using the lightest percussion that will produce a clear note.

If the client becomes fatigued, encourage frequent rest periods. Adjust the client's position for comfort without compromising the ability to visualize the area of assessment.

The nurse uses the sense of hearing during the physical examination when performing auscultation. A stethoscope allows the nurse to listen to sounds produced in the heart, lungs, abdomen, and blood vessels.

Besides auscultation, the nurse should listen to what clients say relative to their health status during the examination. Throughout the entire examination, the nurse uses the senses of hearing and smell. Smell is used to investigate any environmental, body, or fluid odors, such as drainage from a wound. Also, the nurse can often detect the use of alcohol or tobacco products through the sensation of smell.

INTEGUMENT

The **integumentary system** (skin, hair, scalp, and nails) provides the body with external protection, regulates temperature, and is a sensory organ for pain, temperature, and touch. The sebaceous and sweat glands are considered appendages of the skin. Nurses should routinely assess the skin of older and debilitated clients for primary lesions that may lead to the development of secondary lesions such as pressure ulcers. See Chapter 37 for a complete discussion of skin integrity.

To facilitate learning and psychomotor proficiency, the integumentary system is assessed separately. However, once skills are established, the integumentary system assessment can be integrated into the examination of other systems.

Skin

The skin is the largest organ system of the body, with its surface area covering approximately 20 square feet in the average adult. Skin assessment provides a noninvasive observation of the body's physiological functions. See Table 27-3 on pages 547–548, which presents information on assessing the skin.

See the Respecting Our Differences display on page 546 for ways to detect color changes in light and dark skin.

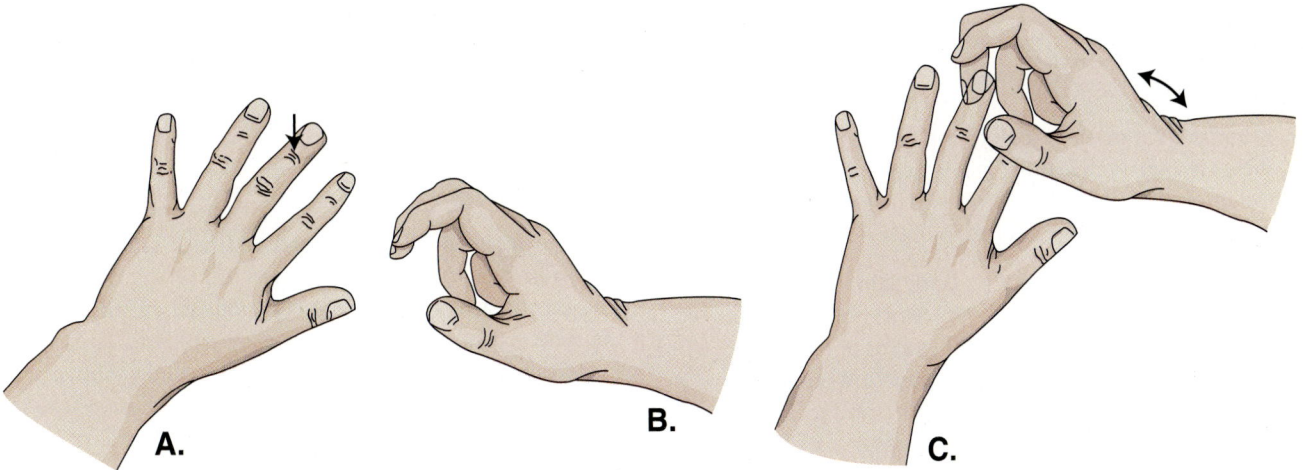

FIGURE 27-2 Percussion. A. Hyperextend the pleximeter finger and press the distal phalanx and joint firmly on the surface to be percussed. **B.** Cock the dominant hand upward with the middle finger partially flexed and poised to strike. **C.** Strike the pleximeter finger with the tip of the right plexor finger. DELMAR/CENGAGE LEARNING

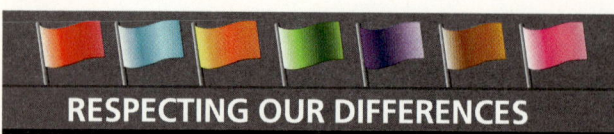

RESPECTING OUR DIFFERENCES

Skin Color Variations in Light Skin and Dark Skin

Carotenemia: Yellow-orange tinge; result of increased amount of carotene in bloodstream; caused by ingestion of foods high in carotene (e.g., carrots, sweet potatoes), endocrine disorders (e.g., diabetes mellitus), and anorexia nervosa

Light Skin
- On forehead, palms, and soles.
- No discoloration of mucous membranes or sclerae.

Dark Skin
- On palms and soles.
- No discoloration of mucous membranes or sclerae.

Cyanosis: Mottled bluish color; result of reduced oxygenated hemoglobin; may be caused by anxiety, exposure to cold, and chronic heart and lung disease

Light Skin
- Dusky blue.

Dark Skin
- Dark, dull, and lifeless.
- Most noticeable in conjunctivae, oral mucosa, and nail beds.

Erythema: Redness; result of increased visibility of oxygenated hemoglobin; may be caused by emotions (blushing, hearty laughter), fever, warm ambient temperature, local inflammation, consumption of alcohol, and carbon monoxide poisoning

Light Skin
- Generalized red or bright pink.
- Generalized or in local areas (i.e., inflammation, pressure on bony prominence).

Dark Skin
- Difficult to detect.
- Check for redness in lips.
- Localized areas of inflammation appear darker than surrounding skin.

Note: Bright cherry-red coloration in face and neck occurs with carbon monoxide poisoning.

Jaundice: Yellowish discoloration as result of increased serum bilirubin; may be caused by liver inflammation or hemolytic disease (e.g., after severe burns)

Light Skin
- Yellow sclera.
- Discoloration may be generalized; seen in sclera, hard palate, and mucous membranes.

Dark Skin
- Most noticeable in palms of hands and juncture between hard and soft palates.

Pallor: Loss of color in skin; result of absence of oxygenated hemoglobin; may be caused by

smoking, cold environment, stress, shock, hypotension, anemia, and prolonged elevation of body part

Light Skin
- Skin looks dull.
- Loss of rosy tone in white skin.
- Yellow-toned skin appears more yellow.

Dark Skin
- Skin appears dull.
- Brown skin has yellowish hue.
- Yellow-toned skin appears more yellow.
- Black skin appears ashen gray.

Data from D'Amico, D., and Barbarito, C. (2007). *Health & physical assessment in nursing.* Upper Saddle River, NJ: Pearson Prentice Hall; Jarvis, C. (2007). *Physical examination & health assessment* (5th ed.). Philadelphia: Elsevier.

Lesions of the skin vary from superficial, involving only the epidermis, to penetrating the dermis or subcutaneous layers of the skin. Tables 27-4 on page 548 and 27-5 on page 550 describe the common skin lesions.

Hair

Hair is distributed over the body except for the palmar and plantar surfaces, lips, nipples, and the glans penis. The amount and texture of hair vary with age, gender, and race. Men have coarser, thicker chest and facial hair growth than women. The two types of body hair are:

- Vellus: Fine, unpigmented hair that covers most of the body.
- Terminal hair: Coarser, darker hair of scalp, eyebrows, and eyelashes; axillary and pubic hair become terminal with the onset of puberty.

See Table 27-6 on page 552 for details on assessing the hair and scalp.

Nails

The nail plate is the translucent protective tissue that covers the distal portion of the digits. See Tables 27-7, on page 552, and 27-8, on page 553, for a description of nail assessment. Careful assessment of nails and nail beds elicits valuable information because they may exhibit changes indicative of systematic diseases.

HEAD AND NECK

Areas to be included in the head and neck examination are the skull, face, eyes, ears, nose, mouth, pharynx, and neck. The carotid artery assessment is conducted either as part of the neck examination or with peripheral artery assessment. Inspection and palpation are used throughout this assessment. Auscultation is used if the carotid arteries are assessed as part of the head and neck examination.

Skull and Face

Assessment of the skull and face involves inspection and palpation. During inspection, observe the shape of the skull and

TABLE 27-3 Assessment of the Skin

AREA OF ASSESSMENT	NORMAL FINDINGS	SIGNIFICANT FINDINGS AND POSSIBLE CAUSES
Color: Inspect under natural light to ensure accurate findings.	Uniform color except in sun-exposed areas. In dark-skinned people, nail beds, palms, and lips are lighter than surrounding areas.	Redness (inflammation). Bluish coloration (hypoxia).
Lesions: Palpate for mobility, contour, and consistency. Note color, size, anatomic location, and distribution.	Freckles. Skin tags (especially in older adults). Some types of moles and birthmarks.	Primary skins lesions (i.e., vesicles) can lead to secondary lesions (i.e., erosion and crusting, as in chickenpox).

Moisture:
Inspect for wetness and oiliness. Note amount and distribution.
	Varies with:
	  Activity
	  Body temperature
	  Ambient temperature
	  Body part (e.g., skinfolds, axillae)
		Excessive perspiration (hyperthermia, infection, hyperthyroidism, menopause, strong emotions).
		Excessive dryness (dehydration).

Temperature:
Palpate with back of hand.
Note uniformity of warmth.
	Warm.	Hyperthermia:
		  Generalized (fever)
		  Localized (infection)
		Hypothermia:
		  Generalized (shock)
		  Localized (impaired circulation)

Texture: Palpate to determine quality, thickness, and suppleness.	Uneven texture (thicker on palms and soles). Wrinkled leathery skin results from normal aging effects (i.e., decreased collagen, subcutaneous fat).	Generalized roughness (hypothyroidism).
Mobility and turgor (elasticity): Apply pressure to dependent areas (e.g., sacrum, ankles, feet). Note areas of indentation (Figure 27-3). If indentation occurs, apply firm pressure for 5 seconds. Note degree of edema based on depth of pitting in millimeters.	Absence of indentation in dependent areas. Resilient: Springs back to its previous state after being pinched.	Stretched, shiny skin of dependent areas (trauma, decreased venous blood return). "Tenting," failure of skin to spring back to normal shape (dehydration).

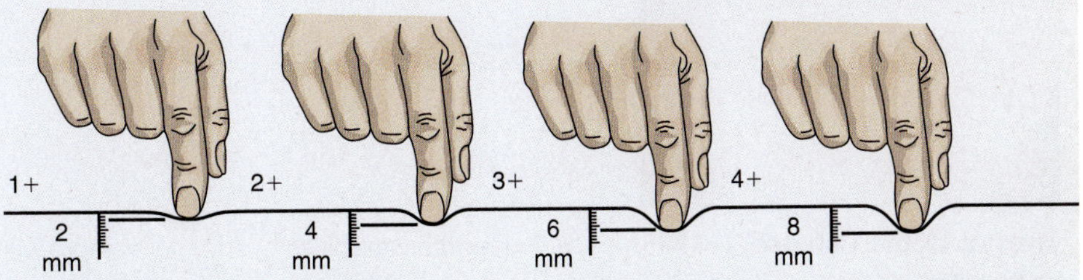

Pitting Edema Scale

1+ Indentation up to 2 mm

2+ Indentation of 4 mm

3+ Indentation of 6 mm

4+ Indentation of 8 mm

FIGURE 27-3 Assessing for Edema DELMAR/CENGAGE LEARNING

(Continues)

TABLE 27-3 (Continued)

AREA OF ASSESSMENT	NORMAL FINDINGS	SIGNIFICANT FINDINGS AND POSSIBLE CAUSES
To assess turgor: Use thumb and forefinger to pinch a fold of skin on sternal area (Figure 27-4). Note speed at which skin returns to place. 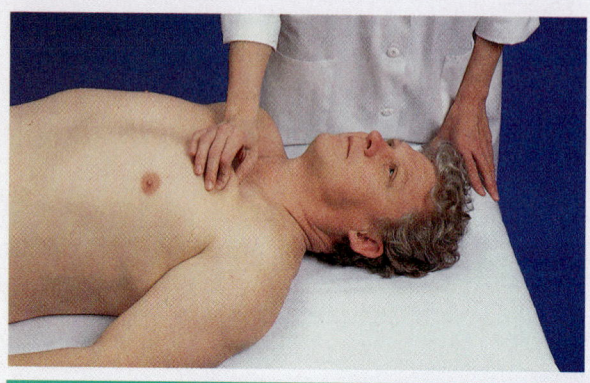 **FIGURE 27-4** Assessing Skin Turgor DELMAR/CENGAGE LEARNING.		

Data from D'Amico, D., and Barbarito, C. (2007). *Health & physical assessment in nursing.* Upper Saddle River, NJ: Pearson Prentice Hall; Estes, M. E. Z. (2010). *Health assessment and physical examination* (4th ed.). Clifton Park, NY: Delmar/Cengage Learning.

TABLE 27-4 Vascular and Purpuric Lesions of the Skin

FINDINGS	BODY AREA ASSESSED	KEY POINTS
Vascular Lesions		
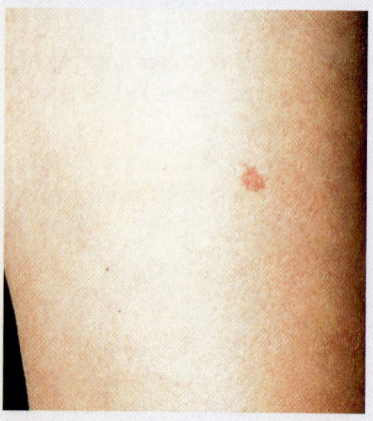 Cherry angioma: Ruby red, 1–3 mm, round lesion.	Trunk and extremities	Pressure with a pinpoint edge causes partial blanching. Increase in size and number and may become brownish with age.

(Continues)

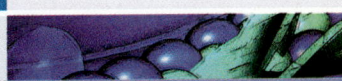

TABLE 27-4 (Continued)

FINDINGS	BODY AREA ASSESSED	KEY POINTS
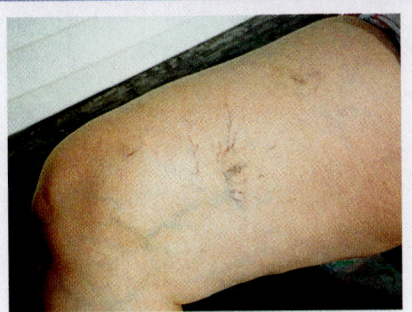 Spider angioma: Fiery red lesion with a central body surrounded by erythema and radiating legs.	Face, neck, arms, and upper trunk	Occurs normally in some people. May occur with pregnancy, vitamin B deficiency, or liver disease.
Venous star: Bluish coloration may resemble a spider or be linear, irregular, and cascading.	Areas with superficial veins: legs and anterior chest	Indicates an increased pressure in superficial veins, for example, varicose veins.

Purpuric Lesions

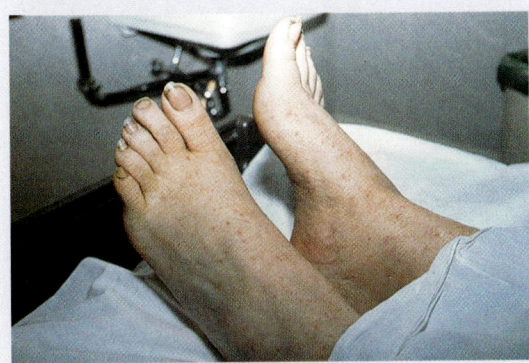 Petechia: Reddish purple, flat round lesion, 1–3 mm in size.	Variable distribution in areas with superficial blood supply	May indicate vitamin C deficiency, blood clotting disorders, liver disease, or drug reactions.
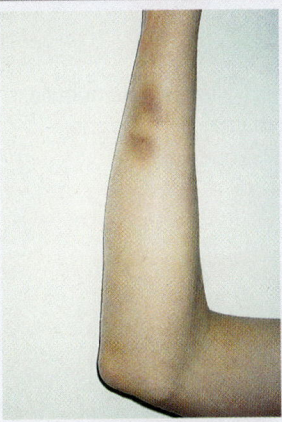 Ecchymosis (bruise): Purplish blue, fading to green, yellow, and brown in time.	Area of blood vessel trauma	Results from injury or with bleeding disorders.

Data from D'Amico, D., & Barbarito, C. (2007). *Health & physical assessment in nursing.* Upper Saddle River, NJ: Pearson Prentice Hall; Jarvis, C. (2007). *Physical examination & health assessment* (5th ed.). Philadelphia: Elsevier.

TABLE 27-5 Common Skin Lesions

PRIMARY LESIONS

| NONPALPABLE | PALPABLE | FLUID-FILLED CAVITIES WITHIN THE SKIN |

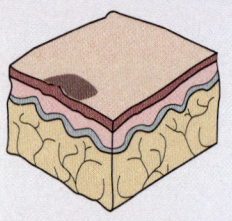

Macule: Localized changes in skin color greater than 1 cm in diameter (e.g., freckles, measles)

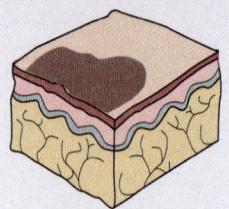

Papule: Solid, elevated lesion 0.5 cm in diameter (e.g., elevated nevi)

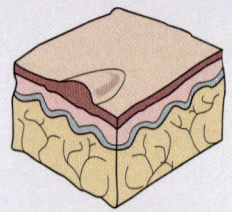

Vesicle: Elevated mass containing serous fluid accumulation between the upper layers of the skin (e.g., herpes simplex and zoster, chickenpox, second-degree burns)

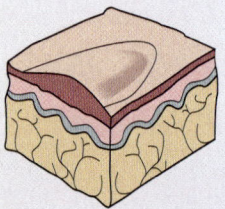

Plaque: Solid, elevated lesion wider than 1 cm in diameter (e.g., psoriasis)

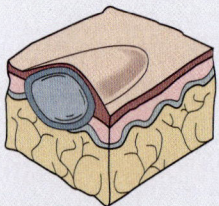

Patch: Localized changes in skin of 1 cm (e.g., vitiligo, stage 1 pressure ulcer)

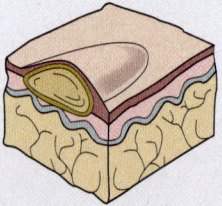

Bullae: Same as vesicle, larger than 1 cm (e.g., contact dermatitis, large second-degree burns, bulbous impetigo, pemphigus)

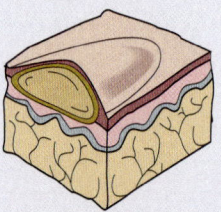

Nodule: Solid and elevated; extends deeper than papule into the dermis or subcutaneous tissues, 0.5–2.0 cm (e.g., lipoma, erythema, cyst)

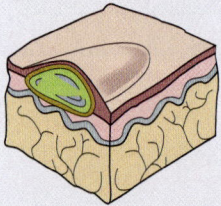

Pustule: Pus-filled vesicle or bulla, 0.5 cm in diameter (e.g., acne, impetigo, carbuncles)

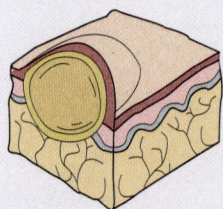

Cyst: Subcutaneous or dermis mass (e.g., sebaceous or epidermoid cyst)

(Continues)

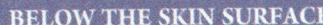

TABLE 27-5 (Continued)

| SECONDARY LESIONS | | |
| ABOVE THE SKIN SURFACE | BELOW THE SKIN SURFACE | BELOW THE SKIN SURFACE |

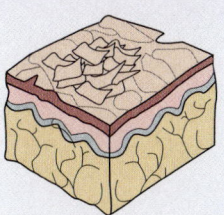

Scales: Flaking of the skin's surface (e.g., dandruff, psoriasis)

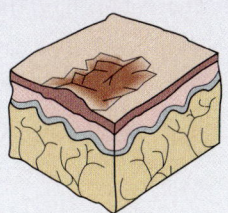

Erosion: Loss of epidermis (e.g., ruptured chickenpox vesicle)

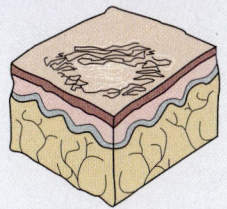

Atrophy: Thinning of skin surface and loss of markings (e.g., striae, aged skin)

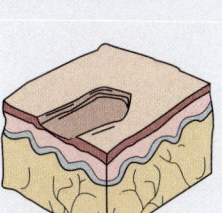

Crust: Dried serum, blood, or pus on skin's surface (e.g., impetigo)

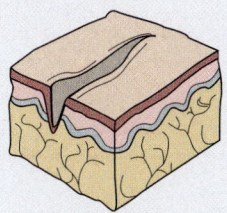

Fissure: Linear crack in the epidermis that can extend into the dermis (e.g., chapped hands or lips, athlete's foot)

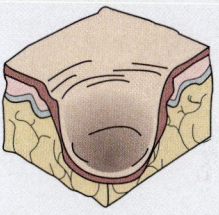

Ulcer: Depressed lesion of the epidermis and upper papillary layer of the dermis (e.g., stage 2 pressure ulcer)

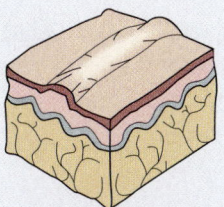

Scar: Fibrous tissue that replaces dermal tissue after injury (e.g., surgical incision)

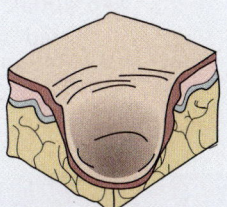

Keloid: Enlarging of a scar past wound edges due to excess collagen formation (more prevalent in dark-skinned persons)

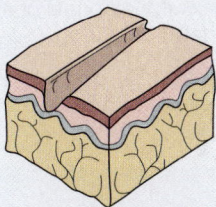

Excoriation: Loss of epidermal layers exposing the dermis (e.g., abrasion)

Delmar/Cengage Learning

determine whether the size of the head is proportionate to body size. Normally, the skull is rounded with a smooth contour; see the Safety First display.

When inspecting facial features, look for symmetry and involuntary muscle movements. Palpate for presence of edema and masses. The normal skull and face will have no abnormal movements (i.e., tics), and there will be neither edema nor masses detected during palpation. Note that sunken eyes, cheeks, and temples are often seen with malnutrition and dehydration. The client's face has its own unique characteristics influenced by factors such as race, emotions, and health status. Facial

▼ SAFETY FIRST ▼

An enlarged skull may indicate hydrocephalus, which occurs with increased intracranial pressure. This finding must be reported immediately to the primary care provider.

TABLE 27-6 Assessment of Hair and Scalp

AREA OF ASSESSMENT	NORMAL FINDINGS	SIGNIFICANT FINDINGS AND POSSIBLE CAUSES
Inspect and palpate scalp to determine quality, distribution, and pattern of hair loss.	Thick and even distribution	Thin and brittle (hypothyroidism) Alopecia (aging, chemotherapeutic drugs, hair grooming products) Hirsutism (genetic, some medications)
Inspect for parasitic infestation.	Free of infestation	White ovoid nits (*Pediculus capitis*, *P. corporis*, and *P. pubis*)
Part the hair all over the scalp; inspect for scales and scars.	Shiny and smooth without lesions, lumps, or masses	Masses or lumps (sebaceous cysts, trauma, tumors)
Beginning at front of scalp, palpate down midline and each side. Note any tenderness, pain, lesions, lumps, or masses.	Absence of pain, redness, or scales	Dry flaking scales (seborrhea) Red patches covered by thick, dry, silvery, adherent scales (psoriasis)

Data from Estes, M. E. Z. (2010). *Health assessment and physical examination* (4th ed.). Clifton Park, NY: Delmar/Cengage Learning.

anomalies provide information relevant to the overall health status and many indicate the presence of disease, for example:

- An elongated head with prominent forehead, nose, and lower jaw and enlarged nose, lips, and ears (acromegaly) results from excessive amounts of growth hormone.
- A round "moon" face with excessive hair growth occurs with Cushing's syndrome, which is caused by excessive amounts of adrenal hormones (i.e., corticosteroids).

- Protrusion or bulging of the eyes (exophthalmos) results from increased pressure in the eye orbit, often caused by inflammation or tumor.
- Pale, edematous tissue around the eyes occurs in people with chronic renal failure.
- Decreased facial mobility and expressions (a masklike facies) result from progressive degenerative neurological disorders, for example, Parkinson disease.

TABLE 27-7 Assessment of the Nails

AREA OF ASSESSMENT	NORMAL FINDINGS	SIGNIFICANT FINDINGS AND POSSIBLE CAUSES
Inspect and palpate nails and nail beds, noting color, shape, and texture.	Firm when palpated. Pinkish color in light-skinned people. Longitudinal streaks of brown or black pigmentation in dark-skinned people. Angle between nail and base of finger is 160°.	See Table 27-8 on page 553 for variations and abnormalities of nail bed.
Test for capillary refill: Press nail between your thumb and index finger. Note degree of blanching and return of normal color.	Nail promptly returns to its normal color when pressure is released.	Delayed return of color to nail bed (circulatory impairment).
Inspect tissue surrounding nails. Note any lesions.	Tissue is intact.	Paronychia (inflammation of skin around the nails).

Data from Estes, M. E. Z. (2010). *Health assessment and physical examination* (4th ed.). Clifton Park, NY: Delmar/Cengage Learning.

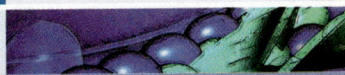

TABLE 27-8 Variations of the Nail Bed

NORMAL NAIL ANGLE

Normal nail angle

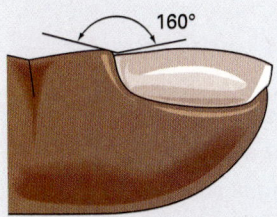

160°

Normal nail: Has an angle of approximately 160° between the fingernail and nail base; nail feels firm when palpated.

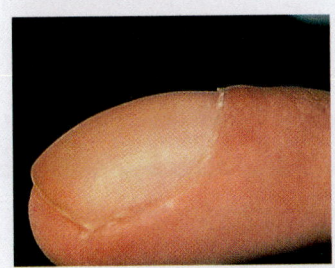

Clubbing: Hypoxia causes an angle greater than 180° between the fingernail and nail base; nail feels springy when palpated. (Robert A. Silveman, MD, Pediatric Dermatology, Georgetown University)

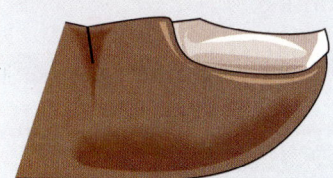

Koilonychia (spoon nail): Characterized by concave curves; associated with iron-deficiency anemia.

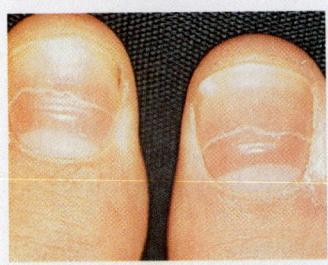

Beau's line: Characterized by transverse depression in the nails; associated with injury and severe systemic infections. (Robert A. Silveman, MD, Pediatric Dermatology, Georgetown University)

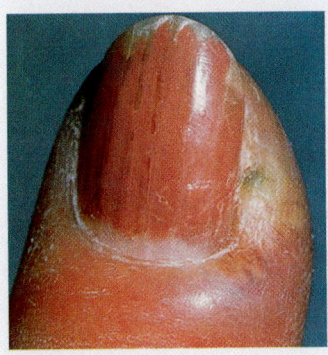

Paronychia: Characterized by an inflammation at the nail base (may be swollen, red, or tender); associated with trauma and local infection.

Delmar/Cengage Learning

Eyes

Active client participation is necessary for assessment of vision. Age-related physiological change is one factor that affects vision; see the accompanying Respecting Our Differences and Safety First displays. A complete eye assessment examines both visual acuity and anatomic structures. Visual acuity should be assessed prior to physically examining the eye. Every nurse uses the technique of inspection; however, the use of the ophthalmoscope falls within the scope of advanced nursing practice.

Assessment of visual acuity is a simple, noninvasive procedure that uses the Snellen chart, a chart that contains various-sized letters with standardized numbers at the end of each line of letters; see Figure 27-5. The standardized numbers (denominators) indicate the degree of visual acuity when the client is able to read the line of letters at a distance of 20 feet. Visual acuity of 20/20 is considered normal. A value of 20/40 indicates that the client can read the Snellen chart from a distance of 40 feet. See the Nursing Checklist for visual acuity assessment guidelines.

Testing of visual fields is done to determine what the client can see when looking straight ahead; see the accompanying Nursing Checklist on page 558. Loss of peripheral vision may be a gradual process that occurs as a physiological, age-related change or may be indicative of glaucoma. Glaucoma is a circulatory disturbance that increases intraocular (aqueous fluid) pressure.

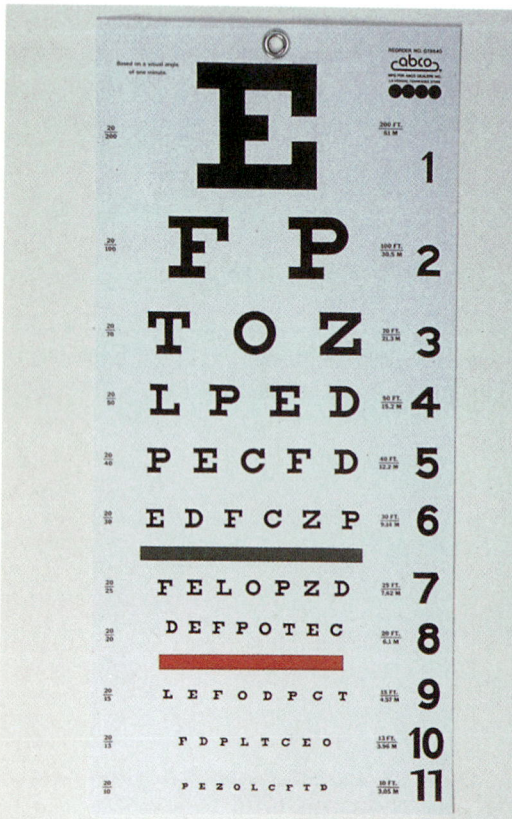

FIGURE 27-5 Snellen Chart DELMAR/CENGAGE LEARNING

RESPECTING OUR DIFFERENCES

Effects of Aging on Vision

Dryness and burning as a result of decreased tear production

Decreased elasticity of lens leads to decreased accommodation of lens (presbyopia)

Floaters as a result of debris in vitreous

Cataract formation (lens opacity)

Increased ocular pressure (glaucoma)

Macular degeneration (loss of central vision)

Data from Jarvis, C. (2007). *Physical examination & health assessment* (5th ed.). Philadelphia: Elsevier.

▼ SAFETY FIRST ▼

Aging people often need more light in order to see because of decreased adaptation to darkness. Clients should be informed of this age-related change, which may impair night driving.

✓ NURSING CHECKLIST

Assessing Visual Acuity

- Position the client 20 feet away from and facing the Snellen chart.
- Remove any corrective lenses.
- Instruct client to cover one eye and read as many lines as possible.
- Note the number of the last line that the client reads correctly.
- Repeat the test with the other eye.
- Document findings as "s-c" (without correction) or "c-c" (with correction).

Visual acuity may be affected by many types of refractive errors, including:

- Astigmatism: An unequal spherical curve of the cornea that prevents the light rays from being focused directly in a point on the retina
- Hyperopia (farsightedness): Refraction error in which rays of light are brought into focus behind the retina
- Myopia (nearsightedness): Elongation of the eyeball that causes the parallel rays to focus in front of the retina
- Presbyopia (farsightedness): Refraction error that results from loss of elasticity of the lens; occurs with aging

See Table 27-9 on pages 555–557 for guidelines on assessing the anatomic structures of the eye.

TABLE 27-9 Assessment of Eye Structures and Function

STRUCTURE/FUNCTION ASSESSED	NORMAL FINDINGS	SIGNIFICANT FINDINGS AND POSSIBLE CAUSES
Extraocular Muscle Function Instruct client to let eyes follow your finger, which is held 6–10 inches in front of client's face. Move your finger through the eight visual fields (Figure 27-6).	Movements are symmetrical and controlled. Both eyes follow direction of the gaze. Upper eyelids cover only the uppermost part of the iris. Eye movement is steady and controlled.	**Nystagmus**, involuntary rhythmical oscillation of eyes (localized injury, cranial nerve disorder)

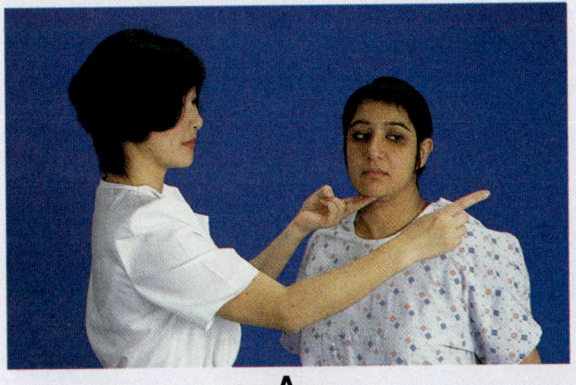
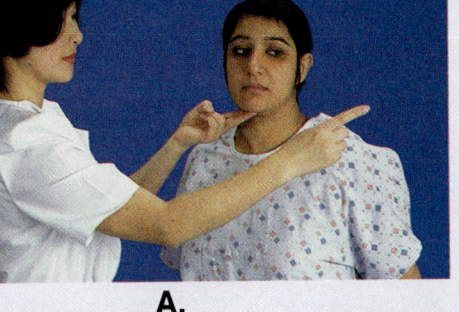
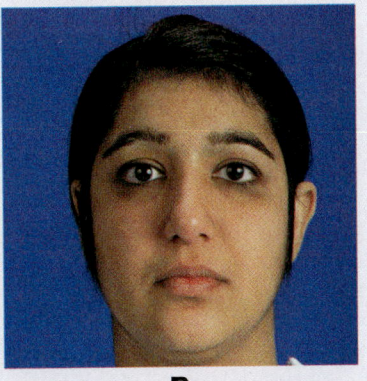

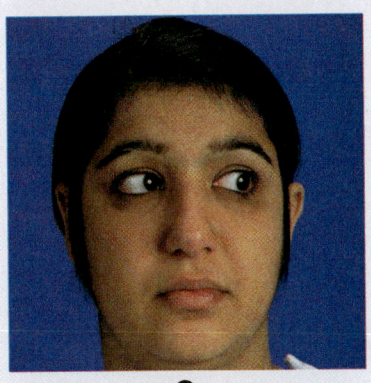
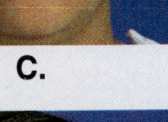
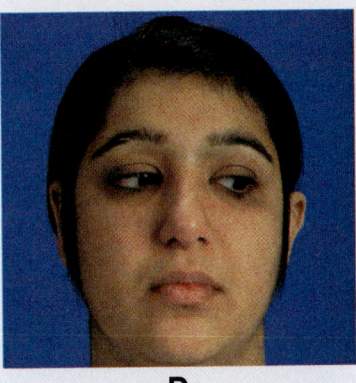
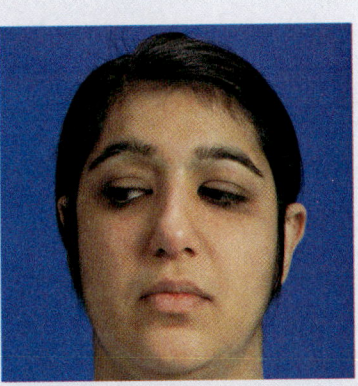
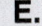

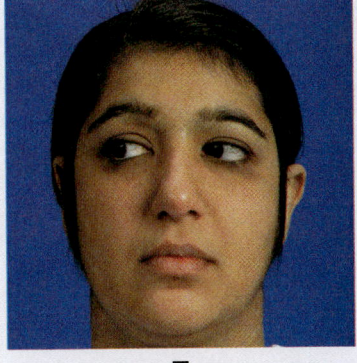
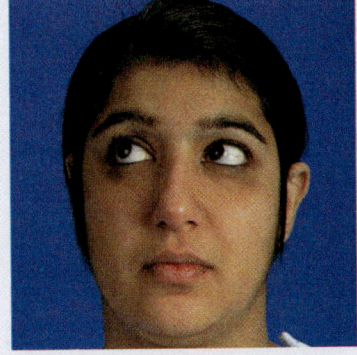
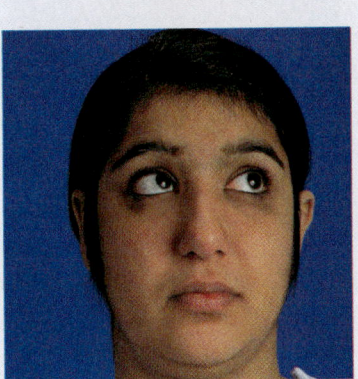

FIGURE 27-6 Testing Extraocular Muscle Function. A. Basic Position. **B.** Normal Resting Position. **C.** Conjugate Left Lateral Gaze. **D.** Left Down and Lateral Gaze. **E.** Right Down and Lateral Gaze. **F.** Conjugate Right Lateral Gaze. **G.** Right Up and Lateral Gaze. **H.** Left Up and Lateral Gaze. DELMAR/CENGAGE LEARNING

(Continues)

TABLE 27-9 (Continued)

STRUCTURE/FUNCTION ASSESSED	NORMAL FINDINGS	SIGNIFICANT FINDINGS AND POSSIBLE CAUSES
Observe for parallel eye movement. Pause during upward and lateral gaze to detect involuntary movement of eyes. Note any lags in eye movement as client follows finger.		

External Anatomic Structures
(see Figure 27-7)

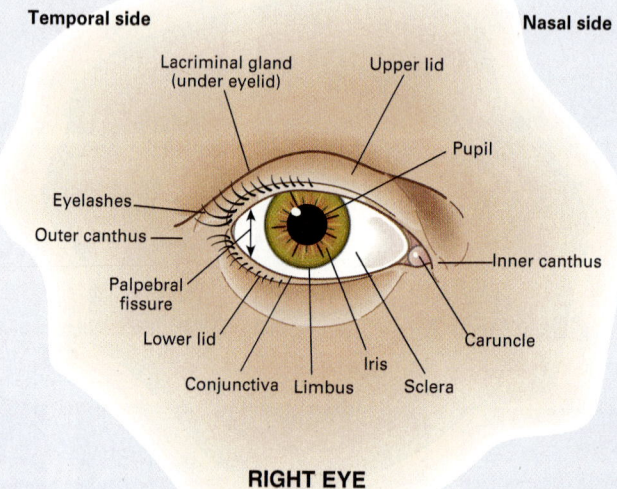

Temporal side   Nasal side

Lacriminal gland (under eyelid)   Upper lid   Pupil   Inner canthus   Caruncle   Sclera   Iris   Limbus   Conjunctiva   Lower lid   Palpebral fissure   Outer canthus   Eyelashes

RIGHT EYE

FIGURE 27-7 **External Structures of the Eye** DELMAR/CENGAGE LEARNING

Observe upper eyelid. Inspect eyes and lids for inflammation, crusting, edema, or masses.	Overlaps the iris; should not overlap pupil. Free from inflammation, crusting, edema, or masses.	Inflammation, crusting, edema, or masses (blepharitis, inflammation of eyelids; hordeolum or sty; chalazion, chronic inflammatory lesion of meibomian gland) Papule with a pearly border and ulcerated center (basal cell carcinoma)
Lacrimal glands and sacs: Inspect for edema. Palpate lacrimal sac and observe for regurgitation of tears.	Lacrimal gland not palpable. Tears flow freely over cornea and conjunctiva.	Edema of lacrimal sac (inflammation, tumor) Regurgitation of tears through the puncta (blocked lacrimal duct)
Conjunctivae and sclera: Instruct client to look upward while you depress lower lid with your thumb.	Conjunctiva should be transparent. In people with light skin, sclerae are a white porcelain color. In people with dark skin, sclerae have a pale yellow hue.	Bright red conjunctiva with rusty drainage (conjunctivitis) Pale conjunctiva (anemia) Bright red patch on the exposed bulbar conjunctiva indicating subconjunctival hemorrhage (trauma, sudden increase in venous pressure)

(Continues)

TABLE 27-9 (Continued)

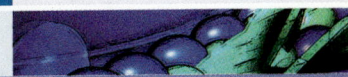

STRUCTURE/FUNCTION ASSESSED	NORMAL FINDINGS	SIGNIFICANT FINDINGS AND POSSIBLE CAUSES
Cornea, lens, pupil, and iris: Inspect.	Pupils are black, round, and equal in size; 3–7 mm in diameter (see Figure 27-8). Margins of iris are intact.	Cloudy pupils and lens opacity (cataracts)

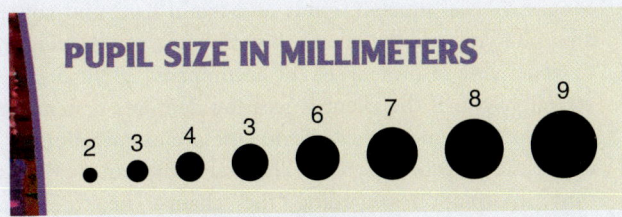

FIGURE 27-8 Pupil Size in Millimeters DELMAR/CENGAGE LEARNING

Pupillary response and reaction: Dim lights. Instruct client to look straight ahead. Move penlight from side of client's face directly in front of pupil (Figure 27-9A). Note quickness of response to light. Shine light into same eye, observing response of opposite pupil for equality of size (Figure 27-9B).	Pupil constricts quickly in direct response to light; opposite pupil should also constrict. Pupils are equal in size. Pupillary accommodation causes constriction in response to objects that are near. Dilation occurs to accommodate distant vision.	Altered papillary reaction time and inequality (increased intracranial pressure, lesions on third cranial nerve, trauma, some medications) Pupillary constriction (inflammation of the iris, medications) Pupillary dilation (trauma, neurological disorders, glaucoma, some medications)

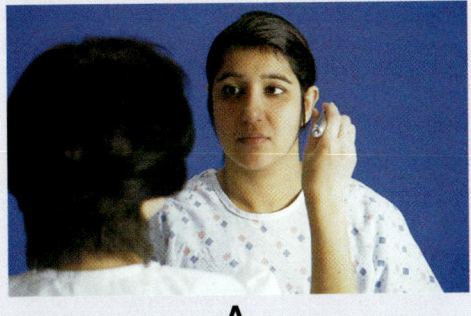 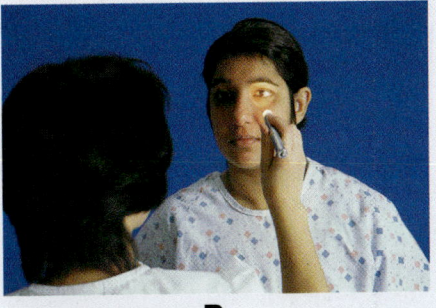

A.   B.

FIGURE 27-9 A. Move penlight from side of client's face to eye. **B.** Shine penlight into the eye and observe response of the opposite pupil. DELMAR/CENGAGE LEARNING

Instruct client to gaze at your finger held 4–6 inches from client's nose, then to glance at a distant object while you note papillary reflex. Move finger toward the bridge of client's nose, noting response of both pupils.	Normal responses are documented as: **P** upils **E** qual **R** ound and **R** eactive to **L** ight **A** ccomodation

Data from Estes, M. E. Z. (2010). *Health assessment and physical examination* (4th ed.). Clifton Park, NY: Delmar/Cengage Learning.

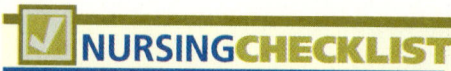

NURSINGCHECKLIST

Testing the Visual Field

- Stand 2 feet in front of the client.
- Instruct the client to cover the right eye while you cover your left eye.
- Ask the client to look into your eye directly opposite to create one visual field.
- Using the eight directions of gaze (as shown in Figure 27-6), move your finger outside the vision field and slowly bring your finger back to the midpoint of the vision field for each direction of gaze.
- Instruct the client to state when your finger becomes visible.
- Note if you see the finger before the client does.
- Repeat for each visual field.

Note: Consensual peripheral vision should occur when the nurse's finger comes into the client's visual field.

Ears

Physical assessment of the ears consists of auditory screening, inspection and palpation of the external ear, and otoscopic examination; see Table 27-10 on page 559, which lists guidelines for assessing the ears.

The nurse must observe the client for signs of hearing difficulty, such as turning the head, lipreading, and speaking in a loud voice. See the accompanying Nursing Process Highlight and Table 27-11 on pages 560–561.

Nose and Sinuses

Assessment is limited to inspection and palpation of the external nose and nasal passages using a penlight. An examination with a nasal speculum to inspect the nasal chambers is usually performed by an advanced nurse practitioner because the nasal chambers are lined with respiratory mucosa. Clients with nasal impairments are at risk of developing respiratory infections. Sinus assessment is limited to palpation of the frontal and maxillary sinuses. Transillumination of the sinuses is usually performed by advanced practitioners. See Table 27-12 on page 562 for a description of nose and sinus assessment.

Mouth and Pharynx

Physical assessment of the oral cavity includes the lips, tongue, buccal mucosa, gums and teeth, hard and soft palates, pharynx, and the breath. Breath odors can provide clues to underlying disorders; see the accompanying Nursing Process Highlight. If the client is wearing dentures or removable orthodontia, remove these devices before examination to visualize and palpate the gums. The oral cavity can yield significant information regarding the client's health because systemic diseases may manifest initially in the oral cavity; see Table 27-13 on page 563.

See the accompanying Nursing Process Highlight for a description of lesions that commonly affect the lips.

NURSING PROCESS HIGHLIGHT

Assessment

Abnormal Breath Odors

- A "fruity" smell (acetone breath) indicates ketoacidosis and is present in malnutrition (e.g., dietary fasting) and diabetes.
- A musty smell is caused by breakdown of nitrogen and may indicate liver disease.
- An ammonia smell occurs with accumulation of urea during end-stage renal disease.

NURSING PROCESS HIGHLIGHT

Assessment

Assessing Clients with Hearing Impairments

If the client uses a hearing aid, asking these questions can be helpful:

How long has the client used the device?

Does the client use the device continuously or only on certain occasions?

Is the hearing aid turned on?

When were the batteries last changed?

Is the device comfortable?

If pain is associated with use of the device, is the pain on the outer ear or in the ear canal?

NURSING PROCESS HIGHLIGHT

Assessment

Common Lip Lesions

Herpes simplex: Painful vesicular lesions that rupture and crust over, for example, cold sores or fever blisters

Chancre: Reddish, round, painless lesion with a depressed center and raised edges; often appears on lower lip; primary lesion of syphilis

Squamous cell carcinoma: A thickened plaque, ulcer, or wartlike growth; usually involves lower lip; most common form of oral cancer

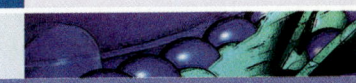

TABLE 27-10 Assessing Structural Components of the Ears

AREA ASSESSED	NORMAL FINDINGS	SIGNIFICANT FINDINGS AND POSSIBLE CAUSES
External ear (Figure 27-10): Inspect for placement, symmetry, and color.	Symmetrical, with upper attachment at same level as eye's corner (lateral canthus). Flesh colored.	Ears set below lateral canthus (congenital anomalies, e.g., Down syndrome). Erythema (inflammation, fever). Clear drainage may be cerebrospinal fluid; **if present, stop the examination and notify the primary care provider immediately.**

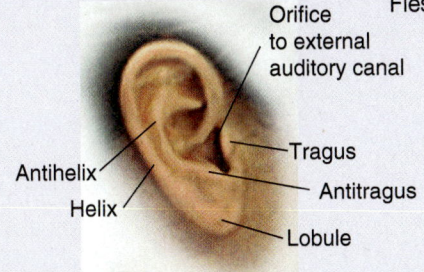

Orifice to external auditory canal

Antihelix

Helix

Tragus

Antitragus

Lobule

FIGURE 27-10 External Structures of the Ear DELMAR/CENGAGE LEARNING

Auricle: Observe for discharge, edema, and erythema. Palpate for lesions or tenderness.	Firm, smooth, free from lesions and pain.	Flaky, scaly skin (seborrhea). Keloids, or scar tissue, on lobe (piercing). Yellow or green discharge, itching, or pain (otitis media).
Ear canal: Select the largest speculum that can comfortably fit in the ear canal. Attach speculum to otoscope to inspect canal and eardrum. Tilt client's head slightly toward opposite shoulder. Pull the pinna up and back on an adult and older child. Pull the pinna down on infants and young children. Insert speculum and look for ear wax, foreign bodies, discharge, scaling, erythema, or edema. Inspect tympanic membrane. Identify the color, light reflex, umbo, and short process and long handle of malleus (see Figure 27-11). Look for perforations, lesions, bulging, or retraction of membrane; dilation of blood vessels; bubbles; or fluid level. Gently withdraw speculum and repeat procedure in opposite ear. Clean speculum before inserting into other ear.	Canal is pink and dry. Cerumen (yellow-brown waxy substance) is normal. Intact tympanic membrane is translucent or pearly gray. Light reflex is seen at 5 o'clock position in right ear and 7 o'clock position in left ear.	Accumulation of cerumen may cause temporary hearing loss due to impaction. **If foreign body is present, stop the examination and notify primary care provider.** Red, bulging membrane (otitis media). Nontender, nodular swelling deep in ear canal (osteoma, a tumor composed of bone tissue). Whitish appearance on tympanic membrane (pus in the middle ear). Perforation of eardrum (infection, trauma).

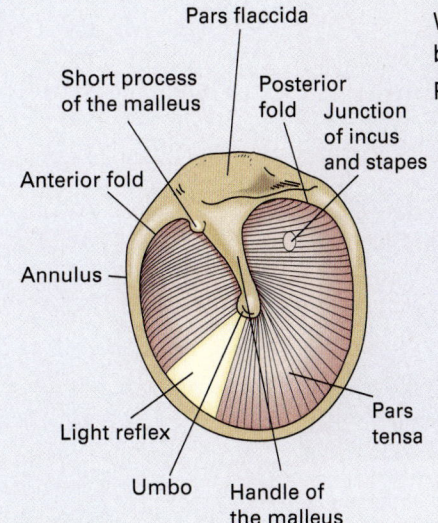

Pars flaccida

Short process of the malleus

Posterior fold

Junction of incus and stapes

Anterior fold

Annulus

Light reflex

Pars tensa

Umbo

Handle of the malleus

FIGURE 27-11 Tympanic Landmarks DELMAR/CENGAGE LEARNING

Data from Estes, M. E. Z. (2010). *Health assessment and physical examination* (4th ed.). Clifton Park, NY: Delmar/Cengage Learning.

TABLE 27-11 Assessing Auditory Acuity

EXAMINATION PROCEDURE	NORMAL FINDINGS	SIGNIFICANT FINDINGS AND POSSIBLE CAUSES
Whispered voice test: Instruct client to tightly cover one ear and repeat words when heard. Stand 1–2 feet away form client, out of view to avoid client lipreading. Stand on side of open ear and softly whisper words. Increase volume until client identifies words correctly. Repeat procedure on other ear.	Able to repeat whispered words correctly.	Inability to hear words may indicate high-frequency hearing loss (excessive exposure to loud noises).
Weber test: Strike tuning fork against your fist or pinch the prongs together. Hold the base of the vibrating fork with thumb and index finger. Center base of fork on top of client's head (see Figure 27-12). Ask client to describe the sound. Repeat test on opposite ear.	Sound perceived equally in both ears = a negative Weber test.	A positive Weber occurs when sound lateralizes to affected ear with a unilateral conductive hearing loss (cerumen impaction, perforated tympanic membrane). Sound can also be lateralized to unaffected ear with sensorineural hearing loss (inner ear disorder, auditory nerve damage, ototoxic drugs, prolonged exposure to excessive noise levels).

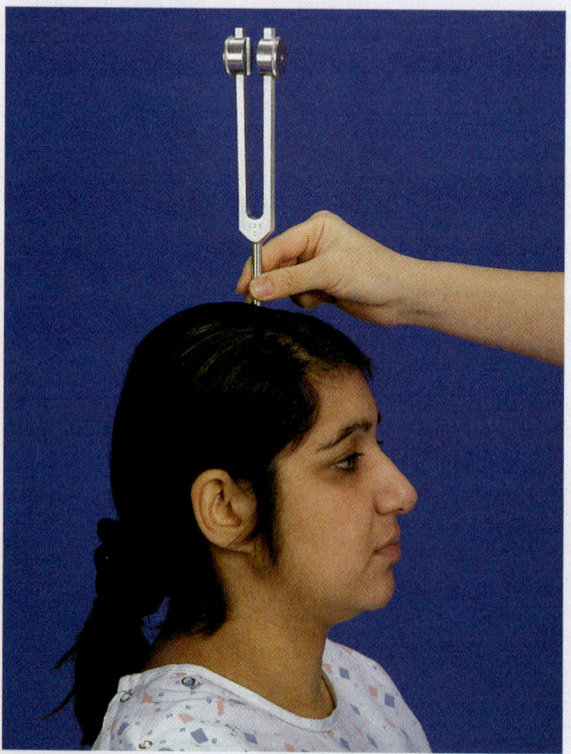

FIGURE 27-12 Weber Test: Place the base of the tuning fork on top of the client's head. DELMAR/CENGAGE LEARNING

(Continues)

TABLE 27-11 (Continued)

EXAMINATION PROCEDURE	NORMAL FINDINGS	SIGNIFICANT FINDINGS AND POSSIBLE CAUSES
Rinne test: Vibrate prongs of tuning fork, place base of fork on mastoid process of ear being tested, and note time until client no longer hears sound (see Figure 27-13A). Move the vibrating fork in front of ear canal, noting length of time sound is heard (see Figure 27-13B).	Sound is heard longer in front of auditory meatus than on mastoid process because air conduction is twice as long as with bone.	Bone conduction that is equal to or greater than air conduction occurs with conductive hearing loss (disease, obstruction, trauma).

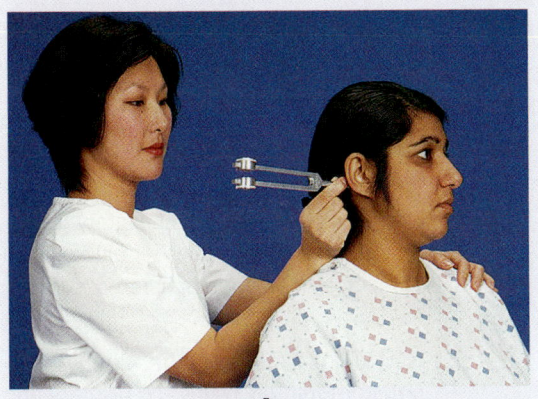

A.

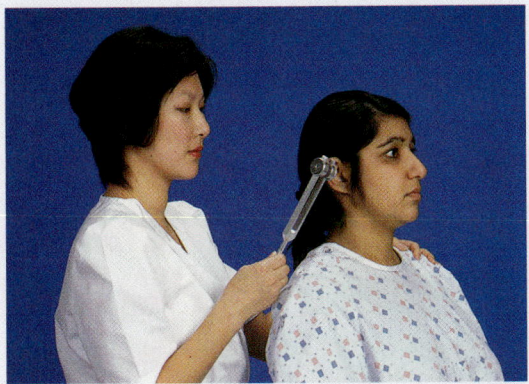

B.

FIGURE 27-13 Rinne Test: A. Place the base of the fork on the mastoid process. **B.** Place tuning fork in front of ear canal. DELMAR/CENGAGE LEARNING

Delmar/Cengage Learning

Neck

Physical examination of the neck includes the neck muscles, lymph nodes of the head and neck, thyroid gland, and trachea. The lymph nodes are normally not easily palpable unless infection is present. If the client has an enlarged thyroid gland, the blood supply will be increased, causing a fine vibration that can be auscultated with the diaphragm of the stethoscope. Frequently, assessment of the neck is done in conjunction with pharyngeal assessment; see Table 27-14 on pages 565–566.

TABLE 27-12 Assessing the Nose and Sinuses

AREA OF ASSESSMENT	NORMAL FINDINGS	SIGNIFICANT FINDINGS AND POSSIBLE CAUSES
Inspect nose for symmetry, edema, inflammation, and discharge.	Located symmetrically, midline of face. Absence of edema, bleeding, lesions, or masses.	Edema (surgery, trauma, e.g., fracture).
Test patency of each nostril: Instruct client to close mouth, apply pressure on one naris, and breathe. Repeat test on opposite naris.	Each nostril is patent.	Inability of air to move through nostril (deviated septum, foreign body, upper respiratory infection, allergies, nasal polyps).
Inspect nasal cavities with a penlight. Extend client's head back and lift tip of nose. Inspect mucosa of each nostril for edema and discharge. Inspect nasal septum for deviation, perforation, lesions, or bleeding.	Mucosa is pink or dull red with no edema or polyps. A small amount of clear watery discharge is normal. Septum is midline and intact.	Red, swollen mucosa with copious clear, watery discharge (common cold). Purulent discharge (bacterial infection). Pale, edematous mucosa with clear, watery discharge (allergies). Normal mucosa with clear, watery discharge that tests positive for glucose usually indicates leakage of cerebrospinal fluid. **NOTE: If present, stop the examination and immediately notify the primary care provider.**
Palpate nasal sinuses (see Figure 27-14). Apply gentle upward pressure on frontal and maxillary areas. Percuss area and note the sound.	Nontender, air-filled cavities, resonant to percussion.	Pain or tenderness (allergy, viral or bacterial infection). Dull sound on percussion (obstruction, e.g., congestion).

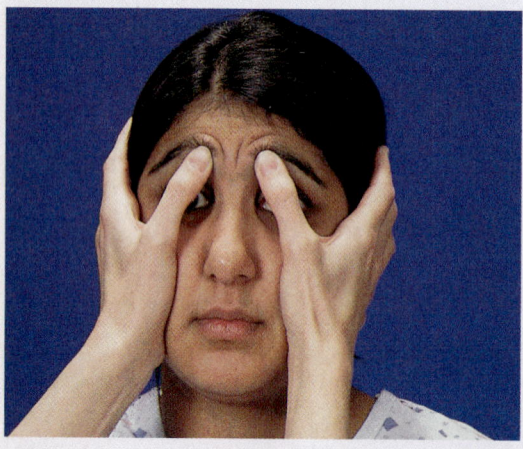

A.

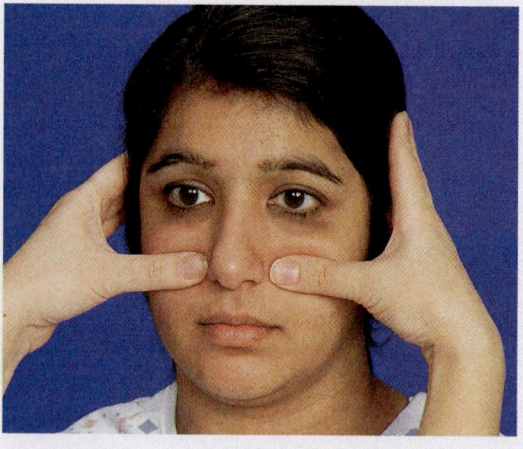

B.

FIGURE 27-14 **Palpating Sinuses: A.** Frontal; **B.** Maxillary DELMAR/CENGAGE LEARNING

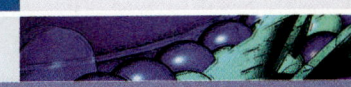

TABLE 27-13 Assessing the Mouth and Pharynx

ASSESSMENT	NORMAL FINDINGS	SIGNIFICANT FINDINGS AND POSSIBLE CAUSES
Stand 12–18 inches in front of client and smell the breath.	Fresh smell.	Halitosis (tooth decay, gum disease, tonsillitis, sinusitis, poor oral hygiene).
Inspect lips and mucosa: Instruct client to open mouth. Retract buccal mucosa with tongue depressor. Inspect color and hydration. Look for lesions or signs of inflammation (see Figure 27-15). Invert lower lip with your thumbs on inner oral mucosa; note muscle tone. Repeat with upper lips using thumbs and index fingers.	Pink, firm, and moist with no lesions or inflammation.	Pale or cyanotic lips (hypoxia). Dry, cracked lips (dehydration, exposure to weather). Angioneurotic edema, i.e., swollen lips (allergic reactions).
Inspect cheeks: Remove dentures, if present. Retract cheeks with a tongue depressor and inspect gingivae (gums). Note color, edema, bleeding, retraction, and lesions.	Pink, smooth, moist, and firm.	Pale gums that bleed easily (periodontal disease, vitamin C deficiency).
Inspect teeth: Instruct client to lightly clench teeth. Note position and alignment. Use tongue depressor to expose the molars. Note color, tartar, cavities, and extractions.	Properly aligned, smooth, white, and shiny.	Chalky discoloration of enamel (early formation of dental caries). Brown or black discoloration (caries).
Inspect tongue: Instruct client to protrude tongue. Inspect dorsum of tongue. Note color, hydration, symmetry, texture, and presence or absence of fasciculation (see Figure 27-16 on page 564). Using a penlight, inspect sides and ventral surface. Note size, texture, nodules, or ulcerations. Grasp tongue with gauze. Gently pull it to one side and palpate the full length of tongue.	Medium red or pink. Midline position when protruded. Moist and smooth along lateral margins. Moves freely. Ventral surface is lightly rough (taste buds).	Enlarged tongue (acromegaly, amyloidosis, stomatitis). Glossitis, deep red with smooth surface (chemotherapy, deficiencies of vitamin B_{12}, niacin, or iron). Thick, white coating with red, raw surface, i.e., candidiasis (immunosuppression).

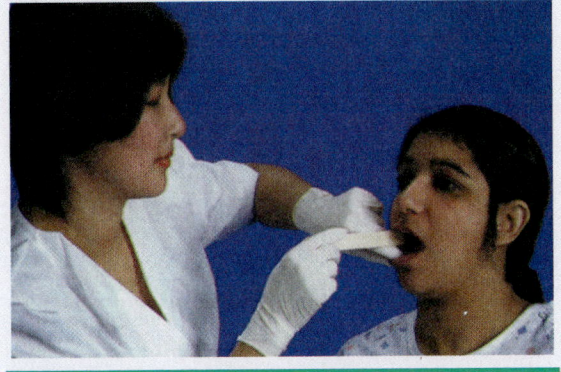

FIGURE 27-15 Inspecting Buccal Mucosa DELMAR/CENGAGE LEARNING

(Continues)

TABLE 27-13 (Continued)

ASSESSMENT	NORMAL FINDINGS	SIGNIFICANT FINDINGS AND POSSIBLE CAUSES
Using a penlight, inspect floor of mouth, salivary glands, and duct openings.		Lesions on ventral surface or hardened areas or ulcerations on lateral surface (cancer).

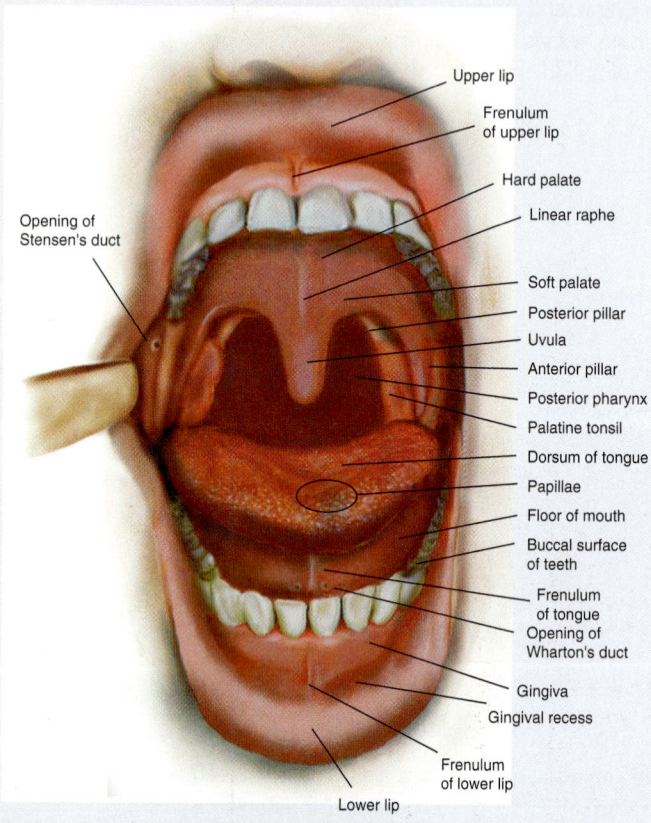

Upper lip
Frenulum of upper lip
Hard palate
Linear raphe
Opening of Stensen's duct
Soft palate
Posterior pillar
Uvula
Anterior pillar
Posterior pharynx
Palatine tonsil
Dorsum of tongue
Papillae
Floor of mouth
Buccal surface of teeth
Frenulum of tongue
Opening of Wharton's duct
Gingiva
Gingival recess
Frenulum of lower lip
Lower lip

FIGURE 27-16 Structures of the Tongue DELMAR/CENGAGE LEARNING

Inspect hard and soft palates: Instruct client to extend head backward and hold mouth open. Using a penlight, inspect the hard palate (roof of mouth) and soft palate. Note color, shape, and lesions.	Both palates are concave and pink. Hard palate has ridges. Soft palate is smooth.	Cleft palate (incomplete fusion of maxillary processes) is a congenital defect. Red, edematous, tender palates (infection). Eroded lesion on hard palate (cancer).
Inspect pharynx: Instruct client to tilt head back and open mouth. Place tongue depressor on middle third of tongue and shine penlight into back of throat. Instruct client to say "ah." Note the position, size, and appearance of tonsils and uvula. If palate and uvula fail to rise symmetrically with phonation, elicit the gag reflex and have client say "ah."	Pharynx is pink, vascular, and lesion free. With phonation, the soft palate and uvula rise symmetrically.	Reddened, edematous uvula and tonsillar pillars with yellow exudate (pharyngitis). Swollen, gray membranes and tonsillar enlargement (acute tonsillitis, mononucleosis, diphtheria).

TABLE 27-14 Assessment of the Neck

ASSESSMENT	NORMAL FINDINGS	SIGNIFICANT FINDINGS AND POSSIBLE CAUSES
Inspect for symmetry and musculature. Instruct client to flex chin to chest and to each side and shoulder. Instruct client to hyperextend neck backward.	Movement through full range of motion (ROM) with no limitation or discomfort.	Pain upon flexion or rotation of head (muscle spasm, inflammation of muscles or meninges, vertebral diseases). Torticollis, i.e., prominent lateral deviation of sternocleidomastoid muscle (inflammation, trauma, sleeping with head in one position). Decreased ROM (degenerative osteoarthritis).
Palpate lymph nodes: Instruct client to relax and flex neck slightly forward. Stand in front of client and systematically palpate anterior cervical nodes and posterior cervical nodes (see Figure 27-17). Note size, shape, mobility, consistency, and tenderness.	Palpable lymph nodes. Small, movable nodes are insignificant.	Palpable nodes (infection, malignancy).

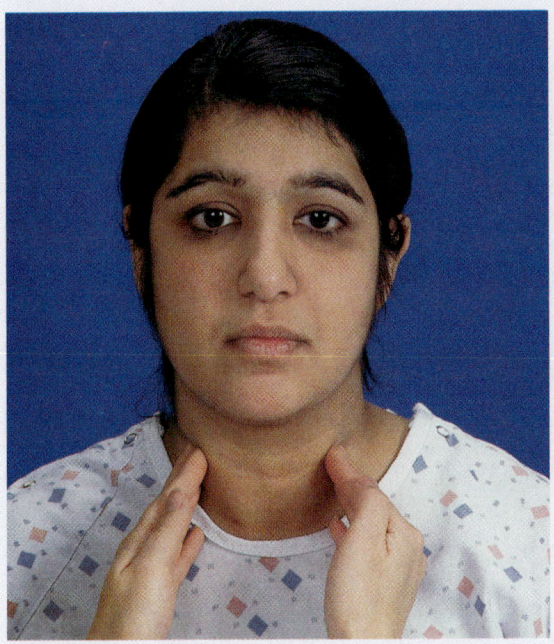 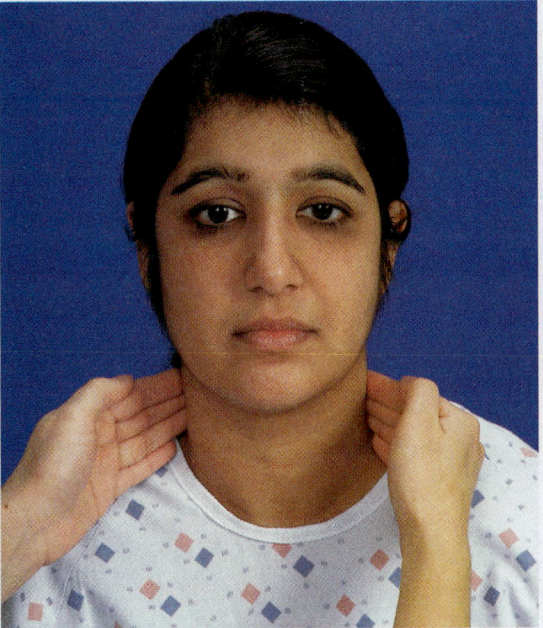

A. **B.**

FIGURE 27-17 **Palpating the Cervical Lymph Nodes: A.** Anterior Approach; **B.** Posterior Approach

DELMAR/CENGAGE LEARNING

Inspect and palpate trachea: Note position. Place thumbs and index fingers on sides of trachea. Apply gentle pressure and palpate.	Midline position in suprasternal notch.	Lateral displacement (neck mass, mediastinal mass, pulmonary disorders).

(Continues)

TABLE 27-14 (Continued)

ASSESSMENT	NORMAL FINDINGS	SIGNIFICANT FINDINGS AND POSSIBLE CAUSES
Palpate thyroid gland: Stand behind or in front of client (see Figure 27-18). Instruct client to slightly extend neck. Rest thumbs on nape of neck, and place index and middle fingers of both hands on thyroid isthmus and anterior surfaces of lateral lobes. Ask client to swallow and to flex neck forward and to left. Gently move thyroid cartilage to the right. Note any bulging of gland. Place your thumb deep into and behind sternocleido-mastoid muscle with index and middle fingers in front. Ask client to swallow. Note any enlargement of glands. If gland is enlarged, place stethoscope diaphragm over gland. Note on auscultation presence of bruit (soft vibration or rushing sound).	Thyroid cannot be visualized. Smooth, soft, nontender, and not enlarged. Isthmus is palpable when swallowing occurs. No bruit.	Masses or enlargements during swallowing (goiter, thyroid disease). Bruits heard on auscultation (enlarged toxic goiter).

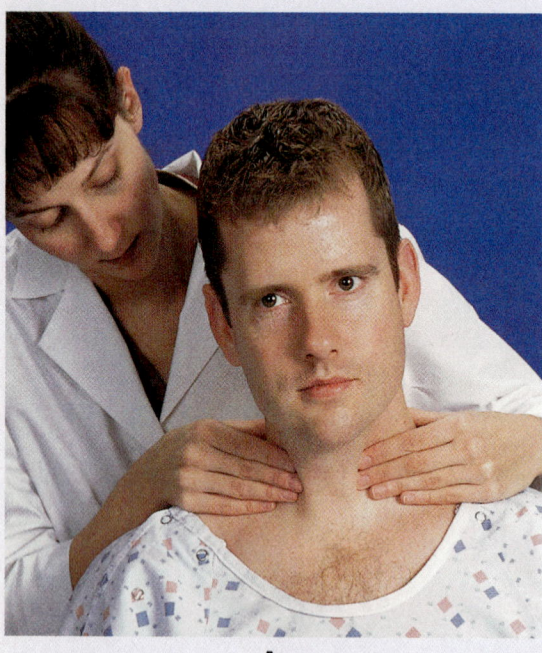

A.

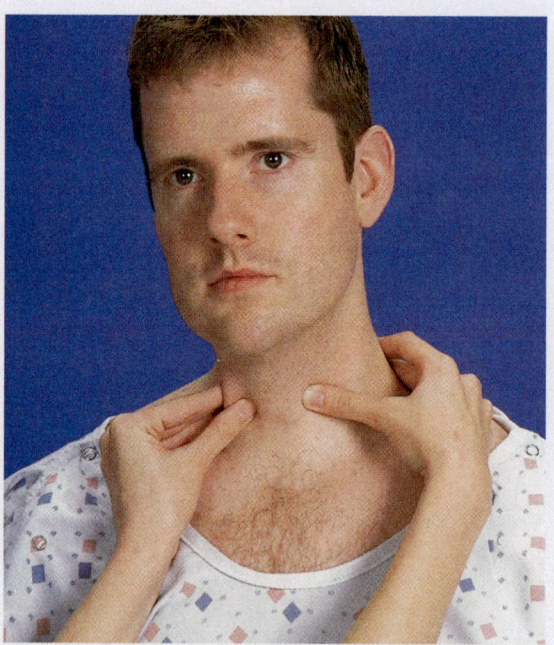

B.

FIGURE 27-18 Palpating the Thyroid: **A.** Posterior Approach; **B.** Anterior Approach DELMAR/CENGAGE LEARNING

Delmar/Cengage Learning

THORAX AND LUNGS

Physical assessment includes inspection, palpation, percussion, and auscultation of the posterior, lateral, and anterior thorax and lungs. Figure 27-19 depicts the landmarks of the thorax. Landmarks are imaginary lines that are based on anatomic structures such as the spine and sternum. These landmarks assist with locating the underlying organs for percussion and auscultation and for accurate documentation of findings. The angle of Louis is a landmark for identifying the ribs in the midclavicular line. Each intercostal space (ICS) is named for the number of the rib directly above it; that is, the space between the third and fourth ribs is the third ICS. When used together, landmarks and ICSs identify the specific lobes of the lungs for percussion and auscultation. See Chapter 32 for a description of structural changes that may occur in the thorax.

Respiratory auscultation reveals the presence of normal and abnormal breath sounds. During auscultation, the client should be instructed to breathe only through the mouth because mouth breathing decreases air turbulence that could interfere with an accurate assessment. Figure 27-20 on page 568 shows the anterior, posterior, and right lateral positions of the lung lobes. Table 27-15 on page 568 (containing Figures 27-21 through 27-26) presents the specific areas of the thorax and lungs to be examined and the normal and key findings of this assessment.

Auscultation of breath sounds is a skill that develops with practice. There are many factors that may interfere with correctly assessing breath sounds; see the accompanying Nursing Process Highlight.

There are three distinct types of normal breath sounds with their own unique pitch, intensity, quality, location, and relative duration in the inspiratory and expiratory phases of respiration. These normal breath sounds are:

- **Vesicular sounds:** soft, breezy, and low-pitched sounds heard longer on inspiration than expiration that result from air moving through the smaller airways over the lung's periphery, with the exception of the scapular area
- **Bronchovesicular sounds:** medium-pitched and blowing sounds heard equally on inspiration and expiration

---

NURSING PROCESS HIGHLIGHT

Assessment

Factors Affecting Auscultation of Breath Sounds

- **Rustling of paper drapes or gowns.** Ask client to remain still while you are listening to the breath sounds.
- **Chest hair:** Course or dense hair may sound like crackles. Dampen the hair to prevent distortion of findings.
- **Shivering or chattering of teeth.** Determine why client is shivering or chattering, and correct the problem.
- **Mechanical ventilator tubing:** A gurgling sound can be caused by water condensing in mechanical ventilator tubing. Clear all tubing of moisture prior to auscultation.
- **Secretions in upper airway:** Oropharyngeal secretions may cause respirations to be loud and gurgling. Ask client to clear throat, or perform oropharyngeal or nasopharyngeal suctioning if necessary.

Data from Estes, M. E. Z. (2010). Health assessment and physical examination (4th ed.). Clifton Park, NY: Delmar/Cengage Learning.

---

from air moving through the large airways, posteriorly between the scapula and anteriorly over bronchioles lateral to the sternum at the first and second ICSs
- **Bronchial sounds:** loud and high-pitched sounds with a hollow quality heard longer on expiration than inspiration from air moving through the trachea

These normal breath sounds must be auscultated over the correct location, for example, bronchial sounds over the trachea. Otherwise, bronchial sounds in clients with emphysema are heard in the peripheral lung areas where normal vesicular sounds should be heard.

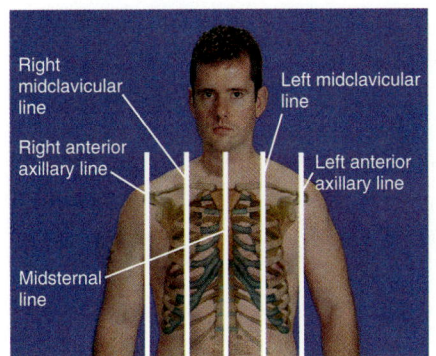

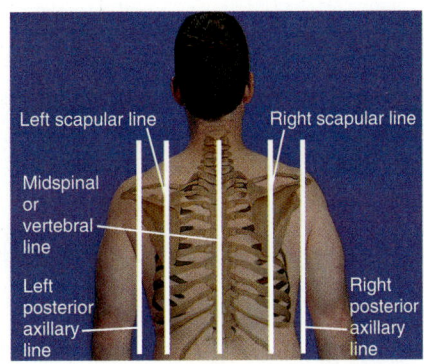

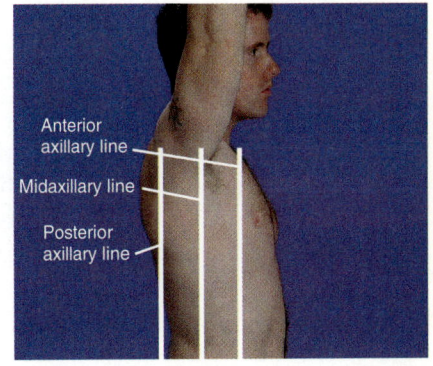

A.   **B.**   **C.**

FIGURE 27-19 Landmarks of the Thorax: A. Anterior Thorax; **B.** Posterior Thorax; **C.** Right Lateral Thorax DELMAR/CENGAGE LEARNING

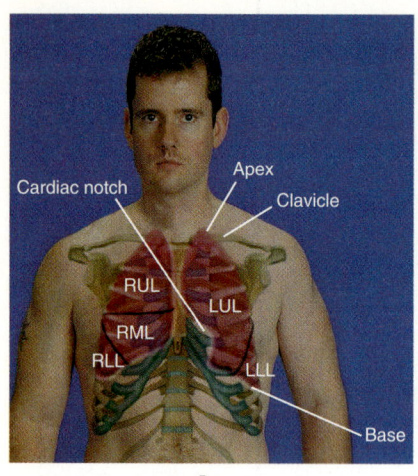
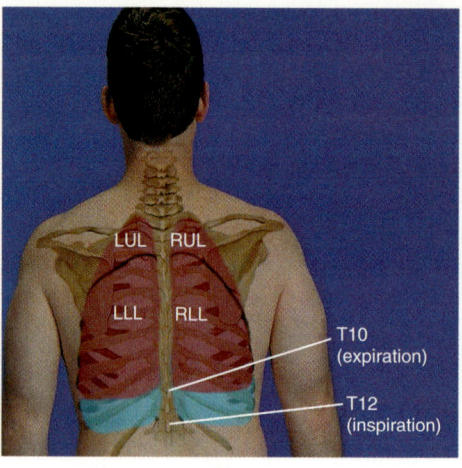
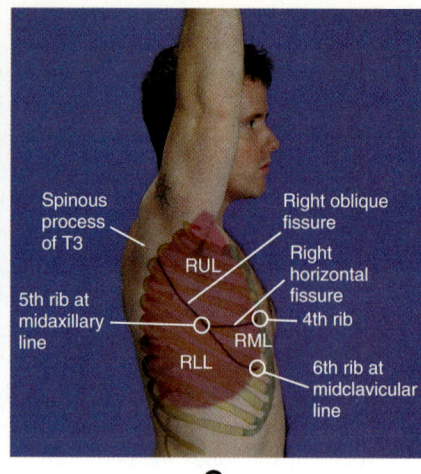

A.   **B.**   **C.**

FIGURE 27-20 Positions of the Lung Lobes: **A.** Anterior View with Ribs; **B.** Posterior View with Ribs; **C.** Right Lateral View with Ribs
DELMAR/CENGAGE LEARNING

TABLE 27-15 Assessment of Thorax and Lungs

ASSESSMENT AREA/TECHNIQUES	NORMAL FINDINGS	SIGNIFICANT FINDINGS AND POSSIBLE CAUSES
Inspect posterior thorax: Place client in a sitting position, with arms folded across chest (to separate scapulae) and back exposed. Inspect shape and symmetry of chest. Note respiratory rate, rhythm, and movement of chest wall. Note any signs of distress. Estimate the anteroposterior diameter in proportion to lateral diameter.	Respirations are quiet, regular, and effortless, with rate of 12–20 per minute. Thorax rises and falls in unison with respiratory cycle. Ribs slope across and downward, without movement or bulging in the intercostal space (ICS). The adult ratio of anteroposterior to lateral chest diameter ranges form 2:2 to 5:7.	Horizontal slope of ribs (emphysema). Bulging in ICS (increased respiratory effort). Retraction of ICS during inspiration (airway obstruction, e.g., asthma). Impaired respiratory movement (diseases of lungs or pleurae). Increased anteroposterior diameter (barrel chest as a result of chronic obstructive pulmonary disease).
Palpate posterior thorax: Palpate lesions or areas of tenderness. Palpate thoracic expansion at 10th rib: Place thumbs close to client's spine and spread hands over thorax (see Figure 27-21 on page 569). Note divergence of thumbs; feel for range and symmetry of movement during deep inhalation and full exhalation. Place ulnar aspect of open hand on each location as shown in Figure 27-22 on page 569. Instruct client to say "99" and palpate for tactile fremitus (vibrations created by sound waves). Note areas of increased or decreased fremitus. Move hands from side to side, with client repeating "99" with same intensity every time hands are placed on back.	Posterior thorax is free from tenderness, lesions, and pulsations. Thumbs should separate an equal distance (approximately 3–5 cm) and in the same direction during inhalation and meet at the midline on expirations. Fremitus is equal on both sides of thorax, strongest at level of tracheal bifurcation.	Tenderness (trauma, e.g., fractured rib). Unilateral decreased thoracic expansion (pneumonia, pneumothorax). Bilateral decreased expansion (emphysema, pleurisy). Absent or decreased fremitus (decreased voice tone; bronchial obstruction; accumulation of fluid, air, or solid tissue in pleural space). Fremitus is increased over consolidated areas of lungs.

(Continues)

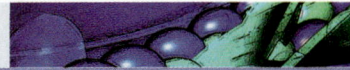

TABLE 27-15 (Continued)

ASSESSMENT AREA/TECHNIQUES	NORMAL FINDINGS	SIGNIFICANT FINDINGS AND POSSIBLE CAUSES

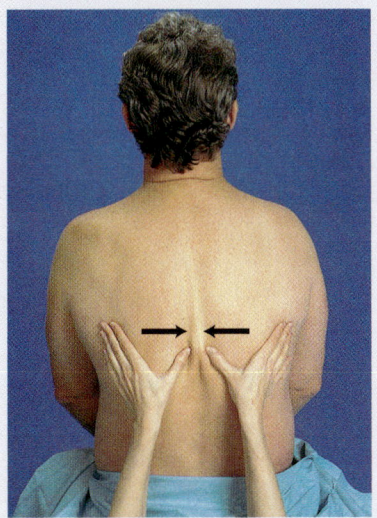

FIGURE 27-21 Palpating Posterior Thoracic
Expansion DELMAR/CENGAGE LEARNING

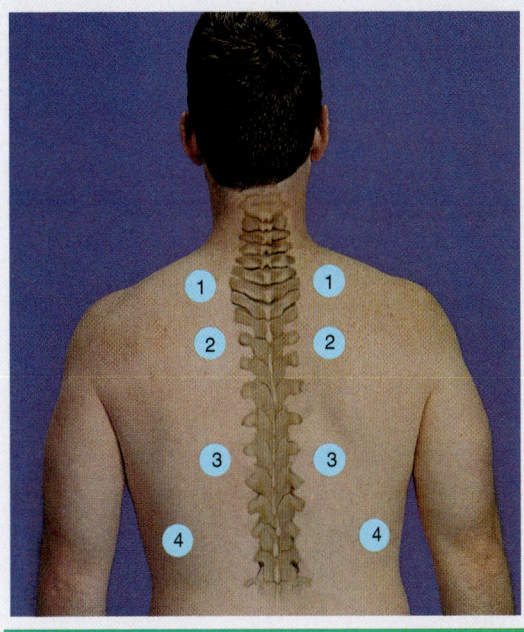

FIGURE 27-22 Palpation Pattern for Tactile Fremitus: **Posterior Thorax** DELMAR/CENGAGE LEARNING

Percuss chest systematically
(see Figure 27-23):

Start at lung apices. Move hands from side to side across top of each shoulder. Note sound produced from each percussion strike and compare with contralateral sound.

Continue downward in posterior lateral movement, palpating over every other ICS (see Figure 27-24). Note intensity, pitch, duration, and quality of percussion.

Air-filled lungs create a resonant sound.

Identify contralateral sound; bones (e.g., ribs, spine) create a flat sound.

Thorax is more resonant in children and thin adults.

Hyperresonance in adults (pneumothorax, asthma, emphysema).

Dull sound (pneumonia, pleural effusion, tumors).

NOTE: Pleural fluid sinks to lowest part of pleural space (fluids collect in posterior lobes in supine client).

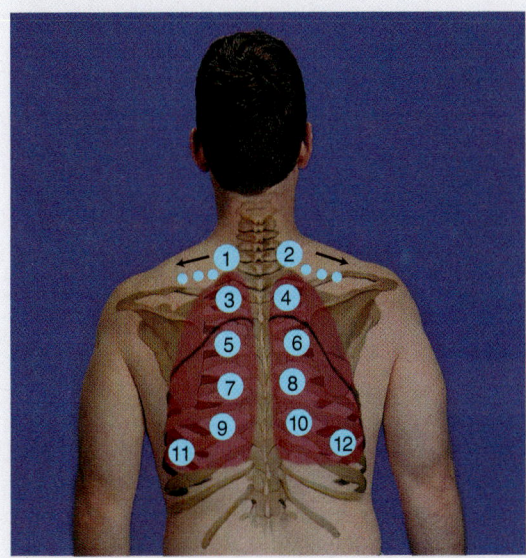

FIGURE 27-23 Percussion Pattern of Posterior **Thorax** DELMAR/CENGAGE LEARNING

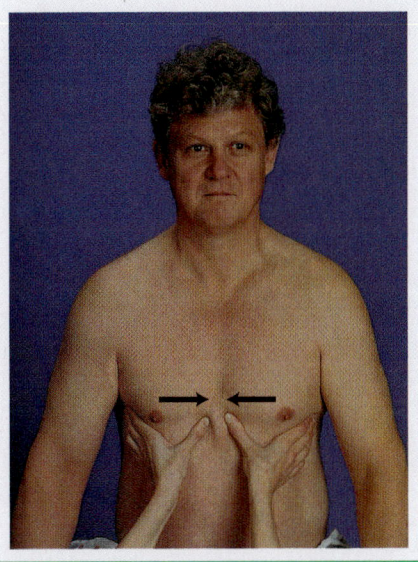

FIGURE 27-24 Palpating Anterior **Thoracic Expansion** DELMAR/CENGAGE LEARNING

(Continues)

TABLE 27-15 (Continued)

ASSESSMENT AREA/TECHNIQUES	NORMAL FINDINGS	SIGNIFICANT FINDINGS AND POSSIBLE CAUSES
Auscultate posterior and lateral surfaces: Place stethoscope diaphragm on right lung apex. Instruct client to inhale and exhale deeply and slowly when stethoscope is felt on the back. Repeat on left lung apex. Move downward every other ICS and auscultate, placing stethoscope in the same position on both sides of chest. Auscultate the lateral aspect by placing the stethoscope directly below the right axilla. Instruct client to breathe only through the mouth and to inhale and exhale slowly. Proceed downward, every other ICS on the same side.	A large chest produces decreased breath sounds.	Decreased breath sounds (obstruction, e.g., foreign object, emphysema, atelectasis). Absent breath sounds (empyema, hemothorax, pneumothorax, pneumonectomy).
Inspect anterior thorax: Place client in sitting or supine position. Inspect for symmetry and depth of respiration, rhythm of respirations, slope of ribs, and presence of musculoskeletal deformities.	Scapulae at same height. Thorax rises and falls in unison with respiratory cycle; ribs are at a 45° angle with sternum. Inhalation breath sounds inaudible at a distance of more than 2–3 cm from the mouth.	One scapula higher than the other (scoliosis). Rib angle of less than 45° (emphysema, cystic fibrosis). Chest retraction on inspiration obstructs free inflow of air (asthma, tracheal/laryngeal obstruction, tumor).
Palpate anterior thorax: Place fingerpads on right lung apex, above the clavicle. Move downward to each rib and ICS. Note tenderness, pulsation, masses, and crepitus (a grating or crackling sensation caused by two rough surfaces rubbing together). Repeat on left side. Assess respiratory expansion by placing thumbs along each costal margin with hands on lateral rib cage. Instruct client to inhale deeply. Note divergence of thumbs on expansion; feel range and symmetry of respiratory movement. Palpate for tactile fremitus (see Figure 27-25 on page 571).	Same as normal findings for posterior palpation. Note that fremitus is usually decreased or absent over the precordium (chest wall).	Pulsations (thoracic aortic aneurysm). Pain or tenderness (fractured rib). Unilateral decreased thoracic expansion (pneumonia, pneumothorax). Crepitus occurs when air escapes the lung and is trapped in subcutaneous tissue (any condition that interrupts the pleurae, e.g., pneumothorax, thoracic surgery).
Percuss anterior thorax: Percuss symmetrically (see Figure 27-26 on page 571). Percuss 2–3 strikes along right lung apex; repeat on left lung apex. Proceed downward and percuss in every other ICS going from right to left in same position on both sides. Gently lift breast tissue as necessary.	Resonant sound over lung tissue (hyperresonance in children and thin adults). Cardiac, liver, and gastric silhouettes emit dull sound. Ribs emit flat sound.	Dullness over lung tissue (pneumonia, tumors).

(Continues)

TABLE 27-15 (Continued)

ASSESSMENT AREA/TECHNIQUES	NORMAL FINDINGS	SIGNIFICANT FINDINGS AND POSSIBLE CAUSES

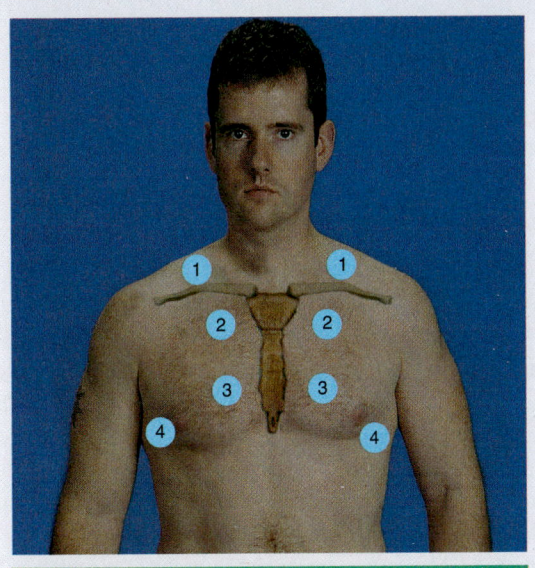

FIGURE 27-25 Palpation Pattern for Tactile Fremitus: Anterior Thorax DELMAR/CENGAGE LEARNING

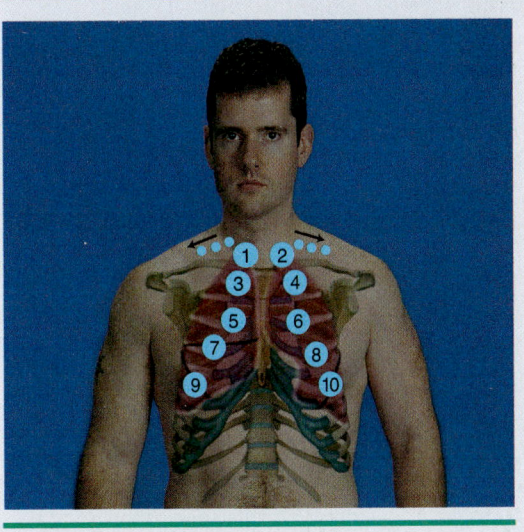

FIGURE 27-26 Percussion Pattern for Anterior Thorax DELMAR/CENGAGE LEARNING

In each thoracic area, assess for:

  a. Resonant lung field
  b. Cardiac dullness: third to fifth ICS left of sternum
  c. Liver dullness: Place pleximeter finger parallel to upper border of expected liver dullness in right mid-clavicular line; percuss downward.
  d. Gastric air bubble: Repeat procedure performed for liver dullness on left side.

Auscultate anterior thorax: Instruct client to breathe through mouth. Compare symmetrical areas of the lungs while moving stethoscope downward. Listen to breath sounds. Note intensity, and identify abnormal variations. If breath sounds are diminished, ask client to breathe hard and fast with mouth open.	A large chest wall will normally produce decreased breath sounds.	Absent breath sounds (empyema, hemothorax, pneumothorax, pneumonectomy).

Delmar/Cengage Learning

Breath sounds that are not normal are described as either abnormal or **adventitious breath sounds** (superimposed sounds on the normal vesicular, bronchovesicular, and bronchial breath sounds). Abnormal breath sounds are characterized by decreased or absent sounds. The five types of adventitious breath sounds are:

- **Crackles:** heard predominantly on inspiration over the base of the lungs as an interrupted fine crackle (dry, high-pitched crackling, popping sound of short duration) that sounds like a piece of hair being rolled between the fingers in front of the ear or a coarse crackle (moist, low-pitched crackling, gurgling sound of long duration) that sounds like water going down the drain after the plug has been pulled on a full tub of water

- **Rhonchi:** heard predominantly on expiration over the trachea and bronchi as a continuous, low-pitched musical sound
- **Wheezes:** heard predominantly on expiration all over the lungs as a continuous sonorous wheeze (low-pitched snoring) or sibilant wheeze (high-pitched musical sound)
- **Pleural friction rub:** heard on either inspiration or expiration over the anterior lateral lungs as a continuous creaking, grating sound
- **Stridor:** heard predominantly on inspiration as a continuous crowing sound

During the assessment of the thorax and lungs, the nurse should monitor the client for symptoms of hyperventilation (light-headedness or dizziness). If this occurs, continue the assessment when the client's dizziness is gone and breathing is normal.

HEART AND VASCULAR SYSTEM

Heart and vascular system assessment techniques consist of inspection, palpation, and auscultation. The nurse should review the client's health history for cardiac risk factors such as family history, cigarette smoking, and dietary and exercise habits. Many people can reduce their risk of cardiac problems by making lifestyle alterations. Nurses are key in providing information that helps clients promote cardiovascular health and wellness; see the accompanying Client Teaching Checklist.

Heart

Inspection, palpation, and auscultation are performed in a systematic manner using specific cardiac landmarks. The cardiac landmarks (see Figure 27-27) are defined as follows:

- Aortic area is the second ICS to the right of the sternum.
- Pulmonic area is the second ICS to the left of the sternum.

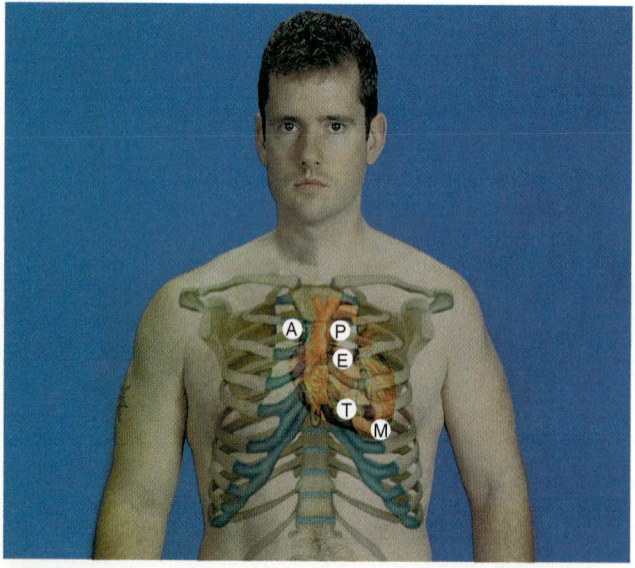

FIGURE 27-27 Cardiac Landmarks: A, aortic area; P, pulmonic area; E, Erb's point; T, tricuspid area; and M, mitral area.

DELMAR/CENGAGE LEARNING

✓ **CLIENT TEACHING CHECKLIST**

Promoting Cardiovascular Health

- Determine risk as a result of family history.
- Avoid cigarette smoking and passive smoke inhalation.
- Control hypertension and hyperlipidemia through diet, exercise, and prescribed medications.
- Control glucose intolerance/diabetes through diet, exercise, and prescribed medications.
- Engage in physical activity.
- Maintain healthy body weight and body mass index.
- Engage in stress management/relaxation techniques regularly.

- Erb's point is located in the third ICS to the left of the sternum.
- Tricuspid area (right ventricular area or septal area) is the fifth ICS to the left of the sternum.
- Mitral area (left ventricular or apical area) is the fifth ICS at the left midclavicular line.

The mitral area is correlated anatomically with the apex of the heart, and the aortic and pulmonic areas are correlated anatomically with the base of the heart. Assessment proceeds either from the base of the heart to the apex or from the apex to the base.

The first heart sound (S_1) occurs with closure of the atrioventricular valves, signaling the beginning of systole. S_1, which sounds like "lub," can be heard across the left chest but is loudest at the apex. The second heart sound (S_2) indicates the end of systole and sounds like "dub." Additional heart sounds (S_3 and S_4) may also be heard during auscultation. S_3 (also called a ventricular gallop) may be heard in the tricuspid and mitral areas during the early to mid-diastole following the S_2 sound. S_3 is heard best when the client is in the left lateral recumbent position. S_4 (also called atrial diastolic gallop) may be heard in the tricuspid and mitral areas during the late phase of diastole, before S_1 of the next cardiac cycle. S_4 is heard best when the client is in the supine position.

An S_3 can be a normal physiological sound in children and young adults; in adults it may be indicative of cardiac dysfunction (Estes, 2010). An S_4 may occur with or without any evidence of cardiac decompensation, or it can be indicative of coronary artery disease and heart failure (Estes, 2010).

There are distinct abnormal findings found on palpation and auscultation of the chest and heart. During palpation, the nurse should assess for **thrills** (vibrations that feel similar to what one feels when a hand is placed on a purring cat) and **heaves** (lifting of the cardiac area secondary to an increased workload and force of left ventricular contraction). Abnormal heart sounds relative to **stenosis** (a narrowing or constriction of a blood vessel or valve) or **regurgitation** (the backward flow of blood through a diseased heart valve, also known as insufficiency) can be heard during auscultation as a click (a high-pitched systolic sound created by the opening of the valve) or a **murmur** (swishing or blowing sounds of long duration heard during the systolic and diastolic phases created by turbulent blood flow through a valve). Other abnormal sounds heard on auscultation are a pericardial friction rub (high-pitched, multiphasic, scratchy, or grating sound that does not change with respirations) and **bruits** (blowing sounds that are heard when the blood flow becomes turbulent as it rushes past an obstruction).

Murmurs are characterized by their:

- Location: area where the murmur is heard loudest (e.g., mitral, pulmonic).
- Radiation: transmission of sound from a specific valve to other adjacent structures (mitral murmurs can radiate to the axilla).
- Timing: phase in the cardiac cycle. If the murmur occurs simultaneously with the pulse, it is a systolic murmur. If the murmur is not related to the pulse, it is a diastolic murmur.
- Intensity: the loudness or character.

- Quality: sound produced (harsh, rumbling, blowing, or musical).
- Pitch: high, medium, or low (auscultated with the bell of a stethoscope for low-pitched murmurs and the diaphragm for high-pitched murmurs).
- Configuration: pattern that the murmur makes over time; described as crescendo (soft to loud), decrescendo (loud to soft), crescendo-decrescendo (soft to loud to soft), and plateau (sustained sound) (Estes, 2010).

See the accompanying Nursing Process Highlight on page 574 for a classification scale for murmurs. Table 27-16 presents the specific areas to be examined and the normal and key findings of assessment of the heart. Some common terms associated with cardiac assessment are:

- **Aneurysm:** localized (aortic) abnormal dilation of a blood vessel wall
- **Angina:** pain in chest, neck, or arm resulting from myocardial ischemia
- Arteriosclerosis: buildup of plaques in the inner layers of the walls of large to medium-sized arteries

TABLE 27-16 Assessing the Heart

ASSESSMENT	NORMAL FINDINGS	SIGNIFICANT FINDINGS AND POSSIBLE CAUSES

Heart:
 Inspect, palpate, and auscultate.
 Place client in supine position with head elevated 30°–45°.
 Drape to expose anterior thorax.
 Inspect anterior thorax and precordium. Note presence of pulsations, heaves, or retractions.
 Simultaneously inspect and palpate each of the cardiac landmarks for apical impulses. Use fingerpads to palpate pulsations and ball of hand to palpate thrill or heaves.
   a. Aortic area (second ICS to right of sternum)
   b. Pulmonic area (second left ICS)
   c. Third left ICS
   d. Right ventricular area (left, lower half of sternum and parasternal area)
   e. Apex of heart (fifth ICS medial to midclavicular line)
	Absence of visible pulsations, heaves, or retractions.	Visible pulsations, heaves, or retractions require additional inspection with palpation to identify exact location and timing in relation to cardiac cycle (systole or diastole).
		   a. Thrill (aortic stenosis or regurgitation).
		   b. Thrill (pulmonic stenosis or regurgitation).
		   c. Pulsations (left ventricular aneurysm, enlarged right ventricle).
		   d. Thrill and heave (tricuspid stenosis or regurgitation).
		   e. Thrill (mitral stenosis or regurgitation). Heave (left ventricular hypertrophy).

Aortic area: Note pulsation, thrill, or vibration of aortic valve closure. *Pulmonic area:* Third left ICS: Note pulsation, thrill, or vibration for pulmonic valve closure. *Right ventricular area:* Assess for a diffuse lift (heave) or thrill.		

(Continues)

TABLE 27-16 (Continued)

ASSESSMENT	NORMAL FINDINGS	SIGNIFICANT FINDINGS AND POSSIBLE CAUSES
Apex of heart: Note pulsation, thrill, or heave. Palpate high in epigastric region for pulsations, bruits, or masses.	Pulsations thrusting upward against the fingerpads are caused by aorta. No bruits or masses.	Bruit (aneurysm). A mass and strong pulsations (abdominal aortic aneurysm). **Notify primary care provider immediately if signs of aneurysm are detected.**
Auscultate heart sounds: In every area auscultated, distinguish S_1 and S_2 sounds.	S_1: Usually auscultated at all sites; louder at apical area. S_2: Usually heard at all sites; louder at base of heart. S_3: In children and young adults. S_4: In many older adults.	Increased or decreased intensity. Varying intensity with different beats. Increased intensity at aortic area. Increased intensity at pulmonic area. S_3 in older adults. S_4 may be a sign of hypertension.

Delmar/Cengage Learning

- Atrial fibrillation: rapid, random contractions of the atria with irregular ventricular beats
- Bundle branch block: conduction abnormality of the cardiac impulse through the bundle of His fibers
- Heart failure: circulatory congestion caused by a cardiac disorder
- Coronary artery disease: any abnormal condition that may affect the arteries of the heart
- Ischemia: local and temporary lack of blood supply to the heart
- Myocardial infarction: necrosis of the heart muscle
- Thrombophlebitis: inflammation of a vein with a formed blood clot

NURSING PROCESS HIGHLIGHT

Assessment

Classification of Murmurs

Grade I: Barely audible
Grade II: Audible immediately
Grade III: Moderate intensity
Grade IV: Loud, may be associated with a thrill
Grade V: Loud, with palpable thrill, audible with stethoscope in contact with chest wall
Grade VI: Louder, heard without stethoscope, palpable thrill

Vascular System

Both the central vessels (carotid arteries and jugular veins) directly affect brain functioning by transporting nutrients and waste products. The carotid arteries must be carefully assessed for patency since they are the only source of blood to the brain. During auscultation, determine the presence of a bruit; if a bruit is discovered, palpate for a thrill. Both thrills and bruits at the carotid arteries indicate turbulent blood flow, which results from obstruction of the vessels; see the Safety First display.

The jugular veins return blood from the brain to the superior vena cava and right side of the heart. By assessing the jugular veins for distention and pulsations, the nurse can assess the adequacy of function of the right side of the heart. Bilateral jugular vein distention (JVD) is usually an indicator of right-sided heart failure. See Table 27-17 on page 575 for assessment of the vascular system.

▼ SAFETY FIRST ▼

ASSESSING CAROTID ARTERIES
Never palpate both carotid arteries simultaneously as this may occlude blood flow to the brain. Palpate first one artery, then the other, to avoid impeding adequate circulation.

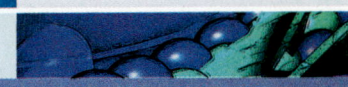

TABLE 27-17 Assessing the Vascular System

ASSESSMENT AREAS/TECHNIQUES	NORMAL FINDINGS	SIGNIFICANT FINDINGS AND POSSIBLE CAUSES
Inspection, palpation, and auscultation: Assist client to supine position with head elevated 30°–45° and drape to expose only areas being assessed.		
Carotid arteries: Inspect right carotid artery along margin of sterno-cleidomastoid muscle. Palpate carotid artery at lower half of neck (to avoid carotid sinus). Instruct client to turn head toward right side. Place fingerpads of index and middle fingers around medial edge of sternoclei-domastoid muscle. Instruct client to hold breath. Auscultate carotid artery, and listen for bruits. Repeat on left side.	1. Absence of kinks or bulging. 2. Pulses are equal in rate and rhythm. 3. No bruits.	1. Kinks or bulges (hypertension, arteriosclerosis). 2. Decreased pulsations (arterial narrowing or occlusion). 3. Bruits (narrow or obstructed artery).
Jugular veins: Inspect and palpate. Assist client to supine with head elevated 30°–45°. Avoid neck hyperextension or flexion. Inspect right internal jugular vein. Measure the vertical distance in centimeters from the sternal angle (angle of Louis) to top of dis-tended neck vent to obtain an indirect jugular venous pressure. Repeat on left side.	Measurement of 1–2 cm above the angle of Louis with head of bed elevated 45°.	Distended jugular veins (greater than 2 cm) with client in sitting position (fluid volume overload, e.g., rapid infusion of intravenous solution). Increased jugular venous pressure accompanied by a third heart sound (heart failure).
Peripheral pulses: Inspect and palpate. Starting with temporal artery, palpate pulses in sequential pattern (upper extremities to lower extremities). Note rhythm, rate, quality, and volume at each pulse site. If unable to palpate a pulse, use an ultrasound stethoscope (Doppler) to amplify sound.	Bilateral equality and symmetry of peripheral pulses.	Markedly diminished or absent pulses indicate arterial occlusion and inadequate circulation.
Tissue perfusion: Inspect and palpate. Perform the Allen test to determine patency of radial and ulnar arteries (see Figure 27-28 on page 576).	Palms should turn pinkish color promptly when pressure is removed.	Persistence of pallor when one ar-tery is manually compressed indi-cates occlusion of the other artery. Edema or ulceration (venous stasis).

(Continues)

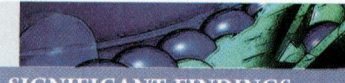

TABLE 27-17 (Continued)

ASSESSMENT AREAS/TECHNIQUES	NORMAL FINDINGS	SIGNIFICANT FINDINGS AND POSSIBLE CAUSES

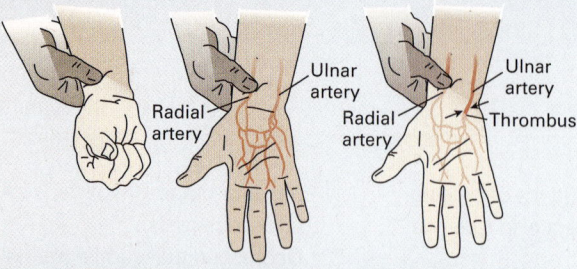

FIGURE 27-28 Allen Test: **A.** Pallor is initiated by compressing the radial artery with client's fist clenched. **B.** A patent ulnar artery reveals the return of palm perfusion despite radial artery compression. **C.** An occluded ulnar artery results in continued pallor of the hand while the radial artery is still compressed. DELMAR/CENGAGE LEARNING

a. Firmly compress arteries and instruct client to open the hand.
b. Note color of palms.
c. Repeat on other hand. Inspect both legs from groin and buttocks to feet. Note venous enlargement, redness or discoloration, and ulcers over saphenous veins.

Tenderness, pain, warmth, redness, or discoloration (thrombophlebitis).

Dilated, tortuous veins are varicosities.

Data from D'Amico, D., & Barbarito, C. (2007). *Health & physical assessment in nursing.* Upper Saddle River, NJ: Pearson Prentice Hall; Estes, M. E. Z. (2010). *Health assessment and physical examination* Clifton Park, NY: Delmar/Cengage Learning (4th ed.).; Jarvis, C. (2007). *Physical examination & health assessment* (5th ed.). Philadelphia: Elsevier.

To assess blood perfusion of peripheral vessels and skin, the nurse should note changes in skin temperature, color, sensation, and the pulses. Because the position of the extremities can affect the skin temperature and appearance, always assess extremities at heart level and at normal room and body temperature. Feeling the toes for warmth and color provides important information relative to peripheral circulation and tissue perfusion. Peripheral pulses should be compared bilaterally, and changes in strength and quality should be noted (Estes, 2010).

BREASTS AND AXILLAE

Inspection and palpation are used to assess breasts of both males and females. Palpation is used for assessment of the axillae and lymph nodes of all clients.

The breasts are divided into four quadrants, inclusive of the tail of Spence, by lines crossing at the nipples (see Figure 27-29 on page 577). These quadrants are used in a sequential fashion during assessment. Figure 27-30 on page 577 shows a cross section of breast tissue.

See Table 27-18 on page 577, which presents specific areas of the female breast and axillae to be examined and the normal and significant findings with possible causes. This table does not describe the physiological changes associated with pregnancy.

The technique for assessing male breasts and axillae are similar to those used in assessing females; see the accompanying Nursing Checklist on page 581. The inspected areas should be free of erythema, edema, rashes, and nodules. A firm disc at the areolar area may indicate gynecomastia (glandular enlargement of the male breast). Rashes may indicate allergies to soap or deodorant. Indicators of possible carcinoma include enlarged tender nodes and distortion of nipple and areola.

Palpation of the supraclavicular, infraclavicular, and axillary nodes is included in the assessment of the breasts. The

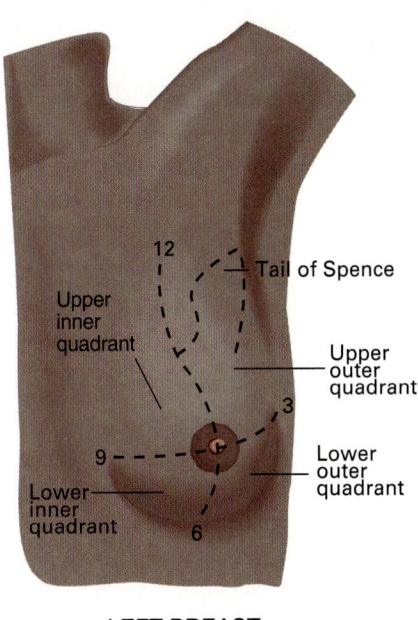

FIGURE 27-29 Quadrants of the Left Breast DELMAR/CENGAGE LEARNING

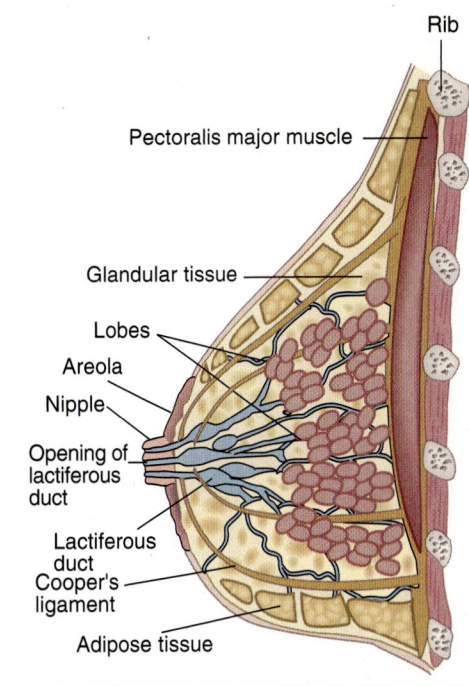

FIGURE 27-30 Cross Section of the Left Breast DELMAR/CENGAGE LEARNING

TABLE 27-18 Assessment of Breasts and Axillae, Female

AREA OF ASSESSMENT	NORMAL FINDINGS	SIGNIFICANT FINDINGS AND POSSIBLE CAUSES
Breasts, Areolar Area, Nipples, and Axillae		
Inspection: Assist client to sitting position on edge of exam table or bed facing you. Have client disrobe to waist. Inspect breasts for color, vascularity, thickening or edema, size, symmetry, contour, lesions, masses, or exudate. Inspect for each of the above with the client: a. Raising arms on each side above the head (accentuates retraction if present). b. Pressing hands into hips (contracts pectoral muscles and accentuates any retraction). c. Leaning forward to allow breasts to hang freely away from chest.	Flesh-colored breasts. Areolar areas and nipples have darker pigmentation. Moles, nevi, and terminal hair may be present on areolar areas. Superficial vascular patterns are diffuse and symmetrical. Breast on same side as dominant arm is usually larger. Nipples should point upward and laterally or outward and downward. **Supernumerary nipples** (extra nipples) appear as pigmented moles along the "milk line." Convex breast without flattening, retractions, or dimpling.	Reddened areas (inflammation, infection, inflammatory carcinoma). **Striae**, red or silvery-white streaks (rapid stretching of skin with resultant damage to elastic fibers of dermis; see Figure 27-31A on page 578). Local or unilateral superficial vascular patterns may indicate tumor formation (see Figure 27-31B). Thickening or edema of breast tissue or nipple causes enlarged skin pores, giving the appearance of orange rind (peau d'orange), which may indicate obstruction of lymphatic drainage (e.g., tumor) (Figure 27-31C). Significant differences in size or symmetry may indicate tumor (Figure 27-31D). Asymmetrical nipple direction or recent nipple inversion, flattening, or depression indicates nipple retraction (Figure 27-31E).

(Continues)

TABLE 27-18 (Continued)

AREA OF ASSESSMENT	NORMAL FINDINGS	SIGNIFICANT FINDINGS AND POSSIBLE CAUSES

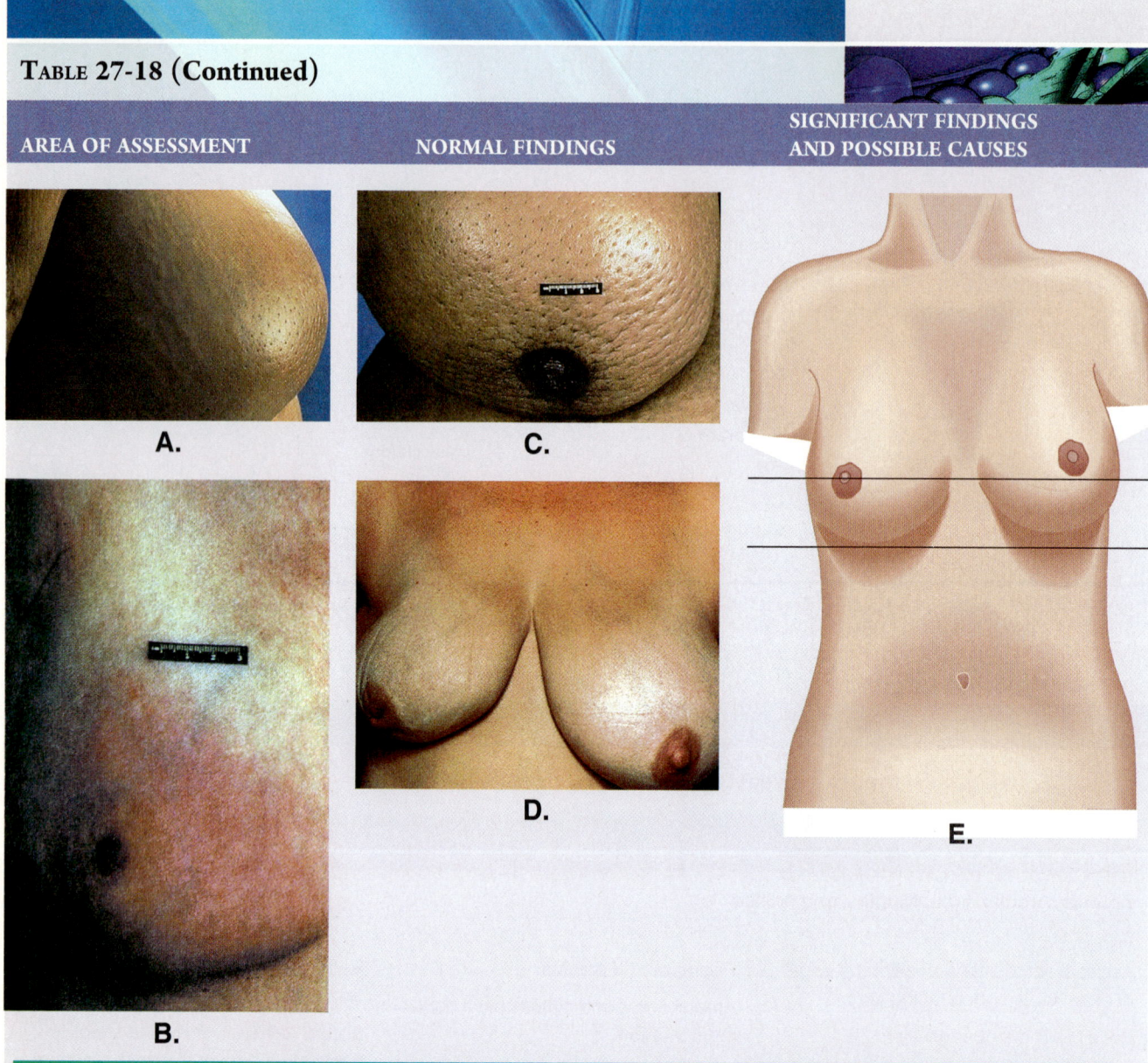

FIGURE 27-31 Abnormal Breast Findings: **A.** Striae; **B.** Superficial Vascular Patterns; **C.** Peau d'Orange; **D.** Asymmetry of Breasts; **E.** Asymmetry of Nipples with Deviation COURTESY OF DR. S. EVA SINGLETARY, MD, UNIVERSITY OF TEXAS, M. D. ANDERSON CANCER CENTER

Thickening of a previously inverted nipple may indicate a tumor.

Unilateral reduction of breast tissue or structures (trauma, surgery).

Scaly, eczema-like nipple erosion or persistent dermatitis may indicate Paget's disease (malignant neoplasm).

Nipple discharge in nonpregnant or non-lactating woman (oral contraceptives, tranquilizers, manual stimulation, infection, or benign breast disease).

(Continues)

Table 27-18 (Continued)

AREA OF ASSESSMENT	NORMAL FINDINGS	SIGNIFICANT FINDINGS AND POSSIBLE CAUSES
Palpation of axillae: Palpate in sequential manner. Stand in front of client. Instruct client to place arms at side. Place client's head in a flexed position (relaxes sternocleidomastoid muscle). Simultaneously palpate supraclavicular nodes (see Figure 27-32A on page 580). Place fingerpads over client's clavicles, lateral to sternocleidomastoid muscle. Proceed with a rotary motion of the palmar surfaces of index fingers. Probe deeply in scalene triangles to palpate nodes. Using rotary motion, palpate infraclavicular nodes (see Figure 27-32B).	Palpable lymph nodes should be less than 1 cm in diameter with no enlargement of axillary lymph nodes.	Fixed, firm, immobile lymph nodes greater than 1 cm in diameter (metastasis, i.e., spread of malignant cancer cells to other body parts). Enlarged, painful, or tender nodes that are matted together (systemic infection, carcinoma).
Palpate breasts: Stand at right side facing client. Instruct client to place arms at side. Support the inferior aspect of the breast. Begin palpation at outer quadrant of breast. NOTE: For small-breasted clients, use dominant hand to palpate tissue against chest wall. Use both hands with pendulous breasts. Palpate in a downward, sweeping manner from outer quadrants to sternal border of each breast. Repeat with client's arms raised above the head (enhances retraction).	Tissue consistency or elasticity varies with age, menses, pregnancy, and breast size. Firm elasticity of young breasts and a less firm, granular feel of older breasts. Premenstrual fullness, nodules, and tenderness are common. Large breasts may have a firm transverse ridge of compressed tissue along the lower edge; not to be confused with a tumor.	Significant tenderness may indicate benign inflamed lactiferous duct. Hard, poorly circumscribed nodules, loss of elasticity, and bloody discharge (cancer). Breast augmentation surgery produces a feeling of being fluid-filled or firmness throughout the tissue, with inferior suture line scars.
Lymph Nodes: Palpate and Inspect 1. *Client in sitting position:* Note any rash, unusual pigmentation, or nodes. Instruct client to take a deep breath and relax shoulders and arms. Use left hand to adduct client's left arm close to chest wall, and place client's left forearm on your right shoulder or arm.	Painless palpation of one or two soft, nontender nodes less than 1 cm in diameter without enlarged lymph nodes in other regions.	Rashes (allergic response, e.g., soap, deodorant). Redness and inflammation (infection of sweat glands). Enlarged, painful, or tender nodes that are matted together (systemic infection, carcinoma). Fixed, firm, immobile, irregular lymph nodes greater than 1 cm in diameter (metastasis). Loss of nipple elasticity or nipple thickening (tumor).

(Continues)

TABLE 27-18 (Continued)

AREA OF ASSESSMENT	NORMAL FINDINGS	SIGNIFICANT FINDINGS AND POSSIBLE CAUSES

Place fingerpads of right hand into apex of client's axilla (behind pectoral muscles), and gently roll the tissue against chest wall and axillary muscles.

Work downward to locate and palpate the four axillary lymph node groups (see Figure 27-32C):

a. Posterior (subscapular) at anterior edge of latissimus dorsi muscle

b. Central (midaxillary) at thoracic wall of axilla

c. Anterior (pectoral) behind lateral edge of pectoralis major muscle

d. Lateral (brachial) on inner aspect of upper aspect of humerus close to axillary vein
Repeat on client's right axilla.

2. *Supine position:*
Place client in supine position (spreads breast tissue thinly and evenly over chest wall).

Stand on client's right side, and place client's left arm above head.

With fingerpads, palpate left breast by compressing mammary tissue gently against chest wall by either (a) concentric circles that move from periphery to nipple or (b) in wedge sections from periphery to nipple.

Proceed with palpation to include tail of Spence, periphery, and areola.

Compress the nipple to express any discharge. If present, palpate breast along wedge radii to distinguish from which lobe the discharge originates.

Repeat on opposite breast.

White, milky discharge in nonpregnant, nonlactating, woman (hormone-induced discharge from lesions or anterior pituitary, or drug-induced).

Nonmilky discharge from nipple (benign or malignant breast disorder).

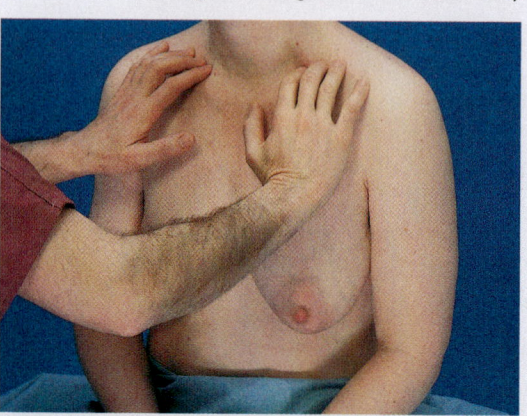

A.

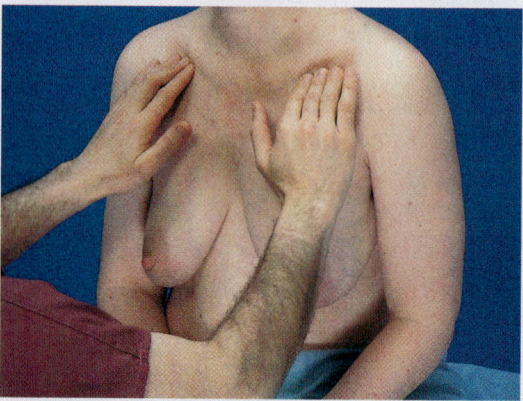

B.

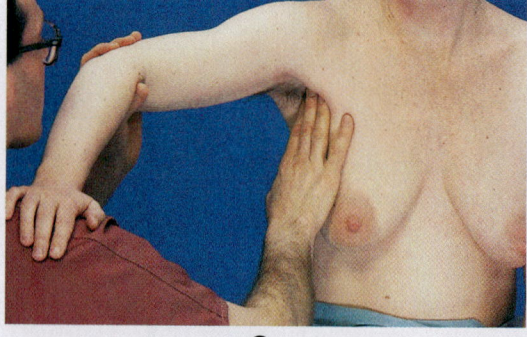

C.

FIGURE 27-32 **Palpating Lymph Nodes: A.** Palpation of Supraclavicular Nodes; **B.** Palpation of Infraclavicular Nodes; **C.** Palpation of the Axillary Lymph Nodes DELMAR/CENGAGE LEARNING

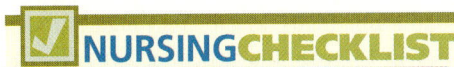

NURSING CHECKLIST

Assessing Male Breasts and Axillae

- Place client in sitting position facing you.
- Have client disrobe to the waist.
- Inspect nipple and areola, looking for nodules, edema, or ulcerations.
- Palpate the areola and note nodules.
- Inspect and palpate the axillae for presence of rash, erythema, and nodes.
- Repeat on other side.

pattern of lymph drainage is illustrated in Figure 27-33. Note that not all the lymphatics drain into the axilla; therefore, depending on the location of a malignant lesion, the spread of cancer cells may occur directly to the infraclavicular nodes, deep into the chest or abdomen, or to the opposite breast.

The American Cancer Society (ACS, 2009) reports that breast cancer is the second-leading cause of cancer death of American women. The chance that breast cancer will be the cause of a woman's death is about 1 in 35 (about 3%). The rate of deaths from breast cancer continues to decline, primarily as a result of early screening and treatment (ACS, 2009).

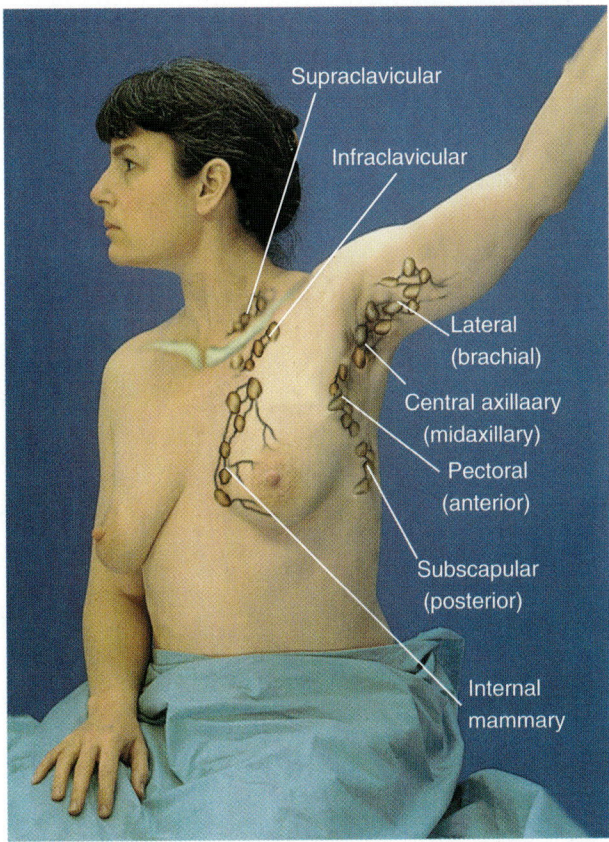

FIGURE 27-33 Lymph Drainage Patterns: Left Breast

DELMAR/CENGAGE LEARNING

Breast Self-Examination

Long-term survival rates for breast cancer have a direct correlation to early detection of the disease. Nurses play a major role in women's health by teaching breast self-examination (BSE) and by supporting women in achieving healthier lifestyles believed to decrease the risk factors of breast cancer (Estes, 2010).

The nurse should use the time during the assessment to educate the client about BSE and encourage the client to ask questions. See the Client Teaching Checklist for Breast Self-Examination.

ABDOMEN

Physical examination of the abdomen provides essential data relative to the various functions of the gastrointestinal and genitourinary systems and the abdominal aorta. The sequence of abdominal assessment is inspection, auscultation, percussion, and palpation. Auscultation is performed as the second step because palpation and percussion may alter the frequency of bowel sounds. The abdominal landmarks used for assessment are presented in Figure 27-35 on page 582.

CLIENT TEACHING CHECKLIST

Breast Self-Examination

1. Lie down and place your right arm behind your head. Slightly elevate your shoulders.
2. Use the fingerpads of the three middle fingers on your left hand to feel for lumps in the right breast, making overlapping, dime-sized circular motions of the fingerpads to feel the breast tissue; see Figure 27-34A on page 582.
3. Apply three different levels of pressure to feel all the breast tissue: light pressure to feel tissue closest the skin, medium pressure to feel deeper tissue, and firm pressure to feel tissue closest to the chest and ribs. A firm ridge in the lower curve of each breast is normal.
4. Move your hand in an up-and-down pattern from the underarm to the sternum or a vertical pattern from the clavicle to the ribs, checking the entire breast area.
5. Repeat the exam on your left breast, using the fingerpads of the right hand.
6. Stand in front of the mirror with your hands pressing firmly down on your hips (contracts the chest wall muscles and enhances any breast changes), and look at your breasts for any changes in size, shape, contour, or dimpling; see Figure 27-34B.
7. While sitting or standing and with your arm slightly raised, examine each underarm. (Raising your arm up straight tightens the tissue in this area and makes it difficult to examine.)

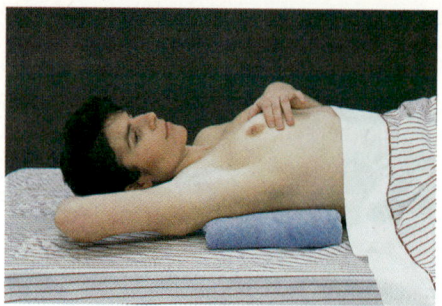

A.

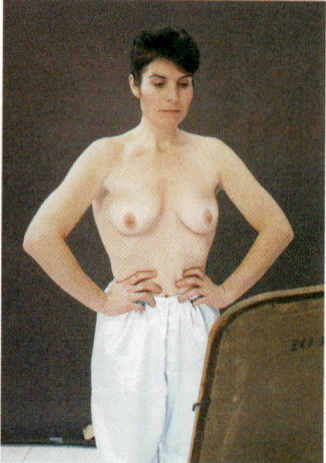

B.

FIGURE 27-34 **Breast Self-Examination: A.** Lying Down: Palpating Breast; **B.** Before Mirror: Hands Pressed into Hips DELMAR/ CENGAGE LEARNING

During inspection, note the presence of abdominal distention, for which there are many causes. A mnemonic device for remembering the possible causes of abdominal distention is shown in the accompanying Nursing Process Highlight.

Auscultate the four quadrants, as shown in Figure 27-36, when assessing bowel sounds and listening for vascular bruits. Assessment should always begin in the right lower quadrant (RLQ). Table 27-19 on page 583 presents the specific areas of the abdomen to be examined and the normal and key findings of this assessment.

The nurse should percuss all four quadrants in the same systematic fashion. During percussion of the abdomen, note when **tympany** (a musical drumlike sound that occurs over air-filled cavities) changes to **dullness** (a muffled thudlike sound that occurs over dense tissue). Tympany usually occurs over the stomach, which is filled with gas; dullness is heard over thicker organs, such as the liver.

Light palpation of the abdomen is done in all four quadrants, beginning in the RLQ, for resistance, tenderness, and

NURSING PROCESS HIGHLIGHT

Assessment

The Seven Fs of Abdominal Distention: Etiological Factors

Fat
Fluid (ascites, excessive fluid accumulation in abdominal cavity)
Flatus
Feces
Fetus
Fatal growth (malignancy)
Fibroid tumor

Estes, M. E. Z. (2010). *Health assessment and physical examination* (4th ed.). Clifton Park, NY: Delmar/Cengage Learning.

Right hypochondriac region	Epigastric region	Left hypochondriac region
Right lumbar region	Umbilical region	Left lumbar region
Right iliac region	Hypogastric region	Left iliac region

FIGURE 27-35 **Abdominal Landmarks** DELMAR/CENGAGE LEARNING

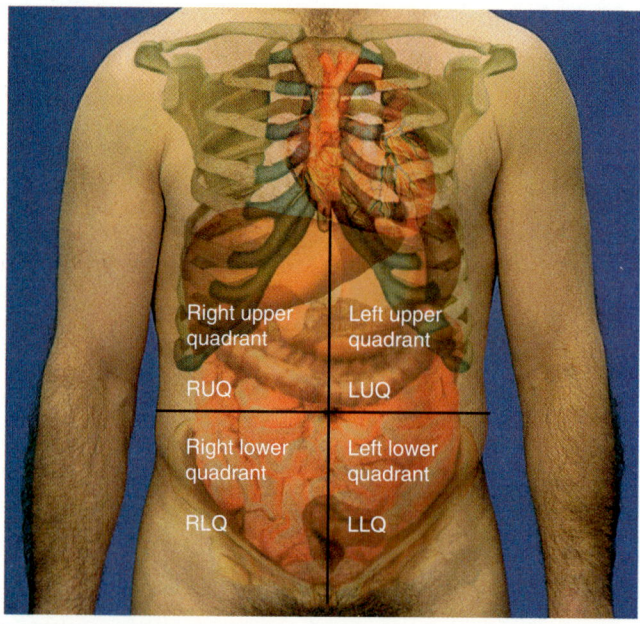

Right upper quadrant — RUQ
Left upper quadrant — LUQ
Right lower quadrant — RLQ
Left lower quadrant — LLQ

FIGURE 27-36 **Abdominal Quadrants** DELMAR/CENGAGE LEARNING

TABLE 27-19 Assessing the Abdomen

ASSESSMENT AREA/TECHNIQUES	NORMAL FINDINGS	SIGNIFICANT FINDINGS AND POSSIBLE CAUSES
Inspect, auscultate, percuss, and palpate.		
Place client in supine position, with knees flexed over a pillow. Use sheets and drapes to expose only the abdomen. *Inspection and palpation:* Inspect from rib margin to pubic bone. Note contour, symmetry, and presence of peristalsis, pulsations, scars, striae, or masses. Observe for smooth, even respiratory movement. Observe for surface motion (peristalsis). Inspect umbilicus for contour, location, and signs of inflammation or hernia. Inspect epigastric area for pulsations.	Contour is flat or rounded and bilaterally symmetrical. Abdomen rises with inhalation and falls with exhalation. Visible peristalsis slowly traverses the abdomen in a downward-slanting movement; observed in thin clients. Umbilicus is depressed and beneath abdominal surface. Pulsations of abdominal aorta are visible in thin clients.	A protuberant abdomen (poor muscle tone, e.g., inadequate exercise, obesity). Taut stretching of skin across abdominal wall is distension. Striae (*linea alba*) (obesity, pregnancy, ascites, tumors). Uneven respiratory movement with retraction (appendicitis). Strong peristaltic movement (intestinal obstruction). Bulging of umbilicus (hernia). Marked pulsations in epigastric area (aortic aneurysm).
Auscultation: Use stethoscope diaphragm. Auscultate at each of the four abdominal quadrants for bowel sounds. Listen for a full minute to the frequency and character of bowel sounds. Listen at least 5 minutes before determining absence of bowel sounds.	High-pitched sound, heard every 5 to 15 seconds as intermittent gurgling sounds. Bowel sounds in all four quadrants. Bowel sounds audible at ileocecal valve area.	Absence of bowel sounds, none heard for 3–5 minutes (paralytic ileus, peritonitis, obstruction). Hypoactive or diminished bowel (low pitch, one or two occurring in a 2-minute interval) Normal in first few hours postanesthesia. May indicate decreased bowel motility (e.g., peritoneal irritation, paralytic ileus). Hyperactive, loud, audible, gurgling sounds (hunger, diarrhea). Rushed, high-pitched, or tingling sounds (intestinal blockage).
Listen with bell of stethoscope over aorta, epigastric area, renal arteries, and femoral arteries. Note bruits over each area.	Absence of bruits.	A bruit over an abdominal vessel (aortic aneurysm or partial obstruction).
Percussion: Percuss all four quadrants in a systematic fashion (see Figure 27-37 on page 584). Begin percussion in RLQ, move up to RUQ, cross over to LUQ, and move down to LLQ. Note when tympany changes to dullness.	Tympany is heard because of gas in stomach and intestines. Dullness is heard over organs (e.g., liver).	Dullness over stomach or intestines (tumor, ascites, or fecal-filled intestines).

(Continues)

TABLE 27-19 (Continued)

ASSESSMENT AREA/TECHNIQUES	NORMAL FINDINGS	SIGNIFICANT FINDINGS AND POSSIBLE CAUSES
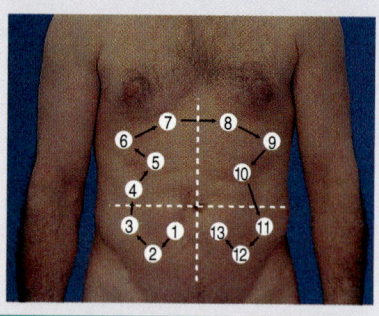 **FIGURE 27-37** Directional Pattern of **Abdominal Percussion** DELMAR/CENGAGE LEARNING		

Palpation:

Perform light palpation.

Never palpate over areas where bruits are auscultated.

Instruct client to cough. If client experiences pain in a quadrant, palpate that area last.

Depress abdominal wall 2 cm in each quadrant.

Note texture and consistency of underlying tissue.

Smooth texture with consistent softness.

Tenderness, accompanied by warm skin (inflammation).

Large masses (feces, tumors).

Delmar/Cengage Learning

---

rebound tenderness. Deep palpation is not addressed because this assessment technique usually requires supervision during the learning process. Detection of abdominal organs (gallbladder, liver, spleen, fecal-filled colon, flatus-filled cecum) by palpation is an abnormal finding and, thus, should be reported.

MUSCULOSKELETAL SYSTEM

The musculoskeletal system provides clients with the ability to maintain and change their positions in response to both internal and external stimuli. Muscle tone and bone strength allow the client to maintain an erect position. The musculoskeletal system consists of bones, joints, skeletal muscles, and supportive connective tissue (see Figure 27-38 on page 585).

Inspection, palpation, range of motion (ROM), and muscle testing are performed on the major skeletal muscles and joints. Table 27-20 on page 587 presents the specific areas of the musculoskeletal system to be examined and the normal and key findings of this assessment.

Assessment may reveal several findings indicative of musculoskeletal dysfunction. The following are some of these findings:

- Pain and limited ROM in the vertebrae may be caused by herniation of vertebral discs, arthritis, or degenerative joint disease.
- Hard, painless nodules on the dorsolateral aspects of the interphalangeal joints (Heberden's nodes) indicate osteoarthritis.
- Flexion contracture of the little, ring, and middle fingers (Dupuytren's contracture) is associated with arthritis.
- Bilateral swelling of the wrists occurs with rheumatoid arthritis. A painful, asymmetrical elbow with a misaligned forearm occurs with subluxation (dislocation) of the elbow. Localized tenderness and pain with impaired ROM of the elbow indicate epicondylitis, resulting from repetitive motion of the joint.

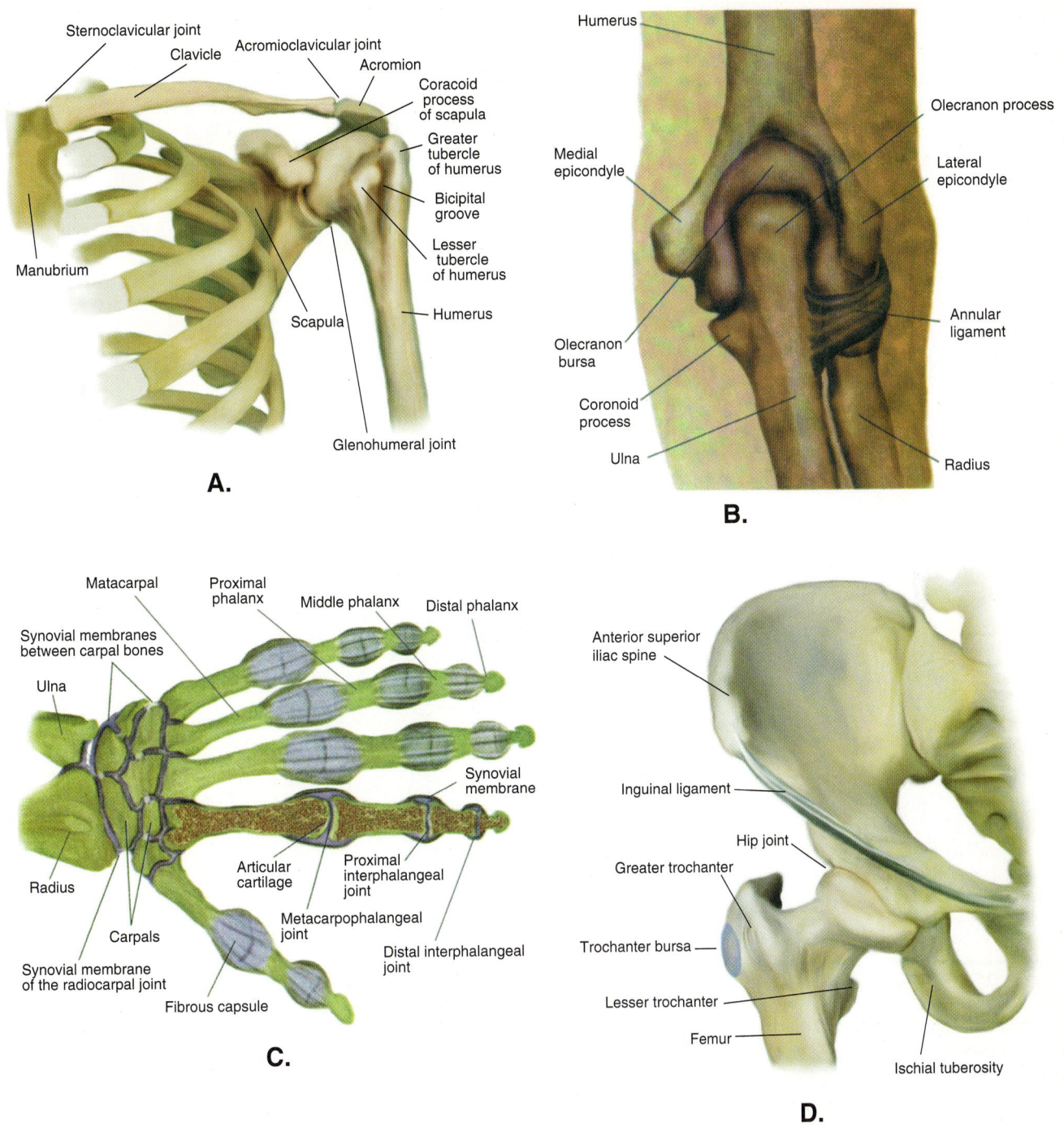

A.

B.

C.

D.

FIGURE 27-38 **Musculoskeletal System: A.** Shoulder; **B.** Elbow; **C.** Wrist and Hand; **D.** Hip; **E.** Leg; **F.** Knee; **G.** Ankle and Foot

DELMAR/CENGAGE LEARNING

- Pain, swelling, and redness of the first metatarsophalangeal joint usually indicate gouty arthritis.

A complete musculoskeletal examination requires the full assessment of ROM. A **goniometer** is a protractor with two movable arms (see Figure 27-39 on page 587) used to measure the angle of a skeletal joint during ROM.

Skeletal muscles provide contour for the body and promote joint mobility. Muscle contour is affected by the exercise and activity patterns of the client. **Hypertrophy** refers to an increase in muscle size and shape due to an increase in muscle fiber. **Atrophy** refers to thin, flabby muscles due to a reduction in muscle size and shape. Increased muscle tone (**hypertonicity**) causes resistance with joint movement. **Hypotonicity** refers to a flabby muscle with poor tone.

Joints are normally nontender and move freely. **Arthritis** is an inflammation of the joints that causes pain and swelling. Degenerative joint disease or **osteoarthritis** (the most common type of degenerative arthritis, in which the joints

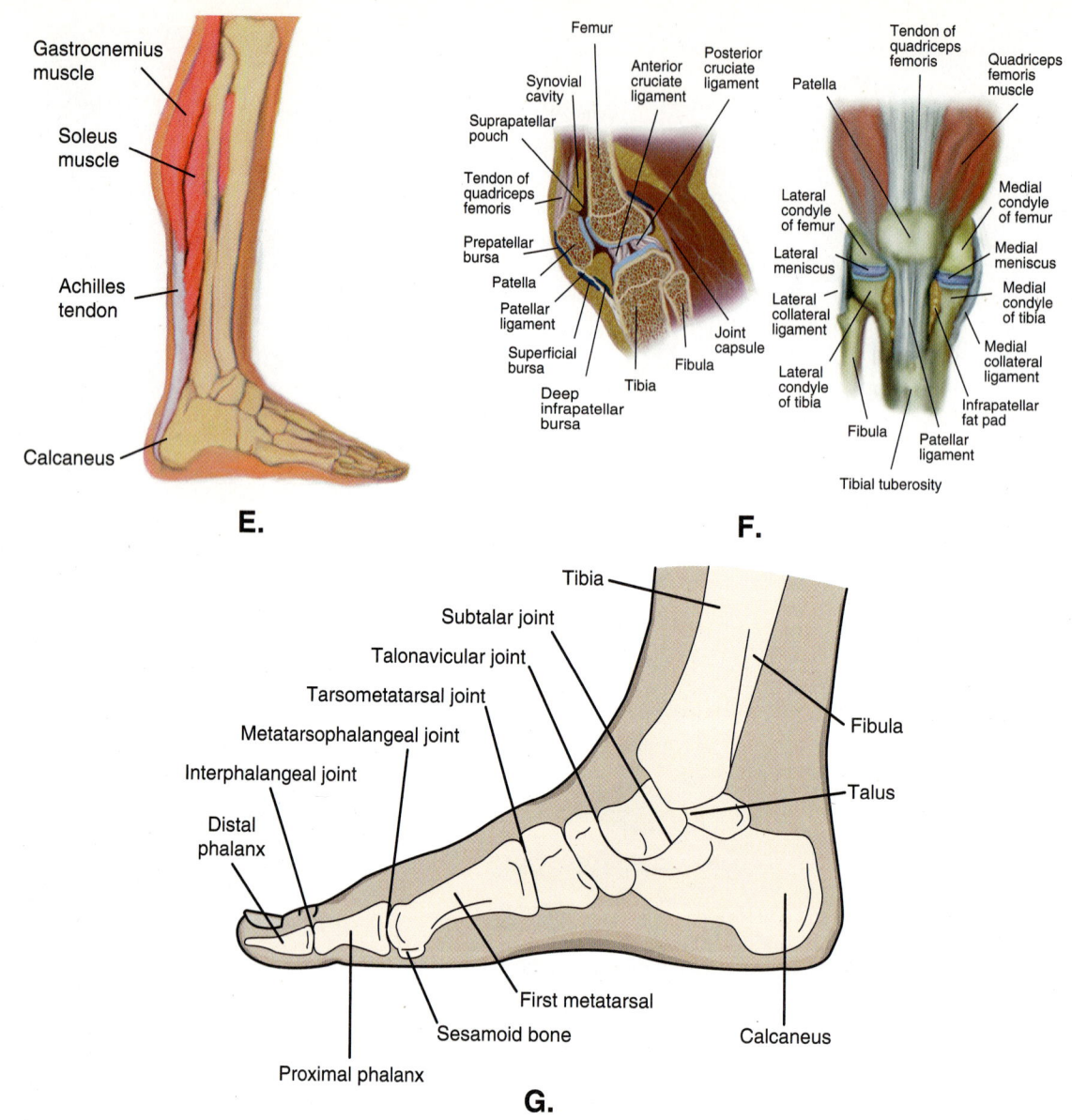

E.

F.

G.

FIGURE 27-38 (Continued)

become stiff and tender to touch) causes the joints to undergo degenerative changes. ROM and activities of daily living are compromised by the loss of joint mobility. Crepitus is often palpated in joints affected by degenerative joint disease. See Chapter 36 for information on nursing care of clients with mobility problems.

NEUROLOGICAL SYSTEM

A complete neurological examination includes an assessment of mental status, sensation, cranial nerves, motor functioning, cerebellar function, and reflexes. See Chapter 38 for a complete discussion of cranial nerve function. Clients with minor or intermittent neurological symptoms may require only a screening assessment; see Table 27-21 on page 588.

Mental Status

The mental status assessment should be done during the interview and health history. A complete assessment should

be performed if the client exhibits any signs of neurological deficit, such as:

- Known brain lesion (stroke, tumors, trauma)
- Suspected brain lesion (new seizures, headaches, behavioral changes)
- Memory deficits
- Confusion
- Vague behavioral complaints (by significant others if client unaware of or denies behavioral changes)
- Aphasia
- Irritability
- Emotional lability
- Change in level of consciousness

PHYSICAL APPEARANCE AND BEHAVIOR Pertinent information relative to mental status is assessed by observing the client's posture and movements, dress and grooming, and facial expressions. The nurse should note the client's gait and posture to determine whether it is relaxed, slumped, or rigid.

TABLE 27-20 Assessment of Musculoskeletal System

ASSESSMENT AREA/TECHNIQUE	NORMAL FINDINGS	SIGNIFICANT FINDINGS AND POSSIBLE CAUSES
Muscles—Inspection and palpation: 1. Compare muscles on one side of body to corresponding muscles on opposite side. Inspect for size, using a tape measure for accuracy. 2. Inspect muscles for tremors and shortening (i.e., contractures). 3. To assess muscle tone, palpate muscles at rest. 4. Test muscle strength on both sides of body.	1. Equal on both sides of body. 2. Absence of contractures and tremors. 3. Firm muscles. 4. Strength equal on both sides.	1. Asymmetry, atrophy, or hypertrophy. 2. Misalignment of body part (e.g., foot drop occurs with plantar flexion). 3. Lack of muscle tone. 4. Spasticity or flaccidity.
Bones—Inspection and palpation: 1. Inspect skeleton for alignment and structure. 2. Palpate bones for tenderness and edema.	1. Skeletal alignment with intact bones. 2. Absence of swelling, tenderness, or pain.	1. Fractures, misalignment (e.g., scoliosis). 2. Swelling, tenderness, or pain (fracture, osteoporosis, arthritis, cancer).
Joints—Inspection and palpation: Inspect and palpate for size, tenderness, swelling, crepitus, nodules, or masses. Assess ROM in each joint.	No swelling, tenderness, nodules, or masses. Absence of crepitation. Joints move smoothly. ROM will vary according to individual's usual degree of physical activity.	Tenderness, crepitus, and limited ROM (arthritis, bursitis, bone misalignment).

Delmar/Cengage Learning

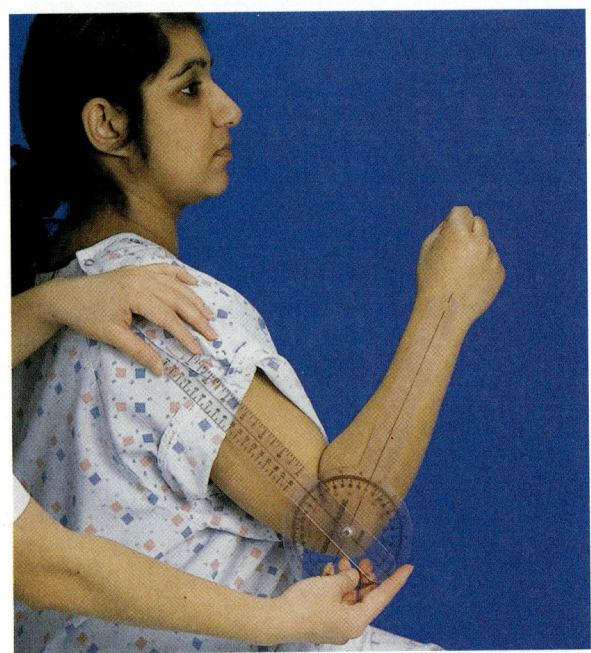

FIGURE 27-39 Use of Goniometer to Measure Joint ROM

DELMAR/CENGAGE LEARNING

The client should appear relaxed but with the appropriate amount of concern regarding the assessment. The client should exhibit an erect posture, smooth gait, and symmetrical body movements.

Dress and grooming are influenced by the client's economic status, age, home situation, and cultural background. Information obtained from the health history assists the nurse in determining appropriate dress and grooming for each client. It is also helpful to ask clients directly about their grooming and hygiene routines.

Facial expressions should be symmetric and appropriate to the content of the conversation. Facial expressions may demonstrate anxiety or depression. The nurse should observe the client's verbal and nonverbal behaviors and note if the client's affect appears labile, blunted, or flat. Affect refers to the emotional feeling tone that is reflected by one's facial expression.

COMMUNICATION   Client communication should be assessed throughout the entire interview, health history, and physical examination. The client should be able to produce spontaneous, coherent speech with an effortless flow and normal inflections, volume, pitch, articulation, rate, and rhythm. The message

TABLE 27-21 Neurological Screening Assessment

AREA OF ASSESSMENT	ASSESSMENT PARAMETER	OUTCOME FINDINGS
Mental status/level of consciousness	Note general appearance, affect, speech content, memory, logic, judgment, and speech patterns during the health history. Perform the Glasgow Coma Scale (GCS) with motor assessment component and pupil assessment.	If any abnormalities are evident, perform a full mental status assessment. If the GCS < 15, perform a full assessment of mental status. If motor assessment is abnormal or asymmetrical, perform a complete motor and sensory assessment.
Sensation	Assess pain and vibration in the hands and feet with light touch on the limbs.	If deficits are identified, perform a complete sensory assessment.
Cranial nerves (CNs)	Assess CN II, III, IV, VI: visual acuity, gross fields, funduscopic, pupillary reactions, and extraocular movements. Assess CN VII, IX, X, XII: facial expression, gross hearing, voice, and tongue.	If any abnormalities exist, perform complete assessment of all 12 CNs.
Motor system	Assess muscle tone and strength, abnormal movements, and grasps.	If deficits are noted, perform a complete musculoskeletal assessment.
Cerebellar function	Observe the client's gait and ability to walk heel to toe and to perform shallow knee bends. Perform Romberg's test: Ask the client to stand erect, feet together and arms at side, first with eyes open, then closed. The nurse should stand close to the client to catch the client in the event of a fall. Note the client's ability to maintain balance with eyes open and closed for 20 seconds with minimum swaying.	If any deficits exist, perform a complete cerebellar assessment.
Reflexes	Assess the muscle stretch reflexes and the plantar response.	If an abnormal response is elicited, perform a complete reflex examination.

Delmar/Cengage Learning

should make sense. Comprehension of language should be intact, and the client's ability to read and write should be commensurate with educational level.

Aphasia is an impairment of language functioning that results from injury to the cortex. Aphasia is classified as sensory (receptive), motor (expressive), or global (mixed sensory and motor). In receptive aphasia, auditory comprehension is impaired as well as the content of speech. The client is unaware of the deficits, and his or her ability to name people and objects is severely impaired. With expressive aphasia, speech is slow, repetitive, and hesitant. The client has difficulty selecting and organizing words, and writing is impaired. Oral and written comprehension are severely impaired with global aphasia.

LEVEL OF CONSCIOUSNESS
Consciousness is the level of awareness of the self and the environment. Conscious behavior requires arousal (or wakefulness) and awareness (or cognition and affect). Awareness is a higher-level function of the cerebral cortex that includes judgment and thinking, which are usually assessed as part of the cognitive assessment.

The Glasgow Coma Scale (GCS) is an international scale used in grading neurological responses to determine the client's level of consciousness; see Chapter 38 for a detailed discussion.

Cognitive Abilities and Mentation

Assessment of cognitive function includes testing for attention, memory, judgment, insight, spatial perception, calculation, abstraction, thought process, and thought content. See Chapter 38 for a complete discussion about assessment of these abilities.

Sensation

Sensation should be tested early in the neurological assessment because of the detail involved and the need for client cooperation. If the client becomes fatigued, the findings may be unreliable. The assessment is divided into three sections:

- Exteroceptive sensations: superficial sensations that originate in the sensory receptors in the skin and mucous membranes (light touch, pain, heat, and cold)

- Proprioceptive sensations: deep sensations that originate in the sensory receptors in the muscles, joints, tendons, and ligaments (motion, position, and vibration sense)
- Cortical sensations: sensations that compose cerebral integration and discrimination abilities

Some examples of impaired cortical sensations are **stereognosis** (ability to identify objects by manipulation and touch), **graphesthesia** (ability to identify numbers, letters, or shapes drawn on the skin), and **extinction** (ability to discriminate the points of distance when two body parts are simultaneously touched).

The sensory **dermatome map** (cutaneous area whose sensory receptors and axons feed into a single dorsal root of the spinal cord) is used to assess the major sensory nerves (see Figure 27-40). The map of dermatomes is helpful in identifying the areas of pain and altered sensation. Although several dorsal roots may receive input from a single dermatome, the map is helpful in identifying where a neurological lesion may exist. For example, pain localized in the posterior area of the neck would suggest a possible lesion in the third cervical spinal cord segment.

The neurological assessment is performed with the client's eyes closed so that the client's ability to perceive the stimulus can be determined. The nurse should observe the client's reactions by watching for facial grimacing or with-

drawal of the stimulated extremity. Compare the client's sensation on the corresponding areas bilaterally. The nurse should note the proximal to distal sensory differences on all four extremities, evaluate whether any sensory deficits follow a dermatome distribution, and map the borders of any area exhibiting changes in sensation.

Cranial Nerves

A complete assessment of the 12 cranial nerves is necessary for a baseline assessment, if a tumor of a specific cranial nerve is suspected, or when periodic assessment is required after surgery or radiation treatments. An abbreviated cranial nerve assessment is an integral part of a neurological screening. Pupil assessment (cranial nerve III, oculomotor) is included in the screening assessment and is tested with the trochlear and abducens (cranial nerves IV and VI) because all three cranial nerves supply the muscles of the eye.

Motor Function

Assessment of the motor system involves testing for muscle size, tone, and strength under voluntary movements. Cerebellar assessment can be done either with motor testing or separately as follows.

Cerebellar Function

Assessment of cerebellar function includes observation of coordination, balance, and gait. Cerebellar muscular activity requires the motor coordination of various muscle groups to execute smooth, precise, and harmonious movements. Coordination is an integrated process that involves complicated neural integration of the motor and premotor cortex, basal ganglia, cerebellum, vestibular system, posterior columns, and peripheral nerves.

COORDINATION Equilibratory coordination is concerned with maintenance of an upright stance and depends on the vestibular, cerebellar, and proprioceptive systems. Nonequilibratory coordination is concerned with smaller movements of the extremities and involves the cerebellar and proprioceptive mechanisms.

To test coordination, the nurse should position the client comfortably with eyes open. Clients who wear glasses should be wearing their glasses before coordination is assessed. Instruct the client to first touch the index finger to the nose, then to alternate rapidly with the index finger of the opposite hand. Ask the client to close the eyes and continue to rapidly touch the nose with alternate index fingers. Tell the client to open the eyes, touch the finger to the nose, and touch the nurse's index finger, which is held about 18 inches away from the client. The test is repeated with the client using the opposite hand. Throughout testing, the nurse should observe for intention tremor or over- or undershooting of the client's finger.

To assess rapid alternate movements of the upper extremities, ask the client to alternately pat the knees with rapid supinating and pronating of the hands. Test the lower extremities for rapid alternating movement by asking the

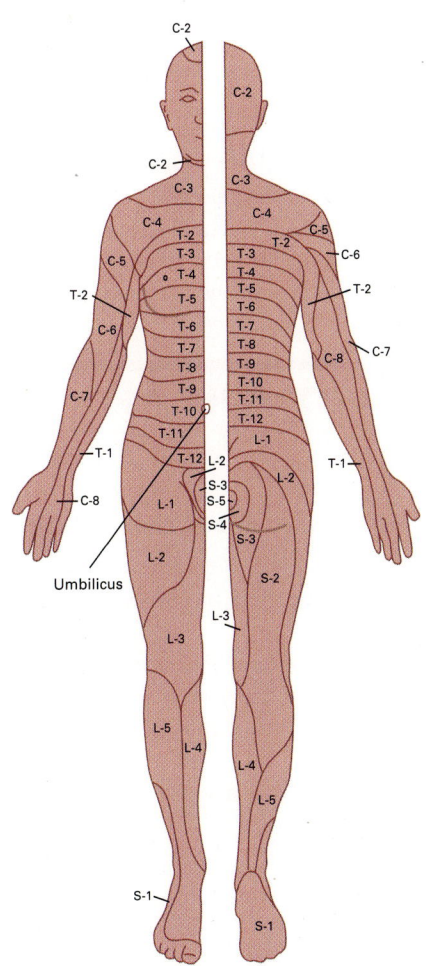

FIGURE 27-40 Dermatome Map DELMAR/CENGAGE LEARNING

client to rapidly extend the ankle ("tap your foot") and to place the heel just below the knee on the shin of the opposite leg and slide it down to the foot.

The client should be able to rapidly alternate touching finger to nose and moving finger from nose to the nurse's finger in a coordinated fashion. Also, the client should be able to perform alternating movements in a purposeful, rapid, coordinated manner. The client should demonstrate the ability to purposefully and smoothly run the heel down the shin.

BALANCE AND GAIT   The performance of Romberg's test is previously described in Table 27-21. A positive Romberg sign exists if the client becomes unsteady and tends to fall when the eyes are closed.

Assessment of gait begins when the client enters the room and continues throughout the examination. The nurse must consider the client's age, activity level, and degree of alertness. The tandem walk is tested by having the client walk in a straight line touching the ground heel to toe. The arms should be held at the side, and the eyes should be open. Note the client's posture and ability to maintain balance. Posture should be upright with a narrow base and the gait smooth with arms swinging opposite the movement of the legs. Heel-to-toe walk should be in a straight line without losing balance.

Reflexes

A reflex action is a specific, involuntary response to an adequate stimulus. The stimulus can occur in a joint, a muscle, or the skin and is transmitted through the sensory and motor pathways of the reflex arc and specific spinal cord segments. To elicit a muscle stretch reflex, the nurse should briskly tap the client's tendon with a reflex hammer.

Normal reflexes are classified into two main categories: muscle stretch (deep tendon) reflexes (DTR) and superficial (cutaneous) reflexes. During reflex testing, clients should be relaxed and positioned so that their extremities are symmetrical. The nurse should hold the reflex hammer loosely between the thumb and index finger and strike the tendon with a brisk motion from the wrist. The reflex hammer should make contact with the correct point on the tendon in a quick, direct manner.

Table 27-22 on pages 591–592 discusses the assessment of common DTRs: biceps, triceps, brachioradialis, patellar, Achilles, and plantar (Babinski). When testing the reflexes, the nurse should observe the degree and speed of response of the muscle after the reflex hammer makes contact. The reflex responses between the right and left sides should be compared. The normal response to taps in the correct area should elicit a brisk ($++$ or $+++$) contraction of the muscles involved; see the accompanying Nursing Process Highlight.

REPRODUCTIVE SYSTEM

Assessment of the genitalia may produce feelings of fear, anxiety, indignity, and loss of control in some clients. These feelings may be reduced by the sensitivity of the nurse before,

during, and after the assessment. The nurse must respect the client's wishes regarding privacy and take into consideration cultural issues concerning this aspect of health assessment. For example, many Middle Eastern women will remain veiled during an assessment. By using techniques to diminish client discomfort and by empowering the client through education and participation in the assessment process, nurses offer a path for clients in the management of their own health care; see the accompanying Spotlight On display. Many states require that a male nurse be accompanied by a female nurse or assistant during a gynecologic examination.

See Chapter 19 for discussion of physiological changes of aging that affect sexuality in both men and women.

FEMALE GENITALIA

Assessment of the female genitalia uses the techniques of inspection and palpation. Table 27-23 on page 593 presents specific areas of the female external genitalia to be examined and the normal and key findings of this assessment. Speculum

---

NURSING PROCESS HIGHLIGHT

Assessment

Reflex Grading Scale

Scale	Response
0	Absent
+	Present but diminished
++	Normal
+++	Mildly increased but not pathologic
++++	Markedly hyperactive; clonus may be present

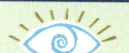 **SPOTLIGHT ON...**

Caring

Physical Examination of the Female Genitalia

- Encourage client to verbalize any concerns about the examination.
- Be nonjudgmental while listening to the client.
- Inform client that the examination should not be painful, even though it may be uncomfortable at times.
- Assure client that privacy will be maintained during the examination.
- Provide explanation of interventions prior to performing them.
- Ask client if she has any questions before, during, and after the examination.

assessment of the internal genitalia is not discussed because this function is usually within the scope of advanced practice registered nurses or other registered nurses prepared in expanded roles.

In preparation for the examination, place the client in the lithotomy position with knees flexed perpendicular to bed. Instruct client to relax thighs in order to allow each leg to abduct to the sides. Elevate the client's head for comfort, and drape to expose only the area being examined. Wash hands and don gloves prior to examining the genitalia.

There are many types of abnormal lesions that affect the female genitalia; some of the more common ones are:

- Chancre: A reddish, round ulcer with a depressed center and raised edges that appears during the primary phase of

TABLE 27-22 Assessment of Common Deep Tendon Reflexes

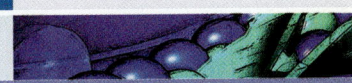

TYPE	ASSESSMENT	NORMAL REFLEX
Biceps 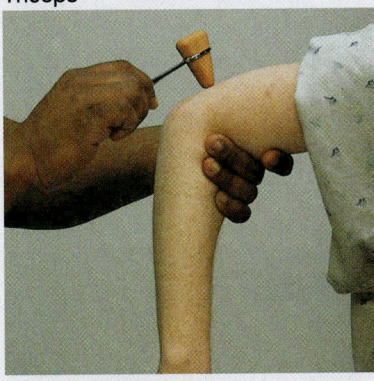	Flex client's arm between 45° and 90°. Place your thumb firmly on the biceps tendon just above the crease of antecubital fossa and tap thumb with reflex hammer.	Flexion of arm at elbow
Triceps	Flex client's arm between 45° and 90°. Tap triceps tendon just above elbow.	Extension of elbow
Brachioradialis 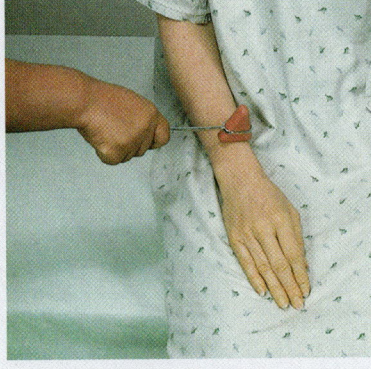	Flex client's arm 45° and place in lap with the arm in semipronation. Tap brachioradialis tendon on thumb side of wrist.	Flexion of forearm

(Continues)

TABLE 27-22 (Continued)

TYPE	ASSESSMENT	NORMAL REFLEX
Patellar 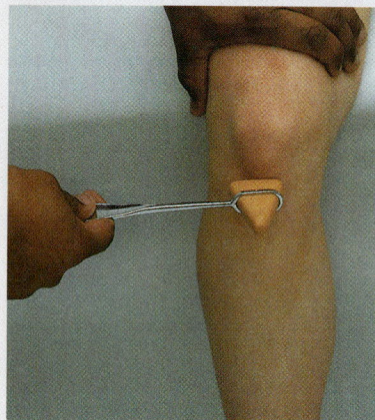	Ask client to sit in a chair or on edge of bed with legs hanging freely or in a supine position with knee flexed. Tap patellar tendon just below the patella.	Extension of leg below the knee
Achilles 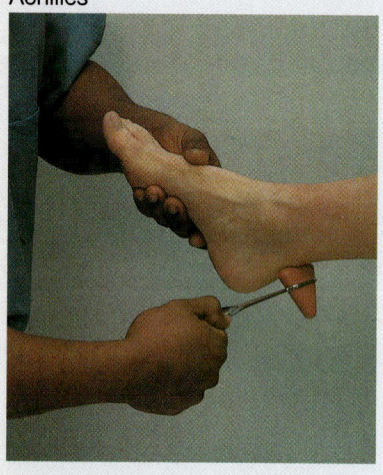	Ask client to sit with feet dangling and partially dorsiflexed or in a supine position with leg flexed at knee and thigh externally rotated. Tap the Achilles tendon just above heel.	Plantar flexion of foot
Plantar (Babinski) 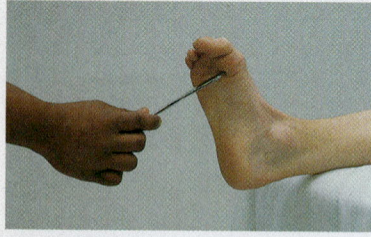	Position the client's ankle firmly against the bed and slowly stroke client's sole with the handle of the reflex hammer.	Bending of the toes downward

Delmar/Cengage Learning

syphilis at the site where the treponema enters the body. It lasts for 4 weeks, then disappears.

- Condyloma acuminatum: White, dry, painless growth (wart) that has a narrow base that is caused by the human papillomavirus.

- Condylomata lata: Raised, round, wartlike plaque with a moist surface covered by a gray exudate that appears during the secondary stage of syphilis.

- Herpes simplex: Small, red vesicles that fuse together to form a large ulcer that may be painful and itchy.

TABLE 27-23 Assessment of Female Genitalia

ASSESSMENT AREA/ TECHNIQUE	NORMAL FINDINGS	SIGNIFICANT FINDINGS AND POSSIBLE CAUSES
Inspection Look for distribution, amount, and characteristics of pubic hair. Inspect skin for color, edema, and lesions. Separate labia majora and labia minora for a thorough inspection.	Even hair distribution. Clear skin except for nevi. Labia majora and minora are symmetrical, with a smooth to wrinkled surface that is intact. Skin of vulva is slightly darker than surrounding areas. No nodules, ecchymosis, edema, lesions, or rashes. Sebaceous cysts (nontender, yellow-colored nodules smaller than 1 cm) may be present.	Scant pubic hair (hormonal changes). Ecchymosis over mons pubis or labia (trauma, e.g., accidental injury, intentional abuse). Rash over mons pubis or labia (dermatitis, parasitic infestation). Labial edema (hematoma, Bartholin's cyst, or obstruction of lymphatic system). Painless mass with pruritus or a cauliflower-like growth (malignancy). Varicose veins (pregnancy, prolonged standing, or congenital disposition).
Inspect clitoris, urethral meatus, and vaginal introitus when separating labia minora.	Free from lesions. Clitoris is less than 1 cm in width and less than 2 cm in length. Urethral meatus appears as a small slit and is same color of surrounding tissue. Absence of discharge, redness, and edema. Introitus mucosa is pink and moist with a clear to white discharge. Free of odor and bulging.	Clitoral hypertrophy (androgen excess). Foul-smelling discharge of any color (urinary tract infection, vaginitis, or cervicitis). Redness or edema around the urethra meatus (infection of Skene's glands, urethral carcinoma, prolapse of urethral mucosa). Pale color and dryness occur with atrophy (topical steroids, aging). External tear of vaginal introitus (trauma). Bulging of anterior vaginal wall may indicate a cystocele (protrusion of urinary bladder through the wall of the vagina) due to weak ligaments.

Delmar/Cengage Learning

MALE GENITALIA

Assessment of the male genitalia includes the essential organs (testes and gonads), the accessory organs (seminal vesicles and bulbourethral glands), several ducts (epididymis, ductus [vas] deferens, ejaculatory), and the urethra. The supporting structures include the scrotum, penis, and spermatic cord. Table 27-24 on page 594 presents the specific areas of the male genitalia to be examined and the normal and key findings of this assessment.

In preparation for the examination, place the client in the supine position with legs slightly spread apart. If the client is unable to tolerate the supine position, the standing position also allows for a thorough examination of the genitalia. Wash hands and don gloves prior to the examination. It is important to be sensitive to the client's feelings during the examination; see the accompanying Respecting Our Differences display and Table 27-24.

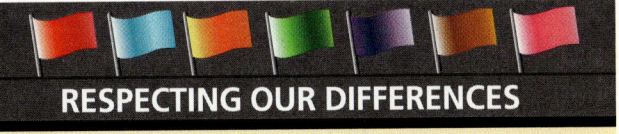

RESPECTING OUR DIFFERENCES

Before beginning the examination, consider the client's cultural background. What are his beliefs, attitudes, and feelings about the examination? Does the client's culture prohibit a female nurse from examining a male client? Are there cultural prohibitions on a male nurse examining a male client?

TABLE 27-24 Assessment of Male Genitalia

ASSESSMENT AREA/TECHNIQUE	NORMAL FINDINGS	SIGNIFICANT FINDINGS AND POSSIBLE CAUSES
Pubic hair: Look for distribution, amount, and characteristics.	Triangular distribution, often spreading up the abdomen.	Scant amount or absence of hair (hormonal problems).
Penis: Inspect the anterior and posterior surfaces by lifting the penis. Retract foreskin on uncircumcised clients. Note lesions, edema, and inflammation. Palpate the penile shaft. Note pulsations, tenderness, swelling, masses, or plaques. Inspect the urethral meatus. Note location, color, and presence of discharge.	Foreskin retracts easily. Glans penis varies in size and shape. A small amount of smegma (oily, pasty material consisting of desquamated epidermal cells and sebum). Pulsations are present on dorsal sides of penis. Meatus is centrally located on tip of penis and pink.	Phimosis (inability of foreskin to be retracted over glans penis) may develop in uncircumcised males. Paraphimosis occurs when retracted foreskin causes proximal constriction to glans; penis distal to foreskin becomes edematous and gangrenous. Priapism is a continuous penile erection. Absent pulsations indicate vascular insufficiency. Varied placement of meatus may result from congenital defects, epispadias (meatus opens on dorsal side of penis), and hypospadias (meatus opens on underside of penis).
Scrotum: Gently move penis to one side to assess scrotal skin. Lift up posterior side. Note lesions, inflammation, and edema. Begin scrotal palpation at right testicle. Proceed to the epididymis, then to the spermatic cord and the external ring. Note consistency and presence of tenderness or masses.	Scrotal skin is thin and wrinkled. Scrotal skin hugs testicles firmly in young males; becomes elongated and flaccid in older adults. Left scrotal sac is lower than the right. Testicles are sensitive to pressure and are firm, ovoid, smooth, and equal in size bilaterally.	Unilateral edema with a hard, fixed nodule (malignancy). Enlarged testicle with extreme sensitivity (testicular torsion, i.e., "twisting"). Swollen, indurated, tender (inflammation, i.e., epididymis). Warm scrotal skin, tenderness, and acute onset of edema indicate orchitis, i.e., testicular inflammation (associated with the mumps).
Inguinal area: Have client stand, if possible. Inspect first while client is at rest, then instruct client to bear down. Observe for bulges. Begin palpation on client's right side. Invaginate (telescope) loose scrotal skin with index finger. Follow spermatic cord upward to opening of external inguinal ring. Ask client to cough or bear down to check for mass or bulging. Bearing down may make hernia visible.	Inguinal area is smooth and free from edema or bulges.	Swelling above the inguinal ligament may indicate presence of inguinal hernia (protrusion of portion of the bowel through the external inguinal ring). A mass medial to the femoral vessels and inferior to the inguinal ligament indicates a femoral hernia (protrusion of portion of the bowel or omentum through the femoral wall).

Common abnormal lesions of the external male genitalia are:

- Candidiasis: Multiple, discrete, flat pustules with scaling and surrounding edema that are superficial mycotic infections of moist cutaneous sites associated with diabetes mellitus, deficiencies in systemic immunity, and antibiotic therapy
- Chancroid: Tender, ulcerated, exudative, papular lesion with an erythematous halo surrounding edema and a friable base that results from small breaks in epidermal tissue and inoculation of *Haemophilus ducreyi*
- Tinea cruris: Erythematous plaques with scaling, papular lesions with sharp margins caused by fungal infections of the groin

Chancre, condyloma acuminatum, and herpes simplex are also common abnormal lesions of the external male genitalia. These lesions are described in the section for common abnormal lesions of the external female genitalia.

Many nurses may feel anxious about examining the male genitalia. Nurses who feel uncomfortable about this assessment need to work through their feelings about sexuality and reproduction in order to communicate effectively with clients; see the accompanying Spotlight On display.

Assessment of the genitalia provides an opportunity for client teaching. For example, uncircumcised clients often need information on proper hygiene. Instruct the client to retract the foreskin daily so that the underlying skin can be washed with warm water and soap. Tell the client to return the foreskin to its original position once the underlying skin is thoroughly dried.

Some health care agencies do not allow nurses to perform a digital examination of the anus and rectum. Nurses must check the agency's policies relative to this part of the physical examination. Nursing students should have a qualified registered nurse with them the first time they perform a digital examination. After this procedure has been done, the color of feces on the gloved finger should be noted. Bright red or tarry black stools are indicative of bleeding and should be reported. Usually a sample of the feces is tested for occult blood.

Early detection and treatment decrease testicular cancer mortality rates. Monthly testicular self-examination (TSE) allows for early detection of testicular cancer. During the scrotal examination, the client needs to be taught how to perform a TSE; see the accompanying Client Teaching Checklist.

ANUS AND RECTUM

The anorectal examination is an important part of a comprehensive physical assessment.

The assessment includes the anus and rectum in clients of both genders; for males, the prostate gland is also examined. These assessments should be performed on a regular basis as they provide screening for diseases such as cancer.

Prior to the actual examination, the nurse should assess the client's degree of apprehension and reassure the client that some anxiety over this part of the examination is normal. The anorectal examination is usually done as the last part of the complete physical examination, after trust has been established between client and nurse. A step-by-step explanation, description of the expected sensations, reassurance, and a gentle technique will minimize client embarrassment and discomfort; see the accompanying Spotlight On display on page 596.

It is important to use a systematic approach to examination. For females, proceed from the anus to the rectum; with

---

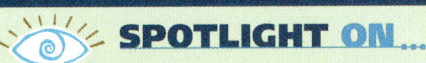

SPOTLIGHT ON...

Professionalism

Demonstrating Confidence while Examining the Male Genitalia

Nurses, both male and female, may feel anxious about examining the male genitalia. It is important that you work through your own feelings in order to help clients discuss their concerns. Some ways to increase your confidence are to:

- Practice interviewing with a male friend or classmate.
- Practice using correct terminology.
- Familiarize yourself with lay terminology, as many clients do not know the correct anatomic terms for body parts.

✓ **CLIENT TEACHING CHECKLIST**

Testicular Self-Examination

- Ask the client if monthly TSE is performed.
- Explain to the client that monthly TSE will allow for early detection of testicular cancer.
- Review the anatomy of the scrotum by describing that the testicles are ovoid structures that feel firm and rubbery and that the epididymis, located behind the testicles, is softer and feels ropelike.
- Instruct the client to perform the examination during a warm shower using the thumb and first two fingers to gently feel each testicle and the epididymis. The testicles should move freely within the scrotum and have a smooth surface; the epididymis should be softer.

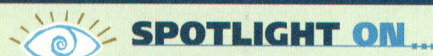

SPOTLIGHT ON...

Professionalism

It is important to maintain a professional, nonjudgmental approach while performing the anorectal examination. How would you respond if the following situations occurred during the assessment?

Prior to the examination, the client is unable to sit still on the exam table.

The client develops an erection.

The client passes flatus.

The client loses bowel control.

RESPECTING OUR DIFFERENCES

Incidence of Prostate Cancer Rates by Race

African American: 248 per 100,000 men

Caucasian: 156 per 100,000 men

Hispanic: 138 per 100,000 men

Asian/Pacific Islander: 93 per 100,000 men

American Indian/Alaska Native: 73 per 100,000 men

Data from National Cancer Institute. (2008). *Surveillance Epidemiology and End Results*. Retrieved January 26, 2009, from http://seer.cancer.gov/statfacts/html/prost.html.

males, proceed from the anus to the prostate. See Table 27-25 which presents the specific areas of the anus and rectum to be examined.

In 2008, more than 186,000 men died from prostate cancer, which primarily affects older males (National Cancer Institute, 2008). The median age at diagnosis for cancer of the prostate is 68 years. In addition to age, race is also a risk factor; see the Respecting Our Differences display.

TABLE 27-25 Assessment of the Anus and Rectum

ASSESSMENT AREA/TECHNIQUE	NORMAL FINDINGS	SIGNIFICANT FINDINGS AND POSSIBLE CAUSES
Assist client to side-lying position. Drape to expose only areas to be examined. Spread client's buttocks.		
Inspect perineum and anus. Observe for excoriation, inflammation, rashes, and nodes. Palpate any nodules for tenderness. Lubricate gloved index finger of dominant hand. Instruct client to inhale and exhale deeply. Inspect anus for hemorrhoids, fissures, excoriation. As sphincter relaxes, insert fingertip into the anal canal. Note sphincter tone, tenderness, or nodules. Insert finger further and palpate as much of rectal wall as possible, noting nodules or tenderness.	Perineum is smooth, intact, and slightly darker than surrounding skin. Anus is dark, puckered, and pink to dark brown. Skins tags usually present. Strong rectal sphincter tone. Smooth rectal wall.	Fissure or tear (abscess, trauma). Venous prominence on anus (external hemorrhoids).
With males: Palpate surface of prostate gland. Extend fingertip above prostate gland, and instruct client to bear down. Note size, shape, consistency, and mobility of prostate.	Prostate gland is small, smooth, and mobile.	Firm, hard, or indurated nodules on prostate (cancer). Firm, tender mass (abscess). A tender, warm prostate may indicate acute bacterial prostatitis associated with a bladder infection.

Data from Estes, M. E. Z. (2010). *Health assessment and physical examination* (4th ed.). Clifton Park, NY: Delmar/Cengage Learning; Jarvis, C. (2007). *Physical examination & health assessment* (5th ed.). Philadelphia: Elsevier.

POSTASSESSMENT CARE OF THE CLIENT

A physical examination is taxing on the client, especially if the complete assessment is performed in one session. The nurse should assess the client's needs after this process and respond appropriately. The nurse should also dispose of soiled articles in the proper container and clean and store equipment. Thanking the client for cooperating during the physical examination demonstrates concern and caring.

Outpatient Setting

If the physical examination is conducted in the community, the nurse should acknowledge the client's rights to privacy and confidentiality; see the accompanying Community Considerations display. The client should be offered assistance, for example, with toileting or dressing. If a family member is in the home, the nurse should notify that person when the assessment is completed. If the client is home alone, the nurse should verify that the client is capable of meeting his or her own needs before leaving. Listen carefully to the client's remarks, and provide information regarding the assessment.

Inpatient Setting

Nursing students should check with their instructors before conducting the assessment to ascertain the amount of information that they can share with the client during and after the examination. This varies in different agencies and according to the primary care provider. It is best to secure this information before beginning the examination.

After concluding the assessment, dispose of soiled articles and clean and store the equipment. The bed should be returned to a low position, with side rails up and call light in place. Check on the client after assessment to monitor the client's condition.

COMMUNITY CONSIDERATIONS

Nurses who practice in community settings provide the same essential services to clients as those performed in inpatient settings. Essential services include:

- Advocacy for clients unable to do so for themselves
- Delivery of legal and ethical care (e.g., respect for client rights, use of standard precautions)
- Health promotion (client education)
- Medication education
- Pain management

DATA DOCUMENTATION

Reporting information is a critical part of documentation. If findings require immediate attention (e.g., bright red blood or a change in the nature and character of a previous symptom), report the findings and document in the medical record the actions taken.

Health care agencies have specific forms for recording the assessment findings. Review these forms before initiating the assessment, and record the findings on the appropriate form as the data are gathered. Some data (e.g., vital signs) may need to be recorded on more than one form.

Documentation should reflect the objective data obtained from the examination regarding the client's current condition. Avoid phrases such as *client appears lethargic*; instead, record the GCS score. Abnormal assessment findings must be documented and reported.

KEY CONCEPTS

- The physical examination provides a complete picture of the client's physiological functioning; when combined with a health and psychosocial assessment, it forms a database to direct decision making.
- Because the client will experience some anxieties regarding the examination, it is important for the nurse to keep the client informed while performing the examination.
- The purposes of draping the client are to prevent unnecessary exposure and chilling during the examination.
- The physical examination is done in a sequential, head-to-toe fashion to ensure a thorough assessment of each system.
- Assessment begins with initial contact with the client.

- Use the landmarks and visualize the internal organs when assessing the thorax, heart, and abdomen.
- The order of abdominal assessment is inspection, auscultation, percussion, and palpation because palpation and percussion can alter the bowel sounds.
- Nurses play a major role by teaching breast self-examination (BSE) and testicular self-examination (TSE) and by supporting clients in achieving healthy lifestyles.
- Nurses must be aware of their own feelings in order to communicate with clients effectively during the physical examination.
- Reporting information is a critical part of documentation; if assessment findings require immediate attention, report the findings and document actions in the medical record.

- Know the agency's policies relative to performing and documenting a physical assessment.

- Documentation should reflect the objective data obtained from the examination.

REVIEW QUESTIONS

1. A nurse is performing assessment of a client's vascular system. Which of the following actions must the nurse avoid?
   a. Auscultate for bruits at the carotid arteries.
   b. Check nail beds for capillary refill.
   c. Palpate both carotid arteries simultaneously.
   d. Perform the Allen test.

2. Which of the following methods is useful for assessing skin turgor?
   a. Indenting the ankle
   b. Pinching a skin fold
   c. Touching to determine degree of moisture
   d. Using the goniometer

3. List the order in which assessment techniques should be performed during physical examination of the abdomen.
   a. _____ Auscultation
   b. _____ Inspection
   c. _____ Palpation
   d. _____ Percussion

4. A client becomes irritable, has labile emotions, and experiences sudden onset of headache. Which of the following assessments is most important for the nurse to perform?
   a. Cardiovascular
   b. Integumentary
   c. Neurological
   d. Visual

5. The client is a 72-year-old African American male. He weighs 235 pounds, and his current blood pressure is 178/102. Which of the following is a modifiable risk factor for cardiovascular disease presented by this client?
   a. Family history
   b. Gender
   c. Obesity
   d. Race

6. The nurse is performing a physical assessment of the heart. Which of the following assessment findings should be reported immediately to the primary care provider?
   a. A mass and strong pulsations in the epigastric region
   b. Absence of bruits
   c. Absence of heaves
   d. Slight pulsations over the aorta

7. Which of the following assessment findings indicates cyanosis in a client with dark skin?
   a. Blue nail beds
   b. Bluish coloration on lips
   c. Dark, dull, lifeless-looking skin
   d. Generalized mottled, dusky-blue hue

8. Which of the following tests would the nurse perform to test cerebellar function?
   a. Allen
   b. Romberg
   c. Rinne
   d. Weber

9. The nurse is caring for a client who is on steroid therapy. Which of the following assessment findings would the nurse expect this client to exhibit?
   a. Enlarged skull
   b. Masklike facial expression
   c. Round, moon face
   d. Sunken eyeballs

10. Which assessment finding should the nurse report when assessing a client with light skin?
    a. Bright cherry-red cheeks and neck
    b. Pigmented areas on breast nipples that are darker than surrounding skin
    c. Pink nail beds
    d. White sclera

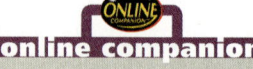

online companion

Visit the DeLaune and Ladner online companion resource at **www.delmar.cengage.com** for additional content and study aids. Click on Online Companions, then select the Nursing discipline.

If the nurse is an intelligent being, and not a mere carrier of diets to and from the patient, let her exercise her intelligence in these things.

—FLORENCE NIGHTINGALE (IN SKRETKOWICZ, 1992)

CHAPTER 28

Diagnostic Testing

COMPETENCIES

1. Discuss the relevant client teaching guidelines for the care of the client before, during, and after diagnostic testing.
2. Describe the common specimen collection methods.
3. Describe common invasive and noninvasive diagnostic procedures.
4. Discuss nursing interventions for the common diagnostic procedures.

KEY TERMS

agglutination	echocardiogram	phagocytosis
agglutinins	electrocardiogram	phlebotomist
agglutinogens	electroencephalogram	pneumothorax
Allen test	electrolyte	polyp
amniocentesis	endoscopy	Port-a-Cath
analytes	enzymes	predictive value
aneurysm	erythrocytes	radiofrequency ablation
angiography	general anesthesia	radiography
anions	hematuria	red cell indices
antibodies	hemoconcentration	regional anesthesia
antigens	hemoglobin electrophoresis	sensitivity
ascites	hemolysis	signal-averaged
aspiration	incidence	electrocardiography
atherosclerotic plaque	invasive	specificity
biopsy	ketones	spherocytes
cardiac catheterization	late potentials	stress test
cations	leukocytes	thallium
central line	lipoproteins	thoracentesis
cholinesterase	local anesthesia	thrombus
computed tomography	lumbar puncture	transducer
conscious procedural sedation	magnetic resonance imaging	trocar
contrast medium	mammography	type and crossmatch
culture	necrosis	ultrasound
digital subtraction angiography	noninvasive	urobilinogen
disseminated intravascular	occult	venipuncture
coagulation	Papanicolaou test	void
Doppler	paracentesis	

With the arrival of health care reform, reimbursement practices such as managed care, and medicolegal concerns, health care is redefining the importance of history taking and physical examinations with a decreasing reliance on diagnostic tests. In the last two decades, before reform acts, health care relied heavily on the use of diagnostic testing to determine the nature of the client's condition.

Health care providers are using the findings from a thorough history and physical to determine the need for diagnostic testing. The client's history and presenting symptoms determine which diagnostic procedures are necessary to formulate a medical diagnosis and the course of treatment. The challenge of cost-effective health care pushes practitioners to rely on basic assessment and to be selective with expensive diagnostic tests. To reflect the emphasis on cost containment, the nurse's role has changed from doing for the client to teaching clients to do for themselves. The role of the nurse is to teach the client, family, and significant others about the procedures involved with diagnostic testing, the steps to be taken in preparation for the specific test, and the care that will follow the procedure. Although the primary focus is on teaching, the nurse may assist in performing various noninvasive and invasive procedures. Nurses must be aware of the implications of diagnostic testing so as to deliver appropriate nursing care to the client.

To understand the nature of diagnostic tests, nurses need to review anatomy and physiology. Knowing the anatomical and physiological functions of the body will assist nurses in relating certain diagnostic tests to specific disease processes.

This chapter discusses the most common diagnostic tests. The terms *test* and *procedure* are used interchangeably throughout the chapter. The term *prescribing practitioner* is used in this chapter to refer to either the physician or other authorized prescribers. Most state boards of nursing allow advanced practice registered nurses to order and perform certain diagnostic tests. See Chapter 11 for a discussion of professional responsibility.

OVERVIEW OF NONINVASIVE AND INVASIVE DIAGNOSTIC TESTING

Diagnostic tests are either noninvasive or invasive. Noninvasive means the body is not entered with any type of instrument. The skin and other body tissues, organs, and cavities remain intact. Invasive means accessing the body's tissue, organ, or cavity through some type of instrumentation procedure.

NURSING CARE OF THE CLIENT

Diagnostic testing is a critical element of assessment (see Chapters 6 and 27). Assessment data are used to formulate nursing diagnoses, a plan of care, and outcome measures in collaboration with the client. Ongoing client assessment and evaluation of the client's expected outcomes require the incorporation of diagnostic findings.

Preparing a Client for Diagnostic Testing

The nurse plays a key role in scheduling and preparing the client for diagnostic testing. "The emphasis of pretest is on appropriate test selection, proper patient preparation, individualized patient education, and emotional support" (Fischbach & Dunning, 2008, p. 9). When tests are not scheduled correctly, the client is inconvenienced. It may also delay interventions, which places the client's health status at risk. The institution is also at risk to lose money. Table 28-1 presents a sample protocol of the nursing care to prepare a client for diagnostic testing.

The nursing care contained in the protocol provides a systemic format, based on the nursing process, to prepare the client for most diagnostic studies. During the assessment of the client, make sure the client is wearing an identification band (see Figure 28-1). The identification band is a key factor to ensure client safety in all health care settings.

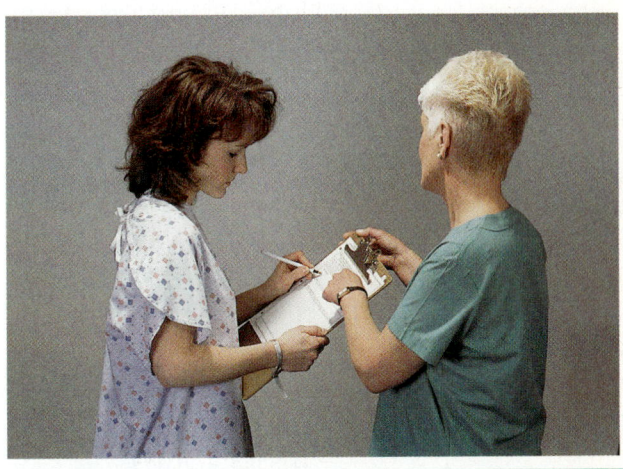

FIGURE 28-1 Nurse and client prepare for diagnostic testing.
DELMAR/CENGAGE LEARNING

TABLE 28-1 Protocol: Preparing the Client for Diagnostic Testing	
Purpose	To increase the reliability of the test by providing client teaching on why the test is being performed, what the client can expect during the test, and the outcomes and side effects of the test
	To decrease the client's anxiety about the test and the associated risk
Level	Independent
Supportive data	Increasing the client's knowledge promotes cooperation, enhances the quality of the testing, and decreases the time required to perform the study with an outcome of increased cost-effectiveness.
	Proper physical preparation prevents delays.
Assessment	Check to be sure the client is wearing an identification band.
	Review the medical record for herbal supplements, allergies, and previous adverse reactions to dyes and other contrast media; a signed consent form; and the recorded findings of diagnostic tests relative to the procedure.
	Assess for presence, location, and characteristics of physical and communicative limitations or preexisting conditions.
	Monitor the client's knowledge of why the test is being performed and what to expect during and after testing.
	Monitor vital signs for clients scheduled for invasive testing to establish baseline data.
	Assess client outcome measures relative to the practitioner's preferences for preprocedure preparations.

(Continues)

TABLE 28-1 (Continued)

	Monitor level of hydration and weakness for clients who are NPO (nothing by mouth), especially geriatric and pediatric populations.
Report to practitioner	Notify practitioner of herbal supplements, allergies, previous adverse reactions, or suspected adverse reactions following administration of drugs.
	Notify practitioner of any client or family concerns you were not able to alleviate.
Interventions	Clarify with practitioner if regularly scheduled medications are to be administered.
	The NPO status is determined by the type of test.
	Administer cathartics or laxatives as denoted by the test's protocol; however, there must be a specific practitioner order to give children and infants a laxative. Instruct clients who are weak, especially geriatric clients, to call for assistance to bathroom.
	Teach relaxation techniques, such as deep breathing and imagery.
	Establish intravenous (IV) access if necessary for procedure.
Evaluation	Evaluate client's knowledge of what to expect.
	Evaluate client's anxiety level.
	Evaluate client's level of safety and comfort.
	Monitor that someone will accompany a child to the department where the test is to be performed and remain with the child during the tests if not at risk of harmful exposure.
Client teaching	Discuss the following with the client and family as appropriate to the specific test:
	• Explain reason for test and what to expect
	• An estimation of how long the test will take
	• NPO (if oral medication to be taken, how much water to drink)
	• Cathartics or laxative: how much, how often
	• Sputum: cough deeply, do not clear throat
	• Urine: voided, clean-catch specimen, time to collect
	• No objects (jewelry or hair clips) to obscure x-ray film
	• Barium: taste, consistency, aftereffects (stools lightly colored for 24–72 hours, can cause obstruction or impaction)
	• Iodine: metallic taste, delayed allergic reaction (itching, rashes, hives, wheezing and breathing difficulties)
	• Positioning during the test
	• Positioning posttest (e.g., angiography)—immobilize limb
	• Posttest, encourage fluids if not contraindicated
Documentation	Record the following in the client's medical record:
	• Practitioner notification of allergies or suspected adverse reactions to contrast media
	• Presence, location, and characteristics of symptoms
	• Teaching and the client's response to teaching
	• Response to interventions (client's outcomes)

Delmar/Cengage Learning

Other key nursing measures to ensure client safety are to establish baseline vital signs, identify known allergies, and assess the effectiveness of teaching. As more Americans increase their usage of herbal products, nurses need to identify and report these herbal supplements when ordering laboratory tests. Some herbal products may cause abnormal test results and confusion in proper diagnosis (e.g., Dan Shen, ginseng, devil's claw, and dong quai may interact with warfarin, an anticoagulant with a narrow therapeutic range). In the ambulatory and outpatient centers, the nurse might have only one opportunity to assess and record the vital signs; it is important for the nurse to confirm that these findings are *normal values* for the client. To accurately assess the client's response to anesthetic agents and the procedure, the nurse has to compare the vital signs taken during and after the procedure with the baseline data.

The client needs to know what to expect during the procedure. Teaching can increase the client's level of cooperation and should decrease the degree of anxiety. The client's family should also know what will happen during the procedure and approximately how long the procedure normally lasts.

 SAFETY FIRST

DIAGNOSTIC TESTING: SAFETY MEASURES
Use Standard Precautions whenever performing invasive and noninvasive testing to protect your health and safety as well as that of other health care providers and the client.

Reference is made to Table 28-1 throughout this chapter. This protocol provides the nurse with the direction and guidance needed to plan nursing care. Nurses must also know the institution's protocols and procedures because these are not standardized in all practice settings.

Care of the Client during Diagnostic Testing

Although the care of the client needs to be individualized for a specific procedure, general guidelines for client care during a procedure are given in Table 28-2. Protocols are used to assist the nurse with client care.

Standard Precautions are initiated when exposure to body fluids presents a threat to the safety of the caregiver. Protective barriers, such as gloves and a gown, should be used during invasive procedures. The nurse is responsible for labeling any specimen with the client's name, room number (hospitalized clients), date, time, and source of the specimen. Some specimens may need to be taken immediately to the laboratory or placed on ice (e.g., arterial blood gases).

In order to promote the client's comfort and cooperation during diagnostic tests, nurses must consider the management of procedural pain. Although not all procedures are painful, advances in diagnostic and therapeutic studies have placed clients at risk for painful procedures. Clients who are repeatedly subjected to painful procedures without adequate analgesia become anxious and anticipate pain; if pain is experienced during one procedure, the client is reluctant to return for the same procedure or other tests.

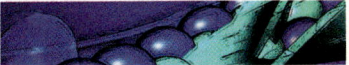

TABLE 28-2 Protocol: Care of the Client during Diagnostic Testing

Purpose	To increase cooperation and participation by allaying the client's anxiety and to provide the maximum level of safety and comfort during a procedure
Level	Interdependent
Supportive data	Increasing the client's participation and comfort encourages relaxation of muscles to facilitate instrumentation.
	Proper preparation of the client ensures efficient use of time during the test and reliable results.
Assessment	Check the client's identification band to ensure the correct client.
	Review the medical record for allergies.
	Assess the preprocedure sedatives administered to the client before the administration of anesthesia during the procedure.
	Assess airway maintenance and gag reflex if a local anesthetic is sprayed into the client's throat.
	Assess vital signs throughout the procedure and compare with baseline data.
	Assess the client's ability to maintain and tolerate the prescribed position.
	Assess the client's comfort level to ensure the effectiveness of the anesthetic agent.
	Assess for related symptoms indicating complications specific to the procedure (e.g., accidental perforation of an organ).
Report to practitioner	Notify the practitioner if the client has any concerns or questions that you were not able to resolve.
	Notify the practitioner if the client has family members present and where they are waiting during the procedure.
	Notify the practitioner when the client is positioned properly and the anesthetic agent has been administered to the client.

(Continues)

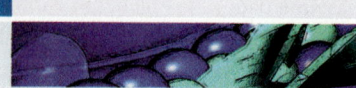

TABLE 28-2 (Continued)

Interventions	Institute Standard Precautions or appropriate aseptic technique for the specific test.
	Report to all personnel involved with the test any known client allergies.
	Place client in the correct position, drape, and monitor to ensure that breathing is not compromised.
	Remain with the client during the administration of anesthesia.
	If the procedure requires the administration of a dye, ensure the client is not allergic to the dye; if the client has not received the dye before, perform the skin allergy test according to the drug manufacturer's instructions that accompany the medication.
	Maintain the client's airway and keep resuscitative equipment available.
	Assist the client to relax during insertion of the instrument by telling the client to breathe through the mouth and to concentrate on relaxing the involved muscles.
	Explain what the practitioner is doing so that the client will know what to expect.
	Label and handle the specimen according to the type of materials obtained and the testing to be done.
	Report to the practitioner any symptoms of complications.
	Secure client transport from the diagnostic area.
	Posttest in the diagnostic area:
	1. Assist client to a comfortable, safe position.
	2. Provide oral hygiene and water to clients who were NPO for the test if they are alert and able to swallow.
	3. Remain with the client awaiting transport to another area.
Evaluation	Evaluate client's ventilatory status and tolerance of the procedure.
	Evaluate client's need for assistance.
	Evaluate client's understanding of what was performed during the procedure.
	Evaluate client's understanding of findings identified during the procedure.
	Evaluate client's knowledge of what to expect after the procedure.
Client teaching	Discuss the following with the client and family as appropriate to the specific test:
	• Explain what occurred during the procedure.
	• Answer questions and concerns of the client or family member.
	• Explain what to expect during the immediate recovery phase.
	• Explain what to report to the nurse during the immediate recovery phase.
Documentation	Record in the client's medical record:
	• Who performed the procedure
	• Reason for the procedure
	• Type of anesthesia, dye, or other medications administered
	• Type of specimen obtained and where it was delivered
	• Vital signs and other assessment data, such as client's tolerance of the procedure or pain and discomfort level
	• Any symptoms of complications
	• Who transported the client to another area (designate the names of persons who provided transport and place of destination)

Delmar/Cengage Learning

Recognizing that diagnostic procedures are performed in various settings, conscious procedural sedation (conscious sedation) is often used to manage pain during diagnostic testing.

Conscious procedural sedation is a minimally depressed level of consciousness during which the client retains the ability to maintain a continuously patent airway and respond appropriately to physical stimulation or verbal

DIAGNOSTIC PROCEDURES THAT MAY REQUIRE ANALGESIA OR SEDATION

- Bone marrow aspiration or biopsy
- Cardioversion
- Endoscopy
- Lumbar puncture
- Paracentesis
- Placement of catheters, lines, and tubing
- Radiologic procedures (CT and MRI)
- Thoracentesis
- Tissue biopsies
- Venipuncture

symptoms of accidental perforation of an organ (e.g., sudden changes in vital signs).

The nurse has additional responsibilities:

- Preparing the room (e.g., adequate lighting)
- Gathering and charging for supplies used during the procedure
- Testing the equipment to ensure it is functional and safe
- Securing proper containers for specimen collection

Practitioners usually have *preference cards* within the diagnostic testing area that specify the type of equipment to be used, the position to place the client, and the type of sedation or anesthesia.

Care of the Client after Diagnostic Testing

Nursing care postprocedure is directed toward restoring the client's prediagnostic level of functioning (see Table 28-3). Nursing assessment and interventions are based mainly on the nature of the test and whether or not the client received anesthesia. Anesthesia can be administered in one of three ways:

- **Local anesthesia**—client loses sensation to a localized body part—spraying the back of the throat with lidocaine to decrease the gag reflex
- **Regional anesthesia**—client loses sensation in an area of the body—laparoscope for a tubal sterilization
- **General anesthesia**—client loses all sensation and consciousness—major surgical procedures

See Chapter 40 for additional discussion of anesthesia.

commands (Fischbach & Dunning, 2008). The nurse managing conscious sedation is usually functioning in an expanded role that requires additional education and demonstrated ability beyond basic education. See the accompanying display for some procedures that may require analgesia or sedation.

Ongoing assessment of the client's status is required during the procedure. Always assess the patency of the client's airway, which may be compromised by the client's position, anesthesia, or the procedure itself. During an invasive procedure, the nurse needs to monitor for signs and

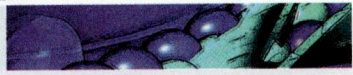

TABLE 28-3 Protocol: Care of the Client after Diagnostic Testing

Purpose	To restore the client's prediagnostic level of functioning by providing care and teaching relative to what the client can expect after a test and the outcomes or side effects of the test
Level	Interdependent
Supportive data	Increasing the client's participation and knowledge of expected outcome measures after a diagnostic test. Proper postprocedure care and client teaching alerts the client to what signs and symptoms need to be reported to the practitioner.
Assessment	Check the identification band, and call the client by name. Assess the client closely for signs of airway distress, adverse reactions to anesthesia or other medications, and other signs that may indicate accidental perforation of an organ. Assess body area(s) where a biopsy was performed for bleeding. Assess the client's color and skin temperature. Assess vascular access lines or other invasive monitoring devices. Assess the client's ability to expel air if air was instilled during a gastrointestinal test. Assess the client's knowledge of what to expect during the recovery phase.

(Continues)

Table 28-3 (Continued)

Report to practitioner	Notify the practitioner of any signs of respiratory distress, bleeding, or changes in vital signs; adverse reactions to anesthetic, sedative, or dye; and other signs of complications.
	Notify the practitioner regarding client or family concerns or questions that you are not able to answer.
	Notify the practitioner when any results are obtained from the diagnostic test.
	Notify the practitioner when the client is fully alert and recovered for an order to discharge.
Interventions	Implement the practitioner's orders regarding the postprocedure care of the client.
	Institute Standard Precautions or surgical asepsis as appropriate to the client's care needs.
	Position the client for comfort and accessibility to perform nursing measures.
	Monitor vital signs according to the frequency required for the specific test.
	Observe the insertion site for a hematoma or blood loss; replace pressure dressing as needed.
	Monitor the client's urinary output and drainage from other devices.
	Enforce activity restrictions appropriate to the test.
	Schedule client appointments as directed by the practitioner.
Evaluation	Evaluate the client's respiratory status to any anesthetic agents.
	Evaluate the client's tolerance of oral liquids.
	Evaluate the client's understanding of procedural findings or the time frame that written results should be reported to the practitioner.
	Evaluate the client's knowledge of what to expect after discharge.
Client teaching	Based on client assessment and evaluation of knowledge, teach the client or family about the following: • Dietary or activity restrictions • Signs and symptoms that should be reported immediately to the practitioner • Medications
Documentation	Record in the client's medical record on the appropriate forms: • Assessment data, nursing interventions, and achievement of client expected outcomes • Client or family teaching and demonstrated level of understanding • Written instructions given to the client or family members

Delmar/Cengage Learning

The client is monitored closely for signs of respiratory distress and bleeding. Some diagnostic procedures require that the vital signs be measured every 15 minutes for the first hour, then gradually decreased in frequency until the client is stable (alert and vital signs within the client's normal range).

Some diagnostic tests require the use of medications that are excreted through the kidneys; the nurse monitors the client's intake and output for 24 hours. The client is taught how to monitor intake and output. Instruct the client to report **hematuria**, the presence of blood in the urine. Clients receiving radioactive iodine must have their urine collected and properly discarded in a special container, according to agency policy for handling radioactive medical wastes.

When clients are discharged after diagnostic tests, they should receive written instructions. Most agencies have discharge forms for the nurse to document teaching regarding medications, dietary and activity restrictions, and signs and symptoms to be reported immediately to the practitioner. Clients may also need to have follow-up appointments made for them.

LABORATORY TESTS

Common laboratory studies are usually simple measurements to determine how much or how many **analytes** (a substance dissolved in a solution, also called a solute) are present in a specimen. Laboratory tests are ordered by prescribing practitioners to:

• Detect and quantify the risk of future disease
• Establish and exclude diagnoses

- Assess the severity of the disease process and determine the prognosis
- Guide the selection of interventions
- Monitor the progress of the disorder
- Monitor the effectiveness of the treatment

Nurses are often the first to view results of laboratory studies, and they need to know the terminology regarding laboratory tests: purpose, process, procedure, and normal test values. The clinical value of a test is related to (Fischbach & Dunning, 2008):

1. **Specificity**—the ability of a test to correctly identify those individuals who do not have the disease.
2. **Sensitivity**—the ability of a test to correctly identify those individuals who have the disease.
3. **Incidence**—the prevalence of a disease in a population or community; the predictive value of the same test can be different when applied to people of differing ages, genders, and geographic locations.
4. **Predictive value**—the ability of screening test results to correctly identify the disease state; a true positive correctly identifies persons who actually have the disease, whereas a true negative correctly identifies persons who do not actually have the disease.

Laboratory test results are based on normal range values. Le Système International d'Unités (SI), the International System of Units, is an international normal range reference established for reporting laboratory results (Pagana & Pagana, 2006). For example, the SI reference range for reporting red blood cell count for a woman is 4.0 to 5.2×10^{12}/L; the conventional range would appear as 4,000,000 to 5,200,000/mm^3 of blood.

SPECIMEN COLLECTION

The scheduling and sequencing of laboratory tests is an important function of the nurse. All tests requiring **Venipuncture**, the puncturing of a vein with a needle to aspirate blood, are grouped together so that the client is subjected to only one venipuncture. Fasting laboratory and radiologic studies are scheduled on the same day so that the client has to fast for only one day. Appropriate scheduling increases the client's comfort level and satisfaction.

"Communication errors account for more incorrect results than do technical errors" (Fischbach & Dunning, 2008, p. 13). Accuracy in laboratory testing requires that:

- The practitioner's order is transcribed onto the correct requisition form.
- All information requested should be written onto the form (e.g., the client's full name and medical number).
- Pertinent data that could influence the test's results, such as medication taken or herbal supplements, must be included.
- Collection of the specimen from the correct client is confirmed by the identification band.
- Laboratory results are placed on the correct client's medical record.

The risk for error increases when clients have the same last name. To improve client safety in health care settings, the Joint Commission has established annual safety goals based on sentinel events associated with errors. The Joint Commission *2009 Hospitals' National Patient Safety Goals* address the need to:

- Improve the accuracy of client identification by using two client identifiers and conducting a verification process before starting procedures.
- Improve the effectiveness of communications among caregivers by reading back verbal orders, creating a list of abbreviations not to be used, and reporting critical tests and critical results in a timely manner.
- Reduce the risk of health care–associated infections by meeting hand hygiene guidelines and sentinel events resulting from infection.
- Encourage clients' active involvement in their own care as a client safety strategy (Joint Commission, 2008).

Point-of-care testing (POCT) is a common practice in critical care settings and is proving to be a cost-effective, quality intervention for both clients and agencies. With advances in POCT technology over the past two decades, critical care nurses can perform a blood analysis and within seconds to minutes have a measurement upon which to change or implement an intervention. Nurses should be involved in the implementation and evaluation process of POCT since accuracy of the test is contingent on correct calibration and correct usage by the test performer. The following advantages are inherent in POCT (McConnell, 1999; Schallom, 1999):

- Prompt client diagnosis, treatment, and monitoring by decreasing turnaround time (TAT)
- Decreasing the risk for error by eliminating many of the steps in conventional laboratory testing
- Decreasing prolonged hospital stays and avoiding unnecessary hospitalizations by facilitating appropriate triage from emergency departments and prehospital settings
- Decreasing delays or cancellations of surgical procedures due to unavailable laboratory results, and the actual time the client spends in surgery
- Minimizing blood loss due to phlebotomy since POCT devices usually require only a few microliters or drops of blood versus 25 to 125 microliters per day for the critically ill client due to laboratory testing

Studies regarding POCT's clinical and financial value have revealed positive results: improved overall day-stay unit operations

▼ SAFETY FIRST ▼

DOCUMENTATION
Document on the laboratory requisition slip and in your nurses' notes any difficulty you experience while collecting the specimen. Such problems may be indicative of adverse effects that clients may experience due to the nature of the test and are conditions that must be reported and treated immediately.

and client services as well as earlier therapeutic decision-making time when blood test results are required for emergency room clients. Although studies have proven positive results in settings where the client's condition is acute and unstable, critical care applications may be quite different from those on a general medical or surgical unit. Studies will need to document the usefulness of POCT as a quality intervention in nonacute care settings.

Venipuncture

Venipuncture can be performed by various members of the health care team. Laboratories employ a **phlebotomist**, an individual who performs venipuncture, to collect blood specimens; however, it is the responsibility of a nurse to know *how* to perform a venipuncture. Nurses routinely perform venipuncture in the home, long-term care settings, and hospital critical care units.

Venipuncture can be performed by using either a sterile needle and syringe or a vacuum tube holder with a sterile two-sided needle. Test tubes are used to collect blood specimens. Test tubes have different colored stoppers to indicate the type of additive in the test tube. Collecting tubes are universally color coded as follows:

- Red—no additive
- Lavender—EDTA (ethylenediaminetetraacetic acid)
- Light blue—sodium citrate
- Green—sodium heparin
- Gray—potassium oxalate
- Black—sodium oxalate

There are three sources of venipuncture variability that can cause inaccurate results. **Hemoconcentration** is the reduced volume of plasma water and the increased concentration of blood cells, plasma proteins, and protein-bound constituents. It occurs with increased capillary hydrostatic pressure that causes water to shift from the intravascular into the interstitial space.

Hemoconcentration can be caused by prolonged standing or a prolonged time of application of a tourniquet during venipuncture. Alterations in the circulating blood volume can also cause hemoconcentration, such as occurs with dehydrated and burned clients.

Hemolysis is the breakdown of red blood cells and the release of hemoglobin. Hemolysis occurs with the rapid flow of blood through small-bore needles and exposure to large negative pressures. A negative pressure exists inside the collecting test tubes and syringe. To minimize the possibility of hemolysis, use a large-bore needle, moderate flow rates, and moderate negative pressures.

The third source of variability occurs when a blood specimen is drawn from a site above an intravenous (IV) infusion. The specimen is contaminated with IV solutions. Blood should be drawn from the client's other arm or below the infusion site.

Venipuncture is an invasive procedure. Health care providers performing venipuncture are at risk for the transmission of bloodborne organisms, such as human immunodeficiency virus (HIV) and hepatitis. HIV is the causative agent for

▼ **SAFETY FIRST** ▼

PREVENTING HEMOCONCENTRATION
Keep to a minimum both the length of time a client stands before venipuncture and the length of time of tourniquet application during venipuncture. These actions lower the risk of hemoconcentration and increase the rate of accuracy in laboratory tests.

acquired immunodeficiency syndrome (AIDS). Health care providers with weeping dermatitis or other exudative lesions should avoid handling all invasive equipment because the pathogens from these conditions can contaminate the equipment and spread infection to clients.

Correct selection (see Figure 28-2) and preparation of equipment and vein provides for a safe and efficient venipuncture (see Procedure 28-1). The gauge of the needle should be appropriate to the size of the vessel to prevent hemolysis. Review of the client's health history and physical assessment data will assist in identifying special client considerations. Venipuncture should not be performed on a flaccid arm of clients who have suffered a stroke. The normal muscle contraction, known as the venous pump, helps force blood back to the heart. These muscle contractions also help prevent blood backflow by forcing upper vein valves to open and lower valves to close. If an arm is paralyzed, the venous pump is lost, greatly increasing the risk of vein thrombosis ("Advice P.R.N.," 2008). If the client has a bleeding disorder or is taking anticoagulant therapy, apply pressure to the puncture site for 3 to 5 minutes after the removal of the needle.

Arterial Puncture

Assessment of arterial blood gases (ABG) reveals the ability of the lungs to exchange gases by measuring the partial

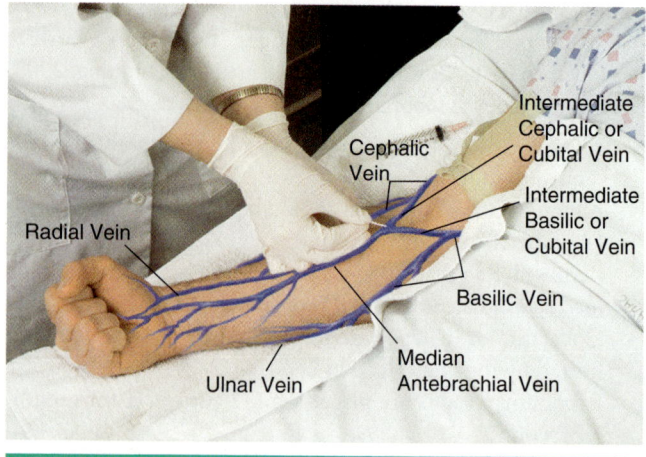

FIGURE 28-2 Nurse selects site for venipuncture. DELMAR/CENGAGE LEARNING

pressures of oxygen (Po_2) and carbon dioxide (Pco_2) and evaluates the pH of arterial blood. Blood gases are ordered to evaluate:

- Oxygenation
- Ventilation and the effectiveness of respiratory therapy
- Acid-base level of the blood

Arterial blood samples are drawn from a peripheral artery (e.g., radial or femoral) or from an arterial line. The arterial blood sample is collected in a 5-mL heparinized syringe. The syringe is then rotated to mix the blood with the heparin to prevent clotting. The blood sample is placed on ice to reduce the rate of oxygen metabolism.

In some agencies it is within the scope of nursing practice to perform radial artery puncture; however, femoral artery puncture is usually performed only by an advanced practitioner. An increased risk of hemorrhage exists with a femoral puncture. Although it is not common practice for student nurses to draw ABG samples, students often have to assist with the procedure and care for the client after the procedure.

Arterial punctures should not be performed:

- If the client is hyperthermic
- Immediately after breathing and suctioning treatments (wait 20 minutes)
- If there have been changes on ventilator settings

Arterial samples are also contraindicated in the following conditions:

- Anticoagulant therapy
- Clotting disorders
- Symptomatic peripheral vascular disease
- Negative Allen test

An **Allen test** is performed to measure the collateral circulation to the radial artery. See Chapter 27 for the Allen test procedure.

Regardless of who performs the arterial puncture, the nurse is responsible for assessing the client for symptoms of bleeding or occlusion postpuncture. Direct pressure must be applied to the puncture site until all bleeding has stopped, a minimum of 5 minutes if the radial artery is used and 10 minutes for the femoral. Ensure that all bleeding has stopped before releasing the pressure. Symptoms of impaired circulation include:

- Numbness, tingling, and pain
- Bluish color
- Absence of a peripheral pulse

Capillary Puncture

Skin punctures are performed when small quantities of capillary blood are needed for analysis or when the client has poor veins. Capillary puncture is also commonly performed for blood glucose analysis, discussed later in this chapter.

The common sites for capillary punctures are the:

- Heel—most common site for neonates and infants
- Fingertip—the inner aspect of palmar fingertip used most commonly in children and adults
- Earlobe—when the client is in shock or the extremities are edematous

To perform a skin puncture, assemble the equipment, prepare the client, and select the appropriate site (see Procedure 28-2).

Central Lines

Blood samples can be collected from central lines. A **central line** refers to a venous catheter inserted into the superior vena cava through the subclavian, internal, or external jugular vein. A central line is inserted when a peripheral route cannot be obtained, for treatment, and to withdraw blood for analysis. Central lines are used to treat alterations in fluid or electrolytes. The client's nursing diagnoses may include the following: *Deficient fluid volume related to nausea and/or vomiting* or *Imbalanced nutrition, less than body requirement related to anorexia.*

Nurses need to know the type and location of the central line catheter. There are various types of central lines. Central lines can have either one or more lumens inside the catheter. For example, a central venous catheter has either one or two lumens, whereas a Hickman multilumen catheter may have either two or three catheters contained in one sheath.

It is standard practice to mark each lumen of a multilumen catheter with the name of the infusion (e.g., fluid or medication). Lumens are marked to prevent the mixing of medications. Lumens without continuous infusion of fluids are capped with an infusion plug and flushed with a heparin solution every 8 hours according to agency protocol. Heparin prevents obstruction of the catheter lumen with a blood clot. The first sample of blood drawn from the central line cannot be used for diagnostic testing; it must be discarded. The amount of discard volume is directly related to the dead space (catheter size). The agency's protocol should indicate the volume to discard relative to the type and size of catheter.

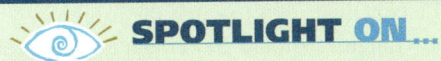 **SPOTLIGHT ON...**

Diagnostic Testing and Confidentiality

Mr. Takahashi comes to the Ambulatory Surgery Clinic for his preoperative diagnostic testing. You overheard the staff saying that Mr. Takahashi has had a history of hepatitis. Your instructor gathers all the student nurses and asks, "Who needs the experience of performing a venipuncture?" Two of your classmates indicate to the instructor that they have not had the opportunity to perform this procedure. Should you say anything to the instructor? Would you share with your classmates Mr. Takahashi's history? If you said something, would this be a breach of client confidentiality?

Delmar/Cengage Learning

The nursing care of central lines requires strict sterile technique (see Chapter 29). The prescribing practitioner has to write an order to allow a blood sample to be obtained from a central line. See the Nursing Checklist for how to draw a blood sample from a central line.

Implanted Port

Some clients have a Port-a-Cath (a port that has been implanted under the skin) over the third or fourth rib. The port has a catheter that is inserted into the superior vena cava or right atrium through the subclavian or internal jugular vein. The implanted port is used for the same purpose as the central lines.

Blood can be withdrawn for sampling by accessing the port using strict sterile technique. Accessing a port should be performed only by a nurse with proper education. Students are not usually taught how to access an implanted port.

Urine Collection

The kidneys are responsible for maintaining homeostasis of the body's buffering systems and the volume and ionic and osmotic composition of its fluid compartments; see Chapter 39 for a complete discussion of the composition of fluid compartments. As with blood, all urine collection requires the use of Standard Precautions to prevent the transmission of microorganisms among clients, nurses, and other health care providers.

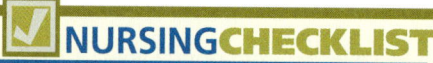

NURSINGCHECKLIST

Obtaining a Blood Sample from a Central Line

- Gather equipment (the sizes of the needle and syringe to obtain the blood sample are determined by the amount of blood needed for the test and the type and size of central line catheter).
- Check the client's identification band.
- Wash hands and don gloves to prevent exposure to bloodborne organisms.
- Select a port that is not used routinely for an infusion.
- Cleanse the port of the lumen with an antiseptic.
- Insert the needle into the port and aspirate the discard volume according to agency protocol; dispose of the syringe containing the discard blood into a sharps container.
- Access the port and withdraw the blood sample.
- Apply the same principles used in venipuncture to prevent the hemoconcentration and hemolysis of blood when withdrawing the sample.
- Transfer the sample into the correct collection tubes, and discard the contaminated needle and syringe into the sharps container.
- Instill the required heparin solution to prevent the lumen from clotting.
- Transport specimen to the laboratory.
- Remove gloves, and wash hands.

Urine can be collected for various studies. The type of testing determines the method of collection. The different methods of urine collection are:

- Random collection (routine analysis)
- Timed collection
- Collection from a closed urinary drainage system
- Clean-voided specimen

The urine from a closed urinary drainage system is a sterile specimen. Client teaching depends on the client's age and the method of collection. Initiate the protocol for preparing the client for testing (see Table 28-1). The method of collection should be written on the laboratory requisition.

RANDOM COLLECTION The prescribing practitioner usually writes the order for a UA (routine urine analysis), which is also called a random collection. It can be collected at any time using a clean cup. The urine does not have to be collected in a sterile container. Instruct the client to urinate into the specimen cup or into a clean bedpan or urinal. Wearing gloves, transfer the urine into a clean container. Seal the lid tightly, label, and place in a biohazard bag for transport to the laboratory. Urine should be refrigerated if the specimen cannot be sent to the laboratory within 1 hour; after an hour, unrefrigerated urine becomes alkaline because bacteria begin to split urea into ammonia.

TIMED COLLECTION Timed collection is done over a 24-hour period. The urine is collected in a plastic gallon container that contains preservative(s), some of which are caustic. The laboratory usually adds the preservatives to the container. If the analyte to be studied is light sensitive, a dark plastic container is necessary.

Provide the client with specific instructions. The client is told to void (the process of urine evacuation) and discard the specimen at the beginning of the collection. The 24-hour collection begins with the first discarded voiding. For example, if the client is instructed to void at 1000 hours (24-hour clock time frame), discard the urine and save all other voided specimens until 1000 hours the following day. The client can void throughout the test into a clean container, then pour the urine into the collection bottle. Toilet tissue should not be dropped into the container used to catch the urine.

The collection container should be refrigerated or kept on ice throughout the 24 hours. This retards bacterial growth and stabilizes the analytes. The last urine collection, at 1000 hours, should be a complete, forced voiding at the exact timed period. Seal the labeled container tightly, and take it immediately to the lab.

COLLECTION FROM A CLOSED DRAINAGE SYSTEM A sterile specimen can be collected from a client with an indwelling Foley catheter with a closed drainage system. A sterile specimen is used to culture the urine. *The urine specimen should not be obtained from the drainage bag.* The analytes in the urine drainage bag change; this will cause inaccurate results. Bacteria grow quickly in the drainage bag. The catheter's closed drainage tubing has an aspiration port that is used for a sterile specimen collection (see Procedure 28-3).

CLEAN-VOIDED SPECIMEN Clean-voided (clean-catch, or midstream) specimen collection is done to secure a specimen uncontaminated by skin flora. A clean-voided specimen should be obtained on first voiding in the morning. Most adult clients are capable of following instructions to perform this test.

Different aseptic techniques are used for women and men. Poor technique in cleaning the perineum can contaminate the specimen. Instruct the female client to cleanse from the front to the back (see Procedure 28-4).

Instruct the male client to perform the same procedure except for the cleansing of the perineal area; men should cleanse from the tip of the penis downward (see Procedure 28-4). The Nursing Checklist describes the procedure for obtaining a clean-voided specimen from a man.

When obtaining a clean-voided specimen from infants and small children, secure assistance. Follow the Nursing Checklist that describes the procedure for obtaining a clean-voided specimen from an infant or child.

Stool Collection

Explain to the client why the stool specimen is being collected. Instruct the client to defecate into a clean bedpan or

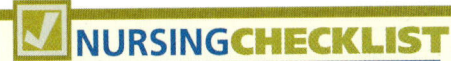
NURSINGCHECKLIST

Clean-Voided Specimen, Male

- Check the client's identification band.
- Instruct the client on the procedure.
- Wash hands and don gloves if the client needs assistance with the procedure.
- If uncircumcised, retract the foreskin, and hold retracted.
- Cleanse the head of the penis with a towelette using a circular motion. Cleanse the meatus and glans beginning with the urethral opening, and make one complete circle around the penis, moving down the glans shaft.
- Discard the towelette.
- Repeat the procedure until all three towelettes have been used.

NURSINGCHECKLIST

Clean-Voided Specimen, Infant and Child

- Check the identification band.
- Explain the procedure to family member present with infant or child. If the child can cooperate, tell child what to do before having someone hold him or her in position.
- Wash hands and don gloves.
- Place in a supine position with hips externally rotated.
- Have parent or assistant flex and abduct the knees, and hold the knees throughout the procedure.
- Cleanse the perineal area as you would for an adult.
- Place a sterile collection bag over the perineum or penis and scrotum, and apply a diaper.
- Remove the collection bag immediately after voiding.
- Transfer the urine into the labeled collection container, close lid tightly, and place in biohazard bag for immediate transport to the laboratory.

container, discarding tissue into the toilet. Stools can be collected for either a one-time defecation or over 24, 48, or 72 hours. If a specimen is needed over a prolonged period of time, all stools must be placed into a container and refrigerated. Once collected, label the container with the client's name, date, time, and the test to be performed on the specimen. All stool specimens are placed in a biohazard bag before transport to the laboratory.

HEMATOLOGIC SYSTEM

Understanding the hematologic system requires a knowledge of the blood's composition and its functions. Table 28-4 discusses the origin, normal range values, and the major function for each of the three types of cells found in blood:

TABLE 28-4 Types of Blood Cells

CELL	ORIGIN	NORMAL VALUES	MAJOR FUNCTION
Erythrocytes	Bone marrow	F: 4.0–5.2 × 10^{12}/L M: 4.5–5.9 × 10^{12}/L	Transport hemoglobin
Leukocytes	Granulocytes and monocytes from bone marrow Lymphocytes and plasma cells from lymph tissue	5.0–10.0 × 10^9/L	The body's protective system
Platelets	Megakaryocytes in bone marrow	140–400 × 10^3/mm^3	Vascular repair

Fischbach, F., & Dunning, M. (2008). *A manual of laboratory and diagnostic tests* (8th ed.). Philadelphia: Lippincott, Williams & Wilkins.

- Red blood cells (**erythrocytes**)
- White blood cells (**leukocytes**)
- Platelets

About 40% to 45% of the blood's volume is composed of blood cells; the remaining blood volume is plasma, as shown in Figure 28-3. Plasma is part of the body's extracellular fluid system, consisting of water and analytes. Blood proteins form the largest portion of the plasma analytes. The average plasma volume for a normal adult is 3 L.

Red Blood Cells

Red blood cells (RBCs), in embryonic life, are produced first in the yolk sac until the middle trimester; then the liver becomes the main organ of RBC production. RBC production becomes the exclusive function of the bone marrow by the end of gestation, after birth, and throughout life. RBC bone marrow site production changes with age:

- From birth to age 5—all bone marrow
- From 5 to 20 years—the shaft of the long bones (tibia and femur)
- After 20 years—the membranous bones (ilia, ribs, sternum, and vertebrae). As part of the normal aging process, the production of RBCs decreases with age.

    Functions of the RBCs include:

- Transporting oxygen-carrying hemoglobin
- Transporting carbon dioxide in the form of sodium bicarbonate
- Being an acid-base buffer for whole blood

White Blood Cells

There are six types of white blood cells (WBCs, leukocytes) found in the blood.

- Neutrophils
- Eosinophils
- Basophils
- Monocytes
- Lymphocytes
- Plasma cells

The polymorphonuclear cells, neutrophils, eosinophils, and basophils have a granular appearance, hence, the name granulocytes or polys. The granulocytes and monocytes are responsible for **phagocytosis**, the process by which certain cells engulf and dispose of foreign bodies. The lymphocytes and plasma cells function mainly as the body's immune system.

 SAFETY FIRST

STOOL FROM A CLIENT WITH HEPATITIS
When collecting a stool specimen from a client with hepatitis, write on the lab requisition form that the client has hepatitis. This increases the laboratory personnel's awareness to be extra careful when handling the specimen.

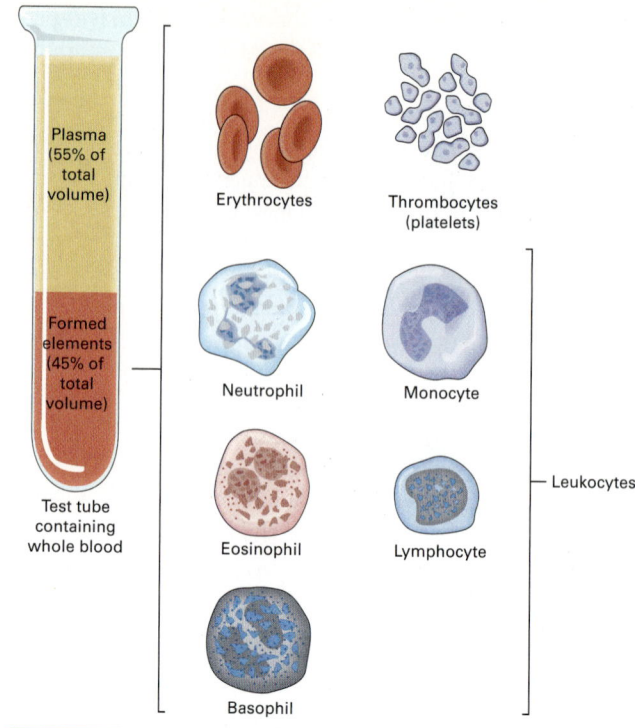

FIGURE 28-3 Blood Cells DELMAR/CENGAGE LEARNING

The WBCs are formed and stored in the bone marrow until needed by the body. Table 28-5, on page 615, presents laboratory studies for a complete blood count with SI values and when each analyte is either increased or decreased in clinical situations.

Red Cell Indices

Red cell indices measure the size and hemoglobin content of the RBCs. The RBC indices are:

- Mean red cell hemoglobin (MCH)
- Mean red cell hemoglobin concentration (MCHC)
- Mean red cell volume (MCV)

The indices are diagnostic in determining the type of anemia. For example, an elevated MCHC means that **spherocytes** (smaller, thicker red cells) are present; this occurs in acquired hemolytic anemia.

Platelets

Platelets are fragments of a seventh type of WBC found in the bone marrow, the megakaryocytes. Platelets maintain hemostasis and blood coagulation by being the active mechanism of the blood in vascular repair. The active factors necessary for blood to coagulate are found in the cytoplasm of platelets. Blood coagulation is a comprehensive, sequential process of the body's response to injury.

The blood coagulation flow chart (see Figure 28-4 on page 616) reviews the key elements of vascular constriction and coagulation. Prothrombin (factor II) is a plasma protein, formed in the liver, and requires vitamin K for synthesis. It is activated when blood vessels are damaged. Prothrombin

TABLE 28-5 Complete Blood Count with Clinical Significance

ANALYTE	NORMAL VALUES	INCREASED	DECREASED
Red blood cell count	F: $4.0–5.2 \times 10^{12}$/L M: $4.5–5.9 \times 10^{12}$/L	Dehydration, induced hypoxia, polycythemia	Anemias, hypothyroidism, leukemias
Hemoglobin (Hb) Whole blood Fetal plasma	F: 120–150 g/L M: 139–163 g/L 0–75 mg/L <0.01	Chronic obstructive lung disease, polycythemia, high altitudes, burns, shock	Anemia, severe hemorrhage
Hematocrit (Hct)	F: 0.36–0.46 M: 0.41–0.53	Dehydration, polycythemia	Leukemia, hemorrhage
Mean red cell Hb	26–34 pg/RBC	Macrocytosis	Microcytic hypochromic anemia
Mean red cell Hb concentration	310–370 g/L	Spherocytosis	Chronic iron deficiency anemia
Mean red cell volume	80–100 fL	Aplastic anemia, cirrhosis, folic acid, vitamin B_{12}	Chronic iron deficiency, thalassemias, chronic anemia
White Blood Cell (WBC)			
Total count	$5.0–10.0 \times 10^9$/L	Acute leukemia, infections, surgery, trauma	Acute chronic leukemias, aplastic anemia, agranulocytosis
WBC Differential	% of total WBC		
Band neutrophils	3–6	Severe bacterial disease	
Segmented neutrophils	50–62	Diabetic acidosis, infarctions, inflammatory diseases, malignancies	
Lymphocytes	25–40		
Monocytes	3–7	Chronic lymphocytic leukemia	Lupus erythematosus, Hodgkin's disease
Eosinophils	0–3	Chronic inflammatory diseases	
Basophils	0–1	Allergies, parasites Myelofibrosis	

Fischbach, F., & Dunning, M. (2008). *A manual of laboratory and diagnostic tests* (8th ed.). Philadelphia: Lippincott, Williams & Wilkins.

activator causes the conversion of prothrombin into thrombin, which then causes fibrinogen to form threads. This whole process takes 10 to 15 seconds. Prothrombin activator is the governing element in blood coagulation. Prothrombin time (PT) measures the defects in this extrinsic clotting mechanism, specifically fibrinogen (factor I), prothrombin (factor II), and factors V, VII, and X (Pagana & Pagana, 2009).

Drugs can either increase or decrease the PT. Common drugs that increase the PT include salicylates, steroids, sulfonamides, oral anticoagulants, antibiotics, quinidine, Dilantin, Aldomet, Tagamet, cathartics, and alcohol. Other drugs can decrease the PT: digitalis, oral contraceptives, corticosteroids,

chloral hydrate, barbiturates, vitamin K, Placidyl, Doriden, griseofulvin, Alupent, and rifampin. Be sure to list the drugs the client is taking on the laboratory requisition for the PT test.

Partial thromboplastin (PTT) or activated partial thromboplastin time (APTT) measures the intrinsic clotting mechanism factors (I, II, V, X, XI, and XII). There are five primary screening tests to diagnose suspected coagulation disorders (Fischbach & Dunning, 2008; Pagana & Pagana, 2009):

1. Platelet count, size, and shape
2. Bleeding time—the ability of platelets to function normally and the ability of capillaries to constrict their

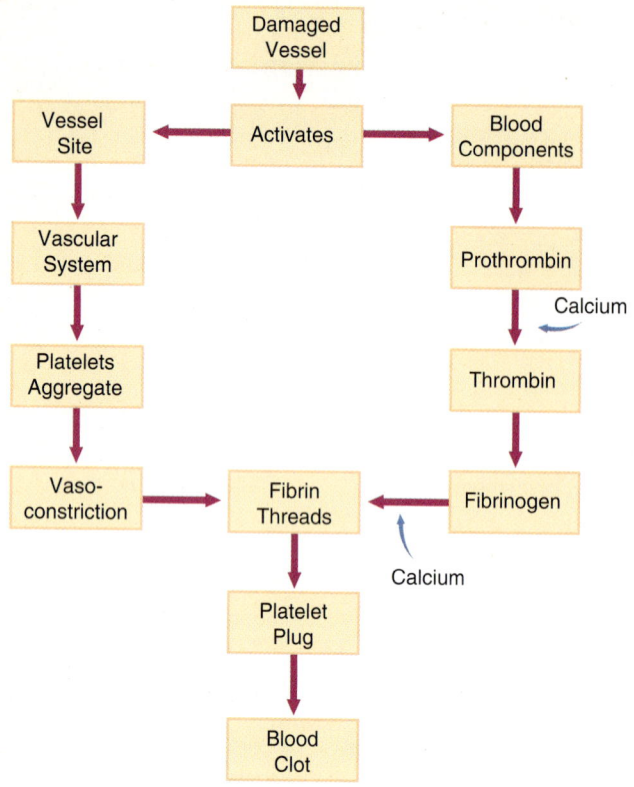

FIGURE 28-4 Blood Coagulation Flow Chart DELMAR/CENGAGE LEARNING

walls; prolonged with deficiencies in platelets and other clotting factors

3. PTT—measures the ability of the blood to clot; prolonged with any intrinsic factor deficiencies such as hemophilia A (factor VIII) and hemophilia B (factor X)

4. PT—measures the total quantity of prothrombin in the blood, monitors the effectiveness of coumarin therapy; prolonged with deficiencies in the extrinsic factors and vitamin K

5. Fibrinogen level—investigates abnormal PT and APTT, and screens for **disseminated intravascular coagulation** (DIC) (an acquired hemorrhagic syndrome characterized by uncontrolled formation and deposition of thrombi) and fibrin-fibrinogenolysis; levels increase with acute inflammatory reactions, trauma, coronary heart disease, and cigarette smoking and decrease in liver disease, DIC, cancer, primary fibrinolysis, and congenital hypofibrinogenemia.

Thrombin time (TT) measures the fibrinogen portion of the hemostatic mechanism; it is infrequently used today to evaluate the fibrinogen-to-fibrin reaction. Direct measurements of fibrinogen level and the increasing use of other tests have decreased the usefulness of TT (Pagana & Pagana, 2009).

Sickle Cell Test

The sickle cell test (hemoglobin S) is used to identify the sickle cell trait and sickle cell disease. A negative result, which is normal, indicates the absence of hemoglobin S. The presence of sickle cells causes a positive result, thus requiring

hemoglobin electrophoresis to determine the presence of the genetically transmitted deficit.

Hemoglobin electrophoresis refers to a laboratory test that uses an electromagnetic field (an anode [+] and a cathode [−], which are separated by cellulose acetate or starch gel) to identify various types of hemolytic anemia. Electrophoresis distinguishes between genetically transmitted homozygous and heterozygous hemoglobin S, which is responsible for sickle cell anemia. For example, if both genes carry hemoglobin S, it is called homozygous and the client has sickle cell disease; however, if only one gene has the abnormal hemoglobin S and the other gene has the normal hemoglobin A, the client is heterozygous, having the sickle cell trait. Electrophoresis is also used to identify fetal hemoglobin and distinguishes between thalassemia minor and major.

Sickle cell anemia is a blood disorder with multiple, recurring symptoms that not only causes the client pain from the clumping of RBCs in the joints but has widespread effects on other systems. Figure 28-5, on page 617, demonstrates the pathologic changes in the body and the resulting effects of sickle cell anemia.

Other common laboratory tests that measure hematologic functions are presented in Table 28-6 on page 618.

TYPE AND CROSSMATCH

A **type and crossmatch** is a laboratory test that identifies the client's blood type and determines the compatibility of blood between a potential donor and recipient (client). There are four basic blood types (A, B, AB, and O) that are determined by the presence or absence of A or B antigens, as shown in Figure 28-6 on page 619. **Antigens** are substances, usually proteins, that cause the formation of and react specifically with antibodies. **Antibodies** are immunoglobulins produced by the body in response to bacteria, viruses, or other antigenic substances. Type A and type B are antigens that are classified as **agglutinogens**, which are substances that cause **agglutination** (clumping of RBCs). **Agglutinins** are specific kinds of antibodies whose interaction with antigens is manifested as agglutination.

Blood types are also designated as either positive or negative, depending on the presence or absence of the Rh factor. Rh factor refers to an antigen found on the RBC. Rh positive means the antigen is present; Rh negative means the antigen is absent.

When factoring the four basic blood types with either the Rh-positive or Rh-negative factor, there are eight possible combinations (see the accompanying display on basic blood types). An individual's blood type is determined by heredity.

BASIC BLOOD TYPES

- A positive
- B positive
- AB positive
- O positive
- A negative
- B negative
- AB negative
- O negative

Sickle Cell Anemia

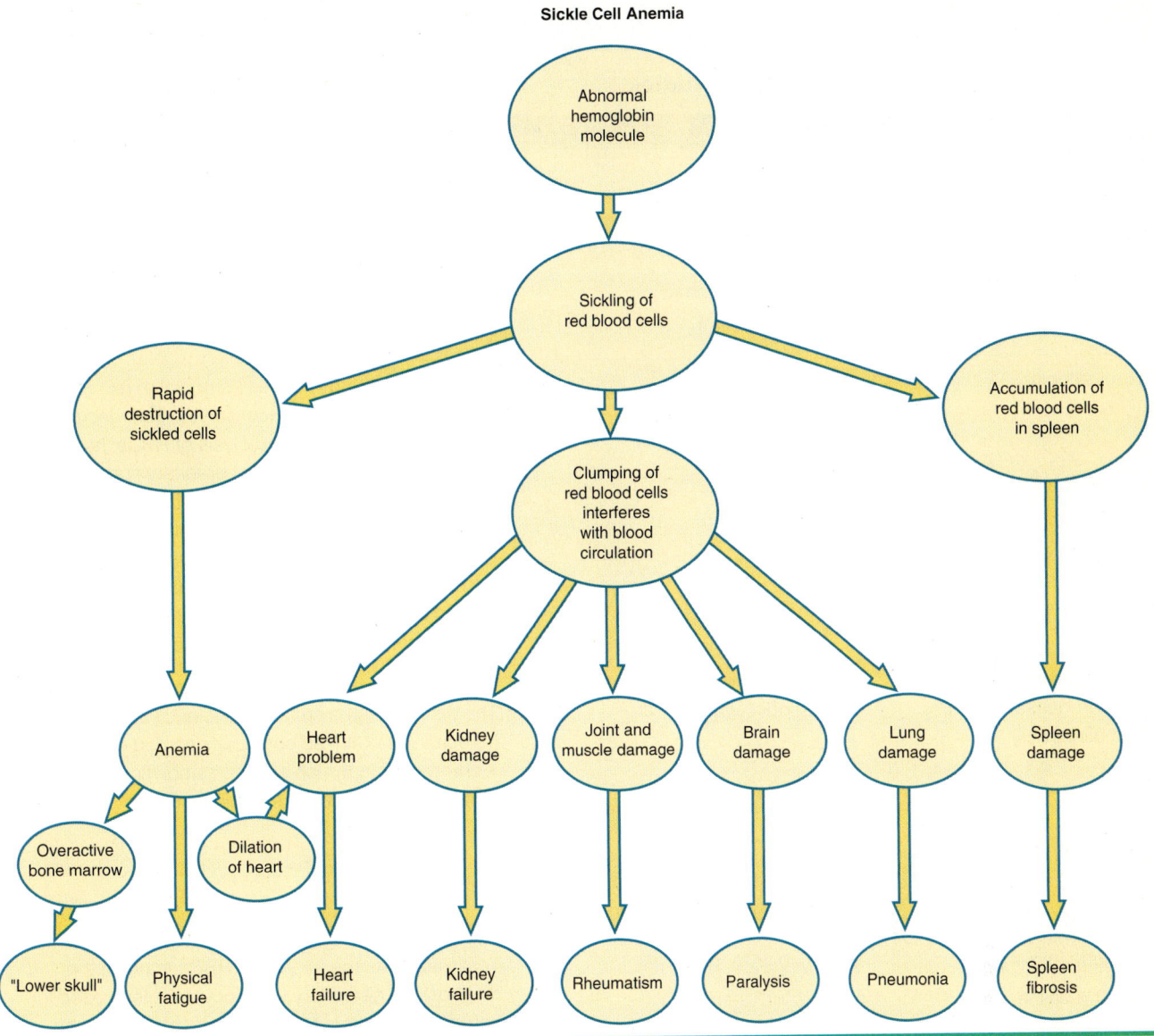

FIGURE 28-5 Sickle cell anemia: the clumping of red blood cells with their resulting effects on the body. DELMAR/CENGAGE LEARNING

Crossmatch determines the compatibility of the donor's blood with that of the recipient. In the laboratory, a sample of the recipient's blood is mixed with the blood of a possible donor. If the blood sample is compatible, the mixed sample does not agglutinate. For example, blood type A negative means that the person's blood contains the A antigen but does not contain the anti-Rh agglutinins. The first time the person is exposed to A-positive blood, either through a transfusion or by giving birth to an Rh-positive child, agglutination does not occur because the body has no antibodies against the antigen. However, once the body has had time to build up antibodies (agglutinins), agglutination will occur.

Blood Chemistry

Sophisticated automated instrumentation makes it possible to conduct a wide variety of blood chemistry testing identifiers on a single sample of blood. The tests are grouped under such headings as electrolytes, blood sugar, lipids, hormones, vitamins, minerals, and drug investigation. By measuring several blood chemicals at one time, a pattern of abnormalities is established, which allows for unsuspected diseases to be identified and which can lead to early diagnosis when symptoms are vague or absent (Fischbach & Dunning, 2008). The results may be reported as normal, low, high, panic, or toxic.

Blood Glucose

Glucose is a simple sugar formed from the digestion of carbohydrates and used by the cells for energy. Insulin is needed to transport glucose into the cells. Advances in technology have enabled the nurse, client, or caregiver to perform some laboratory tests at the bedside and in the home environment. Blood glucose monitoring, using either reagent strips or glucose meters, combined with a skin puncture lancet, is an example of

TABLE 28-6　Hematologic Function Studies

TEST	NORMAL RANGES	DIAGNOSTIC VALUE
Erythrocyte sedimentation rate (ESR or sed rate)	Westergren: F: <50 yr 0–25 mm/h >50 yr 0–30 mm/h M: <50 yr 0–15 mm/h >50 yr 0–20 mm/h	Alterations in the plasma proteins cause aggregation of the RBCs with an elevated ESR: moderately, with inflammatory diseases; high, with multiple myeloma, macroglobulinemias, hyperfibrinogenemias.
Haptoglobin	0.10–0.30 g/L 12–35 μmol/L	Haptoglobins bind with free hemoglobin released from the destruction of RBCs, conserving iron; decreased in any condition causing hemolysis of RBCs: hemolytic anemias (sickle cell anemia, hereditary spherocytosis, erythroblastosis fetalis), thalassemia, liver disease, transfusion reactions, systemic lupus erythematosus, prosthetic heart valve implants; increased with acute and chronic infections, inflammation, malignancies, steroid therapy, rheumatoid arthritis, ulcerative colitis, peptic ulcer, oral contraception, pregnancy.
Glucose-6-phosphate dehydrogenase (G6PD) (red blood cell)	F: 7.4–9.4 International Units/g hemoglobin, whites 6.5–9.3 International Units/g hemoglobin, African Americans M: 7.4–9.4 International Units/g hemoglobin, whites 6.6–10.8 International Units/g hemoglobin, African Americans	G6PD is an enzyme in RBCs that metabolizes glucose. The test measures enzyme deficiencies that are hereditary, sex-linked conditions carried on the female X chromosome, which causes hemolytic anemia. Clinical disease traits are found in males.
Osmotic fragility <0.30% saline >0.50% saline	0.30%–0.45% saline	Test measures the fragility of RBCs to aid in the diagnosis of hereditary spherocytosis. Increased in hereditary spherocytosis, spherocytosis resulting from autoimmune hemolytic anemia, severe burns, chemical poisoning, erythroblastosis fetalis, transfusion reactions, prosthetic heart valve transplantation. Decreased in sickle cell and iron deficiency anemia, polycythemia vera, hemoglobin C disease, thalassemia major, liver disease, obstructive jaundice, splenectomy.
Reticulocyte count (results reported in % of total erythrocytes)	Adults 0.5%–2.0% Children 0.5%–2.0% Infants 0.5%–3.5% Newborns 2.5%–6.0%	Used to differentiate between hypoproliferative and hyperproliferative anemias; to assess blood loss and bone marrow response to therapy. Increased in hemolytic and sickle cell anemia; hereditary spherocytosis; treatment of anemias from iron, vitamin B$_{12}$, and folic acid deficiencies. Decreased in aplastic, iron deficiency, and untreated pernicious anemias; chronic infection; radiation therapy.

Delmar/Cengage Learning

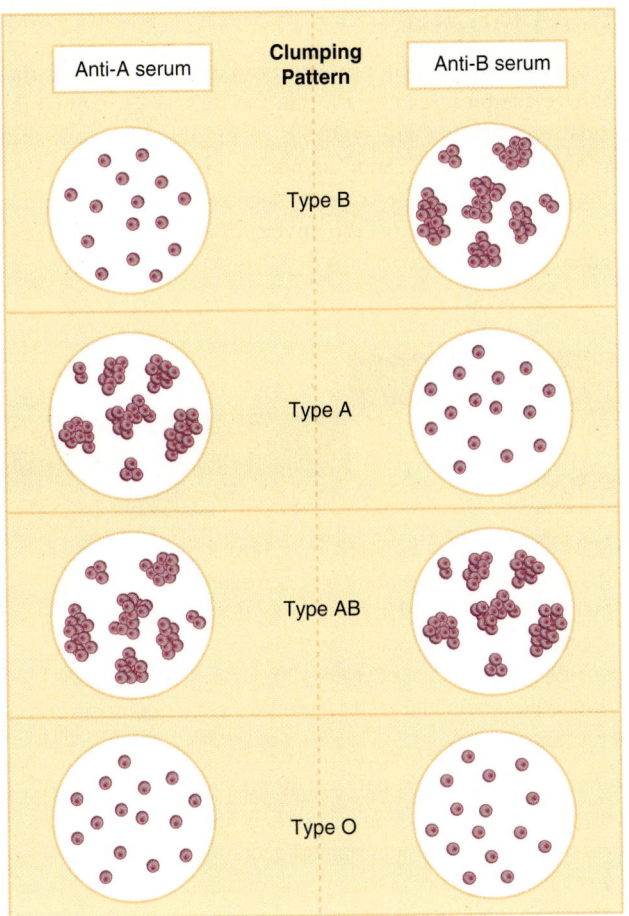

FIGURE 28-6 Blood Types DELMAR/CENGAGE LEARNING

Elite (Bayer), Glucometer (Bayer), OneTouch II (Life-Scan), SureStep Pro (LifeScan), InDuo (LifeScan), and Precision (MediSense). With the variety of meters available, it is essential that the nurse and client using the device review the specific manufacturer's operating instructions and be familiar with the equipment. Failure to do so could compromise the test results.

Glucose measurement is also performed by venipuncture: fasting blood sugar (FBS) or nonfasting (usually 2 hours postprandial). The normal fasting value is 70 to 115 mg/dL and less than 120 mg/dL postprandial. The 2-hour postprandial blood sugar is drawn 2 hours after the client eats a meal. This test is used to screen for diabetes mellitus; if the results are abnormal, the practitioner may order a glucose tolerance test.

A glucose tolerance test is the most accurate test for diagnosing hypoglycemia and hyperglycemia (diabetes mellitus). The client is asked to fast until the test begins. The test is conducted as follows:

- Initial blood and urine specimens are obtained.
- An oral loading dose of glucose is administered.
- Blood and urine specimens are obtained at 30 minutes, 1 hour, 2 hours, 3 hours, and sometimes 4 hours after loading dose.

Figure 28-7 is a graphic presentation of the results of a glucose tolerance test, showing results that indicate hyperglycemia, normal glucose, and hypoglycemia.

Glucose results reveal deficits in either the digestion of carbohydrates or glucose metabolism (e.g., diabetes mellitus). Drugs, especially diuretics and steroids, can cause physiological changes resulting in elevated blood glucose values. Clients receiving IV fluids with a high glucose content need to have their glucose levels monitored for hyperglycemia.

Serum Electrolytes

An **electrolyte** is an element or compound that when dissolved in water or another solvent, separates into ions and provides for cellular reactions. Some electrolytes act on the cell membrane and allow for the transmission of electrochemical impulses in nerve and muscle fibers. Other electrolytes determine the activity of different enzymatically catalyzed reactions that are necessary for cellular metabolism.

such technology. The convenience of these tests has changed the clinical management of many clients with diabetes.

Obtaining a capillary blood sample through skin puncture is the preferred method of testing when frequent blood glucose monitoring is needed. There are primarily two methods used to measure capillary blood glucose. Both methods require a large drop of capillary blood obtained through skin puncture with a sterile lancet and a reagent strip. The first method requires that a drop of blood be applied to a special chemical reagent strip. The participant visually compares the reagent strip to a color chart on the reagent container. Accuracy may be compromised if the result falls between two colors and the participant must estimate the blood glucose level. Examples of reagent strips include Chemstrip BG, Glucostix, and TrendStrips.

A second method of blood glucose monitoring replaces the visual comparison method with the use of a portable meter. Once the blood is placed on the reagent strip, the meter provides an accurate measurement of the blood glucose level. Depending on the type of meter, some reagent strips must be inserted into the meter by the participant while other meters require that the blood droplet be applied to the strip that is already in the meter; see Procedure 28-5. Examples of meters include Accu-Chek Advantage (Accu-Chek), Accu-Chek Active (Accu-Chek), Bayer

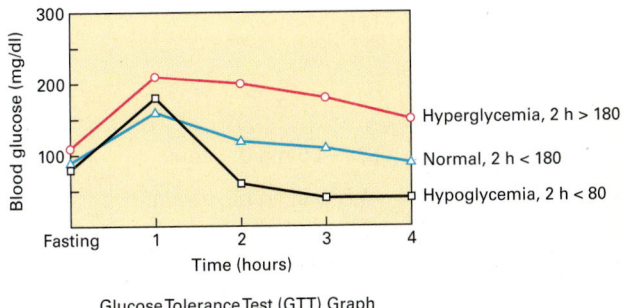

FIGURE 28-7 Glucose Tolerance Test (GTT) Graph DELMAR/CENGAGE LEARNING

Cations are ions that have a positive charge: sodium (Na^+), potassium (K^+), calcium (Ca^{++}), and magnesium (Mg^{++}). **Anions** are ions that have a negative charge: chloride (Cl^-) and phosphate (HPO_4^{--}).

The routine electrolyte laboratory tests are presented in Table 28-7. These tests measure the serum concentration of sodium, potassium, calcium, chloride, magnesium, and phosphate. See Chapter 33 for a detailed discussion of the intracellular and extracellular functions of electrolytes.

Blood Enzymes

Enzymes are globular proteins produced in the body that catalyze chemical reactions within the cells by promoting the oxidative reactions and synthesis of various chemicals, such as lipids, glycogen, and adenosine triphosphate (ATP). Enzyme tests play a key role in diagnosing the degree of tissue damage mainly to the myocardium and, to a lesser degree, to the brain.

TABLE 28-7 Routine Serum Electrolytes

ELECTROLYTE	NORMAL RANGES	CLINICAL SIGNIFICANCE
Sodium	135–148 mEq/L, adult 138–144 mEq/L, children 133–144 mEq/L, newborns	• *Increased:* excessive intake of sodium without water; salt water drowning; high solute concentration (tube feeding, IV, hyperalimentation) without fluid correction; diarrhea; diabetes insipidus; primary aldosteronism; renal failure. • *Decreased:* excessive intake of water without sodium (oral, IV therapy, tap water enemas); heart failure; cirrhosis; nephrosis and massive diuretic therapy.
Potassium (serum)	3.5–5.0 mEq/L, adult 3.4–4.7 mEq/L, children 3.7–5.9 mEq/L, newborns	• *Increased:* high potassium intake (oral, IV therapy, rapid infusion of aged blood); renal disease; drugs (adrenal steroids, potassium-conserving diuretics, potassium penicillin, chemotherapeutic agents); Addison's disease; burns and other massive tissue trauma; metabolic and respiratory acidosis. • *Decreased:* drugs (diuretics, digitalis); metabolic alkalosis; primary aldosteronism; Cushing's disease; vomiting and gastric suction.
Calcium	Total 8.4–10.5 mg/dL Ionized 1.13–1.32 mmol/L	• *Increased:* hyperparathyroidism; bone catabolism (multiple myeloma, leukemia, bone tumors); immobility. • *Decreased:* renal failure; sprue; pancreatitis; Crohn's disease; hyperphosphatemia; drugs (aminoglycosides, antacids containing aluminum, caffeine, cisplatin, corticosteroids, loop diuretics, Mithracin, phosphate).
Chloride	96–109 mEq/L, adult 98–105 mEq/L, children 94–112 mEq/L, newborn	• *Increased:* hyperparathyroidism; drugs (ammonium chloride, ion exchange resin, phenylbutazone); metabolic acidosis; respiratory acidosis; dehydration. • *Decreased:* prolonged vomiting and gastric suction; diarrhea; diuretics (ethacrynic acid and furosemide).
Magnesium	1.3–2.0 mEq/L, adult 1.6–2.6 mEq/L, children 1.4–2.9 mEq/L, newborn	• *Increased:* chronic renal failure, drugs (magnesium sulfate, antacids, enemas containing magnesium, sedatives); acute adrenocortical insufficiency. • *Decreased:* chronic diarrhea and alcoholism; nontropical sprue; steatorrhea; hereditary malabsorption; starvation; bowel resection; diuretics (mannitol, urea, glucose); hypoparathyroidism.
Phosphate	2.7–4.5 mg/dL, adult 4.5–5.5 mg/dL, children 4.5–6.7 mg/dL, newborn	• *Increased:* renal insufficiency; intake, IV solutions and enemas; blood transfusion; muscle necrosis; hypoparathyroidism. • *Decreased:* alcohol withdrawal; hyperventilation; diabetic ketoacidosis; phosphate-binding antacids.

Fischbach, F., & Dunning, M. (2008). *A manual of laboratory and diagnostic tests* (8th ed.). Philadelphia: Lippincott, Williams & Wilkins.

Elevations in plasma levels of intracellular enzymes occur during myocardial necrosis (tissue death as the result of disease or injury). Enzymes are released into the bloodstream in proportion to the degree of cellular damage.

Enzymes are not used as single diagnostic values in determining a diagnosis but are viewed in relation to other diagnostic studies. The results from several diagnostic procedures will assist the practitioner in determining the cause of clinical symptoms.

Creatine phosphokinase (CPK) is an enzyme used to convert creatine to phosphocreatine and adenosine diphosphate (ADP) to ATP. ATP provides energy to the cells to carry on metabolism. CPK levels indicate the degree of normal tissue catabolism. Elevated values of CPK reflect the damage that has occurred in tissue with a high CPK content. For example, the myocardium has a high CPK content; when the client has a myocardial infarction (MI), CPK is elevated because the heart's tissue has been damaged, requiring ATP to repair the damaged myocardium.

CPK has three isoenzymes of differing molecular structure that are present in different tissue (see Table 28-8). The isoenzymes provide clinical data to the practitioner in diagnosing the site and extent of tissue injury.

Aspartate aminotransferase (AST) is one of two enzymes that catalyze the transfer of the nitrogenous portion of an amino acid to an acid residue. It is an intracellular enzyme found mainly in the liver, heart, skeletal muscles, kidney, pancreas, and RBCs. The normal range is:

- Adults and children: 4–36 International Units/L
- Newborns: 4 times as high as those of adults

Blood for AST is drawn to determine:

- A recent MI (together with the CPK and lactic dehydrogenase levels)
- Acute hepatic disease

- The client's progress and prognosis in cardiac and hepatic diseases

Certain drugs may increase the AST (see the accompanying display). Remember to note drugs on the laboratory requisition when a client is taking a drug that can influence the results of testing.

Lactate dehydrogenase (LDH), a cellular enzyme that contributes to carbohydrate metabolism, catalyzes the reversible conversion of muscle pyruvic acid into lactic acid. The diagnostic value of serum LDH is limited because it is present in almost all body tissue; however, through electrophoresis, five isoenzymes can be related to specific tissue (see Table 28-9).

The percentage of isoenzymes changes with tissue damage. For example, in an acute MI the LHD_1 becomes greater than LDH_2 12 to 48 hours postinfarction.

DRUGS THAT CAN ELEVATE ASPARTATE AMINOTRANSFERASE (AST)

- Antibiotics
- Contraceptives
- Cortisone
- Digitalis
- Flurazepam
- Guanethidine
- Indomethacin
- Isoniazid
- Mithramycin
- Narcotics
- Pyridoxine
- Rifampin
- Salicylate
- Theophylline
- Vitamin A

TABLE 28-8 CPK Isoenzymes

ISOENZYME	NORMAL RANGES	TISSUE SOURCE
CPK_1 (BB)	0%	Primarily in brain; indicative of cerebrovascular accident
CPK_2 (MB)	0%–4%	Exclusively in myocardium; indicative of myocardial infarction
CPK_3 (UU)	96%–100%	Found in skeleton and myocardium/skeletal muscle disorders

Fischbach, F., & Dunning, M. (2008). *A manual of laboratory and diagnostic tests* (8th ed.). Philadelphia: Lippincott, Williams & Wilkins.

TABLE 28-9 LDH Isoenzymes

ISOENZYME	RANGES OF % OF TOTAL LDH	TISSUE SOURCE
LDH_1	17–27	Primarily in heart, kidneys, RBCs
LDH_2	29–39	Primarily in heart, kidneys, RBCs
LDH_3	19–27	Primarily in lungs, to a lesser extent in pancreas, thyroid, adrenal glands, lymph nodes
LDH_4	8–16	Liver and skeletal tissue
LDH_5	6–16	Liver and skeletal tissue

Fischbach, F., & Dunning, M. (2008). *A manual of laboratory and diagnostic tests* (8th ed.). Philadelphia: Lippincott, Williams & Wilkins.

α-Hydroxybutyrate dehydrogenase (HBD) is the total LDH forced to act on α-ketobutyric acid rather than lactic or pyruvic acid. It is a serum measurement used when the assay of isoenzymes of LDH is not available in the laboratory. Once an MI has been diagnosed, the HBD has clinical significance by indicating the duration of tissue injury. HBD will remain elevated up to 2 weeks after infarction.

Alkaline phosphatase (a zinc-dependent enzyme) influences bone calcification and lipid and metabolite transport. The normal plasma range is 30 to 120 International Units/L. Alkaline phosphatase is used to detect:

- Osteoblastic activity
- Hepatic tumors or abscess
- Impaired zinc status
- The response of vitamin D in the treatment of deficiency-induced rickets

Certain drugs can cause a mild to moderate elevation in the alkaline phosphatase (see the accompanying display).

Acid phosphatase is an enzyme found primarily in the adult male prostate gland. It is used clinically to distinguish between encapsulated and metastatic carcinoma of the prostate gland. If the cancer cells are contained within a capsule, the acid phosphatase levels remain normal (0.2 to 0.8 International Units/L).

Glucose-6-phosphate dehydrogenase is an RBC enzyme. The normal range and the clinical significance are shown in Table 28-6.

The main proteolytic enzymes for digestion are contained in the pancreatic juices (trypsin, chymotrypsin, and carboxypeptidase). The common laboratory tests for measuring the digestive enzymes are presented in Table 28-10. Client must fast 1 to 2 hours before having a serum amylase drawn. If the client has eaten and receives a narcotic at the same time, the serum results could be invalidated.

DRUGS THAT CAN ELEVATE ALKALINE PHOSPHATASE

- Allopurinol
- Antibiotics
- Ergosterol
- Estrogen
- Isoniazid
- Methyldopa
- Methyltestosterone
- Oral contraceptives
- Phenothiazine tranquilizers
- Procainamide
- Propranolol
- Sulfonamides
- Tolbutamide

Cholinesterase is an enzyme manufactured in the liver that is responsible for the breakdown of acetylcholine and other choline esters. The normal range for cholinesterase in adults and children is 8 to 18 International Units/L. It is elevated in diabetes, hyperthyroidism, and nephrotic syndrome. Decreases in cholinesterase can result from severe anemias and infections, exposure to some insecticides, liver disease, malnutrition, shock, and uremia.

Prostate-Specific Antigen

Prostate-specific antigen (PSA) is a glycoprotein found in the prostate tissue. PSA is used in combination with digital rectal examinations to detect prostate cancer; see Chapter 27 for a discussion regarding digital rectal examinations. The normal values are: men less than 40 years, <2.0 ng/mL (<2.0 mcg/L) and men 40 years and older, <2.8 ng/mL (<2.8 mcg/L). PSA may fluctuate over time, and therefore the test results should be confirmed several weeks after the initial testing before proceeding with further invasive testing such as prostate biopsy.

TABLE 28-10 Digestive Enzymes

ENZYMES	NORMAL RANGES	CLINICAL SIGNIFICANCE
Alanine aminotransferase	10–60 units/L	Hepatocellular damage
Aldolase	1.5–8.1 units/L	Anemia (hemolytic and megaloblastic); granulocytic leukemia; metastatic carcinoma; skeletal muscle tissue damage
Amylase	25–125 units/L	Pancreatitis
Aspartate aminotransferase	5–40 units/L	Hepatitis; infectious mononucleosis; cirrhosis
Lipase	10–140 units/L	Acute pancreatitis
5'-Nucleotidase	0–17 units/L	Biliary cirrhosis; extrahepatic obstruction; hepatic carcinoma; metastatic neoplasia of liver

Fischbach, F., & Dunning, M. (2008). *A manual of laboratory and diagnostic tests* (8th ed.). Philadelphia: Lippincott, Williams & Wilkins.

Blood Lipids

Coronary heart disease (CHD) is the number one killer of both men and women in the United States. According to the National Center for Health Statistics (1999), some 7 million Americans suffer from CHD and more than 500,000 Americans die of heart attacks caused by CHD each year. The National Cholesterol Education Program and the American Heart Association have published guidelines and recommendations regarding the need to improve laboratory detection of hypercholesterolemia and treatment. Total blood cholesterol is the most common measurement of blood cholesterol. Cholesterol is measured in milligrams per deciliter of blood (mg/dL). Blood cholesterol for adults is classified by levels.

Exogenous cholesterol is present in the diet and absorbed into the gastrointestinal tract. Endogenous cholesterol is formed in the liver and other cells in the body. As much as 80% of cholesterol is converted into cholic acid to form bile salts. Cholesterol is also needed:

- Throughout the body for the formation of membranes
- By the adrenal glands to form adrenocortical hormones
- By the ovaries to form progesterone and estrogen
- By the testes to form testosterone
- By the skin to provide a water-soluble barrier

Cholesterol and other fats cannot dissolve in the blood; they have to be transported to and from the cells by special carries called lipoproteins (blood lipids bound to protein). The types of lipoproteins are described in the following, but the ones to be most concerned about are low-density lipoprotein (LDL) and high-density lipoprotein (HDL).

- Chylomicrons—mainly ingested triglycerides
- Very low-density lipoproteins (VLDLs)—mainly endogenous triglycerides
- LDLs—moderate amounts of phospholipids with 50% cholesterol
- HDLs—50% protein

LDL is the major cholesterol carrier in the blood. When too much LDL circulates in the blood, it can slowly build up in the walls of the arteries feeding the heart and brain. The buildup of LDL and other substances causes the formation of atherosclerotic plaque, a thick, hard deposit that can clog the arteries in the heart and brain. A thrombus (a blood clot) can develop around the plaque that blocks the flow of blood to part of the heart muscle and causes an MI. If the thrombus blocks the flow of blood to part of the brain, it results in a cerebrovascular accident (CVA). High levels of LDL cholesterol (more than 130 mg/dL) increase the risk for CHD; this type of cholesterol is often called bad cholesterol.

HDL accounts for one-third to one-fourth of blood cholesterol and carries the cholesterol away from the arteries and back to the liver, where it is removed from the blood. HDL removes excess cholesterol from atherosclerotic plaques, slowing their growth. HDL is known as good cholesterol because a high level of HDL seems to decrease the risk of CHD.

Triglycerides are the chemical form in which most fat exists in food as well as in the body; they account for more than 90% of dietary intake and comprise 95% of fat stored in tissues. Triglycerides are insoluble in water and are the main plasma glycerol ester. An increase in triglyceride levels can be detected by plasma measurements; this test evaluates suspected atherosclerosis and measures the body's ability to metabolize fat.

Table 28-11 shows the relationship of lipids to a client being at risk for CHD. The practitioner must examine all of the lipid levels together. For instance, a client whose total cholesterol, LDL cholesterol, and triglycerides are all slightly elevated and whose HDL is slightly decreased is at a greater risk for CHD than someone whose cholesterol is elevated but whose HDL is also high.

The nurse must prepare clients for the lipid level testing by teaching them to:

- Eat a regular diet 3 to 7 days before the test
- Fast 12 to 14 hours before the test
- Refrain from vigorous exercise 24 hours before the test
- Refrain from caffeine and nicotine 24 hours before the test
- Per practitioner order, withhold drugs 24 hours before the test (many drugs affect the serum triglyceride level)
- Be aware that repeat tests may be necessary to confirm elevated levels because results can vary 15% or more from day to day

Diurnal variation causes triglycerides to be lowest in the morning and highest around noon (Fischbach & Dunning, 2008).

TABLE 28-11 Relationship of Lipids to Coronary Heart Disease Risk

LIPID	DESIRABLE LEVELS	BORDERLINE CHD RISK	HIGH CHD RISK
Cholesterol	<200 mg/dL	200–239 mg/dL	>240 mg/dL
LDL cholesterol	<130 mg/dL	130–159 mg/dL	>160 mg/dL
HDL cholesterol	>40 mg/dL	35–40 mg/dL	<35 mg/dL
Triglyceride	<250 mg/dL	250–500 mg/dL	>500 mg/dL

Fischbach, F., & Dunning, M. (2008). *A manual of laboratory and diagnostic tests* (8th ed.). Philadelphia: Lippincott, Williams & Wilkins.

Several factors can affect the test results. The client's position, such as lying down, causes a redistribution between vascular and extravascular compartments. For instance, after 5 minutes in a recumbent position, total plasma cholesterol may be significantly reduced (10%–15% decrease after 20 minutes). Recent trauma and severe infections may decrease the cholesterol level by 10% to 30%. Because pregnancy increases the HDL, LDL, and VLDL levels 20% to 30%, postpone testing 3 to 4 months postdelivery.

Therapeutic Drug Monitoring

Therapeutic drug monitoring is performed when a quantitative relationship exists between the drug concentration and drug response or toxicity is known. For a drug concentration to be significant:

- It must be determined in a blood sample drawn after the drug has been completely absorbed from the oral or intramuscular route.
- It has had an opportunity to be distributed to its site of action.
- Its steady state has been reached (e.g., four to five half-lives must have passed).

For instance, with digoxin (a cardiac medication, administered on a daily schedule) the absorption and distribution phases may take 6 to 12 hours to complete. For a meaningful interpretation, the blood specimen should be drawn at least midway through the elimination phase (6 hours before the next dose). If the specimen is drawn just before the next dose, one obtains a trough concentration, whereas a specimen drawn 6 to 12 hours after dosing yields a peak concentration. For digoxin, the swing between peak and trough would be expected to be minimal because the drug is given at intervals that are less than the drug's terminal half-life (42 ± 19 hours). Generally, such sampling is most significant after steady state has been reached (about 8 days for digoxin). Trough and peak sampling help the practitioner to determine the dose rate, keeping the drug level below toxic value.

Arterial Blood Gases

Blood gas results are reported in millimeters of mercury (Hg). Normal ABG ranges are:

- P_{O_2} 75–100 mm Hg
- P_{CO_2} 35–45 mm Hg
- pH 7.35–7.45

The clinical interpretation of gases studies the relationship between the gases. For example, a low P_{O_2} combined with a high P_{CO_2} may indicate bronchiole obstruction or that the alveoli are filled with fluid. In both situations, there is an impairment of gaseous exchange. See Chapter 32 for a complete discussion.

URINE ANALYSIS

Urine is an ultrafiltrate of plasma that contains many of the substances carried in the blood. Urine samples are easy to obtain and provide the practitioner with information to evaluate the client's health status.

Reagent dipsticks provide the nurse with a means of simple and quick testing for routine screening urinary evaluations of protein, glucose, ketones, hemoglobin, urobilinogen, nitrates, and pH. The sticks contain a reagent that changes colors in the presence of specific substances; the color change is observed and compared to a chart for the presence of abnormal levels of substances.

The components of the routine urinalysis are identified, and certain components are described; urine studies that measure electrolytes, enzymes, hormones, and other substances are not presented in this chapter. Urine is examined for cytology to detect cell changes caused by malignancies or inflammation. Toxicological analysis of urine is performed to detect drugs that have been used and abused.

Routine Urinalysis

The two major components of a routine urinalysis (UA) are macroscopic analysis and microscopic analysis. Macroscopic analysis includes color, appearance, odor, specific gravity, pH, protein, glucose, ketones, blood, bilirubin and urobilinogen, nitrite, and leukocyte esterase. Microscopic analysis includes RBCs, WBCs, epithelial cells, casts and crystals, and other substances such as bacteria, yeast, mucus, spermatozoa, and parasites. See the accompanying display for some of the normal urine values.

The best time to collect urine for a UA is in the morning after the first voiding; urine that has accumulated in the bladder overnight is concentrated and may lead to invalid results. The urine sample should be evaluated within 1 hour of collection or refrigerated until it can be examined; allowing the sample to be exposed to room temperature may alter the components (e.g., the glucose level may drop or bacteria may grow).

The pH is governed by the hydrogen ion concentration of the urine. Disorders such as diabetes mellitus, dehydration, diarrhea, emphysema, and starvation make the urine acidic. Chronic renal failure, renal tubular acidosis, urinary tract infections, and salicylate poisoning cause the urine to be alkaline.

Urine specific gravity (USG) measures the density and concentration of particles in the urine with the density of water, which is 1.000. USG measurement provides information regarding the client's hydration status and functional ability of the kidneys. Nurses measure USG as part of an assessment of fluid balance using one of three methods:

- The refractometer, which resembles a small telescope, is the most accurate method (Flasar, 2008). Place a drop of urine on a slide at the end of the scope, keeping the instrument level; hold the refractor up to a light. The beam of light deviates when it enters the solution, giving the refractive index; for example, if the light beam is at the 1.022 mark, this figure is recorded as the USG. The refractor also measures the protein content in the same drop of urine; protein in the urine can cause the USG to be falsely high.
- The multiple-test dipstick has a separate area with a reagent USG. As the indicator changes color, compare it with the chart that accompanies the dipstick for the numeric value of the USG.

- The urinometer or hydrometer is the oldest method of bedside monitoring of USG. Put a sample of 10 to 20 mL in the small cylinder, then float the bulb-shaped instrument in the urine; read the USG at the meniscus, using the calibrated scale as shown in Figure 28-8.

When questions arise regarding the accuracy of the USG, obtain a urine osmolality test. The osmolality test is more accurate because it measures the total number of particles in a solution.

When the blood levels of glucose exceed the renal threshold (180 mg/dL), glucose spills into the urine. Multiple agents are available for measuring the glucose content of urine. These agents are not as accurate a test method as blood glucose levels.

Some of the reducing agents can measure other products, such as protein and blood, along with the glucose (Clinitest and Clinistix). Each product has specific step-by-step instructions for performing the test and reading the results. Teach the client how to perform these urine tests.

Ketones are products of fatty acid metabolism and are completely metabolized by the liver under normal conditions. The most common cause of ketonuria is diabetes. However, with strenuous exercise, starvation, and sustained febrile and hypoxic conditions, an increase in fatty acid metabolism causes ketoacidosis, resulting in ketone bodies in the urine.

Normally the urine is free from blood cells and casts. When the renal system is impaired as in renal damage or failure, nephritis, and stones and infections in the urinary tract, the following can occur:

- Bleeding with resulting RBCs in the urine
- Accumulation of epithelial cells with cast formation
- WBCs, which indicate infections

STOOL ANALYSIS

Stool analysis is used to determine the various constituents of the stool for diagnostic purposes such as diseases of the gastrointestinal tract, the liver, and the pancreas. The normal constituents found in stool include epithelial cells shed from the gastrointestinal tract, small amounts of fats, bile pigments in the form of urobilin, gastrointestinal and pancreatic secretions, and electrolytes. The bacterial degradation of bile pigments to stercobilin causes the brown color of feces, and the characteristic odor is caused by bacterial action on proteins and other residues. The distal portion of the colon causes the shape and caliber of normal stools, and the normal consistency is described as "plastic." The nurse may observe alterations in color, odor, shape, or consistency; these changes may indicate the presence of disease.

Urobilinogen is derived from the normal bacterial action of intestinal flora on bilirubin. It is increased with severe hemolysis of RBCs and decreased with most biliary obstructions.

Occult Blood

Chemical screening for occult blood is the most commonly performed test of feces. When blood is invisible on inspection, it is said to be **occult**; it is blood that can be detected only through a microscope or by chemical means. In the gastrointestinal tract, the digestive process acts on blood, making it occult. Random sampling for occult blood is done to diagnose gastrointestinal bleeding, ulcers, and malignant tumors. Colorectal cancer is a leading cause of cancer deaths in the United States. Most colorectal cancers begin as a **polyp**, a small abnormal growth of tissue, in the wall of the colon. As the polyp grows, it may cause bleeding from the rectum, blood in the stool, or a change in the shape of the stool. Screening for colorectal cancer begins with fecal occult blood testing. The American Cancer Society (ACS, 2008) recommends that people over 50 who are at average risk have a fecal occult blood test every year.

See Chapter 27 for the complete set of guidelines for colorectal screening as developed by the ACS. (See Table 28-14 later

NORMAL URINE VALUES

- pH   4.6–8.0   Adults and children
                   5.0–7.0   Newborns
- Color   Amber-yellow
- Specific gravity   1.010–1.020
- Protein:
  Qualitative   None
  Quantitative   10–100 mg/24 h
- Glucose   None
- Ketones   None
- Blood   0–2 RBCs

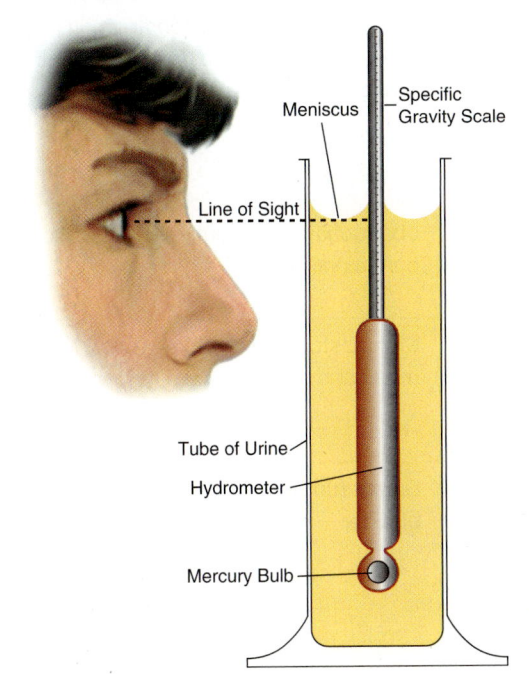

Meniscus · Specific Gravity Scale · Line of Sight · Tube of Urine · Hydrometer · Mercury Bulb

FIGURE 28-8 Urinometer DELMAR/CENGAGE LEARNING

TABLE 28-12 Common Contrast-Mediated Studies

STUDY	VISUALIZATION/TECHNIQUE	INDICATIONS
Barium swallow (esophagography)	Esophageal; swallowing a barium solution, using fluoroscopic and cineradiographic techniques	Dysphagia, heartburn, or regurgitation of food, esophageal reflux, stricture, polyps, and other diseases
Upper gastrointestinal series (UGI)	Lower esophagus, stomach, duodenum, and upper jejunum; ingestion of a solution of barium sulfate using x-ray and fluoroscopic techniques	Pain, heartburn, diarrhea, weight loss, anorexia, nausea or vomiting of unknown etiology, strictures and varices in lower esophagus, ulcer, inflammation of stomach or small bowel, tumor, obstructions
Barium enema (BE) or lower gastrointestinal series (LGI)	Colon; x-ray and fluoroscopic techniques after rectal instillation of both air and barium (double-contrast study)	Rectal bleeding, weight loss, anemia of unknown etiology, small lesions and polyps, suspected abnormality in bowel motility or obstruction, diverticula, megacolon, or other structural changes
Oral cholecystography (OCG)*	Gallbladder; 12 to 14 hours after oral ingestion of dye, usually iopanoic acid the evening before	Pain of unknown etiology, suspected gallstones, tumor, or a fistula between the biliary system and GI tract
Intravenous cholangiography (IVC)*	Hepatic and common bile ducts for stones and stricture; IV contrast medium iodipamide with plain and tomographic films taken 15 minutes after the injection and periodically for up to 8 hours	Gallbladder not visualized on an OCG, if the client is unable to absorb the oral dye for an OCG, or if the symptoms persist after cholecystectomy
T-tube cholangiogram*	Common bile ducts and gallbladder; during surgery after placement of the tube in the duct or 7 to 10 days after gallbladder surgery, injection of an iodinated contrast medium into the T-tube with x-ray and fluoroscopic techniques	Patency of the common bile duct before T-tube removal, detection of stones, duct fistula, or biliary tract strictures and neoplasms
Percutaneous transhepatic cholangiogram (PTHC)*	Intrahepatic, extrahepatic, and biliary ducts, and gallbladder; an iodinated contrast medium is injected into the liver and, with the aid of fluoroscopy, into the bile duct	Jaundice to determine obstruction to biliary flow caused by stones, tumor, stricture, or anatomic abnormalities
Antegrade pyelography	Kidneys' collecting system; injection of an iodinated contrast medium into the renal pelvis with the aid of fluoroscopy or ultrasound and a pressure reading within the kidney, measured by a manometer	Kidneys are unable to excrete dye given for intravenous pyelography, if ureteral obstruction is present, or if a cystoscopy is contraindicated
Retrograde urethrography	Male urethral membranous, bulbar, and penile areas or female urethra; instillation of an iodinated contrast medium into a catheter with films and fluoroscopy techniques	Men postoperatively to evaluate urethral repair and to detect urethral abnormalities
Retrograde cystography*	Urinary bladder; air or an iodinated contrast medium is instilled into a bladder catheter, the catheter is clamped, and films are taken while the catheter is clamped (if films are taken during emptying of the bladder, the test is called a voiding cystourethrogram)	Detect rupture and pathology of the urinary bladder

(Continues)

TABLE 28-12 (Continued)

STUDY	VISUALIZATION/TECHNIQUE	INDICATIONS
Retrograde ureteropyelography* (retrograde pyelogram)	Ureters and renal collecting system; diatrizoate sodium is injected via ureteral catheters inserted by cystoscopy, x-rays are taken with the catheters in place and during and after their removal	Detect presence and location of a ureter or kidney stone, abnormalities or pathology of the renal system, when the client is allergic to iodinated contrast medium
Intravenous pyelogram (IVP)* (excretory urogram [EUG])	Calyces and pelves of the kidneys, ureters, and urinary bladder (KUB); an abdominal x-ray is taken (KUB), followed by an injection of an iodinated contrast medium and serial x-rays	Abnormalities of the kidneys, ureter, or bladder
Sialography	Salivary ducts: sublingual, submaxillary, submandibular, and parotid; injection of an iodinated contrast medium into the duct with films taken with the client placed in various positions	Persistent pain and edema in the salivary glands, detect inflammation of the gland or stones, tumors, or strictures that obstruct the salivary ducts
Arthrography	Joint and soft tissues: meniscus, cartilage, ligaments, and structures of the joint capsule; rotator cuff, subacromial bursa; joint site anesthetized and injected with a contrast medium and various x-ray views of the joint site	Unexplained joint pain, traumatic ligament disorders (tears and lacerations), dislocations, and to detect abnormalities of the synovial membrane or shoulder, evaluate injury following onset of arthritis, or perform minor surgical procedures on a joint
Bronchography	Tracheobronchial tree; injection of an iodinated oil contrast medium via a catheter inserted into the trachea and bronchi with x-rays taken with the client placed in various positions	Detect obstructions caused by tumors, cyst, or foreign object; determine cause of persistent hemoptysis and recurring pneumonia
Hysterosalpingography	Uterine cavity and fallopian tube; injection of a water-soluble or oil-based iodinated contrast medium via a cannula inserted into the cervix, the flow of the medium is viewed fluoroscopically and x-rays are taken	Abnormalities of the female reproductive system such as tubal patency, obstructions, adhesions; to detect cause of repeated spontaneous abortions; and to evaluate tubal ligation or tubal reanastomosis
Myelogram	Spinal subarachnoid space or the spinal canal; injection of a contrast medium into the spinal canal via lumbar puncture under fluoroscopy to view the flow of the medium toward the head as the table is tilted and x-rays are taken	Determine abnormalities and cause of persistent, chronic pain, and to detect lesions of the spinal cord (meningeal tumors, cysts, or ruptured intervertebral disks)

Note: *Test should be performed before any study using barium as the contrast medium.
Delmar/Cengage Learning

in this chapter for the diagnostic procedures: colonoscopy and proctosigmoidoscopy.)

When the practitioner is using occult blood to confirm suspicions of a gastrointestinal disorder, the client is placed on a 3-day diet free of meat, poultry, and fish to decrease the possibility of a false-positive result. Common drugs that can cause a positive test for occult blood are salicylate, steroids, and indomethacin.

Parasites

The gastrointestinal tract can harbor parasites and their eggs (ova). Some of these parasites are harmless, whereas others cause clinical symptoms. With the exception of pinworms (which can enter the body through both the oral and anal routes), all other common parasites gain portal entry through the mouth by ingesting contaminated water or food. Roundworm, hookworm, whipworm, tapeworm, *Trichinella spiralis*, and *Entamoeba histolytica* are common parasites found in the United States.

CULTURE AND SENSITIVITY TESTS

Culture refers to the growing of microorganisms to identify the pathogen. Any secreted or excreted body fluid, drainage, or tissue sample can be cultured for microorganism identification: blood, eye and ear, nose and throat, skin, nails, hair, genital and rectal areas, sputum, bronchial washings, feces, urine, tissue biopsy, cerebrospinal tissue, semen, gastrointestinal fluid, and other body fluids. In combination with the culture, microorganisms are tested for sensitivity to specific antibiotics. Culture and sensitivity (C&S) tests are performed to identify both the nature of the invading organisms and their susceptibility to commonly used antibiotics. Sensitivity allows the practitioner to select the appropriate antibiotic therapy.

The nurse is usually responsible for collecting specimens for C&S testing; refer to Table 28-1. Standard precautions are used to collect the specimen from the site at a time when the microorganisms are present in large numbers, before the initiation of antibiotic therapy. The specimens are collected in sterile, disposable containers that take into consideration the microorganism's special needs for survival, such as anaerobic environment or special media requirements such as liquid (broth), solid (agar), or cell culture lines. Label the specimens with all pertinent information such as the client's history and status (e.g., temperature), site, time, and test ordered; take the specimen to the laboratory immediately to avoid overgrowth or death of the microorganisms.

PAPANICOLAOU TEST

Papanicolaou test (smear method of examining stained exfoliative cells), commonly called a Pap smear, is done to evaluate the cell maturity, metabolic activity, and morphologic variations of the cervical tissue. Papanicolaou testing can also be used for tissue specimens from other organs, such as bronchial aspirations and gastric secretions.

The ACS recommends the revised clinical guidelines of the American College of Obstetricians and Gynecologists for the frequency of Pap tests other cervical screening and still recommends an annual gynecology exam that includes an annual pelvic examination for women age 21 and older. ACOG guidelines are evidence based and incorporate new tests for detecting cervical changes as well as improved understanding of the pathology and evolution of cancer. The ACS (2008) recommends:

- First screen: First Pap test approximately 3 years after first intercourse or at age 21, whichever occurs first
- Up to age 30: annual cervical cytology because women under 30 are at higher risk for acquiring human papillomavirus (HPV) that may cause precancerous changes
- Women age 30 and older: Two options are available:
  1. Cervical cytology testing alone: If a woman age 30 or older has negative results on three consecutive annual cervical cytology tests, then she may be rescreened with cervical cytology alone every 2 to 3 years.

2. Women who test negative on a cervical cytology test and an FDA-approved test for HPV should be rescreened with both tests every 3 years; women who test negative on only one of the tests should be screened more frequently.

Exceptions are women who are infected with HIV, are immunosuppressed, were exposed to diethylstilbestrol (DES) in utero, or were previously diagnosed with cervical cancer; such women may require more frequent cervical screening. Women who have had a hysterectomy but have a history of abnormal cell growth should be screened yearly until they have three consecutive negative vaginal cytology tests, after which time routine screening may be discontinued.

Screening may be discontinued in women who have had a hysterectomy with removal of the cervix for benign reasons and with no history of abnormal or cancerous cell growth. The ACS calls for cessation of testing in the not-high-risk groups at age 70 and the U.S. Prevention Services Task Force by age 65.

To increase the accuracy of a cervical specimen, the client should be told to avoid intercourse, douches, and vaginal creams for 24 hours before the test. The vaginal speculum should not be lubricated. This test should not be performed if the client is menstruating because the specimen will be unsuitable for cytologic study.

RADIOLOGIC STUDIES

Radiography (the study of x-rays or gamma ray–exposed film through the action of ionizing radiation) is used by the prescribing practitioner to study internal organ structure. Radiographic procedures can be either noninvasive or invasive, and client preparation varies accordingly. Although noninvasive procedures such as plain-film x-rays, tomography, and barium sulfate as a contrast medium do not require a signed consent form, the clients should be told what to expect. The exception is mammography, which uses xeroradiography; these clients are required to sign consent forms. Invasive radiographic procedures such as IV cholangiography, antegrade pyelography, and bronchography use an iodinated dye that is administered intravenously or directly into an organ or tissue to be examined; these studies require the client to sign a consent form and are performed under sterile conditions using Standard Precautions.

Tomography is an imaging technique in which a selected body plane is isolated from the tissues on either side. It is particularly useful in visualizing air-filled structures such as the lungs, paranasal sinuses, and kidneys. Fluoroscopy is an imaging technique that allows the viewer to observe movement on a fluorescent viewing screen in the area being filmed while the study is in progress. It is valuable in evaluating movement of the diaphragm, heart, and digestive system; it is also used in catheter placement during angiography, needle insertion for biopsy or removal of fluid from a body cavity, and nasogastric tube insertion for precise placement in the stomach or small bowel. Cineradiography is a rapid-sequence filming technique similar to that used in motion pictures; it creates a photographic record of the motion under study, such as swallowing.

Xeroradiography is an x-ray imaging technique that uses a photoelectric process rather than the photochemical process of conventional x-rays; the images are printed on paper like that of a typical office copier. While distinct images are produced with excellent contrast, this process reduces the amount of radiation exposure to the client. It is most useful in studying soft tissues for small-point abnormalities and is used primarily for x-rays of the breasts.

CONTRAST-MEDIATED STUDIES

Contrast-mediated studies use a **contrast medium** to enhance the viewing of soft tissue details. The contrast medium may be administered orally, rectally, by IV, intrathecally, or by insufflation; when injected to visualize blood vessels and lymphatics, the studies are called angiography. Barium sulfate and the organic iodides are the most commonly used contrast media. These radiopaque substances block the passage of the x-rays, resulting in the images on film; see Table 28-12 for the most common contrast-mediated studies. Barium solutions should not be used if perforation of the bowel is suspected. Barium studies should be sequenced as follows: barium enema before the upper gastrointestinal series (UGI) and the UGI before the barium swallow, if the UGI series and barium swallow are performed as separate studies. Iodine injections may cause the client to experience temporary symptoms of shortness of breath, nausea, and a warm or hot, flushed sensation.

PLAIN FILMS

Plain films are radiologic (x-ray and roentgenogram) studies that use external beams to evaluate bones and soft tissues of the body. X-rays are produced by applying an electron beam to a vacuum tube containing tungsten; the resulting rays have a shorter wavelength than that of visible light rays and are able to penetrate many substances that are opaque to visible light.

Chest X-Ray

The most common radiologic study is the noninvasive, noncontrasted chest x-ray. The best results are obtained when the films are taken in the radiology department; however, a portable chest x-ray can be performed at the bedside.

Radiographic projection positions of chest x-ray films are taken from various views (see Figure 28-9). Multiple views of the chest are necessary for the practitioner to assess the entire lung field. To prepare the client for a chest x-ray, remove metal objects (jewelry) and all clothing from the waist up and replace with a gown. Metal will appear on the x-ray film, thereby obscuring visualization of parts of the chest. Pregnant women are draped with a metal apron to protect the fetus.

Chest films can indicate the following alterations and diseases:

- Lesions (tumors, cysts, masses) in the lung tissue, chest wall, bony thorax, or heart
- Inflammation of lung tissue (pneumonia, atelectasis, abscesses, tuberculosis); pleura (pleuritis); and pericardium (pericarditis)
- Fluid accumulation in the lung tissue (pulmonary edema, hemothorax); pleura (pleural effusion); and pericardium (pericardial effusion)
- Bone deformities and fractures of the rib and sternum
- Air accumulation in the lungs (chronic obstructive pulmonary disease, emphysema) and pleura (pneumothorax)
- Diaphragmatic hernia

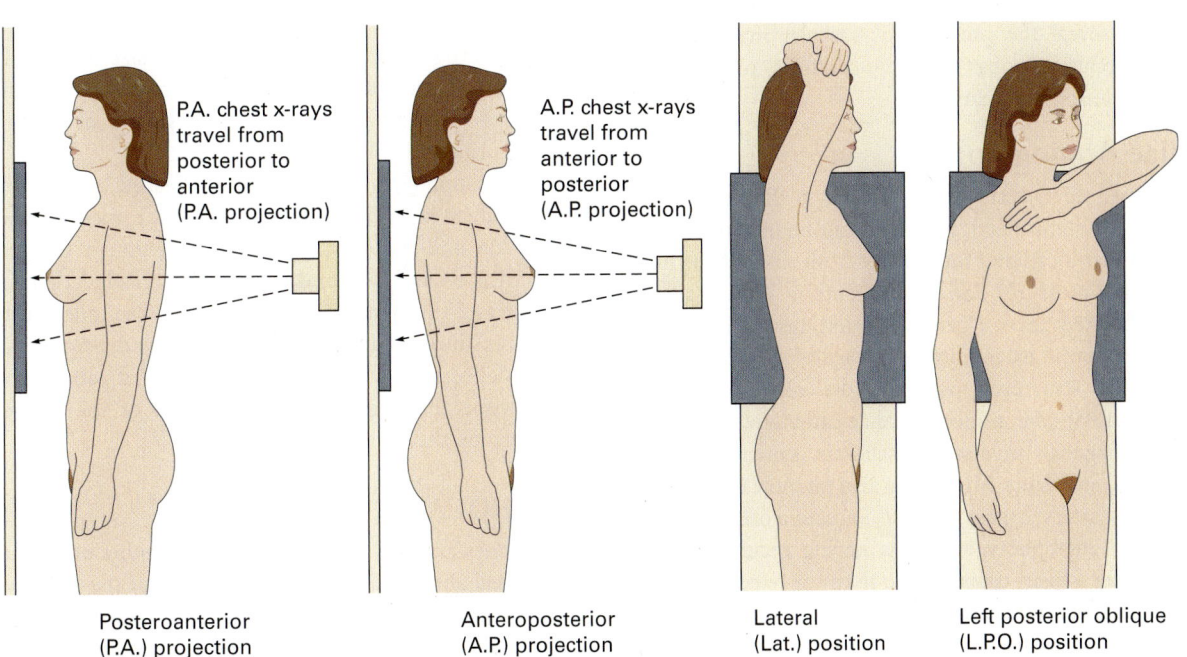

Posteroanterior (P.A.) projection — P.A. chest x-rays travel from posterior to anterior (P.A. projection)

Anteroposterior (A.P.) projection — A.P. chest x-rays travel from anterior to posterior (A.P. projection)

Lateral (Lat.) position

Left posterior oblique (L.P.O.) position

FIGURE 28-9 **Radiographic Projection Positions** DELMAR/CENGAGE LEARNING

RISKS OF EXPOSURE TO RADIATION

All radiation studies carry risks of exposure to radiation. Certain cells are at greater risk for adverse effects (e.g., gonadal and somatic cells). Children should be exposed to x-rays only when absolutely necessary for diagnostic purposes. Women who are pregnant should not be x-rayed because the cells of the developing embryo are sensitive to radiation. The adverse effects of radiation therapy include genetic mutations, cancer, and congenital anomalies.

MAMMOGRAPHY

Mammography (a low-dose radiographic study of breast tissue) is used to reveal congenital abnormalities and lesions. The ACS (2008) recommends that women age 40 and older at average risk should have an annual screening mammogram and clinical breast examination (CBE) by a health professional. Women at increased risk should talk with their health professional regarding individualized approaches to screening; see Chapter 27 for a discussion of breast cancer screening.

ANGIOGRAPHY STUDIES

Angiography allows visualization of the vascular structures through the use of fluoroscopy with a contrast medium. Films are taken in rapid sequence after the injection of an iodinated contrast medium into the vessel or vascular system to be examined. Angiograms are serial radiographs of blood vessels that are used to evaluate the size, shape, and patency of the veins (venograms); arteries (arteriograms) of organs and tissues; or lymph vessels and nodes (lymphograms). Angiography is also useful in diagnosing an aneurysm (weakness in the wall of a blood vessel).

Digital subtraction angiography is a computerized imaging of the vasculature with visualization on a monitor screen after the IV injection of iodine through a catheter. The results reveal the presence of vascular malformations (stenosis, occlusion, obstruction, ulceration, plaques, and aneurysms), lesions, and emboli.

Cardiac Angiography

Cardiac catheterization reveals defects in the heart chambers, valves, and coronary arteries. Using fluoroscopy, a cardiologist inserts a catheter into one or both sides of the heart and measures pressures and cardiac output; blood samples may be obtained for oxygen saturation testing. With the injection of a contrast medium the cardiologist can further define cardiac structures, including the coronary arteries, and assess cardiac wall motion. Cardiac catheterization is performed to diagnosis myocardial ischemia, syncope, valvular heart disease, and acute MI; it may also be indicated after an MI, coronary artery bypass surgery, percutaneous transluminal coronary angioplasty in clients having recurring symptoms, and after a heart transplant to monitor rejection.

Prepare the client as described in Table 28-1. The femoral and brachial arteries are common catheter insertion sites; the radial artery is also an option. Mark pulses on the arm or leg that will be used to assist with pulse assessment postprocedure. The procedure lasts 30 minutes to 1 hour, but the entire test, including pre- and postcatheterization care, may take up to 4 hours.

Postcatheterization the nurse should:

- Place the client on telemetry.
- Apply manual pressure (for 30 minutes or longer) when the catheter sheath is removed, and then apply a pressure dressing.
- Keep the client on bed rest with the involved extremity straight and immobile.
- Monitor and record vital signs to include the presence, quality, and character of peripheral pulses and the color, temperature, and tactile sensation of the involved extremity.
- Encourage oral fluids and record intake and output.
- Instruct the client to report any warm, tickling sensations at the puncture site that would indicate bleeding.
- Monitor for procedural complications: bleeding or hematoma formation at the site; allergic reactions; and cardiovascular, pulmonary, and neurologic changes.

Other Angiographic Procedures

See Table 28-13, on page 631, for a description of other angiographic procedures that are named for the type of vessel and the method or route of the injection.

ULTRASONOGRAPHY

Ultrasound (echogram) is a noninvasive study that uses high-frequency sound waves to visualize deep body structures. This test should be scheduled before any studies using a contrast medium or air to ensure accuracy because an ultrasound *does not* require any contrast medium. The client is instructed to lie still during the procedure.

Ultrasound is used to evaluate the brain, thyroid gland, heart, vascular structure, abdominal aorta, spleen, liver, gallbladder, pancreas, and pelvis. An ultrasound is commonly done during pregnancy to evaluate the size of the fetus and placenta; a full bladder is needed to ensure visualization. Instruct the mother to drink 6 to 8 glasses of water and to avoid urination before testing.

A coupling agent (lubricant) is placed on the surface of the body area to be studied to increase the contact between the skin and the transducer, an instrument that converts electrical energy to sound waves. The transducer emits waves that travel through the body tissue and are reflected back to the transducer and recorded. The varying density of body tissues deflects the waves into a differentiated pattern on an oscilloscope. Photographs can be taken of the sound wave pattern on the oscilloscope.

ECHOCARDIOGRAMS

An echocardiogram is an ultrasonographic procedure used to reveal abnormal structure or motion of the heart wall and thrombi. This test is also used after radiofrequency ablation (the delivery of low-voltage, high-frequency alternating electrical current to cauterize the abnormal myocardial tissue) to identify the potential complications of pericardial effusion.

TABLE 28-13 Angiographic Procedures

ANGIOGRAM	DESCRIPTION	MAJOR INDICATIONS
Cerebral	Cerebral vessels, the carotid and vertebral arteries	Detection of vessel displacement caused by tumors, abscess, edema, hematoma, narrowing or occlusion of vessels, aneurysm, increased intracranial pressure
Adrenal	Adrenal gland arteries or veins	Arteriogram: detect tumors or hyperplasia. Venogram: secure blood samples for testing cortisol, catecholamines, and hormone levels
Pulmonary	Pulmonary vessels	Arterial and venous abnormalities and pulmonary embolism
Hepatic and portal	Hepatic artery and portal vein	Hepatic: malignant tumor. Portal: hepatocellular carcinoma from hepatitis and cirrhosis
Renal	Large and small arteries of the renal vasculature and parenchyma or of the veins and their branches	Detect tumors and other abnormalities and prospective renal donors
Mesenteric	Gastrointestinal vasculature	Abnormalities of the aorta, stomach, pancreas, and small and large intestines to identify acute bleeding source and perform perfusion or embolization to control hemorrhage
Fluorescein	Retinal vasculature and circulation	Eye abnormalities caused by changes in the retinal vascularity
Lymphangiography	Lymphatic flow and nodal patterns	Detect pathologic nodes identified by enlargement or filling defects and the presence of obstructed lymphatic flow patterns
Upper extremity	Hand or arm	Detect obstruction, ischemia vasospasms, lesions, or trauma
Lower extremity	Leg or foot	Filling defects, vasospasms, lesions, stenosis, and occlusion associated with aortic, arterial, or venous disease

Delmar/Cengage Learning

DOPPLER ULTRASONOGRAPHY

Doppler, a handheld transducer, transmits high-frequency sound waves to the artery or vein being studied. The sound waves strike the moving RBCs and are reflected back to the transducer, which amplifies the sound and produces a graphic recording. Doppler ultrasonography reveals blood clots and peripheral vascular disease.

NONNUCLEAR SCAN STUDIES

Nonnuclear scan studies are noninvasive and use a special machine and scanning system as opposed to radiopharmaceuticals. Computed tomography and magnetic resonance imaging use computer-generated images on a screen for viewing and recording. A signed informed consent form is required for MRI procedures and CT studies if a contrast medium is used.

COMPUTED TOMOGRAPHY

Computed tomography (CT; computed axial tomography or computed transaxial tomography) uses x-ray combined with a special scanning machine, detectors that determine the amount of radiographic beams absorbed by tissues, and a computer that processes these readings and reconstructs a body region by calculating the differences in tissue absorption of the radiographic beams. CT scanning produces a series of three-dimensional, cross-sectional anatomic views of the tissue structure of solid organs and the difference between soft tissue and water. Figure 28-10, on page 632, demonstrates the direction of sagittal, transverse, and coronal planes taken during CT scanning. Figure 28-11, on page 633, shows the direction of CT scan waves. Contrast media may be used to further clarify or enhance findings such as to determine tissue density, differentiate a specific organ from other structures, or identify small tumors. It is primarily used in diagnosing tumors and inflammatory disorders.

UNCOVERING THE
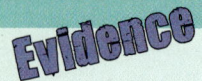

TITLE OF STUDY
"Predictors of Time from Hospital Arrival to Initial Brain-Imaging among Suspected Stroke Patients. The North Carolina Collaborative Stroke Registry."

AUTHORS
K. Rose, W. Rosamond, S. Huston, C. Murphy, and C. Tegeler

PURPOSE
To examine the client demographics, hospital characteristics, and clinical predictors of delay time from hospital arrival until CT among 20,374 clients enrolled in the North Carolina Collaborative Stroke Registry (January 2005 to April 2008).

METHODS
Delay time was log-transformed in linear regression analyses and dichotomized (<25 minutes, >25 minutes) in logistic regression analyses to correspond to the 1999 National Institute of Neurological Disorders and Stroke (NINDS) guidelines.

FINDINGS
In multiple linear regression analyses, prehospital delay time, mode of transport, race, gender, presumptive diagnosis, time of day, weekday versus weekend arrival, and hospital type were significantly associated with CT delay. Among clients arriving within 2 hours of symptom onset, the strongest independent predicators of meeting the NINDS guidelines were arrival by emergency medical services versus other modes of transportation and a presumptive diagnosis of transient ischemic attack versus unspecified stroke type.

IMPLICATIONS
Although most clients do not arrive at the hospital in a timely manner and cannot be considered for time-dependent therapies, among those who do, disparities exist in the time to receipt of CT scan, suggesting room for improvement in hospital-level stroke systems of care.

Rose, K., Rosamond, W., Huston, S., Murphy, C., & Tegeler, C. (2008). Predictors of time from hospital arrival to initial brain-imaging among suspected stroke patients. The North Carolina Collaborative Stroke Registry. *Stroke*, 39(12), 3262–3267. Retrieved August 26, 2008, from http://stroke.ahajournals.org/cgi/content.

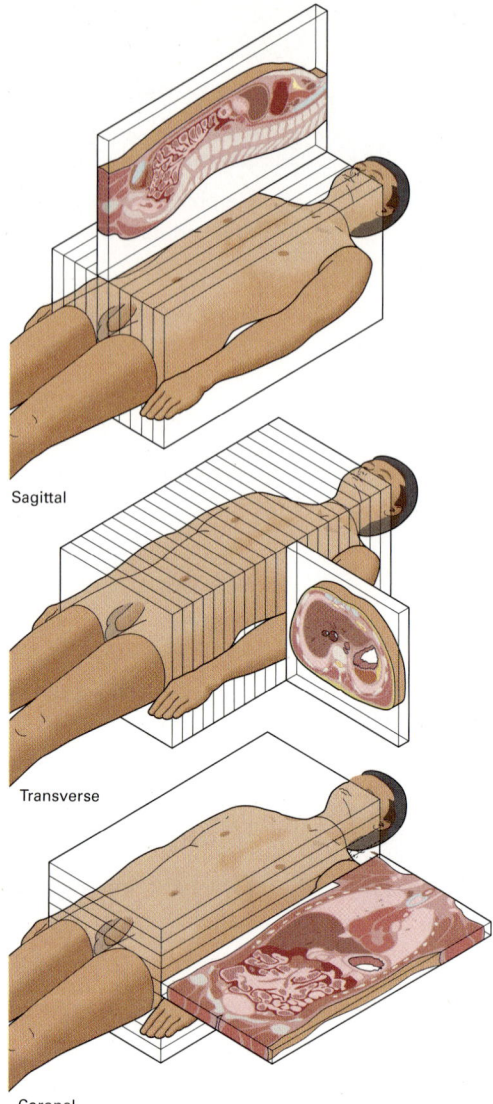

Sagittal

Transverse

Coronal

FIGURE 28-10 Computed Tomography DELMAR/CENGAGE LEARNING

client is instructed to wear earphones to decrease the discomfort from the machine's clanging sound. A noniodine IV paramagnetic contrast agent may be used during the study. The study reveals lesions and changes in the body's organs, tissues, vascular, and skeletal structures.

RADIOACTIVE STUDIES

Radionuclide imaging (nuclear scanning) uses radionuclides (or radiopharmaceuticals) to image the morphologic and functional changes in the body's structure. A scintigraphic scanner is placed over the area of study to detect the radiation emission and to produce a visual image of the structure on film. Radiopharmaceutical agents are administered by various routes with consideration given to time delays of absorption. The results reveal congenital abnormalities,

MAGNETIC RESONANCE IMAGING

Magnetic resonance imaging (MRI) is an imaging technique that uses radio waves and a strong magnetic field to make continuous cross-sectional images of the body. The

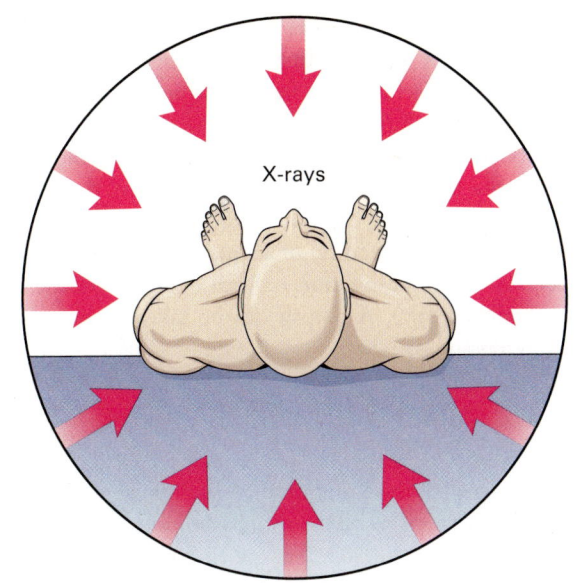

FIGURE 28-11 Direction of Computed Tomography Scan Rays DELMAR/CENGAGE LEARNING

lesions, skeletal changes, infections, and gland and organ enlargement.

ELECTRODIAGNOSTIC STUDIES

These diagnostic tests use devices to measure the electrical activity of the heart, brain, and skeletal muscles. Electrical sensors (electrodes) are placed at certain anatomic points to measure the tone, velocity, and direction of the impulses. The impulses are then transmitted to an oscilloscope or printed on graphic paper.

ELECTROCARDIOGRAPHY

An electrocardiogram (ECG or EKG) is a graphic recording of the heart's electrical activity. The client may be asked not to smoke or drink caffeinated beverages 24 hours before the test. Nicotine and caffeine can affect the heart rate.

Electrodes are applied to the chest wall and extremities. A lubricating gel applied to the electrodes increases the conduction of electrical activity between the skin and electrode. The client is instructed to lie still during the pain-free test. The test can reveal abnormal transmission of impulses and electrical position of the heart's axis.

A portable cardiac monitor (Holter monitor) is a device that records the heart's electrical activity. It produces a continuous recording over a specified period of time (e.g., 24 hours). The portable unit allows the client to ambulate and perform regular activities. Clients are instructed to maintain a log of activities that occur when they feel their heart beating faster or irregularly. The practitioner reviews the ECG tracing in relation to the client's log to determine if certain activities, such as walking, are associated with abnormal transmission of impulses.

Signal-Averaged Electrocardiography

Signal-averaged electrocardiography (SAECG) is a surface ECG that amplifies late potentials, the electrical activity that occurs after normal depolarization of the ventricles. The test requires a specialized ECG machine and small computer to detect the late potentials. It is performed on clients who have had an MI. The test reveals the client's risk for ventricular tachycardia.

Stress Test

A stress test measures the client's cardiovascular response to exercise tolerance. It demonstrates the ability of the myocardium to respond to increased oxygen requirements (the result of exercise) by increasing the blood flow to the coronary arteries.

The client walks on a treadmill while connected to an ECG machine, and the heart rate and blood pressure are monitored. The speed and grade of the treadmill are increased every 3 minutes until the client tires or achieves the target heart rate, or until clinical signs develop (e.g., angina or an arrhythmia). The test is suited for clients who can exercise and who are not taking cardiac medications such as beta blockers that prevent the heart rate from increasing (King, 2004).

RADIONUCLIDE STUDIES. Radionuclide studies, thallium-201 scintigraphy, and technetium-99m sestamibi use isotopes to highlight differences in coronary perfusion at rest and with stress (King, 2004). Thallium, a radionuclide that is the physiological analogue of potassium, is normally absorbed into normal myocardial tissue from the circulating blood. During the test, thallium is administered intravenously to detect damaged myocardial tissue (necrotic or ischemic). Because thallium is not absorbed by the damaged tissue, the degree of heart damage can be estimated.

There are two types of thallium tests: resting imaging or stress imaging. Resting imaging is performed a few hours after MI. The thallium is injected and an ECG tracing is performed. Stress imaging (thallium stress test) is performed while the client is on the treadmill with ECG monitoring. At peak stress the IV thallium is injected; scanning is done 3 to 5 minutes postinjection. The test is stopped immediately if the client becomes symptomatic for ischemia.

ELECTROENCEPHALOGRAPHY

An electroencephalogram (EEG) is the graphic recording of the brain's electrical activity. The procedure is painless and takes about an hour. The test is performed in a quiet, nonstimulating environment. It can reveal the presence and type of seizure disorder and intracranial lesion. The absence of brain's electrical activity is used to confirm death.

During the procedure, electrodes are placed on the client's scalp. The electrodes transmit the impulses from the brain to an EEG machine. The machine amplifies the brain's impulses and makes a recording of the waves on strips of paper.

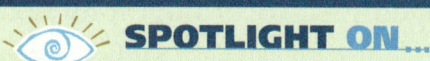

SPOTLIGHT ON...

Participating in Diagnostic Testing

A client comes to an outpatient clinic for a laparoscopy to retrieve an egg for in vitro fertilization. You are to assist the practitioner with this procedure. How would you handle this situation if your own religious beliefs were in conflict with the procedure being performed? Would it make any difference if the client had had an abortion as a teenager?

ENDOSCOPY

Endoscopy is the visualization of a body organ or cavity through a scope. The procedure is performed with an endoscope (a metal or fiberoptic tube) being inserted directly into the body structure to be studied (see Figure 28-12). A light at the end of the scope allows the practitioner to assess for lesions and structural problems. The endoscope has an opening at the distant tip that allows the practitioner to administer an anesthetic agent, lavage, and suction as well as biopsy tissue. Common endoscopic procedures are presented in Table 28-14 on page 635.

General client preparation and positioning depend on the structure being studied, as discussed in Table 28-14. As with all invasive procedures, the client needs to sign a consent form and the nurse needs to establish baseline vital signs before administering sedative agents.

Postprocedure the nurse monitors the vital signs, observes for bleeding, and assesses for procedural risks (e.g., return of the gag and swallowing reflexes following an esophagogastroduodenoscopy with local anesthesia).

ASPIRATION AND BIOPSY

Aspiration is performed to withdraw fluid that has abnormally collected or to obtain a specimen. Aseptic technique and Standard Precautions are used during aspiration. Aspiration diagnostic studies are invasive; implement the protocols for diagnostic tests. A local anesthetic is administered in the area being studied to decrease the client's discomfort when the skin is pierced by the needle.

A stylet needle with an outer, hollow-bore needle is used to pierce the skin. Once the needle is in place, the stylet is withdrawn, leaving only the outer needle to aspirate the fluid. A tissue **biopsy**, the excision of a small amount of tissue, can be obtained during aspiration or with other diagnostic tests (e.g., bronchoscopy). A biopsy can be taken from most of the body's tissue.

AMNIOCENTESIS

Amniocentesis is the withdrawal of amniotic fluid to obtain a sample for specimen examination. The amniotic fluid increases during pregnancy from 50 mL at the end of the first trimester to an average of 1000 mL near term. This test is indicated when:

- Maternal age exceeds 35.
- A spontaneous abortion occurred with a previous pregnancy.
- There is a family history of genetic, chromosomal, or neural tube defects.

The amniocentesis is performed when the amniotic fluid volume reaches 150 mL, usually after the 16th week of pregnancy.

There are no restrictions on fluids or food. The procedure usually lasts 10 to 15 minutes. Instruct the mother to void to prevent the risk of puncturing a full bladder. Position the client supine and assesses the fetal heart tones.

The abdomen is prepped and injected with lidocaine hydrochloride, a local anesthetic agent. The practitioner withdraws 10 to 20 mL amniotic fluid by transabdominal needle aspiration. Postprocedure the nurse monitors the client's vital signs and fetal heart tones and assesses for signs of labor. Instruct the client to notify the practitioner of any signs of labor or infection.

BONE MARROW ASPIRATION AND BIOPSY

The sternum and iliac crest are the common sites for bone marrow puncture. During a bone marrow puncture, a fluid specimen (aspiration) or a core of marrow cells (biopsy) can be obtained. Both tests are commonly done concurrently to obtain the best marrow specimen. The test can reveal anemias or cancer, such as leukemia, multiple myeloma, or Hodgkin's disease, or the client's response to chemotherapy.

There are no restrictions on fluids or food before the puncture. The nurse should explain the procedure to elicit the client's support during the procedure. The client must lie perfectly still throughout the procedure. The client is usually fearful; allay the client's fear with relaxation methods or sedation. Infants and small children are restrained by holding them throughout the procedure.

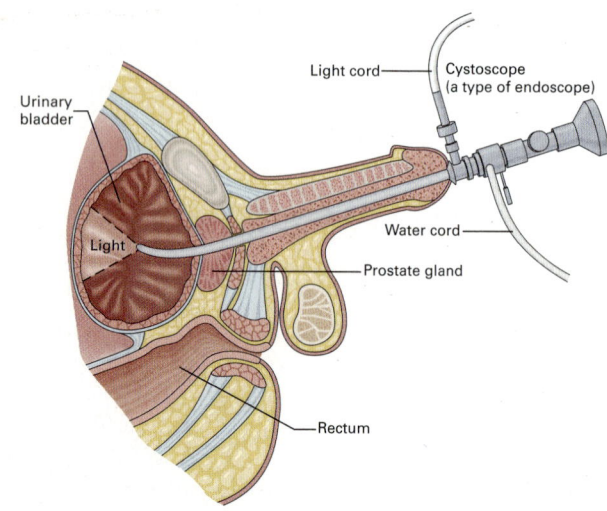

FIGURE 28-12 Cystoscope DELMAR/CENGAGE LEARNING

TABLE 28-14 Endoscopic Procedures

PROCEDURE AND AREA STUDIED	PREPARATION/POSITION	CLINICAL SIGNIFICANCE
Arthroscopy—examines joint structures, primarily the knee	Instruct client to fast after midnight; test is usually performed under local anesthesia, may be done under spinal or general anesthesia if surgery is necessary. Position the joint for accessibility.	Diagnose torn meniscus, patellar, condylar, and synovial disorders; perform surgery. Also used to monitor the progression of a disease or effectiveness of therapy.
Bronchoscopy—examines the bronchus and bronchial tree	Instruct client to fast 6–12 hours before the test; test is usually done under local anesthesia. Position client supine or sitting upright.	Identify the origin of bleeding, lesions, or obstruction; collect a specimen for bacteriologic and cytologic examination (diagnose abnormal cells); remove foreign bodies, lesions, mucus plugs, or excessive secretions.
Colonoscopy—examines the large intestine	Instruct client to maintain a clear liquid diet for 48 hours before the test and to take the prescribed laxative the evening before the examination; place client on left side with knees flexed and drape.	Identify origin of bleeding or lesions; evaluate inflammatory and ulcerative bowel disease and recurrence of polyps or malignant lesions.
Colposcopy—examines the cervix and vagina following a positive Pap smear	No restriction on food or liquids. Place client in lithotomy position.	Evaluate abnormal cytology or grossly suspicious lesions and perform a biopsy or take photographs of suspicious lesions.
Cystoscope (see cystourethroscopy)		
Cystourethroscopy—uses two instruments: a cystoscope to examine the bladder and ureter openings, and a urethroscope to examine the bladder neck and the urethra	Food and fluids are restricted only if the client is to receive general anesthesia; regional anesthesia is usually given. Place client in a lithotomy position.	Identify bladder lesions and urethral strictures, ulcers, inflammation, and an enlarged prostate gland.
Esophagogastroduodenoscopy (EGD)—examines the esophagus, stomach, and upper duodenum	Instruct client to fast 6–12 hours before the test. An intravenous tranquilizer may be given, then a local anesthetic is sprayed into the back of the throat to decrease the gag reflex (swallowing will seem difficult). Place client in a sitting position.	Identify diverticula, varices, Mallory-Weiss syndrome, esophageal rings and hiatal hernia, and esophageal and gastric stenoses. When combined with histologic and cytologic tests, may indicate acute or chronic ulcers, benign or malignant tumors, and inflammatory disease.
Laparoscopy—examines the peritoneal cavity: pelvis and abdomen	Instruct client to fast 8 hours before the surgery; the test is performed either with a local or general anesthetic agent. Place the client in a lithotomy position; catheterize the client to ensure the bladder is empty (avoids puncture of the bladder during the test with the laparoscope).	Used to detect cysts, adhesions, fibroids, and infections of the uterus, fallopian tubes, and ovaries; ectopic pregnancies; and liver lacerations and cirrhosis. May also be used for lysis of adhesions, ovarian biopsy, tubal sterilization, foreign body removal, and fulguration of endometriotic implants.

(Continues)

TABLE 28-14 (Continued)

PROCEDURE AND AREA STUDIED	PREPARATION/POSITION	CLINICAL SIGNIFICANCE
Proctosigmoidoscopy—three steps: 1. Digital examination to dilate the anal sphincters to detect obstruction that might hinder passage of the endoscope. 2. A sigmoidoscope to examine the distal sigmoid colon and rectum. 3. A proctoscope to examine the lower rectum and anal canal.	Instruct client according to prescribing practitioner orders relative to dietary restrictions and bowel preparation (these are usually based on prescribing practitioner preference). If the client has rectal inflammation, a local anesthetic agent is applied to decrease discomfort. Secure the client to a tilting table that rotates into horizontal and vertical positions.	Identify internal hemorrhoids, hypertrophic anal papillae, polyps, fissures, fistulae, and rectal and anal abscesses.

Delmar/Cengage Learning

Client positioning is determined by the site to be used, supine (sternum) or side-lying (iliac crest). The site is prepped for puncture to decrease the skin's normal flora. Explain to the client that pressure may be experienced as the specimen is withdrawn. The client should not move when the specimen is being withdrawn; a sudden movement may dislodge the needle.

Postprocedure the client should be on bed rest for an hour. The nurse monitors vital signs to assess for bleeding (rapid pulse rate, low blood pressure). Instruct the client to report to the practitioner any bleeding or signs of inflammation.

PARACENTESIS

Paracentesis is the aspiration of fluid from the abdominal cavity. This test can either be diagnostic, therapeutic, or both. For instance, with end-stage liver or renal disease there is **ascites**, an accumulation of fluid in the abdomen. Pressure caused from the ascites can interfere with breathing and gastrointestinal functioning. Aspiration in this instance is therapeutic. If a culture specimen is taken, it is also diagnostic.

Have the client void and obtain a body weight before the procedure. Place the client in a high Fowler's position in a chair or sitting on the side of the bed. The skin is prepped, anesthetized, and punctured with a **trocar**, a large-bore abdominal paracentesis needle. The trocar is held perpendicular to the abdominal wall and advanced into the peritoneal cavity. When fluid appears, the trocar is removed, leaving the inner catheter in place to drain the fluid. Observe the client for pressure changes that can result from the rapid removal of fluid.

Postprocedure apply a sterile dressing to the puncture site. Monitor the client for changes in vital signs and electrolytes. Instruct the client to record the color, amount, and consistency of drainage on the dressing after discharge.

THORACENTESIS

Thoracentesis is the aspiration of fluids from the pleural cavity. The pleural cavity normally contains a small amount of fluid to lubricate the lining between the lungs and pleura. Infection, inflammation, and trauma may cause an increased production of fluid, which can impair ventilation.

Position the client with arms crossed and resting on a bedside table to allow access to the rib cage (see Figure 28-13). Instruct the client not to cough during insertion of

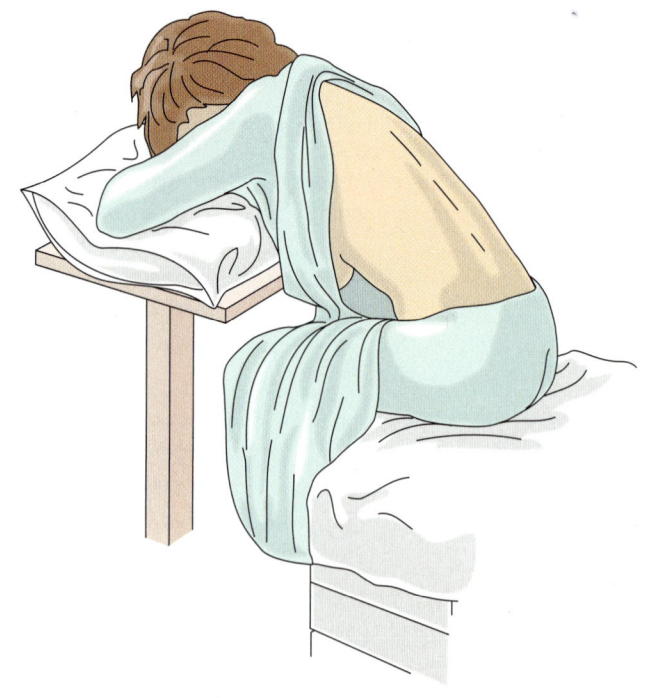

FIGURE 28-13 Client Position for Thoracentesis DELMAR/CENGAGE LEARNING

the needle. The practitioner selects, preps, and anesthetizes the puncture site. The needle is usually inserted into the intercostal space at the location of maximum dullness to percussion. Posteriorly, the site should be above the ninth rib, and laterally, above the seventh rib.

During the procedure, monitor the client for symptoms of a **pneumothorax** (collection of air or gas in the pleural space causing the lungs to collapse), such as dyspnea, pallor, tachycardia, vertigo, and chest pain. Postprocedure observe for cardiopulmonary changes and a mediastinum shift as assessed by vital signs and bloody sputum.

CEREBROSPINAL FLUID ASPIRATION

Lumbar puncture ("spinal tap") is the aspiration of cerebrospinal fluid (CSF) from the subarachnoid space. The specimen is examined for organisms, blood, and tumor cells. A spinal tap is also performed:

- To obtain a pressure measurement when blockage is suspected
- During a myelogram, as discussed earlier
- To instill medications (anesthesia, antibiotics, or chemotherapy)

A spinal tap is contraindicated in clients with increased intracranial pressure, hemorrhagic diathesis, and an infection at the proposed puncture site.

Place the client in a lateral recumbent position with the craniospinal axis parallel to the floor and flat of the back perpendicular to the procedure table. Have the client assume a flexed knee-chest position to bow the back. This position separates the vertebrae. Most clients will require assistance in maintaining this position throughout the procedure. To assist, the nurse stands facing the client with one hand across the client's posterior shoulder blades and the other hand over the buttocks.

The practitioner selects, preps, and anesthetizes the puncture site (usually interspace L_3-L_4, L_4-L_5, or L_5-S_1). The needle and stylet are inserted into the midsagittal space and advanced through the longitudinal subarachnoid space (see Figure 28-14).

Once in the subarachnoid space, the stylet is removed, leaving the needle in place. An initial CSF pressure reading is taken:

- A three-way stopcock with a manometer (calibrated column) is securely connected to the spinal needle.
- The stopcock is opened toward the manometer to allow the CSF to rise in the column. Under normal conditions, the CSF will fluctuate in the column with respirations.
- When the CSF stabilizes, a pressure reading is taken.

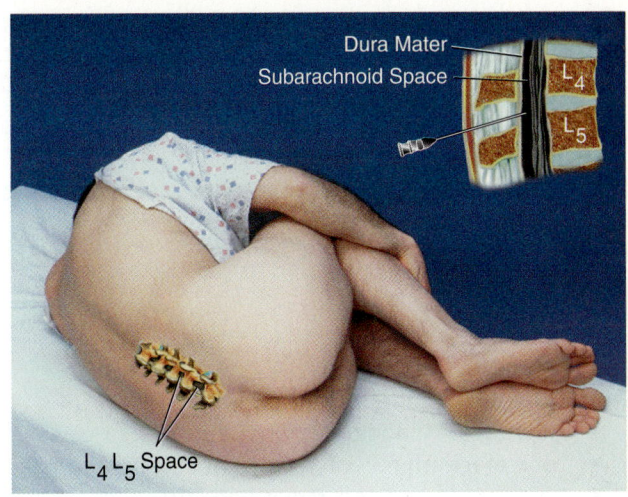

Dura Mater
Subarachnoid Space
L_4
L_5

L_4 L_5 Space

FIGURE 28-14 Lumbar puncture: position of client and insertion of the needle into the subarachnoid space. DELMAR/CENGAGE LEARNING

If the pressure reading is greater than 200 mm H_2O or falls quickly, only 1 or 2 mL CSF is obtained for analysis. If the pressure is less than 200 mm H_2O, an adequate specimen sampling is withdrawn slowly.

After the pressure reading is taken, the stopcock is turned to allow the CSF to slowly flow into a sterile test tube. A sterile cap is placed on the test tube, and the sample is transported to the laboratory for analysis. Rapid withdrawal of CSF can cause a transient postural headache. Throughout the procedure, monitor the client's cardiorespiratory status.

Postprocedure, pressure is applied and then a sterile bandage. Assess the bandage for leakage of CSF and the client's neurologic and cardiorespiratory status. A postural headache is the most common complication of a lumbar puncture; using a small-bore spinal needle minimizes the chances of a headache.

▼ SAFETY FIRST ▼

TAKING THE PRESSURE READING
The client should be relaxed and quiet during the initial pressure reading; straining increases the CSF.

PROCEDURE 28-1

Performing Venipuncture

EQUIPMENT
- Disposable gloves
- Alcohol swabs
- Rubber tourniquet
- Sterile 2 × 2 gauze pads
- Band-Aid or adhesive tape (precut)
- Appropriate blood collection tubes
- Labels for each collection tube with the appropriate client information included
- Completed laboratory requisition forms
- Needle/equipment disposal container
- Small pillow or folded towel to support the extremity if needed
- Syringe method: sterile needles: 20 to 21 gauge for adults, 23- to 25-gauge butterfly for older adults, 23- to 25-gauge butterfly for children
- Vacutainer method: Vacutainer tube with needle holder; sterile double needles (20 to 21 gauge for adults, 23 to 25 gauge for children)

ACTION	RATIONALE
1. Greet client by name and validate client's iden-tification.	1. Proper client identification ensures safety for the client and the nurse.
2. Explain the procedure to the client.	2. Client rights dictate that any action be explained to the client. The client always has the right to refuse a procedure. Information decreases anxiety.
3. Wash hands/hand hygiene.	3. Reduces transmission of microorganisms.
4. Bring equipment to bedside or client exam room. Transfer client to the procedure room, especially for small children, as it is important to keep their hospital room a "safe haven."	4. Provides an organized approach to the procedure.
5. Close curtain or door.	5. Provides privacy.
6. Raise or lower bed and table to comfortable working height.	6. Maintains good body mechanics for the nurse during the procedure.
7. Position client's arm; extend arm to form a straight line from shoulder to wrist. Place pil-low or towel under upper arm to enhance extension. Client should be in a supine or semi-Fowler's position.	7. Helps stabilize the arm. The bed should sup-port the client's body (when possible) in case client should feel faint during the procedure.
8. Apply disposable gloves.	8. Reduces the risk of infection to both the client and the nurse (Standard Precautions).
9. Apply the tourniquet 3 to 4 inches above the venipuncture site. Most often the antecubital fossa site is used. The tourniquet should be able to be removed by pulling the end with a single motion.	9. Tourniquet provides improved visibility of the veins as they dilate in response to decreased venous return of blood flow from the extrem-ity to the heart.
10. Check for the distal pulse. If there is no pulse felt, then the tourniquet is applied too tightly and must be reapplied more loosely.	10. If the pressure is too tight, it may impede arte-rial flow to the extremity.
11. Have client open and close fist several times, leaving fist clenched prior to venipuncture.	11. Increases the venous distension and enhances visibility of the vein. Vigorous motion, however, may result in hemoconcentration of the specimen.

(Continues)

PROCEDURE 28-1
Performing Venipuncture (Continued)

ACTION	RATIONALE
12. Maintain tourniquet for only 1 to 2 minutes.	12. Prolonged time may increase client discomfort and alter some laboratory results (i.e., falsely elevated serum potassium).
13. Identify the best venipuncture site through palpation; the ideal site is a straight prominent vein that feels firm and slightly rebounds when palpated. Palpate potential site.	13. Straight, intact veins are easier to puncture. A thrombosed vein is rigid, or rolls easily, and is difficult to stick.
14. Select the vein for venipuncture. (If the tourniquet has been on too long, release it and let the client rest for 1 to 2 minutes before reapplying the tourniquet.)	14. Allowing the client to rest increases client comfort and ensures accurate laboratory results.
15. Prepare to obtain the blood sample. Technique varies depending on equipment used: • Syringe method: Have syringe with appropriate needle attached. • Vacutainer method: Attach double-ended needle to Vacutainer tube and have the proper blood specimen tube resting inside the Vacutainer. Do not puncture the rubber stopper yet.	15. • A needle with a very small bore can damage the red cells as the blood is drawn and lead to inaccurate test results. • The long end of the needle is used to puncture the vein, and the short end enters the blood tube.
16. Cleanse the venipuncture site with alcohol swab or chlorhexidine alcohol using a circular method at the site and extending the motion 2 inches beyond the site (see Figure 28-15). Allow the alcohol to dry.	16. The alcohol solution and mechanical cleaning motion cleans the skin surface of bacteria that may cause infection at the site. Allowing the alcohol to dry reduces the stinging sensation that the client may experience.

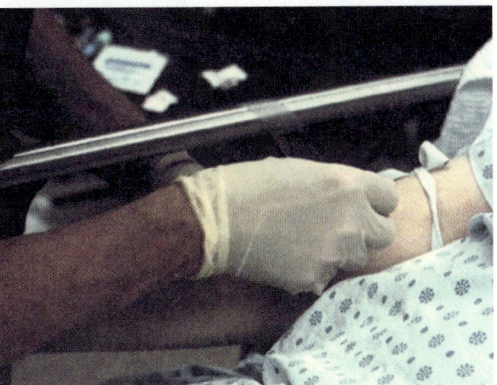

FIGURE 28-15 After applying the tourniquet, cleanse the skin at the venipuncture site. Do not let the tourniquet stay on longer than 2 minutes. If you need more time, remove the tourniquet for a couple of minutes to allow the client to rest and begin again. DELMAR/CENGAGE LEARNING

ACTION	RATIONALE
17. Remove the needle cover and warn that client will feel the needle stick for a few seconds.	17. Clients will be better able to control their reaction if they know what to expect.
18. Place the thumb or forefinger of the nondominant hand 1 inch below the site and pull the skin taut.	18. Helps stabilize the vein during insertion.
19. Hold syringe needle or Vacutainer at a 15° to 30° angle from the skin with the bevel up.	19. This angle reduces the chance of penetrating through the vein during insertion. The needle causes less trauma to the skin and vein when the bevel is up during insertion.

(Continues)

PROCEDURE 28-1
Performing Venipuncture (Continued)

ACTION	RATIONALE
20. Slowly insert needle/Vacutainer (see Figure 28-16).	20. Prevents puncture through the other side of the vein.
21. Technique varies depending on equipment used: • Syringe method: Gently pull back on syringe plunger and look for blood return. Obtain desired amount of blood into the syringe. • Vacutainer method: Hold Vacutainer securely and advance specimen tube into needle of holder. Be careful not to advance the needle into the vein. The blood should flow into the collection tube. After the collection tube is full, grasp the Vacutainer firmly, remove the tube, and insert additional specimen collection tubes as indicated (see Figures 28-16 and 28-17).	21. • If blood does not appear, the needle is not in the vein. • Pushing the needle through the stopper breaks the vacuum and causes the flow of blood into the collection tube. Failure of blood to appear in the collection tube indicates the vacuum in the tube has been lost or the needle is not in the vein.

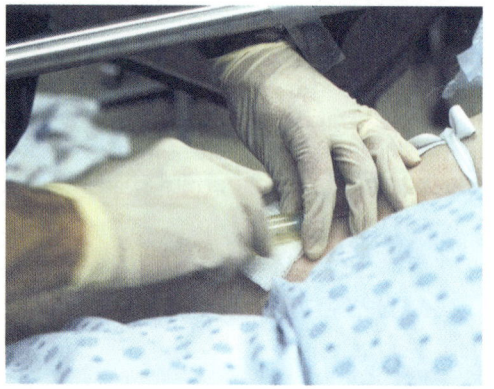

FIGURE 28-16 Hold the Vacutainer and needle assembly securely and press the specimen tube into the holder. The needle inside the holder will pierce the specimen tube and blood should begin to flow into the tube. DELMAR/CENGAGE LEARNING

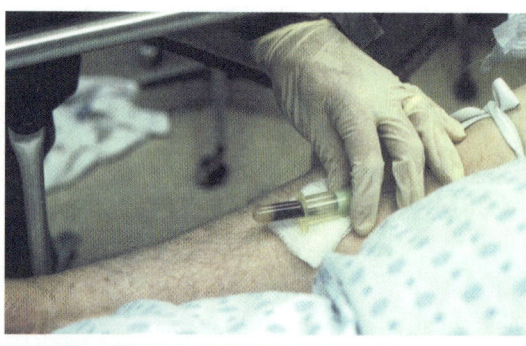

FIGURE 28-17 Allow the tube to fill with blood. When it is full, remove the tube and insert additional tubes as needed. DELMAR/CENGAGE LEARNING

22. After the specimen collection is completed, release the tourniquet.	22. Reduces bleeding from pressure when the needle is removed.
23. Apply 2 × 2 gauze over the puncture site without applying pressure and quickly withdraw the needle from the vein.	23. Positions the gauze for removal and helps to gently prevent the skin from pulling with the needle removal.
24. Immediately apply pressure over the venipuncture site with the gauze for 2 to 3 minutes or until the bleeding has stopped. Tape the gauze dressing over the site (or apply the Band-Aid).	24. Direct pressure stops the bleeding and minimizes formation of a hematoma. You may avoid using tape or a Band-Aid if after applying pressure no bleeding is present. Many clients are sensitive to tape, and its removal can be painful.

(Continues)

PROCEDURE 28-1
Performing Venipuncture (Continued)

ACTION	RATIONALE
25. Syringe method: Using one hand, insert the syringe needle into the appropriate collection tube and allow vacuum to fill. • You may also remove the stopper from each Vacutainer collection tube, remove the needle from the syringe, fill the tube, and replace the stopper.	25. Using a one-handed method to fill the syringe helps reduce the chance of needlestick injury. • This alternative method allows you to control the speed and amount of fill in the collection tubes.
26. If any of the blood tubes contain additives, gently rotate back and forth 8 to 10 times.	26. Ensures that the additive is properly mixed throughout the specimen.
27. Inspect the client's puncture site for bleeding. Reapply clean gauze and tape if necessary.	27. Keeps site clean and dry.
28. Assist client into a comfortable position. Return bed to low position with side rails up if appropriate.	28. Provides comfort and safety for the client.
29. Check tubes for any external blood and decontaminate with alcohol as appropriate.	29. Prevents contamination to other equipment and personnel.
30. Check tubes for proper labeling. Place tubes into appropriate bags and containers for transport to the laboratory.	30. Ensures the specimens are properly identified.
31. Dispose of needles, syringe, and soiled equipment into proper container.	31. Prevents spread of disease and needlestick injury.
32. Remove and dispose of gloves.	32. Reduces transmission of microorganisms.
33. Wash hands/hand hygiene.	33. Reduces transmission of microorganisms.
34. Send specimens to the laboratory.	34. Facilitates timely handling of specimens and accurate results.

delegation tip

The procedure of performing a venipuncture for the purposes of blood drawing is frequently delegated to properly trained ancillary personnel. Documentation of their competency and skill should be available to the nurse, and periodic reevaluation should occur according to agency and state policy. The ancillary personnel should be reminded to not obtain blood specimens from an extremity above the site of infusing fluids and to report to the nurse any complications or concerns the client might express postprocedure.

nursing tips

Clients with a depressed white blood cell count are susceptible to infection. Whenever you have to puncture the skin of a client with a depressed white blood cell count, cleanse the puncture site for 2 to 3 minutes.

PROCEDURE 28-2
Performing a Skin Puncture

EQUIPMENT
- Antiseptic 70% isopropanol or povidone-iodine
- Microhematocrit tubes or micropipette (collection tubes)
- Sterile 2 × 2 gauze
- Sterile lancet
- Nonsterile gloves
- Hand towel or absorbent pad

(Continues)

PROCEDURE 28-2
Performing a Skin Puncture (Continued)

ACTION	RATIONALE
1. Wash hands/hand hygiene.	1. Reduces transmission of microorganisms.
2. Check the client's identification band if appropriate.	2. Ensures the correct client.
3. Explain the procedure to the client.	3. Allays anxiety and encourages cooperation.
4. Prepare supplies: • Open sterile packages. • Label specimen collection tubes. • Place in easy reach.	4. Ensures efficiency.
5. Apply gloves.	5. Decreases the health care provider's exposure to bloodborne organisms.
6. Select site: lateral aspect of the fingertips in adults and children; heel for neonates and infants.	6. Avoids damage to nerve endings and calloused areas of the skin.
7. Place the hand or heel in a dependent position; apply warm compresses if fingers or heel are cool to touch.	7. Increases the blood supply to the puncture site.
8. Place hand towel or absorbent pad under the extremity.	8. Prevents soiling the bed linen.
9. Cleanse puncture site with an antiseptic and allow to dry. Use 70% isopropanol if the client is allergic to iodine (see Figure 28-18).	9. Reduces skin surface bacteria; povidone-iodine must dry to be effective.
10. With nondominant hand, apply gentle milking pressure above or around the puncture site. Do not touch the puncture site.	10. Increases blood to puncture site and maintains asepsis.
11. Read directions carefully before using the lancet. • With the sterile lancet at a 90° angle to the skin, use a quick stab to puncture the skin (about 2 mm deep) (see Figure 28-19). • With the automatic Unistik, push the lancet into the body of Unistik until it clicks. Hold the body of the Unistik and twist off the lancet cap. Place the end of the Unistik tightly against the client's finger and press the lever. The needle automatically retracts after use.	11. Provides a blood sample with minimal discomfort to the client.

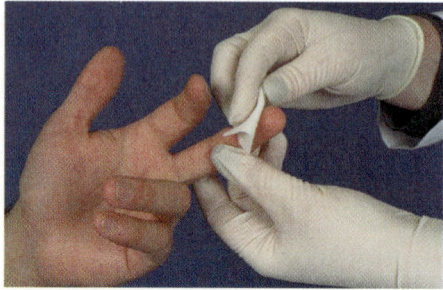

FIGURE 28-18 Cleanse the puncture site and allow it to dry. DELMAR/CENGAGE LEARNING

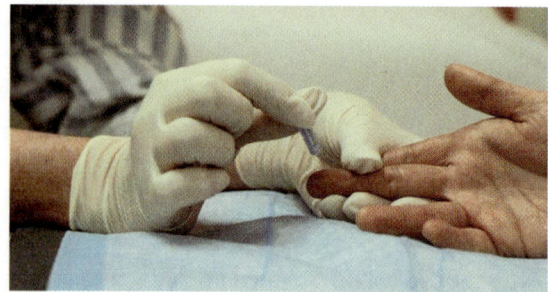

FIGURE 28-19 Use a quick stab to puncture the skin. DELMAR/CENGAGE LEARNING

(Continues)

PROCEDURE 28-2
Performing a Skin Puncture (Continued)

ACTION	RATIONALE
12. Wipe off the first drop of blood with sterile 2 × 2 gauze; allow the blood to flow freely (see Figure 28-20).	12. The first drop may contain a large amount of serous fluid, which could affect the results. Pressure at the puncture site can cause hemolysis.
13. Collect the blood into the tube(s). If blood for a platelet count is to be collected, obtain this specimen first (see Figure 28-21).	13. Allows blood collection; avoids aggregation of platelets at the puncture site.
14. Apply pressure to the puncture site with a sterile 2 × 2 gauze (see Figure 28-22).	14. Controls bleeding.
15. Place contaminated articles into a sharps container.	15. Reduces the risk of needlestick.
16. Remove gloves; wash hands.	16. Reduces transmission of microorganisms.
17. Position client for comfort with call light in reach.	17. Provides for comfort and communication.
18. Wash hands/hand hygiene.	18. Reduces transmission of microorganisms.

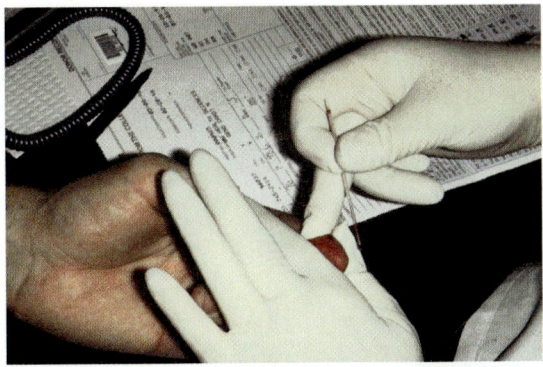

FIGURE 28-20 Allow the blood to flow from the puncture site to ensure an adequate amount can be obtained. DELMAR/CENGAGE LEARNING

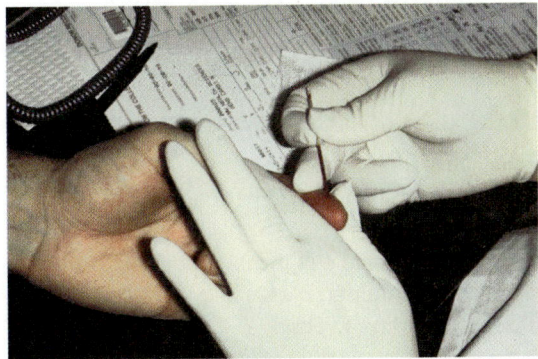

FIGURE 28-21 Collect a small sample of blood. DELMAR/CENGAGE LEARNING

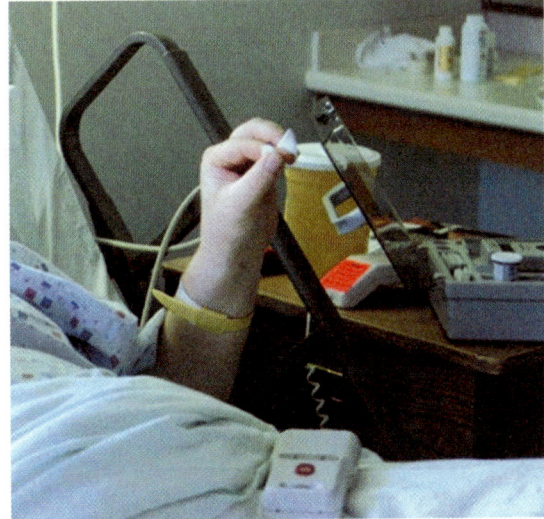

FIGURE 28-22 Apply pressure to the puncture site to stop further bleeding. DELMAR/CENGAGE LEARNING

(Continues)

PROCEDURE 28-2
Performing a Skin Puncture (Continued)

delegation tip

Properly trained ancillary personnel may perform skin puncture. Agency policy usually dictates certification and recertification requirements for this skill. Proper client and specimen identification are of the utmost importance and must be consistently demonstrated by the ancillary personnel.

nursing tips

- *Visualize urine before tests to look for contamination.*
- *Read instructions before dipping stick or test tape in urine.*
- *Have at least 20 cc of urine for urinometer.*
- *Verify that the urine is second-voided specimen and explain this need to the client.*

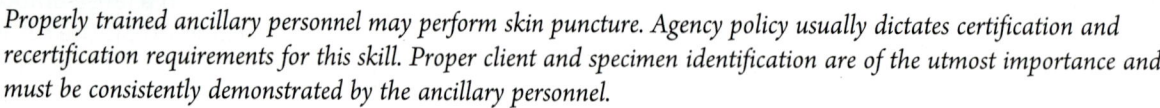

PROCEDURE 28-3

Obtaining a Residual Urine Specimen from an Indwelling Catheter

EQUIPMENT
- Nonserrated clamp or rubber band
- Nonsterile gloves
- Syringe with needle (1 inch), 10 cc
- Specimen container, plastic bag, and labels
- Povidone-iodine swabs

ACTION	RATIONALE
1. Wash hands/hand hygiene.	1. Reduces transmission of microorganisms.
2. Check health care provider's order.	2. Determines test and container needed for the specimen.
3. Explain procedure to the client and provide privacy.	3. Informs client and maintains client dignity.
4. Check for urine in the tubing.	4. Determines if there is sufficient urine in the collecting tubing for a specimen. Urine from the collection bag should not be used for sterile specimens.
5. If more urine is needed, clamp the tubing using a nonserrated clamp or a rubber band for 10 to 15 minutes (see Figure 28-23 on page 645).	5. Collects 10 cc of urine, which is needed for most urinalyses.
6. Put on clean gloves.	6. Practices Standard Precautions.
7. Clean sample port with a povidone-iodine swab.	7. Prevents entrance of microorganisms into the system.
8. Insert sterile needle and syringe into the sample port or catheter at a 45° angle and withdraw 10 mL of urine (see Figure 28-24 on page 645).	8. Obtains specimen with sufficient volume for most urine tests.
9. Put urine into sterile container and close tightly, taking care not to contaminate the lid of the container.	9. Prevents contamination of specimen and spill of urine.

(Continues)

PROCEDURE 28-3
Obtaining a Residual Urine Specimen from an Indwelling Catheter (Continued)

ACTION	RATIONALE

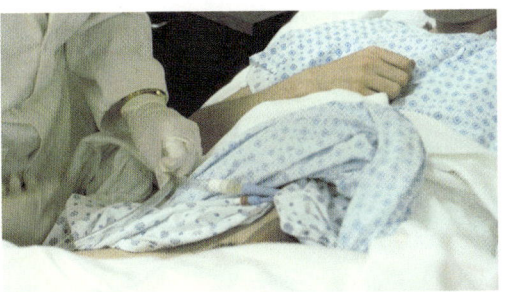

FIGURE 28-23 Clamp the tubing by folding it over and securing it with a rubber band to collect an adequate sample. DELMAR/CENGAGE LEARNING

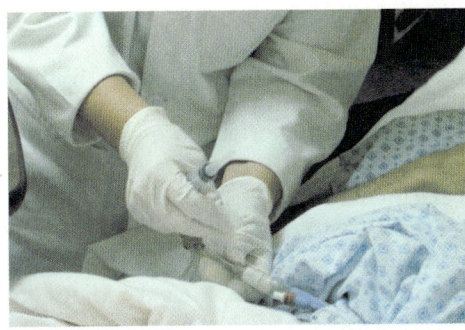

FIGURE 28-24 Cleanse the sample port and insert a sterile needle and syringe into the port. DELMAR/CENGAGE LEARNING

ACTION	RATIONALE
10. Remove clamp and rearrange tubing, avoiding dependent loops.	10. Reestablishes urine flow and drainage into the system.
11. Label specimen container, put it in a plastic bag, and send to the laboratory.	11. Ensures right test and controls transfer of pathogens.
12. Wash hands/hand hygiene.	12. Reduces transmission of microorganisms.

delegation tip

Obtaining a urine specimen from an indwelling catheter requires the skill and problem-solving ability of a nurse. This task cannot be delegated to ancillary personnel.

nursing tips

When doing catheter care, do not allow urine to drain back into the bladder.

PROCEDURE 28-4

Collecting a Clean-Catch Midstream Urine Specimen

EQUIPMENT
- Sterile collection container with lid and label
- Toilet paper
- Nonsterile latex-free gloves
- Sterile midstream kit, antiseptic towelettes, or cotton balls with antiseptic solution
- Sterile gauze (optional)

ACTION	RATIONALE
1. Wash hands/hand hygiene.	1. Provides for organization and reduces the transmission of microorganisms.
2. Assess the client's ability to complete the procedure, including understanding, mobility, and balance.	2. Improves compliance and likelihood of obtaining sterile specimen.
3. Assess the client for signs and symptoms of urinary abnormalities.	3. Improves compliance and provides baseline data.

(Continues)

PROCEDURE 28-4
Collecting a Clean-Catch Midstream Urine Specimen (Continued)

ACTION	RATIONALE
4. Check the client's identification.	4. Ensures accuracy.
5. If the client is to complete the procedure in privacy, explain the procedure, give equipment to the client, and wait for specimen. If the client has decreased personal hygiene, perform the procedure after a bath or have the client wash the perineal area before the procedure.	5. Increases compliance. Protects client from embarrassment.
6. If the nurse is to perform the procedure, wash hands and apply gloves. If the client is to perform the procedure, instruct the client to wash hands before and after the procedure. If the client is more comfortable, allow him or her to wear gloves.	6. Decreases transmission of microorganisms.
7. Provide privacy.	7. Decreases embarrassment.
8. Instruct the client. Female client: Sit with legs separated on the toilet. Male client: Sit down to help control splashing.	8. Increases compliance and understanding.
9. Using sterile procedure, open kit or towelettes (see Figure 28-25). Open sterile container, placing the lid with sterile side up on a firm surface (see Figure 28-26).	9. Prevents contamination of the specimen.
10. Female client: Use the thumb and forefinger to separate the labia, or have the client separate the labia with fingers (see Figure 28-27 on page 647). With the labia separated, use a downward stroke (from the top of the labia down toward the rectal area), and cleanse one side of the labia with the towelette (see Figure 28-28 on page 647). Discard the towelette and repeat the procedure on the other side with another towelette, keeping the labia separated at all times. With a third towelette, use a downward stroke from the top of the urethral opening to the bottom. Discard the towelette.	10. Provides access for cleaning the labia. Cleanses area and prevents contamination of clean area. Prevents contamination by feces. Keeping labia separated avoids contamination and decreases microorganisms in specimen.

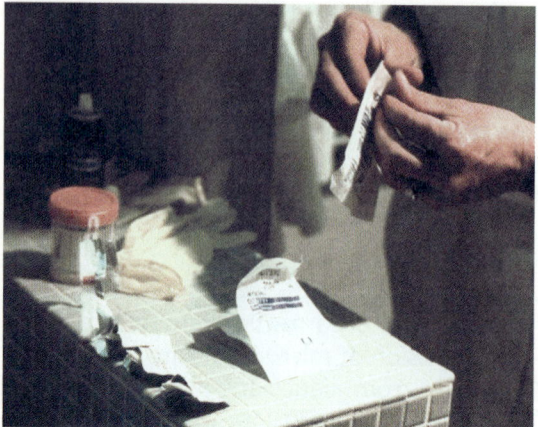

FIGURE 28-25 Open specimen cup and kit or cleansing towel packages prior to beginning the procedure. DELMAR/CENGAGE LEARNING

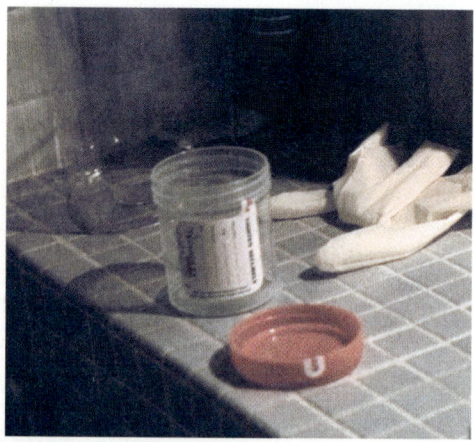

FIGURE 28-26 Place the lid on a firm surface, sterile side up. Do not touch the inside of the lid. DELMAR/CENGAGE LEARNING

(Continues)

PROCEDURE 28-4
Collecting a Clean-Catch Midstream Urine Specimen (Continued)

ACTION	RATIONALE

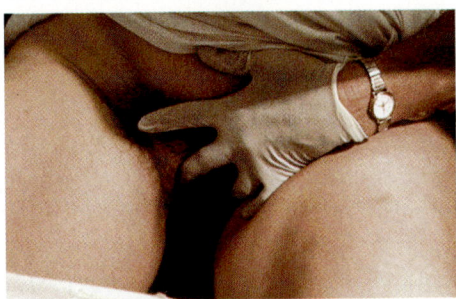

FIGURE 28-27 Separate the labia with the fingers of the nondominant hand. DELMAR/CENGAGE LEARNING

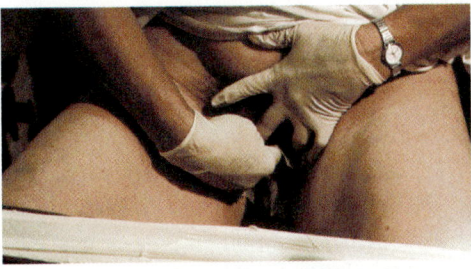

FIGURE 28-28 Cleanse each side and down the middle using a single downward stroke for each towelette. Keep the labia separated. DELMAR/CENGAGE LEARNING

11. Male client: Pull back the foreskin (if present in uncircumcised male) and clean with a single stroke around meatus and glans. Use a circular motion starting with the head of the penis at the urethral opening, moving down the glans shaft. Discard the towelette and repeat the procedure with another towelette, keeping the foreskin retracted. Cleanse the head of the penis three times using a circular motion. Use a new towelette each time.

11. Prevents contamination of microorganisms from foreskin. Single strokes and moving away from opening prevent contamination of the urethral opening.

12. Ask the client to begin to urinate into the toilet. After the stream starts with good flow, place the collection cup under the stream of urine. Avoid touching the skin with the container. Fill the container with 30 to 60 cc of urine and remove the container before urination ceases. Wipe with toilet paper.

12. The specimen is collected midstream to avoid contamination of urine that touches the labia. The initial urine flushes bacteria from the orifice, and the end urine may have contact with the meatus or labia and, hence, be contaminated.

13. Place the sterile lid back onto the container and close tightly (see Figure 28-29). Clean and dry the outside of the container with a towelette. Wash hands. Label and enclose in a plastic biohazard bag (see Figure 28-30), and follow facility policy for transporting specimen to the laboratory.

13. Prevents contamination of sterile specimen, prevents spillage, and ensures accuracy.

14. Remove and dispose of gloves and perform hand hygiene.

14. Decreases transmission of microorganisms.

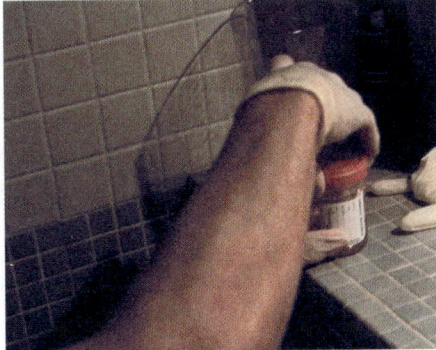

FIGURE 28-29 Replace the lid and close tightly. DELMAR/CENGAGE LEARNING

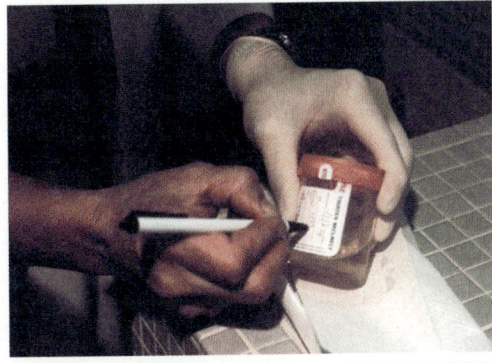

FIGURE 28-30 Label the container with the name of the client, date, and time the specimen was collected. DELMAR/CENGAGE LEARNING

(Continues)

PROCEDURE 28-4
Collecting a Clean-Catch Midstream Urine Specimen (Continued)

delegation tip

Collection of a clean-catch specimen may be delegated to ancillary personnel properly trained in the technique of cleaning the client and obtaining the voided specimen.

nursing tips

- *Labia may be slippery after cleansing; therefore, use sterile dry gauze to hold apart during urination.*
- *Clients often do not understand the need to remove the specimen container before completing urination; therefore, carefully explain the purpose for midstream collection.*
- *If the client is unable to void, run tap water within hearing distance or place a warm compress over the bladder.*

PROCEDURE 28-5

Measuring Blood Glucose Levels

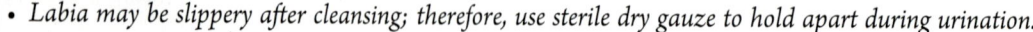

EQUIPMENT
- Reagent strips
- Disposable latex-free gloves
- Lancet or automatic lancing device
- Paper towels
- Alcohol wipe
- 2 × 2 gauze
- Cotton ball
- Blood glucose meter

ACTION	RATIONALE
1. Review orders, identify the client, and review the manufacturer's instructions for meter usage.	1. Prevents performing an invasive procedure on the wrong client and promotes accuracy of results.
2. Wash hands/hand hygiene.	2. Reduces transmission of microorganisms.
3. Assemble the equipment at the bedside (see Figure 28-31 on page 649).	3. Allows for a smooth procedure.
4. Have the client wash hands with soap and water, and position the client comfortably in a semi-Fowler's position or upright in a chair.	4. Reduces transmission of microorganisms and increases blood flow to the puncture site. Avoids having the client stand during the procedure, as some clients may be prone to fainting.
5. Remove a reagent strip from the container and reseal the container cap. Then, turn on meter.	5. Tight closure of the container keeps strips from discoloring from environmental factors. Activates meter for test.
6. Following the manufacturer's instructions, calibrate the meter by inserting the strip into the meter.	6. Some meters need to be calibrated; others require the timer to be adjusted; each meter has different requirements when setting it up for use.

(Continues)

PROCEDURE 28-5
Measuring Blood Glucose Levels (Continued)

ACTION	RATIONALE

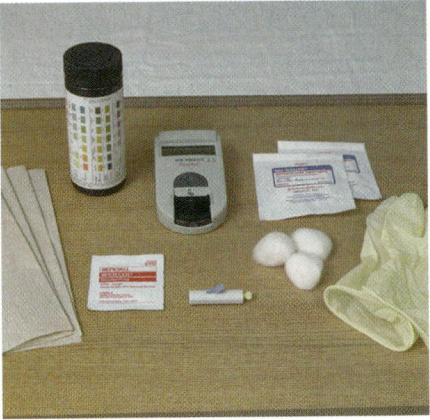

FIGURE 28-31 Supplies for blood glucose testing. DELMAR/
CENGAGE LEARNING

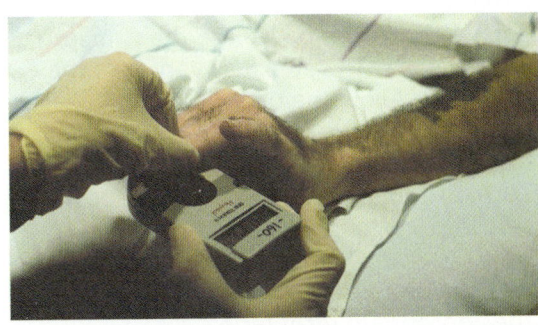

FIGURE 28-32 Perform the skin puncture. DELMAR/CENGAGE
LEARNING

7. Remove the unused reagent strip from the meter and place it on a clean, dry surface (paper towel) with the test pad facing up.
8. Apply disposable gloves.
9. Select appropriate puncture site and perform skin puncture (see Figure 28-32).
10. Wipe away the first drop of blood from the site.
11. Gently squeeze the site to produce a large droplet of blood.

12. Transfer the drop of blood to the reagent strip by carefully moving the site over the strip. The droplet should transfer without smearing (see Figure 28-33).
13. Quickly press the timer on the meter and lay the strip next to the meter on a clean, dry surface.

14. Apply pressure to the puncture site (see Figure 28-34).

7. Moisture may alter the test results.

8. Protects from contamination by blood.
9. Collects blood necessary for the test.

10. This drop may impede accurate results because it may contain a large amount of serous fluid.
11. Do not contaminate the site by touching it; the droplet of blood needs to be large enough to cover the test pad on the reagent strip.
12. The test pad must absorb the droplet of blood for accurate results. Smearing of the blood will alter results.

13. Timing is critical to produce accurate results. Always check the manufacturer's instructions because the technique varies between meters.
14. This will stop the bleeding at the site.

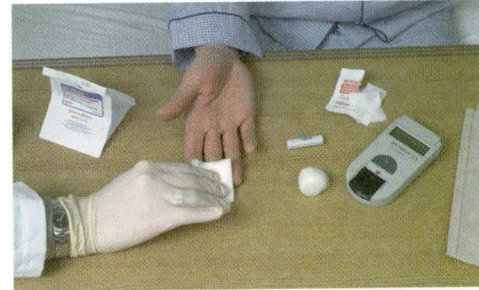

FIGURE 28-34 Apply pressure to the site. DELMAR/CENGAGE
LEARNING

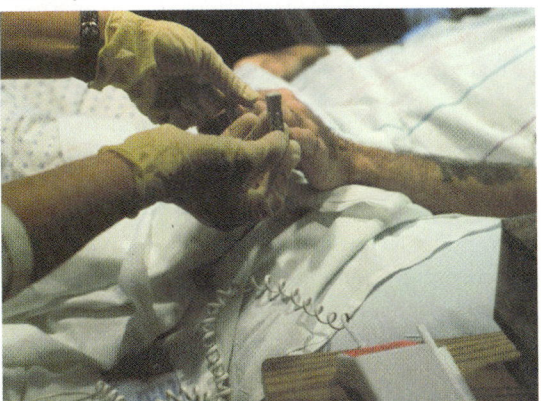

FIGURE 28-33 Transfer a drop of blood to the test strip. DEL-
MAR/CENGAGE LEARNING

(Continues)

PROCEDURE 28-5
Measuring Blood Glucose Levels (Continued)

ACTION	RATIONALE
15. After 60 seconds, wipe the blood from the test pad with a cotton ball; place the strip into the meter. (*Note:* This step may vary with the type of meter.) Allow the timer to continue.	15. This step is specific to certain meters (e.g., Accu-Chek III) that require the strip to enter the meter dry.
16. Read the meter for results found on the unit display.	16. Each meter has a specified time for the reading to occur.
17. Turn off the meter and properly dispose of the test strip, cotton ball, and lancet.	17. Reduces contamination by blood to other individuals; sharps must always be handled properly to protect others from accidental injury.
18. Remove disposable gloves and place them in the appropriate receptacle.	18. Reduces transmission of microorganisms.
19. Wash hands/hand hygiene.	19. Reduces contamination by microorganisms.
20. Review tests results with the client.	20. Promotes participation in health care.
21. Notify the health care provider of the test results.	21. Results will be used to determine the client's treatment plan.
22. Wash hands/hand hygiene.	22. Reduces transmission of microorganisms.

delegation tip

Properly trained ancillary personnel may measure blood glucose levels. Agency and state health department policies usually dictate certification and recertification requirements for this skill. Proper client and specimen identification are of the utmost importance and must be consistently demonstrated by the ancillary personnel. Proper recording of results and prompt reporting to the nurse of abnormal findings are essential.

nursing tips

- *Have client hold hand in a dependent position while you are setting up the equipment to promote venous engorgement in the fingertips.*
- *Be sure client's hands are warm.*
- *Use client's nondominant hand, if possible.*

KEY CONCEPTS

- Most invasive procedures require the client's written consent and a thorough understanding of the reasons the test is being performed. Nurses explain the purpose of the diagnostic test and the reasons it has been ordered.

- Nurses prepare clients for diagnostic testing by ensuring client understanding and compliance with preprocedural requirements.

- Clients, families, and significant others need to be involved in the testing process; advise them of the estimated time the procedure requires.

- Nurses teach the client how to perform relaxation and imagery techniques to cope with the discomfort and anxiety experienced during procedures.

- After a procedure, the nurse provides care and teaches the client what to expect following a diagnostic test and the outcomes or side effects of the test.

- Specimen collection methods include punctures such as venipuncture, arterial puncture, capillary puncture, catheter insertion, and bone marrow aspiration. Specimens collected by noninvasive methods include urine, stool, sputum, throat tissue, and cervical tissue.

- Invasive procedures include endoscopy, angiography, aspiration, biopsy, and other procedures in which body cavities are punctured.

- Noninvasive procedures include radiography, fluoroscopy, mammography, computed tomography, radioisotope scanning, ultrasonography, magnetic resonance imaging, and electrodiagnostic studies.

- The role of the nurse in diagnostic procedures is to facilitate the scheduling of diagnostic tests, perform client teaching, perform or assist with procedures, and assess the client for adverse responses to the procedures.

- Nurses should schedule diagnostic procedures to promote client comfort and cost containment.
- Standard Precautions are used when obtaining a specimen for diagnostic examination or assisting with an invasive procedure.

- Before the procedure, the nurse is responsible for obtaining baseline vital signs and assessing the client's preparation for testing.
- Nurses may assist the practitioner in performing invasive procedures.
- After the procedure, the nurse assesses the client for secondary procedural complications and provides any necessary nursing interventions.

REVIEW QUESTIONS

1. Preparing the client for diagnostic testing includes which of the following? Select all that apply.
   a. Appropriate preparation
   b. Individualized education
   c. Placing in the correct position
   d. Initiating Standard Precautions
   e. Providing emotional support
   f. Documenting the diagnostic outcomes

2. The purpose of the Joint Commission's *2009 Hospitals' National Patient Safety Goals* is to do which of the following?
   a. Improve the hospital's rating
   b. Decrease client error
   c. Increase hospital revenues
   d. Increase the image of nursing

3. Decreasing the length of time a client stands prior to venipuncture and the length of time the tourniquet is left on the client's arm helps to prevent which of the following?
   a. Hemoconcentration
   b. Hemorrhage
   c. Homeostasis
   d. Hypoxemia

4. After drawing arterial blood gases (ABG), the nurse should
   a. Pack the blood sample in ice for transport to the laboratory.
   b. Keep pressure on the radial artery puncture site for at least 1 minute.
   c. Transfer the blood sample to a heparinized test tube.
   d. Draw the second sample in 10 minutes.

5. When there is a delay in sending a urine sample to the laboratory for analysis, the nurse should
   a. Notify the prescribing practitioner.
   b. Discard the urine sample.
   c. Place the sample in a plastic bag and refrigerate.
   d. Write "stat" on the requisition and demand that the laboratory pick up the sample.

6. Which best defines culture and sensitivity?
   a. It is a common screening test.
   b. It allows the bacteria to grow and multiply so that the exact organism can be identified by various methods of analysis.
   c. It identifies both the nature of the invading organism(s) and their susceptibility to commonly used antibiotics.
   d. It evaluates the cell maturity, metabolic activity, and morphologic variations.

7. Which of the following are contrast-mediated studies? Select all that apply.
   a. Barium swallow
   b. Bronchography
   c. Intravenous cholangiography
   d. Mammography
   e. Myelogram
   f. Ultrasonography

8. List the following steps in the correct order for instructing a male client to obtain his own clean-catch midstream urine specimen.
   a. Wash hands.
   b. Pull back the foreskin (uncircumcised) and clean with a single stroke around the meatus and glans with a towelette using a circular motion starting with the head of the penis at the urethral opening, moving downs the glans shaft. Discard the towelette and cleanse the head of the penis three times using a circular motion and new towelette each time.
   c. Open the sterile procedure kit and place the lid face down on a firm surface.
   d. Begin to urinate into the toilet; after the stream starts to flow, place the collection cup under the stream of urine, and collect 30 to 60 cc of urine without touching the skin with the container.
   e. Tightly place the lid on the container.
   f. Label the container and place in a plastic biohazard bag.

online companion

Visit the DeLaune and Ladner online companion resource at **www.delmar.cengage.com** for additional content and study aids. Click on Online Companions, then select the Nursing discipline.

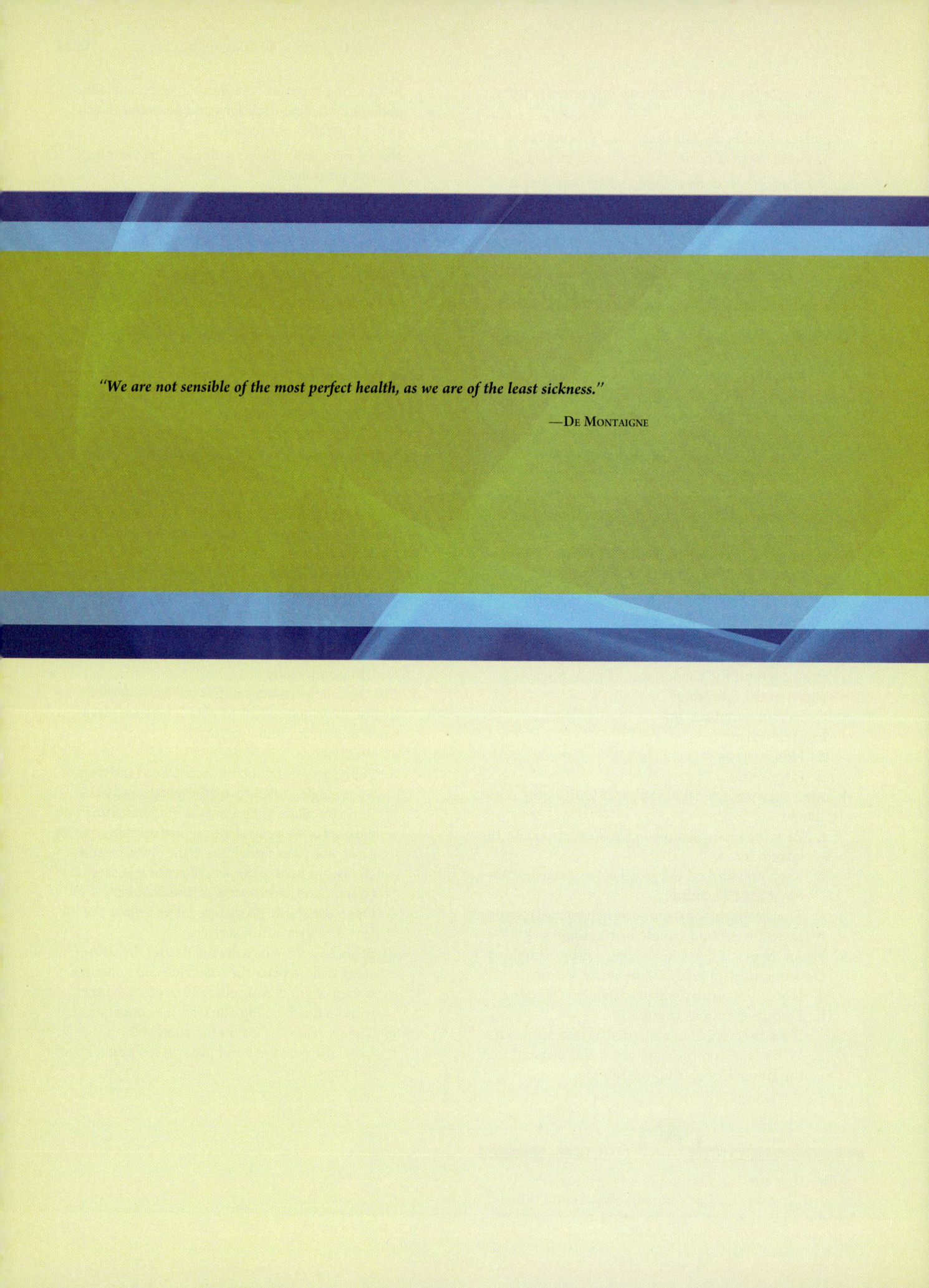

"We are not sensible of the most perfect health, as we are of the least sickness."

—DE MONTAIGNE

CHAPTER 29

Safety, Infection Control, and Hygiene

COMPETENCIES

1. Describe the factors affecting environmental safety.
2. Describe the chain of infection.
3. Explain the principles of medical and surgical asepsis.
4. Contrast the various types of isolation precautions.
5. Discuss the factors that influence a client's personal hygiene practices.
6. Explain the role of assessment in maintaining a safe environment.
7. Discuss the nursing interventions that can be used to resolve environmental hazards in institutional and home settings.
8. Describe the nursing interventions that promote a client's personal hygiene.

KEY TERMS

acquired immunity
agent
airborne transmission
anthropogenic
antibodies
antigens
antiseptic hand rub
antiseptic handwash
asepsis
aseptic technique
autoimmune disorders
biological agents
body image
cavities
chain of infection
chemical agents
chemical restraints
clean objects
cleansing
client behavior accidents
colonization
communicable agents
communicable diseases
compromised host
contact transmission
convalescent stage
dirty (soiled) objects

disinfectants
disinfection
equipment accidents
erythema
floras
germicide
gingivitis
halitosis
hand hygiene
handwashing
health care–associated infections
   (HAIs)
hospital-acquired conditions
   (HACs)
host
humoral immunity
hygiene
illness stage
incubation period
infection
infectious agents
inflammation
localized infections
lymphokines
medical asepsis
mode of transmission
pathogenicity

pathogens
perineal care
physical agents
physical restraints
poison
prodromal stage
pyorrhea
resident floras
restraints
risk for infection
sebum
self-care deficit
sensory overload
spores
sterilization
stomatitis
surgical asepsis
surgical hand antisepsis
susceptible host
systemic infections
therapeutic procedure accidents
transient floras
vaccination
vectorborne transmission
vehicle transmission
virulence

Safe care is a basic need of all clients, regardless of the setting. Registered nurses (RNs) are responsible for providing the client with a safe environment through the delivery of professional, quality nursing care that incorporates safety precautions, infection control practices, and hygiene assistance. This chapter describes the RN's role in each of these areas.

CREATING A CULTURE OF CLIENT SAFETY

A culture of safety pertains to environmental safety in health care settings, including the home. A landmark report published by the Institute of Medicine (IOM) of the National Academy of Sciences in 1999, *To Err Is Human: Building a Safer Health Care System*, brought national attention to the problem of hospital medical errors. Historical, medical error review was based on the underlying assumption that most injuries were the result of incompetent, negligent behavior or corporate greed; therefore, error and error analysis focused

on humans as the unreliable sources of error. However, the IOM report found that most medical errors did not result from individual carelessness but from basic flaws in the health care delivery systems.

The IOM report served as a catalyst of reform in health care organizations, educational institutions, and regulatory and accrediting agencies to remove the blame from health care providers and to improve health care systems. Client safety is defined as "freedom from accidental injury" and error as a "failure of a planned action to be completed as intended or the use of a wrong plan to achieve an aim" (Kohn, Corrigan, & Donaldson, 1999, pp. 13–14). In a later report, client safety practices were defined as "a type of process or structure whose application reduces the probability of adverse events resulting from exposure to the health care system across a range of diseases and procedures" (Shojania, Duncan, & McDonald, 2001, p. 13).

The challenge to current health care organizations is to create a culture of client safety and to focus on change rather than blame. The Patient Safety and Quality Improvement Act of 2005 amended the Public Health Service Act to encourage a culture of safety in health care organizations. The act provides legal protection of information voluntarily reported to the client safety organizations. The National Patient Safety Foundation of the American Medical Association, the U.S. Department of Veterans Affairs, and the Joint Commission have made a commitment to develop polices, conduct research, and establish standards that foster a culture of client safety.

Professional nursing has initiated an agenda of developing evidenced-based practices promoting health care cultures of client safety. A key role for nurse administrators is to help improve RN access to evidence-based literature to enable RNs to interact more proactively for safety.

In 2003, the Joint Commission established the first National Patient Safety Goals (NPSGs) to promote specific improvements in client safety. Based on the data collected annually, the Joint Commission publishes and revises the NPSGs as evidence-based recommendations. The 2009 NPSGs are to:

- Identify clients correctly
- Improve staff communications
- Use medicines safely
- Prevent infection
- Check client medicines
- Prevent clients from falling
- Help clients to be involved in their care
- Identify client safety risks
- Watch clients closely for changes in their health and respond quickly if they need help
- Prevent errors in surgery

To improve the quality of care during a hospital stay, the Centers for Medicare and Medicaid Services (CMS) identified certain **hospital-acquired conditions (HACs)** that are deemed reasonably preventable by following evidence-based guidelines and are either costly or common. The HACs are called "never events" because they are events that should never happen in a hospital. The Medicare Modernization Act and Deficit Reduction Act of 2005 granted the CMS the right to reduce, withhold, or refuse reimbursement

to hospitals for certain HACs. The Medicare law went into effect in October 2008. Medicare will no longer reimburse hospitals at a higher rate for the increased costs that result from HACs; however, Medicare will continue to pay for prescribing practitioner and other covered items or services that are needed to treat the HAC, including postacute care. The HACs include:

- Foreign object (e.g., sponge or needle) inadvertently left in clients after surgery
- Air embolism
- Transfusion with the wrong type of blood
- Severe pressure ulcers
- Falls and trauma
- Catheter-associated urinary tract infection
- Vascular catheter–associated infection
- Manifestations of poor control of blood sugar levels
- Surgical site infection following coronary artery bypass graft
- Surgical site infection following certain orthopedic procedures
- Surgical site infection following bariatric surgery for obesity
- Deep vein thrombosis and pulmonary embolism following certain orthopedic procedures (CMS, 2008)

It is the intent of Medicare to add documents to the list of HACs as needed to ensure client safety. "If at discharge, there is a selected condition that was either not identified by the hospital as present on admission, or could not be identified based on data and clinical judgment at admission, it is considered hospital-acquired" (CMS, 2008, p. 2). Emerging is a number of different lists by hospital and private insurers that expands the Medicare list.

FACTORS AFFECTING SAFETY

Client safety is influenced by several factors such as age, lifestyle, sensory and perceptual alterations, mobility, emotional state, and staffing.

Age

Risk for injury varies with chronological age and developmental stage. Health education about preventive measures can facilitate injury prevention for various age groups.

As infants mature, their potential for injury increases. Infants, toddlers, and preschoolers are explorers of their environment. Most accidents involving these age groups are avoidable with careful adult supervision to prevent falls from bed, burns, electrical hazards, choking on small objects, and drowning.

As school-age children explore their environment outside of the home, their risk for injury increases. Prevention measures during this stage focus on not accepting candy, food, gifts, or rides from strangers; bicycle, skating, and swimming safety; and substance abuse.

Adolescents and young adults usually enjoy good physical health; however, their lifestyles put them at risk for injury. Since this age group spends much time away from home, collaborative educational efforts among parents, schools, and

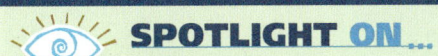

SPOTLIGHT ON...

Legal and Ethical

Reporting Errors

Registered nurses are taught in nursing school to safeguard our clients and do them no harm. When mistakes occur, nurses are reluctant to report the error. Nurses worry about resultant harm to clients, families, their career, and themselves. No matter how hesitant a nurse may be to report an error, the ethical response is to inform the client and family. What can nurses do to create a culture of support when a nursing colleague is involved in errors that have unintentionally caused harm?

community health care providers need to focus on environmental safety. High-risk factors for injury and death are automobile accidents, substance abuse, violence, unwanted pregnancies, and sexually transmitted diseases.

Studies indicate that adolescents who initiate substance use in middle school and continue into high school are likely to become multisubstance users (tobacco, alcohol, and drugs). The progression from lighter to heavier use of illicit substances during adolescence leads to more serious multisubstance use careers.

Adult risk for injury is generally related to lifestyle, work practices, and behaviors. Prevention measures during this period emphasize nutrition, exercise, and occupational safety. High-risk factors for this age group include fatigue, anxiety, sleep pattern disturbances, caregiver role strain, and altered health maintenance.

The older adult is prone to falls, especially in the bathroom, bedroom, and kitchen, because of a loss of agility and visual acuity, a predisposition to dizziness and syncope, and side effects from medications. Every year one in three Americans over the age of 65 years experiences a fall and, of these, 30% cause injury requiring medical treatment (Cassels, 2008). Prevention measures for this age group emphasize slow positional changes, good lighting, hand rails, and skidproof strips in the bathtub or shower and under rugs and carpets.

Lifestyle

Lifestyle practices can increase a person's risk for injury and potential for disease. Individuals who operate machinery; experience stress, anxiety, and fatigue; use alcohol and drugs (prescription and nonprescription); and live in high-crime neighborhoods are at risk for injury. Risk-taking behaviors such as daredevil activities, driving vehicles at high speeds, and smoking are factors associated with accidents (Figure 29-1).

Sensory and Perceptual Alterations

Sensory functions are essential for the accurate perception of environmental safety. If one of the senses is altered, then the other senses compensate to facilitate perception of the environment. For instance, a blind person usually will develop a keen sense of touch and hearing. Clients who have visual, hearing, taste, smell, communication, or touch perception impairments are at increased risk for injury. These clients are often not able to perceive a potential danger. See Chapter 38 for a complete discussion on sensory or perceptual alterations.

Mobility

Clients who have impaired mobility are at increased risk for injury, especially falls. Mobility impairments may be a result of poor balance or coordination, muscle weakness, or paralysis. Immobility may also precipitate physiological and emotional complications such as decubitus and depression, respectively. See Chapter 36 for a complete discussion on mobility.

Emotional State

Emotional states such as depression and anger affect a client's perception of environmental hazards and degree of risk-taking

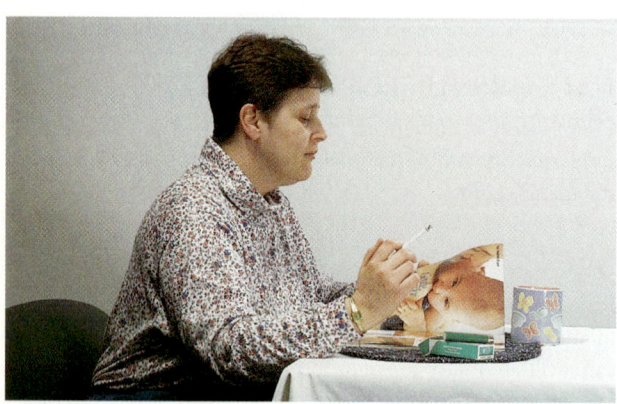

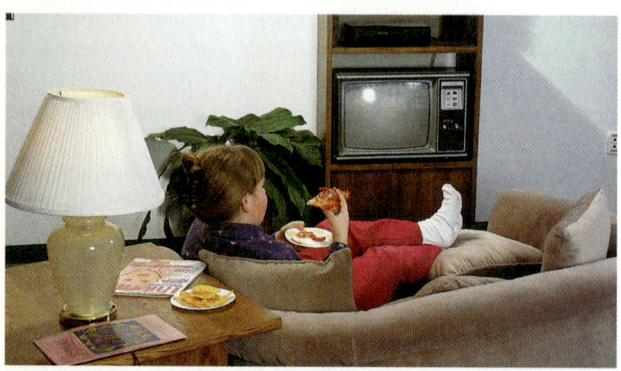

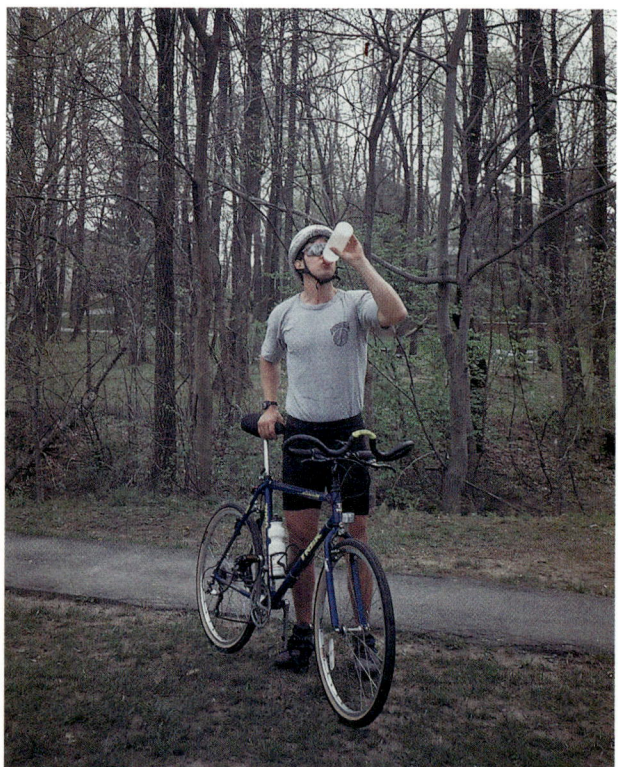

FIGURE 29-1 Lifestyle practices that can either increase or decrease a client's risk of injury. Can these practices be easily reversed, in terms of risky behavior, or adopted, in terms of promoting healthy approaches, by clients? DELMAR/CENGAGE LEARNING

behavior. These emotional states alter a client's thinking patterns and reaction time. Usual safety precautions may be forgotten during periods of emotional stress. Self-confidence decreases when older adults fall; they tend to limit their activities because they fear falling again.

TYPES OF ACCIDENTS

In the health care setting, accidents are categorized by their causative agent: client behaviors, therapeutic procedures, or equipment:

1. **Client behavior accidents** occur when the client's behavior or actions precipitate the incident, for example, poisonings, burns, and self-inflicted cuts and bruises.
2. **Therapeutic procedure accidents** occur during the delivery of medical or nursing interventions, for example, medication errors, client falls during transfers, contamination of sterile instruments or wounds, and improper performance of nursing activities.
3. **Equipment accidents** result from the malfunction or improper use of medical equipment, for example, electrocution and fire.

National and institutional policies establish safety standards; for example, the risk for equipment accidents can be reduced by having the biomedical engineering department check the equipment inspection label prior to use. All accidents and incident reports must be fully documented according to institutional protocol.

Staffing

As Hinshaw describes nurse staffing and client safety, "balancing the development of cultures of safety with nursing workforce challenges is similar to navigating the perfect storm" (2008, p. S4). The perfect storm is characterized as a tempest of extreme intensity that rarely happens and is a result of multiple factors that end in a situation worse than previously experienced. The climate of change is demanding client safety (the Joint Commission, NPSGs, the CMS) while nursing is being confronted with a shortage of nurses and nursing faculty. The response to this storm from health care organizations is to create cultures of safety, recognizing the importance of public policy for client safety, the need for health systems reforms, and the use of appropriate evidence-based practice. Nursing will be held more and more accountable for assessment and client advocacy skills and for incorporating solid scientific evidence into practice.

POTENTIAL OCCUPATIONAL HAZARDS

Nurses and other health care providers are at risk for injury in the workplace. The Occupational Safety and Health Administration (OSHA), a division of the Department of Labor, has the power to enforce safety standards and to cite and discipline agencies that are not in compliance with the standards. Numerous hazards exist in today's workplace, such as latex allergies, bloodborne pathogens, work-related musculoskeletal disorders (MSDs), chemotherapeutic agents, environmental pollution, and violence. Nurses who prepare or administer chemotherapeutic agents are exposed to occupational hazards from dermal absorption, ingestion, and inhalation from aerosolization of powder or liquid during reconstitution or from spillage. The salient points regarding latex allergy and MSDs are discussed here; bloodborne pathogens are discussed later in this chapter.

Latex Allergy

The National Institute for Occupational Safety and Health (NIOSH, 1997) issued an *Alert* titled *Preventing Allergic Reactions to Natural Rubber Latex in the Workplace.* Latex products are manufactured from a milky fluid derived from the Brazilian rubber tree, *Hevea brasiliensis.* The allergic response is attributed to the proteins contained in the milky fluid and to the chemicals that are added during the processing and manufacture of commercial latex. There are three types of latex reactions: irritant contact dermatitis; allergic contact dermatitis, the most common type of reaction; and immediate hypersensitivity, a systemic reaction, also called type I IgE–mediated reaction.

Since 1992, when OSHA issued regulations requiring health care workers to wear gloves and other protective devices such as surgical masks and goggles as a safeguard against bloodborne pathogens, health care workers have been placed at risk for developing latex allergy. Commercial latex is in more than 20,000 medical products such as blood pressure cuffs, stethoscopes, catheters, and wound drains, to name a few, as well as in many household items. Reports indicate that 1%–6% of the general population and about 8%–12% of regularly exposed health care workers are sensitive to latex (NIOSH, 1997).

The NIOSH (1997) recommends that employers and employees take a commonsense approach based on current knowledge to protect workers from latex exposure and allergy in the workplace; refer to the accompanying display on page 658 on the NIOSH's recommendations to prevent latex exposure. The NIOSH recommends that if latex gloves are worn, they should be powder free and low allergen because these gloves are less likely than powdered ones to produce allergic responses. Latex-allergic clients should wear MedicAlert identification, carry two doses of epinephrine, and carry several pairs of nonlatex gloves for use by emergency medical personnel (Ricci, 2008).

Work-Related Musculoskeletal Disorders

Work-related back pain affects 38% of nurses. The predominant cause of nurse back pain is lifting clients. OSHA has recommendations for nursing home employers to help reduce the number and severity of MSD conditions such as low back pain, sciatica, rotator cuff injuries, epicondylitis, and carpal tunnel syndrome. The recommendations in these guidelines are based on a review of existing practices and programs, state OSHA programs, and available scientific information. These guidelines are also available to hospitals and other health care providers to reduce of the risk of MSD. OSHA ergonomic standards state that a 51-pound stable object with handles is the heaviest amount that can be safely lifted. Health care providers are being challenged, in the midst of personnel cutbacks, to develop and implement safety policies that protect the provider and support OSHA's ergonomic regulations.

NIOSH RECOMMENDATIONS TO PREVENT LATEX EXPOSURE

EMPLOYERS

- Provide workers with nonlatex gloves.
- Provide appropriate barrier protection for workers handling infectious materials; if latex gloves are chosen, provide reduced-protein, powder-free gloves to protect workers from infectious materials.
- Provide good housekeeping to remove latex-containing dust, and ensure that workers change ventilation filters and vacuum bags frequently in latex-contaminated areas.
- Provide education programs regarding latex allergy.
- Periodically screen high-risk workers for latex allergy symptoms.
- Evaluate current policies whenever a worker is diagnosed with a latex allergy.

WORKERS

- Use nonlatex gloves for contact with noninfectious materials.
- Use CDC-appropriate barrier protection when handling infectious materials; if latex gloves are chosen, use reduced-protein, powder-free gloves to reduce exposure and reactions to latex chemical additives (allergic contact dermatitis).
- Use appropriate work practices when wearing latex gloves: Avoid oil-based hand creams or lotions that can cause glove deterioration unless they have been shown to reduce latex-related problems and maintain glove barrier protection; wash hands with a mild soap and dry thoroughly after removing latex gloves; use good housekeeping practices to remove latex-containing dust.
- Attend latex allergy educational programs to become knowledgeable about procedures and to recognize the symptoms of a latex allergy: skin rashes; hives; flushing; itching; nasal, eye, or sinus symptoms; asthma; and shock.
- Avoid direct contact with latex gloves and other products if you develop symptoms until you have been seen by a prescribing practitioner experienced in treating latex allergies.
- If you have a latex allergy, consult your prescribing practitioner regarding exposure precautions, contact with gloves and other latex-containing products, and areas that contain latex powder from gloves worn by other workers; inform your employer and health care providers that you have a latex allergy.
- Carefully follow your prescribing practitioner's instructions regarding allergic latex reactions.

Adapted from National Institute for Occupational Safety and Health Centers for Disease Control and Prevention. (1997). *Preventing allergic reactions to natural rubber latex in the workplace* (DHHS [NIOSH] Publication No. 97-135U). Washington, DC: U.S. Department of Health and Human Services, Public Health Service, Centers for Disease Control and Prevention, National Institute for Occupational Safety and Health.

The ergonomic standards require that all employers must provide workers with the following information: common MSD hazards, signs and symptoms of MSDs and the importance of reporting them early, how to report MSD signs and symptoms, and a summary of the requirement of OSHA standards. The standards require the employer to ensure pay and benefits in the event that an employee needs to take time off or go on lighter duty because of a work-related MSD.

INFECTION CONTROL PRINCIPLES

Client safety in the health care environment requires the reduction of microorganism transmission. Infection control practices are directed at controlling or eliminating sources of infection in the health care agency or home. Nurses are responsible for protecting clients and themselves by using infection control practices. Nurses and clients must be educated about the types of infections, modes of transmission, risks for susceptibility, and infection control practices required to control or prevent further transmission.

PATHOGENS, INFECTION, AND COLONIZATION

Pathogenicity is the ability of a microorganism to produce disease. Microorganisms that cause diseases in humans are called **pathogens**. Five types of microorganisms can be pathogenic: bacteria, viruses, fungi, protozoa, and *Rickettsia*. **Virulence** is the degree of pathogenicity of an infectious microorganism (pathogen).

Infection and colonization are not synonymous. **Infection** is an invasion and a multiplication of microorganisms in body tissue that result in cellular injury. These microorganisms are called **infectious agents**. Infectious agents that are capable of being transmitted to a client by direct or indirect contact through a vehicle (or vector) or airborne route are also called **communicable agents**. Diseases produced by these agents are referred to as **communicable diseases**. **Colonization** is the multiplication of microorganisms on or within a host that does not result in cellular injury. However, microorganisms that are colonized on a host may be a potential source of infection, especially if host susceptibility declines or if the microorganism's virulence increases.

Some microorganisms reside on the human body as normal flora. This is synonymous with colonization. **Floras** are microorganisms on the human body. There are two types of flora: resident and transient. **Resident floras** are microorganisms that are always present, usually without altering the client's health. Handwashing with soap and water alone is not sufficient to remove resident flora; there must be considerable friction, which is created by rubbing the hands and scrubbing the nails. **Transient floras** are microorganisms that are episodic. They attach to the skin for a brief period of time but do not continually live on the skin. Transient flora is usually acquired from direct contact with the microorganisms on environmental surfaces. Handwashing with soap and water is an effective means of removing transient flora.

CHAIN OF INFECTION

A susceptible host or the presence of a pathogen alone does not mean that an infectious process will occur. The **chain of infection** describes the phenomenon of developing an infectious process. There must be an interactive process that involves the agent, host, and environment. This interactive process must involve several essential elements, or links in the chain, for transmission of microorganisms to occur. Figure 29-2 on page 660 identifies the six essential links (elements) in the chain of infection. Without the transmission of microorganisms, an infectious process cannot occur. Therefore, knowledge about the chain of infection for an infectious process permits control or elimination of the microorganism by breaking the links in the chain of infection. Breaking the chain of infection occurs by altering the interactive process of agent, host, and environment, as shown in Figure 29-2.

Agent, Host, and Environment

An **agent** is an entity that is capable of causing disease. Agents that cause disease may be:

- **Biological agents**: Living organisms that invade the host, such as bacteria, viruses, fungi, protozoa, and *Rickettsia*
- **Chemical agents**: Substances that can interact with the body, such as pesticides, food additives, medications, and industrial chemicals
- **Physical agents**: Factors in the environment that are capable of causing disease, such as heat, light, noise, radiation, and machinery

In the chain of infection, the main concern is biological agents and their effect on the host.

A **host** is a simple or complex organism that can be affected by an agent. Generally, a human being is considered a host. A **susceptible host** is a person who lacks resistance to an agent and is thus vulnerable to disease. A **compromised host** is a person whose normal defense mechanisms are impaired and who is therefore susceptible to infection.

Interaction between agent and host occurs in the environment; the environment consists of everything other than the agent and host. Environmental factors that affect the chain of infection are water, food, plants, animals, housing conditions, noise, meteorological conditions, and environmental chemicals. Many of the conditions that promote the transmission of microorganisms are **anthropogenic**, reflecting changes in the relationship between humans and their environments.

The causes of most emerging infectious diseases are the same today as throughout recorded history: the transfer and dissemination of existing agents to new host populations (a process called "global microbial traffic"). For instance, cholera probably originated in Asia in ancient times; in the nineteenth century it spread to Europe and the New World because of increased global travel. Cholera entered South America for the first time in 1992 through the possible contaminated bilge water released from a Chinese freighter. The causes of emerging infectious diseases and outbreaks require careful consideration of environmental changes and especially of anthropogenic factors.

Modes of Transmission

The **mode of transmission** is the process that bridges the gap between the portal of exit of the biological agent from the reservoir or source and the portal of entry of the susceptible "new" host. Most biological agents have a primary mode of transmission; however, some microorganisms may be transmitted by more than one mode. Almost anything in the environment can become a potential means of transmitting infection, depending on the agent.

The most important and frequent mode of transmission is **contact transmission**, which involves the direct physical transfer of an agent from an infected person to a host through direct contact with a contaminated object or close contact with contaminated secretions. Sexually transmitted diseases are examples of diseases spread by direct contact.

Airborne transmission occurs when a susceptible host contacts droplet nuclei or dust particles that are suspended in the air. Vehicle and vectorborne transmission are indirect modes of transmission, because transmission occurs by an intermediate source. **Vehicle transmission** occurs when an agent is transferred to a susceptible host by contaminated inanimate objects such as water, food, milk, drugs, and blood. **Vectorborne transmission** occurs when an agent is transferred to a susceptible host by animate means such as mosquitoes, fleas, ticks, lice, and other animals.

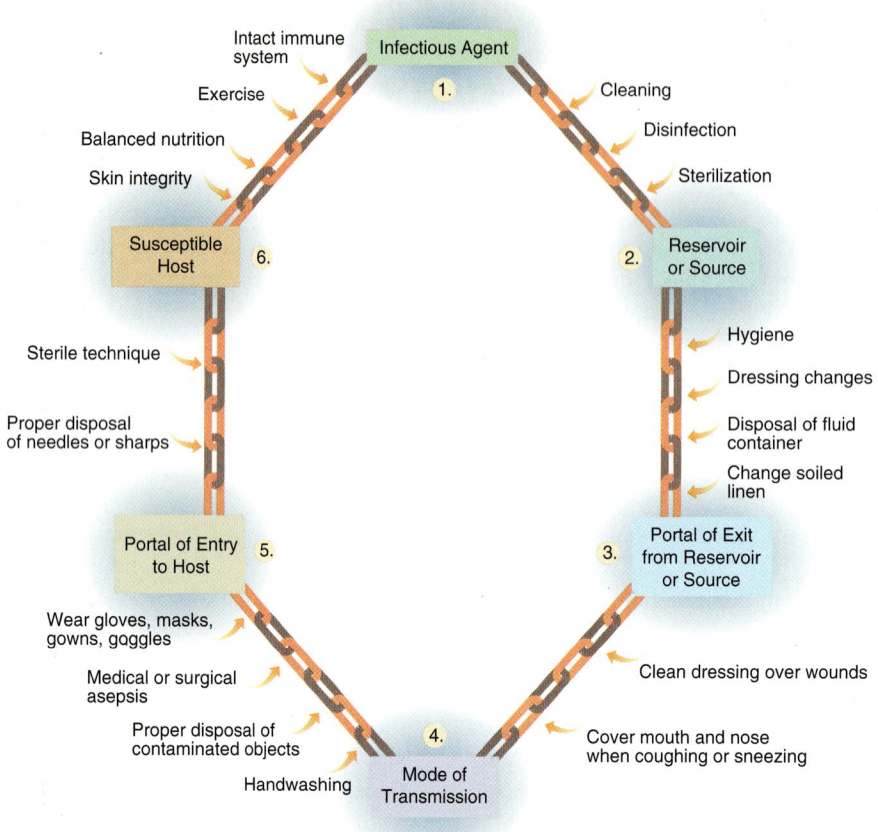

FIGURE 29-2 Breaking the chain of infection. Preventive measures follow each critical link in the chain of infection. DELMAR/CENGAGE LEARNING

Breaking the Chain of Infection

Nurses focus on breaking the chain of infection by applying proper infection control practices to interrupt the mode of transmission. The chain of infection can also be broken by interrupting or blocking the agent, portal of exit, or portal of entry or by destroying the agent or decreasing the host's susceptibility. Refer to Figure 29-2, which shows preventive measures that break the chain of infection. Host susceptibility is dependent on the immune system to function as a defense mechanism.

NORMAL DEFENSE MECHANISMS

A host's immune system serves as a normal defense mechanism to resist the transmission of infectious agents. A unique feature of the immune system is its ability to recognize "self" and "nonself"; that is, the immune system recognizes which agents are not consistent with the genetic composition of the host (self). These agents are usually referred to as antigens (nonself). **Antigens** are foreign proteins. An immune response is mounted against an antigen, which is recognized as nonself, to protect the body from infection. The immune defenses are categorized as nonspecific and specific immune defenses. Nonspecific and specific immune defenses work in harmony to defend the host from pathogens.

Nonspecific Immune Defense

The nonspecific immune defense mounts a response to protect the host from all microorganisms; it is not dependent on prior exposure to the antigen. Nonspecific immune defenses are skin and normal flora; mucous membranes; sneeze, cough, and tearing reflexes; elimination and acidic environment; and inflammation.

SKIN AND NORMAL FLORA   Intact skin is the first line of defense against infection, serving as a physical barrier to infectious agents. Skin cells are shed along with potentially harmful microorganisms. **Sebum** is produced by the skin and contains fatty acids that kill some bacteria. The normal flora that resides on the skin competes with pathogenic flora for food and inhibits their multiplication. The balance of normal flora may become disrupted as a result of the inappropriate use of antibiotics, which allows pathogenic organisms to proliferate and causes infection or superinfection.

MUCOUS MEMBRANES AND SNEEZE, COUGH, AND TEARING REFLEXES   Mucous membranes also function as a physical barrier to infectious agents. Mucus produced by these membranes entraps infectious agents and contains substances such as antibodies, lactoferrin, and lysozyme, which inhibit bacterial growth. Cilia of the respiratory tract trap and propel mucus and microorganisms away from the lungs. The sneeze and cough reflexes physically expel mucus and microorganisms from the respiratory tract and oral cavity with force. Tears protect the eyes by continually flushing away microorganisms.

ELIMINATION AND ACIDIC ENVIRONMENT Elimination patterns and an acidic environment normally prevent the microbial growth of pathogenic organisms. Resident flora of the large intestines prevents the growth of pathogens. The mechanical process of defecation evacuates the bowel of feces and microorganisms. Acidity of the urine prevents microbial growth. The flushing action of urination cleanses the bladder neck and urethra of microorganisms and prevents microorganisms from ascending into the urinary tract.

Normal vaginal flora prevents growth of several pathogens. At puberty, lactobacilli ferment and produce sugars in the vagina that lower the pH to an acidic range. The acidic environment of the vagina prevents pathogenic growth. Inappropriate use of antibiotics destroys the lactobacilli and their protective function.

INFLAMMATION **Inflammation** is a nonspecific cellular response to tissue injury or infection. Tissue injury caused by bacteria, trauma, chemicals, heat, or any other phenomenon releases multiple substances that produce dramatic secondary changes in the injured tissue. This entire complex of tissue changes and response to injury is referred to as the inflammatory process (see Table 29-1). The inflammatory process has five stages, facilitating the localization, neutralization, and resolution of the offending agent within the damaged tissue. The result of the body's response to injury produces the characteristic local and systemic signs of inflammation, discussed in the assessment section of this chapter.

The intensity of the inflammatory process is usually in proportion to the degree of tissue injury. For example, when staphylococci invade the tissues, they release lethal cellular toxins that cause the inflammatory process to develop quickly; the staphylococcal infection is characteristically walled off rapidly before the organism can multiply and spread. Streptococci, on the other hand, do not cause such intense local tissue destruction, and the walling-off process develops slowly, allowing the organism to reproduce and migrate. Therefore, the streptococci have a far greater tendency than do staphylococci to spread throughout the body and cause death, even though staphylococci are far more destructive to the tissue.

Specific Immune Defense

The specific immune defense mounts an immune response that is specific to the invading antigen. Unfortunately, the specific immune defense sometimes inappropriately reacts to the host's own tissue (**autoimmune disorders**).

The specific immune defense is activated by the failure of phagocytes to completely destroy the antigen; this causes the production of T lymphocytes (T cells) that regulate the immune response by activating other cells. Stimulated T cells

TABLE 29-1 Stages of the Inflammatory Process

STAGE	DESCRIPTION	RESULT
1	Initial injury precipitates release of chemicals: histamine, bradykinin, serotonin, prostaglandins (reaction products of the complement and blood-clotting systems), and lymphokines (hormonal substances released by sensitized T cells).	Activates the inflammation process.
2	Increased blood flow to the inflamed area (**erythema**).	Produces characteristic signs of redness and increased warmth.
3	Increased capillary permeability with leakage of large quantities of plasma out of the capillaries into the damaged tissue; tissue spaces and lymphatics blocked by fibrinogen clots.	Initiates the inflammation process; infection is "walled off," and nonpitting edema occurs.
4	Damaged tissue infiltrated by leukocytes, which engulf the bacteria and necrotic tissue. After several days, these leukocytes eventually die and form a cavity of necrotic tissue and dead leukocytes (mainly neutrophils and some macrophages).	Produces purulent exudate (pus).
5	Destroyed tissue cells are replaced with identical or similar structural and functioning cells and/or fibrous tissue.	Promotes tissue healing or the formation of fibrous (scar) tissue, which may reduce the functional capacity of the tissue.

Delmar/Cengage Learning

are referred to as sensitized T cells. T cells migrate to the area of injury and release chemical substances called lymphokines. Lymphokines attract other phagocytes and lymphocytes to the area of injury and assist in antigen destruction.

T cells also stimulate the production of B cells that differentiate into plasma cells, producing antibodies specific to the antigen. Antibodies are protein substances that counteract and neutralize the effects of antigenic toxins and destroy bacteria and other cells. Antibodies destroy the antigen. Stimulation of B cells and antibody production are referred to as humoral immunity.

B-cell activation causes formation of memory B cells. Memory B cells remember the antigen and prepare the host for future antigen invasion. Therefore, when the antigen enters the body again, the immune response will occur more rapidly by producing antibodies faster. The formation of these antibodies is referred to as acquired immunity, which protects the individual against invading agents such as lethal bacteria, viruses, toxins, and even foreign tissues from other animals.

The process of vaccination provides acquired immunity against specific diseases. There are three ways an individual can be vaccinated:

1. By injection of dead organisms that are no longer capable of causing disease but still have their chemical antigens, such as typhoid fever, whooping cough, and diphtheria.
2. By toxins that have been treated with chemicals so that their toxic nature has been destroyed even though their antigens for causing immunity are still intact, such as tetanus and botulism.
3. By infection with live organisms that have been attenuated (grown in a special culture media or passed through a series of animals for mutation; the organisms then do not cause the disease but still carry the specific antigen). Attenuated vaccines protect against poliomyelitis, yellow fever, measles, smallpox, and many other viral diseases.

See Chapter 18 for a detailed discussion on vaccination and immunization schedules for children, teens, and adults.

STAGES OF THE INFECTIOUS PROCESS

Activation of the immune response indicates the occurrence of infection. Infection results from tissue invasion and damage by an infectious agent. There are two types of infectious responses:

1. Localized infections are limited to a defined area or single organ with symptoms that resemble inflammation (redness, tenderness, and swelling).
2. Systemic infections affect the entire body and involve multiple organs.

Localized or systemic infections progress through four stages of infection:

- Incubation
- Prodromal
- Illness
- Convalescence

The incubation period is the time interval between entry of an infectious agent in the host and the onset of symptoms. During this time period, the infectious agent invades the tissue and begins to multiply to produce an infection.

The prodromal stage is the time interval from the onset of nonspecific symptoms until specific symptoms of the infectious process begin to manifest. During this period, the infectious agent continues to invade and multiply in the host. A client may also be infectious to other persons in this time period.

The illness stage is when the client is manifesting specific symptoms of an infectious process. The period of time from the beginning of the disappearance of acute symptoms until the client returns to the previous state of health is referred to as the convalescent stage.

EMERGING INFECTIONS

Homelessness is an increasing social and public health problem, with an estimated 100 million persons homeless worldwide (Badiaga, Raoult, & Brouqui, 2008). Without physical shelter or with a compromised physical shelter that does not meet basic standards of health and safety, such as access to safe water and sanitation, personal safety, and protection from the elements, homeless persons are at risk for many communicable infections. The primary health concerns for this population are the overcrowded living conditions that expose the homeless to airborne infections, especially tuberculosis (TB). The lack of personal hygiene and clothing changes can cause exposure to scabies, body lice infestations, and louseborne disease.

The incidence of TB is higher in the homeless populations than in the general population. Most TB cases occurring in the homeless are primary infections caused from recent person-to-person transmission leading to outbreaks. Frequently, the homeless are injection drug users and engage in risky sexual behavior, which cause exposure to bloodborne and sexually transmitted infections such as human immunodeficiency virus (HIV), hepatitis C virus (HCV), and hepatitis B virus (HBV; Badiaga et al., 2008).

The outbreak in 2003 of SARS-CoV, a coronavirus that causes severe acute respiratory distress syndrome, was characterized by nonspecific symptoms that included fever, discomfort, and mild respiratory symptoms. Although no new cases of SARS have been reported, the 2003 outbreak prompted the Centers for Disease Control and Prevention (CDC) to implement new measures of infection control at the first point of encounter within a health care setting, such as emergency departments. These new measures are discussed later in this chapter.

The major hepatitis viruses are HAV, HBV, HCV, HDV, HEV, and HGV. HAV is a virus that is most commonly transmitted by close contact with an infected person, after eating items contaminated with infected feces. Children in diapers or those who come into contact with other children in diapers are at risk for HAV because of inadequate handwashing in day care centers. HAV causes mild flulike symptoms, jaundice, severe stomach pains, and diarrhea. The hepatitis A vaccine is not administered to children 2 years of age and under.

HCV is the most common bloodborne pathogen in the United States. An estimated 4 million Americans have tested positive for HCV, with 25,000 new HCV infections occurring annually. HCV is a member of the *Flaviviridae* family, which also causes the West Nile virus; it mutates rapidly and evades the body's attempts to develop an effective antibody response. No vaccine is available. Transmission is primarily by exposure to blood, including illicit intravenous (IV) drug use; occupational exposure to blood by needlestick injury; perinatal exposure, HCV-infected mother; blood transfusion or organ transplant before 1990; exposure to contaminated equipment; and sexual contact with an infected person. Persons infected are usually asymptomatic or have general flulike symptoms. In 80% of HCV-infected persons, the disease becomes chronic and progresses to chronic liver disease, liver cancer, and liver transplantation. Nurses need to recognize the higher risk of HCV than HIV infection from an accidental needlestick.

The West Nile virus was first isolated in 1937; the first cases in the Western Hemisphere were reported in New York in 1999. This *Flavivirus* is usually transmitted when a mosquito feeds on an infected bird and then bites a human; however, data released from the CDC show that with the West Nile virus, the most common pathogens are transmitted through transfusions. It is similar to the virus that causes St. Louis encephalitis, and if it crosses the blood-brain barrier and causes encephalitis, it may be fatal.

Viral hemorrhagic fevers (VHFs), such as Ebola hemorrhagic fever, belong to the family of RNA viruses, the *Filoviridae*. The largest Ebola outbreak occurred in Uganda in 2000, resulting in more than 400 cases and 110 deaths. The disease is transmitted through direct contact with blood, secretions, and excretions of acutely ill persons or with tissues during autopsy. The only reported incidence in the United States occurred with a shipment of infected monkeys from the Philippines; although the virus did not cause illness, several workers became infected with and developed antibodies. This incident occurred in Reston, Virginia; therefore, it was named the Ebola-Reston hemorrhagic fever virus.

HIV infection or acquired immunodeficiency syndrome (AIDS) is present in most body fluids. HIV is a bloodborne pathogen that is transmitted with some exchange of body fluid, mainly blood. Transmission occurs by contaminated IV needles, anal intercourse, vaginal intercourse, oral-genital sex, and transfusion of blood and blood products. Vulnerable populations include gay men, IV drug users, their partners, their children, and those who receive contaminated blood, such as clients with hemophilia. Research continues for treatments and vaccines. The disease is usually fatal.

HEALTH CARE–ASSOCIATED INFECTIONS

Health care–associated infections (HAIs) are infections acquired in the hospital or other health care facilities that were not present or incubating at the time of the client's admission. HAIs are also referred to as health care–acquired infections. HAIs include those infections that become symptomatic after the client is discharged as well as infections

among medical personnel. Most HAIs are transmitted by health care personnel who fail to practice proper handwashing procedures or to change gloves between client contacts.

Hospitalized clients are at risk for HAIs because the environment provides exposure to a variety of virulent organisms that the client has not been exposed to in the past; therefore, the client has not developed any resistance to these organisms. In addition, illness, often the reason for hospital admission, impairs the body's normal defense mechanisms. According to the CDC (2008), HAIs are one of the top 10 leading causes of death in the Unites States.

The most common endemic infections in hospitals affect the urinary tract, upper and lower respiratory tracts, gastrointestinal tract, conjunctiva, and skin. Hospitalized clients have multiple comorbidities that increase their risk of infection. For example, urologic abnormalities (prostatic hypertrophy) are associated with urinary tract infections. Chronic obstructive lung disease and congestive heart failure increase a client's risk of developing pneumonia. Diabetes or vascular insufficiency may lead to more frequent and severe skin infections (pressure ulcers, cellulitis, and vascular ulcers). Since these high-risk clients are housed together, the transmission of pathogens is increased among residents. For instance, organisms may be transmitted through the air (e.g., TB, influenza), on the hands of staff members (e.g., *Staphylococcus aureus* or uropathogens), and by contaminated items (e.g., *Escherichia coli*).

HAIs are receiving increased attention because of the development of multiple-drug–resistant organisms (MDROs). The two most common MDROs are bacteria—methicillin-resistant *Staphylococcus aureus* (MRSA) and vancomycin-resistant enterococcus (VRE)—in both hospital and long-term care clients; other drug-resistant organisms include TB bacilli and *Clostridium difficile* (*C. difficile*).

MRSA has become a prevalent pathogen in the United States. In the hospital setting, the most important reservoirs of MRSA are infected or colonized clients. MRSA is transmitted mainly through the hands of health care workers who may have become contaminated by contact with colonized or infected clients or body sites of the personnel themselves, or devices, items, or environmental surfaces contaminated with body fluids containing MRSA. When a hospitalized client gets an MRSA infection, it is difficult to treat and often leads to serious problems such as pneumonia, wound, and blood infections (Holcomb, 2008). According to the CDC (2007), approximately 18,650 persons died during a hospital stay because of related MRSA infections. The main way to prevent the spread of MRSA is to utilize Standard Precautions, discussed later in this chapter.

C. difficile causes diarrhea that may range from mild diarrhea to severe colitis. It is transmitted by factors that cause an overgrowth of *C. difficile* and by contact with the organism. According to Harris (2006), antibiotics such as cephalosporins, ampicillin, amoxicillin, and clindamycin and invasive bowel procedures such as surgery or colonoscopy disrupt normal bowel flora and cause an overgrowth of *C. difficile*. Clients may also acquire *C. difficile* from a health care provider's poor hand hygiene, direct contact with environmental surfaces contaminated with *C. difficile*, and ineffective disinfection practices (Todd, 2006). *C. difficile* A and B bacteria are diagnosed in the stool; two or three stool specimens are required for the enzyme-linked immunosorbent assay (ELISA).

There is controversy regarding the use of alcohol-based hand rubs when dealing with *C. difficile*. An anaerobic spore-forming organism, *C. difficile* is not susceptible to alcohol in the spore state; however, most *C. difficile* organisms released in disease outbreaks are in the vegetative form, and these can be killed by alcohol ("Advice P.R.N.," 2008). The CDC has no clear guidelines regarding the use of alcohol-based hand rubs but recommends not using them during *C. difficile* outbreaks. Nurses need to adhere to agency policies, which should be based on the CDC's recommendations on the latest evidence-based practices.

Hand hygiene is the most important intervention in preventing and controlling the transmission of infection. Clients at risk for infection must understand the measures needed to reduce or prevent the spread and growth of microorganisms. Because hygienic care requires close contact with the client, the nurse promotes a caring therapeutic relationship by using this time for assessment, teaching, and counseling.

HYGIENE

Hygiene is the science of health. Hygienic care promotes cleanliness, provides for comfort and relaxation, improves self-image, and promotes healthy skin. Client hygiene is an extension of providing client safety and protecting the client's defense mechanisms. The health of the body's first line of defense (skin and mucous membranes) is promoted by client hygiene. Nurses are responsible for ensuring that the client's hygienic needs are met. The type of hygienic care provided depends on the client's ability, needs, and practices.

FACTORS INFLUENCING HYGIENIC PRACTICE

Hygienic needs and practices are unique to each client; nurses should provide individualized care based on these needs and practices. Hygienic practices are influenced by several factors, including body image, social and cultural practices, personal preferences, socioeconomic status, and knowledge.

Body Image

Body image is the client's subjective belief about his or her own physical appearance. Body image is associated with the client's emotions, mood, attitude, and values. See Chapter 22 for a complete discussion of this concept. A client's body image directly affects the type of personal hygiene practiced; this may change if the client's body image is altered because of illness or surgical procedures. During this time, the nurse should help the client maintain hygienic practices in accordance with the client's pre-illness level of hygiene and personal preferences.

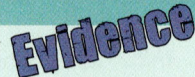

UNCOVERING THE Evidence

TITLE OF STUDY
"Invasive Methicillin-Resistant *Staphylococcus aureus* Infections in the United States"

AUTHORS
R. Klevens, M. Morrison, J. Nadle, S. Petit, K. Gershman, S. Ray, L. Harrison, R. Lynfield, G. Dumyati, J. Townes, A. Craig, E. Zell, G. Fosheim, L. McDougal, R. Carey, and S. Fridkin

PURPOSE
To describe the incidence and distribution of invasive MRSA disease in nine U.S. communities and to estimate the burden of invasive MRSA infections in the United States in 2005.

METHODS
Active, population-based surveillance was performed for invasive MRSA in nine sites participating in the Active Bacterial Core surveillance (ABCs)/Emerging Infections Program Network from July 2004 through December 2005.

FINDINGS
Most MRSA infections were health care associated. There were 8987 observed cases of invasive MRSA reported: 5250 (58.4%) were community-onset infections, 2389 (26.6%) were hospital-onset infections, 1234 (13.7%) were community-associated infections, and 114 (1.3%) could not be classified. Incidence rates were highest among persons 65 years and older, blacks, and males. There were 1598 in-hospital deaths among clients with MRSA infections during the study.

IMPLICATIONS
MRSA infection is a major public health problem related mainly to health care but no longer limited to intensive care units, acute care hospitals, or any health care institution. Invasive MRSA infection affects certain populations disproportionately.

Klevens, R., Morrison, M., Nadle, J., Petit, S., Gershman, K., Ray, S., et al. (2007). Invasive methicillin-resistant *Staphylococcus aureus* infections in the United States. *Journal of the American Medical Association, 298*(15), 1763–1771.

Social and Cultural Practices

Social and cultural practices also directly influence hygienic practices. Clients are socialized to their hygienic practices by family practices in early childhood. As a person ages, hygienic practices are influenced by maturational development and socialization with people outside of the family. For example, teenagers are usually concerned with peer acceptance and follow the latest trends in personal hygiene. In later adulthood, hygienic practices may be influenced by coworkers and social networks.

Cultural practices and beliefs are derived from family, religious, and personal values developed during maturation. See Chapter 20 for a complete discussion of cultural diversity. Clients from diverse cultural backgrounds will have differing hygienic practices. For example, some cultures do not permit women to submerge their bodies in water during the time of menstruation because of the fear that the woman may drown. In North America, people typically bathe daily and use numerous deodorant products. In Europe, people do not bathe daily and seldom use deodorant products. Europeans do not consider the smell of human perspiration as offensive as do North Americans. Nurses should have a nonjudgmental attitude when assessing or providing hygienic care to clients from different social or cultural backgrounds.

Personal Preferences

Personal preferences influence when bathing occurs, what products are used, and what type of bath is performed. For example, some male clients may shave before bathing, while others prefer to wait until after the bath. Some clients prefer to bathe in the morning to facilitate waking, while others prefer to bathe before bedtime to encourage relaxation and sleep. Unless a client's health is affected, the nurse should permit clients to practice their usual routine and use the hygienic products that they prefer. Individualized nursing care should incorporate the client's personal hygiene preferences.

Socioeconomic Status

A client's hygienic practices may be influenced by socioeconomic status. Limited economic resources may affect the type, frequency, and extent of hygiene practiced. Assessment of socioeconomic status provides information about the availability of

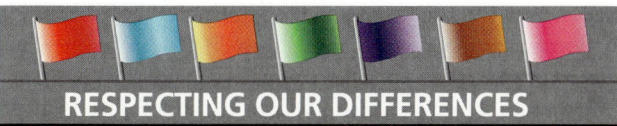

RESPECTING OUR DIFFERENCES

Hygiene and Personal Preferences

What role do values have in relation to self-care needs? Do you believe that a client's hygienic activities demonstrate personal preferences and idiosyncrasies that are based on family, culture, religion, and other factors? What should you do to avoid projecting your own values onto the client? If the client states, "I feel uncomfortable about you bathing me," what should you do? Another area that requires sensitivity on your part deals with a client's use or failure to use hygienic products, for example, deodorant. How do you feel about caring for a client who does not use deodorant or whose hygiene habits differ greatly from your own?

hygiene supplies. Some clients may not be able to afford deodorants, perfumes, soaps, shampoo, and toothpaste. The nurse can function as an advocate for the client by making referrals to community agencies that provide assistance to needy persons, for example, Catholic Charities or a local chapter of the American Association of Retired Persons.

Knowledge

Knowledge level influences the client's understanding about the relationship between hygiene and health. Thus, knowledge should influence a client's hygienic practices. In addition to being knowledgeable, before clients perform basic hygiene, they must be motivated and believe that they are capable of self-care.

Frequently, an illness or a surgical procedure results in deficient knowledge about basic hygienic practices. In these situations, the client may not know the correct procedures or types of hygiene that can be performed. The nurse is responsible for providing the necessary education about hygiene during an illness. Sometimes the nurse may have to perform all hygienic practices for a client during an illness until the client is able to regain this ability.

ASSESSMENT

The nursing process facilitates an understanding of the scope of challenges inherent in the nursing care of clients at risk for injury, infections, or a self-care deficit. The assessment data should direct the prioritization of the client's problem and accompanying nursing diagnoses. Clients at risk for injury or infection require frequent reassessment of their status with appropriate changes in the plan of care and expected outcomes.

The assessment and physical examination data are correlated with the laboratory indicators to identify those clients who are at risk for problems relating to safety, infection, or hygiene. One of the assessment models should be used to provide structure to the assessment. See Chapter 6 for a complete discussion of assessment models. Appropriate risk appraisals may be incorporated into the nursing health history interview. These core elements of assessment are discussed in relation to clients in ambulatory, institutional, and home settings. Refer to the accompanying display on page 666 for a sample format for developing minimum safety standards applicable to all health care settings.

HEALTH HISTORY

The nursing health history interview is the first part of assessment; it provides the client's subjective, specific health data. Key elements of relevant data regarding the client at risk for safety and infection are obtained in the health history. See Chapter 6 for a sample of a nursing health history tool.

The client is often asked to complete a health history questionnaire; however, depending on the client's status, the nurse may have to perform an interview to obtain these data. If the client is unable to provide the subjective data, the nurse must designate on the questionnaire or in the nursing progress notes who provided the information.

STANDARD OF CARE: SAFETY

CLIENT OUTCOME

The client will receive care in a safe health care environment and remain free of preventable injuries.

NURSING PRACTICE STANDARDS

1. Perform a client injury risk appraisal upon admission and prior to therapeutic nursing interventions. Risk factors for injury include, but are not limited to, age, altered mental status, previous history of falls, impaired mobility, sensory deficits, perceptual deficits, and inability to communicate.
2. Eliminate or modify risk elements when possible, such as assisting with mobility and placing bed rails up with bed in the lowest position.
3. Implement environmental precautions, such as hand rails, nonslip mats or rugs, and adequate lighting.
4. Use infection control practices that prevent or control the transmission of pathogens.
5. Maintain IV access according to IV protocols.
6. Implement emergency measures in accordance with American Heart Association guidelines for cardiopulmonary resuscitation (CPR) and advanced life support.
7. Know and comply with the institution's Environmental Health and Safety guidelines.
8. Implement emergency measures during fires and disasters.
9. Use mechanical, radiant, chemical, and thermal equipment according to the manufacturer's guidelines and the institution's policy and procedures.
10. Use a multidisciplinary approach to enhance client safety, as indicated.

KEY INTERVIEW QUESTIONS ABOUT SAFETY, INFECTION CONTROL, AND HYGIENE

- Describe the things you do to stay healthy.
- How do you typically spend a day (e.g., home or work)?
- What are your health care concerns?
- Do you need assistance with bathing and dressing?
- Do you regularly visit the dentist and eye doctor?
- Do you use dental floss on a regular basis?
- Have you recently come into contact with someone who has an infectious disease?
- Do you wash your hands when preparing food?
- Do you keep meats and dairy products refrigerated until ready to use?
- Is there a smoke detector or fire extinguisher in your home?
- Are emergency phone numbers readily available?

During the nursing health history interview, assess the client's general health perception and management status to determine how the client manages self-care. This information will provide data regarding the client's routine self-care and health promotion needs. Sample questions that relate specifically to habits that foster safe, healthy patterns of behavior are presented in the accompanying display. These questions are appropriate for home health and ambulatory care settings as well as inpatient settings.

PHYSICAL EXAMINATION

A complete health assessment includes a systematic physical examination, generally conducted from head to toe, in order to obtain objective data relative to the client's health status

and presenting problems. See Chapter 27 for a complete discussion of a physical examination.

When assessing the client to determine the level of risk for injury or infection and hygienic deficits, focus the physical examination on the following areas and signs:

- Level of consciousness, using the Glasgow Coma Scale to evaluate this attribute (see Chapter 38 for discussion of this tool)
- Range of motion or total immobilization of an extremity
- Localized infection: Redness, swelling, warmth, tenderness, pain, and loss of movement in a specific body part
- Systemic infection: Fever, with a corresponding increase in pulse and respirations; weakness; anorexia, with possible accompanying findings of nausea, vomiting, and diarrhea; enlarged and/or tender lymph nodes
- Secretions or exudate of the skin or mucous membranes and detection of crackles, rhonchi, or wheezes in the lungs on auscultation

The condition of the skin is a good indicator of a client's general health status. Assessment of skin integrity provides data concerning a client's nutritional and hydration status, continuity of intact skin, hygienic practices, and overall physical abilities. Similarly, a client with limited mobility is at risk for developing joint contractures, skin breakdown, and muscle atrophy.

Risk Factors

A comprehensive nursing assessment involves using specifically developed risk assessment tools and appraising the client's environment to detect potential hazards. The client's self-care abilities, used for determining the level of assistance needed in providing hygienic care, are appraised during the health history. The analysis of relevant risk factors alerts the nurse to actual or possible risks. Skin integrity is usually compromised when a person is placed on bed rest.

A skin integrity risk appraisal such as the Braden scale (see Chapter 37) should be completed to assist with planning care.

Client in an Inpatient Setting

Inpatient clients should be assessed for fall and infection risk factors. The hospitalized or institutionalized client's risk for falls is identified after compiling specific assessment data that are correlated with contributing factors. Each of these indicators carries a specific weight, as shown in the accompanying display, Fall Risk Appraisal, to determine the client's risk. The inpatient client should be assessed for falls every shift or as designated by institutional policy. To minimize the chance of falls, make sure the client's environment is safe: The bed is kept in a low position, side rails are up, personal belongings are in easy reach, and assistive devices (e.g., walker) are nearby, as shown in Figure 29-3 on page 668.

To determine risk for infection, review or listen to the client's response to the health history and interview questions related to "exposure to infectious diseases," "invasive procedures," and "behaviors you think you should change." An infection risk appraisal is based on the defining characteristics that place a client at risk for an infection. These factors are listed in the section titled Nursing Diagnosis.

Client in the Home

An injury risk appraisal will provide the nurse with assessment data to determine the client's level of safety knowledge, as previously discussed in the standard of care for safety. Injuries in the home are primarily the result of falls, fires, electrical malfunctions, suffocation, weapons, and household and medication poisonings. Home health nurses may use a safety risk appraisal; refer to the accompanying display on fall risks.

The safety risk data assessed in the home environment direct the nurse in planning for the client's and caregiver's education. The home health nurse needs to prioritize these data when planning the client's care. Assessment, teaching, and outcome evaluation of all safety hazards can take several home visits.

DIAGNOSTIC AND LABORATORY DATA

Appraising the client's risk for injury should also include an evaluation of laboratory findings relative to an abnormal blood profile (e.g., altered clotting factors, anemic conditions, or leukocytosis). See Chapter 28 for a complete discussion of abnormal blood profiles. Malnourished clients are at risk for injury.

The laboratory indicators for an infection are:

1. An elevated leukocyte (white blood cell [WBC]) and WBC differential:
   - Neutrophils: Increased in acute, severe inflammation

FALL RISK APPRAISAL

Area of Assessment	Score
General Factors	1
Restraint (Posey, arm, leg)	
Orthostatic changes	
History of falls/crawling out of bed/syncope (brief loss of consciousness)	
Seizure disorder	
Elimination Function	2
Decreased bladder/bowel tone	
Urgency/frequency	
Incontinence	
Nocturia (excessive urination at night)	
Age	3
Over 65	
Level of Consciousness/ Mental Status	4
Lethargic (slow to respond)	
Inability or refusal to follow directions	
Inability or refusal to call for help	
Impaired judgment, memory, awareness	
Confused, disoriented	
Sensory Deficits	5
Diminished visual acuity, blind, blurred vision	
Slow reaction time	
Mobility/Physical Limitations	6
Decreased mobility in lower extremities	
Up with assistance	
Amputee/joint difficulties	
Weakness, dizziness, fatigability, vertigo (dizziness), syncope	
Cast, splint	
Use of crutches, cane, walker	
Hemiparesis (one-sided paralysis), paraparesis (loss of function), hemiplegic, paraplegic (loss of function in lower limbs)	
Ataxia (unsteady gait)	
Improper-fitting/smooth-soled/no footwear	
Unsteady gait, decreased balance, imbalance	
Medications	7
Sedatives/hypnotics/tranquilizers	
Diuretics/antihypertensives/laxatives	
Narcotics/analgesics/anesthetics	
Antihistamines	
Antiseizures	
Barbiturates/phenothiazines	
Eye drops	
Antipsychotics/antidepressants	

Scoring: If the client is over 65 years of age, the indicator has a weight of 3. If the client is also receiving a diuretic, which has a weight of 7, the total risk factor for this client is 10. This would place the client at high risk for falls and would require the implementation of special fall measures.

Adapted from the Patient Care Documentation Sheet, courtesy of Tulane University Hospital & Clinic, New Orleans, LA

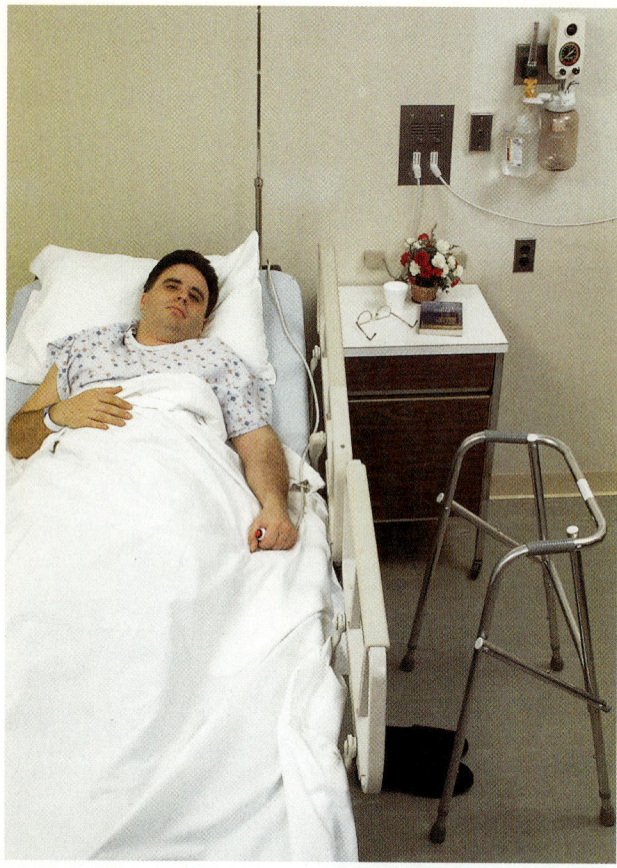

FIGURE 29-3 This client's risk of falls has been assessed and responded to through the measures shown here. Do all clients within the hospital setting need to be assessed for the risk of falls, regardless of their health status or reason for hospitalization? DELMAR/CENGAGE LEARNING

- Lymphocytes: Increased in chronic bacterial and viral infections
- Monocytes: Increased in some protozoan and rickettsial infections and TB
- Eosinophils and basophils: Unaltered in an infectious process
2. An elevated erythrocyte sedimentation rate (ESR): Increased in the presence of inflammation
3. An elevated pH of involved body fluids (gastric, urine, or vaginal secretions): Indicates the presence of microorganisms
4. Positive cultures of involved body fluids (blood, sputum, urine, or other drainage): Indicates the growth of microorganisms

Refer to Chapter 28 for the age-related normal laboratory values for each of the preceding tests.

NURSING DIAGNOSIS

After data collection and analysis, the nurse is able to formulate a nursing diagnosis. If Gordon's Functional Health Patterns model is used to conduct the assessment, the nurse can use the classification of nursing diagnoses by functional health patterns that relate to safety, infection, and hygienic deficits, for example:

I. Health perception–health management pattern
- *Risk for injury*
- *Risk for infection*
II. Activity-exercise pattern
- *Bathing/hygiene self-care deficit*
- *Dressing/grooming self-care deficit*
- *Toileting self-care deficit*

RISK FOR INJURY

The primary nursing diagnosis *risk for injury* exists when the client is at risk for injury as a result of environmental conditions interacting with the individual's adaptive and defensive resources (North American Nursing Diagnosis Association [NANDA], 2009-2011). Although this diagnostic label does not have defining characteristics as set forth by NANDA, it is categorized as having either internal or external potential hazards. An internal biochemical risk factor for a client with impaired vision would be stated as *risk for injury* related to sensory dysfunction. In contrast, a home health nurse's assessment data that identify drugs on a nightstand with a toddler in the home as creating an external chemical risk factor for the toddler would be stated as *risk for injury* related to drugs (pharmaceutical agents).

NANDA (2009-2011) has six defined subcategories of specific risk factors for this diagnostic labeling:

1. *Risk for suffocation:* An accentuated risk of accidental suffocation
2. *Risk for poisoning:* An accentuated risk of accidental exposure to, or ingestion of, drugs or dangerous products in doses sufficient to cause poisoning
3. *Risk for trauma:* An accentuated risk of accidental tissue injury (e.g., wound, burn, fracture)
4. *Risk for aspiration:* Risk for entry of gastrointestinal secretions, oropharyngeal secretions, solids, or fluids into the tracheobronchial passages
5. *Risk for disuse syndrome:* Risk for deterioration of body or body systems as the result of prescribed or unavoidable musculoskeletal inactivity
6. *Risk for latex allergy response:* Risk for allergic response to natural latex rubber products

These six subcategories of nursing diagnoses provide the nurse with the opportunity to relate specific nursing interventions to the diagnosed problem. For example, the specific nursing diagnosis for the situation of a toddler in the home environment encountering medications on a nightstand would be *risk for poisoning* related to medicines not stored in locked cabinets and accessible to children. The level of risk would be increased if the medications on the client's nightstand were in open containers or the closed containers failed to have childproof caps. The subcategory diagnosis provides specific nursing interventions directed at the level of risk for the toddler and the need for client teaching.

HOME SAFETY RISK APPRAISAL

INFANT

- Crib has side rails that stay in the up position while infant is in the crib.
- Infants are not left unattended, especially on elevated surfaces or in the bath.
- Bath water temperature is 37.8°C–40.6°C (100°F–105°F). Check temperature for comfort with wrist.
- Environment is kept warm and draft-free at bath time.
- Bottles are sterilized and formula is refrigerated.
- Toys are soft without detachable pieces.
- Car seat has restraint strap and is used consistently.
- Stroller and carry seat are sturdy with a restraint strap.
- Fire, police, and poison control numbers are posted by telephones.
- Caregivers know infant CPR.

TODDLER/PRESCHOOLER

- Sharp objects are placed out of reach and out of sight.
- Poisons are labeled and placed in a locked cabinet.
- Medications and other toxins have childproof lids and are stored in a locked cabinet.
- Small, hard food objects (peanuts, candy) are kept in locked cabinets.
- Stairs and floor furnaces have gates or barriers.
- Safety locks are on doors and windows.
- Electrical outlets are covered.
- Burners on the stove are not left on and unattended.
- Pots with hot liquids are placed on back burners with handles facing toward the back wall.
- Home and yard are free from poisonous plants.
- Play equipment is kept in proper functioning condition; toys have no small parts; crayons are nontoxic.
- Outdoor play is supervised in a fenced area with locks on gates.
- Car seat/belt is used consistently.
- Supervision is given to child when she or he is crossing the street.
- Caregivers know child CPR and the Heimlich maneuver.

SCHOOL-AGE CHILD

- Play and sports are supervised.
- Play equipment is kept in proper functioning condition and free from hazards.
- Outdoor play is limited to soft surfaces.
- Bicycle helmet is worn consistently.

- Child is taught to not open the door or speak to strangers while at play.
- Firearms are kept unloaded in locked cabinets.
- Caregivers know child CPR and the Heimlich maneuver.
- Seat belt is worn at all times.

ADOLESCENT

- Firearm safety is taught.
- Seat belt is worn at all times.
- Teenagers take drivers' education and are cautioned about drinking and driving.
- Caregivers know adult CPR and the Heimlich maneuver.

ADULT

- Firearms have safety latches.
- A smoke detector and a fire extinguisher are installed in the home.
- Sharp-edged objects are safely stored.
- A nondrinking designated driver is chosen.
- Emergency phone numbers are readily available.
- Caregivers know adult CPR and the Heimlich maneuver.

OLDER ADULT

- Stairs have adequate lighting and nonskid surfaces, and rails are in good condition.
- Throw rugs are not present.
- Hallways are uncluttered.
- Carpets are free from frayed ends/pieces.
- Phone and other cords are behind furniture.
- Bathtub has rails and a nonslip surface.
- Shower stall has a seat.
- Bathroom is free from drafts.
- Shoes fit properly, with nonskid soles.
- Home is adequately ventilated and heated.
- Home is free of space heaters.
- Pilot lights are functional for gas appliances.
- Electrical appliances are in good working condition.
- Food is properly refrigerated.
- Medications are kept in properly labeled containers with readable print.
- Emergency phone numbers are readily available.
- Fire and police departments are aware of older adult at home alone.
- Caregivers know adult CPR and the Heimlich maneuver.

RISK FOR INFECTION

Risk for infection is the state in which an individual is at increased risk for being invaded by pathogenic organisms (NANDA, 2009–2011). The risk factors that increase the client's vulnerability to infections are:

- Inadequate primary defenses (broken skin, traumatized tissue, decrease in ciliary action, stasis of body fluids, change in pH of secretions, and altered peristalsis)
- Inadequate secondary defenses, acquired immunity, and immunosuppression
- Tissue destruction and increased environmental exposure
- Chronic diseases and malnutrition
- Invasive procedures and pharmaceutical agents
- Trauma
- Rupture of amniotic membranes
- Insufficient knowledge to avoid exposure to pathogens (NANDA, 2009–2011)

SELF-CARE DEFICITS

A self-care deficit exists when the client is not able to perform one or more of the activities of daily living (ADL). NANDA (2009–2011) identifies three self-care deficits related to hygienic practices. These diagnostic labels, together with their defining characteristics and related factors, are presented in Table 29-2.

OTHER NURSING DIAGNOSES

Clients who are at risk for injury and infection or who have a self-care deficit may have other problems. These associated physiological and psychological problems are discussed in detail in other chapters in this unit. The common nursing diagnoses that often accompany diagnostic labels for risk or self-care deficits are:

- *Imbalanced nutrition (specify less than body requirements or more than body requirements)*
- *Ineffective protection*
- *Impaired tissue integrity*
- *Impaired oral mucous membrane*
- *Impaired skin integrity*
- *Social isolation*
- *Risk for loneliness*
- *Ineffective coping*
- *Impaired physical mobility*
- *Hopelessness*
- *Powerlessness*
- *Deficient knowledge (specify)*
- *Acute pain*
- *Anxiety*
- *Fear*

This list is not all-inclusive but indicates the number of related problems that need to be considered when planning care.

TABLE 29-2 Self-Care Deficits

NURSING DIAGNOSIS AND DEFINITION	DEFINING CHARACTERISTICS	RELATED FACTORS
Bathing/hygiene self-care deficit: A state in which the individual experiences an impaired ability to perform or complete bathing/hygiene activities for self	Inability to wash body or body parts, obtain water from a water source, or regulate the temperature or flow of water	Intolerance to activity; decreased strength and endurance; pain and discomfort; impairment of perception or cognition, neuromuscular activity, and musculoskeletal function; and depression or severe anxiety
Dressing/grooming self-care deficit: A state in which the individual experiences an impaired ability to perform or complete dressing and grooming activities for self	Impaired ability to put on or take off necessary items of clothing, obtain or replace articles of clothing, fasten clothing, or maintain appearance at a satisfactory level	Intolerance to activity; decreased strength and endurance; pain and discomfort; impairment of perception or cognition, neuromuscular activity, and musculoskeletal function; and depression or severe anxiety
Toileting self-care deficit: A state in which an individual experiences an impaired ability to perform or complete toileting activities for self	Unable to get to toilet or commode, sit on or rise from toilet or commode, manipulate clothing for toileting, carry out proper toilet hygiene, or flush toilet or commode	Impaired transfer ability and mobility status; intolerance to activity; decreased strength and endurance; pain and discomfort; impairment of perception or cognition, neuromuscular activity, and musculoskeletal function; and depression or severe anxiety

North American Nursing Diagnosis Association. (2009–2011). © 2009, 2007, 2005, 2003, 2001, 1998, 1996, 1994 NANDA International. Used by arrangement with Wiley-Blackwell Publishing, a company of John Wiley & Sons, Inc.

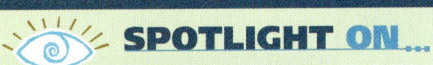

SPOTLIGHT ON...

Caring and Compassion

Self-Care Deficits

Imagine that you are unable to feed yourself, you cannot dress yourself, and you are incontinent and must rely on others to clean you. You are completely dependent on caregivers since you have no family or friends to assist you. How do you feel about being dependent on caregivers to meet your basic needs? What happens if the caregivers do not respond when you ask for help? How do you feel when others make decisions for you?

OUTCOME IDENTIFICATION AND PLANNING

The primary nursing goal is to provide safe care through the identification of actual or potential hazards and the implementation of safety measures. The assessment data are reviewed with the client, and the nurse records the areas in which the client indicates a need for change and health teaching, for example, age-related exercise or maintaining a safe environment. These findings are incorporated into the plan of care, reflecting the individualized needs of each client.

During the planning phase, the nurse collaborates with the client and other health care providers to determine the goals, outcomes, and interventions and manipulates the external environment to reduce the risk of injury and infection. Identified outcomes provide direction for the nursing care that is implemented to reduce the risk of injury and infection.

Another critical element of the care plan is client/caregiver education related to the identification of potential hazards and health promotion practices. The nursing care plan should include safety measures that educate clients about preventive actions and modification of an unsafe environment, for example, proper use of a call light or the side effects of medications.

Table 29-3 on page 672 discusses the basic components of care planning and measurements for clients at risk of or with a self-care deficit. Sample statements of goals are included in the table. The nursing interventions are statements taken from the Nursing Intervention Classification system. For each of these nursing interventions, there are specific actions taken by the nurse to individualize the care for each client. The nurse could use Gordon's Functional Health Patterns to plan care. These may be used for clients at risk of or with a self-care deficit, including health perception–health management; activity-exercise pattern; and cognitive-perceptual pattern. Nursing actions are discussed in detail in the following section.

IMPLEMENTATION

Nursing care implemented for clients with alterations in health perception–health management or activity and exercise involves continual assessment of client health risks and prioritization of risk reduction nursing interventions, such as:

- Administration of prescribed medications (see Chapter 30)
- Provision of balanced nutritional intake (see Chapter 34)
- Promotion of adequate rest and exercise (see Chapters 35 and 36)
- Decreasing the spread of infection

Implementation of safety measures may require an alteration in the physical environment as directed by the fall prevention protocol or Standard Precautions; see Table 29-4 on page 674. Chapter 36 provides additional information on fall prevention.

Nursing measures to counter common physical hazards that impair environmental safety are maintaining electric beds in the low position with side rails up and call light within easy reach and keeping the bedroom and bathroom uncluttered to prevent falls. Some states consider side rails a form of restraint. Nurses must be knowledgeable about statutory provisions relative to health care in their state.

The implementation of Standard Precautions is the most effective nursing measure to prevent and control the spread of infections. Standard Precautions are discussed in detail later in this chapter.

RAISE SAFETY AWARENESS AND KNOWLEDGE

Nurses in all settings must demonstrate an awareness of safety hazards and teach clients accordingly. Clients must be aware of and knowledgeable about safety precautions in order to prevent injuries. Clients may also need specific safety information on oxygen, IV equipment, use of heating devices, and automatic bed controls.

A Food and Drug Administration (FDA) safety alert addressed entrapment hazards with side rails on hospital beds. The FDA received 102 reports of head and body entrapment incidents that resulted in 68 deaths, 22 injuries, and 12 entrapments without injury that occurred in hospitals, long-term care facilities, and private homes. All reported that entrapments occurred in one of the four ways identified in Figure 29-4 on page 673.

PREVENT FALLS

Falls occur among clients who are weak, fatigued, uncoordinated, paralyzed, confused, or disoriented. Since falls are often due to more than one cause, no single intervention will prevent all clients from falling (Ferris, 2008). Capezuti and colleagues (2008) studied the difference between lower leg length of frail nursing home clients and the height of the toilets and beds in the lowest position and found that bed and toilet height was greater than the clients' lower leg lengths, thereby increasing the risk for falls. Tinetti and associates (2008) studied the utilization of fall prevention tools and

TABLE 29-3 **Planning the Care of Clients at Risk for Injury or Infection and/or with a Self-Care Deficit**

NURSING DIAGNOSIS AND DEFINITION	GOALS	NURSING OUTCOMES	NURSING INTERVENTIONS
Risk for injury	1. The client will identify factors that increase the potential for injury. 2. The client will remain free of bodily injury.	• Safe home environment: Physical arrangements to minimize environmental factors that might cause physical harm or injury in the home	• Risk identification: Analysis of potential risk factors, determination of health risks, and prioritization of risk reduction strategies for an individual • Fall prevention: Instituting special precautions with client at risk for injury
Risk for infection	1. The client will remain free of health care–associated infections. 2. The client will reduce exposure to known infectious agents.	• Infection severity: Severity of infection and associated symptoms	• Infection protection: Prevention and early detection of infection in a client at risk • Infection control: Minimizing the acquisition and transmission of infectious agents
Bathing/hygiene self-care deficit	1. The client will maintain an optimum functional level of hygienic practices in a safe and an effective manner. 2. The client's skin will remain clean and intact.	• Self-care: Bathing: Ability to cleanse own body independently with or without assistive device • Self-care: Hygiene: Ability to maintain own personal cleanliness and kempt appearance independently with or without assistive device	• Bathing: Cleaning of the body for the purpose of relaxation, cleanliness, and healing • Dressing: choosing, putting on, and removing clothes for a person who cannot do this for self • Skin surveillance: Collection and analysis of client data to maintain skin and mucous membrane integrity • Perineal care: Maintenance of perineal skin integrity and relief of perineal discomfort
Deficient knowledge: related to health hazard	The client will not sustain injuries.	• Risk control: Personal actions to prevent, eliminate, or reduce modifiable health threats	• Teaching, individualized: Planning, implementation, and evaluation of a teaching program designed to address a client's particular needs

Moorhead, S., Johnson, M., & Maas, M. (Eds.). (2008). *Nursing outcomes classification (NOC)* (4th ed.). St. Louis, MO: Elsevier Health Sciences; McCloskey Dochterman, J. C., & Bulechek, G. M. (Eds.). (2008). *Nursing interventions classification (NIC)* (5th ed.). St. Louis, MO: Elsevier Health Sciences.

found that dissemination of evidence about fall prevention, coupled with interventions to change clinical practice, may reduce fall-related injuries in elderly clients. The data obtained from the client's fall risk appraisal will identify which clients require special nursing measures to prevent falls. The risk for falls can be reduced by:

- Good supervision
- Orienting clients to the environment and call system
- Providing ambulatory aids (wheelchairs or walkers)
- Placing personal belongings on tables near the bed
- Keeping hospital beds in lowest position with side rails up
- Using nonslip mats and rugs
- Illuminating the environment

Although falls do not necessarily constitute malpractice, they are a major reason nurses are involved in lawsuits.

Restraints

Restraints are protective devices used to limit the physical activity of a client or to immobilize a client or extremity. They are used to protect the client, allow for treatment in a safe environment, and reduce the risk of injury to others.

The use of restraints has become very controversial because of resultant client injuries. The Omnibus Budget Reconciliation Act of 1987 and the Health Care Financing Administration regulations of 1999 governing clients' rights are forcing a reexamination of how clients are cared for in acute and critical care settings. In response to more individualized care regarding the use of restraints, the Joint Commission revised its standards for restraint use with nonpsychiatric clients; see the accompanying display on Joint Commission–revised standards on page 675.

Nurses must document, according to the institutional protocol, the application and care of the client in restraints (see the accompanying display on restraints). Refer to Chapter 12 for additional information regarding the use of restraints and their legal implications.

Restraints used to either limit physical activity or immobilize a client can be physical or chemical. **Physical restraints**

reduce the client's movement through the application of a device. Most states require a prescribing practitioner's order for the application of physical restraints. **Chemical restraints** are medications used to control the client's behavior. Commonly used chemical restraints are anxiolytics and sedatives.

This chapter limits discussion to the common types of physical restraints:

- Jacket (body restraint): A sleeveless vest with straps that cross in front or back of the client and are tied to the bed frame or chair legs (see Figure 29-5A on page 676).
- Belt: Straps or belts applied across the client to secure him or her to the stretcher, bed, or wheelchair (see Figure 29-5B).
- Mitten or hand: Enclosed cloth material applied over the client's hand to prevent injury from scratching (see Figure 29-5C).
- Elbow: A combination of fabric and plastic or wooden tongue blades that immobilize the elbow to prevent flexion (see Figure 29-5D).
- Limb or extremity: Cloth devices that immobilize one or all limbs by securely tying the restraint to the bed frame or chair (see Figure 29-5E).
- Mummy: A blanket or sheet that is folded around the child to limit movement. Mummy restraints are used to perform procedures on children (see Figure 29-5F).

KEY ELEMENTS OF RESTRAINT DOCUMENTATION

- Reason for the restraint
- Method of restraint
- Application: Date, time, and client's response
- Duration
- Frequency of observation and client's response
- Safety: Release from restraint with periodic, routine exercise and assessment for circulation and skin integrity
- Assessment of the continued need for restraint
- Client outcome

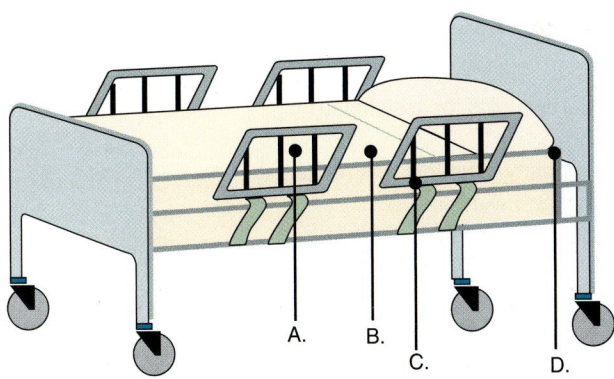

FIGURE 29-4 Entrapment hazards with hospital bedside rails. A. Through the bars of an individual side rail; B. through the space between split side rails; C. between the side rail and mattress; or D. between the headboard or footboard, side rail, and mattress. FROM FOOD AND DRUG ADMINISTRATION, *SAFETY ALERT*, AUGUST 23, 1995.

▼ SAFETY FIRST ▼

RESTRAINTS
Jacket or belt restraints should not restrict respiratory effort. Placing a restraint too tight on the diaphragm will inhibit the expansion of the lungs.

TABLE 29-4 Adult Fall Prevention Protocol

Purpose	To direct the nursing management of the client at risk for falls
Level	Interdependent nursing function
Supportive Data	Assessment of risk factors from falls and/or a history of falls is a prerequisite of intervention. Risk factors for falls include age, dizziness, confusion, use of medications (prescribed and over the counter), and physical or mental alterations. Fall prevention is used to increase staff awareness of clients at risk for falls and to provide preventive safety measures.

Content

Assessment	1. Perform client injury risk appraisal and identify fall risks. Update status of fall risks daily and as needed on nursing care plan. 2. Perform a balance and gait screening on those clients who report a single fall. 3. Assess effects of medications administered that increase risk of falling. 4. Implement institution's fall prevention program.
Report to prescribing practitioner	5. Notify prescribing practitioner of previous fall history and identify risk factors for a fall. 6. Notify prescribing practitioner of adverse effects of medications that may increase the client's risk of falling.
Client teaching	7. Orient client to environmental surroundings on admission and as necessary. 8. Instruct client and significant others on safety measures. 9. Instruct client and significant others on correct use of hospital equipment. 10. Instruct client with risk for falls to call for assistance when ambulating or performing activities of daily living (ADL).
Environmental interventions	11. Install an electronic sensing device on beds that measures and signals when a client shifts to a rising position. 12. Keep bed in lowest position, brakes locked, and side rails up. 13. Keep call light and frequently used objects within easy reach at the bedside. 14. Keep environment clean and clutter free. 15. Provide adequate lighting at all times. 16. Lock wheels on wheelchair, bed, and stretcher at all times. 17. Provide nonslip footwear, mats, and rugs. 18. Keep hospital furniture in the same place throughout hospital stay. 19. Provide call cord in bathroom. 20. Encourage use of handrails in bathroom and hallways. 21. Provide nonslip mats in the tub or shower. 22. Place high-risk clients in a room near the nurses' station. 23. Request an environment assessment of the older client's home by a qualified professional prior to discharge.
Direct nursing care	24. Respond promptly to call lights and verbal requests for assistance. 25. Provide assistance with ADL. 26. Maintain close supervision by performing hourly safety assessments. 27. Encourage significant others to stay with high-risk clients. 28. Provide proper equipment for ambulation and elimination needs. 29. Communicate client's injury risk status in shift report.
Evaluation	30. Evaluate client's knowledge of safety measures. 31. Evaluate effectiveness of environmental interventions. 32. Evaluate changes in client's injury risk status. 33. Evaluate effectiveness of direct nursing care. 34. Provide focused training based on each incident.

(Continues)

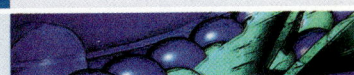

TABLE 29-4 (Continued)

Documentation	35. Document the following in the client's medical record:
	a. Assessment of client's injury risk status
	b. Nursing plan of care
	c. Safety measures implemented
	d. Client education performed
	e. Client outcomes

Adapted from American Geriatrics Society (2001). *Guidelines for the prevention of falls in older persons*, *49*, 664–672; Farmer, B. (2003). Try this: Best practices in nursing care of older adults. *Dermatology Nursing, 15*(4), 375–376; Jackson, L., & Gleason, J. (2004). Proactive management breaks the fall cycle. *Nursing Management, 35*(6), 37–38.

JOINT COMMISSION RESTRAINT STANDARDS FOR NONPSYCHIATRIC CLIENTS

ORGANIZATIONAL PERSPECTIVE

- Design a system to achieve a restraint-free environment.

POLICIES/PROCEDURES/PROTOCOLS

- Clients are allowed to refuse restraints.
- Informed consent is obtained.

PREVENTIVE STRATEGIES

- Alternative treatments are not effective.
- It is absolutely necessary to ensure safety.

PLAN OF CARE

- Individualized, and ensure client's assessed needs are met.
- Preserve client's rights, dignity, and well-being.

EDUCATION

- Is ongoing for staff and client.
- Is provided to families when appropriate.

INITIATION AND MONITORING OF RESTRAINT USE

- Based on state law.
- Initiated on individual orders of a licensed independent practitioner.
- Applied/monitored/assessed/reassessed by qualified staff.
- Time limitations are predetermined.
- Restraints are periodically removed or released.
- Orders are reviewed as defined by the organization, not to exceed 30 days.
- Medication to control behavior is part of the therapeutic plan.

DOCUMENTATION

- Includes all restraint episodes according to organizational policies and procedures.
- Occurs, at a minimum, every 2 hours.
- Indicates that alternatives were tried before restraints were applied.
- Is entered into the client's medical record.

Joint Commission. (2008). *Provisions of care, treatment, and services*. Retrieved September 22, 2008, from http://www.jointcommission.org/NR/rdonlyres.

The nursing plan of care should include safety measures to reduce the potential for injury from restraints (see Procedure 29-1 on pages 695–699). Additional safety measures to observe when using restraint devices:

- Restraints can be changed and released easily, using only a clove hitch knot (see Figures 29-6 and 29-7 on page 677).
- Restraints should not interfere with any treatments (e.g., IV therapy) or aggravate the client's health problem.

- There should be enough slack on the straps so that the client can move both arms and legs and for range-of-motion exercises.
- At least once every 2 hours, the nurse must perform circulation and neurological exams, assessing the color, sensation, temperature, motion, and capillary refill in the area distal to the restraint.
- There should be a provision for psychological support of client and significant others.

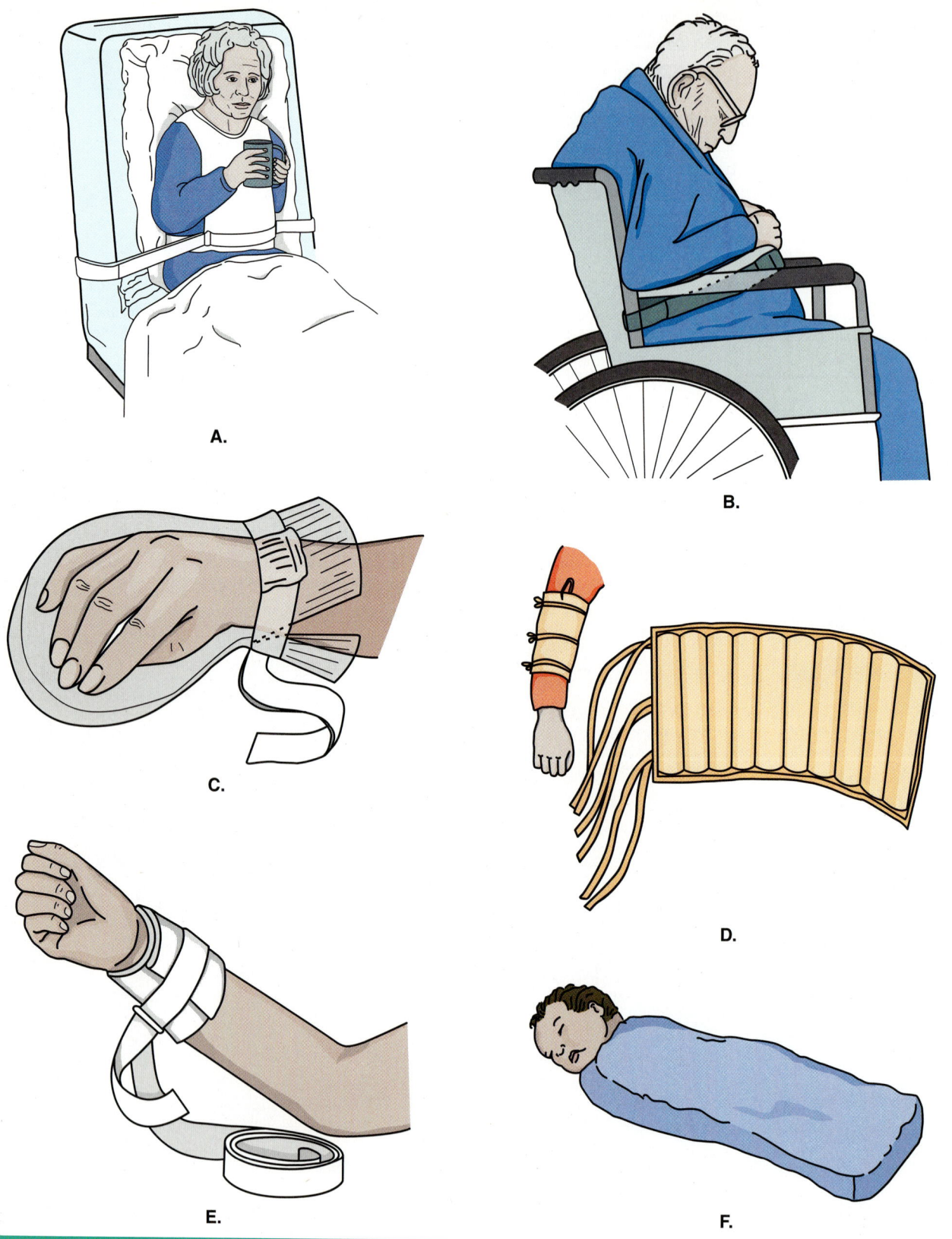

FIGURE 29-5 Types of Physical Restraints: A. Jacket; B. Belt; C. Mitten or Hand; D. Elbow; E. Limb or Extremity; and F. Mummy.

DELMAR/CENGAGE LEARNING

Figures 29-6 and 29-7 demonstrate how to make a clove hitch knot used in applying restraints. Note how the clove hitch restraint, made from a strip of gauze, does not tighten when force is applied against it. The restraint strap is secured to the bed frame, *not to the side rail*, so as to avoid accidental injury to the extremity in the event that the side rail is released while the restraint strap is attached to it.

Environment

Adequate lighting assists in the visualization of environmental hazards. Rooms should be adequately lit so the client can safely perform ADL and health care providers can perform procedures. Lighting can be supplemented by lamps and night-lights. It can also assist in protecting the home against crime.

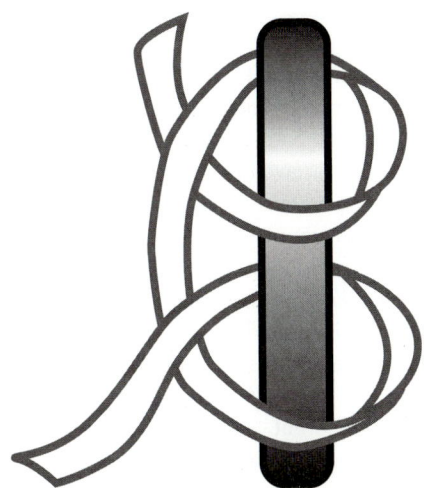

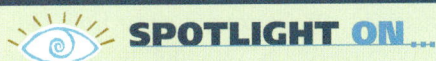

FIGURE 29-6 **Clove Hitch Knot** DELMAR/CENGAGE LEARNING

☁ SPOTLIGHT ON...

Caring and Compassion

Use of Restraints

Gloria Hernandez is an 83-year-old widow who fractured her hip when she fell in the bathtub. She had hip replacement surgery yesterday. Tonight she is very confused and is trying to dislodge the bandage and stitches. Mrs. Hernandez is now being restrained for protection. What other nursing activities could have been implemented prior to the use of restraints? Do you think that restraints will affect Mrs. Hernandez's mental status? If so, in what ways? What are some other effects Mrs. Hernandez may experience as a result of being restrained? How would you feel about the use of restraints if Mrs. Hernandez were your grandmother?

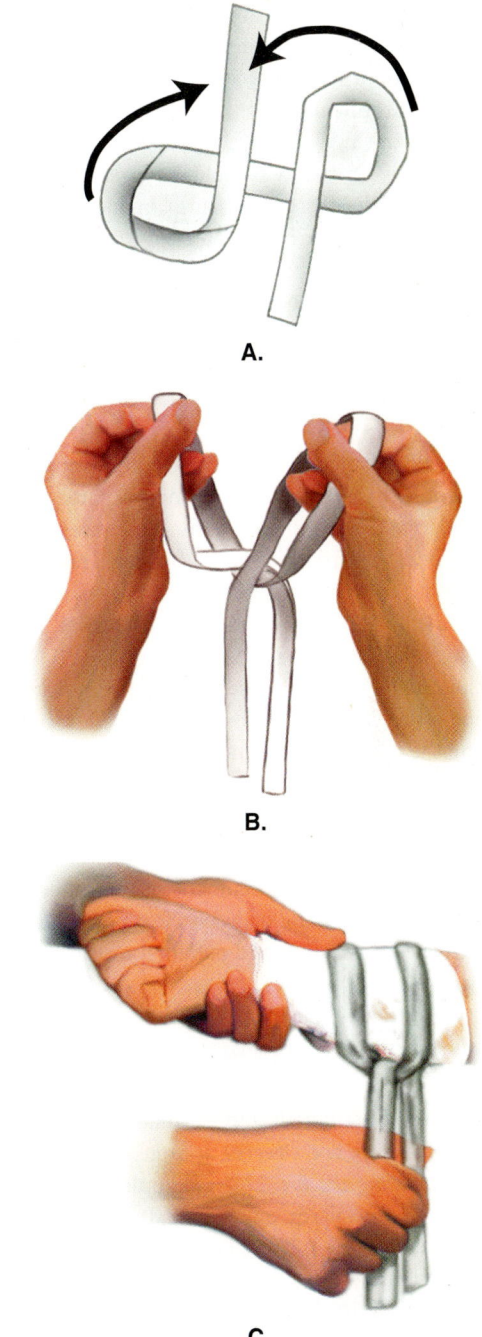

FIGURE 29-7 **Making a Clove Hitch Knot: A. Make a figure-eight; B. Pick up the loops; and C. Put the limb through the loops and secure.** DELMAR/CENGAGE LEARNING

Obstacles in heavily traveled areas of health care facilities or homes are a risk to the client's safety. Older adults or persons who are unfamiliar with the environment are at greatest risk of injury from obstacles. The risk that obstacles pose can be reduced by keeping hallways clear, removing excess furniture from heavily traveled areas, removing all electrical cords or taping them securely to the floor, removing throw rugs, applying nonslip pads to rugs, cleaning up spills immediately, and removing objects that could fall from the tops of appliances.

Bathrooms pose a threat to the client in the home because of the presence of water and storage of medication. Common bathroom accidents are falls, scalds or burns, and poisonings. Bathroom accidents can be reduced by the use of grab bars near the tub, shower, and toilet; nonslip mats in the tub and shower; and a secured bathroom rug near the tub or shower. Other safety measures include checking the temperature of the water before entering the tub or shower; checking the thermostat setting on the water heater; and storing medications in a locked cabinet, out of reach of children or disoriented or confused adults.

PREVENT FIRE

Fire is a potential danger to all people in an institutional or a home environment. Immobilized or incapacitated clients are at increased risk during a fire. Common causes of fire are smoking in bed, discarding cigarette butts in trash cans, and faulty electrical equipment. Fire occurs with the interaction of three elements: sufficient heat to ignite the fire, combustible material, and oxygen to support the fire.

Nursing goals are fire prevention and protection of clients during a fire. Nursing interventions aimed at preventing or reducing the risk of fire include:

- Clearly marking fire exits
- Knowing locations of fire extinguishers and their operation
- Practicing fire evacuation procedures
- Posting emergency phone numbers by all telephones
- Keeping open spaces and hallways clear of clutter
- Checking electrical cords and outlets for exposed or damaged wires
- Reporting identified electrical hazards
- Educating clients about fire hazards

In the event of a fire, follow institutional policy and procedures for fire containment and evacuation. Nursing interventions during a fire are directed at *protecting the client from injury and containing the fire.* Nurses should be familiar with the locations of fire alarm pull boxes. If a fire occurs, the nurse should utilize the nearest fire box for notification and move clients to safety.

Nurses should be familiar with the use of fire extinguishers and their locations. The fire extinguisher should be directed toward the base of the fire. The four types of fire extinguishers used are water, carbon dioxide, regular dry chemical, and multipurpose dry chemical. Each type of fire extinguisher is used for a specific class of fire, as discussed in Table 29-5.

ENSURE SAFE OPERATION OF ELECTRICAL EQUIPMENT

Clients have contact with a variety of electrical equipment in the hospital environment, such as bed controls and IV and client-controlled analgesia pumps. All electrical equipment should have a three-pronged electrical plug that is grounded. A grounded plug transmits any stray electrical current from equipment to the ground. To protect the client from electri-

TABLE 29-5 Fire Extinguishers

TYPE	CLASS OF FIRE
Water (Type A)	Paper, wood, draperies, upholstery, or rubbish
Carbon dioxide or dry chemical (Types B and C)	Flammable liquids, flammable gases, or electrical fires
Multipurpose dry chemical (Types A, B, and C)	Any type of fire

Delmar/Cengage Learning

cal injury, the nurse should read the warning labels on all equipment, use only grounded electrical equipment, check for frayed electrical cords, avoid overloading circuits, and report any shocks received from equipment to the biomedical department (see Figure 29-8).

If a client receives an electrical shock, the nurse should turn off or remove the electric source before touching the client. Then, the client's pulse should be checked. If the client has no pulse, CPR should be initiated. If the client has a pulse, the nurse should assess vital signs, mental status, and skin integrity for burns. A prescribing practitioner should be notified of the event. The nurse should note points of entry and exit of electrical current to assess for potential complications.

REDUCE EXPOSURE TO RADIATION

Clients are exposed to radiation during diagnostic testing and therapeutic interventions. Injury can occur from radiation if there is overexposure or exposure to untargeted tissues. Exposure to untargeted tissues can occur with radiation implants that become dislodged. General principles of

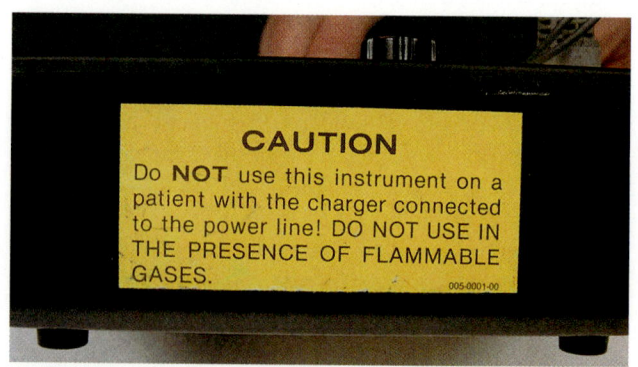

FIGURE 29-8 Warning Label on Electrical Equipment DELMAR/
CENGAGE LEARNING

radiation exposure and protection are based on time, distance, and shielding. Protection from radiation therapy includes:

- Minimizing time in contact with radiation source (implants or client)
- Maximizing distance from radiation source (implants or client)
- Using appropriate radiation shields
- Monitoring radiation exposure with a film badge
- Labeling all potentially radioactive material
- Never touching dislodged implants or body fluids of client

Both the client and the nurse are at risk for radiation injury. The client's risk for injury can be reduced by education about radiation treatment and necessary precautions, placing the client in a private room, and providing a lead apron when necessary to protect nontargeted body tissues. The nurse's risk for injury can be reduced by observing all radioactive labels, wearing gloves when handling radioactive body discharges, washing hands, wearing a lead apron, disposing of radioactive substances in special containers, reducing time of client contact, and wearing a badge that measures the amount of radiation exposure.

PREVENT POISONING

A poison is any substance that causes an alteration in the client's health, such as injury or death, when inhaled, injected, ingested, or absorbed by the body. Antidotes and treatments are available for some but not all types of poisonings. Direct and indirect causes of poisonings are:

- Inadequate supervision of children
- Ingestion of household plants
- Improper storage of toxic substances
- Insect or snake bites
- Accidental ingestion of a toxic substance or medication overdose

The poison control center should be notified when poisoning is suspected. The person reporting the poisoning should be prepared to state the amount and type of poison ingested, inhaled, or injected; the client's age; and the symptoms. Clients who have ingested poison should be turned on their side to prevent aspiration while awaiting further treatment. Client education about safety measures can prevent some accidental poisonings. The following Client Teaching Checklist provides some safety measures to prevent accidental poisoning. Keep syrup of ipecac available at all times.

REDUCE NOISE POLLUTION

Noise pollution, a situation that results when the noise level becomes uncomfortable for the client or staff, frequently occurs in the health care setting as a result of visitor traffic, medical equipment, and personnel. It can result in a disorganized environment, hearing loss, and sensory overload. Sensory overload is an increased perception of the intensity of auditory and visual stimuli. Sensory overload can alter a client's recovery by increasing anxiety, paranoia, hallucinations, and depression. Safety measures include maintaining a quiet

environment, controlling traffic, and providing earplugs. Taylor-Ford, Catlin, LaPlante, and Weinke (2008) conducted a study regarding sound levels in a hospital and concluded that the use of sound-absorbing materials in the hospital's physical structure may be the most effective measure in reducing sound levels. See Chapter 38 for a discussion of sensory overload.

ENSURE ASEPSIS

Nurses are responsible for providing the client with a safe environment, which includes preventing the transmission of HAIs. Asepsis is the absence of microorganisms. Providing nursing care using aseptic technique decreases the risk and spread of HAIs. Aseptic technique is the infection control practice used to prevent the transmission of pathogens. Two types of asepsis are medical and surgical.

Medical Asepsis

Medical asepsis uses practices to reduce the number, growth, and spread of microorganisms. Medical asepsis is also referred to as "clean technique." Objects are generally referred to as "clean" or "dirty" in medical asepsis. Clean objects are considered to have the presence of some microorganisms that are usually not pathogenic. Dirty (soiled) objects are considered to have a high number of microorganisms, with some that are potentially pathogenic. Common medical aseptic measures used for clean or dirty objects are handwashing, gloves, changing linens daily, and cleaning floors and hospital furniture daily.

HAND HYGIENE   The CDC (2002) published new handwashing guidelines: *Hand Hygiene in Health-Care Settings: Recommendations of the Healthcare Infection Control Practice Advisory Committee and the HICPAC/SHEA/APIC/IDSA Hand Hygiene Task Force*. These guidelines provide new terminology and definitions:

✔ CLIENT TEACHING CHECKLIST

SAFETY MEASURES TO PREVENT ACCIDENTAL POISONINGS

- Store medications in child-resistant containers.
- Do not take medications in front of children.
- Never call medicine candy.
- Limit the number of tablets in a medicine container.
- Place toxic substances in a locked cabinet out of reach of children.
- Never remove labels from containers.
- Do not place poisonous substances in food or beverage containers.
- Place poison stickers on toxic substances.
- Display poison control center phone numbers near telephones.

- **Hand hygiene.** "A general term that applies to either handwashing, antiseptic handwash, antiseptic hand rub, or surgical hand antisepsis" (CDC, 2002, p. 4).
- **Handwashing.** "Washing hands with plain (i.e., nonantimicrobial) soap and water" (CDC, 2002, p. 4).
- **Antiseptic handwash.** "Washing hands with water and soap or other detergents containing an antiseptic agent" (CDC, 2002, p. 4).
- **Antiseptic hand rub.** "Applying an antiseptic hand rub product to all surfaces of the hands to reduce the number of microorganisms" (CDC, 2002, p. 4).
- **Surgical hand antisepsis.** "Antiseptic handwash or antiseptic hand rub performed preoperatively by surgical personnel to eliminate transient and reduce resident hand flora. Antiseptic detergent preparations often have persistent antimicrobial activity" (CDC, 2002, p. 4).

The CDC guidelines are evidenced based, with more than 230 references and research studies (see the accompanying Safety First display for a summary of these guidelines). The report stresses the common mode of transmission of health care–associated pathogens from frequently colonized areas of normal intact skin with such bacteria as *Staphylococcus aureus* and *Klebsiella*. These organisms are identified during activities such as lifting the client; taking a pulse, blood pressure, or oral temperature; and touching the client's hands or shoulders or an inanimate object in the room. When hands are visibly soiled, showing dirt or contaminated with proteinaceous material, blood, or other body fluids, such as fecal material or urine, the CDC recommends handwashing (see Procedure 29-2 on pages 699–701).

The Task Force reviewed clinical trails using various products for hand hygiene (alcohols, chlorhexidine, hexachlorophene, iodophors, PCMZ, and triclosan, as well as plain or antibacterial soap and water; see the accompanying display on CDC hand hygiene). The Task Force acknowledged the efficacy of alcohol-based products. Alcohol-based hand rubs reduce the number of microorganisms on the skin, are fast acting, and cause less skin irritation. Although gloves reduce hand contamination by 70% to 80%, prevent cross-contamination, and protect clients and health care providers from infection, hand hygiene is still required.

The CDC recommends evaluation of hand hygiene products based on the efficacy of antiseptic agents against various pathogens and the acceptability for usage (smell, consistency, color, and effect of dryness on hands). Accordingly, health care agencies need to develop and implement a system for measuring improvements in adherence to hand hygiene recommendations, such as periodic monitoring of personnel adherence to hand hygiene recommendations and focused assessment of the adequacy of practice when outbreaks of infection occur. Health care providers should be encouraged to report contact dermatitis due to alcohol hand rubs, although this occurrence is rare.

Surgical Asepsis

Surgical asepsis, or sterile technique, consists of those practices that eliminate all microorganisms and spores from an

▼ SAFETY FIRST ▼

CDC HAND HYGIENE
- Adhere to hand hygiene using alcohol-based hand rubs by health care personnel before and after each client encounter.
- Use handwashing for visibly soiled hands.
- Use soap and water for hand hygiene in non–health care settings.
- Use hand hygiene when wearing gloves.
- Apply an alcohol-based product to the palm of the hand and rub hands together, covering all surfaces of hands and fingers until hands are dry (the volume needed to reduce the number of bacteria on hands varies by product) after client contact.
- Avoid wearing artificial nails, and keep natural nails less than one-quarter of an inch long if providing client care.

object or area. **Spores** are single-celled microorganisms or microorganisms in the resting or inactive stage. Surgical asepsis refers to handwashing, the donning of surgical attire (caps, masks, and eyewear), the handling of sterile instruments and equipment, and establishing and maintaining sterile fields.

Surgical asepsis is practiced by the nurse in the operating room, during labor and delivery, and for many diagnostic and therapeutic interventions at the client's bedside. Common nursing procedures that require sterile technique are:

- All invasive procedures, either intentional perforation of the skin (injections, insertion of IV needles or catheters) or entry into a bodily orifice (tracheobronchial suctioning, insertion of a urinary catheter)
- Nursing measures for clients with disruption of skin surfaces (changing a surgical wound or IV site dressing) or destruction of skin layers (trauma and burns)

DONNING STERILE GLOVES There are two methods for applying sterile gloves: open and closed. The open method is used most frequently when performing procedures that require the sterile technique, such as dressing changes (see Procedure 29-3 on pages 701–705 for applying sterile gloves

▼ SAFETY FIRST ▼

HAND HYGIENE
Perform hand hygiene before and after every client contact. The most common cause of HAIs is contamination from the hands of health care providers.

by the open method). The closed method is used when the nurse wears a sterile gown.

DONNING SURGICAL ATTIRE Surgical nurses are required to wear a surgical mask and a clean cloth or paper cap that covers all of the hair. After the cap is applied, the nurse positions the mask to cover the nose and mouth (see Procedure 29-4 on pages 705–709). Protective eyewear (glasses or goggles) is worn during all procedures that pose a threat of splashing body fluids into the eyes.

SURGICAL HAND ANTISEPSIS Surgical hand antisepsis or scrub is used to remove soil and most transient microorganisms from the skin. Nurses working in the operating room perform surgical hand antisepsis to decrease the client's risk for an infection. The skin on the nurse's hands and arms should be intact (free of lesions). Agency policy determines how to perform the scrub with regard to method and timing (see Procedure 29-5 on pages 710–713 for the basic principles of performing surgical hand antisepsis).

GOWNING AND CLOSED GLOVING Nurses in the operating room and special procedure areas such as cardiac catheterization labs use the closed gloved method when donning a sterile gown. After the surgical scrub, the nurse proceeds to don the sterile gown and gloves using the closed method (see Procedure 29-6 on pages 714–716). The sterile gown serves as a barrier to decrease the risk of wound contamination. The sterile gown also allows the nurse to move freely in the environment with sterile drapes and objects.

REDUCE OR ELIMINATE INFECTIOUS AGENTS

Transmission of microorganisms to clients may also occur through contact with inanimate objects. Cleansing, disinfecting, and sterilizing can break this link in the chain of infection by reducing or destroying microorganisms on objects. Cleansing, disinfection, and sterilization are usually the responsibility of nursing, housekeeping, and central supply departments. These infection control practices can and should also be practiced in the home care setting.

Cleansing

Cleansing is the removal of soil or organic material from instruments and equipment used in providing client care. Nurses are involved in cleansing instruments after assisting in or performing an invasive procedure. Reusable objects are cleansed prior to sterilization and disinfection to reduce the amount of contamination and loosen the material on the object. Cleansing involves the use of water, mechanical action, and sometimes a detergent. Contaminated objects are cleaned using a soft-bristled brush to scrub the surface. The steps for proper cleansing are:

1. Rinse object under cold water, since warm water causes proteins in organic material to coagulate and stick.
2. Apply detergent and scrub object under running water with soft-bristled brush.
3. Rinse the object under warm water.
4. Dry the object prior to sterilization or disinfection.

Cleansing presents a potential hazard to the nurse through the splashing of contaminated material onto the body. Nurses should wear gloves, masks, and goggles during cleansing.

Disinfection

Disinfection is the elimination of pathogens, except spores, from inanimate objects. **Disinfectants** are chemical solutions used to clean inanimate objects. Bedpans, blood pressure cuffs, linens, stethoscopes, thermometers, and some types of endoscopes are disinfected in the hospital setting. The U.S. Environmental Protection Agency licenses (registers) disinfection products and monitors the products to ensure that they work as claimed on the label. Common disinfectants are alcohol, sodium hypochlorite, quaternary ammonium, phenolic solutions, and glutaraldehyde. In the home, Lysol and bleach are common disinfectants that are capable of eliminating several pathogens. A **germicide** is a chemical that can be applied to both animate and inanimate objects to eliminate pathogens. Antiseptic preparations such as alcohol and silver sulfadiazine are germicides and may be used on skin.

Sterilization

Sterilization is the total elimination of all microorganisms, including spores. Instruments that are used for invasive procedures must be sterilized. Methods of achieving sterilization are moist heat or steam, radiation, chemicals, and ethylene oxide gas. The method of sterilization depends on the type of contamination, amount of contamination, and object to be sterilized.

Autoclaving sterilization, which uses moist heat or steam, is the most common sterilization technique used in the hospital setting. Boiling water is not an effective sterilization measure, as some viruses and spores can survive boiling water. Objects that have been boiled in water for 15 to 20 minutes at 121°C (249.8°F) are considered clean but not sterilized. However, boiling water is still the best and most common sterilization measure used in the home. For example, boiling baby bottles and nipples makes them safe for use.

Home Health Care

Home care and hospice nurses are faced with significant challenges when adapting acute care infection control practice to the home care setting, such as cleaning and disinfecting equipment and using clean versus sterile technique. Common practice of home care organizations requires special practice regarding the handling of the *nursing supply bag;* see the accompanying display on page 682 on a basic nursing bag technique procedure that may be followed in the home.

Disposal of Infectious Waste

All health care facilities must have guidelines for the disposal of infectious waste materials as deemed by the OSHA Act of

NURSING SUPPLY BAG TECHNIQUE PROCEDURE

- Place the bag on a clean, dry surface.
- Wash hands with soap and running water prior to direct client contact. For MRSA or VRE clients, wash hands with antibacterial soap and running water. Cleanse hands with a waterless product if running water is not available.
- Remove the necessary supplies from the nursing bag, and place them on a clean, dry surface.
- Perform client care.
- Clean and disinfect semicritical equipment such as an oral thermometer with a 70% isopropyl alcohol prep pad, and return the equipment to the supply bag.
- Clean noncritical equipment such as a blood pressure cuff, stethoscope, or scale, if soiled, and return to the bag. If the client is infected or colonized with multidrug-resistant (MDR) bacteria, and equipment has not been designated for the client's individual use, clean and disinfect the equipment with a disinfectant of the home care or hospice organization's choice prior to replacing the noncritical items in the bag.
- Remove personal protective items such as a gown and gloves if worn.
- Wash hands with soap and running water prior to direct client contact. For MRSA or VRE clients, wash hands with antibacterial soap and running water. Cleanse hands with a waterless product if running water is not available, and wash hands with soap and running water as soon as possible.

Adapted from Friedman, M., & Rhinehart, E. (2000). Improving infection control home care: From ritual to science-based practice. *Home Healthcare Nurse, 18*(2), 99–106.

DISPOSAL OF BIOLOGICAL MATERIALS

- Laboratory wastes
- Blood, blood products, and all other body fluids
- Client care items: soiled bed linens and protection pads soiled with visible blood, urinals, and bedpans
- Disposable instruments
- Medication and soiled treatment items
- Surgical waste

1991 (see the accompanying display on the disposal of biological materials). Always observe the biological hazard symbol, and handle all infectious materials as a hazard. OSHA regulations mandate that "immediately after use, sharps shall be disposed of in closable, puncture-resistant, disposable containers that are leakproof on the sides and bottom and are labeled or color coded." Dispose of soiled and infectious items in the home; do not place in car to dispose elsewhere.

When disposing of infectious waste:

- Wear gloves.
- Use the proper containers (red or one labeled with the biological hazard symbol as required by the facility); leakproof plastic bags for waste from client areas (soiled dressings, gloves, linens); and sharps containers for needles, scalpels, and other sharp instruments or devices (see Figure 29-9 on page 683).
- Ensure that all infectious waste is properly labeled.
- Use care when handling plastic bags to avoid punctures and tearing.
- Disinfect carts used to carry infectious waste.
- Dispose of waste in designated areas only.
- Wash hands after disposing of hazardous materials.

Containers for contaminated sharps should be readily accessible to personnel and maintained in an upright position.

Sharps-Related Hazards

The Needlestick Safety and Prevention Act of 2000 and the 2001 revised OSHA Bloodborne Pathogens Standards (BPS) require implementation of safety-engineered sharp devices. Although these mandates require institutions to convert to safety products, sharps-related hazards to health care workers persist. According to a study conducted by the American Nurses Association (ANA) regarding workplace safety and needlestick injuries, nurses stated that needlestick injuries and bloodborne infections remain major concerns. The study also revealed that 55% of the nurses experienced needlestick injuries from needles contaminated by blood or body fluids (ANA, 2008). The CDC estimates that 384,325 health care workers are injured annually by needles and other sharps. Of these injuries, about 44% are sustained by nurses, according to Exposure Prevention Information Network (EPINet) data for 2001. The EPINet is a computer-based sharps injury surveillance program that provides for agencies to track injuries by individual departments such as the operating room. Health care workers can file

▼ SAFETY FIRST ▼

NEEDLE DISPOSAL
Used needles should not be recapped, bent, or broken. Needles should be placed in a puncture-resistant marked or color-coded container close to the work site. Correct disposal decreases the risk of needle punctures to caregivers.

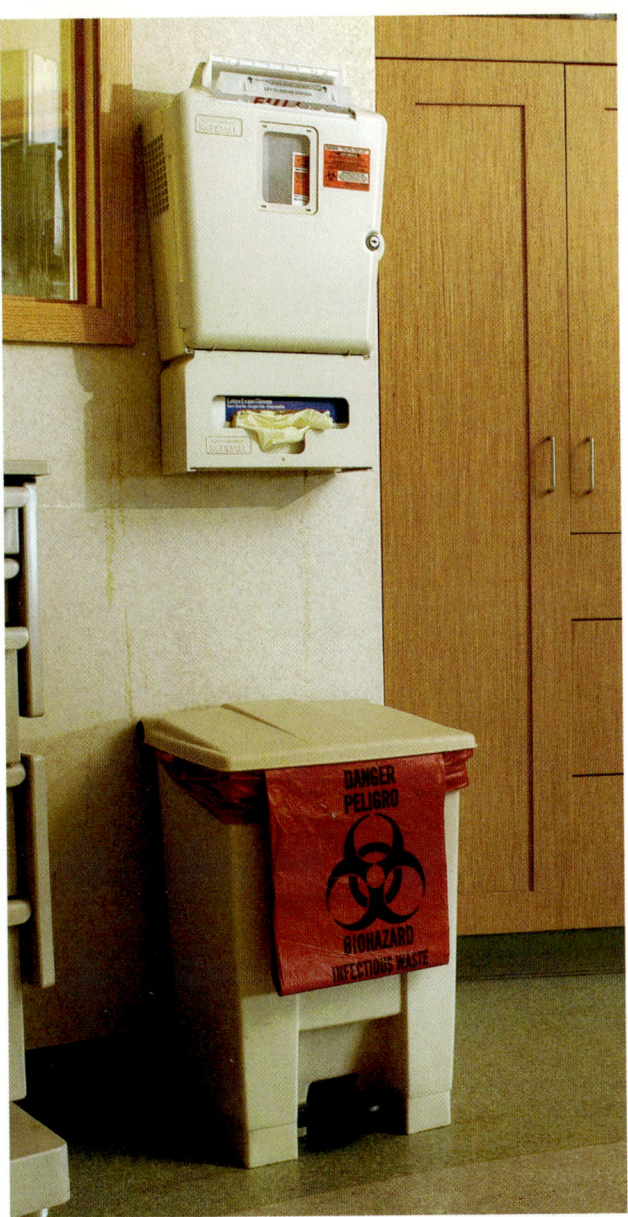

FIGURE 29-9 Sharps Disposal and Infectious Waste Containers
DELMAR/CENGAGE LEARNING

complaints regarding the violation of either the Occupational Safety and Health Act or the BPS with OSHA (see http://www.osha.gov/as/opa/worker/complain.html).

PRACTICE STANDARD AND ISOLATION PRECAUTIONS

In 2007 the CDC issued revised isolation guidelines that contain a two-tiered approach established in the 1996 guidelines. The first tier is Standard Precautions (see Front Page). Standard Precautions include a group of infection prevention practices that are based on the assumption that every person is potentially infected or colonized with an organism that could be transmitted in the health care setting. These practices include hand hygiene; personal protective equipment (PPE), which is the use of gloves, gown, mask, eye protec-

tion, or face shield, depending on the anticipated exposure; and safe injection practices. Items or equipment in the client's environment that may have been contaminated with infectious body fluids must be handled in a manner to prevent transmission of infectious agents. Three new practices were added to the revised 2007 guidelines that focus on protection of clients: respiratory hygiene/cough etiquette; safe infection practices; and use of masks for insertion of catheters or injections of material into spinal or epidural spaces through lumbar puncture procedures. The safe injection practices apply to the use of needles, cannulas that replace needles, and, where applicable, IV delivery systems.

The Transmission-Based Precautions are the second tier of the CDC's revised guidelines. These guidelines are used when the route of transmission is not completely interrupted using the Standard Precautions. There are three categories of Transmission-Based Precautions: contact, droplet, and airborne transmission (see Figure 29-10A–C on pages 684-686). Transmission-based precautions are to be used for specific syndromes that are highly suspicious for infections until a diagnosis is confirmed (see Table 29-6 on page 687). Immunosuppressed clients require transmission-based precautions, as described in Table 29-6.

Nurses use isolation precautions to protect the host's normal defense mechanisms by preventing the transmission of pathogens (HAIs). Isolation precautions include barrier protection that breaks the chain of infection.

When the nurse cares for a client in isolation, additional precautions are used along with handwashing and gloves. A mask and eye protection (or face shield) are worn to protect the mucous membranes of the eyes, nose, and mouth during interventions that are likely to produce splashes or sprays of blood, body fluids, secretions, and excretions. A nonsterile gown is also worn to protect the skin and clothing against splashes or sprays.

Nurses caring for clients with TB (an infectious disease caused by the tubercle bacillus *Mycobacterium tuberculosis*) are required to wear special masks since transmission occurs between individuals through respiratory contact. There are two types of TB masks: the high-efficiency particulate air (HEPA) mask used for suspected or confirmed MDR TB and the disposable submicrometer mask used for confirmed TB. These masks form a tight-fitting seal against particulates 1 to 5 mm.

Isolation precautions are usually ordered by the prescribing practitioner; however, nurses may initiate these precautions whenever there is a nursing diagnosis related to the infectious process, for example, *risk for infection* related to decreased resistance of the immune system. Most agencies require nurses to obtain a culture from a draining body area and to initiate isolation precautions when positive cultures are reported. Once isolation precautions have been instituted, visitors and all personnel should comply with the agency's policy regarding isolation precautions. Signs should be posted in a prominent location outside of the client's room, indicating the type of isolation precautions, preparation prior to entering the room, and necessary supplies that should be readily available.

CONTACT PRECAUTIONS

(in addition to Standard Precautions)

 **VISITORS: Report to nurse before entering.**

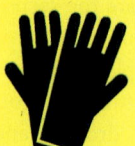

Gloves

Don gloves upon entry into the room or cubicle.
Wear gloves whenever touching the patient's intact skin or surfaces and articles in close proximity to the patient.
Remove gloves before leaving patient room.

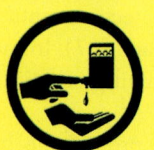

Hand Hygiene

Hand Hygiene according to Standard Precautions.

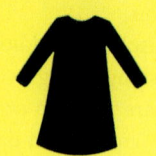

Gowns

Don gown upon entry into the room or cubicle.
Remove gown and observe hand hygiene before leaving the patient-care environment.

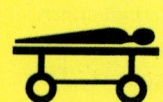

Patient Transport

Limit transport of patients to medically necessary purposes.
Ensure that infected or colonized areas of the patient's body are contained and covered.
Remove and dispose of contaminated PPE and perform hand hygiene prior to transporting patients on Contact Precautions.
Don clean PPE to handle the patient at the transport destination.

Patient–Care Equipment

Use disposable noncritical patient-care equipment or implement patient-dedicated use of such equipment.

Form No. **CPR7**   BREVIS CORP., 225 West 2855 South, SLC, UT 84115   © 2007 Brevis Corp.

FIGURE 29-10A Transmission-Based Precautions: Contact Precautions FROM BREVIS CORPORATION, 3310 S. 2700, SALT LAKE CITY, UT 84109, COPYRIGHT © 2007 BREVIS CORPORATION.

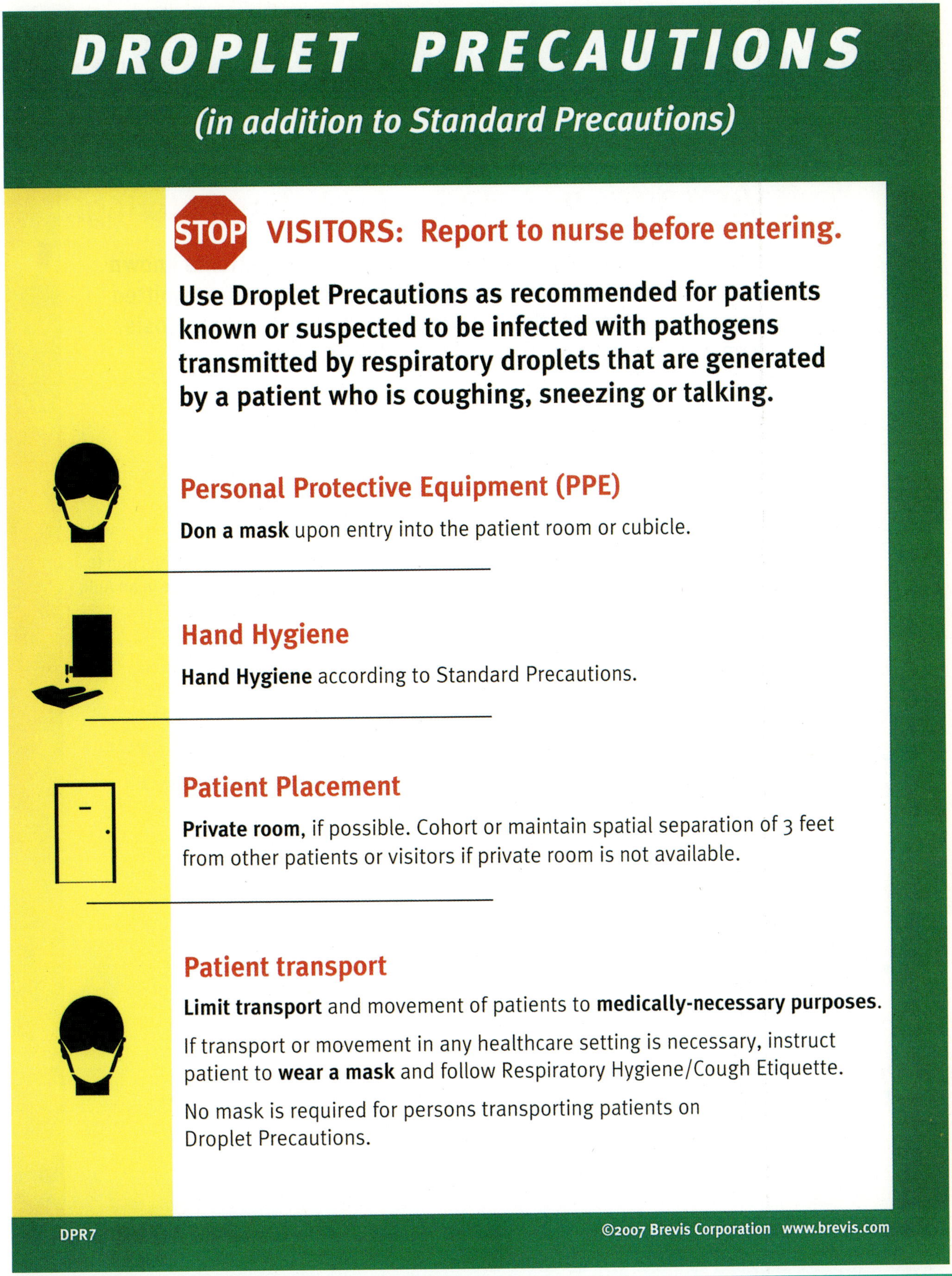

DROPLET PRECAUTIONS

(in addition to Standard Precautions)

 **VISITORS: Report to nurse before entering.**

Use Droplet Precautions as recommended for patients known or suspected to be infected with pathogens transmitted by respiratory droplets that are generated by a patient who is coughing, sneezing or talking.

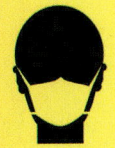

Personal Protective Equipment (PPE)

Don a mask upon entry into the patient room or cubicle.

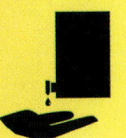

Hand Hygiene

Hand Hygiene according to Standard Precautions.

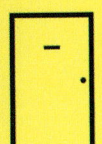

Patient Placement

Private room, if possible. Cohort or maintain spatial separation of 3 feet from other patients or visitors if private room is not available.

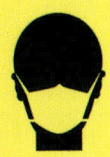

Patient transport

Limit transport and movement of patients to **medically-necessary purposes**.

If transport or movement in any healthcare setting is necessary, instruct patient to **wear a mask** and follow Respiratory Hygiene/Cough Etiquette.

No mask is required for persons transporting patients on Droplet Precautions.

DPR7

©2007 Brevis Corporation www.brevis.com

FIGURE 29-10B Transmission-Based Precautions: Droplet Precautions FROM BREVIS CORPORATION, 3310 S. 2700, SALT LAKE CITY, UT 84109, COPYRIGHT © 2007 BREVIS CORPORATION.

AIRBORNE PRECAUTIONS

(in addition to Standard Precautions)

VISITORS: Report to nurse before entering.

Use Airborne Precautions as recommended for patients known or suspected to be infected with infectious agents transmitted person-to-person by the airborne route (e.g., M. tuberculosis, measles, chickenpox, disseminated herpes zoster).

Patient placement

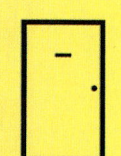

Place patients in an **AIIR** (Airborne Infection Isolation Room).
Monitor air pressure daily with visual indicators (e.g., flutter strips).

Keep door closed when not required for entry and exit.

In ambulatory settings instruct patients with a known or suspected airborne infection to wear a surgical mask and observe Respiratory Hygiene/Cough Etiquette. Once in an AIIR, the mask may be removed.

Patient transport

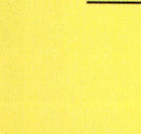

Limit transport and movement of patients to **medically-necessary purposes.**

If transport or movement outside an AIIR is necessary, instruct patients to **wear a surgical mask,** if possible, and observe Respiratory Hygiene/Cough Etiquette.

Hand Hygiene

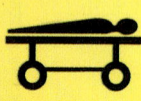

Hand Hygiene according to Standard Precautions.

Personal Protective Equipment (PPE)

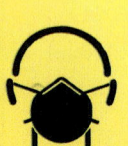

Wear a fit-tested NIOSH-approved **N95** or higher level respirator for respiratory protection when entering the room of a patient when the following diseases are suspected or confirmed: Listed on back.

APR

©2007 Brevis Corporation www.brevis.com

FIGURE 29-10C Transmission-Based Precautions: Airborne Precautions FROM BREVIS CORPORATION, 3310 S. 2700, SALT LAKE CITY, UT 84109, COPYRIGHT © 2007 BREVIS CORPORATION.

TABLE 29-6 Transmission-Based Precautions

CATEGORY	PRIVATE ROOM	GLOVES	GOWNS	MASKS
Contact precautions	If possible; cohort if not available	Required	If anticipate contact with soiled items; client is incontinent; or there is diarrhea, ileostomy, colostomy, or wound drainage	Not required
Droplet precautions	If possible; cohort or maintain separation of 3 feet	Not required	Not required	Required when within 3 feet
Airborne precautions	Required. Negative air pressure, 6–12 air changes per hour, keep door closed, discharge air outdoors or HEPA filter	Not required	Not required	N95 respirator required for known or suspected tuberculosis and measles or varicella if not immune

Delmar/Cengage Learning

Clients should be placed in a private room with adequate ventilation and have their own supplies. Personal belongings should be kept to a minimum, and health care providers should use disposable supplies and equipment. All articles leaving the room, such as soiled linens and collected specimens, should be labeled and either placed in impermeable bags or double bagged (see Procedure 29-7 on pages 718–719). Home health nurses should provide the client and family with appropriate written isolation instructions relative to the specific precautions.

Isolation precautions are for the client's protection; however, clients who are placed on isolation precautions may experience psychological discomfort (see Figure 29-11). Nurses should be alert for symptoms of anxiety, depression, rejection, guilt, or loneliness. Clients should be educated on which isolation precautions will be practiced and their purposes. Nurses should encourage clients to verbalize their feelings regarding the isolation precautions and provide clients with intellectual stimulation. Visitors should be encouraged to prevent the clients' feelings of isolation and loneliness. The Nursing Checklist lists some psychological interventions.

COMPLEMENTARY AND ALTERNATIVE THERAPIES

The ANA, in its 1995 *Social Policy Statement*, recognizes holistic, complementary, and alternative practices for the client. More and more clients are seeking alternative therapy

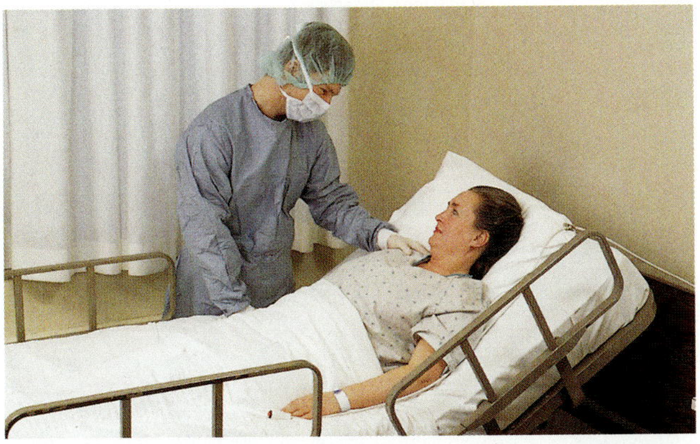

FIGURE 29-11 This nurse is interacting with a client who requires isolation precautions. Although both the client and nurse are observing isolation precautions, they are still able to communicate with one another. In planning the care of this client, what would the nursing outcomes be regarding these interventions? DELMAR/CENGAGE LEARNING

✓ NURSINGCHECKLIST

Psychological Interventions for Clients Requiring Isolation Precautions

- Explain isolation procedure and rationale.
- Discuss client's feelings about isolation procedures.
- Convey a sense of empathetic understanding.
- Permit visitors in accordance with isolation precautions.
- Support existing coping mechanisms.
- Visit with the client.

for common medical conditions, mainly chronic conditions. Hospitals are becoming more responsive to client demands by incorporating new practice models to allow the client choices and requests for alternative options as part of a holistic approach to both curing and healing. The Massachusetts and Louisiana state boards of nursing have issued statements regarding the role and scope of RN practice and holistic care.

Documentation of the client's alternative or complementary practices should be included in the health history to ensure an integration of alternative and conventional care. Nurses need to have a knowledge of herbal products and their effects to avoid possible adverse reactions when prescribed drugs are used in combination with the client's herbal regimen. A brief discussion regarding herbal baths and the use of herbs for infections is presented; see Chapter 31.

Herbal Baths

Herbal baths are a safe home method of treatment for all clients, especially infants and the elderly, and can be made just for the specific part of the body, such as the hands, hips, or feet, or can be a full body bath. A bath made from freshly grated ginger root tea stimulates circulation, alleviates aches and pains, breaks a cold, helps arthritis, and warms the body. To calm the mind and relax the body, combine equal parts of lavender, rose, chamomile, and skullcap in the bath water. To stimulate circulation and relieve fever and chills, combine equal parts bayberry bark, ginger, and prickly ash and one-fourth part cayenne pepper in the bath water. Clients using herbs in bath water for the first time should do a simple patch test to rule out a possible allergic response.

Herbs for Infections

Herbs are used in two ways for infections. Through their antimicrobial action, they work directly against microbes. They also augment and vitalize the body's own defenses. Although research may not always be available to explain exactly how herbs work, many plants have a direct toxic effect upon microbes. Common antimicrobials to combat infections safely include echinacea, eucalyptus, garlic, myrrh, nasturtium, thyme, wild indigo, and wormwood.

PROVIDE FOR CLIENT BATHING NEEDS

Bathing clients is an essential component of nursing care. Whether the nurse performs the bath or delegates the activity to another health care provider, the nurse retains the responsibility for ensuring that the hygienic needs of the client are met. The type of bath provided will depend on the purpose of the bath and the client's self-care ability. The two general categories of baths are cleaning and therapeutic.

Cleaning Baths

Cleaning baths are provided as routine client care. The purpose of a cleaning bath is personal hygiene. The five types of cleaning baths are shower, tub, self-help or assisted bed bath, complete bed bath, and partial bath.

SHOWER Most ambulatory clients are capable of taking a shower. Clients with limited physical ability can be accommodated by placing a waterproof chair in the shower (see Figure 29-12). The nurse provides minimal assistance with a shower. The Nursing Checklist, on page 689, discusses guidelines for helping clients with tub or shower baths.

TUB BATH Clients frequently prefer and enjoy tub baths. A tub bath permits washing and rinsing in the tub. Tub baths can also be therapeutic. Clients with limited physical ability should be assisted with entering and exiting the tub.

SELF-HELP BATH A self-help, or assisted, bed bath is used to provide hygienic care for clients who are confined to bed. In the self-help bed bath, the nurse prepares bath equipment but provides minimal assistance. This assistance is usually limited to washing difficult-to-reach body areas such as the feet and back.

COMPLETE BED BATH A complete bed bath is provided to dependent clients confined to bed. The nurse washes the client's entire body during a complete bed

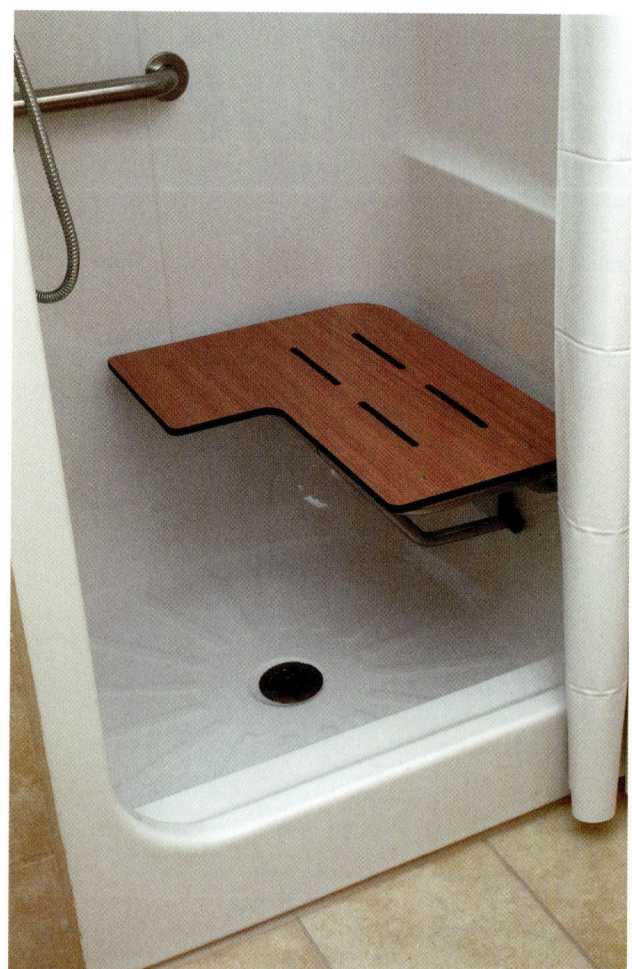

FIGURE 29-12 Shower Seat for Client Safety DELMAR/CENGAGE LEARNING

✓ NURSING CHECKLIST

Tub or Shower Bath

- Schedule use of tub or shower, and provide necessary equipment.
- Assist with ambulation to and from tub or shower.
- Place bath mat in tub or shower. Provide shower seat if necessary.
- Place "occupied" sign on door.
- Adjust room temperature and temperature of water.
- Half fill the tub with water. Do not allow the client to soak longer than 20 minutes.
- Assist the client with getting into and out of the tub or shower. Provide with a call system.
- Assist with cleaning as necessary.
- Clean tub or shower after use according to agency policy.

bath. Procedure 29-8 on pages 720–723 outlines the actions involved in giving a complete bed bath.

PARTIAL BATH A partial (or an abbreviated) bath consists of cleaning only body areas that would cause discomfort or odor if not washed thoroughly. These areas are the face, axillae, hands, and perineal area. The nurse or client may perform a partial bath depending on the client's self-care ability. Partial baths may be performed with the client lying in bed or standing at the sink.

Therapeutic Baths

Therapeutic baths require a prescribing practitioner's order stating the type of bath, temperature of water, body surface to be treated, and type of medicated solutions to use. A therapeutic bath is usually performed in a tub and lasts about 20 to 31 minutes. Therapeutic baths are classified as hot or warm water, cool or tepid water, soak, sitz, oatmeal or Aveeno, cornstarch, or sodium bicarbonate, depending on the prescribed type of bath.

Hot or warm-water tub baths are used to reduce muscle spasms, soreness, and tension; however, they have the potential for causing skin burns. Cool or tepid baths are used to relieve tension or lower body temperature. The nurse needs to prevent chilling and rapid temperature fluctuations during a cool or tepid bath.

A soak can include the entire body or can be limited to only one body part. A soak consists of applying water, with or without a medicated solution, to reduce pain, swelling, or irritation or to soften or remove dead tissue.

Sitz baths cleanse and reduce inflammation in the perineal and anal areas. They are commonly used for hemorrhoids or anal fissures and after perineal or rectal surgery. Skin irritations can be soothed with oatmeal or Aveeno, cornstarch, or sodium bicarbonate baths.

PROVIDE CLEAN BED LINENS

After a bath, clean linens are placed on the bed to promote comfort. If the client is able to get out of the bed, assist the client to a chair and proceed with making the bed. Procedure 29-9 on pages 724–728 describes the steps involved with making an unoccupied bed. After surgery, the client should be returned to a clean bed with the linens folded to the foot of the bed to promote easy client transfer.

If the client is unable to get out of the bed, refer to Procedure 29-10 on pages 729–732 for a description of the steps involved in making an occupied bed. Assistance will be needed if the client is in traction or cannot be turned. Care must be taken to avoid disturbing the traction weights. If the client cannot be turned, change the linens from head to toe. Place a waterproof drawsheet on the beds of clients who are incontinent or have profuse drainage.

PROVIDE SKIN CARE

The skin functions as a protective barrier between the internal and external environments. In addition, it functions to regulate body temperature, secrete sebum, excrete sweat, transmit sensations, and facilitate the absorption of vitamin D.

Skin care provides cleansing and conditioning to promote the optimal functioning of the skin. It consists of providing adequate nutrition, baths, perineal care, and back rubs. Excessive or abrasive skin care can damage skin and result in loss of function. Performing skin care provides an excellent opportunity for the nurse to assess skin integrity.

Perineal Care

Perineal care is the cleansing of the external genitalia, perineum, and surrounding area. Perineal care is also referred to as "peri-care" or "perineal-genital" care. The purposes of perineal care are to prevent or eliminate infection and odor, promote healing, remove secretions, and provide comfort. Perineal care can be provided alone or as part of the bed bath.

Perineal care may be an embarrassing procedure for both the client and the nurse, especially if the client is of the opposite sex. Clients who are embarrassed may elect to perform their own perineal care. In this situation, the nurse should provide the client with warm water, a moistened washcloth, soap, a dry towel, and privacy. If the client is unable to perform perineal care, the nurse is responsible for providing this care in a professional and private manner (see Procedure 29-11 on pages 732–734).

Back Rubs

Back rubs and massages stimulate the client's circulation, relax muscles, and relieve muscle tension as well as provide the nurse with an opportunity for skin assessment. Emollient creams and lotions are used to facilitate the rubbing and lubrication of the skin during a back rub or massage.

The client is positioned prone or on the side. Nurses create friction and pressure by rubbing their hands on the client's skin. The friction creates heat, which dilates the peripheral circulation and increases the blood supply to the skin. The pressure provides manual stimulation to muscle fibers, which relaxes the muscles. Chapter 31 presents the technique for performing a back rub.

Prior to performing a back rub or massage, the nurse must assess for contraindications. Caution should be exercised when massaging limbs. Massaging limbs, especially the lower limbs, could dislodge a thrombus (blood clot), creating an embolus (circulating blood clot). Bony prominences should be massaged lightly to avoid damaging underlying tissue.

PROVIDE FOOT AND NAIL CARE

Proper foot and nail care is essential for ambulation and standing. This is often ignored until problems exist. Common problems with feet and nails may be a direct result of abuse and neglect, such as from inadequate foot and nail hygiene, fingernail and cuticle biting, incorrect nail trimming, poorly fitted shoes, and exposure to harsh chemicals. These problems result in alterations of skin integrity with the potential for infection.

The first signs of foot and nail problems are usually pain or tenderness. These symptoms affect a client's posture and may result in limping with subsequent strain on certain muscle groups. Clients with illnesses such as diabetes mellitus need special foot and nail care. Clients with diabetes mellitus experience alterations in circulation that predispose them to foot problems.

The purposes of foot and nail care are to prevent infection and soft tissue trauma from ingrown or jagged nails and to eliminate odor. Hygienic care of feet and nails consists of regular trimming of nails; cleaning under nails; cleaning, rinsing, and drying feet and nails; and wearing properly fitted shoes. The Nursing Checklist discusses the specific interventions that should be taken in providing foot and nail care.

Soaking nails assists with their cleaning if they are dirty or thickened. An orangewood stick is used to clean under nails since a metal instrument can roughen the nail and cause it to harbor dirt. The safest instrument to trim nails is the nail clipper; however, some clients feel that cutting the nails makes them brittle. If the client chooses not to cut the nails, the nails should be filed straight across. Special attention should be given to drying the areas between the toes. An emollient, such as cold cream, helps keep nails and cuticles soft.

Callused areas should never be cut. Repeated soaking usually facilitates the removal of calluses. Lotion should be applied to the foot to maintain moisture and soften callused areas. If the client's feet retain excessive moisture (sweat), then water-absorbent powder should be applied between the toes.

The client should wear clean, properly fitted shoes. The fit should not be extremely tight but should be snug enough to provide support to the foot. An arch support should be in each shoe. Shoe size should be large enough so that the shoe is one-half inch longer than the longest toe. Common foot problems can often be alleviated by assessing footwear and providing proper education on footwear and foot and nail care.

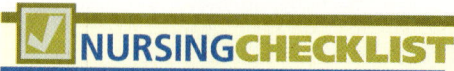

NURSINGCHECKLIST

Foot and Nail Care

- Soak feet in warm water and a detergent or in warm oil.
- Use an orangewood stick to clean the nails and release the cuticle growth from the nail.
- File or cut the nails straight across to prevent ingrown nails.
- Trim the cuticles as necessary.
- Pat all areas dry with a clean towel.
- Apply an emollient.

PROVIDE ORAL CARE

The oral cavity functions in mastication, secretion of mucus to moisten and lubricate the digestive system, secretion of digestive enzymes, and absorption of essential nutrients. Common problems occurring in the oral cavity are:

- Bad breath (**halitosis**)
- Dental caries (**cavities**)
- Plaque
- Periodontal disease (**pyorrhea**)
- Inflammation of the gums (**gingivitis**)
- Inflammation of the oral mucosa (**stomatitis**)

Poor oral hygiene and loss of teeth may affect a client's social interaction and body image as well as nutritional intake. Daily oral care is essential to maintain the integrity of the mucous membranes, teeth, gums, and lips (see Procedure 29-12 on pages 735–740). Through preventive measures, the oral cavity and teeth can be preserved. Preventive oral care consists of fluoride rinsing, flossing, and brushing.

Fluoride

Researchers have determined that fluoride can prevent dental caries. This finding has led to the fluoridation of water supplies in many communities. Fluoride is a common component of mouthwashes and toothpastes. However, persons with excessive dryness or irritated mucous membranes should avoid commercial mouthwashes because of the alcohol content, which dries out mucous membranes.

Fluoride supplements are available without a prescription. Infants can be given fluoride drops as early as 2 weeks of age to prevent dental caries. Nurses should educate clients about fluoride as an excellent preventive measure against dental caries. However, excessive fluoride usage can affect the color of tooth enamel. To prevent discoloration, fluoride should be administered with a dropper directed toward the back of the throat.

Flossing

Flossing should be performed daily in conjunction with brushing teeth. Flossing prevents the formation of plaque, removes plaque between the teeth, and removes food debris. Dental caries and periodontal disease can be prevented by regular flossing. Flossing is best performed after toothpaste is applied to the teeth but before brushing (see Procedure 29-12). This order permits the fluoride in the toothpaste to come into direct contact with the tooth surfaces, thus preventing dental caries. Flossing can also be performed after brushing, but brushing first does not maximize the fluoride's contact with the tooth surfaces.

Brushing

Brushing teeth should follow flossing. Teeth should be brushed after each meal. Brushing should be performed using a dentifrice (toothpaste) that contains fluoride to aid in preventing dental caries. An effective homemade dentifrice is the combination of two parts salt and one part baking soda. Brushing removes plaque and food debris and promotes blood circulation of the gums. Dentures should be brushed using the same brushing motion as that used for brushing teeth. Refer to Procedure 29-12 for brushing teeth and denture care.

Oral Care for the Unconscious Client

Oral care for the unconscious client maintains a clean oral cavity and intact mucous membranes (see Procedure 29-12). Special care should be exercised when performing oral care for unconscious clients to prevent client aspiration or injury to the nurse (client biting because of gag reflex).

PROVIDE HAIR CARE

Hair affects a client's personal appearance and body image. It functions to maintain the body temperature and as a receptor for the sense of touch. Assessment of hair texture, growth, and distribution provides information on a client's general health status.

Common hair problems are dandruff, hair loss, tangled or matted hair, and infestations such as pediculosis and lice. Hair problems can be reduced by daily hair care, which helps promote hair growth; prevent hair loss, infections, or infestations; promote circulation of the scalp; evenly distribute oils along hair shafts; and maintain the client's physical appearance. Hair care consists of brushing and combing, shampooing, shaving, and mustache and beard care.

Brushing and Combing

Hair should be brushed or combed daily according to the client's preferred hairstyle. Brushing and combing stimulate circulation to the scalp, distribute oils along hair shafts, and arrange the placement of hair. A clean brush or comb should be used. Hair should be brushed from the scalp toward the hair ends. Sensitive scalps should be brushed or combed gently. Wetting the hair with water before brushing or combing can prevent damage to the hair and painful pulling of the scalp.

Clients who are immobilized may have tangled or matted hair. Care should be taken to prevent pain when combing by holding the tangled hair near the scalp while combing. If the client permits, the hair can be braided to avoid tangling

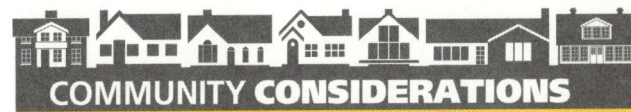

COMMUNITY CONSIDERATIONS

Cultural Influences on Hygiene

Keep in mind that all self-care and hygiene practices are influenced by the client's background and cultural values. Always ask clients about preferences prior to performing care, and show sensitivity to those practices that may differ from your own.

or matting, but braiding the hair tightly should be avoided since tight braids may cause pain and hair loss. A nurse must receive written, informed consent to cut a client's hair.

Shampooing

When soiled, hair should be shampooed according to the client's usual routine. The purposes of shampooing are to stimulate scalp circulation, remove soil from hair, and facilitate brushing and combing. Hair can be shampooed in the tub, in the shower, at the sink, or in the bed, depending on the client's abilities and preferences.

Clients confined to bed can have their hair shampooed with water or with shampoos that do not require water (see Nursing Checklist: Shampooing Hair in Bed, on page 692). Hair is shampooed by thoroughly wetting all hair, applying about a teaspoon of shampoo, lathering shampoo, and gently massaging the scalp with the pads of the fingertips. Hair should be rinsed thoroughly after shampooing, then dried with an absorbent towel. Brush or comb in the client's preferred hairstyle.

Shaving

Shaving is the removal of hair from the skin surface. Males often shave to remove facial hair, and women may shave to remove leg and/or axillary hair. Operative procedures may also require skin preparation for shaving an area of the body.

Shaving may be performed before, during, or after the bath. Care should be used to avoid cutting the skin. Prior to shaving, the area should be washed with soap and warm water to soften the hair. A warm washcloth may be placed over the area for a few minutes to assist with softening. A shaving cream or mild soap is applied to the area to ease hair removal. To shave, the skin should be pulled taut. The razor is held at a 45° angle and moved over the skin in short, firm strokes in the direction of hair growth. After the skin is shaved, it should be washed, rinsed, and patted dry.

Mustache and Beard Care

Mustaches and beards require daily care, consisting of keeping the hair clean, trimmed, and combed. Mustaches and beards can be washed with soap or shampoo. Frequently, they require only a gentle wiping with a moist washcloth. A mustache or beard should never be shaved by the nurse without written, informed consent.

✅ NURSINGCHECKLIST

Shampooing Hair in Bed

- Remove pillow. Position the client with head and shoulders near edge of bed. Cotton may be placed in the external ear canal.
- Place a linen protector or plastic head-washing tray under the head to protect the bed from becoming wet and to facilitate the draining off of water and shampoo.
- Offer the client a towel to cover eyes, if desired (see Figure 29-13).
- Shampoo hair beginning at the hair line and working toward the back of the head.
- Rinse thoroughly to remove all residue from the scalp. Repeat washing and rinsing until hair squeaks when fingers move through hair.
- Squeeze excess water from hair. Wrap a towel around client's head and rub hair and scalp with towel. Remove linen protector or plastic tray and complete drying of hair.

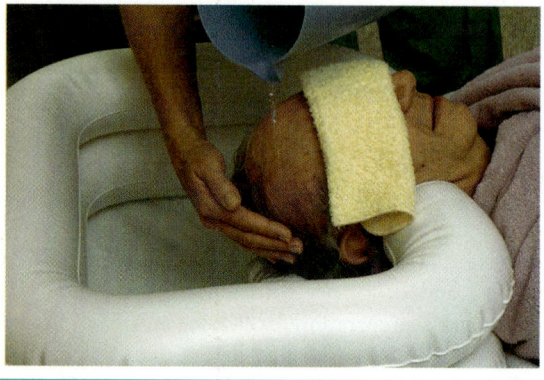

FIGURE 29-13 Shampooing Hair in Bed DELMAR/CENGAGE LEARNING

▼ SAFETY FIRST ▼

SHAVING

Review the client's medical record and the facility's policy regarding the use of razors for shaving. Clients prone to bleeding, such as those on anticoagulants, should be instructed to use only electric razors for shaving.

PROVIDE EYE, EAR, AND NOSE CARE

Eye, ear, and nose care should be included in routine hygienic care.

Eyes

Eyes are continually cleansed by the production of tears and the movement of eyelids over the eyes. Eyelids should be washed daily with a warm washcloth from the inner to outer canthus. Eyelashes function to prevent foreign material from entering the eyes and conjunctival sacs. Eyelashes and eyebrows should be washed as necessary.

A client's artificial eye (prosthetic) may require daily cleaning. The eye must be removed from the eye socket and washed (see Procedure 29-13 on pages 741–745). Some artificial eyes are permanently implanted.

Comatose clients have special eye care needs since they lack a blink reflex. These clients require frequent instillations of lubricants or eyedrops to prevent corneal abrasions. The accompanying Nursing Checklist describes eye care for the comatose client.

CONTACT LENSES The nursing history should indicate whether the client wears contact lenses, and the routine care and level of assistance should be recorded on the client's care plan. Clients who can insert, remove, and manage the care of their lenses will require minimal assistance from the nurse. If the client is unable to assist with lens care and also has corrective eyeglasses, suggest that he or she wear the eyeglasses during hospitalization. There are two types of contact lenses: hard and soft. Each type requires different cleaning and care (see Procedure 29-13). During emergency situations, the nurse should remove the lenses and place them in the appropriate solution.

Ears

Hearing can be affected by foreign material or wax in the external ear canal. Cleaning the ears involves cleaning the external ear canal and auricles. Objects should not be inserted into the ear canal. Excess wax or foreign material should be

✅ NURSINGCHECKLIST

Eye Care for the Comatose Client

- Cleanse eyelids, eyelashes, and eyebrows with warm washcloth at least every 4 hours. Clean from inner to outer canthus.
- If eyes remain open and blink reflex is absent, liquid tear solutions should be applied to prevent corneal drying and ulcerations.
- Eyes can be closed and covered with an eye patch or a protective shield. The eye patch or a protective shield should be removed at least every 4 hours to assess eyes and provide eye care.

removed by gently washing the external ear and auricles with a warm washcloth while pulling the ear downward in the adult client. Irrigation of the ear may be necessary to remove dried wax. The prescribing practitioner should be notified prior to irrigation of the ear.

HEARING AIDS Hearing aids amplify sound. The health history should indicate whether the client is wearing a hearing aid, and the plan of care should address the cleaning schedule of this aid. Clients with hearing aids should clean the ear mold regularly to ensure proper functioning. There are four types of hearing aids: bodyworn, eyeglass, behind the ear, and in the ear. Some hearing aids have a telephone switch that can be turned on and off.

If the hearing aid is not functioning properly, check the on-off switch and volume control, battery (replace as necessary),

NURSING CARE PLAN

Client at Risk for Injury

CASE PRESENTATION
Mr. Simon, age 75, is admitted to the hospital with coronary heart disease (CHD). He has a family history of CHD. He smokes two packs of cigarettes a day, has diabetes mellitus, and is obese.

ASSESSMENT
- Weight gain of 7 pounds in past month
- Blood cholesterol 320 mg/dL
- High-density lipoproteins (HDL) 28 mg/dL
- Blood pressure 186/116
- Diminished visual acuity
- Decreased bladder tone
- Weakness and syncope
- Glasgow Coma Scale (GCS) score of 12

NURSING DIAGNOSIS 1
Risk for injury related to sensory dysfunction and altered level of consciousness.

EXPECTED OUTCOME
The client will be protected from injury during the hospitalization.

INTERVENTIONS/RATIONALES
1. Initiate the fall prevention protocol. Identifies and reduces risk for injury.
2. Reassess the client's injury status every 4 hours. Identifies changes and highlights need to modify plan of care.
3. Place the client in a room as close as possible to the nurses' station. Facilitates faster response time to client's needs.
4. Place fall alert signs on the client's door and head of bed. Alerts other health care workers to client's risk status.
5. Turn on the bed alarm. Helps monitor client status and facilitates prompt response if client tries to get out of bed unassisted.
6. Monitor the client and the environment every 2 hours and whenever a caregiver passes by the client's room. Provides information on status, progress, and needs of client; encourages team approach to client care.
7. Instruct all caregivers to respond promptly to call light. Ensures rapid response to client's needs.
8. Teach the client to use the call light; reinforce teaching each time before leaving the client alone. Ensures that client has means and knowledge to call for assistance if necessary.

EVALUATION
Fall prevention protocol implemented; client discharged on third day of hospitalization free from injury.

plastic tubing for cracks and loose connections, and telephone switch, which should be in the off position unless the client is using the phone. The hearing aid should be handled carefully since dropping or bumping it can damage its delicate mechanisms. When not in use, the hearing aid should be stored in a container because dust and dirt can damage the mechanism.

When communicating with a client who has a hearing aid, the nurse should address her or him by name and then wait for the client to face the nurse before speaking further. Always face the client and speak in a slow, natural voice. Shouting causes distortion of sound and usually makes the client feel uncomfortable.

Nose

The nose provides the sense of smell, prevents entrance of foreign material into the respiratory tract, humidifies inhaled air, and facilitates breathing. Excessive or dried secretions may impair nasal function. Excessive nasal secretions are removed by inserting a cotton-tipped applicator moistened with water or saline into the nostrils. The applicator should not be inserted beyond the cotton tip. Infants may have excessive nasal secretions removed by a suction bulb. Clients with a nasogastric tube should receive meticulous skin care to the nose area to prevent skin breakdown.

EVALUATION

Evaluation is based on the achievement of goals and client expected outcomes, regardless of the setting. Clients with alterations in the health perception–health management pattern or activity-exercise pattern are at risk for injury, infection, and self-care deficits. Keeping clients free from injury and infection requires frequent reassessment through the use of risk appraisals, with timely adjustments made in the plan of care in order for nursing interventions to be effective. When falls occur, every client warrants a postfall assessment to identify new risk factors and suggest new interventions to prevent the next fall (Ferris, 2008).

It is imperative that clients not only be free of injury during hospitalization but also develop a true awareness of

▼ SAFETY FIRST ▼

The use of restraints or other protective devices on confused clients usually increases clients' confusion, placing them at a greater risk for injury. Restraints should be used only when all other nursing measures are ineffective in providing client safety.

the internal and external factors that increase the risk for injury. Achievement of this outcome measure is directly related to the behaviors clients observe while in the hospital and through client teaching. Modification of a home to a safe environment is evidence for the home health nurse that learning has taken place.

Adherence to barrier precautions is critical in preventing the spread of infectious agents, especially HAIs, to clients, self, and other health care workers. The nurse needs to correlate the client's diagnostic laboratory results and temperature in evaluating the expected outcome of remaining free of signs and symptoms of infection. If the nurse is caring for a client with an infection, the evaluation should indicate the stage of the inflammatory process (see Table 29-1).

The therapeutic value of hygiene is maximized when the client can participate and is kept free from infection and alterations in skin integrity. Evaluation should identify the client's level of functioning in self-care activities.

At the time of discharge from the hospital, appropriate referrals should be made to home health care agencies to assist the client in achieving optimum functioning levels for safety and hygienic practices. Clients at risk for infection should have follow-up visits by the home health nurse to measure the effectiveness of client teaching and resources in the home to prevent the transmission of infections.

PROCEDURE 29-1 — Applying Restraints

EQUIPMENT (See Figures 29–14, 29–15, and 26–16)
• Restraints appropriate to the client's condition and type of restraint required
• Cotton batting or foam padding

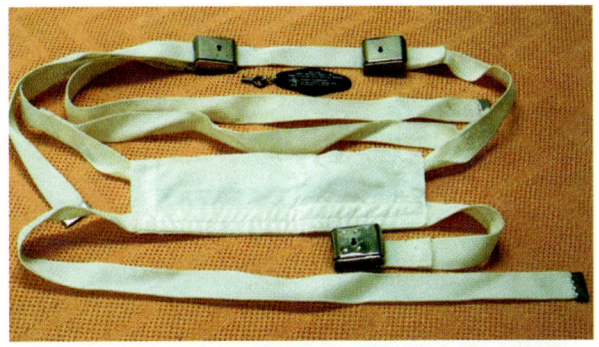

FIGURE 29-14 **Locking Belt Restraint** DELMAR/CENGAGE LEARNING

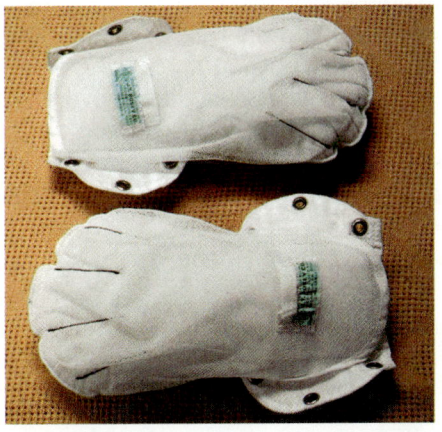

FIGURE 29-15 **Mitten Restraints** DELMAR/CENGAGE LEARNING

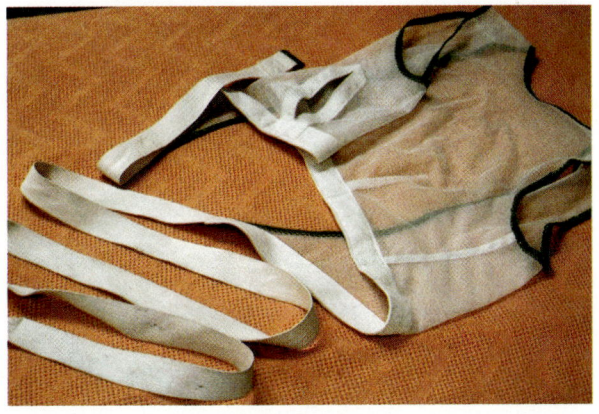

FIGURE 29-16 **Jacket Restraint** DELMAR/CENGAGE LEARNING

ACTION	RATIONALE
CHEST RESTRAINT	
1. Wash hands/hand hygiene.	1. Prevents the spread of microorganisms.
2. Explain that the client will be wearing a jacket attached to the bed. Explain that this is for safety.	2. Promotes client cooperation.
3. Place the restraint over the client's hospital gown or clothing.	3. Provides for client privacy and prevents the restraint from rubbing the client's skin.
4. Place the restraint on the client with the opening in the front (see Figure 29-17 on page 696).	4. Allows movement but restricts freedom.
5. Overlap the front pieces, threading the ties through the slot/loop on the front of the vest.	5. Secures the restraint.

(Continues)

PROCEDURE 29-1
Applying Restraints (Continued)

ACTION	RATIONALE
6. If the client is in bed, secure the ties to the movable part of the mattress frame with a half-knot (see Figure 29-18).	6. Allows the restraint to move with the bed if the head of the bed is raised or lowered.
7. If the client is in a chair, cross the straps behind the seat of the chair and secure the straps to the chair's lower legs, out of the client's reach (see Figure 29-19). If it is a wheelchair, be sure the straps will not get caught up in the wheels.	7. Provides support for the client to sit up while restricting freedom.
8. Step back and assess the client's overall safety. Be sure the restraint is loose enough not to be a hazard to the client but tight enough to restrict the client from getting up and harming himself or herself.	8. Looking at the overall picture can allow the nurse to see dangers that might have been missed.
9. Wash hands/hand hygiene.	9. Prevents the spread of microorganisms.

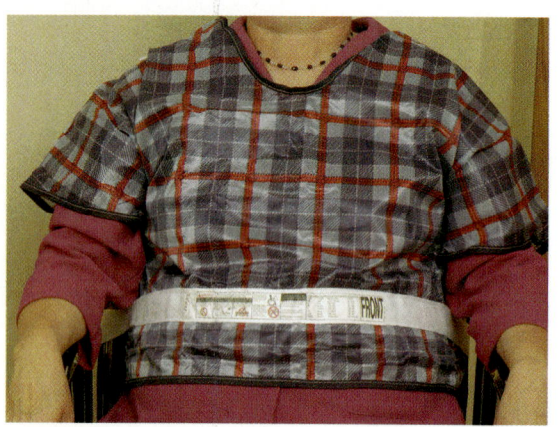

FIGURE 29-17 Place the jacket restraint on the client. Make sure the restraint is the proper size for the client and has been applied correctly. DELMAR/CENGAGE LEARNING

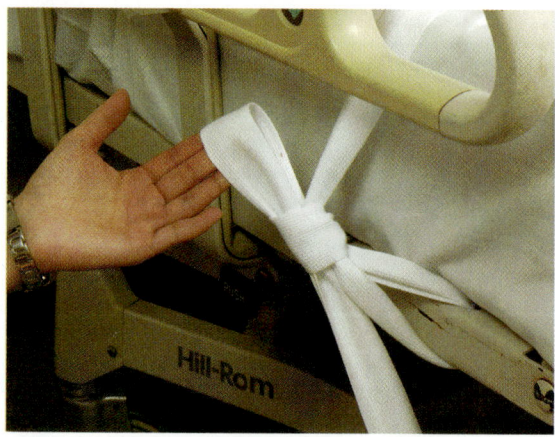

FIGURE 29-18 Secure ties to the movable part of the frame.
DELMAR/CENGAGE LEARNING

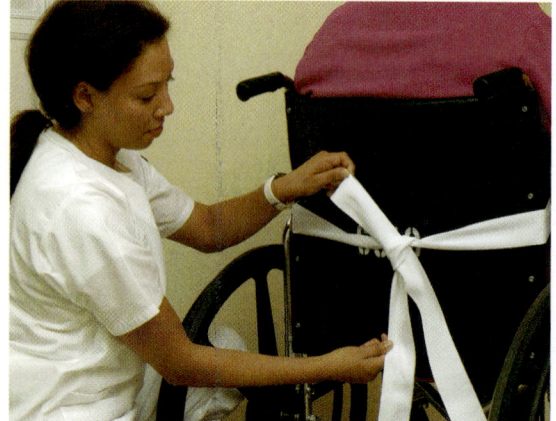

FIGURE 29-19 Secure restraining straps out of the client's reach. DELMAR/CENGAGE LEARNING

(Continues)

PROCEDURE 29-1
Applying Restraints (Continued)

ACTION	RATIONALE
APPLYING WRIST OR ANKLE RESTRAINTS	
10. Wash hands/hand hygiene.	10. Prevents the spread of microorganisms.
11. Explain to the client that you will be placing a wrist or ankle band that will restrict movement.	11. Promotes client cooperation.
12. Place padding around the client's wrist/ankle.	12. Prevents the restraint from chafing the skin.
13. Wrap the restraint around the client's wrist/ankle, pull the tie through the loop in the restraint, and tie a square knot (see Figure 29-20).	13. Secures the restraint and prevents the restraint from overtightening at the wrist.
14. Tie the restraint ties to the movable portion of the mattress frame.	14. When the head or foot of the client's bed is moved, the restraint will move with it.
15. Slip two fingers under the restraint to check for tightness. Be sure the restraint is tight enough that the client cannot slip it off but loose enough that the neurovascular status of the client's extremity is not impaired.	15. If the restraint is too tight, the client's neurovascular status may be impaired, causing injury.
16. Step back and assess the client's overall safety. Be sure the restraint is loose enough not to be a hazard to the client but tight enough to restrict the client from getting up and harming himself or herself (see Figure 29-21 on page 698).	16. Looking at the overall picture can allow the nurse to see dangers that might have been missed.
17. Place the call light within the client's reach.	17. Allows the client to contact the nurse to have any needs met. Provides the client with an increased sense of safety.
18. Check on the client every half hour while restrained. Assess the safety of the restraint placement and the client's neurovascular status.	18. Assures that the client remains safe. Clients may try to escape from restraint and injure themselves in the attempt. States and institutions may have regulations outlining the frequency of client checks if the client is in restraints. Be aware of any regulations that apply.
19. Wash hands/hand hygiene.	19. Prevents the spread of microorganisms.

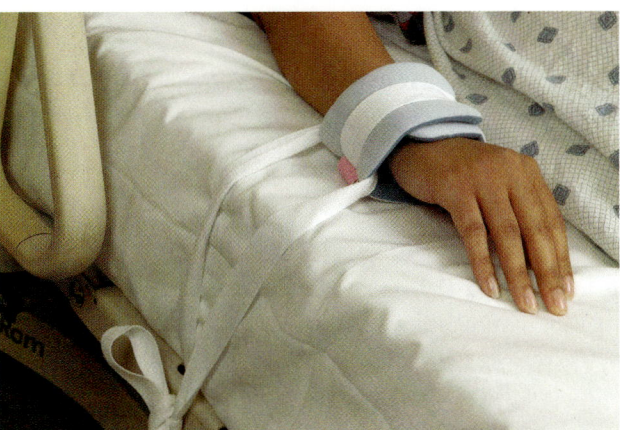

FIGURE 29-20 Wrap restraint around the client's wrist. DELMAR/CENGAGE LEARNING

(Continues)

PROCEDURE 29-1
Applying Restraints (Continued)

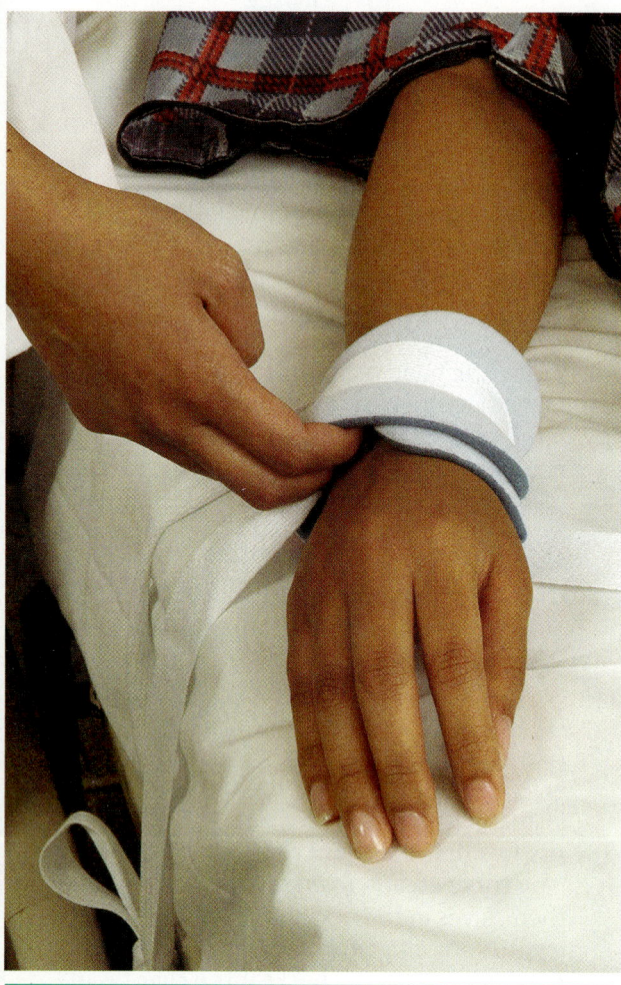

FIGURE 29-21 Restraints should not be too tight or loose. Check frequently. DELMAR/CENGAGE LEARNING

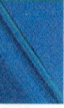

delegation tip

Delegation of the application of restraints to ancillary personnel is acceptable if appropriate orders are in place and proper training has occurred. The assessment of the need for and the type of restraints required and their proper application and maintenance requires the professional nurse's observation and documentation per facility policy.

nursing tips

- *Know facility policies and state laws that govern the use of restraints. Determine whether treatment plan authorizes a client to be restrained or monitored in accordance with medical orders and regulations. Know the laws regarding specified person to prescribe restraints. Reassess according to regulations.*
- *Become familiar with restraint equipment: vest, limb, mitt, belt, body (Posey), and leather restraints.*

(Continues)

PROCEDURE 29-1
Applying Restraints (Continued)

nursing tips

- *Be safe and efficient when applying restraints. Always have organized and available assistance when placing restraints on a client. A team effort can provide simultaneous client teaching by one health care professional while another applies the restraint.*
- *Ensure that client comfort is not compromised. Provide frequent checks. Assess need for padding bony prominences to avoid pressure ulcers. Provide assistance with nutrition, elimination, repositioning, and general care.*
- *Always keep the client and family well informed regarding the rationale for restraints and the associated care required.*
- *Continuously assess client need for restraints. Allow changes in condition to dictate withdrawing or maintaining restraints.*
- *Restraints must be sized properly and according to the client's body build and weight. If restraints are loose, and smaller ones are unavailable, use gauze pads or soft towels to build them up, and then tape securely.*
- *If leather restraints are used, have a key that fits the locks readily available.*
- *Pad bony prominences before applying protective devices.*
- *Attach the device to the movable bed frame, not the side rails.*
- *Check client's respiratory status if a chest device is used.*
- *Check position of chest device so it is not constricting the client's neck.*
- *Restrain client on side if risk of aspiration is assessed.*
- *Do not secure four restraints to one side of the bed.*
- *When applying two-point restraints, restrain one arm and the opposite leg.*
- *Never apply restraint above an IV site.*
- *Do not restrain a client in the prone position.*
- *Provide frequent repositioning, massage, and surveillance of bony prominences.*
- *Be sure to place the client's call light within reach.*

PROCEDURE 29-2

Handwashing: Visibly Soiled Hands

EQUIPMENT
- Soap
- Sink
- Paper or cloth towels
- Running water

ACTION	RATIONALE
1. Remove jewelry. Wristwatch may be pushed up above the wrist (midforearm). Push sleeves of uniform or shirt up above the wrist at mid-fore-arm level.	1. Provides access to skin surfaces for cleaning. Facilitates cleaning of fingers, hands, and fore-arms.

(Continues)

PROCEDURE 29-2
Handwashing: Visibly Soiled Hands (Continued)

ACTION	RATIONALE
2. Assess hands for hangnails, cuts, or breaks in the skin and areas that are heavily soiled.	2. Intact skin acts as a barrier to microorganisms. Breaks in skin integrity facilitate development of infection and should receive extra attention during cleaning.
3. Turn on the water. Adjust the flow and temperature. Temperature of the water should be warm.	3. Running water removes microorganisms. Warm water removes less of the natural skin oils.
4. Wet hands and lower forearms thoroughly by holding under running water. Keep hands and forearms in the down position with elbows straight. Avoid splashing water and touching the sides of the sink.	4. Water should flow from the least contaminated to the most contaminated areas of the skin. Hands are considered more contaminated than arms. Splashing of water facilitates transfer of microorganisms. Touching of any surface during cleaning contaminates the skin.
5. Apply about 5 mL (1 tsp) of liquid soap. Lather thoroughly.	5. Lather facilitates removal of microorganisms. Liquid soap harbors less bacteria than bar soap.
6. Vigorously rub hands together for about 10 to 15 seconds. Interlace fingers and thumbs, and move back and forth to wash between digits. Rub palms and back of hands with circular motion (see Figure 29-22). Special attention should be provided to areas such as the knuckles and fingernails, which are known to harbor organisms (see Figure 29-23).	6. Friction mechanically removes microorganisms from the skin's surface and loosens dirt from soiled areas.
7. Rinse with hands in the down position, elbows straight. Rinse in the direction of forearm to wrist to fingers.	7. Flow of water rinses away dirt and microorganisms.
8. Blot hands and forearms to dry thoroughly. Dry in the direction of fingers to wrist and forearms. Discard the paper towels in the proper receptacle.	8. Blotting reduces chapping of skin. Drying from cleanest (hand) to least clean area (forearms) prevents transfer of microorganisms to cleanest area.
9. Turn off the water faucet with a clean, dry paper towel (see Figure 29-24 on page 701).	9. Prevents contamination of clean hands by a less clean faucet.

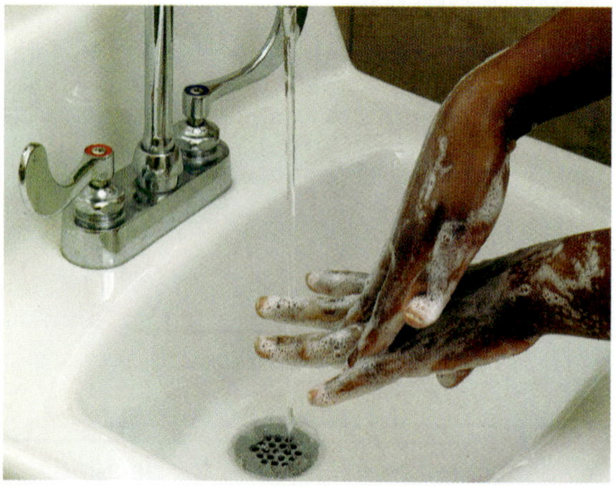

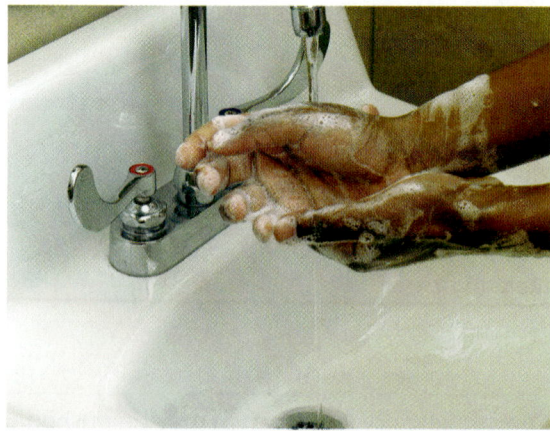

FIGURE 29-22 Lather thoroughly, and rub hands together.
DELMAR/CENGAGE LEARNING

FIGURE 29-23 Give special attention to fingernails and knuckles. DELMAR/CENGAGE LEARNING

(Continues)

PROCEDURE 29-2
Handwashing: Visibly Soiled Hands (Continued)

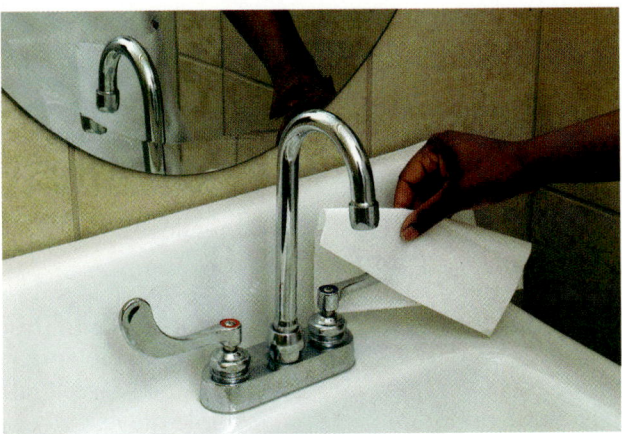

FIGURE 29-24 Turn off faucet with a clean, dry paper towel. DELMAR/CENGAGE LEARNING

delegation tip

All hospital personnel are expected to maintain proper handwashing technique and routinely apply Standard Precautions.

nursing tips

- *If in doubt, it is dirty.*
- *Wash hands before and after every client contact. The most common cause of HAIs is contaminated hands of health care providers.*
- *When you turn on the faucet of a sink with which you are unfamiliar (especially in the home care setting), you might get wet! Be a bit tentative the first time until you investigate the water pressure and the faucet.*

PROCEDURE 29-3

Applying Sterile Gloves via the Open Method

EQUIPMENT (See Figure 29-25)
- Package of proper-size sterile gloves

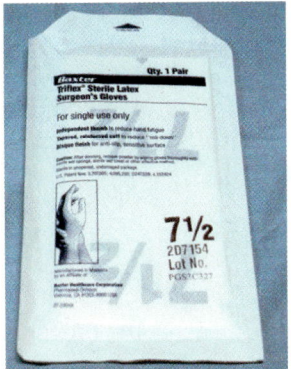

FIGURE 29-25 Sterile Gloves DELMAR/CENGAGE LEARNING

(Continues)

PROCEDURE 29-3
Applying Sterile Gloves via the Open Method (Continued)

ACTION	RATIONALE
1. Wash hands/hand hygiene.	1. Prevents the spread of microorganisms.
2. Read the manufacturer's instructions on the package of sterile gloves; proceed as directed in removing the outer wrapper from the package (see Figure 29-26 on page 703), placing the inner wrapper onto a clean, dry surface (see Figure 29-27 on page 703). Open inner wrapper to expose gloves (see Figure 29-28 on page 703).	2. Manufacturers package gloves differently; the instructions will indicate how to open properly to avoid contamination of the inner wrapper; any moisture on the surface will contaminate the gloves.
3. Identify right and left hand; glove dominant hand first.	3. Dominant hand should facilitate motor dexterity during gloving.
4. Grasp the 2-inch- (5-cm-) wide cuff with the thumb and first two fingers of the nondominant hand, touching only the inside of the cuff (see Figure 29-29 on page 703).	4. Maintains sterility of the outer surfaces of the sterile glove.
5. Gently pull the glove over the dominant hand, making sure the thumb and fingers fit into the proper spaces of the glove (see Figure 29-30 on page 703).	5. Prevents tearing the glove material; guiding the fingers into proper places facilitates gloving.
6. With the gloved, dominant hand, slip your fingers under the cuff of the other glove, gloved thumb abducted, making sure it does not touch any part on the nondominant hand (see Figure 29-31 on page 703).	6. Cuff protects gloved fingers, maintaining sterility.
7. Gently slip the glove onto your nondominant hand, making sure the fingers slip into the proper spaces (see Figures 29-32 and 29-33 on page 704).	7. Contact is made with two sterile gloves.
8. With gloved hands, interlock fingers to fit the gloves onto each finger. If the gloves are soiled, remove by turning inside out as described in the following steps.	8. Promotes proper fit over the fingers.
9. Slip gloved fingers of the dominant hand under the cuff of the opposite hand, or grasp the outer part of the glove at the wrist if there is no cuff.	9. Contact is made with two sterile gloves.
10. Pull the glove down to the fingers, exposing the thumb (see Figure 29-34 on page 704).	10. Frees the thumb for the next step.
11. Slip the uncovered thumb into the opposite glove at the wrist, allowing only the glove-covered fingers of the hand to touch the soiled glove (see Figure 29-35 on page 704).	11. Contact is made with two sterile gloves.
12. Pull the glove down over the dominant hand almost to the fingertips, and slip the glove onto the other hand (see Figure 29-36 on page 704).	12. Removes glove without contact with soiled surfaces.
13. With the dominant hand touching only the inside of the other glove, pull the glove over the dominant hand so that only the inside (clean surface) is exposed.	13. Exposes only the clean surface of the gloves.
14. Dispose of soiled gloves according to institutional policy (see Figure 29-37 on page 704).	14. Prevents the transfer of microorganisms.
15. Wash hands/hand hygiene.	15. Prevents the spread of microorganisms.

(Continues)

PROCEDURE 29-3
Applying Sterile Gloves via the Open Method (Continued)

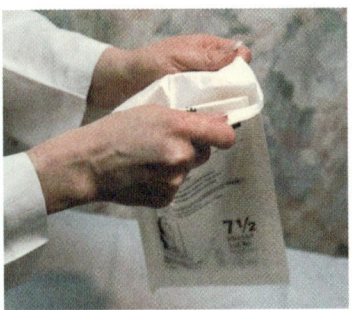

FIGURE 29-26 **Remove the outer wrapper of the sterile glove package.** DELMAR/CENGAGE LEARNING

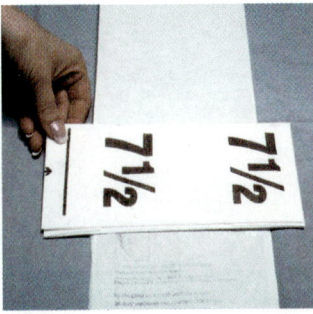

FIGURE 29-27 **Place the gloves in the inner wrapper on a clean, dry surface.** DELMAR/CENGAGE LEARNING

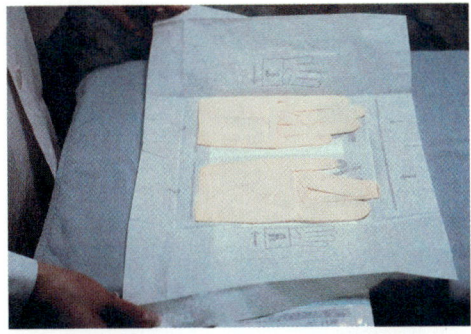

FIGURE 29-28 **Open the inner wrapper to expose gloves.** DELMAR/CENGAGE LEARNING

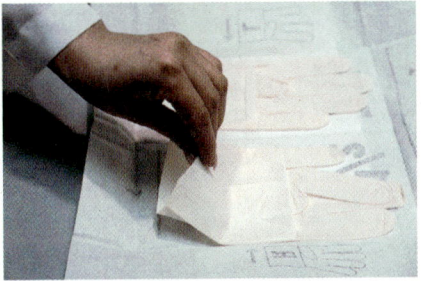

FIGURE 29-29 **Grasp first cuff with the nondominant hand.** DELMAR/CENGAGE LEARNING

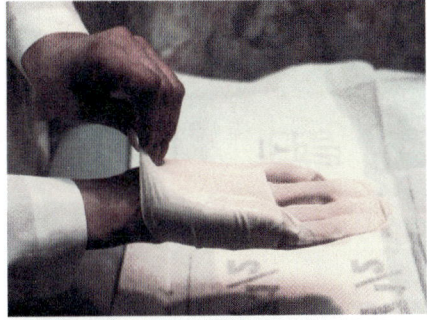

FIGURE 29-30 **Pull the glove over the dominant hand.** DELMAR/CENGAGE LEARNING

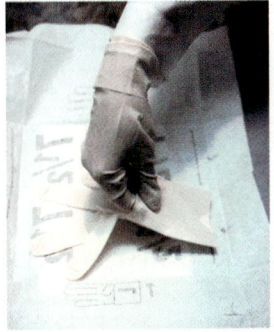

FIGURE 29-31 **Slip fingers under the cuff of the second glove.** DELMAR/CENGAGE LEARNING

(Continues)

PROCEDURE 29-3
Applying Sterile Gloves via the Open Method (Continued)

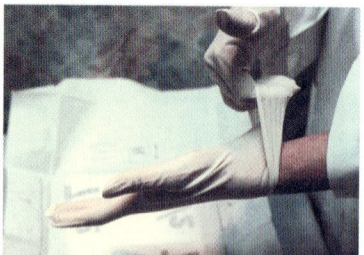

FIGURE 29-32 Pull on the second glove. DELMAR/CENGAGE LEARNING

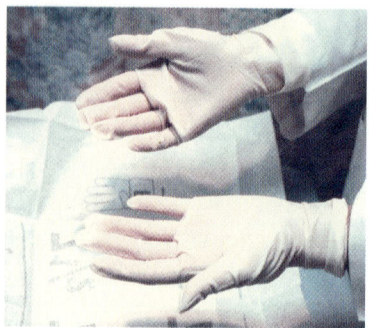

FIGURE 29-33 Make sure all fingers are in the proper spaces. DELMAR/CENGAGE LEARNING

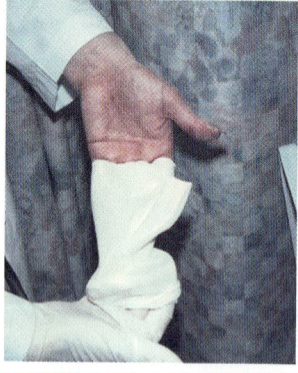

FIGURE 29-34 Peel glove down to fingers, exposing one thumb. DELMAR/CENGAGE LEARNING

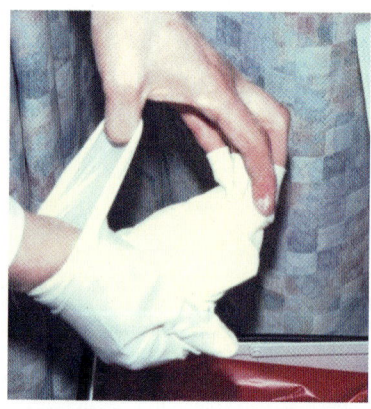

FIGURE 29-35 Slip uncovered thumb into the opposite glove. DELMAR/CENGAGE LEARNING

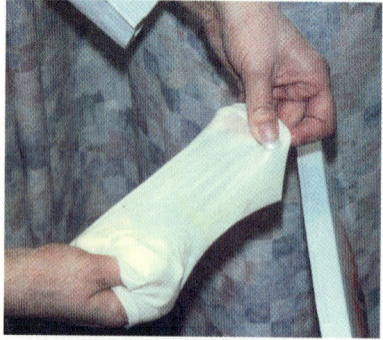

FIGURE 29-36 When soiled gloves are removed correctly, only the inside, clean surface of one glove is exposed. DELMAR/CENGAGE LEARNING

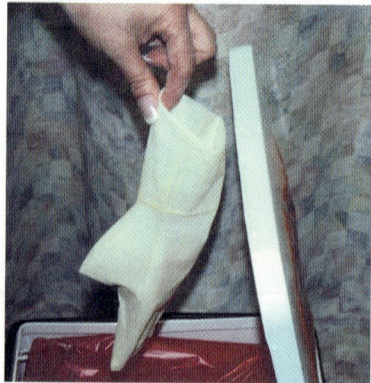

FIGURE 29-37 Dispose of gloves in appropriate receptacle. DELMAR/CENGAGE LEARNING

(Continues)

PROCEDURE 29-3
Applying Sterile Gloves via the Open Method (Continued)

delegation tip

Sterile gloving is delegated only if personnel are specifically trained, such as in a surgical suite or a testing laboratory setting.

nursing tips

- *Touch only dirty to dirty, clean to clean, and sterile to sterile.*
- *Be aware of the immediate environment when applying sterile gloves to avoid accidental contamination.*
- *Be sure to have everything you need ready before donning sterile gloves.*

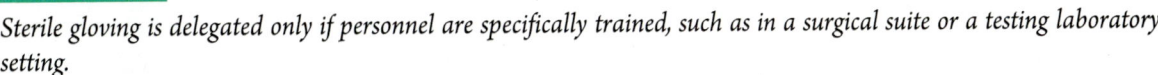

PROCEDURE 29-4

Donning and Removing Clean and Contaminated Gloves, Cap, and Mask

EQUIPMENT
- Gloves, clean—sterile, if necessary
- Gown, sterile or clean
- Cap
- Mask

ACTION	RATIONALE
1. Wash hands/hand hygiene. Gather equipment (see Figure 29-38 A–D on page 706).	1. Prevents the spread of microorganisms.
2. The first item of apparel donned should be the cap or surgical hat/hood. Hair should be tucked in a manner so that all hair is covered (see Figure 29-39 on page 706).	2. "Hair acts as a filter when left uncovered and collects bacteria in proportion to its length, curliness, and oiliness. Strands of hair may fall in the surgical area. Shedding from hair has been shown to lead to surgical wound infection" (Association of periOperative Registered Nurses [AORN], 2004).
3. Apply a mask around mouth and nose, and secure in a manner that prevents venting. For masks with strings (see Figure 29-40 on page 706): a. Hold mask by top, and pinch center (metal strip) over bridge of nose. b. Pull top two strings over ears, and secure at top, back of head. c. Tie two lower ties around back or nape of neck so bottom of mask fits snugly under chin (see Figure 29-41 on page 707).	3. Masks are worn to contain and filter droplets of microorganisms that are expelled when talking, sneezing, or coughing. Masks prevent the transmission of oral and nasopharyngeal organisms between the nurse and client.
4. Open gown, slip arms into sleeves, and secure at neck and side (see Figure 29–42 A and B on page 708).	4. Gowns act as a protective barrier and should be worn to reduce exposure to blood, body fluid, or other potentially infectious liquids.

(Continues)

PROCEDURE 29-4
Donning and Removing Clean and Contaminated Gloves, Cap, and Mask (Continued)

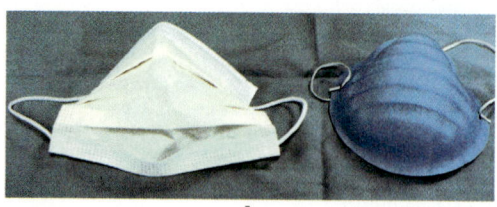

A.

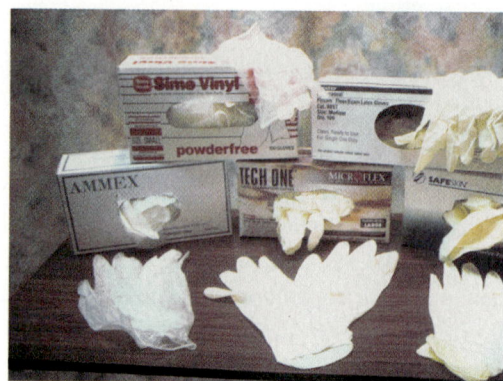

C.

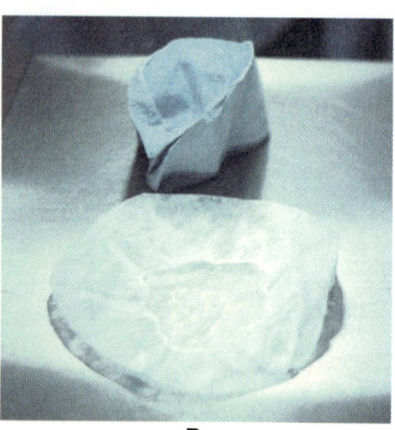

B.

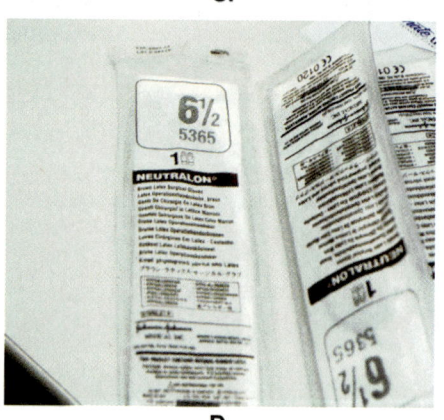

D.

FIGURE 29-38 A. Masks; B. Caps; C. Clean Gloves; D. Sterile Gloves. DELMAR/CENGAGE LEARNING

ACTION	RATIONALE
5. Protective eyewear should be worn whenever the health care provider or client is at risk for splash and contamination. Eyewear is applied as goggles/glasses or face shields, which have elastic ties for around the ears.	5. Protective eyewear reduces the incidence of contamination to the eyes. If eyewear or face shields become contaminated, they should be discarded immediately and replaced with a clean barrier.

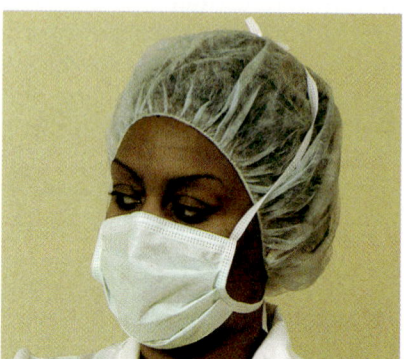

FIGURE 29-39 Caps and surgical caps should cover the head, and hair should be tucked in. DELMAR/CENGAGE LEARNING

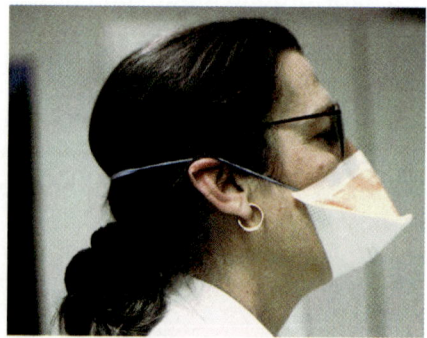

FIGURE 29-40 Secure mask around mouth and nose. DELMAR/CENGAGE LEARNING

(Continues)

PROCEDURE 29-4
Donning and Removing Clean and Contaminated Gloves, Cap, and Mask (Continued)

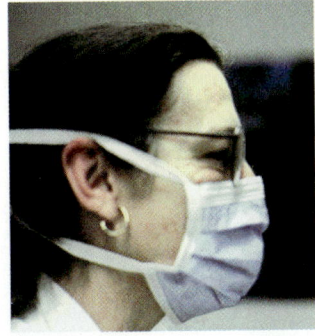

FIGURE 29-41 **Bottom of the mask should fit snugly under chin.** DELMAR/CENGAGE LEARNING

ACTION	RATIONALE
6. Don clean gloves. If sterile gloves are required for a procedure, use the open or closed method.	6. Gloves are worn to prevent gross contamination of the hands. They should be changed between clients, and hands should be washed. The open method is used when performing procedures that require sterile technique but do not require donning a sterile gown, or when both gloves need to be changed without assistance during a surgical procedure. The closed method is used by scrubbed personnel in the operating room (see Procedure 29-6).
7. The open glove technique: a. Slide the hands into the gown all the way through the cuffs on the gown. b. Pick up the cuff of the left glove using the thumb and index finger of the right hand. c. Pull the glove onto the left hand, leaving the cuff of the glove turned down. d. Take the gloved left hand and slide the fingers inside the cuff of the right glove, keeping the gloved fingers under the folded cuff. e. Pull the glove onto the right hand. f. Rotate the arm as the cuff of the glove is pulled over the gown.	7. The open glove method is commonly used for sterile procedures or when both gloves need to be changed without assistance during a surgical procedure.
8. The closed glove technique: a. Slide the hands into the gown all the way through the cuffs on the gown. b. Use right hand to pick up left glove. c. Place the glove on the upward-turned left hand—palm side down thumb to thumb with the fingers extending along the forearm and pointing toward the elbow. d. Hold the glove cuff and sleeve cuff together with the thumb of the left hand.	8. The closed glove technique is used by the scrubbed personnel in the operating room. This is preferred, as the possibility of the glove touching the skin is eliminated.

(Continues)

PROCEDURE 29-4
Donning and Removing Clean and Contaminated Gloves, Cap, and Mask (Continued)

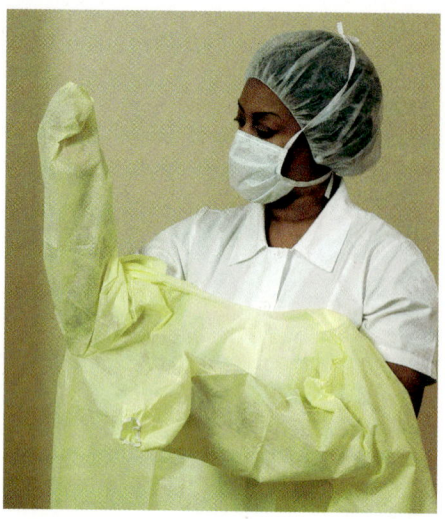

A.

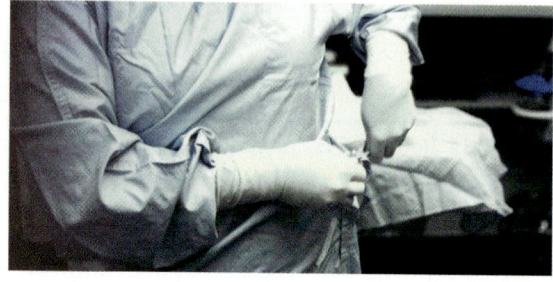

B.

FIGURE 29-42 A. Put on the gown before putting on gloves; B. Tie the gown at the neck and waist. DELMAR/CENGAGE LEARNING

ACTION	RATIONALE
e. The right hand stretches the cuff of the left glove over the opened end of the sleeve.	
f. Work the fingers into the glove as the cuff is pulled onto the wrist.	
g. The left glove is done in the same manner.	
9. Enter the client's room, and explain the rationale for wearing isolation attire.	9. Minimizes anxiety and feelings of isolation.
10. After performing necessary tasks, remove gown, gloves, mask, and cap before leaving the room.	10. Reduces transmission of organisms.
11. Removal of gown: Untie gown and remove from shoulders. Fold and roll gown down in front into a ball so contaminated area is rolled onto center of gown. Dispose in approved receptacle.	11. Reduces transmission of organisms.
12. Removal of gloves: a. Grasp outside cuff of one glove and pull off, turning inside out. Hold it with the remaining gloved hand (see Figure 29-43 on page 709). b. Pull the second glove off without touching the outside of the second glove. Turn the second glove as it is removed (see Figure 29-44 on page 709). Dispose into receptacle with first glove.	12. a. Reduces risk of contamination. b. Reduces risk of contamination.
13. Removal of mask: Untie bottom strings of mask first, then top strings, and lift off face. Hold mask by strings and discard.	13. Prevents contaminated surface of mask from contacting uniform.
14. Removal of cap: Grasp top surface of cap and lift from head.	14. Minimizes contact of hands to hair.
15. Wash hands/hand hygiene.	15. Prevents the spread of microorganisms.

(Continues)

PROCEDURE 29-4
Donning and Removing Clean and Contaminated Gloves, Cap, and Mask (Continued)

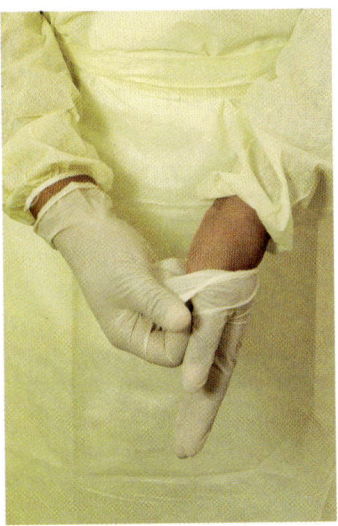

FIGURE 29-43 Grasp the outside cuff, and turn the glove inside out. DELMAR/CENGAGE LEARNING

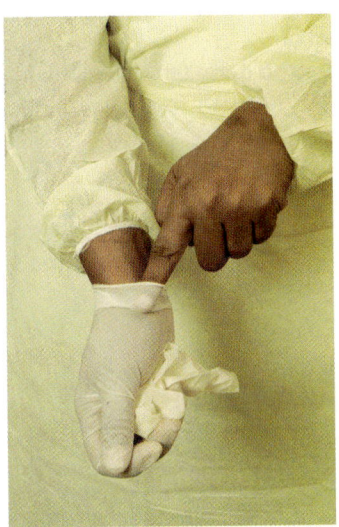

FIGURE 29-44 Turn the second glove over the first glove. DELMAR/CENGAGE LEARNING

delegation tip

Donning and removing gloves, caps, and masks is a skill that is required of all personnel, including ancillary personnel. Proper technique should be monitored by the nursing staff.

nursing tips

- *Post signs on the doors of clients who require specific barrier methods using words and/or pictures that are clear and understandable.*
- *Review isolation procedures regularly.*
- *Provide a supply of the appropriate barrier at the doorway of the client's room.*
- *If you need equipment such as an item you are carrying in your pocket, you will not be able to reach your pocket after you don your gown. You will not be able to touch needed items if your gloves and gown are contaminated. Think ahead. Plan.*
- *Remember, masks become ineffective if worn too long, become wet, or are not changed between clients.*
- *Remember that anything you touch with a contaminated glove will be contaminated. Think: Sterile can touch sterile; clean can touch clean.*

Surgical Hand Antisepsis

EQUIPMENT
- Surgical scrub items (antimicrobial soap, two brushes, and nail file)
- Surgical shoe covers (booties) and cap, face mask, sterile gown, and proper-size gloves
- Sterile towel

ACTION	RATIONALE
1. Rings, watches, and bracelets should be removed prior to beginning the surgical scrub.	1. Decreases resident and transient microorganisms. The Association of periOperative Registered Nurses recommends washing and rinsing moistened hands and forearms with an approved surgical scrub agent before beginning the surgical scrub procedure.
2. Use a deep sink with side or foot pedal to dispense antimicrobial soap and control water temperature and flow.	2. Prevents hands and forearms from touching a soiled surface.
3. Have two surgical scrub brushes and nail file (see Figure 29-45).	3. Enhances mechanical friction during the scrub.
4. Apply surgical shoe covers and cap to cover hair and ears completely.	4. Prevents introduction of contaminants into environment.
5. Apply mask (see Figure 29-46).	5. Provides a respiratory barrier.
6. Before beginning the surgical scrub:	6. Preparing the sterile items prior to the scrub decreases the risk of contaminating scrubbed hands.
a. Open the sterile package containing the gown; using aseptic technique, make a sterile field with the inside of the gown's wrapper.	
b. Open the sterile towel, and drop it onto the center of field.	
c. Open the outer wrapper from the sterile gloves, and drop the inner package of gloves onto the sterile field beside the folded gown and towel.	
7. At a deep sink with foot or knee controls (see Figure 29-47 on page 711), turn on warm water; under flowing water, wet hands, beginning at tips of fingers, to forearms—keeping hands at level above elbows. Prewash hands and forearms to 2 inches above the elbow.	7. Water should flow from the hands to the elbow to promote elimination of contaminants from the hands.

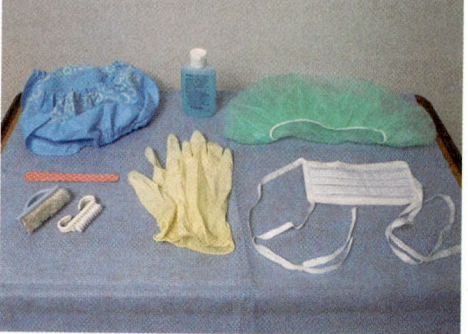

FIGURE 29-45 Surgical Scrub Items. DELMAR/CENGAGE LEARNING

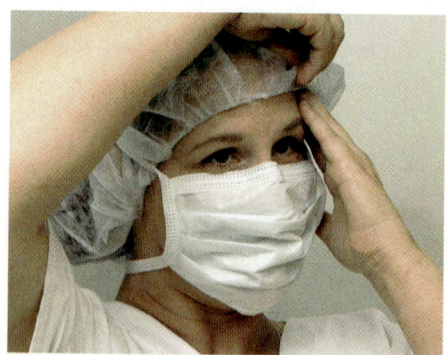

FIGURE 29-46 Apply cap and mask. DELMAR/CENGAGE LEARNING

PROCEDURE 29-5
Surgical Hand Antisepsis (Continued)

ACTION	RATIONALE
8. Apply a liberal amount of soap onto hands, and rub hands and arms to 2 inches above elbows (see Figures 29-48 on page 711 and 29-49 on page 711).	8. Reduces number of microorganisms on hands.
9. Using nail file under running water, clean under each nail of both hands, and drop file into sink when finished (see Figure 29-50 on page 711).	9. Removes dirt that harbors microorganisms.
10. Wet and apply soap to scrub brush, if needed. Open prepackaged scrub brush if available (see Figure 29-51 on page 712). With brush in dominant hand, using a circular motion, scrub nails and all skin areas of nondominant hand and arm (10 strokes to each of the following areas): a. Nails b. Palm of hand and anterior side of fingers	10. Removes resident bacteria from the skin's surfaces; the circular motion mechanically removes microorganisms. Scrubbing the nondominant hand first sets a routine you can remember if you should get interrupted during the scrub.
11. Rinse brush thoroughly, and reapply soap.	11. Decreases transfer of microorganisms.
12. Continue with scrub of nondominant arm with a circular motion for 10 strokes each to the lower, middle, and upper arm; drop brush into the sink.	12. Decreases transfer of microorganisms from the arm; dropping the brush avoids contamination.

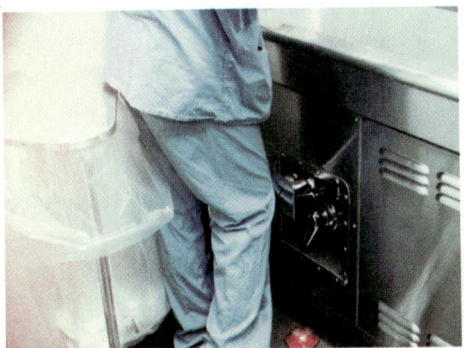

FIGURE 29-47 Handwashing Sink with Knee Controls. DELMAR/CENGAGE LEARNING

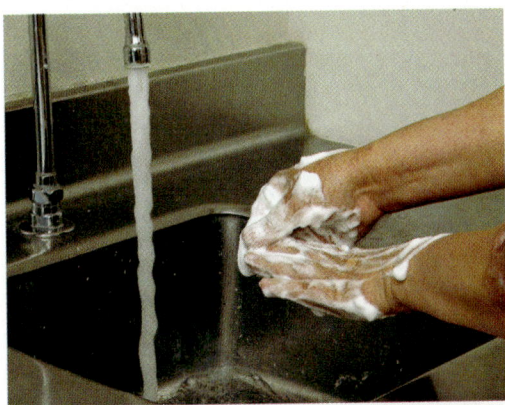

FIGURE 29-48 Apply a liberal amount of soap. DELMAR/CENGAGE LEARNING

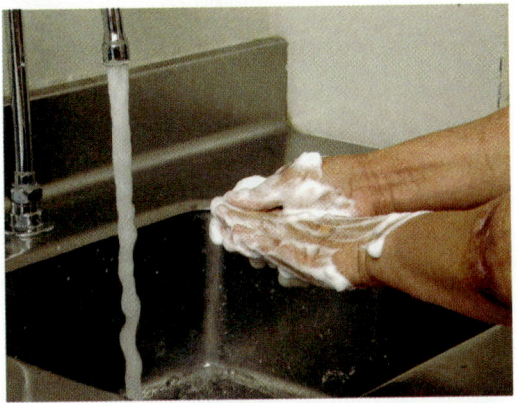

FIGURE 29-49 Scrub hands and arms. DELMAR/CENGAGE LEARNING

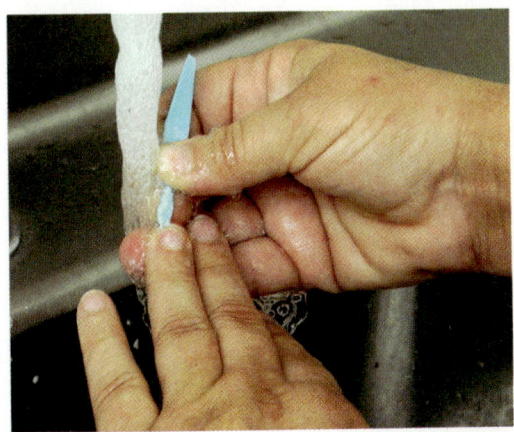

FIGURE 29-50 Use a nail file under running water to clean fingernails. DELMAR/CENGAGE LEARNING

(Continues)

PROCEDURE 29-5
Surgical Hand Antisepsis (Continued)

ACTION	RATIONALE
13. Maintaining the hands and arms above elbow level, place the fingertips under running water, and thoroughly rinse the fingers, hands, and arms (allow the water to run off elbows into the sink); take care not to get uniform wet (see Figure 29-52.	13. Allows flow of water to cleanse from the area of least contamination to the area of most contamination. Water conducts microorganisms, and keeping uniform dry aids in maintaining sterility of gown.
14. Take the second scrub brush and repeat Actions 10–13 on dominant hand and arm.	14. See Rationales 10–13.
15. Keep arms flexed and proceed to area (operating or procedure room) with sterile items (see Figure 29-53).	15. Prevents water from flowing from least (elbows) to most (hands) clean area.
16. Secure sterile towel by grasping it on one edge, opening the towel, full length, making sure it does not touch uniform.	16. Maintains the sterility of the towel.
17. Dry each hand and arm separately; extend one side of the towel around fingers and hand, and dry in a rotating motion up to the elbow (see Figure 29-54 and Figure 29-55 on page 713).	17. Prevents contamination by drying from cleanest to least clean area.
18. Reverse the towel and repeat the same action on the other hand and arm, thoroughly drying the skin.	18. Prevents contamination of the gown.
19. Discard the towel into a linen hamper.	19. Keeps the environment clean.

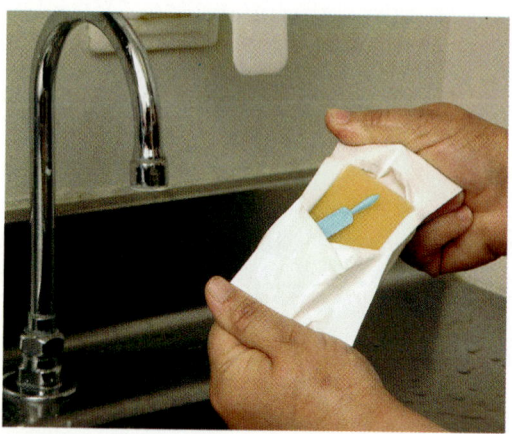

FIGURE 29-51 Prepackaged Scrub Brush. DELMAR/CENGAGE LEARNING

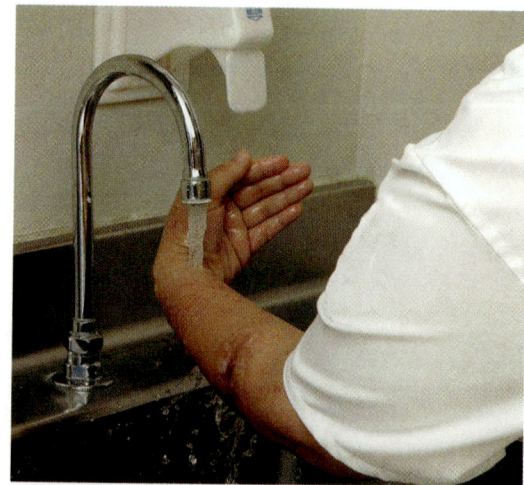

FIGURE 29-52 Thoroughly rinse fingers, hands, and arms. DELMAR/CENGAGE LEARNING

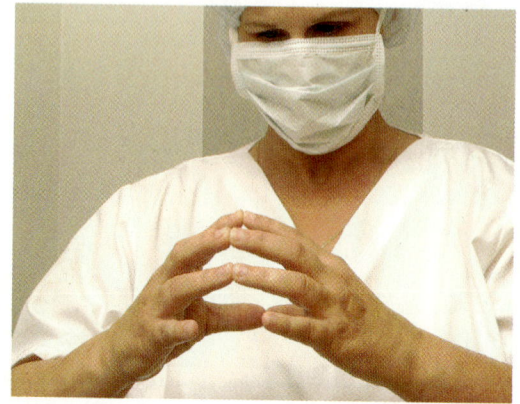

FIGURE 29-53 Keep arms flexed, and proceed to area. DELMAR/CENGAGE LEARNING

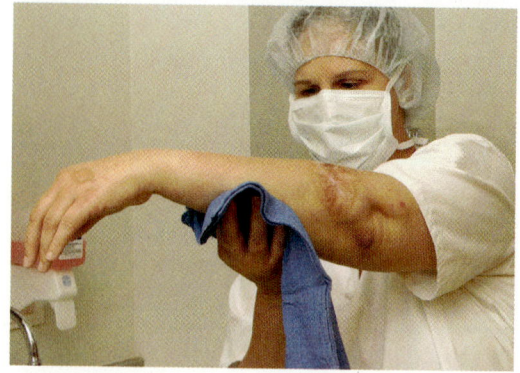

FIGURE 29-54 Dry arms in a rotating motion. DELMAR/CENGAGE LEARNING

(Continues)

PROCEDURE 29-5
Surgical Hand Antisepsis (Continued)

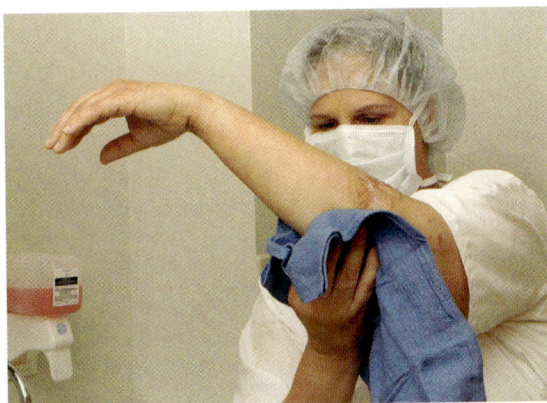

FIGURE 29-55 **Dry arms up to the elbows.** DELMAR/CENGAGE LEARNING

delegation tip

Surgical scrubbing is delegated only if the personnel are specifically trained, such as in a surgical suite or a testing laboratory.

nursing tips

- *Be sure to keep hands and forearms above elbow level.*
- *Avoid products with iodine if an allergy is present.*
- *Make sure you are not splashed by another person washing his or her hands.*

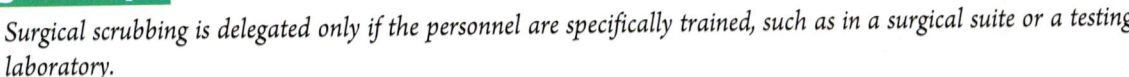

PROCEDURE 29-6
Applying Sterile Gloves and Gown via the Closed Method

EQUIPMENT
- Sterile gown
- Sterile and proper-size gloves

ACTION	RATIONALE
GOWNING	
1. Wash hands/hand hygiene.	1. Prevents the spread of microorganisms.
2. The sterile gown is folded inside out.	2. Allows ungloved hands to touch only the inside.
3. Grasp the gown inside the neckline, step back, and allow the gown to open in front of you; keep the inside of the gown toward you; do not allow it to touch anything (see Figure 29-56 on page 714).	3. Keeps the outside of the gown sterile.

(Continues)

PROCEDURE 29-6
Applying Sterile Gloves and Gown via the Closed Method (Continued)

ACTION	RATIONALE
4. With hands at shoulder level, slip both arms into the gown; keep your hands inside the sleeves of the gown (see Figure 29-57).	4. Prevents the gown from touching nonsterile objects; allows sterile items to come into contact only with other sterile items.
5. The circulating nurse will step up behind you and grasp the inside of the gown, bring it over your shoulders, and secure the ties at the neck and waist.	5. Prevents any part of the gown from touching a nonsterile object; provides complete coverage of undergarments.

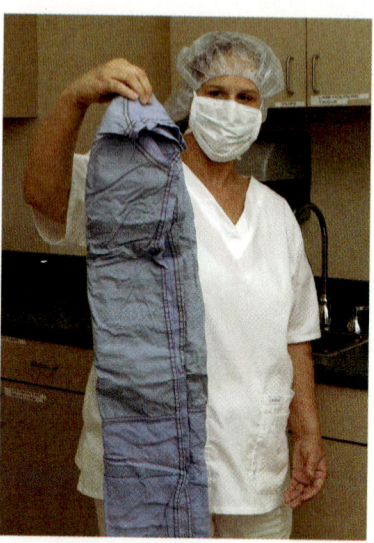

FIGURE 29-56 Allow the gown to fall open. DELMAR/CENGAGE LEARNING

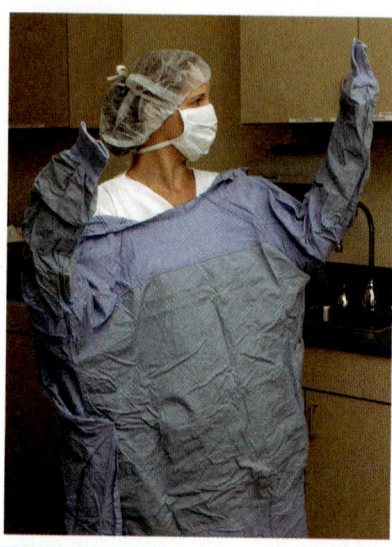

FIGURE 29-57 Slip both arms into the gown. DELMAR/CENGAGE LEARNING

CLOSED GLOVING

6. With hands still inside the gown sleeves, open the inner wrapper of the gloves on the sterile gown field (see Figure 29-58 on page 715).	6. Maintains sterility of the gloves.
7. With nondominant sleeved hand, grasp the cuff of the glove for the dominant hand and lay it on the extended dominant forearm (see Figure 29-59 on page 715); with palm up, place the palm of the glove against the sleeved palm, with fingers of the glove pointing toward elbow (see Figure 29-60 on page 715).	7. Only sterile items come into contact with each other.
8. Manipulate the glove so the sleeved thumb of dominant hand is grasping the cuff; with nondominant hand, turn the cuff over the end of dominant hand and gown's cuff.	8. Prevents the hands from contaminating the sterile glove.
9. With sleeved nondominant hand, grasp the cuff of the glove and the gown's sleeve of the dominant hand; slowly extend the fingers into the glove, making sure the cuff of the glove remains above the cuff of the gown's sleeve (see Figure 29-61 on page 715).	9. Provides a closed sterile method for gloving; the glove cuff over the gown prevents contamination of the operative field with microorganisms.
10. With the gloved dominant hand, repeat Actions 8 and 9 (see Figures 29-62 and 29-63 on page 716).	10. Only sterile items can touch each other.
11. Interlock gloved fingers; secure fit.	11. Promotes dexterity of gloved hands.
12. Wash hands/hand hygiene.	12. Prevents the spread of microorganisms.

(Continues)

PROCEDURE 29-6
Applying Sterile Gloves and Gown via the Closed Method (Continued)

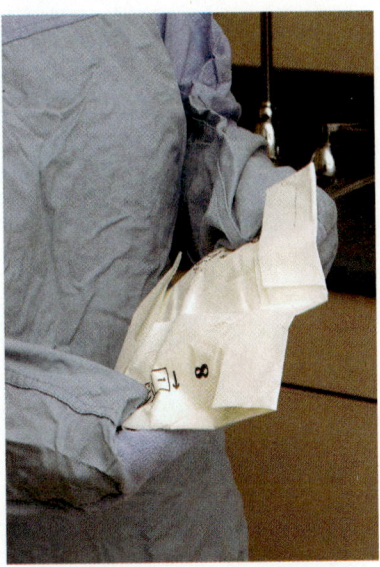

FIGURE 29-58 Keep hands inside the gown sleeves when opening gloves. Handle the gloves through the fabric of the gown. DELMAR/CENGAGE LEARNING

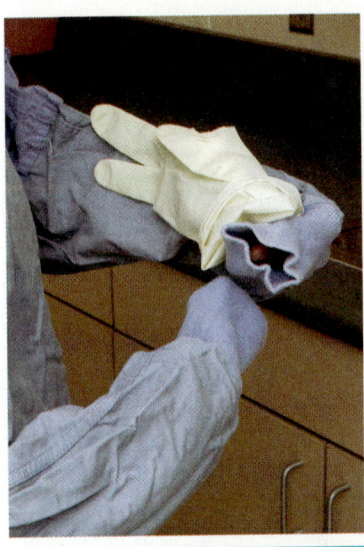

FIGURE 29-59 Grasp the cuff of the glove. DELMAR/CENGAGE LEARNING

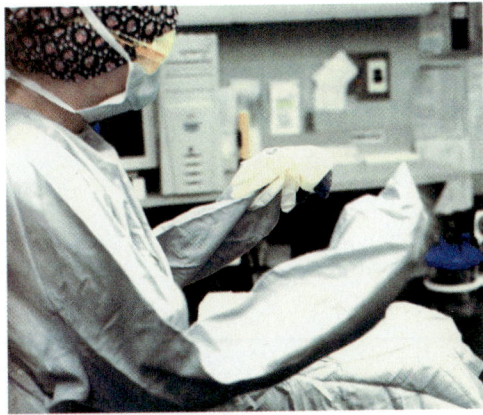

FIGURE 29-60 Keep the fingers of the glove facing the elbow. DELMAR/CENGAGE LEARNING

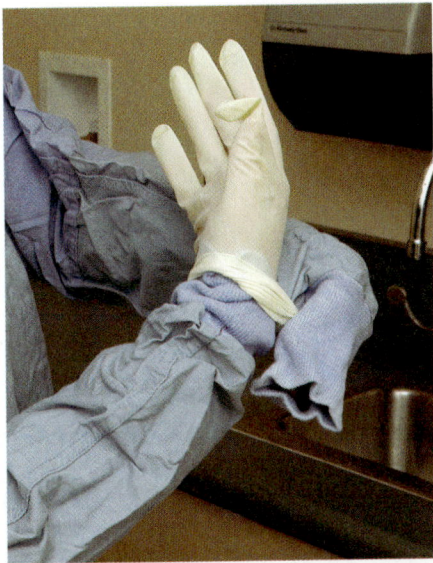

FIGURE 29-61 Extend fingers into the glove. DELMAR/CENGAGE LEARNING

(Continues)

PROCEDURE 29-6
Applying Sterile Gloves and Gown via the Closed Method (Continued)

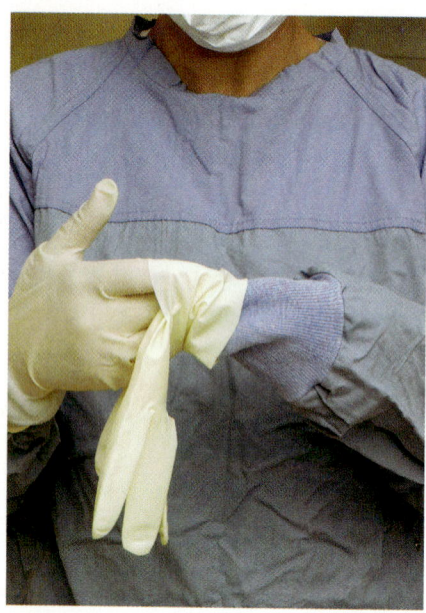

FIGURE 29-62 Place the second glove on the gown. DELMAR/
CENGAGE LEARNING

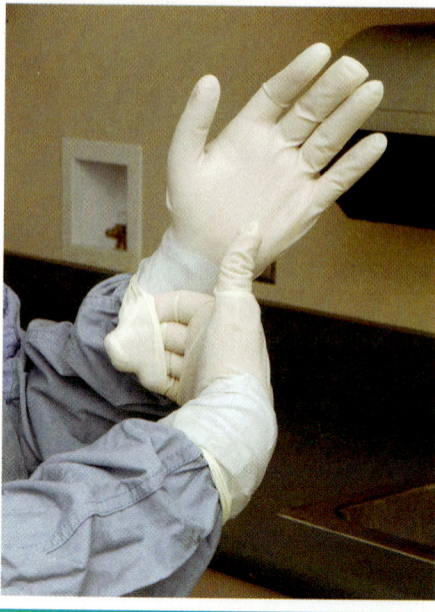

FIGURE 29-63 Extend the fingers into the second glove.
DELMAR/CENGAGE LEARNING

delegation tip

Sterile gloving and gowning is delegated only if the personnel are specifically trained, such as in a surgical suite or a testing laboratory setting.

nursing tips

- *Touch only sterile to sterile.*
- *Do not lean against the scrub sink.*
- *Be careful not to get scrub uniform wet. This will contaminate the sterile gown.*

PROCEDURE 29-7
Removing Contaminated Items

EQUIPMENT
- Disposable gloves
- Labeled bag for disposal of soiled linens; bag should be hot-water soluble; bag may also be colored (red) for easy identification. (*Note:* Some agencies may require linens to be double bagged for removal.)
- Self-supporting stand for linen bag
- Second linen bag if double-bagging technique used

(Continues)

PROCEDURE 29-7
Removing Contaminated Items (Continued)

ACTION	RATIONALE
REMOVAL OF SOILED LINEN	
1. Wash hands/hand hygiene when entering the client's room or use an alcohol-based hand rub.	1. Prevents the spread of microorganisms.
2. Wear disposable gloves; wear other protective items (gowns, goggles) as determined by the situation and agency's policies.	2. Protects the nurse from contamination from blood and body fluids.
3. Place labeled linen bag in stand (see Figure 29-64).	3. Proper labeling or identification of the linen bag ensures proper handling by other agency personnel. Check agency policy for issues of confidentiality with regard to labeling.
4. Gather linens and separate from disposable items.	4. Prevents waste from being placed in linen bag.
5. Do not allow any linens to touch the floor.	5. The floor is always considered a contaminated area.
6. Place soiled linens in the linen bag; keep clean linens in a different area (see Figure 29-65).	6. It is important to prevent cross-contamination to clean supplies and linen.
7. Take care not to shake the linens when removing items from the bed or bathroom.	7. Minimizing movement of the linens through the air helps reduce the risk of transmission of microorganisms.
8. Do not allow the soiled linens to come into contact with clothing. Carry linens with arms extended outward.	8. Prevents contamination of the nurse and cross-contamination to other clients.
9. Do not overfill the bag.	9. Ensures proper closure of bag.
10. Tie ends of the bag securely.	10. Prevents linens from spilling out of the bag.
11. Check for any punctures or tears in the bag.	11. The linen bag must be intact to prevent transmission of microorganisms.
12. Double bag items if there is concern that the outside of the bag is contaminated or torn.	12. This is necessary to prevent cross-contamination and transmission of microorganisms to other personnel or other areas.
13. Wash hands/hand hygiene.	13. Prevents the spread of microorganisms.

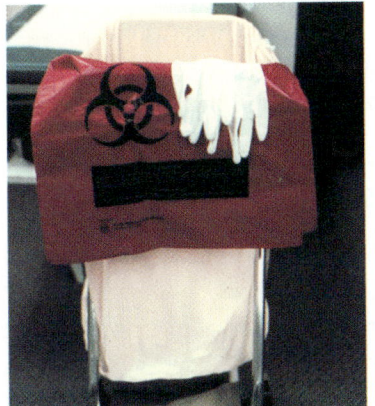

FIGURE 29-64 Biohazard bags and gloves are used to handle and dispose of contaminated items. DELMAR/CENGAGE LEARNING

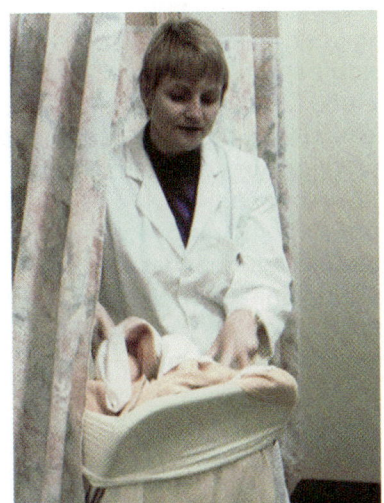

FIGURE 29-65 Place soiled linen in a bag. DELMAR/CENGAGE LEARNING

(Continues)

PROCEDURE 29-7
Removing Contaminated Items (Continued)

ACTION	RATIONALE
DOUBLE-AGGING TECHNIQUE	
14. With double bagging of linens, follow Actions 1–11. Then place the first bag into a second bag. Either a second nurse holds the second bag, or it is in a stand immediately outside of the room.	14. Some agencies require double bagging of linens to reduce the possibility of transmission of microorganisms. In most situations, it is not necessary unless the single bag is not sturdy enough to hold the items or if the outside of the single bag has become contaminated.
15. The second bag is properly labeled and secured.	15. Proper labeling or identification of the linen bag ensures proper handling by other agency personnel. Most agencies will have bags marked *biohazardous.*
16. The linens are then ready for the laundry.	16. Linens should be disposed of as soon as possible per agency policy.
17. Wash hands/hand hygiene.	17. Prevents the spread of microorganisms.
REMOVAL OF OTHER CONTAMINATED ITEMS	
18. Removal and bagging of trash bag follow the same procedure as for linens (see Figure 29-66 on page 719).	18. Check agency policy to determine whether double bagging is required.
19. Sharps containers need to be removed when three-quarters full or if the outside of the container becomes contaminated. Lock down the lid if available, and follow hospital policy for removal (see Figure 29-67 on page 719). Never reach into a container with your hand.	19. Overfilling a sharps container can lead to injuries to staff members.
20. Perform hand rub.	20. Proper hand hygiene reduces transmission of microorganisms.
21. Use disposable equipment when able (see Figure 29-68 on page 719).	21. Reduces the possibility of transmission of microorganisms.
22. Properly bag, label, and remove any nondisposable equipment that will require special cleaning (disinfection and sterilization).	22. Proper handling and labeling of items will ensure proper handling by other agency personnel.
23. Disassemble special procedure trays into disposable and nondisposable parts. Send nondisposable items (after proper bagging) to central services for decontamination.	23. Some agencies require that items that can be sterilized by autoclave (glass, metal) be separated from rubber and plastic items.
24. Laboratory specimens should be placed in a leakproof container and require no other precautions. Check to see that containers are not visibly contaminated on the outside (see Figure 29-69 on page 719).	24. Personnel handling laboratory specimens must utilize Standard Precautions.
25. Wash hands/hand hygiene.	25. Prevents the spread of microorganisms.

(Continues)

PROCEDURE 29-7
Removing Contaminated Items (Continued)

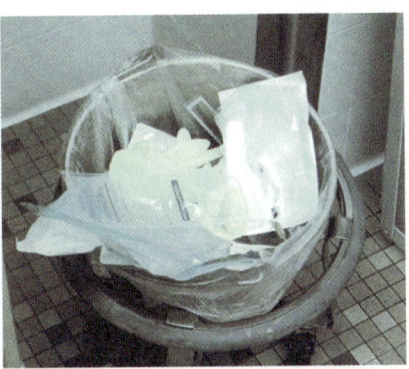

FIGURE 29-66 Bag all trash prior to removal. DELMAR/CENGAGE LEARNING

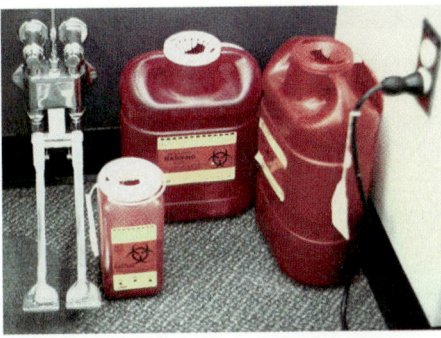

FIGURE 29-67 Remove and replace full sharps containers to avoid needlestick injuries from pushing sharp items into a full container. DELMAR/CENGAGE LEARNING

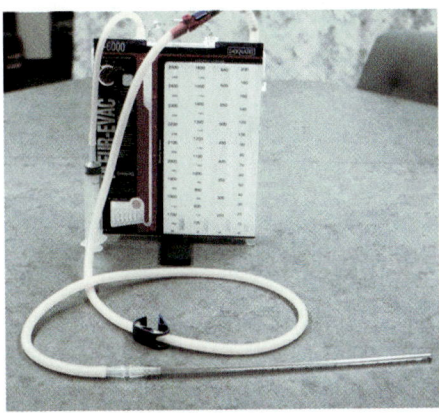

FIGURE 29-68 Using disposable equipment reduces contamination risks. DELMAR/CENGAGE LEARNING

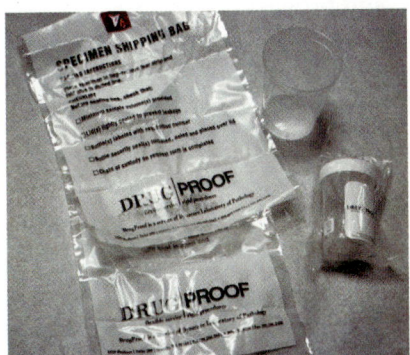

FIGURE 29-69 Place specimens in leakproof containers to avoid contamination. DELMAR/CENGAGE LEARNING

delegation tip

Infection control measures are used for all clients. Careful handling of all contaminated items from the client's environment is the responsibility of all personnel involved in the client's care. The registered nurse may delegate these activities but is responsible for adhering to Standard Precautions.

nursing tips

- *Check supplies (bags, labels) before beginning bagging of items for removal.*
- *Always wash hands before and after entering a room and bagging soiled items, even when wearing gloves.*
- *Use disposable equipment and supplies when possible.*
- *Do not take items such as a stethoscope into another client's room for use without proper cleaning when there is risk of transmission of infection.*
- *Review your agency's policies for specific guidelines. Some institutions may require double bagging for some items.*
- *Recheck labels and restock special bags as needed so that supplies are readily available for other caregivers and personnel.*

PROCEDURE 29-8

Bathing a Client in Bed

EQUIPMENT

- Bath towels
- Washcloths
- Bath blanket
- Washbasin
- Soap
- Soap dish
- Lotion
- Deodorant
- Clean gown
- Clean linens
- Disposable, latex-free gloves

ACTION	RATIONALE
1. Assess the client's preferences about bathing.	1. Provides client with the opportunity to participate in care.
2. Explain procedure to client. Gather supplies (see Figure 29-70).	2. Enhances cooperation.
3. Prepare environment. Close doors and windows, adjust temperature, provide time for elimination needs, and provide privacy (see Figure 29-71).	3. Protects from chills during bath and increases sense of privacy.
4. Wash hands/hand hygiene. Apply gloves. Gloves should be changed when emptying water basin.	4. Prevents the spread of microorganisms.
5. Lower side rail on the side close to you. Position client in a comfortable position close to the side near you.	5. Prevents unnecessary reaching. Facilitates use of good body mechanics.
6. If bath blankets are available, place over top sheet. Remove top sheet from under bath blanket. Remove client's gown. Bath blanket should be folded to expose only the area being cleaned at that time. (Top sheets or towels may also be used for bath blankets.)	6. Prevents exposure of client. Promotes privacy. Protects from chills.
7. Fill washbasin two-thirds full. Permit client to test temperature of water with hand. Water should be changed when a soap film develops or water becomes soiled.	7. Prevents accidental burns or chills.
8. Wet the washcloth and wring it out (see Figure 29-72 on page 721).	8. Prevents unnecessary wetting of the client.

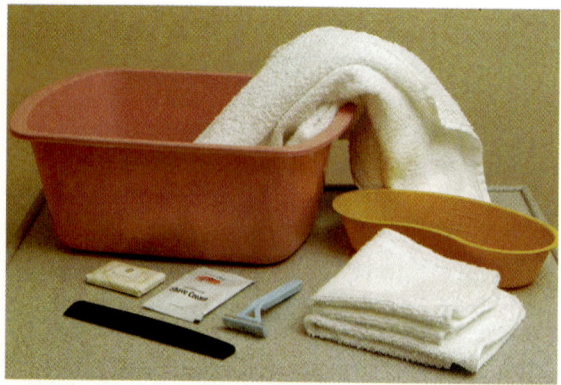

FIGURE 29-70 Emesis and bath basins, soap, towels, and lotion are used to bathe the client. A razor and shaving cream are used to groom the male client. DELMAR/CENGAGE LEARNING

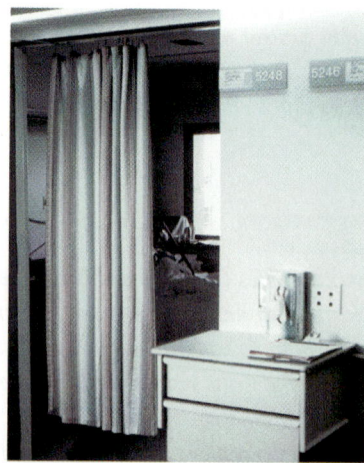

FIGURE 29-71 Close doors and/or curtains, and provide privacy prior to beginning the bath. DELMAR/CENGAGE LEARNING

(Continues)

PROCEDURE 29-8
Bathing a Client in Bed (Continued)

ACTION	RATIONALE
9. Make a bath mitten with the washcloth. To make a mitten, grasp the edge of the washcloth with the thumb; fold a third over the palm of the hand; wrap remainder of cloth around hand and across palm, and grasp the second edge under the thumb; and fold the extended end of the washcloth onto the palm, and tuck under the palmar surface of the cloth.	9. Prevents ends of washcloth from dragging across skin. Promotes friction during bath.
10. Wash the face (see Figure 29-73). Ask about the client's preference for using soap on the face. Use a separate corner of the washcloth for each eye, wiping from inner to outer canthus. Wash neck and ears. Rinse and pat dry. Male clients may want to shave at this time. Provide assistance with shaving as needed.	10. Some clients may not use soap on the face. Using separate corners of the washcloth reduces the risk of transmitting microorganisms. Patting dry reduces skin irritation and drying.
11. Wash arms, forearms, and hands (see Figure 29-74). Wash forearms and arms using long, firm strokes in the direction of distal to proximal (see Figure 29-75 on page 722). Arm may need to be supported while being washed. Wash axilla. Rinse and pat dry. Apply deodorant	11. Long strokes promote circulation. Soaking hands softens nails and loosens soil from skin and nails. Strokes directed distal to proximal promote venous return.

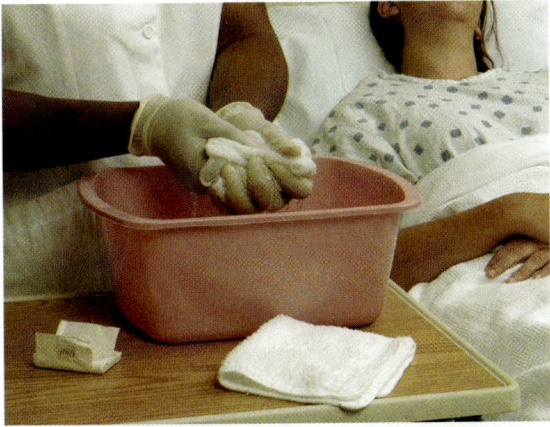

FIGURE 29-72 Wet the washcloth and wring out the excess water. The nurse is wearing a mask and gown because the client is in isolation. DELMAR/CENGAGE LEARNING

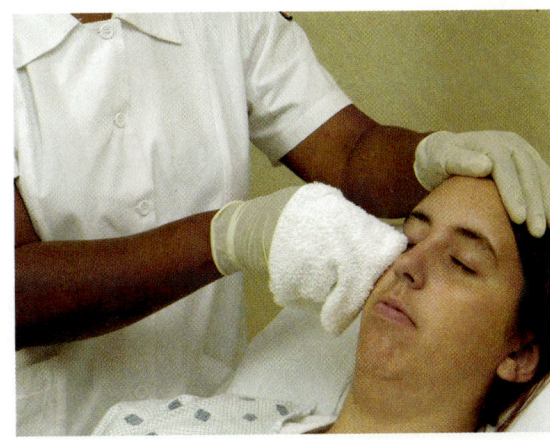

FIGURE 29-73 Wash the client's face first. DELMAR/CENGAGE LEARNING

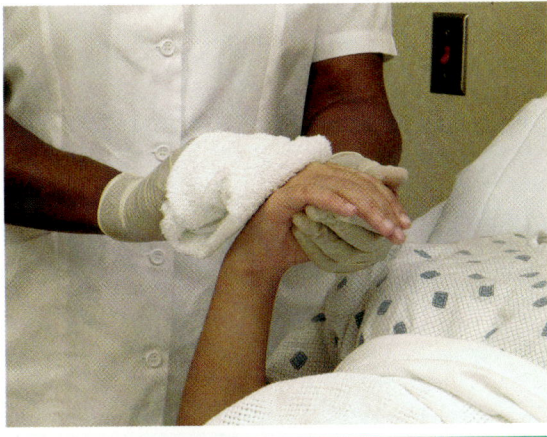

FIGURE 29-74 Wash the hands and arms next. DELMAR/CENGAGE LEARNING

(Continues)

PROCEDURE 29-8
Bathing a Client in Bed (Continued)

ACTION	RATIONALE
or powder if desired. Immerse client's hand into basin of water. Allow hand to soak about 3 to 5 minutes. Wash hands, interdigit area, fingers, and fingernails. Rinse and pat dry.	
12. Wash chest and abdomen. Fold bath blanket down to umbilicus. Wash chest using long, firm strokes. Wash skin fold under the female client's breast by lifting each breast. Rinse and pat dry. Fold bath blanket down to suprapubic area. Use another towel to cover chest area. Wash abdomen using long, firm strokes. Rinse and pat dry. Replace bath blanket over chest and abdomen. Cover chest or abdomen area in between washing, rinsing, and drying to prevent chilling.	12. Promotes privacy and prevents chills. Long strokes promote circulation. Perspiration and soil collect within skin folds.
13. Wash legs and feet. Expose leg farthest from you by folding bath blanket to midline. Bend the leg at the knee. Grasp the heel, elevate the leg from the bed, and cover bed with bath towel. Place washbasin on towel. Place client's foot into washbasin (see Figure 29-76). Allow foot to soak while washing the leg with long, firm strokes in the direction of distal to proximal. Rinse and pat dry. Clean soles, interdigits, and toes. Rinse and pat dry. Perform same procedure with the other leg and foot.	13. Supports joints to prevent strain and fatigue. Soaking foot loosens dirt, softens nails, and promotes comfort.

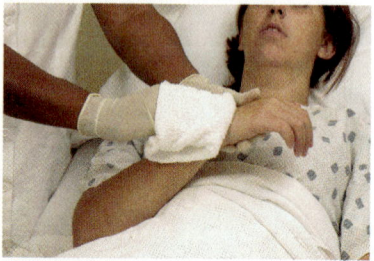
A.

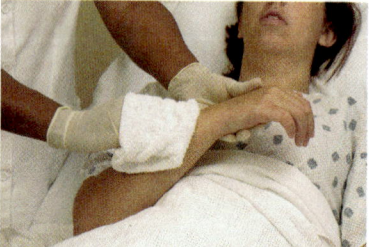
B.

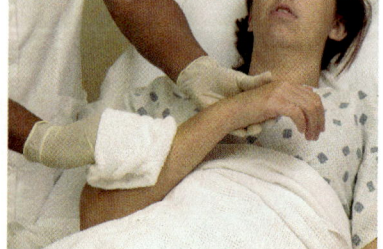
C.

FIGURE 29-75 (A–C) Wash from distal to proximal—from hands to forearms to upper arms. DELMAR/CENGAGE LEARNING

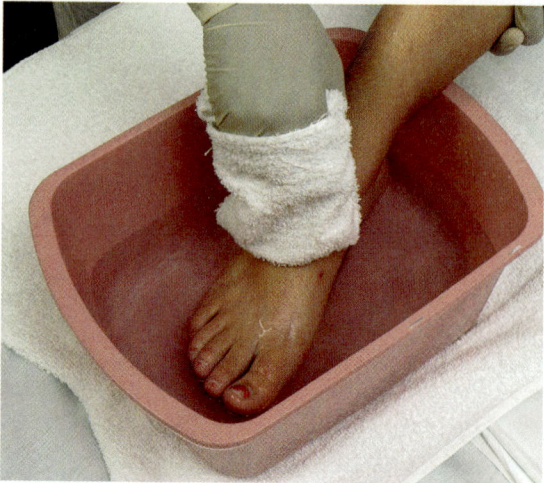

FIGURE 29-76 Place feet in basin. Clean interdigits and soles of feet. DELMAR/CENGAGE LEARNING

(Continues)

PROCEDURE 29-8
Bathing a Client in Bed (Continued)

ACTION	RATIONALE
14. Wash back. Assist client into prone or side-lying position facing away from you. Wash the back and buttocks using long, firm strokes. Rinse and pat dry. Give back rub and apply lotion.	14. Exposes back and buttocks for washing. Back rub promotes relaxation and circulation.
15. Perineal care: Assist client to supine position. Perform perineal care (see Figures 29-77 and 29-78).	15. Removes genital secretions and soil.
16. Apply lotion as desired or needed. Apply clean gown.	16. Lotion lubricates skin. Powder absorbs excess perspiration.
17. Document skin assessment, type of bath given, and client outcomes and responses.	17. Provides evidence of nursing care.
18. Wash hands/hand hygiene.	18. Prevents the spread of microorganisms.

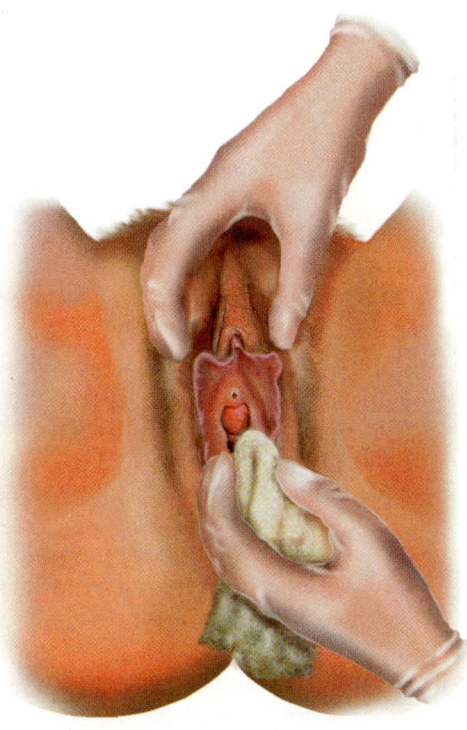

FIGURE 29-77 Clean the female perineal area. DELMAR/CENGAGE LEARNING

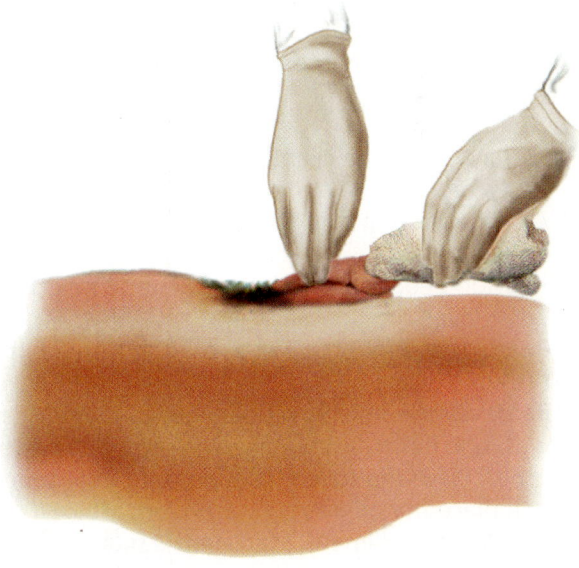

FIGURE 29-78 Clean the male perineal area. DELMAR/CENGAGE LEARNING

delegation tip

This skill is routinely delegated to ancillary personnel, who should allow the client to perform as much of the bath as possible or permitted. The caregiver employs Standard Precautions, properly positions the client, and observes and reports the client's skin condition and color to the nurse. The nurse retains the responsibility to assess the client.

nursing tips

- *Be sure to thoroughly rinse soap off the client. Soap can cause drying and chafing.*
- *Be sure to thoroughly dry the client, especially skin folds and areas that rub together often. Leaving water in these areas can cause cracking and irritation.*
- *Use this time to assess the client's skin integrity. Are there any rashes or open or reddened areas?*
- *Encourage clients to assist in the bath as much as they are able. Self-care for basic needs is a way to maintain a sense of self-control and self-esteem during illness.*

PROCEDURE 29-9

Changing Linens in an Unoccupied Bed

EQUIPMENT
- Bottom sheet (fitted, if available)
- Top sheet
- Mattress pad
- Pillowcase (each pillow on the bed)
- Drawsheet (regular top sheet may be used)

ACTION	RATIONALE
1. Wash hands/hand hygiene.	1. Prevents the spread of microorganisms.
2. Place hamper by client's door if linen bags are not available (see Figure 29-79 on page 725). Explain procedure to client. Assess condition of blanket and/or bedspread.	2. Provides for proper disposal of soiled linens. Encourages client cooperation. Allows for organization of supplies.
3. Gather linens and gloves. Place linens on a clean, dry surface in reverse order of usage at the client's bedside (pillowcases, top sheet, drawsheet, bottom sheet).	3. Provides easy access to items.
4. Apply gloves.	4. Reduces risk of infection from soiled, contaminated linens.
5. Inquire about the client's toileting needs and attend as necessary.	5. Provides for client comfort and prevents interruptions during bed making.
6. Assist client to a safe, comfortable chair.	6. Increases client's comfort and decreases risk of falls.
7. Position bed: flat, side rails down, and height adjusted to waist level.	7. Promotes good body mechanics and decreases back strain.
8. Remove and fold blanket and/or bedspread. If clean and reusable, place on clean work area.	8. Keeps reusable bed linens clean.
9. Remove soiled pillowcases by grasping the closed end with one hand and slipping the pillow out with the other. Place the soiled cases on top of the soiled sheet, and place the pillows on clean work area.	9. Allows easy removal of the pillowcases without contamination of uniform by soiled linens and keeps pillows clean.
10. Remove soiled linens: Start on the side of the bed closest to you; free the bottom sheet and mattress pad by lifting the mattress and rolling soiled linens to the middle of the bed. Go to the other side of the bed. Repeat action.	10. Prevents tearing and fanning of linens. Linens are folded from cleanest to most soiled area to prevent contamination.
11. Fold (do not fan or flap) soiled linens: head of bed to middle, foot of bed to middle. Place in linen bag or hamper, keeping soiled linens away from uniform.	11. Fanning or flapping linens increases the number of microorganisms in the air. Folding linens reduces the risk of transmission of infection to others.
12. Check mattress. If mattress is soiled, clean it with an antiseptic solution and dry it thoroughly.	12. Reduces the transmission of microorganisms.
13. Remove gloves, wash hands, and apply a second pair of clean gloves (when appropriate).	13. Reduces the transmission of microorganisms to clean linens.
14. Open the clean mattress pad lengthwise onto the bed with the seamed side of the sheet toward the mattress. Unfold half of the pad's width to the center crease, and smooth the pad flat. If there are elastic bands to hold the pad in place, slide them under the corners of the mattress.	14. Facilitates making bed in an organized, time-saving manner by not having to go from one side of the bed to the other.
15. Proceed with placing the bottom sheet onto the mattress. Linens differ from facility to facility. Bottom sheets may be fitted or they may be flat. Proceed to the appropriate action for the linens available.	15. Use linens available at the facility.

(Continues)

PROCEDURE 29-9
Changing Linens in an Unoccupied Bed (Continued)

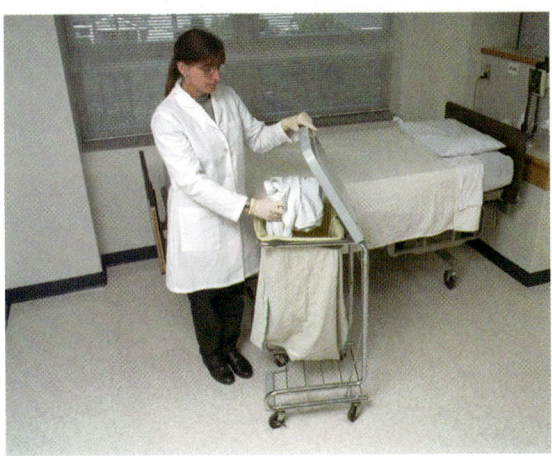

FIGURE 29-79 Clean linens and a laundry hamper for used linens are brought to the bedside to make the unoccupied bed. Gloves help reduce the transmission of microorganisms. DELMAR/CENGAGE LEARNING

FITTED BOTTOM SHEET

16. Position yourself diagonally toward the head of the bed.

17. Start at the head with seamed side of the fitted sheet toward the mattress.

18. Lift the mattress corner with your hand closest to the bed; with your other hand, pull and tuck the fitted sheet over the mattress corner; secure at the head of the bed.
19. Pull and tuck the fitted sheet over the mattress corners at the foot of the bed.

16. Ensures good body mechanics and efficient procedure.
17. Placement of seamed side toward mattress prevents irritation of the client's skin.
18. Prevents straining of back muscles; decreases the chance that the sheet will pull out from under the mattress.
19. Prevents straining of back muscles; decreases the chance that the sheet will pull out from under the mattress.

FLAT REGULAR SHEET

20. Unfold the bottom sheet with the seamed side toward the mattress. Align the bottom edge of the sheet with the edge of the mattress at the foot of the bed.

21. Allow the sheet to hang 10 inches (25 cm) over the mattress on the side and at the top of the bed.

22. Position yourself diagonally toward the head of the bed. Lift the top of the mattress corner with the hand closest to the bed, and smoothly tuck the sheet under the mattress.
23. Miter the corner at the head of the bed using the information in the steps that follow.

24. Face the side of bed and lift and lay the top edge of the sheet onto the bed to form a triangular fold.
25. With your palms down, tuck the lower edge of sheet (hanging free at the side of the mattress) under the mattress.

20. Placement of the seamed side toward the mattress prevents irritation to the client's skin. Ensure proper placement of the sheet so that it can be tightly secured at the top and on both sides of the bed.
21. Proper placement of linens ensures adequate sheeting for all sides of the bed.
22. Prevents straining of back muscles; decreases the chance that the sheet will pull out from under the mattress.
23. Secures sheet tightly to the mattress, with the triangular fold providing a smooth tuck to keep the linen in place.
24. Forms the base for the tuck.

25. Forms the first half of the tuck.

(Continues)

PROCEDURE 29-9
Changing Linens in an Unoccupied Bed (Continued)

26. Grasp the triangular fold, and bring it down over the side of the mattress. Allow the sheet to hang free at the side of the mattress.

27. Place the drawsheet on the bottom sheet, and unfold it to the middle crease (see Figure 29-80 on page 727).

28. Face the side of the bed, palms of hands down. Tuck both the bottom and drawsheets under the mattress. Ensure that the bottom sheet is tucked smoothly under the mattress all the way to the foot of the bed.

29. Go to the other side of the bed, unfold the bottom sheet, and repeat the actions used to apply the mattress pad and bottom sheet.

30. Unfold the drawsheet, if used, and grasp the free-hanging sides of both the bottom and drawsheets. Pull toward you, keeping your back straight, and with a firm grasp (sheets taut) tuck both sheets under the mattress. Use your arms and open palms to extend the linen under the mattress. Place the protective pad on the bottom sheet.

31. Place the top sheet on the bed and unfold lengthwise, placing the center crease (width) of the sheet in the middle of the bed. Place the top edge of the sheet (seam up) even with the top of the mattress at the head of the bed. Pull the remaining length toward the bottom of the bed.

32. Unfold and apply the blanket or spread. Follow the same technique used in applying the top sheet (see Figure 29-81 on page 727).

33. Miter the bottom corners. With your palms down, tuck the lower edge of the sheet under the mattress. Grasp the triangular fold and bring it down over the side of the mattress. Allow the sheet to hang free at the side of the mattress (see Figures 29-82, 29-83, and 29-84 on page 727).

34. Face the head of the bed and fold the top sheet and blanket over 6 inches (15 cm). Fanfold the sheet and blanket (from the foot to the middle of the bed) (see Figure 29-85 on page 727).

35. Apply a clean pillowcase on each pillow (see Figure 29-86 on page 728). With one hand, grasp the closed end of the pillowcase. Gather the pillowcase and turn it inside out overhand. With same hand, grasp the middle of one end of the pillow. With the other hand, pull the case over the length of the pillow. The corners of the pillow should fit snugly into the corners of the case.

36. Return the bed to the lowest position and elevate the head of the bed 30° to 45°. Put side rails up on side farthest from client.

37. Inquire about toileting needs of the client; assist as necessary.

38. Assist the client back into the bed and pull up the side rails; place call light in reach; take vital signs.

26. Will form the final portion of the mitered corner when tucked in.

27. Provides a sheet to lift and move the client in bed without having to use the bottom sheet and remake the bed. Helps keep the bottom sheet clean.

28. Keeps sheet taut, in place, and wrinkle free, thereby decreasing the risk of skin irritation.

29. Unfolding decreases air current; air currents can spread microorganisms.

30. Uses your body's weight in pulling the sheet taut and prevents strain on your back muscles.

31. Making one side of the bed at a time saves time and movement. Seam will be folded down to prevent contact with the client's skin, which can result in irritation.

32. Provides warmth.

33. Secures linen at the foot of the bed.

34. Allows the client easy access to the bed.

35. Keeps clean pillowcase away from uniform.

36. Provides for client safety.

37. Saves client energy and provides time to care for client's needs.

38. Promotes client safety and a means to call for assistance. Sitting up in a chair and movement may cause changes in the client's vital signs.

(Continues)

PROCEDURE 29-9
Changing Linens in an Unoccupied Bed (Continued)

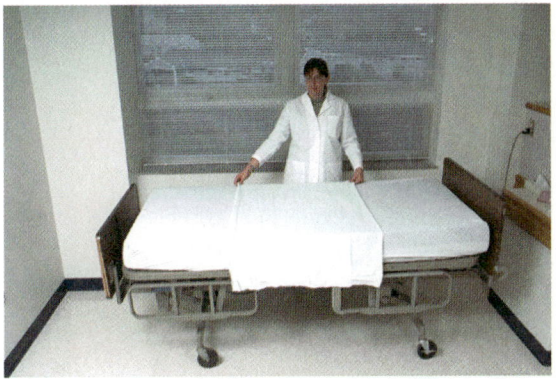

FIGURE 29-80 The clean drawsheet is placed on top of the bottom sheet. DELMAR/CENGAGE LEARNING

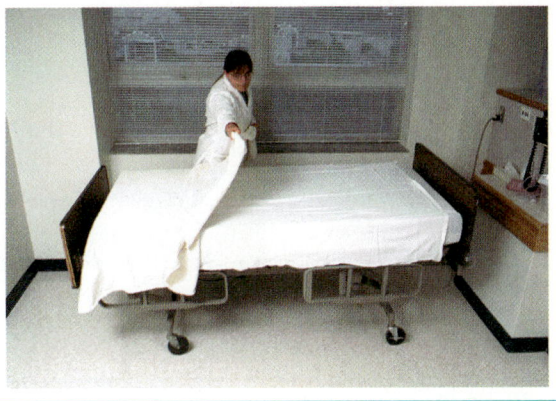

FIGURE 29-81 Place the blanket or spread over the top sheet. DELMAR/CENGAGE LEARNING

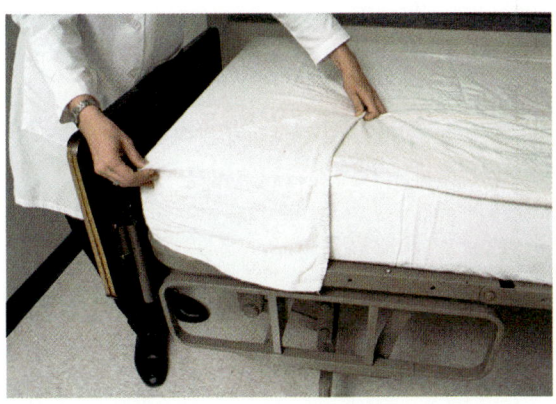

FIGURE 29-82 Lift and lay the hem of the sheet and blanket on the bed to form a triangular fold. DELMAR/CENGAGE LEARNING

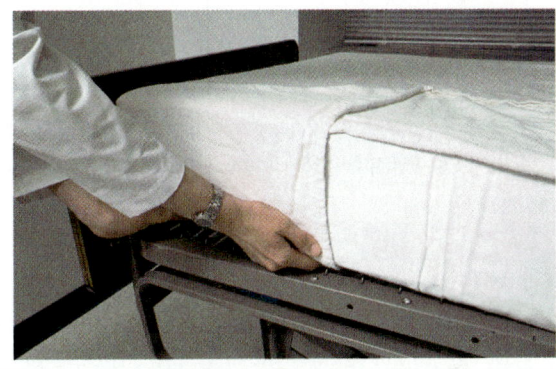

FIGURE 29-83 Tuck the lower edge of the sheet and blanket under the mattress. DELMAR/CENGAGE LEARNING

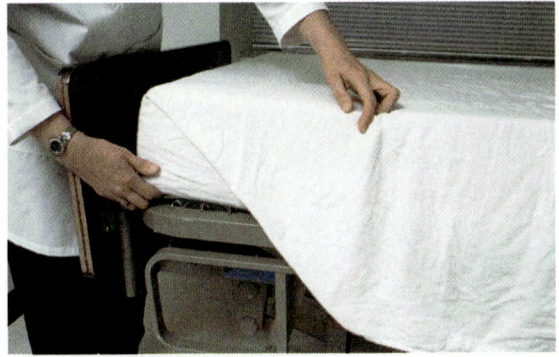

FIGURE 29-84 Bring the triangular fold down, and let it hang freely at the side of the mattress. DELMAR/CENGAGE LEARNING

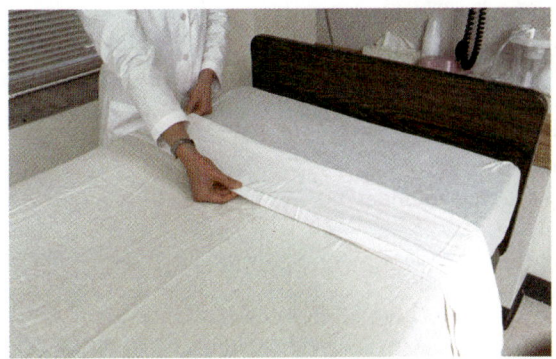

FIGURE 29-85 Fold the top sheet and blanket 6 inches. DELMAR/CENGAGE LEARNING

PROCEDURE 29-9
Changing Linens in an Unoccupied Bed (Continued)

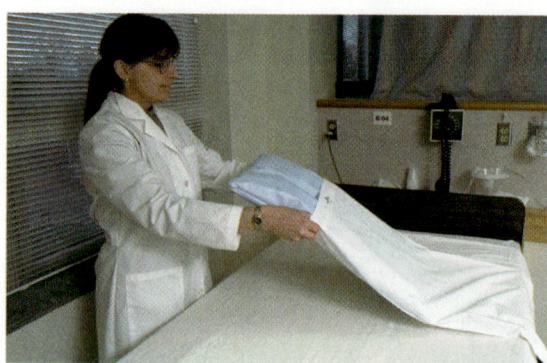

FIGURE 29-86 Place a clean pillowcase on each pillow while keeping the clean pillowcase away from uniform. DELMAR/CENGAGE LEARNING

ACTION	RATIONALE
39. Remove gloves; wash hands/hand hygiene.	39. Prevents the spread of microorganisms.
40. Document your actions and the client's response during the procedure and to sitting up in a chair.	40. Documents completion of procedure and assessment findings of client's tolerance.

delegation tip

Bed making is usually delegated to ancillary personnel. Their instruction should include safety precautions for themselves and the client and understanding the appropriate use of Standard Precautions.

nursing tips

- *If the bed raises and lowers, raise it up to a comfortable height to prevent back strain.*
- *Make one side of the bed completely, and then move to the other side to save time and steps.*
- *Be careful not to carry the dirty linens close to your uniform to prevent contamination.*

PROCEDURE 29-10
Changing Linens in an Occupied Bed

EQUIPMENT
- Linen hamper
- Top sheet, drawsheet, bottom sheet
- Pillowcase
- Blanket
- Bath blanket

ACTION	RATIONALE
1. Explain procedure to client. Gather equipment (see Figure 29-87 on page 729).	1. Promotes client cooperation.
2. Wash hands/hand hygiene.	2. Prevents the spread of microorganisms.
3. Bring equipment to the bedside (see Figure 29-88 on page 729).	3. Facilitates a smooth procedure.

(Continues)

PROCEDURE 29-10
Changing Linens in an Occupied Bed (Continued)

ACTION	RATIONALE

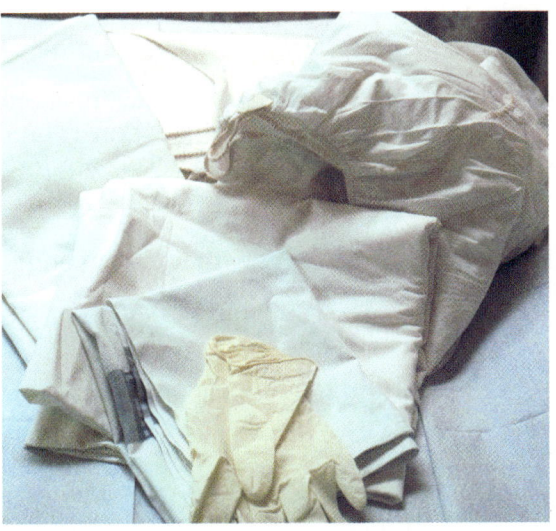

FIGURE 29-87 Top and bottom sheets, drawsheet, and pillowcase are used to make the occupied bed. Gloves reduce the transmission of microorganisms. DELMAR/CENGAGE LEARNING

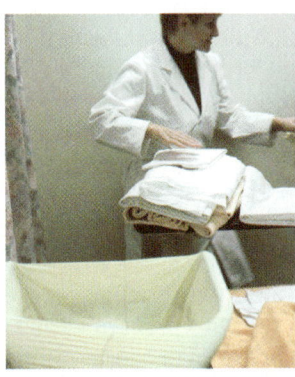

FIGURE 29-88 Bring clean linens and empty linen hamper to the bedside. DELMAR/CENGAGE LEARNING

4. Remove top sheet and blanket. Loosen bottom sheet at foot and sides of bed. Lower side rail nearest the nurse, if necessary, for access. Client may be covered with a bath blanket (see Figure 29-89 on page 730).

5. Position client on side, facing away from you. Reposition pillow under head.

6. Fanfold or roll bottom linens close to client toward the center of the bed (see Figure 29-90 on page 730).

7. Smooth wrinkles out of mattress. Place clean bottom linens with the center fold nearest the client. Fanfold or roll clean bottom linens nearest client and tuck under soiled linens (see Figure 29-91 on page 731). Maintain an adequate amount of sheet at head and foot of bed for tucking.

8. Miter bottom sheet at head of bed, then at foot of bed. To miter, lift the mattress and tuck the sheet over the edge of the mattress, lift edge of sheet that is hanging to form a triangle, and lay upper part of sheet back onto bed; tuck the lower hanging section under the mattress. Repeat for each corner. Tuck the sides of the sheet under the mattress.

9. Fold the drawsheet in half. Identify the center of the drawsheet, and place it close to the client. Fanfold or roll drawsheet closest to client and tuck under soiled linens (see Figure 29-92 on page 731). Smooth linen. Add protective padding if needed. Tuck drawsheet under mattress, working from the center to the edges. drawsheet should be positioned under the lower back and buttocks.

10. Logroll client over onto side facing you. Raise side rail.

4. Facilitates easy removal of linens. Lowering only side rail close to nurse reduces client's risk of falls. Bath blanket prevents exposure and chills.

5. Provides space to place clean linens.

6. Keeps soiled linens together. Promotes comfort when client later rolls to other side.

7. Provides for maximum fit of sheets and decreases chance of wrinkles.

8. Holds linens firmly in place.

9. drawsheet facilitates moving and lifting clients while in bed.

10. Positions client off of soiled linens. Protects client from falling.

(Continues)

PROCEDURE 29-10
Changing Linens in an Occupied Bed (Continued)

ACTION	RATIONALE
11. Move to other side of bed. Remove soiled linens by rolling into a bundle, and place in linen hamper without touching uniform.	11. Prevents cross-contamination.
12. Unfold/unroll bottom sheet, then drawsheet. Look for objects left in the bed. Grasp each sheet with knuckles up and over the sheet and pull tightly while leaning back with body weight (see Figure 29-93 on page 731). Client may be positioned supine.	12. Tight sheets keep linens wrinkle free and decrease the risk of skin irritation. Leaning back uses body weight for good body mechanics.
13. Place top sheet over client with center of sheet in middle of bed. Unfold top of sheet over client. Remove bath blankets left on client to prevent exposure during bed making. Place top blanket over client, same as the top sheet.	13. Provides client with top sheet and blanket to prevent chilling.
14. Raise foot of mattress and tuck the corner of the top sheet and blanket under. Miter the corner. Repeat with other side of mattress. Bend the knees and not the back for proper mechanics.	14. Secures top sheet and blanket into place.
15. Grasp top sheet and blanket over client's toes and pull upward, then make a small fanfold in the sheet.	15. Permits client to move feet under the sheets. Provides room under the tight top sheet and blanket. Prevents toe decubitus and sheet burns from pressure.
16. Remove soiled pillowcase. Grasp center of clean pillowcase, and invert pillowcase over hand/arm. Maintain grasp of pillowcase while grasping center of pillow. Use other hand to pull pillowcase down over pillow. Place pillow under client's head. While changing pillowcase, client can be instructed to rest head on bed, or place a blanket under client's head.	16. Provides clean pillowcase without shaking pillow or pillowcase. Promotes comfort.
17. Document procedure used to change linens and client's condition during the procedure.	17. Provides documentation of nursing care and assessment of client's status.
18. Wash hands/hand hygiene.	18. Prevents the spread of microorganisms.

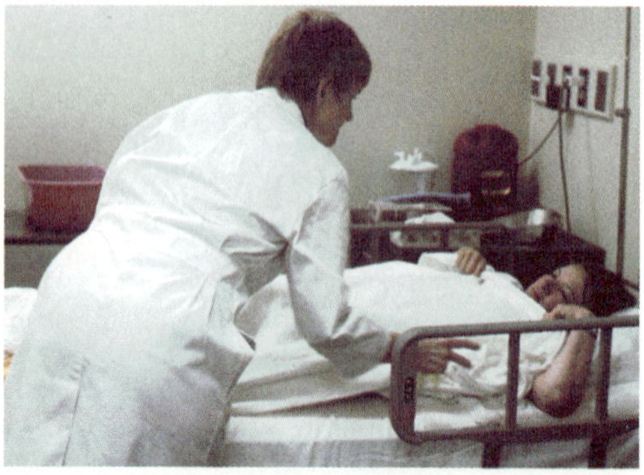

FIGURE 29-89 Client may be covered with a bath blanket for warmth and modesty while top sheet and blanket are removed. DELMAR/CENGAGE LEARNING

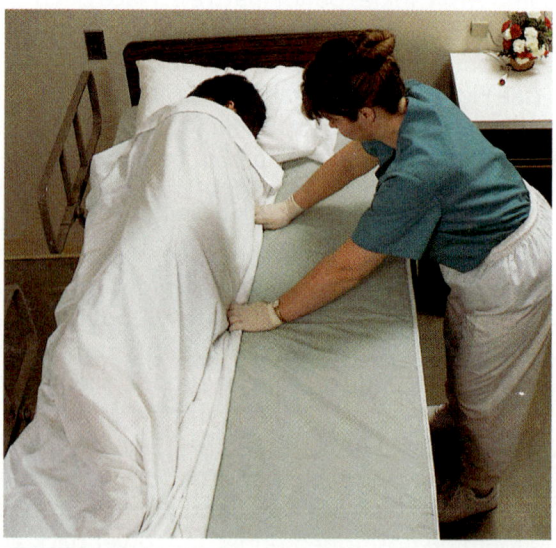

FIGURE 29-90 Fanfold the bottom linens close to the client toward the center of the bed. DELMAR/CENGAGE LEARNING

(Continues)

PROCEDURE 29-10
Changing Linens in an Occupied Bed (Continued)

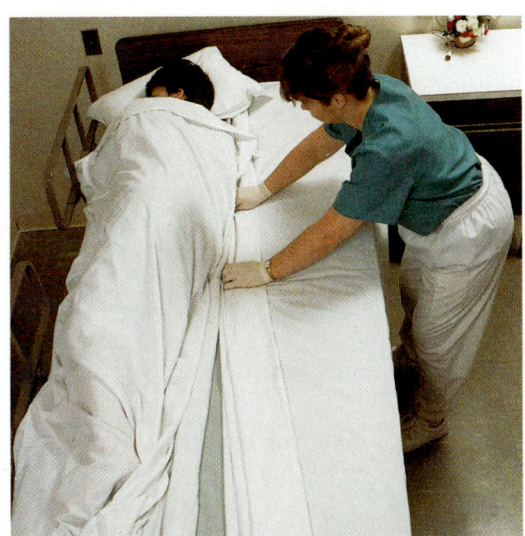

FIGURE 29-91 Fanfold the clean bottom linens nearest the client, and tuck under the soiled linens. DELMAR/CENGAGE LEARNING

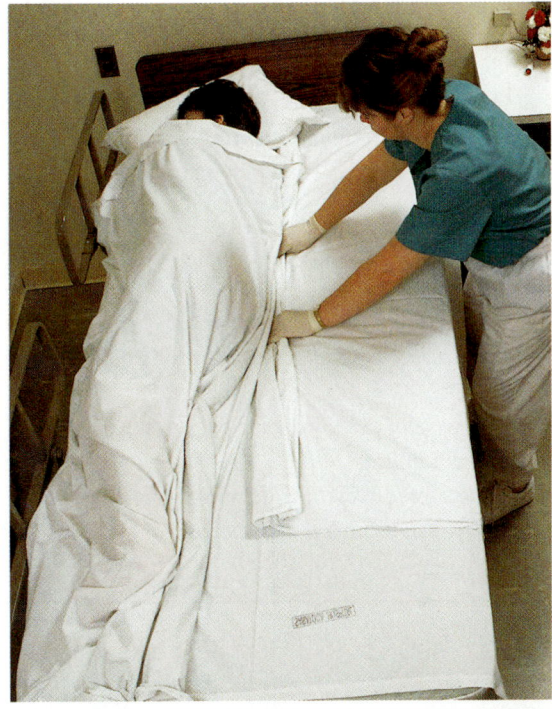

FIGURE 29-92 Fanfold the drawsheet close to the client, and tuck under the soiled linens. DELMAR/CENGAGE LEARNING

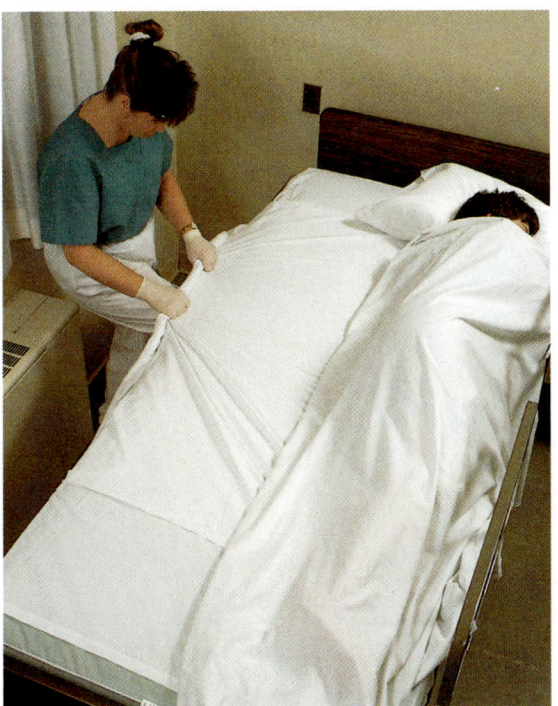

FIGURE 29-93 Grasp the bottom sheet and drawsheet and pull tightly. DELMAR/CENGAGE LEARNING

(Continues)

PROCEDURE 29-10
Changing Linens in an Occupied Bed (Continued)

delegation tip

Bed making is usually delegated to ancillary personnel. Their instruction should include the appropriate use of Standard Precautions and safety precautions for themselves and the client, such as the proper movement of the client in bed, how to manage drains and dressings, and the use of proper body mechanics. In certain situations where the client is in critical condition and multiple tubes, especially chest tubes, are present, the nurse should assist.

nursing tips

- *Roll or fold the linens under the client. Do not put them underneath the client.*
- *Be aware of wrinkles and seams upon which the client may be lying. They can cause pressure areas on the client's skin.*
- *Check for personal belongings in the client's bed when changing the linens. Clients may keep important items near them in bed.*
- *Be sure to keep the side rails up on the opposite side of the bed.*
- *Get help from another caregiver if the client is combative or difficult to move.*

PROCEDURE 29-11

Perineal and Genital Care

EQUIPMENT
- Personal protective equipment (gloves, gown)
- Toilet paper/washcloths
- Waterproof pads
- Cleansing solution if needed
- Perineal wash bottle (fill with plain, warm water)
- Water receptacle (bedpan or toilet if client is ambulatory)
- Dry towels
- Perineal treatment (i.e., ointment or lotions) if necessary
- Linen receptacle
- Room deodorizer

ACTION	RATIONALE
1. Wash hands/hand hygiene, and wear gloves. Gather equipment (see Figure 29-94 on page 733). If appropriate and splashing is likely, wear gown, mask, and goggles.	1. Prevents the spread of microorganisms.
2. Close privacy curtain or door.	2. Provides privacy.
3. Position client.	3. If client is ambulatory, perineal care may be done either with client on or standing at the toilet. If perineal care is to be performed in the bed, place the client on the side or over a deep bedpan.
4. Place waterproof pads under the client in the bed or under bedpan if used.	4. Protects bed linens.

(Continues)

PROCEDURE 29-11
Perineal and Genital Care (Continued)

ACTION	RATIONALE
5. Remove fecal debris with disposable paper, and dispose in toilet.	5. May require several attempts. If performing at the bedside, may collect paper in disposable pad or linens until end of procedure.
6. Spray perineum with washing solution if indicated. Alternatively, plain water may be used.	6. Several perineal solutions are available, which may or may not require rinsing. Carefully evaluate this requirement. Solutions that require rinsing may cause skin breakdown if left on the skin.
7. Cleanse perineum with wet washcloths (front to back on females), changing to clean area on washcloth with each wipe. Cleanse the penis on the male (see Figure 29-95).	7. Maximizes cleansing; prevents spread of rectal flora to vagina.
8. Carefully examine gluteal folds and scrotal folds for debris. Gently examine vulva for debris.	8. Fecal material causes irritation and skin breakdown rapidly when left in contact with skin.
9. If soap is used, spray area with clean water from the peri-bottle.	9. Rinses soap, which can irritate the skin, from the area.
10. Change gloves.	10. Reduces the transmission of microorganisms.
11. Dry perineum carefully with towel.	11. Residual moisture provides an ideal environment for the growth of microorganisms.
12. If indicated, apply barrier lotion or ointment.	12. Barrier ointments may be used if client is incontinent or skin folds tend to harbor moisture.
13. Reposition or dress client as appropriate.	13. Promotes client comfort.
14. Dispose of linens and garbage according to hospital policy.	14. Prevents spread of disease or bacteria.

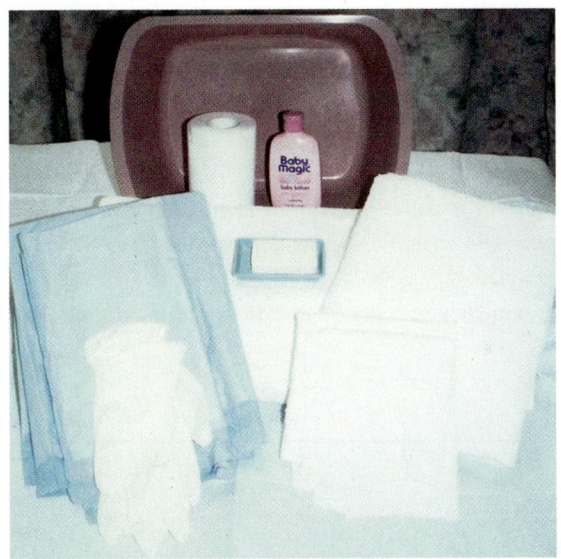

FIGURE 29-94 Toilet paper, soap, lotion, towels, gloves, and a basin are all used to provide perineal care. DELMAR/CENGAGE LEARNING

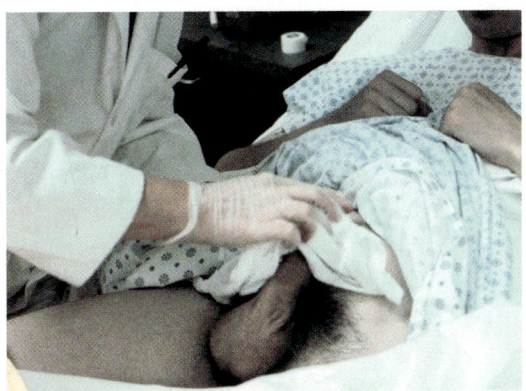

FIGURE 29-95 Cleanse the penis with a warm, wet washcloth. DELMAR/CENGAGE LEARNING

(Continues)

PROCEDURE 29-11
Perineal and Genital Care (Continued)

ACTION	RATIONALE
15. Deodorize room if appropriate.	15. Promotes client comfort. This may also be done at the beginning of the procedure.
16. Wash hands/hand hygiene.	16. Reduces the transmission of microorganisms.

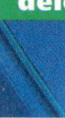

delegation tip

This skill is routinely delegated to ancillary personnel, who should be trained in Standard Precautions and proper client positioning and to report color, odor, and amount of any discharge, if present, to the nurse.

nursing tips

- *When performing perineal care on a client in bed, make sure bed height is adjusted to permit proper body mechanics.*
- *Perineal care and bed linen changes may be performed at the same time. Begin by performing peri-care, then wrap soiled linens under the client, and place clean linens to the edge of soiled linens. Roll the client to the other side, and proceed with linens change.*
- *Always wash hands after performing perineal care. Gloves do not provide a flawless barrier.*
- *When performing peri-care for an adult or a child, it is important to be sensitive to developmental considerations. Peri-care is usually learned early, and inability or difficulty performing this basic task for oneself can evoke feelings of embarrassment, worthlessness, and incompetence. It is critical that the nurse convey respect in an age-appropriate and a culturally sensitive manner. Perineal care should be performed as often as necessary. Some procedures will necessitate a schedule. If peri-care is necessary after elimination, do not delay. Even short delays can result in unnecessary suffering.*
- *Ask the client about soap/iodine allergies. Often, clients will not disclose this upon admission. Some perineal procedures will require use of iodine preparations.*
- *In uncircumcised males, gently retract the foreskin to clean smegma and other debris from the area around the glans. This procedure is not universal, however, and it is appropriate to ask the client whether this is acceptable. Care should be taken to replace the foreskin as soon as possible to prevent edema of the glans.*
- *Many cultures prescribe cleansing from the "front to the back" of the female perineum to prevent rectal debris and germs from coming into contact with the vulva. Be aware that this is also a cultural preference and if necessary may be followed for medical reasons (for example, interruptions in vaginal or perineal integrity).*
- *If possible, have a same-sex health care provider perform peri-care.*
- *Some clients may prefer to perform their own peri-care; however, they may not be able to complete adequate care and may require assistance.*

PROCEDURE 29-12

Oral Care

EQUIPMENT

BRUSHING AND FLOSSING
- Toothbrush
- Toothpaste with fluoride
- Emesis basin
- Towel
- Cup of water

- Nonsterile gloves
- Dental floss
- Mirror
- Lip moisturizer

DENTURE CARE
- Denture brush
- Denture cleaner
- Emesis basin
- Towel

- Cup of water
- Nonsterile gloves
- Tissue
- Denture cup

SPECIAL CARE ITEMS FOR CLIENTS WITH IMPAIRED PHYSICAL MOBILITY OR WHO ARE UNCONSCIOUS (COMATOSE)
- Soft toothbrush or toothette
- Tongue blade
- 3 × 3 gauze sponges
- Cotton-tip applicators

- Prescribed solution
- Plastic Asepto syringe
- Suction machine and catheter

ACTION	RATIONALE
SELF-CARE CLIENT: FLOSSING AND BRUSHING	
1. Assemble articles for flossing and brushing (see Figure 29-96 on page 736).	1. Promotes efficiency.
2. Provide privacy.	2. Relaxes the client.
3. Place client in a high Fowler's position (see Figure 29-97 on page 736).	3. Decreases risk of aspiration.
4. Wash hands/hand hygiene. Apply gloves.	4. Prevents the spread of microorganisms.
5. Arrange articles within client's reach.	5. Facilitates self-care.
6. Assist client with flossing and brushing as necessary. Position mirror, emesis basin, and water with straw near the client and a towel across the chest (see Figure 29-98 on page 736).	6. Flossing and brushing decrease microorganism growth in the mouth. Use of mirror permits cleaning back and sides of teeth.
7. Assist client with rinsing mouth.	7. Removes toothpaste and oral secretions.
8. Reposition client, raise side rails, and place call button within reach.	8. Promotes comfort, safety, and communication.
9. Rinse, dry, and return articles to proper place.	9. Promotes a clean environment.
10. Remove gloves, wash hands/hand hygiene, and document care.	10. Reduces the transmission of microorganisms and documents nursing care.
SELF-CARE CLIENT: DENTURE CARE	
11. Assemble articles for denture cleaning (see Figure 29-99 on page 736 and Figure 29-100 on page 737).	11. Promotes efficiency.
12. Provide privacy.	12. Relaxes the client.
13. Assist client to a high Fowler's position.	13. Facilitates removal of dentures.

(Continues)

PROCEDURE 29-12
Oral Care (Continued)

ACTION	RATIONALE

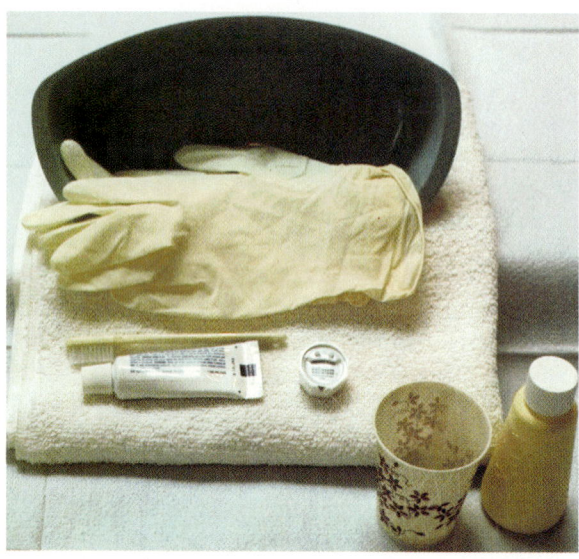

FIGURE 29-96 Toothbrush, dental floss, mouthwash, and emesis basin are all used in providing oral care. DELMAR/CENGAGE LEARNING

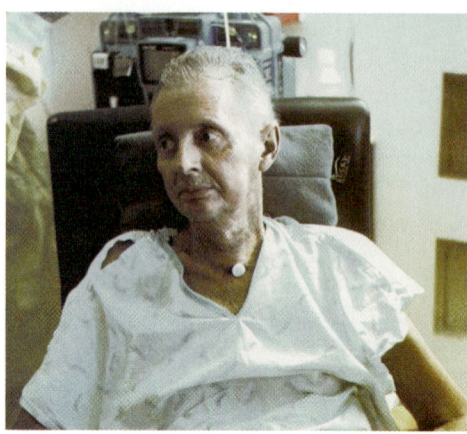

FIGURE 29-97 Place the client in a sitting position in a chair or in bed if possible. DELMAR/CENGAGE LEARNING

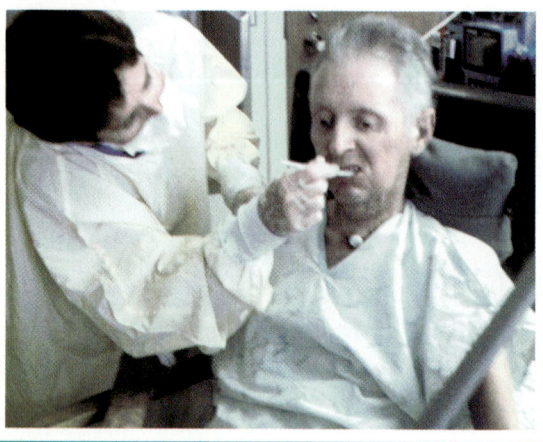

FIGURE 29-98 Promote independence, but assist with flossing or brushing as necessary. DELMAR/CENGAGE LEARNING

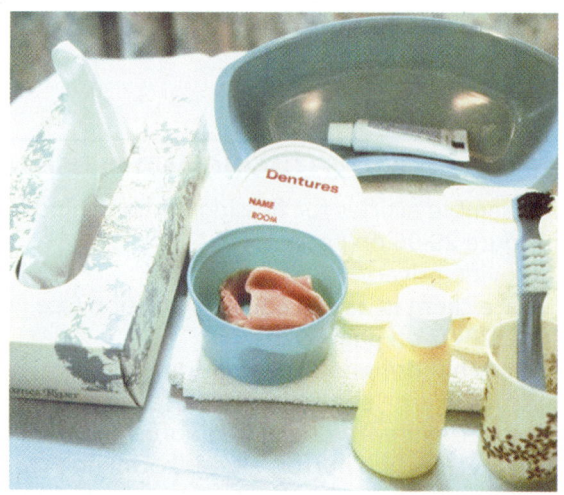

FIGURE 29-99 Denture brush and denture cup are added to oral care equipment when the client has full or partial dentures. DELMAR/CENGAGE LEARNING

14. Wash hands/hand hygiene, and apply gloves.

15. Assist client with denture removal:
   a. Top denture:
      • With tissue, grasp the denture with thumb and forefinger and pull downward.
      • Place in denture cup.
   b. Bottom denture:
      • Place thumbs on the gums and release the denture. Grasp denture with thumb and forefinger and pull upward.
      • Place in denture cup.

14. Reduces the transmission of microorganisms and exposure to body fluids.
15. Breaks seal created with dentures without causing pressure and injury to oral membranes. Prevents breaking of dentures.

(Continues)

PROCEDURE 29-12
Oral Care (Continued)

ACTION	RATIONALE

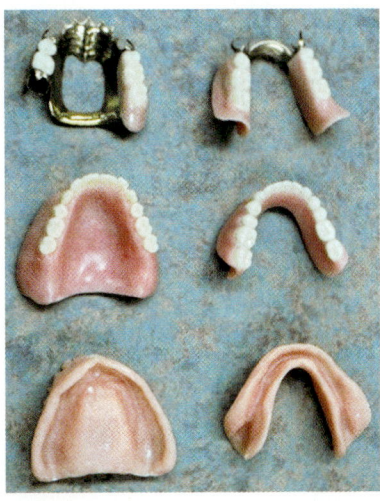

FIGURE 29-100 Dentures may include full upper or lower plates, or partial plates. DELMAR/CENGAGE LEARNING

ACTION	RATIONALE
16. Apply toothpaste to brush, and brush dentures either with cool water in the emesis basin or under running water in the sink. Pad sink with towel to protect dentures in case they are dropped.	16. Facilitates removal of microorganisms.
17. Rinse thoroughly.	17. Removes toothpaste.
18. Assist client with rinsing mouth and replacing dentures.	18. Freshens mouth and facilitates intake of solid food.
19. Reposition client with side rails up and call button within reach.	19. Promotes comfort, safety, and communication.
20. Rinse, dry, and return articles to proper place.	20. Maintains a clean environment.
21. Remove gloves, wash hands, and document care.	21. Reduces the transmission of microorganisms and documents nursing care.

FULL-CARE CLIENT: BRUSHING AND FLOSSING

ACTION	RATIONALE
22. Assemble articles for flossing and brushing.	22. Promotes efficiency.
23. Provide privacy.	23. Relaxes client.
24. Wash hands/hand hygiene, and apply gloves.	24. Reduces the transmission of microorganisms and exposure to body fluids.
25. Position client as condition allows: high Fowler's; semi-Fowler's; or lateral position, head turned toward side (see Figure 29-101 on page 738).	25. Decreases risk of aspiration.
26. Place towel across client's chest or under face and mouth if head is turned to one side.	26. Catches secretions.
27. Moisten toothbrush or toothette, apply small amount of toothpaste, and brush teeth and gums.	27. Moistens mouth and facilitates plaque removal.

(Continues)

PROCEDURE 29-12
Oral Care (Continued)

ACTION	**RATIONALE**

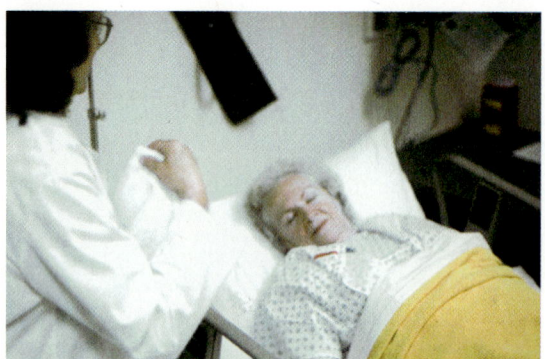

FIGURE **29-101** If client is unable to sit up, turn head to the side. DELMAR/CENGAGE LEARNING

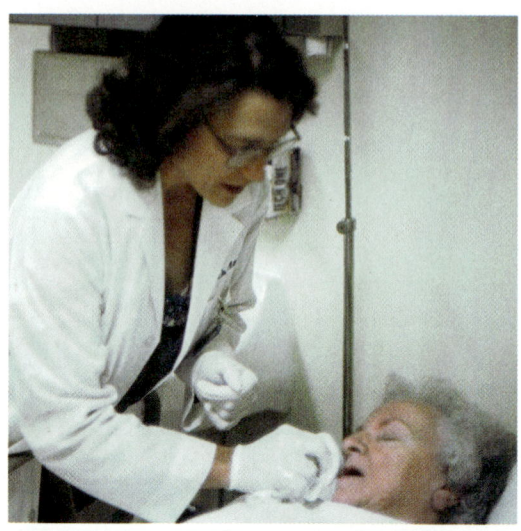

FIGURE **29-102** After completing oral care, dry the lips and face gently and carefully. DELMAR/CENGAGE LEARNING

28. Grasp the dental floss in both hands or use a floss holder and floss between all teeth; hold floss against tooth while moving floss up and down sides of teeth.

28. Removes plaque and prevents gum disease.

29. Assist the client in rinsing mouth.

29. Removes toothpaste and oral secretions.

30. Reapply toothpaste and brush the teeth and gums using friction in a vertical or circular motion. On inner and outer surfaces of teeth, hold brush at 45° angle against teeth and brush from sulcus to crowns of teeth. On biting surfaces, move brush back and forth in short strokes. All surfaces of teeth should be brushed from every angle.

30. Permits cleaning of back and sides of teeth and decreases microorganism growth in mouth.

31. Assist the client in rinsing and drying mouth (see Figure 29-102).

31. Removes toothpaste and oral secretions.

32. Apply lip moisturizer, if appropriate.

32. Maintains skin integrity of lips.

33. Reposition client, raise side rails, and place call button within reach.

33. Promotes comfort, safety, and communication.

34. Rinse, dry, and return articles to proper place.

34. Provides an orderly environment.

35. Remove gloves, wash hands/hand hygiene, and document care.

35. Reduces the transmission of microorganisms and documents nursing care.

CLIENTS AT RISK FOR OR WITH AN ALTERATION OF THE ORAL CAVITY

36. Assemble articles for flossing and brushing.

36. Promotes efficiency.

37. Provide privacy.

37. Relaxes client.

38. Wash hands/hand hygiene, and apply gloves.

38. Reduces the transmission of microorganisms and exposure to body fluids.

39. Bleeding:
   a. Assess oral cavity with a padded tongue blade and flashlight for signs of bleeding.

39.
   a. Determines whether bleeding is present, amount, and specific areas.

(Continues)

PROCEDURE 29-12
Oral Care (Continued)

ACTION	RATIONALE
b. Proceed with the actions for oral care for a full-care client except: • Do not floss. • Use a soft toothbrush, toothette, or a tongue blade padded with 3 × 3 gauze sponges to gently swab teeth and gums. • Dispose of padded tongue blade into a biohazard bag according to institutional policy. • Rinse with tepid water.	b. • Decreases risk of bleeding and trauma to gums. • Decreases risk of bleeding and trauma to gums. • Promotes proper disposal of contaminated waste. • Cleanses mouth.
40. Infection: a. Assess oral cavity with a tongue blade and flashlight for signs of infection. b. Culture lesions as ordered. c. Proceed with the actions for oral care for a full-care client except: • Do not floss. • Use prescribed antiseptic solution. • Use a tongue blade padded with 3 × 3 gauze sponges to gently swab the teeth and gums. • Dispose of padded tongue blade into a biohazard bag according to institutional policy. • Rinse mouth with tepid water. • Apply additional solution as prescribed.	40. a. Determines appearance, integrity, and general condition. b. Identifies growth of specific microorganisms. c. • Prevents irritation, pain, and bleeding. • Antiseptic solutions decrease growth of microorganisms. • Promotes proper disposal of contaminated materials. • Cleanses mouth. • Provides a coating that promotes healing of the tissue.
41. Ulceration: a. Assess oral cavity with a tongue blade and flashlight for signs of ulceration. b. Culture lesions as ordered. c. Proceed with actions for oral care for a full-care client except: • Do not floss. • Use prescribed antiseptic solution. • Use a tongue blade padded with 3 × 3 gauze sponges to gently swab the teeth and gums. • Dispose of padded tongue blade into a biohazard bag according to institutional policy. • Rinse mouth with tepid water. • Apply additional solution as prescribed.	41. a. Determines appearance, integrity, and general condition. b. Identifies growth of specific microorganisms. c. • Prevents irritation, pain, and bleeding. • Antiseptic solutions decrease growth of microorganisms. • Promotes proper disposal of contaminated materials. • Cleanses mouth. • Provides a coating that promotes healing of the tissue.

UNCONSCIOUS (COMATOSE) CLIENT

ACTION	RATIONALE
42. Assemble articles for flossing and brushing.	42. Promotes efficiency.
43. Provide privacy.	43. Relaxes client.
44. Wash hands/hand hygiene, and apply gloves.	44. Reduces the transmission of microorganisms and exposure to body fluids.
45. Explain the procedure to the client.	45. Demonstrates respect for the client.

(Continues)

PROCEDURE 29-12
Oral Care (Continued)

ACTION	RATIONALE
46. Place the client in a lateral position, with the head turned toward the side.	46. Prevents aspiration.
47. Use a floss holder, and floss between all teeth.	47. Prevents transfer of microorganisms from a client bite.
48. Moisten toothbrush or toothette, and brush the teeth and gums using friction in a vertical or circular motion. Do not use toothpaste. On inner and outer surfaces of teeth, hold brush at 45° angle against teeth and brush from sulcus to crowns of teeth. On biting surfaces, move brush back and forth in short strokes. All surfaces of teeth should be brushed from every angle.	48. Permits cleaning of back and sides of teeth and decreases microorganism growth in mouth. Toothpaste may foam and cause aspiration.
49. After flossing and brushing, rinse mouth with an Asepto syringe (do not force water into the mouth), and perform oral suction.	49. Promotes cleansing and removal of secretions and prevents aspiration.
50. Dry the client's mouth.	50. Prevents skin irritation.
51. Apply lip moisturizer.	51. Maintains skin integrity of lips.
52. Leave the client in a lateral position with head turned toward side for 30 to 60 minutes after oral hygiene care. Suction one more time. Remove the towel from under the client's mouth and face.	52. Prevents pooling of secretions and aspiration.
53. Dispose of any contaminated items in a biohazard bag and clean, dry, and return all articles to the appropriate place.	53. Promotes proper disposal of contaminated materials.
54. Remove gloves, wash hands/hand hygiene, and document care.	54. Reduces the transmission of microorganisms and documents nursing care.

delegation tip

Oral care is routinely delegated to ancillary personnel, who should allow the client to perform as much of the oral care as possible or permitted. The caregiver should be trained to employ Standard Precautions, to properly position the client, and to observe and report the condition and color of the client's mucous membranes to the nurse.

nursing tips

- *Never place your fingers in a client's mouth. A bite block or padded tongue blade can be used to hold the client's mouth open.*
- *The unconscious client's head should be turned to one side, with a basin placed under the mouth. Oral suction should be available. Only small amounts of water should be used.*
- *Be careful when handling and cleaning dentures or other oral appliances. They can be slippery when wet and may break if dropped into the sink or onto the floor.*
- *Clients with orthodontic appliances may have special oral care needs. Ask the client or the client's family about any special cleaning needs or special appliance care.*
- *Avoid using oil-based products around oxygen and oxygen equipment because oil and grease are flammable. Petroleum jelly may be used on clients receiving oxygen, but it should not be used on oxygen equipment.*
- *Avoid breathing directly on client to avoid transmission of microorganisms.*
- *Wear a mask and goggles if within distance of splashes or sprays from the client's coughing.*

PROCEDURE 29-13

Eye Care

EQUIPMENT

ARTIFICIAL EYE
- Storage container
- Mild soap
- 3 × 3 gauze sponges
- Cotton balls
- Towel
- Emesis basins
- Eye irrigation syringe (optional)
- Running water
- Sterile gloves
- Biohazard bag
- Saline solution

CONTACT LENSES
- Lens container
- Soaking solution—type used by client
- Nonsterile gloves
- Towel
- Suction cup (optional)
- Scotch tape (optional)

ACTION	RATIONALE

ARTIFICIAL EYE REMOVAL

1. Inquire about client's care regimen, and gather equipment accordingly (see Figure 29-103 on page 742).

2. Provide privacy.
3. Wash hands/hand hygiene. Apply gloves.

4. Place client in a semi-Fowler's position.
5. Place the cotton balls in an emesis basin filled halfway with warm tap water.
6. Place 3 × 3 gauze sponges in bottom of second emesis basin, and fill halfway with mild soap and tepid water.
7. Grasp and squeeze excess water from a cotton ball. Cleanse the eyelid with the moistened cotton ball, starting at the inner canthus and moving outward toward the outer canthus. After each use, dispose of cotton ball in biohazard bag. Repeat procedure until eyelid is clean (without dried secretions).
8. Remove the artificial eye:
   a. Using dominant hand, raise the client's upper eyelid with index finger, and depress the lower eyelid with thumb.
   b. Cup nondominant hand under the client's lower eyelid.
   c. Apply slight pressure with index finger between the brow and the artificial eye, and remove it. Place it in an emesis basin filled with warm, soapy water.

1. Promotes continuity of care.

2. Relaxes the client.
3. Prevents the spread of microorganisms.

4. Facilitates procedure and client participation.
5. Dry cotton balls could cause irritation.

6. Gauze serves as padding to prevent breakage of the prosthesis.

7. Eliminating the excess water prevents water from running down the client's face. Cleansing the eyelid prevents contamination of the lacrimal system (inner canthus area). Disposal of cotton balls reduces transmission of microorganisms to other health care workers.

8. Cleanses the artificial eye.
   a. Promotes removal of the artificial eye.
   b. Cupping reduces dropping and possible breaking of the eye.
   c. Applying pressure will help the prosthesis slip out.

(Continues)

PROCEDURE 29-13
Eye Care (Continued)

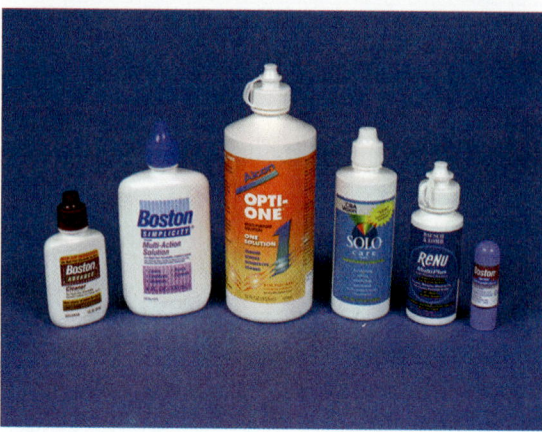

FIGURE 29-103 Commercial soaking and eye care solutions. Many types of soaking solutions are available. Select the type normally used by the client whenever possible. DELMAR/CENGAGE LEARNING

ACTION	RATIONALE
9. Grasp a moistened cotton ball and cleanse around the edge of the eye socket. Dispose of the soiled cotton ball in biohazard bag.	9. Cleanses the eye socket. Disposal of cotton ball reduces transmission of microorganisms to other health care workers.
10. Inspect the eye socket for any signs of irritation, drainage, or crusting. *Note:* If the client's usual care regimen or a prescribing practitioner's order requires irrigation of the socket, proceed with Action 11; otherwise, go to Action 12.	10. Indicates an infection.
11. Eye socket irrigation:	11. Cleanses the eye socket and removes secretions.
a. Lower the head of the bed and place the client in a supine position. Place protector pad on bed. Turn head toward socket side, and slightly extend neck.	a. Positioning of client facilitates ease in performing the procedure and client's comfort.
b. Fill the irrigation syringe with the prescribed amount and type of irrigating solution (warm tap water or normal saline).	b. Ensures compliance with client's regimen or prescribed orders.
c. With nondominant hand, separate the eyelids with your forefinger and thumb while resting fingers on the brow and cheekbone.	c. Keeps the eyelid open and the socket visible.
d. Hold the irrigating syringe in dominant hand several inches above the inner canthus; with thumb, gently apply pressure on the plunger, directing the flow of solution from the inner canthus along the conjunctival sac.	d. Prevents injury to the client.
e. Irrigate until the prescribed amount of solution has been used.	e. Ensures compliance with client's regimen of prescribed orders.
f. Wipe the eyelids with a moistened cotton ball after irrigating. Dispose of soiled cotton ball in biohazard bag.	f. Reduces the transmission of microorganisms to prosthesis.
g. Pat the skin dry with the towel.	g. Prevents maceration of the skin.
h. Return the client to a semi-Fowler's position.	h. Promotes client's comfort.
i. Remove gloves, wash hands/hand hygiene, and apply clean gloves.	i. Reduces the transmission of microorganisms.

(Continues)

PROCEDURE 29-13
Eye Care (Continued)

ACTION	RATIONALE
12. Rub the artificial eye between index finger and thumb in the basin of warm, soapy water.	12. Creates cleaning with friction and prevents breakage of the prosthesis.
13. Rinse the prosthesis under running water or place in the clean basin of tepid water. Do not dry the prosthesis. *Note:* Either reinsert the prosthesis (Action 14) or store in a container (Action 15).	13. Removes soap and secretions. Keeping the artificial eye wet prevents irritation from lint or other particles that might adhere to it and facilitates reinsertion.
14. Reinsert the prosthesis:	14. Allows for client comfort.
a. With the thumb of the nondominant hand, raise and hold the upper eyelid open.	a. Facilitates reinsertion of the prosthesis without discomfort to the client.
b. With the dominant hand, grasp the artificial eye so the indented part is facing toward the client's nose, and slide it under the upper eyelid as far as possible.	b. Positions the prosthesis for insertion.
c. Depress the lower lid.	c. Allows the prosthesis to slide into place.
d. Pull the lower lid forward to cover the edge of the prosthesis.	d. Holds the prosthesis in place.
15. Place the cleaned artificial eye in a labeled container with a saline or tap water solution.	15. Protects the prosthesis from scratches and keeps it clean.
16. Grasp a moistened cotton ball and squeeze out excessive moisture. Wipe the eyelid from the inner to the outer canthus. Dispose of the soiled cotton ball in a biohazard bag.	16. Squeezing the cotton ball removes moisture. Cleansing the eyelid prevents contamination of lacrimal system. Disposal of cotton ball reduces the transmission of microorganisms to other health care workers.
17. Clean, dry, and replace equipment.	17. Promotes a clean environment.
18. Reposition the client, raise side rails, and place call light in reach.	18. Promotes client's comfort, safety, and communication.
19. Dispose of biohazard bag according to institutional policy.	19. Reduces the transmission of microorganisms to other health care workers.
20. Remove gloves. Wash hands/hand hygiene.	20. See Rationale 19.
21. Document procedure, client's response and participation, and client teaching and level of understanding.	21. Demonstrates that the procedure was done and the level of client participation and learning.

CONTACT LENS REMOVAL

22. Assemble equipment for lens removal.	22. Promotes efficiency.
23. Assess level of assistance needed, provide privacy, and explain the procedure to the client.	23. Level of assistance determines level of intervention. Privacy reduces anxiety. Explanation of procedure promotes cooperation.
24. Wash hands/hand hygiene.	24. Prevents the spread of microorganisms.
25. Assist the client to a semi-Fowler's position if needed.	25. Facilitates removal of lens.
26. Drape a clean towel over the client's chest.	26. Provides a clean surface and facilitates the location of a lens if it falls out during removal.

(Continues)

PROCEDURE 29-13
Eye Care (Continued)

27. Prepare the lens storage case with the pre-scribed solution.

28. Instruct the client to look straight ahead. Assess the location of the lens. If it is not on the cornea, either you or the client should gently move the lens toward the cornea with the pad of the index finger (see Figure 29-104 on page 745).

29. Remove the lens.
    a. Hard lens:
       • Cup nondominant hand under the eye.
       • Gently place index finger on the outside corner of the eye and pull toward the temple. Ask client to blink. Catch the lens in your nondominant hand.
    b. Soft lens:
       • With nondominant hand, separate the eyelid with your thumb and middle finger.
       • With the index finger of the dominant hand gently placed on the lower edge of the lens, slide the lens downward onto the sclera and gently squeeze the lens.
       • Release the top eyelid (continue holding the lower lid down), and remove the lens with your index finger and thumb.
       • *Note:* If Action 29 is unsuccessful, secure a suction cup to remove the contact lens. If you are unable to remove the lens, notify the prescribing practitioner or qualified practitioner.

30. Store the lens in the correct compartment of the case ("right" or "left"). Label with the client's name.
31. Remove and store the other lens by repeating Actions 29 and 30.
32. Assess eyes for irritation or redness.
33. Store the lens case in a safe place.
34. Dispose of soiled articles, and clean and return reusable articles to proper location.
35. Reposition the client, raise side rails, and place call light in reach.
36. Remove gloves. Wash hands/hand hygiene.
37. Document procedure, client's response and assessment findings, and the storage place of the lenses.

27. Hard lenses can be stored dry or in a special soaking solution. Soft lenses are stored in sterile normal saline without a preservative.
28. Client's position promotes easy removal of lens. Positioning lens on the cornea aids removal. Use of the finger pad of the index finger prevents damage to cornea and lens.

29. Provides for cleaning and storage of the lens.
    a.
       • Cupping the hand under the eye helps catch the lens to prevent breakage.
       • Pulling the corner of the eye tightens the eyelid against the eyeball. Pressure on the upper edge of the lens causes the lens to tip forward.
    b.
       • Separating the eyelid exposes the lower edge of the lens.
       • Positions the lens for easy grasping with the pad of the index finger, which prevents injury to the cornea and lens. Squeezing the lens allows air to enter and release the suction.
       • Ensures control of the lens.
       • Suction cup is used to remove a lens from an unconscious or a dependent client.

30. Storage prevents damage to the lenses and ensures that each lens will be reinserted into the correct eye.
31. See Rationales 29 and 30.

32. Reveals signs of corneal irritation.
33. Prevents damage or loss.
34. Reduces the transmission of infection.

35. Promotes client comfort, safety, and communication.
36. Prevents the spread of microorganisms.
37. Documents the removal of lenses, condition of the cornea, and where the lenses are stored.

(Continues)

PROCEDURE 29-13
Eye Care (Continued)

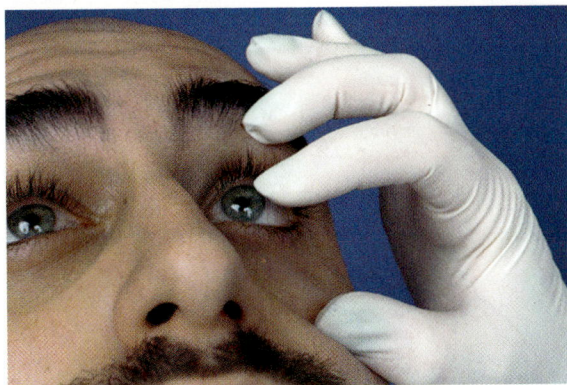

FIGURE 29-104 If the lens is not on the cornea, gently move it toward the cornea with the pad of the index finger. DELMAR/CENGAGE LEARNING

delegation tip

Eye care requires the assessment and intervention of the nurse. Delegation to ancillary personnel is inappropriate.

nursing tips

- Be aware of right and left. Take care not to mix up a client's contacts.
- Prostheses are slippery. Be careful not to drop while handling them.
- Place a towel or washcloth over the bottom of the sink when cleaning contacts or a prosthesis to prevent breakage if dropped and to prevent loss down the drain.
- If the client has glasses as well as contacts, encourage the client to send the contacts home with family and to wear glasses while in the hospital.
- Place a towel in front of the client when an eye prosthesis is removed to catch it if it slips out of your hand.

KEY CONCEPTS

- Factors influencing client safety are age, lifestyle, sensory and perceptual alterations, mobility, and emotional state.

- Types of accidents that can occur in the health care setting are client behavior, therapeutic procedure, and equipment.

- Assessment of a safe environment consists of performing an injury risk appraisal.

- Nurses can help clients maintain a safe environment by resolving or alleviating hazards related to falls, lighting, obstacles, bathroom hazards, fire, electricity, radiation, poisoning, and noise pollution.

- The chain of infection involves a biological agent, a reservoir of the agent, a portal of exit, a mode of transmission, a portal of entry of the agent into the host, and a susceptible host.

- Medical and surgical asepsis prevents the transfer of microorganisms by implementation of practices to reduce the number, growth, or spread of microorganisms from an object or area.

- The guidelines from the CDC require that transmission-based precautions be used for specific syndromes that are highly suspicious for infections until a diagnosis is confirmed.

- Hygienic practices are influenced by body image, social and cultural practices, personal preference, socioeconomic status, and knowledge.

- Basic hygienic practices include bathing, skin care, perineal care, back rubs, foot and nail care, oral care, hair care, and eye, ear, and nose care.

REVIEW QUESTIONS

1. Which action provided for legal protection of information voluntarily reported to an organization regarding safety issues?
   a. Public Health Service Act
   b. Report of the Institute of Medicine in 1999
   c. Centers for Disease Control and Prevention
   d. Patient Safety and Quality Improvement Act of 2005

2. The physiological changes of aging increase the risk for which of the following
   a. Choking
   b. Electrical hazards
   c. Falls
   d. Substance abuse

3. When an infectious disease is transmitted to a person by direct or indirect contact, it is called a:
   a. Portal of entry to a host
   b. Susceptible host
   c. Communicable disease
   d. Portal of exit from a reservoir

4. The family member of a client diagnosed with hepatitis A asks the nurse how to avoid infecting other family members. The nurse's response would be based on the understanding that hepatitis A is primarily spread by:
   a. Sexual contact with an infected person who does not show symptoms of the disease
   b. Contaminated needles from a person who has some form of hepatitis
   c. Blood transfusions of improperly prepared blood
   d. Fecal contamination or contaminated food or water from person to person

5. One of the major concerns of nurses in the workforce is:
   a. The threat of malpractice
   b. Job security
   c. Exposure to bloodborne infection by needlestick injuries
   d. Exposure to contaminated equipment

6. What kills bacteria most effectively?
   a. Warm water scrub
   b. Soap and water handwash
   c. Alcohol-based hand rubs
   d. Antiseptic handwash

7. When performing a venipuncture, which Standard Precaution should be implemented?
   a. Gloves
   b. Face shield
   c. Goggles
   d. Gloves, face shield, and goggles

8. Which hospitalized client does the nurse identify to be at greatest risk for the development of a urinary tract HAI?
   a. A 48-year-old male suspected of Parkinson's disease who had been jogging prior to admission
   b. A 75-year-old male who has pancreatic cancer
   c. A 34-year-old male who drinks 2500 mL of fluid daily, following a fracture of the fibula
   d. A 60-year-old obese female with cholecystitis

9. When considering the client's personal preferences for hygiene, which factor should the nurse deem as primary?
   a. Keep the nursing aides on schedule.
   b. Hygiene is a routine procedure.
   c. No two persons perform hygiene in the same manner.
   d. Get all hygiene procedures performed before the family comes to visit.

10. The primary goal in providing oral hygiene to an unconscious client is to prevent:
    a. Mouth odors
    b. Mouth ulcers
    c. Aspiration
    d. Dental caries

online companion

Visit the DeLaune and Ladner online companion resource at **www.delmar.cengage.com** for additional content and study aids. Click on Online Companions, then select the Nursing discipline.

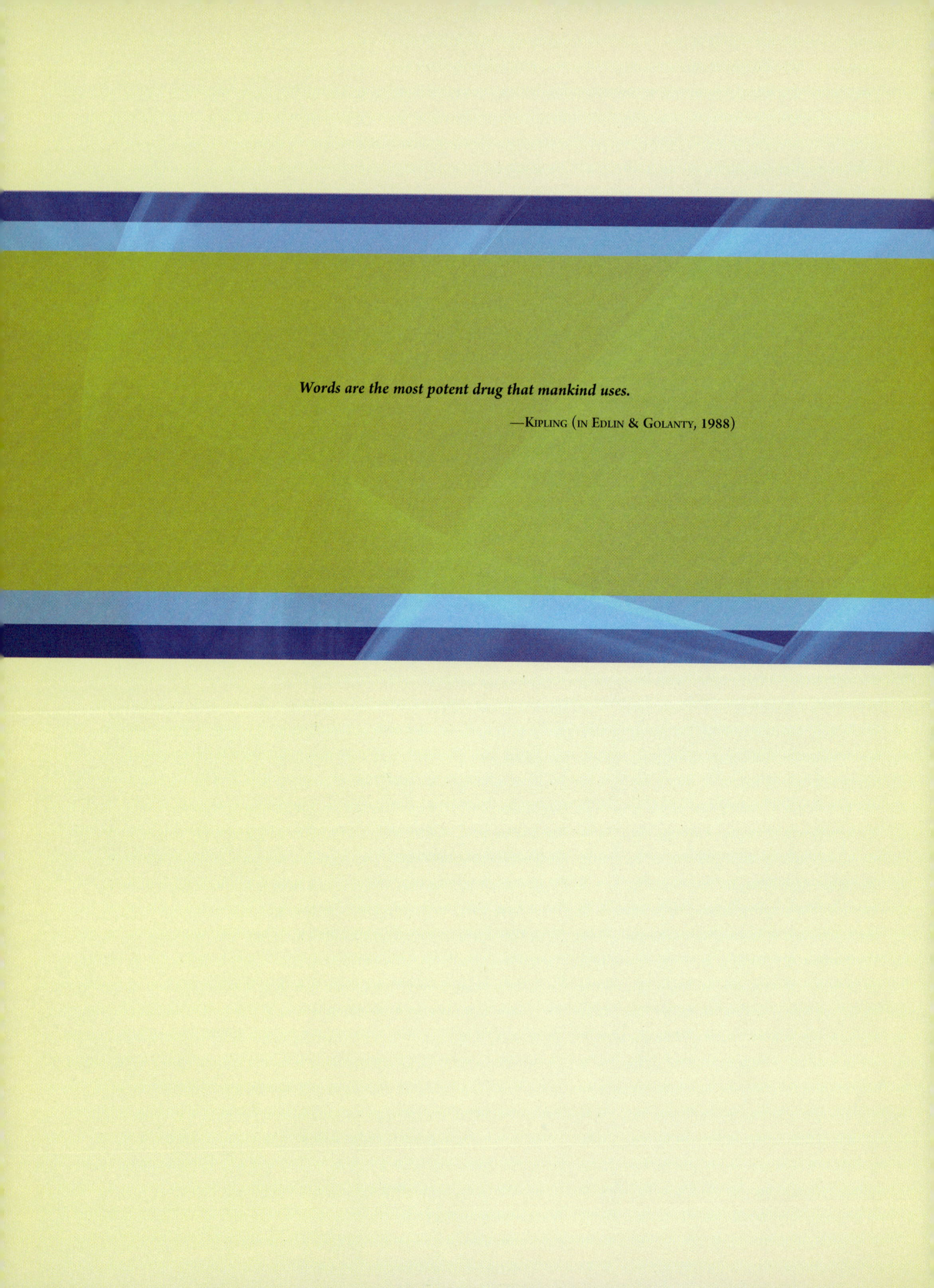

Words are the most potent drug that mankind uses.

—Kipling (in Edlin & Golanty, 1988)

CHAPTER 30

Medication Administration

COMPETENCIES

1. Define the key terms and abbreviations frequently used in medication administration.
2. Describe the influence of drug standards and legislation on medication administration.
3. Discuss the nurse's legal responsibilities in preparation and administration of medications.
4. Explain the principles of pharmacokinetics, including absorption, distribution, metabolism, and excretion of drugs.
5. Describe the factors that can affect a drug's action.
6. Identify the responsibilities of the nurse for each type of medication order.
7. Differentiate between allergic reaction, side effect, toxic effect, and idiosyncratic reaction to medications.
8. Correctly calculate appropriate dosage for medications as prescribed.
9. Discuss principles of safe medication administration including the five rights of medication administration.
10. Correctly explain procedures for the different methods of medication administration including the choice of route and site.
11. Discuss potential liabilities for the nurse administering medications.
12. Develop teaching guidelines for clients regarding medication in the home.

KEY TERMS

absorption	enteral instillation	pharmacokinetics
addiction	excretion	phlebitis
adverse reactions	half-life	plateau
aspiration	idiosyncratic reaction	prn
bioavailability	infiltration	side effect
buccal	intradermal (ID)	stat order
dependence	intramuscular (IM)	stock supplied
dissolution	intravenous (IV)	subcutaneous
distribution	metabolism	sublingual
drug allergy	onset of action	therapeutic range
drug incompatibility	parenteral	toxic effect
drug interaction	patency	trough
drug tolerance	peak plasma level	unit-dose form
duration	pharmacognosy	Z-track (zigzag) technique

Alterations in health related to acute or chronic conditions lead clients to seek relief of their symptoms through various treatment options. One modality frequently used to help alleviate symptoms and restore health is a medication regime. Medications are substances prescribed by the client's prescribing practitioner to help in the treatment, relief, or cure of the cause of the client's health alterations or in the prevention of such alterations. The term *prescribing practitioner* refers to any health care provider who is authorized to prescribe medications (e.g., physicians, dentists, advanced practice nurses).

Medication management requires the collaborative efforts of many health care providers. Once prescribed, pharmacists are licensed to prepare and dispense medications. Nurses are responsible for administering medications. Dietitians are often involved in identifying possible food and drug interactions.

Nurses play an essential role in the administration of, education about, and evaluation of the effectiveness of prescribed medications. The nurse's role changes with the setting of the client. In the home care community setting, clients take their own medication as prescribed by the prescribing practitioner. Nurses are responsible for educating clients about their medications and the possible side effects as well as for evaluating the outcome of the prescribed therapy in restoring and maintaining clients' health. In the acute care setting, nurses spend a great deal of time administering medications and evaluating their effectiveness. Nurses are responsible for teaching clients how to take their medications safely upon discharge.

Medication administration requires specialized knowledge, judgment, and nursing skill based on the principles of pharmacology. The focus of this chapter is to assist the student in applying principles of pharmacology and in acquiring skills in the safe administration of medications. The nursing process is used to direct nursing decisions relative to safe drug administration and to ensure compliance with standards of practice.

DRUG STANDARDS AND LEGISLATION

A drug is a chemical substance intended for use in the diagnosis, treatment, cure, mitigation, or prevention of a disease. When a drug is given to a client, there is an intended specific effect. An assumption made by nurses before administration of any medication is that the drug will be safe for the client to consume if the dose, frequency, and route are within the therapeutic range for that drug. This assumption is implied in accord with standards that are set to ensure drug uniformity in strength, purity, efficacy, safety, and bioavailability (readiness to produce a drug effect).

STANDARDS

Standards have been developed to ensure drug uniformity so that effects are predictable. The *United States Pharmacopeia* and *National Formulary* (USP and NF) are books of drug standards for usage in the United States. The USP and NF list drugs that have been recognized as being in compliance with legal standards of purity, quality, and strength.

The USP has been providing standards for pharmaceutical preparations since its first edition in 1820. The NF was published in 1898 by the American Pharmaceutical Association to provide a listing of drugs that complied with established standards. The *British Pharmacopoeia* is the British complement to the USP, and the *Canadian Formulary* provides a listing of drugs commonly used in Canada.

FEDERAL LEGISLATION

The Pure Food and Drug Act of 1906 designated the USP and the NF as the official references to establish drug standards. It also gave the federal government the authority to enforce these standards.

The federal Food, Drug, and Cosmetic Act of 1938 empowered the Food and Drug Administration (FDA) to test all new drugs for toxicity before granting a pharmaceutical company approval to market a drug. The federal Food, Drug, and Cosmetic Act of 1938 was amended in 1952 to distinguish prescription (legend) drugs from nonprescription (over-the-counter) drugs and to regulate the dispensing of prescriptions. Testing for drug effectiveness materialized with the Kefauver-Harris Act of 1962.

The Harrison Narcotic Act of 1914 classified habit-forming drugs as narcotics and began regulating these substances. This law and other drug abuse laws have been replaced with the Comprehensive Drug Abuse Prevention and Control Act (Controlled Substance Act) of 1970. This act defines a *drug-dependent person* in terms of physical and psychological dependence and provides for strict regulation of narcotics and other controlled drugs such as barbiturates through the establishment of five categories of scheduled drugs (see the accompanying display on controlled substances). Any controlled substance must be recorded by the dispensing pharmacist. The Drug Enforcement Administration employs pharmacists to inspect all types of records, including prescriptions, to detect the illicit distribution of these substances.

STATE AND LOCAL LEGISLATION

Within an individual state, the nurse's functions and responsibilities are defined by the state nurse practice act. The wording of a state's practice act may be general so that it gives the nurse a broad range of responsibilities, or it may be very specific in the limitations it sets. The nurse is responsible for knowing the boundaries set by the state practice act in the particular state of practice. A health care institution may develop policies that are more restrictive than the nurse practice act but cannot expand the scope of practice outlined by the state legislation. The primary intent of all state practice acts is to protect the public by defining required education and skill levels of all state-licensed nurses.

State and local regulations of medications must conform with federal legislation. States, however, have the power to enforce additional regulations that impose stricter control of substances. For example, the Controlled Substance Act has codeine in antitussives as a schedule V drug, but an individual state that identifies abuse of antitussives with codeine may place this drug in the schedule II category, which is more restrictive.

HEALTH CARE INSTITUTION REGULATIONS

All health care institutions are required to meet minimum standards set by federal, state, and local agencies. In addition to these standards, most institutions have established specific policies that regulate administration of medication within the institution. Institutional policies are typically more restrictive and more specific than federal and state regulations. Health care institutions are trying to prevent problems stemming from medication administration. For example, institutional policies may set the times for medication administration (e.g., medications ordered for every 8 hours are given at 0600 [6 AM], 1400 [2 PM], and 2200 [10 PM]) or may mandate discontinuation of medications unless reordered by the prescribing practitioner (e.g., antibiotics must be reordered every 5 days).

PHARMACOKINETICS

For a drug to achieve a therapeutic effect, it must proceed from the point of entry into the body to the tissue with which it will react. The effectiveness is further affected by the dosage of the drug and the amount of time the drug spends in the body before it is excreted.

Pharmacokinetics refers to the study of the absorption, distribution, metabolism, and excretion of drugs to determine the relationship between the dose of a drug and the drug's concentration in biological fluids. The knowledge of pharmacokinetics is used by prescribing practitioners in medication management.

The prescribing practitioner, when ordering a drug, is concerned mainly with dose and route to produce the most therapeutic effects; prescribing practitioners, pharmacists, and nurses are all involved in identifying appropriate times for drug administration and for avoiding interactions with other substances that could alter the drug's actions. Prescribing practitioners and nurses monitor the client's response to the drug's action. Drug actions are dependent on four properties: absorption, distribution, metabolism, and excretion.

CONTROLLED SUBSTANCES

- Schedule C-I: High abuse potential, no current accepted medical use (e.g., heroin, marijuana, LSD)
- Schedule C-II: High abuse potential for severe dependence (e.g., narcotics, amphetamines, dronabinol, some barbiturates)
- Schedule C-III: Less abuse potential than schedule II drugs for moderate dependence (e.g., nonbarbiturate sedatives, nonamphetamine stimulants, limited amounts of certain narcotics)
- Schedule C-IV: Lower abuse potential than schedule III drugs for limited dependence (e.g., sedatives, antianxiety agents, nonnarcotic analgesics)
- Schedule C-V: Limited abuse potential (e.g., codeine used as antitussive, antidiarrheals)

ABSORPTION

The degree and rate of **absorption**, or passage of a drug from the site of administration into the bloodstream, depend on several factors: the drug's physicochemical effects, its dosage form, its route of administration, its interactions with other substances in the digestive system, and various client characteristics such as age. Oral preparations, such as tablets and capsules, must first disintegrate into smaller particles for gastric juices to dissolve and prepare the drug for absorption in the small intestines. **Dissolution** is the rate at which a drug becomes a solution. After ingestion, a pill, capsule, or caplet must disintegrate before it can be dissolved and then absorbed by the body for therapeutic use. The more rapid the rate of dissolution, the more quickly the drug can be absorbed. Oral drugs in liquid form are more readily absorbed by the gastrointestinal tract than are tablets. Figure 30-1 shows the process of absorption of solid drugs.

Drugs administered intramuscularly are absorbed through the muscle into the bloodstream. Suppositories are absorbed through the mucous membranes into the blood. Intravenous drugs are immediately bioavailable because of their direct injection into the blood to produce a drug effect.

Blood flow to the absorption site is a major factor in drug absorption. A rich blood supply facilitates absorption, whereas a poor blood supply will slow absorption. **Sublingual** (under the tongue) medications, such as Nitrostat (for angina), are absorbed more quickly than are medications such as insulin that are injected into subcutaneous tissue. A person in shock, which results in poor peripheral circulation, may not absorb intramuscular medications as well as a person with normal circulation. Circulation is enhanced by exercise, so a diabetic who has exercised hard may experience low blood sugar (hypoglycemia) because of more rapid absorption of the insulin from increased peripheral circulation.

The solubility of the drug is also a factor in absorption. To be absorbed, the drug must be in a liquid form. The more soluble the drug, the faster it will be absorbed. Because cells have a fatty acid layer, drugs that are more lipid in content

are absorbed more rapidly. Chemicals and minerals that are insoluble in the gastrointestinal tract, such as barium salts, are not absorbed. When given parenterally, drugs with an oily base such as streptomycin (an anti-infective) are absorbed more slowly than are drugs dissolved in a water base.

The pH of the drug is another factor in absorption. A drug that is acidic (e.g., aspirin) can be more easily absorbed in an acidic environment such as gastric content. A drug that is more basic in composition is not absorbed in the stomach but passes on to the small intestine, where it is absorbed.

Drugs that are highly concentrated (e.g., epinephrine) tend to be absorbed more quickly than drugs that are lower in concentrations. Less well researched is the effect ethnicity and culture have on the therapeutic effects of medications. Some studies have identified differences in required drug levels as well as responses to medications (e.g., antihypertensive drugs and the African American client). Drugs do not have the same effect in all people. Diet is a factor as well as adherence to herbal and homeopathic remedies (e.g., the herb ginseng can act as an accelerant or inhibitor of certain medications). Prescribing practitioners need to be aware of and sensitive to these cultural variations that may affect clients in their care (Institute for Safe Medication Practices [ISMP], 2003).

Another factor affecting absorption is the ingestion of food before taking oral medications. Interactions of some medications with food change the chemical structure of the drug, thereby affecting absorption. For example, tetracycline (an anti-infective) should not be taken with dairy products. Clients taking warfarin (an anticoagulant) should avoid or limit their intake of food high in vitamin K, which is an antidote for warfarin. Some medications, when given together, interact with each other to impair absorption.

The administration time of dosages needs to be regulated to ensure adequate absorption of drugs. For example, it may be best to take certain medications a half hour before meals. The nurse needs to use this knowledge to be sure prescribed medications are administered properly.

DISTRIBUTION

Distribution refers to the movement of drugs from the blood into various body fluids and tissues. The rate at which the drug reaches the specific site of action is affected by blood flow, cell membrane permeability, and the protein-binding capacity of the medication.

How fast the drug reaches the organs and tissues depends on the cardiac output (blood flow) of the person. When conditions exist that decrease blood flow (e.g., cardiogenic shock) or when circulation to the tissue is poor (e.g., peripheral vascular disease from atherosclerosis), the distribution of the drug will be slowed. When conditions exist that increase blood flow (e.g., strenuous exercise), distribution will be facilitated.

To be distributed to the tissue, the drug must cross the cell membrane. Some membranes act as a barrier for distribution of medications. The blood-brain barrier, for example, allows only fat-soluble medications to pass through (e.g., alcohol, general anesthetics, penicillin G).

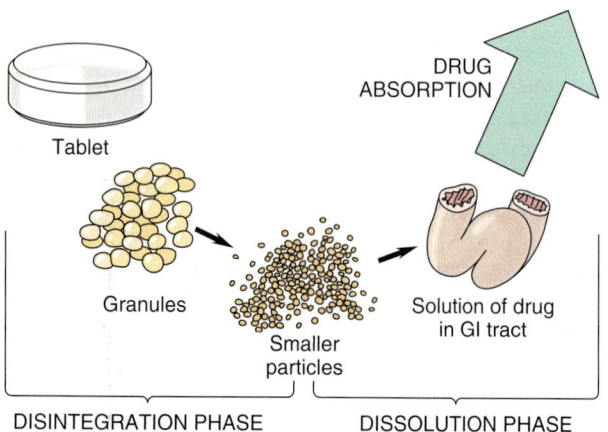

FIGURE 30-1 Phases of Solid Drug Absorption DELMAR/CENGAGE LEARNING

Once the drug enters the circulation, it may become attached to proteins, mostly albumin. This protein binding decreases the amount of free drug available to reach the site of action. This is because the protein–drug molecule is trapped in the blood flow, as it is too large to diffuse through the cell membrane. While medications vary in the extent to which they bind with proteins, most drugs have some protein-binding properties. Some diseases (e.g., malnutrition, liver disease) cause a decrease in circulating albumin that results in more free drug. This can result in increased distribution of the drug (enhanced pharmacologic effect) and toxicity if not carefully monitored.

Body composition also affects the distribution of medications. Many drugs are prescribed based on body weight. An increase in body fat (in an obese person, for example) causes longer drug duration because of slower distribution. The less a person weighs, the higher the concentration of medication in the circulation, which results in a more powerful drug effect. This needs to be monitored very closely in older adults who have changes in body composition naturally related to aging and often lose weight due to a decreased appetite.

METABOLISM

After the medication is absorbed and distributed, the body eliminates the drugs. The process of metabolism (also known as biotransformation) refers to the physical and chemical processing of the drug. In metabolism, the drug is inactivated and changed into a water-soluble compound that can be excreted by the body. The liver is the primary source of biotransformation. The rate of metabolism is determined by the presence of enzymes in the liver cells that detoxify the drugs. Diseases that affect the liver (e.g., cirrhosis) affect the body's ability to biotransform medications. Other conditions that affect metabolism are blood flow to the liver, the presence of other substances that affect liver function, and age. If drug metabolism is inhibited, there will be a buildup of the medication, causing a cumulative effect. This will be exhibited as a prolonged response to a normal dose of medication. If metabolism is enhanced (as in high blood flow states), the medications will be inactivated faster than expected, resulting in a shorter response to medications. A client's race and ethnic heritage can influence how drugs are metabolized (see the section on cultural diversity).

EXCRETION

Excretion is the process in which drugs are eliminated from the body. Excretion occurs primarily through hepatic biotransformation and renal excretion; it refers to the movement of a drug or its metabolites from the tissues back into circulation and from the circulation into the organs of excretion.

Factors that affect the kidneys' ability to excrete drugs include maturity of the kidneys, circulation, and disease. As kidney function decreases, there can be an accumulation of drugs, which can result in toxicity. If the kidneys are not functioning normally, a decreased dosage of medications may be needed. Adequate fluid intake aids in the elimination

of drugs in a healthy individual. Other organs, such as exocrine glands, the skin, the gastrointestinal tract, and the lungs, contribute to the elimination of some drugs.

DRUG NOMENCLATURE

A drug may be used as an aid in the diagnosis, treatment, or prevention of disease; in abnormal conditions for the relief of pain or suffering; or to improve any physiological or pathologic condition. The terms *drug, medication,* and *medicine* are often used interchangeably by health care providers and laypersons.

Drugs can be identified by their chemical, generic, official, or trade names. The *chemical name* is a precise description of the drug's composition (chemical formula). The *nonproprietary,* or *generic, name* in the United States is the name assigned by the U.S. Adopted Names Council to the manufacturer who first develops the drug. When the drug is approved, it is given an *official name* that may be the same as the nonproprietary name. Drugs with a proven therapeutic value are listed in the USP and NF by their official names. When pharmaceutical companies market the drug, they assign a *proprietary name,* also called a *trade* or *brand name;* therefore, one generic drug may have several trade names based on the number of companies marketing the drug. For example, ibuprofen is a generic name; common trade names for this drug are Advil, Excedrin IB, Motrin, and Nuprin. See the accompanying display on trade and generic drug names for additional examples.

DRUG ACTION

Drug action refers to a drug's ability to combine with a cellular drug receptor. Depending on the location of different cellular receptors affected by a given drug, a drug can have a local effect, a systemic effect, or both local and systemic effects. For example, when diphenhydramine hydrochloride (Benadryl) cream is applied to the skin, it elicits only a local effect; however, when this drug is administered in a tablet or injectable form, it causes both systemic and local effects.

PHARMACOLOGY

Pharmacology is the study of the effects of drugs on living organisms. This section discusses the pharmacologic activities

---

SAMPLE TRADE AND GENERIC DRUG NAMES

TRADE NAME	GENERIC NAME
Bayer	Aspirin
Benadryl	Diphenhydramine hydrochloride
Robitussin	Guaifenesin
Zovirax	Acyclovir

of drug action as it relates to medication management, drug classification, drug preparation, and routes of administration.

Medication Management

The purpose of medication management is to produce the desired drug action by maintaining a constant drug level. Drug action is based on the half-life of a drug.

A drug's **half-life** refers to the time it takes the body to eliminate half of the blood concentration level of the original drug dose. For example, if a drug has a half-life of 6 hours, 50% of the drug's original dose is present in the blood 6 hours after administration; in 12 hours after administration, 25% of the original drug is present. Because of a drug's half-life, repeated doses are often required to maintain the drug level over a 24-hour interval.

The nurse should understand other terms used to describe drug action: onset, peak plasma level, trough, duration, and plateau. **Onset of action** is the time it takes the body to respond to a drug after administration. Onset is affected by route of administration and pharmacokinetic factors already discussed. A **peak plasma level** is the highest blood concentration of a single drug dose before the elimination rate equals the rate of absorption. Once the peak plasma level is achieved, the blood concentration level will decrease steadily unless another drug dose is given. **Trough** is the lowest blood serum concentration of a drug in a person's system. This is measured immediately before the next scheduled dose. Trough levels help adjust dosage to prevent toxicity or drug buildup. **Duration** is the time a drug remains in the system in a concentration great enough to have a therapeutic effect. The accompanying display defines the common terms associated with the medical management of medication administration. If a series of scheduled drug doses are administered, the blood

concentration level is maintained; maintenance of a certain level is called a **plateau**.

Classification

Drugs are commonly classified by the body system that they interact with (e.g., cardiovascular) or in accord with the drug's approved therapeutic usage (e.g., antihypertensive). Drugs with multiple therapeutic uses are usually classified in accordance with their most common usage.

Preparation and Route

Drugs are available in many forms for administration by a specific route. (See the accompanying display on drug preparations on page 755.) The route refers to how the drug is absorbed: oral, buccal, sublingual, rectal, parenteral (hypodermic routes), topical, and inhalation.

Drugs prepared for administration by one route should not be substituted by other drug forms. For example, when a client has difficulty swallowing a large tablet or capsule, *the nurse should not administer an oral solution or elixir of the same drug without first consulting the prescribing practitioner because a liquid may be more easily and completely absorbed, producing a higher blood level than a tablet.*

The nurse should be aware of the various drug forms and how they are administered. Certain drug preparations require special consideration regarding administration. For example:

- Chewable tablets are designed to be chewed before swallowing because chewing enhances gastric absorption.
- Buccal and sublingual medications must be allowed to dissolve completely before the client can drink or eat.
- Suspensions and emulsions should be administered immediately after shaking and pouring from the bottle.

ORAL ROUTE Most drugs are administered by the oral route because it is the safest, most convenient, and least expensive method. The disadvantage of the oral route is that it is slower acting than the other routes, such as injectables. Drugs may not be given orally to clients with gastrointestinal intolerance or those on NPO (nothing by mouth) status. Oral drugs should be given with caution to clients who have difficulty swallowing, such as a client who has had a cerebrovascular accident (stroke). Oral administration is also precluded by unconsciousness.

When small amounts of drugs are required, the **buccal** (cheek) or sublingual route is used. Drugs administered through these routes act quickly because of the oral mucosa's thin epithelium and large vascular system, which allows the drug to quickly be absorbed by the blood.

Certain oral drugs are prepared for sublingual or buccal administration to prevent their destruction or transformation in the stomach or small intestines. Buccal drugs are designed to be placed in the buccal pocket (superior-posterior aspect of the internal cheek next to the molars) for absorption by the mucous membrane of the mouth. Sublingual medications are designed to dissolve quickly when placed under the tongue. For example, erythrityl tetranitrate (an antianginal) can be given either sublingually or buccally as prescribed,

---

COMMON TERMS ASSOCIATED WITH MEDICAL MANAGEMENT

- Half-life: The time it takes the body to eliminate half the blood concentration level of the original drug dose
- Onset: The time it takes the body to respond after medication administration
- Peak plasma level: The time it takes for a drug to reach the highest blood concentration after a single dose before the elimination rate equals the rate of absorption
- Trough: The lowest blood serum concentration immediately before the next scheduled dosage
- Duration: The time a drug remains in the system in a therapeutic concentration
- Plateau: Blood concentration level maintained after a series of scheduled drug doses is administered

whereas isoproterenol hydrochloride (a bronchodilator) and nitroglycerin (an antianginal) are given sublingually, and methyltestosterone (an androgen) is given only buccally.

PARENTERAL ROUTE By definition, **parenteral** means introduction of a medication by any route other than the oral-gastrointestinal route. However, medical usage of this term refers to injecting medication into body tissue. Sterile technique is always used for any medication injection. The four routes that nurses commonly use to administer parenteral medications are as follows:

- **Intradermal (ID)** is an injection into the dermis.
- **Subcutaneous** is an injection into the subcutaneous tissue.
- **Intramuscular (IM)** is an injection into the muscle.
- **Intravenous (IV)** is an injection into a vein.

Other parenteral routes (e.g., intrathecal or intraspinal, intracardiac, intrapleural, intra-arterial, and intra-articular) are used by prescribing practitioners and in some cases by advanced practice registered nurses for medication administration.

TOPICAL ROUTE Most topical drugs are given to deliver a drug at, or immediately beneath, the point of application. Although a large number of topical drugs are applied to the skin, other topical drugs include eye, nose and throat, ear, rectal, and vaginal preparations. Drugs applied directly to the skin are absorbed through the epidermal layer into the dermis, where they create local effects or are absorbed into the bloodstream. Drug action varies with the vascularity of the skin, usually requiring several applications over a 24-hour period to cause the desired therapeutic effect.

DRUG PREPARATIONS

ORAL SOLIDS

- Tablets: compressed or molded substances to be swallowed whole, chewed before swallowing, or placed in the buccal pocket or under the tongue (sublingual)
- Capsules: substances encased in either a hard or a soft soluble container or gelatin shell that dissolves in the stomach
- Caplets: gelatin-coated tablets that dissolve in the stomach
- Powder and granules: finely ground substances
- Troches, lozenges, and pastilles: similar preparations of drugs designed to dissolve in the mouth
- Enteric-coated: coated tablets that dissolve in the intestines
- Time-release capsules: encased substances that are further enclosed in smaller casings that deliver a drug dose over an extended period of time
- Sustained-release: compounded substances designed to release a drug slowly to maintain a steady blood medication level

TOPICAL

- Liniments: substances mixed with an alcohol, oil, or soapy emollient that are applied to the skin
- Ointments: semisolid substances for topical use
- Pastes: semisolid substances, thicker than an ointment, that are absorbed slowly through the skin
- Transdermal patches: contain medication that is absorbed through the skin over an extended period of time
- Suppositories: gelatin substances designed to dissolve when inserted in the rectum, urethra, or vagina

INHALANTS

- Inhalations: drugs or dilution of drugs administered by the nasal or oral respiratory route for a local or systemic effect

SOLUTIONS

- Solutions: contain one or more soluble chemical substances dissolved in water
- Enemas: aqueous solutions for rectal instillation
- Douches: aqueous solutions that function as a cleansing or antiseptic agent that may be dispensed in the form of a powder with directions for dissolving in a specific quantity of warm water
- Suspensions: particle or powder substances that must be dissolved in a liquid (shaken vigorously) before administration
- Emulsion: a two-phase system in which one liquid is dispersed in the form of small droplets throughout another liquid
- Syrups: substances dissolved in a sugar liquid
- Gargles: aqueous solutions
- Mouthwashes: aqueous solutions that may contain alcohol, glycerin, and synthetic sweeteners and surface-active flavoring and coloring agents
- Nasal solutions: aqueous solutions in the form of drops or sprays
- Optic (eye) and otic (ear) solutions: aqueous solutions that are instilled as drops
- Elixirs: nonaqueous solutions that contain water, varying alcohol content, and glycerin or other sweeteners

Transdermal patches, another type of topical preparation, are used to deliver medications such as nitroglycerin (antianginal) and certain supplemental hormone replacements for absorption by the blood to produce systemic effects. An adhesive disk secures the medication ointment to the skin. The frequency for changing the patch varies with the specific drug. The medication can last from 24 hours to 7 days.

Some topical drugs, such as eye and nasal drops and vaginal and rectal suppositories, can be applied directly to the mucous membranes. These drugs are absorbed quickly into the bloodstream, and, depending on the drug's dose (strength and quantity), may cause systemic effects.

The client may complain of a burning sensation when the nurse instills eye or nasal drops because the cornea of the eye and nasal mucous membranes are often sensitive to medications. Eyedrops should never be applied onto the sensitive cornea.

Inhalants   Inhalants (e.g., oxygen and most general anesthetics) deliver gaseous or volatile substances that are almost immediately absorbed into the systemic circulation. The inhalants are delivered into the alveoli of the lungs, which promote fast absorption owing to:

- The permeability of the alveolar and vascular epithelia
- An abundant blood flow
- A very large surface area for absorption

Oropharyngeal handheld inhalers deliver topical drugs to the respiratory tract to create local and systemic effects. There are three types of inhaler: metered-dose inhaler or nebulizer, turbo-inhaler, and nasal inhaler. They are explained later in this chapter.

Intraocular Route   Intraocular medications are administered by applying a clear, flexible, elliptical-shaped disk similar to a contact lens to the conjunctival sac. This provides continuous treatment of diseases such as open-angle glaucoma. Pilocarpine, a medication to treat glaucoma, can be administered in this manner. The disk can remain in the client's eye for up to a week. This route increases compliance and decreases the number of times a client must administer medication.

Drug Interaction

Drug interaction refers to the effect one drug can have on another. Drug interactions may occur when one drug is administered in combination with a second drug or when a short time interval exists between the administration of two different drugs. Drugs can be combined deliberately to produce a positive effect, as when hydrochlorothiazide (a potassium-depleting diuretic) is combined with spironolactone (a potassium-sparing diuretic) to maintain a normal blood level of potassium.

A positive drug combination can also occur when one drug, such as a preoperative medication, is deliberately given to potentiate the action of another drug.

Not all drug combinations are therapeutic. Some drug combinations can interfere with the absorption, effect, or excretion of other drugs. For example, calcium products and magnesium-containing antacids can cause inadequate absorption of tetracycline (an antibiotic) in the digestive tract.

Side Effects and Adverse Reactions

Drug effects other than those that are therapeutically intended and expected are called **adverse reactions**. A nontherapeutic effect may be mild and predictable (**side effect**) or unexpected and potentially hazardous (adverse effect). There are several types of adverse reactions: drug allergy, drug tolerance, toxic effect, and idiosyncratic reactions.

Drug allergy (hypersensitivity) is an antigen-antibody immune reaction that occurs when an individual who has been previously exposed to a drug has developed antibodies against the drug. The type of reaction may be mild (skin rash, urticaria, headache, nausea, or vomiting) or severe (anaphylaxis). Drug reactions are often manifested in the skin because of its abundant blood supply.

Anaphylaxis is an immediate, life-threatening reaction to a drug (e.g., penicillin) characterized by respiratory distress, sudden severe bronchospasm, and cardiovascular collapse. If emergency measures (administration of epinephrine, bronchodilators, and antihistamines) are not instituted immediately, anaphylaxis can be fatal.

Drug tolerance occurs when the body becomes so accustomed to a specific drug that larger doses are needed to produce the desired therapeutic effect. For example, cancer clients with severe pain may require larger and larger doses of morphine (narcotic analgesic) to control the pain as the body builds up a tolerance to the morphine.

A **toxic effect** occurs when the body cannot metabolize a drug, causing the drug to accumulate in the blood. Toxic reactions can result after prolonged intake of high doses of medication or after only one dose.

An **idiosyncratic reaction** is a highly unpredictable response that may be manifested by an overresponse, underresponse, or atypical response. For example, 1 of 40,000 clients will develop aplastic anemia after receiving chloramphenicol (an antibiotic).

Food and Drug Interactions

Medication management requires avoidance of possible food and drug interactions. There are three primary types of food and drug interaction:

1. Certain drugs may interfere with the absorption, excretion, or use in the body of one or more nutrients.
2. Certain foods may increase or decrease the absorption of a drug into the body.
3. Certain foods may alter the chemical actions of drugs, preventing their therapeutic effect on the body.

Most interaction problems occur with the use of diuretics, oral antibiotics, and anticoagulant and antihypertensive drugs (see the accompanying display on common food and drug interactions on page 757). Clients on sodium-restricted diets should be advised to consult with a pharmacist regarding the sodium content in prescription and over-the-counter drugs. Some drugs can contain almost one-half the total daily allowance of sodium. Alcohol is also considered a drug. Small amounts of alcohol interact with many drugs (e.g., antibiotics, antihistamines, anticoagulants, sleeping pills). Food and drug interactions can vary depending on the dose and the form in which the drug is taken and the client's age, sex, body weight, nutritional status, and specific medical condition.

FACTORS INFLUENCING DRUG ACTION

Individual client characteristics such as genetic factors, age, height and weight, and physical and mental conditions can influence the action of drugs on the body. Sometimes mistaken for drug allergies, genetic factors can interfere with drug metabolism and produce an abnormal sensitivity to certain drugs.

The nurse should consider age-related factors that can influence drug action and dosing. For example, neonates and infants have underdeveloped gastrointestinal systems, muscle mass, and metabolic enzyme systems and inadequate renal function; older adults clients often experience decreased hepatic or renal function and diminished muscle mass.

The prescribing practitioner often correlates the client's age, height, and weight when determining the dosage for many drugs. The nurse should make sure that this information is recorded accurately in the client's medical record. The amount of body fat may also alter drug distribution because some drugs such as digoxin (inotropic) are poorly distributed to fatty tissues.

The client's physical condition can also alter the effects of drugs. For example, in an edematous client, the drug must be distributed to a larger volume of body fluids than for a nonedematous client; therefore, the edematous client may require a larger drug dose to produce the drug action, whereas a dehydrated client would require a smaller dosage. Diseases that affect liver and renal functions can alter the metabolism and elimination of most drugs.

PROFESSIONAL ROLES IN MEDICATION ADMINISTRATION

The prescribing practitioner determines the therapeutic drug plan and conveys the plan to others by initiating orders or a prescription. In health care settings (long-term care facilities and hospitals), medication orders are written on a prescribing practitioner's order form. Prescribing practitioners can also write medication orders on legal prescription pads or through the computer terminal. When allowed by organizational policy, the prescribing practitioner may also give medication orders via telephone or as verbal orders.

When the prescribing practitioner gives a medication order orally, either directly or over the telephone, the nurse enters the information on the medical record. This information includes the name of the prescribing practitioner who ordered the medication, the name of the medication, the

COMMON FOOD AND DRUG INTERACTIONS

DRUG EFFECTS ON NUTRITIONAL STATUS

- Abuse of antacids can lead to phosphate depletion, which can cause a vitamin D deficiency, resulting in osteomalacia, or softening of the bones due to loss of calcium.
- Excessive use of diuretics may result in the loss of electrolytes, especially potassium, that places clients with cardiac conditions at a higher risk for serious rhythm problems. Potassium loss is greatest in clients taking digitalis as well as diuretics, making the heart more sensitive to the drug.
- Prolonged use of oral contraceptives by women may cause folacin and vitamin C deficiencies if their diets are inadequate in these nutrients.
- Hydralazine (antihypertensive drug) can deplete the body's supply of vitamin B_6.

FOOD EFFECTS ON DRUG ABSORPTION

- Calcium in milk and milk products may decrease the absorption of certain antibiotics such as tetracycline.
- Certain liquids (e.g., soda pop and high-acid fruit or vegetable juices) can cause an increase in the stomach acidity that can dissolve some drugs

before they reach the intestine. Because most drugs are absorbed in the intestines, this interaction will decrease the amount of drug that can be absorbed into the body.
- Certain foods such as fatty foods can increase the rate of absorption of some drugs (e.g., griseofulvin, an antifungal).

FOOD EFFECTS ON DRUG UTILIZATION

- The effects of anticoagulants can be decreased by certain foods in the liver such as green leafy vegetables that contain vitamin K, which is used by the body to promote blood clotting.
- Aged or fermented foods (e.g., aged cheese, chicken livers) and other foods can decrease the metabolism in the body of monoamine oxidase inhibitors that are used to treat depression and high blood pressure.
- Long-term use of licorice and licorice-flavored candy or drugs can counteract the effect of high blood pressure medication.

dosage, the frequency, the route of administration, and the nurse's name. Most institutions require the prescribing practitioner to confirm oral orders within 24 hours; the nurse is responsible for ensuring that the verbal order is clear. The verbal or telephone orders should be verified (i.e., read back) verbatim by the person receiving the order. See Chapter 13 for a complete discussion of written and verbal orders and the role of the nurse in transcribing orders.

The pharmacist processes the prescribing practitioner's orders, clarifies any entries that are unclear, and prepares the medications for administration. The pharmacist is responsible for filling prescriptions and for making sure they are valid entries. Pharmacists also assess medication plans, monitoring for incompatibilities and, at times, recommending the best time to administer a medication to obtain therapeutic benefit (e.g., Lovastatin, a cholesterol-lowering drug, is most effective if taken in the evening). The pharmacist participates in calculating the appropriate dosage of certain medications such as anti-infective drugs (e.g., gentamicin). These dosages are based on the client's body weight and kidney function and may be adjusted during the course of therapy by the pharmacist with the prescribing practitioner's consent. Nurses frequently consult with pharmacists in determining compatibility if IV medications are to be administered simultaneously. Pharmacists also answer medication-related questions for both nurses and clients.

Nurses spend a great deal of time with their clients and have specific knowledge and skills that qualify them to administer medication and to evaluate a medication's effectiveness. Nurses understand why particular medications are ordered for clients and what physiological changes may result from the medications that cause therapeutic effects. Because of their knowledge, skills, and frequent client contact, nurses can readily assess changes in a client's condition and can determine whether it is appropriate to administer a medication on the basis of the client's condition.

Nurses are responsible for teaching clients to self-administer medications (e.g., insulin) and for assessing the client's ability to self-administer correctly. Before discharge, nurses teach clients about the medications they will be taking at home and how to assess for side effects and adverse reactions. Client education includes demonstration by the nurse and return demonstration by the client on how to prepare and administer the medication (e.g., an insulin injection). Even though time may be a limiting factor, it is only the nurse's observation of client performance by demonstration that ensures that clients can safely and successfully administer their own medications.

Most agencies have policies relative to medication administration, such as stop dates for certain types of drugs, regularly scheduled times to administer medications as specified in the drug order, and a listing of abbreviations officially accepted for use in the agency. The agency's medical records department maintains the official listing of abbreviations adopted by the medical staff; only abbreviations from the official list can be used in any part of the client's medical record. See the accompanying display for a list of common abbreviations used in medication orders.

The ISMP and the National Coordinating Council for Medication Error Reporting and Prevention (NCC MERP), with the support of accrediting and professional organizations, stress the importance of avoiding dangerous abbreviations and dosage expressions when communicating information about medications. For example, the apothecary symbol for dram (3) is often misunderstood or misread for "3." Only the metric system should be used when communicating a medication dose, since abbreviations can be confusing. The Latin abbreviation for ear (AU, *aurio uterque*), for example, may be mistaken for the Latin abbreviation for eye (OU, *oculo uterque*). Ear or eye should be spelled out, not abbreviated. Besides the ISMP and the NCC MERP, the Joint Commission's National Patient Safety Goals specify that certain abbreviations must appear on a "do not use" list. For example, the use of U or u can easily be mistaken for a zero (4 U can be misread as 40), causing a 10-fold (or more) overdose. See Table 30-1 on page 759 for the NCC MERP listing of dangerous abbreviations that should be avoided.

TYPES OF MEDICATION ORDERS

The prescribing practitioner prescribes medications in different ways, depending on their purpose. Medications can be prescribed as stat, single-dose, standing, and prn orders.

COMMON ABBREVIATIONS USED IN MEDICATION ORDERS

ABBREVIATION	MEANING
a.c.	before meals
ad lib	freely, as desired
b.i.d.	two times a day
c̄	with
cap	capsule
elix	elixir
h	hour
hrly	hourly
ID	intradermal
IM	intramuscular
IV	intravenous
IVPB	intravenous piggyback
p.c.	after meals
per	by
PO	by mouth
prn	as needed
q	every
q2h	every 2 hours
q.i.d.	four times a day
qs	sufficient quantity
stat	immediately
supp	suppository
susp	suspension
tab	tablet
t.i.d.	three times a day
Tr or tinct	tincture

TABLE 30-1 Dangerous Abbreviations

ABBREVIATION	INTENDED MEANING	COMMON ERROR
U	Units	Mistaken for a zero (0) or a four (4), resulting in overdose. Also mistaken for "cc" (cubic centimeters) when poorly written.
μg	Micrograms	Mistaken for "mg" (milligrams), resulting in a 1000-fold overdose.
Q.D., QD, q.d., qd	Latin abbreviation for every day	The period after the "Q" has sometimes been mistaken for an "I," and the drug has been given "QID" (four times daily) rather than daily.
Q.O.D., QOD, q.o.d., qod	Latin abbreviation for every other day	Misinterpreted as "QD" (daily) or "QID" (four times daily). If the "O" is poorly written, it looks like a period or "I."
SC or SQ	Subcutaneous	Mistaken for "SL" (sublingual) when poorly written.
T I W	Three times a week	Misinterpreted as "three times a day" or "twice a week."
D/C	Discharge; also discontinue	Clients' medications have been prematurely discontinued when D/C (intended to mean "discharge") was misinterpreted as "discontinue" because it was followed by a list of drugs.
HS	Half strength	Misinterpreted as the Latin abbreviation "HS" (hour of sleep).
cc	Cubic centimeters	Mistaken for "U" (units) when poorly written.
AU, AS, AD	Latin abbreviations for both ears; left ear; right ear	Misinterpreted as Latin abbreviations "OU" (both eyes), "OS" (left eye), or "OD" (right eye).
MgSO$_4$	Magnesium sulfate	Mistaken for morphine sulfate.
MS, MSO$_4$	Morphine sulfate	Mistaken for magnesium sulfate.

National Coordinating Council for Medication Error Reporting and Prevention (NCC MERP). © 1998–2008. All Rights Reserved.

Stat Orders

When the prescribing practitioner writes orders, the nurse should read all of the orders to determine if any stat orders have been prescribed. A **stat order** is an order for a single dose of medication to be given immediately. Stat drugs are often prescribed in emergency situations to modify a serious physiological response; a stat dose of nitroglycerin may be ordered for a client experiencing chest pain. The nurse should assess and document the client's response to all stat medications.

Single-Dose Orders

Single-dose orders are one-time medications or may require the administration of drops or tablets over a short period of time. The nurse should administer single-dose orders only once, either at a time specified by the prescribing practitioner or at the earliest convenient time. These drugs are often prescribed in preparation for a diagnostic or therapeutic procedure; for example, radiopaque tablets may be administered in preparation for a gallbladder test, or a one-time order may be given for a preoperative medication.

Standing Orders

Standing orders are also referred to as *scheduled orders* because they are administered routinely as specified until the order is canceled by another order. The standing orders stay in effect until the prescribing practitioner discontinues or modifies the dosage or frequency with another order or until a prescribed number of days has elapsed as determined by agency policy. The purpose of a standing medication order is to maintain the desired blood level of the medication.

Agency policy determines the actual times for administering medications for a 24-hour time interval. For example, t.i.d. drugs may be administered at 0800, 1400, and 2000 or at 0900, 1500, and 2100. Medications ordered every day may have a specified time identified in the order, such as isophane (NPH) insulin 10 units subcutaneously at 0600, or they may be given at the agency's designated time, for example, Lanoxin 0.25 mg PO every day at 0900.

When the order specifies the number of days or the number of dosages of the drug the client is to receive, the order has an automatic stop date to discontinue the drug. For example, the order may read tetracycline 250 mg PO q6h for 5 days. The nurse should execute this order by administering 250 mg tetracycline orally every 6 hours for 5 days for a total of 20 doses. Day 1 begins with the administration of the drug and the time the first dose is given. If the first dose of tetracycline is given on a Tuesday at 1200, and then every 6 hours, the last dose will be given on Sunday at 0600. Although the medication is given over 6 consecutive days, it totals 20 doses as ordered. Most agencies have an automatic stop date to discontinue certain medications, such as 5 or 7 days for antibiotics and 48 or 72 hours for narcotics.

prn Orders

A drug may be ordered on a **prn** (as needed) basis as circumstances indicate. The drug is administered when, in the nurse's judgment, the client's condition requires it. Before administering a prn medication, the nurse must thoroughly assess the client, using both objective and subjective data in determining the appropriateness of administering the medication. This type of order is commonly written for analgesics, antiemetics, and laxatives.

The order written by the prescribing practitioner indicates how frequently a prn medication can be given. A nurse cannot administer a prn medication more frequently than the order indicates without consulting with the prescribing practitioner for a change in that order. Examples of prn orders are meperidine (a narcotic analgesic) 75 mg IM q3–4 hours prn incisional pain and Tylenol 650 mg q4 hours prn headache. When the prn medication has been administered, the nurse documents the assessment and the time of administration. In addition, the nurse is responsible for monitoring the effectiveness of the medication and documenting the effect in the client's medical record. The nurse administers the pain medication on the basis of the assessment of the client's pain and as specified in the order.

PARTS OF THE DRUG ORDER

All orders should be written clearly and legibly, and the drug order should contain seven parts:

1. The name of the client
2. The date and time when the order is written
3. The name of the drug to be administered
4. The dosage
5. The route by which it is to be administered and special directives about its administration
6. The time of administration and frequency
7. The signature of the prescribing practitioner writing the order (e.g., the prescribing practitioner or advanced practice registered nurse)

Drug prescriptions written in settings other than acute care facilities may also specify whether the generic or trade name of the drug is to be dispensed, the quantity to be dispensed, and how many times the prescription can be refilled.

SYSTEMS OF WEIGHT AND MEASURE

Medication administration requires the nurse to have a knowledge of weight and volume measurement systems. In North America, three systems of measurement are used in medication management: metric, apothecary, and household.

METRIC SYSTEM

The metric system of weights and measures was adopted by the USP in 1890 and the *British Pharmacopoeia* in 1914 to the exclusion of all other systems except for equivalent dosages. The Council on Pharmacy and Chemistry of the American Medical Association adopted the metric system exclusively in 1944. Resistance to changing established customs interfered with the exclusive adoption of the metric system. Today, the metric system is used in every major country of the world and is used almost exclusively in U.S. medical practice.

The metric, or decimal, system is a simple system of measurement based on units of 10. The basic units can be multiplied or divided by 10 to form secondary units. The decimal point is moved to the right for calculating multiples, and the decimal point is moved to the left for division.

The basic units of measurement in the metric system are the meter (linear), the liter (volume), and the gram (mass). The metric system uses prefixes derived from Latin to designate subdivisions of the basic units and prefixes derived from Greek to designate multiples of the basic units (see the accompanying display on metric system prefixes). When the metric system is used, a zero is always placed in front of the decimal for values less than 1 (e.g., 0.5) to prevent error.

APOTHECARY SYSTEM

The apothecary system, which originated in England, is based on the weight of one grain of wheat. Therefore, the basic unit of weight is the grain (gr), and the basic unit of volume is the minim (the approximate volume of water that weighs a grain). The grain is expressed in fractions such as morphine gr 1/4. The minim (*m*) is the smallest unit of

---

METRIC SYSTEM PREFIXES

LATIN PREFIXES—SUBDIVISIONS OF THE BASIC UNIT
deci (1/10, or 0.1)
centi (1/100, or 0.01)
milli (1/1000, or 0.001)

GREEK PREFIXES—MULTIPLES OF THE BASIC UNIT
deka (10)
hecto (100)
kilo (1000)

volume, followed in ascending order by the fluid dram (D), fluid ounce (Z), pint (pt), quart (qt), and gallon (gal).

HOUSEHOLD SYSTEM

The household system of measurement is similar to the apothecary system of liquid measures and is the least accurate of the three systems. The units of liquid measure are drop (gtt), teaspoon (tsp), tablespoon (Tbsp), cup, and glass. Household units are often used to inform clients of the size of a liquid dose.

The USP recognizes the use of the teaspoon as the ordinary practice for household medication administration and states that the teaspoon may be regarded as representing 5 mL. Household spoons are not appropriate when accurate measurement of a liquid dose is required; therefore, the USP recommends that a calibrated oral syringe or dropper be used for accurate measurement of liquid drug doses.

APPROXIMATE DOSE EQUIVALENTS

The conversion of metric doses with the apothecary and household systems are *approximate dose equivalents* (see the accompanying display on approximate metric system equivalents on page 762). The approximate dose equivalents represent the quantities usually ordered by prescribing practitioners when using either the metric or apothecary system of weights and volumes for drug doses. If the prepared dosage form is prescribed in the metric system, the pharmacist may dispense the corresponding approximate equivalent in the apothecary system and vice versa. For example, if the prescribing practitioner prescribes morphine gr 1/4, the pharmacist may dispense morphine 15 mg. The USP and NF reference *exact equivalents* that must be used to calculate quantities in pharmaceutical formularies and prescription compounding.

CONVERTING UNITS OF WEIGHT AND VOLUME

The nurse has to apply the knowledge of measurement systems and their conversions when the prescribing practitioner prescribes a drug dosage in one system and the pharmacy dispenses the equivalent dose in another. Given the above example of morphine, if the prescribing practitioner orders morphine gr 1/4 and the pharmacist dispenses morphine 15 mg, the nurse is responsible for ensuring the correct dose. The nurse knows that 1 grain equals 60 milligrams; to convert the ordered dose to milligrams, the nurse should use the following calculation:

$$1 gr = 60 mg$$
$$x = 1/4 \ gr \times 60 \ mg/gr$$
(the grains cancel out)
$$x = 60/4 \ mg$$
$$x = 15 \ mg$$

Measurement Conversions within the Metric System

Because the metric system is based on units of 10, dose equivalents within the system are computed by simple arithmetic, either dividing or multiplying. For example, to change milligrams to grams (1000 mg equals 1 g) or milliliters to liters (1000 mL equals 1 L), divide the number by 1000:

$$250 \ mg = x \ g$$
(move the decimal point three places to the left)
$$x = 0.25 \ g$$
or
$$500 \ mL = x \ L$$
(move the decimal point three places to the left)
$$x = 0.5 \ L$$

To convert grams to milligrams or liters to milliliters, the nurse multiplies the number by 1000:

$$0.005 \ g = x \ mg$$
(move the decimal point three places to the right)
$$x = 5 \ mg$$
or
$$0.725 \ L = x \ mL$$
(move the decimal point three places to the right)
$$x = 725 \ mL$$

The nurse may need to convert the volumes of liters and milliliters for enemas and irrigating solutions such as for bladder and wound irrigations. IV solutions are sterile, prepackaged solutions dispensed in volumes as ordered by the prescribing practitioner, such as 50 mL, 100 mL, 250 mL, 500 mL, and 1000 mL (1 liter).

Measurement Conversions between Systems

When converting grains to milligrams, the nurse must multiply by 60. For example, if the prescribing practitioner orders nitroglycerin (an antianginal) 1/150 gr PO for chest pain, the dispensed dose will be 0.4 mg:

$$1 \ gr = 60 \ mg$$
$$x = 1/150 \ gr \times 60 \ mg/gr$$
(the grains cancel out)
$$x = 1/150 \times 60/1 \ mg$$
$$x = 60/150 \ mg$$
(divide 60 by 150)
$$x = 0.4 \ mg$$

The nurse converts between pounds and kilograms (2.2 lb = 1 kg) by dividing or multiplying by 2.2. For example, if the ordered dose is 10 mg/kg and the client weighs 150 lb:

$$\frac{150 \ lb}{2.2 \ lb/kg} \times \frac{10 \ mg/kg}{x}$$

APPROXIMATE METRIC SYSTEM EQUIVALENTS

LIQUID MEASURE (VOLUME)

METRIC	APOTHECARY	HOUSEHOLD
5 mL	= 1 fluid dram	= 1 teaspoonful
10 mL	= 2 fluid drams	= 1 dessertspoonful
15 mL	= 4 fluid drams	= 1 tablespoonful
30 mL	= 1 fluid ounce	= 1 ounce
60 mL	= 2 fluid ounces	= 1 wineglassful
120 mL	= 4 fluid ounces	= 1 teacupful
240 mL	= 8 fluid ounces	= 1 tumblerful
500 mL	= 1 pint	= 1 pint
1000 mL	= 1 quart	= 1 quart
4000 mL	= 1 gallon	= 1 gallon

WEIGHT

METRIC	APOTHECARY
1 mg	= 1/60 grain
4 mg	= 1/15 grain
10 mg	= 1/6 grain
15 mg	= 1/4 grain
30 mg	= 1/2 grain
60 mg	= 1 grain
1 g	= 15 grains
4 g	= 1 dram
30 g	= 1 ounce
500 g	= 1.1 pound
1000 g (1 kg)	= 2.2 pounds

(the lb and kg cancel out)

$$x = 68.2 \times 10 \text{ mg}$$
$$x = 682 \text{ mg}$$

In clinical settings, household measures are used for bedside recording of intake so that the client or family member can record the volume ingested by the client. Agencies have a legend on their intake form with the approximate conversions from household to metric volume measures based on the type of containers used in that specific agency. See Chapter 33 for the procedure for measuring intake and output. Home health nurses often have to convert a liquid dose to an approximate household unit.

DRUG DOSE CALCULATIONS

Several formulas may be used by the nurse when calculating drug doses. One formula uses ratios based on the *dose on hand* and the *dose desired*. For example, cephalexin (anti-infective cephalosporin) 500 mg PO q.i.d. (dose desired) is ordered by the prescribing practitioner; the dose on hand is 250 mg/5 mL. The formula is as follows:

$$\frac{250 \text{ mg (dose on hand)}}{5 \text{ mL (dose on hand)}} = \frac{500 \text{ mg (dose desired)}}{x \text{ (dose desired)}}$$

(cross-multiply)

$$250x = 5 \times 500$$
$$x = \frac{5 \times 500}{250}$$
$$x = 10 \text{ mL}$$

The ratio formula can be used in calculating dosages. For example, the prescribing practitioner orders heparin (anticoagulant) 10,000 units SC; the dose on hand is 40,000 units/mL:

$$\frac{40,000 \text{ units}}{1 \text{ mL}} \times \frac{10,000 \text{ units}}{x}$$
(units cancel out)
$$40,000x = 10,000$$
$$x = \frac{10,000}{40,000}$$
$$x = {}^1\!/_4$$
$$x = 0.25 \text{ mL}$$

Pediatric Dosages

Several rules have been devised to calculate infants' and children's dosages (e.g., *Young's rule, Clark's rule,* and *Fried's rule*), but these rules give only approximate dosages. Even when pediatric drug dosages are calculated on body surface area, weight, and age of the child, they are based on a proportion of the usual adult dose (approximate). Regardless of the method used in calculating pediatric drug dosages, the nurse should realize that dosages are approximate and often need adjustment based on the child's response.

The body surface area method of determining pediatric doses is based on the body surface area of an adult weighing 150 lb. The body surface area of an adult weighing 150 lb is 1.73 square meters. The approximate child dose is calculated as follows:

$$\frac{\text{Body surface area of child}}{\text{Body surface area of adult}} \times \text{adult dose}$$
$$= \text{aproximate child dose}$$

$$\frac{\text{Body surface area of child (m}^2)}{1.73 \text{ m}^2} \times \text{adult dose}$$
$$= \text{approximate child dose}$$

Nomograms based on height and weight are used to compute the body surface area (see Figure 30-2 on page 763). A straight line is drawn from the client's height in the left column to the client's weight in the right column. The point at which this line intersects the body surface area column (designated SA) indicates the body surface area. Nomograms are used primarily in calculating pediatric drug dosages; however, they are also used when calculating some adult drug dosages (e.g., aminoglycosides and antineoplastic agents).

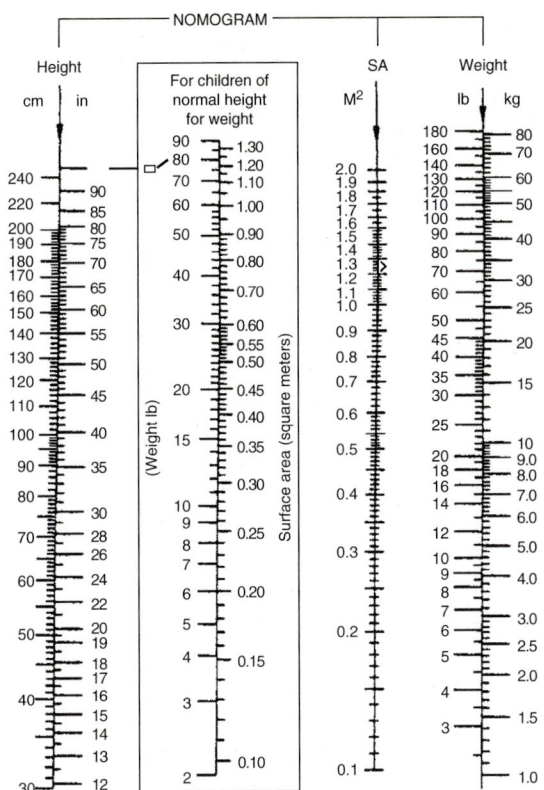

Directions for use: (1) Determine client height. (2) Determine client weight. (3) Draw a straight line to connect the height and weight. Where the line intersects on the SA line is the derived body surface area (m²).

FIGURE 30-2 Nomogram for Estimating Body Surface Area
REPRINTED WITH PERMISSION FROM BEHRMAN, R. E., KLIEGMAN, R., & ARVIN, A. M. (EDS.). (1996). *NELSON TEXTBOOK OF PEDIATRICS* (15TH ED.). PHILADELPHIA: ELSEVIER.

SAFE DRUG ADMINISTRATION

Nurses must administer numerous drugs daily in a safe and efficient manner. The nurse should administer drugs in accord with nursing standards of practice and agency policy. The safe storage and maintenance of an adequate supply of drugs are other responsibilities of the nurse.

The nurse documents the actual administration of medications on the medication administration record, or MAR. The MAR is a medical record form that contains the drug's name, dose, route, and frequency of administration. Drug data are entered either by the nurse when transcribing the order (handwritten onto the form) or by the pharmacist when dispensing the order (a computer-generated pharmacy MAR form is shown in Figure 30-3 on page 764).

GUIDELINES FOR MEDICATION ADMINISTRATION

To protect the client from medication errors, nurses have traditionally used as a guideline the "5 rights" of drug administration. The 5 rights help prevent medication error; however, errors can still occur even when nurses diligently follow the

5 rights. Sometimes other system failures occur; for example, during the ordering, transcribing, and dispensing process, errors may occur. In an effort to further reduce medication errors, some institutions have enlarged the 5 rights to 7 or 10 rights, such as right reason or right documentation. Standards of nursing practice still refer to the basic right 5s, as shown in the accompanying display.

Right Drug

Before administering any medication, the nurse compares the medications listed on the MAR, other recording forms, or computer orders against the prescribing practitioner's order. When administering a medication, the nurse should check the label written on the container against the MAR at least three times before giving the drug. The nurse should:

1. Check the label when removing the drug container from the client's medication drawer.
2. Check the drug when removing it from the container.
3. Check the drug before returning it to the client's medication drawer.

Some medications come in a unit-dose prepackaged form. The nurse should check the medication a third time even though there would be no container to return to the drawer. This third check should be done at the bedside before opening the unit-dose medication.

The nurse should give only medications that the nurse has prepared and checked. The nurse who administers the medication is the responsible party should an error occur. If a client questions a medication to be administered, the nurse should never ignore the question. Clients are active participants in their care and usually know when a medication is different from that usually taken. The nurse should withhold this medication until the order can be rechecked. Frequently, the medication order has changed, but the client question can stop an error before it occurs.

If the client refuses a medication, it should be discarded rather than returned to the original container. Unit-dose medications that have not been opened can be saved.

Right Dose

The unit-dose system was implemented to help decrease medication errors. However, there are times when medications on hand are in a larger volume or strength than needed. Careful calculation is especially important when the prescribing

---

FIVE RIGHTS OF DRUG ADMINISTRATION

1. Right drug
2. Right dose
3. Right client
4. Right route
5. Right time

PHARMACY MAR

START STOP	MEDICATION	SCHEDULED TIMES	OK'D BY	0001 HRS. to 1200 HRS.	1201 HRS. to 2400 HRS.
08/31/xx 1800 SCH	PROCAN SR 500 MG TAB-SR 500 MG Q6H PO	0600 1200 1800 2400	JD	0600 GP 1200 GP	1800 MS 2400 JD
09/03/xx 0900 SCH	DIGOXIN (LANOXIN) 0.125 MG TAB 1 TAB QOD PO ODD DAYS-SEPT.	0900	JD	0900 GP	
09/03/xx 0900 SCH	FUROSEMIDE (LASIX) 40 MG TAB 1 TAB QD PO	0900	JD	0900 GP	
09/03/xx 0845 SCH	REGLAN 10 MG TAB 10 MG AC&HS PO GIVE ONE NOW!	0730 1130 1630 2100	JD	0730 GP 1130 GP	1630 MS 2100 MS
09/04/xx 0900 SCH	K-LYTE 25 MEQ EFFERVESCENT TAB 1 EFF. TAB BID PO DISSOLVE AS DIR. START 9-4	0900 1700	JD	0900 GP	1700 GP
09/03/xx 1507 PRN	NITROGLYCERIN 1/50 GR 0.4 MG TAB-SL 1 TABLET PRN* SL PRN CHEST PAIN		JD		
09/03/xx 1700 PRN	DARVOCET-N 100* 1 TAB Q4-6H PO PRN MILD-MODERATE PAIN		JD		
09/03/xx 2100 PRN	MEPERIDINE*(DEMEROL) INJ 50 MG Q4H IM PRN SEVERE PAIN W PHENERGAN		JD		2200 (H) MS
09/03/xx 2100 PRN	PROMETHAZINE (PHENERGAN) INJ 50 MG Q4H IM PRN SEVERE PAIN W DEMEROL		JD		2200 (H) MS

Gluteus		Nurse's Signature	Initial	Allergies: NKA		Patient:	Patient, John D.
A. Right	H. Right					Patient #:	3-81512-3
B. Left	I. Left	7-3 G. Pickar, R.N.	GP			Admitted:	08/31/xx
Ventro Gluteal				Diagnosis: CHF		Physician:	J. Physician, MD
C. Right	J. Right	3-11 M. Smith, R.N.	MS				
D. Left	K. Left					Room:	PCU-14 PCU
E. Abdomen	1|2 3|4	11-7 J. Doe, R.N.	JD				

FIGURE 30-3 Computerized Pharmacy Medication Administration Record (MAR) DELMAR/CENGAGE LEARNING

practitioner orders a unit of measurement different from what is supplied by the pharmacy.

The nurse must know how to reduce the risk of error by correctly calculating doses and having them double-checked before administration. Policy in some agencies, for instance, mandates that two nurses check insulin dosages to ensure accuracy. After calculations have been completed, the nurse should prepare the medication using appropriate measurement devices such as graduated measuring cups, syringes, and droppers.

To prepare scored or crushed medications, the nurse should make sure scored tablets are broken evenly. This practice will prevent overdosage or underdosage of a medication. If the medication has to be crushed with a mortar and pestle, the nurse should thoroughly cleanse the pestle after each use. Cleansing the pestle will avoid mixing of different medications and will prevent the client from receiving minute amounts of a medication that may cause serious adverse effects.

Right Client

The nurse should correctly identify the client by using at least two client identifiers. Compare the client's name and one other identifier, usually the hospital identification number on the identification bracelet with the MAR (see Figure 30-4 on page 765). Ask the client to state his or her name, if possible, for a third identifier. Identification bracelets that become blurred or are missing for any reason should be replaced. The nurse needs to obtain a new identification band for the client. Verify the identification by asking the client to state his or her full name before placing the new band on the client's arm.

Right Route

The route of the medication is specified in the written order. The nurse should consult the prescribing practitioner whenever a route is not identified in the prescription, when the route indicated differs from the recommended one, or when the

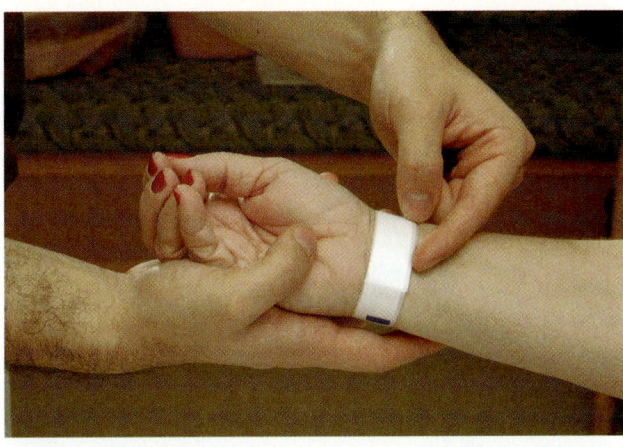

FIGURE 30-4 Check a client's identification band before administering medication. DELMAR/CENGAGE LEARNING

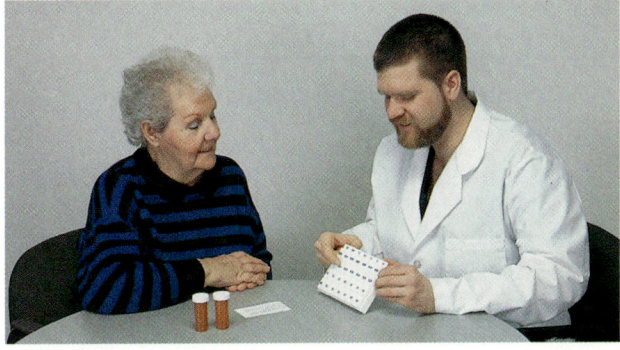

FIGURE 30-5 A pill box correlated to the days of the month can help the client follow her medication regimen. DELMAR/CENGAGE LEARNING

nurse questions the choice of route prescribed. For example, the nurse should not substitute an oral medication for an IM medication simply because the oral medication is available and the IM one is not.

Injecting a medication designed to be administered orally can cause adverse reactions such as a sterile abscess at the injection site. Medications for parenteral injections should be prepared from medications designed for this purpose. Manufacturers of medications label medications that can be used for parenteral injections as "for parenteral use only."

Right Time

Medications are generally ordered on a schedule. Nurses are responsible for knowing why a medication is ordered on a certain schedule and for following that schedule as closely as possible. A drug should not be given more than a half hour before or after the scheduled time (according to organizational policy) without first checking with the prescribing practitioner. Some computerized programs, such as bar coding, discussed later in this chapter, have increased the window for administering medications from 1 hour to 2 hours to provide the nurse with additional time to avoid having to document a "late" dose of medication.

To maintain the drug's effect, the nurse has to give the medication in a timely manner. Some medications must be given at a certain time for proper therapeutic effect; for example, insulin should be given at a set time before meals. These types of drugs should be administered as ordered. See the Nursing Checklist on page 766 for guidelines that ensure the safe administration of medications.

In the home health and community care settings (e.g., a retirement home), the nurse has different responsibilities regarding drug safety (see Figure 30-5). The nurse should promote drug safety measures that are appropriate to the environment and inherent risk factors (see the accompanying display on drug safety considerations on page 766).

DOCUMENTATION OF DRUG ADMINISTRATION

A critical element of drug administration is documentation. The standard is "if it was not documented it was not done." Many drug errors can be avoided with appropriate documentation. The nurse responsible for administering the medication must initial the medication on the MAR near the time the drug is scheduled after the client has taken the drug. Usually there is a space available for a full signature on the record.

If the client refuses to take a medication once it has been prepared, the nurse must indicate that a dose was missed. In some hospitals, a circle is placed around the time the medication was scheduled to be given. The nurse should write in the record why the dose was missed and notify the prescribing practitioner. The client may have refused because the tablet was too large. The medication may be supplied as a liquid so an alternate form of the medication can be given; the nurse must request that the prescribing practitioner change the order to a liquid. Clients do have the right to refuse medications. However, if clients understand the actions of the medication, they may be willing to take the medication. Clients who are scheduled for various diagnostic tests or treatments at the time the medication is to be administered will need to have the medication times rescheduled.

DRUG SUPPLY AND STORAGE

Drugs are dispensed by the pharmacy to nursing units through various methods to accommodate the agency's medication system. Once the pharmacy delivers the drugs to a nursing unit, the nurse is responsible for their safe storage.

Scheduled drugs for each client are usually dispensed in a **unit-dose form**. Unit dose is a system of packaging and labeling each dose of medication by the pharmacy, often to supply a 24-hour time period. The pharmacy usually delivers the drugs and stores the drugs in the designated area for each client. Unit-dose drugs are usually stored in a medication cart that contains individual drawers for each client's medication supply or in the medication room in a separate, organized

☑ **NURSING**CHECKLIST

Guidelines for Safe Administration of Medications

- Never administer medications that are prepared by another nurse. The nurse is responsible for a medication error when administering a medication that was inaccurately prepared by another nurse.

- Nurses should listen carefully to the client who questions the addition or deletion of a medication. Most clients are aware of their prescribed medications. If a client questions the drug or dose the nurse is preparing to administer, the nurse should recheck the order.

- If a medication is withheld, indicate the exact reason why in the client's record. Legally the nurse is accountable for giving ordered medications to the client; however, circumstances may prevent the nurse from giving a medication as ordered. Medications may be held for some diagnostic tests, or the client receiving antihypertensive medications may have a blood pressure that is lower than normal. If the nurse gave the antihypertensive, the blood pressure would decrease, causing further hypotension.

- *Do not leave medications at the client's bedside for any reason.* The client may forget to take the medication, medications can accumulate, and the client could take two or more of the same medication, causing an overdose, or another client who is confused could take the medicine.

- Initial the MAR only for those medications actually administered. This practice ensures accurate charting by clearly indicating which actions the nurse has performed.

- Advise clients not to take medications belonging to others and not to offer their medications to others. Medications are ordered for each client on the basis of the history, physical examination, and effectiveness of the medication.

DRUG SAFETY CONSIDERATIONS IN HOME HEALTH AND COMMUNITY CARE SETTINGS

- Help the client remove outdated prescriptions and over-the-counter drugs from medication cabinets. The chemical composition may change over time, causing a different drug action. Over-the-counter drugs may interact with prescription drugs, either by decreasing or potentiating the effects of the prescription medication.

- Encourage the client or caregivers to maintain drug refills to decrease the risk of missing scheduled medications.

- Use a mechanism such as a paper clock, reminder calendar, or pill box to help the client or caregiver remember to take or administer prescribed medications as scheduled.

Certain drugs are **stock supplied** (dispensed and labeled in large quantities) and stored in the medication room or other area on the nursing unit. Stock supplies are kept together in a secured area.

Certain IV fluids and medications must be stored in the medication refrigerator to preserve the integrity of the drug. The Public Health Department and accrediting agencies mandate that only drugs can be stored in the medication refrigerator.

Narcotics and Controlled Substances

Health care agencies have forms to record the supply on hand and the administration of narcotics and controlled substances in accord with federal regulations. These forms usually require the recording of the following information for each drug administered:

- Name of the client receiving the drug
- Amount of the drug used
- Time the drug was administered
- Name of the prescribing practitioner
- Name of the nurse administering the drug

Nursing practice usually requires that nurses count the narcotics and controlled substances at specified intervals. For example, at the change of shifts, one nurse who is going off duty counts the drugs with a nurse coming on duty. Each drug used must be accounted for on the narcotic record. When the narcotic count does not check, the nurse must report the discrepancy immediately. Narcotics and controlled substances are kept in a double-locked drawer, box, room, or medication-dispensing cart. The law requires these safety precautions in the use of narcotics and controlled substances to aid in the control of drug misuse. If for any reason a narcotic has to be discarded, a second person should act as a witness and that person should also sign the narcotic sheet.

container for each client. The unit-dose system has made it easier for nurses to administer the correct dose, thereby reducing the number of medication errors.

The nurse, usually at the beginning of each shift, checks the medications in each client's drawer. Some medication carts are locked, and the nurse keeps the key. Medication drawers should be removed only one at a time from the cart when the nurse is preparing the medication for administration. The client's drawer should never be left unattended on top of the cart. Drugs should not be removed from one client's supply for administration to another client.

DRUG ABUSE

Federal, state, and local rules regulate the appropriate use of drugs. Despite these rules, some people use drugs for purposes other than their proper use, seriously jeopardizing their health. Misuse of drugs also creates problems for family members and the community as a whole. "The American Medical Association and the World Health Organization have both recognized addiction as an illness, not a lack of willpower" (Dossey & Keegan, 2008, p. 514). **Addiction** is defined as a physiological or psychological dependence on a substance, such as alcohol or morphine, or a behavior such as eating, gambling, working, or engaging in sexual intercourse. The rest of this discussion focuses only on substance abuse.

Nursing practice requires the nurse to be knowledgeable about the addictive process in order to assess and care for clients with drug toxicity or overdose and withdrawal. Continual or periodic use of drugs may lead to **dependence** (reliance on or need to take a drug). The term *chemical dependence* is often used as a more inclusive term than *drug dependence* because it includes problems with *all mind-altering substances that have the potential of creating dependence* (Crosby & Bissell, 1989).

Addiction implies more than a physical dependence alone, and it does not refer exclusively to illicit drugs. Illicit drugs are substances sold illegally, such as cocaine, PCP (angel dust), hallucinogenic agents (LSD and peyote), and cannabinoids (marijuana and hashish). There are two types of drug dependence that can occur separately or together:

- Physiological dependence: the biochemical changes in body tissues that occur when the tissue depends on a substance for normal functioning; cessation of the substance causes physical withdrawal symptoms.
- Psychological dependence: the emotional reliance on a substance to maintain a sense of well-being; the degree of psychological dependence can vary from a mild desire to an intense craving or compulsion for the substance.

Although there are many types of addictions to various substances, alcohol addiction is the most prevalent one in the United States, afflicting at least 11 million people (Dossey & Keegan, 2008). The nurse should be able to identify the characteristics of substance abuse (see the accompanying display on the characteristics of alcoholism) and work together with other health care team members in planning the care for clients experiencing the disorder.

Nurses and other health care providers (prescribing practitioners, dentists, and pharmacists) are at risk for substance abuse because of their access to drugs such as benzodiazepines (Valium, Librium), sedative hypnotics (Nembutal, Placidyl), amphetamines (Dexedrine, Benzedrine), and narcotics (meperidine, morphine). The actual incidence of chemical dependence among nurses and other health care professionals is difficult to document; however, it is estimated that 6% to 16% of registered nurses in the United States are chemically dependent (Crosby & Bissell, 1989). The difficulty of obtaining factual data for the number of chemically addicted nurses is often related to the reluctance of professionals to report one another.

COMMON CHARACTERISTICS OF ALCOHOLISM

- Denial that there is a drinking problem
- Rationalization
- Restlessness, impulsiveness, anxiety
- Selfishness, self-centeredness, lack of consideration
- Irritability, anger, rage
- Physical cruelty; child, spouse, or older adult abuse
- Depression, isolation, self-destruction
- Low self-esteem, shame, guilt, remorse, loneliness
- Susceptibility to disease

From Dossey, B. M., & Keegan, L. (2008). *Holistic nursing: A handbook for practice* (5th ed.). Sudbury, MA: Jones & Bartlett.

Although it may be uncomfortable to report an addicted colleague, nurses have a moral responsibility to report the situation to the appropriate authority. Nurses who are addicted may display suspicious behaviors such as insisting on carrying the narcotic keys and volunteering to administer all of the narcotics during the shift. See the accompanying display for other behavioral characteristics of drug-addicted nurses on page 768.

In 1983, Florida was the first state to enact a "diversion" law as an alternative to disciplinary proceedings against substance abusers. Florida's diversion program is called the Intervention Project for Nurses and has served as a model for other states to create similar programs such as impaired nurse programs. "A structured recovery program which identifies the problem, helps restore the individual to a state of biological, psychological, social and spiritual well-being, and provides monitoring during recovery can contribute to the return to safe practice" (Tallant, 2008, p. 6). These programs provide support, confidentiality, and stringent on-the-job monitoring and allow the nurse to maintain licensure as long as the nurse complies with the program. An impaired nurse program is a welcomed alternative for nurses with addictive behaviors and has increased the reporting of nurses with addiction problems. (Contact the state board of nursing office to inquire about alternative programs to disciplinary measures.)

More recently, some hospitals have taken a proactive role in combating the problem of drug abuse among nurses with the use of a computer-controlled dispensing system (see Figure 30-6 on page 768). With this system, the likelihood of the nurse's abusing narcotics is markedly decreased. The nurse enters a private security code. The system will provide the nurse with a printout of the medications given to the client and will charge the client. This dispensing system eliminates stock supplies of narcotics and controlled drugs, decreasing the nurse's access to these drugs.

CHARACTERISTICS OF DRUG-ADDICTED NURSES IN THE WORKPLACE

- Exhibit extreme and rapid mood swings
- Always wear long sleeves
- Sign out more controlled drugs than anyone else
- Report frequent spills and breakage of controlled drugs
- Commit multiple medication errors
- Practice illogical or sloppy charting
- Are frequently absent from work
- Come to work early and stay late
- Frequently use sick leave

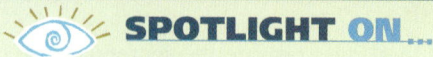

SPOTLIGHT ON...

Legal and Ethical

Chemical Dependence

If you were practicing in a state where the only action from the state board of nursing in the situation of an addicted nurse was license suspension or revocation, would you report a fellow nurse? If you did not, what could happen to the clients under the nurse's care, and what would be the legal implications for you? Likewise, if you were addicted, what would be the implications for your continued nursing practice?

MEDICATION COMPLIANCE

Medication compliance can be associated with the client's understanding of why a medication was ordered and how a medication can decrease the likelihood of getting a disease or how it can lessen the effects of an existing disease. When clients do not consistently take their prescribed medications, or when they adjust the scheduling or dose of the medication, they are *noncompliant.*

There are several reasons why clients choose not to take ordered medications. If a hypertensive client is asymptomatic (without distress), it may be difficult for the client to understand the need to take prescribed medications. If medications are taken, the dose may be altered at the discretion of the client. Medications are costly, and the client may be on a fixed income or unemployed. If the medication does not provide prompt relief, the client may consider the medication useless and discontinue it. The medication may be discontinued if the client experiences undesirable side effects, such as dizziness, impotence, or weight gain.

Compliance can be enhanced if the client is given information on the medication to take home when discharged from the hospital. Large-type print or illustrations should be used with older clients. Caregivers should be included when educating the client. Scheduling the medications around certain activities of daily living may serve as a reminder to the client that the medication must be taken. Providing the client with a telephone number and the name of a nurse to call if questions arise can ensure compliance.

The nurse in the community has an opportunity to see how medications are arranged in the client's home. Outdated medications must be discarded. After consulting with the client and caregiver, the nurse can make suggestions that may improve compliance.

Nurses have to remember that many older clients take a multitude of drugs. Some drugs actually cancel each other out when taken together, thus eliminating the therapeutic response. A client taking BuSpar and digoxin may experience digoxin toxicity. BuSpar may displace the serum binding of digoxin and increase the toxic levels of that drug. Nurses must sort through the medications with the client and report back to the prescribing practitioner the drugs taken in addition to those ordered by that practitioner.

LEGAL ASPECTS OF ADMINISTERING MEDICATIONS

Clients are awarded settlements in malpractice suits when nurses are negligent in their practice. Negligence exists any time the nurse fails to do something that a reasonable nurse would do under similar circumstances or does something that a reasonable nurse would not do. Malpractice is any professional misconduct or unreasonable lack of skill in professional duties. See Chapter 12 for related information on legal issues.

MEDICATION ERRORS

Nurses have learned the five rights as a guideline to safe administration of medications. If the nurse gives the wrong medicine to the wrong person, an error has been made. If the

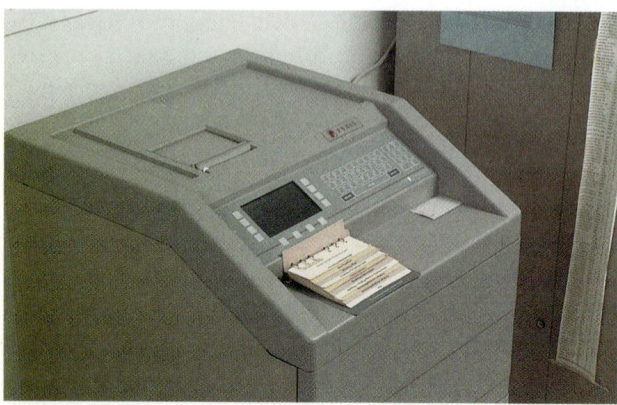

FIGURE 30-6 Computer-Controlled Dispensing System DELMAR/
CENGAGE LEARNING

nurse has the right medicine but wrong dose or wrong route, a medication error has been made. If the nurse gives the medication at the wrong time, an error has been made. Nurses must inform the prescribing practitioner of the error made. If an antidote must be given, the prescribing practitioner needs accurate information to make appropriate care decisions.

Medication errors must be reported in a timely manner. Knowing the actions and the side effects of drugs will help the nurse assess the client's response and health status. Event reports are required in some institutions to document medication errors. A report of a medication error must include the name of the medication, the dose given, the route, the time the medication was administered, the specific error that occurred, the time the prescribing practitioner was contacted about the error, and what countermeasures were taken. Sometimes nurses discover errors made by other nurses. These must also be documented and reported. Brooke (2008) recommends documentation of all nursing care associated with the error, including interventions and any follow-up care, in the client's medical record, stating only the facts without blaming anyone or expressing one's opinion. The event report should not be mentioned in the medical record, or it may become admissible in court if a lawsuit develops.

Questioning the Medication Order

The nurse is responsible and held accountable for questioning any medication order if, in the nurse's judgment, the order is unclear or in error. The nature of the error may be in any part of the drug order, and the nurse should seek clarification from the prescribing practitioner. A drug error has serious legal implications if the nurse involved could have been expected, on the basis of knowledge and experience, to have noted the error.

If the prescribing practitioner disregards the nurse's query, another line of authority must be pursued by the nurse to prevent a drug error. The medication in question should not be administered until the order has been clarified. The nurse should withhold any drug when the client's health may be jeopardized. Notify the prescribing practitioner of the need to withhold the medication and the reason withholding it is necessary. Document the reason for withholding the drug (e.g., withholding a dose of an antihypertensive medication due for a client who is currently experiencing hypotension) on the MAR and the nurse's notes.

When the nurse is not able to read or understand the order, the prescriber should be contacted for clarification. The nurse should not *guess* what the prescriber who wrote the order is trying to communicate; the only safe nursing action is to validate the order with the prescribing practitioner.

Preventing Medication Errors

In the United States, medication errors are responsible for one death every day and injure an estimated 1.3 million people annually. The number of serious drug errors continues to increase. According to the FDA:

- Errors doubled between 1998 (34,966) and 2005 (89,842).

- The number of fatal adverse drug events increased 2.7-fold during the same period.
- The medications most frequently implicated in deaths included oxycodone, fentanyl, clozapine, morphine, acetaminophen, infliximab, interferon beta, and etanercept (Moore, 2007).

The public's awareness of medication errors in health care has been heightened by media coverage in recent reports; the public's response has been a demand for a safe health care system. The NCC MERP defines *medication error* as follows:

> A medication error is any preventable event that may cause or lead to inappropriate medication use or patient harm while the medication is in the control of the health care professional, patient, or consumer. Such events may be related to professional practice, health care products, procedures, and systems, including prescribing; order communication; product labeling, packaging, and nomenclature; compounding; dispensing; distribution; administration; education; monitoring; and use. (2008, p. 1)

The NCC encourages the use of their medication error definition by researchers, software developers, and institutions to ensure a common taxonomy.

In 1999 the Institute of Medicine (IOM) released its report *To Err Is Human: Building a Safer Health System.* Two consecutive IOM reports, *Crossing the Quality Chasm* and *Priority Areas for National Action: Transforming Health Care,* positioned medication errors as a priority and recommended that immediate action be taken to improve this aspect of health care. The IOM reports recommended the creation of a center for client safety within the Agency for Healthcare Research and Quality (AHRQ). In 2001 Congress established a new Center for Quality Improvement and Patient Safety in the AHRQ. This center is responsible for monitoring medication errors.

Since the publication of the IOM reports, health care providers, policy makers, and accreditation and professional organizations (e.g., the Joint Commission and the American Nurses Association [ANA]) have reviewed the process of medication administration to identify the true incidence of errors and to assist with the development of national standards to promote safe medication practices. Although many of the studies regarding medication errors recognize that the systems in place or the lack of these systems, and not the prescribing practitioners, account for many of the errors, the nurse has an obligation to provide safe client care in accordance with standards of practice.

Besides the dangers inherent in certain abbreviations or dose designations for medications, discussed previously, errors may also occur as a result of misreading drugs, drug abbreviations, and decimals. These errors are a result of similar brand and generic names, compounded by illegible handwriting, new drugs, and similar packing or labeling of drugs. The abbreviation for magnesium sulfate is $MgSO_4$; however, it may be misinterpreted for morphine sulfate (MSO_4). The use of decimals and zeros is another cause of errors. For example, a zero used after the decimal in 1.0 mg may cause the dose to be misread as 10 mg if the decimal point is not seen; likewise, when a zero is not used before the decimal in a dose of .5 mg, the dose may be misread as 5 mg. Zeros should always be used before a decimal when the dose is less than a whole unit, and terminal zeros should not be used for doses expressing whole numbers.

Many of the solutions under study to create a safer health care system for medication administration rely on computer programs. In 2003, the FDA proposed regulation requiring drug manufacturers to place bar codes on the labels of all prescription and over-the-counter drugs that are frequently used in hospitals; pharmaceutical manufacturers, drug repackagers, and distributors would have 3 years to comply. According to the FDA, the bar code would have the drug's national drug code (NDC) that uniquely identifies the drug, its strength, and its dosage form. The FDA indicated that a bar-coding system coupled with a computerized order entry system would promote compliance of the five rights of medication administration for all health care workers. A client's medical regimen and MAR would be entered into the hospital's database and encoded in the client's identification armband and would be accessible to a nurse through a handheld device. When the armband was scanned by the device, the client's MAR would be displayed from the hospital's database. The nurse would scan the bar code, the client's identification armband, and the code on his or her identification badge; the mainframe computer would process the scanned information, updating the MAR and regimen appropriately.

The Veterans Health Administration (VHA) pioneered a computer-based bar-coding system, Bar Coding in Medication Administration (BCMA), in one of its facilities in 1995. Although only 2% of U.S. hospitals use bar codes, in 2000 all 173 VHA facilities nationwide were directed to have bar codes on all medications that could be scanned by a nurse using a handheld device. Although the VHA nurses documented this new system for medication administration as being safer, it is more time consuming. Reports generated by the bar-coding system identify all "late" entries as an error; errors are tracked by the system. Therefore, the VHA adjusted the "right time" to provide medication from the standard 30 minutes to an hour before or after the prescribed time. The warning for avoiding errors caused by the use of terminal zeros with doses expressed in whole numbers is applicable with computer prescribing as well as handwritten entries.

ASSESSMENT

Drug administration is based on assessment data obtained by reviewing the client's medical history, eliciting a drug history, performing a physical examination, and obtaining and interpreting relevant laboratory results. Assessment is an ongoing process and requires the knowledge, skills, and abilities of a licensed professional.

MEDICAL HISTORY

The client's medical history is obtained by the nurse when conducting the interview assessment and by reviewing the client's medical record. The nurse should identify all chronic diseases and disorders and correlate these data with the drugs prescribed by the prescribing practitioner. Because the client may have more than one prescribing practitioner, the admitting prescribing practitioner might not be aware of all the drugs the client is taking, including over-the-counter medications. It is the nurse's responsibility to gather this information and document it on the client's chart.

Preexisting conditions such as liver and kidney dysfunction may require drug alteration because they prolong drug action, thereby increasing the potential for toxicity. The nurse needs to elicit this type of information during the medical history so that these clients can be closely monitored for signs of adverse reactions to drugs.

DRUG HISTORY

A drug history is obtained on admission to a health care facility. The drug history should contain specific questions about the client's background: allergies, prescription and over-the-counter drugs, herbal supplements, medical history, biographical data, lifestyle and beliefs, and sensory and cognitive status. See Chapter 6 for a complete discussion of taking a health history. If the client is unable to answer the questions, the nurse should contact a family member to obtain the data. Drug history data are used by nurses in determining the client's plan of care and learning needs.

Allergies

The nurse should inquire about all food and drug allergies. If the client has had an allergic reaction to a drug, the nurse should have the client describe the details of the reaction: name of the drug; dosage, route, and number of times the drug was taken before the reaction; onset of the reaction; and manifestations of the reaction. The nurse should question the client about possible contributing factors to the allergic reaction, such as concurrent use of stimulants (tobacco, alcohol, or illegal drugs) or significant changes in nutritional status.

👁 SPOTLIGHT ON...

Legal & Ethical

Medication Error

While monitoring a client who has an order for Solu-Cortef (an anti-inflammatory drug) intravenously, you notice that Solu-Medrol (an anti-inflammatory drug) is in the client's room. You recheck the order to make sure that the original order was for Solu-Cortef and that the order was not changed. What should your next action be? How do you feel about the nurse who made the medication error but did not recognize it?

The nurse should also ask about allergies to foods because drugs may contain the same elements or nutrients that cause allergic reactions to some foods. For example, clients who are allergic to shellfish may also experience a reaction to drugs containing iodine. Vaccines are commonly derived from chick embryos and would be contraindicated in clients with allergies to eggs.

Allergies to food and drugs, including over-the-counter drugs and herbal supplements, should be noted in the client's record, in the admission note, on the MAR, and on the history and physical examination forms. The pharmacy should be notified of any drug or food allergies. In hospitals, clients wear allergy alert bands that list all medications to which the person is allergic. Nurses in all settings should discuss the use of medical alert bracelets by clients with allergies. These bracelets inform prescribing providers of allergies should the person not be able to speak.

Prescription Drugs

The nurse should have the client identify all current prescription drugs and describe:

- Why the drug was prescribed and by whom
- The drug's dosage, route, and frequency
- The client's knowledge of the drug's action: side and adverse effects, when to notify the prescribing practitioner, and special administration considerations such as with or without foods

If the client is receiving any drug that requires monitoring before administration such as insulin (antidiabetic hormone), the nurse needs to make sure the client is checking blood sugar and that the results are within normal limits.

Over-the-Counter Drugs

Clients usually have to be questioned separately about nonprescription drugs because they often fail to identify these drugs when asked to list all the medications they take routinely. For example, the nurse must determine if the client takes aspirin, antacids, or laxatives routinely. The client should describe the dosage, route, and frequency of these drugs. Because many drugs are available in topical form, the nurse should also inquire about the use of creams, ointments, patches, or sprays. Clients admitted to inpatient facilities should be asked if they have any over-the-counter drugs with them.

The nurse should explain to the client in a sensitive manner why these questions are necessary in order to allay any anxieties that might arise from this nature of questioning. Depending on the dosage and frequency, nonprescription drugs may have a profound effect on the client's treatment.

Complementary Therapy

The practice of healing has always incorporated the use of herbs as medicines. The World Health Organization recognizes that of 119 plant-derived pharmaceutical medicines, about 74% are used in modern medicine in ways that are correlated directly with their traditional uses as plant medicines by native cultures. An estimated 25% of all pharmaceuticals are derived directly from plants (White & Foster, 2007): For example, quinine (an extract from the South American *cinchona*) is used to treat malaria; digitalis, which comes from foxglove, is an inotropic drug used to treat congestive heart failure; and the active components of periwinkle, vinblastine, and vincristine are used in the treatment of certain cancers.

Herbal medicine, also known as botanical medicine (and in Europe, as phytotherapy or phytomedicine), refers to the use of a plant or plant part to make medicine, food flavors, or aromatic oils for soaps and fragrances. An herbal medicine can come from a leaf, flower, stem, seed, root, fruit, bark, or any other plant part. Herbs are often used to season foods (culinary herbs) or to maintain or restore health (medicinal herbs).

The traditional use of herbs was based on trial and error. The process of discovery produced both positive and negative results, since many herbs contain poisonous substances that counteract the main ingredients for which they might be taken. **Pharmacognosy**, the study of the biochemical aspects of natural products, seeks to standardize herbal products so that they consistently include the same amount of active ingredients and are free of any harmful components that the plant may contain.

Herbs are classified by the U.S. government as dietary supplements (vitamins, minerals, enzymes, hormones, amino acids, and other nutritional products). Congress passed the Dietary Supplement Health and Educational Act of 1994 and "grandfathered" most botanical products as a new class of products known as dietary supplements. Although dietary supplements are not regulated by the FDA, product labeling of herbal medicines is restricted to structure and function claims. Manufacturers can indicate on a product label how the herb can affect a normal body structure or function, but promotional material and packaging cannot claim to treat or prevent a disease. For example, a product label for ginkgo can say "increases microcirculation in the brain," but it cannot say "cures early-stage Alzheimer's" or "alleviates tinnitus" even though there is research to support the effectiveness of standardized ginkgo extracts in the treatment of these diseases.

Herbs and supplements are regulated by other organizations such as the American Botanical Council (ABC), the American Herbal Products Association (AHPA), and the Natural Nutritional Foods Association (NNFA). The ABC promotes the safe and effective use of medicinal plants by educating the public, government agencies, research institutions, industry, and the media on the scientific research that can guide decisions about producing and consuming herb-based products that benefit health and well-being. The AHPA is a group of herbalists, researchers, and manufacturers that created a code of ethics that members adhere to and releases product safety alerts regarding adulteration—that is, contamination with an unlabeled substance—of herbal products. The AHPA publishes the *Botanical Safety Handbook,* a reference on the safe and effective use of herbs. The NNFA is a group of manufacturers and retailers concerned with product quality and truth in packaging and advertising. The NNFA supports a True Label Program to ensure that products produced by its members actually contain what their labels claim.

It is estimated that 1 out of every 3 Americans uses one or more herbal products (White & Foster, 2007). Although herbal medicines generally have fewer and far milder side effects than drugs, problems can arise if they are used improperly or in combination with drugs. Nurses need to know which herbs can alter the activity of certain drugs. For example, garlic and ginkgo may increase the effects of blood thinners, whereas goldenseal, Oregon graperoot, and barberry may counteract short-acting blood thinners. Refer to Chapter 31 for additional information on the safe, effective use of herbal medicines.

HERBAL SUPPLEMENTS As the use of herbal products increases in the United States, nurses must have their clients identify these products and indicate their usage when performing certain laboratory tests (e.g., therapeutic drug monitoring, trough and peak plasma levels). Certain herbal supplements may interfere with the desired effects of drugs; for example, St. John's wort may cause a decrease of trough serum digoxin concentration by 33% and peak concentration by 26% (Dasgupta, 2003). Other herbs (e.g., Chan Su, Dan Shen, Uzara root, Siberian and Asian ginseng) may also interfere in the therapeutic drug monitoring of digoxin.

BIOGRAPHICAL DATA

The client's biographical data, including age, education, occupation, and insurance coverage, may influence the nursing care plan and teaching plan. These data are also used by the nurse when helping a client develop a drug regimen that complements the client's daily routine.

CULTURAL DIVERSITY

The large number of ethnic cultures in the United States challenges professional nurses to be culturally competent. One in 4 Americans are of a race other than white (e.g., African American, Hispanic, Asian). In order for nurses to properly assess and teach clients regarding their medications, they need an understanding of cultural differences, as they may enhance compliance and minimize adverse events.

Ethnic culture affects one's beliefs about health, illness, and medications; how one interacts with health care providers; compliance with treatment regimens; and how one responds physiologically to medications. Studies have shown that a person's race or ethnic background affects the metabolism of drugs; common genetic polymorphisms, enzymes used for drug metabolism, influence the metabolism of many medications. For example, Asians and Eskimos require lower doses of anxiolytics than whites, while African Americans respond faster to neuroleptics and anxiolytics; and Asians, Indians, and Pakistanis need lower doses of lithium and antipsychotic drugs, while Hispanics usually require lower doses of antidepressants than whites. Since certain drugs within the same class are often cleared by different metabolic pathways, ethnic differences may impair metabolism, increasing or decreasing the expected drug effect.

Ethnic beliefs also play a role in the early discontinuation of prescribed drugs. When symptoms abate, African and Native Americans and Hispanics question the continued need for the drug, often discontinuing use of drugs such as antibiotics and antidepressants before the disease is cured. Diabetes is rare among Asians, so it is difficult for Asian Americans to grasp the relationship between blood sugar and diet. See Chapter 20 for additional information regarding cultural variances of drugs.

LIFESTYLE AND BELIEFS

The client's lifestyle and beliefs affect attitudes toward health, use of the health care system, and daily activity patterns. These factors often determine the client's dietary habits and nontherapeutic use of drugs such as tobacco, alcohol, and illegal drugs.

SENSORY AND COGNITIVE STATUS

The nurse should assess for and inquire about sensory deficits such as vision or hearing impairments, weakness or paralysis, or loss of sensation in one or more extremities. These deficits may impair a client's ability to comply with a prescribed drug plan, administer a subcutaneous injection, break a scored tablet, or open a medication container.

The nurse should assess the client's cognitive abilities throughout the drug history interview by noting whether the client is alert and oriented and interacts appropriately. Clients who are not able to express their thoughts coherently or who exhibit impaired memory function will require special consideration by the nurse when planning the client's care and teaching plan. See Chapter 38 for a complete discussion of sensory and cognitive impairments.

PHYSICAL EXAMINATION

The nurse conducts a physical assessment to identify those body systems that may be affected by a particular drug the client is currently taking or will be taking. The nurse assesses the client's condition before administering any drug to establish the client's baseline, or normal, health status. For example, the nurse assesses the client's apical pulse before administering Lanoxin (an inotropic) so that the heart rate after receiving the drug can be compared with the baseline measurement. During the physical examination, the nurse should carefully inspect the skin of those clients who self-administer medications such as insulin and heparin to ensure they are using proper technique.

DIAGNOSTIC AND LABORATORY DATA

Common laboratory values, such as electrolytes, blood urea nitrogen, creatinine, glucose, complete blood count, and a white blood cell count, are usually monitored over a period of time to identify trends and to measure the body's response to medications. Laboratory results are evaluated on the basis of the client's clinical condition, physical assessment, and drug therapies. See Chapter 28 for a complete discussion of laboratory testing.

NURSING DIAGNOSIS

The nurse analyzes the assessment data to determine the client's ability to self-administer medications and to identify any potential or actual drug-related problems. Once the nurse identifies the actual or potential problems, relevant nursing diagnoses can be formulated. The common nursing diagnoses specifically related to medication administration are (North American Nursing Diagnosis Association, 2009):

- *Deficient knowledge*
- *Ineffective health maintenance*
- *Impaired physical mobility*
- *Disturbed sensory perception*
- *Readiness for enhanced knowledge*

The addictive client may have a different set of nursing diagnoses, such as:

- *Imbalanced nutrition*
- *Impaired verbal communication*
- *Disabled family coping*
- *Impaired social interaction*
- *Social isolation*
- *Spiritual distress*
- *Readiness for enhanced spiritual well-being*

Selecting the most appropriate nursing diagnosis will identify the client's teaching needs. For example, the nursing diagnosis for clients who inquire about the side effects of their medications would be *Readiness for enhanced knowledge: Expresses an interest in learning*.

PLANNING AND OUTCOME IDENTIFICATION

Nurses need to carefully plan nursing care activities to ensure safe administration of medications. Reviewing scheduled diagnostic tests, laboratory results, and the overall plan of care helps to ensure that clients receive medications at the appropriate time and that medications that should not be given are withheld until their administration can be clarified with the prescribing practitioner. For example, digoxin might be withheld if the lab test indicates an above-normal level.

Medication administration is a good time for nurses to incorporate client teaching. Adequate planning provides for questions and discussion by the client and demonstration of skills learned (as in self-administration of insulin injections).

The nurse develops goals and plans the care on the basis of the nursing diagnosis. Nursing interventions are identified and incorporated into the plan of care to promote the attainment of goals and to assist the client in achieving outcomes. See the accompanying display for the nursing outcomes classification (NOC) defined for medication administration. The NOC outcome Self-Care: Parenteral Medication is discussed in Chapter 33.

Most clients admitted to a hospital or a long-term care facility have one or more nursing diagnoses related to alterations that precipitated the admission. Inherent in their nursing care plans are outcomes related to medication administration. For example, the nursing diagnosis *Ineffective breathing pattern* related to decreased energy may have as a client outcome "demonstrates correct use of a metered-dose inhaler."

IMPLEMENTATION

The primary nursing interventions related to medication management are assessment, administration, and teaching. *Medication administration* is defined as "preparing, giving, and evaluating the effectiveness of prescription and nonprescription drugs" (Bulechek, Butcher, McCloskey, & Dochterman, 2008, p. 477). The nurse should use the time spent with the client during medication administration to assess the client's knowledge and response to the drug's action and adverse reactions.

The administration of medication requires the implementation of safety guidelines, following the five rights. Medications are administered in accordance with set procedures based on the prescribed route. This section presents procedures and guidelines for medication administration by the following routes: oral, including sublingual, buccal, and enteral; parenteral; site-specific topical applications; and inhalation.

Once the teaching plan has been developed, the nurse should initiate discharge teaching of drug therapy. Assessment data, especially the client's history, help the nurse in determining who should be included in the teaching session. For example, an older client living alone is physically capable

---

NOC—MEDICATION ADMINISTRATION

1. *Knowledge: Medication.* Definition: Extent of understanding conveyed about the safe use of medication; Sampling of indicators: Description of actions of medication(s); Descriptions of precautions for medication(s); Description of self-monitoring technique; Description of proper use of alert identification.
2. *Medication response.* Definition: Therapeutic and adverse effects of prescribed medication; Therapeutic indicators: Expected therapeutic effects; Expected change in blood chemistries; Expected change in symptoms; Maintenance of therapeutic blood levels of medication; Adverse indications: Allergic reaction; Adverse effects; Drug interaction; Drug intolerance.
3. *Self-care: Nonparenteral Medication.* Definition: Ability to administer oral and topical medications to meet therapeutic goals independently with or without assistance; Sampling of indicators: Identifies medication; Monitors therapeutic response; Uses monitoring equipment accurately; Stores medications properly; Obtains needed laboratory tests.

Moorhead, S., Johnson, M., Maas, M., & Swanson, E. (2008). *Nursing outcomes classification (NOC)* (4th ed.). St. Louis, MO: Elsevier Health Sciences.

of self-administering but may have short-term memory loss. In this situation the nurse should obtain the client's permission to include a family member, neighbor, or friend in the teaching session.

Drug teaching usually occurs in two phases. The first phase involves a formal teaching session. The nurse explains the drug's action, route, side and adverse effects, and the specific signs of a drug reaction that require prescribing practitioner notification. Clients often need assistance in developing a drug schedule that promotes compliance and complements their lifestyle. Self-administration may require the nurse to teach the client specific procedural techniques, such as subcutaneous injection.

The second phase of client teaching is ongoing, occurring whenever the nurse administers a drug. The nurse should assess and reinforce the client's knowledge of drugs at each interaction. If the client is being taught self-administration, the drug teaching plan should identify the dates for teaching, and expected outcomes should identify a date for client achievement of targeted goals.

MEDICATION ADMINISTRATION: ORAL

Oral administration of drugs is the most common route; however, there are potential risk factors that the nurse must consider. Before administering oral drugs, the nurse should assess the client's ability to take the medication as prescribed. This assessment includes the client's gag reflex, state of consciousness, and presence of nausea and vomiting.

The nurse should protect the client against aspiration when administering any form of oral drug. **Aspiration** refers to the inhalation of regurgitated gastric contents into the pulmonary system. If a client has a weak gag reflex or difficulty swallowing water, medication can be inhaled during medication administration. To prevent aspiration, the nurse confirms the client's gag reflex and ability to swallow. When administering an oral drug, the nurse prepares the medication, correctly identifies the client, and provides some form of liquid. See Procedure 30-1 for administering an oral medication. The nurse should remain with the client until *all* of the medications have been swallowed. If there is doubt that the client has swallowed the pill, the nurse should don a nonsterile glove and visually inspect the client's mouth with a tongue depressor (see Figure 30-7).

Medication Administration: Sublingual and Buccal

Sublingual and buccal drugs are types of oral medications. Certain drugs are given by these routes to prevent their destruction or transformation in the stomach or small intestines. The nurse should assess the integrity of the mucous membranes by inspecting underneath the client's tongue and in the buccal cavity. If the membranes are excoriated or painful, the nurse should withhold the medication and notify the prescribing practitioner. Some buccal drugs may irritate the mucosa, requiring the nurse to use alternate sides of the mouth to prevent irritation of the mucosa.

Sublingual and buccal administration of drugs (see Figure 30-8 on page 775) requires the nurse to use Standard Precautions because the nurse's hand may come into contact with oral secretions. Drugs given by these routes are quickly absorbed by the mucosa's thin epithelium and the abundant blood supply.

MEDICATION ADMINISTRATION: ENTERAL

Enteral instillation refers to the delivery of drugs through a gastrointestinal tube. Enteral tubes provide a means of direct instillation of medications into the gastrointestinal system of clients who cannot ingest them orally.

COMMUNITY CONSIDERATIONS

The American Nurses Association and various governing bodies support written medication information for clients that is "scientifically accurate, unbiased in content and tone, sufficiently specific and comprehensive, presented in an understandable and legible format, timely, up to date, and useful." Written medication information should:

- Be appropriate to client literacy levels
- Reflect print size appropriate to client's visual abilities
- Give straightforward instructions
- Include brand and trade names
- Prominently display drug warnings
- Outline indications for use, contraindications, and precautions
- List possible adverse reactions and risks, storage, and use

From American Nurses Association. (1997, March/April). *American Nurse, 29*(2), 11.

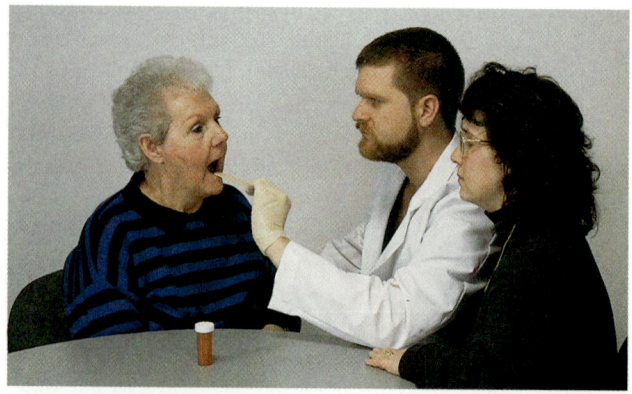

FIGURE 30-7 Check the client's mouth to ensure that medications have been swallowed. DELMAR/CENGAGE LEARNING

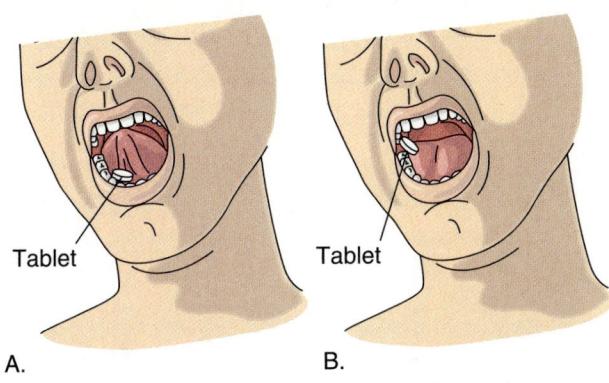

Tablet

Tablet

A.   B.

**FIGURE 30-8 A. Sublingual Administration of a Tablet;
B. Buccal Administration of a Tablet** DELMAR/CENGAGE LEARNING

There are several types of enteral tubes. A *nasogastric tube* (NG) is a soft rubber or plastic tube that is inserted through a nostril and into the stomach. The *gastrostomy tube* is surgically inserted into the stomach through the creation of an artificial fistula. The prescribing practitioner uses an endoscope to insert a *percutaneous endoscopic gastrostomy* (PEG) tube into the stomach.

The nurse should assess the client for the presence of bowel sounds and check the tube for **patency** (openness) and placement before administering a medication. The most reliable method for verification of placement of enteral tubes is x-ray examination. The measurement of pH secretions withdrawn from the feeding tube helps differentiate the location of the tube (see the Nursing Checklist on verifying placement of an enteral tube). The instillation of drugs is contraindicated when the tube is obstructed or improperly placed, when the client is vomiting, or if bowel sounds are absent. See Chapter 34 for a complete discussion of the purpose, insertion, and nursing care of clients with enteral tubes.

The nurse prepares the medication for instillation as prescribed by the prescribing practitioner once the patency and placement of the tube have been determined. It is preferable to instill liquid medications into tubes, especially PEG tubes that have a small lumen. Tablets can clog the tube unless they are finely crushed. When the prescribing practitioner orders a drug in the tablet or capsule form, the nurse should crush the tablet into minute particles and dissolve the crushed tablet in 15 to 30 mL of warm water before instillation. Some tablets cannot be crushed without altering their therapeutic effect. The nurse should check with the pharmacist if unsure. The instillation of cold solution may cause abdominal cramps. Capsules are prepared for administration by opening the capsule and emptying the contents into a liquid. When the drug is prepared, the nurse is ready to instill the medication (see the Nursing Checklist, on page 776, on instilling drugs into enteral tubes).

The nurse should question the prescribing practitioner if oily medications and enteric-coated or sustained-release tablets are ordered because these drug forms should not be given through a tube. Oily preparations may cling to the sides of the tube and resist mixing with the irrigating solution. Crushing

enteric-coated or sustained-release tablets destroys their intended effect. Do not crush buccal or sublingual tablets. Never attempt to give whole or undissolved medications through an enteral tube. See the accompanying display, on page 776, on special considerations for enteral tube management.

MEDICATION ADMINISTRATION: PARENTERAL

Parenteral medications are given through a route other than the alimentary canal; these routes are ID, subcutaneous, IM, or IV. The angle of injection and the depth of penetration will indicate the type of injection. Many clients have broadly classified the parenteral route into one category: "injections" or "shots." The nurse should provide the client with an explanation of the various routes used when administering parenteral drugs. To prepare and administer parenteral medications, the

✓ NURSINGCHECKLIST

Verifying Placement of an Enteral Tube
The nurse checks the patency and placement of a nasogastric tube before adding any water or medications by performing the following actions:

- Wash hands/hands hygiene, and don nonsterile gloves.
- Unclamp the tube.
- Draw 20 mL of air into syringe.
- Aspirate approximately 10 mL of gastric contents.
- Check the contents and obtain pH level: pH below 4 means tube is in stomach; pH range of 6 to 7 means tube is in intestines.
- Assess the color of aspirate.
- If unable to aspirate contents or unsure of pH results, call prescribing practitioner for order to obtain x-ray verification.
- Wash hands/hand hygiene.
- Document results.

Do not administer the medication until placement in the stomach is verified.

▼ SAFETY FIRST ▼

RISK FOR ASPIRATION
Clients, especially those with an NG tube, are at risk for aspiration from esophageal reflux. Position the client as directed in the Nursing Checklist on instilling drugs into enteral tubes to minimize the risk of esophageal reflux and aspiration.

nurse must have knowledge of the special equipment, use manual dexterity and sterile technique, and follow Standard Precautions. An injection is an invasive procedure because it breaks the skin barrier. As such, it must be performed using proper aseptic technique to prevent risk of infection.

✓ NURSING**CHECKLIST**

Instilling Drugs into Enteral Tubes

- Wash hands/hand hygiene, and don nonsterile gloves.
- Place the client in a high or semi-Fowler's position, as the client's condition allows; for an NG tube, unpin the tube from the client's gown to allow manipulation of the tube's free end. Place a linen saver over the bed linens to prevent soilage during administration of the medication.
- Dissolve crushed tablets, gelatin capsules, and powders in 15 to 30 mL of warm water. Dissolve each medication separately. Do not give whole or undissolved medications through the tube.
- Attach the syringe to the free end of the tube, pour the medication into the syringe barrel, and open the clamp; for NG tube instillation, hold the NG tube at the client's nose level.
- Hold the syringe barrel at a slight angle and allow the medication to flow at a steady, slow rate; add more medication before the syringe empties to prevent air from entering the stomach. If necessary, adjust the height of the NG tube to achieve a steady flow rate. Never push medications into the tube.
- Flush the tube with 15 to 30 mL of warm water, and add the next medication; repeat this process until all medications have been administered.
- As the syringe barrel begins to empty with the last of the medication, slowly add 30 to 60 mL of warm water into the syringe to clear the medication from the sides and distal end of the tube to prevent clogging.
- Before the syringe empties of water, clamp the tube, and detach and dispose of the syringe.
- Position the client as appropriate; clients with an NG tube should be placed on the right side with the head of the bed slightly elevated for at least 30 minutes after the instillation.
- Clean area, remove and dispose of gloves in the proper receptacle, and wash hands/hand hygiene.
- Document the instillation of the medication on the MAR, and record on the intake and output sheet the total amount of fluid instilled.

SPECIAL CONSIDERATIONS FOR ENTERAL TUBE MANAGEMENT

- When a client is receiving intermittent tube feedings, schedule the medications to prevent the two solutions from being given together.
- An adult client should not receive more than 400 mL of liquid at one time. If the administration of feedings and medication coincide, give the medication first to ensure that the client receives the prescribed dosage on time; the feeding may not be given in its entirety.
- When the client is receiving a continuous feeding, stop the feeding and aspirate the gastric contents. If the gastric contents are greater than 150 mL, withhold the medication and notify the prescribing practitioner.
- Never put tablets into tube feeding bags.
- For clients who have an NG tube for decompression (removal) of gastric contents, turn off the suction for 20 to 30 minutes after the instillation of the medication to allow time for the gastric contents to be emptied into the intestines, where most drugs are absorbed.
- For clients who have a nasogastric tube, never use the pigtail air vent for irrigation or administration of fluids.

The Centers for Disease Control and Prevention (CDC) issued revised Standard Precautions in 2007 that include new guidelines for safe injection practices. These guidelines address sterile technique and the need to use safe practice when preparing and administering medications, such as the following: Use each piece of sterile equipment once and discard, use single-dose vials for parenteral medications whenever possible, and do not use bags or bottles of IV solution as a common source of supply for multiple clients (CDC, 2007).

Equipment

Nurses use special equipment such as syringes, needles, ampules, and vials when administering parenteral medications.

SYRINGES   A syringe has three basic parts: the hub, which connects with the needle; the barrel, or outside part, which contains measurement calibrations; and the plunger, which fits inside the barrel and has a rubber tip (see Figure 30-9 on page 777). The nurse must ensure that the hub, inside of the barrel, and shaft and rubber plunger tip are kept sterile. When handling the syringe, the nurse should touch only the outside of the barrel and the plunger's handle.

Most syringes are disposable, made of plastic, and individually packaged for sterility. There are several types of syringes, such as the hypodermic, insulin, and tuberculin syringes (see Figure 30-10 on page 777). When a medication

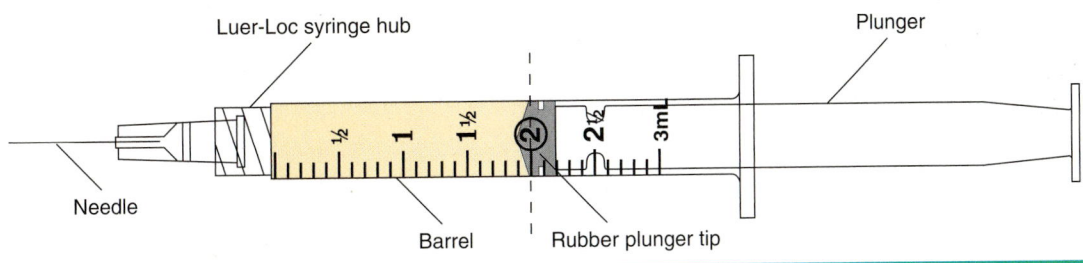

Luer-Loc syringe hub   Plunger

Needle   Barrel   Rubber plunger tip

FIGURE 30-9 Parts of Syringe DELMAR/CENGAGE LEARNING

is incompatible with plastic, it is usually prefilled in a single-dose glass syringe. Syringes are often prepackaged with the commonly used needle size and gauge and are referred to as *disposable plastic syringes.*

The *hypodermic syringe* comes in 2-, 2.5-, 3-, 5-, 10-, and 12-mL sizes. The measurement calibrations (scales) are usually printed in milliliters and minims. Most syringes are marked in cubic centimeters (cc), and most drugs are ordered in milliliters; these are equivalent measurements (1 cc = 1 mL). The hypodermic syringe is used most often when a medication is ordered in milliliters. When the order is written in minims, it is safer to prepare the drug in a tuberculin syringe.

The *insulin syringe* is designed specially for use with the ordered dose of insulin. For example, if the prescribing practitioner writes the order for 30 units of U-100 insulin, the nurse will use an insulin syringe that is calibrated on the 100-unit scale. Insulin syringes are calibrated on the U-100 (100-unit) scale, which is based on 100 units of insulin contained in 1 mL of solution. Insulin syringes come in sizes that hold 0.5 mL (50 units) to 1.0 mL (100 units). Insulin syringes that hold 0.5 mL are the easiest to read and are therefore used for low dosages. There are other sizes of insulin syringes that complement the ordered dose, such as U-30 and U-50, although these dosages are seldom prescribed. The nurse should always compare the size of insulin syringe and the dose indicated on the insulin bottle with the prescribing practitioner's order; all three unit doses must be the same.

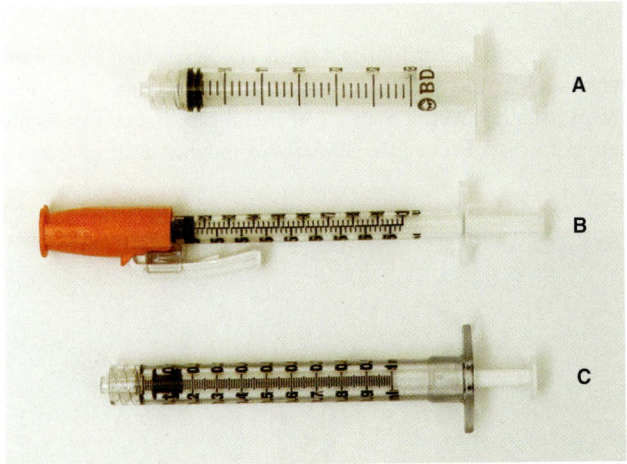

The *tuberculin syringe* is a narrow syringe, calibrated in tenths and hundredths of a milliliter (up to 1 mL) on one scale and in sixteenths of a minim (up to 1 minim) on the other scale. Originally this syringe was designed to administer the tuberculin drug, but it is commonly used today to administer small or precise doses, such as pediatric dosages. The tuberculin syringe should be used for doses 0.5 mL or less.

Prefilled single-dose syringes should not be confused with a unit dose. The nurse must be careful to check the prescribed dose against that in the prefilled syringe and discard excess medication. For example, if the prescribing practitioner orders diazepam (Valium) 5 mg IM as a preoperative sedative and the prefilled single-dose contains 10 mg/2 mL, the nurse must calculate dosage (5 mg/1 mL) and destroy 1 mL from the syringe before administration.

The Joint Commission requires labeling of all syringes. Not all medications are dispensed by the pharmacy in ready-to-administer injectable products in labeled syringes as prescribed for each client. Unlabeled syringes increase the risk for medication errors; see the accompanying Uncovering the Evidence display on page 778. Historically, nurses have used tape for labeling syringes, but this is not considered safe practice since the tape may obscure the contents and the graduations on the syringe barrel. Cohen (2008) suggests that providing commercially available syringe labels in all drug preparation areas and letting nurses choose a standard format can help reduce risks associated with unlabeled syringes.

NEEDLES Most needles are disposable, made of stainless steel, and individually packaged for sterility. Reusable needles are seldom used, except in certain areas such as surgery and special procedure rooms; reusable needles require frequent inspection to ensure that the needle is sharp, and resterilization is necessary between uses.

The needle has four basic parts: the hub, which fits onto the syringe; the cannula, or shaft, which is attached to the hub; the bevel, which is the slanted part at the tip of the shaft; and the safety cap. Needles come in various sizes, from 1/4 inch to 5 inches, and with gauges that range from 28 to 14 (see Figure 30-11 on page 778).

The *gauge* of the needle refers to the diameter of the shaft; the larger the gauge number, the smaller the diameter of the shaft. Large-gauge needles produce less trauma to the body's tissue; however, the nurse has to consider the viscosity of a solution when selecting the gauge.

The *shaft of the needle* determines its length. The nurse selects the length of the needle on the basis of the client's

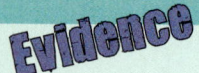

UNCOVERING THE Evidence

TITLE
"2007 Study of Injectable Medication Errors"

AUTHOR
American Nurses Association

PURPOSE
To identify opinions, concerns, and experiences about challenges related to labeling on syringes.

METHODS
A nationwide online survey of nurses was conducted by the Atlanta-based Arketi Group and sponsored by the ANA and Inviro Medical Devices. Of the 1039 nurses, 22% of those surveyed had been a nurse for 1 to 5 years, 12% had been a nurse for 6 to 10 years, 15% had been a nurse for 11 to 15 years, and 51% had been a nurse for more than 15 years.

FINDINGS
Nearly all (97%) nurses worry about medication error, and two-thirds (68%) believe medication error could be reduced with more consistent syringe labeling.

IMPLICATIONS
The study indicates a need for the right safety equipment in regard to injectables in order to reduce the risk of medication errors and sharps-related injuries.

American Nurses Association. (2008). 2007 Study of Injectable Medication Errors. Retrieved September 29, 2008, from http://psnet. ahrq.gov/resource.aspx?resourceID=5503.

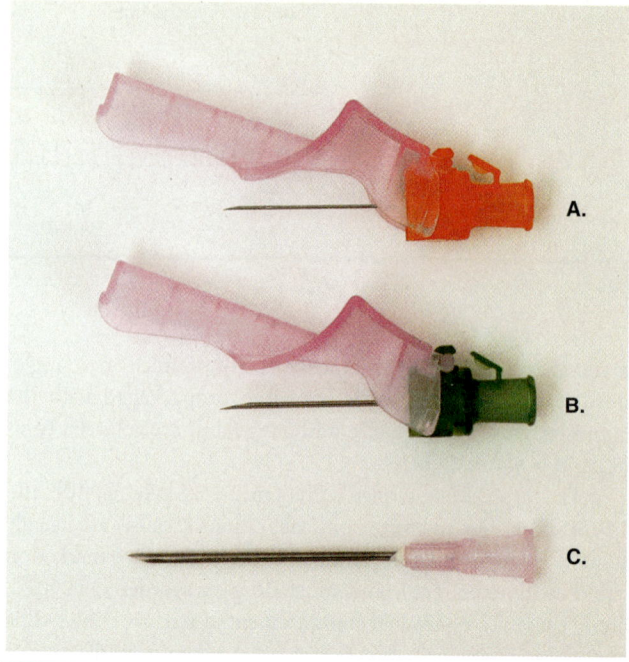

FIGURE 30-11 Examples of some various gauges and lengths of needles: A. 25-gauge, 1-inch needle with safety cap; **B.** 21-gauge, 1-inch needle with safety cap; **C.** 18-gauge, 11/2-inch needle DELMAR/CENGAGE LEARNING.

muscle development and weight and the type of injection, such as ID versus IM.

The needle may have a short or long *bevel*. The length of bevel selected is based on the type of injection. Long bevels are sharp and produce less pain when injected into the subcutaneous or muscle tissues; however, a short-bevel needle must be used for ID and IV injections to prevent occlusion of the bevel either by the tissue or by a blood vessel wall.

When the nurse removes a needle from its sterile wrapper, the hub of the needle should be immediately attached to the hub of the syringe to prevent contamination. Likewise, the protective cover should remain on the needle's shaft until the nurse is ready to use the needle.

After an injection, the nurse should not recap the needle; used needles should be disposed of in the proper receptacles, such as a sharps container, to prevent needlesticks. See Chapters 29 and 33 for details on how to prevent needlestick injuries. Most agencies have sharps containers in all client care areas. Chapter 33 provides a complete discussion of the needleless system.

AMPULES AND VIALS Drugs for parenteral injections are sterile preparations. Drugs that deteriorate in solution are dispensed as tablets or powders and dissolved in a solution immediately before injection. Drugs that remain stable in a solution are dispensed in ampules and vials in an aqueous or oily solution or suspension.

Ampules are glass containers of single-dose drugs (see Figure 30-12). The glass container has a constriction in the stem to facilitate opening the ampule. See Procedure 30-2 for removing a drug from an ampule. The medication is aspirated into a syringe with a filter needle to prevent small glass fragments from entering the syringe. Because many drugs are irritating to the subcutaneous tissue, the nurse should change the needle on the syringe after withdrawing a drug from an ampule.

Glass, single- or multiple-dose, rubber-capped drug containers are called vials (see Figure 30-13 on page 779). The vial is usually covered with a soft metal cap that can be easily removed. See Procedure 30-3 for removing a drug from a

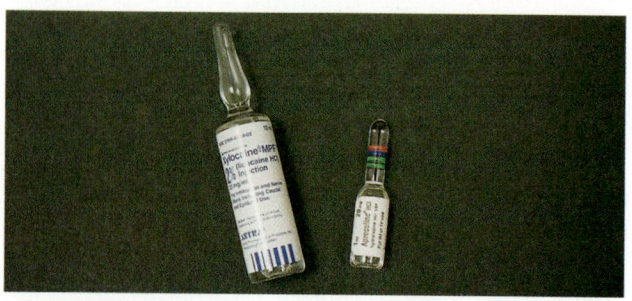

FIGURE 30-12 Ampules DELMAR/CENGAGE LEARNING

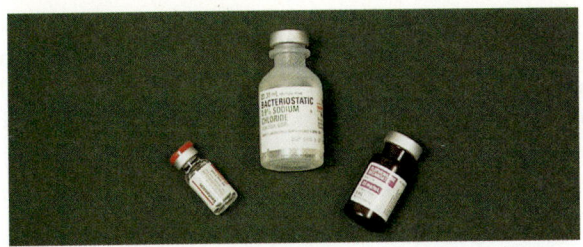

FIGURE 30-13 Vials DELMAR/CENGAGE LEARNING

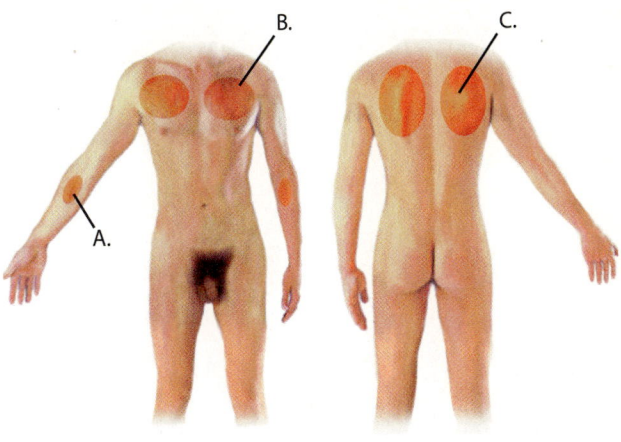

FIGURE 30-15 Intradermal Injection Sites: A. Inner Aspect of the Forearm; **B.** Upper Chest; **C.** Upper Back DELMAR/CENGAGE LEARNING

vial. The nurse should change the needle on the syringe after withdrawing a drug from a vial. Inserting the needle through the rubber cap of the vial can dull the needle or remove the needle coating that helps it glide through the skin.

Compatible medications can be mixed in the same syringe. Refer to compatibility charts or check with the pharmacist to determine if the medications can be mixed. If medications are going to be mixed, care must be exercised not to contaminate one medication with the other in their respective vials. See Procedure 30-4 for mixing insulins in one syringe. The nurse must calculate and measure carefully to be sure the final dose is accurate.

Angle of Injection

The angle of insertion depends on the type of injection. Figure 30-14 illustrates the angle of insertion for each type of parenteral injection.

Medication Administration: Intradermal

ID or intracutaneous injections are typically used to diagnose tuberculosis, identify allergens, and administer local anesthetics. The site below the epidermis is the location for administering ID injections; drugs are absorbed slowly from this site. The sites commonly used for ID injection are the inner aspect of the forearm (if it is not highly pigmented or covered with hair), upper chest, and upper back beneath the scapula (see Figure 30-15). Only small amounts of water-soluble medication should be used for subcutaneous injections.

The drug's dosage for an ID injection is usually contained in a small quantity of solution (0.01 to 0.1 mL). A 1-mL tuber-

culin syringe with a short bevel, 25- to 27-gauge, 3/8- to 1/2-inch needle is used to provide accurate measurement. If repeated doses are ordered, the site should be rotated. ID injections are administered into the epidermis layer by angling the needle 10° to 15° to the skin. See Procedure 30-5 for administering ID injections.

Medication Administration: Subcutaneous

Subcutaneous injections are commonly used in the administration of medications such as insulin and heparin because these drugs are absorbed slowly, to produce a sustained effect. Subcutaneous injections place the medication into the subcutaneous tissue, between the dermis and the muscle. Clients who administer frequent subcutaneous injections should rotate sites regularly. An administration chart can help them keep track of the sites used. The amount of medication given varies but should not exceed 1.0 mL; if repeated drug doses are given, rotate the sites. Subcutaneous tissues are sensitive to irritating medications. Hard painful lumps can develop beneath the skin if the sites are not rotated.

Common sites for subcutaneous injections are the abdomen, the lateral and anterior aspects of the upper arm or thigh, the scapular area on the back, and upper ventrodorsal gluteal areas (see Figure 30-16 on page 780). The nurse should select a sterile 0.5- to 3-mL syringe with a 25- to 29-gauge, 3/8- to 1/2-inch needle. The medication is administered by angling the needle 45° or 90° to the skin. The client's body weight will influence the angle used for injection. As a general rule, to reach subcutaneous tissue, the nurse grasps 2 inches of tissue between two fingers and inserts the needle at a 90° angle. If only 1 inch of tissue can be grasped between the fingers, use a 45° angle to administer the medication.

The length of the needle may also vary with body weight. Normally for subcutaneous injections, a 25-gauge, 5/8-inch needle is used. A child will require a short needle, and an obese person may require a longer needle to ensure placing the medication in the subcutaneous tissue. The length of the needle should be approximately half the width of the

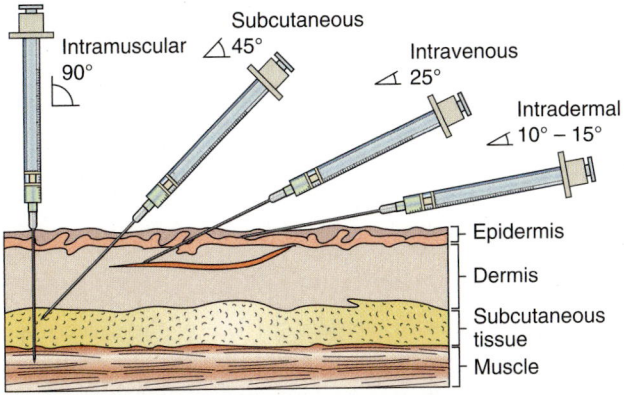

FIGURE 30-14 Angles of Insertion for Parenteral Injections
DELMAR/CENGAGE LEARNING

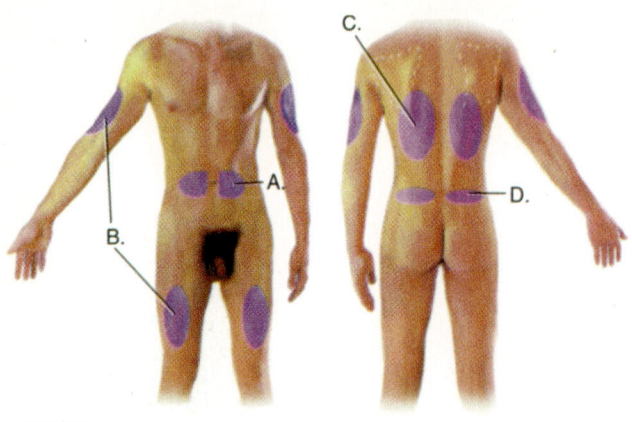

FIGURE 30-16 **Subcutaneous Injections Sites: A.** Abdomen;
B. Lateral and Anterior Aspects of the Upper Arm and Thigh;
C. Scapular Area on Back; **D.** Upper Ventrodorsal Gluteal Area
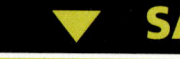

SAFETY FIRST

ASPIRATING THE SYRINGE
Do not aspirate on the plunger when giving heparin; *doing so may cause tissue damage.*

COMMON INTRAMUSCULAR INJECTION SITES AND MUSCLES

SITE	MUSCLE
Ventrogluteal	Gluteus medius
Anterolateral aspect of thigh	Vastus lateralis
Upper arm	Deltoid

pinched skinfold. See Procedure 30-6 for the technique used in administering a subcutaneous injection.

Medication Administration: Intramuscular

IM injections are used to promote rapid drug absorption and to provide an alternate route when the drug is irritating to subcutaneous tissue. The IM route enhances the absorption rate because there are more blood vessels in the muscles than in subcutaneous tissue; however, the absorption rate may be affected by the client's circulatory status.

Since the 1920s over 90 research studies related to IM injections have been reported in the literature (Beyea & Nicoll, 1995). Researchers have studied the medication volume and appropriate size of the syringe and needle for administering an IM injection to a particular site. "Research on the maximum volume to be drawn up for a single injection is still inconclusive" (Beyea & Nicoll, 1996, p. 34). The nurse should determine the maximum volume to inject on the basis of the site and the client's muscle development:

- 3 mL for a large muscle (gluteus medius) in a well-developed adult
- 1 to 2 mL for less developed muscles in children and in older and thin clients
- 0.5 to 1.0 mL for the deltoid muscle

When more than 3 mL is ordered, the medication can be divided into two different sites.

There are three common sites for administrating IM injections (see the accompanying display on common IM injection sites). Injection sites are identified by using appropriate anatomic landmarks (see Figure 30-17 on page 781).

The primary site for administering an IM injection in clients over 7 months old is the ventrogluteal (VG) site. The gluteus medius is a well-developed muscle, free of major nerves and large blood vessels. Research shows that injuries—including fibrosis, nerve damage, abscess, tissue necrosis, muscle contraction, gangrene, and pain—have been associated with all the common sites (e.g., dorsogluteal, deltoid, vastus lateralis) *except* the VG site (Beyea & Nicoll, 1996, p. 35). Recent research has suggested that the dorsogluteal muscle, which was once the first choice for adult IM injections, is no longer a safe site for IM injections (Hunt, 2008). These studies have demonstrated that the exact location of the sciatic nerve varies from one person to another. If the sciatic nerve is damaged by a needle, the person may experience adverse outcomes, such as pain or temporary or permanent paralysis of the lower extremities. Accidental injection into the superior gluteal artery may cause increased absorption or hemorrhage.

The nurse should avoid using the deltoid site in children. The deltoid muscle is not well developed in infants, children, and many adults. This site should be used only for small medication volumes.

The nurse will need to decide on the gauge and length of the needle on the basis of the consistency of the solution, the site, and how far the needle must be injected to reach the muscle. A 21- to 23-gauge needle will accommodate the consistency of most drugs and will minimize tissue injury and subcutaneous leakage. The needle's length is determined by the site:

- 11/2-inch needle, VG site for average-sized adults
- 1-inch needle, VG site for children
- 1-inch needle, deltoid or vastus lateralis

An obese client usually requires a 2-inch needle to ensure that the needle will reach a large muscle such as the gluteal muscle. For example, for a client weighing 100 pounds, use a needle 1 to 11/2 inches long; usually for a child, use only a 1-inch needle. It is important to consider the size of the client when determining the needle length; some children are large, and some adults are small. The nurse should administer an IM injection at a 90° angle. See Procedure 30-7 for administering an IM injection.

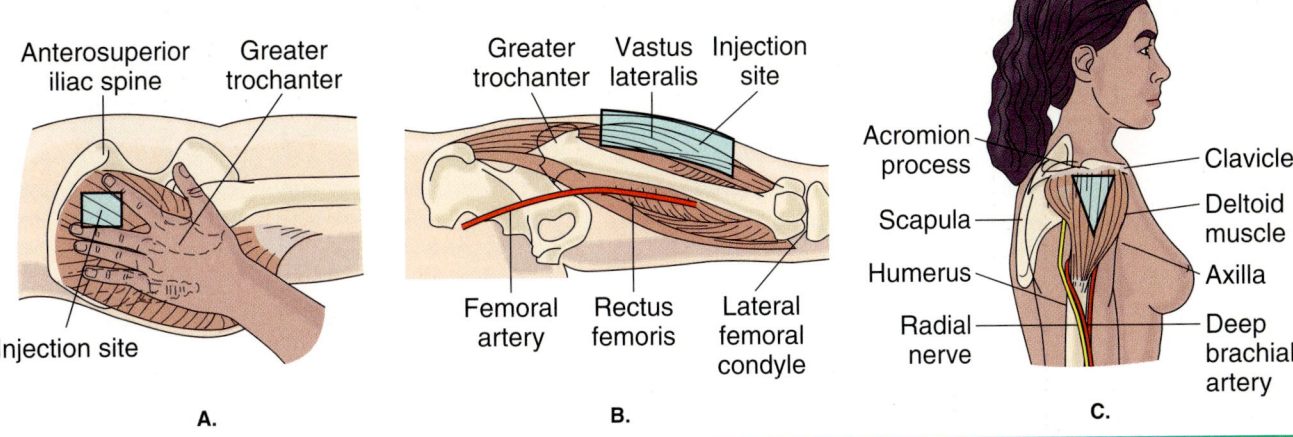

FIGURE 30-17 Intramuscular Injection Sites: A. Ventrogluteal: Place palm of left hand on right greater trochanter so index finger points toward anterosuperior iliac spine; spread first and middle fingers to form a V; the middle of the V is the injection site; **B.** Vastus lateralis: Identify greater trochanter; place hand at lateral femoral condyle; injection site is middle third of anterior lateral aspect. **C.** Deltoid: Locate the lateral side of the humerus from two to three finger widths below the acromion process in adults or one finger width below the acromion process in children. DELMAR/CENGAGE LEARNING

Z-TRACK INJECTION The **Z-track (zigzag) technique** refers to a method used in administering IM injections (see Procedure 30-7). This technique was traditionally used when administering Imferon, an iron preparation, which can cause permanent discoloration in the subcutaneous tissue. Today, the technique is used commonly when administering VG injections.

When administering a Z-track injection, the nurse should place the client in the prone position; then pull the skin to one side, insert the needle at a 90° angle, and administer the medication (see Figure 30-18). Spreading the skin, a common method formerly used for IM injections, increases the risk that medication will leak into the needle track and the subcutaneous tissue; this risk is virtually eliminated using the Z-track technique, making it the technique of choice (Beyea & Nicoll, 1996). The nurse waits 10 seconds and withdraws the needle at the same angle used for insertion; the site should not be massaged because massaging can cause tissue irritation.

Table 30-2 on page 782 summarizes the basics of ID, subcutaneous, and IM injections.

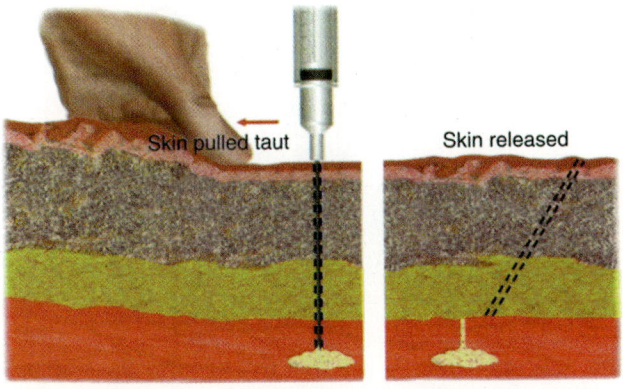

FIGURE 30-18 Administering Intramuscular Injection Using Z-Track Technique: Pulling skin taut and then releasing it after the needle is withdrawn seals the site DELMAR/CENGAGE LEARNING

Medication Administration: Intravenous

The IV route is used when a rapid drug effect is desired or when the medication is irritating to tissue. IV administration provides immediate release of medication into the bloodstream; consequently, it can be dangerous. IV medications are administered by one of the following methods:

- IV fluid container (Figure 30-19 on page 782) and infusion pump
- Volume-control administration set
- Intermittent infusion by piggyback or partial fill
- Intravenous push (IVP or bolus)

See Chapter 33 for a discussion of other IV delivery systems.

When administering IV medications, regardless of the method used, the nurse should assess the patency of the infusion system and the condition of the injection site for signs of complications such as **infiltration** (swelling and discomfort at the IV site) and **phlebitis** (inflammation of a vein). See Chapter 33 for a complete discussion of these IV complications. Some IV medications or solutions with high or low pH or high osmolarity are irritating to veins and can cause phlebitis.

INFUSION PUMP An infusion pump is used to regulate fluids intravenously by exerting positive pressure on the tubing or on the fluid (see Figures 30-20 and 30-21 on pages 782 and 783). When the fluid flow is unrestricted, the pump pressure is comparable to that of gravity flow; however, if restrictions develop (increased venous resistance), the pump can maintain the fluid flow by increasing the pressure applied to the fluid. (See Chapter 33 for additional information.) Whenever electronic devices are used to regulate medication administration, nurses must avoid at-risk behaviors related to technology, such as overriding alerts on the infusion pumps.

TABLE 30-2 **Summary of Intradermal, Subcutaneous, and Intramuscular Injections**

TYPE OF INJECTION	PURPOSE	SITE	NEEDLE SIZE	MAXIMUM DOSE	ANGLE OF INSERTION
Intradermal	Injects medication below the epidermis; drugs are absorbed slowly; typically used for diagnosis of tuberculosis and allergens	Inner aspect of forearm; upper chest; upper back	Syringe with short bevel; 25- to 27-gauge; 3/8- to 1/2-inch	0.01–0.1 mL	10°–15°
Subcutaneous	Injects medication between dermis and muscle; absorbed slowly; typically used for insulin and anticoagulants	Abdomen; lateral and anterior aspects of upper arm and thigh; scapular area on back; ventrogluteal area	25-gauge, 5/8-inch needle (varies by size of person)	0.5–1.0 mL	45° or 90°
Intramuscular	Used to promote rapid drug absorption and to provide an alternate route when drug is irritating to subcutaneous tissue	Ventrogluteal; dorsogluteal; anterolateral aspect of thigh (vastus lateralis); upper arm (deltoid)	The gauge and length of needle are selected on the basis of medication volume and viscosity and client's body size	Well-developed adults: 4 mL in a large muscle; infants and small children: 0.5–1.0 mL; children and older adults: 1–2 mL; deltoid muscle: 0.5–1 mL	90°

Delmar/Cengage Learning

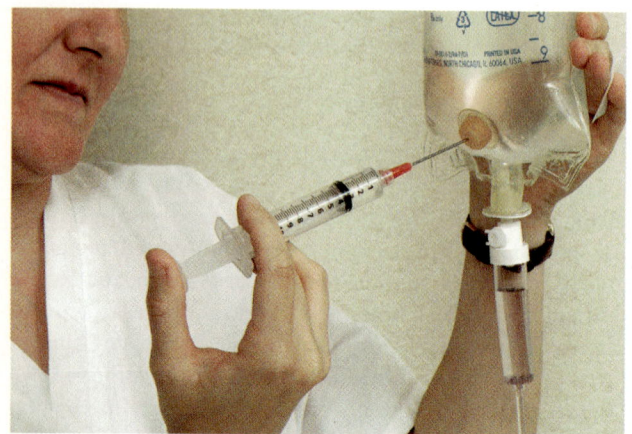

FIGURE 30-19 Adding a Medication to an Intravenous Fluid Container DELMAR/CENGAGE LEARNING

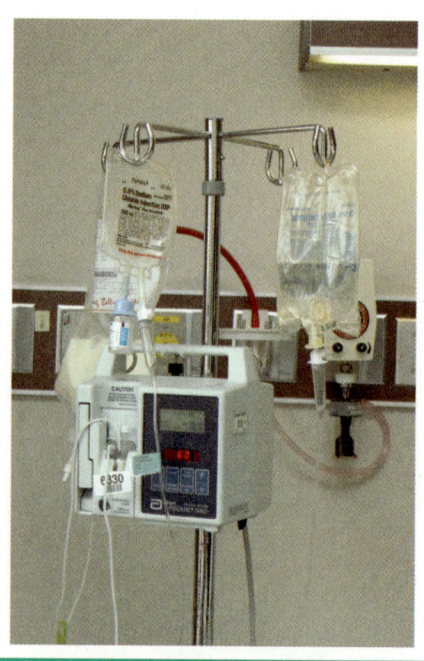

FIGURE 30-20 Infusion Pumps DELMAR/CENGAGE LEARNING

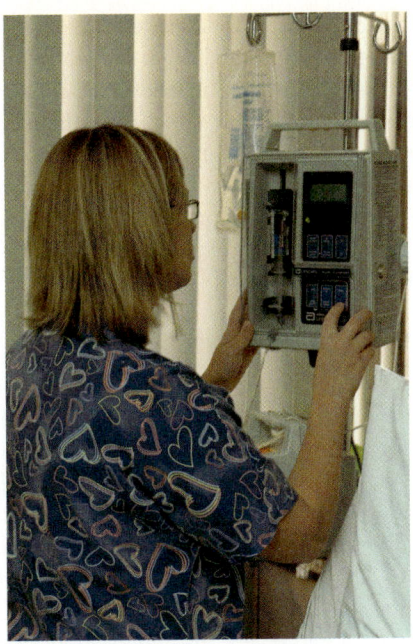

Figure 30-21 A nurse regulates intravenous fluids on an infusion pump DELMAR/CENGAGE LEARNING

ADDING DRUGS TO A VOLUME-CONTROL ADMINISTRATION SET

A volume-control set is used to administer small volumes of IV solution. These devices have various names as determined by the manufacturer, such as Soluset, Metriset, VoluTrol, or Buretrol. To administer a drug by this method, the nurse should:

- Withdraw the prescribed amount of medication into a syringe that is to be injected into the volume-control set.
- Cleanse the injection port of a partially filled volume-control set with an alcohol swab.
- Inject the prepared medication into the port of the volume-control set.
- Gently mix the solution in the volume-control chamber.

After injecting the medication into the volume-control chamber, the nurse should check the infusion rate and adjust as necessary to the prescribed rate of infusion.

ADMINISTERING MEDICATIONS BY INTERMITTENT INFUSION

A common method of administering IV medications is by using a secondary, or partial-fill, additive bag, often referred to as an IV piggyback (IVPB). A secondary line is a complete IV set (fluid container and tubing with either a microdrip or a macrodrip system) connected to a Y-port of a primary line (see Procedure 30-8). The primary line maintains venous access. The IVPB is used for medication administration. See Chapter 33 for a complete discussion of primary and secondary lines. When the IVPB medication is incompatible with the primary IV solution, the nurse must flush the primary IV tubing with normal saline before and after administering the medication.

INTERMITTENT INFUSION DEVICES

When the client requires only the administration of IV medications without the infusion of solutions, an intermittent infusion device is inserted into a peripheral needle or catheter in the client's vein (see Figure 30-22). This device is commonly referred to as a heparin or saline lock, depending on the agency's policy regarding the device's maintenance. A lock provides continuous access to venous circulation, eliminating the need for a continuous IV, and it increases the client's mobility.

The device can be used to infuse intermittent IVPB or IVP medications, or it can be converted to a primary IV. A major consideration for inserting a heparin lock device is that it provides venous access in case of an emergency. Lock devices are routinely used with cardiac clients.

Locks are generally flushed every 8 hours to maintain patency (patency refers to being freely opened). Some agencies require a diluted dose of heparin (100 units/mL) to be injected into the lock; other agencies use normal saline to keep the device patent. See Chapter 33 for a complete discussion of heparin and saline locks. When heparin is used, the device must be flushed with normal saline solution before and after administration of a medication.

ADMINISTERING IVP MEDICATIONS

The method of medication administration by IV bolus or IVP injection is determined by the type of IV system. For example, an IVP medication can be injected into a saline or heparin lock (see Figure 30-23) or into a continuous infusion line. When giving an IVP medication into a continuous infusion line, the nurse must stop the fluids in the primary line; the nurse usually pinches the IV tubing closed to inject the drug (see Figure 30-24 on page 784). This technique is safe and prevents the nurse from having to recalculate the drip rate of the primary infusion line.

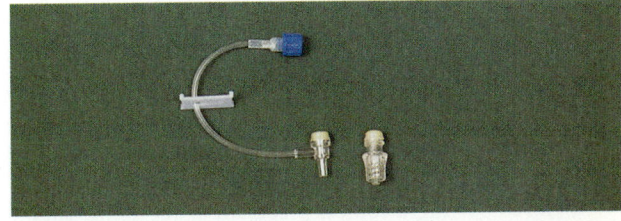

Figure 30-22 Heparin Locking Device DELMAR/CENGAGE LEARNING

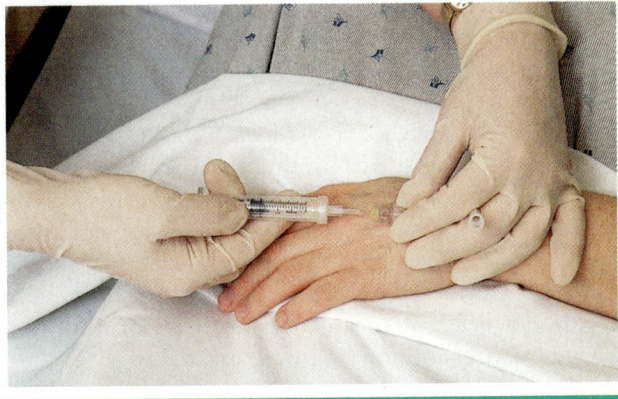

Figure 30-23 Injecting a Bolus of Medication into a Peripheral Saline Lock DELMAR/CENGAGE LEARNING

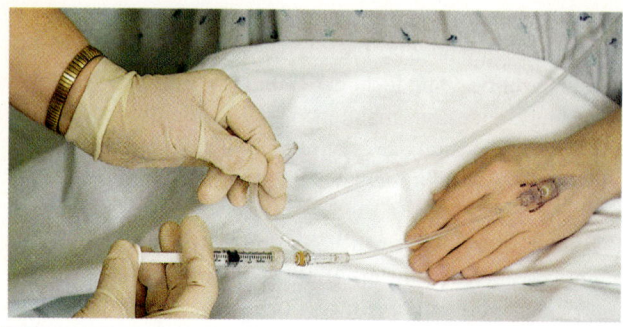

FIGURE 30-24 Pinch the IV tubing of a primary infusion line to administer an IVP medication DELMAR/CENGAGE LEARNING

IVP medications can also be given into a central line or directly into the vessel by venipuncture. The five rights of medication administration are implemented when administering an IV bolus. The nurse must know the specific time interval to inject the medication and the specific reactions of the infused drug. The client must be monitored closely during and after injection for drug reactions.

MEDICATION ADMINISTRATION: TOPICAL

Topical medications may be administered to the skin, eyes, ears, nose, throat, rectum, and vagina. The medication generally provides a local effect but can also cause systemic effects. Drugs directly applied to the skin to produce a local effect include lotions, pastes, ointments, creams, powders, and aerosol sprays. The rate and degree of the drug's absorption are determined by the vascularity of the area.

Topical drugs are usually given to provide continuous absorption to produce different effects: to relieve pruritus (itching), to protect the skin, to prevent or treat an infection, to provide local anesthesia, or to create a systemic effect. Topical medications are usually ordered two or three times a day to achieve their therapeutic effect.

Before applying a topical preparation, the nurse should assess the condition of the skin for any open lesions, rashes, or areas of erythema and skin breakdown. Because secretions are produced by the skin and mucous membranes, the nurse should always implement Standard Precautions when applying a topical drug. The medication can be transferred to the nurse if gloves are not worn or an applicator, such as a sterile tongue depressor, is not used. The nurse should check with the client and the medical record for any known allergies.

Body oils may interfere with the adhesive properties of the patch, disk, or tape. The skin harbors microorganisms, and lesions can cause encrustation. The nurse should cleanse the area by washing with soap and warm water, unless contraindicated by a specific order. The skin should be thoroughly dry before a topical medication is applied. Open wounds require the nurse to use surgical asepsis.

When the skin is dry, the nurse can apply the medication. When applying a paste, a cream, or an ointment, the nurse should use a sterile tongue depressor to remove the medication

from the container; this method prevents cross-contamination. The medication is transferred from the tongue blade to a gloved hand for application. The medication should be applied in long, smooth strokes in the direction of the hair follicles to prevent the medication from entering the hair follicles. A new sterile tongue depressor should be used whenever more medication is removed from the container. Two to 4 hours after the application, the nurse should assess the area for signs of an allergic reaction.

Medication Administration: Eye

Eye medications, often referred to as ophthalmic medications, refer to drops, ointments, and disks. These drugs are used for diagnostic and therapeutic purposes—to lubricate the eye or socket for a prosthetic eye and to prevent or treat eye conditions such as glaucoma (elevated pressure within the eye) and infection. Diagnostically, eyedrops can be used to anesthetize the eye, dilate the pupil, and stain the cornea to identify abrasions and scars.

The nurse should review the abbreviations used in medication orders to ensure that the medication is instilled in the correct eye. Cross-contamination is a potential problem with eyedrops. The nurse should adhere to the following safety measures to prevent cross-contamination:

- Each client should have a bottle of eyedrops. Clients should never share eye medications.
- Discard any solution remaining in the dropper after instillation.
- Discard the dropper if the tip is accidentally contaminated, as by touching the bottle or any part of the client's eye. The risk of transferring infection from one eye to the other is increased if the tip touches any part of the client's eye.

See Procedure 30-9 for administering eye medications. The nurse should insert medication disks at bedtime because they usually cause blurring of the eyes on insertion. Standard Precautions are used when eye care and medications are being administered because of the potential contact with bodily secretions.

Medication Administration: Ear

Solutions ordered to treat the ear are often referred to as *otic* (pertaining to the ear) drops or irrigations. Eardrops may be instilled to soften ear wax, to produce anesthesia, to treat infection or inflammation, or to facilitate removal of a foreign body, such as an insect. External auditory canal irrigations are usually performed for cleaning purposes and less frequently for applying heat and antiseptic solutions. The internal ear is very sensitive to changes in temperature. Sudden changes can cause nausea and dizziness. Eardrops and irrigation fluids should be at room temperature.

Before instilling a solution into the ear, the nurse should inspect the ear for signs of drainage, an indication of a perforated tympanic membrane. Eardrops are usually contraindicated when the tympanic membrane is perforated. If the tympanic membrane is damaged, all procedures must be performed using sterile aseptic technique; otherwise, medical asepsis is used when instilling medications into the ear (see

Procedure 30-9). Medication should never be forced into the ear canal, especially if it is occluded (as by wax). Forcing medication into an occluded eardrum can injure the eardrum.

Certain conditions have contraindications for specific drugs; for example, hydrocortisone eardrops are contraindicated in clients with a fungal infection or a viral infection such as herpes.

Medication Administration: Nasal

Nasal instillations can be performed with different preparations: drops or nebulizers (atomizer or aerosol). Nasal drugs are administered to produce one or more of the following effects: to shrink swollen mucous membranes, to loosen secretions and facilitate drainage, and to treat infections of the nasal cavity or sinuses. Because many of these products are nonprescription drugs, clients should be taught their correct usage. For example, nasal decongestants are common over-the-counter drugs used to shrink swollen mucous membranes; however, when these drugs are used in excess, they may have a reverse or rebound effect by increasing nasal congestion.

The nasal sinuses (frontal, ethmoid, maxillary, and sphenoid sinuses) communicate with the nasal fossae and are lined with mucous membranes similar to those that line the nose. Nose drops can be instilled to remain in the nasal passage, to reach the ethmoid and sphenoid sinuses, or to reach the frontal or maxillary sinuses. Location is determined by the degree of hyperextension and position of the head during instillation (see Figure 30-25). Although the nose is considered a clean (not sterile) cavity, because of its connection with the sinuses, the nurse uses medical asepsis when performing nasal instillations. See Procedure 30-10 for administering nasal instillations.

Nebulizers (inhalers) are used to deliver a fine mist containing medication droplets. The nurse should administer or assist clients with the usage of atomizers and aerosols:

- Instruct the client to clear the nostrils by blowing the nose.
- Client should be in an upright position with head tilted back slightly.

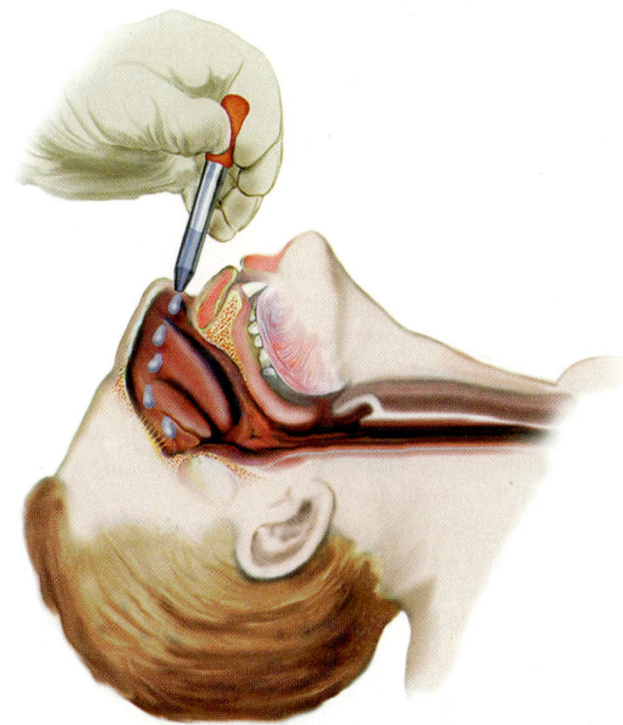

FIGURE 30-25 Positioning a Client for Nose Drop Instillation
DELMAR/CENGAGE LEARNING

Atomizer

- Occlude one nostril to prevent air from entering the nasal cavity and to allow the medication to flow freely in the open nostril.
- Insert the atomizer tip into the open nostril and instruct the client to inhale, then squeeze the atomizer once, and instruct the client to exhale.

Aerosol

- Shake the aerosol well before each use.
- Grasp between thumb and index finger and insert the adapter tip into one nostril while occluding the other nostril with a finger, then press the adapter cartridge firmly to release one measured dose of medication.
- Repeat the above steps as ordered for the other nostril.
- Instruct the client to keep head tilted backward for 2 to 3 minutes and to breathe through the nose while the medication is being absorbed.

When the client is discharged with a nasal inhaler, the nurse should teach the client how to store and use the device.

Respiratory inhalants are delivered by devices that produce fine droplets that are inhaled deep into the respiratory tract. A nebulizer is a device that is used to aerosolize medications into a mist for delivery directly into the lungs. These medication droplets are absorbed almost immediately through the alveolar epithelium into the bloodstream.

Oropharyngeal handheld inhalers deliver medications that produce both local and systemic effects, such as bronchodilators and mucolytics. Bronchodilators improve airway

▼ **SAFETY FIRST** ▼

SYSTEMIC EFFECTS OF EYEDROPS

The nurse should apply pressure to the inner canthus when instilling eyedrops that have potential systemic effects such as atropine and timolol maleate (Timoptic). Gentle pressure over the inner canthus prevents the medication from flowing into the tear duct, thereby decreasing the absorption rate of the drug.

patency and are used to prevent or treat bronchospasms, asthma, and allergic reactions. Mucolytics are used to liquify tenacious (thick) bronchial secretions. There are three types of oropharyngeal handheld inhalers: the metered-dose inhaler, the turbo-inhaler, and the nasal inhaler (previously discussed).

Clients must be able to form an airtight seal around the inhaling devices and be able to assemble the turbo-inhaler. This requirement prevents some clients, such as clients with visual or coordination impairments, from using these devices. Bronchodilators are contraindicated in clients who have a history of tachycardia.

The nurse should ensure that the client knows how to use the inhaler correctly so that the prescribed medication dose is delivered. See Procedure 30-11 for teaching a client how to use the nebulizer.

A metered-dose inhaler delivers a measured dose of the medication with each push of the canister. The nurse needs to evaluate the client's ability to adequately compress the inhaler to deliver a full dose and to inhale at the same time as the dose is expressed. Failure to do either could prevent the client from receiving the full benefit of the inhaler. The ability to compress the inhaler for dose delivery can be affected by hand strength (which diminishes with age), flexibility (as in arthritic changes), and disease related to weakness (such as chronic respiratory disease). Careful discharge instructions and observation of the client performing the task are important to continued therapeutic effect at home (see the accompanying Client Teaching Checklist for home care application).

Medication Administration: Rectal

Rectal instillations can be in the form of enemas, suppositories, and ointments. See Chapter 39 for a complete discussion of enema administration. Rectal ointments are used to treat local conditions and symptoms such as pain, inflammation, and itching caused by hemorrhoids. Rectal suppositories are cone-shaped masses of substances designed to melt at body temperature and to produce the intended effect at a slow and steady rate of absorption.

Suppositories provide a safe and convenient route for administering drugs that interact poorly with digestive enzymes or have a bad taste or odor. They are also used to provide temporary relief for clients who cannot tolerate oral preparations: for example, to relieve nausea and vomiting. Suppositories are also used to induce relaxation, relieve pain and local irritation, reduce fever, and stimulate peristalsis and defecation in clients who are constipated.

Rectal suppositories are contraindicated in cardiac clients because insertion may stimulate the vagus nerve, causing cardiac dysrhythmias (abnormal heart patterns). These drugs are also avoided in clients recovering from rectal or prostate surgery because they may cause pain on insertion and trauma to the tissues.

The nurse should assess the rectum for irritation or bleeding and check sphincter control. Some clients may

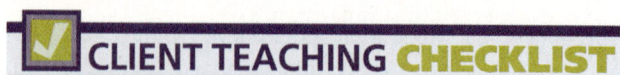

CLIENT TEACHING CHECKLIST

HOME CARE

Considerations for Use of Nasal Inhalers

- Provide the client with the manufacturer's directions for the specific type of inhaler, such as how to replace a medication cartridge for a nasal aerosol.
- Inhalers should be stored at room temperature.
- Aerosols are prepared under pressure and should not be punctured or placed in an incinerator.
- Instruct the client not to allow other people to use the inhaler.
- Caution the client about overuse that could cause a rebound effect, making the condition worse.
- Ensure that the client is knowledgeable about the expected and adverse effects of the drug. Some of these drugs do not produce therapeutic effects for several days, and some require 2 weeks of continuous use before the drug effects appear.
- Provide the client with a telephone number to call if assistance is needed.

experience problems in retaining the suppository. The nurse should instruct such a client to remain in the Sims' position for at least 15 minutes or should place the client on the abdomen, if the condition allows, and hold the buttocks closed. The prescribing practitioner should be notified when the client is unable to retain a suppository so that another route can be ordered.

Suppositories are often stored in the refrigerator to preserve the integrity of the drug form. A softened suppository is difficult to insert; to harden a suppository, place it under cold running water while it is still in its original wrapper. The nurse should follow the five rights of medication administration and Standard Precautions when administering rectal instillations. See Procedure 30-12 for the procedure on inserting a rectal suppository.

Medication Administration: Vaginal

Medications inserted into the vagina are in the form of suppositories, creams, gels, ointments, foams, or douches. These medications may be used to treat inflammation, infections, and discomfort, or as a contraceptive measure.

Vaginal creams, gels, and ointments usually come with a disposable tubular applicator with a plunger to insert the drug. Standard Precautions are always used by the nurse when inserting suppositories. Body temperature causes the suppository to melt and be absorbed. Suppositories are usually inserted with the index finger of a gloved hand; however, small suppositories may come with an applicator, and the suppository is placed in the applicator's tip. Many clients prefer to insert their own vaginal suppository. In this case, provide privacy for the client. See Procedure 30-13 for the procedure on instilling a vaginal suppository. After insertion of these preparations, the client may notice drainage and should be informed that this is expected. If a suppository is given to treat infection, tell the client that the drainage may be foul smelling. The nurse should advise the client to wear a perineal pad to prevent soiling of the underpants. Clients should be instructed not to use tampons after the insertion of vaginal medications because the tampon can absorb the medication and decrease the drug's effect.

Sterile technique is usually required by agency policy, especially if there is an open wound when administering a vaginal douche (irrigation). Douches are ordered to apply antimicrobial solutions, to remove offensive or irritating discharge, to reduce inflammation, and to prevent hemorrhage with warm or cold irrigations. The nurse should ensure that the client does not have an allergy to iodine because many vaginal preparations contain povidone-iodine.

NURSING CARE PLAN

The Client with Deep Vein Thrombosis

CASE PRESENTATION

Mrs. Landry, a 45-year-old, was admitted to your floor with a diagnosis of deep vein thrombosis. The client noticed swelling of her left leg about a week ago but decided to treat it at home. Four days later, the lower leg was very edematous, warm, and painful to move. After an office visit, the client was admitted to the hospital. This is Mrs. Landry's first hospitalization. On examination you find that the left leg is warmer than the right. The left thigh circumference is 3 inches larger than the right. The prescribing practitioner ordered a heparin IV drip after a loading dose bolus was given. The drip contained 10,000 units heparin in 500 mL of D5W at 10 mL/h (200 units/h). The prescribing practitioner anticipates that Mrs. Landry will be weaned off of the heparin drip and started on subcutaneous heparin within 5 days. At the time of discharge, she will be given Coumadin.

ASSESSMENT

- Edematous left thigh
- Left leg warmer to touch than right
- Left thigh circumference 3 inches larger than right

NURSING DIAGNOSIS 1: *Impaired tissue perfusion* related to the development of venous thrombi in the deep femoral vein.
NOC: Medication response
NIC: Maintenance of therapeutic blood levels of medication

EXPECTED OUTCOMES

The client will:

1. Report an absence of pain.
2. Demonstrate an absence of edema.
3. Experience the same degree of skin temperature in both legs.

INTERVENTIONS/RATIONALES

1. Maintain on bed rest. Reduces the possibility of embolus; may decrease the pain and swelling.
2. Elevate the legs above the heart. Elevation facilitates venous return and decreases the edema.

(Continues)

NURSING CARE PLAN (Continued)

3. Measure the circumference of the left thigh and compare with that of the right thigh. Measuring the circumference provides a quantitative reference point that can be used to evaluate the swelling.
4. Apply moist heat to the affected extremity. Heat provides an analgesic effect; it decreases venospasms and pain.
5. Administer the heparin as prescribed. Heparin prevents the conversion of fibrinogen to fibrin and prothrombin to thrombin, thereby limiting the extension of the thrombus.
6. Monitor the partial thromboplastin time (PTT). The PTT is used to monitor heparin therapy because heparin, a short-acting anticoagulant, increases the PTT.

NURSING DIAGNOSIS 2: *Injury, risk for,* bleeding related to the administration of an oral anticoagulant.
NOC: Medication response
NIC: Maintenance of therapeutic blood levels of medication

EXPECTED OUTCOMES
The client will:

1. Not demonstrate evidence of bleeding from gums or nose, in urine or stool, or under the skin.
2. Maintain the prothrombin time (PT) or international normalized ratio (INR) within therapeutic range.

INTERVENTIONS/RATIONALES
1. Advise the client to withhold the medication in the event that bleeding occurs and to notify the prescribing practitioner immediately. The dose may need to be adjusted.
2. Encourage the client to discontinue smoking. Smoking has a tendency to increase the metabolism of the medication, necessitating an increase in the dose.
3. Provide dietary education. Foods high in fat and foods rich in vitamin K can interfere with the PT.
4. Warn against taking oral contraceptive medication. There may be a decrease in anticoagulant effect due to the increased production of clotting factors with oral contraceptives.
5. Warn against taking aspirin and other over-the-counter medications. Aspirin may increase the risk of bleeding; it inhibits platelet formation.

EVALUATION
Resolution of the signs and symptoms of deep vein thrombus is a measurement of success. The client will be able to ambulate without difficulty, and the swelling, temperature difference, and pain will disappear. The client will be knowledgeable about taking the oral anticoagulant on discharge. Discharge follow-up will be needed to monitor the client's progress on the oral anticoagulant.

EVALUATION

The nurse is responsible for the ongoing evaluation of the client's response to medication. This evaluation requires knowledge of the therapeutic action of drugs and of the side effects and adverse reactions that can occur. Changes in a client's health status can change the way a client responds to medications. For example, clients who develop renal failure do not excrete medications well, and medications can build up within their system. Nurses need to assess for changes in clients' responses to medication. Nurses in the community setting need to evaluate their clients' ongoing ability to manage their own medication regimens. They can discuss the regimen with the client and the family, observe client technique (as in self-administration of injections), and take physiological measures such as blood pressure readings. The nurse uses all information gathered through any source as a way of determining if the intended interventional outcomes are met.

The nurse who identifies a potential medication risk and initiates actions to prevent client injury is performing another form of evaluation. For example, if the client in the home setting cannot remember if the prescribed medications have been taken, providing the client with a daily or weekly pill box that is filled when the nurse is present prevents the client from taking too much medication or failing to take the dose as ordered.

PROCEDURE
30-1

Medication Administration: Oral, Sublingual, and Buccal

EQUIPMENT

- Prescribing practitioner's order for the medication
- Medication administration record (MAR)
- Medication cart or dispensing computer
- Medication tray
- Disposable medication cups
- Glass of water, juice, or other liquid
- Drinking straw
- Mortar and pestle, if needed
- Paper towels

ACTION	RATIONALE
1. Wash hands/hand hygiene; put on clean gloves.	1. Reduces the number of microorganisms.
2. Arrange the medication tray and cups in the medication room or on the medication cart outside the client's room (see Figure 30-26). Most hospitals use a computerized, limited-access medication cart. Follow institutional protocol.	2. Organizing medications and equipment saves time and reduces the possibility of error.

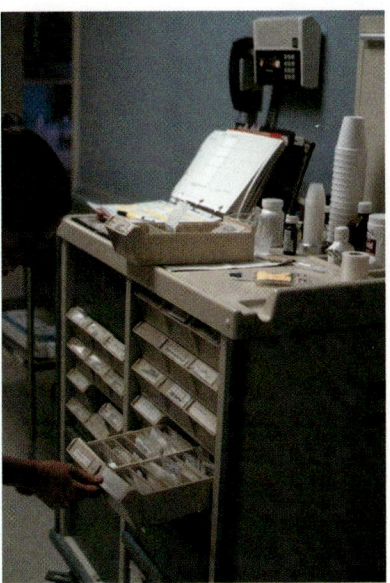

FIGURE 30-26 In some settings, medications are prepared at the medication cart. DELMAR/CENGAGE LEARNING

3. Unlock the medication cart, or log on to the computer.	3. Medications need to be safeguarded.
4. Prepare the medication for one client at a time following the five rights. Select the correct drug from the medication drawer according to the MAR (see Figure 30-27 on page 790). Calculate the drug dosage if needed.	4. The five rights are right client, right time, right medication, right dose, and right route. Comparing the MAR with the label reduces error. Double-checking reduces error in calculation.

(Continues)

PROCEDURE 30-1
Medication Administration: Oral, Sublingual, and Buccal (Continued)

ACTION	RATIONALE

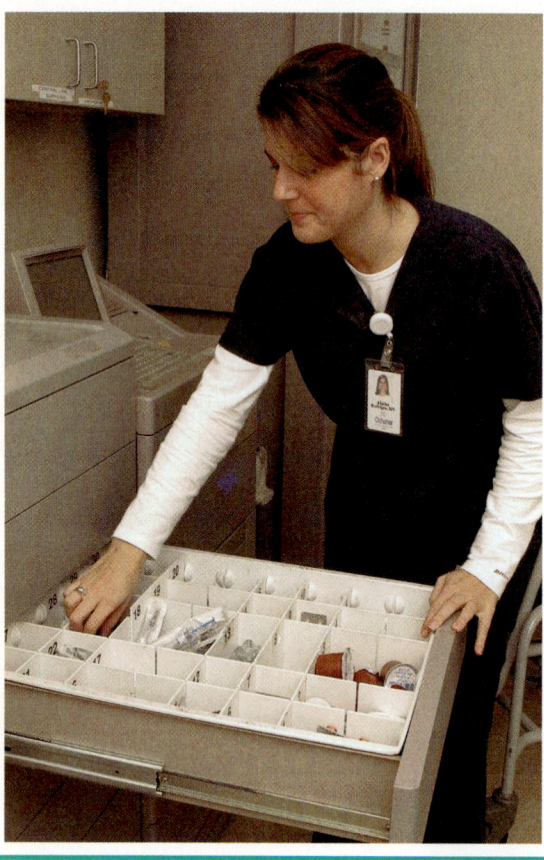

FIGURE 30-27 Select the correct drug from the medication drawer. DELMAR/CENGAGE LEARNING

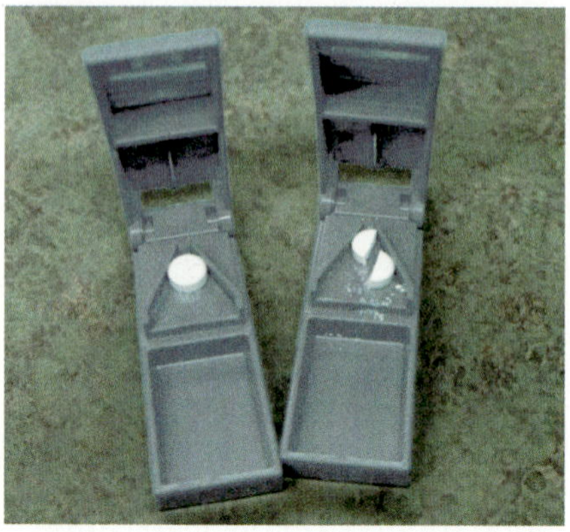

FIGURE 30-28 Scored tablets may be broken, if necessary.
DELMAR/CENGAGE LEARNING

5. To prepare a tablet or capsule: Pour the required number of tablets or capsules into the bottle cap, and transfer the medication to a medication cup without touching them.
   - Scored tablets may be broken, if necessary, using gloved hands or with a pill-cutting device (see Figure 30-28).
   - A unit-dose tablet should be placed directly into the medicine cup *without* opening it until it is administered to the client.
   - For clients with difficulty in swallowing, some tablets may be crushed into a powder using a mortar and pestle or by being placed between two paper medication cups and ground with a blunt object, then mixed in a small amount of applesauce or custard. Be aware that time-released or specially coated medications must not be crushed. Check with the pharmacy if you are uncertain (see Figure 30-29 on page 791).

5. Avoids wasting expensive medications and avoids contamination of medication.
   - Tablets that are not scored are not meant to be broken. The medication's effectiveness would be diminished if the tablet were broken or crushed.
   - The wrapper maintains cleanliness and identification until it is administered.
   - A large tablet is usually easier to swallow if it is ground and mixed with soft food.

(Continues)

PROCEDURE 30-1
Medication Administration: Oral, Sublingual, and Buccal (Continued)

ACTION	RATIONALE

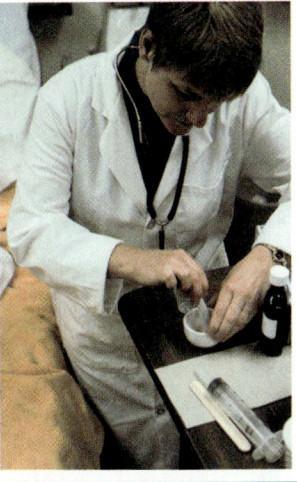

FIGURE 30-29 Some medications may be crushed and mixed with soft food, such as applesauce, for clients with difficulty in swallowing. DELMAR/CENGAGE LEARNING

6. To prepare a liquid medication: Remove the bottle cap from the container, and place cap upside down on the cart. Hold the bottle with the label up and the medication cup at eye level while pouring (see Figure 30-30). Fill the cup to the desired level using the surface or base of the meniscus as the scale, not the edge of the liquid on the cup. Wipe lip of bottle with paper towel.

6. Placing the bottle cap upside down on the cart prevents contamination of the inside of the container. Holding the bottle with the label up keeps spilled liquid from obliterating the label. Holding the medication cup at eye level ensures an accurate dose. Wiping the lip of the bottle prevents the bottle cap from sticking.

7. To prepare a narcotic, obtain the key to the narcotic drawer and check the narcotic record for the drug count when signing out the dose (see Figure 30-31). If the drug count does not agree with records, report to charge nurse immediately. Institution may require an incident report be filed.

7. Controlled substance laws require records of each dose dispensed. Early identification of errors assists in corrective action.

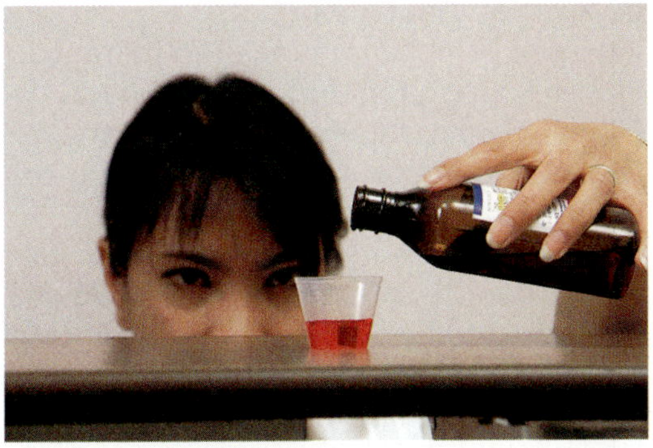

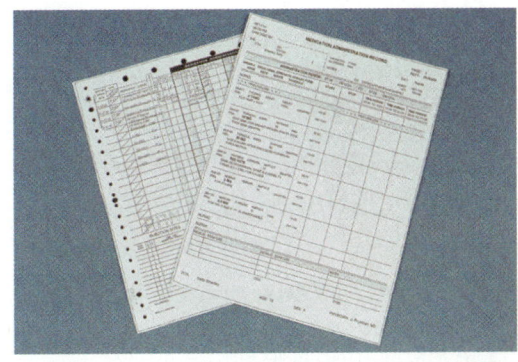

FIGURE 30-31 Controlled substance laws require records of each narcotic dose administered. DELMAR/CENGAGE LEARNING

FIGURE 30-30 Measure oral medications at eye level. DELMAR/CENGAGE LEARNING

(Continues)

PROCEDURE 30-1
Medication Administration: Oral, Sublingual, and Buccal (Continued)

ACTION	RATIONALE
8. Check expiration date on all medications. • Double-check the MAR with the prepared drugs. • Return stock medications to their shelf or drawer. • Place MARs with the client's medications. • Do not leave drugs unattended.	8. Expired medications may lose their effectiveness. • Reduces risk of error. • Ensures safety of stock medications. • Ensures identification of medications. • Drugs are safeguarded by nurse.
9. Administer medications to client: Observe the correct time to give the medication. • Identify the client by reading the client's name bracelet, repeating the name, and asking client to state name (see Figure 30-32). Additionally, check the hospital number if name alert or client is not reliable.	9. Ensures the therapeutic effect of the drug when given within 30 minutes of the prescribed time. *(Right time.)* • Identification bracelets made at the time of admission are the most reliable source of identification even if the client is unable to state name. *(Right client.)*

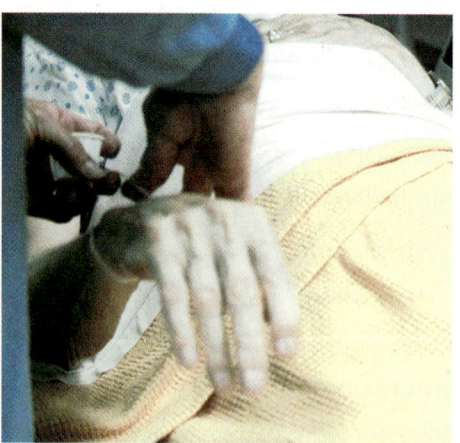

FIGURE 30-32 Identify the client by reading the client's name bracelet and asking his or her name before administering medication. DELMAR/CENGAGE LEARNING

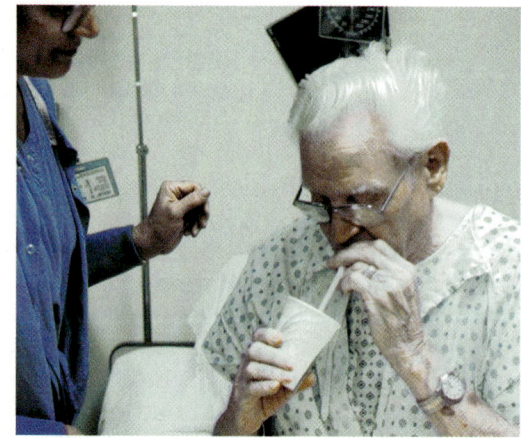

FIGURE 30-33 Allow the client to hold the tablet, and give water or juice to help the client swallow the medication. DELMAR/CENGAGE LEARNING

• Check the drug packaging if it is present to ensure the medication type and dosage. • Assess the client's condition and the form of the medication. • Perform any assessment required for specific medications such as a pulse or blood pressure. • Explain the purpose of the drug, and ask if the client has any questions. • Assist the client to a sitting or lateral position. • Allow client to hold the tablet or medication cup. • Give a glass of water or other liquid, and straw if needed, to help the client swallow the medication (see Figure 30-33). • For *sublingual* medications, instruct client to place medication under the tongue and allow it to dissolve completely.	• Prevents giving the wrong medication or wrong dose. *(Right medication, right dose.)* • Allows you to assess the route of the medication and if this route is appropriate. *(Right route.)* • Determines whether the medication should be given at that time or not. • Improves compliance with drug therapy. • Prevents aspiration during swallowing. • Client becomes familiar with medications. • Promotes client comfort in swallowing and can improve fluid intake. • Drug is absorbed through the mucous membranes into the blood vessels. If swallowed, the drug may be destroyed by gastric juices or detoxified in the liver too quickly so that its intended effects will not occur. • Promotes local activity on mucous membranes.

(Continues)

PROCEDURE 30-1
Medication Administration: Oral, Sublingual, and Buccal (Continued)

ACTION	RATIONALE
• For *buccal* administration of drugs, instruct the client to place the medication in the mouth against the cheek until it dissolves completely.	• Allows medication administration via NG or feeding tube. Ensures that the medication is absorbed and utilized correctly.
• For oral medications given through a *nasogastric tube,* crush tablets or open capsules and dissolve powder with 20 to 30 mL of warm water in a cup. Be sure medication will still be properly absorbed if crushed and dissolved. Check placement of the feeding tube or nasogastric tube before instilling anything but air into the tube.	• Nurse is responsible for ensuring that the client receives the dose and does not save it or discard it. • Maintains client's comfort.
• Remain with the client until each medication has been swallowed or dissolved.	
• Assist the client into a comfortable position.	
10. Dispose of soiled supplies; wash hands/hand hygiene.	10. Reduces transmission of microorganisms.
11. Record the time and route of administration on the MAR, and return it to the client's file.	11. Prevents administration error.
12. Return the cart to the medicine room; restock the supplies as needed. Clean the work area.	12. Assists other staff in completing duties efficiently.

delegation tip

The skill of medication administration and assessment of effects is not delegated to ancillary personnel in acute care settings. This may vary in state or federal institutions. Ancillary personnel are generally informed about the medications the client is receiving if adverse effects are anticipated or are being monitored.

nursing tips

Some medications require monitoring of blood levels to determine their effectiveness. When reviewing these laboratory values, notice if the levels are higher (toxic) or lower (subtherapeutic) than the recommended therapeutic range for that medication. Adjustments in the medication dose by the prescribing practitioner may be warranted to reach the recommended therapeutic level.

PROCEDURE 30-2

Withdrawing Medication from an Ampule

EQUIPMENT
- Medication ampule
- Sterile gauze pad or alcohol pad
- Syringe with filter needle
- Replacement needle
- Clean workspace
- Medication administration record (MAR)

(Continues)

PROCEDURE 30-2
Withdrawing Medication from an Ampule (Continued)

ACTION	RATIONALE
1. Wash hands/hand hygiene; secure supplies (see Figure 30-34).	1. Decreases transmission of microorganisms.
2. Select appropriate ampule (see Figure 30-35).	2. Ensures client receives correct medication.
3. Select syringe with filter needle (see Figure 30-36).	3. Filter needle entraps any glass fragments.
4. Obtain a sterile gauze pad.	4. Using a gauze pad prevents the nurse from being cut on the jagged edge of the broken ampule.
5. Select and set aside the appropriate length of safety needle for planned injection.	5. Accurate needle length ensures the medication is administered where it is intended.
6. Clear a workspace.	6. Prevents contamination of microdroplets that may spill when the ampule is broken.
7. Observe ampule for location of the medication.	7. The medication frequently becomes trapped in the top of the ampule.
8. If the medication is trapped in the top, flick the neck of the ampule repeatedly with your fingernail while holding the ampule upright (see Figure 30-37 on page 795).	8. Flicking the neck and top of the ampule moves the medication into the body of the ampule.

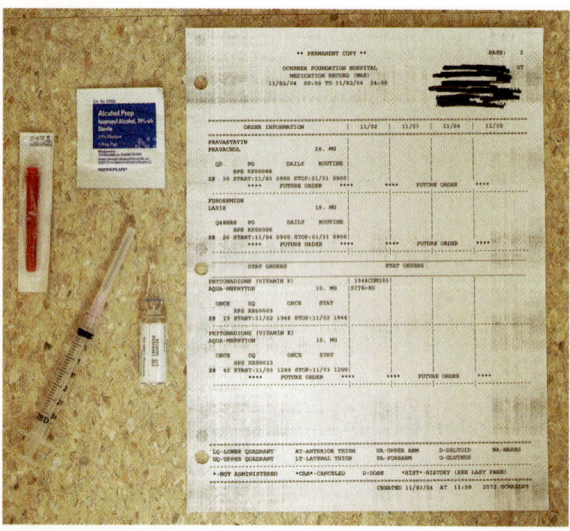

FIGURE 30-34 Syringes, needles, alcohol wipes, and medication ampules are used to withdraw medication from an ampule. DELMAR/CENGAGE LEARNING

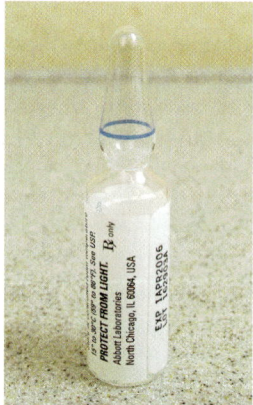

FIGURE 30-35 Medication Ampule DELMAR/CENGAGE LEARNING

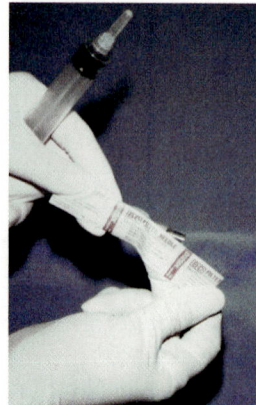

FIGURE 30-36 Select a syringe and a filter needle.
DELMAR/CENGAGE LEARNING

(Continues)

PROCEDURE 30-2
Withdrawing Medication from an Ampule (Continued)

ACTION	RATIONALE

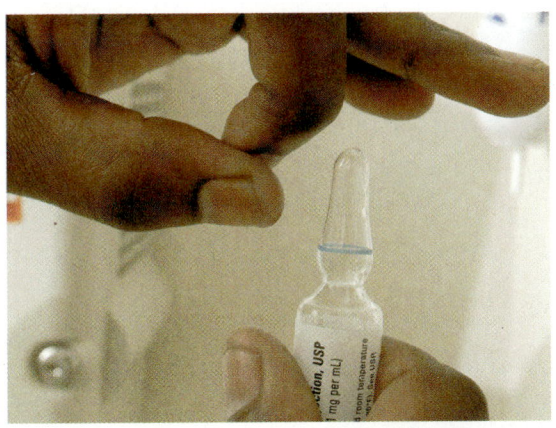

FIGURE 30-37 Flick the neck of the upright ampule to dislodge medication from the top of the vial. DELMAR/CENGAGE LEARNING

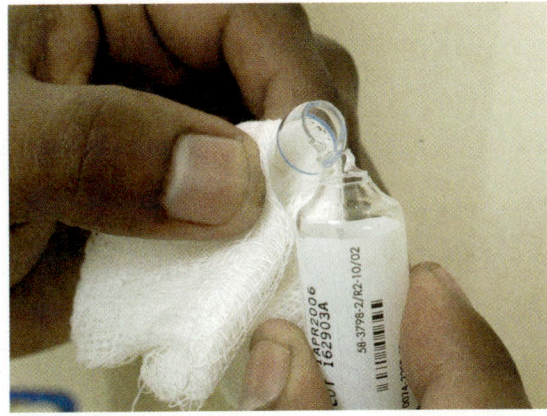

FIGURE 30-38 Wrap gauze or alcohol pad around the neck to protect fingers. Snap off the top in a quick outward motion. DELMAR/CENGAGE LEARNING

9. Wrap the sterile gauze pad around the neck and snap off the top in an outward motion directed away from self (see Figure 30-38).

9. The gauze prevents the nurse from being cut by the jagged edge of the broken ampule. The outward motion provides added safety for the nurse.

10. Invert ampule and place the needle into the liquid. Gently withdraw medication into the syringe (see Figure 30-39).

10. Inverting the ampule allows all the medication to be withdrawn into the syringe. Surface tension will hold the medication in the ampule until the negative pressure of the syringe barrel draws it into the syringe.

11. Alternately, place the ampule on the counter, hold and tilt slightly with the nondominant hand. Insert the needle below the level of liquid and gently draw liquid into the syringe, tilting the ampule as needed to reach all the liquid.

11. While it is more difficult to read the syringe calibrations, it is easier to hold the ampule steady. Choose the method most comfortable for you.

12. Remove the filter needle and replace with the safety injection needle (see Figure 30-40).

12. The filter needle is designed to trap glass particles and must not be used for client injections.

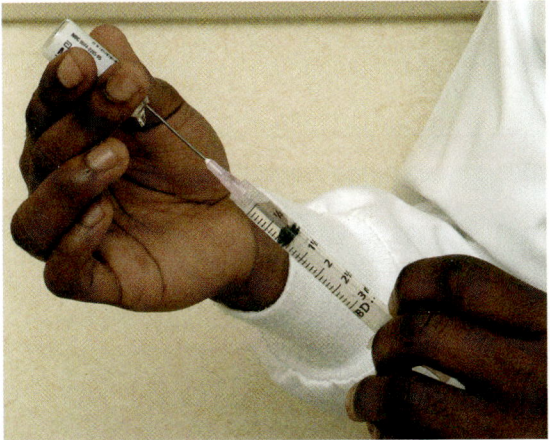

FIGURE 30-39 Invert ampule and gently draw the liquid into the syringe. DELMAR/CENGAGE LEARNING

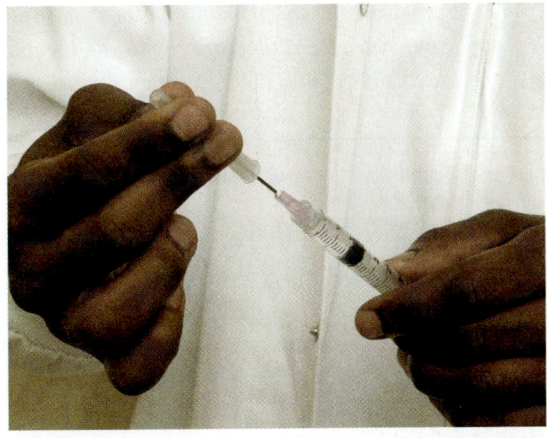

FIGURE 30-40 Remove the filter needle and replace with the injection needle. DELMAR/CENGAGE LEARNING

(Continues)

PROCEDURE 30-2
Withdrawing Medication from an Ampule (Continued)

ACTION	RATIONALE

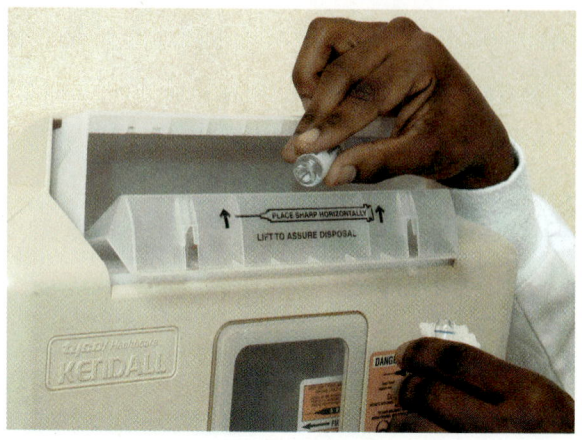

FIGURE 30-41 Dispose of the filter needle, ampule, and ampule top in an appropriate container. DELMAR/CENGAGE LEARNING

13. Dispose of filter needle and glass ampule (including lid) in appropriate sharps container (see Figure 30-41).

14. Label the syringe with drug, dose, date, and time.

15. Wash hands/hand hygiene.

13. Needles or sharp glass objects must always be disposed of in puncture and leak-proof containers in order to provide safety for clients and health care workers.

14. Prevents medication errors from taking place.

15. Decreases transmission of microorganisms.

delegation tip

The skill of medication administration is not delegated to ancillary personnel in acute care settings. This may vary in state or federal institutions. Ancillary personnel are generally informed about the medications the client is receiving if adverse effects are anticipated or are being monitored.

nursing tips

- *Double-check the vial for the appropriate medication. Be certain that a medication error does not happen.*
- *Verify that the generic name on the vial is the same trade medication that is desired.*
- *Many new medications are coming on the market, often with similar names. Always verify that the medication you are about to use is the medication desired.*

PROCEDURE 30-3
Withdrawing Medication from a Vial

EQUIPMENT
- Medication vial
- Syringe with needle
- Clean workspace

- Alcohol sponge pad
- Gloves (optional)
- Medication administration record (MAR)

(Continues)

PROCEDURE 30-3
Withdrawing Medication from a Vial (Continued)

ACTION	RATIONALE
1. Wash hands/hand hygiene; secure supplies (see Figure 30-42). Apply gloves (optional).	1. Decreases transmission of microorganisms.
2. Select the appropriate vial (see Figure 30-43).	2. Prevents medication errors.
3. Verify prescribing practitioner's orders.	3. Prevents medication errors.
4. Check expiration date.	4. Avoids giving expired medication, which may have altered potency.
5. Determine the route of medication delivery, and select the appropriate size syringe and needle.	5. The route of medication delivery is essential to knowing what size syringe and needle will be needed.
6. While holding the syringe at eye level, withdraw the plunger to the desired volume of medication.	6. Holding the syringe at eye level makes it easier to read the syringe calibrations and increases accuracy.
7. Clean the rubber top of the vial with a 70% alcohol pad. Use a circular motion starting at the center and working out.	7. Ensures that the center of the rubber top is the cleanest area for needle entry. Reduces potential contamination with microorganisms.
8. Using sterile technique, uncap the needle (see Figure 30-44).	8. Prevents spread of microorganisms.
9. Lay the needle cap on a clean surface.	9. Prevents spread of microorganisms.

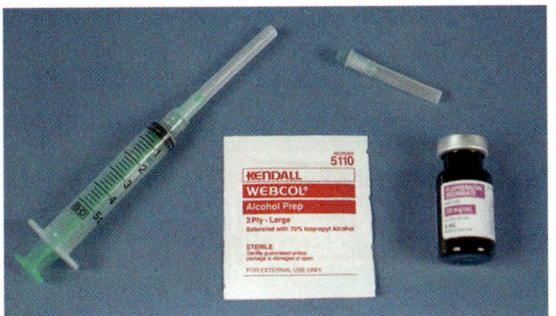

FIGURE 30-42 Syringe, needle, vial of medication, and alcohol wipe are used to withdraw medication from a vial. DELMAR/CENGAGE LEARNING

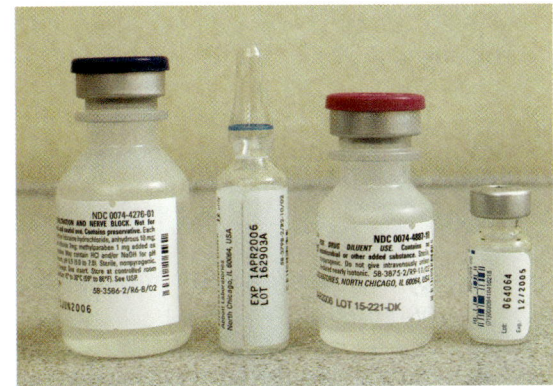

FIGURE 30-43 Carefully select the medication ordered. DELMAR/CENGAGE LEARNING

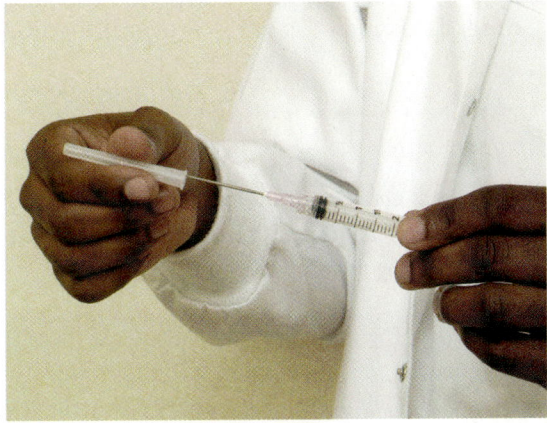

FIGURE 30-44 Using sterile technique, uncap the needle. DELMAR/CENGAGE LEARNING

(Continues)

PROCEDURE 30-3
Withdrawing Medication from a Vial (Continued)

ACTION	RATIONALE

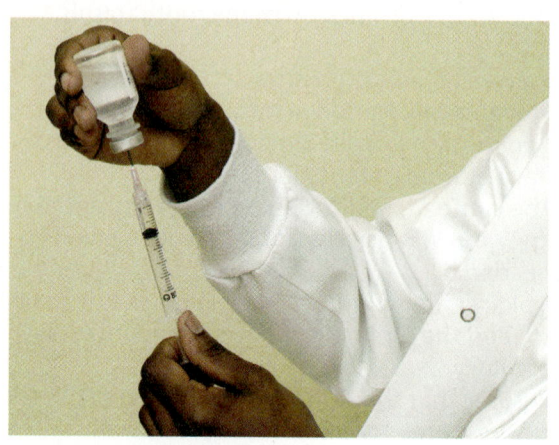

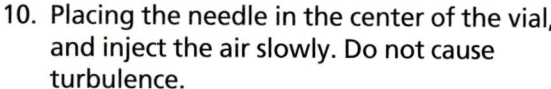

FIGURE 30-45 Invert the vial and slowly withdraw the medication until the appropriate dosage has been reached. DELMAR/CENGAGE LEARNING

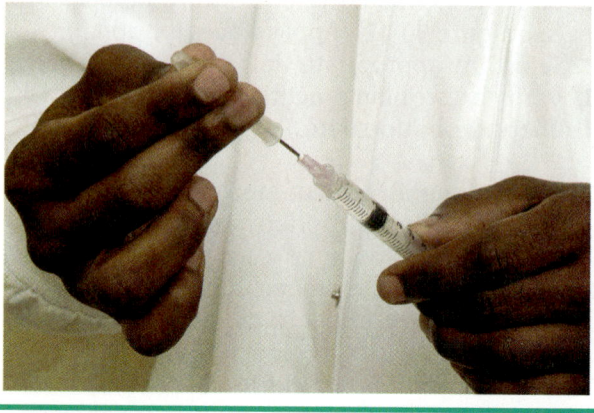

FIGURE 30-46 Follow the institutional policy regarding recapping needles. DELMAR/CENGAGE LEARNING

ACTION	RATIONALE
10. Placing the needle in the center of the vial, and inject the air slowly. Do not cause turbulence.	10. Adding air prevents the buildup of negative pressure in the vial. Injecting quickly may cause turbulence, which can result in air bubbles forming within the vial, which could affect the accuracy of the volume of liquid being withdrawn.
11. Invert the vial and slowly, using gentle negative pressure, withdraw the medication. Keep the needle tip in the liquid.	11. Decreases the number of air bubbles that tend to form with unsteady, fast, jerky motions. Keeping the needle tip in the liquid prevents drawing in air.
12. With the syringe at eye level, determine that the appropriate dose has been reached by volume (see Figure 30-45).	12. Ensures client receives the ordered dose of medication.
13. Slowly withdraw the needle from the vial. Follow the institution's policy regarding recapping and changing needles (see Figure 30-46).	13. Avoids splatter of medication and potential contamination of nearby supplies. Keeps the needle sterile.
14. Using ink, mark the current date and time and initials on the vial.	14. Prevents using a medication that has been opened too long per institutional protocol.
15. Label the syringe with drug, dose, date, and time.	15. Prevents medication errors.
16. Wash hands/hand hygiene.	16. Decreases transmission of microorganisms.

delegation tip

The skill of medication administration is not delegated to ancillary personnel in acute care settings. This may vary in state or federal institutions. Ancillary personnel are generally informed about the medications the client is receiving if adverse effects are anticipated or are being monitored.

nursing tips

- *Use the Z-track method routinely.*
- *Palpate your landmarks. Do not just visualize them.*
- *At times the medication itself causes pain for the client. Giving the medication slowly will decrease the client's discomfort.*

PROCEDURE 30-4

Mixing Medications from Two Vials into One Syringe

EQUIPMENT

- Medication administration record (MAR)
- Medication vials
- Syringe
- Alcohol wipes

ACTION	RATIONALE
1. Check MAR against the prescribing practitioner's written orders.	1. Ensures accuracy in the administration of the medication.
2. Check for drug allergies.	2. Decreases risk of allergic reaction such as hives, urticaria, or anaphylactic shock.
3. Wash hands/hand hygiene.	3. Decreases transmission of microorganisms.
4. Gather the equipment needed (see Figure 30-47). Prepare the medication for one client at a time.	4. Promotes organization. Ensures that the right client receives the right medications.
5. Check need for one medication to be drawn up before the other.	5. Determines the order in which medications will be drawn up.
6. Determine the total medication volume (in milliliters) you will have in the syringe when you have finished drawing both medications into the syringe.	6. Determines how much of the second medication will need to be drawn into the syringe.
7. Swab the top of each vial with alcohol (see Figure 30-48).	7. Decreases the transmission of microorganisms.
8. Draw air into the syringe equal to the amount of medication to be drawn up from the second vial (see Figure 30-49 on page 800). Inject air into the second vial, and remove the syringe and needle from the vial (see Figure 30-50 on page 800). Some protocols require changing needles.	8. Avoids creating a vacuum in the second vial. When you draw medication from the second vial, you will not be able to inject air at that time because your syringe will already contain medication from the first vial. If you inject air, you will risk injecting medication and contaminating the second vial.

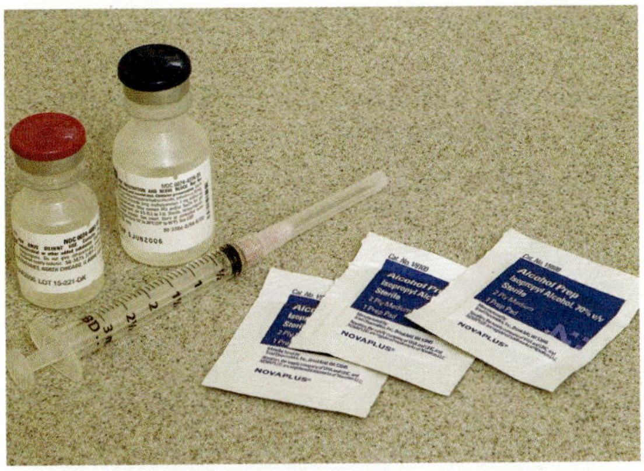

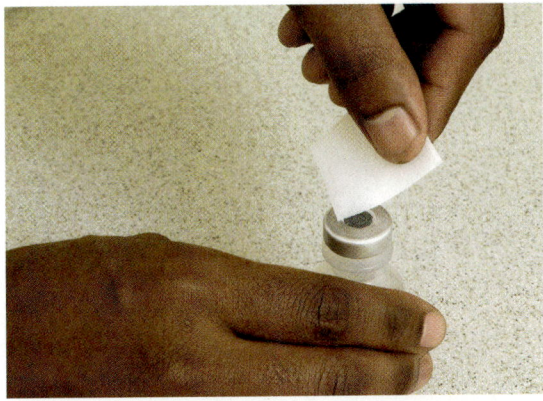

FIGURE 30-47 Syringe with needle, vials, and alcohol wipes are used to draw two medications into one syringe. DELMAR/CENGAGE LEARNING

FIGURE 30-48 Swab the top of each vial with alcohol. DELMAR/CENGAGE LEARNING

(Continues)

PROCEDURE 30-4
Mixing Medications from Two Vials into One Syringe (Continued)

ACTION	RATIONALE

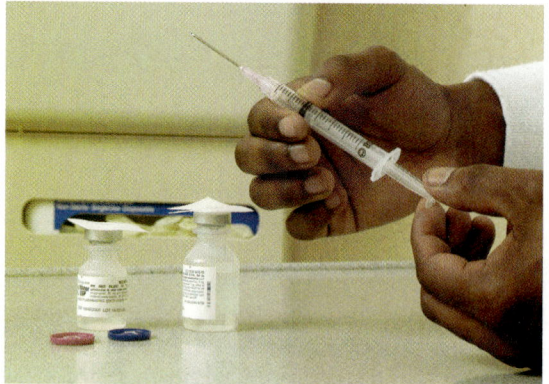

FIGURE 30-49 Draw air into the syringe equal to the amount of medication to be drawn up from the second vial. DELMAR/CENGAGE LEARNING

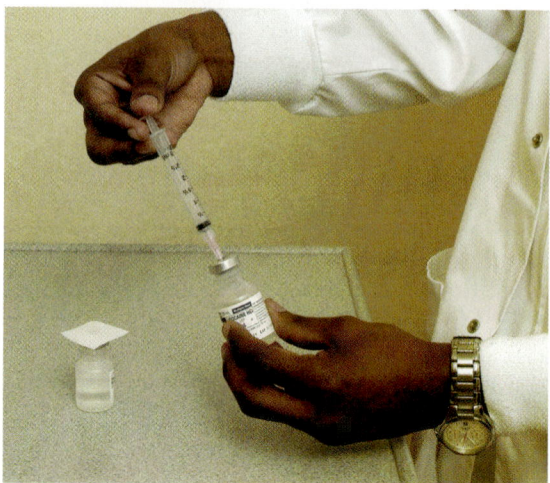

FIGURE 30-50 Inject air into the second vial. DELMAR/CENGAGE LEARNING

9. Draw air into the syringe equal to the amount of medication to be drawn up from the first vial. Inject air into the first vial. Keep the needle and syringe in the vial (see Figure 30-51).

10. Pulling back on the plunger, withdraw the correct amount (in milliliters) of medication from the first vial (see Figure 30-52).

11. Remove the syringe from the first vial, and insert it into the second vial. Withdraw medication from the second vial to the volume (in milliliters) total of both medications summed together (see Figures 30-53 and 30-54 on page 801).

9. Avoids creating a vacuum in the first vial.

10. Draws up the first medication.

11. Draws up the second medication. Drawing up medication equal to the total of both medications ensures the correct amount of second medication is withdrawn.

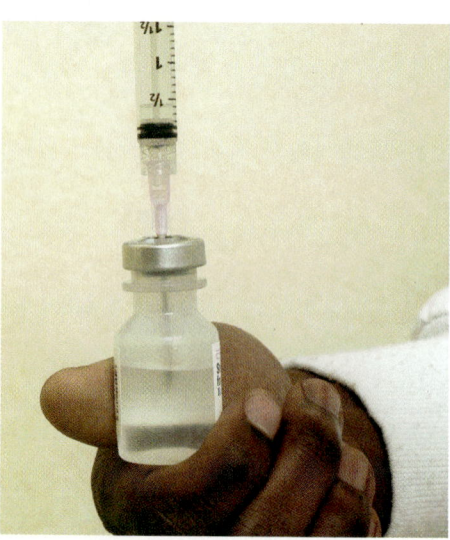

FIGURE 30-51 Inject air into the first vial. DELMAR/CENGAGE LEARNING

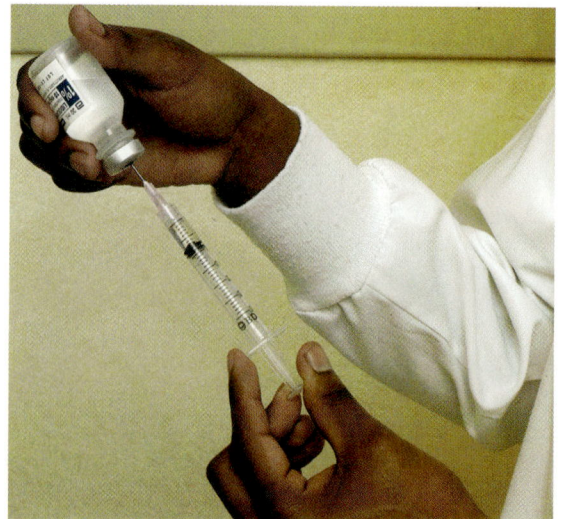

FIGURE 30-52 Withdraw the correct amount of medication from the first vial. DELMAR/CENGAGE LEARNING

(Continues)

PROCEDURE 30-4
Mixing Medications from Two Vials into One Syringe (Continued)

ACTION	RATIONALE

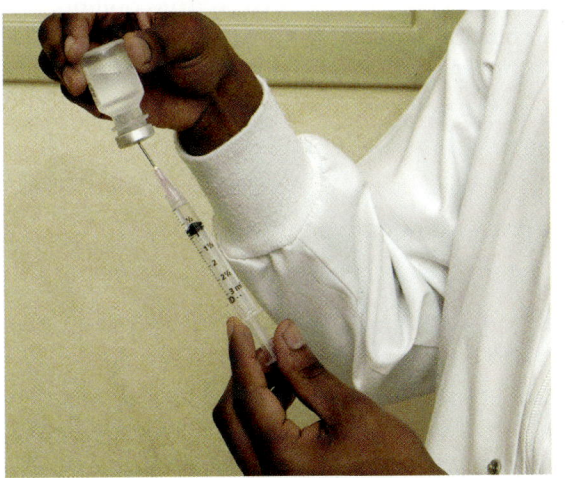

FIGURE 30-53 Withdraw medication from the second vial to the volume of both medications summed together. DELMAR/CENGAGE LEARNING

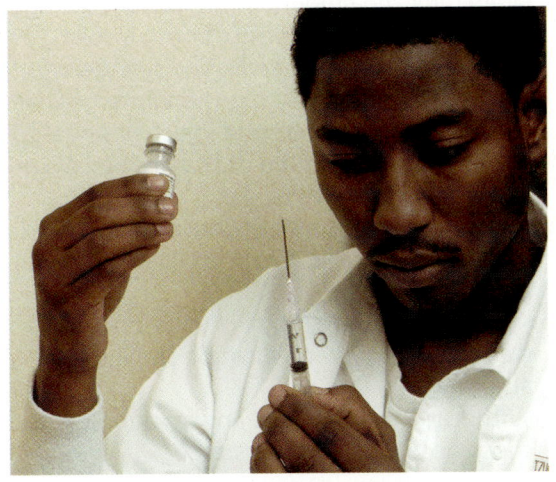

FIGURE 30-54 Double-check the syringe to make sure it contains medication equal to the total volume of both medications summed together. DELMAR/CENGAGE LEARNING

ACTION	RATIONALE
12. Either leave the needle in the second vial until just prior to injecting the medication or follow the institution's policy regarding recapping needles.	12. Prevents needlestick injuries.
13. Wash hands/hand hygiene.	13. Reduces transmission of microorganisms.

MIXING INSULIN

Insulin solutions come premixed and in insulin pens; however, if these are not available, certain insulin solutions can be mixed. The clear insulin (regular, short-acting) is generally drawn up first, and then the cloudy solution (intermediate or long-acting). Mixing insulin can change time of action, absorption, and bioavailability; therefore, check the manufacturers' information regarding types of insulin, and carefully assess response of client. Before administering insulin, dosage must be double-checked by two professionals. An inaccurate dose of insulin can be life threatening.

ACTION	RATIONALE
14. Check client's most recent blood glucose level, dietary intake, oral intake status (e.g., NPO), and signs and symptoms related to glucose level.	14. Prevents hypoglycemic episodes. May need to check with prescribing practitioner regarding insulin dosage. Prevents wasting of insulin if not to be given.
15. Repeat Actions 1–4.	15. See Rationales 1–4.
16. Remove caps from insulin vials (if necessary). Gently rotate (never shake) the suspension insulin (e.g., NPH, intermediate, or long-acting insulin) until no sediment is at the bottom of the vial.	16. Long-acting insulin is a cloudy suspension and needs to be completely and gently mixed to ensure that all particles are distributed equally in suspension.
17. Wipe off tops on insulin vials with alcohol sponge.	17. Removes surface microorganisms.

(Continues)

PROCEDURE 30-4
Mixing Medications from Two Vials into One Syringe (Continued)

ACTION	RATIONALE
18. Draw back the amount of air into the syringe that equals the total dose of both insulin solutions. Insert the needle and syringe into the vial with the cloudy, suspension (intermediate or long-acting insulin), and inject air equal to the amount to be given of that insulin. Do not touch solution with needle.	18. Prevents negative pressure from pulling solution into vial for next use. Prevents contamination with different types of insulin.
19. Insert needle and syringe into vial of short-acting or regular insulin, and inject air equal to the amount to be given.	19. Prevents negative pressure in vial.
20. Keep needle and syringe in solution. Invert vial and withdraw medication slowly and accurately.	20. Slow withdrawal can help prevent air trapping and ensure accuracy.
21. Withdraw needle, expel any air bubbles, and check dose with another nurse.	21. Insulin must be double-checked for accuracy because of the dangers of administration of an inaccurate dose.
22. Invert the vial with longer-acting insulin, holding plunger carefully, and withdraw long-acting insulin, being careful not to inject any regular insulin into vial. Check dose with another nurse.	22. Prevents withdrawal of air and too much insulin. If too much insulin is withdrawn, the solution must be discarded and the procedure repeated. If regular insulin is accidentally injected into a vial of cloudy insulin, the vial must be discarded.
23. Store insulin properly according to manufacturer's specifications.	23. Ensures effective product.
24. Wash hands/hand hygiene; prepare to administer injection.	24. Prevents transmission of microorganisms.

delegation tip

The skill of medication administration is not delegated to ancillary personnel in acute care settings. This may vary in state or federal institutions. Ancillary personnel are generally informed about the medications the client is receiving if adverse effects are anticipated or are being monitored.

nursing tips

Manufacturers are required by law to put the expiration date on all drugs. The nurse should check the expiration date to ensure that the drug is current. Outdated drugs should be returned to the pharmacy for proper disposal.

PROCEDURE 30-5
Medication Administration: Intradermal

EQUIPMENT
- Tuberculin syringe, 1 mL
- Needle (25- to 27-gauge, 1/4- to 5/8-inch)
- Antiseptic or alcohol swabs
- Medication ampule or vial
- Medication card or medication administration record (MAR)
- Disposable gloves

(Continues)

PROCEDURE 30-5
Medication Administration: Intradermal (Continued)

ACTION	RATIONALE
1. Wash hands/hand hygiene; put on clean gloves.	1. Reduces transmission of microorganisms.
2. In the inpatient setting, close door or curtains around bed and keep gown or sheet draped over body. In the outpatient setting, close door to exam or treatment room. Identify client.	2. Provides privacy. Ensures medication is given to right client.
3. Select injection site. • Inspect skin for bruises, inflammation, edema, masses, tenderness, and sites of previous injections. • Forearm site should be 3 to 4 finger widths below antecubital space and one hand width above wrists on inner aspect of forearm.	3. Injection site should be free of lesions. Repeated daily injections should be rotated. Ensures a clear site for interpreting results.
4. Select 1/4- to 5/8-inch, 25- to 27-gauge needle (see Figure 30-55).	4. Ensures that needle will be injected into the intradermis.
5. Assist client into a comfortable position. Forearm site: Relax the arm with elbow and forearm extended on a flat surface. Distract client by talking about an interesting subject.	5. Relaxation minimizes discomfort. Distraction reduces anxiety.
6. Use antiseptic swab in a circular motion to clean skin at site.	6. Circular motion and mechanical action of swab remove secretions containing microorganisms.
7. While holding the swab between fingers of nondominant hand, pull cap from needle.	7. Swab remains accessible during procedure. Prevents contamination of needle.
8. Administer injection: • With nondominant hand, stretch skin over site with forefinger and thumb. • Insert needle slowly at a 10° to 15° angle, bevel up, until resistance is felt; then advance to no more than 1/8 inch below the skin. The needle tip should be seen through the skin. • Slowly inject the medication. Resistance will be felt. • Note a small bleb, like a mosquito bite, forming under the skin surface (see Figure 30-56).	8. • Needle penetrates tight skin easier than loose skin. • Ensures needle tip is in the dermis. • Dermal layer is tight and does not expand easily when fluid is injected. • Indicates the medication was deposited in the dermis.

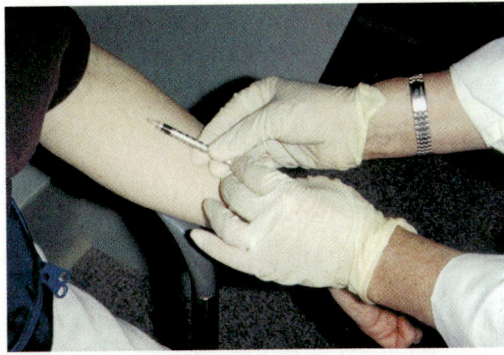

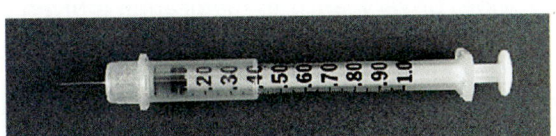

FIGURE 30-55 Syringes come in many sizes. Select a 1-mL tuberculin safety syringe for intradermal injections. DELMAR/CENGAGE LEARNING

FIGURE 30-56 Note a small bleb, like a mosquito bite, forming under the skin surface as the medication is injected. DELMAR/CENGAGE LEARNING

(Continues)

PROCEDURE 30-5
Medication Administration: Intradermal (Continued)

ACTION	RATIONALE
9. Withdraw the needle while applying gentle pressure with the antiseptic swab.	9. Supporting tissue around injection site minimizes discomfort.
10. Do not massage the site.	10. Prevents medication from being dispersed into the tissue and altering test results.
11. Assist the client to a comfortable position.	11. Promotes comfort.
12. Discard the uncapped needle and syringe in a safe receptacle.	12. Decreases risk of needlestick.
13. Remove gloves; wash hands/hand hygiene.	13. Reduces transmission of microorganisms.

delegation tip

The skill of medication administration is not delegated to ancillary personnel in acute care settings. This may vary in state or federal institutions. Ancillary personnel are generally informed about the medications the client is receiving if adverse effects are anticipated or are being monitored.

nursing tips

- *Remember to inject the needle with the bevel up so the medication is not injected into the subcutaneous tissue.*
- *Remember when documenting the site of the injection to indicate left or right arm, as markings often wash off.*
- *Mark sites with skin marking pen, if appropriate. This avoids confusion when evaluating results.*
- *If a bleb or wheal does not appear after an intradermal injection, select another site and repeat injection.*

PROCEDURE 30-6
Medication Administration: Subcutaneous

EQUIPMENT
- Syringe appropriate for the medication being given
- Needle (25- to 27-gauge, 3/8- to 5/8-inch)
- Antiseptic or alcohol swabs
- Medication ampule or vial
- Medication administration record (MAR)
- Disposable gloves

ACTION	RATIONALE
1. Wash hands/hand hygiene; put on clean gloves. Select the appropriate syringe for the mediation being given (see Figure 30-57 on page 805).	1. Reduces number of microorganisms.
2. Close door or curtains around bed, and keep gown or sheet draped over client. Identify client.	2. Provides privacy. Ensures medication is given to right client.
3. Select injection site. • Inspect skin for bruises, inflammation, edema, masses, tenderness, and sites of previous injections and avoid these areas. • Use subcutaneous tissue around the abdomen, lateral aspects of upper arm or thigh, or scapular area.	3. Injection site should be free of lesions. • Repeated daily injections should be rotated. • Avoids injury to underlying nerves, bones, and blood vessels.

(Continues)

PROCEDURE 30-6
Medication Administration: Subcutaneous (Continued)

ACTION	RATIONALE

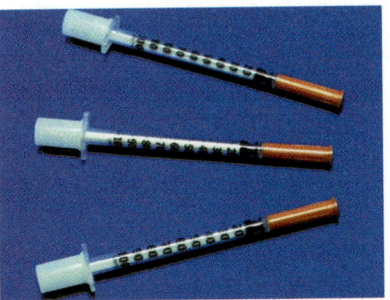

FIGURE 30-57 100-unit insulin syringes are used to administer insulin subcutaneously. DELMAR/CENGAGE LEARNING

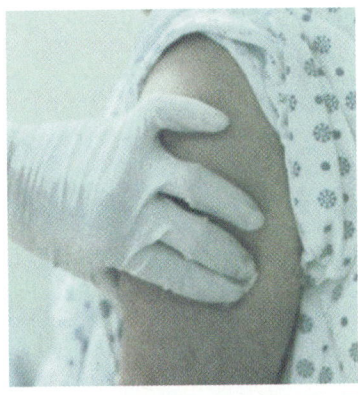

FIGURE 30-58 Pinch the skin with the nondominant hand.
DELMAR/CENGAGE LEARNING

ACTION

4. Select needle size:
   • Measure skinfold by grasping skin between thumb and forefinger.
   • Be sure needle is one-half the length of the skinfold from top to bottom.
5. Assist client into a comfortable position:
   • Relax the arm, leg, or abdomen.
   • Distract client by talking about an interesting subject or explaining what you are doing step by step.
6. Use antiseptic swab to clean skin at site.

7. While holding swab between fingers of nondominant hand, pull cap from needle.
8. Administer injection:
   • Hold syringe between thumb and forefinger of dominant hand like a dart.
   • Pinch skin with nondominant hand (see Figure 30-58).
   • Inject needle quickly and firmly (like a dart) at a 45° to 90° angle (see Figure 30-59 on page 806).
   • Release the skin.
   • Grasp the lower end of the syringe with non-dominant hand, and position dominant hand to the end of the plunger. Do not move the syringe.
   • Pull back on the plunger to ascertain that the needle is not in a vein. If no blood appears, slowly inject the medication. (Aspiration is contraindicated with some medications; check with the pharmacy if you are unclear.)

RATIONALE

4. Ensures that needle will be injected into subcutaneous tissue.

5. Relaxation minimizes discomfort. Distraction reduces anxiety.

6. Circular motion and mechanical action of swab remove microorganisms.
7. Swab remains accessible during procedure. Prevents contamination of needle.
8.
   • Quick, smooth injection is easier with proper position of syringe.
   • Needle penetrates tight skin easier than loose skin. Pinching skin elevates subcutaneous tissue.
   • Quick, firm injection minimizes discomfort. Angle depends on amount of subcutaneous tissue present and the site used.
   • Injection requires smooth manipulation of syringe parts. Movement of syringe may cause discomfort.
   • Aspiration of blood indicates intravenous placement of needle, so procedure may have to be abandoned.

(Continues)

PROCEDURE 30-6
Medication Administration: Subcutaneous (Continued)

ACTION	RATIONALE

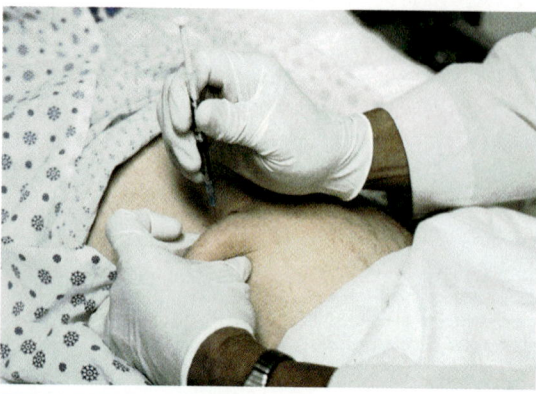

FIGURE 30-59 When injecting at a 90° angle, hold the syringe like a dart and pierce the skin quickly and firmly. DELMAR/CENGAGE LEARNING

ACTION	RATIONALE
9. Remove hand from injection site and quickly withdraw the needle. Apply pressure with the antiseptic swab. Do not push down on the needle with the swab while withdrawing it, as this will cause more pain.	9. Supporting tissue around injection site minimizes discomfort. Removing hand before withdrawing needle reduces chance of needlestick.
10. Apply pressure. Some medications should not be massaged. Ask the pharmacy if you are unclear.	10. Stimulates circulation and improves drug distribution and absorption.
11. Assist the client to a comfortable position.	11. Promotes comfort and encourages client to remain still.
12. Discard the uncapped needle and syringe in a disposable needle receptacle.	12. Decreases risk of needlestick.
13. Remove gloves; wash hands/hand hygiene.	13. Reduces transmission of microorganisms.

delegation tip

The skill of medication administration is not delegated to ancillary personnel in acute care settings. This may vary in state or federal institutions. Ancillary personnel are generally informed about the medications the client is receiving if adverse effects are anticipated or are being monitored.

nursing tips

- *A simple rule to follow: If 2 inches of tissue can be grasped, the needle should be inserted at a 90° angle. If 1 inch of tissue can be grasped, the needle should be inserted at a 45° angle.*
- *Do not push a needle through the skin; insert it quickly and smoothly.*
- *Divert the client's attention by engaging in conversation.*

PROCEDURE 30-7

Medication Administration: Intramuscular

EQUIPMENT

- Safety syringe (1- to 3-mL)
- Safety needle (19- to 23-gauge, 11/4 to 11/2 inches)
- Antiseptic or alcohol swabs
- Medication ampule or vial
- Medication administration record (MAR)
- Disposable gloves

ACTION	RATIONALE
1. Wash hands/hand hygiene; put on clean gloves.	1. Reduces number of microorganisms.
2. Close door or curtains around bed, and keep gown or sheet draped over client. Identify client.	2. Provides privacy. Ensures medication is given to the right client.
3. Select injection site. • Inspect skin for bruises, inflammation, edema, masses, tenderness, and sites of previous injections. • Use anatomic landmarks.	3. Injection site should be free of lesions. • Repeated daily injections should be rotated. • Avoids injury to underlying nerves, bones, and blood vessels. Site should be selected based on muscle development, type and amount of medication, and comfortable access to site.
4. Select needle size: Assess size and weight of client and site to be used. If appropriate, select prefilled syringe plunger, barrel, and needle cartridge (see Figures 30-60 and 30-61).	4. Ensures that needle will be injected into the muscle.
5. Assist client into a comfortable position: • For vastus lateralis, lying flat or supine with knee slightly flexed. • For ventrogluteal, lying on side or back with knee and hip slightly flexed. • For deltoid, standing with arm relaxed at side, sitting with lower arm relaxed on lap, or lying flat with lower arm relaxed across abdomen. • Distract client by talking about an interesting subject.	5. Relaxation minimizes discomfort. Distraction reduces anxiety.
6. Use antiseptic swab to clean skin at site.	6. Circular motion and mechanical action of swab remove secretions containing microorganisms.
7. While holding swab between fingers of nondominant hand, pull cap from needle.	7. Swab remains accessible during procedure. Prevents contamination of needle.

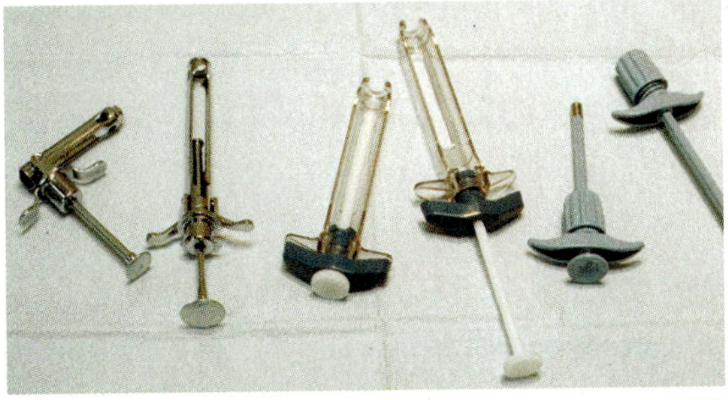

FIGURE 30-60 There are many types of prefilled syringe plungers in use today. DELMAR/CENGAGE LEARNING

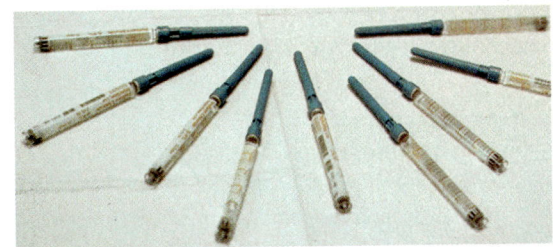

FIGURE 30-61 Prefilled Barrel and Needle Cartridges
DELMAR/CENGAGE LEARNING

(Continues)

PROCEDURE 30-7
Medication Administration: Intramuscular (Continued)

ACTION	RATIONALE

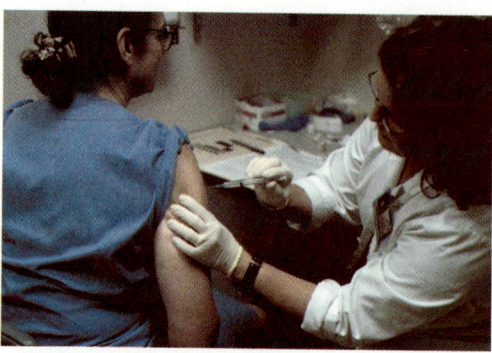

FIGURE 30-62 Inject needle quickly and firmly at a 90° angle. DELMAR/CENGAGE LEARNING

8. Administer injection:
   • Hold syringe between thumb and forefinger of dominant hand like a dart.
   • Spread skin tightly or pinch a generous section of tissue firmly—for cachectic clients.
   • Inject needle quickly and firmly (like a dart) at a 90° angle (see Figure 30-62).
   • Release the skin.
   • Grasp the lower end of the syringe with nondominant hand, and position dominant hand to the end of the plunger. Do not move the syringe.
   • Pull back on the plunger and aspirate to ascertain if needle is in a vein. If no blood appears, slowly inject the medication.
9. Remove nondominant hand, and quickly withdraw the needle. Apply pressure with the antiseptic swab.
10. Apply pressure. Certain protocols suggest gentle massage action.

11. Assist the client to a comfortable position.
12. Close the safety cap, and discard the uncapped needle and syringe in a specified biohazard sharps container.
13. Remove gloves, and wash hands/hand hygiene.

8.
   • Quick, smooth injection is easier with proper position of syringe.
   • Needle penetrates tight skin more easily than loose skin.
   • Quick, firm injection minimizes discomfort.
   • Injection requires smooth manipulation of syringe parts. Movement of syringe may cause discomfort.
   • Aspiration of blood indicates intravenous placement of needle, so procedure may have to be abandoned.

9. Supporting tissue around injection site minimizes discomfort. Removing hand prior to withdrawing needle prevents needlestick.
10. Pressure prevents medication from leaking out of site. Gentle massage stimulates circulation and improves drug distribution and absorption.
11. Promotes comfort.
12. Decreases risk of needlestick.

13. Reduces transmission of microorganisms.

delegation tip

The skill of medication administration is not delegated to ancillary personnel in acute care settings. This may vary in state or federal institutions. Ancillary personnel are generally informed about the medications the client is receiving if adverse affects are anticipated or are being monitored.

(Continues)

PROCEDURE 30-7
Medication Administration: Intramuscular (Continued)

nursing tips

The nurse should not draw an air bubble when using a plastic disposable syringe, as doing so can dramatically affect the medication dosage.

PROCEDURE 30-8
Medication Administration via Secondary Administration Sets (Piggyback)

EQUIPMENT
- Disposable gloves
- Medication prepared in a labeled infusion bag
- Short microdrip or macrodrip tubing set for piggy-back (needleless system preferred); see Figure 30-63
- Safety sterile needles, 21- or 23-gauge, if needleless system not available
- Antiseptic swab
- Adhesive tape
- IV pole
- Medication administration record (MAR)

ACTION	RATIONALE
1. Check prescribing practitioner's order.	1. Ensures accurate administration of medication.
2. Wash hands/hand hygiene. *Gloves are not necessary if you are adding fluids to an existing infusion line.* Secure IV tubing for piggyback administration (see Figure 30-63).	2. Reduces transmission of microorganisms.
3. Check client's identification bracelet.	3. Ensures medication is given to correct client.
4. Explain procedure and reason drug is being given.	4. Information decreases anxiety.

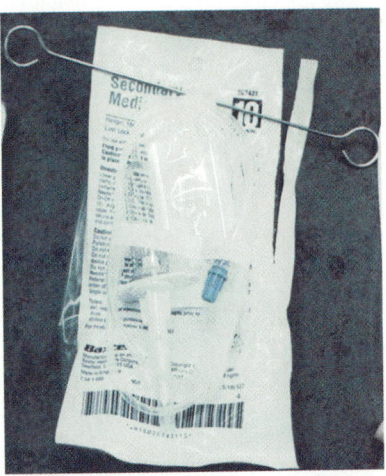

FIGURE 30-63 IV Tubing Set for Piggyback Administration. DELMAR/CENGAGE LEARNING

(Continues)

PROCEDURE 30-8
Medication Administration via Secondary Administration Sets (Piggyback) (Continued)

ACTION	RATIONALE
5. Prepare medication bag: • Close clamp on tubing of infusion set. • Spike medication bag with infusion tubing (see Figure 30-64). • Open clamp (see Figure 30-65). • Allow tubing to be filled with solution to evacuate air from tubing (see Figure 30-66).	5. • Prevents leakage of solution. • Provides a method of infusing the medication into the system. • Allows the solution to fill the tubing. • Prevents air embolus.

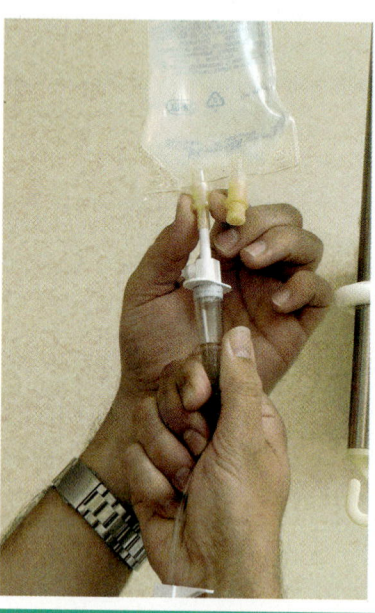

FIGURE 30-64 Spike the medication bag with the infusion tubing. DELMAR/CENGAGE LEARNING

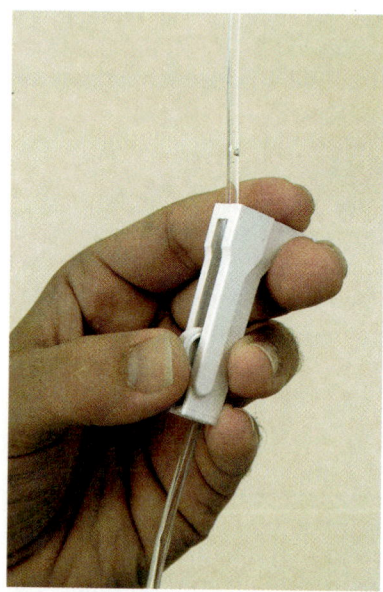

FIGURE 30-65 Open the clamp on the IV tubing. DELMAR/CENGAGE LEARNING

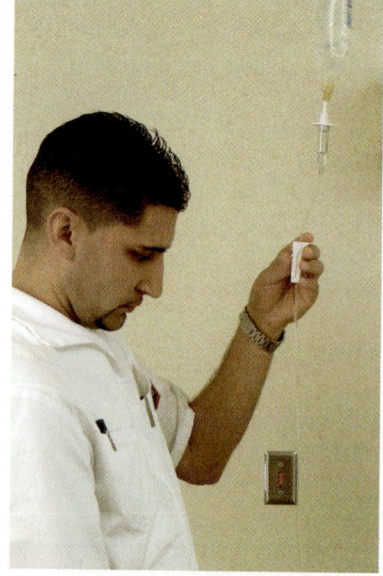

FIGURE 30-66 Allow the tubing to fill with solution. DELMAR/CENGAGE LEARNING

(Continues)

PROCEDURE 30-8
Medication Administration via Secondary Administration Sets (Piggyback) (Continued)

ACTION	RATIONALE

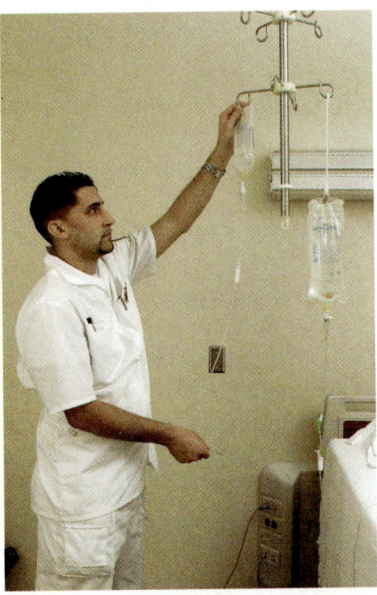

FIGURE 30-67 Hang the piggyback bag higher than the primary IV bag. DELMAR/CENGAGE LEARNING

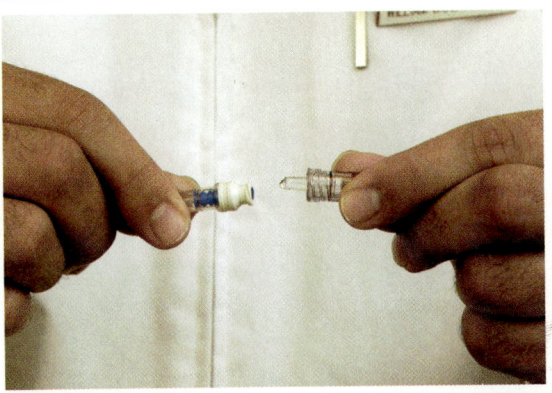

FIGURE 30-68 Remove cap on the needleless system port and connect the needleless system tubing. DELMAR/CENGAGE LEARNING

6. Hang piggyback medication bag above level of primary IV bag. One way to do this is to lower the primary bag using an extender (found in the piggyback tubing package) (see Figure 30-67).
7. Connect piggyback tubing to primary tubing at Y-port:
   - For needleless system, remove cap on port and connect tubing (see Figure 30-68).
   - If a needle is used, clean port with antiseptic swab and insert small-gauge needle into center of port.
   - Secure tubing with adhesive tape.
8. Administer the medication:
   - Check the prescribed length of time for the infusion.
   - Regulate the flow rate of the piggyback by adjusting the regulator clamp (see Figure 30-69 on page 812).
   - Observe whether backflow valve on piggyback has stopped flow of primary infusion during drug administration.
9. Check primary infusion line when medication is finished:
   - Regulate primary infusion rate.
   - Leave secondary bag and tubing in place for next drug administration.
10. Dispose of all used materials, and place needles in needle biohazard sharps container.
11. Wash hands/hand hygiene.

6. Relationship between height of the bags affects the flow rate to the client.

7. Ensures medication in piggyback bag is infused.
   - A needleless system is preferred to prevent accidental needlesticks.
   - A small-gauge needle does less damage to the rubber stopper on the port.
   - Prevents accidental removal of tubing.

8.
   - Each medication has a recommended rate for IV piggyback administration.
   - Medication infuses through primary line.
   - Prevents backup of medication into primary infusion line.

9.
   - Reestablishes primary infusion.
   - Reduces risk for entry of microorganisms by repeated changes of tubing.

10. Reduces transmission of microorganisms.
11. Reduces transmission of microorganisms.

(Continues)

PROCEDURE 30-8
Medication Administration via Secondary Administration Sets (Piggyback) (Continued)

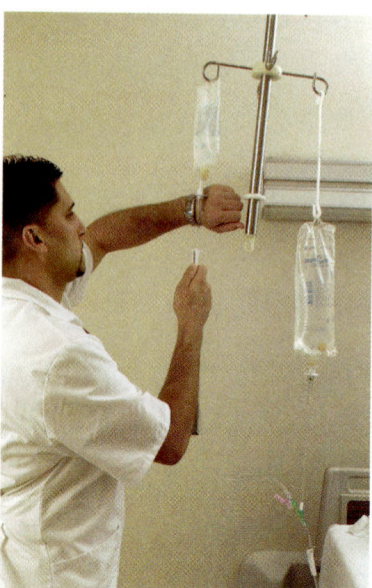

FIGURE 30-69 Regulate the flow rate of the piggyback by adjusting the regulator clamp. DELMAR/CENGAGE LEARNING

delegation tip

The skill of medication administration is not delegated to ancillary personnel in acute care settings. This may vary in state or federal institutions. Ancillary personnel are generally informed about the medications the client is receiving if adverse effects are anticipated or are being monitored.

nursing tips

- *Prepare medication and label in the medication room before approaching the client.*
- *Some IV solutions should be prepared by the pharmacist under the laminar air flow hood to ensure a sterile solution.*
- *Check with the pharmacist or drug text regarding drug compatibility.*

PROCEDURE 30-9
Medication Administration: Eye and Ear

EQUIPMENT
EYE MEDICATION
- Medication administration record (MAR)
- Eye medication
- Tissue or cotton ball
- Nonsterile latex-free gloves (if needed)

EAR MEDICATION
- Medication administration record (MAR)
- Ear medication
- Nonsterile latex-free gloves
- Tissue

(Continues)

PROCEDURE 30-9
Medication Administration: Eye and Ear (Continued)

ACTION	RATIONALE
EYE MEDICATION	
1. Check with the client and the chart for any known allergies or medical conditions that would contraindicate use of the drug.	1. Prevents occurrence of adverse reactions.
2. Gather the necessary equipment.	2. Promotes efficiency.
3. Follow the five rights of drug administration.	3. Promotes safety.
4. Take the medication to the client's room and place on a clean surface.	4. Decreases risk of contamination of bottle cap.
5. Check client's identification armband.	5. Accurately identifies client.
6. Explain the procedure to the client; inquire if the client wants to instill medication. If so, assess the client's ability to do so.	6. Reduces client's anxiety and enhances collaboration; some clients are used to instilling their own medication.
7. Wash hands/hand hygiene; don nonsterile latex-free gloves if needed.	7. Decreases contact with bodily fluids.
8. Place client in a supine position with the head slightly hyperextended.	8. Minimizes drainage of medication through the tear duct.
INSTILLING EYEDROPS	
9. Remove cap from eye bottle, and place cap on its side.	9. Prevents contamination of the bottle cap.
10. Squeeze the prescribed amount of medication into the eyedropper.	10. Ensures correct dose.
11. Place a tissue below the lower lid.	11. Absorbs the medication that flows from the eye.
12. With dominant hand, hold eyedropper 1/2–3/4 inch above the eyeball; rest hand on client's forehead to stabilize.	12. Reduces risk of dropper touching eye structure and prevents injury to the eye.
13. Place hand on cheekbone and expose lower conjunctival sac by pulling down on cheek.	13. Stabilizes hand and prevents systemic absorption of eye medication.
14. Instruct the client to look up, and drop prescribed number of drops into center of conjunctival sac (see Figure 30-70 on page 814).	14. Reduces stimulation of the blink reflex; prevents injury to the cornea.
15. Instruct client to gently close eyes and move eyes. Briefly place fingers on either side of the client's nose to close the tear ducts and prevent the medication from draining out of the eye (see Figure 30-71 on page 814).	15. Distributes solution over conjunctival surface and anterior eyeball.
16. Remove gloves; wash hands/hand hygiene.	16. Reduces transmission of microorganisms.
17. Record on the MAR the route, site (which eye), and time administered.	17. Provides documentation that medication was given.
EYE OINTMENT APPLICATION	
18. Repeat Actions 1–8.	18. See Rationales 1–8.
19. Lower lid:	19.
• With nondominant hand, gently separate client's eyelids with thumb and finger and grasp lower lid near margin immediately below the lashes; exert pressure downward over the bony prominence of the cheek.	• Provides access to the lower lid. • Reduces stimulation of the blink reflex and keeps cornea out of the way of the medication. • Ensures drug is applied to entire lid.

(Continues)

PROCEDURE 30-9
Medication Administration: Eye and Ear (Continued)

ACTION	RATIONALE

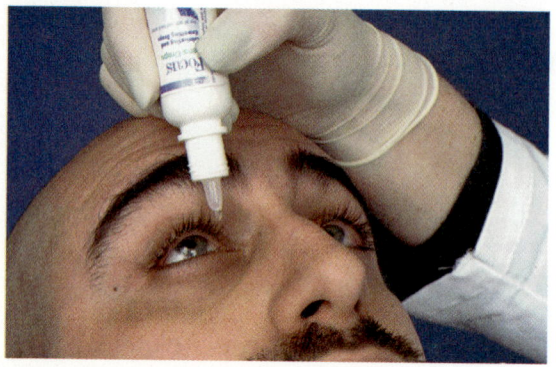

FIGURE 30-70 Instruct the client to look up. Administer prescribed number of drops into the center of the conjunctival sac. DELMAR/CENGAGE LEARNING

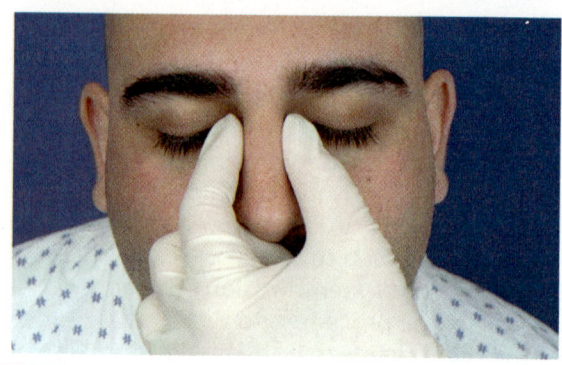

FIGURE 30-71 Placing the fingers on the sides of the client's nose closes the tear ducts and prevents the medication from draining out of the eye. DELMAR/CENGAGE LEARNING

- Instruct client to look up.
- Apply eye ointment along inside edge of the entire lower eyelid, from inner to outer canthus.
20. Upper lid:
- Instruct client to look down.
- With nondominant hand, gently grasp client's lashes near center of upper lid with thumb and index finger, and draw lid up and away from eyeball.
- Squeeze ointment along upper lid starting at inner canthus.
21. Repeat Actions 16 and 17.

MEDICATION DISK
22. Repeat Actions 1–8.
23. Open sterile package and press dominant, sterile gloved finger against the oval disk so that it lies lengthwise across fingertip.
24. Instruct the client to look up.

25. With nondominant hand, gently pull the client's lower eyelid down and place the disk horizontally in the conjunctival sac.
- Then pull the lower eyelid out, up, and over the disk.
- Instruct the client to blink several times.
- If disk is still visible, repeat steps.
- Once the disk is in place, instruct the client to gently press the fingers against the closed lids; do not rub eyes or move the disk across the cornea.
- If the disk falls out, pick it up, rinse under cool water, and reinsert.

20.
- Keeps cornea out of the way of the medication.
- Ensures medication is applied to entire length of lid.

21. See Rationales 16 and 17.

22. See Rationales 1–8.
23. Promotes sticking of disk to fingertip.

24. Reduces stimulation of the blink reflex and keeps cornea out of the way of the medication.
25. Allows the disk to automatically adhere to the eye.
- Secures the disk in the conjunctival sac.
- Allows the disk to settle into place.
- Ensures correct placement of the disk.
- Secures disk placement. Prevents corneal scratches.
- Preserves medication. This is not a sterile procedure. Health care provider must wear gloves to pick up disk.

(Continues)

PROCEDURE 30-9
Medication Administration: Eye and Ear (Continued)

ACTION	RATIONALE
26. If the disk is prescribed for both eyes, repeat Actions 23–25.	26. Ensures both eyes are treated at the same time.
27. Repeat Actions 15–17.	27. See Rationales 15–17.

REMOVING AN EYE MEDICATION DISK

28. Repeat Actions 3 and 5–8.	28. See Rationales 3 and 5–8.
29. Remove the disk:	29.
• With nondominant hand, invert the lower eyelid and identify the disk.	• Exposes the disk for removal.
• If the disk is located in the upper eye, instruct the client to close the eye, and place your finger on the closed eyelid. Apply gentle, long, circular strokes; instruct client to open the eye. Disk should be located in corner of eye. With your fingertip, slide the disk to the lower lid, and then proceed.	• Safely moves the disk to the lower conjunctival sac. • Safely removes the disk without scratching the cornea.
• With dominant hand, use the forefinger to slide the disk onto the lid and out of the client's eye.	
30. Remove gloves; wash hands/hand hygiene.	30. Reduces transmission of microorganisms.
31. Record on the MAR the removal of the disk.	31. Provides documentation that the disk was removed.

EAR MEDICATION

1. Check with client and chart for any known allergies.	1. Prevents the occurrence of hypersensitivity reactions.
2. Check the MAR against the prescribing practitioner's written orders.	2. Ensures accuracy in identification of the medication.
3. Wash hands/hand hygiene.	3. Reduces transmission of microorganisms.
4. Calculate the dose (see Figure 30-72).	4. Ensures administration of correct dose.
5. Use the identification armband to properly identify the client.	5. Ensures correct client.

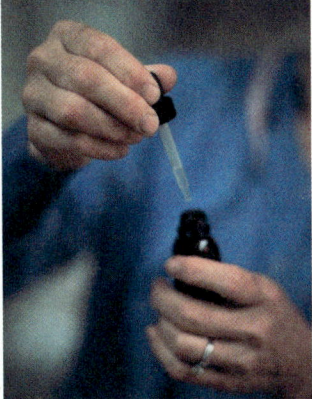

FIGURE 30-72 Calculate the correct dose and draw medication into the ear dropper. DELMAR/CENGAGE LEARNING

(Continues)

PROCEDURE 30-9
Medication Administration: Eye and Ear (Continued)

ACTION	RATIONALE

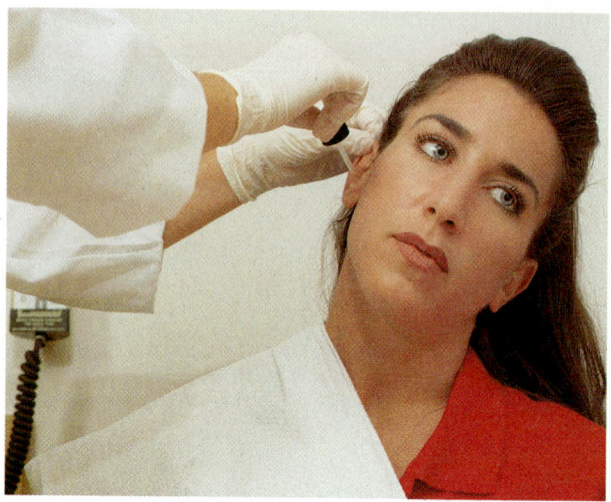

FIGURE 30-73 Slowly instill the drops, holding the dropper at least 1/2 inch above the ear canal. DELMAR/CENGAGE LEARNING

ACTION	RATIONALE
6. Explain the procedure to the client.	6. Enhances cooperation.
7. Place the client in a side-lying position with the affected ear facing up.	7. Facilitates administration of the medication.
8. Straighten the ear canal by pulling the pinna down and back for children less than 3 years of age or upward and outward in adults and older children.	8. Opens the canal and facilitates introduction of the medication.
9. Slowly instill the drops into the ear canal by holding the dropper at least 1/2 inch above the ear canal (see Figure 30-73).	9. Prevents injury to the ear canal.
10. Ask the client to maintain the position for 2 to 3 minutes.	10. Allows for distribution of the medication.
11. Place a cotton ball on the outermost part of the canal.	11. Prevents the medication from escaping when the client changes to a sitting or standing position.
12. Wash hands/hand hygiene.	12. Reduces transmission of microorganisms.
13. Document the drug, number of drops, time administered, and ear medicated.	13. Documenting actions of the nurse will reduce the number of medication errors.

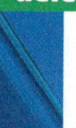

delegation tip

The skill of medication administration is not delegated to ancillary personnel in acute care settings. This may vary in state or federal institutions. Ancillary personnel are generally informed about the medications the client is receiving if adverse effects are anticipated or are being monitored.

nursing tips

It is a common error in household units to equate one drop to one minim. Because drops are variable, calibrated droppers should be used to administer medications by this method.

PROCEDURE 30-10

Medication Administration: Nasal

EQUIPMENT
- Medication in spray, drops, or aerosolized form
- Latex-free gloves
- Tissue as needed
- Dropper as needed

ACTION	RATIONALE
1. Wash hands/hand hygiene. Wear a mask if the client is coughing or sneezing. Don latex-free gloves (see Figure 30-74).	1. Reduces transmission of microorganisms. Respiratory-related microorganisms are easily transferred by the hands and air droplets. Gloves prevent absorption of medication through the skin of health care worker.
2. Explain the purpose of the medication and the position desired for the client (see Figure 30-75).	2. Clients will be more compliant with medication if they understand the purpose and proper use of medication. Proper positioning is necessary with nose drops so the drops will reach the area of treatment by gravity with the client assuming a dependent position.
3. Explain to the client the sensation of the local effects of the medications, such as burning, tingling, and effect on taste buds. If drops are used, explain to the client that a sensation of medications may be felt in the posterior oral pharynx.	3. Some nasal medications cause undesirable tastes. If this occurs, the prescribing practitioner may order other medications or encourage mouthwashes after treatment. Warning of postnasal sensations of the medication will prepare the client. Some clients may feel a quick sensation of choking. This can be frightening if the client has not been alerted to this consequence.
4. If a nasal inhaler is prescribed, explain the manufacturer's directions and how inhalers work. Follow the five rights of drug administration (check identification and orders at five different stages of administration).	4. Clients will be more compliant if they understand the use of the inhalers and that a fine cold mist will be released into the nasal passage via a pressurized container. Nasal medications that are prescribed must be considered to have the same safety precautions of administration as any medication.

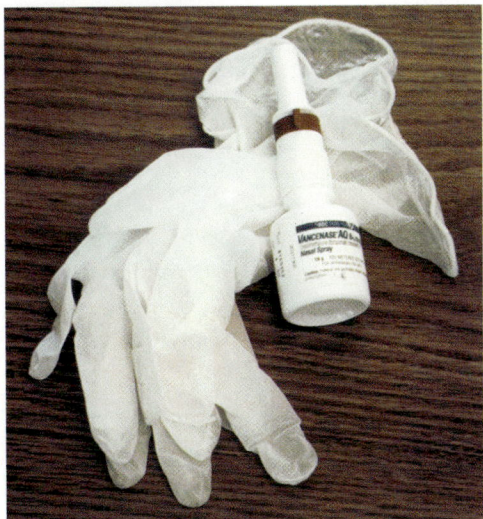

FIGURE 30-74 Nasal medication spray. Wear latex-free gloves when administering nasal medication to a client. DELMAR/ CENGAGE LEARNING

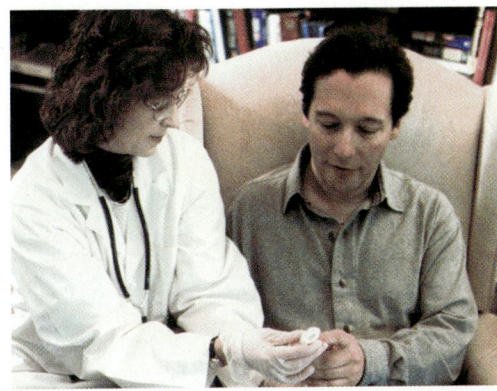

FIGURE 30-75 Explain the purpose of the medication to the client. DELMAR/CENGAGE LEARNING

(Continues)

PROCEDURE 30-10
Medication Administration: Nasal (Continued)

ACTION	RATIONALE
5. Have the client assume a comfortable position. If inhalers are to be used, this will generally be an upright position. If drops are to be instilled, the client should assume the appropriate position as mentioned earlier to medicate specific sinuses that need treatment. Before the instillation of drops or the use of an inhaler, ask the client to blow nose and clear nostrils of discharge as much as possible. Squeeze nose drops into dropper.	5. Nose drops are effective only if they reach the areas to be medicated. The client should be as comfortable as possible; otherwise, the client may not stay in desired position an adequate time. If the client is in a position with the neck hyperextended, a pillow or support by the nurse's hand under the neck may be necessary. Medications can be effective only if they are in contact with the mucous membranes. If large amounts of discharge are present, medications cannot be effective.
6. Have the client exhale and close one nostril.	6. The client will be asked to inhale with the use of nasal medications, so exhalation first is necessary.
7. Ask the client to inhale while the spray is pumped or sprayed into the first nostril (see Figure 30-76). If nose drops are used, insert nasal dropper only about 3/8 inch into the nostril, keeping the tip of the dropper away from the sides of the nostril. Insert the prescribed dosage of medication into the nostril. Discard any unused medication in dropper.	7. Nasal medications are more effective if instilled during inhalation as they will be carried and distributed farther into the nasal passages. Droppers should be kept away from the nostril to avoid inserting bacteria into the medication bottle. Excess medication is discarded for the same reason.
8. Ask the client to blot excess drainage from the nostril; however, do not have the client blow nose.	8. Blowing the nose will remove medication and therefore should not be done. However, excess medication should be removed from dripping out of the nostrils onto the facial areas in order to avoid discomfort.
9. Repeat the procedure on the other nostril.	9. Most often both nostrils contain congestion and therefore need to be treated.
10. Help the client resume a comfortable position. If nose drops are used, the client should stay in the appropriate position as indicated by manufacturer's suggestions, generally 5 minutes. Ask the client to breathe through the nose after the decongestion administration. It may be necessary to occlude one nostril at a time and breathe deeply.	10. Nose drops need positions that by gravity will allow medications to reach areas of desired treatment. (*Note:* If client will be self-administering medication, have client demonstrate administration; see Figure 30-77 on page 819.)

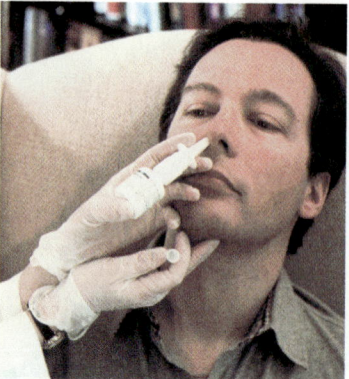

Figure 30-76 Ask the client to inhale while the spray is administered into the nostril.
DELMAR/CENGAGE LEARNING

(Continues)

PROCEDURE 30-10
Medication Administration: Nasal (Continued)

ACTION	RATIONALE

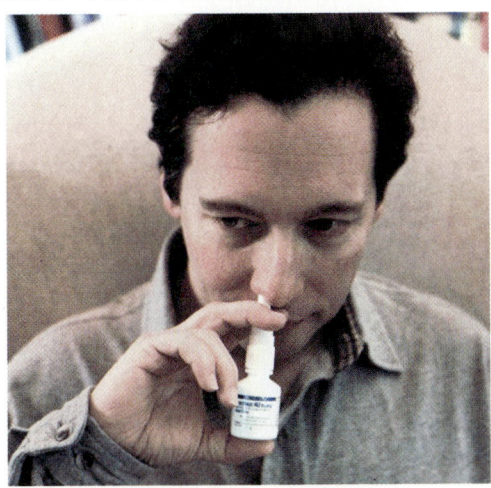

FIGURE 30-77 If the client will be self-administering the medication, have the client demonstrate how to administer the medication. DELMAR/CENGAGE LEARNING

11. Remove all soiled supplies and dispose according to Standard Precautions. Remove gloves. Wash hands/hand hygiene.	11. Use of gloves and proper disposal decreases the chance of transmission of microorganisms. Respiratory diseases are especially easily transmitted.
12. Evaluate the effect of the medication in 15 to 20 minutes.	12. It is necessary to note if the medication is effective without adverse side effects; otherwise, other medications may be considered. If the client experiences bothersome or unpleasant symptoms, such as a bad taste, other medications may be considered. Clients generally will not comply with medications that have too many unpleasant side effects.

delegation tip

The skill of medication administration is not delegated to ancillary personnel in acute care settings. This may vary in state or federal institutions. Ancillary personnel are generally informed about the medications the client is receiving if adverse effects are anticipated or are being monitored.

nursing tips

- *If the nasal route of administration is used for medications with systemic effects, evaluate the patency of nasal passage before administration of the medication.*
- *Certain nasal medications may cause an unpleasant taste. Using a mouthwash after administration of the medications may aid in compliance with the prescribed regimen.*
- *Some clients may feel nauseated or even vomit after use of nasal medication, such as with nose drops or sprays that drip into the oral pharynx.*

Medication Administration: Nebulizer

EQUIPMENT

HANDHELD NEBULIZER

- Medication administration record (MAR)
- Nebulizer set (cup, tubing, cap, T-shaped tube, mouthpiece, or mask) or prepackaged nebulizer and applicator

- Medication(s)
- Saline
- Air compressor, wall air, or wall oxygen

METERED-DOSE INHALER

- Metered-dose inhaler

- Aerochamber, if appropriate

ACTION	RATIONALE
HANDHELD NEBULIZER	
1. Assess client's ability to use the nebulizer.	1. Ensures client compliance.
2. Check the MAR against the prescribing practitioner orders.	2. Ensures accuracy in the administration of medication. *(Right drug)*
3. Check for drug allergies and hypersensitivity.	3. Decreases the risk of allergic reaction such as hives, urticaria, or anaphylactic shock.
4. Wash hands/hand hygiene before setting up the nebulizer; gather equipment (see Figure 30-78).	4. Reduces transmission of microorganisms.
5. Set up the medication(s) for one client at a time.	5. Ensures that client receives the right medication(s). *(Right drug)*
6. Look at the medication at eye level if using droppers to dispense the solution into the nebulizer.	6. Increases accuracy. *(Right dose)*

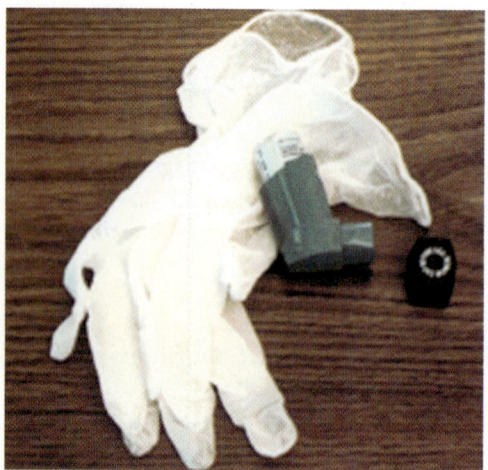

A

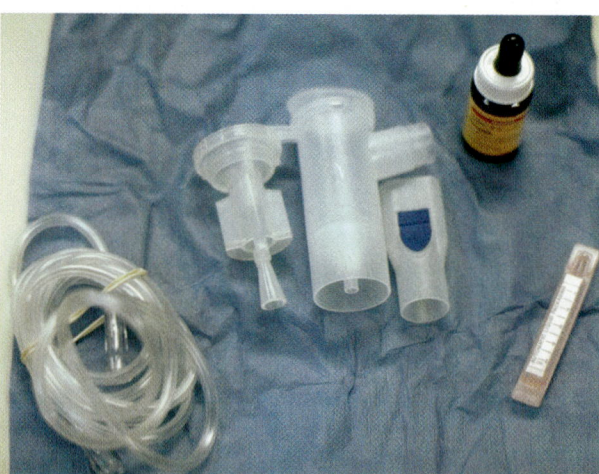

B

FIGURE 30-78 A. Handheld Nebulizer and Gloves; B. Nebulizer Cup, Tubing, Cap, T-Shaped Tube, Medication, and **Mouthpiece** DELMAR/CENGAGE LEARNING

(Continues)

PROCEDURE 30-11
Medication Administration: Nebulizer (Continued)

ACTION	RATIONALE
7. Pour the entire amount of the drug(s) into the nebulizer cup carefully. • Avoid touching the drug while pouring into the nebulizer cup.	7. Determines the correct amount of medicine and ensures accurate dosage. *(Right dose)* • Reduces transmission of microorganisms.
8. Cover the cup with the cap and fasten.	8. Prevents spillage of the medication.
9. Fasten the T-piece to the top of the cap.	9. Provides a connector for the mouthpiece.
10. Fasten a short length of tubing to one end of the T-piece.	10. Provides dead space to prevent room air from entering the system and medicated aerosol from escaping.
11. Fasten the mouthpiece or mask to the other end of the T-piece. • Avoid touching the nebulizer mouthpiece or the interior part of the mask.	11. Provides a portal for the client to inhale the aerosolized medication. • Reduces transmission of microorganisms.
12. Identify the client prior to administration of medication(s).	12. Ensures the right client gets the medication. *(Right client)*
13. Identify the medication(s) to the client, and clearly explain the therapeutic purpose(s) of the medication.	13. Promotes client's cooperation and awareness of the medication's effects.
14. Advise the client to sit in an upright position.	14. Promotes better expansion of the lungs.
15. Attach tubing to the bottom of the nebulizer cup, and attach the other end to the air compressor or wall air. • Before turning it on, adjust the wall oxygen valve to 6 L/min (or less per prescribing practitioner's orders). • Leave the air on for about 6 to 7 minutes until the medications get used up.	15. Provides a conduit for the compressed air. • Drives the medication into a mist or wet aerosol form. • Allows the client to receive the entire dose of medication.
16. Instruct the client to breathe in and out slowly and deeply through the mouthpiece or mask. • The client's lips should be sealed tightly around the mouthpiece.	16. Promotes better deposition and efficacy of the medication in the airways.
17. Remain with the client long enough to observe the proper inhalation-exhalation technique.	17. Ensures the correct use of the nebulizer to get the full effects from the medications administered.
18. Wash hands/hand hygiene.	18. Reduces transmission of microorganisms.
19. Record the medications administered along with the date, time, and dosages on the chart.	19. Provides documentation of administration of drugs.
20. When the nebulizer cup is empty, turn off the compressor or wall air. • Detach the tubing from the compressor and the nebulizer cup. • If the nebulizer is disposable, dispose of the nebulizer in the appropriate container. • If the nebulizer is to be reused for this client, carefully wash, rinse, and dry the nebulizer components.	20. Stops the aerosolization. • Prepares components for cleaning or disposal. • Prevents transmission of microorganisms. • Prevents transmission of microorganisms.

(Continues)

PROCEDURE 30-11
Medication Administration: Nebulizer (Continued)

ACTION	RATIONALE
21. Assess the client immediately following the treatment for results or adverse effects from the treatment.	21. Allows the nurse to determine the effectiveness of the treatment.
22. Reassess the client 5 to 10 minutes following the treatment.	22. Some effects may be delayed.
23. Wash hands/hand hygiene.	23. Reduces transmission of microorganisms.

METERED-DOSE NEBULIZER (SEE FIGURE 30-79)

ACTION	RATIONALE
24. Assess the client for ability to use the metered-dose nebulizer.	24. Ensures client compliance.
25. Check the MAR against the prescribing practitioner's orders.	25. Ensures accuracy in the administration of medication.
26. Check for drug allergies and hypersensitivity.	26. Decreases the risk of allergic reaction, such as hives, urticaria, or anaphylactic shock.
27. Wash hands/hand hygiene before administering medication; don latex-free gloves.	27. Decreases risk of transmission of microorganisms and prevents reaction to latex.
28. Shake the prepackaged nebulizer.	28. Thoroughly mixes the medication.
29. Place the nebulizer into the applicator (see Figure 30-80).	29. Allows for proper administration of the medication.
30. Place the aerochamber onto the nebulizer if needed.	30. The aerochamber provides dead space for the medicated mist while the client inhales.
31. Have client place mouthpiece in mouth.	31. Delivers medication to lungs through the proper route.
32. Have the client press down on the prepackaged dispenser as the client simultaneously inhales.	32. Allows delivery of the medication to the lungs.
33. If there is an aerochamber attached to the nebulizer, have the client inhale slowly and deeply.	33. Allows proper delivery of the medication.
34. Observe the client for several minutes to assess for possible adverse effects from the medication.	34. Nebulized medication is delivered into the bloodstream almost immediately and reactions can occur right away.
35. Wash hands/hand hygiene.	35. Prevents transmission of microorganisms.
36. Record the medication administration and your observations.	36. Provides a record of care and ensures continuity of care.

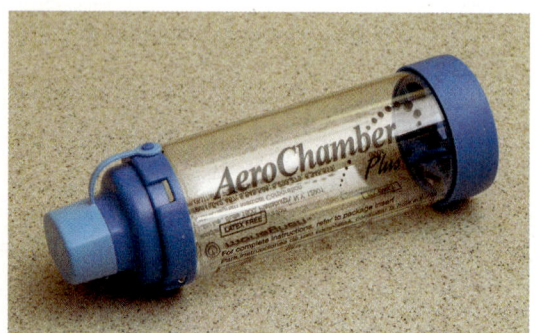

FIGURE 30-79 Metered-Dose Nebulizer DELMAR/CENGAGE LEARNING

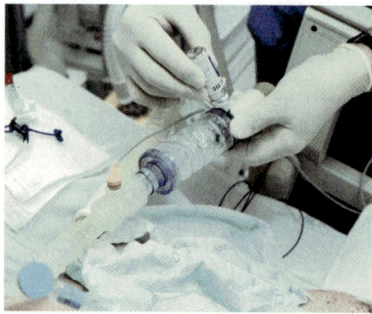

FIGURE 30-80 Preparation of a Metered-Dose Nebulizer and Medication DELMAR/CENGAGE LEARNING

(Continues)

PROCEDURE 30-11
Medication Administration: Nebulizer (Continued)

delegation tip

The skill of medication administration is not delegated to ancillary personnel in acute care settings. This may vary in state or federal institutions. Ancillary personnel are generally informed about the medications the client is receiving if adverse effects are anticipated or are being monitored.

nursing tips

- *Evaluate the client's need for medication delivery. Some clients, such as young clients (usually less than 5 years old), clients with coordination problems, and clients with severe or acute asthma, will benefit more from using a nebulizer. Some clients, such as school-aged children, active adults, and clients with exercise-induced asthma, will benefit more from the ease and portability of a metered-dose inhaler.*
- *Be aware of the client's ability to use the nebulizer device. Young children and clients with acute or severe exacerbation may not be able to use the mouthpiece for the nebulizer. A mask may provide better delivery of the medication(s).*
- *Measure the medication accurately by looking at the medicine dropper at eye level, and pour the exact amount of medication needed into the cup.*
- *Familiarize yourself with all the asthma medications in order to be aware of any outcomes the client may have from treatment. Some medications that the client might be taking can interact with each other. Beta blockers (propranolol, atenolol, and labetalol) can antagonize the beta agonists, increasing asthma symptoms. The nurse needs to be familiar with the medications in order to anticipate possible reactions.*

PROCEDURE 30-12
Medication Administration: Rectal

EQUIPMENT
- Medication (suppository or medicated enema)
- Water-soluble lubricant
- Latex-free gloves
- Tissue or washcloth
- Bedpan if client physically immobile
- Medication administration record (MAR)
- Towels or pads (e.g., disposable "blue pads")

ACTION	RATIONALE
1. Assess the client's need for the medication.	1. Allows nurse to determine effectiveness of the medication.
2. Check prescribing practitioner's written order.	2. Ensures safe and accurate administration of medication.
3. Check the MAR against the medication order, verifying correct client, medication, dose, route, and time.	3. Ensures accuracy and decreases chance of medication error.
4. Check for any drug allergies.	4. Decreases risk of allergic reaction.
5. Review the client's history for any previous surgeries or bleeding.	5. Contraindications for rectal administration may be discovered.
6. Gather the equipment needed for the procedure before entering the client's room (see Figure 30-81 on page 824).	6. Prevents numerous trips to gather supplies and helps the procedure flow smoothly.

(Continues)

PROCEDURE 30-12
Medication Administration: Rectal (Continued)

ACTION	RATIONALE

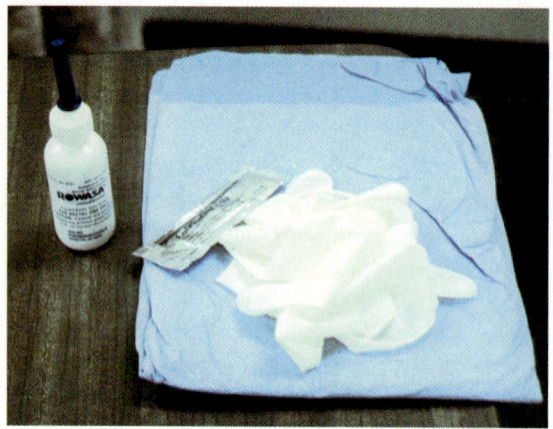

FIGURE 30-81 Protective Pad, Latex-Free Gloves, Lubricant, and Rectal Medication DELMAR/CENGAGE LEARNING

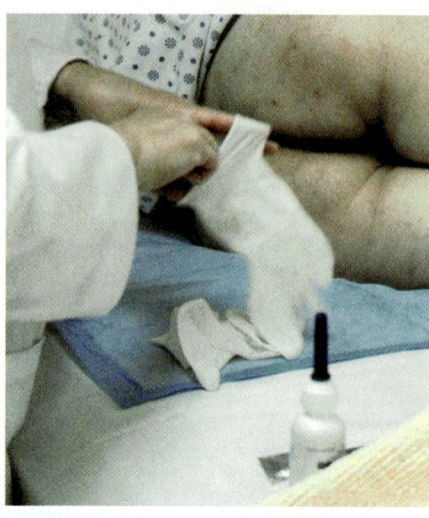

FIGURE 30-82 Don latex-free gloves before administering rectal medications. DELMAR/CENGAGE LEARNING

7. Assess the client's readiness to receive the medication. Encourage visitors to leave until the procedure is completed, and close door or curtain.
8. Wash hands/hand hygiene.
9. Apply disposable gloves (see Figure 30-82).
10. Ask the client's name and check identification band.
11. Assist client into correct position: side-lying Sims' position, preferably the left side with upper leg drawn up toward chest. Provide protection under client such as towel or pad.

12. Visually assess the client's external anus.
13. Remove suppository from wrapper, and lubricate rounded end along with insertion finger. If a medicated enema is used, lubricate the enema tip if it is not prelubricated (see Figure 30-83).

7. Promotes privacy and maintains self-image.

8. Reduces transmission of microorganisms.
9. Prevents contact with fecal material.
10. Ensures correct client.
11. The descending colon is on the left side; this is a more anatomically correct position. This position exposes the anus to identify placement. Pads can provide comfort to client who may fear soiling linen.
12. Determines presence of any active bleeding.
13. Lubrication decreases friction and decreases discomfort.

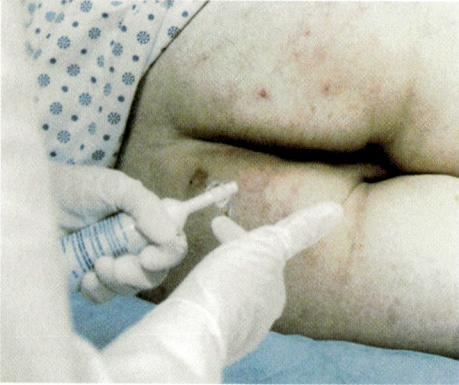

FIGURE 30-83 Lubricate the enema tip if necessary. DELMAR/CENGAGE LEARNING

(Continues)

PROCEDURE 30-12
Medication Administration: Rectal (Continued)

ACTION	RATIONALE
14. Tell client he or she will experience a cool sensation and pressure during administration. Encourage slow deep breaths.	14. Prepares client for administration. Relaxes the rectal sphincter.
15. Retract buttocks with nondominant hand, visualizing the anus (see Figure 30-84). Using the dominant index finger, slowly and gently insert the suppository through the anus, past the internal sphincter, and against the rectal wall. Depth of insertion will differ if client is a child or infant. If instilling a medicated enema, gently insert the enema tip past the internal sphincter and instill the contents by slowly squeezing (see Figure 30-85).	15. Slow insertion minimizes pain. Correct placement ensures adequate absorption and less chance for expulsion of medication.
16. Remove finger or enema tip, and wipe client's anal area with a washcloth or tissue.	16. Removes lubricant externally. Promotes cleanliness and comfort.
17. Discard gloves.	17. Reduces transmission of microorganisms.
18. Discuss with client a 10-minute time frame to remain in bed or on side.	18. Keeps suppository or medicated fluid in place for better absorption.
19. Place call light in client's reach if administering suppository containing laxative to assist once client has sensation to defecate.	19. Gives client control over situation and nurse response once sensation to defecate occurs.
20. Record administration of medication.	20. Provides documentation of administration of medication.
21. Document effectiveness or any side effects of treatment on nursing flow sheet or progress note if applicable.	21. Communicates with other caregivers the effectiveness of treatment.
22. Wash hands/hand hygiene.	22. Reduces transmission of microorganisms.

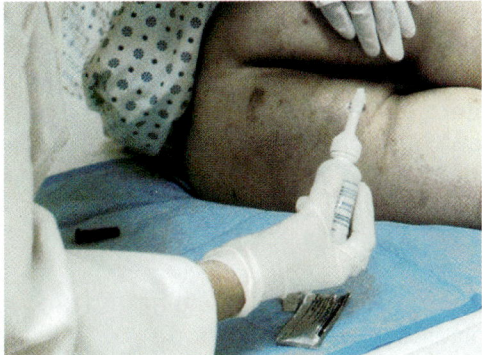

FIGURE 30-84 Retract the buttock and visualize the anus.
DELMAR/CENGAGE LEARNING

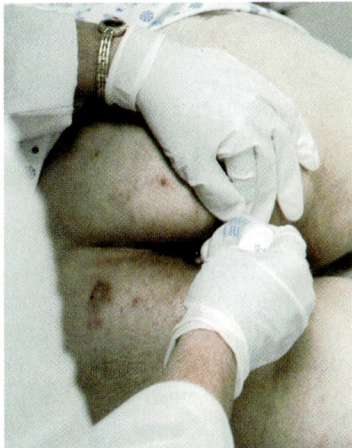

FIGURE 30-85 Gently insert the enema tip and instill the contents by slowly squeezing the bottle. DELMAR/CENGAGE LEARNING

(Continues)

PROCEDURE 30-12
Medication Administration: Rectal (Continued)

delegation tip

The skill of medication administration is not delegated to ancillary personnel in acute care settings. This may vary in state or federal institutions. Ancillary personnel are generally informed about the medications the client is receiving if adverse effects are anticipated or are being monitored.

nursing tips

- *Adjust the height of the bed to decrease back strain during insertion.*
- *Communication helps decrease anxiety and promotes cooperation.*
- *Observe the client's nonverbal and verbal cues during the procedure.*
- *Provide for privacy: Close the door, pull the curtains, and ask visitors to leave until the procedure is complete.*

PROCEDURE 30-13

Medication Administration: Vaginal

EQUIPMENT

- Vaginal medication: cream, foam, jelly, or suppository
- Applicator (if needed)
- Water-soluble lubricating jelly (for suppository)
- Nonsterile latex-free gloves
- Perineal pad
- Paper towel, toilet tissue, or tissue paper
- Washcloth and warm water (optional)

ACTION	RATIONALE
1. Verify orders.	1. Prevents medication errors.
2. Ascertain if the client has ever had vaginal medications before and understands the procedure.	2. Enables client understanding and compliance.
3. Ask the client to void.	3. Provides for client comfort during the procedure.
4. Wash hands/hand hygiene.	4. Reduces transmission of microorganisms.
5. Arrange equipment at client's bedside.	5. Promotes organization.
6. Provide complete privacy by closing door and curtains.	6. This procedure can be embarrassing, and this protects the client's privacy.
7. Assist the client into a dorsal-recumbent or Sims' position (see Figure 30-86 on page 827).	7. Allows positioning for administration and for medication to remain in vagina.
8. Drape the client as appropriate, such as over the client's abdomen and lower extremities. Provide towel or protective pad on bed.	8. Provides privacy. Prevents linen from becoming soiled.
9. Position lighting to illuminate vaginal orifice.	9. Assists in visualization of vagina and proper administration of medication.
10. Don latex-free gloves and assess the perineal area for redness, inflammation, discharge, or foul odor.	10. Decreases risk of transmission of microorganisms. Provides baseline data. Decreases risk of reaction to latex.

(Continues)

PROCEDURE 30-13
Medication Administration: Vaginal (Continued)

ACTION	RATIONALE

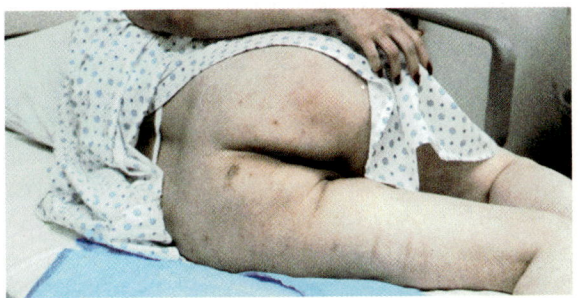

FIGURE 30-86 This client is placed in Sims' position for administering vaginal medications. DELMAR/CENGAGE LEARNING

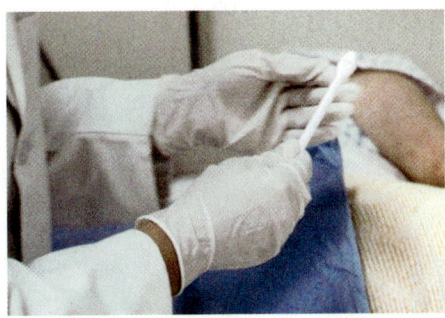

FIGURE 30-87 Place the suppository in the applicator. DELMAR/CENGAGE LEARNING

11. If using an applicator, fill with medication. If using a suppository, remove the suppository from the foil and position in the applicator (applicator is optional) (see Figure 30-87). An applicator may be used for suppositories, or a gloved finger may be used. The foil is discarded. Apply water-soluble lubricant to suppository or applicator (optional for applicator).

11. The medication is prepared for insertion. Lubricant provides comfort and ease of insertion.

12. For suppository, with nondominant hand, retract the labia (see Figure 30-88).

12. Allows visualization of the vaginal orifice and eases insertion of medication.

13. With dominant hand, insert the applicator 2 to 3 inches into the vagina, sliding the applicator posteriorly (see Figure 30-89). Push the plunger to administer the medication (see Figure 30-90 on page 828). With a suppository, insert the tapered end first with the index finger or applicator along the posterior wall of the vagina (approximately 3 inches).

13. Medication must be inserted completely to provide coverage of the entire vagina. When medication is deposited at the posterior end of the vagina, gravity will allow medication to move toward the orifice.

14. Withdraw the applicator and place on a towel.

14. Reduces transmission of microorganisms.

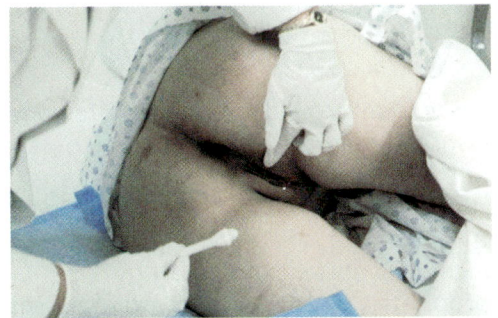

FIGURE 30-88 Retract the labia with the nondominant hand. DELMAR/CENGAGE LEARNING

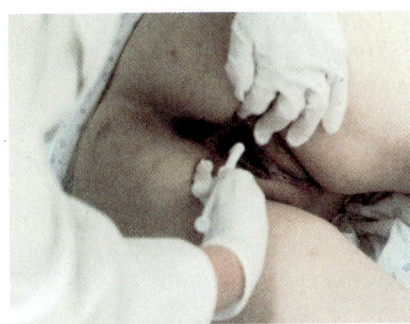

FIGURE 30-89 Slide the applicator 2 to 3 inches into the vagina. DELMAR/CENGAGE LEARNING

(Continues)

PROCEDURE 30-13
Medication Administration: Vaginal (Continued)

ACTION	RATIONALE

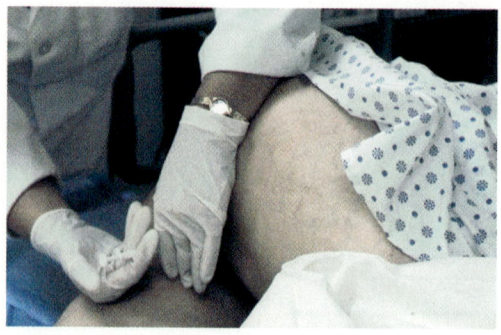

FIGURE 30-90 Push the plunger to administer the medication. DELMAR/CENGAGE LEARNING

15. If administering a douche or irrigation:
    - Warm solution to slightly above body temperature (105°F to 110°F). Check using the back of the hand or the wrist.
    - Position the client in a semirecumbent position on a bedpan, on a toilet seat, or in a tub.
    - Apply lubricant to the irrigation nozzle and insert approximately 3 inches into the vagina.
    - Hang the irrigant container approximately 2 feet above the client's vaginal area.
    - Open the clamp, and allow a small amount of solution to flow into the vagina.
    - Move the nozzle and rotate around the entire vaginal area. If the labia are inflamed, allow the solution to flow over the labia as well. If the client is on the toilet seat, alternate between closing off the labia and allowing solution to be expelled.

16. Wipe and clean client's perineal area, including the labia (from front to back) with toilet tissue. Some clients may prefer that the perineal area is also cleaned with a washcloth and warm water.

17. Apply a perineal pad.

18. Wash the applicator (if reusable) with soap and warm water and store in appropriate container in client's room.

19. Remove gloves; wash hands/hand hygiene.

15.
    - Avoids burning the client. The mucous membranes of the vagina are sensitive.
    - Provides comfort during procedure and allows for appropriate drainage of irrigation solution.
    - Provides comfort.
    - Height is necessary for drainage by gravity. If the container is too high, the flow will be too forceful and uncomfortable.
    - Allows the client to evaluate the temperature.
    - Rotation allows for irrigation throughout vagina. Closing off labia allows medication to stay in and flush total vagina.

16. Provides comfort for client and avoids spread of infective agents to perineal area.

17. Protects client from discomfort of drainage and spread of infection or irritation to perineal area.

18. Applicator can be used only for individual clients; however, some applicators and inducers are reusable and must be appropriately cleaned and stored to prevent reinsertion of infective agents.

19. Reduces transmission of microorganisms.

(Continues)

PROCEDURE 30-13
Medication Administration: Vaginal (Continued)

ACTION	RATIONALE
20. Instruct the client to remain flat for at least 30 minutes.	20. Allows maximum contact between the medication and the vaginal mucous membranes.
21. Raise side rails and place the call light in reach.	21. Provides for client comfort and safety.
22. Wash hands/hand hygiene.	22. Reduces transmission of microorganisms.

delegation tip

The skill of medication administration is not delegated to ancillary personnel in acute care settings. This may vary in state or federal institutions. Ancillary personnel are generally informed about the medications the client is receiving if adverse effects are anticipated or are being monitored.

nursing tips

- *Insert medication 2 to 3 inches.*
- *Clean client carefully after inserting medication to avoid perineal irritation.*

KEY CONCEPTS

- The *United States Pharmacopeia* and *National Formulary* (USP and NF) outline drug standards for usage in the United States.
- The Food and Drug Administration (FDA) tests all drugs for toxicity before granting a company the right to market a drug.
- Drugs are usually referred to by their trade (company) or generic (nonproprietary) name.
- The oral administration route is the safest and least expensive administration route, although it is also the slowest to act.
- Parenteral drugs are injected through intradermal (ID), subcutaneous, intramuscular (IM), or intravenous (IV) routes and are typically fast-acting drugs.
- The pharmacokinetics of drugs includes absorption, distribution, metabolism, and excretion.
- Safe drug administration is facilitated by following the five rights: right drug, right dose, right client, right route, and right time.
- Nurses are both morally and legally responsible for correct administration of medications; this includes following institutional policy, considering clients' desires and abilities, fostering compliance, and cor-

rectly documenting all actions related to medication administration and medication errors.
- Drug abuse is a common problem, both in society and in the health care professions; nurses have a responsibility to report addicted colleagues so that they can find resources to help overcome their addictions.
- Before administering medications, the nurse must thoroughly assess the client's drug history, medical history, and psychosocial and cultural factors that may affect drug acceptance and compliance.
- Oral medications should be poured and measured at eye level to ensure accuracy.
- Although the prescribing practitioner will determine the dose and route of a parenteral drug, the nurse is responsible for choosing the correct gauge and length of the needle to be used.
- The nurse must always carefully monitor client reactions to medications and ensure that clients are appropriately educated as to the actions, side effects, and contraindications of all medications they are receiving.

REVIEW QUESTIONS

1. The purpose of medication management is to produce the desired drug action by maintaining a constant drug level. The highest blood concentration of a single drug dose before the elimination rate equals the rate of absorption is called _____.
   a. Onset of action
   b. Peak plasma level
   c. Half-life
   d. Plateau

2. The nurse cannot understand the prescribing practitioner's standing orders. What should she do?
   a. Contact the unit manager to interpret the order.
   b. Have the unit secretary call the prescribing practitioner.
   c. Call the prescribing practitioner to have the order clarified.
   d. Send the order to pharmacy, and let the pharmacist fill the order.

3. The prescribing practitioner has order 2 teaspoonsful of Milk of Magnesia. The nurse converts this dose to the metric system and administers

   _____.
   a. 5 mL
   b. 10 mL
   c. 15 mL
   d. 30 mL

4. What information should be obtained from the drug history?
   a. Prescription drugs
   b. Allergies
   c. Herbal supplements
   d. Over-the-counter drugs
   e. Client's sensory and cognitive status
   f. Lifestyles and beliefs

5. What is the appropriate method to administer medications through a nasogastric tube?
   a. Mix all medications together that are compatible, and flush with 20 to 30 mL warm water at the end.
   b. Administer those medications that are compatible, and flush with 60 mL warm water at the end.
   c. Administer each medication individually, and flush with 100 mL warm water at the end.
   d. Administer each medication individually, flush with 15 to 30 mL warm water between each medication, and flush with 30 to 60 mL at the end.

6. What is the usual dosage range for intradermal injections?
   a. 0.01 to 0.1 mL
   b. 0.1 to 0.15 mL
   c. 1.15 to 0.2 mL
   d. 0.2 to 0.25 mL

7. The prescribing practitioner ordered 5 mL of a medication to be given deep IM for a 45-year-old female who weighs 140 pounds and is 5'7" tall. What is the most appropriate method to administer this injection?
   a. A 5-mL syringe, 20–23-gauge, 1-inch needle
   b. Two 3-mL syringes, 20–23-gauge, 1½-inch needle
   c. Two 3-mL syringes, 23–25-gauge, 1-inch needle
   d. Two 2-mL syringes, 20–23-gauge, 1½-inch needle

8. The correct way to administer eardrops to an adult client is to _____.
   a. Pull the pinna straight back
   b. Pull the pinna down and back
   c. Pull the pinna upward and outward
   d. Pull the pinna straight down

9. Which of the following is the correct way to administer eyedrops to an adult client?
   a. Hold eye dropper in dominant hand, hold ½–¾ inch above the eyeball, and rest hand on client's forehead to stabilize. Use fingers of nondominant hand to separate the eyelids, instruct client to look up, and drop prescribed number of drops into center of the eye. Instruct the client to close eyes and move them around. Briefly place fingers on either side of the client's nose to close the tear ducts and prevent the medication from draining out of the eye.
   b. Hold eye dropper in dominant hand, hold ½–1 inch above the eyeball, and rest hand on client's forehead to stabilize. Instruct the client to look up, and drop the prescribed number of drops into the center of the conjunctival sac. Instruct the client to gently close eyes and move eyes. Use a tissue to apply gentle pressure and absorb excess medication.
   c. Hold eyedropper in dominant hand, hold ½–⅗ inch above the eyeball, and rest hand on client's forehead to stabilize. Place nondominant hand on cheekbone, and expose lower conjunctival sac by pulling down on cheek. Instruct the client to look up, and drop the prescribed number of drops into the center of the conjunctival sac. Instruct client to gently close eyes and move eyes. Place fingers briefly on either side of the client's nose to close the tear ducts and prevent the medication from draining out of the eye.
   d. Hold eyedropper in dominant hand; with nondominant hand, gently separate client's eyelids with thumb and finger, and grasp lower lid near margin immediately below lashes; exert pressure downward over the bony prominence of the cheek. Instruct the client to look up, and drop

the prescribed number of drops into the center of the conjunctival sac.

10. An RN has just received word of a new admission to the unit with the diagnosis of shortness of breath and indigestion-type pain. The RN needs to delegate procedures to other personnel and retain certain nursing functions. Which nursing functions can be delegated?

a. Delegate to an LPN the administration of a prn IM injection for pain.
b. Delegate to an LPN the assessment of the new admission.
c. Delegate to an ancillary person the vital signs of the new admission.
d. Delegate to an ancillary person the observation of a client self-administering a metered-dose nebulizer.

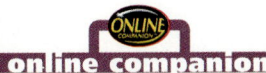

online companion

Visit the DeLaune and Ladner online companion resource at **www.delmar.cengage.com** for additional content and study aids. Click on Online Companions, then select the Nursing discipline.

Only nature heals.

—Hippocrates

CHAPTER 31

Complementary and Alternative Modalities

COMPETENCIES

1. Describe historical events influencing the use of complementary and alternative treatment modalities.

2. Discuss the effect of the mind-body relationship on a person's health.

3. Explain the concept of the nurse as an instrument of healing in holistic nursing practice.

4. Identify the various mind-body, body-movement, energetic-touch healing, spiritual, nutritional, and other modalities that can be used as complementary therapies in client care.

5. Discuss the use of complementary and alternative modalities throughout the life cycle.

KEY TERMS

acupressure
acupuncture
allopathic
alternative therapies
aromatherapy
Ayurveda
biofeedback
bodymind
centering
chakra
chiropractic
complementary therapies

effleurage
endorphins
energetic-touch therapies
friction
healing touch
imagery
integrative therapy
meditation
music-thanatology
neuropeptides
neurotransmitters
nutraceuticals

petrissage
phytonutrients
psychoneuroimmunology
relaxation response
shaman
shamanism
tapotement
therapeutic massage
therapeutic touch
touch
vibration

Western society tends to think of healing in terms of medical, surgical, and other technological interventions. However, in many other cultures—both past and present—healing has been promoted by faith, magic, ritual, and other nonmedical approaches.

The use of alternative therapies (treatment approaches that are not accepted by mainstream medical practice) and complementary therapies (treatment approaches that can be used in conjunction with conventional medical therapies) is becoming more prevalent among the general public. This chapter discusses complementary and alternative medicine (CAM) treatment methods that are currently being used in holistic nursing practice. Nurses are encouraged to think critically before recommending or implementing these approaches and to also be open to the possibilities that are available to help people live to their fullest potential. It is important to remember that what is considered "alternative" to one culture may be viewed as "traditional" in another (e.g., traditional Chinese medicine and Ayurvedic medicine). The classification of CAM therapies changes according to research findings. "The list of what is considered to be CAM changes continually, as those therapies that are proven to be safe and effective become adopted into conventional health care and as new approaches to health care emerge" (National Center for Complementary and Alternative Medicine [NCCAM], 2007b).

HISTORICAL INFLUENCES ON CONTEMPORARY PRACTICES

For as long as history has been recorded, people have tried to cure ills and relieve pain. Early cave drawings depict healers practicing their art. Primitive healers attributed the cause of diseases to magic and superstition; as a result, religious beliefs and health practices became intertwined.

FROM ANCIENT TRADITION TO EARLY SCIENCE

Remedies and practices that are based in ancient traditions are being rediscovered and used by contemporary holistic

healers. This section discusses the impact of ancient healing practices on current use of CAM modalities.

Ancient Greece

The ancient Greek culture perceived health as maintenance of balance in all dimensions of life. In Greek mythology, Asclepius was the god of healing. Temples (called Asclepions) were beautiful places for people (regardless of ability to pay) to rest, restore themselves, and worship. The elaborate healing system consisted of myths, symbols, and rites administered by rigorously trained priest-healers.

The Far East

Healing systems of the Far East have traditionally integrated mind, body, and spirit into a system of balanced energy between the individual and the universe. The concept of a life force or life energy permeates Eastern philosophies. The accompanying Respecting Our Differences display lists the names of the life force in various cultures.

China

The traditional Chinese healing system is based on the belief in the oneness of all things in nature. Life energy (*chi*) flows through both the universe and the person, thus creating a

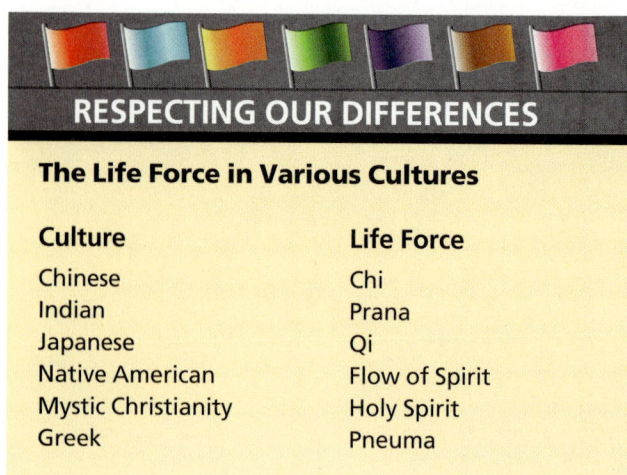

RESPECTING OUR DIFFERENCES

The Life Force in Various Cultures

Culture	Life Force
Chinese	Chi
Indian	Prana
Japanese	Qi
Native American	Flow of Spirit
Mystic Christianity	Holy Spirit
Greek	Pneuma

wholeness among all things and people. Chi provides warmth, protection from illness, and vitality. Chi flows along an invisible system of meridians (pathways) that link the organs together and connect them to the external environment and, therefore, to the universe. Illness and injury can alter the flow of this energy. The energy flow can be influenced by stimulating points along the meridians. Both acupuncture and acupressure are based on this concept of energy meridians.

Herbalism is an essential component of traditional Chinese healing practice. In seeking to promote balance, healers use herbs for dual purposes. For example, the herb *dong quai* relaxes the uterus when it is contracted and tightens it if it is too relaxed. A complete discussion of the use of herbs in contemporary health practices appears later in this chapter.

Many contemporary Western health care providers are studying and now using traditional Chinese medicine (TCM). These healing techniques have been used in various situations, such as with clients who are experiencing chronic pain associated with illness or injury. Acupuncture, one technique used in TCM, is the application of needles to various points on the body to alter the energy flow (see Figure 31-1).

India

Ayurveda, a healing system based on Hindu philosophy, embraces the concept of an energy force in the body that seeks to maintain balance or harmony. From the Ayurvedic perspective, the body and mind are filled with a vital energy (*prana*) that is the life force. The life energy (prana) is transported through the body by a "wind" or *vata*. Vata regulates every type of movement.

The Hindu concept of chakras refers to seven primary energy centers in the physical body. A chakra is a concentrated area of energy. The chakras are vertically aligned through the center of the body from the crown of the head to the pelvis. Chakras influence the physical body, emotions, mental patterns, and spiritual awareness. Each chakra has specific functions and a corresponding relationship to body structures and organs; see Figure 31-2.

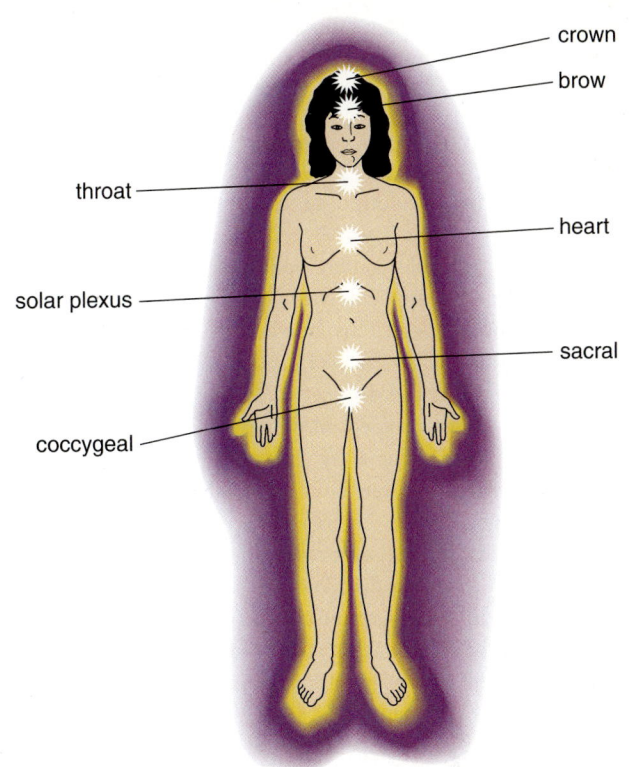

FIGURE 31-2 Locations of the Seven Major Chakras DELMAR/ CENGAGE LEARNING

Prevention of illness and restoration of health through introspection and spiritual growth are the primary goals in the Ayurvedic system. Union of the Divine and the Truth occurs through the physical and meditative practice of yoga. In contemporary practice, Ayurvedic intervention may consist of yoga, herbs, diet, exercise, steam baths, cathartics, and detoxifying massage.

SHAMANISTIC TRADITION

A need to understand and explain life processes (i.e., birth, health, illness, and death) is part of being human. Ritualized practices have been used to keep peace with the great spirits, to harness their power, to promote power, and to prevent death.

Shamanism refers to the practice of entering altered states of consciousness with the intent of helping others. The shaman, a folk healer-priest who uses natural and supernatural forces to help others, has an extensive knowledge of herbs, is skilled in many forms of healing, and serves as guardian of the spirits. Illness is considered to be the result of spirit loss. Shamans have the power to heal by working with the spirits to encourage their full return to the individual. The shaman functions as both healer and priest and one who has access to the supernatural.

Seeking wisdom about the universe, a relationship with the creator, and avoidance of death are all accomplished through ritualized processes that are performed by the shaman. The shaman's practice incorporates special objects such as power animals, totems, and fetishes as well as ritual songs, dances, food, and clothing. Sleep deprivation, ritual chants, isolation, imagery, drumming, and hallucinogenic drugs may

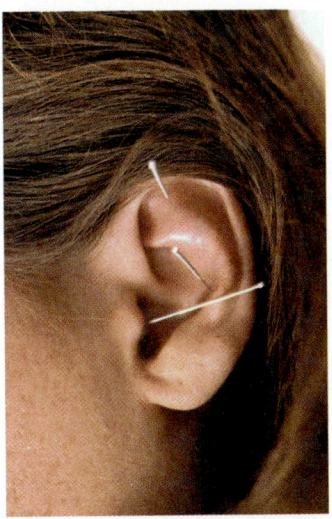

FIGURE 31-1 Acupuncture Needles Inserted for Treatment of Depression COURTESY OF JACK STAR/PHOTOLINK/GETTY IMAGES

be used to create a trancelike state that is the vehicle through which the shaman contacts the spirit world.

ALLOPATHIC MEDICINE

Western medicine, referred to as **allopathic** medicine, is relatively new in that it was begun about 200 years ago. Its fundamental principle is that body and mind are separate entities. Allopathic medicine views the human as a collection of separate body parts. This conventional medical approach views health as the absence of disease and sees the goal of treatment as curing the disease or "fixing" the problem (e.g., trauma). The Western medical model focuses on ridding the body of symptoms induced by disease or injury.

The allopathic system is effective when aggressive treatment is needed for an emergency situation. State-of-the-art technology and advanced surgical techniques have become true lifesavers for many in modern Western societies. However, with its emphasis on curing symptoms, allopathic medicine overlooks the crucial role of energy, emotions, and thoughts. Allopathic medicine has been less effective in treating chronic conditions such as hypertension and arthritis. "The value of alternative medicine is especially effective for people with chronic, debilitating illnesses for which conventional medicine has few, if any, answers" (Fontaine, 2004, p. 10). See Table 31-1 for a comparison of allopathic and alternative perspectives.

CONTEMPORARY TRENDS

The public perception of CAM treatment methods has been changing over the past few decades. In the late 1960s and early 1970s, the "natural," "new age," and "self-help" movements began to attract adherents, first among consumers and later among health care practitioners. During that time, there was a growing trend toward rejection of traditional medicine because of its perceived invasiveness, painfulness, cost, and ineffectiveness. A rekindled interest in Eastern religions, lifestyle, and medicine has fueled the development of contemporary holistic, CAM modalities. CAM therapy has a major tenet—holism—that is, the connection among mind, body, and spirit.

Ever-increasing numbers of consumers who are seeking natural and safe approaches to health care are using CAM. The goals of CAM are numerous, including pain relief and treatment of chronic illness.

There is an increasing prevalence of the use of CAM in the United States. According to a nationwide, government-sponsored survey released in December 2008, approximately 38% of U.S. adults and 12% of children use some type of CAM. The use of CAM is greatest among individuals aged 30–69 years (NCCAM, 2008). Benson (2008) states that over 35 million U.S. adults use CAM therapies to improve health. The growing interest in complementary therapies is evidenced by the increased sale of natural substances, such as herbs and vitamins, which has become a multimillion dollar industry over the last decade.

Health care consumers who want to be more involved in their own healing view CAM as a way to promote their

TABLE 31-1 Comparison of Allopathic and Alternative Medicine

ALLOPATHIC PERSPECTIVE	ALTERNATIVE PERSPECTIVE
Health is absence of disease.	Health is a state of well-being characterized by mind/body balance.
Focus is on cure of disease.	Emphasis is on health maintenance and disease prevention through lifestyle choices.
Mind and body are treated as separate entities.	Mind and body are one; what affects one affects the other.
Disease results from causative agents, usually external.	Disease originates from within and is the result of imbalances that occur in response to an unhealthy lifestyle or inner disharmonies.
Healing depends on outside agents to cure the disease.	The body has a natural ability to heal itself.
Treatment consists of drugs, surgery, and radiation.	Treatment consists of diet, exercise, herbal medicines, social support, and stress management.
Healing is aggressive, quick, and seeks to destroy the invading agents.	Healing is a slow, natural process.
The physician plays the central role in healing.	The client has the most important role in healing (i.e., lifestyle choices).

Data from Fontaine, K. L. (2004). *Healing practices: Alternative therapies for nursing* (2nd ed.). Upper Saddle River, NJ: Prentice-Hall.

autonomy. Nurses are encouraged to teach clients to use the best of all systems in order to promote positive health outcomes. **Integrative therapy**, a clinical approach that combines Western technological medicine with techniques from Eastern medicine, is becoming more prevalent in the United States.

In 1992, the U.S. government established the Office of Alternative Medicine (OAM) at the National Institutes of Health (NIH) to study the efficacy of unconventional, alternative treatment methods. The OAM is now the NIH NCCAM. Its mission is to conduct and support research and training and to disseminate information on CAM to the public and health care practitioners.

MIND-BODY MEDICINE AND RESEARCH

The Western medical model is founded on the dualistic belief that the mind, body, and spirit are separate entities. However, psychoneuroimmunology (PNI), a relatively new field of science, is studying the complex relationship between the cognitive, affective, and physical aspects of humans. Psychoneuroimmunologists are investigating how the brain transmits signals along the nerves to enhance the body's normal immune functioning. PNI research supports the idea that the human mind can alter physiology. As stated by Briones:

The nervous system as well as the endocrine system maintain extensive communication with the immune system through the influence of hormones and neurotransmitters and also by way of the hardwiring of sympathetic and parasympathetic nerves to the lymphoid organs. There is now convincing evidence that the communication between these three body systems is bidirectional. (2007, p. 256)

All body cells have receptor sites for neuropeptides (amino acids produced in the brain and other sites in the body that act as chemical communicators) that are released when neurotransmitters (chemical substances produced by the body that facilitate nerve transmission) signal emotions in the brain. Thus, it is possible for cells to be directly affected by emotions. In other words, people can affect their health by what they think and feel. The intermeshed complex system of psyche and body chemistry is now referred to as the bodymind, an inseparable connection and operation of thoughts, feelings, and physiological functions.

HOLISM AND NURSING PRACTICE

The growth of the holistic health movement is based on the concept that body, mind, and spirit are interconnected. Holism refers to the concept that the whole is greater than the sum of its parts. Nursing in its broadest sense (theory, concept, and practice) is truly holistic in nature. Holism encompasses consideration of the physiological, psychological, sociocultural, intellectual, and spiritual aspects of each individual. Holistic nursing can be described as the art and science of caring for the whole person, knowing that each person is unique in all expressions of self. As holistic healers, nurses often employ CAM techniques to promote clients' well-being. The accompanying Spotlight On display lists concepts basic to a holistic philosophy of caring.

THE NATURE OF HEALING

The word *healing* is derived from the Anglo-Saxon word *hael*, which means to make whole, to move toward, or to become whole. It is important to establish that healing is not the same as curing (ridding one of disease) but rather is a process that activates the individual's healing forces from within. As a healing facilitator, the nurse enters into a relationship

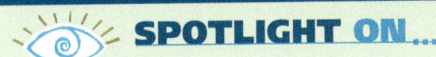

SPOTLIGHT ON...

Caring

Holistic Concepts

- Mind and body are one, not separate.
- People are responsible for their own choices.
- People have the power to solve their own problems.
- Well-being is multifaceted—physical, emotional, mental, and spiritual.

with the client and can assist the client by offering to be a guide, change agent, or instrument of healing (a means by which healing can be achieved, performed, or enhanced).

COMPLEMENTARY AND ALTERNATIVE INTERVENTIONS

Many CAM interventions are used in holistic nursing practice. These interventions are categorized as mind-body, body-movement, energetic-touch, spiritual, nutritional, and other methodologies (see Table 31-2 on page 838). Although different in technique, many of the CAM therapies have common ideological threads, including:

- The whole system must be considered if the *parts* of the individual are to be helped to function.
- The person is integrated and related to his or her surroundings.
- There exists some life force or energy that can be used in the healing process.
- Ritual, prescribed practice, and skilled practitioners are integral parts of holistic healing interventions.

MIND-BODY: SELF-REGULATORY TECHNIQUES

Self-regulatory techniques are methods by which an individual can consciously control some functions of the sympathetic nervous system (e.g., heart rate, respiratory rate, and blood pressure). Self-regulatory techniques include relaxation, meditation, imagery, biofeedback, and hypnosis.

Relaxation

As a result of the flight-or-fight response (see Chapter 23 for details), the body releases epinephrine, speeds up metabolism, and increases heart and respiratory rates. Relaxation techniques offer a way for a person to reduce stress and return to a normal physiological state.

Cardiologist Herbert Benson (1975) studied the effects of meditation on individuals. He then incorporated the basic elements of meditation into the therapeutic process he called

TABLE 31-2 Categories of Complementary and Alternative Interventions

MIND-BODY	BODY-MOVEMENT	ENERGETIC-TOUCH	SPIRITUAL	NUTRITIONAL AND MEDICINAL	OTHER
• Hypnosis • Imagery • Biofeedback • Meditation • Relaxation	• Chiropractic therapy • Yoga • Tai chi	• Therapeutic touch • Healing touch • Massage • Acupuncture • Acupressure • Reflexology	• Faith healing • Prayer • Laying on of hands • Shamanism: sand painting, sweat lodges, drumming	• Herbs • Antioxidants • Macrobiotic diet	• Humor • Pet therapy • Music • Aromatherapy

Delmar/Cengage Learning

the **relaxation response**, a state of increased arousal of the parasympathetic nervous system, which leads to a relaxed physiological state. Benson employed the relaxation response with individuals experiencing high blood pressure and heart disease. While initially trying to avoid a mystical flavor in his work, Benson later discovered that the techniques were more effective if individuals focused on an inspirational prayer or phrase.

One method for achieving relaxation is progressive muscle relaxation (PMR), which is the alternate tensing and relaxing of muscles (see Chapter 23 for a complete discussion of PMR). PMR is used to exert positive effects on heart rate and anxiety levels (Mayo Clinic, 2007). Aids to relaxation training include music or nature sounds, hypertonic saline relaxation tanks, isolation chambers, yoga, and imagery.

Nurses can use relaxation techniques in their work with clients to reduce pain and stress. Relaxation techniques are also an essential aspect of cognitive behavioral therapy when treating people with phobias, fear, and depression.

Meditation

The practice of **meditation**, quieting the mind by focusing one's attention, can bring about remarkable physiological changes. People who meditate strive for a sense of oneness within themselves and a sense of relatedness to a greater power and the universe. One form of meditation is mindfulness, in which individuals focus their complete attention on the present moment. This process temporarily stops negative thinking and related anxiety.

Some therapeutic benefits of meditation are:

• Stress relief
• Relaxation
• Reduced levels of lactic acid
• Decreased oxygen consumption
• Slowed heart rate
• Decreased blood pressure
• Improved functioning of immune system

As stated by Cuellar (2008), mindfulness meditation can be useful in improving health outcomes and quality of life.

To evoke the relaxation response through meditation, repeat a word or short phrase, preferably one that has special meaning to the individual. For example, some individuals repeat a short prayer or relaxing phrase.

Imagery

Imagery is a type of thinking without words in which the senses are used to evoke one's imagination. The practitioner encourages the client to use as many of the senses as possible in order to enhance the formation of vivid images. See Table 31-3, which presents examples of images that can be evoked by the five senses.

Imagery is not a new concept in nursing. In the mid-1800s, Nightingale wrote in *Notes on Nursing* (1860) about nurses helping the ill to alter their thoughts through images of nature, such as a bouquet of flowers.

Guided imagery can be used with clients who are capable of hearing and understanding the nurse's suggestions of

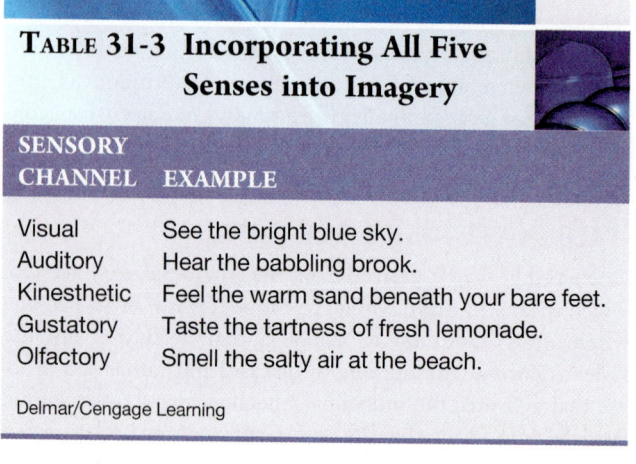

TABLE 31-3 Incorporating All Five Senses into Imagery

SENSORY CHANNEL	EXAMPLE
Visual	See the bright blue sky.
Auditory	Hear the babbling brook.
Kinesthetic	Feel the warm sand beneath your bare feet.
Gustatory	Taste the tartness of fresh lemonade.
Olfactory	Smell the salty air at the beach.

Delmar/Cengage Learning

meaningful and physiologically correct images. For example, a nurse can show a chart of the stages of bone healing to a client who has suffered a fracture and ask the client to imagine this activity occurring in his or her body.

In addition to being a tool for distraction when a person is confronting pain, discomfort, and fear, imagery is a powerful mechanism for making decisions and for altering behaviors. Imagery is also used to reduce pain and anxiety before and during procedures and to promote comfort. Imagery is described by Reed as being "time- and cost-effective, and creat[ing] a healing partnership between nurse and patient" (2007, p. 276). However, imagery is not suitable for use with every client; see the accompanying Safety First display. See Chapter 23 for directions on performing imagery and PMR exercises.

Biofeedback

Biofeedback is a measurement of physiological responses that yields information about the relationship between the mind and the body and helps clients change those responses through mental activity. Biofeedback allows a person to see the effect of the mind on the body. While attached to sensitive devices that measure such bodily responses as skin temperature, blood pressure, galvanic skin resistance, and electrical activity in the muscles, the individual imagines stressful experiences. The person's physiological responses are then measured and recorded. Subsequent physiological responses to the relaxation response are also recorded. The individual receives an interpretation of these responses and is taught methods for practicing relaxation.

Biofeedback is used as a restorative method in rehabilitation settings to help clients who have lost sensation and function as the result of illness or injury. Biofeedback also enhances relaxation in tense muscles, relieves tension headaches, reduces bruxism (grinding of the teeth), reduces the pain of temporomandibular joint syndrome, and relieves backache. Temperature biofeedback is useful in training people to purposefully warm their hands to treat Raynaud's disease (a circulatory disorder), to lower blood pressure, and to prevent or relieve migraine headaches.

Hypnosis

Misconceptions about the practice of hypnosis were once very common. Currently hypnosis is becoming more accepted as a therapeutic intervention. Therapeutic hypnosis induces altered states of consciousness or awareness (a trance) during which the person is more receptive to suggestion. It also enhances the client's ability to form images. In 1955, the British Medical Association approved hypnotherapy as a valid medical intervention. The American Medical Association did likewise in 1958. Therapeutic use of suggestion is the heart of hypnosis. Suggestions can be phrased directly ("You will feel more comfortable") or indirectly ("You may feel different"). Hypnosis is a potentially effective and powerful tool for altering pain, anxiety, and some physiological processes. Although hypnosis is useful as an adjunct to treatment, it does not magically cure problems such as nicotine addiction, alcoholism, and eating disorders and should be used in conjunction with other modalities.

Nurses wishing to use hypnosis in their practice must be aware of the guidelines concerning this modality in the scope of practice as defined by the respective state boards of nursing. Advanced training in hypnosis is also necessary.

BODY-MOVEMENT: MANIPULATION STRATEGIES

As the name implies, body-movement therapies employ techniques for moving or manipulating various body parts to achieve therapeutic outcomes. Methods such as movement and exercise, yoga, tai chi, and chiropractic treatment are discussed in the following sections.

Movement and Exercise

Movement, as a therapeutic intervention and health-promoting activity, is associated with athletic exercise, dance, celebration, and healing rituals. Although the primary goal of exercise is fitness (muscle strength, flexibility, endurance, and cardiovascular and respiratory health), there are many other positive outcomes of exercise (see Chapter 23 for a complete discussion of the benefits of exercise).

Nurses can help clients use movement as therapy in a variety of ways, including range-of-motion exercises, water exercises, physical therapy, and stretching exercises. Physical activity is an effective method through which people of all ages can improve their level of functioning. Some of the therapeutic benefits of exercise are as follows:

- Improves circulation
- Enhances respiratory function
- Promotes elimination
- Stimulates the release of endorphins (brain chemicals that boost mood and help fight depression)
- Helps regulate metabolism
- Enhances immune function

YOGA Many cultures believe that particular forms of movement keep the body's life forces in correct balance and flow. Yoga and tai chi are examples of ancient ritual movements that enhance overall health, including spiritual enlightenment and well-being. Both of these approaches require concentration, strength, flexibility, and use of symbolic movements. The three main elements of yoga are breathing, movement, and posture. Yoga involves completing a series of postures carried out in sequential order; see Figure 31-3 on page 840, which illustrates some basic yoga postures.

▼ SAFETY FIRST ▼

PRECAUTION FOR IMAGERY
Imagery is not recommended for clients who are emotionally unstable. The thoughts could become overwhelming and thus increase anxiety.

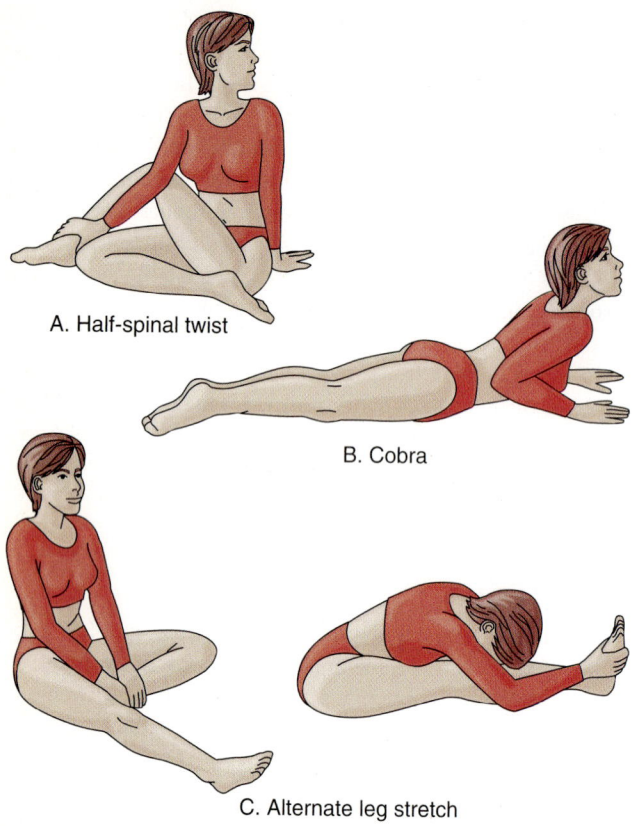

A. Half-spinal twist

B. Cobra

C. Alternate leg stretch

FIGURE 31-3 **Yoga Postures** DELMAR/CENGAGE LEARNING

Yoga rejuvenates, promotes longevity and self-realization, and speeds up the natural evolution of the person toward self-enlightenment. Yoga, a form of meditative exercise, originated in India and is an essential component of Ayurvedic healing.

TAI CHI Tai chi is based on the philosophy of the quest for harmony with nature and the universe through the laws of complementary (yin and yang) balance. When perfect harmony exists, the body functions effortlessly, spontaneously, perfectly, and in accordance with the laws of nature. If one moves to the right, then one must also move to the left. Tai chi consists of a series of sequential dancelike moves connected in a smooth, flowing process.

People who regularly perform tai chi believe it enhances stamina, agility, and balance and that it boosts energy and confers a sense of well-being. Tai chi has been shown to lower blood pressure and heart rate in people in cardiac rehabilitation programs, and it is also a method for improving balance and, thus, reducing falls, which is especially helpful for older adults (Leddy, 2006). Tai chi also helps reduce symptoms of individuals experiencing fibromyalgia, a musculoskeletal disorder associated with pain and functional impairment.

Chiropractic

The major principle underlying **chiropractic** therapy is that the brain sends vital energy to every organ in the body via the nerves originating in the spinal column. Disease

results from interferences along that pathway; therefore, manipulation of the spinal column is useful in alleviating a variety of ills. Removing the blocks with quick thrusts and adjustments allows the body to restore its innate recuperative power.

Chiropractic is widely accepted by the medical community. Chiropractors are staff members of some medical centers and hospitals. As with any CAM intervention, nurses should encourage clients considering the use of chiropractic services to undergo comprehensive health assessments first to rule out any contraindications. Many insurance companies pay for chiropractic services.

ENERGETIC-TOUCH HEALING

A category of CAM therapies that has been incorporated into nursing for decades is the **energetic-touch therapies**, a group of techniques that work with the body's energy field by the use of the hands to direct or redirect energy to enhance balance within the field. These modalities are effective interventions for many client problems and can be used to restore harmony in all aspects of a person's health. Energetic-touch therapies can be used with persons of all ages.

Energetic-touch therapies have their roots in traditional Chinese, ancient Eastern, and Native American philosophies. The fundamental concept is that individuals are composed of a life force, a source of energy that is not confined to physical skin boundaries. Another fundamental belief underlying energetic-touch therapies is that life depends on the movement of energy. Figure 31-4 on page 841 illustrates the energy field that extends beyond a person's physical body.

An individual's energy field consists of layers of energy that are in constant flux. The energy layers can be diminished or otherwise adversely affected by any type of illness, trauma, or distress. The energy system can also be positively affected by the intentionally directed use of the hands of a practitioner.

Holistic nurses were integral in helping the North American Nursing Diagnosis Association International (NANDA, 2009) to establish the diagnosis *Disturbed energy field*. NANDA considers this to be a disturbed energy field that leads to an imbalance of body, mind, or spirit.

There are many energetic-touch therapies being used by nurses today. These therapies are being effectively integrated into holistic practice. Massage, therapeutic touch, healing touch, Reiki, Jin Shin Jyutsu, and J Shin Do are some examples. Three of those therapies—massage, therapeutic touch, and healing touch—are discussed in more detail.

Touch

One of the most universal CAM modalities is touch. **Touch**, simply defined, is the means of perceiving or experiencing through tactile sensation. According to anthropologist Montague (1986), touch is the earliest sense to develop in humans and, thus, it provides a basic means of interacting with others and the environment. Tactile stimulation is necessary for survival and the healthy behavioral development of an individual (Bowlby, 1984). Touch has been used in all ancient cultures and shamanistic traditions for healing.

recipient's well-being. It involves kneading, rubbing, and using friction. The primary techniques used to perform a massage are described in Table 31-4.

Many touch therapies have been assimilated into mainstream nursing practice. Massage therapy is now recognized as a highly beneficial modality and is prescribed by a number of health care practitioners. In addition, many states now have licensing requirements for massage practitioners.

Traditionally, back rubs have been administered by nurses to provide comfort to hospitalized clients. Massage techniques can be used with all age groups and are especially beneficial to those who are immobilized. A back rub or massage can achieve many results, including relaxation, increased circulation of the blood and lymph, and relief from musculoskeletal stiffness and pain. "Massage is an applicable, noninvasive, therapeutic modality that can be integrated safely as

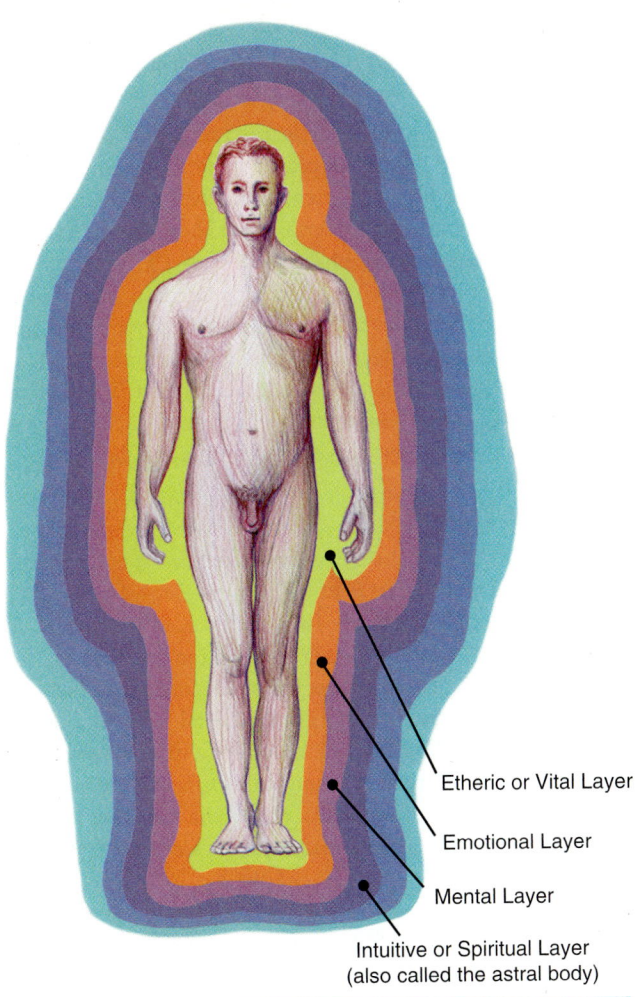

FIGURE 31-4 Layers of Human Energy Field Extending Beyond the Physical Boundaries DELMAR/CENGAGE LEARNING

Etheric or Vital Layer

Emotional Layer

Mental Layer

Intuitive or Spiritual Layer (also called the astral body)

The advent of scientific medicine and Puritanism led many healers away from the purposeful use of touch. Some cultures are very comfortable with physical touch; others specify that touch may be used only in certain situations within specified parameters. See Chapter 20 for a complete discussion about cultural aspects of touch.

Because touch involves personal contact, the nurse must be sure to convey positive intentions. When in doubt, the nurse should withhold touch until effective communication with the client has been established. Touch has several important uses in nursing practice in that it:

- Is an integral part of assessment
- Promotes bonding between nurse and client
- Is an important means of communication, especially when other senses are impaired
- Assists in soothing, calming, and comforting
- Helps keep the client oriented

See the Safety First Display on page 842.

Therapeutic Massage

Therapeutic massage is the application of pressure and motion by the hands with the intent of improving the

TABLE 31-4 Basic Massage Techniques	
TECHNIQUE	**DESCRIPTION**
Effleurage	The entire hand is used. Gliding and long rhythmic strokes are used. Firm, even-pressured strokes are directed toward the heart to assist blood return. Lighter pressure is used when moving away from the heart.
Petrissage	Pressing, squeezing, kneading, and rolling movements by both hands; entire hands are used. Deep circulation is enhanced. C-shaped motions stimulate muscle bodies. Promotes muscular relaxation.
Friction	Thumb pads, heel of hand, or fingertips are used. Focused, deep, circular motions are used. Penetrates deeper muscle layers. Is done after effleurage and petrissage.
Tapotement	Palm, fingertips, and knuckles are used. Brisk, vigorous, rhythmic, percussive movements are used. Hands alternately tap, cup, slap, and pummel muscles. Invigorates and stimulates tired muscles.
Vibration	Very fine, rapid, shaking movements are administered by entire hand. Stimulates or relaxes muscles.

Delmar/Cengage Learning

▼ SAFETY FIRST ▼

CONTRAINDICATIONS FOR TOUCH

It is important to know when not to touch. It may be difficult for persons who have been neglected, abused, or injured to accept touch therapy. Touching those who are distrustful or angry may escalate negative behaviors.

an adjunct intervention for managing side effects and psychological conditions associated with anticancer treatment in children. Massage may support immune function during periods of immunosuppression" (Hughes, Ladas, Rooney, & Kelly, 2008, p. 442).

Massage should be used with caution for people with heart disease, diabetes, hypertension, or kidney disease because increased circulation in these conditions may be harmful. Massage should never be attempted in areas of circulatory abnormalities such as aneurysm, varicose veins, necrosis, phlebitis, or thrombus or in areas of soft-tissue injury, open wounds, inflammation, joint or bone injury, dermatitis, recent surgery, or sciatica. See the Safety First display.

Procedure 31-1 describes the techniques involved in performing a massage. Almost half of all state boards of nursing recognize CAM as being within the scope of nursing practice (S. S. Kim, Erlen, Kim, & Sok, 2006). The National Association of Nurse Massage Therapists (NANMT) was established in 1990 to promote professional ethical standards for nurse massage therapists. The standards established by the NANMT reflect those of the American Nurses Association.

Therapeutic Touch

Therapeutic touch (TT), which is based on ancient healing practices (e.g., the laying on of hands), consists of assessing alterations in a person's energy field and using the hands to direct energy to achieve a balanced state. The practice of TT was developed in the early 1970s by Dolores Krieger, PhD, RN, then professor of nursing at New York University, and Dora Kunz, a noted healer. TT is based on four concepts:

- A human being is an open energy system.
- Anatomically, a human being is bilaterally symmetrical.
- Illness is an imbalance in an individual's energy field.

▼ SAFETY FIRST ▼

Do not massage areas with visible redness or edema, which may be indicators of a thrombus (blood clot). Rubbing such an area may release the thrombus into the bloodstream, resulting in a circulatory problem.

- Human beings have natural abilities to transform and transcend their conditions of living (Kunz & Krieger, 2004).

The TT process is readily learned in workshops, can be done with hands either on or off the body in the energy field, complements medical treatments, and has reasonably consistent and reliable results (see Figure 31-5). Table 31-5 on page 843 presents the five-phase process of TT.

The relaxation response may be apparent in the client as quickly as 2 to 5 minutes after a TT treatment has begun, and some clients may fall asleep or require less pain medication after a treatment. A clinical study indicates that TT reduces both pain and anxiety in clients with cancer (Jackson et al., 2008). Healing is enhanced when body energy is balanced.

Healing Touch

Healing touch (HT) is an energy-based therapeutic modality that alters the energy field through the use of touch. HT was developed by Janet Mentgen, a nurse, in the 1980s. In 1993, HT was established as a certification program of the American Holistic Nurses Association. Its curriculum includes varied techniques for use of HT in general balancing of the body's energy field, relaxation, and specific problems such as headaches, spinal problems, and pain. One study indicates that the use of HT reduced anxiety and the length of hospital stay in clients with coronary artery bypass surgery (MacIntyre et al., 2008).

Table 31-6 on page 844 lists the five steps of HT. HT recognizes the need for follow-up or sequential treatments as well as discharge planning and referral to assist the client in adequately meeting goals.

In both TT and HT, the practitioner uses **centering**, a process of bringing oneself to an inward focus of serenity, before initiating treatment. Centering is a useful tool to employ before performing any treatment or before any situation that may be stressful or difficult (e.g., an important school examination).

In addition to therapeutic massage, TT, and HT, there are many other touch modalities that can be integrated into

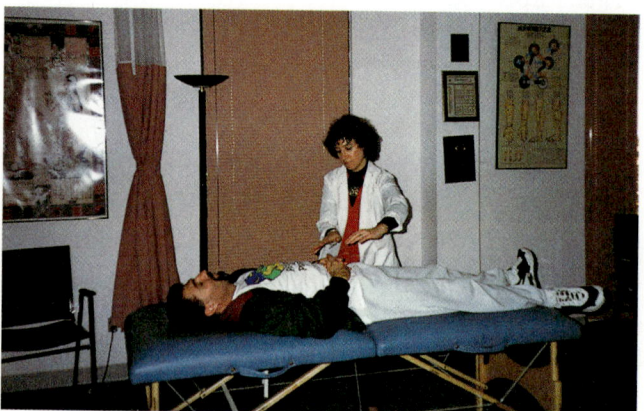

FIGURE 31-5 A nurse administers therapeutic touch to a client. Is there a relationship between the use of TT as a therapeutic modality and the healing systems that can be traced to Far Eastern cultures? DELMAR/CENGAGE LEARNING

TABLE 31-5 Phases of Therapeutic Touch

PHASE	DEFINITION	TECHNIQUES
Centering	• Bringing body, mind, and emotions to a quiet, focused state of consciousness • Being still • Being nonjudgmental	Become centered by use of: • Controlled breathing • Imagery • Meditation
Assessment ("scanning")	• Using the hands to determine the nature of the client's energy field • Being attuned to sensory cues (e.g., warmth, coolness, static, pressure, tingling) to detect changes in client's energy	• Hold hands 2 to 6 inches away from person's energy field while moving the hands from the head to the feet in a rhythmic, symmetrical manner.
Unruffling ("clearing")	• Facilitating the symmetrical and rhythmic flow of energy through the field	• Use slightly more vigorous hand movements from midline while continuing to move in a rhythmic and symmetrical manner from the head to the feet.
Treatment ("balancing," "rebalancing," or "intervention")	• Projecting, directing, and modulating energy on the basis of the nature of the living energy field • Assisting to reestablish order in the system	• Because each practitioner experiences the living energy field uniquely, the law of opposites serves as a guideline for intervening (e.g., if a pulling or drawing sensation is detected, then direct energy to the depleted area until it feels replenished). • Continue to assess, clear, and balance the field while remaining centered.
Evaluation	• Using professional, informed, and intuitive judgment to determine when to end the session	• Reassess the field. • Elicit feedback from the client. • Give the client an opportunity to rest and integrate the process.

Note: The phases, although learned sequentially by beginners, are dynamic and often are performed concurrently and repetitively by experienced practitioners. Data from Macrae, J. (2005). *Therapeutic touch: A practical guide.* New York: Alfred A. Knopf.

nursing practice. Some of the more common types of touch therapies are reflexology and acupressure with its many variations. These techniques involve deep-tissue bodywork and require advanced training for practitioners.

Shiatsu Acupressure

Shiatsu acupressure is based on East Asian philosophy and Japanese methodology. *Shiatsu,* from the word meaning "finger pressure," differs from acupuncture, a procedure that uses needles and heat to deliver treatment. In Shiatsu, blocked energy within the client is released by application of the practitioner's fingers, thumbs, and heels of the hands along certain pressure points (meridians). Acupressure, which is a noninvasive technique, has been used to successfully treat nausea and vomiting associated with pregnancy (Can Gurkan & Arslan, 2008; Shin, Song, & Seo, 2007). Acupressure is also recommended as an effective, noninvasive method for decreasing agitated behavior in people with dementia (Yang, Wu, Lin, & Lin, 2007). When practicing shiatsu, nurses need to be self-aware and grounded—that is, focused on their

inner energy. This focus enables the practitioner to concentrate completely on promoting the client's comfort.

Acupuncture

Acupuncture is the use of needles inserted at specific points on the body (energy pathways) to promote healing. Acupuncture is done to manipulate the energy flow throughout the body; treatment focuses on correcting the flow of *chi* (energy) when imbalances (blockages) occur. TCM practitioners believe that meridians conduct chi between the body's surface and internal organs. Acupuncture points are believed to stimulate the central nervous system to release chemicals into the muscles, spinal cord, and brain. These chemicals either alter the experience of pain or produce other chemicals that lessen pain.

Acupuncture is one of the oldest, most commonly used medical procedures in the world. It originated in China over 2,000 years ago and is effective in treating a variety of health problems. Extensive research is currently being done to determine the efficacy of acupuncture. This CAM method

TABLE 31-6 Steps of Healing Touch

STEP	DESCRIPTION	NURSING GUIDELINES
Initial interview	• Provides the working base for energetic interventions and functions as an intake assessment.	• Introduce yourself. • Explain the HT modality so that a feeling of confidence can begin to develop. • Determine the main problem or reason for treatment. • Identify relevant health history: hospitalizations, diseases, injuries, diagnoses, medications (past and present) including use of recreational drugs, nicotine, alcohol, caffeine, vitamins, and herbs. All these factors can influence the energy field.
Assessment	• In wellness, the energy flows evenly from head to toe without blocks, breaks, unevenness, or temperature variations. Any disruption of the flow reflects disharmony in that area.	• Approach the client from a centered state. • Begin by determining the shape of the energy field by slowly scanning its outer edges. • Start 3 to 4 feet away from the body and move toward it using the palms until you can determine the actual outline of the energy field. • Continue the assessment by feeling the vital layer 1 to 6 inches off the skin. • Identify areas in relation to the physical body where the field is different, perhaps not as vibrant or as smooth as in other areas.
Documentation	• Begins with the initial client contact.	• Mentally take note of all sensations, even subtle ones. • A picture of the energy pattern is usually easy to execute by drawing the perceived pattern on a simple outline of the body. • Areas of energetic differences can be drawn in, as can injuries, swelling, scars, or the track of a pain ridge.
Intervention	• The healer can choose many healing interventions in this sequence: therapeutic touch, full-body techniques, and localized and specific techniques.	• During the intervention, which may last 20 to 30 minutes, all of the healer's skill and experience are used.
Completion and grounding	• After completion of the interventions, carefully ground the client to help restore balance and promote integration. • Determine that the client is fully alert if the client will leave after the session.	Grounding can be done in a variety of ways, including: • Hold the feet until you sense a flow and a connection with the client and sense that the client's energy is back in the feet. • Brush down the body from head to toe and down the arms toward the ground. Repeat briskly several times. • Give a suggestion: "Feel your fingers and your toes; now gently move them until you return to full awareness in this room." • Reassess the energy field at this time and document the changes. • Spend some time with the client to obtain feedback. Focus on what the client experienced. Talking helps the client to feel grounded.

has been shown to be effective for management of symptoms (i.e., pain, dyspnea, nausea, and vomiting) in clients receiving palliative and hospice care (Standish, Kozak, & Congdon, 2008). Other studies indicate the efficacy of acupuncture in pain reduction, in children with cancer (Rheingans, 2007), and in adults with pain resulting from osteoarthritis of the knee (Maa, Sun, & Wu, 2008). The use of acupuncture in effectively treating insomnia is documented in other research studies (Kalavapalli & Singareddy, 2007; K. B. Kim & Sok, 2007). Findings of another study indicate that acupuncture is helpful in reducing hot flashes for women receiving hormonal treatment for breast cancer (Walker, de Valois, Davies, Young, & Maher, 2007).

Reflexology

Reflexology is rooted in ancient healing arts. Egyptian wall paintings from approximately 2300 BC show the use of reflexology. Contemporary use of reflexology is credited to the work of William H. Fitzgerald, an American physician who, in the early 1900s, discovered that applying pressure to certain parts of the fingers could relieve pain in other body parts. In the 1930s, Eunice Ingham discovered that certain points on the feet were more responsive to pressure and provided better pain relief than points on the hand.

The fundamental concept of reflexology is that the body is divided into 10 equal, longitudinal zones that run the length of the body from the top of the head to the tip of the toes. These 10 zones are correlated with the 10 fingers and toes. The foot is viewed as a microcosm of the entire body. Reflexology theory posits that illness manifests itself in calcium deposits and acids in the corresponding part of the person's foot. Pressing specific points on the foot stimulates energy movement and produces relaxation, reduces stress, and promotes health by relieving pressures and accumulation of toxins in the corresponding body part (see Figure 31-6).

Reflexology can be used as a complementary method for managing chronic conditions such as asthma, sinus infections, migraines, irritable bowel syndrome, kidney stones, and constipation. Other symptoms that have responded well to reflexology sessions are phantom limb pain (experienced by individuals with amputated limbs) and anxiety (Brown & Lido, 2008; McVicar et al., 2007).Once the pressure points are learned, the nurse can massage the areas of the client's foot to relieve pain and produce relaxation. See the Community Considerations display.

SPIRITUAL THERAPIES

A state of wholeness or health is dependent not only on one's relationship to the physical and interpersonal environment but also to the spiritual aspects of self. The idea that there is a relationship between spirituality and health is not new. Spirituality is the core of many holistic modalities.

The role of the spirit in healing is witnessed in all cultures. The inseparable link between the state of one's soul (life energy or spirit) and the state of one's health is accepted by many cultures. Psychoneuroimmunologists are validating that there are inner mechanisms of healing within individuals. Many of the major religions have ideologies relating to health, illness, and healing. Health maintenance implies having a balanced spiritual life. Refer to Chapter 24 for more information on spirituality.

Faith Healing

At the heart of spiritual or faith healing is the practitioner's belief that one has to purify one's self and reach a state of unity with God or a Higher Power. This process, based on religious belief, is usually done through prayer. During preparation for healing, the practitioner adapts a passive and receptive mood in order to be a channel for divine power. To benefit from the healer's intervention, the ill person's belief enhances, but is not crucial to, the success of healing.

Individuals with strong spiritual beliefs rely on faith for support, comfort, and assistance. For example, "in contemporary Navajo society, traditional Navajo ceremonies, Native American Church prayer meetings, and Navajo Christian

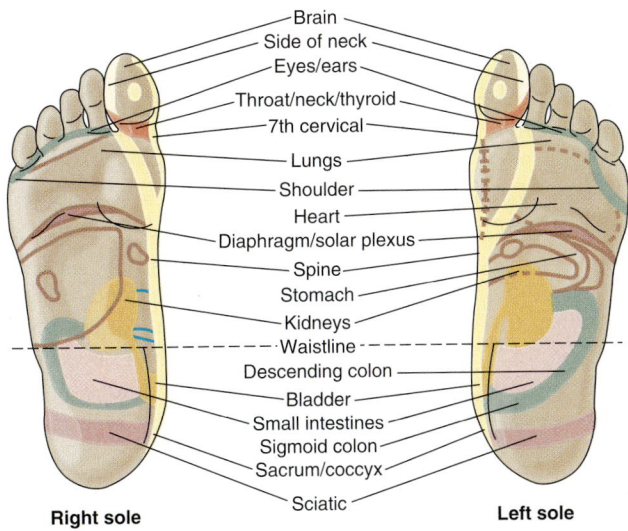

Right sole **Left sole**

FIGURE 31-6 Foot Reflexology Charts REPRODUCED WITH PERMISSION FROM BETTER HEALTH WITH FOOT REFLEXOLOGY; COPYRIGHT © 1983 BY DWIGHT C. BYERS. INGHAM PUBLISHING, INC., POB 12642, ST. PETERSBURG, FL 33733-2642. WWW.REFLEXOLOGY-USA.NET

COMMUNITY CONSIDERATIONS

Application of Touch

Is there a group of people whom you can identify as being socially isolated or in distress who could benefit from one or more of the touch therapies? Consider residents of extended care facilities, caregivers of chronically ill children or elderly parents, and hospice clients. Do you think that touch therapies can be used as routine preventive care for healthy populations?

faith healing are all highly sought-after resources in the everyday pursuit of health and well-being" (Csordas, Storck, & Strauss, 2008, p. 595). According to Mehl-Madrona (2008), people with cancer who sought out aboriginal healers perceived a sense of forgiveness, release of anger and blame, and refusal to accept death as imminent. A study by Tanyi and Werner (2007) indicates that African American women with end-stage renal disease had several sources of spiritual support, including perceptions of God's concern for them, a sense of life's purpose, and satisfaction with life.

Healing Prayer

When individuals pray, they believe they are communicating directly with God or a Higher Power. Prayer is an integral part of a person's spiritual life and, as such, can affect well-being. Florence Nightingale (1860) recognized that prayer helps connect individuals to nature and the environment. Many religions adhere to established rituals for organized prayer. For example, Tibetan Buddhists use prayer wheels—wooden and metal cylinders with prayers written on them. Islam has five periods of prayer scheduled daily. Some religious groups, such as Christian Scientists, rely on prayer in lieu of conventional medical therapy due to the belief that prayer alone can heal disease. "Chronic illnesses such as cancer are very stressful events and prayer is a valuable coping strategy for Muslim cancer patients" (Rezaei, Adib-Hajbaghery, Seyedfatemi, & Hoseini, 2008, p. 96). Results from another study indicate that prayer was preferred by the majority of older home care clients experiencing depression (Fyffe, Brown, Sirey, Hill, & Bruce, 2008).

NCCAM (2007a) is currently investigating the effects of prayer on physical health. The exact mechanism for the effect of prayer on healing is not known; see Figure 31-7. "Prayer has been used for persons with every type of illness, of all age groups, and from all cultures" (Snyder, 2006, p. 149). Prayer provides comfort and support to many individuals experiencing pain and anxiety as a result of illness and/or treatment procedures.

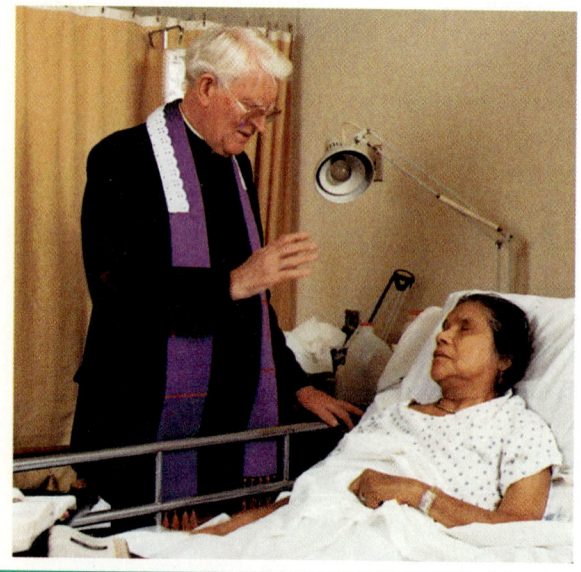

FIGURE 31-7 Prayer brings a sense of peace and healing to many individuals. DELMAR/CENGAGE LEARNING

NUTRITIONAL THERAPIES

In the last 40 years, nutritional interventions for prevention and treatment of disease have received increased interest from consumers and health care providers. This section addresses the CAM nutritional approaches.

Nutraceuticals

Currently, many foods are being studied for their medicinal value. The term **nutraceuticals** refers to any natural substances found in plant or animal foods that act as protective or healing agents. **Phytonutrients** are those chemicals found in plants; see Table 31-7 on page 847 for a listing of the major phytonutrients and their actions.

The best source of nutrients is fresh whole foods, preferably eaten in their natural form. The standard Western diet lacks many essential nutrients and contains many harmful additives due to processing. In contrast, the TCM diet contains fresh, semiraw, and slightly cooked ingredients. Foods that are being investigated by the National Cancer Institute (2007) for possible cancer preventive qualities include carrots, celery, citrus fruits, flaxseed, garlic, licorice root, parsley, and soybeans.

Antioxidants and Free Radicals

Antioxidants exert several beneficial effects, including prevention of cancer, reduction of heart disease, and decreased allergy symptoms (Lukan, Racz, Mocnejova, & Tkac, 2008). Antioxidants react with free radicals, preventing them from damaging cells and from altering DNA. Dietary antioxidants have been shown to be effective in protecting the body from free radicals. The antioxidants devour free radicals (unstable molecules that alter genetic codes and trigger the development of cancer growth in cells).

Sources for dietary antioxidants include vitamin C (in fruits and vegetables), beta-carotene (yellow-orange pigment in fruits and vegetables), and vitamin E (in polyunsaturated oils, butter, and eggs). Other vitamins, minerals, trace elements, and enzymes are being investigated for possible therapeutic value. See Chapter 34 for a through discussion of the essential vitamins, their functions, and major sources.

Macrobiotic Diet

In the 1960s, macrobiotic diets (from the Greek *makro,* meaning long, and *bios,* meaning life) became popular because of the heightened interest in "natural" and more spiritual approaches to managing health and illness. The basis for macrobiotics is the Taoist concept of balance between opposites that is achieved through food intake. Food has the qualities of *yin* (associated with death, cold, and darkness) and *yang* (associated with immortality, heat, and light). For example, tropical and sweet foods are yin, and meat and eggs are yang. Overindulgence in either type causes difficulties; too much yin yields worry and resentment whereas too much yang leads to hostility and aggression. People need balance and, therefore, should consume foods that are neither too yin nor too yang.

Because brown rice and whole grains are categorized as balanced foods, they are major staples in a macrobiotic diet.

The diet should be flexible and related to the season; it should consist of foods indigenous to the area in which the individual lives. Foods to be avoided include processed and treated foods, red meat, sugar, dairy products, eggs, and caffeine. See the Safety First display.

Herbal Therapy

Herbal medicine has been a powerful tool in folk healing for centuries. Medicinal herbs have been catalogued for thousands of years and have probably existed in every culture. Many drugs commonly used today were once folk remedies derived from plants. For example, salicin, the active chemical ingredient found in white willow bark, has been used by TCM practitioners and Native Americans for pain relief. This same salicin is a precursor to salicylic acid, an ingredient in aspirin. Herbal medicine, also known as botanical medicine or phytotherapy, uses plant extracts for therapeutic outcomes. Many holistic practitioners incorporate the use of herbs into their practice.

Learning about herbal treatment is similar to learning pharmacology. Herbs work because of their chemical composition. Different herbs contain different compounds that can strengthen the immune system, alter the blood chemistry, or protect specific organs against disease. For example, peppermint oil may help relieve the symptoms of irritable bowel syndrome by exerting a relaxant effect on the muscles of the gastrointestinal tract. Echinacea is frequently used for its immune-enhancing properties. However, it should not be taken longer than 8 to 10 consecutive weeks due to the potential for liver toxicity.

Herbs are not cure-alls, and many take time to exert their healing properties. Generally, it is wise to use herbs for treating conditions one would ordinarily self-treat; see the Safety First display on page 848. Conditions that generally respond well to herbal therapy are:

▼ SAFETY FIRST ▼

MACROBIOTIC DIETS
Children and pregnant women should use the macrobiotic diet with caution. It may not have sufficient variety and, therefore, could be deficient in vitamins D and B$_{12}$.

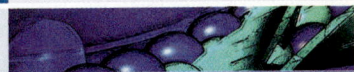

TABLE 31-7 Actions and Sources of Major Phytonutrients

PHYTONUTRIENT	SOURCES	ACTIONS
Ascorbic acid	Citrus fruits, broccoli, most fruits and vegetables	Binds iron, preventing it from becoming a cancer-causing preoxidant
Capsaicin	Red chili peppers	Helps prevent carcinogens from binding with DNA at the cellular level
Catechins	Green tea, black tea	Reduces the risk of gastrointestinal cancers
Fiber lignans	Soybeans, flaxseed, nuts	Inhibits growth of tumors
Fiber pectins	Apples, pears, plums, prunes	Improves colon health; encourages growth of beneficial intestinal flora
Lycopene	Tomatoes, tomato sauce	Protects against prostate cancer; helps block UVA and UVB rays
Phytoestrogens	Soy products, alfalfa sprouts	Helps reduce menopausal symptoms; may block some cancers (e.g., breast, prostate)
Phytosterols	Plant oils, corn, sesame, soy, safflower, pumpkin, wheat	Inhibits uptake of cholesterol from foods; blocks hormonal role in cancer production
Protease inhibitors	Soybeans and soy products, eggs, cereals, potatoes	Protects against negative effects of radiation and free radical damage; prevents activation of certain genes that cause cancer
Sulfur compounds	Onions, garlic	Lowers blood pressure; improves immune system response; fights infections; has antimicrobial effect; lowers cholesterol; reduces triglycerides

Data from Balch, P. (2008). *Prescription for nutritional healing: The A-to-Z guide to supplements.* New York: Penguin; Weil, A. (2007). *8 weeks to optimum health: A proven program for taking full advantage of your body's natural healing power* (rev. ed.). New York: Random House.

▼ SAFETY FIRST ▼

USE OF MEDICINAL PLANTS
Avoid casual treatment of self or others with plants. Just because the substance is "natural" does not mean it is harmless. If not processed properly, many plants (including some herbs) can be poisonous.

- Allergies
- Arthritis
- Digestive problems (indigestion, diarrhea)
- Headache
- Insomnia
- Kidney and urinary tract infections
- Menopausal symptoms
- Menstrual problems
- High or low blood pressure
- Skin disorders

Table 31-8 on page 849 lists medicinal uses of commonly used herbs.

In the past decade, several thousand natural products were tested by the National Cancer Institute. Many contemporary cancer therapies are derived from natural sources.

Herbs are not to be used indiscriminately, as their use may result in some negative outcomes. Some individuals may experience allergic reactions to certain botanicals; see Table 31-9 on page 850 for possible allergic reactions to herbs. Consumers need to be taught the following regarding herbs and allergies: to recognize the potential for developing allergic reactions to herbs, to identify the indicators of such reactions, and to immediately stop using the herb if allergic symptoms occur.

Individuals using herbs need to understand that problems can occur when taking herbal products and medications concurrently. The chemical constituents of herbs may alter the effects of some medications; see Table 31-10 on page 850. To ensure client safety, nurses should:

- Ask clients about their use of herbals in a nonjudgmental manner.
- Discuss the risks and benefits of the herbs taken.
- Suggest that clients purchase and use only herbal products labeled "standardized" for quality checks.

OTHER CAM METHODOLOGIES

The mind-body, body-movement manipulation, energetic-touch, spiritual, and nutritional treatment modalities are not the only available CAM therapies. Others, such as aromatherapy, humor, pet therapy, and music therapy, are also being used as methods to improve health status.

Aromatherapy

Aromatherapy is the therapeutic use of concentrated essences or essential oils that have been extracted from plants and flowers. When diluted in a carrier oil for massage or in warm water for inhalation, essences may be stimulating, uplifting, relaxing, or soothing. Essential oils help relax the mind and the body by promoting balance between the sympathetic and parasympathetic nervous systems. Oils can be absorbed through the skin or enter the body through inhalation.

Aromatherapists use concentrated oils derived from roots, bark, or flowers of herbs and other plants to treat specific ailments. The aromas cause physical and emotional responses within a person. Aromatherapy is used to treat a variety of conditions and promote a sense of well-being, including:

- Stress and anxiety-related problems
- Muscular and rheumatic pains
- Digestive disorders (e.g., nausea)
- Female sexual health conditions (e.g., PMS, postpartal problems, and menopausal symptoms)
- Dermatological conditions

According to a literature review by Buckle (2007), numerous pilot studies have indicated the efficacy of aromatherapy on radiation burns, slow-healing wounds, Alzheimer's disease, and end-of-life agitation.

Some essential oils have antibacterial properties and are found in a wide variety of pharmaceutical preparations. Essential oils should be used intelligently and with caution; see the Nursing Checklist and the accompanying Safety First display.

Humor

Of all the complementary interventions presented in this chapter, humor is the one that can be used most often to

✓ NURSING CHECKLIST

Guidelines for Using Aromatherapy

- Always dilute essential oils in a carrier oil.
- Do a skin patch test for sensitivity before applying essential oils to the skin.
- Avoid contact with the eyes.
- Inhale essential oils only for short periods of time.
- Store in dark glass bottles, tightly capped and away from heat and sunlight.
- Store only in glass containers, not plastic.
- Use only pure essential oils, not synthetics.

▼ SAFETY FIRST ▼

PRECAUTIONS WITH ESSENTIAL OILS
Some essential oils can trigger asthma attacks or epileptic seizures, cause harm to people with cancer, or elevate or depress blood pressure. Instruct clients with asthma, cancer, epilepsy, or hypertension and those who are pregnant to avoid the use of essential oils.

TABLE 31-8 Medicinal Value of Herbs

HERB	MEDICINAL USES (SEE NOTE)	HERB	MEDICINAL USES (SEE NOTE)
Aloe vera (*Aloe vera*)	• Promotes wound healing • Minor cuts and abrasions • Burns		sickness associated with pregnancy) • Stimulates circulation in feet and hands • Expectorant • Helps relieve indigestion and flatulence • Diarrhea
Calendula (*Calendula officinalis*)	• Promotes wound healing • Cuts, abrasions • Minor burns • Sunburn • Acne • Athlete's foot • Oral thrush (as a mouthwash) • Vaginal thrush (as a douche)	Ginkgo (*Ginkgo biloba*)	• Enhances cerebral blood flow • Mild depression • Dementia • Impotence • Peripheral vascular insufficiency • PMS • Memory impairment
Celery seed (*Apium graveolens*)	• Cholesterol-lowering effect • Dizziness, headache • Diuretic effect		
Chamomile (*Matricaria chamomilla; Anthemis nobilis*)	• Produces a calming effect • Nausea • Tension headache	Lavender (*Lavandula angustifolia*)	• Headache • Reduces muscle spasms • Increases relaxation
Dandelion (*Taraxacum officinale*)	• Produces a diuretic effect • Helps decrease edema (especially that of premenstrual fluid retention) • Indigestion	Milk thistle (*Silybum marianum*)	• Liver disorders • Hepatitis • Cirrhosis • Gallstones
Eucalyptus (*Eucalyptus globulus*)	• Antibacterial • Produces a decongestant effect	Peppermint (*Mentha × Piperita*) Sage (*Salvia officinalis*)	• Headache • Sinus congestion • Digestive aid • Nausea • Antibacterial properties
Evening primrose (*Oenothera biennis*)	• Atopic eczema • Asthma • Migraine • PMS symptoms (e.g., mood swings, breast pain, and tenderness) • Arthritis	Saint John's wort (*Hypericum perforatum*)	• Mild to moderate depression • Sleep disorders • Viral infections
Feverfew (*Tanacetum parthenium*)	• Migraine headache	Thyme (*Thymus vulgaris, T. serpyllum*)	• Antimicrobial properties • Helps relieve symptoms of common cold • Antispasmodic effect on bronchioles • Relieves cystitis • Antifungal effect (especially athlete's foot)
Garlic (*Allium sativum*)	• Decreases cholesterol and blood pressure • Helps protect against and treat respiratory infections • Expectorant	White willow (*Salix alba*)	• As a mouthwash for oral thrush • Sedative effect • Counters insomnia • Headache • Fever • Muscular aches and pains
Ginger (*Zingiber officinale*)	• Nausea (especially effective with motion sickness and morning		

Note: This information is not intended to be a guide for self-medication or the treatment of others. Consult a health care practitioner trained in the use of herbs before consuming any herb for medicinal purposes.

Data from Garran, T. A. (2008). *Western herbs according to traditional Chinese medicine.* Rochester, VT: Inner Traditions/Bear; Gladstar, R. (2008). *Rosemary Gladstar's herbal recipes for vibrant health.* North Adams, MA: Storey Books; Hoffman, D. (2007). *Herbal prescriptions after 50: Everything you need to know to maintain vibrant health* (2nd ed.). Rochester, VT: Inner Traditions International; Khalsa, K. P. S., & Tierra, M. (2009). *The way of Ayurvedic herbs: A contemporary introduction and useful manual for the world's oldest healing system.* Twin Lakes, WI: Lotus Press.

TABLE 31-9 Possible Reactions to Certain Botanicals

BOTANICAL	REACTION
Apricot (*Prunus armeniaca*)	Contact allergy
Arnica (*Arnica montana*)	Contact allergy
Celery (*Apium graveolens*)	Photosensitivity
Garlic (*Allium sativum*)	Systemic reaction
Motherwort (*Leonurus cardiaca*)	Photosensitivity
Tansy (*Tanacetum vulgare*)	Systemic reaction

Data from Skidmore-Roth, L. (2009). *Mosby's handbook of herbs and natural supplements* (4th ed.). St. Louis, MO: Elsevier.

TABLE 31-10 Interactions between Herbs and Medications

HERBAL PRODUCT	DRUG	EFFECT WHEN COMBINED
Aloe	Thiazide diuretics and corticosteroids	Enhanced potassium loss
	Cardiac glycosides and antiarrhythmic agents	Potentiated by potassium loss
Belladonna	Tricyclic antidepressants, amantadine, quinidine	Increased anticholinergic effect
Brewer's yeast	MAO inhibitor antidepressants	Increased blood pressure
Dan Shen	Warfarin	Increased warfarin bioavailability; increased prothrombin time
Ginkgo	Warfarin, heparin	Increased risk of bleeding
Licorice root	Acetaminophen	Speeds acetaminophen excretion
	Antihypertensives	Decreased antihypertensive effect
	Estrogens	Increased estrogenic effect
	Fludrocortisone	Increased blood pressure
	Thiazide diuretics and corticosteroids	Enhanced potassium loss

Data from Gladstar, R. (2008). *Rosemary Gladstar's herbal recipes for vibrant health*. North Adams, MA: Storey Books; Skidmore-Roth, L. (2009). *Mosby's handbook of herbs and natural supplements* (4th ed.). St. Louis, MO: Elsevier.

promote wellness. Humor is a frequently used modality with clients of all ages in a variety of health care settings. Humor has many therapeutic outcomes, including:

- Increased ability to cope with pain
- Enhanced immune functioning
- Reduced preprocedural anxiety

Former chair of the Task Force in Psychoneuroimmunology at the School of Medicine at UCLA, Norman Cousins (1979), related how he enhanced his recovery from an incurable connective tissue disorder, ankylosing spondylitis, by the daily watching of films and movies that made him laugh. Humor can be used effectively to relieve anxiety and promote relaxation, improve respiratory function, enhance immunological function, and decrease pain by stimulating the production of endorphins.

It is important to determine the client's perception of what is humorous in order to avoid offending. Differentiation between humorous and offensive situations varies greatly from culture to culture and person to person. Nurses can use humor with clients in a variety of ways. A humor cart (portable cart or carrier filled with joke books, magic tricks, and funny videos) is easy to use and allows clients to select their own humor tools for health. The type of humor should be age appropriate and culturally sensitive. See the Nursing Checklist on this page.

Pet Therapy

The use of animals to enhance health status has a long history. In Britain in the eighteenth and nineteenth centuries, pets were used in institutions to give a sense of meaning and purpose to people institutionalized due to developmental delays (mental retardation). Florence Nightingale (1860) noted the value of pets as companions for individuals with chronic illness.

✔ NURSINGCHECKLIST

Using Humor as a Therapeutic Intervention

- Establish a trusting nurse-client relationship.
- Conduct a humor assessment to determine the type of humor appreciated by the client and the client's usual response to humor.
- Follow the client's lead in the type of humorous strategies used (e.g., jokes, satire, puns).
- Involve the family and significant others in the humor.
- Use humor as an adjunct, not a substitute, for pain medication.
- Continually evaluate the humor strategy for its effectiveness.

The therapeutic use of pets may be particularly helpful with older adults. Playing with and petting animals can help people feel less isolated; see Figure 31-8. Pet therapy is currently used as adjunctive treatment for people in both acute and long-term care settings. There are many uses for pet therapy. It can be implemented to help cope with physical limitations, improve mood, decrease blood pressure, and improve socialization skills and self-esteem.

Music

Music enters the bodymind through the auditory sense. Therapeutic use of music consists of playing music to elicit positive changes in behavior, emotions, or physiological response. Music complements other treatment modalities and encourages clients to become active participants in their health care and recovery.

Music is a good adjunct to use with imagery as it can add to the relaxation response and, therefore, heighten images; see Figure 31-9. Music can be used to relax or stimulate. Music is used for celebrations, spiritual ceremonies, entertainment, and recreation.

The basic elements of music—rhythm, pitch, and intensity—are transmitted by sensory impulses from the cochlea to the thalamus, and then to the cerebral cortex, affecting the autonomic nervous system. Here are some ways in which music has been used as a therapeutic intervention:

- Music can reduce postoperative pain in women following gynecologic surgery (Good & Ahn, 2008).
- As a group intervention, music can improve depression, anxiety, and relationships in clients with mental illness (Choi, Lee, & Lim, 2008).

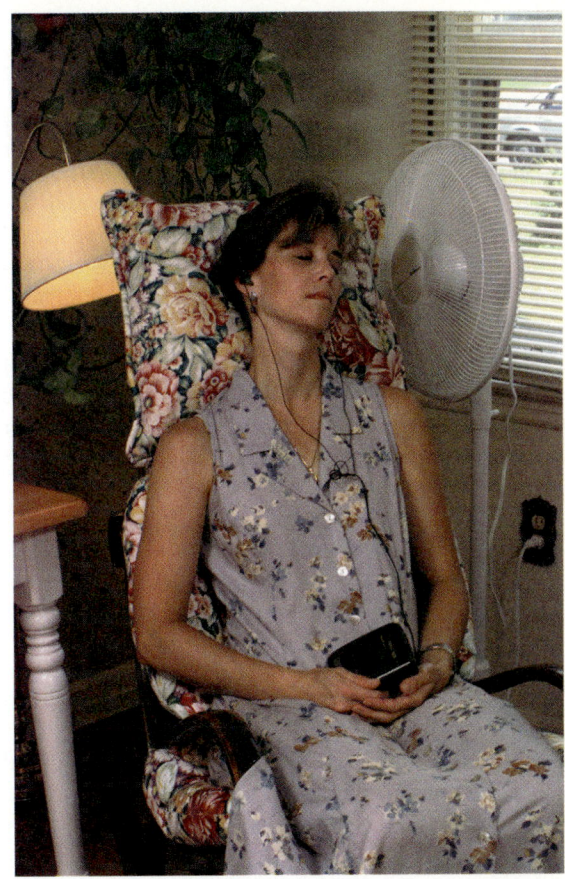

FIGURE 31-9 This individual is experiencing the combined effects of music and imagery, which potentiate the relaxing effects of each modality. DELMAR/CENGAGE LEARNING

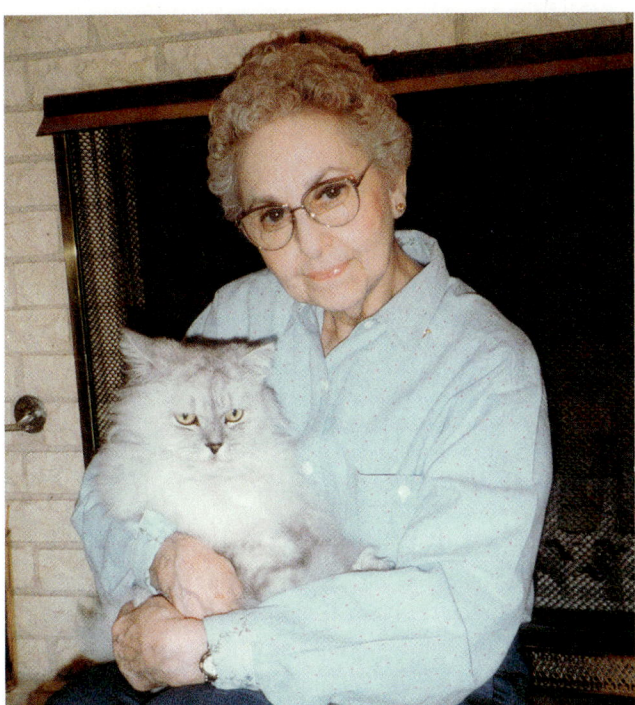

FIGURE 31-8 Interacting with pets can lead to therapeutic benefits. DELMAR/CENGAGE LEARNING

- When used with clients experiencing moderate to severe dementia, music had a positive effect on anxiety, agitation, irritability, and nighttime disturbances (Raglio et al., 2008).
- Music improved intraoperative relaxation and postoperative relaxation for clients who had cardiac surgery (Ikedo, Gangahar, Quader, & Smith, 2007).

Music can be a very useful tool for clients who may be immobilized, who must wait for diagnostic tests, or who undergo the perioperative experience. Pleasurable sounds and music can reduce stress, perception of pain, anxiety, and feelings of isolation. To promote relaxation, select music that is repetitive and low-pitched. Rhythm is most soothing when it has a 3/4 beat. Relaxation is induced by repetition of music, such as lullabies and chants. Music can also be especially useful in helping adolescent clients relax.

Although music is therapeutic for people at all stages of the life cycle, **music-thanatology** is a holistic and palliative method for use of music with dying clients. Music-thanatology is used to help dissipate obstacles to the client's peaceful transition to death. When used with clients who have advanced-stage cancer, music helps reduce anxiety, pain, and isolation and provides the potential for a more peaceful dying experience (Magill & Berenson, 2008).

NURSING AND COMPLEMENTARY/ALTERNATIVE APPROACHES

Nurses play an important role in educating consumers about unconventional interventions by providing information about the safety and efficacy of such methods. Working as advocates and educators, nurses help clients to integrate CAM modalities with conventional treatment methods (Eliopoulos, 2009).

Education is a major function of nursing and is greatly needed as consumers try to determine which CAM methods to use. Consumers should be taught to recognize the signals of fraudulent practice and to avoid healers who:

- Promise immediate relief or success
- State that their way is the only sure therapy
- Refuse to work with other health care providers
- Claim to have all the answers
- Use testimonials that claim amazing results

Other nursing interventions are to provide clients with information about the appropriate use of CAM, to protect clients from unsafe practices and practitioners, and to assist colleagues in being informed of the ever-changing knowledge base about CAM. Many clients and family members obtain health care information from the World Wide Web. See the accompanying Client Teaching Checklist for information on helping clients evaluate Web resources.

Holistic nurses individualize every intervention on the basis of the client's unique needs. From the time before birth until the moment of death, people of all ages experience trauma, stress, and life challenges and have needs in all dimensions. Nurses are challenged to discover and meet those needs. Table 31-11 on page 853 provides suggestions for the use of CAM modalities throughout the life cycle. See the accompanying Respecting Our Differences displays.

CLIENT TEACHING CHECKLIST

Evaluating Health Resources on the Web

Encourage clients to answer these questions:

- Who runs the site?
- Who pays for the site?
- What is the purpose of the site?
- Where does the information come from?
- How is the information selected?
- How current is the information?
- How does the site choose links to other sites?
- What information about you does the site collect, and why?

Data from National Center for Complementary and Alternative Medicine. (2006). *Get the facts: 10 things to know about evaluating medical resources on the Web.* Retrieved August 12, 2009, from http://nccam.nih.gov/health/webresources

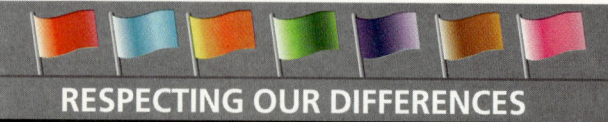

RESPECTING OUR DIFFERENCES

You are assigned to care for a 6-year-old boy who does not speak your language, who is confined to bed, and whose parents must leave him for periods of time because of work obligations. During these periods he cries and is uncooperative with staff. The parents feel guilty, and everyone on your unit finds his behavior unsettling. Your nurse manager asks you to devise a care plan to meet the child's needs and help him cope. What CAM treatment modalities can you employ to deal with his anxieties? Do you need a prescribing practitioner's order to use them?

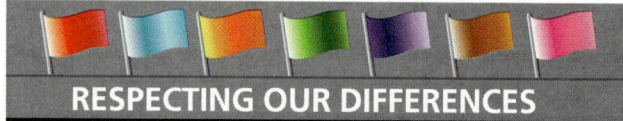

RESPECTING OUR DIFFERENCES

Complementary and Alternative Treatment: To Seek It or Not?

Your close friend has AIDS and is experiencing a great deal of pain and discouragement. She wants to find alternative methods to ease the pain. She confides in you that she believes there may be a cure available at the holistic health center. How do you best help your friend with this situation? What do you advise? Evaluate the same scenario by changing the friend to a client. Is your approach different? Do you give the same advice?

NURSE AS INSTRUMENT OF HEALING

When nurses serve as instruments of healing, the objective is to help clients call forth their inner resources for healing. In order to accomplish this goal, nurses must develop the following attributes:

- Knowledge base: Initially established in nursing school and then continuously expanded through lifelong learning
- Intentionality: A conscious direction of goals that is essential in helping the healer to focus
- Respect for differences: Demonstrated by honoring clients' culturally based health beliefs
- Ability to model wellness: Tending to one's own needs and attempting to stay as healthy and balanced as possible

In order to assist client healing, it is imperative that nurses take care of themselves. Self-nurturing enables nurses to be effective in caring for others because they have met their own needs. See the Uncovering the Evidence display on page 853.

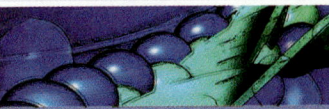

TABLE 31-11 Complementary and Alternative Therapies throughout the Life Cycle

POPULATION	RECOMMENDED CAM THERAPIES	POPULATION	RECOMMENDED CAM THERAPIES
Premature infants	• Massage (with modifications) • Energetic-touch therapies • Sound (e.g., recorded human heartbeat) • Gentle movement • Touch (stroking, skin-to-skin contact)		• Hypnosis • Yoga • Tai chi • Pet therapy
Infants	• Massage (with modifications) • Energetic-touch therapies • Music (e.g., lullabies) • Movement (e.g., rocking)	Adolescents	All modalities discussed in this chapter, as appropriate to condition
Toddlers and preschoolers	• Massage • Energetic-touch therapies • Music (e.g., playing and listening to songs, singing) • Movement • Play (all activities should be age appropriate) • Humor • Imagery • Storytelling • Art/drawing • Aromatherapy (with precautions)	Adults	All modalities discussed in this chapter, as appropriate to condition
		Women during childbirth	• Massage (emphasis on lower back and legs) • Energetic-touch therapies • Breath coaching • Imagery • Hypnosis
School-age children	• Massage • Energetic-touch therapies • Music (playing and listening) • Movement (e.g., dance) • Play (all activities should be age appropriate) • Humor (e.g., riddles, jokes) • Imagery • Storytelling • Art/drawing • Aromatherapy (with precautions)	Older adults	• Massage (lighter pressure and modifications for body's status) • Aromatherapy (with precautions) • Heat and cold applications (with precautions) • Any other modalities discussed in this chapter, as appropriate to condition and with precautions
		Terminally ill persons	• Massage • Reflexology • Energetic-touch therapies • Music-thanatology • Prayer • Any other modalities discussed in this chapter, as appropriate to condition and with precautions

Delmar/Cengage Learning

UNCOVERING THE

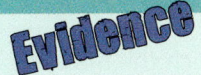

TITLE OF STUDY

"The Effect of Aromatherapy Massage with Music on the Stress and Anxiety Levels of Emergency Nurses: Comparison between Summer and Winter"

AUTHORS

M. Cooke, K. Holzhauser, M. Jones, C. Davis, and J. Finucane

(Continues)

UNCOVERING THE (Continued)

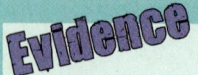

PURPOSES

(1) To evaluate the use of aromatherapy massage and music as interventions to cope with the occupational stress and anxiety experienced by emergency department nurses and (2) to compare any difference in results between massage sessions performed in the summer and the winter.

METHODS

The study used a one-group, pretest-posttest, quasi-experimental design with random assignment of participants. Nursing occupational stress was assessed before and after 12 weeks of aromatherapy massage with music. Anxiety was measured before and after each massage session.

FINDINGS

Emergency nurses were significantly more anxious in winter than in summer. Aromatherapy massage with music significantly reduced emergency nurses' anxiety.

IMPLICATIONS

High stress levels can be detrimental to the health of emergency nurses. The provision of a support mechanism such as on-site massage may be used as an effective strategy for reducing anxiety experienced by emergency nurses.

Cooke, M., Holzhauser, K., Jones, M., Davis, C., & Finucane, J. (2007). The effect of aromatherapy massage with music on the stress and anxiety levels of emergency nurses: Comparison between summer and winter. *Journal of Clinical Nursing, 16*(9), 695–703.

PROCEDURE 31-1 — Administering Therapeutic Massage

EQUIPMENT
- Flat sheet
- Towel
- 1 or 2 pillows
- Lotion or oil
- Bath blanket or light coverlet

ACTION	RATIONALE
1. Set room temperature at approximately 75°F. Provide low or indirect lighting, privacy, and background music.	1. Maintains client's body heat, protects privacy, and promotes relaxation.
2. Prepare the massage table or hospital bed by placing a clean sheet on the surface. Adjust the surface height.	2. Both the massage table and hospital bed are adjustable so that the height of the work surface can be raised or lowered as necessary to prevent back strain.
3. Remove rings and watch. Wash hands/hand hygiene.	3. Avoids scratching the client and prevents transmission of microorganisms.
4. Explain the procedure to the client.	4. Prepares the client for the treatment.
5. Assist the client to assume either a prone, Sims', supine, or sitting position, depending on client's condition.	5. Appropriate position enables the nurse to apply the necessary amount of pressure without causing discomfort for the client.
6. Loosen or remove clothing from the client's back and arms. Drape the client with a sheet to cover areas not being treated directly.	6. Exposes parts of the back on which the massage will be performed. Draping untreated parts of the back helps keep the client warm and provides privacy.
7. Squeeze a small amount of lotion or oil into the palm of the hand to warm before applying to the client.	7. Cold lotion or oil can cause discomfort to the client.

(Continues)

PROCEDURE 31-1
Administering Therapeutic Massage (Continued)

ACTION	RATIONALE
8. Begin with light to medium effleurage (see explanation in text) at lower back and continue upward following muscle groups, being careful to avoid the spine and spinal processes (see Figure 31-10). Move hands up toward the base of the neck and continue outward over the trapezius muscles with circular motions, over and around shoulders and upper arms, and return with lighter downward strokes laterally over the latissimus dorsi to the upper gluteals. Use slow rhythmical movements, keeping in contact with the skin at all times. Check pressure. Continue the effleurage for approximately 3 minutes.	8. Prevents damage to internal structures, stimulates circulation, and promotes relaxation.
9. Continue treatment if appropriate with gentle petrissage (see explanation in text) to major muscle groups in the back, shoulders, and upper arms (see Figure 31-11).	9. Enhances circulation, stimulates muscles, and promotes relaxation.
10. Use friction (see explanation in text) to particular muscle groups where tension is being held.	10. Penetrates deeper muscle layers, thus promoting further relaxation.
11. Use tapotement (see explanation in text) to stimulate any muscle groups that may be fatigued.	11. Invigorates and stimulates tired muscles.
12. Finish treatment with effleurage.	12. Assists with relaxation and provides a sense of completion.
13. Wipe any excess lotion or oil from skin with towel, or use small amount of warm soap and water to clean client's skin, taking care to dry completely.	13. Promotes and maintains skin integrity.
14. Assist client into comfortable position for a period of rest or sleep.	14. Allows client to fully experience therapeutic benefit of massage.
15. Document treatment, client's response, and skin assessment data.	15. Communicates pertinent data to other members of treatment team; promotes continuity of care.
16. Wash hands/hand hygiene.	16. Reduces transmission of microorganisms.

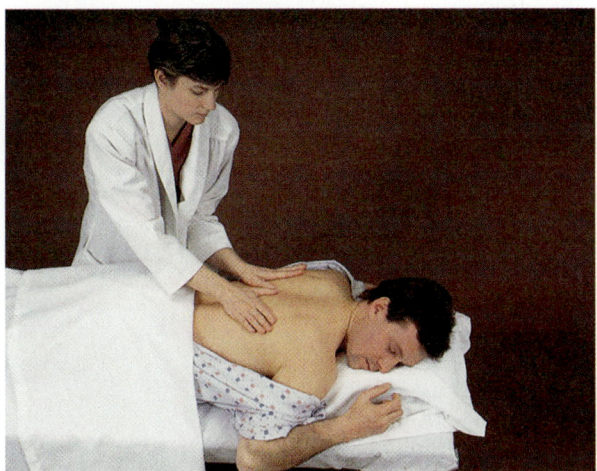

FIGURE 31-10 Effleurage from Lower Back to Base of Neck
DELMAR/CENGAGE LEARNING

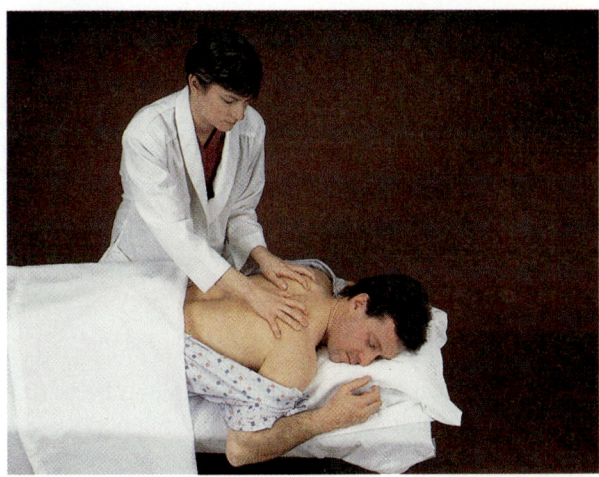

FIGURE 31-11 Petrissage of Shoulders DELMAR/CENGAGE LEARNING

(Continues)

PROCEDURE 31-1
Administering Therapeutic Massage (Continued)

delegation tip

Therapeutic massage may be delegated to any individual properly trained in performing the techniques.

nursing tips

- *Keep the client covered as much as possible to provide privacy and promote comfort.*
- *Be sure to determine client preference when using lotions or oils. Some fragrances may be unpleasant to a client.*
- *Ask client for input regarding the use of music during massage.*
- *Use this time as an opportunity to assess the client's skin integrity and psychological comfort level.*

KEY CONCEPTS

- Ever-increasing numbers of health care consumers are using CAM modalities.
- Psychoneuroimmunology is the study of how the body and mind are connected and how beliefs, thoughts, and emotions affect health.
- Holistic nursing practice encompasses consideration of each client as a unique and whole being with many aspects: physiological, psychological, sociocultural, intellectual, and spiritual.
- Healing is not curing but rather is regaining balance and finding harmony and wholeness as changes take place from within the individual.
- No one person can heal another, but a nurse can act as a guide, support system, or instrument of healing for a client.
- Some of the mind-body modalities that nurses use are meditation, relaxation, imagery, biofeedback, and hypnosis.

- Body-movement modalities include movement, exercise, and chiropractic therapy.
- Energetic-touch therapies can be used with persons of all ages and in various stages of illness and wellness.
- Energetic-touch therapies include massage, therapeutic touch (TT), healing touch (HT), shiatsu acupressure, and reflexology.
- Spiritual therapies such as faith healing, healing prayer, and laying on of hands are helpful modalities.
- Nutritional therapies include antioxidants, macrobiotic diets, and herbal therapy.
- Other modalities, such as aromatherapy, humor, pet therapy, and music therapy, are valuable adjuncts to conventional treatment.

REVIEW QUESTIONS

1. Which of the following CAM interventions should be avoided when working with toddlers?
   a. Art/drawing
   b. Hypnosis
   c. Massage
   d. Music
2. A nurse is working with a client who uses herbs to promote health. Which of the following herbs is useful in treating nausea?
   a. Aloe vera
   b. Calendula

   c. Ginger
   d. Sage
3. Native American healing practices are strongly rooted in which of the following?
   a. Allopathic medicine
   b. New Age concepts
   c. Spiritual beliefs
   d. Yoga techniques
4. Which of the following nursing responses is most therapeutic for a client who expresses interest in using herbal remedies?

a. "I use lavender and valerian to help me relax at night."

b. "My herbalist recommends the use of St. John's wort to promote healing."

c. "Since they are natural, herbs are completely safe."

d. "What have you been doing to promote your health?"

5. When planning care for a client with chronic pain, the nurse establishes a diagnosis of *Disturbed energy field*. Which of the following CAM approaches would be of most use for this client?

a. Aromatherapy

b. Healing touch

c. Herbals

d. Humor

6. Which of the following foods are dietary sources of antioxidants? Select all that apply.

a. Butter

b. Carrots

c. Flaxseed

d. Garlic

e. Parsley

f. Red meat

7. Which of the following is a reason why many people seek out and use CAM therapies?

a. CAM therapies are cost-effective.

b. Cultural beliefs usually prohibit the use of "folk remedies."

c. Insurance companies reimburse for most CAM therapies.

d. They are satisfied with allopathic treatment methods.

8. Which of the following best describes the Ayurvedic perspective of health?

a. Absence of disease equals health.

b. Harmony is maintained through use of natural and supernatural forces.

c. Prana in the body maintains a state of balance.

d. Use of totems, fetishes, dance, and chanting promotes health.

9. A nurse is caring for a Buddhist client who asks that his priest be allowed to conduct chanting and healing prayers in his hospital room. Which of the following nursing actions is most appropriate?

a. Check with the nursing supervisor about the client's request.

b. Explain that the client may go to the hospital chapel for prayer and chanting.

c. Provide privacy for the client and priest to pray and chant.

d. Tell the client that chanting is not allowed because it will disturb other clients.

10. Which of the following statements accurately describes CAM? Select all that apply.

a. CAM considers the whole person through use of body-mind interventions.

b. CAM is most effective in treating acute, emergency situations.

c. The American public has a negative view of CAM approaches.

d. The U.S. federal government supports research into the efficacy of CAM modalities.

e. There has been little scientific research to support the use of CAM modalities.

f. Use of CAM modalities is increasing in the United States.

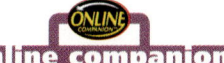

online companion

Visit the DeLaune and Ladner online companion resource at **www.delmar.cengage.com** for additional content and study aids. Click on Online Companions, then select the Nursing discipline.

"And what nursing has to do in either case, is to put the patient in the best condition for nature to act upon him."

—FLORENCE NIGHTINGALE (IN SKRETKOWICZ, 1992)

CHAPTER 32

Oxygenation

COMPETENCIES

1. Describe the basic physiological mechanisms of ventilation, circulation, and oxygenation.
2. Assess the client's ventilatory, circulatory, and oxygenation status.
3. Explain potential client outcomes when oxygenation is impaired.
4. State common client knowledge deficits related to oxygenation impairment.
5. Develop nursing interventions that promote oxygenation.
6. Describe actions for emergency support of airway, ventilation, and circulation.

KEY TERMS

aerobic metabolism	deadspace	oxygen uptake
anaerobic metabolism	diastole	oxyhemoglobin dissociation curve
anemia	diffusion defect	paroxysmal nocturnal dyspnea
angina pectoris	external respiration	postural drainage
atelectasis	gallops	precapillary sphincters
atherosclerosis	heart failure	restrictive pulmonary disease
autoregulation	Heimlich maneuver	shunting
cardiac conduction system	hypercapnia	sleep apnea
cardiac cycle	hypoxemia	surfactant
cardiac output	hypoxia	systole
cardiopulmonary resuscitation (CPR)	infarction	tachypnea
	intermittent claudication	tracheotomy
chest physiotherapy (CPT)	internal respiration	ventilation
chronic obstructive pulmonary disease (COPD)	ischemia	ventilation-perfusion (V/Q) mismatching
	murmurs	
cyanosis	obstructive pulmonary disease	work of breathing

Oxygenation, the delivery of oxygen to the body's tissues and cells, is necessary to maintain life and health. Clients with compromised oxygenation status need careful assessment and thoughtful nursing care to achieve an adequate and comfortable level of oxygenation function. The purpose of this chapter is to explore the elements of the process of oxygenation, common mechanisms by which it may be impaired, and interventions that are aimed at improving oxygen delivery to the cells.

PHYSIOLOGY OF OXYGENATION

The delivery of oxygen to the body's cells is a process that depends upon the interplay of the pulmonary, hematologic, and cardiovascular systems. Specifically, the processes involved include ventilation, alveolar gas exchange, oxygen transport and delivery, and cellular respiration. The basic anatomy of the lungs is shown in Figure 32-1.

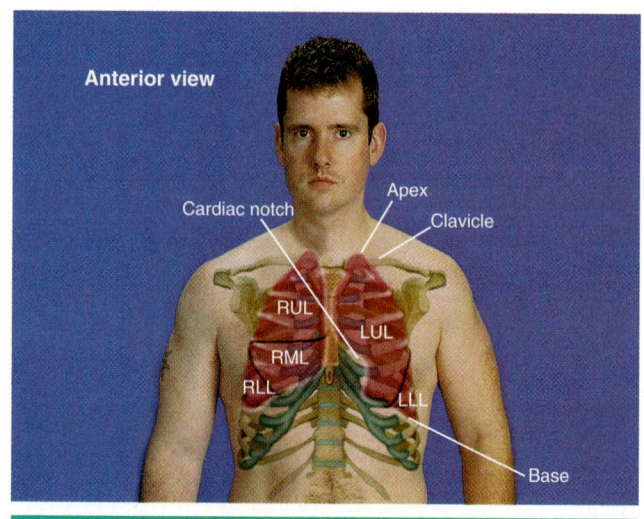

FIGURE 32-1 Lungs. RUL = right upper lobe, RML = right middle lobe, RLL = right lower lobe, LUL = left upper lobe, LLL = left lower lobe. DELMAR/CENGAGE LEARNING

VENTILATION

The first step in the process of oxygenation is **ventilation**, which is the movement of air into and out of the lungs for the purpose of delivering fresh air into the lung's alveoli (see Figure 32-2 on page 861). Ventilation is regulated by respiratory control centers in the pons and medulla oblongata, which are located in the brain stem. The rate and depth of ventilation are constantly adjusted in response to changes in the concentrations of hydrogen ion (pH) and carbon dioxide (CO_2) in the body's fluids. For instance, an increase in carbon dioxide in the blood or a decrease in pH in the body's fluids will stimulate faster and deeper ventilation. A decrease

in blood oxygen concentration (**hypoxemia**) will also stimulate ventilation, but to a lesser degree.

Inhalation of air is initiated when the diaphragm contracts, pulling it downward and thus increasing the size of the intrathoracic space (see Figure 32-3 on page 861). This space is also increased by contraction of the external intercostal muscles, which elevate and separate the ribs and move the sternum forward. The effect of increasing the space inside the thorax is to decrease the intrathoracic pressure so that air will be drawn in from the atmosphere. Stretch receptors in the lung tissue send signals back to the brain to cause cessation of inhalation, preventing overdistension of the lungs. Exhalation

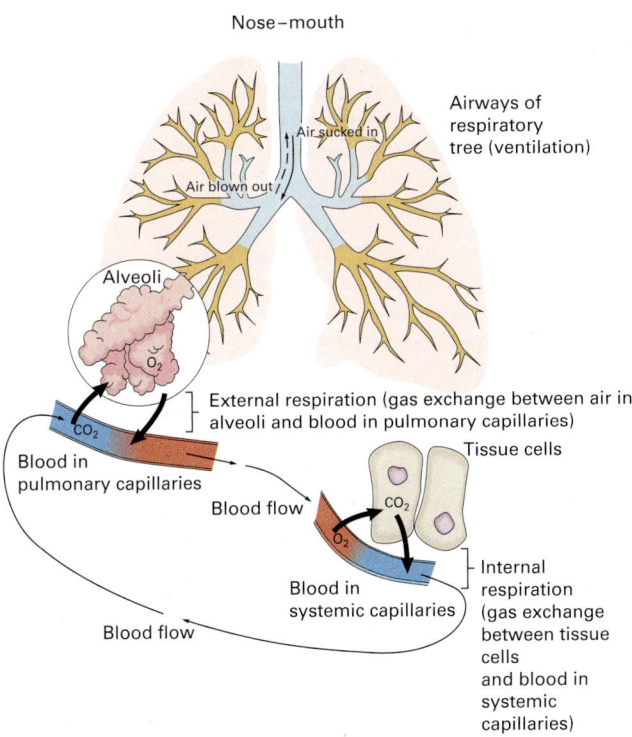

Nose–mouth

Airways of respiratory tree (ventilation)

Air sucked in

Air blown out

Alveoli

O_2

CO_2

External respiration (gas exchange between air in alveoli and blood in pulmonary capillaries)

Blood in pulmonary capillaries

Tissue cells

CO_2

O_2

Blood flow

Blood in systemic capillaries

Internal respiration (gas exchange between tissue cells and blood in systemic capillaries)

Blood flow

FIGURE 32-2 Elements of Oxygenation of the Pulmonary and Hematologic Systems DELMAR/CENGAGE LEARNING

occurs when the respiratory muscles relax, thus reducing the size of the intrathoracic space, increasing the intrathoracic pressure, and forcing air to exit the lungs. Under normal conditions, exhalation is a passive process.

When the movement of air is impeded, additional muscles may be used to increase the ventilatory ability. These accessory muscles of ventilation include the sternocleidomastoid muscle, the abdominal muscles, and the internal intercostal muscles. In some disease states, exhalation is impaired, requiring that the individual actively force air out of the lungs rather than passively exhaling. Forced expiration is aided by the intercostal muscles and the abdominal recti. When additional muscular force is required for breathing, the **work of breathing** is said to be increased.

Several mechanisms exist to keep the airways clear of microorganisms and debris. As air is inhaled through the nose, the larger particles are filtered out through hairs lining the nasal passages. The mucous membranes of the nasopharynx and sinuses warm and humidify the inspired air, and the film of mucus lining these membranes traps smaller particles. Closure of the glottis protects the airway from aspiration of food and fluids during swallowing. In the trachea and larger bronchi, tiny hairlike cilia continually produce wavelike movements to propel mucus and particles upward, where they can be coughed out. If any invaders manage to reach the alveoli, specialized alveolar macrophages will engulf and destroy the offending organism. Disease processes can interfere with any of these protective mechanisms, increasing the individual's vulnerability to infection and injury.

ALVEOLAR GAS EXCHANGE

Once fresh air reaches the lung's alveoli, the next step in the process of oxygenation begins. The exchange of oxygen from the alveolar space into the pulmonary capillary blood is

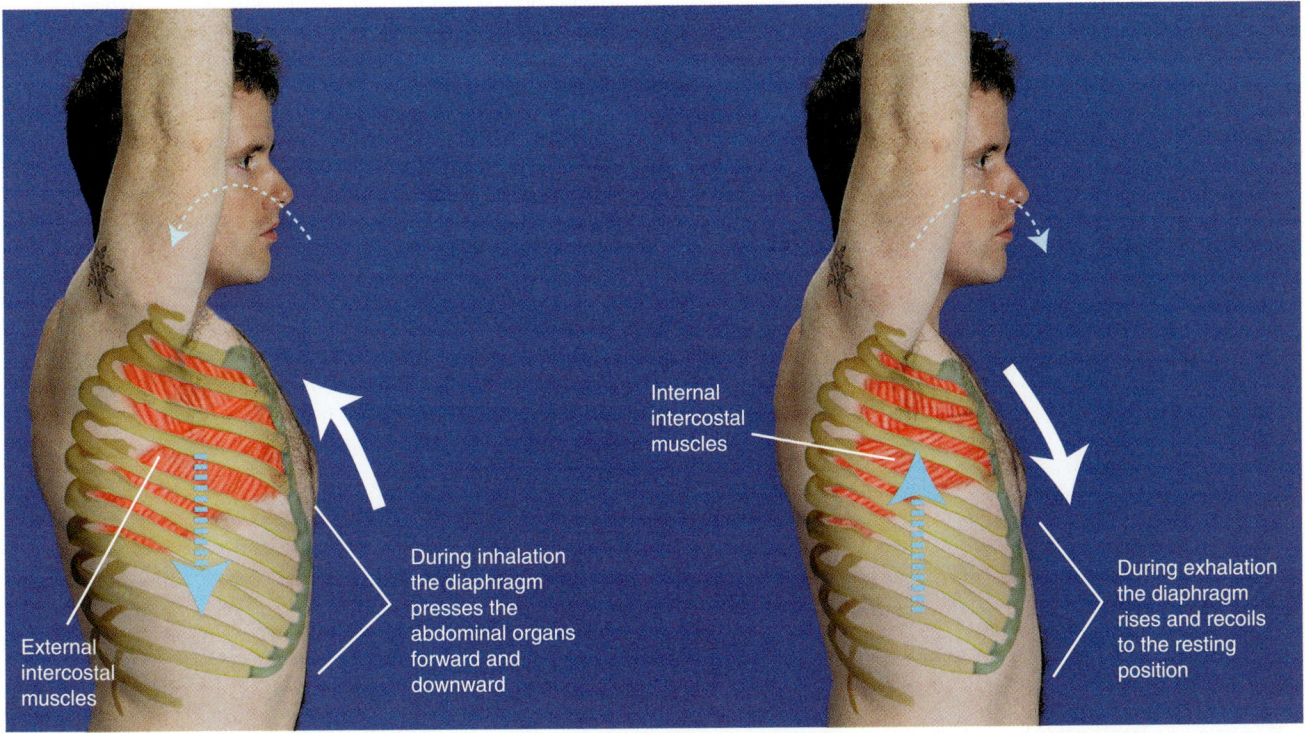

Internal intercostal muscles

During inhalation the diaphragm presses the abdominal organs forward and downward

During exhalation the diaphragm rises and recoils to the resting position

External intercostal muscles

FIGURE 32-3 Mechanics of breathing. Inhalation increases the volume of the thorax by diaphragmatic excursion and elevation of the sternum. Exhalation is normally accomplished by passive elastic recoil. DELMAR/CENGAGE LEARNING

referred to as oxygen uptake; it may also be called external respiration. Oxygen diffuses across the alveolar membrane in response to a concentration gradient; that is, it moves from an area of higher concentration (the alveoli) to an area of lower concentration (the pulmonary capillary blood), seeking equilibrium. At the same time, carbon dioxide diffuses from the blood to the alveolar space, also in response to a concentration gradient (see Figure 32-4).

OXYGEN TRANSPORT AND DELIVERY
Oxygen Transport in the Blood

Once the diffusion of oxygen across the alveolar-capillary membrane occurs, the oxygen molecules are dissolved in the blood plasma. Three factors influence the capacity of the blood to carry oxygen: the amount of dissolved oxygen in the plasma, the amount of hemoglobin, and the tendency of the hemoglobin to bind with oxygen. However, the plasma is not able to carry nearly enough dissolved oxygen to meet the metabolic needs of the body. The oxygen-carrying capacity of the blood is greatly enhanced by the presence of hemoglobin in the erythrocytes.

The amount of oxygen carried in a sample of blood is measured in two ways. Oxygen dissolved in plasma is expressed as the partial pressure of oxygen (PaO_2). The normal PaO_2 in arterial blood is about 80 to 100 mm Hg. The oxygen dissolved in plasma, however, represents only about 1% to 5% of the total oxygen content of the blood. The vast majority of oxygen

in the blood is carried bound to the hemoglobin molecule. The amount of oxygen bound to hemoglobin is expressed as the percentage of hemoglobin that is saturated with oxygen (SaO_2), with 100% being fully saturated. Since the SaO_2 is a percentage indicating the relationship between oxygen and hemoglobin, the nurse should interpret the client's SaO_2 measurement with the hemoglobin level. Normal saturation of arterial blood (SaO_2) is about 96% to 98%.

Hemoglobin molecules have the ability to form a reversible bond with oxygen molecules, so that the hemoglobin readily takes up oxygen in the lungs, while it also readily releases oxygen to the body's cells in the systemic capillary beds. This seemingly paradoxical shift in hemoglobin's affinity for oxygen is represented by the oxyhemoglobin dissociation curve, which is a graphic representation of the relationship between the PaO_2 and oxygen saturation.

The affinity of hemoglobin for oxygen is highest when the PaO_2, the measure of oxygen dissolved in the arterial blood plasma, is 70 mm Hg or higher; in this portion of the curve, further increases in PaO_2 result in very little change in SaO_2 (see Figure 32-5A on page 863). This characteristic of the oxyhemoglobin dissociation curve accounts for the rapid uptake of oxygen by hemoglobin in the pulmonary circulation and allows for some decrease in PaO_2, such as might occur with disease or in high altitudes, without significantly sacrificing SaO_2.

As the oxygen-saturated blood is circulated to the peripheral capillary beds, dissolved oxygen diffuses out of blood. This decrease in dissolved oxygen causes hemoglobin to lose its affinity for oxygen, so the oxygen is then released to the body's cells. Once the PaO_2 in the blood drops below 60 mm Hg, hemoglobin releases oxygen very easily. This release is represented in the lower left portion of the curve, also known as the venous portion, and permits rapid unloading of oxygen to the cells (see Figure 32-5B on page 863).

Several physiological factors may alter the affinity of hemoglobin for oxygen, and these shifts can be represented on the oxyhemoglobin dissociation curve. A shift to the left occurs when affinity is increased so that for a given PaO_2, the associated SaO_2 will be higher. This means that although the arterial blood may be carrying adequate oxygen, little of it is being released to the tissues. A shift to the left may be caused by increased pH (alkalosis), hypothermia, or a decrease in the red blood cell enzyme 2,3-diphosphoglycerate (2,3-DPG), which may occur after massive transfusions of banked blood.

A shift to the right of the oxyhemoglobin dissociation curve means that for a given PaO_2, the SaO_2 will be lower. This phenomenon represents a decreased affinity of hemoglobin for oxygen so that oxygen is more readily released to the tissues. This shift occurs in response to acidosis, hyperthermia, and hypoxia (which induces increased production of 2,3-DPG) and results in improved delivery of oxygen to the tissues.

Circulation

Once oxygen is bound to hemoglobin, the oxygen is delivered to the cells of the body by the process of circulation. Circulation of the blood is the function of the heart and blood vessels.

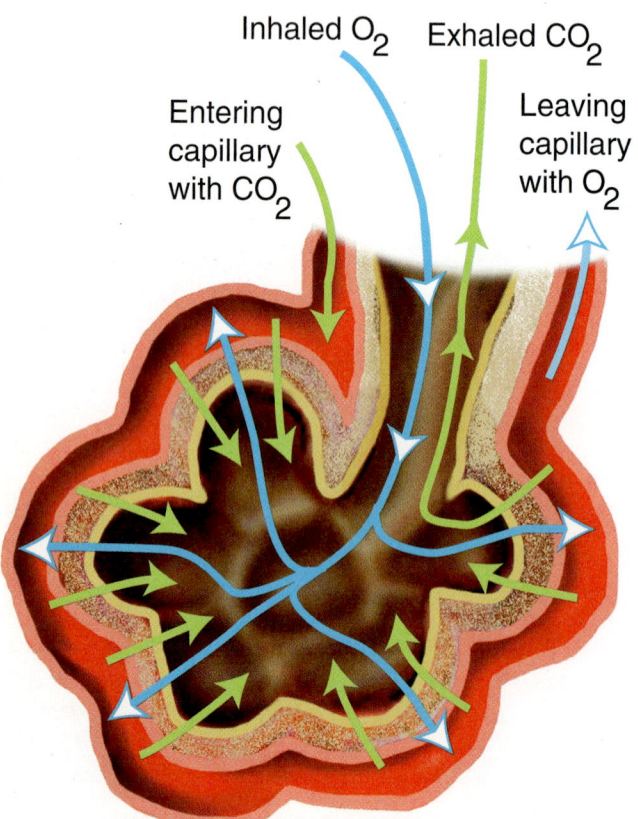

Inhaled O_2 Exhaled CO_2

Entering capillary with CO_2 Leaving capillary with O_2

FIGURE 32-4 Alveolar Gas Exchange DELMAR/CENGAGE LEARNING

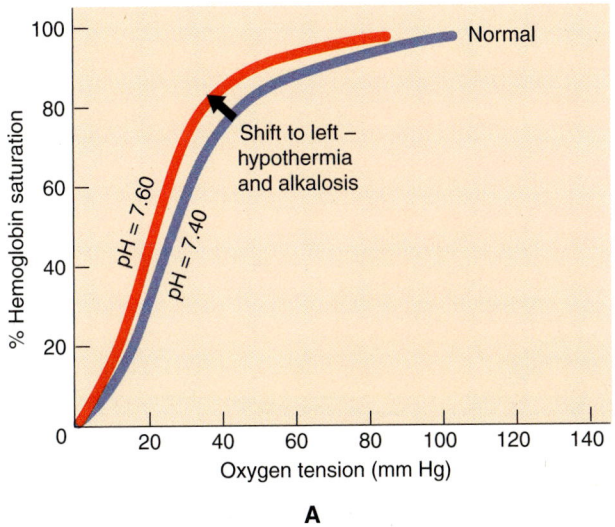 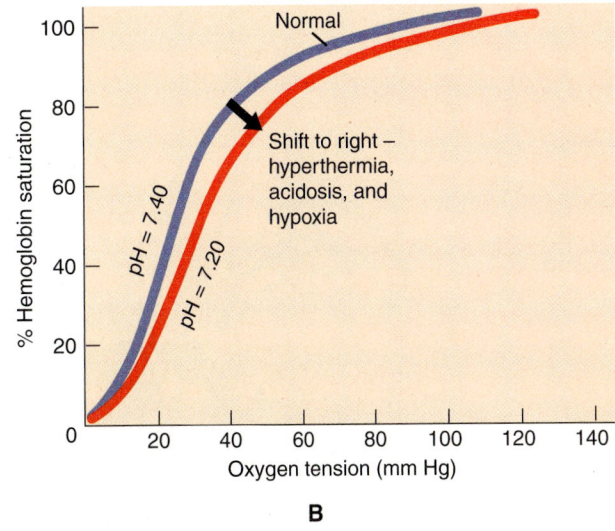

A   **B**

FIGURE 32-5 Oxyhemoglobin Dissociation Curve: **A.** Effect of increase in pH; **B.** Effect of decrease in pH. DELMAR/CENGAGE LEARNING

The heart is a muscular pump that is divided into four chambers: the right and left atria and the right and left ventricles (see Figure 32-6 on page 864). A series of valves allows for unidirectional blood flow through the chambers, which is driven by the sequential contraction and relaxation of the heart muscle.

A single cycle of atrial and ventricular contraction and relaxation is referred to as a **cardiac cycle**, which is the product of the interplay of electrical and mechanical events. The electrical activity of the heart involves the generation and transmission of electrical current by specialized cardiac cells known as the **cardiac conduction system** (see Figure 32-7 on page 864). A small mass of cells in the right atrium, the *sinoatrial node*, or *SA node*, normally controls the heart rate by rhythmically generating electrical impulses. For this reason, the SA node is often referred to as the heart's "pacemaker." The impulses created by the SA node travel along specialized internodal pathways to spread throughout the atria, resulting in mechanical muscular contraction. The electrical activity is then transmitted down to the ventricles via the *atrioventricular (AV) node* and spreads through the ventricular tissue along the *bundle of His, right and left bundle branches,* and *Purkinje fibers.* Again, the result is muscular contraction. The sequential contraction and relaxation of the atria and ventricles are essential factors in the cyclical filling and emptying of the chambers, which produce circulation.

The process of a chamber filling is referred to as **diastole**, and the process of a chamber emptying is **systole**. Atrial diastole occurs as the right and left atria relax and blood flows into the right and left atrial chambers from the venae cavae and pulmonary veins, respectively. As pressure rises in the atria, the atrioventricular valves (the mitral and tricuspid) open, permitting the blood to begin flowing into the ventricles. Ventricular filling is further augmented by contraction of the atrial muscle (atrial systole), forcing additional blood into the ventricles. This contribution to ventricular filling is sometimes called "atrial kick."

Filling of the ventricles causes the intraventricular pressure to rise. When the intraventricular pressure exceeds the pressure in the atria, the atrioventricular valves close. The ventricular muscle then begins to contract, further increasing intraventricular pressure until it is sufficient to force open the two semilunar valves (the pulmonic and aortic valves). As contraction of the ventricular walls proceeds, blood is forced out of the ventricles and into the circulation (ventricular systole).

Blood leaving the right ventricle is pumped into the pulmonary artery, which quickly branches into the right and left pulmonary arteries. Further division of the pulmonary arterial tree culminates in the pulmonary capillary bed. Blood in the pulmonary capillaries is in very close contact with the alveolar air; it is here that alveolar-capillary gas exchanges take place. From the pulmonary capillaries, the freshly oxygenated blood flows into the pulmonary veins and to the left atrium, which delivers it to the left ventricle (see Figure 32-8 on page 865).

Blood leaving the left ventricle enters the aorta. The aorta serves as the "trunk" of the arterial tree, with branches leading to every organ and tissue group in the body. Blood flow through the arterial system is driven by the pressure generated during ventricular systole and is influenced by the volume and viscosity of the blood and the amount of resistance within the arterial system. Blood flow to specific organs and tissues may be increased or reduced by the relaxation or contraction of **precapillary sphincters**, which are rings of smooth muscle surrounding the arterioles. This mechanism allows for redistribution of blood flow to the areas of greatest need, a process known as **autoregulation**.

Blood return through the venous system is also driven by pressure gradients, although the venous system operates under lower pressure than the arterial system does. In order to boost venous return, many veins (particularly in the lower extremities) are equipped with valves that prevent backward flow of blood (regurgitation); as the veins are compressed by their surrounding skeletal muscles, blood is forced along toward the vena cava and ultimately to the right atrium.

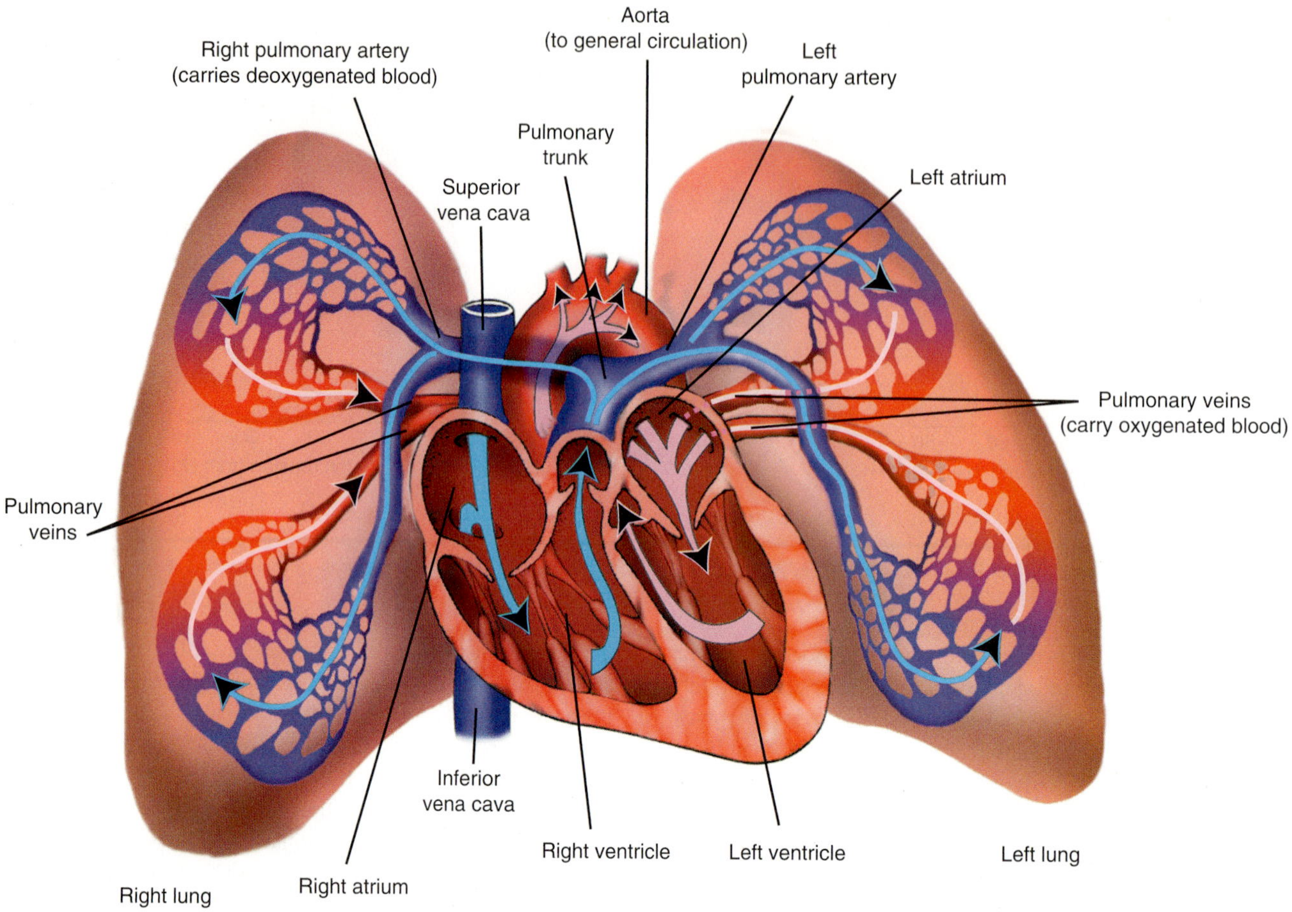

Right pulmonary artery
(carries deoxygenated blood)

Aorta
(to general circulation)

Left
pulmonary artery

Pulmonary
trunk

Superior
vena cava

Left atrium

Pulmonary veins
(carry oxygenated blood)

Pulmonary
veins

Inferior
vena cava

Right ventricle

Left ventricle

Left lung

Right lung

Right atrium

FIGURE 32-6 **Major Structures of the Heart and Pulmonary Circulation** DELMAR/CENGAGE LEARNING

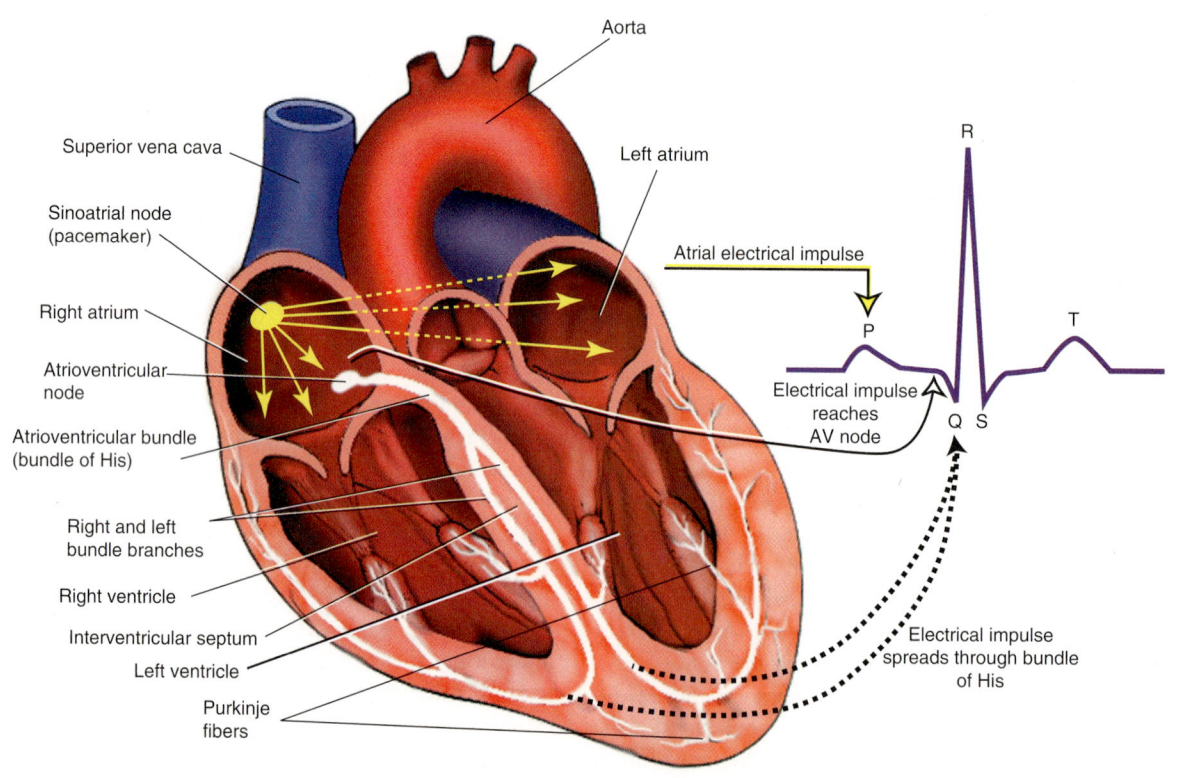

Aorta

Superior vena cava

Left atrium

Sinoatrial node
(pacemaker)

Atrial electrical impulse

Right atrium

Atrioventricular
node

Electrical impulse
reaches
AV node

Atrioventricular bundle
(bundle of His)

Right and left
bundle branches

Right ventricle

Interventricular septum

Left ventricle

Electrical impulse
spreads through bundle
of His

Purkinje
fibers

R

P

T

Q S

FIGURE 32-7 **Cardiac Conduction System** DELMAR/CENGAGE LEARNING

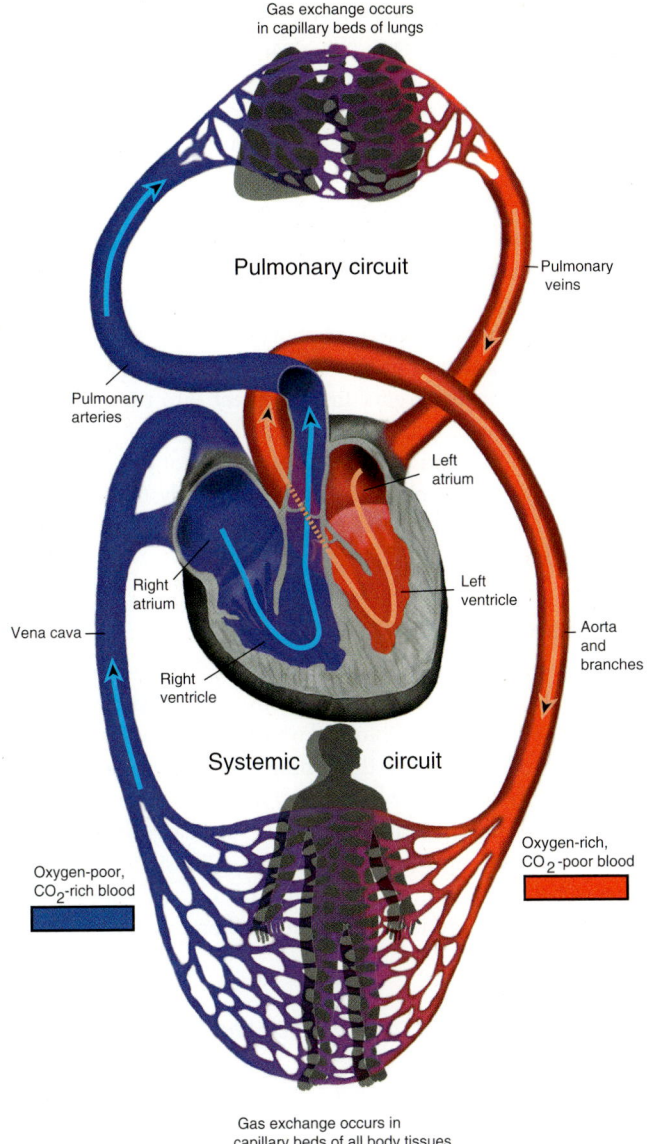

Gas exchange occurs
in capillary beds of lungs

Pulmonary circuit

Pulmonary
veins

Pulmonary
arteries

Left
atrium

Right
atrium

Left
ventricle

Vena cava

Aorta
and
branches

Right
ventricle

Systemic   circuit

Oxygen-poor,
CO_2-rich blood

Oxygen-rich,
CO_2-poor blood

Gas exchange occurs in
capillary beds of all body tissues

FIGURE 32-8 Systemic and Pulmonary Circuits DELMAR/CENGAGE LEARNING

CELLULAR RESPIRATION

Gas exchange at the cellular level, like that at the alveolar level, takes place via diffusion in response to concentration gradients. Oxygen diffuses from the blood to the tissues, while carbon dioxide moves from the tissues to the blood; the blood is then reoxygenated by the lungs. This process is referred to as **internal respiration**.

FACTORS AFFECTING OXYGENATION

Adequate oxygenation is influenced by many factors, including age, environmental and lifestyle factors, and disease processes.

AGE

Oxygenation status can be influenced by age. Older adults may exhibit a barrel chest and require increased effort to expand the lungs. Loss of alveolar gas exchange is accompanied by a decrease in the Pa_{O_2}. Older adults are also more susceptible to respiratory infection because of decreased activity in the cilia, which normally are an effective defense mechanism.

ENVIRONMENTAL AND LIFESTYLE FACTORS

Environmental and lifestyle factors can significantly affect a client's oxygenation status. Clients who are exposed to dust, animal dander, asbestos, or toxic chemicals in the home or workplace are at increased risk for alterations in oxygenation. Individuals who experience significant physical or emotional stress or who are obese or underweight are also subject to changes in oxygenation status; see the accompanying Uncovering the Evidence display on page 866. Smokers and those exposed to secondhand smoke should be questioned as to the type and amount of tobacco and number of years of exposure.

DISEASE PROCESSES

Oxygenation alterations can often be traced to disease states related to alterations in ventilation, alveolar gas exchange, oxygen uptake, or circulation. There are many disease states that may affect oxygenation, including obstructive pulmonary disease, restrictive pulmonary disease, diffusion defects, ventilation-perfusion mismatching, atherosclerosis, heart failure, anemia, and alterations in oxygen uptake.

Obstructive Pulmonary Disease

Alterations in ventilation may be related to obstructive or restrictive pulmonary disease. **Obstructive pulmonary disease** occurs when the airways become partially or completely blocked, diminishing airflow, or the lungs lose some of their elastic recoil, trapping stale air, which should be exhaled. In both cases, the end result is impaired exhalation, air trapping, and difficulty bringing fresh air into the alveoli (see Figure 32-9 on page 867). The most common obstructive pulmonary diseases are asthma, emphysema, and chronic bronchitis, collectively known as **chronic obstructive pulmonary disease (COPD)**.

Restrictive Pulmonary Disease

Restrictive pulmonary disease represents pathologies that impair the ability of the chest wall and lungs to expand during the inspiratory phase of ventilation. This impairment increases the work of breathing and also reduces airflow to the alveoli. A wide variety of disorders causes restrictive lung disease, including pneumonia and pulmonary fibrosis (scarring). The following compromise a client's respiratory health, increasing the susceptibility to pneumonia:

- Smoking
- Emphysema
- Intoxication
- Weak cough reflex

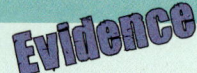

UNCOVERING THE

TITLE OF STUDY
"Importance of Aerobic Fitness in Cardiovascular Risks in Sedentary Overweight and Obese African-American Women"

AUTHOR
T. Gaillard

PURPOSE
To examine the clinical and metabolic risk factors of cardiovascular disease (CVD) in nondiabetic, sedentary, overweight or obese African American women with varying degrees of aerobic fitness.

METHODS
Forty-eight African American women, with mean age of 43 years and body mass index of 32.3, participated in the study. Fasting and 2-hour postprandial serum glucose, insulin, and C-peptide levels were obtained during an oral glucose tolerance test. Insulin sensitivity was calculated by homeostasis model assessment of insulin resistance (HOMA-IR). Aerobic fitness was categorized empirically as very low aerobic fitness (VLAF; n = 17, Vo_{2max} < 21 mL/kg/min), low aerobic fitness (LAF; n = 12, Vo_{2max} 21–24.4 mL/kg/min), and moderate aerobic fitness (MAF; n = 19, Vo_{2max} > 24.4 mL/kg/min).

FINDINGS
Significant differences were found in serum glucose, insulin, and C-peptide levels as well as the HOMA-IR in the VLAF versus LAF and MAF groups. Mean HOMA-IR was statistically greater in the VLAF and LAF groups when compared to the MAF group.

IMPLICATIONS
Modest aerobic fitness has a significant impact on insulin sensitivity, atherogenic lipids, lipoprotein parameters, and the overall risks for CVD in sedentary overweight or obese African American women. Whether modest physical fitness translates into prevention of type 2 diabetes and CVD in African American women remains to be determined by additional research.

Gaillard, T. (2007). Importance of aerobic fitness in cardiovascular risks in sedentary overweight and obese African-American women. *Nursing Research, 56*(6), 407–415.

- Immunosuppressed status
- Medicated or unconscious status

Traumatic injury to the thorax or a break in the pleural membrane that surrounds the lungs may also produce restrictive pulmonary dysfunction. The stability of the chest depends upon the rib cage; multiple rib fractures may produce a type of paradoxical chest wall movement called "flail chest" that impedes normal airflow. The dual-layer pleural membrane also has an important structural function; it helps maintain a negative pressure between its two layers that keeps the lungs from collapsing upon themselves. A break in either layer of the membrane or an abnormal collection of fluid between them interferes with this function, permits alveoli to collapse, and increases the work of breathing. Common pleural defects are described in Table 32-1 on page 867.

Alveolar collapse, known as **atelectasis**, can be caused by pleural defects as described above, by compression from a mass such as a tumor, or by occlusion of the small airways by secretions, which prevents air movement into the associated alveoli. Failure of a client to breathe deeply after abdominal surgery may result in atelectasis. Regardless of the cause, atelectasis results in restrictive pulmonary dysfunction and reduces the amount of alveolar-capillary surface area engaged in gas exchange.

Diffusion Defects

Another mechanism of oxygenation impairment is a decrease in the efficiency of gas diffusion from the alveolar space into the pulmonary capillary blood, known as a **diffusion defect**. This may be caused by thickening of the alveolar-capillary basement membrane or by marked increases in the speed of blood flow through the pulmonary capillary beds, which reduce contact time with the alveoli. Diffusion defects by themselves are uncommon but may coexist with obstructive or restrictive pulmonary disease such as emphysema, pulmonary edema, or fibrosis.

Ventilation-Perfusion Mismatching

Gas exchange across the alveolar-capillary membrane is also influenced by **ventilation-perfusion (V/Q) mismatching**, or the balance between ventilation and perfusion. The amount of fresh air entering the alveoli (alveolar ventilation) and the amount of blood flow to various regions of the pulmonary capillary network (perfusion) are not uniform throughout the lungs. Due to alterations in position and the effect of gravity, certain zones of lung tissue may have better ventilation or perfusion than others at any given time.

An important mechanism of compensation in healthy lung tissue is to produce vasoconstriction or bronchoconstriction as needed to better match ventilation to perfusion or vice versa. Many disease states, however, produce areas of V/Q mismatching that cannot be overcome by compensatory responses. When mismatching occurs, some alveolar regions will be well ventilated but poorly perfused (a condition known as **deadspace**), while others may be well perfused but poorly ventilated (known as **shunting**). This phenomenon is illustrated in Figure 32-10 on page 868.

Alterations in circulation may occur in either the pulmonary or the systemic vasculature and may be localized or generalized. Generalized decreases in pulmonary circulation may be caused by right-sided heart failure or by pathologies in the pulmonary vascular system such as pulmonary hypertension and the resultant pulmonary artery sclerosis. Regional

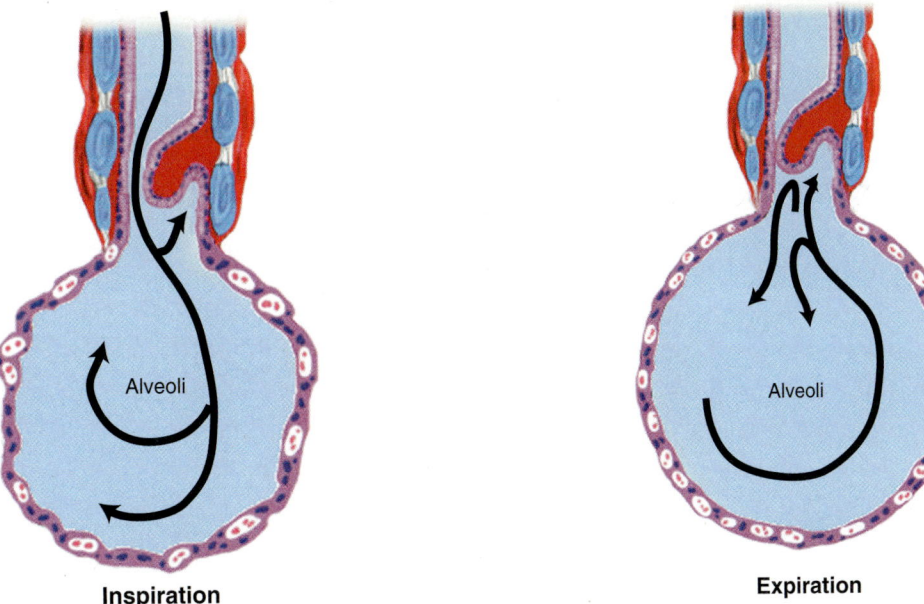

Inspiration

Expiration

FIGURE 32-9 One mechanism of air trapping in COPD. During inspiration, the airway widens and opens. During exhalation, the airway closes, trapping air distal to the obstruction and preventing fresh air from entering the alveoli. DELMAR/CENGAGE LEARNING

TABLE 32-1 Common Pleural Defects

PLEURAL DEFECT	DESCRIPTION
Pleural effusion	Collection of fluid between the pleural layers. May consist of serous fluid (hydrothorax), purulent fluid (empyema), or chyle (chylothorax).
Hemothorax	Collection of blood between the pleural layers.
Pneumothorax	A collection of air between the pleural layers caused by a hole in one or both layers of the pleural membrane. May be classified as open (communicating with a chest wall wound) or closed (no exterior wound).
Tension pneumothorax	A pneumothorax that rapidly expands with each respiratory cycle, compressing the lungs and heart and pushing the great vessels and trachea toward the opposite side of the chest. A tension pneumothorax is a medical emergency requiring immediate intervention.

Delmar/Cengage Learning

decreases in pulmonary circulation may be related to blockage of a pulmonary artery by an embolus or by regional vasoconstriction.

Atherosclerosis

Alterations in systemic circulation may also be generalized or localized. A common cause of altered arterial circulation is atherosclerosis. This disease is characterized by narrowing and eventual occlusion of the lumen (opening of the arteries) by deposits of lipids, fibrin, and calcium on the interior walls of the arteries (see Figure 32-11 on page 868). The reduction in blood flow with accompanying oxygen deprivation leads to ischemia (deprivation of blood flow) and even-

tual infarction (necrosis or death) of the affected tissue. Atherosclerosis in the coronary arteries (coronary heart disease) and the arteries of the brain (cerebral vascular disease) causes myocardial infarction and stroke, respectively, two of the leading causes of death in our society.

Heart Failure

Generalized decreases in tissue perfusion may be caused by left-sided heart failure or by loss of circulating blood volume as may occur with shock or hemorrhage. Heart failure is a condition in which the heart is unable to pump enough blood to meet the metabolic needs of the body; typically, this is accompanied by a backup of blood in the venous circuits

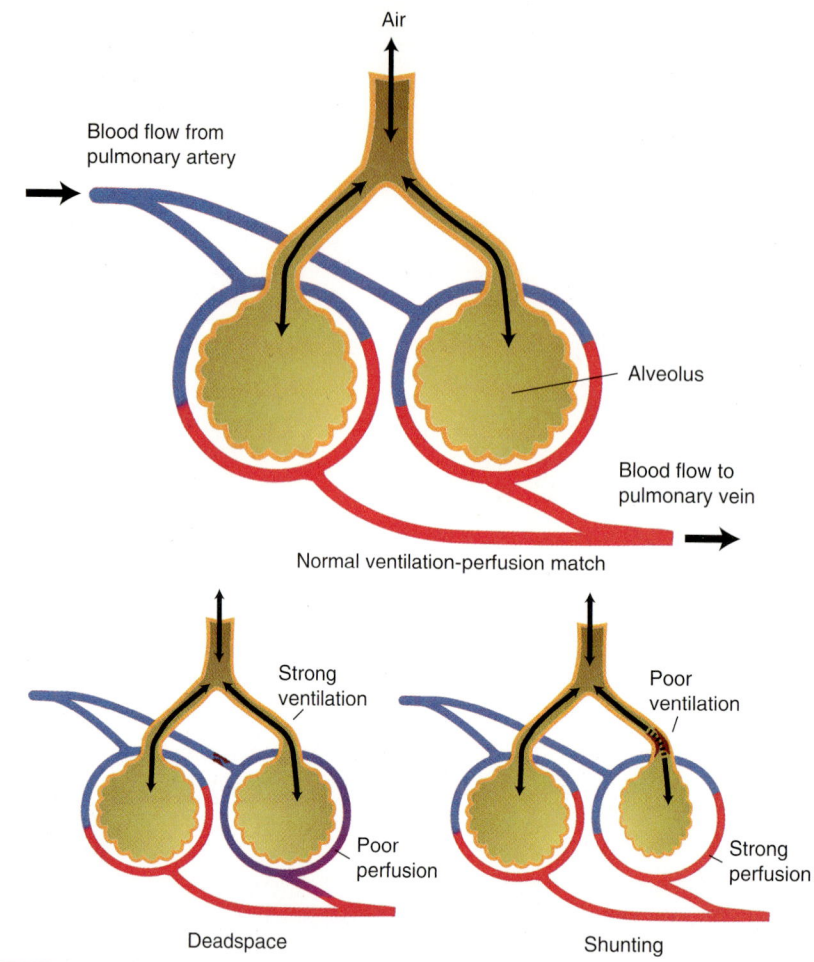

Air

Blood flow from
pulmonary artery

Alveolus

Blood flow to
pulmonary vein

Normal ventilation-perfusion match

Strong
ventilation

Poor
perfusion

Deadspace

Poor
ventilation

Strong
perfusion

Shunting

FIGURE 32-10 Types of Ventilation-Perfusion Abnormalities DELMAR/CENGAGE LEARNING

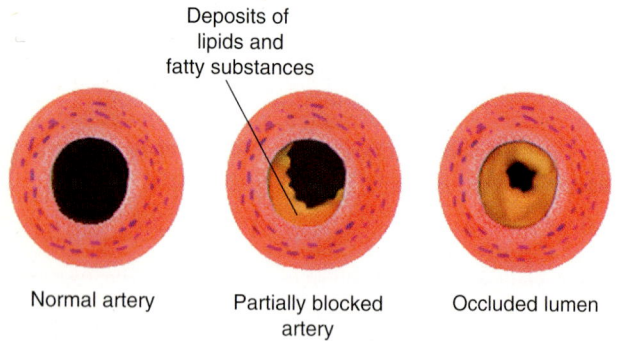

Deposits of
lipids and
fatty substances

Normal artery

Partially blocked
artery

Occluded lumen

FIGURE 32-11 Progression of Atherosclerosis DELMAR/CENGAGE LEARNING

(pulmonary and systemic veins), leading to the condition known as congestive heart failure. The increased pressure of the blood in the engorged veins causes fluid to leak out of the associated capillary beds, causing edema in the tissue, including the lungs (pulmonary edema). See the accompanying Client Teaching display on page 869 for special considerations regarding sexual activity.

Congestive heart failure results in poor arterial perfusion to the body's tissues. This reduction in **cardiac output** (amount of blood pumped by the heart) may be mild, causing only vague symptoms, or may be profound enough to cause death. Causes of congestive heart failure include myocardial infarction, hypertensive heart disease, and valvular disorders, among others.

Loss of circulating blood volume (hypovolemia) may result from massive bleeding, loss of fluid through a wound (such as an extensive burn injury), or severe dehydration.

Anemia

Another factor that influences oxygenation is the amount of hemoglobin in the blood available to bind with oxygen. A deficiency of hemoglobin (**anemia**) may decrease the oxygen-carrying capacity of the blood. A person who is anemic may have normal SaO_2 levels but still continue to experience inadequate tissue oxygenation at the cellular level. Certain poisoning syndromes, most notably carbon monoxide poisoning, mimic anemia in that they reduce oxygenation by competing with oxygen for binding sites on the hemoglobin molecule.

Alterations in Oxygen Uptake

A final factor to consider in the process of oxygenation involves the uptake of oxygen by the body's cells. Certain conditions may impair the cells' ability to take up and utilize

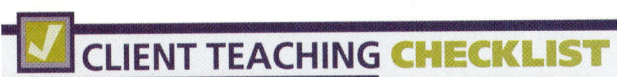

✓ **CLIENT TEACHING CHECKLIST**

Special Considerations regarding Sexual Activity

Clients recovering from acute cardiac compromise, such as congestive heart failure or myocardial infarction, need sensitive nursing care and education regarding sexual activity. Help alleviate their concerns by sharing the following American Heart Association recommendations:

- Check with your health care provider.
- Resume sexual activity when you feel ready; most cardiac-compromised clients can safely resume sexual activity within 2 to 4 weeks.
- Take it slow and establish your comfort level; begin with lower energy forms of sexual expression, such as touching and holding.
- Continue taking prescribed cardiac medications; report to your health care provider any impact of these medications on sexual desire and performance.
- Experiencing an increased awareness of breathing, heartbeat, and muscle tightening during sexual activity is normal.

---

oxygen, particularly when the mitochondria are damaged. Cyanide poisoning and severe sepsis impair mitochondrial functioning, rendering the oxygen in arterial blood useless to the cells.

PHYSIOLOGICAL RESPONSES TO REDUCED OXYGENATION

When oxygen delivery is inadequate to meet the metabolic needs of the body, various responses to this deficit can be expected, including changes in metabolic pathways and efforts to increase the extraction of available oxygen. If these efforts fail, cells will be damaged and ultimately die.

Increased Oxygen Extraction

Under normal conditions, the cells of the body do not extract all of the oxygen carried in the arterial blood. In fact, blood returning to the heart via the venous circulation is typically about 75% saturated with oxygen. In response to poor oxygen delivery or increased oxygen need, the cells can extract more oxygen from the arterial blood.

Anaerobic Metabolism

The utilization of food (glucose) for cellular energy occurs via metabolic pathways that use oxygen; this is known as **aerobic metabolism**. Many cells are also capable of utilizing alternate metabolic pathways in the absence of oxygen for short periods of time; this is referred to as **anaerobic metabolism**. Anaerobic metabolism is limited by several factors:

1. Not all cells are capable of significant anaerobic metabolism (most notably brain cells).
2. Anaerobic metabolism yields less energy per unit of fuel than does aerobic metabolism.
3. Anaerobic metabolism results in the accumulation of acid by-products, such as lactate, which upset the chemical environment of the cell and induce the release of cell-damaging (lysosomal) enzymes.

Tissue Ischemia and Cell Death

Prolonged oxygen deprivation (**hypoxia**) will lead to a syndrome ending in cellular death. The decreased production of adenosine triphosphate (ATP) resulting from anaerobic metabolism reduces the amount of energy available for cellular metabolic functions and results in a breakdown in all cellular functions. The integrity of the cell membrane becomes impaired, and the cell begins to swell. Cellular organelles may become damaged and lysosomal enzymes released, killing the cell. The destruction of tissues or organs as a result of oxygen deprivation is known as an infarction. Widespread cellular death resulting from oxygenation disturbances is the underlying characteristic of a devastating syndrome known as *multiple organ dysfunction syndrome* (MODS).

Carbon Dioxide Transport and Excretion

Carbon dioxide is a natural by-product of glucose metabolism. Like oxygen, it exists normally as a gas and can be dissolved in the plasma as well as loosely bound to the hemoglobin molecule, although carbon dioxide attaches to a different binding site on the hemoglobin molecule than does oxygen. In the lungs, carbon dioxide is released into the alveoli by diffusion, and when the individual exhales, the carbon dioxide exits to the atmosphere.

In the body fluids, carbon dioxide functions as an acid because, combined with water, it produces carbonic acid. The hydrogen ions that are liberated in this process stimulate the respiratory control centers in the pons and medulla to increase the rate and depth of breathing; more carbon dioxide is then released by the lungs, and the pH of the body is brought back to normal. Likewise, increased production of carbon dioxide, as may be associated with fever or exercise, is often a cause of increased ventilatory rate (**tachypnea**) and depth. Elevated blood levels of carbon dioxide (**hypercapnia**) indicate inadequate alveolar ventilation.

ASSESSMENT
HEALTH HISTORY

The health history of the individual experiencing oxygenation deficits is important in the development of the plan of care. The health history should begin with a thorough exploration of the presenting problem (see Table 32-2), including how long it has been present and whether it has recently gotten worse, then should proceed to explore the medical history, impact of the illness on activities of daily living (ADL), and the client's knowledge level and coping abilities.

PHYSICAL EXAMINATION

Inspection will begin when the nurse first encounters the client. This is a time to make general notes of the client's efforts at ventilation, especially anxious or distressed appearance, flaring of nostrils, position preferences, and general chest configuration (see Figure 32-12). While counting the respiratory rate, also note the rhythm or pattern of the breathing for regularity or irregularity (see Figure 32-13). The signs and symptoms of hypoxia are relative to the onset. Early clinical manifestations of hypoxia include restlessness,

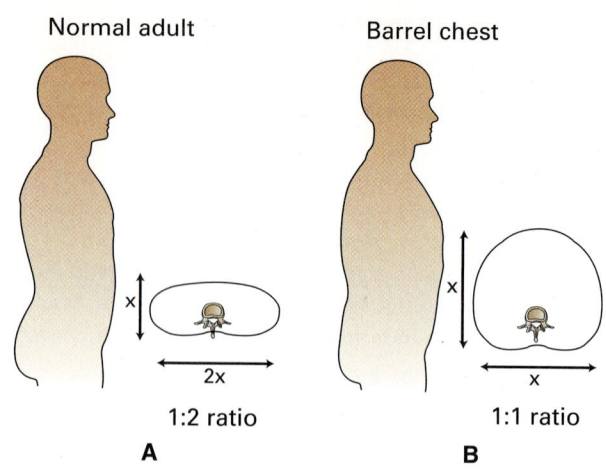

FIGURE 32-12 Changes in chest configuration and posture.
A. The normal ratio of the anterior-posterior diameter to the lateral diameter is 1:2. **B.** With a barrel chest, the ratio between the diameters is 1:1. DELMAR/CENGAGE LEARNING

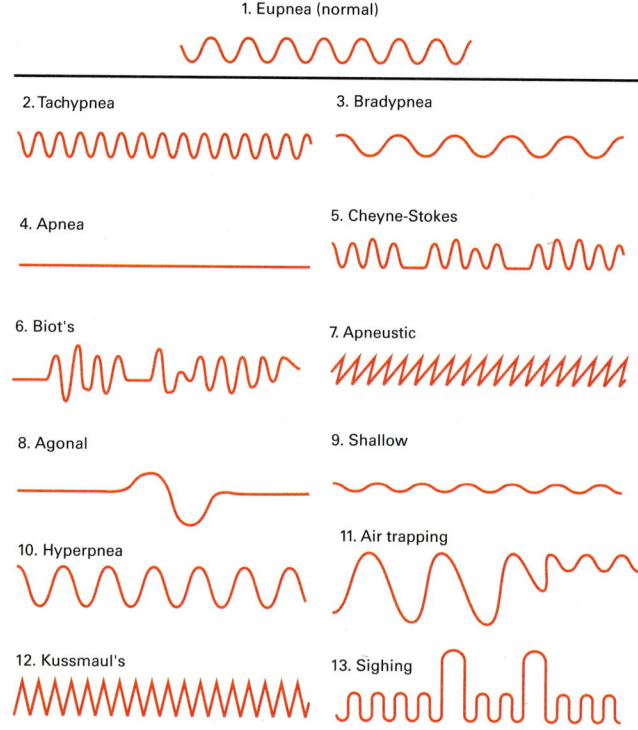

FIGURE 32-13 Respiratory Patterns DELMAR/CENGAGE LEARNING

TABLE 32-2	Health History Related to Oxygenation 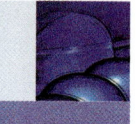	
PRESENTING PROBLEM	**QUALIFIERS**
Cough	• Onset: sudden or gradual, how long ago • Nature: dry, moist, barking, hacking, productive, nonproductive • Pattern: continuous, occasional, related to time of day, position or activity, weather • Severity • Associated symptoms: pain, shortness of breath, wheezing • Alleviating factors: vaporizers, OTC medications
Sputum	• Amount, color, odor • Presence of blood in sputum
Shortness of breath	• Onset: sudden or gradual • Nature: precipitated by choking or gagging • Pattern: associated with activity or position; continuous or intermittent • Associated symptoms: pain, cough, diaphoresis • Alleviating factors
Pain	• Location and radiation • Nature: stabbing, dull, aching, burning, squeezing, crushing • Associated symptoms: dizziness, nausea, diaphoresis, palpitations • Aggravating factors • Alleviating factors

Delmar/Cengage Learning

apprehension, anxiety, dizziness, inability to concentrate, confusion, agitation, increased pulse rate, increased rate and depth of respiration, and elevated blood pressure (unless the hypoxia is caused by shock). If the hypoxia goes untreated, the respiratory rate may decline and changes in the level of consciousness progress to stupor or coma, indicating ischemia of neuronal cells resulting from oxygen deprivation. Perfusion deficits resulting in poor circulation can be visually noted in mottled skin, **cyanosis** (bluish coloration of the skin), and edema. The bluish discoloration of cyanosis is the result of the presence of desaturated hemoglobin in capillaries that may occur from either hypoxia or stagnant blood flow. When cyanosis is observed in the tongue, soft palate, and conjunctiva of the eye, it indicates hypoxemia, whereas cyanosis of the extremities, nail beds, and earlobes is often a result of vasoconstriction and stagnant blood flow. Clubbing of the fingers, which manifests as a flattened angle of the nailbed and a rounding of the fingertips, is a sign of chronic hypoxia (see Figure 32-14). Regardless of the mechanism behind it, it is important to remember that cyanosis is often a late development in clients with poor oxygenation and may be further delayed in those with dark skin pigmentation or low blood hemoglobin (anemia). Therefore, the absence of cyanosis should not be taken as an assurance that oxygenation is adequate. However, the presence of cyanosis, especially central cyanosis, should be considered an indicator of a hypoxic emergency.

Common palpation findings related to compromised ventilation include vocal fremitus and displacement of the

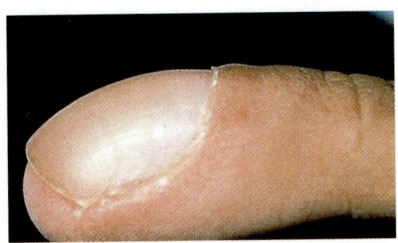

FIGURE 32-14 Clubbing of the Fingers as a Result of Chronic Hypoxia COURTESY OF ROBERT A. SILVERMAN, MD, PEDIATRIC DERMATOLOGY, GEORGETOWN UNIVERSITY

trachea. Perfusion deficits are noted in changes in pulse rate or character, clammy skin, and ulcers in the lower extremities.

Percussion may reveal hyperresonance, dull percussion tone, or changes in the density of the lungs and surrounding tissues.

Auscultation may reveal adventitious breath sounds (e.g., crackles [rales], wheezes, rhonchi, pleural friction rub, or stridor), all indicators of alterations in ventilation (see Table 32-3). Circulation deficits will be noted upon auscultation by **gallops**, or extra heart sounds, and **murmurs**, or sounds produced by blood flowing through a malfunctioning valve.

DIAGNOSTIC AND LABORATORY DATA

There are many tests to measure oxygenation status. Pulse oximetry uses light waves to measure oxygen saturation (SaO_2) noninvasively (see Figure 32-15 on page 872). See Chapter 40, Procedure 40-2: Pulse Oximetry. Arterial blood gases (ABGs) measure a number of indicators that can affect oxygenation status; these factors and their values are listed in Table 32-4 on page 872. Sputum collection is another valuable tool in assessing a client's oxygenation functioning; this procedure is outlined in Table 32-5 on page 873, and common findings and their indications are listed in Table 32-6 on page 873. Measurements of lactic acid, hemoglobin, and hematocrit are also useful in determining the effectiveness of the body's oxygen delivery to tissues.

TABLE 32-3 Characteristics of Adventitious Breath Sounds

BREATH SOUND	RESPIRATORY PHASE	DESCRIPTION	CONDITIONS
Fine crackle	Predominantly inspiration	Dry, high-pitched crackling, popping; short duration; roll hair by ears between your fingers to simulate this sound	Chronic obstructive pulmonary disease, congestive heart failure, pneumonia, pulmonary fibrosis, atelectasis
Coarse crackle	Predominantly inspiration	Moist, low-pitched crackling, gurgling; long duration	Pneumonia, pulmonary edema, bronchitis, atelectasis
Sonorous wheeze	Predominantly expiration	Low-pitched; snoring	Asthma, bronchitis, airway edema, tumor, bronchiolar spasm, foreign body obstruction
Sibilant wheeze	Predominantly expiration	High-pitched; musical	Asthma, chronic bronchitis, emphysema, tumor, foreign body obstruction
Pleural friction rub	Inspiration and expiration	Creaking, grating	Pleurisy, tuberculosis, pulmonary infarction, pneumonia, lung abscess
Stridor	Predominantly inspiration	Crowing	Croup, foreign body obstruction, large airway tumor

Delmar/Cengage Learning

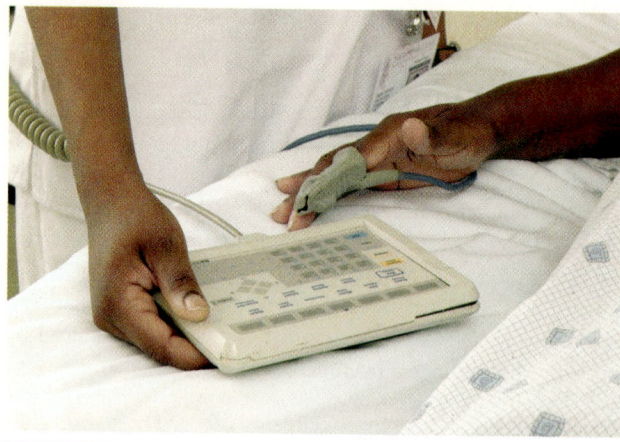

FIGURE 32-15 Client with Pulse Oximeter DELMAR/CENGAGE LEARNING

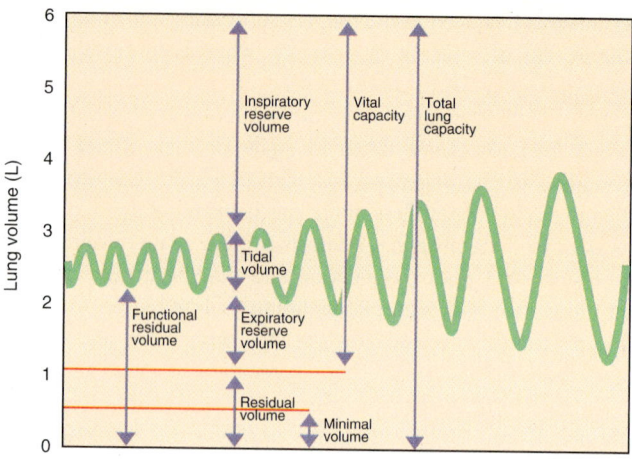

FIGURE 32-16 Graphic Representation of Lung Volumes and Capacities DELMAR/CENGAGE LEARNING

Selected tests to determine oxygenation status are discussed in Table 32-7 on page 874. (See Figure 32-16 for ventilatory function.) Clients undergoing these tests are often apprehensive and need nursing care and education directed at their knowledge levels. Refer to Chapter 28 for further diagnostic information.

NURSING DIAGNOSIS

Nursing care of the client experiencing oxygenation problems should be prioritized on the basis of the A-B-C format used in basic life support; that is, consider the *airway, breathing,* and *circulation* first and foremost. The primary nursing diagnoses are related to these priorities. Pertinent North American Nursing Diagnosis Association–approved nursing diagnoses regarding oxygenation are discussed in the sections that follow.

INEFFECTIVE AIRWAY CLEARANCE

Ineffective airway clearance exists when the client has difficulty maintaining a patent (open) airway at any point along the airway. This occlusion of the airway may be partial or complete. Causes of ineffective airway clearance include:

- Obstruction of the airway by the tongue (as may occur in the comatose or anesthetized client)
- Obstruction of airway by secretion (as may occur with excessive sputum production and ineffective or absent cough)
- Upper airway obstruction caused by edema of the larynx or glottis
- Obstruction of the trachea or a bronchus by foreign body aspiration
- Partial occlusion of the bronchi and bronchioles by infection (bronchitis, bronchiolitis), inflammation and smooth muscle spasm (asthma), or occlusion or compression by a tumor mass
- Occlusion of the more distal airways by the changes associated with emphysema

Assessment findings in the client with ineffective airway clearance include a complaint of feeling short of breath or

TABLE 32-4 Arterial Blood Gases		
MEASUREMENT	**NORMAL ARTERIAL VALUES**	**CLINICAL SIGNIFICANCE**
pH	7.35–7.45	Indicates acid-base balance
P_{CO_2}	35–45 mm Hg	Partial pressure of carbon dioxide; indicates adequacy of alveolar ventilation; represents respiratory component of acid-base balance
HCO_3-	22–26 mEq/L	Bicarbonate level; indicates metabolic component of acid-base balance
Pa_{O_2}	80–100 mm Hg	Partial pressure of oxygen; represents oxygen dissolved in plasma
Sa_{O_2}	96%–98%	Saturation of hemoglobin with oxygen

Delmar/Cengage Learning

TABLE 32-5 Protocol: Assisting a Client with Sputum Collection

Purpose	• To collect an adequate sample of sputum for laboratory analysis or culture • To minimize contamination of the sample with oral or other secretions
Level	• Independent
Supportive data	• Increasing the client's knowledge promotes cooperation and increases the diagnostic value of the sample obtained.
Assessment	• Verify the type of test to be performed: Cytology studies should be collected into a cup containing a preservative solution; cultures must be collected into a sterile container. • Assess the client's level of consciousness and ability to follow instructions. • Assess the client's breath sounds; coarse rales indicate the presence of sputum in the airways.
Interventions	• Obtain correct specimen container. • Wash hands and don clean gloves. • Assist the client to rinse the mouth with water (not mouthwash). • Instruct client to raise sputum from the lungs, not the throat or nose. • Instruct client to expectorate sputum into the cup without touching the inside of the container. • Replace cap on container as soon as sample is obtained. Label container and wash the outside if indicated. • Place in a bag with a biohazard label for transport. • Provide mouth care for the client and assist to a comfortable position. • Remove gloves and wash hands. Send specimen to lab immediately.
Documentation	• Document amount, color, character, and odor of sputum obtained and time the specimen was sent to the lab.

Delmar/Cengage Learning

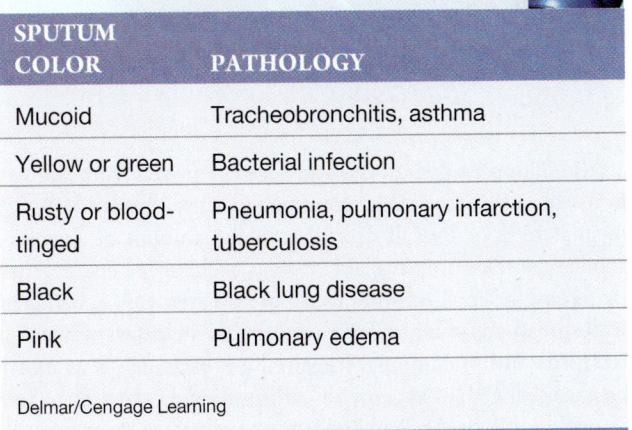

TABLE 32-6 Pathologies Associated with Different Colors of Sputum

SPUTUM COLOR	PATHOLOGY
Mucoid	Tracheobronchitis, asthma
Yellow or green	Bacterial infection
Rusty or blood-tinged	Pneumonia, pulmonary infarction, tuberculosis
Black	Black lung disease
Pink	Pulmonary edema

Delmar/Cengage Learning

suffocating, a condition sometimes referred to as "air hunger." The use of accessory muscles of ventilation may be noted, and the client may complain of fatigue. Shortness of breath may be noted on observation, and the client may have difficulty speaking because of it.

A cough may be noted, and on auscultation crackles and rhonchi may be heard. Poor aeration of the alveoli, as can occur with emphysema and severe asthma, will cause diminished breath sounds over the peripheral lung fields. Complete obstruction of a large or medium-sized airway will result in a loss of breath sounds over the affected lung segment.

INEFFECTIVE BREATHING PATTERNS

Ineffective breathing pattern is commonly a problem for clients with restrictive pulmonary disease or central nervous system disorders that affect breathing. Those with restrictive pulmonary disease, in an effort to decrease their work of breathing, tend to adopt a pattern of rapid, shallow respirations. This respiratory pattern does not deliver adequate fresh air to the alveoli, resulting in chronic air hunger while contributing to muscle fatigue. Central nervous system disorders, including the effects of anesthetics and narcotics, may reduce both the rate and the depth of ventilation. Lesions affecting the brain stem in particular may reduce ventilation to dangerous levels.

Another group of clients at risk for ineffective breathing patterns are those who have had major abdominal or thoracic surgery or whose mobility is restricted. These individuals

TABLE 32-7 Selected Tests for Oxygenation Status

TEST	INDICATIONS/POSSIBLE FINDINGS
Ventilatory function tests	• Volume of air in the lungs at various phases of the ventilatory cycle • Speed and ease of airflow through the airways • Strength of the respiratory muscles
Chest x-ray	• Areas of fluid accumulation (infiltrates) • Solid masses (suggestive of tumors) • Abnormal accumulations of calcium, areas of necrosis (as seen in tuberculosis) • Excessive air trapping (suggestive of emphysema) • Abnormal accumulations of air or fluid in the pleural space (suggestive of pleural effusion or pneumothorax) • Gross abnormalities in size, shape, position of thoracic structures
Computerized tomography (CT) scan, spiral CT scan, magnetic resonance imaging (MRI)	• Detailed pictures of thoracic structures • Spiral CT provides a three-dimensional representation of lesions and normal tissue
Ventilation perfusion (V/Q) scan	• Areas of impaired airflow (suggestive of pulmonary emboli)
Bronchoscopy	• Sputum collection • Examination of tissue
Thoracentesis	• Tissue sample collection
Echocardiography	• Size and motion of cardiac structures • Accumulation of fluid in the pericardial sac (suggestive of pericardial effusion)
Electrocardiography	• Heart rate and rhythm • Abnormal sites of impulse formation (ectopic pacemakers) • Areas of blocked or delayed impulse transmission • Chamber enlargement (as seen in heart failure) • Areas of ischemia, injury, or infarction
Stress test	• Changes in ECG tracings (may indicate ischemic heart disease)

Delmar/Cengage Learning

have a tendency to take shallow breaths and to avoid sighing and coughing, both necessary to maintain airway integrity.

Neuromuscular diseases that weaken the respiratory muscles may also result in ineffective breathing patterns as well as impaired airway clearance. Examples of such disorders include Guillain-Barré syndrome and myasthenia gravis. Alterations in thoracic structures that interfere with breathing patterns include abnormal curvatures of the spine (scoliosis, kyphosis), chest wall injury, and pleural defects.

IMPAIRED GAS EXCHANGE

Impaired gas exchange occurs when, despite the delivery of fresh air to the alveoli, adequate oxygen does not enter the arterial blood or carbon dioxide is not removed from the venous blood. Often this condition is the result of V/Q mismatching or overall decreases in the amount of alveolar-capillary surface area available for gas exchange, a characteristic of emphysema. Another cause of impaired gas exchange is widespread shunting, as may occur with atelectasis (alveolar collapse) and pneumonia. Impaired gas exchange is assessed by measuring the oxygen and carbon dioxide content in the arterial blood via ABG analysis, pulse oximetry, or both.

DECREASED CARDIAC OUTPUT

Decreased cardiac output impairs oxygen delivery to the tissues and may also be a factor in impaired gas exchange, as when congestive heart failure causes pulmonary edema. Causes of decreased cardiac output include heart failure and various types of shock. The assessment findings associated with decreased cardiac output may include low blood pressure; cool, clammy skin; weak, thready pulses; low urine output; and a diminished level of consciousness. If pulmonary edema is present, crackles will be heard over the lung bases and the client may produce frothy pink or white sputum.

INEFFECTIVE TISSUE PERFUSION

Ineffective (decreased) tissue perfusion may be widespread, as in the case of decreased cardiac output, or it may be confined to one or more tissues or organs of the body. A common cause of regional decreases in tissue perfusion is atherosclerosis, which may impair perfusion to the heart, brain, kidneys, or extremities. Assessment findings depend upon the organ or tissue involved, but one common finding is pain. The tissue that is deprived of oxygen will in many cases be painful, as the accumulation of lactic acid and the chemical mediators of the inflammatory response stimulate local pain receptors.

OTHER NURSING DIAGNOSES

The relationship between the primary nursing diagnoses discussed earlier and the secondary nursing diagnoses in the client with oxygenation problems is reciprocal; that is, the primary diagnoses both influence and are influenced by the secondary diagnoses. A holistic approach to nursing care requires that all diagnoses affecting the client be considered and prioritized in developing the plan of care.

Deficient Knowledge

Deficient knowledge may exist to varying degrees in the client with either acute or chronic oxygenation problems. Involving the client in the plan of care requires that the client be informed regarding the disease process, diagnostic procedures, and treatment modalities. Assessment for deficient knowledge involves questioning the client and family with regard to their understanding and perceptions of these subjects. It is a mistake to assume that a client with a long-standing chronic illness has a good understanding of that illness.

Activity Intolerance

Activity intolerance reflects the impact of the illness on the client's ability to perform ADL; the degree of this impairment may range from mild to severe, but it is important that this judgment be based on the client's, not the nurse's, perception of the activity intolerance. Activity restrictions that may be a mere annoyance for one individual can be viewed as catastrophic by another.

To assess activity intolerance, both interview and observation are useful. Ask the client to compare the current level of activity with the previous level and desired level. In addition, observe the client performing activities such as moving about in bed, ambulating, and performing personal care activities; note the point at which fatigue or dyspnea occurs and the amount of rest required. Objective tests of exercise tolerance, such as stress tests, may be performed in certain cases.

Insomnia

Insomnia is common in people with both cardiac and pulmonary disease. As mentioned earlier, many people with restrictive and obstructive pulmonary diseases find that breathing is easiest in an upright position; this position is also more comfortable for those with congestive heart failure. Sudden attacks of dyspnea during sleep, called **paroxysmal nocturnal dyspnea**, may interrupt the sleep of these clients, resulting in chronic fatigue. Complaints of poor sleep, along with daytime sleepiness and fatigue, are common assessment findings. Insomnia can result in personality changes, hallucinations, and delusions.

A particular sleep problem associated with airway obstruction is **sleep apnea**. It is often seen in males who are overweight and have short, thick necks and is commonly associated with loud, heavy snoring. The soft tissues of the upper airways collapse during sleep, resulting in periods of absence of breathing (apnea). The individual then rouses enough to resume breathing, interrupting the normal sleep cycle. These individuals may complain of persistent daytime fatigue despite what seems to be adequate nighttime sleep.

Imbalanced Nutrition

Nutritional alterations are also commonly associated with both cardiac and pulmonary disease. The client with dyspnea may have difficulty consuming adequate food because of the effort involved; in turn, the malnutrition contributes to respiratory muscle weakness. The client with a productive cough may have an unpleasant taste in the mouth, interfering with appetite. Congestive heart failure may cause a poor appetite (anorexia) because of decreased perfusion to the gut. On the other hand, obesity can affect oxygenation by increasing the work of breathing as well as the cardiac workload.

Acute Pain

Acute pain may be present in the client with ischemia to the heart or to the extremities due to inadequate perfusion; chest wall or pleuritic pain may also be a feature of many pulmonary disorders. Adequate pain control can influence the effectiveness of breathing patterns and coughing, making pain control a priority in these cases. Pain assessment should address the nature of the pain, its intensity, its location and radiation, factors that make it better or worse, and any associated symptoms. For instance, pain caused by myocardial ischemia is called **angina pectoris** and is often described as crushing or squeezing in nature; it may be confined to the chest or it may radiate to the neck, shoulder, jaw, arm, or hand. Ischemia to the extremities (most often the legs) produces a pain known as **intermittent claudication**, which is typically brought on by exercise and relieved by rest. See Chapter 35 for further discussion of pain assessment.

Anxiety

Anxiety is often a prominent finding in individuals who are experiencing breathing difficulties or acute cardiac problems, such as chest pain. The anxious client may have difficulty answering questions and focusing on the instructions being given and may expend excessive amounts of precious energy in the process. Therefore, recognition and control of anxiety bring both psychological and physiological benefits.

PLANNING AND OUTCOMES

In identifying goals and planning nursing care for the client with oxygenation disorders, carefully consider individual goals for each nursing diagnosis and each client; the goals should be individualized to reflect the client's capabilities and limitations. In many cases, identifying desired outcomes of care is best accomplished in small steps, progressing from one level of functioning to the next until the ultimate objective is attained. Such an approach prevents the client from feeling overwhelmed with the magnitude of the task at hand while allowing for the satisfaction of reaching intermediate outcomes. Outcomes may be based on physiological parameters such as respiratory rate or ABG values, on activity tolerance and client comfort levels, or on identified learning needs.

The outcomes for a particular client should be based upon the assessment findings that led to the nursing diagnoses at hand. For example, if a respiratory rate of 30 breaths per minute with a shallow breathing pattern and suprasternal retraction led to a diagnosis of ineffective breathing pattern, then the desired outcome of intervention might be a respiratory rate of 20 breaths per minute or less and the absence of retractions. Achievement of the outcome indicates resolution of the problem.

COLLABORATION

The management of care for a client with impaired oxygenation requires a dynamic and systematic collaborative approach to providing and coordinating health care services. It is the participative process of a multidisciplinary team that facilitates options and services for meeting the client's health needs in a way that decreases fragmentation and duplication of care and enhances quality, cost-effective outcomes. Refer to the clinical pathway for a client with pneumonia in the Nursing Care Plan at the end of this chapter for an example of collaborative practice among various disciplines.

IMPLEMENTATION

Interventions for promoting and maintaining adequate oxygenation include airway clearance, breathing patterns, oxygen update and delivery, cardiac output and tissue perfusion, and emergency interventions. Other interventions address the associated nursing diagnoses for maintaining the client's optimal level of health. The interventions for acid-base management are discussed in Chapter 33.

INTERVENTIONS TO PROMOTE AIRWAY CLEARANCE

Interventions to promote airway clearance focus on clearing the airways of secretions, relieving bronchospasm, and, when necessary, bypassing the natural airway structures with an artificial airway. All of these procedures are facilitated when the client has been well informed of the purpose for the interventions and knows what to expect.

Teach Effective Coughing

Effective coughing techniques may need to be taught to the client experiencing either short-term or chronic airway obstruction. Coughing is an important element of postoperative care in order to prevent pulmonary complications. Effective coughing should be preceded by a series of slow, deep breaths. One technique that may be useful is "huffing," or delivering a series of short, forceful exhalations, prior to actual coughing. The intent is to raise the sputum to the level where it can then be coughed out. If the client is recovering from thoracic or abdominal surgery, splinting the incision by holding a pillow firmly against it will reduce the pain caused by coughing. In most cases, assisting the client to a sitting position will increase the effectiveness of the cough. Assess the sputum produced by coughing, noting the amount, color, and odor. Recognize that the client may become fatigued after coughing and need a rest period; also offer oral care such as a mouth rinse after sputum has been expectorated.

Initiate Postural Drainage and Chest Physiotherapy

Postural drainage and **chest physiotherapy (CPT)** are techniques intended to promote the drainage of secretions from the lungs. Positioning for drainage of each of the lung lobes is accompanied by percussion or vibration applied to the chest wall to loosen secretions (see Figure 32-17 on page 877). Percussion involves using a cupped hand to beat firmly on the chest wall (see Figure 32-18 on page 877); a firm rubber cup of a size appropriate to the client's body size may also be used. Vibration is done using a special vibrator applied to the chest wall. Inhalation treatments containing bronchodilator or mucolytic drugs may be administered before CPT and postural drainage.

Measures should be taken to minimize the client's anxiety and discomfort during these procedures. Pain medications, if indicated, should be timed so that their effectiveness peaks at the time of the treatment. Also, the nurse must recognize that some clients may be unable to tolerate certain postural drainage positions, and the treatment must be modified. Those with congestive heart failure or increased intracranial pressure particularly will not be able to tolerate a head-down position.

...

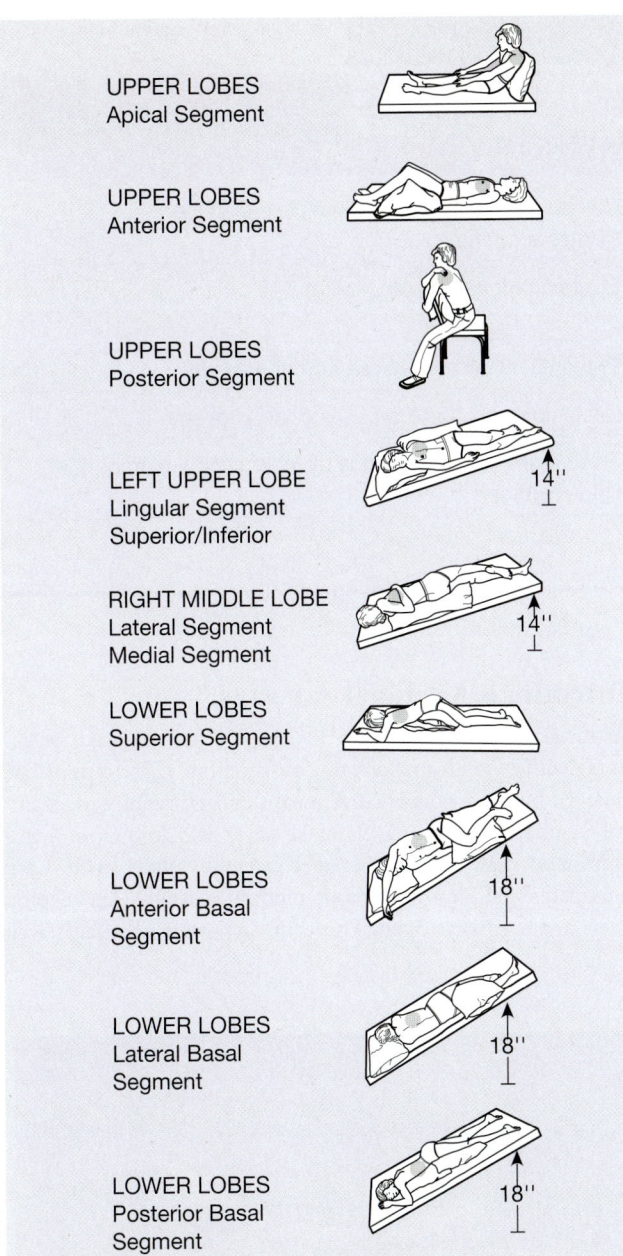

UPPER LOBES
Apical Segment

UPPER LOBES
Anterior Segment

UPPER LOBES
Posterior Segment

LEFT UPPER LOBE
Lingular Segment
Superior/Inferior
14"

RIGHT MIDDLE LOBE
Lateral Segment
Medial Segment
14"

LOWER LOBES
Superior Segment

LOWER LOBES
Anterior Basal
Segment
18"

LOWER LOBES
Lateral Basal
Segment
18"

LOWER LOBES
Posterior Basal
Segment
18"

FIGURE 32-17 Postural Drainage Positions DELMAR/CENGAGE LEARNING

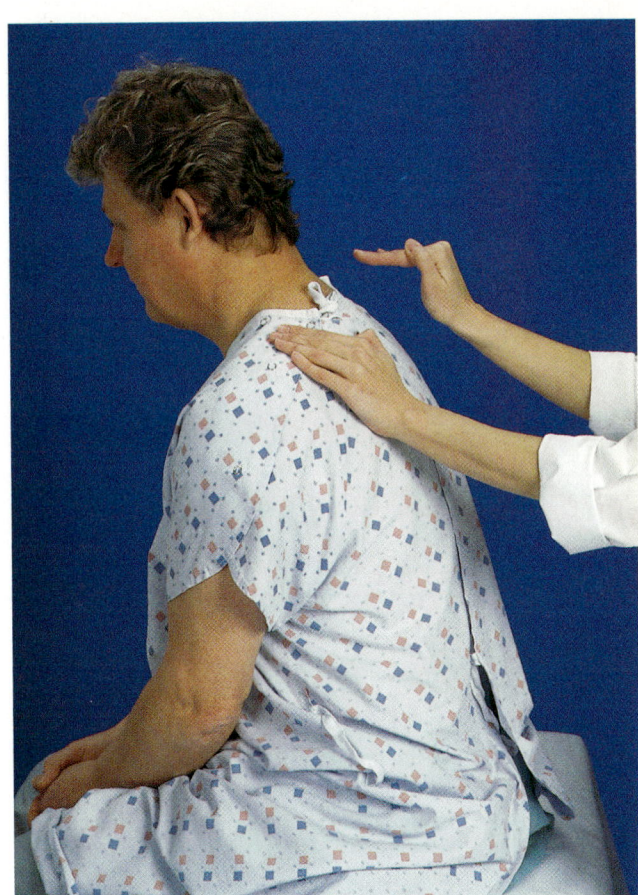

FIGURE 32-18 Chest Wall Percussion: Positions of Hands to Strike DELMAR/CENGAGE LEARNING

Monitor Hydration

Hydration, that is, the provision of adequate fluid intake, is important in thinning the pulmonary secretions so that they may be more easily expectorated. This may be beneficial in cases of pneumonia, bronchitis, and asthma. Clients experiencing congestive heart failure, on the other hand, may require limitation of fluid intake to reduce pulmonary congestion due to fluid volume overload.

Each exhalation contains not only carbon dioxide and other gases but also water vapor. This "insensible fluid loss" will be increased in those who are tachypneic as well as in clients receiving supplemental oxygen if the oxygen is not adequately humidified. Artificial airways that bypass the natural humidification processes of the nose and oropharynx also contribute to increased insensible fluid losses. Drying and inflammation of the respiratory mucosa may result. For this reason, humidification of inspired oxygen, especially that which is delivered through an artificial airway, is very important.

Administer Medications

Medications that assist in airway clearance include expectorants, mucolytics, and bronchodilators. It may be beneficial to administer the medications before CPT or postural drainage treatments in order to maximize the treatment's effectiveness. Clients must be taught the name of the medication they are receiving, the purpose of the medication, the dose, and how it is to be taken. The most common and most significant side effects should also be reviewed with the client. A summary of medications used for airway clearance is presented in Table 32-8 on page 878.

Monitor Environmental and Lifestyle Conditions

Environmental and lifestyle conditions may greatly influence the client's long-term recovery. Allergic conditions such as asthma may improve dramatically if the allergens to which the client is sensitive are identified and removed from the client's environment. Certain allergens such as animal dander

TABLE 32-8 Medications Used for Airway Clearance

DRUG TYPE	COMMON EXAMPLES	ACTIONS
Beta-adrenergic sympathomimetic	Epinephrine, isoproterenol, albuterol, metaproterenol, terbutaline	Causes bronchial smooth muscle relaxation (dilates bronchi)
Corticosteroid	Beclomethasone, prednisone, prednisolone, hydrocortisone	Elicits anti-inflammatory action
Mast cell stabilizer	Cromolyn sodium	Prevents histamine release from mast cells
Methylxanthine	Aminophylline, theophylline	Dilates bronchi and increases ciliary movement
Mucolytic/ expectorant	Mucomyst (acetylcysteine), guaifenesin	Thins respiratory secretions by increasing the amount of fluid produced

Delmar/Cengage Learning

or feather pillows may be relatively easy to eliminate; others, such as house dust and pollen, may be impossible to eliminate but can be reduced using devices such as air filters.

Smoking is a significant contributing factor in both heart and lung disease. Smoking cessation may not reverse advanced disease but will often reduce the client's symptoms and improve the quality of life. Smoking cessation programs and support groups, along with nicotine replacements such as transdermal patches, may help the client succeed in quitting smoking.

Introduce Artificial Airways

Artificial airways (see Figure 32-19A–D) may be used for clients with significant airway obstruction that cannot be relieved by more conservative means or who require mechanical ventilatory support. Nasal airways, also known as nasal trumpets, may be placed in conscious adults who have adequate breathing ability but require assistance in keeping their upper airways open. These airways are usually fairly well

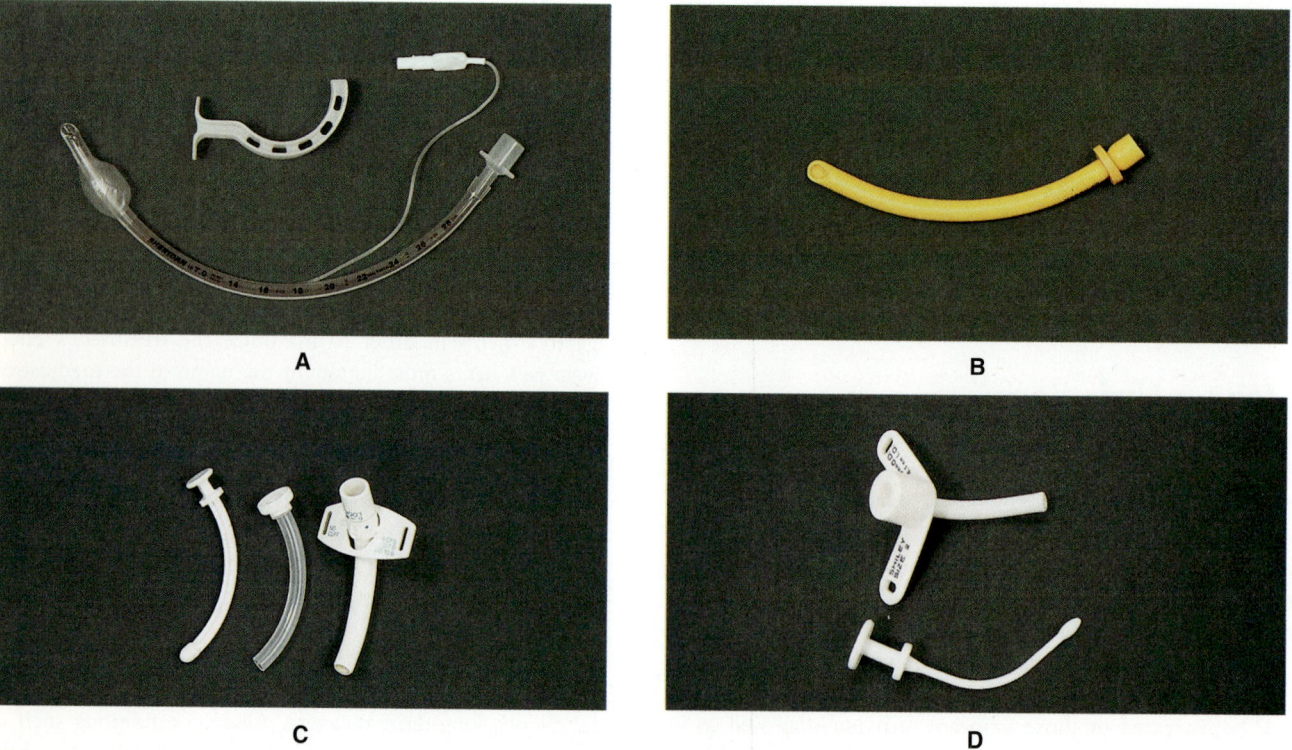

A

B

C

D

FIGURE 32-19 **Types of Artificial Airways: A.** Oral airway and endotracheal tube; **B.** Nasal trumpet; **C.** Tracheostomy tube; **D.** Pediatric tracheostomy tube. DELMAR/CENGAGE LEARNING

tolerated and can provide a conduit for frequent nasotracheal suctioning while minimizing trauma to the nasal mucosa.

The oral airway is used to maintain the tongue away from the posterior oropharynx in the unconscious client. It is essential to choose the correct size, since an airway that is too large may actually cause occlusion, while one that is too small may compress the tongue, stimulating the vomiting center. Oral airways are not well tolerated in conscious individuals, who may gag and vomit if an oral airway is in place.

Endotracheal tubes bypass the upper airway structures altogether; they may be inserted via the nose or mouth and are passed beyond the vocal cords into the trachea. An inflatable cuff near the distal end of the tube serves to seal off the airway, allowing for mechanical ventilatory assistance and protecting the airway from aspiration.

Since endotracheal tubes bypass the filtration and humidification normally provided by the nose and oropharynx, care must be taken to humidify the inspired air and to prevent introduction of pathogenic organisms into the lungs. Meticulous attention to aseptic technique when caring for clients with endotracheal tube and ventilator circuits is mandatory.

Mouth care must be provided for the client with an endotracheal tube. The tube prevents adequate swallowing, so the client will be unable to eat. Frequent cleansing and suctioning of the oral cavity (every 2 hours) reduces discomfort and the risk of breakdown and infection of the oral mucosa.

Nutritional needs for the client with an endotracheal tube must be addressed by providing enteral feeding (via nasogastric or gastrostomy tube) or total parenteral nutrition (hyperalimentation). Whatever the means, adequate nutrition is necessary to maintain and improve respiratory muscle strength.

A **tracheotomy** is a surgical procedure done to provide long-term airway support or as an emergency procedure when an endotracheal tube cannot be passed successfully. An opening (stoma) is made in the trachea below the cricoid cartilage, and a semirigid plastic tube (tracheostomy tube) is passed through the opening and into the trachea. A cuff, similar to that in an endotracheal tube, is inflated near the distal airway. The cuff of an endotracheal tube or tracheostomy tube must be deflated before removing the tube; removal of a tube with an inflated cuff may cause laryngeal edema and damage to the vocal cords. For this reason, the tube must be taped securely in place, and confused or agitated clients may require sedation or wrist restraints to prevent them from pulling at the tube.

Many tracheostomy tubes consist of two tubes or *cannulae*: an outer cannula that stays in place and an inner cannula that can be removed to be cleaned or replaced. This permits thorough removal of encrusted secretions to prevent occlusion of the airway. The outer cannula is connected to a flange that permits the tubes to be secured around the neck with twill tape or a cloth strap. See Procedure 32-1 for tracheostomy care.

Like an endotracheal tube, a tracheostomy tube bypasses the upper airways, so humidification and prevention of infection must be considered. Because both types of airways prevent the movement of air through the vocal cords, which produce speech, the client will not be able to talk while these tubes are in place (some long-term tracheostomy clients may be outfitted with a tracheostomy tube that has slits, or "fenestrations," that permit speech). If possible, reviewing an alternate method of communication prior to tube insertion can reduce the anxiety and isolation that may be felt by the intubated client. Writing of messages and use of an alphabet board are two possible methods of communication. Significant others should also be advised that the intubated client will not be able to speak but can hear and understand what is being said.

Suction the Airway

Suctioning of the airway, whether a natural or artificial airway, may be necessary to clear secretions the client cannot remove by coughing. Suctioning becomes especially important when an endotracheal tube or tracheostomy tube is present because coughing is significantly impaired by these devices.

Nasotracheal suctioning involves passing a suction catheter or nasal trumpet through the naris and into the oropharynx. See Procedures 32-2 and 32-3 regarding suctioning. Once the tip is in the oropharynx, a strong cough reflex may be elicited. At this time suction is applied to the catheter, and it is withdrawn while a twisting motion is applied to the catheter.

Endotracheal suctioning involves passing the suction catheter through the endotracheal tube or tracheostomy into the trachea and applying suction as the catheter is withdrawn.

INTERVENTIONS TO IMPROVE BREATHING PATTERNS
Properly Position Client

Client positioning to improve breathing patterns may begin by taking cues from the client. If the client finds that breathing is easier in an upright or sitting position, the nurse should allow that position to be maintained. Supporting the client with elevation of the head of the bed or with pillows can reduce the client's workload and minimize fatigue. Maintaining proper body alignment and preventing slouching or slumping in the bed increase the efficiency of ventilatory efforts.

As previously stated, clients with obstructive respiratory disease may find that leaning forward, with the clavicles elevated, is most comfortable. Providing an overbed table for the client on which to rest the elbows may facilitate this position, *provided the wheels are locked or removed to prevent the table from rolling away and placing the client at risk for a fall.*

Teach Controlled Breathing Exercises

Controlled breathing exercises may also improve breathing efficiency for the client with obstructive respiratory disease. One technique that is especially useful is *pursed-lip breathing.* This technique involves forced exhalation against pursed (partially closed) lips, which maintains positive pressure in the lungs during the expiratory phase and prevents collapse of the smaller airways. This in turn reduces the amount of air trapping characteristic of obstructive disease.

Deep-breathing exercises encourage the client to take slow, deep breaths instead of the rapid, shallow breathing pattern that may be present in restrictive lung disease and in those who are anxious. Abdominal breathing involves the use of the abdominal muscles to pull the diaphragm downward. Placing one's hand on the client's abdomen and instructing the client to watch it rise give a visual aid to teaching the technique.

Apical and basal expansion exercises direct the client to focus on achieving maximal expansion of the upper lung lobes (apices) and lower lobes (bases), respectively. To perform these techniques, place one's hands flat against the chest wall just below the clavicles for apical exercises or over the lower ribs along the midaxillary lines for basal exercises and apply gentle pressure. Instruct the client to push the nurse's hands away with the chest wall by breathing. These exercises should be repeated several times a day.

Incentive spirometry is another technique used to encourage deep breathing. The client draws air through the spirometry device, which measures the volume of air displaced by moving a float ball or similar device up a column. Goals (incentives) can be marked on the spirometer, and clients can compare their progress with the desired goal. Instruct the client to hold the inspired breath for 2–3 seconds before exhaling. Incentive spirometry is often performed in the care of postoperative clients and is usually done every 1 to 2 hours while awake.

Deep breathing may also be augmented using intermittent positive-pressure breathing (IPPB). An IPPB machine delivers a volume of air under pressure through a mouthpiece when the client draws air through the mouthpiece. IPPB requires the client's cooperation, so preparatory teaching is essential. IPPB may include the administration of aerosolized medications and may be followed by coughing exercises, CPT, and postural drainage.

Introduce Chest Drainage Systems

Chest drainage systems (chest tubes) improve breathing patterns by removing accumulations of air and fluid from the pleural space, permitting the lungs to return to normal expansion. The tubes are inserted through the chest wall via a stab wound; multiple holes in the tip of the tube collect drainage from the pleural space. This drainage is then collected into a drainage system by either suction control or gravity. A special feature called a water seal prevents the reintroduction of air into the pleural space through the chest tube.

INTERVENTIONS TO IMPROVE OXYGEN UPTAKE AND DELIVERY

Administer Oxygen

Oxygen uptake in the pulmonary capillary beds can be improved by increasing the concentration of oxygen in the alveolar air; this increase in the Pa_{O_2} in the alveoli increases the driving pressure for gas diffusion across the alveolar-capillary membrane.

The percentage of oxygen in the inspired air is referred to as the fraction of inspired oxygen, or F_{IO_2}, expressed as a percentage; normal atmospheric air has an F_{IO_2} of 21%. Supplemental oxygen delivery systems are capable of increasing the F_{IO_2} to anywhere from 24% to nearly 100% oxygen (see Figures 32-20 on page 881 and 32-21 on page 882 and Procedure 32-4).

Oxygen administration, like the administration of any drug, is not without hazards. Clients who have chronic pulmonary disease associated with carbon dioxide retention (hypercapnia) may become insensitive to carbon dioxide levels to drive their respiratory rate. Instead, these clients may depend upon a chronic low oxygen level in the blood (hypoxemia) to stimulate their respiratory drive. While low-flow oxygen may be beneficial to these clients, excessive oxygen administration may obliterate that hypoxic drive, resulting in apnea.

Another possible hazard of oxygen administration is oxygen toxicity. Prolonged administration of high F_{IO_2} (greater than 50% for more than 24 hours) may actually damage lung tissue and produce severe respiratory difficulties. The mechanisms by which oxygen toxicity occurs are twofold. First, it should be understood that 78% of the inspired air consists of the gas nitrogen. Although nitrogen is (under normal conditions) physiologically inert, it does serve an important function in the lung: It keeps the alveoli open simply by occupying space. High concentrations of oxygen displace nitrogen from the alveoli; as this oxygen is absorbed by the alveolar capillary blood, the volume of gas in the alveolar space is reduced and the alveoli collapse. Once the alveoli have collapsed (atelectasis), no airflow occurs and the work of breathing increases dramatically.

Second, oxygen in high concentrations is toxic to the type II alveolar cells, which are responsible for the production of **surfactant**. Surfactant is a substance that assists in keeping the alveoli open by reducing the alveolar surface tension (the tendency of the alveolar walls to collapse upon themselves). Atelectasis results when surfactant is insufficient.

Widespread atelectasis due to oxygen toxicity may result in a syndrome known as the adult respiratory distress syndrome (ARDS), which is characterized by diffuse pulmonary edema, severe stiffness of the lung tissue, and profound hypoxemia.

COMMUNITY CONSIDERATIONS

Oxygen increases the risk of fire. Although oxygen itself is not a flammable gas, it is a necessary catalyst for fire to occur. The presence of any fuel (bed linens, paper) along with any source of ignition (a lighted cigarette, an electrical spark) will lead to fire more rapidly, and the fire will burn more vigorously, in an oxygen-rich environment. Instruct clients on oxygen administration to caution all family members and visitors to the home to avoid lighting matches, cigarettes, or any other substances in the presence of the oxygenation equipment. Also advise clients receiving therapy in the home to inspect all electrical equipment prior to use.

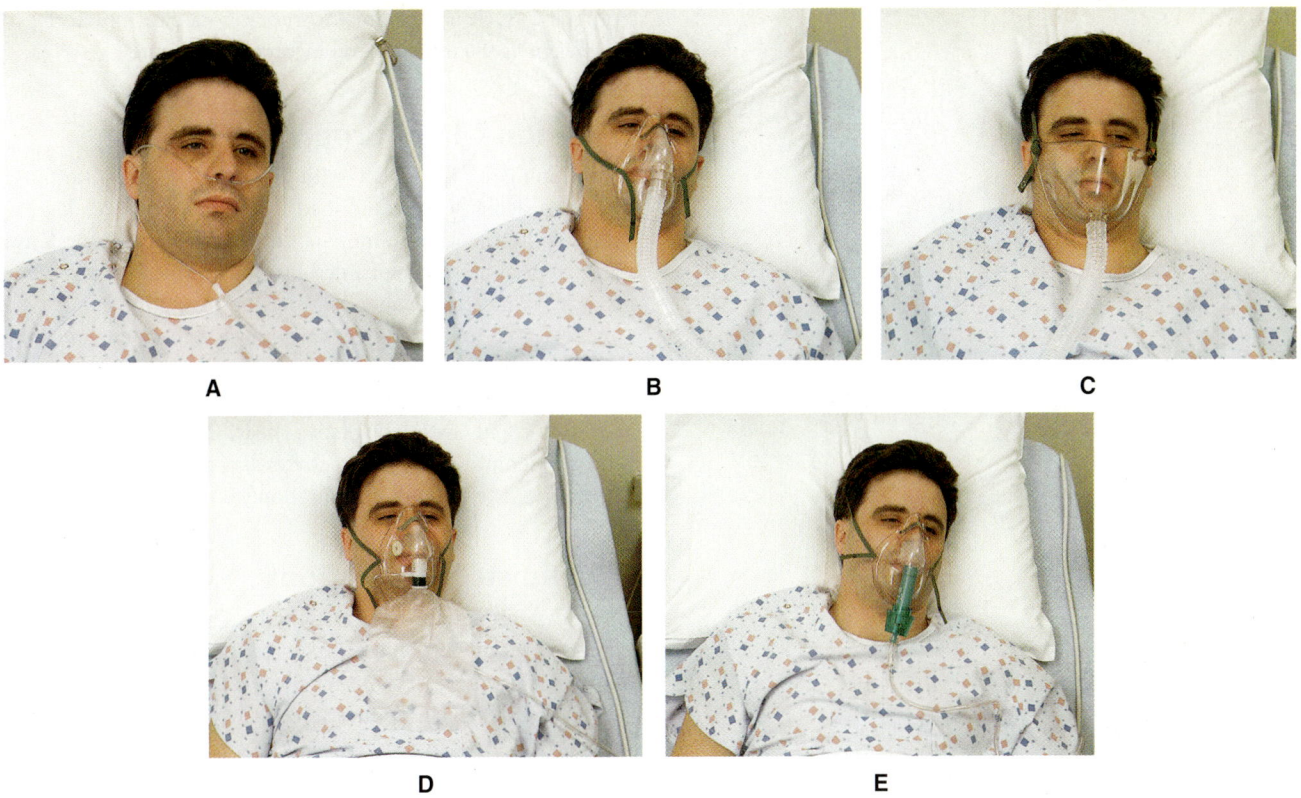

FIGURE 32-20 **Oxygen Delivery Systems: A.** Nasal cannula; **B.** Single face mask; **C.** Open face tent; **D.** Reservoir mask; **E.** Venturi mask.
DELMAR/CENGAGE LEARNING

Administer Blood Components

Blood component administration is indicated when the client's oxygenation is impaired because of decreased circulating blood volume, decreased hemoglobin concentration in the blood (anemia), or hemorrhage. Red blood cells may be administered. Since a blood transfusion is really a type of tissue transplant, extreme care must be taken to decrease the possibility of an immune system rejection response known as a transfusion reaction.

INTERVENTIONS TO INCREASE CARDIAC OUTPUT AND TISSUE PERFUSION

The client with impaired cardiac output and tissue perfusion is likely to be experiencing edema of the lower extremities and the lungs, fatigue, activity intolerance related to poor tissue oxygenation, and possibly angina and intermittent claudication. Interventions are aimed at reducing symptom severity while optimizing cardiac performance.

Manage Fluid Balance

Management of fluid balance is a cornerstone in the care of the client with reduced cardiac output. If congestive heart failure is present, fluid intake may be restricted to prevent edema and circulatory overload. Often, sodium intake is also limited because sodium promotes fluid retention. Diuretics may also be given to increase fluid excretion by the kidneys.

▼ **SAFETY FIRST** ▼

BLOOD ADMINISTRATION
To minimize the risk of a serious transfusion reaction when administering blood components, be sure to:

- Follow institutional policy regarding client identification for each transfusion.
- Assess and record client vital signs (temperature, pulse, blood pressure, respirations) before initiating the transfusion and within 1 hour of completing the transfusion.
- Instruct the client to report any unusual feelings, including flushing, itching, headache, or back pain.
- Reassess vital signs after the first 10 to 15 minutes of slowly infusing the blood component. Stop the transfusion immediately if fever, tachycardia, hypotension, dyspnea, or any reports of the previously listed symptoms occur. Notify the client's prescribing practitioner and the blood bank for further instructions.

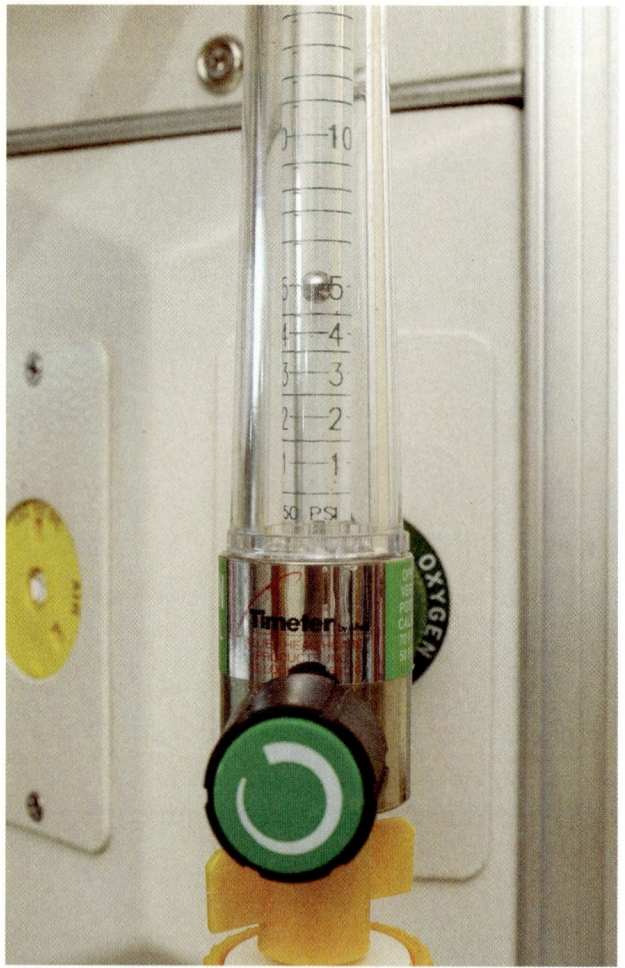

FIGURE 32-21 Oxygen Flow Meter Attached to Wall DELMAR/
CENGAGE LEARNING

Monitoring of fluid balance by the nurse may involve the measurement of fluid intake and output (I&O) and measurement of daily weights. I&O measurement involves teaching the client the importance of accounting for all I&O and providing a container for the measurement of urine. Daily weights should be performed at the same time each day (usually early in the morning), with the same amount of clothing on, and on the same scale to maximize accuracy.

Clients receiving diuretics may also require monitoring for electrolyte imbalances. Potassium, particularly, may become depleted in the client receiving loop diuretics such as furosemide. Encouraging the consumption of potassium-rich foods such as bananas, and perhaps potassium supplementation, is often required.

Suggest Activity Restrictions and Assistance with Activities of Daily Living

Activity restrictions and assistance with ADL should be based upon the client's activity tolerance. The purpose of activity assistance is to decrease the oxygen demands of the body. The client's activity tolerance may be gradually increased through a sequence of exercise protocols as part of a cardiac rehabilitation

program. Such a program incorporates careful monitoring of the client as the exercise level increases over time.

Position Client Properly

Positioning of the client with decreased cardiac output is done to decrease the fluid load to the heart and to decrease the development of pulmonary edema. The venous system is able to pool blood when aided by gravity; this "venous capacitance" is increased when the client's head and upper body are elevated and the legs are in a dependent position. Although it is customary in the hospital environment to place clients in a supine position, this position may be detrimental for the client with congestive heart failure, as evidenced by worsening dyspnea, tachycardia and tachypnea, and decreased arterial oxygen saturation.

Administer Medications

Medications to improve cardiac output and perfusion include diuretics as mentioned earlier, cardiac glycosides, and other inotropic agents. Antihypertensives, nitrates, and vasodilators may also be given to increase cardiac oxygen supply and reduce the myocardium's demand for oxygen. Table 32-9 on page 883 lists the drugs most commonly used.

EMERGENCY INTERVENTIONS

Complete airway obstruction, cardiac arrest, and respiratory arrest are emergency situations that will result in death if not immediately rectified. Nurses receive regular training in the basic life support techniques described in the following text; hands-on practice is an essential component of that training, and this text is not intended to serve as a substitute.

Remove Airway Obstruction

Complete airway obstruction is often the result of aspiration of food or some other foreign object into the trachea. The presence of a complete airway obstruction is characterized by an inability to speak or cough; the victim may also raise the hands to the throat and will likely appear very anxious. The rescuer should verify that obstruction is present by asking the victim, "Are you choking?"

Relief of the obstruction is attempted by way of the **Heimlich maneuver**, which is described in Procedure 32-5.

Initiate Cardiopulmonary Resuscitation

Cardiac and respiratory arrest require artificial support of circulation and ventilation if the victim is to survive. **Cardiopulmonary resuscitation (CPR)** is the accepted technique of basic life support, as described in Procedure 32-6. The technique described is used for adult victims; different techniques are applied for children and infants and can be learned through courses such as those offered by the American Heart Association or the American Red Cross.

TABLE 32-9 Medications Used to Improve Cardiac Function

DRUG TYPE	COMMON EXAMPLES	ACTIONS
Diuretic	Furosemide (Lasix), bumetanide (Bumex), hydrochlorothiazide (HydroDIURIL, HCTZ), spironolactone (Aldactone)	Affects renal tubules, resulting in increased excretion of water and certain electrolytes; lowers blood pressure and decreases cardiac workload
Cardiac glycoside	Digoxin (Lanoxin)	Increases force of cardiac contraction and slows heart rate
Inotropic agent	Dobutamine (Dobutrex), amrinone (Inocor), dopamine (Intropin), isoproterenol (Isuprel)	Increases force of cardiac contraction
Antihypertensive	ACE inhibitors (captopril, enalapril), beta-adrenergic blockers (labetalol, propranolol, atenolol), calcium channel blockers (nicardipine, diltiazem), centrally acting alpha-adrenergics (clonidine, methyldopa), ganglionic blockers (trimethaphan), peripherally acting antiadrenergics (guanethidine, prazosin), vasodilators (minoxidil, hydralazine)	Lowers blood pressure by various mechanisms, decreasing the heart's workload
Nitrate	Nitroglycerin, isosorbide dinitrate (Isordil)	Dilates the coronary arteries and peripheral vessels, increasing cardiac oxygen supply while decreasing cardiac workload

Delmar/Cengage Learning

INTERVENTIONS TO ADDRESS ASSOCIATED NURSING DIAGNOSES
Explore Lifestyle and Activity Adaptations

Lifestyle and activity adaptations may be necessary for the client with chronic alterations in oxygenation. Interventions related to lifestyle and activity have three general purposes:

- To minimize energy and oxygen consumption
- To reduce factors that contribute to the disease process
- To systematically increase activity tolerance

Measures to reduce energy and oxygen consumption are chosen after a careful assessment of the client's activity tolerance. Clients may need assistance with ADL, including hygiene and toileting; however, it should be noted that complete bed rest is not always the best option. Many clients find that using a bedside commode or toilet is less physically taxing than using a bedpan, especially for bowel movements.

Occupational roles may also need to be modified. If the client is not able to continue working in the old job, it may be possible to take on a new job that is less taxing or to reduce the number of hours worked. If such changes are not possible, the client may have to quit working altogether. All of these possibilities may cause much distress to the client and family, who must grapple with role issues, authority and autonomy issues, and possibly financial concerns. Signs of inadequate family coping, such as marital discord, anger or

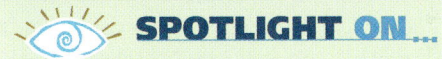

SPOTLIGHT ON...

Professionalism

Mouth-to-Mouth Breathing

In recent years, increased concern over the possibility of disease transmission during mouth-to-mouth breathing has led to the development of newer variations on this technique. Several styles of masks that fit over the victim's mouth and contain a one-way valve through which the rescuer breathes are available for both in-hospital and community use. Have you ever performed mouth-to-mouth breathing through one of these masks? Knowing that there is a possibility of disease transfer, would you be willing to administer mouth-to-mouth breathing without a mask?

hostility, sleep disturbances, and depression, should be noted and appropriate interventions, such as a referral for counseling, should be instituted.

Lifestyle adaptations aimed at reducing factors that contribute to the disease process include removal of allergens

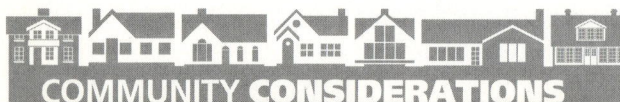

COMMUNITY CONSIDERATIONS

Activity adaptations in the home setting may involve alterations in the physical environment of the home, changes in family roles, or changes in work roles. The client who cannot climb stairs may need to have sleeping quarters moved to the first floor of the house. Clients may also need to give up household chores that cause distress and perhaps take on other, less physically taxing roles. Changes such as these can be trying for the entire family, and they will need support during the period of transition. Home health nurses are a tremendous resource for families facing role changes related to illness.

☑ CLIENT TEACHING CHECKLIST

Following a Healthy Diet

Reduction of total dietary fat, saturated fat, and cholesterol can be a challenge and requires careful client teaching. Use food labels and reference charts to help clients follow these dietary outlines:

- Reduce fat intake to no more than 30% of the total caloric intake.

- Keep saturated fats down to no more than 10% of the total caloric intake. Saturated fats include those from animal sources such as milk and dairy products. Palm and coconut oils, although from vegetable sources, have the same effect as animal fats in terms of raising serum cholesterol.

- Limit cholesterol intake to no more than 300 mg per day.

- Eat less meat and dairy products and more fresh fruits, vegetables, and whole grains.

- Avoid processed foods, especially those with sauces or fillings. When eating out, choose baked or grilled dishes rather than fried, sautéed, or stewed.

- Enjoy treats such as rich desserts only occasionally; choose low-fat desserts such as low-fat frozen yogurt, fruit sorbets, or angel food cake whenever possible.

from the environment, smoking cessation, and control of modifiable risk factors for heart disease. Allergen control and smoking cessation were discussed in the section Interventions to Promote Airway Clearance. Modification of cardiac risk factors includes smoking cessation as well as dietary alterations and weight control, control of diabetes and hypertension if present, exercise, and stress management. A comprehensive cardiac rehabilitation program addresses all of these issues while monitoring the client's progress toward individualized goals.

Encourage Dietary and Nutritional Modifications

Dietary modifications for cardiovascular disease may include reduction of sodium intake and reduction of total fat, saturated fat, and cholesterol intake. Sodium consumption may be reduced by decreasing or eliminating salt used in cooking and added at the table and avoiding highly processed foods such as prepared meats, canned meat or fish, and many prepared sauces. The client should be taught to examine food labels for sodium content per serving; see the Client Checklists on this page and page 883 regarding a healthy diet and general reminders.

The client who is not receiving adequate nutrient intake because of poor appetite or severe dyspnea will need assistance in finding ways to increase intake of calories and essential nutrients. Eating small, frequent meals of high nutritional value and using dietary supplements are often helpful.

Promote Comfort

Promoting comfort for the client with oxygenation disturbances can be a challenge but is extremely important. Comfort influences the client's ability to eat, sleep, learn, and cope with the illness and the care being provided.

Altered comfort related to pain is best approached by removing or modifying the cause of the pain if possible and administering analgesics if indicated. The use of analgesics in the postoperative client is particularly important in allowing the

client to participate fully in deep-breathing and coughing exercises. See Chapter 35 for more discussion of pain management.

Pain related to tissue ischemia is best relieved by improving the oxygen delivery to the tissues while reducing the oxygen demand. The first response to ischemic pain should be to rest the affected tissue. If the pain is in the legs, for example, the client should sit down. Improving delivery of oxygen to the legs in the client with peripheral vascular disease may involve positioning the legs lower than heart level (elevating the legs will often make the pain worse).

Heart pain related to ischemia (angina pectoris) should also be dealt with first and foremost by resting. Resting will decrease the heart's workload and in some cases is sufficient to relieve the pain. Improving oxygen delivery to the heart may be accomplished by providing supplemental oxygen or by using medications, such as nitrates, that improve coronary blood flow. In some cases, narcotic analgesics such as morphine are necessary.

COMPLEMENTARY THERAPIES

Many complementary therapies that enhance oxygenation originate in ancient healing traditions of China and India. For example, the practice of meditation and yoga produces a

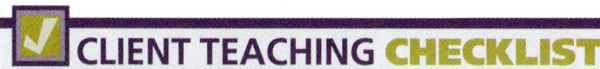

CLIENT TEACHING CHECKLIST

General Reminders

- Assess the client's and family's level of knowledge.
- Focus on identifying misconceptions that need to be clarified.
- Ask open-ended questions, such as "Tell me what your medications are for," instead of simple yes-or-no questions.
- Set goals with the client's input; base goals upon realistic expectations.
- State goals clearly: For example, "Mr. Jones will be able to name all of his medications, the dose, and frequency they are taken and list one major side effect of each."
- Individualize teaching methods, taking into account the client's particular needs and abilities.
- Involve the family in teaching sessions.

HERBS

HERBS FOR THE CIRCULATORY SYSTEM

Broom	Buckwheat	Cayenne
Dandelion	Ginger	Hawthorn
Horse chestnut	Lime blossom	Mistletoe
Yarrow		

HERBS FOR THE RESPIRATORY SYSTEM

Stimulants (expectorants):

Bittersweet	Cowslip	Daisy
Senega	Soapwort	Squill
Thuja		

Relaxants (promote expectoration):

Angelica	Aniseed	Coltsfoot
Elecampane	Flaxseed	Grindelia
Hyssop	Plantain	Thyme
Wild cherry bark	Wild lettuce	

Demulcents (mucilaginous):

Lungwort root	Coltsfoot	Flaxseed
Licorice	Comfrey	Marshmallow
Mullein		leaf

Adapted from Hoffmann, D. (1998). *The new holistic herbal* (3rd ed.). Boston: Element.

sense of serenity and relaxation and other positive physiologic benefits. Harvard Medical School professor Herbert Benson studied the effects of people who practiced transcendental meditation in the 1970s and showed that meditation decreases oxygen consumption and metabolism; lowers blood pressure, heart rate, and respiratory rate; increases the production of alpha brain waves; and relieves stress and enhances overall well-being. Dean Ornish, MD, has successfully reversed coronary artery disease by using yoga with dietary changes, moderate exercise, and support groups.

Herbs

Herbs are often used with relaxation techniques, exercise, and diet to prevent diseases of the cardiovascular and respiratory systems; see the accompanying display for commonly used herbs for these systems. Respiratory stimulants are expectorants that loosen mucus from the respiratory system. *Lobelia* (Indian tobacco) contains lobeline, a nonaddicting substance similar to nicotine, and is often used to quit smoking.

Arnold, Clark, Lasserson, and Wu (2008) assessed the efficacy and safety of herb and plant extracts in the management of chronic asthma. The evidence base for the effects of herbal treatment was hampered by the variety of treatments assessed, poor reporting quality of the studies, and lack of available data. The researchers determined that positive review findings warrant additional well-designed trails in this area.

NURSING CARE PLAN

The Client with Pneumonia

CASE PRESENTATION

Mrs. Johnson is a 72-year-old woman hospitalized for left lower lobe pneumonia. She complains of a persistent cough and occasional pain in her left chest associated with coughing, fever, and shortness of breath. Prior to this admission, she has been healthy and independent. Upon assessment, you find her mildly dyspneic, occasionally pausing in the middle of a sentence to breathe. Her respiratory rate is 28 breaths per minute. Her pulse is 100 per minute and regular; blood pressure is 140/90 mm Hg. Her skin is warm, dry, and pale pink with brisk capillary refill. You do not note any edema. She is receiving oxygen by nasal cannula at 6 L/min.

(Continues)

NURSING CARE PLAN (Continued)

ASSESSMENT
- Dyspnea, tachypnea, and tachycardia
- Cough, chest pain, fever

NURSING DIAGNOSIS 1: *Impaired gas exchange* related to presence of infectious exudate in the left lower lobe of the lung
NOC: Respiratory status: gas exchange
NIC: Airway management: facilitation of patency of air passages

EXPECTED OUTCOMES
The client will:

1. Report relief of dyspnea.
2. Demonstrate return of respiratory rate to 20/min or less and heart rate to 100/min or less.
3. Be able to speak comfortably.

INTERVENTIONS/RATIONALES

1. Teach client effective techniques for coughing, such as sustained maximal inspiration and "huffing." Increases the clearance of exudate.
2. Assist with chest physiotherapy and postural drainage as indicated. Promotes the clearance of exudate by using gravity, percussion, and vibration of the chest wall.
3. Humidify inspired oxygen, and encourage oral fluid intake. Promotes liquefaction of pulmonary secretions, which facilitates expectoration.
4. Encourage client to lie on right side while in bed. Positioning with the unaffected lung down provides the best match of ventilation and perfusion.
5. When assessing for dyspnea, do so not only with the client at rest but also during activities such as talking, eating, and moving. Clients who appear to be breathing comfortably at rest may become dyspneic with minimal activity.

NURSING DIAGNOSIS 2: *Imbalanced nutrition: less than body requirements* related to decreased oral intake and increased metabolic requirements
NOC: Nutritional status: food and fluid intake
NIC: Nutritional management

EXPECTED OUTCOMES
The client will:

1. Maintain usual body weight
2. Consume at least 50% of food provided

INTERVENTIONS/RATIONALES

1. Provide oral care after coughing, after respiratory treatments, and before meals. Coughing and the expectoration of secretions can create an unpleasant taste in the mouth, which interferes with appetite.
2. Assess food intake and provide supplements if intake is insufficient to meet caloric needs. Dietary supplements may provide increased calories and nutrients.
3. Encourage liberal fluid intake. Clients with fever and dyspnea lose excess body fluids through the skin and lungs. Adequate hydration will help liquefy pulmonary secretions and prevent decreases in circulating blood volume. Always check for contraindications such as heart failure, kidney disease, or a prescribing practitioner–ordered fluid restriction before encouraging increased fluids.
4. Weigh daily. Monitors progress to goal so that plan can be modified as needed. Daily gains or losses in excess of 1 pound are often due to fluid balance alterations. Slower gains or losses may be due to nutritional alterations.

(Continues)

NURSING CARE PLAN (Continued)

EVALUATION

Success of the nursing interventions can be measured by a visible increase in the client's comfort and ease of speaking and a decreased effort at the work of breathing. The client will report that dyspnea has been relieved and will have respiratory and heart rates within the normal range. Ongoing evaluation will be needed to monitor client's weight to ensure that intake is adequate to meet client's caloric requirements.

EVALUATION

Clients with compromised oxygenation status need careful nursing care to address both their physical and psychological needs. Evaluation will be based on the outcomes and goals that the nurse and client have established together. In many instances, the evaluation of the success of the specific inter-

ventions will be a matter of degree, that is, the degree to which the client is or can be returned to a satisfactory state of respiratory functioning. It is important when evaluating progress to revisit the initial plan of care to determine if each expected outcome was within reasonable expectations and then to revise the goals, interventions, and plan of care to reflect truly reasonable expectations.

PROCEDURE 32-1

Maintaining and Cleaning the Tracheostomy Tube

EQUIPMENT

- Gloves
- Sterile water or saline
- Tracheostomy dressing (4 × 4 gauze *without* cotton lining)
- Hydrogen peroxide
- Cotton-tip applicators
- Tracheostomy ties (twill tape, intravenous tubing, or commercially available Velcro ties)

ACTION	RATIONALE
CLEANING TRACH TUBE SITE	
1. Wash hands/hand hygiene, apply gloves, and assemble equipment (see Figure 32-22 on page 888).	1. Reduces the transmission of microorganisms.
2. Remove soiled dressing and discard.	2. Prevents contamination of other areas.
3. Cleanse neck plate of tracheostomy tube with cotton applicators moistened with hydrogen peroxide.	3. Removes crusted secretions from neck plate of tracheostomy tube.
4. Rinse neck plate of tracheostomy tube with applicators moistened with sterile water or saline.	4. Removes hydrogen peroxide.
5. Cleanse skin under neck plate of tube with cotton applicator moistened with hydrogen peroxide (see Figure 32-23 on page 888).	5. Removes dried and crusted secretions from under neck plate of tracheostomy tube.

(Continues)

PROCEDURE 32-1
Maintaining and Cleaning the Tracheostomy Tube (Continued)

ACTION	RATIONALE

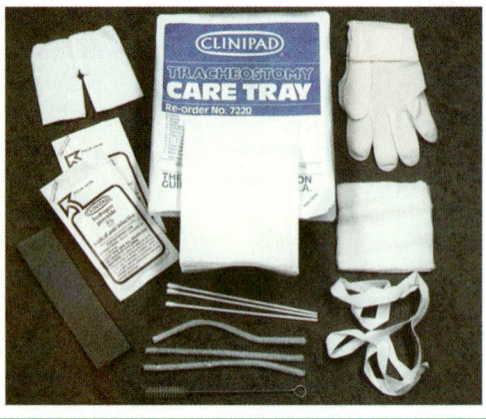

FIGURE 32-22 Tracheostomy care tray, hydrogen peroxide, tape, dressing, sterile and clean gloves. DELMAR/CENGAGE LEARNING

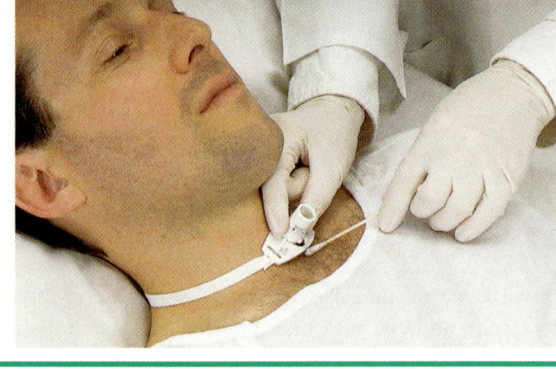

FIGURE 32-23 Clean stoma under faceplate. DELMAR/CENGAGE LEARNING

6. Rinse skin under neck plate with applicators moistened with sterile water or saline.
7. Dry skin under neck plate with cotton applicators.
8. *Using your clean hand,* gently loosen the inner cannula of the tracheostomy tube by twisting the outer ring counterclockwise; then withdraw the inner cannula in a smooth motion. Place the inner cannula into the basin of peroxide.
   Note: Some tracheostomy tubes use disposable inner cannulae that would be replaced at this point in the procedure. If replacing a disposable inner cannula, skip to Action 12.
9. *Using your sterile hand,* pick up the cannula. Using your clean hand, pick up the nylon brush and scrub to remove any visible crusts or secretions from inside and outside the cannula (see Figure 32-24 on page 889).

10. Place the cannula into the container of sterile saline. Agitate so that all surfaces are bathed in saline.
11. Inspect the inner cannula again to be sure it is clean; then remove excess saline from the lumen by tapping the cannula against a sterile surface.
12. Gently replace the inner cannula, following the curve of the tube. When fully inserted, lock the inner cannula in place by rotating the external ring clockwise until it clicks into place.

6. Removes hydrogen peroxide.

7. Removes moisture, which can result in skin irritation.
8. Minimizes trauma to the client's tracheal tissues and reduces reflexive coughing. The hydrogen peroxide serves to dissolve crusted secretions.

9. Any secretions retained on the inner cannula may be aspirated into the client's lungs, causing infection and possible airway obstruction. In some cases, the pipe cleaners may be needed to gain access to the inner surface of the cannula.
10. Rinses the peroxide off the cannula before it is returned to the client.

11. Fluid trapped in the lumen of the cannula can be aspirated by the client.

12. Minimizes tissue trauma and unintentional displacement.

(Continues)

PROCEDURE 32-1
Maintaining and Cleaning the Tracheostomy Tube (Continued)

ACTION	RATIONALE

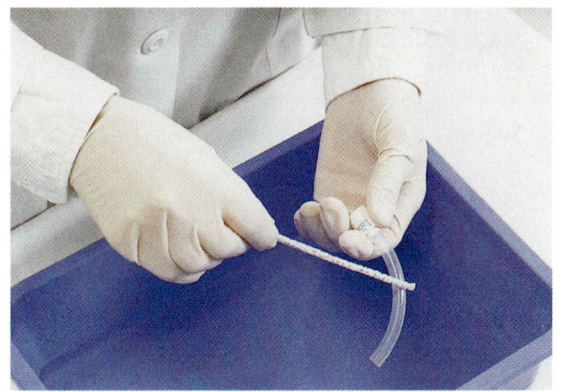

FIGURE 32-24 Clean lumen and inner cannula. DELMAR/CENGAGE LEARNING

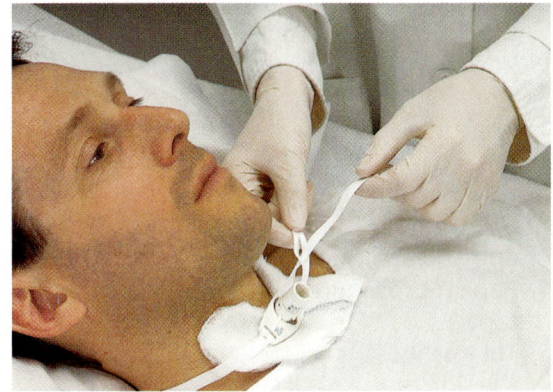

FIGURE 32-25 Change tracheostomy ties. DELMAR/CENGAGE LEARNING

ONE-PERSON TECHNIQUE OF CHANGING TRACHEOSTOMY TIES

ACTION	RATIONALE
13. Prepare clean tracheostomy ties. • Cut a length of twill tape that will fit around the client's neck plus 6 inches. Cut the ends of the twill tape on the diagonal. • Open Velcro ties on continuous neck band.	13. Ensures that all equipment is prepared prior to beginning procedure. A diagonal cut will make the tape easier to thread.
14. Leaving the old tracheostomy ties in place, insert one end of the new tracheostomy tie through the hole in the tracheostomy neck plate from back to front (see Figure 32-25). Pull the ends even, and slide both ends of the tape around the back of the head to the other side.	14. Maintains tube security while tapes are changed.
15. Insert one end of tape through the opening on the other side of the tracheostomy tube neck plate from back to front.	15. Secures tracheostomy tube.
16. Tie the two ends of the new tape with a square knot at side of neck. Keep two fingers under the tape as the knot is tied. Without putting pressure on the neck plate or the tape, pull on the knot to make sure it will stay tied.	16. Secures tracheostomy tube. Fingers under tape prevent the tape from being tied too tightly.
17. Untie and remove old tracheostomy tapes and discard. Hold the neck plate firmly with one hand while untying the old tapes.	17. Old tapes can be removed once the tracheostomy tube has been secured. Holding the plate firmly prevents dislodgment if the new tie is accidentally cut.
18. Place one finger under tracheostomy ties.	18. Checks for tightness and security.

TWO-PERSON TECHNIQUE OF CHANGING TRACHEOSTOMY TIES

ACTION	RATIONALE
19. Cut two pieces of twill tape about 12 to 14 inches in length.	19. Prepares equipment prior to beginning procedure.
20. Make a fold about 1 inch below the end of each piece of twill tape, and cut a half-inch slit lengthwise in the center of the fold.	20. Prepares tape for insertion.

(Continues)

PROCEDURE 32-1
Maintaining and Cleaning the Tracheostomy Tube (Continued)

ACTION	RATIONALE
21. Have a second person gently hold the tracheostomy tube in place with fingers on both sides of the neck plate.	21. Prevents accidental movement of the tracheostomy tube that could result in coughing and accidental decannulation.
22. Untie old tracheostomy ties and discard.	22. Removes tracheostomy ties.
23. Insert the split end of the tracheostomy tape through the opening on one side of the tracheostomy tube neck plate. Pull the distal end of the tracheostomy tie through the cut end and pull tightly.	23. Secures tracheostomy tie within neck plate.
24. Repeat procedure with second piece of twill tape.	24. Secures tracheostomy tube.
25. Tie tracheostomy tapes with a double knot at the side of the neck.	25. Secures tracheostomy tube.
26. Insert one finger under tracheostomy tapes.	26. Ensures that tube has been tied securely.
27. Insert tracheostomy gauze under neck plate of tube.	27. Prevents irritation of skin from secretions and rubbing of tracheostomy tube.
28. Discard all used materials; wash hands/hand hygiene.	28. Reduces transmission of microorganisms.

delegation tip

The maintenance and cleaning of tracheal tubes cannot be delegated by the nurse. Ancillary personnel may assist the nurse in providing care to clients receiving this treatment and should be instructed to report a client experiencing increased secretions, dyspnea, or the need for suctioning to the nurse.

nursing tips

Use sterile equipment and careful technique while performing the procedure to prevent microorganisms from contaminating a new trach wound.

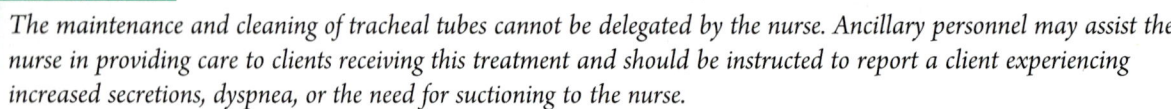

PROCEDURE 32-2
Performing Nasopharyngeal and Oropharyngeal Suctioning

EQUIPMENT
- Suction source (wall suction regulator with collection bottle or portable suction machine)
- Sterile suction kit (contains suction catheter, sterile gloves, sterile solution container; may contain a small container of sterile normal saline)
- Sterile water-soluble lubricant
- Extension tubing connected to suction device
- Small bottle of sterile water or normal saline if not included in kit
- Personal protective devices: gown, mask, and goggles or face shield if splattering is likely (e.g., a client with a vigorous productive cough)

(Continues)

PROCEDURE 32-2
Performing Nasopharyngeal and Oropharyngeal Suctioning (Continued)

ACTION	RATIONALE
1. Assess the client's need for suctioning: inability to effectively clear the airway by coughing and expectoration; coarse bubbling or gurgling noises with respiration.	1. Suctioning is an uncomfortable and traumatic procedure and should be used only when needed.
2. Choose the most appropriate route (nasopharyngeal or oropharyngeal) for your client. If nasopharyngeal approach is considered, inspect the nares with a penlight to determine patency. Alternatively, you may assess patency by occluding each naris in turn with finger pressure while asking the client to breathe through the remaining naris.	2. The oropharyngeal approach is easier but requires that the client cooperate; it may also produce gagging more readily in some persons. The nasopharyngeal route is more effective for reaching the posterior oropharynx but is contraindicated in clients with a deviated nasal septum, nasal polyps, or any tendency toward excessive bleeding (low platelet count, use of anticoagulants, recent history of epistaxis or nasal trauma).
3. Explain the procedure to the client. Advise that suctioning may cause coughing or gagging but emphasize the importance of clearing the airway.	3. Promotes cooperation and reduces anxiety.
4. Wash hands/hand hygiene.	4. Reduces the transmission of microorganisms.
5. Position the client in a high Fowler's or semi-Fowler's position.	5. Maximizes lung expansion and effective coughing.
6. If the client is unconscious or otherwise unable to protect airway, place in a side-lying position.	6. Protects the client from aspiration in the event of vomiting.
7. Connect extension tubing to suction device if not already in place, and adjust suction control to between 80 and 100 mm Hg.	7. Excessive negative pressure can cause tissue trauma, whereas insufficient pressure will be ineffective.
8. Put on gown and mask as well as goggles or face shield if indicated.	8. Protects from splattering with body fluids.
9. Using sterile technique (see Figure 32-26), open the suction kit. Consider the inside wrapper of the kit to be sterile, and spread the wrapper out carefully to create a small sterile field.	9. Produces an area in which to place sterile items without contaminating them.

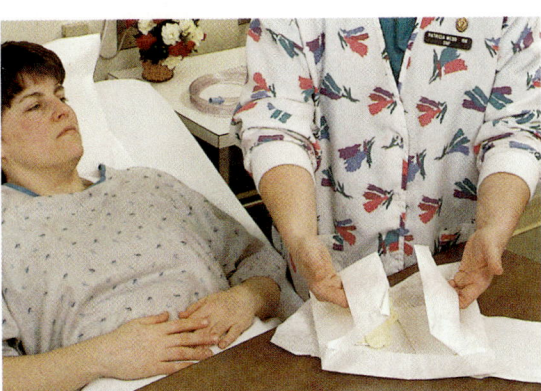

FIGURE 32-26 Sterile Technique DELMAR/CENGAGE LEARNING

(Continues)

PROCEDURE 32-2
Performing Nasopharyngeal and Oropharyngeal Suctioning (Continued)

ACTION	RATIONALE
10. Open a packet of sterile water-soluble lubricant, and squeeze out the contents of the packet onto the sterile field.	10. Lubricant will be used to further lubricate the catheter tip if the nasopharyngeal route is used.
11. If sterile solution (water or saline) is not included in the kit, pour about 100 mL of solution into the sterile container provided in the kit.	11. This solution will be used to lubricate the catheter and to rinse the inside of the catheter to clear secretions.
12. Carefully lift the wrapped gloves from the kit without touching the inside of the kit or the gloves themselves. Lay the wrapped gloves down next to the suction kit, and open the wrapper. Put on the gloves using sterile gloving technique.	12. The gloves should be kept sterile for handling the sterile suction catheter to avoid introducing pathogens into the client's airway.
13. If a cup of sterile solution is included in the suction kit, open it.	13. This solution will be used to lubricate the catheter and to rinse the inside of the catheter to clear secretions.
14. Designate one hand as *sterile* (able to touch only sterile items) and the other as *clean* (able to touch only nonsterile items).	14. Usually, the dominant hand is the sterile hand, while the nondominant hand is clean. This prevents contamination of sterile supplies while allowing you to handle unsterile items.
15. *Using your sterile hand,* pick up the suction catheter. Grasp the plastic connector end between your thumb and forefinger, and coil the tip around your remaining fingers.	15. Prevents accidental contamination of the catheter tip.
16. Pick up the extension tubing *with your clean hand.* Connect the suction catheter to the extension tubing, taking care not to contaminate the catheter (see Figure 32-27).	16. The extension tubing is not sterile.
17. Position your clean hand with the thumb over the catheter's suction port.	17. Suction is activated by occluding this port with the thumb. Releasing the port deactivates the suction.
18. Dip the catheter tip into the sterile solution, and activate the suction. Observe as the solution is drawn into the catheter.	18. Tests the suction device as well as lubricates the interior of the catheter to enhance clearance of secretions.

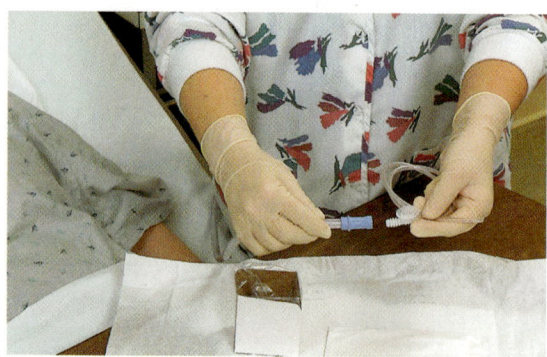

FIGURE 32-27 Attach catheter to tubing. DELMAR/CENGAGE LEARNING

(Continues)

PROCEDURE 32-2
Performing Nasopharyngeal and Oropharyngeal Suctioning (Continued)

ACTION	RATIONALE
19. For oropharyngeal suctioning, ask the client to open mouth. Without activating the suction, gently insert the catheter and advance it until you reach the pool of secretions or until the client coughs.	19. To minimize trauma, do not apply suction while the catheter is being advanced.
20. For nasopharyngeal suctioning, estimate the distance from the tip of the client's nose to the earlobe and grasp the catheter between your thumb and forefinger at a point equal to this distance from the catheter's tip.	20. Ensures placement of the catheter tip in the oropharynx and not in the trachea.
21. Dip the tip of the suction catheter into the water-soluble lubricant to coat the catheter tip liberally.	21. Promotes the client's comfort and minimizes trauma to nasal mucosa.
22. Insert the catheter tip into the naris with the suction control port uncovered. Advance the catheter gently with a slight downward slant. Slight rotation of the catheter may be used to ease insertion. Advance the catheter to the point marked by your thumb and forefinger (see Figure 32-28).	22. Guides the catheter toward the posterior oropharynx along the floor of the nasal cavity.
23. If resistance is met, *do not force the catheter.* Withdraw it and attempt insertion via the opposite naris.	23. Forceful insertion may cause tissue damage and bleeding.
24. Apply suction intermittently by occluding the suction control port with your thumb; at the same time, slowly rotate the catheter by rolling it between your thumb and fingers while slowly withdrawing it. Apply suction for no longer than 15 seconds at a time.	24. Prolonged suction applied to a single area of tissue can cause tissue damage.
25. Repeat Action 24 until all secretions have been cleared, allowing brief rest periods between suctioning episodes.	25. Promotes complete clearance of the airway.
26. Withdraw the catheter by looping it around your fingers as you pull it out.	26. Allows you to maintain control over the catheter tip as it is withdrawn.
27. Dip the catheter tip into the sterile solution and apply suction.	27. Clears the extension tubing of secretions that would promote bacterial growth.

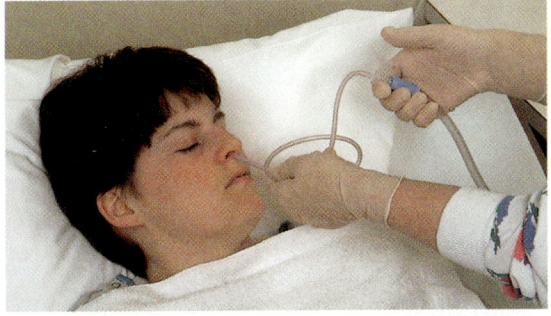

FIGURE 32-28 Insert catheter into nostril. DELMAR/CENGAGE LEARNING

(Continues)

PROCEDURE 32-2
Performing Nasopharyngeal and Oropharyngeal Suctioning (Continued)

ACTION	RATIONALE
28. Disconnect the catheter from the extension tubing. Holding the coiled catheter in your gloved hand, remove the glove by pulling it over the catheter. Discard catheter and gloves in an appropriate container.	28. Contains the catheter and secretions in the glove for disposal.
29. Discard remaining supplies in the appropriate container.	29. Follow institutional policy regarding the disposal of client care supplies.
30. Wash hands/hand hygiene.	30. Prevents the transmission of microorganisms.
31. Provide the client with oral hygiene if indicated or desired.	31. Suctioning and coughing may produce an unpleasant taste.
32. Document the procedure, noting the amount, color, and odor of secretions and the client's response to the procedure.	32. Changes in the amount, color, or odor of pulmonary secretions may indicate infection.

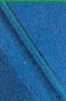

delegation tip

Nasopharyngeal and oropharyngeal suctioning are not delegated by the nurse. Ancillary personnel may assist in providing care to clients receiving these treatments and should be instructed to report a client experiencing a nonproductive cough, dyspnea, or the need for suctioning to the nurse.

nursing tips

Clients with oxygenation impairment may be confused or agitated, making safety a vital concern of the nurse.

PROCEDURE 32-3

Suctioning Endotracheal and Tracheal Tubes

EQUIPMENT

- Sterile gloves
- Mask, eye protection, and gown if appropriate
- Source of negative pressure (suction machine or wall suction)
- Sterile suction catheter
- Oxygen or Ambu bag
- Equipment for tracheostomy care or tracheostomy care tray

ACTION	RATIONALE
SUCTIONING A TRACHEAL TUBE	
1. Assess depth and rate of respirations; auscultate breath sounds.	1. Determines need for suctioning.
2. Assemble supplies on bedside table (see Figure 32-29A and 32-29B on page 895).	2. Organizes work.

(Continues)

PROCEDURE 32-3
Suctioning Endotracheal and Tracheal Tubes (Continued)

ACTION	RATIONALE

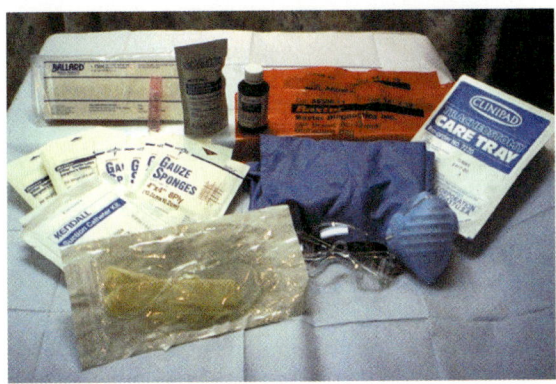

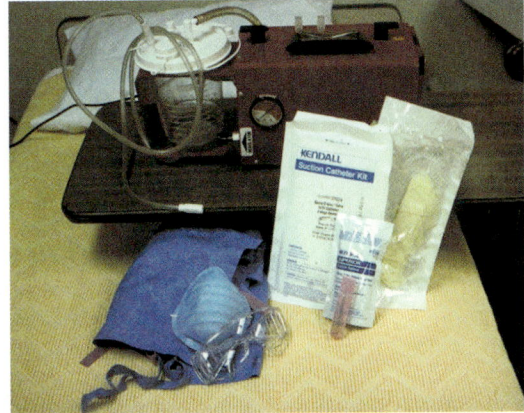

A   B

FIGURE 32-29 **A.** Protective gear, dressing, and a tracheostomy care tray. **B.** Protective gear and suction equipment.
DELMAR/CENGAGE LEARNING

3. Wash hands/hand hygiene.

4. Connect suction tube to source of negative pressure. Set suction control to between 80 and 100 mm Hg.

5. Administer oxygen or use Ambu bag before beginning procedure.

6. Remove inner cannula and place in basin of hydrogen peroxide to loosen secretions, if reusable, or set aside if disposable. Do not dispose of disposable cannula until new inner cannula is securely in place.

7. Apply sterile glove to dominant hand.

8. Open sterile suction catheter or use the reusable closed system catheter. The sterile suction catheter is removed from the package with the dominant, sterile hand. Wrap the catheter tubing around hand from the tip of the catheter down to the port end. Attach catheter to suction.

9. Quickly and gently insert the catheter during inspiration until resistance is met or the client coughs; then pull back 1 cm (1/2 inch).

10. Apply suction intermittently while gently rotating the catheter and removing it (see Figure 32-30 on page 896).

   - In a disposable catheter, suction is applied by placing the thumb of dominant hand over the open port of the catheter connector.
   - In a closed system catheter, suction is applied by depressing the white button at the connector end of the catheter.

3. Reduces transmission of microorganisms.

4. Prepares for suctioning procedure.

5. Hyperoxygenates client and prevents hypoxia during suctioning.

6. Suctioning should be performed after inner cannula has been removed to allow easier passage of the suction catheter. Retain the old cannula until you are sure the new cannula fits correctly.

7. Ensures sterile technique.

8. Maintains catheter sterility and prevents accidental contamination.

9. Minimizes removal of oxygen and trauma to the tracheal mucosa.

10. Increases removal of mucus while minimizing irritation to tracheal mucosa.

(Continues)

PROCEDURE 32-3
Suctioning Endotracheal and Tracheal Tubes (Continued)

ACTION	RATIONALE

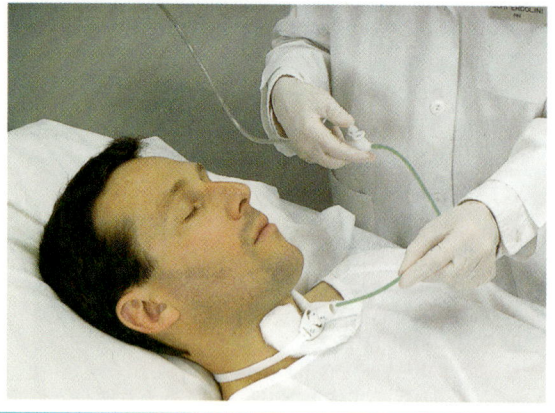

FIGURE 32-30 Suction tracheostomy. DELMAR/CENGAGE LEARNING

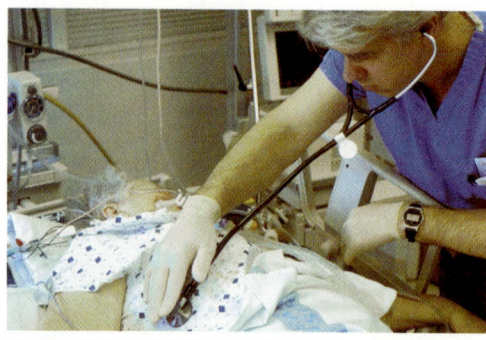

FIGURE 32-31 Assess for respiratory rate and lung sounds. Repeat suctioning if needed. DELMAR/CENGAGE LEARNING

11. Wrap the disposable suction catheter around sterile, dominant hand while withdrawing it from the endotracheal tube.
12. Suction for no more than 10 seconds.
13. Administer oxygen using the sigh function on the ventilator or using an Ambu bag.
14. Assess airway and repeat suctioning as necessary.
15. Clean inner cannula using tracheostomy brush and rinse well in sterile water or sterile saline. Dry (or open new disposable inner cannula).
16. Reinsert inner cannula and lock into place.

17. Apply humidified oxygen or compressed air.
18. Remove gloves and discard.

19. Wash hands/hand hygiene.
20. Record the procedure and client's tolerance of the procedure, including amount and consistency of secretions.

SUCTIONING AN ENDOTRACHEAL TUBE
21. Repeat Actions 1–14 (see Figure 32-31 and Figure 32-32 on page 897).
22. Remove gloves and discard.

23. Wash hands/hand hygiene.
24. Record the procedure and client's tolerance of the procedure, including amount and consistency of secretions.

11. Prevents accidental contamination of the catheter.

12. Prevents hypoxia.
13. Reoxygenates the client.

14. Determines need to continue suctioning.

15. Removes secretions and maintains patent inner cannula.

16. Prevents secretions from obstructing outer cannula.
17. Thins secretions.
18. Prevents transmission of microorganisms to other clients.
19. Reduces the transmission of microorganisms.
20. Provides documentation of the procedure.

21. See Rationales 1–14.

22. Prevents transmission of microorganisms to other clients.
23. Reduces the transmission of microorganisms.
24. Provides documentation of the procedure.

(Continues)

PROCEDURE 32-3
Suctioning Endotracheal and Tracheal Tubes (Continued)

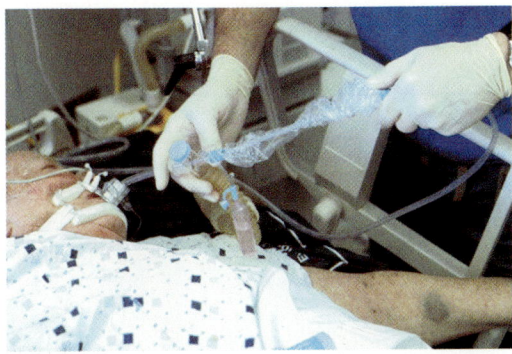

FIGURE 32-32 Endotracheal suctioning. Apply suction while gently rotating the catheter and removing it. Do not suction for more than 10 seconds. DELMAR/CENGAGE LEARNING

delegation tip

The suctioning of endotracheal and tracheal tubes is not delegated by the nurse. Ancillary personnel may assist the nurse in providing care to clients receiving this treatment and should be instructed to report a client experiencing increased secretions, dyspnea, or the need for suctioning to the nurse.

nursing tips

- *Because suctioning removes air (and oxygen) from the client's airways as well as secretions, care must be taken to avoid excessive suctioning and prevent severe oxygen desaturation.*
- *After suctioning, provide mouth care and suction the oropharynx if indicated. Assist the client to a comfortable position and allow for a rest period.*

PROCEDURE 32-4
Administering Oxygen Therapy

EQUIPMENT
- Stethoscope
- Oxygen source—portable or in-line
- Oxygen flow meter
- Oxygen delivery device: nasal cannula, mask, tent, or T-tube with adapter for artificial airway
- Oxygen tubing
- Pulse oximetry
- Humidifier and distilled or sterile water (not needed with low flow rates per nasal cannula)

ACTION	RATIONALE
NASAL CANNULA (SEE FIGURE 32-33 ON PAGE 898)	
1. Wash hands/hand hygiene.	1. Reduces the transmission of microorganisms.
2. Verify the prescribing practitioner's order.	2. Ensures correct dosage and route.

(Continues)

PROCEDURE 32-4
Administering Oxygen Therapy (Continued)

ACTION	RATIONALE

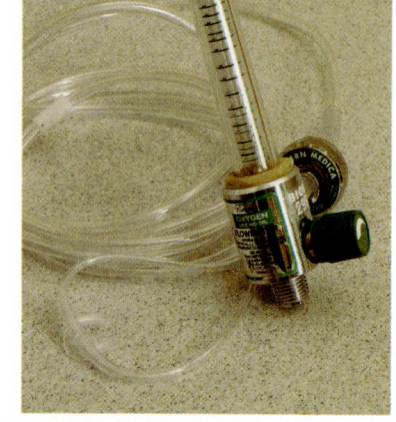

FIGURE 32-33 Nasal cannula and oxygen tubing attached to a flow meter. DELMAR/CENGAGE LEARNING

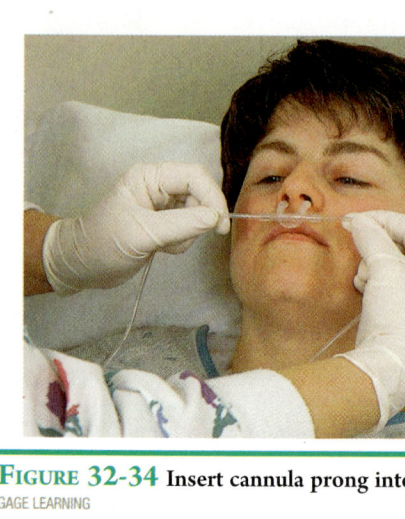

FIGURE 32-34 Insert cannula prong into nostrils. DELMAR/CENGAGE LEARNING

3. Explain procedure and hazards to the client. Remind clients who smoke of the reasons for not smoking while O₂ is in use.

4. If using humidity, fill humidifier to fill line with distilled water and close container.

5. Attach humidifier to oxygen flow meter.

6. Insert humidifier and flow meter into oxygen source in wall or portable unit.

7. Attach the oxygen tubing and nasal cannula to the flow meter and turn it on to the prescribed flow rate (1–5 L/min). Use extension tubing for ambulatory clients so they can get up to go to the bathroom.

8. Check for bubbling in the humidifier.

9. Place the nasal prongs in the client's nostrils (see Figure 32-34). Secure the cannula in place by adjusting the tubing around the client's ears and using the slip ring to stabilize it under the client's chin.

3. Increases compliance with procedures. Oxygen supports combustion.

4. Prevents drying of the client's airway and thins any secretions.

5. Allows the oxygen to pass through the water and become humidified.

6. For access to oxygen. Many institutions also have compressed air available from outlets very similar in appearance to oxygen outlets. Green always stands for oxygen. Be sure to plug the flow meter into the green outlet.

7. Rates above 6 L/min are not efficacious and can dry the nasal mucosa.

8. Ensures proper functioning.

9. Keeps delivery system in place so client receives the amount of oxygen ordered.

(Continues)

PROCEDURE 32-4
Administering Oxygen Therapy (Continued)

ACTION	RATIONALE
10. Check for proper flow rate every 4 hours and when the client returns from procedures.	10. Ensures that client receives proper dose. The nasal cannula is a low-flow system because it administers oxygen while the client also inspires room air. The actual dose of oxygen received by the client will vary depending on the client's respiratory pattern. The delivery rate may be changed during procedures.
11. Assess client's nostrils every 8 hours. If the client complains of dryness or has signs of irritation, use sterile lubricant to keep mucous membranes moist. Add humidifier if not already in place.	11. Dry membranes are more prone to breakdown by friction or pressure from nasal cannula.
12. Monitor vital signs, oxygen saturation, and client condition every 4–8 hours (or as indicated or ordered) for signs and symptoms of hypoxia.	12. Detects any untoward effects from therapy.
13. Wean client from oxygen as soon as possible using standard protocols.	13. Oxygen is not without side effects and should be used only as long as needed. Problems with reimbursement may develop if criteria for therapy are not met.

MASK: VENTURI (HIGH-FLOW DEVICE), SIMPLE MASK (LOW FLOW), PARTIAL REBREATHER MASK, NONREBREATHER MASK, AND FACE TENT

ACTION	RATIONALE
14. Wash hands/hand hygiene.	14. Reduces the transmission of microorganisms.
15. Repeat Actions 2–6.	15. See Rationales 2–6.
16. Attach appropriately sized mask (see Figure 32-35 on page 900) or face tent to oxygen tubing, and turn on flow meter to prescribed flow rate. The Venturi mask will have color-coded inserts that list the flow rate necessary to obtain the desired percentage of oxygen. Allow the reservoir bag of the nonrebreathing or partial rebreathing mask to fill completely. Figure 32-36 on page 900 shows several types of oxygen masks.	16. Ensures proper fit; size needed is based on the client's size. Checks the oxygen source and primes the tubing and mask or tent.
17. Check for bubbling in the humidifier.	17. Ensures proper functioning.
18. Place the mask or tent on the client's face, fasten the elastic band around the client's ears, and tighten until the mask fits snugly.	18. Prevents loss of oxygen from the sides of the mask.
19. Check for proper flow rate every 4 hours.	19. Ensures that client is receiving the proper dose.
20. Ensure that the ports of the Venturi mask are not under covers or impeded by any other source.	20. Air must be entrained to mix room air and oxygen coming from source to ensure proper oxygen percentage (F_{IO_2}).
21. Assess client's face and ears for pressure from the mask, and use padding as needed.	21. Provides client comfort and prevents skin breakdown.
22. Wean client to nasal cannula and then wean off oxygen per protocol.	22. Oxygen is not without side effects and should be used only as long as needed. The nasal cannula provides a lower F_{IO_2} than the mask. Problems with reimbursement may develop if criteria for therapy are not met.

(Continues)

PROCEDURE 32-4
Administering Oxygen Therapy (Continued)

ACTION	RATIONALE

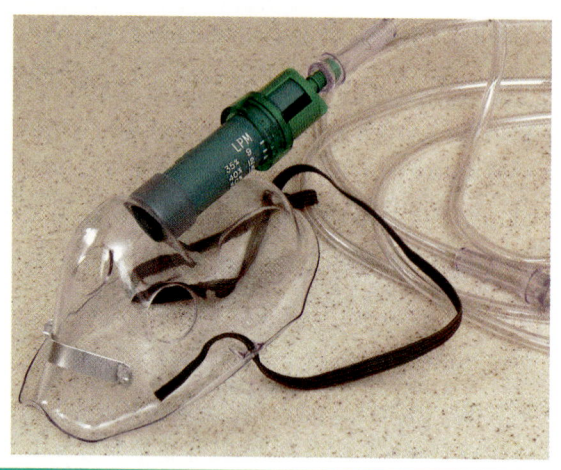

FIGURE 32-35 Make sure the mask used is the appropriate size for the client. DELMAR/CENGAGE LEARNING

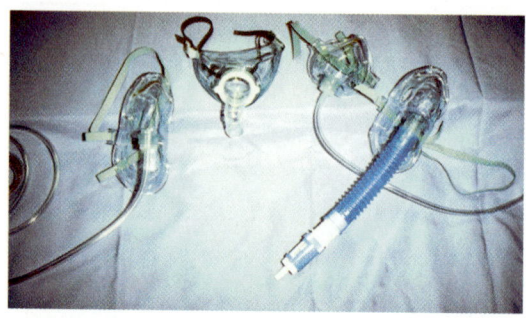

FIGURE 32-36 Different types of oxygen masks: simple oxygen mask, tracheostomy mask, pediatric mask, and Venturi mask. DELMAR/CENGAGE LEARNING

OXYGEN VIA AN ARTIFICIAL AIRWAY (TRACHEOSTOMY OR ENDOTRACHEAL TUBE)

23. Wash hands/hand hygiene.
24. Verify the prescribing practitioner's order.
25. Fill the humidifier with sterile water, and close the container.
26. Attach humidifier and warmer to the oxygen flow meter (see Figure 32-37).

27. Attach the wide-bore oxygen tubing and T-tube adapter or tracheostomy mask to the flow meter, and turn the meter to the flow rate needed to achieve the prescribed oxygen concentration. An oxygen analyzer may be used to check the actual oxygen percentage being delivered.

23. Reduces the transmission of microorganisms.
24. Ensures correct dosage and time.
25. Avoids contamination of the water.

26. Humidification and warming of the air are essential with an artificial airway because the upper airway is bypassed by the tube.
27. Checks the oxygen source and primes the tubing and adapter.

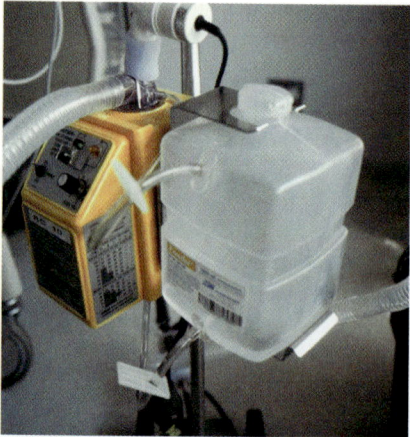

FIGURE 32-37 Oxygen Humidifier and Warmer DELMAR/CENGAGE LEARNING

(Continues)

PROCEDURE 32-4
Administering Oxygen Therapy (Continued)

ACTION	RATIONALE
28. Check for bubbling in the humidifier and a fine mist from the adapter.	28. Ensures proper functioning.
29. Attach the T-piece to the client's artificial airway, or place the mask over the client's airway. Be sure the T-piece is firmly attached to the airway (see Figure 32-38).	29. Ensures that client will not develop complications related to an interrupted oxygen supply.
30. Position tubing so that it is not pulling client's airway.	30. Provides for client comfort and prevents dislodgment of the artificial airway.
31. Check for proper flow rate and patency of the system every 1–2 hours, depending on the acuity of the client. Suction as needed to maintain a patent airway.	31. Ensures that client is receiving proper dose.
32. Monitor airway patency, vital signs, oxygen saturation, and signs and symptoms of hypoxia every 2 hours, or more frequently as necessary or as ordered. Additionally, monitor breath sounds and tube position every 4 hours.	32. Detects response to or any untoward effects from therapy. Determines whether tube is in place.

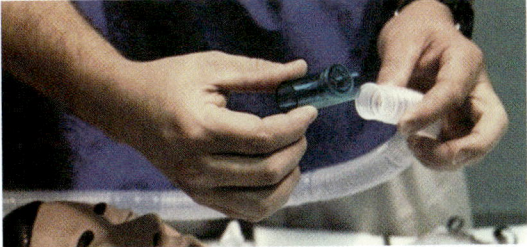

FIGURE 32-38 Attach the T-piece to the oxygen tubing. DELMAR/CENGAGE LEARNING

delegation tip

The initiation of oxygen therapy requires assessment by a nurse or respiratory care practitioner. All personnel are responsible for maintaining fire and safety precautions when oxygen is in use. Ancillary personnel should be instructed to report dyspnea, tachycardia, any changes in the client's activity tolerance, a respiratory rate less than 12 or greater than 20 breaths per minute in the adult client, or changes in mental status. Ancillary personnel should be instructed how to properly reapply respiratory therapy equipment, how to initiate assistance with activities of daily living for the client requiring oxygen therapy, and to report any abnormal client responses.

nursing tips

Promote client comfort by adjusting tubing or padding so that clients are more likely to leave oxygen therapy equipment on.

<table>
<tr><td>

PROCEDURE 32-5

</td><td>

Performing the Heimlich Maneuver

</td></tr>
</table>

EQUIPMENT

- An individual with the training to perform this procedure

ACTION	RATIONALE
FOREIGN BODY OBSTRUCTION—ALL CLIENTS 1. Assess airway for complete or partial blockage (see Figure 32-39).	1. If there is good air exchange and the client is able to forcefully cough, you should not intervene or interfere with the client's attempts to expel the foreign body. Encourage attempts to cough and breathe, as attempts to cough will provide a more forceful effort. If complete airway obstruction is apparent, the Heimlich maneuver or alternative method of subdiaphragmatic thrust should be performed immediately.
2. Activate emergency response assistance if respiratory distress or complete blockage; for example, ask bystander to call 911.	2. Provides follow-up care by professionally trained personnel.
CONSCIOUS ADULT CLIENT—SITTING OR STANDING (HEIMLICH MANEUVER)	
3. Stand behind the client (see Figure 32-40).	3. Proper positioning is necessary to provide an effective subdiaphragmatic thrust.
4. Wrap both arms around the client's waist (see Figure 32-41 on page 903).	4. Proper positioning is necessary to provide an effective subdiaphragmatic thrust.
5. Make a fist with one hand, and grasp the fist with your other hand, placing the thumb side of the fist against the client's abdomen. The fist should be placed midline, below the xiphoid process and lower margins of the rib cage and above the navel (see Figure 32-42 on page 903).	5. Correct hand placement is important to prevent internal organ damage.

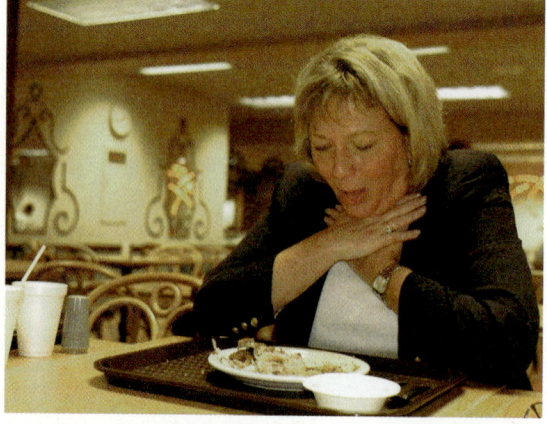

FIGURE 32-39 Assess the client. Assess the airway for blockage. DELMAR/CENGAGE LEARNING

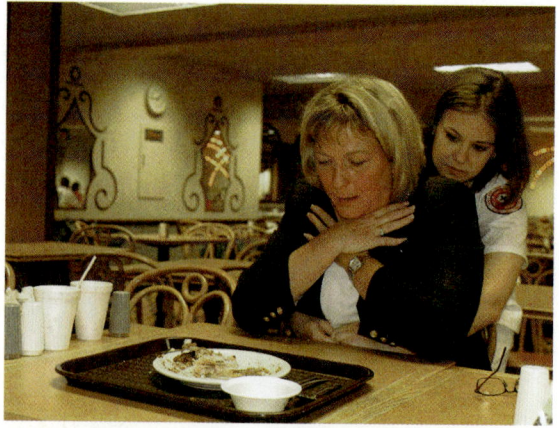

FIGURE 32-40 Stand behind the client. DELMAR/CENGAGE LEARNING

(Continues)

PROCEDURE 32-5
Performing the Heimlich Maneuver (Continued)

ACTION	**RATIONALE**

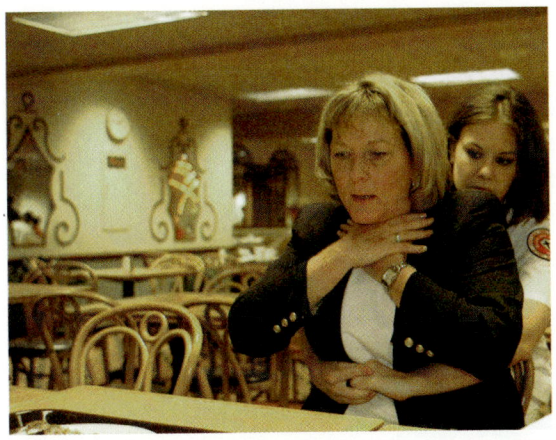

FIGURE 32-41 Wrap both arms around the client's waist.
DELMAR/CENGAGE LEARNING

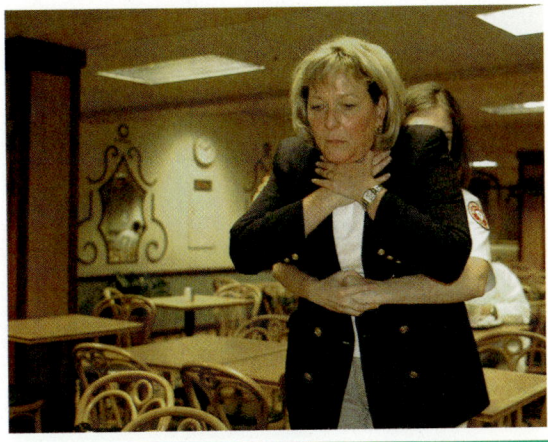

FIGURE 32-42 Make a fist. Place the fist below the xiphoid process, above the client's navel. DELMAR/CENGAGE LEARNING

ACTION	RATIONALE
6. Perform a quick upward thrust into the client's abdomen; each thrust should be separate and distinct.	6. This subdiaphragmatic thrust can produce an artificial cough by forcing air from the lungs.
7. Repeat this process 6 to 10 times until the client either expels the foreign body or loses consciousness.	7. Attempts to dislodge food or a foreign body to relieve airway obstruction should be continued as long as necessary because of the serious consequences of hypoxia.

UNCONSCIOUS ADULT CLIENT OR ADULT CLIENT WHO BECOMES UNCONSCIOUS

ACTION	RATIONALE
8. Repeat Actions 1 and 2.	8. Determines the need for intervention and summons essential help.
9. Position the client supine; kneel astride the client's abdomen.	9. Proper positioning is necessary to provide an effective subdiaphragmatic thrust.
10. Place the heel of one hand midline, below the xiphoid process and lower margin of the rib cage and above the navel. Place the second hand directly on top of the first hand.	10. Proper positioning is necessary to provide an effective subdiaphragmatic thrust.
11. Perform a quick upward thrust into the diaphragm, repeating 6 to 10 times.	11. A client who becomes unconscious may become more relaxed so that the previously unsuccessful Heimlich maneuver may be successful.
12. Perform a finger sweep:	12. Should only be used on the unconscious client, who will not fight the action.
a. Use one hand to grasp the lower jaw and tongue between your thumb and fingers and lift. This will open the mouth and pull the tongue away from the back of the throat.	a. Draw the tongue away from any foreign body lodged in the back of the throat.
b. Using the index finger of the other hand, insert the finger into the client's mouth next to the cheek and, using a hooking motion, dislodge any foreign body. Caution must be used to prevent pushing the foreign body farther down into the airway (see Figure 32-43 on page 904).	

(Continues)

PROCEDURE 32-5
Performing the Heimlich Maneuver (Continued)

ACTION	RATIONALE

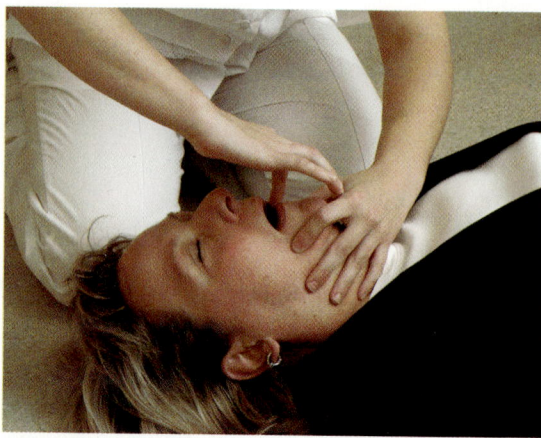

FIGURE 32-43 Use a sweeping, hooking motion to dislodge and remove obstruction. DELMAR/CENGAGE LEARNING

ACTION	RATIONALE
13. Open the client's airway, and attempt ventilation.	13. The brain can suffer irreversible damage if it is without oxygen for over 4–6 minutes.
14. Continue sequence of Heimlich maneuver, finger sweep, and rescue breathing as long as necessary.	14. Life-saving efforts must continue until they are successful or until the rescuer becomes exhausted and cannot go on.

CONSCIOUS ADULT SITTING OR STANDING—CHEST THRUSTS

ACTION	RATIONALE
15. Repeat Actions 1 and 2.	15. Determines the need for intervention and summons essential help.
16. Stand behind the client, and wrap your arms around the client's waist.	16. Proper hand placement should avoid the xiphoid process and rib cage margins to minimize internal organ damage.
17. Make a fist, and place the thumb side of the fist against the client's abdomen. Grasp fist with other hand upward.	17. Proper hand placement should avoid the xiphoid process and rib cage margins to minimize internal organ damage.
18. Perform backward thrusts until either the client becomes unconscious or the foreign body is expelled.	18. Thrusts may not be effective on the first tries. Keep trying. Chest thrusts should be used only for very obese people and women in the late stages of pregnancy.

UNCONSCIOUS ADULT—CHEST THRUSTS

ACTION	RATIONALE
19. Repeat Actions 1 and 2.	19. Determines the need for intervention and summons essential help.
20. Place client in the supine position, and kneel astride the client's thighs.	20. Places the client and the rescuer in the most effective position to apply interventions.
21. Place the heel of one hand against the client's abdomen. This should be slightly above the navel but below the xiphoid process.	21. This is the most effective position for thrust.
22. Perform each thrust in a slow, separate, and distinct manner.	22. Each thrust should be delivered with intention of relieving the airway obstruction.
23. Follow Actions 9–12 for the adult Heimlich maneuver, unconscious client.	23. Performs the life-saving procedure.

(Continues)

PROCEDURE 32-5
Performing the Heimlich Maneuver (Continued)

ACTION	RATIONALE
AIRWAY OBSTRUCTION—INFANTS AND SMALL CHILDREN	
24. Differentiate between infection and airway obstruction.	24. Infectious complications that lead to airway obstruction require immediate medical attention, establishment of a patent airway (intubation or emergency tracheotomy), and treatment of the underlying infection. Food or foreign body airway obstruction also needs immediate attention; however, airway management differs between each scenario.
Infant Airway Obstruction	
25. Straddle infant over forearm in the prone position with the head lower than the trunk. Support the infant's head, positioning a hand around the jaws and chest.	25. Proper positioning is essential for success of the maneuver and prevention of other organ damage.
26. Deliver five back blows between the infant's shoulder blades.	26. Technique for dislodging the obstruction.
27. Keeping the infant's head down, place the free hand on the infant's back and turn the infant over, supporting the back of the child with hand and thigh.	27. Safely rotates the infant's position to continue life-saving procedures.
28. With free hand, deliver five thrusts in the same manner as infant external cardiac compressions.	28. Technique for dislodging the obstruction.
29. Assess for a foreign body in the mouth of an unconscious infant, and utilize the finger sweep *only* if a foreign body is visualized.	29. A blind finger sweep is avoided in infants and children as a foreign object can be pushed back farther into the airway, increasing obstruction.
30. Open airway and assess for respiration. If respirations are absent, attempt rescue breathing. Assess for the rise and fall of the chest; if not seen, reposition infant and attempt rescue breathing again.	30. Many times some air can get around the foreign body causing the airway obstruction. This allows for some oxygenation of the client. Without oxygen, irreversible brain damage can occur within 4–6 minutes.
31. Repeat the entire sequence again: five back blows, five chest thrusts, assessment for foreign body in oral cavity, and rescue breathing as long as necessary.	31. Life-saving efforts must continue until they are successful or until the rescuer becomes exhausted and cannot go on.
Small Child Airway Obstruction (Conscious, Standing, or Sitting)	
32. Assess air exchange, and encourage coughing and breathing. Provide reassurance to the child that you are there to help.	32. Inability to breathe is a distressing event for anyone, especially a small child who may not fully understand the circumstance. Reassurance is important to gain the child's trust and cooperation with the maneuvers necessary to help him or her, especially if the child is conscious.

(Continues)

PROCEDURE 32-5
Performing the Heimlich Maneuver (Continued)

ACTION	RATIONALE
33. Ask the child if he or she is choking. If the response is affirmative, follow the steps outlined below. In addition, if the child has poor air exchange (and infection has been ruled out), initiate the following steps: a. Stand behind the child with arms wrapped around child's waist and administer 6–10 subdiaphragmatic abdominal thrusts. b. Continue until foreign object is expelled or the child becomes unconscious.	33. Many small children are capable of responding to simple questions such as "Are you choking?" a. Proper positioning is essential for success of the maneuver and prevention of other organ damage. b. Life-saving efforts must continue until they are successful or until the rescuer becomes exhausted and cannot go on.

Small Child Airway Obstruction (Unconscious)

ACTION	RATIONALE
34. Position the child supine, kneel at the child's feet, and gently deliver five subdiaphragmatic abdominal thrusts. The subdiaphragmatic thrusts are delivered in the same manner as for an adult but more gently.	34. This is the recommended position for small children; the astride position may be used for larger children. Proper positioning is essential for success of the maneuver and prevention of other organ damage.
35. Open airway by lifting the lower jaw and tongue forward. Perform a finger sweep only if a foreign body is visualized.	35. Opens the airway and allows visualization of the oral cavity. A blind finger sweep can cause increased obstruction by pushing a foreign object farther back into the airway.
36. If breathing is absent, begin rescue breathing. If the chest does not rise, reposition the child and attempt rescue breathing again.	36. Many times some air can get around the foreign body causing the airway obstruction. This allows for some oxygenation of the client. Without oxygen, irreversible brain damage can occur within 4–6 minutes.
37. Repeat this sequence as long as necessary.	37. Life-saving efforts must continue until they are successful or until the rescuer becomes exhausted and cannot go on.
38. Wash hands/hand hygiene.	38. Reduces transmission of microorganisms.

delegation tip

The Heimlich maneuver may be performed by any trained individual. A technique adjustment may need to be demonstrated in pregnant women.

nursing tips

Approach clients with confidence, and reassure clients that you will remain with them throughout the procedure.

<table>
<tr><td>

PROCEDURE 32-6

</td><td>

Administering Cardiopulmonary Resuscitation (CPR)

</td></tr>
</table>

EQUIPMENT

Hospital or Clinical Setting

- Hard, flat surface (e.g., chest compression board)
- Body substance isolation items
  —Gloves
  —Face shield
  —Mask/CPR oral barrier device

- Ambu bag
- Oral airway
- Emergency resuscitation cart (including defibrillator)
- Documentation forms

Outside: Public Environment

- Hard, flat surface (e.g., floor)
- Body substance isolation items, if available
  —Gloves
  —Face shield
  —Mask/CPR oral barrier device

ACTION	RATIONALE
CPR: ONE RESCUER—ADULT, ADOLESCENT 1. Assess responsiveness by tapping or gently shaking client while shouting, "Are you OK?" (see Figure 32-44). 2. Activate emergency medical system (EMS). In the hospital or clinical setting, follow institutional protocol. In the community or home environment, activate the local emergency response system (e.g., 911). According to the CPR guideline for 2005 (American Heart Association, 2005), rescuers should notify the EMS or phone 911 for unresponsive adults before beginning CPR.	1. Prevents injury to a client who is not experiencing cardiac or respiratory arrest. Also assists in assessing level of consciousness and possible etiology of crisis. 2. Activates assistance from personnel trained in advanced life support.

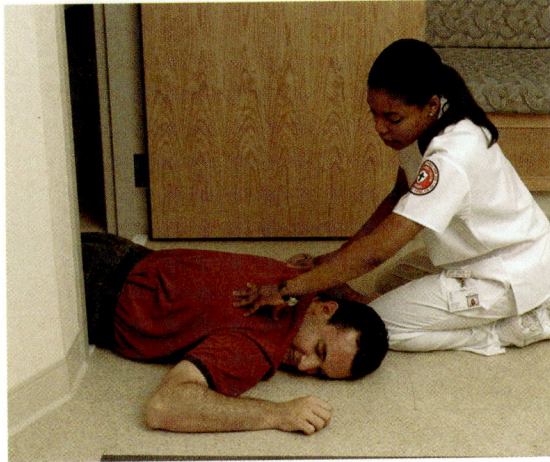

FIGURE 32-44 Assess the client's responsiveness. DELMAR/CENGAGE LEARNING

(Continues)

PROCEDURE 32-6
Administering Cardiopulmonary Resuscitation (CPR) (Continued)

ACTION	RATIONALE
3. Position client in a supine position on a hard, flat surface (e.g., floor or cardiac board). Use caution when positioning a client with a possible head or neck injury.	3. Proper positioning facilitates assessment of the cardiac and respiratory status and successful external cardiac massage. Care must be taken in positioning a client with a potential head or neck injury to prevent further damage.
4. Apply appropriate body substance isolation items (e.g., gloves, face shield) if available.	4. Prevents transmission of disease.
5. Position self. Face the client on your knees parallel to the client, next to the head, to begin to assess the airway and breathing status.	5. Proper positioning prevents rescuer fatigue and facilitates CPR by allowing the rescuer to move from chest compressions to artificial breathing with minimal movement.
6. Open airway. The most commonly used method is the head-tilt/chin-lift method. This is accomplished by placing one hand on the client's forehead and applying a steady backward pressure to tilt the head back while placing the fingers of the other hand below the jaw at the location of the chin and lifting the chin (see Figure 32-45). In the event of a suspected head or neck injury, this lift is modified and the jaw thrust is used. To perform the jaw thrust, place hands at the angles of the lower jaw and lift, displacing the mandible forward while tilting the head backward (see Figure 32-46). Additionally, if available, insert oral airway.	6. A patent airway is essential for successful artificial respirations. The head-tilt/chin-lift assists in preventing the tongue from obstructing the airway. The jaw thrust is used when a head or neck injury is suspected because it prevents extension of the neck and decreases the potential of further injury.
7. Assess for respirations. Look, listen, and feel for air movement (3–5 seconds).	7. Cardiopulmonary resuscitation should not be administered to a client with spontaneous respirations or pulse because of the potential risk of injury.

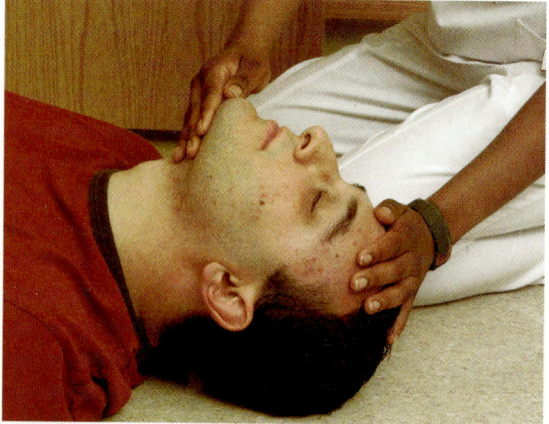

FIGURE 32-45 Use the head-tilt/chin-lift method to open airway. DELMAR/CENGAGE LEARNING

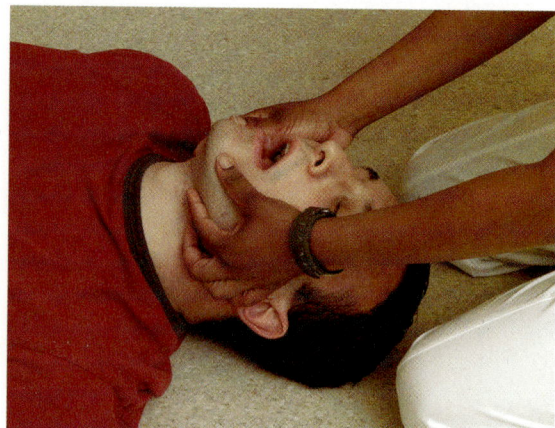

FIGURE 32-46 The jaw-thrust method is used to open the airway if a neck injury is suspected. DELMAR/CENGAGE LEARNING

(Continues)

PROCEDURE 32-6
Administering Cardiopulmonary Resuscitation (CPR) (Continued)

ACTION	RATIONALE
8. If respirations are absent: • Occlude nostrils with the thumb and index finger of the hand on the forehead that is tilting the head back (see Figure 32-47). • Form a seal over the client's mouth using either your mouth or the appropriate respiratory assist device (e.g., Ambu bag and mask) and give two full breaths of 1 second, allowing time for both inspiration and expiration (see Figure 32-48). • In the event of a serious mouth or jaw injury that prevents mouth-to-mouth ventilation, mouth-to-nose ventilation may be used by tilting the head as described earlier with one hand and using the other hand to lift the jaw and close the mouth.	8. Occluding the nostrils and forming a seal over the client's mouth will prevent air leakage and provide full inflation of the lungs. Excessive air volume and rapid inspiratory flow rates can create pharyngeal pressures that are greater than esophageal opening pressures. This will allow air into the stomach, resulting in gastric distention and increased risk of vomiting.
9. Assess for the rise and fall of the chest: • If the chest rises and falls, continue to Action 10. • If the chest does not move, assess for excessive oral secretions, vomit, airway obstruction, or improper positioning.	9. Visual assessment of chest movement helps confirm an open airway. A volume of 800–1200 mL is usually sufficient to make the chest rise in most adults.
10. Palpate the carotid pulse (5–10 seconds) (see Figure 32-49 on page 910): • If present, continue rescue breathing at the rate of 12 breaths/min. Each rescue breath should be given for 1 second. • If absent, begin external cardiac compressions.	10. Performing chest compressions on an individual with a pulse could result in injury. Additionally, the carotid pulse may persist when peripheral pulses are no longer palpable. Hyperventilation assists in maintaining blood oxygen levels. Additionally, a pulse may be present for 6 minutes after respirations have ceased.

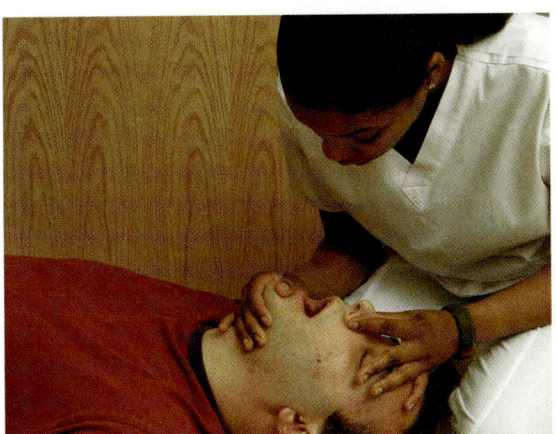

FIGURE 32-47 Occlude both nostrils with fingers. DELMAR/
CENGAGE LEARNING

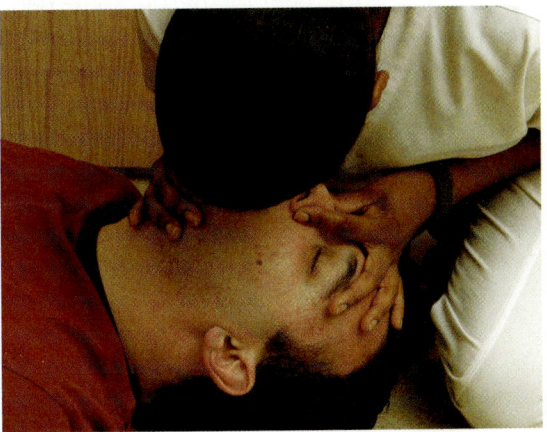

FIGURE 32-48 Give two full breaths. DELMAR/CENGAGE LEARNING

(Continues)

PROCEDURE 32-6
Administering Cardiopulmonary Resuscitation (CPR) (Continued)

ACTION	RATIONALE

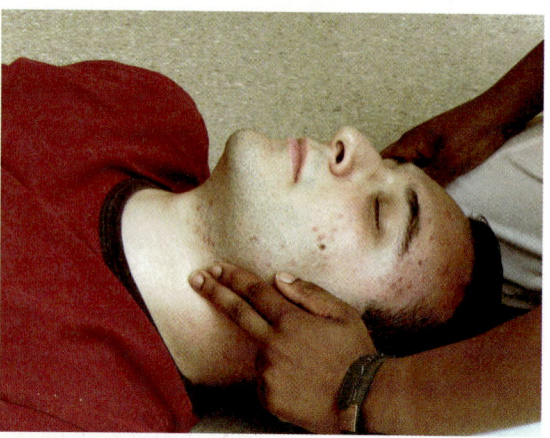

FIGURE 32-49 Palpate for a carotid pulse. DELMAR/CENGAGE LEARNING

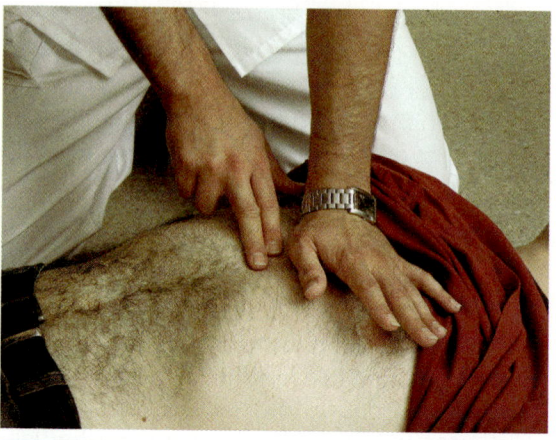

FIGURE 32-50 Place the heel of one hand next to the index finger on the client's sternum. DELMAR/CENGAGE LEARNING

11. Cardiac compressions are performed as follows:

   • Maintain a position on knees parallel to sternum.
   • Position the hands for compressions:

   a. Using the hand nearest to the legs, use the index finger to locate the lower rib margin and quickly move the fingers up to the location where the ribs connect to the sternum.
   b. Place the middle finger of this hand on the notch where the ribs meet the sternum and the index finger next to it.
   c. Place the heel of the opposite hand next to the index finger on the sternum (see Figure 32-50).
   d. Remove the first hand from the notch, and place it on top of the hand that is on the sternum so that they are on top of each other.
   e. Extend or interlace fingers, and do not allow them to touch the chest (see Figure 32-51 on page 911).
   f. Keep arms straight with shoulders directly over hands on sternum, and lock elbows (see Figure 32-52 on page 911).
   g. Compress the adult chest 3.8–5.0 cm (11/2–2 inches) at the rate of approximately 100 compressions per minute.

11. Irreversible brain and tissue damage can occur if a client is hypoxic for over 4–6 minutes. Proper positioning is essential for the following reasons:

   • Allows for maximum compression of the heart between the sternum and vertebrae.
   • Compressions over the xiphoid process can lacerate the liver.
   • Keeping fingers off the chest during compressions reduces the risk of rib fracture.

(Continues)

PROCEDURE 32-6
Administering Cardiopulmonary Resuscitation (CPR) (Continued)

ACTION	RATIONALE

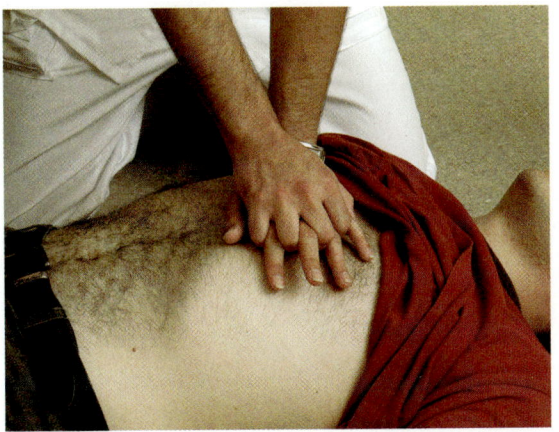

FIGURE 32-51 Extend or interlace the fingers. DELMAR/CENGAGE LEARNING

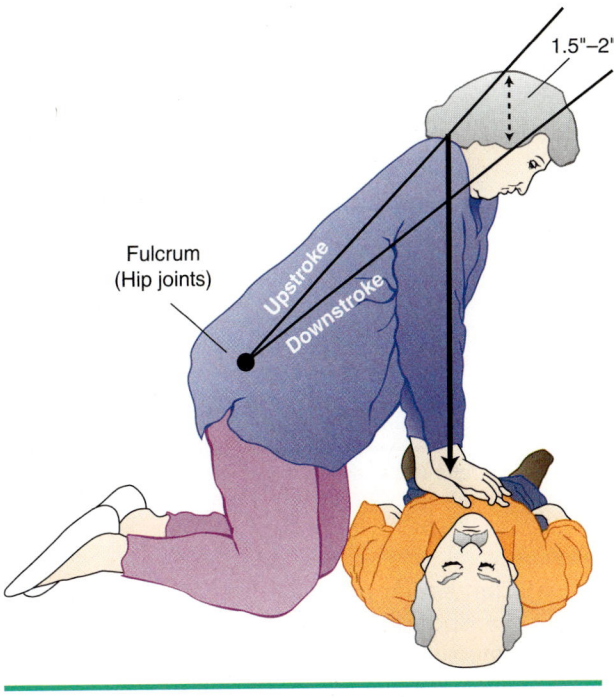

FIGURE 32-52 Proper Position of Rescuer DELMAR/CENGAGE LEARNING

h. The heel of the hand must completely release the pressure between compressions, but it should remain in constant contact with the client's skin.

i. Use the mnemonic "one and, two and, three and . . ." to keep rhythm and timing.

j. Ventilate client as described in Action 8.

12. Maintain a hard and fast compression rate for approximately 100 times/min, interjecting 2 ventilations after every 30 compressions (compression:ventilation rate of 30:2). Each rescue breath should be given for 1 second.

13. Reassess the client after four cycles.

CPR: TWO RESCUERS—ADULT, ADOLESCENT

14. Follow the previous steps with the following changes:

- One rescuer is positioned facing the client parallel to the head while the other rescuer is positioned on the opposite side facing the client parallel to the sternum next to the trunk (see Figure 32-53 on page 912).

- The rescuer positioned at the client's trunk is responsible for performing cardiac compressions and maintaining the verbal mnemonic count. This is Rescuer 1.

12. Faster rate increases blood flow to key organ tissues. Minimizes interruptions in chest compressions. Large and forceful breaths may cause gastric inflation.

13. Determines return of spontaneous pulse and respirations and need to continue CPR.

14.

Proper positioning allows one rescuer to perform artificial respirations while the other administers chest compressions without getting in each other's way. In addition, this facilitates ease in changing positions when one of the rescuers becomes fatigued. Palpating the carotid pulse with each chest compression during the first full minute ensures that adequate stroke volume is being delivered with each compression.

(Continues)

PROCEDURE 32-6
Administering Cardiopulmonary Resuscitation (CPR) (Continued)

ACTION	RATIONALE

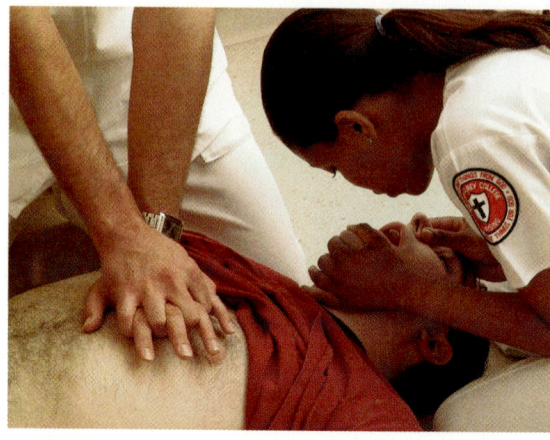

FIGURE 32-53 Two-rescuer positioning. One person kneels on each side of the client. DELMAR/CENGAGE LEARNING

- The rescuer positioned at the client's head is responsible for monitoring respirations, assessing the carotid pulse, establishing an open airway, and performing rescue breathing. This is Rescuer 2.
- Maintain the compression rate at approximately 100 times/min, interjecting 2 ventilations after every 30 compressions (compression:ventilation rate of 30:2).
- Rescuer 2 palpates the carotid pulse with each chest compression during the first full minute.
- Rescuer 2 is responsible for calling for a change when fatigued, following this protocol.
- Rescuer 1 calls for a change and completes the 30 chest compressions.
- Rescuer 2 administers 2 breaths and then moves to a position parallel to the client's sternum and assumes the proper hand position.
- Rescuer 1 moves to the rescue breathing position and checks the carotid pulse for 5 seconds. If cardiac arrest persists, Rescuer 1 says, ''continue CPR'' and delivers 1 breath. Rescuer 2 resumes cardiac compressions immediately after the breath.

Two rescuers are needed because one person cannot maintain CPR indefinitely. When a rescuer becomes fatigued, chest compressions can become ineffective, decreasing the volume of oxygenated blood circulated to key organs and tissue.

(Continues)

PROCEDURE 32-6
Administering Cardiopulmonary Resuscitation (CPR) (Continued)

ACTION	RATIONALE

CPR: ONE RESCUER—CHILD (1–7 YEARS)

15. Assess responsiveness, activate EMS, position the child, apply appropriate body substance isolation, position self, open airway, and assess for respirations as described in Actions 1–7. Remember respiratory arrest is more common in the pediatric population.

16. If respirations are absent, begin rescue breathing:
    - Give two slow breaths (1 sec/breath), pausing to take a breath in between.
    - Use only the amount of air needed to make the chest rise. When you see the chest rise and fall, you are using the right volume of air.

17. Palpate the carotid pulse (5–10 seconds). If present, ventilate at a rate of once every 4 seconds or 15 times/min. If absent, begin cardiac compressions.

18. Cardiac compressions (child 1–7 years):
    - Maintain a position on knees parallel to child's sternum.
    - Position the hands for compressions:
      a. Locate the lower margin of the rib cage using the hand closest to the feet, and find the notch where the ribs and sternum meet.
      b. Place the middle finger of this hand on the notch, and then place the index finger next to the middle finger.
      c. Place the heel of the other hand next to the index finger of the first hand on the sternum with the heel parallel to the sternum (1 cm above the xiphoid process).
      d. Keeping the elbows locked and the shoulders over the child, compress the sternum 2.5–3.8 cm (1–11/2 inches) at the approximate rate of 100 times/min.
      e. Keep the other hand on the child's forehead.

15. See Rationales 1–7.

16. Hypoxia can cause irreversible brain and tissue damage after 4–6 minutes.
    - The volume of air in a small child's lungs is less than an adult's. Excessive air volume and rapid inspiratory rates can increase pharyngeal pressures that exceed esophageal opening pressures. This allows air to enter the stomach, causing gastric distention, increasing the risk of vomiting, and further compromising the client's respiratory status.

17. Performing chest compressions on a child with a pulse could result in injury. Additionally, the carotid pulse may persist when peripheral pulses are no longer palpable. Hyperventilation assists in maintaining blood oxygen levels. Additionally, a pulse may be present for 6 minutes after respirations have ceased.

18. Irreversible brain and tissue damage can occur if a client is hypoxic for over 4–6 minutes. Proper positioning is essential for the following reasons:
    - Allows for maximum compression of the heart between the sternum and vertebrae.
    - The backward tilt of the head lifts the back of small children.
    - Compressions over the xiphoid process can lacerate the liver.
    - Keeping fingers off the chest during compressions reduces the risk of rib fracture.
    - Keeping one hand on the child's forehead helps maintain an open airway.

(Continues)

PROCEDURE 32-6
Administering Cardiopulmonary Resuscitation (CPR) (Continued)

ACTION	RATIONALE
f. Use a compression:ventilation ration of 30:2. Administer a ventilation of 1 second for each breath.	
g. Reevaluate the child after 20 cycles.	
h. According to the guideline published by the American Heart Association (2005), it is recommended that a 1-minute CPR be performed for infants and children up to age 8 before calling 911. In institutions, follow hospital protocol (American Heart Association, 2005).	

CPR: ONE RESCUER—INFANT (1–12 MONTHS)

19. Assess responsiveness, activate EMS, position the child, apply appropriate body substance isolation, position self, open airway, and assess for respirations as described in Actions 1–7. Remember, respiratory arrest is more common in the pediatric population.

19. See Rationales 1–7.

20. If respirations are absent, begin rescue breathing:

- Avoid overextension of the infant's neck.
- Place a small towel or diaper under the infant's shoulders, or use a hand to support the neck.
- Make a tight seal over both the infant's nose and mouth, and gently administer artificial respirations.
- Give two slow breaths (1–11/2 sec/breath), pausing to take a breath in between.
- Use only the amount of air needed to make the chest rise.

20. Irreversible brain and tissue damage can occur if a client is hypoxic for over 4–6 minutes. Proper positioning is essential for the following reasons:

- It is believed that overextension of an infant's head can cause a closing or narrowing of the airway.
- Proper positioning with support allows maximum compression of the heart between the sternum and vertebrae.
- Making a complete seal over the infant's mouth and nose prevents air leakage.
- The volume of air in a small child's lungs is less than an adult's. Excessive air volume and rapid inspiratory rates can increase pharyngeal pressures that exceed esophageal opening pressures. This allows air to enter the stomach, causing gastric distention, increasing the risk of vomiting, and further compromising the client's respiratory status.

21. Assess circulatory status using the brachial pulse:

- Locate the brachial pulse on the inside of the upper arm between the elbow and shoulder by placing your thumb on the outside of the arm and palpating the proximal

21. The carotid pulse is often difficult to locate in the infant; therefore, the brachial artery is the recommended site.

(Continues)

PROCEDURE 32-6
Administering Cardiopulmonary Resuscitation (CPR) (Continued)

ACTION	RATIONALE
side of the arm with the index finger and middle fingers.	
• If a pulse is palpated, continue rescue breathing 20 times/min or once every 3 seconds.	
• If a pulse is absent, begin cardiac compressions.	

22. Cardiac compressions (infant 1–12 months):

- Maintain a position parallel to the infant. Infants can easily be placed on a table or other hard surface.
- Place a small towel or other support under the infant's shoulders and neck.
- Position the hands for compressions:
  a. Using the hand closest to the infant's feet, locate the intermammary line where it intersects the sternum.
  b. Place the index finger 1 cm below this location on the sternum, and place the middle finger next to the index finger.
  c. Using these two fingers, compress in a downward motion 1.3–2.5 cm (1/2–1 inch) at the rate of 100 times/min.
  d. Keep the other hand on the infant's forehead.
  e. At the end of every fifth compression, administer a ventilation (1–11/2 seconds).
  f. Reevaluate infant after 20 cycles.
  g. According to the guideline published by the American Heart Association (2005), it is recommended that a 1-minute CPR be performed for infants and children up to age 8 before calling 911. In institutions, follow hospital protocol (American Heart Association, 2005).

22. Irreversible brain and tissue damage can occur if a client is hypoxic for over 4–6 minutes. Proper positioning is essential for the following reasons:

- Allows for maximum compression of the heart between the sternum and vertebrae.
- A small towel, diaper roll, or some other type of support is necessary for effective cardiac compressions.
- Compressions over the xiphoid process can lacerate the liver.
- Keeping other fingers and hands off the chest during compressions reduces risk of rib fracture.
- Keeping one hand on the infant's forehead helps maintain an open airway.

CPR: TWO RESCUERS—CHILD (1–7 YEARS) AND INFANT (1–12 MONTHS)

23. Follow Action 14 for two-rescuer CPR for adults with the following changes:

- Utilize the child or infant procedure for chest compressions.
- Change the ratio of compressions to ventilation to 5:1 (5 chest compressions to 1 ventilation).
- Deliver the ventilation on the upstroke of the third compression.

23. Improper hand placement can cause internal organ damage or other medical complications in infants or children. Increased rate of ventilation allows for maximum oxygen delivery to prevent tissue hypoxia. Delivering compressions during the upstroke phase allows for full lung expansion during inspiration.

(Continues)

PROCEDURE 32-6
Administering Cardiopulmonary Resuscitation (CPR) (Continued)

CPR—NEONATE OR PREMATURE INFANT

24. Follow the infant guidelines with the following changes for chest compressions:
    - Encircle the chest with both hands.
    - Position thumbs over the midsternum.
    - Compress the midsternum with both thumbs.
    - Compress 1.3–1.8 cm (1/2–3/4 inch) at a rate of 100–120 times/min.

25. If properly trained, use an automated external defibrillator (AED). AEDs are not recommended for children under 8 years of age.
    In hospital setting, use defibrillator as specified by institution protocol. Defibrillator should be placed only by properly trained personnel.

24. Improper hand placement can cause internal organ damage or other medical complications in infants or children.

25. The use of an AED can increase the client's chances for survival by restoring rhythm and circulation. AEDs have not been adequately tested in children, and excessive joules may cause injury.
    Protocol in hospital settings includes the use of defibrillator with codes and can increase survival. Injury to self, staff, or the client may occur with untrained personnel.

delegation tip

The administration of CPR to adults and children is a skill that may be delegated to ancillary personnel and caregivers after proper instruction and CPR certification.

nursing tips

Maintain an ongoing assessment of the cardiac and respiratory status throughout emergency resuscitation efforts.

KEY CONCEPTS

- Adequate tissue oxygenation is essential to survival and may be threatened by deficits in air movement through the lungs to deliver fresh air to the alveoli (ventilation), the exchange of oxygen and carbon dioxide across the alveolar-capillary membrane (diffusion or external respiration), oxygen transport in the blood, the delivery of oxygen to the tissues (circulation), or the uptake of oxygen by the cells (internal respiration).

- Impairment of oxygen delivery to the tissues results first in compensatory efforts such as anaerobic metabolism and increased oxygen extraction; when these efforts fail, tissue ischemia and infarction will ensue.

- Client teaching related to oxygenation impairment involves teaching about the disease process, treatments, and lifestyle alterations that may be indicated; teaching should involve not only the client but also the family.

- Nursing care related to oxygenation focuses on maintaining a patent airway, promoting effective ventilation, promoting optimal circulation and perfusion, and meeting the client's learning, nutritional, activity, and sleep needs.

- A holistic approach to care recognizes that each of the problems experienced by the client with oxygenation deficits is interrelated.

- Emergency support of airway, ventilation, and circulation is achieved by instituting the Heimlich maneuver for airway obstruction and cardiopulmonary resuscitation for cardiopulmonary arrest.

REVIEW QUESTIONS

1. Normal breath sounds heard over both lungs are described as being:
   a. Loud
   b. Intermediate
   c. Soft
   d. Adventitious

2. What is the classic sign of chronic hypoxia?
   a. Cyanosis
   b. Decreased level of consciousness
   c. Clubbing of the fingers
   d. Loss of appetite

3. The breath sound "fine crackle" is indicative of which condition?
   a. Asthma
   b. Bronchitis
   c. Chronic obstructive pulmonary disease
   d. Foreign body obstruction

4. Yellowish-green sputum is indicative of:
   a. Asthma
   b. Bacterial infection
   c. Pneumonia
   d. Pulmonary edema

5. Which client is most prone to problems while receiving oxygen?
   a. Postoperative
   b. Asthmatic
   c. Myocardial infarction
   d. Chronic pulmonary disease

6. Hydration should be restricted in clients experiencing:
   a. Pneumonia
   b. Bronchitis
   c. Asthma
   d. Congestive heart failure

7. Which indicates partial obstruction of the larynx or trachea and demands immediate attention?
   a. Mediastinal crunch
   b. Pleural rub
   c. Rhonchi
   d. Stridor

8. Which should the nurse include when suctioning a client's tracheostomy?
   a. Instill sterile saline down the trachea to stimulate cough, then suction with continuous suctioning.
   b. Insert the catheter until a cough reflex is obtained or until resistance is felt.
   c. Adjust the wall suction to 150 mm Hg for the procedure.
   d. Suction the client's mouth before entering the trachea.

9. Which nursing intervention may not be delegated to ancillary personnel?
   a. Adjusting the rate of oxygen flow
   b. Reapplying a nasal cannula
   c. Providing comfort measures
   d. Reporting a change in the client's condition

online companion

Visit the DeLaune and Ladner online companion resource at **www.delmar.cengage.com** for additional content and study aids. Click on Online Companions, then select the Nursing discipline.

"The most important practical lesson that can be given to nurses is to teach them what to observe—how to observe—what are of importance."

—NIGHTINGALE (IN SKRETKOWICZ, 1992)

CHAPTER 33

Fluids and Electrolytes

COMPETENCIES

1. Review the physiological processes and core concepts relative to body fluid and acid-base balance and imbalances.

2. Relate the common disturbances in body fluid and acid-base balance to their clinical manifestations and nursing interventions.

3. Identify the key elements for assessing clients with body fluid and acid-base alterations.

4. Describe the nursing data that support the common nursing diagnoses and goals for clients with body fluid and acid-base disturbances.

5. Describe the common nursing interventions for clients with alterations in body fluid and acid-base balance.

6. Identify the key indicators to evaluate client achievement of expected outcomes to restore and to maintain body fluid and acid-base balance.

KEY TERMS

acid	homeostasis	infiltration
acid-base balance	hydrostatic pressure	intracath
acid-base buffer system	hypercalcemia	intravenous (IV) therapy
acidosis	hyperchloremia	isotonic
alkalosis	hyperkalemia	osmolality
angiocatheter	hypermagnesemia	osmolarity
arterial blood gases (ABGs)	hypernatremia	osmole
base	hyperphosphatemia	osmosis
butterfly (scalp vein or wing- tipped) needles	hypertonic	osmotic pressure
	hypervolemia	permeability
colloids	hypocalcemia	phlebitis
crystalloids	hypochloremia	piggybacked
cytomegalovirus (CMV)	hypokalemia	semipermeable
diffusion	hypomagnesemia	skin turgor
edema	hyponatremia	solute
electrochemical gradient	hypophosphatemia	solvent
electrolyte	hypotonic	vesicant
flashback	hypoxemia	
flow rate	implantable port	

The physiological functions and alterations of body fluid and acid-base balance are presented in this chapter. The term *body fluid* is used to denote both water and electrolytes, whereas the term *body water* refers to water alone. **Homeostasis**, or equilibrium of the internal environment, refers to the state of balance of body fluid.

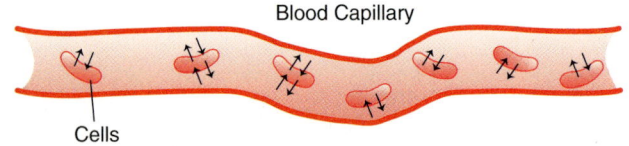

Blood Capillary

Cells

FIGURE 33-1 Movement of Fluid between the Intracellular and Extracellular Compartments DELMAR/CENGAGE LEARNING

PHYSIOLOGY OF FLUID AND ACID-BASE BALANCE

The body normally maintains a balance between the amount of fluid taken in and the amount excreted. Health promotion requires a maintenance of body fluid and acid-base balance.

FLUID COMPARTMENTS

The body's fluid is contained within three compartments: cells, blood vessels, and the tissue space (space between the cells and blood vessels). To understand this concept, visualize cars on a freeway. The cars represent cells; the lanes represent the blood vessels, and the space between the cars in the lanes represents the tissue space. The freeway itself is the body.

Just as traffic is ongoing and continuous, fluids move constantly from one compartment to another to accommodate the cell's metabolic needs (see Figure 33-1). Specific terms are used in describing compartmentalized body fluid. The prefixes (see the accompanying display) used with the root words for the compartments that contain the body fluid give meaning to the following terms:

- *Intracellular fluid: within* the cell
- *Intravascular fluid: within* blood vessels
- *Interstitial fluid: between* cells; fluid that surrounds cells

There are two types of body fluid: intracellular fluid (ICF) and extracellular fluid (ECF). Because intravascular and interstitial fluids are outside the cells, these fluids are extracellular. Key terms used in explaining the movement of molecules in body fluids are:

- **Solute**: Substance dissolved in a solution
- **Solvent**: Liquid that contains a substance in solution
- **Permeability**: Capability of a substance, molecule, or ion to diffuse through a membrane (covering of tissue over a surface, organ, or separating spaces)
- **Semipermeable**: Selectively permeable (All membranes in the body allow some solutes to pass through the membrane without restriction but will prevent the passage of other solutes.)

PREFIXES

Inter-	Between
Intra-	Within
Extra-	Outside
Hypo-	Under, beneath, deficient
Hyper-	Above, beyond, excessive

Cells have permeable membranes that allow fluid and solutes to pass into and out of the cell. Permeability allows the cell to acquire the nutrients it needs from ECF to carry on metabolism and to eliminate metabolic waste products.

Blood vessels have permeable membranes that bathe and feed the cells. The intravascular fluid of arterioles carries oxygen and nutrients to the cells. The venules take in the waste products from the cells' metabolic activity.

Cells and capillaries form a meshlike structure that creates a tissue space between cells and the vascular system to allow cellular access to the vascular system. Interstitial space promotes access of the cells to the arterioles and venules.

BODY WATER DISTRIBUTION

Water is the largest single constituent of the body, representing 45% to 75% of the body's total weight. About two-thirds of the body fluid is intracellular. The remaining one-third is extracellular, with one-fourth of this fluid being intravascular and three-fourths being interstitial fluid. Bones are made up of nearly one-third water, while the muscles and brain cells contain 70% water. Body fat is essentially free of water; therefore, the ratio of water to body weight is greater in leaner people than in obese people.

Water is present in all body tissues and cells and serves two main functions: (1) to act as a solvent for the essential nutrients so that they can be used by the body and (2) to transport nutrients and oxygen from the blood to the cells and remove waste material and other substances from the cells back to the blood so they can be excreted by the body. Water is also needed by the body to:

- Give shape and form to the cells
- Regulate body temperature
- Act as a lubricant in joints
- Cushion body organs
- Maintain peak physical performance

Water loss has a negative effect on the body's ability to function because every 2% to 5% of water loss results in a 30% decrease in work performance (Tierra & Lust, 2008).

ELECTROLYTES

An **electrolyte** is a compound that when dissolved in water or another solvent, forms or dissociates into ions (electrically charged particles) (see Figure 33-2). The electrolytes provide inorganic chemicals for cellular reactions and control mechanisms. Electrolytes have special physiological functions in the body that promote neuromuscular irritability, maintain body fluid osmolarity, regulate acid-base balance, and distribute body fluids between the fluid compartments.

Electrolytes are measured in terms of their electrical combining power, the quantities of cations and anions in a solution, expressed as milliequivalents per liter (mEq/L). Because electrolytes produce either positively charged ions (cations) or negatively charged ions (anions), they are critical regulators in the distribution of body fluid. The main electrolytes in body fluid are sodium (Na^+), potassium (K^+), calcium (Ca^{2+}), and magnesium (Mg^{2+}).

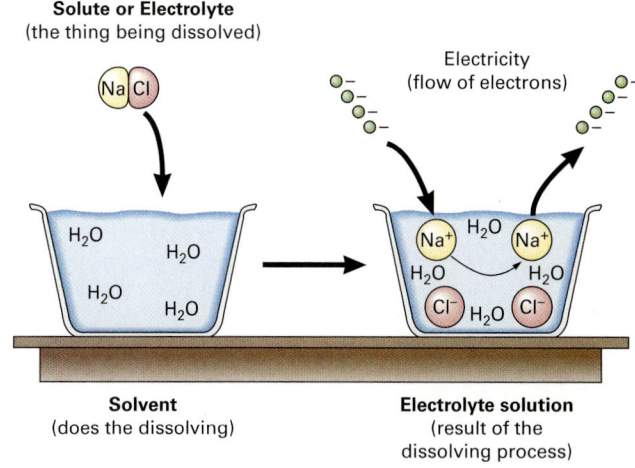

Solute or Electrolyte
(the thing being dissolved)

Electricity
(flow of electrons)

Solvent
(does the dissolving)

Electrolyte solution
(result of the dissolving process)

FIGURE 33-2 Dissolution of Electrolytes DELMAR/CENGAGE LEARNING

Table 33-1 on page 922 discusses the distribution of electrolytes in body fluid, their regulatory functions, and dietary sources. As shown in Table 33-1, the ECF contains the largest quantities of sodium, chloride, and bicarbonate ions, but only small quantities of potassium, calcium, magnesium, phosphate, sulfate, and organic acid ions. The ICF contains only small quantities of sodium and chloride ions and almost no calcium ions. Large quantities of potassium and phosphate ions with moderate quantities of magnesium and sulfate ions are contained within ICF (see Table 33-2 on page 923).

MOVEMENT OF BODY FLUIDS

The physiological forces that affect the movement of body fluids through cell walls and capillaries can be perceived as a mass transportation system that carries traffic between the compartments. These forces transport molecules of water, foods, gases, wastes, and ions to maintain a physiological balance between ECF and ICF volumes. These transport processes account for fluid shifts between the compartments (see Table 33-3 on page 924).

REGULATORS OF FLUID BALANCE

The body has many regulators that maintain fluid balance, including fluid and food intake, skin, lungs, gastrointestinal (GI) tract, and kidneys. When all organs are functioning normally, the body is able to maintain homeostasis.

Fluid and Food Intake and Loss

There are three natural sources by which water enters the body: oral liquids, water in foods, and water formed by oxidation of foods. A normal diet provides the electrolytes required by the body. For example, the typical daily amount of body fluid intake for an adult is:

Ingested liquids	1500 mL
Water in foods	700 mL
Water from oxidation	200 mL
TOTAL	2400 mL

TABLE 33-1   Common Electrolytes

ELECTROLYTE ION	DISTRIBUTION IN BODY FLUID		BASIC FUNCTIONS	DIETARY SOURCES
	EXTRACELLULAR (mEq/L)	INTRACELLULAR (mEq/L)		
Sodium (Na^+)	135–145	15–20	Regulates fluid volume within extracellular fluid (ECF) compartment. Increases cell membrane permeability. Regulates vascular osmotic pressure. Controls water distribution between ECF and intracellular fluid (ICF) compartments. Stimulates conduction of nerve impulses. Maintains neuromuscular irritability.	Table salt (NaCl), 40% of which is sodium; cheese, milk, processed meat, poultry, shellfish, fish, eggs, and foods preserved with salt (e.g., ham and bacon)
Potassium (K^+)	3.5–5	150–155	Regulates osmolality of ICF. Promotes transmission of nerve impulses. Promotes contraction of skeletal and smooth muscles. Promotes enzymatic action for cellular energy production by transforming carbohydrates into energy and restructuring amino acids into proteins. Regulates acid-base balance by cellular exchange of hydrogen ions.	Fruits, especially bananas, oranges, and dried fruits; vegetables, meats, and nuts
Calcium (Ca^{2+})	4.5–5.5	1–2	Provides strength and durability to bones and teeth. Establishes thickness and strength of cell membranes. Promotes transmission of nerve impulses. Decreases neuromuscular excitability. Is essential for blood coagulation. Promotes absorption and utilization of vitamin B_{12}. Activates enzyme reactions and hormone secretions.	Dairy products (milk, cheese, and yogurt), sardines, whole grains, and green leafy vegetables
Magnesium (Mg^{2+})	1.5–2.5	27–29	Activates enzyme systems, mainly those associated with vitamin B metabolism and the utilization of potassium, calcium, and protein. Promotes regulation of serum calcium, phosphorus, and potassium levels. Promotes neuromuscular activity.	Green leafy vegetables, whole grains, fish, and nuts

Delmar/Cengage Learning

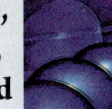

TABLE 33-2	Distribution of Chloride, Bicarbonate, Phosphate, and Sulfate in Body Fluid	
ELECTROLYTE	**EXTRACELLULAR (mEq/L)**	**INTRACELLULAR (mEq/L)**
Chloride (Cl⁻)	98–106	1–4
Bicarbonate (HCO₃⁻)	25–27	10–12
Phosphate (HPO₄⁻)	1.7–4.6	100–104
Sulfate (SO₄⁻)	1	2

Fischbach, F. (2008). *A manual of laboratory and diagnostic tests* (8th ed.). Philadelphia: Lippincott Williams & Wilkins.

Body fluid is replenished by the ingestion of liquids and food products such as meats and vegetables, which contain 65% to 97% water. The third source of body fluid is the metabolism of foods, which yields water of oxidation. The kidneys excrete the largest quantity of fluid; other avenues for water loss are the lungs, skin, and GI tract.

Skin

An estimated water loss of 300 to 400 mL per day occurs by diffusion through the skin of an adult. Because the person is not aware of this water loss, it is called *insensible loss*. Water is also lost through the skin by perspiration; however, the total amount of water lost by perspiration can vary from 1.5 to 3.5 L per hour, depending on environmental factors and body temperature.

Lungs

An estimated insensible water loss of 300 to 400 mL per day occurs in an adult through expired air, which is saturated with water vapor. This amount may vary with the rate and depth of respirations.

Gastrointestinal Tract

Although a large amount of fluid—about 8000 mL per day in the adult—is secreted into the GI tract, almost all of this fluid is reabsorbed by the body. In adults, about 200 mL of water is lost per day in feces. Severe diarrhea can cause a fluid and electrolyte deficit because the GI fluids contain a large amount of electrolytes.

Kidneys

The kidneys play a major role in maintaining fluid balance by excreting 1200 to 1500 mL/day in the adult. The excretion of water by healthy kidneys is proportional to the fluid ingested and the amount of waste or solutes excreted.

When an ECF volume deficit occurs, hormones play a key role in restoring the ECF volume. The release of the following hormones into circulation causes the kidneys to conserve water:

- Antidiuretic hormone (ADH) from the posterior pituitary gland acts on the distal tubules of the kidneys to reabsorb water.
- Aldosterone (produced in the adrenal cortex) causes the reabsorption of sodium from the renal tubules. The increased reabsorption of sodium causes water retention in the ECF, increasing its volume.
- Renin, which is released from the juxtaglomerular cells of the kidneys, promotes vasoconstriction and the release of aldosterone.

The interaction of these hormones with regard to renal functions serves as the body's compensatory mechanism to maintain homeostasis.

Sodium is the main electrolyte that promotes the retention of water. An intravascular water deficit causes the renal tubules to reabsorb more sodium into circulation. Because water molecules go with the sodium ions, the intravascular water deficit is corrected by this action of the renal tubules.

ACID-BASE BALANCE

Acid-base balance refers to the homeostasis of the hydrogen ion concentration in ECF. The slightest variation in the hydrogen ion concentration causes marked alterations in the rate of cellular chemical reactions. The pH symbol is used to indicate the hydrogen ion concentration of body fluids; 7.35 to 7.45 is the normal pH range of ECF. Hydrogen ions (H^+), which carry a positive charge, are protons. Depending on the number of hydrogen ions present, a solution can be either acidic, neutral, or alkaline.

As the number of hydrogen ions increases, the fluid becomes acidic. *Acidity of a solution increases as the pH value decreases.* An **acid** is a substance that donates hydrogen ions. For example, hydrochloric acid (HCl) ionizes in water (a solution) to form hydrogen ions and chloride ions. HCl, which is found in gastric juices, has a strong tendency to form ions, discharging hydrogen ions into the solution; carbonic and acetic acids are considered weak acids because in a solution they provide a low concentration of hydrogen ions.

As the number of hydrogen ions decreases, the fluid becomes alkaline. *Alkalinity of a solution increases as the pH value increases.* A **base** is a substance that accepts hydrogen ions (proton acceptor).

A neutral solution has a pH of 7. In such a solution there are equal numbers of hydrogen ions (H^+) and hydroxyl ions (OH^-), which can combine to form water (H_2O). When the number of hydrogen ions is increased, the solution becomes acidic (pH value below 7); a decrease in the number of hydrogen ions causes the solution to become alkaline (pH value above 7). When the number of free hydrogen ions in a solution increases to the point that the pH value becomes less than 7.35, the body is in a state of **acidosis**. The opposite occurs with **alkalosis**, in which a pH value higher than 7.45 results from a low hydrogen ion concentration.

TABLE 33-3 Movement of Body Fluid

PHYSIOLOGICAL FORCE	PROCESS	RELATED FACTORS
Diffusion Rate of diffusion (continual movement of molecules in a solution or a gas) is influenced by: • Size of the molecule (smaller molecules diffuse faster than larger molecules) • Concentration of the molecules (molecules move from an area of greater concentration to an area of lesser concentration) • Temperature of the solution (higher temperatures increase the rate of diffusion)	Particles move across a permeable membrane and disperse in all directions through a solution or a gas (see Figure 33-3 on page 925).	Particle's electrical charge can also affect the process of diffusion because ions with opposite charges are pulled toward other ions.
Osmosis Process of osmosis, the passage of a solvent from an area of lesser concentration to an area of greater concentration, is influenced by: • Net movement of water • Semipermeability of the membrane	Solvent molecules move across a membrane to an area where there is a higher concentration of solute that cannot pass through the membrane (see Figure 33-4 on page 925).	Osmotic pressure is the force created when two solutions of different concentrations are separated by a selectively permeable membrane. An osmole is the unit of measure of osmotic pressure.
Active transport An electrochemical gradient (sum of all the diffusion forces acting on the membrane, from either a concentration gradient or an electrical or a pressure gradient) exists when there is active transport.	Occurs when a cell membrane moves molecules or ions against an electrochemical gradient from an area of lesser concentration to an area of greater concentration.	For active transport to occur, there must be a carrier and adenosine triphosphate (ATP) molecules inside the cell membrane (see Figure 33-5 on page 925).
Hydrostatic pressure Hydrostatic pressure, the force a liquid exerts on the sides of the container that holds it, is governed by: • Force by which the heart pumps • Rate of blood flow • Arterial blood pressure • Venous blood pressure	The force of fluid presses outward against the blood vessel wall.	Hydrostatic pressure is twice as great at the arterial end than at the venous end, causing fluid and solutes to go from the arterial end of the capillary into the interstitial space.
Filtration Filtration is governed by the presence of a greater hydrostatic pressure in the arterial end capillaries than in the interstitial spaces.	Movement of fluid through a semipermeable membrane from an area with higher hydrostatic pressure to an area with lower hydrostatic pressure creates an outward gain of fluid in the interstitial spaces.	The body achieves total fluid balance when the excess fluid and solutes remaining in the interstitial spaces are returned to the intravascular compartment by the lymphatic system.
Colloid osmotic pressure Created by solutes or colloids (proteins or nondiffusible substances) in the plasma	Movement of fluid between the intravascular and interstitial compartments, based on the number of solute particles on the concentrated side and the presence of a semipermeable membrane.	Because the protein content of intravascular fluid is 16 times as great as that of interstitial fluid, the fluids move into the capillary or intravascular compartment when the heart pumps effectively.

Delmar/Cengage Learning

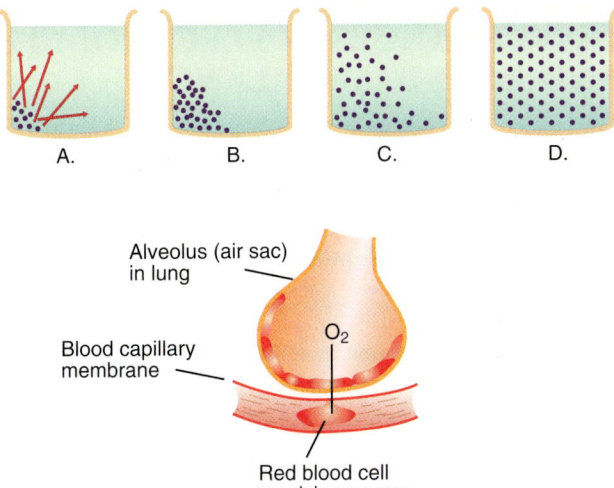

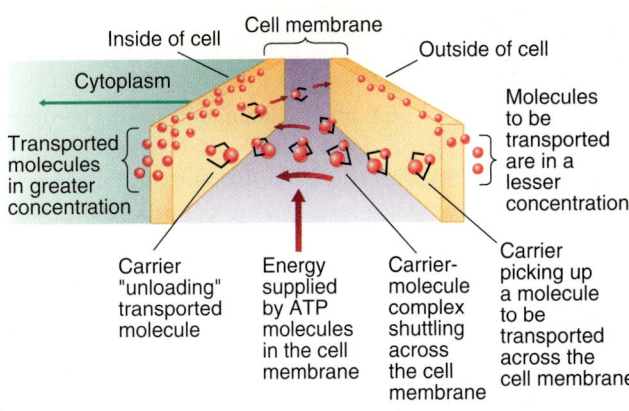

FIGURE 33-5 Active Transport of Molecules from an Area of Lesser Concentration to an Area of Greater Concentration

DELMAR/CENGAGE LEARNING

FIGURE 33-3 Process of diffusion. **A.** A small lump of sugar is placed in a beaker of water; its molecules dissolve and begin to diffuse outward. **B., C.** The sugar molecules continue to diffuse through the water from an area of greater concentration to an area of lesser concentration. **D.** Over a long period of time, the sugar molecules are evenly distributed throughout the water, reaching a state of equilibrium. Example of diffusion in the human body: Oxygen diffuses from an alveolus in a lung, where it is in greater concentration, across the capillary membrane, into a red blood cell, where it is in lesser concentration. DELMAR/CENGAGE LEARNING

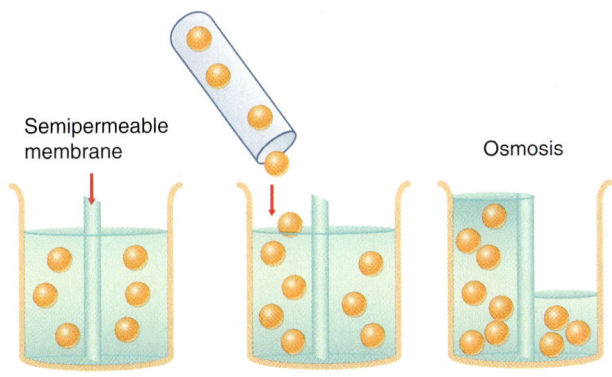

FIGURE 33-4 Process of Osmosis DELMAR/CENGAGE LEARNING

REGULATORS OF ACID-BASE BALANCE

The body has three main control systems that regulate acid-base balance to counter acidosis or alkalosis: the buffer systems, respiration, and renal control of hydrogen ion concentration. These systems vary in their reaction time in regulating and restoring balance to the hydrogen ion concentration of a solution.

Buffer Systems

All body fluids are supplied with an **acid-base buffer system**, a solution containing two or more chemical compounds that prevents marked changes in hydrogen ion concentration when either an acid or a base is added to a solution. The buffer system reacts within a fraction of a second to prevent excessive changes in the hydrogen ion concentration.

There are several *chemical* buffer systems of body fluids, which are activated under different conditions; however, the bicarbonate-carbonic acid system (carbonate system) is the body's primary buffer system. The carbonate system consists of a mixture of carbonic acid (H_2CO_3) and sodium bicarbonate ($NaHCO_3$). The pH of the ECF can be returned to normal limits by this system because carbonic acid is a weak acid, which ionizes to a limited extent, and bicarbonate is a weak base, which yields the hydroxyl ion.

Bicarbonate helps to stabilize pH by combining reversibly with hydrogen ions. Most of the body's bicarbonate is produced in red blood cells (RBCs), where the enzyme carbonic anhydrase accelerates the conversion of carbon dioxide to carbonic acid. The production of bicarbonate is illustrated in the following reversible equation:

$$CO_2 + H_2O \rightleftharpoons H_2CO_3 \rightleftharpoons H^+ + HCO_3^-$$

When the hydrogen ion concentration increases in the extracellular space, the reaction shifts toward the left; a decreased concentration of hydrogen ion drives the reaction to the right.

Respiratory Regulation of Acid-Base Balance

The respiratory buffering system helps to maintain acid-base balance by controlling the content of carbon dioxide in ECF. The *rate of metabolism* determines the formation of carbon dioxide. Carbon dioxide is continually being formed in the body by different intracellular metabolic processes. The carbon in foods is oxidized by oxygen to form carbon dioxide.

It takes the respiratory regulatory mechanism several minutes to respond to changes in the carbon dioxide concentration of ECF. With the increase of carbon dioxide in ECFs, respirations are increased in rate and depth so that more carbon dioxide is exhaled. As the respiratory system removes carbon dioxide, there is less carbon dioxide in the blood to combine with water to form carbonic acid. Likewise, if the blood level of carbon dioxide is low, respirations are depressed to maintain a normal ratio between carbonic acid and basic bicarbonate.

Renal Control of Hydrogen Ion Concentration

The kidneys control ECF pH by eliminating either hydrogen ions or bicarbonate ions from body fluids. If the bicarbonate concentration in the ECF is greater than normal, the kidneys excrete more bicarbonate ions, making the urine more alkaline. Conversely, if more hydrogen ions are excreted in the urine, the urine becomes more acidic. The renal mechanism for regulating acid-base balance cannot readjust the pH within seconds, as can the ECF buffer system, nor within minutes, as can the respiratory compensatory mechanism, but it can function over a period of several hours or days to correct an acid-base imbalance.

FACTORS AFFECTING FLUID AND ELECTROLYTE BALANCE

The balance of fluids and electrolytes in the body is dependent on many factors and will vary with such elements as age and lifestyle.

AGE

Body water distribution is relative to body size. The smaller the body, the larger the fluid content:

- Adult, 60% water
- Child, 60%–77% water
- Infant, 77% water
- Embryo, 97% water

In older adults, body water diminishes because of tissue loss; the percentage of total body weight that is fluid may be reduced to 45% to 50% in persons over age 65. Caution must be used when administering diuretics, especially thiazide diuretics, to older adults to prevent diuretic-induced electrolyte disturbances.

LIFESTYLE

Loss of body fluids can result from stress, exercise, or a warm or humid environment. Stress leads to increased blood volume and decreased urine production, with a subsequent intensification of ADH levels. Sweating and exercise cause the body to lose water and sodium, thus necessitating electrolyte replacement and intensifying the thirst response. Warm climates can exert a similar effect.

An individual's diet will also determine fluid and electrolyte levels. Adequate intake of fluids, carbohydrates, potassium, calcium, sodium, fats, and protein is essential in helping the body maintain homeostasis and function properly. Dehydration is one of the most common yet most serious fluid imbalances that can occur from poor monitoring of diet. One nursing goal is to ensure that all clients understand the role water plays in health and to see that clients understand how to maintain adequate hydration status.

DISTURBANCES IN ELECTROLYTE AND ACID-BASE BALANCE

The clinical management of clients experiencing disturbances in sodium, potassium, calcium, magnesium, and phosphate is presented using the functional health pattern model. See Table 33-4 on page 927 for the causes, clinical manifestations, and nursing interventions for these electrolyte disturbances. Because chloride has several characteristics similar to other ions, a brief discussion of chloride imbalance is also presented. Acid-base imbalances caused by a disturbance in the level of either carbonic acid or bicarbonate are also presented using the functional health pattern model.

ELECTROLYTE DISTURBANCES

In health, normal homeostatic mechanisms function to maintain electrolyte and acid-base balance. In illness, one or more of the regulating mechanisms may be affected, or the imbalance may become too great for the body to correct without treatment. Refer to Chapter 28, Table 28-7, for the normal laboratory values of electrolytes.

Sodium

Sodium is the primary determinant of ECF concentration because of its high concentration and inability to cross the cell membrane easily. As discussed in Table 33-4, alterations in sodium concentration can produce profound central nervous system effects on cognition and sensory perception and on the circulating blood volume. When the kidneys reabsorb sodium ions, chloride and water are reabsorbed with the sodium to maintain the body's fluid volume.

HYPONATREMIA Hyponatremia is a deficit in the extracellular level of sodium. With hyponatremia, there is either a sodium deficit or a water excess; a hypo-osmolar state exists because the ratio of water to sodium is too high. The water moves out of the vascular space into the interstitial space and then into the intracellular space, causing edema. The low extracellular serum sodium causes water to enter the cells in the brain, thereby producing cerebral edema as manifested by the cognitive and sensory changes listed in Table 33-4.

HYPERNATREMIA Hypernatremia is an excess in the extracellular level of sodium. With an excess of sodium or a loss of water, a hyperosmolar state exists because the ratio of sodium to water is too high. This ratio causes an increase in the extracellular osmotic pressure, which pulls fluid out of the cells into the extracellular space. The symptoms of this increase depend on the cause and the location of the edema (see Table 33-4).

Potassium

The normal range of extracellular potassium is narrow (3.5–5.0 mEq/L). The slightest decrease or increase can cause serious or life-threatening effects on physiological

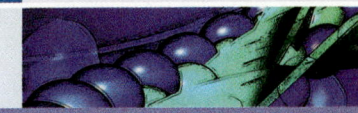

TABLE 33-4 The Clinical Management of Clients Experiencing Common Electrolyte Disturbances

DISTURBANCE AND CAUSES	CLINICAL MANIFESTATIONS	NURSING INTERVENTIONS
Hyponatremia		
Nutrition and metabolism • Low sodium intake • High water intake • Anorexia nervosa • Loss of gastrointestinal (GI) secretions (vomiting, diarrhea, bulimia, suctioning or drainage, tap-water enemas) • Loss of ECF sodium (peritonitis, burns) • Excessive ingestion of water or administration of intravenous (IV) solutions (D5W) • ECF sodium dilution (congestive heart failure [CHF], cirrhosis, nephrosis) Elimination • Advanced renal disorders • Diuretics • Antidiuretic hormone (ADH) • Syndrome of inappropriate antidiuretic hormone (SIADH)	1. Cognitive and sensory • Headaches • Apprehension • Lethargy • Confusion • Depression • Convulsion	Administer comfort measures as needed. Monitor level of consciousness. Institute safety measures for seizures.
	2. Activity and mobility • Muscular weakness	Assist with range of motion.
	3. Skin and mucous membranes • Dry, pale skin • Dry mucous membranes	Administer IV isotonic solution (0.9% NaCl) per order.
	4. Oxygenation and electrocardiogram (ECG) • Tachycardia • Hypotension	Monitor hourly vital signs and intake and output (I&O) (ECF excess, restrict fluids and administer diuretics).
	5. Nutrition and metabolism • Nausea • Vomiting • Diarrhea • Abdominal cramps	Monitor daily intake of sodium, and watch for water intoxication with SIADH (headaches and behavioral changes).
	6. Biochemical • Serum sodium < 135 mEq/L • Specific gravity < 1.008 • Serum osmolality < 280 mOsm/kg	Monitor serum sodium levels. Teach client about adequate intake of sodium, side effects of diuretics, and other causes for hyponatremia.
Hypernatremia		
Nutrition and metabolism • High sodium intake • Low water intake • Severe GI loss (diarrhea and vomiting) • Excessive insensible loss (perspiration) • Salt-water drowning • Administration of IV solutions (hypertonic or isotonic saline, sodium bicarbonate) • Hypertonic saline abortions Elimination • Renal dysfunction (nephritis) • Peritoneal dialysis with glucose solution	1. Cognitive and sensory • Restlessness • Agitation • Delirium • Twitching • Convulsions • Coma	Monitor the client's level of consciousness. Institute safety measures for seizures.
	2. Activity/mobility • ↑ Muscle tone • Hyperreflexia	Maintain body alignment and assist with movement.
	3. Skin and mucous membranes • Flushed, dry skin • Red, dry tongue • Sticky mucous membranes	Administer oral hygiene hourly.
	4. Oxygenation and ECG • Tachycardia	Monitor vital signs hourly.

(Continues)

TABLE 33-4 (Continued)

DISTURBANCE AND CAUSES	CLINICAL MANIFESTATIONS	NURSING INTERVENTIONS
• Uncompensated diabetes insipidus Hemostatic dysfunction • CHF (↓ cardiac output, ↓ renal flow, ↑ sodium retention) • Nephrotic syndrome and cirrhosis (↑ aldosterone leading to ↑ sodium retention)	5. Nutrition and metabolism • Nausea • Vomiting • Anorexia	Administer oral fluids or a parenteral hypotonic solution (0.3% NaCl) as ordered.
	6. Elimination • Polyuria (nephritis and uncompensated diabetes insipidus)	Monitor I&O hourly.
	7. Biochemical • Serum sodium > 146 mEq/L • Urine sodium > 40 mEq/L • Specific gravity < 1.025 • Serum osmolality > 295 mOsm/kg	Monitor laboratory findings. Teach client about foods high in sodium and about sodium-retaining drugs (cough medicines, cortisone, and laxatives with sodium).
Hypokalemia		
Nutrition and metabolism • Malnutrition • Starvation • Crash diets • Alcoholism • Anorexia nervosa • Stress • Licorice abuse • GI loss (vomiting, diarrhea, gastric or intestinal suctioning, intestinal fistula) • Nothing by mouth (NPO) and potassium-free IV fluids • Diabetes mellitus • Hyperaldosteronism • Adrenal tumor, cirrhosis, CHF Elimination • Laxative abuse • Bulimia • Enemas • Potassium-depleting diuretics (thiazide and furosemide) • Diuretic phase of acute renal failure • Dialysis • Steroids • Cushing's syndrome Skin and cellular integrity • Trauma • Tissue injury • Surgery Redistribution of potassium • Insulin • Alkalotic state • Healing phase of burns • Recovery from diabetic acidosis	1. Nutrition and metabolism • ↓ Motility (hypoactive → absent bowel sounds) • Abdominal distention • Paralytic ileus • Nausea • Vomiting	Administer potassium replacement therapy as ordered: • Oral potassium should be diluted in 4–8 oz of water or juice (↓ gastric mucosa irritation). • Dilute IV potassium 20–40 mEq in 1 L of IV fluids (irritating to blood vessels and myocardium). • Never administer bolus IV potassium. Monitor IV site for phlebitis and infiltration.
	2. Cognitive and sensory • Malaise • Disorientation • Coma • Loss of tactile discrimination	Monitor the client's level of consciousness.
	3. Activity and mobility • Muscle weakness • Hyporeflexia	Protect from injury.
	4. Elimination • Constipation • Polyuria	Monitor I&O hourly.
	5. Oxygenation and ECG • Diminished breath sounds • Shallow, rapid, ineffective respirations • Tachycardia • ↓ Peripheral pulses • Postural hypotension • ↑ Sensitivity to digitalis • ST depression • T wave inverted • U wave prominent • Heart block • Cardiac arrest (severe hypokalemia)	Monitor vital signs hourly. Monitor heart rate and rhythm. Monitor client closely for signs of digitalis toxicity (premature atrial and ventricular beats).

(Continues)

TABLE 33-4 (Continued)

DISTURBANCE AND CAUSES	CLINICAL MANIFESTATIONS	NURSING INTERVENTIONS

	6. Biochemical
	  • Serum potassium < 3.5 mEq/L
	  • Serum osmolality < 280 mOsm/L
		Teach client about potassium-rich foods and how to prevent excessive loss (abuse of laxatives and diuretics).

Hyperkalemia		

Nutrition and metabolism
  • Oral potassium supplement
  • IV potassium
Elimination
  • Acute and chronic renal failure
  • Potassium-sparing diuretics
  • Addison's disease
Skin and cellular integrity
  • Massive trauma and crushing injuries
  • Hemolysis
  • Tourniquet application
  • Phlebotomy
  • Burns
	1. Nutrition and metabolism
	  • Abdominal cramps (intermittent GI pain)
	  • Nausea
	  • Diarrhea
		Restrict oral and parenteral potassium intake as ordered. Administer cation-exchange resins (Kayexalate) to reduce serum potassium. Administer glucose and insulin parenteral solutions to facilitate movement of potassium into the cells as ordered.

	2. Activity and mobility
	  • Muscular weakness
	  • Paresthesia
	  • Muscle cramps and pain
		Assess for pain and provide comfort measures as indicated.

	3. Elimination • Oliguria or anuria	Monitor I&O hourly. Monitor client closely if receiving diuretics.

	4. Oxygenation and ECG
	  • Bradycardia → arrest
	  • T wave tented
	  • P wave small → nonvisible
	  • QRS complex widened
	  • Life-threatening dysrhythmias (supra-ventricular or ventricular tachycardia, premature ventricular beats, and ventricular fibrillation → arrest)
		Monitor vital signs and heart rhythm hourly for ECG changes. Institute safety measures when drawing blood:
		  • Leave tourniquet on for 1–2 minutes.
		  • Draw blood from vein away from all infusions.

	5. Biochemical
	  • Serum potassium > 5.3 mEq/L
	  • Serum osmolality > 295 mOsm/L
		If the client is to receive whole blood, indicate on the blood bank requisition the potassium level (blood 10 days or older has an elevated serum potassium due to hemolysis of aging blood). Teach client about potassium-rich foods, potassium-containing salt substitutes, and potassium-conserving diuretics.

Hypocalcemia		

Nutrition and metabolism
  • Inadequate dietary intake of calcium-rich foods (e.g., during pregnancy and lactation, when calcium requirements are high)
  • Poor vitamin D intake and absorption
	1. Cognitive and sensory
	  • Anxiety, irritability
	  • Tingling and numbness of fingers
	  • Tetany
	  • Convulsions
		Monitor client's state of sensorium for safety factors and breathing for laryngeal stridor.

(Continues)

TABLE 33-4 (Continued)

DISTURBANCE AND CAUSES	CLINICAL MANIFESTATIONS	NURSING INTERVENTIONS
• Associated disorders: hypoparathyroidism, pancreatitis, acute metabolic acidosis, and accidental surgical removal of parathyroid glands during a thyroidectomy Elimination • Diarrhea • Wound drainage	2. Activity and mobility • Abdominal and muscle cramps • Positive Trousseau's sign (carpopedal spasm with hypoxia) • Positive Chvostek's sign (contraction of facial muscles when facial nerve is tapped) • Pathologic fractures (persistent deficit)	Administer 10% IV solution of calcium gluconate; observe IV solutions with calcium for infiltration. Teach a diet high in calcium with vitamin D supplement. Administer calcium lactate orally.
	3. Oxygenation and ECG • ↓ Stroke volume • ECG changes: ST segment lengthened and prolonged PR interval	Monitor ECG for changes.
	4. Biochemical • ↓ Prothrombin • Serum calcium < 4.5 mEq/L (total) or < 8.5 mg/dL • Elevated serum phosphorus	

Hypercalcemia

Activity and mobility	1. Cognitive and sensory	Monitor client's state of sensorium
• Excessive movement of calcium out of bones: multiple fractures, bone tumors, immobility Nutrition and metabolism • Overconsumption of milk or dietary salts • Overactivity of parathyroid glands Elimination • Renal impairment • Thiazide diuretics • Steroid therapy	• Depression and lethargy	for safety.
	2. Activity and mobility • ↓ Muscle tone and deep tendon reflexes • Osteoporosis • Osteomalacia • Pathologic fractures • Deep bone pain	Encourage client movement and exercise. Assist client with movement to ↓ pain.
	3. Oxygenation and ECG • Heart block • Arrest (hypercalcemia crisis)	Monitor for ECG changes.
	4. Nutrition and metabolism • Nausea, vomiting, anorexia • Constipation	Teach client to ↓ calcium intake and ↑ fiber.
	5. Elimination • Flank pain from calculi • Polyuria	Encourage oral intake of acid-ash fluids to ↓ deposit of calcium salts.
	6. Biochemical • Serum calcium >5.5 mEq/L (total) or >10.5 mg/dL	Monitor for symptoms of digitalis toxicity; calcium enhances the action of digitalis.

Hypomagnesemia

Nutrition and metabolism	1. Cognitive and sensory	Monitor the client for seizure activity
• Prolonged inadequate dietary intake of magnesium (e.g., malnutrition and alcoholism) • Excessive losses of magnesium (e.g., vomiting, gastric suction)	• Disorientation, confusion • Vertigo • Irritability, tremors	and laryngeal stridor.

(Continues)

TABLE 33-4 (Continued)

DISTURBANCE AND CAUSES	CLINICAL MANIFESTATIONS	NURSING INTERVENTIONS

• Prolonged administration of IV solutions without magnesium additives
Elimination
• Severe renal disease
• Thiazide diuretics
• Aldosterone excess
• Polyuria
	2. Activity and mobility
	  • ↑ Tendon reflexes
	  • Positive Chvostek's & Trousseau's signs	

	3. Oxygenation and ECG
	  • ↑ BP
	  • Tachycardia
	  • Dysrhythmias
	  • T wave flat or inverted
	  • ST segment depressed
		Monitor for ECG changes and assess the client for digitalis toxicity.

	4. Biochemical • Serum magnesium < 1.5 mEq/L	Teach client to eat magnesium-rich foods and to avoid excessive use of laxatives and diuretics.

Hypermagnesemia

Nutrition and metabolism
• Excessive treatment of magnesium deficit
Elimination
• Renal failure
	1. Cognitive and sensory
	  • Lethargy, drowsiness
	  • Coma
		Monitor client for level of consciousness.

	2. Activity and mobility
	  • Muscle weakness, paralysis
	  • ↓ Deep-tendon reflexes
		Assess patellar reflexes; if absent, notify practitioner.

	3. Oxygenation and ECG
	  • ↓ Respirations, 10–12 per minute
	  • ↓ BP
	  • Bradycardia
	  • Atrioventricular block
	  • Respiratory and cardiac arrest (severe hypermagnesemia)
	  • QRS complex widening
	  • QT interval prolonged
		Monitor vital signs q15–30 minutes until stable and for ECG changes. Encourage fluids unless contraindicated to dilute the serum level of magnesium.
		Teach client about over-the-counter drugs with magnesium content.

	4. Biochemical • Serum magnesium > 2.5 mEq/L	

Hypophosphatemia

Nutrition and metabolism
• Inadequate intake: malnutrition, chronic alcoholism
• Prolonged administration of IV solutions that are phosphorus poor or phosphorus free
• Acid-base imbalances (e.g., diabetic ketoacidosis and respiratory alkalosis)
• Increased secretion of parathyroid hormone
• Overuse of aluminum-containing antacids
	1. Cognitive and sensory
	  • Confusion, seizures, coma
	  • Fatigue, memory loss
		Monitor client's level of consciousness.
		Institute safety measures for seizures.

	2. Activity and mobility
	  • Muscle pain, weakness
	  • Paresthesia
	  • Hyporeflexia
	  • Bone pain
	  • Joint stiffness
		Administer pain medications and other comfort measures.
		Assist the client in maintaining proper body alignment.

	3. Oxygenation and ECG
	  • Tissue hypoxia
	  • Hyperventilation
	  • Possible bleeding
	  • Weak pulse
		Monitor for bleeding and respiratory failure.

(Continues)

TABLE 33-4 (Continued)

DISTURBANCE AND CAUSES	CLINICAL MANIFESTATIONS	NURSING INTERVENTIONS
	4. Safety • Possible infection	Institute precautions to prevent infection.
	5. Nutrition and metabolism • Anorexia • Dysphagia	Teach client about phosphorus-rich foods and over-the-counter drugs that contain aluminum hydroxide.
	6. Biochemical • Serum phosphate < 1.7 mEq/L • ↓ Platelet count • ↓ Leukocyte • ↓ Oxygen saturation • ↑ Cardiac enzymes	Administer IV phosphate with caution: Dilute and infuse slowly to avoid phlebitis; infiltration at the IV site may cause tissue sloughing; do not infuse with calcium.
Hyperphosphatemia		
Nutrition and metabolism • Excessive administration of oral and IV solutions containing phosphate substances • Hypoparathyroidism • Laxatives containing phosphate Elimination • Renal insufficiency	1. Activity and mobility • Tetany • Muscle weakness • Flaccid paralysis • Circumoral paraesthesia • Hyperreflexia	Monitor for tetany and other signs of hypocalcemia.
	2. Oxygenation and ECG • Tachycardia • ST segment shortened • QT interval shortened	Monitor heart rate and assess for ECG changes.
	3. Nutrition and metabolism • Nausea, anorexia, vomiting, diarrhea	Administer calcium replacement. Monitor urinary output; 25 mL/hour will increase serum phosphorus level.
	4. Biochemical • Serum level > 2.6 mEq/L • ↓ Serum calcium	Teach client to avoid foods high in phosphorus (to read the labels on canned foods) and excessive use of phosphorus-containing laxatives and enemas.

Delmar/Cengage Learning

functions. A reciprocal relationship exists between sodium and potassium; large sodium intake results in an increased loss of potassium, and vice versa. When potassium is lost from the cells, sodium enters the cells. An intracellular potassium deficit may coexist with an excess of extracellular potassium. There are two main categories of diuretics that can cause hypokalemia: potassium-wasting and potassium-sparing diuretics.

HYPOKALEMIA Hypokalemia is a decrease in the extracellular level of potassium. GI tract disturbances and the use of diuretics can place the client at risk for hypokalemia and

an acid-base imbalance (metabolic alkalosis). Potassium-wasting diuretics can cause hypokalemia. Besides diuretics, other major drug groups that can cause hypokalemia are laxatives, corticosteroids, and antibiotics.

HYPERKALEMIA Hyperkalemia is an increase in the extracellular level of potassium. There are major drug groups that may cause hyperkalemia:

• Potassium-sparing diuretics
• Central nervous system agents
• Oral and intravenous (IV) replacement potassium salts

Hyperkalemia can also inhibit the action of digitalis.

▼ SAFETY FIRST ▼

HYPOKALEMIA

Hypokalemia can cause a cardiac arrest when:

- The potassium level is less than 2.5 mEq/L.
- The client is taking digitalis (a drug that strengthens the contraction of the myocardium and slows down the rate of the heart). *Hypokalemia enhances the action of the drug, causing toxicity.*

Calcium

Most of the body's calcium (99%) is deposited in bone as phosphate and carbonate. The remaining 1% is in the blood plasma (serum). Normally, 50% of the serum calcium is ionized (physiologically active), with the remaining 50% bound to protein. Free, ionized calcium is needed for cell membrane permeability. The calcium that is bound to plasma protein cannot pass through the capillary wall and therefore cannot leave the intravascular compartment. Approximately 50% of the serum calcium level is bound to protein. Correlate the serum calcium level with the serum albumin level when evaluating the laboratory results. *Any change in serum protein will result in a change in the total serum calcium.*

A stable blood level of calcium is maintained by a negative-feedback system controlled by vitamin D, parathyroid hormone, calcitonin (thyrocalcitonin), and the serum concentrations of calcium and phosphate ions. A decreased blood level stimulates the parathyroid gland to secrete parathyroid hormone, which in turn mobilizes the release of calcium from the bone, increases renal reabsorption, and increases intestinal absorption in the presence of vitamin D. Likewise, calcitonin, secreted by the thyroid gland, reduces the blood calcium concentration.

Calcium ions are never completely absorbed from the GI tract. Dietary calcium absorption and utilization require an adequate amount of protein and vitamin D. Besides being needed by the body for bone and tooth formation, calcium is an important ion in the blood-clotting mechanism and for maintaining the integrity of the neuromuscular system.

HYPOCALCEMIA Hypocalcemia is a decrease in the extracellular level of calcium. The rapid administration of citrated blood, alkalosis, and elevated levels of serum albumin

▼ SAFETY FIRST ▼

POTASSIUM CHLORIDE

Never administer more than 10 mEq of intravenous potassium chloride (KCl) per hour; the normal dose of intravenous KCl is 20–40 mEq/L to infuse over an 8-hour period.

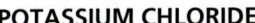

increase the activity of calcium binders, thereby decreasing the amount of free calcium.

HYPERCALCEMIA Hypercalcemia is an increase in the extracellular level of calcium. The clinical symptoms result from a decrease in neuromuscular activity, reabsorption of calcium from bone, and the kidney's response to a high serum calcium concentration. A rapid increase in the extracellular level of calcium (above 8–9 mEq/L) can trigger a hypercalcemic crisis. To prevent a hypercalcemic crisis, provide adequate hydration and administer diuretics, phosphate, or both as prescribed by the prescribing practitioner.

Magnesium

Magnesium plays an important role as a coenzyme in the metabolism of carbohydrates and proteins and as a mediator in neuromuscular activity. Magnesium has the unique characteristic of being the only cation that has a higher concentration in cerebrospinal fluid than in ECF.

HYPOMAGNESEMIA Hypomagnesemia is a decrease in the extracellular level of magnesium and usually occurs with hypokalemia and hypocalcemia. It is probably the most undiagnosed electrolyte deficit because it is asymptomatic until the serum level approaches 1.0 mEq/L; the normal range is 1.5–2.5 mEq/L (Kee, Paulanka, & Polek, 2010).

Drugs that may cause hypomagnesemia include digitalis, potassium-wasting diuretics, cortisone, aminoglycosides, and amphotericin B; the chronic use of laxatives may also cause the condition. The continuous use of total parenteral nutrition (TPN, hyperalimentation) without a magnesium supplement can cause hypomagnesemia. Clinical manifestations are related to the neuromuscular, neurologic, or cardiovascular system (see Table 33-4).

HYPERMAGNESEMIA Hypermagnesemia refers to an increase in the extracellular level of magnesium. It rarely occurs from excessive dietary ingestion; however, overuse of magnesium-containing drugs (antacids, laxatives, and IV magnesium sulfate) can cause hypermagnesemia. The clinical manifestations of hypermagnesemia are nonspecific (see Table 33-4).

Phosphate

Phosphate is the main intracellular anion; it appears as phosphorus in the serum. Phosphorus is similar to calcium in that vitamin D is needed for its reabsorption from the renal tubules.

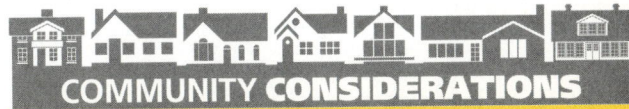

COMMUNITY **CONSIDERATIONS**

Intake of Phosphorus

When the dietary intake of calcium from milk is sufficient to meet minimal requirements, phosphorus needs will also be met. How will you educate clients who either cannot or will not consume an adequate daily intake of milk to meet their calcium and phosphorus needs?

HYPOPHOSPHATEMIA Hypophosphatemia is a decreased extracellular level of phosphorus. An increase in parathyroid hormone causes decreased renal reabsorption and increased excretion of phosphates. The aim of nursing care is to protect the client from injury and to correct the deficit (see Table 33-4).

HYPERPHOSPHATEMIA Hyperphosphatemia is an increased extracellular level of phosphorus. Excessive administration (oral or IV) of phosphate-containing substances can cause hyperphosphatemia. Other causes of hyperphosphatemia are hypoparathyroidism, renal insufficiency, and laxatives containing phosphate.

Chloride

As previously stated, chloride and water move in the same direction as sodium ions, influencing the osmolality of ECF. Although chloride losses usually follow sodium losses, the proportion will differ because a loss of chloride can be compensated for by an increase in bicarbonate. Therefore, signs and symptoms of a chloride imbalance will be similar to those of a metabolic acid-base imbalance, discussed later in this chapter. A deficit of either chloride or potassium will lead to a deficiency of the other electrolyte.

HYPOCHLOREMIA Hypochloremia is a decrease in the extracellular level of chloride. GI tract losses may cause a decrease in chloride because of the acid content of gastric juices, mainly hydrogen chloride. Because the bicarbonate ion compensates for the loss of chloride, the client is at risk for developing metabolic alkalosis. The signs and symptoms of hypochloremia are muscle twitching and slow, shallow breathing. With a severe loss of chloride and ECF volume, there may be a drop in blood pressure.

HYPERCHLOREMIA Hyperchloremia is an increase in the extracellular level of chloride. It usually occurs with dehydration, hypernatremia, and metabolic acidosis. The signs and symptoms of hyperchloremia are muscle weakness; deep, rapid breathing; and lethargy progressing to unconsciousness if untreated.

ACID-BASE DISTURBANCES

The common types of acid-base imbalances are respiratory acidosis and alkalosis and metabolic acidosis and alkalosis.

Laboratory Data

The biochemical indicators of acid-base imbalance are assessed by measurement of arterial blood gases (ABGs). ABGs measure the levels of oxygen and carbon dioxide in arterial blood. The levels of blood pH, bicarbonate ion, sodium, potassium, and chloride are also important in the assessment of acid-base imbalance.

In the determination of whether the acid-base imbalance is caused by a respiratory or a metabolic alteration, the key indicators are bicarbonate and carbonic acid levels (see Figure 33-6).

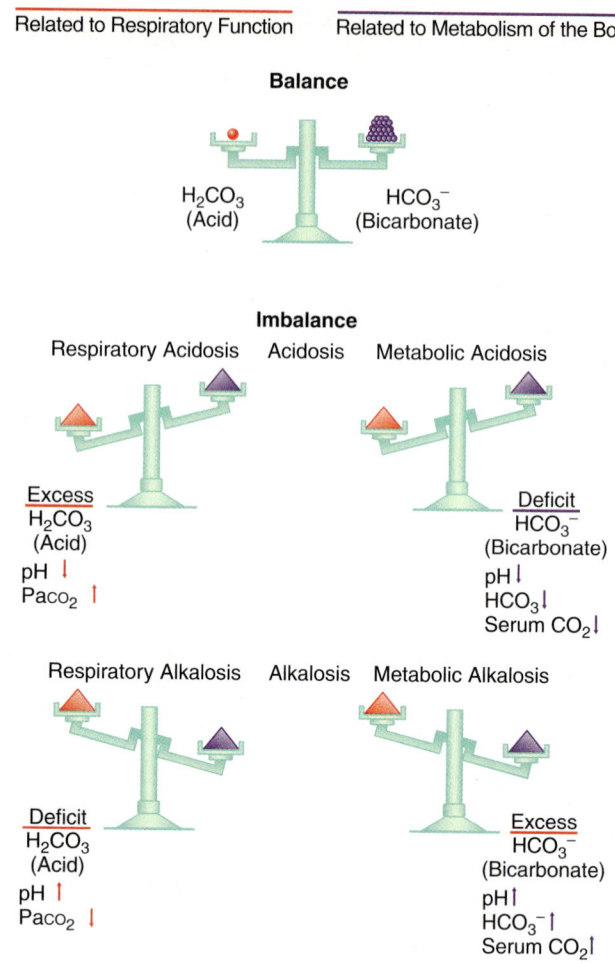

FIGURE 33-6 Acid-Base Balance and Imbalance. DELMAR/CENGAGE LEARNING

With respiratory acidosis and alkalosis, the bicarbonate level is normal and carbonic acid is either increased (acidosis) or decreased (alkalosis). With metabolic acidosis and alkalosis, the carbonic acid is normal and the bicarbonate level is either decreased (acidosis) or increased (alkalosis). Refer to Chapter 28 for a complete discussion of ABG analysis and to Chapter 32, Table 32-4, for normal values for ABGs.

Respiratory Acidosis (Carbonic Acid Excess)

Respiratory acidosis is characterized by an increased hydrogen ion concentration (a blood pH below 7.35), an increased arterial carbon dioxide pressure (greater than 45 mm Hg), and an excess of carbonic acid. Respiratory acidosis is caused by hypoventilation or any condition that depresses ventilation (see the accompanying display on common causes of respiratory acidosis on page 935).

Hypoventilation can begin in the respiratory system, as occurs with respiratory failure, or outside the respiratory system, as occurs with drug overdose. Common drugs that can cause central nervous system depression and place the client at risk for respiratory acidosis are narcotics, barbiturates, and anesthetic agents.

COMMON CAUSES OF ACUTE AND CHRONIC RESPIRATORY ACIDOSIS

Acute	Chronic
Drug-induced CNS depression	Asthma
Pneumonia and atelectasis	Cystic fibrosis
Pulmonary edema	Emphysema
Respiratory distress syndrome	
Pneumothorax	
Hypoventilation	
Poliomyelitis	
Chest trauma	
Brain and spinal cord injury	

Clients with respiratory acidosis experience neurologic changes resulting from the acidity of the cerebrospinal fluid and brain cells. Hypoventilation causes hypoxemia (decreased oxygen levels), which causes further neurologic impairments; refer to Chapter 32 for a complete discussion of hypoxemia. Hyperkalemia may accompany acidosis. See Table 33-5 on page 936 for the clinical manifestations and nursing interventions used to treat respiratory acidosis.

Respiratory Alkalosis (Carbonic Acid Deficit)

Respiratory alkalosis is characterized by a decreased hydrogen ion concentration (a blood pH above 7.45) and a decreased arterial carbon dioxide pressure (less than 35 mm Hg). Respiratory alkalosis is caused by hyperventilation (excessive exhalation of carbon dioxide) resulting in hypocapnia (decreased arterial carbon dioxide concentration). Hyperventilation can be triggered by hypoxia at high altitudes, anxiety, fear, pain, fever, and rapid mechanical ventilation. Other causes of hyperventilation, which involve overstimulation of the respiratory center, include salicylate poisoning, hyperthyroidism, pneumonia, atelectasis, asthma, adult respiratory distress syndrome, congestive heart failure, pulmonary edema and embolus, brain tumors, meningitis, and encephalitis; see Table 33-5 for the clinical manifestations and treatment.

Metabolic Acidosis (Bicarbonate Deficit)

Metabolic acidosis is characterized by a decrease in hydrogen ion concentration (blood pH below 7.35) or a decrease in bicarbonate concentration. Causes of metabolic acidosis can be divided into two categories: loss of base and gain in metabolic acids. Chronic diarrhea causes an excessive loss of bicarbonate and sodium ions from the small intestines. With the loss of sodium ions, chloride ions are in excess and combine with hydrogen to produce a strong acid (hydrochloric acid).

Clients with certain medical diagnoses are at risk for metabolic acidosis. Such conditions include:

1. Diabetic ketoacidosis: The cells are deprived of glucose (decrease or absence of insulin) for metabolism; the liver, in response to the needs of the cells, increases the metabolism of fatty acids, which causes an increase in ketone bodies, making the ECF more acidic.
2. Renal failure: The normal mechanism of the kidneys to conserve sodium and water and excrete hydrogen is compromised.
3. Anaerobic metabolism: Cellular catabolism and acid accumulation occur with starvation, severe malnutrition, infection, fever, trauma, shock, and excessive exercise.
4. Drug overdose: Acid accumulation results from excessive ingestion of salicylate, paraldehyde, and methanol.

In response to metabolic acidosis, the respiratory center is stimulated, causing an increase in the rate and depth of respirations (Kussmaul breathing), to lower the acid concentration in ECF by increasing the exhalation of carbon dioxide. The respiratory compensatory mechanism is usually ineffective in decreasing acids, especially if the client has chronic obstructive pulmonary disease or is in ketoacidosis. Metabolic acidosis causes an electrolyte shift: Hydrogen and sodium ions move into the cell, and potassium moves into the ECF. Hyperkalemia may cause ventricular fibrillation and death. Refer to Chapter 32 for additional information on these diagnoses. The renal compensatory mechanism tries to increase the pH by exchanging sodium ions with hydrogen ions to increase the excretion of hydrogen; refer to Table 33-5 for the clinical manifestations and treatment of metabolic acidosis.

Metabolic Alkalosis (Bicarbonate Excess)

Metabolic alkalosis is characterized by an increased loss of acid from the body or a gain in base (increased levels of bicarbonate). The blood pH is above 7.45. A gain in base may result from excessive ingestion of antacids. These substances neutralize acids, producing alkalosis and hypercalcemia. The excessive oral or parenteral administration of sodium bicarbonate or other alkaline salts (e.g., sodium or potassium acetate, lactate, or citrate) increases the amount of base in ECFs.

The following clinical conditions can place clients at risk for metabolic alkalosis:

1. Vomiting and nasogastric suctioning or lavage cause a loss in hydrochloric acid and chloride; with the loss of the hydrogen and chloride ions, bicarbonate ions are absorbed, unneutralized, into the bloodstream and the pH of the ECF rises (alkalosis).
2. Diarrhea and steroid or diuretic therapy can cause excessive loss of potassium, chloride, and other electrolytes; the potassium deficit causes the kidneys to exchange hydrogen ions (instead of potassium ions) for sodium ions, which promotes the loss of hydrogen, thereby increasing bicarbonate level. Hydrochlorothiazide, a thiazide diuretic, blocks the reabsorption of sodium in the cortex in the distal tubule, causing sodium to be excreted in greater amounts than water (hyponatremia). Thiazides also cause hypokalemia because of the loss of urinary potassium. The secondary effects of thiazides lead to metabolic alkalosis because of a depletion in volume, chloride, potassium, and hydrogen ions (Smeltzer, Bare, Hinkle, & Cheevee, 2008).

TABLE 33-5 Respiratory and Metabolic Acidosis and Alkalosis

IMBALANCE AND CAUSES	CLINICAL MANIFESTATIONS	NURSING INTERVENTIONS
Respiratory acidosis (retention of carbon dioxide)		

• CNS disorders
• Drug overdose
• Pneumonia
• Pulmonary edema
• Pneumothorax
• Restrictive lung disease
	1. Cognitive and sensory
	  • Disorientation
	  • Depression
	  • Weakness → stupor
		1. Institute safety measures.
		  Assist with positioning.

	2. Skin and mucous membranes • Flushed and warm	2. Monitor I&O, and administer fluids as ordered.

	3. Oxygenation and ECG
	  • Dyspnea
	  • Tachycardia
	  • Dysrhythmia
		3. Administer oxygen and medications per order; monitor hourly vital signs and respiratory status (may require mechanical ventilation).

	4. Biochemical
	  • ↓ pH (<7.35)
	  • ↑ $Paco_2$ (>45 mm Hg)
	  • ↑ HCO_3^- (>28 mEq/L, indicating metabolic renal compensation)
		4. Monitor arterial blood gases (ABGs), pH, $Paco_2$, HCO_3^-.

Respiratory alkalosis (hyperventilation)		

• Anxiety, fear
• CNS disorders
• Pain
• Fever
• Pneumonia, atelectasis
• Asthma
• Adult respiratory distress syndrome (ARDS)
• Congestive heart failure, pulmonary edema
• Pulmonary embolus
	1. Cognitive and sensory
	  • Hyperactive reflexes
	  • Tetany
	  • Positive Chvostek's sign
	  • Positive Trousseau's sign
	  • Vertigo
	  • Unconsciousness
		1. Institute safety measures for the client with vertigo or the unconscious client. Encourage the anxious client to verbalize fears. Administer sedation as ordered to relax the client.

	2. Skin and mucous membranes • Sweating (may occur)	2. Keep the client warm and dry.

	3. Oxygenation and ECG
	  • Rapid, shallow breathing
	  • Palpitations
		3. Encourage the client to take deep, slow breaths or breathe into a brown paper bag (inspire CO_2). Monitor vital signs.

	4. Biochemical (uncompensated respiratory alkalosis)
	  • ↑ pH (>7.45)
	  • ↓ $Paco_2$ (<35 mm Hg)
		4. Monitor ABGs, primarily $Paco_2$, a value < 35 mm Hg indicates too little CO_2 (e.g., carbonic acid).

Metabolic acidosis (gain of metabolic acids or loss of base)		

Increased acids:
• Renal failure
• Diabetic ketoacidosis
• Anaerobic metabolism
• Drug overdose (salicylates, methanol)
Loss of base:
• Diarrhea
	1. Cognitive and sensory
	  • Restlessness, disorientation
	  • Stupor, coma
		1. Institute safety measures. Monitor client's sensorium; report alteration in level of consciousness.

	2. Activity and mobility • Weakness, lethargy	2. Assist the client with positioning and proper body alignment.
	3. Skin and mucous membranes • Warm, flushed skin	3. Keep the client comfortable.
	4. Oxygenation and ECG	4. Monitor vital signs and I&O.

(Continues)

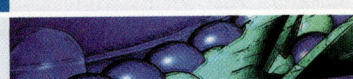

TABLE 33-5 (continued)

IMBALANCE AND CAUSES	CLINICAL MANIFESTATIONS	NURSING INTERVENTIONS
	• Kussmaul breathing (deep, rapid respirations) • Bradycardia, decreased cardiac output • Dysrhythmias	Monitor and report cardiac dysrhythmias. Administer sodium bicarbonate and fluid replacement as ordered.
	5. Nutrition and metabolism • Nausea, vomiting • Abdominal pain	5. Provide comfort measures. Correct metabolic problem as ordered.
	6. Biochemical • ↓ pH (<7.35) • ↓ HCO_3^- (<24 mEq/L) • ↓ BE (base excess <2 mEq/L) • ↓ Serum CO_2 (<22 mEq/L)	6. Monitor ABGs and evaluate the metabolic indicators (HCO_3^- and BE).
Metabolic alkalosis (gain of base or loss of metabolic acids)		
Gain of base: • Excess ingestion of antacids • Excess administration of sodium bicarbonate Loss of metabolic acids: • Vomiting • Nasogastric suctioning or lavage • Low potassium or chloride • Increased aldosterone • Administration of steroids or diuretics	1. Cognitive and sensory • Irritability, confusion	1. Monitor the client's sensorium, and report increasing mental confusion.
	2. Activity and mobility • Tetany • Hypertonic muscles • Hypertonic reflexes	2. Institute safety and comfort measures. Report symptoms of tetany.
	3. Oxygenation and ECG • Depressed rate and depth of respirations	3. Monitor vital signs, and report changes in the client's respiratory status.
	4. Nutrition and metabolism • Vomiting	4. Monitor I&O, recording amount of fluid loss from vomiting and gastric suctioning. Administer intravenous sodium chloride solutions (0.45%–0.9%) as ordered.
	5. Biochemical • ↑ pH (>7.45) • ↑ HCO_3^- (>28 mEq/L) • ↑ BE (base excess <2 mEq/L) • ↓ Serum levels of potassium and chloride	5. Monitor ABGs and evaluate the metabolic indicators (HCO_3^- and BE).

Kee, J., Paulanka, B., & Polek, C. (2010). *Fluids and electrolytes with clinical applications: A programmed approach* (8th ed.). Clifton Park, NY: Delmar/Cengage Learning.

The respiratory and renal compensatory mechanisms respond to an increased bicarbonate–carbonic acid ratio. The rate and depth of respirations are decreased in an effort to retain carbon dioxide. The arterial carbon dioxide concentration rises, creating respiratory acidosis, to counter the pH imbalance of metabolic alkalosis.

A normal serum potassium level is a prerequisite to renal compensation. In alkalosis, potassium ions enter the cells in exchange for hydrogen ions, causing hypokalemia. Hypokalemia further potentiates metabolic alkalosis because the kidneys conserve hydrogen ions by excreting potassium ions in exchange for sodium ions. When hypokalemia is present, the kidneys cannot function as a compensatory mechanism; therefore, they continue to excrete hydrogen, and bicarbonate excess continues. See Table 33-5 for the clinical manifestations and treatment of metabolic alkalosis.

ASSESSMENT

Assessment data are used to identify clients who have potential or actual alterations in fluid volume. Clients receiving certain treatments, such as medications and IV therapy, are at risk for developing imbalances. The key nursing assessment indicators that identify imbalances are daily weights, vital signs, intake and output, and the physical findings of the skin, oral cavity, eyes, venous filling, and neuromuscular system.

Health History

The nursing history should elicit data specific to fluids:

- Lifestyle (sociocultural and economic factors, stress, exercise)
- Dietary intake (recent changes in the amount and types of fluid and food, increased thirst)
- Religion (whether illness has had an effect on beliefs or religion; query whether the client would like a visit from a religious counselor)
- Weight (sudden gain or loss)
- Fluid output (recent changes in the frequency or amount of urine output)
- GI disturbances (prolonged vomiting, diarrhea, anorexia, ulcers, hemorrhage)
- Fever and diaphoresis
- Draining wounds, burns, trauma
- Disease conditions that could upset homeostasis (renal disease, endocrine disorders, neural malfunction, pulmonary disease)
- Therapeutic programs that can produce imbalances (special diets, medications, chemotherapy, administration of IV fluid or TPN, gastric or intestinal suction)

Physical Examination

The nurse performs a complete physical examination and identifies all abnormalities because fluid alterations may affect any body system. The physical assessment of clients with altered fluid status is discussed in this section. Refer to Chapter 26 for procedures on weight and vital sign measurement.

Daily Weight

Changes in the body's total fluid volume are indicated by weight; for instance, each kilogram (2.2 lb) of weight gained or lost is equivalent to 1 L (1000 mL) of fluid gained or lost. Accurate measurement of daily weight requires the nurse to implement the agency's protocol to control certain variables. For example, the nurse should obtain the measurement at the same time each day, using the same scale.

Vital Signs

Measurement of vital signs provides the nurse with information regarding the client's fluid, electrolyte, and acid-base status and the body's compensatory response for maintaining balance. An elevated temperature places the client at risk for dehydration caused by an increased loss of body fluid.

Changes in the pulse rate, strength, and rhythm are indicative of fluid alterations. Fluid volume alterations may cause the following pulse changes:

- Fluid volume deficit (FVD): increased pulse rate and weak pulse volume
- Fluid volume excess (FVE): increased pulse volume and third heart sound

Respiratory changes are assessed by inspecting the movement of the chest wall, counting the rate, and auscultating the lungs. Changes in the rate and depth may cause respiratory acid-base imbalances or may be indicative of a compensatory response in metabolic acidosis or alkalosis, as previously discussed in Table 33-5.

Blood pressure measurements can be used to assess the degree of FVD. FVD can lower the blood pressure with or without orthostatic hypotension. A narrow pulse pressure (less than 20 mm Hg) may indicate FVD that occurs with severe hypovolemia.

Intake and Output

Measure and record the client's intake and output for a 24-hour period to assess for an actual or potential imbalance. A minimum intake of 1500 mL is essential to balance urinary output and the body's insensible water loss. Intake includes all liquids (e.g., ice cream, soup, gelatin, juice, and water) taken by mouth and liquids administered through tube feedings (nasogastric or jejunostomy) and parenterally (IV fluids and blood or its components). Output includes urine, diarrhea, vomitus, and drainage from tubes such as through gastric suction. The recording of intake and output data is usually referred to as the I&O.

Thirst The most common indicator of FVD is thirst. With a decrease in ECF volume or an increase in the plasma osmolality, the hypothalamus triggers a thirst response. Older adults are prone to a FVD (dehydration) because the thirst mechanism in the medulla becomes less responsive with aging.

Food Intake The intake of food also contributes to maintaining ECF volume. One-third of the body's fluid needs are met by ingested food. Food also provides the body with necessary electrolytes. See Chapter 34 for a complete discussion of metabolism.

Edema

Edema, the detectable accumulation of increased interstitial fluid, is the main symptom of FVE. Edema may be localized (confined to a specific area) or generalized (occurring throughout the body's tissue). Localized edema is characterized by taut, smooth, shiny, pale skin. The body may retain 5 to 10 lb of fluid before edema is noticeable. Inspect the dependent body parts—sacrum, back, and legs—to assess peripheral edema. Pitting edema is rated on a 4-point scale:

- +0, no pitting
- +1, 0″–1/4″ pitting (mild)
- +2, 1/4″–1/2″ pitting (moderate)
- +3, 1/2″–1″ pitting (severe)
- +4, greater than 1″ pitting (severe)

Skin Turgor

Skin turgor is the normal resiliency of the skin. When the skin is pinched and released, it springs back to a normal position because of the outward pressure exerted by the cells and interstitial fluid. To measure the client's skin turgor, grasp and raise the skin with two fingers as follows:

- Adults: over the sternum, forehead, or inner aspect of the thigh. With aging, there are fewer elastic fibers in the skin, resulting in reduced skin turgor. Assess the tongue for creases or furrows to monitor dehydration in older adults.
- Children: over the abdominal area or medial aspect of the thigh.

With dehydration there is a decreased skin turgor, as manifested by lax skin that returns slowly to the normal position. Increased skin turgor, which occurs with edema, is manifested by smooth, taut, shiny skin that cannot be grasped and raised.

Buccal (Oral) Cavity

Inspect the buccal cavity. With FVD, there is a decrease in saliva, which causes sticky, dry mucous membranes and dry cracked lips. The tongue has longitudinal furrows.

Eyes

Inspect the eyes. FVD causes sunken eyes, dry conjunctiva, and decreased or absent tearing. Puffy eyelids (periorbital edema, or papilledema) are characteristic of FVE; the client may also have a history of blurred vision.

Jugular and Hand Veins

Circulatory volume is assessed by measuring venous filling of the jugular and hand veins. Place the client in a low Fowler's position. Then:

1. Palpate the jugular (neck) veins: FVE causes a distention in the jugular veins (see Figure 33-7).
2. Place the client's hand below the heart level, and palpate the jugular veins; with FVD there is decreased venous filling (flat neck veins).

Neuromuscular System

Fluid and electrolyte imbalances may cause neuromuscular alterations: The muscles lose their tone and become soft and underdeveloped, and reflexes are diminished. Calcium and magnesium imbalances cause an increase in neuromuscular irritability. To assess for neuromuscular irritability, perform the following tests:

1. Chvostek's sign: Tap the facial nerve 2 cm anterior to the earlobe; unilateral twitching of the facial muscles (inclusive of the eyelids and lips) indicates a positive response (see Figure 33-8).
2. Trousseau's sign: Place a blood pressure cuff on the arm, inflate the cuff slightly above the systolic pressure, leave the cuff inflated 2–3 minutes, and deflate; carpal spasm or tetany indicates a positive response.

A positive Chvostek's sign and Trousseau's sign may occur with hypocalcemia and hypomagnesemia.

Other neurologic signs include inability to concentrate, confusion, and emotional lability, as previously discussed in Tables 5-4 and 5-5.

DIAGNOSTIC AND LABORATORY DATA

Biochemical assessment is another essential source of objective data. Laboratory results can be used to detect imbalances before clinical symptoms are assessed in the physical examination. Laboratory tests used in assessing clients with common alterations in ECF volume are discussed next; refer to Chapter 28 for the normal values presented in this section.

Hemoglobin and Hematocrit Indices

The hematocrit is affected by changes in plasma volume. For instance, with severe dehydration and hypovolemic shock,

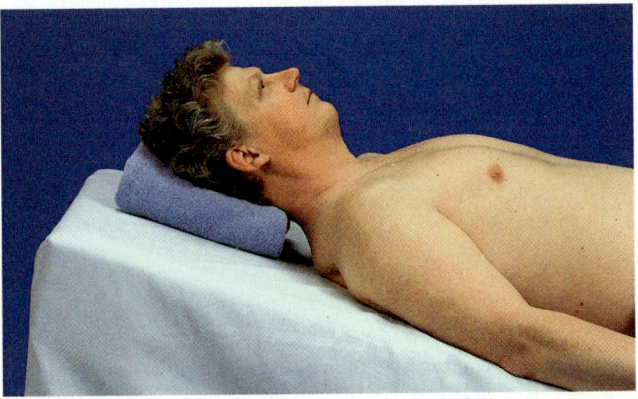

FIGURE 33-7 Positioning the Client to Assess Jugular Vein Distention DELMAR/CENGAGE LEARNING

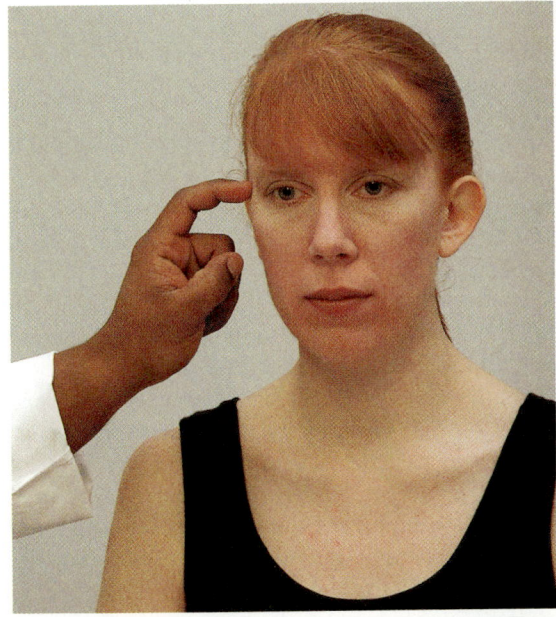

FIGURE 33-8 Assessing for Chvostek's Sign DELMAR/CENGAGE LEARNING

the hematocrit is increased, whereas overhydration decreases the hematocrit. Hemoglobin levels are decreased with severe hemorrhage.

Osmolality

Osmolality is a measurement of the total concentration of dissolved particles (solutes) per kilogram of water. Osmolality measurements are performed on both serum and urine samples to determine alterations in fluid and electrolyte balance. Osmolality can also be explained in relation to the specific gravity of body fluids. Specific gravity expresses the weight of the solution when compared with an equal volume of distilled water; the osmolality of a solution can be estimated by the specific gravity.

SERUM OSMOLALITY   Serum osmolality is a measurement of the total concentration of dissolved particles per kilogram of water in serum, recorded in milliosmoles per kilogram (mOsm/kg). The particles measured in serum osmolality include electrolyte ions, such as sodium and potassium, and electrically inactive substances dissolved in serum, such as glucose and urea. Water and sodium are the main entities that control the osmolality of body fluids. Serum sodium is responsible for 85% to 90% of the serum osmolality.

The normal serum osmolality is 275 to 295 mOsm/kg (Fischbach, 2008). It can increase with dehydration and loss of body water and decrease with water excess.

In clinical practice, the terms *osmolality* and **osmolarity**, the concentration of solutes per liter of cellular fluid, are often used interchangeably to refer to the concentration of body fluid. However, these terms are actually different: Osmolality refers to the concentration of solutes in the total body water (solutes per kilogram of body weight) rather than in cellular fluid. Figure 33-9 relates osmosis to the osmolality of a solution. The appropriate term to use in IV fluid therapy is *osmolarity* (Smeltzer et al., 2008). An osmolar solution is described as:

- **Hypotonic** (hypo-osmolar) when there are fewer solutes in proportion to the volume of water than is the case in the body
- **Isotonic** (iso-osmolar) when body water and solutes (sodium) are in amounts equal to those in the body
- **Hypertonic** (hyperosmolar) when there are more solutes in proportion to the volume of water than is the case in the body

URINE OSMOLALITY   Urine osmolality is a measurement of the total concentration of dissolved particles per kilogram of water in urine, recorded in milliosmoles per kilogram (mOsm/kg). The particles measured in urine osmolality come from nitrogenous waste (creatinine, urea, and uric acid), with urea contributing most. Urine osmolality is a more accurate indicator of hydration than is the specific gravity of urine. Urine osmolality varies greatly with diet and fluid intake and reflects the ability of the kidneys to adjust the concentration of urine in order to maintain fluid balance. Some medications and the presence of protein and glucose

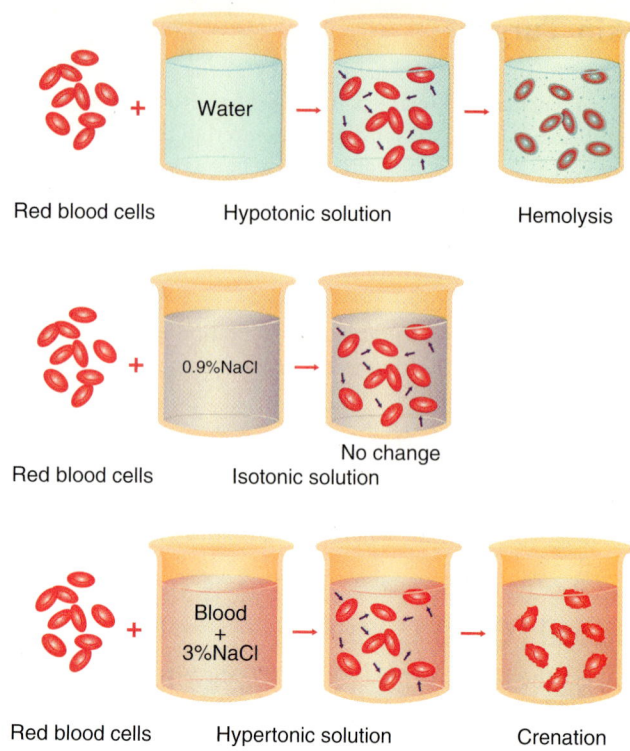

FIGURE 33-9 Osmosis as it relates to the osmolarity of a solution. The movement of water through a membrane from a lower concentration to a higher concentration is called osmosis. In a hypotonic solution, the water moves into the cells, causing them to swell and burst. The cells in the isotonic solution are normal in size and shape because the same amount of water is entering and leaving the cells. Cells in the hypertonic solution are losing water because water moves from a weaker concentration inside the cell to a greater concentration outside the cell membrane.
DELMAR/CENGAGE LEARNING

solutes in the urine can give a false high specific gravity reading. With normal kidney function, a dehydrated client will have an elevated urine osmolality, whereas clients with shock, hyperglycemia, hemoconcentration, and acidosis will have elevations in both urine and serum osmolality.

Urine pH

The measurement of the pH of urine reveals the hydrogen ion concentration of the urine to determine its acid or alkaline status. When the kidney buffering system is compensating for either metabolic acidosis or alkalosis, the pH of the urine should be within normal range (4.6–8.0). This is considered a sign of normal function. However, when the renal compensatory function fails to respond to the pH of the blood, the urine pH will increase with acidosis and decrease in alkalosis.

Serum Albumin

Albumin is synthesized in the liver from amino acids. Serum albumin plays an important role in fluid and electrolyte balance by maintaining the colloid osmotic pressure of blood, which prevents the accumulation of fluid (edema) in the tissues. However, serum albumin has a half-life of 21 days and fluctuates according to the level of hydration; therefore, it is not a good indicator of acute alterations in protein depletion. Clinically, this blood test is used to measure prolonged protein depletion, which occurs in chronic malnutrition. Refer to Chapter 34 for a discussion of serum albumin and prealbumin.

NURSING DIAGNOSIS

"Fluid volume, pressure, and levels of sodium and albumin are keys to maintaining fluid balances between the intracellular and extracellular (intravascular and interstitial) spaces. Capillary permeability and the lymphatic system also play a role" (Holcomb, 2008, p. 50). In order to make a nursing diagnosis, the nurse must be able to interpret assessment and biochemical data and draw conclusions relative to the client's imbalance. The primary nursing diagnoses for clients with fluid imbalances are presented in the accompanying display on nursing diagnoses for fluid alterations.

EXCESS FLUID VOLUME

Excess fluid volume (EFV) exists when the client has increased interstitial and intravascular fluid retention and edema. EFV is related to the excess fluid either in tissues of the extremities (peripheral edema) or in lung tissues (pulmonary edema). Factors that put the client at risk for EFV are:

- Excessive intake of fluids (e.g., IV therapy, sodium)
- Increased loss or decreased intake of protein (chronic diarrhea, burns, kidney disease, malnutrition)
- Compromised regulatory mechanisms (kidney failure)
- Decreased intravascular movement (impaired myocardial contractility)
- Lymphatic obstruction (cancer, surgical removal of lymph nodes, obesity)
- Medications (steroid excess)
- Allergic reaction

Assessment findings in the client with FVE include acute weight gain; decreased serum osmolality (less than 275 mOsm/kg), protein and albumin, blood urea nitrogen (BUN), hemoglobin (hgb), and hematocrit (HCT); increased central venous pressure (greater than 12–15 cm H$_2$O); and signs and symptoms of edema. The clinical manifestations of edema are relative to the area of involvement, either pulmonary or peripheral (see the accompanying display on clinical manifestations of edema).

CLINICAL MANIFESTATIONS OF EDEMA

Pulmonary Edema	Peripheral Edema
Constant cough	Pitting edema in extremities
Dyspnea	Edematous area: tight, smooth, shiny, pale, cool skin
Engorged neck and hand veins	
Moist crackles in lungs	Puffy eyelids
Bounding pulse	Weight gain

DEFICIENT FLUID VOLUME

Deficient fluid volume (DFV) exists when the client experiences vascular, interstitial, or intracellular dehydration. The degree of dehydration is classified as mild, marked, severe, or fatal on the basis of the percentage of body weight lost. There are three types of dehydration based on the proportion of fluid and particles in the intracellular and extracellular spaces:

- *Isotonic dehydration* (hypovolemia) refers to the loss of both fluid and particles in the vascular space that occurs with vomiting, diarrhea, and bleeding; it is the most common form of dehydration, especially in infants and children.
- *Hypertonic dehydration* refers to a greater loss of fluid than particles in the vascular space when the body tries to maintain a normalized isotonic state by pulling fluids from the intracellular space into the vascular space; it occurs in diabetic ketoacidosis, renal insufficiency, and the administration of hypertonic solutions.
- *Hypotonic dehydration* refers to a greater loss of particles than fluid in the vascular space when the body tries to maintain a normal isotonic state by pushing fluids from the vascular space into the intracellular space, causing the cells to swell; it occurs in chronic disease states and with the administration of hypotonic solutions.

Assessment findings in the client with DFV include thirst and weight loss, with the amount varying with the degree of dehydration. With marked dehydration, the mucous membranes and skin are dry. There is poor skin turgor; low-grade temperature elevation; tachycardia; respirations 28 or greater; a decrease (10–15 mm Hg) in systolic blood pressure; slowing in venous filling; a decrease in urine (less than 25 mL per hour); concentrated urine; elevated HCT, hgb, and BUN; and an acid blood pH (less than 7.4).

Severe dehydration is characterized by the symptoms of marked dehydration. Also, the skin becomes flushed. The systolic blood pressure continues to drop (60 mm Hg or below). There are behavioral changes (restlessness, irritability, disorientation, and delirium). The signs of fatal dehydration are anuria and coma that leads to death.

RISK FOR DEFICIENT FLUID VOLUME

Risk for FVD exists when the client is at high risk of developing vascular, interstitial, or intracellular dehydration resulting from active or regulatory losses of body water in excess of needs. Clients who lose excessive amounts of gastric juices, either through vomiting or suctioning, are prone to develop not only DFV but also metabolic alkalosis, hypokalemia, and hyponatremia; gastric juices contain hydrochloric acid, pepsinogen, potassium, and sodium. The multiple factors that can place the client at risk for FVD are listed in the preceding accompanying display, Nursing Diagnoses for Fluid Alterations.

OTHER NURSING DIAGNOSES

The relationship between the primary nursing diagnoses just discussed and the secondary diagnoses in clients with fluid

NURSING DIAGNOSES FOR FLUID ALTERATIONS

Excess Fluid Volume Related to:

- Excessive fluid intake secondary to excess sodium intake
- Compromised regulatory mechanism (renal and cardiac dysfunction)
- Inaccurate intravenous infusion rate

Deficient Fluid Volume Related to:

- Excessive fluid loss secondary to vomiting, blood loss, surgical drains and tubes, diarrhea, and diuretics

Risk for Deficient Fluid Volume Related to:

- Extremes of age (very young or old) and weight
- NPO and fluid restrictions
- Increased fluid output from normal routes: vomiting, diarrhea, urine
- Increased fluid losses from drainage or suction routes: wounds, drains, indwelling tubes (e.g., urine catheter, nasogastric suction)
- Loss of plasma associated with severe trauma and burns
- Disorders that impair fluid intake or absorption (immobility, unconsciousness)
- Chronic disorders: congestive heart failure, pulmonary edema, chronic obstructive lung disease, renal failure, diabetes, cancer, transplant candidates
- Deficient knowledge related to factors influencing fluid requirements (hypermetabolic states, hyperthermia, and dry, hot environment)
- Medications (e.g., diuretics)

imbalances is reciprocal: The primary diagnoses influence and are influenced by the secondary diagnoses. Holistic nursing requires that all diagnoses relative to a client be considered when developing a client's plan of care.

Impaired Gas Exchange

Impaired gas exchange related to a ventilation perfusion imbalance occurs when clients experience a decreased passage of oxygen or carbon dioxide between the alveoli of the lungs and the vascular system. This alteration is assessed by measuring the oxygen and carbon dioxide content through ABG analysis, pulse oximetry, or both. Refer to Chapter 32 for further discussion of oxygenation.

Decreased Cardiac Output

Decreased cardiac output occurs when the blood pumped by a client's heart is reduced so much that it is inadequate to meet the needs of the body's tissue. This alteration may be caused by heart failure and various types of shock. Assessment findings may include low blood pressure; cool, clammy skin; weak, thready pulses; decreased urinary output; and a diminished level of consciousness.

Risk for Infection

Many disorders may place the client at risk for invasion by pathogenic organisms. Clients receiving IV therapy are at risk for an infection because their primary defense, the skin, is broken at the puncture site. Assessment findings indicative of IV site infection are client complaints of soreness around the site, erythema, swelling at the site, and foul-smelling discharge.

Impaired Oral Mucous Membrane

Altered oral mucous membrane occurs when a client experiences disruption in the tissue layers of the oral cavity. It is frequently related to dehydration. Assessment findings may include oral pain or discomfort, stomatitis, and decreased salivation.

Deficient Knowledge

A knowledge deficit may exist to varying degrees in clients with fluid imbalances. Information obtained from a client's health history may indicate the client's level of understanding and perception of these alterations and direct teaching. Clients need to participate actively in their plans of care.

PLANNING AND OUTCOMES

Holistic nursing care for clients experiencing fluid imbalances requires that the nurse, in collaboration with each client, identify specific goals for the nursing diagnosis. These goals should be individualized to reflect the client's capabilities and limitations and should be appropriate to the diagnosis as determined by the assessment data.

The *Nursing Outcomes Classification* (NOC) (Moorhead, Johnson, Swanson, & Maas, 2008) has five outcome classifications in the physiologic health (II) domain regarding fluid and electrolytes:

1. Nutritional Status: Food and Fluid Intake (1008). The rating scale is from not adequate to totally adequate, and the indicators that monitor food and fluid intake (oral, tube feeding, infusions) (p. 413).
2. Electrolyte and Acid/Base Balance (0600). The rating scale is from severely compromised to not compromised, and the indicators that monitor vital signs; serum electrolytes, urine pH, and specific gravity; and cognitive and neuromuscular response (p. 265).
3. Fluid Balance (0601). The rating scale is from severely compromised to not compromised, and the indicators that monitor I&O, weight, pressures, pulses, and serum electrolytes (p. 295).

4. Fluid Overload Severity (0603). The rating scale is from severe to none, and the indicators that monitor for edema, increased blood pressure and weight, and changes in cognition function and serum sodium (p. 297).

5. Hydration (0602). The rating scale is from severely compromised to not compromised, and the indicators that monitor adequate fluid intake, skin turgor, moist mucous membranes, output, serum sodium, and cognitive function (p. 314).

During the planning phase, the nurse also selects and prioritizes nursing interventions to support the client's achievement of expected outcomes based on the goals. For example, if vomiting and diarrhea, with a weight loss of 5% and dry mucous membranes, led to a diagnosis of *Deficient fluid volume*, then goals might include relief from vomiting and diarrhea and achievement of the proper fluid balance of I&O.

COLLABORATION

Infusion therapy in the hospital and other health care facilities usually follows the same format. The prescribing practitioner orders the solution or drug, the pharmacy compounds and dispenses it, and nurses administer it. However, home infusion therapy requires collaborative efforts between pharmacy services and nursing services because many of the responsibilities are shared jointly between pharmacy and nursing. Registered nurses in the home setting administer a wide variety of therapies such as chemotherapy, antibiotics, pain management, and hydration. Oseland and Querciagrossa (2003) address the need for effective communication between pharmacy and nursing and identify the overlapping responsibilities of pharmacy and nursing (see the accompanying display on home infusion therapy).

IMPLEMENTATION

Nurses have the responsibility to collaborate with and advocate for clients to ensure that they receive care that is appropriate, ethical, and based on practice standards. Nurses rely heavily on the data obtained from the history in formulating expected outcomes and selecting appropriate nursing interventions to support the clients' natural patterns as revealed in their histories.

The rationale for interventions related to alterations in either body fluid or electrolytes is based on the goal of maintaining homeostasis and regulating and maintaining essential fluids and nutrients. The nurse capitalizes on clients' adaptive capabilities by selecting interventions based on clients' perceptions of their support, strengths, and options.

The *Nursing Interventions Classification* (NIC) (Bulechek, Butcher, & Dochterman, 2008) has classifications that address three major categories (i.e., Acid-Base Management, Electrolyte Management, and Fluid Management) and a specific classification for the management of each type of alteration (e.g., metabolic acidosis, hypokalemia, hypervolemia). Although the nursing activities are specific for each intervention set, most of these interventions contain the activities of

---

HOME INFUSION THERAPY

Overlapping Responsibilities of Pharmacy and Nursing

Interdisciplinary communication
Review of medical record
Nutritional assessment
Assessment of medication history
Developing a plan of care
Review of lab data
Monitoring therapeutic response
Supply management
24-hour on-call support
Prescribing practitioner follow-up

Oseland, S., & Querciagrossa, A. (2003). Collaboration of nursing and pharmacy in home infusion therapy. *Home Healthcare Nurse, 21*(12), 819.

---

monitoring daily weight, measuring vital signs and I&O, and maintaining patent IV access. The nursing activities relative to assessment and implementation, for example, often require weight and vital sign measurements. Common interventions that promote attainment of expected outcomes to restore and maintain homeostasis are discussed next.

MONITOR DAILY WEIGHT

Daily weight is one of the main indicators of water and electrolyte balance. The nurse is responsible for the accurate measurement and recording of daily weights; the prescribing practitioner uses these data with other clinical findings in determining the client's fluid therapy.

MEASURE VITAL SIGNS

The frequency of measuring the vital signs is dependent upon the client's acuity level and clinical situation. For example, the vital signs of the typical postoperative client might be taken every 15 minutes until stable, whereas a client experiencing shock or hemorrhage should have vital signs monitored continuously. Vital sign measurements and other clinical data are used to determine the type and amount of fluid therapy.

MEASURE INTAKE AND OUTPUT

I&O measurements are initiated to monitor the client's fluid status over a 24-hour period (see Procedure 33-1 for information on how to measure the I&O). Agency policy relative to I&O may vary with regard to:

- The time frames for charting (e.g., every 8 hours versus every 12 hours)
- The time at which the 24-hour totals are calculated
- The definition of "strict" I&O

APPLICATION: HOME CARE

Considerations for Measuring I&O in the Home Care Environment

- Elicit client and family member input when selecting household items to be used for intake measurement.
- Provide containers for measuring output; adapt the urinary container to home facilities, and include teaching relative to proper washing and storage.
- Teach handwashing technique.
- Provide written instructions on what is to be measured.
- Provide sufficient I&O forms to last between the nurse's visits.
- Identify the parameters for evaluating a discrepancy between the I&O and for notifying the nurse or prescribing practitioner.

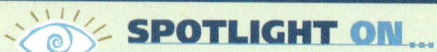

SPOTLIGHT ON...

Oral Hygiene

When you wake up in the morning, do you drink or eat anything before brushing your teeth? If you were sick, hospitalized, and without family or significant other support, would you want to drink or eat if your mouth tasted sour? Many of your clients will feel the same way and will need supportive nursing care to maintain oral hygiene. Muscular weakness and difficulty swallowing are other problems that could compound the client's dependency on you for oral hygiene.

Strict I&O measurement usually involves accounting for incontinent urine, emesis, and diaphoresis and might require weighing soiled bed linens. *Don gloves before handling soiled linen.*

The nurse reviews the client's 24-hour I&O calculations to evaluate fluid status. Intake should exceed the output by 500 mL to account for insensible body losses. I&O and daily weights are critical components of intervention because these measurements are also used to evaluate the effectiveness of diuretic or rehydration therapy. Remove gloves and perform hand hygiene before recording the amount of drainage on the I&O form to prevent the transfer of microorganisms when the form is removed from the client's room.

Securing an accurate I&O requires the full support of the client and the client's family. The client and family members should be taught how to measure and record the I&O (see the accompanying Application display for special home health care considerations).

PROVIDE ORAL HYGIENE

The nurse is responsible for providing oral hygiene to promote client comfort and integrity of the buccal cavity. Refer to Chapter 29 for the procedure on oral hygiene. The frequency of oral hygiene depends on the condition of the client's buccal cavity and the type of fluid imbalance. A client who is dehydrated or NPO for more than 24 hours may have decreased or absent salivation, coated tongue, and furrows on the tongue. These clients are at risk for developing oral diseases such as stomatitis, oral lesions or ulcers, and gingivitis. Avoid the use of alcohol and glycerin mouthwashes and glycerin swabs. These ingredients may feel refreshing, but they have a drying effect on the mucous membranes.

INITIATE ORAL FLUID THERAPY

Oral fluids may be totally restricted—a situation commonly referred to as *nothing by mouth* (NPO, which is from the Latin *non per os*)—or they may be restricted or forced, depending on the client's clinical situation. For example, oral replacement therapy is often used for clients with mild dehydration. According to Hockenberry and Wong (2007), oral rehydration therapy has a very high success rate in the treatment of childhood diarrhea with mild to moderate dehydration, and it has fewer complications when compared to IV replacement therapy. Severe dehydration in children is a medical emergency and must be treated with IV replacement therapy.

Nothing by Mouth

Clients are placed on NPO status as prescribed by the prescribing practitioner. On the basis of agency policy and clarification with the prescribing practitioner, the client may be allowed small amounts of ice chips or medications with a sip of water when NPO. Common clinical situations that may require NPO status include the need to:

- Avoid aspiration in unconscious, perioperative, and preprocedural clients who will receive anesthesia or conscious sedation
- Rest and heal the GI tract in clients with severe vomiting or diarrhea or when the client has a GI disorder (inflammation or obstruction)
- Prevent the further loss of gastric juices in clients with nasogastric suctioning

NPO clients should receive oral hygiene every 1 to 2 hours or as needed for comfort and to prevent alterations of the mucous membranes.

Restricted Fluids

Intake may be restricted to 200 mL over a 24-hour period; intake is commonly restricted in the treatment of EFV related to heart and renal failure. Client and family teaching and collaboration are the main nursing interventions in implementing this measure.

How the nurse limits the fluids should be determined in collaboration with the client. For example:

- Fifty percent of the allowed fluids might be taken at breakfast and lunch.
- The remaining 50% might be taken with the evening meal and before bedtime, unless the client has to be awakened during the night for a medication.

Forced Fluids

Forcing or encouraging the intake of oral fluids, mainly water, may be done when treating older adult clients who are at risk for dehydration and clients with renal and urinary problems (e.g., kidney stones). Compliance is obtained by client education and preference relative to timing and the type of liquids.

A client might, for example, be requested to consume 2000 mL over a 24-hour time period. If the client is intimidated on hearing this amount, which may sound very large, explain that the number of glasses to which this volume equates is only eight. Follow a similar time frame as set forth for restricted fluids, with the largest quantity of fluids administered with meals. Ice, gelatin, and ice cream count as liquid intake.

MAINTAIN TUBE FEEDING

When the client cannot ingest oral fluids and has a normal GI tract, fluids and nutrients can be administered through a feeding tube as prescribed by a prescribing practitioner. Refer to Chapter 34 for a complete discussion of feeding tubes.

MONITOR INTRAVENOUS THERAPY

When fluid losses are severe or the client cannot tolerate oral or tube feedings, fluid volume is replaced parenterally through the IV route. Intravenous (IV) therapy is the administration of fluids, electrolytes, nutrients, or medications by the venous route. The prescribing practitioner prescribes IV therapy to treat or prevent fluid and electrolyte or nutritional imbalances. Prescribing practitioners do not write an order to perform venipuncture. Instead, the order may read "Start IV" and should specify the exact IV therapy ordered; the order to perform the venipuncture is implied. All orders should be questioned if they are not clear. The nurse has specific responsibilities relative to IV therapy (see the accompanying Nursing Process Highlight).

The Infusion Nurses Society (INS, 2006) is the professional organization that establishes standards of practice to promote excellence in IV nursing to ensure the highest quality, cost-effective care for all individuals requiring infusion therapies. Infusion nursing standards of practice direct the development of agency policy and protocols in accordance with state and federal regulations and should complement the manufacturer's direction for usage. The nurse should review the agency's procedures before gathering the equipment. IV therapy requires parenteral fluids (solutions) and special equipment: administration set, IV pole, filter, infusion control device to regulate IV flow rate, and an established venous route.

NURSING PROCESS HIGHLIGHT

Implementation

IV Therapy

- Know why the therapy is prescribed.
- Document client understanding.
- Select the appropriate equipment in accordance with agency policy.
- Obtain the correct solution as prescribed.
- Assess the client for allergies: tape, iodine, latex, ointment, or antibiotic preparations to be used for skin preparation of the venipuncture site.
- Administer the fluid at the prescribed rate.
- Observe for signs of infiltration, the seepage of substances into the interstitial tissue that occurs as a result of accidental dislodgment of the needle from the vein, and other complications that are fluid specific.
- Document implementation of prescribed IV therapy in the client's medical record.

Parenteral Fluids

The nurse confirms the type and amount of IV solution by reading the prescribing practitioner's order in the medical record. IV solutions are sterile and packaged in plastic bags or glass containers. Solutions that are incompatible with plastic are dispensed in glass containers.

Plastic IV solution bags collapse under atmospheric pressure to allow the solution to enter the infusion set. Plastic solution bags are packaged with an outer plastic bag, which should remain intact until the nurse prepares the solution for administration. When the plastic solution bag is removed from its outer wrapper, the solution bag should be dry. If the solution bag is wet, the nurse should not use the solution. The moisture on the bag indicates that the integrity of the bag has been compromised and that the solution cannot be considered sterile. The bag should be returned to the dispensing department that issued the solution. Glass containers are discussed in the section on equipment.

IV solutions are usually packaged in quantities ranging from 50 to 1000 mL. The nurse should select a container that has the prescribed amount of solution closest to the prescribed volume. Crystalloids, electrolyte solutions with the potential to form crystals, are used to replace concurrent losses of water, carbohydrates, and electrolytes. Sodium chloride and Ringer's lactate are commonly used crystalloid solutions.

There are three types of parenteral fluids that are classified in accord with the tonicity of the fluid relative to normal blood plasma. As previously discussed, an osmolar solution can be hypotonic, isotonic, or hypertonic. The type of solution is prescribed on the basis of the client's diagnosis and the goal of therapy. The normal osmolarity of blood is between 280 and 295 mOsm/L, so the desired effect of the tonicity of the fluid is determined as follows:

1. Hypotonic fluid (hypo-osmolar, less than 290 mOsm/L) lowers the osmotic pressure and causes fluid to move into the cells; if fluid is infused beyond the client's tolerance, water intoxication may result.
2. Isotonic fluid (iso-osmolar, 290 mOsm/L) increases ECF volume; if fluid is infused beyond the client's tolerance, cardiac overload may result.
3. Hypertonic fluid (hyperosmolar, greater than 290 mOsm/L) increases the osmotic pressure of the blood plasma, drawing fluid from the cells; if fluid is infused beyond the client's tolerance, cellular dehydration may result (Smeltzer et al., 2008).

Table 33-6 on page 947 discusses the common types of IV solutions in terms of their tonicity, contents, and clinical usage.

Crystalloid solutions can be isotonic (equal to the sodium chloride concentration of blood, 0.9%), hypotonic (less than the sodium chloride concentration of blood), or hypertonic (greater than the sodium chloride concentration of blood) (Kee et al., 2010).

Colloids (nondiffusible substances) function like plasma proteins in blood by exerting a colloidal pressure to replace intravascular volume only. Examples of colloidal solutions are albumin, dextran, Plasmanate, and hetastarch (artificial blood substitute). During the administration of these solutions, the nurse should monitor the client for hypotension and allergic reactions (Kee et al., 2010). Blood transfusions are discussed later in this chapter.

Equipment

IV equipment is sterile, disposable, and prepackaged with user instructions. The user instructions are usually placed on the outside of the package, with a schematic that labels the parts, allowing the user to read the package prior to opening. The following discussion regarding IV equipment, inclusive of the frequency of when to change disposal IV therapy equipment, is based on the revised *2000 Infusion Nursing Standards of Practice* developed by the INS. All IV equipment must be inspected by the nurse to determine the integrity of the IV product before, during, and after use. Product integrity refers to the sterility of the equipment. Products are assessed for integrity by visual examination of the product and checking the expiration date on the equipment. All products identified with a defect must be returned to the appropriate department within the agency with a written report identifying the defect.

Since IV therapy provides a direct access into the vascular system, the nurse must understand the basic epidemiology principles and common organisms that may cause an infection and implement infection control measures to minimize the potential for infectious complications. The nurse uses aseptic technique and Standard Precautions when assembling and changing IV equipment. To decrease the risk of pathogen transmission, hand hygiene is required before and immediately after all IV procedures and upon removal of gloves. The frequency of changing sterile IV equipment reflects not only the national standards of practice but also the agency's established infection control policies. Infection control data may allow the agency to increase the time interval beyond the recommended standard provided the data verify low infection rates. The INS (2006) recommends that an organization that exhibits an increased rate of catheter-related bloodstream infection with the practice of 72-hour administration set changes should return to a 48-hour administration set change interval.

ADMINISTRATION SET The administration set (infusion set) refers to the plastic disposal tubing that provides for the infusion of a solution. There are several types of infusion sets to accommodate the solution and the mode of administration: primary continuous, secondary, primary intermittent, and special tubing for certain solutions such as blood and blood components. There are several add-on devices (e.g., extension sets, filters, stopcocks, PRN adaptor, needleless devices) that are used in conjunction with the administration set and changed whenever the set is changed.

Administration sets are changed at established time intervals and immediately upon suspected contamination or when the integrity of the set has been compromised. The administration set contains an insertion spike with a protective cap, a drip chamber, tubing with a slide clamp and regulating (roller) clamp, a rubber injection port, and a protective cap over the needle adapter (see Figure 33-10 on page 948). The protective caps keep both ends of the infusion set sterile and are removed only just before usage. The insertion spike is inserted into the port of the IV solution container.

Infusion sets can be vented or nonvented. The nonvented type is used with plastic bags of IV solutions and vented bottles. The vented set is used for glass containers that are not vented (see Figure 33-11 on page 948).

Glass containers require an air vent so that air can displace fluid from the container into the IV tubing. Some glass bottles are vented with an inside tube that exits the bottle into a rubber stopper in the neck of the bottle; if the bottle is not vented, then the nurse needs to select a vented infusion set.

The drip chamber is calibrated to allow a predictable amount of fluid to be delivered. There are two types of drip chambers: a macrodrip, which delivers 10 to 20 drops per milliliter of solution, and a microdrip, which delivers 60 drops per milliliter. The drip rate varies with the manufacturer as indicated on the package.

The administration set has a manual flow-control device such as a slide clamp (Figure 33-10), a roller clamp, or a screw to regulate a prescribed infusion rate. Follow the manufacturer's guidelines when using the manual flow-control device to regulate the prescribed infusion rate. The end of the IV tubing contains a needle adapter that attaches to the sterile device inserted in the client's vein. Extension tubing may be used to lengthen the primary tubing.

A primary continuous administration set is used to administer routine solutions prescribed to infuse continuously over a 24-hour period. The primary administration set, inclusive of the add-on devices, is changed every 72 to

TABLE 33-6 Common Intravenous Solutions

TONICITY	SOLUTION	CONTENTS (MEQ/L)	CLINICAL IMPLICATIONS
Hypotonic	Sodium chloride 0.45%	77 Na^+, 77 Cl^-	Daily maintenance of body fluid and establishment of renal function.
Isotonic	Dextrose 2.5% in 0.45% saline	77 Na^+, 77 Cl^-	Promotes renal function and urine output.
	Dextrose 5% in 0.2% saline	38 Na^+, 38 Cl^-	Daily maintenance of body fluids when less Na^+ and Cl^- are required.
	Dextrose 5% in water (D5W)		Promotes rehydration and elimination; may cause urinary Na^+ loss; good vehicle for K^+.
	Ringer's lactate	130 Na^+, 4 K^+, Ca^{2+}, 109 Cl^-, 28 lactate	Resembles the normal composition of blood serum and plasma; K^+ level below body's daily requirement.
	Normal saline (NS), 0.9%	154 Na^+, 154 Cl^-	Restores sodium chloride deficit and extracellular fluid volume.
	Dextran 40 10% in NS (0.9%) or D5W		A colloidal solution used to increase plasma volume of clients in early shock; it should not be given to severely dehydrated clients and clients with renal disease, thrombocytopenia, or active hemorrhaging.
	Dextran 70% in NS		A long-lived (20 hours) plasma volume expander; used to treat shock or impending shock due to hemorrhage, surgery, or burns. It can prolong bleeding and coats the RBCs (draw type and cross-match prior to administering).
Hypertonic	Dextrose 5% in 0.45% saline	77 Na^+, 77 Cl^-	Daily maintenance of body fluid and nutrition; treatment of FVD.
	Dextrose 5% in saline 0.9%	154 Na^+, 154 Cl^-	Fluid replacement of sodium, chloride, and calories (170).
	Dextrose 10% in saline 0.9%	154 Na^+, 154 Cl^-	Fluid replacement of sodium, chloride, and calories (340).
	Dextrose 5% in lactated Ringer's	130 Na^+, 4 K^+, 3 Ca^{2+}, 109 Cl^-, 28 lactate	Resembles the normal composition of blood serum and plasma; K^+ level below body's daily requirement; caloric value 180.
	Hyperosmolar saline 3% and 5% NaCl	856 Na^+, 865 Cl^-	Treatment of hyponatremia; raises the Na^+ osmolarity of the blood and reduces intracellular fluid excess.
	Ionosol B with dextrose 5%	57 Na^+, 25 K^+, 49 Cl^-, 25 lact., 5 Mg^{2+}, 7 PO_4^-	Treatment of polyionic parenteral replacement caused by vomiting-induced alkalosis, diabetic acidosis, fluid loss from burns, and postoperative FVD.
	Ionosol D-CM with dextrose 5%	138 Na^+, 12 K^+, 5 Ca^{2+}, 108 Cl^-, 50 lactate, 3 Mg^{2+}	Treatment of electrolyte losses of duodenal fluids caused by intestinal suction or biliary or pancreatic drainage; treatment of mild acidosis.
	Aminosyn-RF 5.2%	5.4 K^+	Restores fluid and protein and promotes wound healing.
	Aminosyn II 3.5%	18 Na^+	Treatment of malnourished older adult clients and hypoproteinemia; it is not to be given to clients with severe liver damage.

Kee, J. L., Paulanka, B. J., & Polek, C. (2010). *Fluids and electrolytes with clinical applications: A programmed approach* (8th ed.). Clifton Park, NY: Delmar/Cengage Learning.

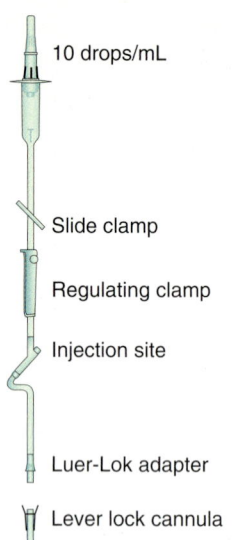

10 drops/mL

Slide clamp

Regulating clamp

Injection site

Luer-Lok adapter

Lever lock cannula

FIGURE 33-10 Basic Administration Set DELMAR/CENGAGE LEARNING

96 hours in conjunction with the peripheral cannula change. A bag of IV solution should not hang longer than 24 hours.

Secondary administration sets are often referred to as "piggyback" administration sets. The secondary tubing is connected into the primary tubing at an injection site (see Figure 33-11) and allows for the administration of a second solution (e.g., medication). Secondary administration sets are also changed every 72 to 96 hours.

Primary intermittent administration sets are used to deliver medications at prescribed intervals through an injection or

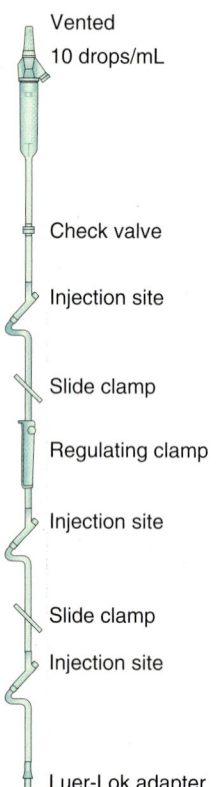

Vented
10 drops/mL

Check valve

Injection site

Slide clamp

Regulating clamp

Injection site

Slide clamp

Injection site

Luer-Lok adapter

FIGURE 33-11 Vented Administration Set DELMAR/CENGAGE LEARNING

access port and are changed every 72 to 96 hours; all add-on devices such as extension sets, filters, PRN adaptors, and stopcocks are changed with the intermittent administration set. A sterile needle or needleless device should be aseptically attached to the intermittent administration set prior to administering the medication and removed immediately after each use.

Neonates, infants, and children are at risk for *Altered fluid balance: Overload, related to rehydration.* IV tubing with a microdrip and special volume-control chambers are used to regulate the amount of fluid to be administered over a specific time interval. Armboards and soft restraints are used to stabilize peripheral infusions by immobilizing the extremity to prevent accidental removal of infusion devices.

Health Hazard A *Health Alert* from Health Care Without Harm (HCWH) (1999) cautioned the public about the potential risks of exposure to diethylhexyl phthalates (DEHP) from medical products such as IV bags and tubing. More than 500 million IV bags are used in the United States every year to deliver blood, medication, and other essential solutions to clients (HCWH, 1999). Eighty percent of the IV bags are made with polyvinyl chloride (PVC), which requires a plasticizer to make the bags soft and flexible. DEHP is the softener used in PVC products. DEHP has been shown to leach from IV bags into the solutions they contain and directly into the client's bloodstream.

The Environmental Protection Agency has classified DEHP as a probable human carcinogen, and HCWH claims that studies have shown that DEHP can damage the heart, liver, testes, and kidneys and interfere with sperm production. Certain drugs such as Taxol (used to treat breast cancer) and Taxotere (used to treat ovarian and breast cancer and AIDS-related Kaposi's sarcoma) have been shown to increase the leaching of DEHP from PVC plastics into the solution; see the accompanying display (on page 949) for additional drugs that can increase leaching of DEHP from PVC IV products. Although one leading producer of vinyl IV bags containing DEHP plans to develop an alternative to PVC for their products, no time frames were given to totally remove these products from the market.

A second health hazard is inherent in the use of DEHP. The disposal of medical products containing DEHP releases highly toxic and endocrine-disrupting dioxins. PVC is the only plastic linked both to phthalate chemical leaching and to the production of dioxin.

INTRAVENOUS FILTERS IV filters prevent the passage of undesirable substances such as particulate matter and air from entering the vascular system. Particulate matter filters are utilized when preparing infusion medications for administration to prevent obstruction in the vascular and pulmonary systems, irritation, and **phlebitis** (inflammation of a vein). Air-eliminating filters are used for the delivery of infusion therapy to decrease the potential of air emboli; the filter should be located as close as possible to the cannula site. IV filters come in various sizes; the finer the filter, the greater is the degree of solution filtration. Although studies have shown that IV filters

DRUGS THAT INCREASE LEACHING OF DEHP FROM PVC PLASTICS

- Chemotherapeutic agents: etoposide (VePesid) and teniposide (Vumon)
- Antianxiety agents: chlordiazepoxide HCl (Librium)
- Antifungal agents: miconazole (Monistat IV)
- Immunosuppressive agents: cyclosporine (Sandimmune) and tacrolimus (Prograf)
- Nutritional solutions: fat emulsions and vitamin A

Stewart, M. (1999, March/April). IV bags pose patient risk. *American Nurse, 31*(2), 12.

reduce the risk of bacteremia and phlebitis as much as 40%, many agencies do not use IV filters because of cost.

NEEDLES AND VENOUS PERIPHERAL-SHORT CATHETERS
Needles and peripheral-short catheters provide access to the venous system. A variety of devices are available in different sizes to complement the age of the client and the type and duration of the therapy and to protect the user from injury (see Figure 33-12).

As with any gauge needle, the larger the number, the smaller the lumen. The nurse considers the client's age, body size, purpose of the infusion, and type of solution to be administered when selecting the gauge of the needle or catheter:

- Infants and small children, 24-gauge
- Preschool through preteen, 24- or 22-gauge
- Teenagers and adults, 22- or 20-gauge
- Geriatric, 22- or 24-gauge

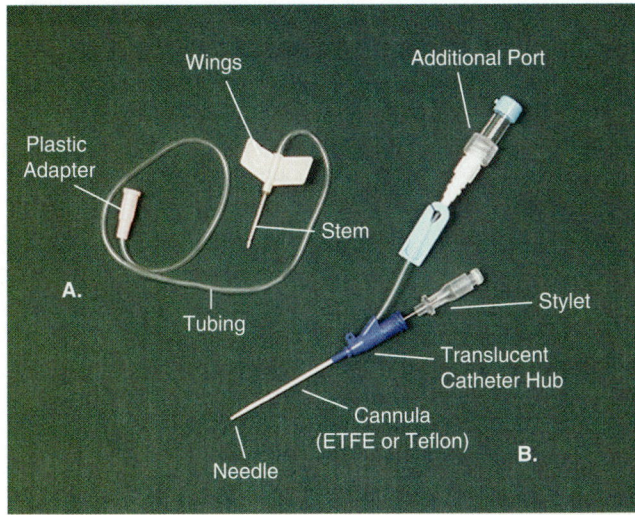

FIGURE 33-12 Peripheral IV Devices: A. Butterfly; B. Angiocatheter DELMAR/CENGAGE LEARNING

Butterfly (scalp vein or wing-tipped) needles are short, beveled needles with plastic flaps attached to the shaft. The flaps, which are flexible, are held tightly together to facilitate ease of insertion and then flattened against the skin to prevent dislodgment during infusion. These needles are commonly used for short-term or intermittent therapy and for infants and children.

There are several types of short catheters used to access peripheral veins. Short peripheral venous catheters vary in length from 3/4 to 11/4 inches. During insertion, some of these catheters are threaded over a needle, and others are threaded inside a needle. **Intracath** is a term used to refer to a plastic tube inserted into a vein. An **angiocatheter** is a type of intracath with a metal stylet to pierce the skin and vein, after which the plastic catheter is threaded into the vein and the metal stylet is removed, leaving only the plastic catheter in the vein. Short venous catheters have a safety mechanism to reduce the risk of accidental needlesticks. These devices are designed to allow for easy insertion of the catheter while providing a built-in safety feature to reduce the potential for exposure to bloodborne pathogens.

PERIPHERAL INTRAVENOUS AND SALINE/HEPARIN LOCKS Peripheral intravenous (PI) and saline/heparin locks are devices that establish a venous route as a precautionary measure for clients whose condition may change rapidly or who may require intermittent infusion therapy. A peripheral catheter is inserted into a vein, and the hub is capped with a Luer-Lok injection or access port (see Figure 33-13).

NEEDLE-FREE SYSTEM Safety is a concern associated with IV therapy; refer to Chapter 29. Accidental needlestick injuries and puncture wounds with contaminated devices increase the employee's risk for infectious diseases such as AIDS, hepatitis (B and C), and other viral, rickettsial, bacterial, fungal, and parasitic infections. Health care agencies now use totally needle-free IV systems (see Figure 33-14 on page 950) to decrease the risk of employee injuries.

VASCULAR ACCESS DEVICES Vascular access devices (VADs) include various catheters and implanted ports that allow for long-term IV therapy or repeated access to the central venous system. The kind of VAD used depends on the client's diagnosis and the type and length of treatment (see Table 33-7 on page 950). Site selection and insertion of central catheters, other than peripherally inserted central catheters, are medical acts performed by a prescribing practitioner. Although there are many types of catheter materials, insertion techniques, and kinds of central catheters, *all central catheters*

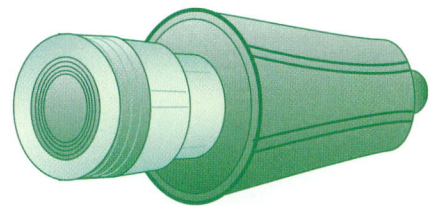

FIGURE 33-13 Luer-Lok Injection Device DELMAR/CENGAGE LEARNING

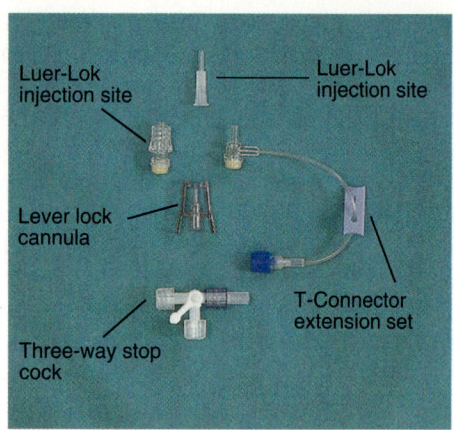

Luer-Lok
injection site

Luer-Lok
injection site

Lever lock
cannula

Three-way stop
cock

T-Connector
extension set

FIGURE 33-14 Needle-Free System DELMAR/CENGAGE LEARNING

*must be radiopaque to allow for radiographic verification of place-
ment of the catheter and its tip prior to the administration of any
solution.*

Central catheters are usually inserted into an upper extremity, the internal jugular veins, and subclavian veins with
the tip located in the distal superior vena cava to minimize
vessel irritation and sclerosis. The femoral vein can be used
for central venous access when there is thrombosis of the internal jugular or subclavian veins; correct tip location should
be in the inferior vena cava. Insertion of a central catheter can
be performed either percutaneously or surgically. Surgically,
either a central catheter is placed entirely under the skin
(implanted) or the catheter partially exits the skin (tunneled).

A tunneled catheter is inserted through the subcutaneous tissue, usually between the nipple and clavicle, with the
catheter tip inserted through the cephalic or external jugular
vein and threaded to the superior vena cava.

An **implantable port** is a device made of a radiopaque silicone catheter and a plastic or stainless steel injection port with a
self-sealing silicone-rubber septum. The prescribing practitioner
inserts the device into a subcutaneous pocket, usually over the
third or fourth rib, lateral to the sternum. The distal tip of the
catheter is surgically tunneled in the cephalic or external jugular
vein, with the proximal end of the catheter tunneled through
the subcutaneous tissue into the injection port of the device.

Implanted ports and pumps are VADs that provide for
the delivery of prescribed parenteral therapies. Accessing
these devices requires the use of aseptic technique. Noncoring
needles such as a Huber needle are used to access an
implanted port or pump and should be changed at least every
7 days. The smallest gauge noncoring needle that can deliver
the prescribed therapy should be used when accessing the
port or pump. Nurses caring for clients with implanted ports
or pumps must have a thorough knowledge of the design features of the device, as explained in the manufacturer's guidelines, to ensure correct access, administration techniques, and
maintenance and to avoid potential complications.

Implanted pumps have a reservoir designed to continuously infuse a specific volume of solution over a preset period of time; the pump must be routinely emptied and
refilled at established intervals. Some pumps have an additional feature, a side port designed for administration of
intermittent medication. The flow rate of some pumps is sensitive to changes in atmospheric pressure, body temperature,
blood pressure, and the viscosity of the medications. Clients
are instructed to report changes in their lifestyle and physical
condition that may affect the pump's flow rate. *Only nurses
who have been specially trained are allowed to access an
implanted port or pump because of the risk of infiltration into
the tissue if needle placement is incorrect.*

TABLE 33-7 Vascular Access Devices

TYPE	BRAND NAME	USE
Nontunneled central venous catheter (single-, dual-, or triple-lumen)	Hohn, Arrow	Short-term fluid or blood administration, obtaining blood specimens, and administering medications
Tunneled central venous catheter (single-, dual-, or triple-lumen)	Hickman, Broviac, Groshong	Long-term (months to years) fluid replacement therapy, medication administration, nutritional supplement, and blood specimen withdrawal
Implanted infusion port (single, dual)	Chemo-Port, Infuse-a-Port, Mediport, Port-a-Cath	Long-term (months to years) fluid replacement therapy, medication administration (especially chemotherapy), blood or blood product administration, and blood specimen withdrawal
Peripherally inserted central catheter (PICC) (single, dual)	PICC, Groshong PICC, Pee-a-Cath, Arrow PICC	Long-term fluid replacement therapy, medication administration (chemotherapy, antibiotics, controlled narcotics), blood or blood product administration, and blood specimen withdrawal

Delmar/Cengage Learning

▼ **SAFETY FIRST** ▼

INSERTING A CVC

When assisting with the insertion of a central venous catheter, observe the client for symptoms of a pneumothorax: sudden shortness of breath or sharp chest pain; increased anxiety; a weak, rapid pulse; hypotension; pallor; or cyanosis. These symptoms indicate accidental puncture of the pleural membrane.

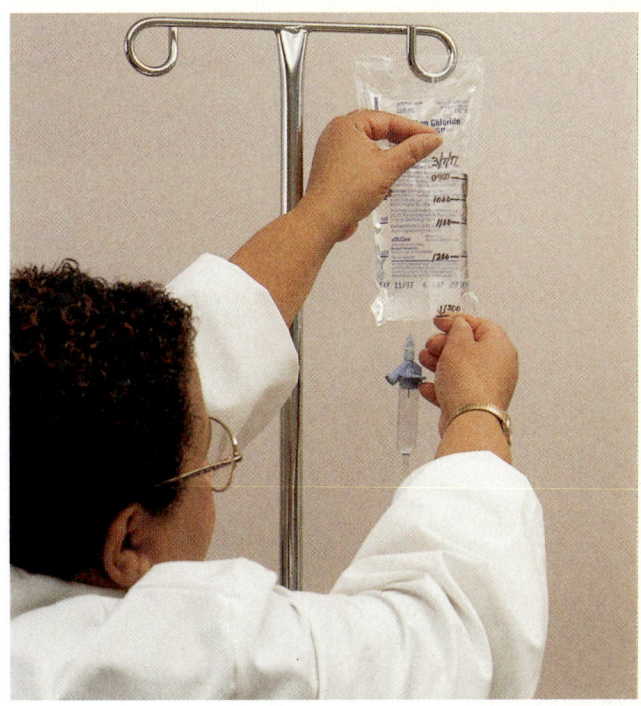

FIGURE 33-15 Apply a time strip to the IV container. DELMAR/ CENGAGE LEARNING

A peripherally inserted central catheter (PICC) is a silicone or polyurethane catheter inserted into one of the major veins in the antecubital fossa or upper extremity with the distal tip terminating in the lower-third section of the superior vena cava. A PICC can be trimmed at the time of insertion to a specific length that is determined by the approximate distance between the insertion site and the superior vena cava. State boards of registered nurses allow specially trained nurses to insert PICCs. Placement of the catheter's tip is confirmed by x-ray prior to the administration of any solution. The registered nurse who inserts the PICC must document the type of PICC inserted and the total length of the inserted catheter and record if the length of the catheter was trimmed prior to insertion.

The recommended way to secure a VAD is with a manufactured catheter stabilization device. These devices contain an adhesive anchoring pad to help reduce catheter dislodgment and the need for removal and reinsertion (Hadaway, 2008). Sterile tape and surgical strips are still acceptable methods of catheter stabilization. The INS (2006) no longer considers dressings as stabilization devices. Although dressings protect the insertion site and skin, there is no evidence that they enhance catheter stabilization (Hadaway, 2008). At each dressing change, document the external catheter length. If the length has changed, the internal tip location has also changed; the altered tip location could increase the risk of complications such as vein thrombosis and dysrhythmias. See Procedure 33-8 on changing the central venous dressing.

Preparing an Intravenous Solution

To prepare an IV solution, read the agency's policy and procedures and gather the necessary equipment. Because IV equipment and solutions are sterile, check the expiration date on the package prior to usage. The solution can be prepared at the nurses' work area or in the client's room (Procedure 33-2 and Procedure 33-3).

The nurse prepares and applies a time strip to the IV solution bag to facilitate monitoring of the infusion rate as ordered by the prescribing practitioner (see Figure 33-15). Use only labels appropriate for IV bags. Do not use a felt-tipped pen to mark an IV bag; the ink from the pen can leak through the plastic and contaminate the solution. Do not label a bag with a time strip made of adhesive silk or paper tape, as the adhesive will leach into the bag. The IV tubing is tagged with the date and time to indicate when the tubing replacement is necessary. IV tubing is changed every 72 to 96 hours in accordance with the agency's policy. The nurse initials the time strip and IV tubing tag.

Initiating IV Therapy

When initiating IV therapy, the nurse should assess for a venipuncture site. Figure 33-16 on page 952 presents the common peripheral sites for starting IV therapy in pediatric, adult, and geriatric clients (see Chapter 28, Procedure 28-1, Venipuncture).

When assessing clients for potential sites, consider their age, body size, clinical status and impairments, and skin condition (see the accompanying display for contraindications when selecting a site on page 952). Lower-extremity veins (e.g., the foot) are common IV sites with children but are avoided in adults because of the danger of thrombophlebitis (INS, 2006). The median vein (see Figure 33-16), usually located between two branches of the median nerve, is difficult to palpate or visualize; venipuncture in this area can be painful and should be avoided whenever possible. Because contact with blood is likely, venipuncture requires the implementation of Standard Precautions. Refer to Chapter 29 for a complete discussion of Standard Precautions.

Select a vein for puncture at its most distal end to maintain the integrity of the vein because venous blood flows with an upward movement toward the heart. The accessory cephalic vein (see Figure 33-16) is a medium- to large-sized vein that is easy to stabilize and palpate and readily accepts large needles; however, valves at the junction with the cephalic vein may prohibit the advancement of a cannula. When

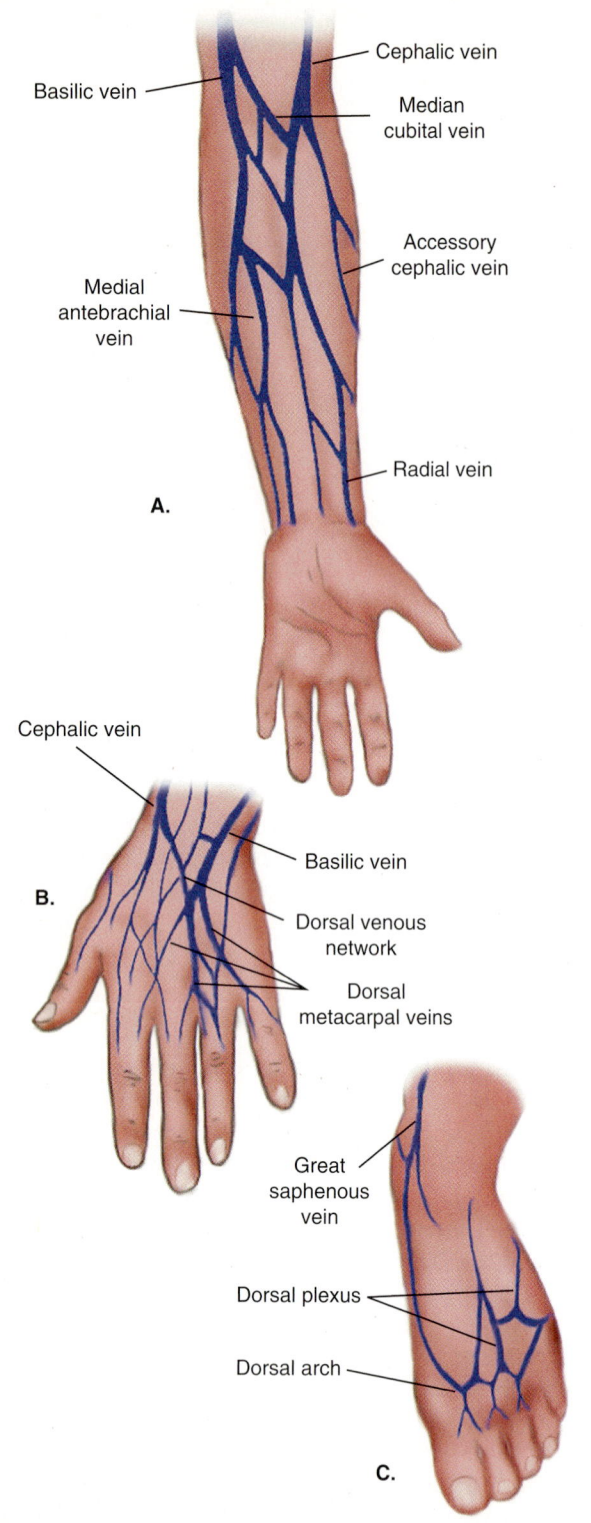

A.
- Basilic vein
- Cephalic vein
- Median cubital vein
- Accessory cephalic vein
- Medial antebrachial vein
- Radial vein

B.
- Cephalic vein
- Basilic vein
- Dorsal venous network
- Dorsal metacarpal veins

C.
- Great saphenous vein
- Dorsal plexus
- Dorsal arch

FIGURE 33-16 Peripheral Veins Used in Intravenous Therapy: **A.** Arm and Forearm; **B.** Dorsum of the Hand; **C.** Dorsal Plexus of the Foot DELMAR/CENGAGE LEARNING

a vein is punctured with an instrument, such as a needle, fluids can infiltrate (leak from the vein into the tissue at the site of puncture). If IV therapy has to be discontinued for any reason, such as infiltration, it can be restarted above the initial puncture site only. No more than two attempts at inserting an IV should be made by a single nurse (INS, 2006).

VENIPUNCTURE SITE CONTRAINDICATIONS

- Signs of infection, infiltration, or thrombosis
- Affected arm of a postmastectomy client
- Arm with a functioning arteriovenous fistula
- Affected arm of a paralyzed client
- Any arm that has circulatory or neurologic impairments

In the 1990s nurses began using ultrasound for PICC insertion, and the technique is now endorsed by the Agency for Healthcare Research and Quality and the Centers for Disease Control and Prevention (CDC). Using ultrasound for PICC insertion raises the rate of successful insertions to more than 90%, compared to about 80% with traditional, non–ultrasound-guided PICC insertion (Moureau, 2008). Ultrasounds not only allow the nurse to easily and accurately locate and identify veins, arteries, and nerve bundles of the upper arm but also let the nurse assess vein characteristics before determining whether the vein is suitable for catheter placement.

When prepping the client's skin for a venipuncture, cleanse the skin with 2% to 3% aqueous chlorhexidine (preferred), tincture of iodine 2%, 10% povidone-iodine, or 70% isopropyl alcohol and wait for it to dry. Do not apply alcohol after the skin has been prepped with povidone-iodine. Allow povidone-iodine to remain on the skin for at least 2 minutes. Chlorhexidine is not approved for use with infants less than 2 months of age. Antiseptic solutions should be allowed to air-dry completely to effectively reduce microbial count (INS, 2006).

Administering IV Therapy

Once the solution is prepared for administration, the nurse calculates the rate and explains the procedure to the client (see Procedure 33-4 for assessing and maintaining an IV insertion site). There are three ways to administer solutions:

1. Initiate the infusion by performing a venipuncture.
2. Use an existing IV system: catheter, saline/heparin or PI lock, central line, or implanted port.
3. Add a solution to a continuous-infusion line (see Procedure 33-35).

Fluid administration can be continuous, ongoing over a 24-hour period, or intermittent (1000 mL ordered once in a 24-hour period). Although fluids may be continuous, the type of fluids can alternate over a 24-hour period; for example, an order might be *add 40 mEq of KCl to first bag of 1000 mL of normal saline*.

The aging process causes physiological changes in the skin, muscles, and veins. The skin loses its durability, making it prone to tears and abrasions. Decrease in muscle mass may cause the vein to roll during puncture. The veins themselves are also more fragile in older adults. When first infusing fluid into the vein, administer it slowly and observe carefully for any sign of infiltration.

IV medications may be **piggybacked**, added to an existing IV solution to infuse concurrently. IV solutions and medications that have been refrigerated should be warmed to room temperature before administration (usually 30 minutes) to increase the client's comfort.

Instead of setting the total volume to be infused (e.g., 1000 mL), set the volume slightly lower (e.g., at 950 mL) so that the alarm will go off before the fluids are absorbed completely. This method will give you time to have the next bag of fluids ready when all 1000 mL have been absorbed. This is especially helpful when dealing with refrigerated fluids that must be warmed to room temperature before administering. If you will be off duty when the volume will be absorbed and you have set the alarm to go off early, tell the oncoming nurse during report.

Flushing

Flushing refers to the instillation of a solution into an IV cannula. Flushing is performed to assess and maintain cannula patency and prevent the mixing of incompatible medications and solutions, following the conversion of continuous IV therapy to intermittent IV therapy, and to maintain intermittent cannula patency following IV medication administration and blood sampling (see Procedure 33-6).

The type of solution and frequency of flushing an intermittent IV cannula are determined by the agency's policy. According to the INS (2006), flushing a cannula at established intervals with saline (0.9% sodium chloride injection) is the accepted solution to ensure and maintain patency of an intermittent PI cannula, while a heparin flush solution is the accepted solution to maintain patency of intermittent central venous devices. The volume of flush is equal to the volume capacity of the cannula and add-on devices times two (INS, 2006). Consideration is also given to the volume and frequency of heparin flush in order to prevent an alteration in the client's clotting factors.

When flushing a cannula, positive pressure within the lumen of the catheter must be maintained to prevent the reflux of blood into the cannula lumen. Use the manufacturer-recommended maximum pressure limits (pounds per square inch) when selecting the size of the syringe to use for flushing, since the smaller the syringe, the greater the pressure generated; excessive internal pressures in the device increase the potential for cannula damage and progressive internal cannula weakening over the life of the device (INS, 2006). If resistance is met when flushing a cannula, do not exert pressure in an attempt to restore patency of an occluded cannula since this action may result in the dislodgment of a clot into the vascular system or rupture of the catheter.

Regulating IV Solution Flow Rates

Infusion sets with macrodrip chambers are often used for adult clients, whereas microdrip chambers are used for volume-sensitive clients, such as geriatric or pediatric clients.

Pediatric and geriatric clients usually require some type of device to regulate the fluids as a safety factor to prevent overload. Devices such as controllers and pumps are commonly used to regulate the rate of infusion.

Calculation of Flow Rate

The **flow rate** is the volume of fluid to infuse over a set period of time as ordered by the prescribing practitioner. The prescribing practitioner will identify either the amount to infuse per hour (such as 125 mL per hour or 1000 mL over an 8-hour period). Calculate the hourly infusion rate as follows:

$$\frac{\text{Total volume}}{\text{Number of hours to infuse}} = \text{mL/hour infusion rate}$$

For example, if 1000 mL is to infuse over 8 hours:

$$\frac{1000}{8} = 125 \text{ mL/hour}$$

Calculate the actual infusion rate (drops per minute) as follows:

$$\frac{\text{Total volume}}{\text{Total time (minutes)}} \times \text{drop factor} = \text{drops per minute}$$

For example, if 1000 mL is to infuse over 8 hours with a tubing drop factor of 10 drops per milliliter:

$$\frac{1000 \text{ mL}}{8(60) \text{ min}} \times 10 \text{ drops/mL}$$

$$= \frac{10,000 \text{ mL}}{480 \text{ min}} = 20.8 \text{ or } 21 \text{ drops/min}$$

Another way to calculate the actual infusion rate is to use the hourly infusion rate; for the example just given:

$$\frac{125 \text{ mL} \times 10 \text{ drops/mL}}{60 \text{ min}} = 20.8 \text{ or } 21 \text{ drops/min}$$

See Procedure 33-7.

Flow-Control Devices

Flow-control devices are used to regulate the infusion at the prescribed administration rate. Safety factors such as the client's age and condition, prescribed therapy, and setting are considered when selecting a flow-control device. There are two basic types of flow-control devices: manual flow-control devices and electronic infusion devices. Manual flow-control devices include roller, screw, and slide clamps and may include volume-control devices such as a buretrol. These devices are used routinely to regulate the accurate delivery of most prescribed IV therapies.

Electronic infusion devices, which are operated either by electricity or battery, are used to administer IV fluids and medications and should be considered on all central access devices (INS, 2006). Electronic infusion pumps have audible alarms that sound when the solution has infused, the infusion tubing contains air or is kinked, or the cannula is clotted. There are two types of electronic infusion devices: controllers and pumps. Controller infusion devices generate flow by gravity and are capable of maintaining a constant preset flow rate either by drop counting or volumetric delivery. The nurse sets the flow rate, and the specific gravity of the solution and the height of the bag determine the maximum delivery pressure. Fluids with low viscosity are usually infused by electronic controllers.

Infusion pumps maintain the flow rate under positive pressure. Pumps counter the effects of resistance in the delivery system and pressure fluctuations at the infusion site. Positive pressure infusion devices are classified as either volumetric or syringe pumps and are used to deliver viscous fluids or large volumes of fluids. Volumetric pumps use either a peristaltic pumping action or a pumping cassette or chamber to deliver a fixed volume over a specified period of time. Syringe infusion pumps rely on a syringe or cartridge to deliver the fluid at a specific set rate.

MANAGING IV THERAPY

IV therapy requires frequent client monitoring by the nurse to ensure an accurate flow rate and other critical nursing actions. These other actions include ensuring client comfort and positioning; checking IV solution for correct solution, amount, and timing; monitoring expiration dates of the IV system (tubing, venipuncture site, dressing) and changing as necessary; and being aware of safety factors.

Coordinate client care with the maintenance of IV lines. Clients with IV therapy usually require assistance with hygienic measures, such as changing a gown. Change IV tubing when doing site care to decrease the number of times the access device is manipulated, thereby decreasing the risk for infiltration and phlebitis. PI devices are changed every 72 to 96 hours as directed by CDC guidelines.

Hypervolemia

Hypervolemia, increased circulating fluid volume, may result from rapid IV infusion of solutions. This causes cardiac overload, which may lead to pulmonary edema and cardiac failure. Monitor the infusion rate hourly, and refer to the Nursing Care Plan "The Client with Excess Fluid Volume" for the assessment and interventions for a client experiencing FVE.

If a solution infuses at a rate greater than prescribed, decrease the rate to *keep vein open* (KVO) and immediately notify the prescribing practitioner. Report the amount and type of solution that infused over the exact time period and the client's response.

Infiltration

Infiltration may be caused by inserting the wrong type of device, using the wrong-gauge needle, or dislodgment of the device from the vein. When a drug or solution is administered under high pressure by a pump, it may also cause infiltration or vein irritation.

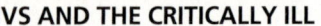

▼ SAFETY FIRST ▼

IVS AND THE CRITICALLY ILL
Never remove a functioning IV device from a critically ill client until another successful venipuncture has been performed; an established IV route may be needed for the administration of solutions, medications, or blood components.

Infiltration results in the leaking of fluids or medications into the surrounding tissue. The client usually complains of discomfort at the IV site. Inspect the site by palpating for swelling, and feel the temperature of the skin (coolness and paleness of skin are indications of infiltration).

The nurse confirms that the needle is still in the vein by pinching the IV tubing; this action should cause a **flashback**: Blood should rush into the tubing if the needle is still in the vein. If a flashback does not occur, aspirate the injection port nearest the device as explained in Procedure 33-4. Discontinue the needle or catheter if it cannot be aspirated, and apply a sterile dressing to the puncture site.

After the IV has been removed, the puncture site may ooze or bleed, especially in clients receiving anticoagulants. If oozing or bleeding occurs, apply pressure and reapply a sterile dressing until it stops. Accurately assess and document the degree of edema.

Clients may be injured by infiltration. If the IV site becomes grossly infiltrated, the edema in the soft tissue may cause a nerve compression injury with permanent loss of function to the extremity. If a **vesicant** (medication that causes blistering and tissue injury when it escapes into surrounding tissue) infiltrates, it may cause significant tissue loss with permanent disfigurement and loss of function.

Phlebitis

Phlebitis may result from either mechanical or chemical trauma. Mechanical trauma may be caused by inserting a device with too large a gauge, using a vein that is too small or fragile, or leaving the device in place for too long. Chemical trauma may result from infusing too rapidly or from an acidic solution, a hypertonic solution, a solution that contains electrolytes (especially potassium and magnesium), or other medications.

Phlebitis may be a precursor of sepsis. Listen for client complaints of tenderness, the first indication of an inflammation. Inspect the IV site for changes in skin color and temperature (a reddened area or pink or red stripe along the vein, warmth, and swelling are indications of phlebitis). Tenderness, not redness, is the earliest sign of PI-site phlebitis.

If phlebitis is present, discontinue the IV infusion. Before removing and discarding the venous device, check the agency's policy to see whether the tip of the device needs to be cultured and sent to the laboratory for a culture and sensitivity test. After removing the device, apply a sterile dressing to the site and moist, warm compresses to the affected area. Document in the nurses' notes the time, symptoms, and nursing interventions.

Hypertonic solutions may cause irritation necessitating frequent IV site changes. Observe the site for symptoms of postinfusion phlebitis following IV removal. This may occur in response to either chemical or mechanical factors of the preexisting IV. Postinfusion phlebitis is treated with warm, moist compresses to the site and elevation of the extremity.

Catheter Sepsis

If the client complains of chills and fever, check the length of time that this IV solution has been hanging and the needle or catheter has been in place; assess the client's vital signs, and assess for other symptoms of pyrogenic reactions, such as backache, headache, malaise, nausea, and vomiting. Unexplained fever may be related to catheter sepsis. Pulse rate increases and temperature is usually above 100°F if IV-related sepsis occurs. Stop infusion, notify the prescribing practitioner, and obtain blood specimens if prescribed.

Intravenous Dressing Change

IV dressing changes require the use of Standard Precautions and aseptic technique; refer to Procedure 33-8. Institutional policy and the type of IV access device and dressing determine the frequency of care:

1. Nontransparent (gauze) dressing may be used for a PI. It is changed every 48 hours.
2. Transparent dressings (Bioclusive, OpSite, Tegaderm) allow visualization of the IV site; these dressings are changed every 3 to 7 days.

Discontinuation of Intravenous Therapy

IV therapy is discontinued on the prescribing practitioner's order as determined by the client's need or response to therapy (Procedure 33-9). The removal of a short peripheral catheter is a nursing intervention to minimize the complication risks related to infusion therapy or to implement the prescribing practitioner's order. Peripheral catheters are removed every 72 to 96 hours and immediately upon suspected contamination or complications. Pressure and a dry sterile dressing are applied to the site upon removal of the catheter; refer to Procedure 33-9. The integrity of the catheter and insertion site should be assessed, with observations and actions documented to the client's medical record.

The removal of a PICC is usually a simple procedure; however, research suggests that in 7% to 12% of PICC removals, difficulties can arise (Macklin, 2000). Only nurses who have been trained in the insertion of a PICC line should remove the catheter. Since the catheter is completely inserted in the vascular system and invisible, the nurse must feel for resistance during removal. If resistance is felt, the nurse stops and assesses for certain complicating factors: venous spasm, vagal reaction, phlebitis, thrombosis, and knotting of the catheter. Prior to removal, the nurse must verify in the client's medical record the type and specific length of the inserted PICC.

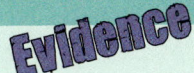

UNCOVERING THE Evidence

TITLE OF STUDY
"The Determination of Record-Keeping Behavior of Nurses Regarding Intravenous Fluid Treatment: The Case of Turkey"

AUTHORS
S. Arslan and A. Karadag

PURPOSE
To determine the record-keeping behavior of nurses regarding intravenous fluid treatment (IVFT).

METHODS
The study was conducted with 150 nurses working in adult clinics of a 936-bed university hospital.

FINDINGS
The most frequently fulfilled record-keeping behaviors were solution type, total solution amount, and date of treatment. The least frequently fulfilled behaviors were the diagnoses of clients and the time of passage for medication added to the solution. The nurses never recorded type of IVFT, complications, and discontinuation of therapy.

IMPLICATIONS
According to the findings of this study, the record-keeping behavior of nurses regarding IVFT is not at the desired level.

Arslan, S., & Karadag, A. (2008). The determination of record-keeping behavior of nurses regarding intravenous fluid treatment: The case of Turkey. *Journal of Infusion Nursing, 31*(5), 287–294.

Blood Transfusion

The purpose of a blood transfusion is to replace blood loss (deficit) with whole blood or blood components. On the basis of the client's unique needs, the prescribing practitioner determines the type of transfusion to administer, either whole blood or a component of whole blood, such as packed RBCs.

WHOLE BLOOD AND BLOOD PRODUCTS Clients with a demonstrated deficiency in either whole blood or a specific component of blood are given a blood transfusion. Whole blood contains RBCs and plasma components of blood. It is used when the client needs all the components of blood to restore blood volume after severe hemorrhage and to restore the capacity of the blood to carry oxygen. Various types of blood components are used in the clinical setting (see Table 33-8 on page 956). Packed RBCs are more commonly prescribed than whole blood.

TABLE 33-8 Blood-Component Therapy

TYPE	USES	SPECIAL CONSIDERATIONS
Fresh or frozen plasma	• Replaces deficient coagulation factors • Increases intravascular compartment	• Use within 6 hours with any straight-line administration set. • Client is at risk for hepatitis.
Platelet	• Corrects bleeding disorders (e.g., thrombocytopenia) • Replaces platelets	• Infuse at rate of 10 minutes a unit with special platelet administration set.
Albumin	• Restores intravascular volume • Treats shock and hypoproteinemia	• Available in 5% and 25% solution. • Infuse slowly with special tubing that accompanies solution.
Granulocyte (white blood cell)	• Restores the leukocyte count, usually depressed in clients receiving radiation or chemotherapy	• Infuse slowly, over 2- to 4-hour interval with Y-type blood filters, and prime with normal saline.
Cryoprecipitate	• Restores factor VIII and fibrinogen in treating hemophilia A	• Infuse with a straight-line administration set. • Observe for febrile reactions.

Delmar/Cengage Learning

Plasma or fresh frozen plasma is separated and frozen within 8 hours after blood collection. Albumin (protein colloid) is a volume expander that maintains the colloid osmotic pressure of the blood. Albumin, hetastarch, and dextran (nonprotein colloids) are agents that increase intravascular volume in order to maintain hemodynamic stability and to provide adequate tissue perfusion. Cryoprecipitate is the most expensive of all blood components because it is constituted from many units of whole blood.

When the prescribing practitioner orders the administration of whole blood or a blood product, the client's blood is typed and cross-matched; refer to Chapter 28 for a complete discussion of blood groups and Rhesus (Rh) factor. Check with the family for donors if time and the client's condition permit. The blood is stored in the blood bank after typing and cross-matching until the nurse is ready to administer it.

Although whole blood has a refrigerated shelf life of 35 days, platelets must be administered within 3 days after they have been extracted from whole blood. If the RBCs and plasma are frozen, their shelf life can be extended up to 3 years (Kee et al., 2010).

INITIAL ASSESSMENT AND PREPARATION
The nurse must perform an initial assessment before administering blood (see the accompanying display on page 957). The viscosity of whole blood usually requires the use of an 18- or 19-gauge needle or catheter to prevent damage to the red cells.

Scheduled IV medications should be infused before blood administration. This sequence prevents a reaction to a medication while blood is infusing; if a reaction were to occur, the nurse would not be able to discern which infusate was causing the reaction.

ADMINISTERING WHOLE BLOOD OR A BLOOD COMPONENT
The agency's blood protocol may require that a licensed person sign a form to release the blood from the blood bank and that a blood product be checked by two licensed personnel prior to infusion. The following information must be on the blood bag label and verified for accuracy: the client's name and identification number, ABO group and Rh factor, donor number, type of product ordered by the practitioner, and the expiration date.

Observe the blood bag for any signs of puncture, gas bubbles, color, and consistency (RBCs clumping). When the information has been verified, both licensed personnel sign the appropriate form. If any of the information does not match exactly or if the product has expired, return the product immediately to the blood bank.

Blood should be administered within 30 minutes after it has been received from the bank to maintain RBC integrity and to decrease the chance of infection. Whole blood should not go unrefrigerated for more than 4 hours. Room temperature will cause RBC lysis, releasing potassium and causing hyperkalemia (see Procedure 33-10).

SAFETY MEASURES
As discussed in Procedure 33-10, the client should be observed for the initial 15 minutes for a transfusion reaction. Vital signs are usually taken every 15 minutes for the first hour, then every hour while the blood is transfusing.

BLOOD TRANSFUSION, INITIAL ASSESSMENT

- Verify that client has signed a blood administration consent form and that this consent matches what the prescribing practitioner has ordered.
- Verify whether the client has an 18- or 19-gauge needle or catheter in the vein; if the blood is to be infused quickly, a 14- or 15-gauge device must be used. Pediatric and older adult clients may require a 23-gauge device because of smaller or thin-walled veins.
- Ensure patency of the existing IV site.
- Establish baseline data for vital signs, especially temperature, and assess skin for eruptions or rashes.
- Check client's blood type against the label on the whole blood or blood component prior to administration, to ensure compatibility.
- Assess client's age. If the client is at risk for circulatory overload (pediatric, older adult, and malnourished clients), notify the blood bank to divide the 500-mL bag of blood into two 250-mL bags or discuss with the prescribing practitioner other alternatives, such as packed RBCs rather than whole blood.

To prevent blood contamination, change the blood tubing and filter every 4 hours or after each unit of blood. Transfuse each unit of blood over a 2- to 4-hour interval.

As a precaution against a blood transfusion reaction, prepare a bag of 0.9% sodium chloride, as directed by policy. The 0.9% sodium chloride is prepared as a secondary infusion system; it should not be connected to the Y-set tubing that is transfusing blood. If the client has a reaction and the blood is discontinued, the secondary bag of 0.9% sodium chloride should be connected and infused. This action prevents the client from receiving all the blood that is in the Y-set tubing, approximately 20 to 30 mL. Even though the procedure for infusing packed cells requires a Y-set for coadministering 0.9%

▼ SAFETY FIRST ▼

TRANSFUSION REACTION
The severity of a transfusion reaction is relative to its onset. Severe reactions may occur shortly after the blood starts to infuse. At the first sign of a reaction, stop the blood infusion immediately.

▼ SAFETY FIRST ▼

BLOOD TRANSFUSION INCOMPATIBILITY
Use only normal saline with a blood product. Blood transfusions are incompatible with dextrose and with Ringer's solution. Together, they cause hemolysis, clumping of RBCs.

sodium chloride, the secondary bag of 0.9% sodium chloride is a precautionary measure for transfusion reactions.

There are three basic types of transfusion reactions: allergic, febrile, and hemolytic. Other complications include sepsis, hypervolemia, and hypothermia. An allergic reaction may be mild or severe, depending on the cause. Hemolytic reactions may be immediate or delayed up to 96 hours, depending on the cause of the reaction. The classic symptoms of a reaction and sepsis are fever and chills.

The immediate nursing actions for all types of reactions and complications are to stop the transfusion, keep the vein open with 0.9% sodium chloride, and notify the prescribing practitioner. Other measures include sending the IV tubing and bag of blood back to the blood bank, obtaining a blood and urine specimen, labeling the specimen "Blood Transfusion Reaction," processing a transfusion reaction report, monitoring vital signs every 15 minutes for 4 hours or until stable, and monitoring the I&O.

A delayed hemolytic reaction results when donor and client anti-A or anti-B agglutinins are mismatched or when there has been improper storage of the blood unit. This reaction causes the cells to clump and form plugs in small blood vessels. Within a few hours or days, the phagocytic white blood cells (WBCs) and the reticuloendothelial system destroy agglutinated cells, releasing hemoglobin into the plasma. The client is monitored for jaundice, persistent anemia or fever, oliguria, flank pain, and abnormal bleeding.

An immediate hemolytic reaction is a rare occurrence. It results from a mismatch of the donor's and client's blood, causing immediate hemolysis of RBCs. The antibodies cause lysis of RBCs, which release proteolytic enzymes that rupture the cell membranes. The clinical manifestations are headache, dyspnea, cyanosis, chest pain, and tachycardia.

Febrile reactions are common and result from the client's sensitivity to WBCs, platelets, or plasma proteins. Warm, flushed skin; headache; muscle pain; and anxiety are the symptoms of a febrile reaction. It is treated with antipyretic medication.

To help prevent a febrile reaction, keep the client warm during the transfusion. Make sure that the tubing has a leukocyte-reduction filter. The leukocyte-reduction filter also reduces the risk of transmitting **cytomegalovirus (CMV)**, a DNA virus that causes intranuclear and intracytoplasmic changes in infected cells. Approximately 10% of seropositive donors are capable of transmitting CMV infection.

Mild allergic reactions are common, resulting from a sensitivity to infusing plasma proteins. Allergic reactions cause a rash, itching, hives (urticaria), and wheezing. Clients with these symptoms should be monitored for anaphylactic shock. Antihistamines may be prescribed to counter the allergic response.

Severe allergic reaction results from an antibody-antigen response as demonstrated by shortness of breath and chest pain; if untreated, it may cause circulatory collapse and cardiac arrest. If this occurs, initiate CPR after the blood has been discontinued.

Sepsis results from the administration of contaminated blood (containing gram-negative bacteria). It is a serious complication. Clinical manifestations include chills and fever, vomiting, abdominal cramping, diarrhea, shock, and renal failure. It is treated with broad-spectrum antibiotics and steroids. Nursing measures are directed toward maintaining hydration and monitoring I&O to evaluate renal function.

Hypervolemia from fluid overload is a preventable complication. Clients at risk for fluid overload are placed in a sitting position. The blood is transfused at a reduced flow rate; request the blood laboratory to divide the unit into two containers of blood so that none of it is unrefrigerated for more than 2 hours during transfusion. Clinical manifestations of hypervolemia are similar to those of fluid overload: dyspnea, cough and rales, distended neck veins, hypertension, tachycardia, and pulmonary edema. Administer oxygen and IV diuretics as prescribed to treat circulatory overload.

Clients needing rapid transfusions are at risk for transfusion-induced hypothermia. Such clients may include neonates needing exchange transfusions and trauma victims who require large volumes of whole blood. A blood-warming device may be prescribed to prevent transfusion-induced hypothermia. The symptoms of transfusion-induced hypothermia result from the rapid transfusion of large amounts of cold blood. If the infusing blood temperature is below 30°C (86°F), the myocardial temperature decreases, causing hypotension and myocardial irritability that may progress to ventricular fibrillation and cardiac arrest. Nursing interventions are directed toward warming the client with temperature-regulating blankets after the transfusion has been stopped. Obtain an electrocardiogram (ECG) to assess for cardiac arrhythmias.

COMPLEMENTARY THERAPY

Herbs and certain foods are used to maintain health and prevent the onset of chronic debilitating diseases such as diabetes mellitus and renal failure. Naturopathic health care practitioners (NDs) use herbs as medicine, and although herbs are the main ingredient of some of the drugs used in conventional medicine, NDs use herbs differently than MDs. MDs prescribe drugs to treat symptoms. For example, in hypertension, the prescribed drug controls the blood pressure but does not correct the reason why the body has increased the pressure in the first place; an ND uses herbs to correct the underlying problem. The following discussion will explain how herbs and foods can be used to treat certain conditions that create disturbances in body fluids and pH.

Traditional Chinese medicine relies on nutrition and dietetic principles to treat certain illnesses and imbalances. Foods are recommended based on their energetic properties such as toxifying, dispersing, heating, cooling, moistening, and drying and eating in tune with seasonal changes. Cooling foods such as watermelon, celery, and cucumber are recommended during the warmer months of spring and summer because they contain a higher percentage of water than warming foods such as meats, garlic, and spices, which are eaten during the cooler months of autumn and winter.

Many plants have a hypoglycemic action; they lower blood sugar levels. Such plants include dandelion root, garlic, ginseng, and nettles. Other plants have also been identified as possessing hypoglycemic action such as allspice, artichoke, banana, barley, bugleweed, lettuce, oats, onion, and spinach, to name a few. When herbs and diet are used in a tailor-made combination for the individual, the amount of glucose entering the blood is kept at a constant level. Tierra and Lust (2008) recommend dandelion root in combination with other tonic herbs such as ginseng and a little ginger for maximum benefit, along with a balanced diet for hypoglycemia.

Herbs such as dandelion and cleavers, which aid the kidneys, not only are useful for renal problems but may aid the cleansing mechanism in treating the whole body, no matter what the problem. The main benefits of dandelion are exerted upon the functions of the liver by clearing obstructions and stimulating and aiding the liver to eliminate toxins from the blood. Dandelion root is helpful in treating hypertension, thus aiding the action of the heart. Dandelion (root and leaf) acts as a diuretic and can be taken for fluid retention, cystitis, and nephritis. Dandelion also contains a high percentage of potassium and actually increases the potassium level, thereby avoiding the loss of potassium caused by synthetic diuretics.

Caution should be used when taking licorice since this herb contains a variety of active ingredients. Glycyrrhizin, an active ingredient of licorice, can produce effects similar to aldosterone. Due to the aldosterone-like effects, whole licorice can cause fluid retention, high blood pressure, and potassium loss in doses that exceed 3 g daily for more than 6 weeks. Clients who take digitalis or a thiazide diuretic or who have hypertension, heart disease, diabetes, or kidney disease should avoid the use of licorice.

EVALUATION

Evaluation is an ongoing process for clients with fluid, electrolyte, and acid-base imbalances. Focus on the client's responses when evaluating whether the time frames and expected outcomes are realistic (such as whether the I&O are within 200 to 300 mL of each other). The client's vital signs should be within normal limits. The IV infusion rate is accurately calculated and reassessed throughout therapy to maintain the client's hydration. The IV site should remain free from erythema, edema, and purulent drainage. The nursing care plan is modified as necessary to support the client's expected outcomes.

NURSING CARE PLAN

The Client with Deficient Fluid Volume

CASE PRESENTATION

Mrs. Gray is a 75-year-old woman with diabetes who has been experiencing flulike symptoms of vomiting and diarrhea for 5 days. She lives alone and does not like to cook. When she got up this morning, she felt weak and dizzy; she called 911 to take her to the clinic. The EMS providers called the practitioner en route, and Mrs. Gray was taken directly to the infusion center.

ASSESSMENT

- Marked thirst
- Temperature 37.2°C
- BP 94/74
- Wt 157 lb (5% loss from 165)
- Dry mucous membranes
- Respirations 30
- Apical pulse 108/min
- ↑ HCT, ↑ hbg, ↑ BUN

NURSING DIAGNOSIS 1: *Deficient fluid volume* related to vomiting and diarrhea
NOC: Hydration
NIC: Fluid/electrolyte management

EXPECTED OUTCOMES

1. The client will
   - Experience relief from vomiting and diarrhea in 2–4 hours.
   - Demonstrate clinical signs of adequate hydration prior to discharge.
   - Understand the reasons for the deficient fluid and the amounts and types of foods and fluids to consume to prevent a recurrence.
2. The client's fluid intake and output will be balanced in 12–24 hours.
3. The client's weight will be stable, and lab values will be within normal limits prior to discharge.

INTERVENTIONS/RATIONALES

1. Assess and document amount, color, and characteristics of vomitus and diarrhea. Determines fluid replacement.
2. Maintain NPO status. Allows the GI tract to heal.
3. Measure vital signs qh. Monitors client status.
4. Assess skin turgor. Indicates hydration status.
5. Administer antiemetics and antidiarrheals. Prevents further fluid loss.
6. Measure and document qh. Assesses fluid balance.
7. Report and document output < 30 mL/h. Alerts to severe fluid imbalance.
8. Administer PO fluids as tolerated 2 hours postvomiting/diarrhea. Gradually reintroduces oral intake.
9. Administer IV lactated Ringer's solution with flow rate as prescribed. Prevents overhydration.
10. Assess and document skin and mucous membrane moisture, skin color and hydration, urine for sugar or acetone, and mental status. Indicates hydration status.
11. Weigh the client on the same scale, in the same clothes, after voiding. Monitor serum glucose, osmolality, HCT, hgb, and BUN. Monitors weight changes and fluid and electrolyte status.

(Continues)

NURSING CARE PLAN (Continued)

12. Assess the client's knowledge level; provide information about causes and why interventions are being performed, and explain actions to take to prevent a recurrence. Educates client as to causes and remedies for fluid volume deficit.

EVALUATION

- Client free from vomiting 2 hours postadmission; diarrhea stopped within 5 hours after being placed NPO.
- Hourly urinary output 30 mL/h; tolerated 4 oz of Gatorade 6 hours postadmission, progressed to clear liquid diet; I&O balanced 20 hours postadmission.
- Mucous membranes moist; good skin turgor and color; absence of thirst; urine was free from sugar and acetone; alert client prior to discharge.
- Client's weight and lab values were within normal limits prior to discharge.
- Client verbalizes knowledge of causes and methods of monitoring fluid status.

NURSING CARE PLAN

The Client with Excess Fluid Volume

CASE PRESENTATION

Mr. Hill, a 68-year-old widower, was taken to the emergency department by his granddaughter and stated, "I can't breathe." He has a history of hypertension and heart disease. He is obese. The practitioner ordered a stat chest x-ray, complete blood cell count (CBC), and electrolytes.

ASSESSMENT

- Shortness of breath (SOB), rales
- Constant cough
- Wt 161.8 lb
- Pitting edema, ankles
- 36.4°C; 186/114; 98; 30 and labored
- Engorged neck veins
- Pulmonary congestion (x-ray)
- ↓ HCT; ↓ hgb

NURSING DIAGNOSIS 1: *Excess fluid volume* related to body fluid overload secondary to heart dysfunction
NOC: Fluid overload severity
NIC: Fluid monitoring

EXPECTED OUTCOMES

1. The client will
   - Have a balanced fluid intake and output (est. 2500 mL/day) for 2 days.
   - Identify a specific amount of weight to lose over the next 6 months.
   - Manifest normal hydration status prior to discharge.
   - Demonstrate understanding of the causes of excess fluid and the role of heart medications, foods, and exercise to assist with weight reduction.
2. The client's skin integrity will be maintained over the edematous areas.

(Continues)

NURSING CARE PLAN (Continued)

INTERVENTIONS/RATIONALES

1. Measure and document hourly I&O; restrict fluids as ordered. Monitors fluid status.
2. Administer diuretics as ordered; document the response. Increases excretion of electrolytes.
3. Weigh daily at the same time with the same clothing. Monitors overall client status.
4. Measure and document vital signs qh until SOB subsides, then q2h. Hourly assessments: Auscultate for third heart sound, breath sounds; assess rate, rhythm, depth of respirations, and the position the client takes to relieve SOB; report changes in respiratory pattern. Monitors client response to therapy and diuretics; gives information to modify plan of care.
5. Inspect and palpate areas of edema. Determines whether edema is localized or generalized and reveals extent.
6. Institute preventive skin measures: Elevate extremities on pillows to ↓ pressure and promote venous circulation; avoid rubbing the skin, apply lotion, pat dry; avoid soap on the area; inspect for redness or blanching. Maintains skin integrity, promotes circulation, and promotes client comfort.
7. Assess client's knowledge of hypertension and decreased cardiac output; digitalis; the effects of a large abdominal girth on breathing; and foods low in sodium, fats, and carbohydrates. Educating client about causes, aggravating and alleviating factors, and effects of fluid excess is the first step in encouraging client in proper self-care.

EVALUATION

- Output for the first 2 hours 2020 mL; Day 2, I&O measurements indicative of fluid balance.
- Client identified need to lose 30 lb over the next 6 months.
- The client's hemodynamic status is within normal levels as demonstrated by HCT, hgb, and BP 156/92 and by the absence of SOB, abnormal breath sounds, jugular engorgement, or peripheral edema.
- The client's skin integrity was maintained.
- The client was unable to verbalize knowledge of how his weight, high-sodium diet, failure to take his heart medications, and chronic alterations caused the fluid excess. Referred to home health for client teaching.

NURSING PROCESS HIGHLIGHT

Implementation

Fluid Replacement

Fluid replacement is based on weight loss. A 2.2-lb (1 kg) loss is equivalent to 1 L (1000 mL) of fluid loss. First, convert Mrs. Gray's weight from pounds to kilograms. Then determine the fluid intake replacement needed on the basis of the weight loss: Include the IV lactated Ringer's solution and PO Gatorade in milliliters. On the basis of the intake, what should have been her output prior to discharge?

NURSING PROCESS HIGHLIGHT

Nursing Diagnosis

Secondary Diagnoses

The nursing diagnosis *EFV: Edema* usually has many accompanying secondary nursing diagnoses: *Breathing pattern: Ineffective,* related to increased capillary permeability causing fluid overload in the lung tissue (pulmonary edema); *Skin integrity: Impaired,* related to edematous tissues (peripheral edema); *Ineffective tissue perfusion* related to hypervolemia as manifested by peripheral (tissue) edema; and *Deficient knowledge: EFV,* related to chronic alterations.

PROCEDURE 33-1

Measuring Intake and Output

EQUIPMENT

- Intake and output (I&O) form at bedside
- I&O graphic record in chart
- Glass or cup
- Bedpan or urinal bedside commode
- Graduated container for output
- Nonsterile gloves
- Sign at bedside stating client is on I&O

ACTION	RATIONALE
1. Wash hands/hand hygiene.	1. Reduces transmission of microorganisms.
2. Explain the rules of I&O record. All fluids taken orally must be recorded on the client's I&O form (sometimes called a fluid balance flow sheet). • Client must void into bedpan or urinal, not into toilet (see Figure 33-17). • Toilet tissue should be disposed of in plastic-lined container, not in bedpan.	2. Elicits client support. • Fluid voided into the toilet cannot be measured. • Liquids absorbed into toilet tissue cannot be measured by volume.
3. Measure all oral fluids in accord with institution policy; for example, cup 150 mL, glass 240 mL. Record all IV fluids as they are infused (see Figure 33-18).	3. Provides for consistency of measurement.
4. Record time and amount of all fluid intake in the designated space on bedside form (oral, tube feedings, IV fluids).	4. Documents fluids.
5. Transfer 8-hour total fluid intake from bedside I&O record to graphic sheet or 24-hour I&O record on client's chart.	5. Provides for data analysis of the client's fluid status.

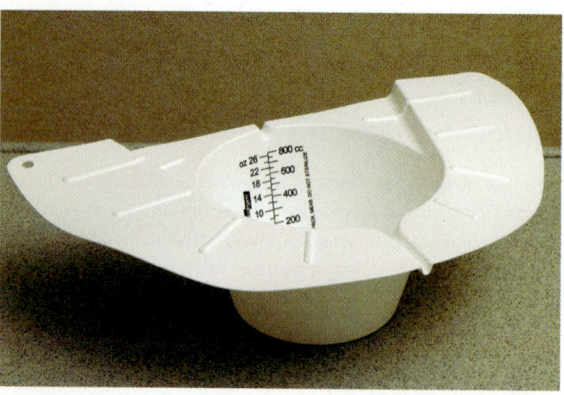

FIGURE 33-17 Graduated specimen container is used to measure urine, drainage, or other output. DELMAR/CENGAGE LEARNING

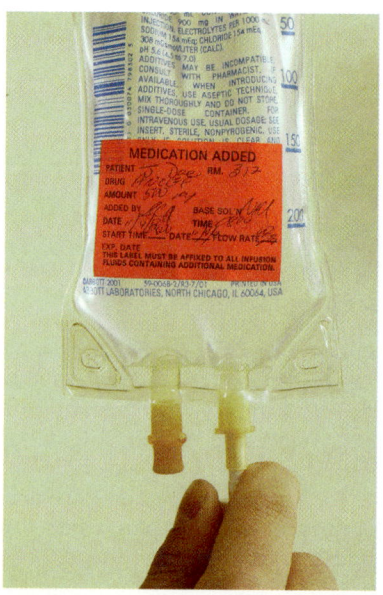

FIGURE 33-18 All IV infused fluids must be measured. DELMAR/ CENGAGE LEARNING

(Continues)

PROCEDURE 33-1
Measuring Intake and Output (Continued)

ACTION	RATIONALE
6. Record all fluid intake in the appropriate column of the 24-hour record.	6. Documents intake by type and amount.
7. Complete 24-hour intake record by adding all 8-hour totals.	7. Provides consistent data for analysis of the client's fluid status over a 24-hour period.

OUTPUT

ACTION	RATIONALE
8. Apply nonsterile gloves.	8. Reduces potential for transmission of pathogens.
9. Empty urinal, bedpan, or Foley drainage bag (see Figure 33-19) into graduated container or commode "hat" (see Figure 33-20).	9. Provides accurate measurement of urine.
10. Remove gloves. Wash hands/hand hygiene.	10. Prevents cross-contamination.
11. Record time and amount of output (urine, drainage from nasogastric tube, drainage tube) on I&O record.	11. Documents output.
12. Transfer 8-hour output totals to graphic sheet or 24-hour I&O record on the client's chart.	12. Provides for data analysis of the client's fluid status.
13. Complete 24-hour output record by totaling all 8-hour totals.	13. Provides consistent data for analysis of the client's fluid status over a 24-hour period.
14. Wash hands/hand hygiene.	14. Reduces transmission of microorganisms.

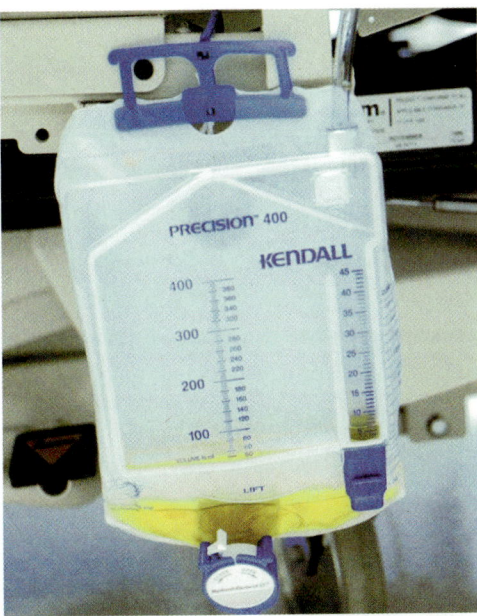

FIGURE 33-19 Urine in Foley drainage bag must be measured. DELMAR/CENGAGE LEARNING

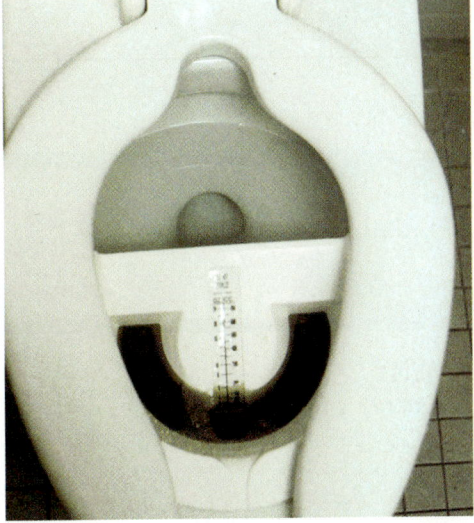

FIGURE 33-20 Empty urine into a graduated container to measure. DELMAR/CENGAGE LEARNING

(Continues)

PROCEDURE 33-1
Measuring Intake and Output (Continued)

delegation tip

I&O measurement may be delegated to ancillary personnel knowledgeable about the following:

- Obtaining accurate measurements and reporting incontinence
- Observing the amount, color, and any odor from the output

- Recording measurements on proper clinical records
- Protecting themselves from contamination from a body fluid and storing collection containers in designated areas

nursing tips

- Keep I&O flow sheet close to the bedside.
- Teach clients about the necessity of keeping accurate I&O records.
- Keep water fresh, and encourage beverages as allowed.
- Record measurements immediately instead of waiting until the end of the shift.
- 240 cc ice chips equal 120 cc fluid.
- Pureed food is not considered to be fluid intake.

- Bottled nutrient tube feedings are liquid and must be considered in I&O.
- All postoperative clients are at risk for fluid loss through blood or plasma from their incision sites. Monitor the dressings.
- Remember that fluids taken to swallow pills must be recorded as intake.
- Do not have visitors or family members empty bedpans, urinals, or catheter bags.

PROCEDURE 33-2
Preparing an IV Solution

EQUIPMENT
- IV solution in a bag
- Medication administration record (MAR)

- IV flow sheet
- IV tubing, if needed

ACTION	RATIONALE
1. Check prescribing practitioner's order for the IV solution (see Figure 33-21 on page 965).	1. Ensures accurate administration of the solution.
2. Wash hands/hand hygiene. Apply gloves if required by institutional policy.	2. Reduces the transmission of microorganisms.
3. Prepare new bag by removing protective cover from bag.	3. Allows for access to the solution container.
4. Inspect the bag for leaks, tears, or cracks. Inspect the fluid for clarity, particulate matter, and color. Check expiration date.	4. Prevents infusing contaminated or outdated solution.

(Continues)

PROCEDURE 33-2
Preparing an IV Solution (Continued)

ACTION	RATIONALE

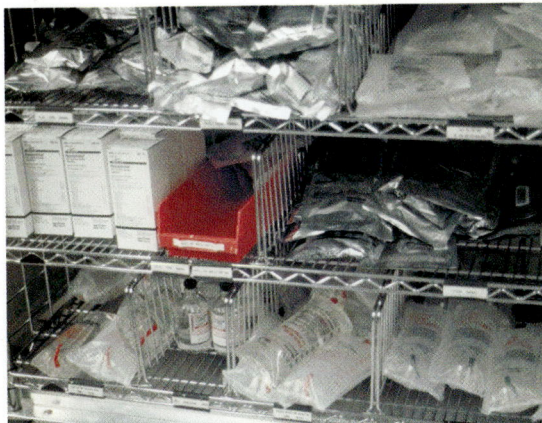

FIGURE 33-21 Many types of prepackaged IV solutions are available. DELMAR/
CENGAGE LEARNING

5. Prepare a label for the IV bag:
   - On the label, note date, time, and your initials.
   - Attach the label to the bag. Keep in mind the bag will be inverted when it is hanging. Make sure the label can be read when the IV is hanging.
6. Store the prepared IV solution in the area assigned by the institution.
7. Remove gloves and dispose of gloves with all used materials.
8. Wash hands/hand hygiene.
9. Document the preparation of the IV solution.

HANGING THE PREPARED IV
10. Wash hands/hand hygiene.
11. Obtain the IV solution for the client as ordered. Check the label on the IV bag to see that it matches the order.
12. Inspect the bag for leaks, tears, or cracks and inspect the fluid for clarity, particulate matter, and color.
13. Check client's identification bracelet.

14. Prepare an IV time label for the IV bag:
   - On the time label, note the rate at which the solution is to infuse.
   - Mark the approximate infusion intervals.
   - Attach the time label to the bag. Keep in mind the bag will be inverted when it is hanging. Make sure the time label can be read when the IV is hanging.

5.
   - Communicates when the bag was opened.
   - Labeling the bag upside down makes identification easier when the bag is hanging.

6. Keeps the prepared solution readily available for when it is needed.
7. Reduces transmission of microorganisms.

8. Reduces transmission of microorganisms.
9. Provides a record to ensure continuity of care.

10. Reduces transmission of microorganisms.
11. Ensures the ordered medication is administered.

12. Prevents infusing contaminated solution.

13. Ensures IV solution is given to the correct client.

14.
   - Communicates how long before the next IV should be hung.
   - Gives a rough estimate of the accuracy of the infusion rate.
   - Placing the time label on the bag upside down makes identification easier when the bag is hanging.

(Continues)

PROCEDURE 33-2
Preparing an IV Solution (Continued)

ACTION	RATIONALE

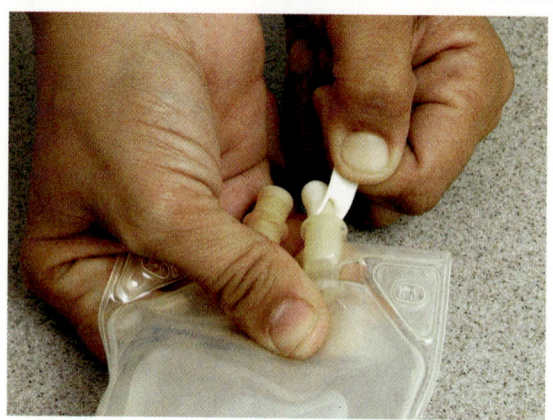

FIGURE 33-22 Open the IV plastic bag and pull down the plastic tab covering the port with one hand while pinching the port with the other hand. DELMAR/CENGAGE LEARNING

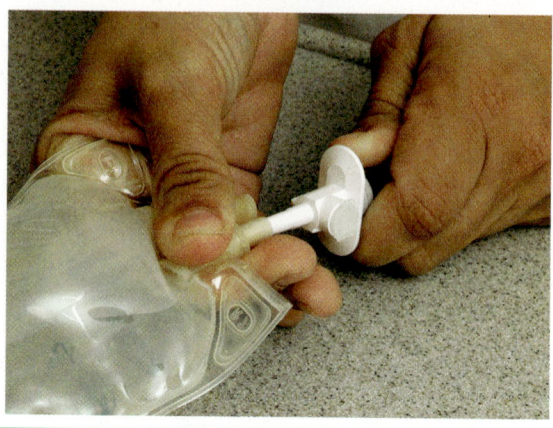

FIGURE 33-23 Remove the cap from the spike, and spike the IV port. DELMAR/CENGAGE LEARNING

15. Make sure the clamp on the tubing is closed. Grasp the port of the IV bag with your nondominant hand, remove the plastic tab covering the port (see Figure 33-22), and insert the full length of the spike into the bag's port (see Figure 33-23).

15. Promotes rapid flow of solution through new tubing without air bubbles.

16. Compress drip chamber to fill halfway.

16. Filling chamber halfway allows the chamber to provide a clear measurement of drip rate when the IV is flowing.

17. Loosen protective cap from the needle or end of the IV tubing, open roller clamp, and flush tubing with solution (see Figure 33-24 on page 967).

17. Removes air from tubing.

18. Close roller clamp and replace cap protector.

18. Prevents fluid from leaking and maintains sterility of needle.

19. When ready to initiate infusion, remove the cap protector from the tubing. Attach the IV tubing to venipuncture catheter.

19. Initiates infusion.

20. Open clamp and regulate flow or, if applicable, attach tubing to infusion device or rate controller if used. Turn on pump and set flow rate (see Procedure 33-7, Setting the IV Flow Rate).

20. Allows flow rate to be regulated.

21. Wash hands/hand hygiene.

21. Reduces transmission of microorganisms.

(Continues)

PROCEDURE 33-2
Preparing an IV Solution (Continued)

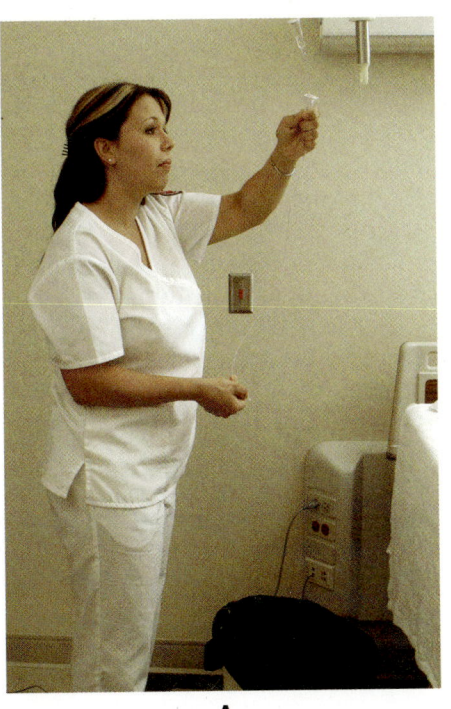
A

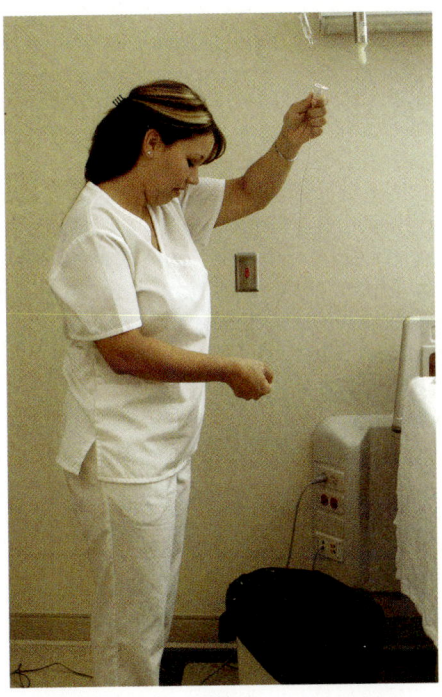
B

FIGURE 33-24 A. Priming the IV tubing. B. Open the roller clamp on the tubing to allow the fluid to enter the tube and expel the air. DELMAR/CENGAGE LEARNING

delegation tip

The skill of IV solution administration is not delegated to ancillary personnel in acute care settings. This may vary in state or federal institutions. Ancillary personnel are generally informed about the medications the client is receiving if adverse effects are anticipated or are being monitored.

nursing tips

- *Anticipate the need for the next bag of IV solution to avoid the risk of an IV clotting caused by the solution running out.*

- *Hold the bag up against both a light and dark solid background to check for discoloration.*

PROCEDURE 33-3
Preparing the IV Bag and Tubing

EQUIPMENT
- Disposable gloves
- IV solution in a bag
- IV tubing as ordered
- Sterile 2 × 2 gauze

(Continues)

PROCEDURE 33-3
Preparing the IV Bag and Tubing (Continued)

ACTION	RATIONALE
1. Check prescribing practitioner's order for the IV solution.	1. Ensures accurate administration of the solution.
2. Wash hands/hand hygiene.	2. Reduces transmission of microorganisms.
3. Check client's identification bracelet. Gather equipment (see Figure 33-25).	3. Ensures medication is given to the correct client.
4. Prepare new bag by removing protective cover. Check the expiration date on the bag and assess for cloudiness or leakage.	4. Allows for quick, smooth preparation. Ensures that the solution is sterile.
5. Open new infusion set. Unroll tubing and close roller clamp.	5. Prevents fluid from leaking after IV bag is spiked.
6. Spike bag with tip of new tubing and compress drip chamber to fill halfway (see Figures 33-26 to 33-28).	6. Promotes rapid flow of solution through new tubing without air bubbles.
7. Open roller clamp, remove protective cap from the end of the tubing, and slowly flush solution completely through tubing.	7. Removes air from tubing. Prevents entry of air into the venous system, a cause of air embolus. If fluid enters tubing too rapidly, air bubbles occur.
8. Close roller clamp and replace cap protector.	8. Prevents fluid from leaking and maintains sterility of tubing.

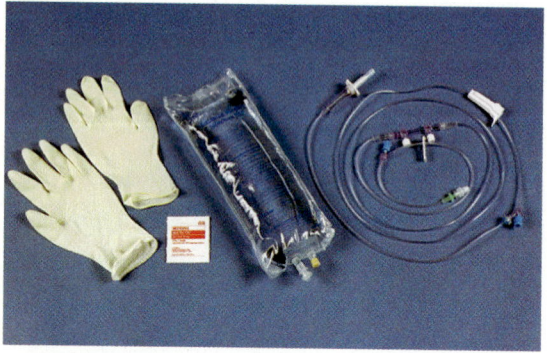

FIGURE 33-25 Gloves, alcohol pad, IV solution, and tubing.
DELMAR/CENGAGE LEARNING

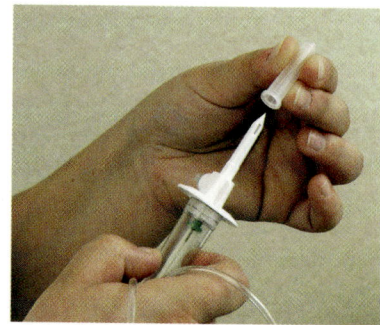

FIGURE 33-26 Remove the protective cap from the end of the IV tubing. DELMAR/CENGAGE LEARNING

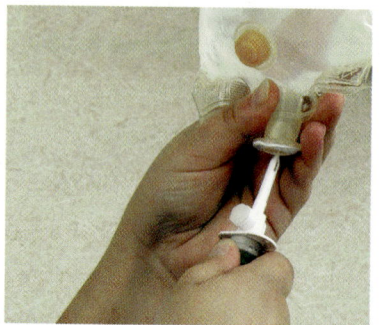

FIGURE 33-27 Spike the bag with the sharp tip of the new tubing. DELMAR/CENGAGE LEARNING

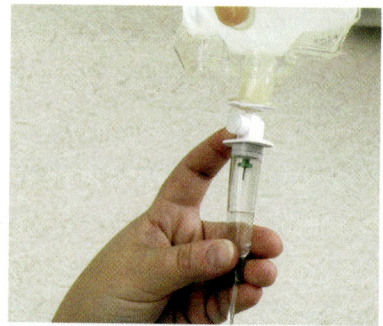

FIGURE 33-28 Compress the drip chamber and allow it to fill halfway with fluid. DELMAR/CENGAGE LEARNING

(Continues)

PROCEDURE 33-3
Preparing the IV Bag and Tubing (Continued)

ACTION	RATIONALE
9. Apply clean gloves.	9. Reduces transmission of microorganisms.
10. Remove old tubing and replace with new tubing:	10.
• Place sterile 2 × 2 gauze under IV catheter or heparin lock.	• Absorbs fluids that may drip during the procedure, preventing contamination of surrounding areas.
• Stabilize hub of catheter or needle and gently pull out old tubing.	• Prevents accidental dislodging of catheter or needle.
• Quickly insert new tubing into hub of catheter or needle.	• Prevents backflow of blood or the entrance of air into the vein.
• Open roller clamp to establish flow of IV solution.	• Prevents catheter occlusion and maintains IV flow at prescribed rate.
• Reestablish drip rate (see Figure 33-29).	• Maintains IV flow at prescribed rate.
• Apply new dressing to IV site.	• Provides protection from infection and accidental dislodgment.
11. Discard old tubing and IV bag.	11. Prevents accidental transmission of microorganisms.
12. Remove gloves and dispose of all used materials.	12. Reduces transmission of microorganisms.
13. Apply a label with date and time of change to tubing. Calculate IV drip rates and begin infusion at prescribed rate.	13. Indicates when tubing replacement is due (every 72–96 hours), in accordance with agency policy. Ensures administration at prescribed rate.
14. Wash hands/hand hygiene.	14. Reduces transmission of microorganisms.

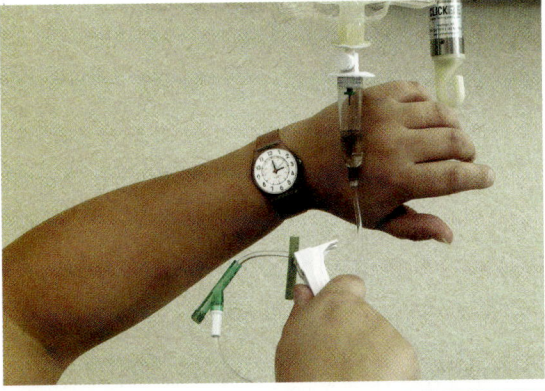

FIGURE 33-29 Establish the drip rate. DELMAR/CENGAGE LEARNING

delegation tip

Initiating IV therapy via IV bag and tubing preparation is a skill involving assessment and the use of medical asepsis. It is a procedure not delegated by the nurse unless other licensed personnel have been trained and certified to perform the procedure.

nursing tips

- *Be sure the tape at the IV site is loosened so it is easier to change the tubing.*
- *Place a towel under the arm of the IV site where the tubing will be changed in order to keep the linen clean in case of blood leaking from the needle during IV tubing change.*

PROCEDURE 33-4

Assessing and Maintaining an IV Insertion Site

EQUIPMENT
- Clean gloves
- Gauze dressing
- Tape
- Nursing documentation record

ACTION	RATIONALE
1. Review prescribing practitioner's order for IV therapy.	1. Ensures accuracy in the administration of IV therapy.
2. Review client's history for medical conditions or allergies.	2. Decreases risk of fluid overload and allergic reactions.
3. Review client's IV site record and intake and output (I&O) record.	3. Assesses for potential problems with fragile IV sites and fluid balance.
4. Wash hands/hand hygiene.	4. Decreases transmission of microorganisms.
5. Assemble equipment and obtain client's vital signs (see Figure 33-30).	5. Assesses for changes in cardiovascular system.
6. Check IV fluid for correct fluid, additives, rate, and volume at the beginning of the shift (see Figure 33-31).	6. Ensures client is receiving correct therapy.
7. Check IV tubing for tight connections every 4 hours.	7. Ensures that no fluid leaks from tubing and connections.
8. Check gauze IV dressing hourly to be sure it is dry and intact (see Figure 33-32 on page 971).	8. Ensures there is no sign of infiltration or infection at IV insertion site.
9. If the gauze is not dry and intact, remove the dressing and observe site for redness, swelling, or drainage.	9. Ensures there is no sign of inflammation or infection at IV site.
10. If an occlusive dressing is used, do not remove the dressing when assessing the site.	10. Ensures there is no sign of inflammation or infection at IV site. Transparent dressings can be left in place up to a week if they remain clean, dry, and intact (Hadaway, 2008).
11. Observe vein track for redness, swelling, warmth, or pain hourly.	11. These are early signs of phlebitis or infiltration.
12. Document IV site findings in the nursing record or flow sheet.	12. Provides documentation of frequent IV site observation.
13. Wash hands/hand hygiene.	13. Decreases transmission of microorganisms.

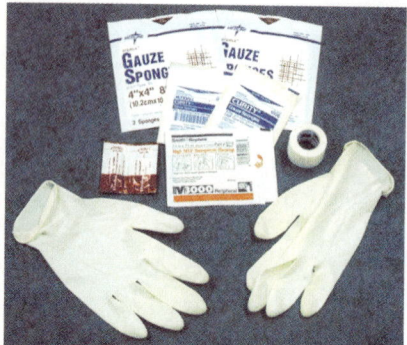

FIGURE 33-30 Transparent dressing, nonsterile gloves, tape, gauze sponges, and topical iodine ointment. DELMAR/ CENGAGE LEARNING

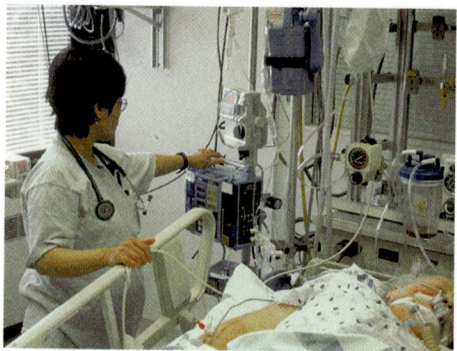

FIGURE 33-31 Check the IV fluid rate, volume, tubing, and additives at the beginning of the shift. DELMAR/CENGAGE LEARNING

(Continues)

PROCEDURE 33-4
Assessing and Maintaining an IV Insertion Site (Continued)

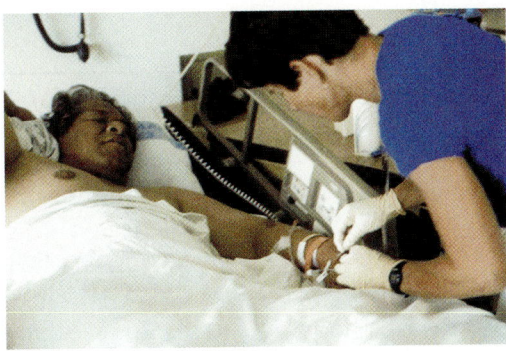

FIGURE 33-32 Check the IV dressing site every hour. DELMAR/CENGAGE LEARNING

delegation tip

Assessing and maintaining the IV after establishing the infusion is the responsibility of the nurse. It is a procedure not delegated unless other licensed personnel have been trained and certified to perform the procedure. Ancillary personnel may be instructed to report an infusion that is dripping too fast or an IV bag that is almost empty. It is the nurse's responsibility to monitor the infusion, but ancillary personnel may also be instructed to report any observations such as swelling, leaking, client concerns about pain, numbness, or tingling at the site or in the extremity used for the infusion. Ancillary personnel may also be involved in monitoring the client's daily weight, if ordered, along with I&O. They should be instructed not to obtain vital signs on an extremity with solutions infusing.

nursing tips

- *Be organized. Review the orders before examining the client's IV so you do not have to go back and check.*
- *Bring supplies with you for the assessment: gauze, tape, scissors, gloves.*

- *As you complete your assessment of the client's IV, incorporate teaching the client the signs and symptoms to report.*

PROCEDURE 33-5

Changing the IV Solution

EQUIPMENT
- Disposable gloves
- IV solution in a bag
- Additives as ordered
- IV tubing
- Alcohol swab (if needed)

(Continues)

PROCEDURE 33-5
Changing the IV Solution (Continued)

ACTION	RATIONALE
1. Check prescribing practitioner's order for the IV solution.	1. Ensures accurate administration of the solution.
2. Wash hands/hand hygiene. Don clean gloves.	2. Reduces transmission of microorganisms.
3. Check client's identification bracelet.	3. Ensures IV solution is given to the correct client.
4. Prepare new bag with additives as ordered by prescribing practitioner (see Figure 33-33).	4. Laboratory tests may reveal a need for potassium, insulin, or magnesium.
• Plan for new bag to be hung at least 1 hour before it is needed.	• Reduces clot formation in vein caused by empty IV bag.
• Change solution when the IV bag is empty but there is still solution in the drip chamber (see Figure 33-34).	• Prevents air from entering tubing and vein from clotting from lack of flow of fluid.
5. Be sure drip chamber is at least half full (see Figure 33-35 on page 973).	5. Prevents entry of air into IV tubing while bag is being changed.
6. Change IV solution:	6.
• Move roller clamp to stop flow of fluid.	• Prevents fluid in drip chamber from emptying while changing solutions.
• Remove old IV bag from IV pole and hang new bag.	• Prepares equipment.
• Spike new bag with tubing (see Figure 33-36 on page 973).	• Maintains sterility of solution.
• Reestablish prescribed flow rate.	• Prevents clotting of vein.

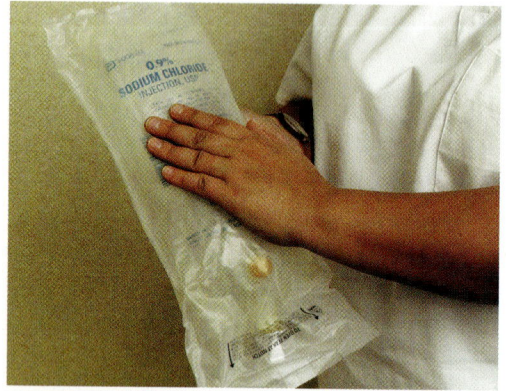

FIGURE 33-33 Prepare new bag. DELMAR/CENGAGE LEARNING

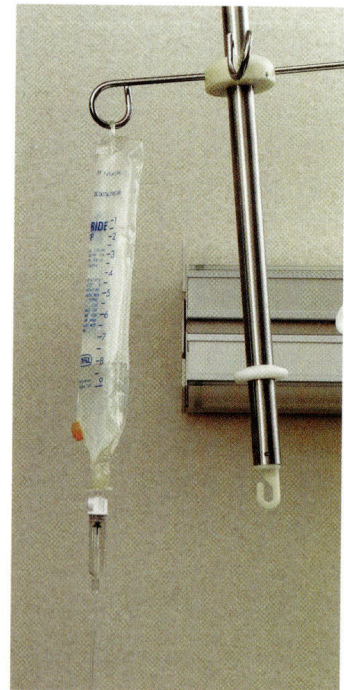

FIGURE 33-34 The IV bag needs to be replaced. DELMAR/CENGAGE LEARNING

(Continues)

PROCEDURE 33-5
Changing the IV Solution (Continued)

ACTION	RATIONALE

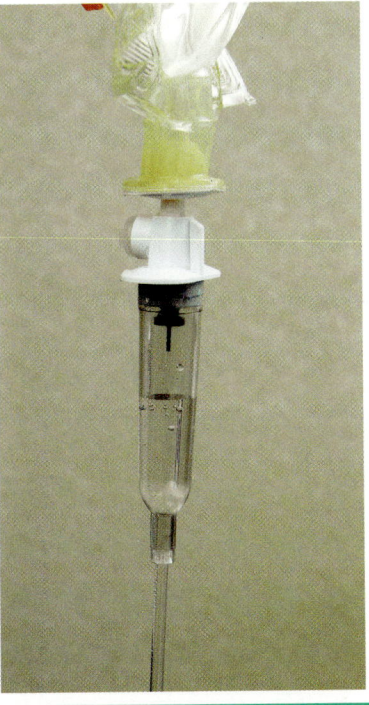

FIGURE 33-35 Make sure the drip chamber is at least half full of fluid. DELMAR/CENGAGE LEARNING

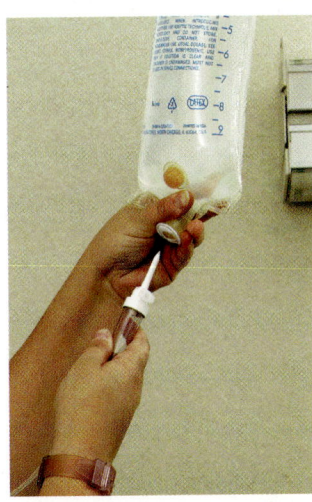

FIGURE 33-36 Spike the new bag with the sharp end of the tubing. DELMAR/CENGAGE LEARNING

7. Check for air in tubing.
   - If air bubbles are present, close the roller clamp. While stretching the tubing, flick the tubing with the finger and watch the bubbles rise to the drip chamber.
   - If a large amount of air is in the tubing, insert a needle with an empty syringe into a port below the air (see Figure 33-37 on page 974) and allow the air to enter the syringe as it flows to the client (see Figure 33-38 on page 974).
8. Empty remaining fluid from old IV if needed (see Figure 33-39 on page 974).
9. Remove gloves and dispose of all used materials.
10. Apply a label with date, time, and type of solution.
11. Wash hands/hand hygiene.

7. Reduces risk of air embolus.

8. Disposes of excess fluid. Reduces risk of spilling large amounts of fluid in waste can.
9. Reduces transmission of microorganisms.

10. Allows for planning of next change.

11. Reduces transmission of microorganisms.

(Continues)

PROCEDURE 33-5
Changing the IV Solution (Continued)

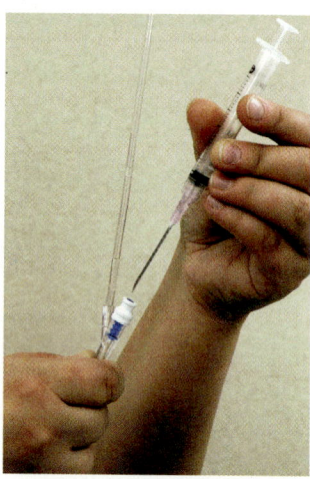

FIGURE 33-37 If there is a large amount of air in the tubing, insert a syringe into a port between the air and the client. DELMAR/CENGAGE LEARNING

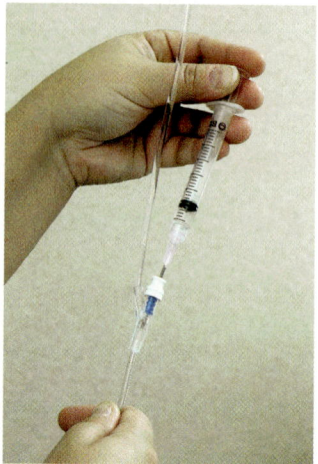

FIGURE 33-38 Allow the air to flow into the syringe. DELMAR/ CENGAGE LEARNING

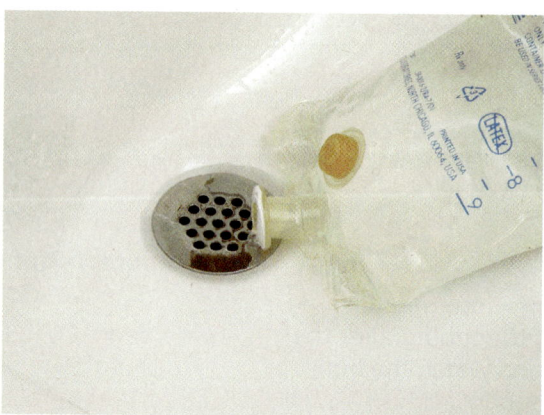

FIGURE 33-39 Drain the remaining fluid from the old IV bag. DELMAR/CENGAGE LEARNING

delegation tip

Changing the IV solution after establishing the infusion is the responsibility of the nurse. It is a procedure not delegated unless other licensed personnel have been trained and certified to perform the procedure. Ancillary personnel may be instructed to report an infusion that is dripping too fast or an IV bag that is almost empty.

nursing tips

- *Anticipate the need for the next bag of IV solution to avoid the risk of an IV clotting because of the solution running out.*

- *Keep in mind the client's laboratory results and need for fluid to be sure the correct solution is given.*

PROCEDURE 33-6
Flushing a Central Venous Catheter

EQUIPMENT
- Chlorhexidine 2% and alcohol swabs
- Syringes (10-mL)
- Vial or ampule of normal saline solution
- Vial of heparin solution (heparin flush or heparin 100 units/mL in saline) (check institution policy on heparin solution use)
- Plastic clamp or metal bull-dog clamp
- Sterile needle (20- to 22-gauge)
- Sterile gloves, gown, and mask

ACTION	RATIONALE
1. Wash hands/hand hygiene. Apply gloves, gown, and other protective equipment as needed.	1. Reduces transmission of microorganisms.
2. Prepare two syringes (see Figure 33-40): one with 10 mL normal saline and one with 5 mL heparin solution.	2. Preparing equipment in advance allows for a smooth procedure.
3. Swab injection cap or catheter hub with alcohol or chlorhexidine 2%.	3. Prevents introduction of microorganisms into catheter.
4. Clamp catheter and remove cap.	4. Prevents entrance of air into catheter.
5. Check catheter for patency:	5. Ensures patency of catheter.
• Attach syringe with normal saline.	• Connects syringe to catheter.
• Release clamp.	• Opens catheter lumen.
• Aspirate heparin solution from catheter (see Figure 33-41).	• Removes old heparin solution.
• Observe blood return.	• Verifies patency of catheter.
• Flush quickly with normal saline (see Figure 33-42 on page 976).	• Ensures that catheter will be cleared of any blood so it will not clot.
• Reclamp.	• Clamping catheter during changes of syringes prevents air from entering catheter.
• Remove empty syringe.	• Continues procedure.
• Attach syringe filled with 5 mL heparin solution to catheter.	• Connects syringe to catheter.
• Release clamp.	• Opens catheter lumen.
• Flush quickly.	• Injects heparin solution into catheter.
• Reclamp.	• Closes catheter lumen.

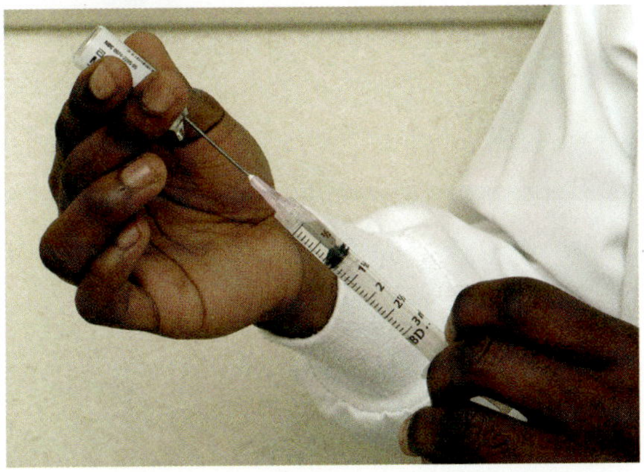

FIGURE 33-40 Prepare two syringes. DELMAR/CENGAGE LEARNING

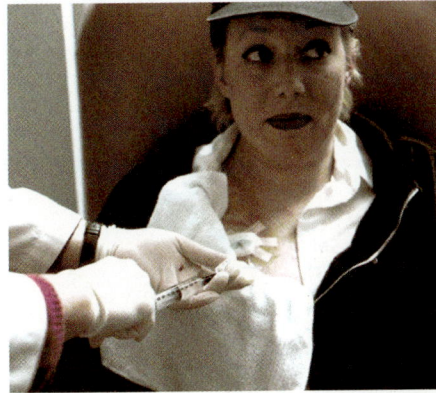

FIGURE 33-41 Aspirate heparin solution from the catheter and flush with saline. DELMAR/CENGAGE LEARNING

(Continues)

PROCEDURE 33-6
Flushing a Central Venous Catheter (Continued)

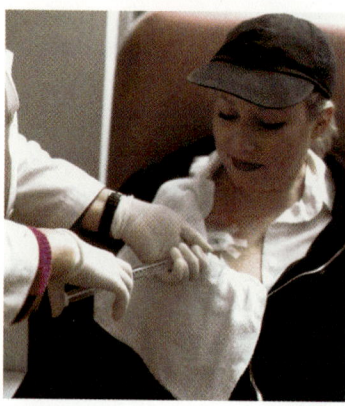

FIGURE 33-42 **Flush with heparin solution.** DELMAR/CENGAGE LEARNING

ACTION	RATIONALE
6. Place new cap on end of catheter, tape all tubing connections, and attach tubing to client's clothing.	6. Maintains sterile seal to catheter.
7. Dispose of soiled equipment and used supplies.	7. Reduces transmission of microorganisms.
8. Wash hands/hand hygiene.	8. Reduces transmission of microorganisms.

delegation tip

Flushing a central venous line is a complex skill requiring assessment and proper technique. It is a procedure not delegated unless other licensed personnel have been trained and certified to perform the procedure.

nursing tips

- *Have all the equipment available for the procedure.*
- *Take advantage of this procedure to assess the client and provide emotional support.*
- *Different catheters require different amounts of heparin or no heparin at all.*

- *Some catheters do not require clamps.*
- *If maneuvers to aspirate blood are not successful, the prescribing practitioner should be notified so fibrinolytic therapy (urokinase) can be ordered and given according to institutional policy.*

PROCEDURE 33-7
Setting the IV Flow Rate

EQUIPMENT
- Watch with a second hand
- IV solution in a bag
- IV tubing
- IV infusion pump
- Volume-control device
- Paper and pencil

ACTION	RATIONALE
1. Check prescribing practitioner's order for the IV solution and rate of infusion.	1. Ensures accurate administration of the solution.
2. Wash hands/hand hygiene.	2. Reduces transmission of microorganisms.

(Continues)

PROCEDURE 33-7
Setting the IV Flow Rate (Continued)

ACTION	RATIONALE
3. Check client's identification bracelet.	3. Ensures medication is given to the correct client.
4. Prepare to set flow rate: • Have paper and pencil ready to calculate flow rate. • Review calibration in drops per milliliter (gtt/mL) of each infusion set.	4. • A nurse unfamiliar with IV fluid rates should calculate the rate at first. • Drops per milliliter vary with manufacturer and tubing type. Macrodrip tubing varies from 10–15 gtt/mL. Microdrip tubing generally delivers 60 gtt/mL.

5. Determine hourly rate by dividing total volume by total hours.
Example 1:
The order reads 1000 mL D5W with 20 mEq KCl over 8 hours:

$$\frac{1000 \text{ mL}}{8 \text{ h}} = 125 \text{ mL/h}$$

Example 2:

Three liters are ordered for 24 hours:

$$\frac{3000 \text{ mL}}{24 \text{ h}} = 125 \text{ mL/h}$$

5. Provides a prescribed hourly rate with no sudden increases or decreases. The formula for calculation is:

$$\frac{m/h}{60 \text{ min}} = mL/min$$

6. Apply a time label to the IV bag with the hourly time periods according to the rate.

6. Provides a visual check of the fluid infused to be sure the rate is correct.

7. Calculate the minute rate based on the drop factor of the infusion set:

$$\text{Drop factor} \times mL/min = gtt/min$$

$$\frac{mL/h \times \text{drop factor}}{60 \text{ min}} = gtt/min$$

$$\frac{\text{hourly rate} \times \text{drop factor}}{\text{infusion time in minutes}} = gtt/min$$

7. The nurse can use the formulas to calculate how many drops per minute will be infused and can adjust the rate for a change in tubing (macrodrip, microdrip).

• Microdrip example:

$$\frac{125 \text{ mL} \times 60 \text{ gtt/mL}}{60 \text{ min}} = \frac{7500 \text{ gtt}}{60 \text{ min}} = 125 \text{ gtt/min}$$

• Macrodrip example:

$$\frac{125 \text{ mL} \times 15 \text{ gtt/mL}}{60 \text{ min}} = 31 \text{ gtt/min}$$

8. Set flow rate using the appropriate device (see Figures 33-43 and 33-44 on page 978).
• For regular tubing without a device: Count drops in drip chamber for 1 minute while

8.
• Ensures that infusion is administered as ordered.
• Pumps the solution through the tubing at the rate set.

(Continues)

PROCEDURE 33-7
Setting the IV Flow Rate (Continued)

ACTION	RATIONALE

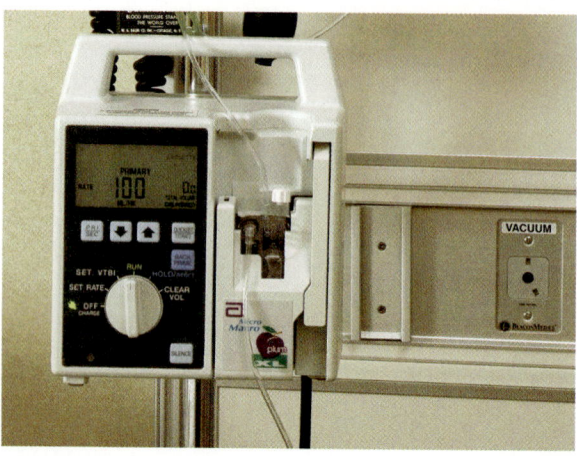

FIGURE 33-43 There are many types of IV pumps available. DELMAR/CENGAGE LEARNING

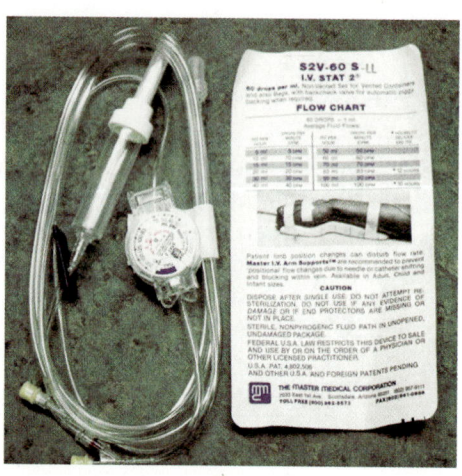

A

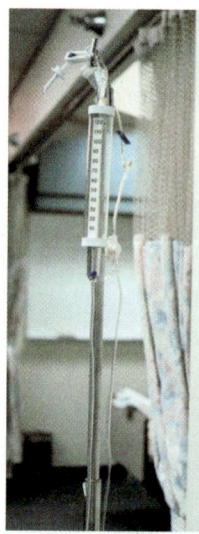

B

FIGURE 33-44 A. IV Tubing and Drip Chamber with a Dial-A-Flo; B. Volume-Control Infusion Chamber DELMAR/CENGAGE LEARNING

watching second hand of watch and adjust the roller clamp as necessary (see Figure 33-45 on page 979).
- For an infusion pump: Insert the tubing into the flow-control chamber, select the desired rate (generally calibrated in cc/min), open the roller clamp, and push the start button.
- For a controller: Place IV bag 36 inches above the IV site, select the desired drops per minute, open the roller clamp, and count drops for 1 minute to verify rate.

- The controller works by gravity.
- The amount of fluid in the volume-control chamber depends on the amount of fluid to be infused per hour:

50 cc/hour = 50 − 100 cc of fluid

100 cc/hour = 100 − 200 cc of fluid

(Continues)

PROCEDURE 33-7
Setting the IV Flow Rate (Continued)

ACTION	RATIONALE
• For volume-control device: Place device between IV bag and insertion spike of IV tubing, fill with 1–2 hours amount of IV fluid, and count drops for 1 minute (see Figure 33-46).	
9. Monitor infusion rates and IV site for infiltration.	9. Infusion devices may fail.
10. Assess infusion when alarm sounds.	10. Alarms on infusion devices signal when a drip has not been sensed. It can be caused by an empty IV bag, a kink in the tubing, a clotted needle, an infiltrated IV, or another malfunction of the device.
11. Wash hands/hand hygiene.	11. Reduces transmission of microorganisms.

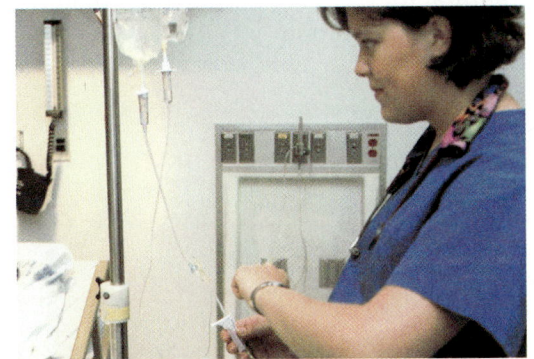

FIGURE 33-45 Count the drips in the drip chamber for 1 minute. DELMAR/CENGAGE LEARNING

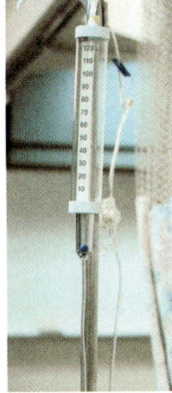

FIGURE 33-46 The controller is placed between the IV bag and the client. It is filled with 1 to 2 hours worth of IV fluid. DELMAR/CENGAGE LEARNING

delegation tip

Setting the rate of the IV after establishing the infusion is the responsibility of the nurse. It is a procedure not delegated unless other licensed personnel have been trained and certified to perform the procedure. Ancillary personnel may be instructed to report an infusion that is dripping too fast or an IV bag that is almost empty. It is the nurse's responsibility to monitor the infusion, but ancillary personnel may also be instructed to report observations such as swelling, leaking, or client concerns about pain, numbness, or tingling at the site or in the extremity used for the infusion.

nursing tips

- *Anticipate the client's need for IV fluid so the next bag is ready to hang before the current one is finished.*
- *Watch for kinks in the IV tubing or other impediments to the infusion of the fluid.*

- *Remember not to depend entirely on an infusion pump or controller as they can fail.*

PROCEDURE 33-8

Changing the Central Venous Dressing

EQUIPMENT

- Chlorhexidine 2% or agency-approved antiseptic solution
- Skin protectant solution
- Sterile gauze, tape, or transparent semipermeable membrane (TSA) dressing
- Label with date and time of dressing change
- Latex-free gloves

ACTION	RATIONALE
1. Wash hands/hand hygiene; don clean gloves. Open dressing tray (see Figure 33-47).	1. Reduces the number of microorganisms.
2. Remove old dressing carefully by pulling up a small section on each side and pulling laterally (see Figures 33-48 and 33-49), being careful not to dislodge the central catheter.	2. Skin integrity may be impaired. The dressing should release from the skin and catheter.
3. Note drainage on dressing.	3. Potential for bleeding or infectious material.
4. Inspect skin at insertion site for redness, tenderness, or swelling (see Figure 33-50).	4. Assesses for infection.

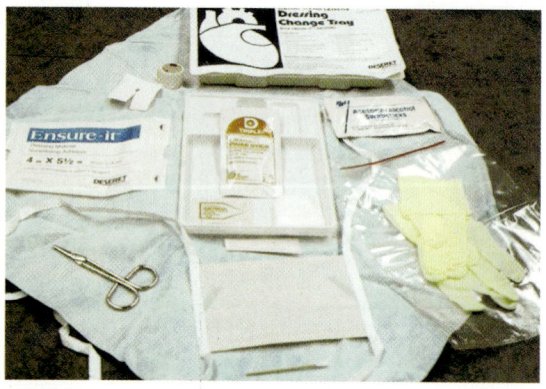

FIGURE 33-47 Central venous catheter dressing change tray, mask, clamp, and nonsterile gloves. DELMAR/CENGAGE LEARNING

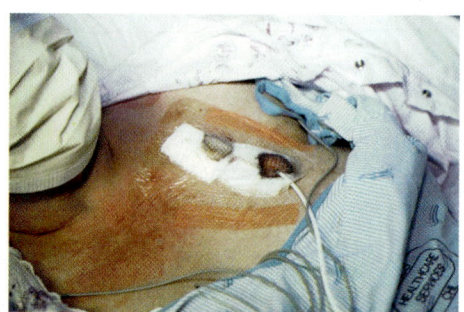

FIGURE 33-48 Inspect the dressing. DELMAR/CENGAGE LEARNING

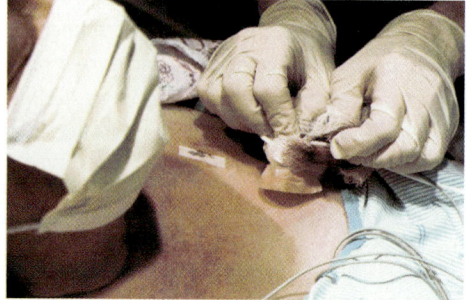

FIGURE 33-49 Remove the old dressing. Be careful not to dislodge the catheter. DELMAR/CENGAGE LEARNING

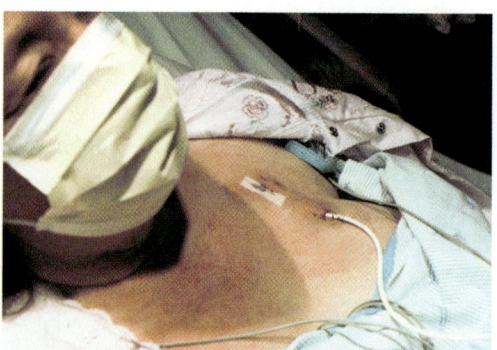

FIGURE 33-50 Inspect the site for redness, tenderness, and swelling. DELMAR/CENGAGE LEARNING

(Continues)

PROCEDURE 33-8
Changing the Central Venous Dressing (Continued)

ACTION	RATIONALE

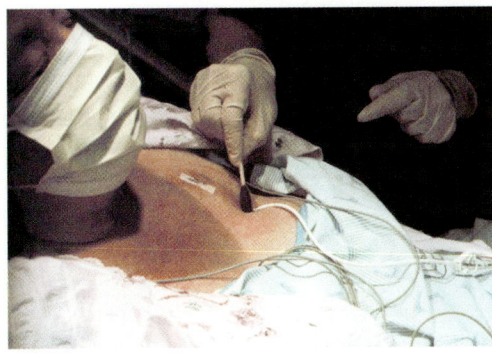

FIGURE 33-51 Clean the site with povidone-iodine swab. DELMAR/CENGAGE LEARNING

ACTION

5. Palpate tunneled catheter for presence of Dacron cuff, using care not to palpate close to the exit site.
6. Visually inspect catheter from hub to skin.

7. Remove gloves and put on sterile gloves.

8. Clean exit site according to institution protocol. Most use chlorhexidine 2% beginning at the catheter and moving out in a circular manner for 3 cm to maintain aseptic technique (see Figure 33-51).

9. Apply a skin protectant solution (check agency policy).

10. Apply transparent dressing (see Figures 33-52, 33-53, and 33-54 on page 982). Some institutions prefer to omit the gauze dressing to allow visualization of the site. In this case, only the TSM dressing is applied.
11. Label with date and time of dressing change (see Figure 33-55 on page 982). Gauze dressings are changed every 48 hours on peripheral and central catheters. TSM dressings are changed at the time of access site rotation or every 3–7 days, whichever occurs first.

RATIONALE

5. Documents proper placement of catheter.

6. Checks whether catheter has a crack or is split or cut.
7. Prevents transmission of microorganisms from skin to exit site.
8. Eliminates microorganisms by chemical and mechanical means. Clinical evidence points to a lower risk of catheter-related bloodstream infections when chlorhexidine gluconate is used to clean the skin during dressing change (Hadaway, 2008).
9. Prevents skin irritation and prolongs dressing integrity. Do not apply antiseptic or antimicrobial ointment to the insertion site unless it is a hemodialysis catheter. According to the CDC, povidone-iodine antiseptic ointment should be applied to a hemodialysis site after catheter insertion and at the end of each dialysis session as long as the ointment does not interact with the catheter material. Check the manufacturer's directions to see if povidone-iodine ointment can be safely used with the client's type of catheter.
10. Prevents bacteria from entering exit site.

11. Documents time to plan for next change.

(Continues)

PROCEDURE 33-8
Changing the Central Venous Dressing (Continued)

ACTION	RATIONALE
12. Secure tubing to client's clothing.	12. Prevents accidental displacement.
13. Remove gloves and dispose of all used materials.	13. Reduces transmission of microorganisms.
14. Wash hands/hand hygiene.	14. Reduces transmission of microorganisms.

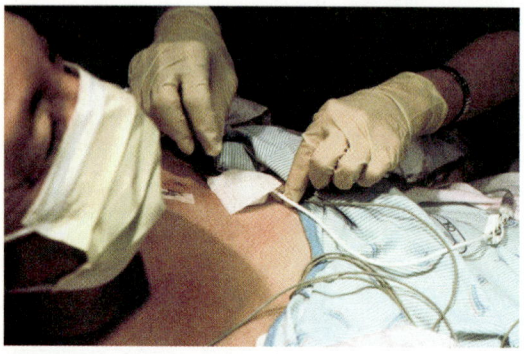

FIGURE 33-52 Slide the first piece of gauze directly over and under the catheter. DELMAR/CENGAGE LEARNING

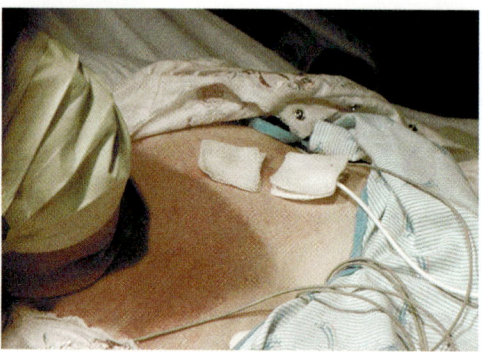

FIGURE 33-53 Place the next piece of gauze directly over the insertion site. DELMAR/CENGAGE LEARNING

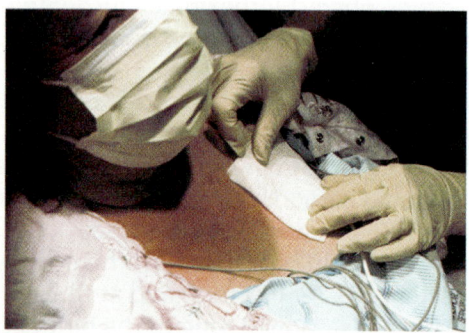

FIGURE 33-54 Place a larger piece of gauze over the area and secure with tape or transparent dressing. DELMAR/CENGAGE LEARNING

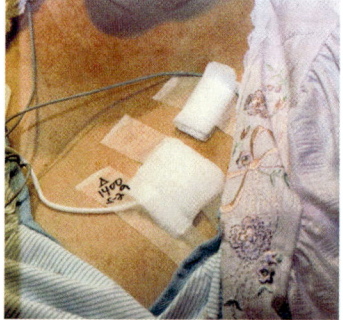

FIGURE 33-55 Write the date and time of the dressing change on the label. DELMAR/CENGAGE LEARNING

delegation tip

Changing the central venous catheter dressing is a skill involving assessment and the use of sterile technique. It is a procedure not delegated by the nurse unless other licensed personnel have been trained and certified to assist with the procedure. Ancillary personnel who will be caring for the client need to be instructed to report any disruption of the closed dressing, along with complaints of pain, redness, or swelling at the insertion site.

(Continues)

PROCEDURE 33-8
Changing the Central Venous Dressing (Continued)

nursing tips

- *A cotton-tipped applicator dipped in normal saline may help loosen exudate on a catheter.*
- *Have a catheter repair kit available if a leak or hole is seen during the dressing change.*
- *In general, never apply alcohol-containing agents directly to the VAD's external portion unless you know it is in accordance with the agency's policy for that specific brand of catheter.*

PROCEDURE 33-9
Discontinuing the IV and Changing to a Saline or Heparin Lock

EQUIPMENT
- Disposable gloves
- Syringe, 3 to 5 mL
- Sterile needles, 25-gauge
- Antiseptic swab (usually alcohol unless control line)
- Syringe with saline flush solution
- Intermittent infusion device
- Transparent dressing, if required

ACTION	RATIONALE
1. Check prescribing practitioner's order to discontinue IV and to insert a saline lock.	1. Ensures accurate placement of saline lock.
2. Wash hands/hand hygiene; don clean gloves.	2. Reduces transmission of microorganisms.
3. Check client's identification bracelet.	3. Ensures correct procedure is performed for the client.
4. Explain procedure and reason for discontinuing IV to client.	4. Information decreases anxiety.
5. Prepare supplies at bedside:	5. Ensures smooth procedure.
• Syringe with saline	
• Syringe with heparin	
• Saline lock (see Figure 33-56 on page 984)	
6. If inserting a new saline lock: Prime the extension tubing with saline and place the saline lock on it. Follow the procedures for starting an IV, including assessing and preparing the site, inserting the over-the-needle-catheter (ONC) (see Figure 33-57 on page 984) or butterfly needle, and obtaining a blood return. Do not attach the needle or ONC to the IV tubing. Instead, attach the ONC to the extension tubing. Dress the site (see Figure 33-58 on page 984) per policy. If inserting a new saline lock, prime extension tubing with solution and place connector in the hub of the angiocatheter. For needleless	6. Priming the extension tubing prevents air from being forced into the vein.

(Continues)

PROCEDURE 33-9
Discontinuing the IV and Changing to a Saline or Heparin Lock (Continued)

ACTION	RATIONALE

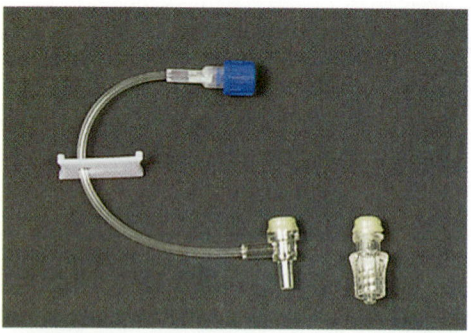

FIGURE 33-56 Saline Lock (Intermittent Infusion Device)
DELMAR/CENGAGE LEARNING

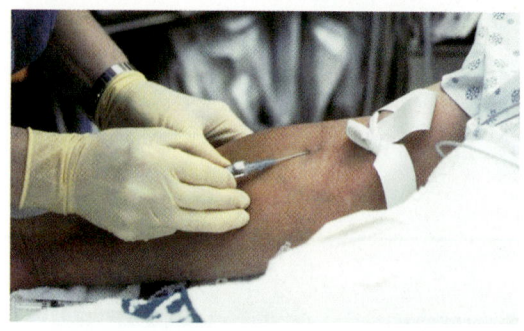

FIGURE 33-57 Insert an over-the-needle catheter. DELMAR/CENGAGE LEARNING

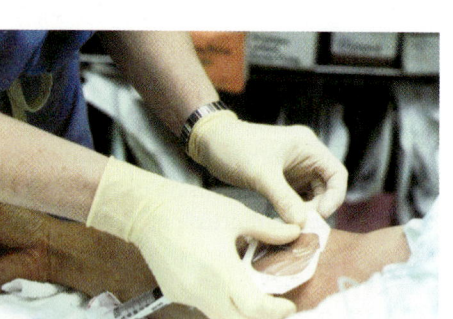

FIGURE 33-58 Cover the site with a transparent dressing.
DELMAR/CENGAGE LEARNING

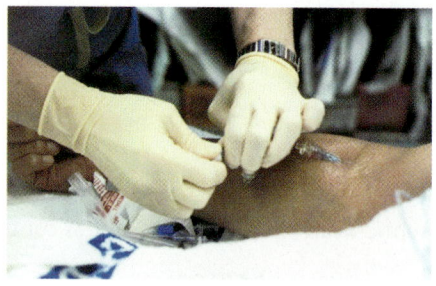

FIGURE 33-59 Screw the saline lock onto the hub of the extension tubing. DELMAR/CENGAGE LEARNING

systems, follow steps of manufacturer. In a spring-loaded, retractable needle system, press the button after a flashback of blood is observed. To ensure needle separation, turn angiocatheter 360° at the hub before inserting the catheter into the vein. Advance the catheter and attach to extension tubing with the addition of a one-way needleless safety valve that has been flushed with solution. Secure with dressing as per institution protocol.

7. If discontinuing an IV and converting to a saline lock: Stop IV infusion.

  • For IV tubing, roll clamp to close IV tubing.
  • For infusion pump, turn switch to off.

8. Place saline lock:

  • Open sterile package with needleless adapter saline lock.
  • For existing IV, loosen IV tubing and remove.
  • Screw saline lock into hub of tubing (see Figure 33-59).

7. Stops the flow of the fluid in the IV tubing.

8. Places the saline lock.

(Continues)

PROCEDURE 33-9
Discontinuing the IV and Changing to a Saline or Heparin Lock (Continued)

ACTION	RATIONALE
• To check for patency, remove cap from one-way valve following vigorous scrubbing with alcohol at the connection site. Connect needleless Luer-Lok syringe to the valve. Inject solution into IV site per protocol, using gentle pulsating motions to create turbulence. Remove syringe and replace sterile cap at end of tubing.	
9. Check for patency of IV:	9. Ensures the IV is patent so that the saline lock will function. Flushing with saline clears the lock.
• Clean saline lock with antiseptic solution (usually alcohol wipe).	• Flushing should be done slowly.
• Insert saline syringe with 25-gauge needle into center of diaphragm. (Needleless system will not require needle.)	• Assess for pain to ensure site is patent.
• Pull back gently on syringe and watch for blood return.	
• Inject saline *slowly* into lock (see Figure 33-60).	
• Assess client's pain at site.	
10. Keep lock patent with normal saline or heparin. Every 8 hours:	10. Ensures patency of saline lock. Only use heparin if prescribed as "flush with heparin" or if institutional policy requires it. Because of the potential for heparin-induced thrombocytopenia, the use of heparin to lock the catheter is becoming more controversial (Hadaway, 2008). The needleless system reduces risk of needlesticks.
• Clean the rubber diaphragm with an antiseptic swab (not applicable if needleless system).	
• Insert the syringe or needleless adapter with saline or heparin into the diaphragm.	
• Inject saline or heparin slowly into lock (see Figure 33-61).	
11. Remove the syringe or needleless adapter from the diaphragm and swab it with an antiseptic swab. Discard needle or adapter in sharps container.	11. Reduces transmission of microorganisms. Reduces risk of needlesticks.
12. Assess the site for any signs of leakage, irritation, or infiltration (see Figure 33-62 on page 986).	12. Detects problems with the site that need additional assessment and intervention.

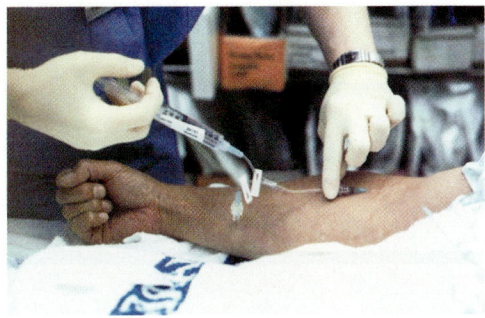

FIGURE 33-60 Inject saline slowly into the lock and extension tubing. DELMAR/CENGAGE LEARNING

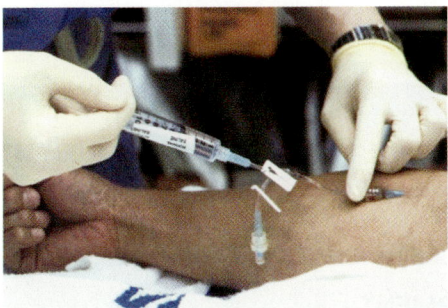

FIGURE 33-61 Maintain the saline lock by injecting saline slowly into the lock, every 8 hours. DELMAR/CENGAGE LEARNING

(Continues)

PROCEDURE 33-9
Discontinuing the IV and Changing to a Saline or Heparin Lock (Continued)

ACTION	RATIONALE
13. Remove gloves and dispose of all used materials.	13. Reduces transmission of microorganisms.
14. Wash hands/hand hygiene.	14. Reduces transmission of microorganisms.

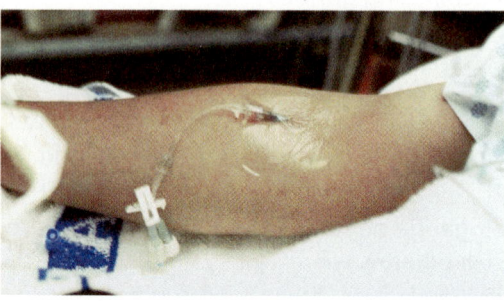

FIGURE 33-62 Assess the site for leakage, irritation, inflammation, or infection. Clean up and dispose of all materials. DELMAR/CENGAGE LEARNING

delegation tip

Discontinuing or changing the IV to a saline lock is the responsibility of the nurse. It is a procedure not delegated unless other licensed personnel have been trained and certified to perform the procedure. Ancillary personnel may be instructed to report any bleeding, leaking, or client concerns after the procedure.

nursing tips

- *Sometimes no blood will return from a saline lock even though it is patent. Removing the screw-on cap, using sterile technique, may result in a blood return if the saline lock is patent. If in doubt, restart the saline lock at a new site.*
- *Be sure the IV site is visible and free of tape or dressing while checking for patency.*

- *Remember, a saline flush must inject enough saline to fill the entire set from the injection port to the needle tip.*
- *In some situations, such as with certain central lines, heparin may be used. Use heparin solution designated for flush, and follow institution protocol.*

PROCEDURE 33-10
Administering a Blood Transfusion

EQUIPMENT
- Blood administration set and filter
- IV solution of 0.9% sodium chloride (normal saline)
- Disposable gloves
- Infusion pump if compatible with the specific blood product
- Tape
- Leukocyte-depleting filter, if ordered
- Pressure bag, if needed
- Blood warmer, if needed

(Continues)

PROCEDURE 33-10
Administering a Blood Transfusion (Continued)

ACTION	RATIONALE
1. Verify the prescribing practitioner's order for the transfusion.	1. Blood must be ordered by a health care provider.
2. If a venipuncture is necessary, see Chapter 28, Procedure 28-1.	2. Ensures a patent and adequate IV for infusion of blood.
3. Explain procedure to the client.	3. Ensures that client understands procedure and decreases anxiety.
4. Review side effects (dyspnea, chills, headache, chest pain, itching) with client and ask client to report these to the nurse.	4. Prompt reporting of a side effect will lead to earlier discontinuation of transfusion and minimize the reaction.
5. Have the client sign consent forms.	5. Most institutions require the client to sign a consent form.
6. Obtain baseline vital signs.	6. Allows detection of a reaction by any change in vital signs during the transfusion.
7. Obtain the blood product from the blood bank within 30 minutes of initiation.	7. Prevents bacterial growth and destruction of red blood cells.
8. Verify and record the blood product and identify the client with another nurse (see Figure 33-63): • Client's name, blood group, Rh type • Cross-match compatibility • Donor blood group and Rh type • Unit and hospital number • Expiration date and time on blood bag • Type of blood product compared with prescribing practitioner's order • Presence of clots in blood	8. Strict verification procedures will reduce the risk of administering blood products to the wrong client. If there is an error during this procedure, notify the blood blank and do not administer the product.
9. Instruct client to empty the bladder.	9. A urine specimen after initiation of the transfusion will be needed if a transfusion reaction occurs.
10. Wash hands/hand hygiene; put on gloves.	10. Reduces transmission of microorganisms and, therefore, risk of transmission of human immunodeficiency virus (HIV), hepatitis, or bloodborne bacteria.
11. Open blood administration kit and move roller clamps to "off" position.	11. Closing the roller clamps prevents accidental spilling of blood.

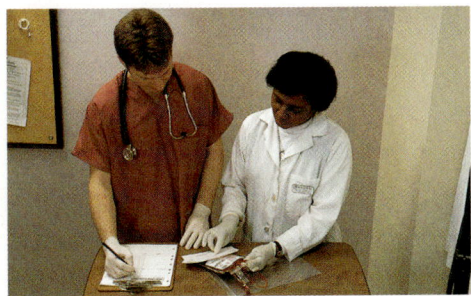

FIGURE 33-63 Verify the blood product with another nurse. DELMAR/CENGAGE LEARNING

(Continues)

PROCEDURE 33-10
Administering a Blood Transfusion (Continued)

ACTION	RATIONALE
12. For Y-tubing set:	12.
• Spike the 0.9% sodium chloride bag and open the roller clamp on the Y-tubing connected to the bag and the roller clamp on the unused inlet tube until tubing from the 0.9% sodium chloride bag is filled. Close clamp on unused tubing.	• The Y-tubing allows the nurse to switch from infusing 0.9% sodium chloride to blood. This is especially helpful when multiple transfusions are given. Follow institutional guidelines for the number of units that can be given before tubing needs to be changed. Dextrose solutions are not used with blood transfusions as they can clot the donor blood.
• Squeeze sides of drip chamber and allow filter to partially fill (see Figure 33-64).	• A correctly filled drip chamber enables an accurate drip count.
• Open lower roller clamp and allow tubing to fill with 0.9% sodium chloride to the hub.	• Removes all air from tubing system.
• Close lower clamp.	• Prevents waste of IV fluid.
• Invert blood bag once or twice. Spike blood bag and open clamps on inlet tube to allow blood to cover the filter completely (see Figures 33-65 and 33-66 on page 989).	• Equal distribution of cells prevents clumping, which can lead to clotting of cells. Fragile blood cells may be damaged if they drop on an uncovered filter.
• Close lower clamp.	• Prevents blood from flowing until tubing is attached to venous catheter.
13. For single-tubing set:	13.
• Spike blood unit.	• Attaches tubing to blood unit.
• Squeeze drip chamber and allow the filter to fill with blood (see Figure 33-67 on page 989).	• A correctly filled drip chamber enables an accurate drip count.
• Open roller clamp and allow tubing to fill with blood to the hub.	• Prevents air from being forced into the vein.
• Prime another IV tubing with 0.9% sodium chloride and piggyback it to the blood administration set with a needle; secure all connections with tape.	• The blood product should not be piggybacked into the 0.9% sodium chloride line to avoid forcing blood cells through both a needle and a venous catheter.

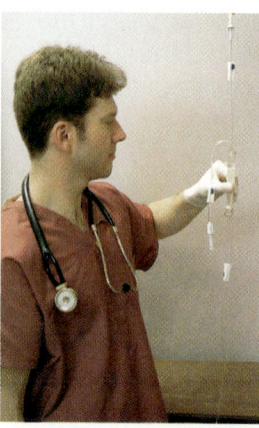

FIGURE 33-64 Close the roller clamp on the administration set and priming drip chamber. DELMAR/CENGAGE LEARNING

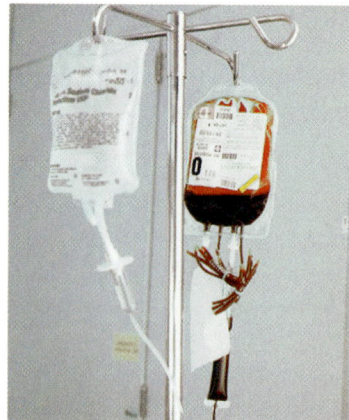

FIGURE 33-65 Blood and 0.9% Sodium Chloride DELMAR/CENGAGE LEARNING

(Continues)

PROCEDURE 33-10
Administering a Blood Transfusion (Continued)

ACTION	RATIONALE

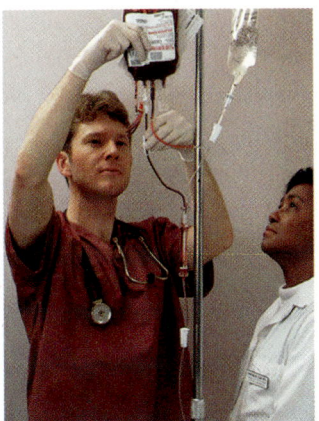

FIGURE 33-66 Close the saline roller clamp and open the blood roller clamp. DELMAR/CENGAGE LEARNING

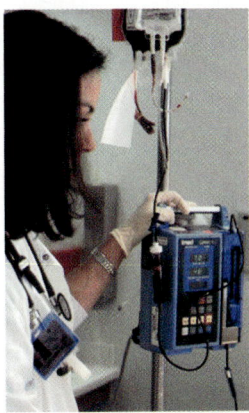

FIGURE 33-67 Allow the filter to fill with blood. DELMAR/CENGAGE LEARNING

14. Attach tubing to venous catheter using sterile precautions, and open lower clamp.
15. Infuse the blood at a rate of 2–5 mL/min according to the prescribing practitioner's order.
16. Remain with client for first 15–30 minutes, monitoring vital signs every 5 minutes for 15 minutes, then every 15 minutes for 1 hour, then hourly until 1 hour after the infusion is completed, or per institution policy.
17. After blood has infused, allow the tubing to clear with 0.9% sodium chloride.
18. Appropriately dispose of blood bag in a biohazard bag, tubing, and gloves, and follow policy regarding disposition. Wash hands/hand hygiene.
19. Document the procedure.

14. Allows the blood product to be infused into the client's vein.
15. Packed red blood cells usually run over 1 1/2–2 hours; whole blood runs over 2–3 hours.
16. If a reaction occurs, it generally happens during the first 15–30 minutes. Changes in vital signs can warn of a transfusion reaction.
17. The client will receive all the blood that is left in the tubing.
18. Reduces transmission of microorganisms.

19. Ensures accurate records.

delegation tip

Initiating a blood transfusion is a skill involving assessment and knowledge regarding blood replacement techniques. It is an invasive procedure not delegated unless other licensed personnel have been trained and certified to perform the procedure. Ancillary personnel who will be caring for the client need to be instructed to handle the transfusion extremity gently and to take vital signs on another extremity. Vital signs should be recorded according to institution policy and the results reported promptly to the nurse. Any client complaints about chills, fever, itching, or the appearance of hives, chest pain, dyspnea, or swelling at the IV site should be immediately reported to the nurse.

(Continues)

PROCEDURE 33-10
Administering a Blood Transfusion (Continued)

nursing tips

Blood components are prescribed to infuse at different rates:

- *Red blood cells: 1 unit over 2–3 hours (<4 hours)*
- *Platelets: 30–60 minutes or more slowly (<4 hours)*

- *Fresh frozen plasma: 200 mL/h or more slowly*
- *Cryoprecipitate: 1–2 mL/min*

KEY CONCEPTS

- Health promotion requires a maintenance of body fluid and acid-base balance.

- There are two types of body fluid: intracellular and extracellular. Because intravascular and interstitial fluids are outside the cells, these fluids are called extracellular fluids (ECFs).

- Water is the largest single constituent of the body, representing 45% to 75% of the body's total weight.

- Electrolytes have special physiological functions in the body that promote neuromuscular irritability, maintain body fluid osmolarity, regulate acid-base balance, and distribute body fluids between the fluid compartments. The body has many regulators that maintain fluid balance: fluid and food intake, skin, lungs, gastrointestinal tract, and kidneys.

- When an ECF volume deficit occurs, hormones play a key role in restoring the ECF volume.

- Sodium is the main electrolyte that promotes the retention of water.

- Acid-base balance refers to the homeostasis of the hydrogen ion concentration in body fluids.

- When the number of free hydrogen ions in a solution increases to lower the pH value below 7.35, the body is in a state of acidosis. The opposite occurs with alkalosis; a pH value higher than 7.45 results from a low hydrogen ion concentration.

- The body has three main control systems to regulate acid-base balance: buffer systems, respiratory regulation, and renal control of hydrogen ion concentration.

- In health, normal homeostatic mechanisms function to maintain electrolyte and acid-base balance; in illness, one or more of the regulating mechanisms may be affected, or the imbalance may become too great for the body to correct without treatment.

- Disturbances in one of the body's electrolytes usually cause changes in other electrolytes and can alter the pH of the blood.

- The slightest decrease or increase in extracellular potassium can cause serious, adverse, or life-threatening effects on physiological functions.

- The client's health history, physical assessment, and biochemical data are used by the nurse in formulating nursing goals, expected outcomes, diagnoses, and interventions.

- Nursing interventions that promote the resolution of alterations in fluid balance are based on the principles of client safety and standards of care.

- Following institutional protocol and established procedures for IV therapy helps ensure client safety.

- Hospitalized clients, especially older adults, are at risk for developing dehydration.

- Clients receiving intravenous therapy and blood transfusions require constant monitoring for complications.

- Evaluation of the achievement of client expected outcomes requires the interrelational analysis of weight, intake and output, vital signs, and biochemical results.

REVIEW QUESTIONS

1. Which client is most at risk for fluid volume deficit?
   a. A 30-year-old woman with a fractured tibia
   b. An 82-year-old woman with a fractured hip
   c. A 58-year-old man with a myocardial infarction
   d. A 35-year-old woman who just delivered a baby

2. The priority nursing action for a client with a serum sodium level of 115 mEq/L is _____.
   a. Frequent oral hygiene
   b. Monitor vital signs every 2 hours
   c. Seizure precautions
   d. Cardiac rhythm monitoring

3. A client receiving D5W at 100 mL/h is most at risk for developing _____.
   a. Hyponatremia
   b. Hypernatremia
   c. Fluid volume deficit
   d. Fluid volume excess

4. The priority nursing assessment for a client with hypokalemia is _____.
   a. Blood pressure
   b. Chvostek's sign
   c. Edema
   d. Heart rhythm

5. The priority nursing action for a client with a serum potassium level of 5.5 mEq/L who has received an oral dose of Kayexalate is to monitor
   _____.
   a. Urine output
   b. Blood pressure
   c. Bowel movement
   d. Seizure activity

6. The priority nursing action for a bedridden client with a serum calcium level of 13 mg/dL is to
   _____.
   a. Provide passive range-of-motion (ROM) exercises and encourage fluids
   b. Teach the client to increase intake of whole grains and nuts
   c. Place a tracheostomy tray at the bedside
   d. Administer calcium gluconate IM as prescribed

7. A client is admitted to the hospital with a history of vomiting for 3 days and decreased oral intake. Which set of arterial blood gases would indicate that the client is in a state of metabolic acidosis?
   a. pH of 7.43, Paco₂ of 36 mm Hg, HCO₃ of 26
   b. pH of 7.41, Paco₂ of 49 mm Hg, HCO₃ of 30
   c. pH of 7.33, Paco₂ of 35 mm Hg, HCO₃ of 17
   d. pH of 7.25, Paco₂ of 56 mm Hg, HCO₃ of 28

8. A client with a small bowel obstruction and a nasogastric tube connected to low intermittent suction for 2 days should be monitored for which acid-base disorder?
   a. Respiratory alkalosis
   b. Respiratory acidosis
   c. Metabolic alkalosis
   d. Metabolic acidosis

9. Which statement about VAD placement reflects best practice?
   a. To maintain patency, infuse 0.9% sodium chloride solution immediately after VAD insertion.
   b. Document the total length of the catheter prior to infusing any solution.
   c. Confirm and document the tip's correct anatomic location from the radiology department before using the VAD.
   d. If the client's VAD was placed at another facility, you don't need to confirm tip location.

10. When priming the IV tubing for a blood transfusion, which type of IV solution should the nurse use?
    a. Dextrose 5% in 0.2% saline
    b. Dextrose 5% in water
    c. Ringer's lactate
    d. Normal saline 0.9%

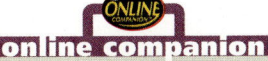

online companion

Visit the DeLaune and Ladner online companion resource at **www.delmar.cengage.com** for additional content and study aids. Click on Online Companions, then select the Nursing discipline.

"The human body is a complex organism with the ability to heal itself—if only you listen to it and respond with proper nourishment and care."

—Balch (2006)

CHAPTER 34

Nutrition

COMPETENCIES

1. Identify the physiological value of nutrients.
2. Describe the processes of digestion, absorption, and metabolism.
3. Describe how diet guidelines and menu planning promote nutrition and health.
4. Explain how culture influences food preferences and eating habits.
5. Explain the impact of age-related changes on nutritional status.
6. Describe the process of assessing a client's nutritional status.
7. Identify common knowledge deficits related to nutrition.
8. Describe the expected outcomes of nursing interventions that promote optimum nutritional status.
9. Describe the role of nutritional support teams in managing the care of clients with nutritional deficits.
10. Identify common nursing interventions for clients experiencing nutritional deficits.

KEY TERMS

absorption
aerobic metabolism
anabolism
anaerobic metabolism
anorexia nervosa
anthropometric measurements
antioxidants
appetite
atherosclerosis
basal metabolic rate (BMR)
body mass index (BMI)
bulimia nervosa
calorie
carbohydrates
catabolism
cholesterol
chylomicrons
deamination
deglutition
diabetes mellitus
dietary fiber
digestion
disaccharides
enteral nutrition
essential amino acids
fat-soluble vitamins

fatty acids
free radical scavengers
free radicals
gluconeogenesis
glycolysis
high-biological-value proteins
  (complete proteins)
hyperglycemia
hyperthyroidism
hypoglycemia
hypothyroidism
insulin
ketogenesis
ketones
kilocalories
lipids
low-biological-value proteins
  (incomplete proteins)
malnutrition
mastication
metabolic rate
metabolism
mid-upper-arm circumference
  (MAC)
minerals
monosaccharides

monounsaturated fatty acids
negative nitrogen balance
nitrogen balance
nonessential amino acids
nutrition
obligatory loss of proteins
parenteral nutrition
peristalsis
phospholipids
polysaccharides
polyunsaturated fatty acids
positive nitrogen balance
prealbumin
proteins
recommended dietary allowances
  (RDAs)
saccharides
satiety
saturated fatty acids
skinfold measurement
total parenteral nutrition (TPN)
transferrin
triglycerides
unsaturated fatty acids
vitamins
water-soluble vitamins

The body requires the consumption of nutrients to support physiological activities of digestion, absorption, and metabolism to maintain homeostasis. The metabolism of nutrients (carbohydrates, proteins, fats, vitamins, and minerals) plays an essential role in providing the body with the necessary substances to maintain internal homeostasis.

PHYSIOLOGY OF NUTRITION

Nutrition is the process by which the body metabolizes and utilizes nutrients. Nutrients are classified as energy nutrients, organic nutrients, and inorganic nutrients; see the accompanying display on classes of nutrients. Energy nutrients release energy for maintenance of homeostasis. Organic nutrients build and maintain body tissues and regulate body processes. Inorganic nutrients provide a medium for chemical reactions, transport materials, maintain body temperature, promote bone formation, and conduct nerve impulses.

In the body, essentially all carbohydrates are converted into glucose before they reach the cells, proteins are converted into amino acids, and fats are converted into fatty acids. These nutrients are digested, absorbed by the blood or

CLASSES OF NUTRIENTS	
DESCRIPTION	**CLASSES**
Energy nutrients	Carbohydrates
	Proteins
	Fats
Organic nutrients	Carbohydrates
	Proteins
	Fats
	Vitamins
Inorganic nutrients	Water
	Minerals

lymphatic system, and transported to the body's cells. Inside the cells' mitochondria, the nutrients react chemically with oxygen and various enzymes to produce energy.

DIGESTION

Digestion refers to the mechanical and chemical processes that convert nutrients into a physically absorbable state.

Figure 34-1 shows the anatomical structures of the gastrointestinal (GI) tract (digestive tract). Figure 34-2 explains the physiological mechanisms that support the digestive process in each anatomical structure.

The mouth prepares foodstuffs for digestion by **mastication**, the chewing, tearing, or grinding of food by the teeth into fine particles and mixing with enzymes in saliva. The salivary glands release lubricating secretions that bind with food particles to facilitate swallowing.

Deglutition, the swallowing of food, begins in the mouth and continues in the pharynx and esophagus. Peristaltic waves and mucous secretions move food down the esophagus. Relaxation of the lower esophageal sphincter (gastroesophageal constrictor muscle) allows food to enter the stomach; contraction of this sphincter muscle prevents regurgitation (reflux) of stomach contents.

Digestion begins in the stomach and is completed in the small intestine. This is accomplished by specific substances entering the duodenum: pancreatic enzymes through the pancreatic duct, bile through the common bile duct, and intestinal enzymes produced in the jejunum. **Peristalsis** (coordinated, rhythmic, serial contraction of the smooth muscle lining of the intestines) forces chyme (an acidic, semifluid paste) through the small intestine to the large intestine and promotes the absorption of vitamins, minerals, and water.

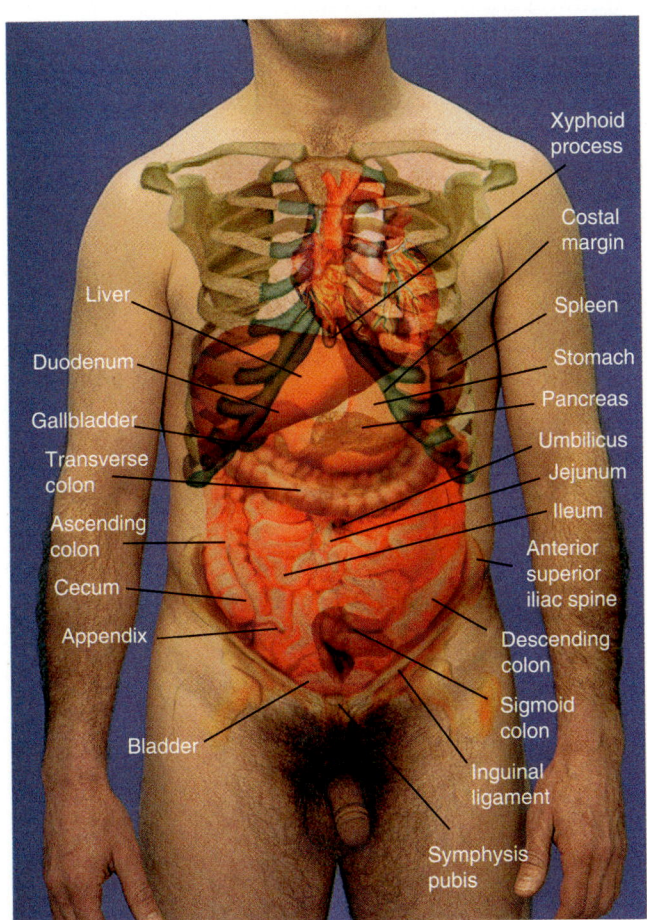

FIGURE 34-1 **Gastrointestinal Tract** DELMAR/CENGAGE LEARNING

A. Carbohydrates

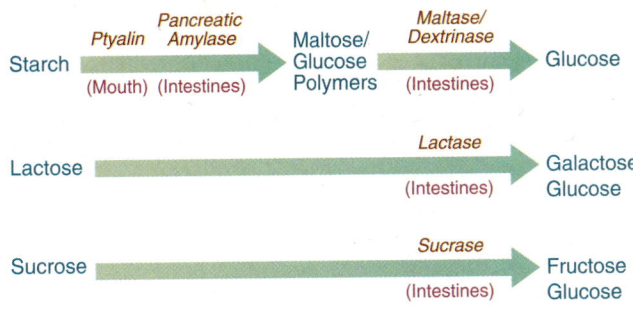

B. Proteins

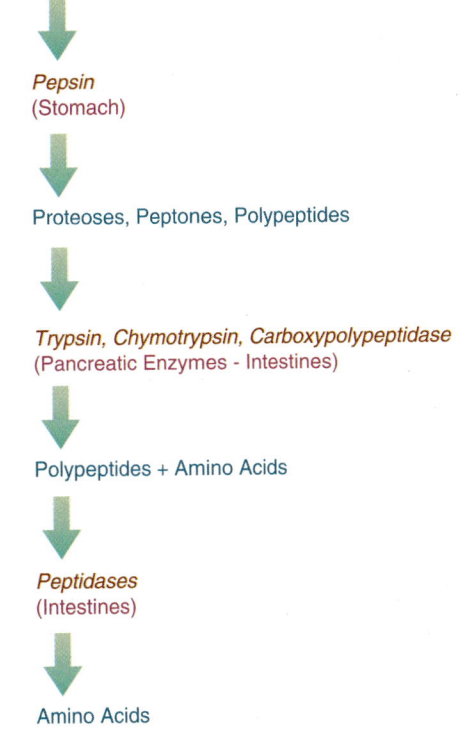

C. Fats

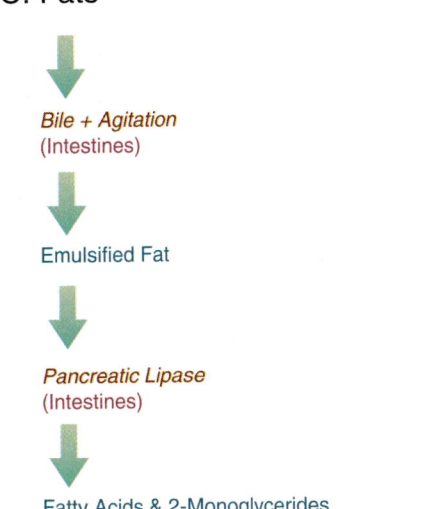

FIGURE 34-2 **Digestion of Proteins, Carbohydrates, and Fats**
DELMAR/CENGAGE LEARNING

Only carbohydrates, proteins, and fats require chemical digestion by enzymatic activity for absorption.

ABSORPTION

Absorption is the process by which the end products of digestion—**monosaccharides** (simple sugars), amino acids, glycerol, fatty acid chains, vitamins, minerals, and water—pass through the epithelial membranes in the small and large intestines into the blood or lymph systems. Most absorption occurs in the small intestine through the processes of osmosis, diffusion, and active transport (see Figure 34-3). Water absorption occurs throughout the digestive tract.

The main function of the large intestine is to absorb water and collect food residue (dietary fiber). **Dietary fiber** is the part of food that body enzymes cannot digest and absorb, such as the outer hulls of corn kernels, grains of wheat, celery strings, and apple skins. Dietary fiber absorbs water in the large intestine, promoting the formation of a soft, bulky stool that moves quickly through the large intestine; some fiber is believed to bind cholesterol in the colon, thus reducing the risk of heart attack (Roth, 2007). In healthy individuals, most of the end products of digestion are absorbed (99% of carbohydrates, 95% of fat, and 92% of protein) and used by the body (Roth, 2007).

METABOLISM

Metabolism is the aggregate of all chemical reactions and processes in every body cell, such as growth, generation of energy, elimination of wastes, and other bodily functions as they relate to the distribution of nutrients in the blood after digestion.

The liver prepares nutrients for their role in energy production. It converts all monosaccharides to glucose and excess amino acids to urea, carbohydrates, or fats. Excess fats are converted in the liver to glycerol and fatty acids, then to acetylcoenzyme A (acetyl CoA).

Glycolysis refers to the breakdown of glucose by enzymes located inside the cell's cytoplasm. This process produces adenosine triphosphate (ATP) and pyruvate, which provide the cell with energy. Pyruvate may be used in two different metabolic functions. In **aerobic metabolism**, pyruvate enters the cell's mitochondria and in the presence of oxygen is converted to acetyl CoA. In **anaerobic metabolism** (metabolism without the presence of oxygen) lactate is produced in the cytoplasm by an enzyme (lactate dehydrogenase); this type of metabolism takes place when the oxygen supply is limited, as in the muscles and red blood cells, which lack mitochondria.

When pyruvic acid is formed by glycolysis, it is then converted into acetyl CoA. This conversion begins a cyclic metabolic pathway called the Krebs cycle (citric acid cycle or tricarboxylic acid cycle). The Krebs cycle extracts energy through oxidation of acetyl CoA within the mitochondria of body cells. The Krebs cycle is a pathway common to all energy nutrients because acetyl CoA may be formed from carbohydrates, proteins, and fats (see Figure 34-4).

Built into the inner mitochondrial membrane is a series of molecules to assist in electron transport during aerobic metabolism. The electron transport system converts energy released from the Krebs cycle into ATP for use by cells in anabolism and catabolism. **Anabolism** refers to the constructive phase of metabolism, in which smaller molecules, such as amino acids, are converted to larger molecules, such as proteins. **Catabolism** is the destructive phase, in which larger molecules, such as glycogen, are converted to smaller molecules, such as pyruvic acid.

The rate of metabolism is governed primarily by the hormones triiodothyronine (T_3) and thyroxine (T_4) secreted by

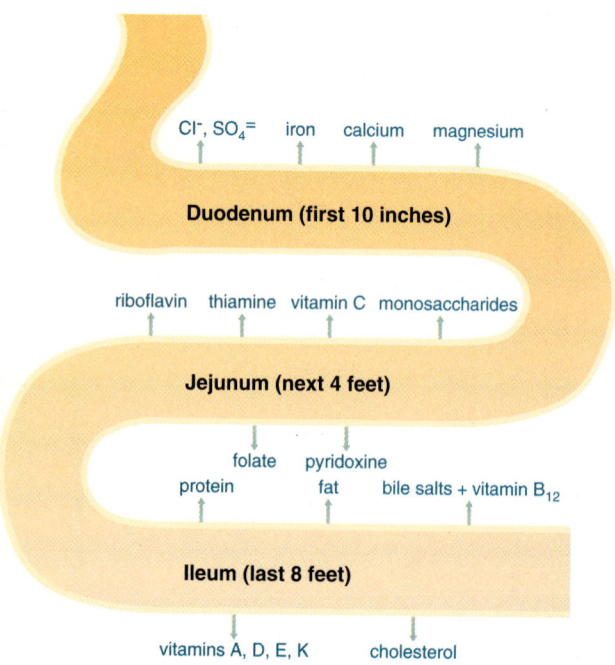

FIGURE 34-3 Nutrient Absorption in the Small Intestine
DELMAR/CENGAGE LEARNING

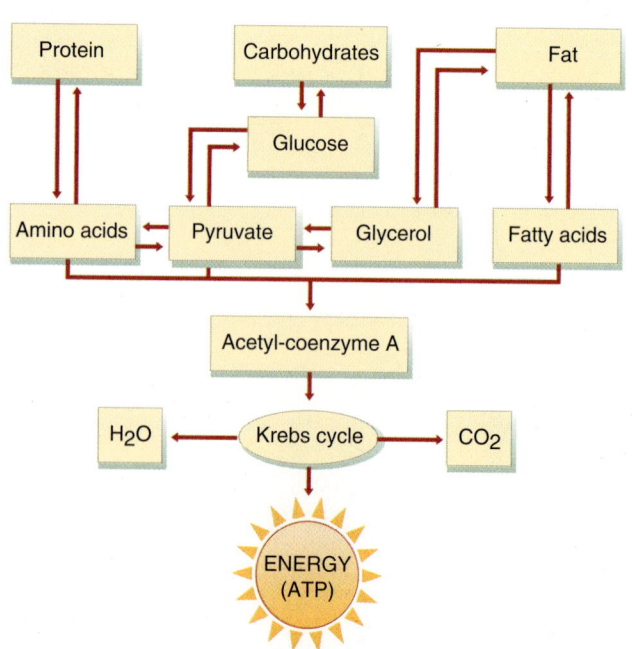

FIGURE 34-4 Energy Nutrients and the Krebs Cycle DELMAR/ CENGAGE LEARNING

the thyroid gland. **Hyperthyroidism** refers to the increased secretion of these thyroid hormones, which increases the rate of metabolism. With **hypothyroidism**, a decrease in the secretion of thyroid hormones, the metabolic rate is decreased.

ENERGY

Metabolic rate refers to the rate of heat liberation during chemical reactions; it is expressed in units called calories. A **calorie** is the quantity of heat required to raise the temperature of 1 gram of water 1°C; it is used to express the quantity of energy released from different foods or expended by different functional processes of the body. Because a large quantity of energy is released during metabolism, the energy is expressed in terms of **kilocalories** (kcal), each of which is equivalent to 1000 calories. The **basal metabolic rate (BMR)** refers to the energy needed to maintain essential physiological functions, such as respiration, circulation, and muscle tone, when a person is at complete rest both physically and mentally.

EXCRETION

Digestive and metabolic waste products are excreted through the intestines and rectum. Other excretory organs are the kidneys, sweat glands, skin, and lungs; see Chapter 39 for a complete discussion of elimination. The skin and sweat glands remove water, toxins, salts, and nitrogen wastes; the lungs remove carbon dioxide and water.

NUTRIENTS

Understanding the role of basic nutrients provides the foundation for selecting foods that promote health. The six categories of nutrients are water, vitamins, minerals, carbohydrates, proteins, and lipids (fats). Selecting the healthiest forms of each of these nutrients and eating them in the proper balance will enable the body to function at its optimal level of health. Nutrients work synergistically; for example, there is a cooperative action between certain vitamins and minerals that work as catalysts, promoting the absorption and assimilation of other vitamins and minerals.

WATER

Water is the most abundant nutrient in the body and accounts for 60% to 70% of an adult's total body weight and 77% of an infant's weight. It is a major component of body fluids, secretions, and excretions. Body water decreases as body fat increases and with aging.

Water and electrolytes are substances that must be acquired from the diet. In the United States, much of water consumption is in the form of beverages (milk, coffee, tea, and soft drinks). The estimated water requirement for infants, children, and adults is 1.5 mL/kcal of energy expenditure. The water and electrolyte requirements for infants correspond to the water-to-energy ratio and the electrolyte composition in human milk and common formulas. Although pregnancy and lactation increase bodily demands for water and electrolytes, these demands are usually met with normal ingested amounts; the one exception is in a lactating woman, who requires, on average, an additional 750 mL/day of water during the first 6 months to match the amount of milk secreted.

Normally the body maintains a balance between the amount of fluid taken in and the amount excreted. The requirements for body water are met through the consumption of liquids and foods and the oxidation of food. Solid foods, especially fruits and vegetables, contain 85% to 95% water. The normal daily turnover of water is 4% of an adult's total body weight and 15% of an infant's total body weight; refer to Chapter 33 for a complete discussion of water's role in maintaining homeostasis.

VITAMINS

Vitamins are organic compounds that regulate cellular metabolism, assisting the biochemical processes that release energy from digested food. Vitamins are called micronutrients because they are needed in small quantities when compared with other nutrients (water, carbohydrates, proteins, and fats). Vitamin requirements are dependent on many factors, such as body size, amount of exercise, rate of growth, and pregnancy.

Of the major vitamins, some are classified as either fat soluble or water soluble. **Fat-soluble vitamins** (vitamins A, D, E, and K) require the presence of fats for their absorption from the GI tract and for cellular metabolism and can be stored for longer periods of time in the body's fatty tissue and the liver. **Water-soluble vitamins** (vitamin C and B complex vitamins) require daily ingestion in normal quantities because these vitamins are not stored in the body.

Certain vitamins, minerals, and enzymes are classified as **antioxidants**, a substance that blocks or inhibits destructive oxidation reactions, such as vitamins C and E, the minerals selenium and germanium, and the enzymes catalase and superoxide dismutase, coenzyme Q_{10}, and some amino acids. Antioxidants help protect the body from the formation of **free radicals**, atoms or groups of atoms that can cause damage to cells. Free radicals can impair the immune system and lead to infections and certain degenerative diseases, such as heart disease and cancer. Free radicals are normally controlled by **free radical scavengers**, substances that remove or neutralize free radicals. Certain enzymes (superoxide dismutase, methionine reductase, catalase, and glutathione peroxidase) are free radical scavengers that are produced by the body. Besides vitamins C, E, A, and beta-carotene, certain herbs also act as antioxidants, such as bilberry, ginkgo, grape seed extract, green tea, and flavonoids. To maintain an effective level of antioxidants, clients should ingest five to nine daily servings of fresh, whole fruits and vegetables. Antioxidants seem to be more effective when obtained from food sources rather than from supplements. Morris (2004) reviewed three prospective studies regarding dietary influences on Alzheimer's disease. The strongest evidence for antioxidant protection against this disease was for ingesting foods high in vitamin E. None of the studies, however, found that vitamin E and vitamin C *supplements* were associated with less risk of Alzheimer's. The functions, clinical significance, and dietary sources of fat-soluble and water-soluble vitamins are presented in Table 34-1. Megadoses of both types of vitamins (fat and water soluble) can cause toxicity. Once the catalytic demands have been met by these vitamins, the remaining vitamins act as free chemicals that may be toxic to the body.

MINERALS

Minerals (inorganic elements) serve as catalysts in biochemical reactions. They are classified according to their daily requirement: macrominerals (quantities of 100 mg or greater)

and microminerals (trace elements, quantities less than 100 mg). The major macrominerals required by the body are calcium, phosphorus, and magnesium; see Chapter 33 for a complete discussion of these minerals (electrolytes).

Microminerals such as copper, fluoride, iodine, iron, selenium, and zinc play essential roles in metabolism. For example:

- Copper and iron are needed for hemoglobin formation.
- Copper is needed for the synthesis of phospholipids and prostaglandin and for the formation of some enzymes.
- Iron is needed for the synthesis of vitamins, purines, and antibodies.
- Fluoride is required for teeth formation and the prevention of dental caries.
- Iodine is the basic component of thyroid hormones.

TABLE 34-1 Fat-Soluble and Water-Soluble Vitamins

VITAMIN	FUNCTIONS	CLINICAL SIGNIFICANCE	DIETARY SOURCES
Fat-Soluble			
Vitamin A (retinol, retinal, retinoic acid)	Epithelial tissue proliferation Retinal pigmentation Immune system (antigen recognition) Antioxidant	Scaly skin, dry mucous membranes Night blindness Increased risk for infections Cancer and other diseases	Whole milk and whole milk products, eggs, fruits and vegetables (green leafy and yellow), fish, animal liver, fish liver oil. Caution: Do not exceed a daily dose of over 10,000 international units if pregnant or history of liver disease
Vitamin D (cholecalciferol, ergosterol)	Bone and tooth development Enhances immunity	Children: rickets and delayed dentition Adults: osteomalacia	Fortified milk, margarine, eggs, fish, cod liver oil, oatmeal, sweet potatoes, vegetable oils
Vitamin E (tocopherol)	Synthesis of heme Antioxidant, prevents oxidation of polyunsaturated fatty acids and of vitamins A and C	Premature infants: macrocytic anemia and hemolysis of RBCs Damage to RBCs, destruction to nerves	Cold-pressed vegetable oils, dark green leafy vegetables, milk, eggs, meats, legumes, nuts, seeds, whole grains
Vitamin K	Formation of prothrombin, blood clotting Bone formation and repair; synthesis of osteocalcin	Newborn: hemorrhagic disease Adults: prolonged clotting times Osteoporosis	Dark green leafy vegetables, asparagus, broccoli, Brussels sprouts, cabbage, cauliflower, egg yolks, liver, oatmeal, oats, rye, safflower oil, soy beans, wheat
Water-Soluble			
B complex Vitamin B₁ (thiamine)	Metabolism of carbohydrates and some amino acids (energy), production of hydrochloric acid, enhances circulation and assists in blood formation	Degeneration of myelin sheath in central nervous system (CNS) (paralysis) and in peripheral nerves (polyneuritis) Weakness of cardiac muscle: heart failure, peripheral vasodilatation, and edema GI: indigestion, severe constipation, anorexia, gastric atony,	Pork, fish, eggs, poultry, dried beans, whole grains, wheat germ, oatmeal, bread, pasta, brown rice, legumes, rice bran, peanuts

(Continues)

TABLE 34-1 (Continued)

VITAMIN	FUNCTIONS	CLINICAL SIGNIFICANCE	DIETARY SOURCES
		hypochlorhydria (referred to as beriberi—all above systems involved)	
Vitamin B$_2$ (riboflavin)	Oxidation and reduction of carbohydrates, fats, and proteins Red blood cell (RBC) formation, antibody production	Digestive disturbances, burning sensations in eyes and skin, headaches, mental depression, forgetfulness (frequently occurs with thiamine or niacin deficiency), skin lesions, eye disorders (cataracts)	Milk, whole grains, green vegetables, liver, cheese, egg yolks, fish, legumes, meat, poultry, yogurt
Vitamin B$_6$ (pyridoxine)	Functions as coenzyme to protein and amino acid metabolism, absorption of fats and protein	Convulsions, dermatitis, nausea and vomiting, anemia, flaky skin	Whole grains, liver, fish, poultry, green beans, meats, nuts, potatoes, eggs, brewer's yeast
Vitamin B$_{12}$ (cobalamin compounds)	Metabolically functions as a coenzyme: hydrogen acceptor and replication of genes	Demyelination of large spinal cord nerves: loss of peripheral sensation and paralysis (usually the result of intrinsic factor deficiency)	Milk, eggs, cheese, meat, fish, poultry, brewer's yeast
Biotin	Synthesis of fatty acids Protein metabolism Utilization of glucose	Infants: seborrheic dermatitis (cradle cap) Adults: rare	Liver, kidneys, dark green vegetables, egg yolk, green beans, brewer's yeast, milk, poultry, saltwater fish, whole grains
Vitamin C (ascorbic acid)	Formation of RBCs Production of collagen (capillary wall integrity) enzyme Metabolism of amino acids Prevention of oxidation of vitamins	Bleeding gums, bruising Poor wound healing, retardation of bone growth, fragile blood vessel walls, gum lesions (referred to as scurvy)	Citrus fruits, strawberries, cantaloupe, fresh vegetables: potatoes, cabbage, tomatoes, broccoli, green peppers
Folic acid (pteroylglutamic acid)	Synthesis of purines and thymine (DNA formation) Maturation of RBCs Functions as coenzyme in DNA and RNA synthesis	Retarded growth Sore red tongue Macrocytic anemia	Liver, green leafy vegetables, meat, fish, poultry, whole grains, barley, bran, brewer's yeast, brown rice
Niacin (nicotinic acid)	Coenzyme in energy metabolism	Muscular weakness, CNS lesions, dementia Skin: cracked, pigmented scaliness Irritation and inflammation of the mucous membranes of GI tract, producing GI hemorrhage (referred to as pellagra)	Meats, dairy products, whole grains, cereals, tuna, broccoli, carrots, cheese, corn flour
Pantothenic acid	Metabolism of carbohydrates and fats	None known	Meats, whole grain cereals, legumes

Delmar/Cengage Learning

- Selenium enhances vitamin E absorption and stimulates antibody response to infection.
- Zinc plays a major role in wound healing, maintains connective tissue integrity, assists with the formation of enzymes and insulin, boosts the immune response, and maintains normal blood concentrations of vitamin E. It also aids in the absorption of vitamin A, has antioxidant properties, and is a constituent of the antioxidant enzyme superoxide dismutase.

Other microminerals are arsenic, cadmium, nickel, silicon, tin, and vanadium; however, the specific roles that these microminerals play in metabolism have not been identified.

CARBOHYDRATES

Carbohydrates are organic compounds composed of carbon, hydrogen, and oxygen. They play a significant role in providing cells with energy and supporting the normal functioning of the body. Table 34-2 on page 1001 identifies the functions of carbohydrates and the problems that result from insufficient intake.

Carbohydrates are classified according to the number of **saccharides** (sugar units):

- Monosaccharides (simple sugars) include glucose, galactose, and fructose.
- **Disaccharides** (double sugars) include sucrose, lactose, and maltose.
- **Polysaccharides** (complex sugars) include glycogen, cellulose (fiber), and starch.

Glucose supplies the major source of energy needed for cellular activity, such as muscle contractions and nerve impulse transmission. When metabolized, every gram of glucose yields 4 kcal. Glucose is also needed for the synthesis of fatty acids and amino acids.

Carbohydrates have a protein-sparing action, based on a minimum daily ingestion of 50 to 100 grams (200–400 kcal) to spare the metabolism of protein. When dietary intake is below the minimum requirement, **triglycerides** (lipid compounds consisting of three fatty acids and a glycerol molecule) and proteins are metabolized to produce energy.

The three major sources of dietary carbohydrates are starches (nonanimal foods, primarily grains), lactose (milk), and sucrose (cane sugar). The ordinary diet contains far more starches than either lactose or sucrose. See Figure 34-2A for information on the digestion of these sugars.

Cells are unable to store large quantities of carbohydrates. The liver converts excess galactose and fructose into glucose and stores it in the form of glycogen. **Insulin** (pancreatic hormone) aids in the diffusion of glucose into the liver and muscle cells and in the synthesis of glycogen. Glucose metabolism is dependent on the availability of insulin (see Figure 34-5 on page 1002).

An increase in blood glucose levels can cause **hyperglycemia**, a blood glucose level greater than 110 mg/dL. This occurs in **diabetes mellitus**, a disease in which the pancreas fails to secrete adequate levels of insulin to accommodate blood glucose levels. When hyperglycemia occurs, **ketones** (the end product of incomplete fat metabolism) build up in the bloodstream, causing metabolic acidosis.

In **hypoglycemia**, the blood glucose level is below normal (less than 80 mg/dL) because the supply of insulin is so high that most of the glucose moves from the blood into the cells. Because brain tissue requires a constant source of glucose for energy, hypoglycemia can alter the normal functions of the brain.

Glucose (dextrose) is a common substance in intravenous therapy (dextrose 5% in water) because it is readily absorbed into the body's cells. This solution provides 170 kcal/L; refer to Chapter 33 for a complete discussion of intravenous replacement therapy.

PROTEINS

Proteins are organic compounds that contain carbon, hydrogen, oxygen, and nitrogen atoms; some proteins also contain sulfur.

After water, proteins are the most abundant intracellular substance. Proteins are essential for almost every bodily function, beginning with the genetic control of protein synthesis, cell function, and cell reproduction (see Table 34-2). The end products of protein digestion are amino acids.

The normal blood concentration of amino acids is between 35 and 65 mg/dL. There are 20 identified amino acids, which are categorized as either essential or nonessential:

- **Nonessential amino acids** can be synthesized (manufactured) in the cells; see the accompanying display on amino acids on page 1002.
- **Essential amino acids** must be ingested in the diet because they cannot be synthesized in the body; see the accompanying display on amino acids.

Proteins are also classified as complete or incomplete. **High-biological-value proteins (complete proteins)** contain all of the essential amino acids. Complete proteins are primarily animal proteins, such as those in meat, poultry, fish, dairy products, and eggs.

Low-biological-value proteins (incomplete proteins) lack one or more of the essential amino acids, usually lysine, methionine, and tryptophan. Most vegetables are incomplete proteins. By properly mixing complementary proteins in the diet, such as corn and beans, one can produce a complete protein.

All essential amino acids are needed by cells for anabolism and repair. The surplus amino acids are sent back to the liver, where they are degraded (nitrogen is split from the amino acid); the remaining parts are used for energy or converted to carbohydrate or fat and stored as glycogen or adipose tissue. Carbon dioxide, water, and nitrogen are the end products of amino acid metabolism.

The degradation of amino acids begins the process of **deamination**, the removal of the amino groups from the amino acids. During protein deamination, several other physiological processes of clinical significance occur:

1. **Gluconeogenesis**, the conversion of amino acids into glucose or glycogen

TABLE 34-2 Normal Function and Deficiencies of Selected Nutrients

NUTRIENT	FUNCTIONS	DEFICIENCIES
Proteins	Growth and replacement: clotting factor production, collagen synthesis, epithelial cell proliferation, fibroblast proliferation	Increased risk of bruising and hemorrhage; muscular wasting; depigmentation of hair and skin; poor wound healing; decreased enzyme production
	Immunity: antibodies, white blood cell production and migration, cell-mediated phagocytosis	Lymphopenia; impaired cellular immunity
	Fluid balance: intracellular osmotic pressure, albumin, maintenance of blood volume	Edema; hypoalbuminemia
	Sodium and potassium balance	Impaired nerve impulse transmission and muscle function
	Buffer action	pH imbalances
	Energy source	Negative nitrogen balance
Carbohydrates	Primary source of energy; sparing of protein.	Impaired brain functions; increased ketone bodies, producing acidosis; poor wound healing
Fats	Source of concentrated energy and essential fatty acids	Inhibited tissue repair
	Cell membrane integrity	Irritated and reddened skin
	Promotes absorption of fat-soluble vitamins; maintains body temperature	Deficit in fat-soluble vitamins; impaired fat digestion
	Synthesis of bile salts, steroid hormones, and vitamin D	Electrolyte depletion
Vitamin A	Collagen synthesis	Poor wound healing
	Epithelialization	Dry, scaly skin
Vitamin C	Collagen synthesis	Poor wound healing
	Maintains capillary integrity	Increased risk of bruising and hemorrhage
Vitamin K	Coagulation	Increased risk of bruising and hemorrhage
Pyridoxine, riboflavin, and thiamine	Cofactors in cellular development	Irritated and reddened skin
	Red blood cell formation	Nerve and muscular weakness; anemia
	Immunity: antibodies and white blood cell formation	Increased risk of infection
Copper	Red blood cell and connective tissue formation	Decreased collagen synthesis; poor wound healing from local tissue ischemia (anemia)
Iron	Collagen synthesis	Impaired collagen cross-linkage
	Enhancement of leukocytic activity	Increased risk of infection
	Hemoglobin synthesis	Anemia
Zinc	Cell proliferation	Poor wound healing
	Cofactor in enzymes	Increased risk of infection; alteration in taste

Adapted from Roth, R. (2007). *Nutrition and diet therapy* (9th ed.). Clifton Park, NY: Delmar/Cengage Learning.

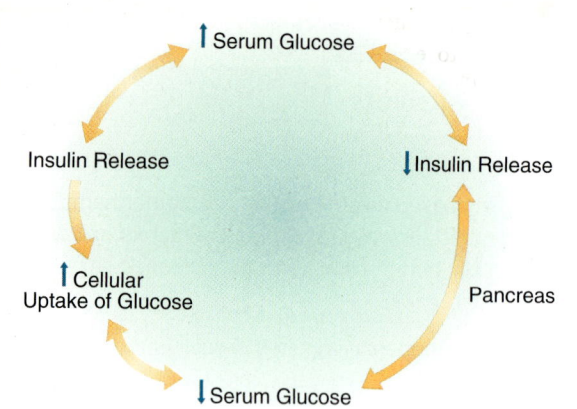

FIGURE 34-5 Serum Glucose–Insulin Feedback System DELMAR/ CENGAGE LEARNING

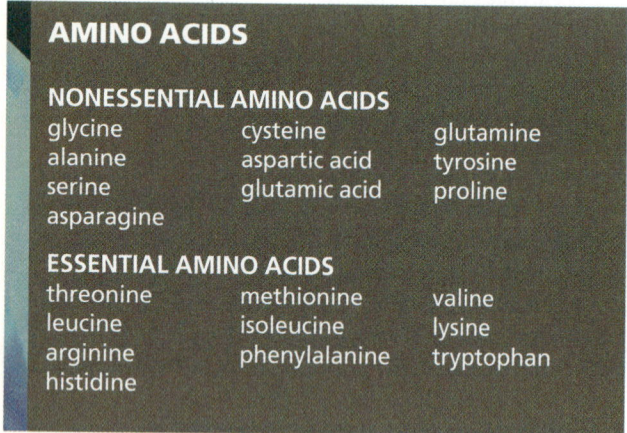

2. **Ketogenesis**, the conversion of amino acids into keto acids or fatty acids
3. **Nitrogen balance**, the net result of intake and loss of nitrogen that measures protein anabolism and catabolism
4. **Positive nitrogen balance**, the condition that exists when nitrogen intake exceeds output (protein anabolism exceeds catabolism)
5. **Negative nitrogen balance**, the condition that exists when nitrogen output exceeds intake (protein catabolism exceeds anabolism)
6. **Obligatory loss of proteins**, the degrading of the body's own proteins into amino acids, which are then deaminated and oxidized (occurs when a person fails to ingest adequate amounts of proteins)

Nitrogen balance measures protein equilibrium and is used to evaluate the client's nutritional status. Clients on bed rest or with a fever are in a catabolic state that produces a negative nitrogen balance. The muscle wasting that occurs with immobility causes negative nitrogen balance. Massive trauma and burns are other common examples of catabolic states that produce a negative nitrogen balance initially upon injury. Diet therapy is directed toward providing adequate amounts of proteins and kilocalories so that the body does not use its own protein as an energy source. A person must ingest a minimum of 20 to 30 grams of protein each day to prevent a net loss of body proteins.

LIPIDS

Lipids (fats) are organic compounds that are insoluble in water but soluble in organic solvents such as ether and alcohol. They are composed of the same elements as carbohydrates (carbon, hydrogen, and oxygen) but have a higher hydrogen concentration. Refer to Table 34-2 for a discussion of the normal functions of fats and the problems that arise from insufficient intake.

Fatty acids are the basic structural units of most lipids. They contain carbon chains and hydrogen. **Saturated fatty acids** form fats, glycerol esters of organic acids whose carbon atoms are joined by single bonds (all of the carbon atoms are saturated with hydrogen). Diets high in saturated fats are associated with a high incidence of coronary heart disease. Foods high in such fats are animal meats (especially beef), whole-milk products, butter, most cheeses, and some plant fats, such as chocolate, coconut, and palm oils.

Unsaturated fatty acids form glycerol esters of organic acids whose carbon atoms are joined by double or triple bonds (at least two carbon atoms in the fatty acid chains in the esters are unattached to hydrogen atoms). **Monounsaturated fatty acids** are fatty acids that form esters with one double or triple bond; foods in this category include nuts, fowl, and olive oil. **Polyunsaturated fatty acids** form esters that have many carbons unbonded to hydrogen atoms. Foods such as fish, corn, sunflower seeds, soybeans, cottonseeds, and safflower oil contain such esters.

The most important lipids follow:

- **Triglycerides** are lipid compounds composed of three fatty acid molecules attached to a glycerol molecule.
- **Phospholipids** are composed of one or more fatty acid molecules and one phosphoric acid radical and usually contain a nitrogenous base.
- **Cholesterol**, a lipid that is produced by the body and used in the synthesis of steroid hormones and excreted in bile, is considered a fat and is found in whole milk and egg yolk.

Phospholipids and cholesterol lipids constitute 2% of the total cell mass; they are basically insoluble in water and are used to form membranous barriers that separate the different intracellular compartments. The cell membrane is composed almost entirely of proteins and lipids (phospholipids and cholesterol).

Besides phospholipids and cholesterol, some cells contain triglycerides, which account for 95% of the fat cell mass. Triglycerides are the body's main storehouse of energy-giving nutrients; when dissolved, they can be used for energy as needed.

Most dietary fats are triglycerides, found primarily in animal food. Most plant foods contain trace elements of triglycerides. Other than butter fat, which is digested by gastric lipase (tributyrase), essentially all fat digestion occurs in the small intestine in the presence of pancreatic juices (see Figure 34-2C).

When free fatty acids, monoglycerides, free cholesterol, and phospholipids are absorbed by the blood and lymph system, they are resynthesized into minute molecules called **chylomicrons** (lipoproteins, synthesized in the intestines, that transport triglycerides to the liver).

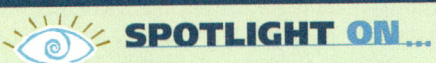

SPOTLIGHT ON...

A Fatty Meal

What impact would it have on a person, especially a teenager, if he or she could see a blood sample drawn 30 minutes after eating a large quantity of fast food? Do you think seeing the blood turn turbid or yellowish after a fatty meal would alter that person's eating habits?

Low-density lipoproteins are responsible for the formation of atherosclerosis, a disease of the arteries in which fatty lesions called atheromatous plaques develop inside the walls of the arteries. A diet high in saturated fats and cholesterol causes the formation of atherosclerosis. Almost half of the deaths in the United States and Europe are attributed to atherosclerosis, usually the result of coronary artery thrombosis.

PROMOTING PROPER NUTRITION

Hunger means a craving for food and is a subjective sensation. For example, when a person has not eaten for hours, the stomach undergoes intense rhythmic contractions called hunger contractions. These contractions sometimes cause pain, in the form of hunger pangs. Hunger not only is a physiological response but also involves psychological sensations. For instance, after a total gastrectomy (surgical removal of the stomach), clients still report a craving for food.

Appetite means the desire for specific types of food instead of food in general. A person's appetite determines the type of foods he or she eats. Satiety means a feeling of fulfillment from food. It is the opposite of hunger and occurs when a person's nutritional stores have been replenished and psychological cravings have been met.

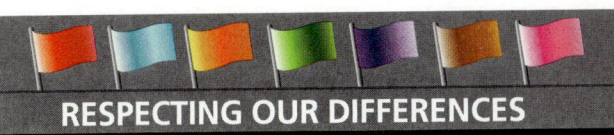

RESPECTING OUR DIFFERENCES

Satiety

How does one know when enough food has been eaten? How do the oral factors of chewing, salivation, swallowing, and tasting contribute to satiety? How true is the saying that healthy eating habits require three meals a day and that each of those meals should be filling? How are lifelong eating habits developed in early childhood?

Daily food guides have been developed by various organizations to establish standards that promote nutrition and health. These guides assist healthy persons in meal planning; however, the guides do not take into account the nutritional needs arising from metabolic and other medical disorders. Besides the American food guides, guidelines have been developed by other countries—for instance, Canada's *Food Guide to Healthy Eating*—and the World Health Organization.

DIETARY REFERENCE INTAKES AND RECOMMENDED DAILY ALLOWANCES

The recommended dietary allowances (RDAs) are recommended allowances of essential nutrients (protein, fat-soluble and water-soluble vitamins, and minerals) by age category, inclusive of weight and height. RDAs are established by the National Nutrition Board of the National Academy of Sciences–National Research Council. RDAs represent the normal nutritional needs of 97% to 98% of the people in each specific category; the RDAs do not take into consideration an individual's specific needs or physiological disorders.

Although RDAs have been in existence for the past 20 years as a nutritional guide to support healthy persons, the Food and Nutrition Board, in partnership with Health Canada, has initiated an effort to define new nutrient reference values. The Dietary Reference Intake (DRI) is a generic term that refers to at least three types of reference values: Estimated Average Requirement (EAR), RDA, and Tolerable Upper Intake Level (UL). EAR is the intake value that is estimated to meet the requirement defined by a specific indicator of adequacy in 50% of an age-specific and a gender-specific group. UL is the maximum level of daily nutrient intake that is unlikely to pose risks of adverse health effects to almost all of the individuals in the group for whom it is designed. The goal of DRI is to set nutrient reference values for all of the nutrients; see the accompanying display on DRIs on page 1004 for the first seven nutrient groups studied.

The Evidence-Based Guidelines issued by the National Institutes of Health call for weight loss by restricting caloric intake and increasing physical activity. Every 5 years the U.S. Department of Agriculture (USDA) and the Department of Health and Human Services are responsible for updating and publishing the *Dietary Guidelines for Americans* (DGA). These guidelines are based on the latest scientific and medical knowledge regarding ways to improve overall health through proper nutrition. The DGA 2005 stresses the need to balance caloric intake with daily physical activity and to choose nutrient-dense foods and beverages from the five major food groups while selecting those foods that limit the intake of saturated and trans fats, cholesterol, added sugar, salt, and alcohol and increasing intake of fruits and vegetables to achieve a healthy weight and prevent certain conditions such as obesity, diabetes, and cardiovascular disease. The DGA is a federal nutrition policy that offers guidelines for federally funded nutrition programs such as school lunch programs. See Figure 34-6 on page 1004 for key recommendations for the general population, as addressed in the DGA 2005.

EVALUATION OF DIETARY REFERENCE INTAKES

EVALUATION OF DIETARY REFERENCE INTAKES

The seven nutrient groups are as follows:

1. Calcium, vitamin D, phosphorus, magnesium, and fluoride
2. Folate and other B vitamins
3. Antioxidants (e.g., vitamins C and E and selenium)
4. Macronutrients (e.g., protein, fat, and carbohydrates)
5. Trace elements (e.g., iron, zinc)
6. Electrolytes and water
7. Other food components (e.g., fiber, phytoestrogens)

THE FOOD GUIDE PYRAMID

The Food Guide Pyramid was first developed by the USDA in 1992 to meet the dietary needs of healthy persons over 2 years of age; it was changed in 2005 to complement the revised DGA and DRI. The pyramid is an educational tool that suggests the number of daily servings from each of the five basic food groups (see Figure 34-6). In addition to the Food Guide Pyramid, pyramids for other cultures include the Native American food pyramid, the Spanish daily food guide flyer, the Mediterranean diet pyramid, the Asian diet pyramid, and Canada's Food Guide to Healthy Eating (see Figure 34-7 on page 1005).

SOCIETAL CONCERNS

Modern society has turned from a diet of whole grains, fruits, and vegetables to one of processed foods, fast foods, additives, preservatives, and hydrogenated oils that can have a damaging effect on a person's health. Processed foods usually contain excessive amounts of sodium that can cause fluid retention and lead to hypertension, aggravating many medical disorders such as congestive heart failure, certain forms of kidney disorders, and premenstrual syndrome (PMS). Additives are placed in foods for one or more of the following reasons: to lengthen shelf life; to make a food more appealing by enhancing color, texture, or flavor; to facilitate food preparation; or to otherwise make the product more marketable. Some additives are derived from natural sources such as sugar, while others are made synthetically, such as aspartame (NutraSweet). Although additives are usually identified on the "ingredient label" of a product, they are initially used without health warnings. For example, monosodium glutamate (MSG) and the artificial sweeteners cyclamate, saccharin, and aspartame are used without warning but have been known to cause headaches, diarrhea, confusion, memory loss, and seizures.

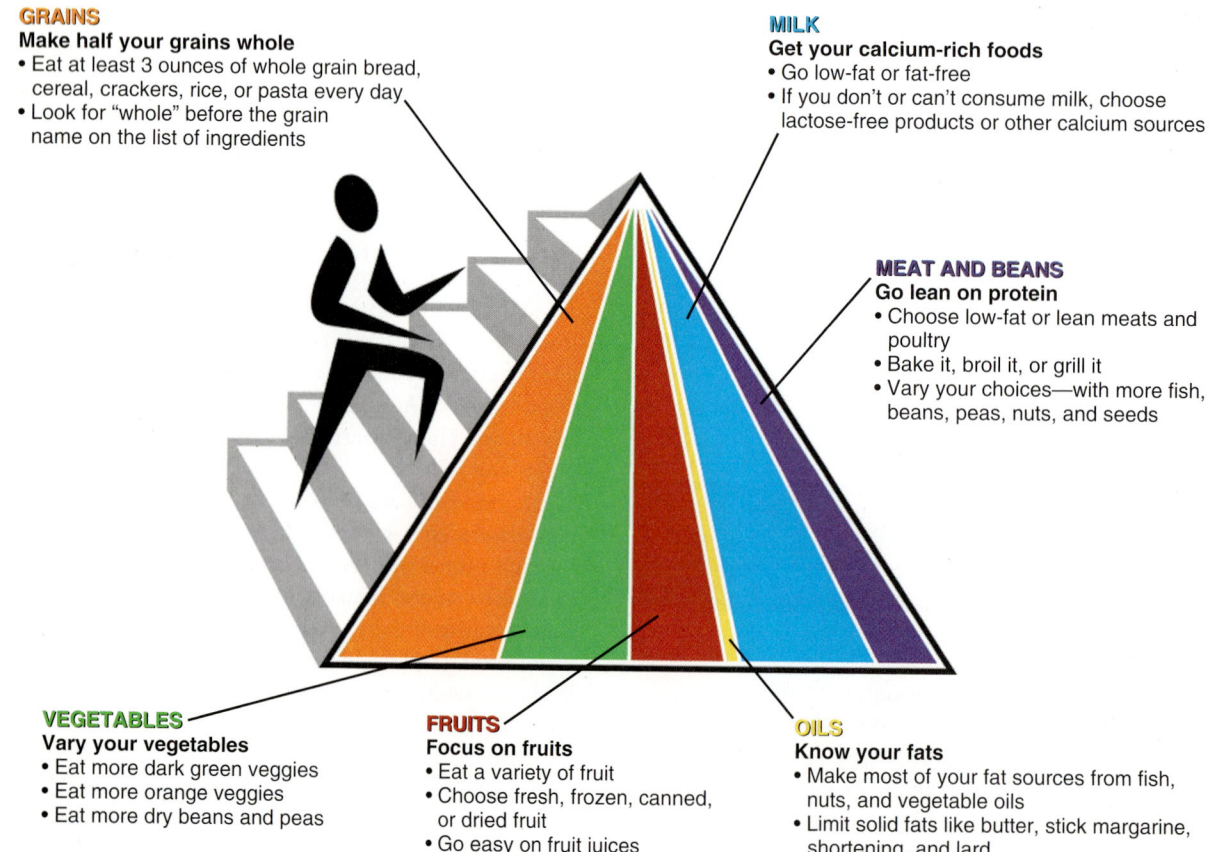

FIGURE 34-6 Steps to a Healthier You: MyPyramid FROM *INSIDE MYPYRAMID*, BY THE U.S. DEPARTMENT OF AGRICULTURE, 2005, RETRIEVED APRIL 21, 2005, FROM HTTP://WWW.MYPYRAMID.GOV/PYRAMID.

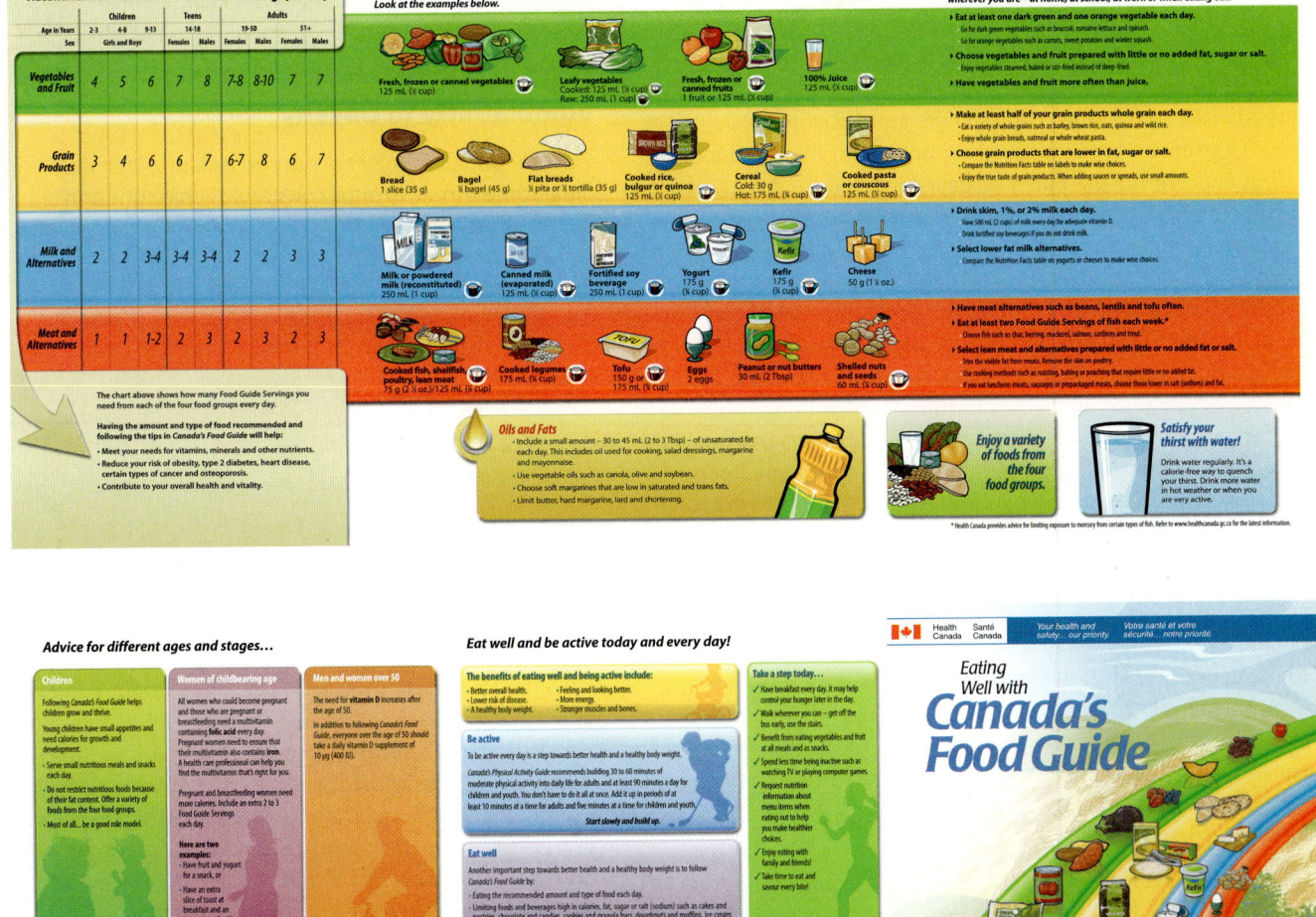

FIGURE 34-7 Canada's Food Guide COURTESY OF CANADA'S FOOD GUIDE TO HEALTHY EATING, HEALTH CANADA, 1992, © REPRODUCED WITH THE PERMISSION OF THE MINISTER OF PUBLIC WORKS AND GOVERNMENT SERVICES CANADA, 2005.

Genetically altering the world's food supply has caused many persons to question the essential ingredients of nutrients and the role of the U.S. Food and Drug Administration (FDA) in regulating safe, healthy food products. Although the FDA in 1993 approved the use of rBGH, a genetically engineered bovine growth hormone that enables dairy cows to produce 100% more milk than normal, Canadian health officials rejected a major U.S. corporation's request for approval of rBGH because the product label acknowledges that it can cause udder infections; painful, debilitating foot disorders; and reduced life span in treated cows. Humans who drink the milk from cows treated with rBGH can develop breast or prostate cancer as well as other reproductive disorders and diseases.

The European Union's Scientific Committee on Veterinary Measures reported that 17 beta-oestradiol, one of the six growth hormones that are used in 90% of all nonorganic beef raised in the United States, is "a complete carcinogen." American beef is banned in Europe because these hormones "may cause a variety of health problems, including cancer, developmental problems, harm to the immune system and brain disease" (Campaign for Food Safety, 1999).

In 1995, no genetically modified crops were grown for commercial sale; however, these statistics have changed rapidly in the past 3 years: By 1998, 73 million acres of genetically modified crops were being grown worldwide, more than 50 million acres of them in the United States; in 1999, an estimated 30,000 genetically modified products were in U.S.

grocery stores; and in 2000, 100% of a major U.S. corporation's soybeans (60 million acres) was genetically modified (Genetically Altering the World's Food, 1999). The FDA's position is that genetically modified foods do not need to be labeled; therefore, the consumer is deprived of the opportunity to make an informed choice in the grocery store.

"Consumers are increasingly choosing organic products out of concern for the purity of their food and the health of the environment" (Long, 1999, p. 44). In 2000, new organic certification rules were passed in the United States. These new regulations prohibit organic farmers from using toxic synthetic pesticides and fertilizers, genetically engineered seeds or other materials, irradiation, and sewage sludge. Organic farmers must adhere to strict standards regarding the use of fresh manure, animal confinement, and antibiotics and hormones. For a product to be labeled "certified organic" on the front of the package, 95% or more of the ingredients must be organically grown. To indicate on the label "made with organic ingredients," the product must contain at least 50% organic ingredients.

WEIGHT MANAGEMENT

Maintaining homeostasis requires a balance between intake of nutrients and energy expenditure. Average weight is relative to energy balance, the situation in which energy intake equals energy output.

Overweight

Overweight is an energy imbalance in which more food is consumed than is needed, causing a storage of fat. Overweight indicates a positive energy balance and is defined as weight 10% to 20% above average; obesity refers to weight 20% above average. Overweight may result from one or more factors: genetic, psychological, social, cultural, economic, or physiological. Genetically linked factors, such as a low BMR, excess fat distribution, and obese parents, place a person at risk for obesity. Some people overeat in response to emotional stress or whenever food is available rather than in response to hunger. Sociocultural norms influence eating habits; some cultures place a high value on excess weight. Hormonal imbalances, such as decreased thyroxin levels, can lower the BMR, causing weight gain if food intake remains constant. Other conditions that may contribute to obesity include some cancers, menopause, smoking cessation, impaired mobility, and some drugs such as antidepressants and glucocorticoids (James & Kohlbry, 2004). The degree of obesity is determined by calculating the body mass index, discussed later in this chapter.

Adult, teenage, and childhood obesity is an epidemic in the United States. Studies of ethnic groups indicate that physical inactivity is a risk factor associated with non–insulin-dependent diabetes (type 2), which is more prevalent in the Unites States in blacks and Native Americans (Gillespie, 2006). Although these populations have a disproportionate number of poor, unemployed, and disadvantaged individuals who lack access to health care, prevention and treatment programs need to focus heavily on exercise that is tailored to the

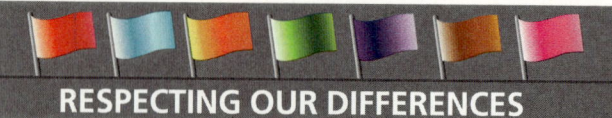

RESPECTING OUR DIFFERENCES

Vulnerability to Obesity

Cultural practices may encourage a calorie-dense diet. Some ethnic groups consider overweight and obesity acceptable or even desirable. An individual's emotional status also affects eating. What implications do these factors have in teaching clients about weight in relation to health?

activity tolerance of each individual. An estimated 80% of adults with type 2 diabetes are overweight or obese (James & Kohlbry, 2004).

Underweight

An underweight person expends more calories than are consumed. Underweight, a negative energy balance, is weight at least 10% to 15% below average. Being underweight decreases the individual's resistance to infection and increases susceptibility to fatigue and sensitivity to cold environments.

Family dynamics and a fear of overweight are psychological conditions that can contribute to eating disorders. **Anorexia nervosa** (self-starvation) disrupts metabolism because of inadequate caloric intake and results in hair loss, low blood pressure, weakness, amenorrhea, brain damage, and even death (Roth, 2007). **Bulimia nervosa** refers to food-gorging binges followed by purging of food, usually through self-induced vomiting or laxative abuse.

Underweight can also be caused by long-term conditions that deplete the body's resources, such as fever, infection, and cancer, or that prevent nutrient absorption, as occurs with diarrhea, metabolic or GI disorders, and laxative abuse. Other causes of underweight are hyperthyroidism and poverty.

FACTORS AFFECTING NUTRITION

Understanding the factors that may influence nutrition is essential in eliciting client and family cooperation in providing optimal nutritional care.

AGE

Infants and children vary in weight and energy requirements. The infant's physiological development has implications for fluid, electrolyte, and food intake that can predispose this age group to various imbalances. These factors are directly related to the infant's total body surface area, immature physiologic development, and the rate of growth and development during the first year of life; refer to Chapter 18 for a complete discussion of growth and development.

✓ CLIENT TEACHING CHECKLIST

Tips to Reduce Dietary Fat

- Read the nutritional labels for fat content on products before buying.
- Substitute plant proteins for meat, and avoid chocolate.
- Use low-fat dairy products such as skim milk instead of whole milk and low-fat yogurt instead of sour cream.
- Use 1/4 cup of egg substitute or two egg whites for one whole egg.
- Substitute margarine that is low in saturated fat for butter on breads, and use low-fat dressings for salads.
- Trim fats from meats and skin from poultry before cooking, and drain fat from meat after cooking.
- Include more fish and less red meat in the diet.
- Use herbs and spices instead of margarine, oil, and salt when cooking to bring out the flavor in foods.
- Cook foods by baking, broiling, boiling, roasting, or stewing to avoid additional fat from frying.
- Avoid adding flour, bread crumbs, and coating mixes when preparing foods.
- Use vegetable oils and sprays instead of shortening, lard, or butter when cooking and baking.
- Eat fresh fruits and vegetables instead of desserts high in fat.

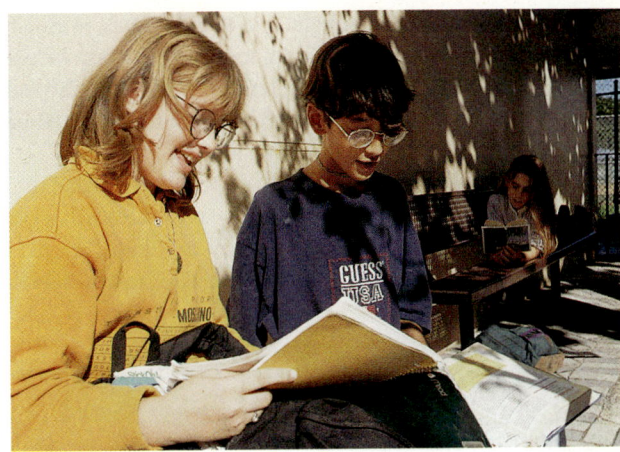

FIGURE 34-8 Adolescents are vulnerable to peer influence
DELMAR/CENGAGE LEARNING

From ages 1 to 6 years, nutritional intake varies in relation to growth rate, making the child's eating habits erratic. The child will usually select foods based on developmental nutritional needs in accordance with:

- High kilocaloric intake to maintain energy requirements
- Adequate levels of protein, vitamin D, calcium, and phosphate to complement teeth eruption and an increase in muscle mass and bone density

School-age children can eat larger meals less frequently because of the digestive system's maturation and the presence of permanent teeth. A diet that supplies the RDAs will promote optimal development and health and at the same time avoid weight gain during the preadolescent period.

Adolescence, a period of rapid growth and sexual maturation, requires guidance in dietary choices. Hormonal changes associated with menstruation make girls prone to fluid imbalance. Teenagers eat many of their meals away from home—for example, in fast-food restaurants.

Peer groups influence a teenager's choices, such as what, when, and where to eat (see Figure 34-8). At the same time, body image is of critical importance for teenagers. The social pressures and other emotional stressors of adolescence may have a negative effect on eating habits, leading to obesity, the use of fad diets, and eating disorders such as anorexia nervosa and bulimia. See the accompanying Spotlight On display for some points on food-related behaviors.

During adulthood, growth stops and metabolism declines, thereby decreasing the need for kilocaloric intake. With pregnancy and lactation, the nutritional needs once again increase. During pregnancy, changes occur that may result in fluid retention (dependent edema), for example, hormonal changes, pressure of the fetus on the inferior vena cava, vascular congestion, and increased capillary filtration pressure.

The aging process brings about structural and functional changes that may put older adults at risk. The older population cannot be classified as a homogeneous group because people do not age physically at the same rate they do chronologically; see the Client Teaching Checklist on page 1008 for dietary guidelines for older clients.

Socioeconomic factors, access to a grocery store, and lifestyle may affect the nutritional status of older adults. Having to prepare their own food and eat alone are other challenges they face. Refer to Chapter 19 for additional information on older adults.

LIFESTYLE

Eating is a social activity in most cultures. A person's lifestyle may have a major impact on food-related behaviors. Families with both parents working or with children involved in

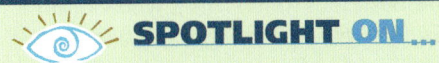

SPOTLIGHT ON...

Food-Related Behaviors

How are food fads developed? What lasting impact do these fads have on health? What role does the media play in forming an individual's food beliefs? Is the statement "Yogurt and vitamin E retard aging" related to a fad or a misconception, or is it a fact based on research? To answer this last question, refer to Table 34-1.

sports and other activities might find it difficult to sit down at the dinner table together for a home-cooked meal. When meals are eaten on the run, they tend to be high in fat and carbohydrates and the family misses the opportunity to come together to share important events of the day.

Food preferences are usually developed in childhood and modified throughout the life span. Lifestyle nutritional behaviors often come from traditional family practices. These practices affect not only food-related behaviors but also an individual's

☑ CLIENT TEACHING CHECKLIST

Special Dietary Considerations for Older Clients

- Special attention must be given to water needs, regardless of physical activity, because the thirst mechanism is less responsive than in younger people.

- Decrease the kilocaloric requirements in relation to activity: 10% for ages 51–75 and 20% to 25% for ages 75 and older. Bedridden and immobilized persons need a further reduction in kilocalories. Limit the quantities of empty kilocaloric foods (sugars, sweets, fats, oils, and alcohol).

- Maintain protein requirements, with 12% to 14% of the kilocalories derived from protein foods (meat, fish, eggs, poultry, milk, and cheese).

- Ensure adequate consumption of fats, especially unsaturated fats, to provide a source of energy, provide the essential amino acids, utilize the fat-soluble vitamins, and serve as a lubricating agent.

- Select carbohydrates as follows: Limit concentrated sweets; use moderate amounts of simple sugars (candy, sugar, jams, jellies, preserves, and syrups); the main source should be complex carbohydrates (fruits, vegetables, cereals, and breads).

- Ensure adequate amounts of vitamin D, calcium, and phosphorus to maintain bone integrity (fortified milk is a good source).

- Ensure high-fiber foods (dried fruits, whole grain cereals, nuts, fresh fruits, and vegetables) to increase satiety and maintain intestinal mobility to avoid constipation.

- Ensure a safe, adequate intake of sodium, avoiding canned foods and salted or cured meats high in sodium content for those with cardiac problems and hypertension.

- Include foods from the food guide pyramid in the amounts that meet the RDAs for ages 51 and older.

NUTRITIONAL BEHAVIORS OF SELECTED ETHNIC GROUPS

- Asians' main food types are rice, green tea, vegetables, and fish. A rice-and-water soup is often fed to the sick.

- The Islamic (Muslim) law does not permit the consumption of pork, alcohol, or meat that has not been slaughtered according to the Islamic code. The main meal is at midday.

- Orthodox Jews are not permitted to eat pig, rabbit, and shellfish; milk and meat are not taken at the same meal. A vegetarian diet is acceptable when kosher meat is not available. Strict guidelines dictate food preparation.

beliefs regarding health and wellness. Lifestyle behaviors can be changed. When understood, people can learn to make healthy nutritional choices. If a person gets sufficient rest, has the self-awareness to recognize stress, exercises regularly, and avoids addictive behaviors such as smoking and alcohol, then he or she will usually make healthy nutritional decisions.

ETHNICITY, CULTURE, AND RELIGIOUS PRACTICES

Dietary customs reflect the socialization and cultural patterns of ethnic groups (see Figure 34-9). Culture is evidenced by patterns of values and behaviors that are characteristic of a particular group. Religious beliefs often dictate which types of foods may be eaten and how they should be prepared.

Although it is not possible to learn the nutritional behaviors for all ethnic groups, recognize the need to comply with the client's routine patterns (see the accompanying display on the nutritional behaviors of selected ethnic groups). Refer to Chapter 20 for additional cultural factors that are evidenced in food behaviors.

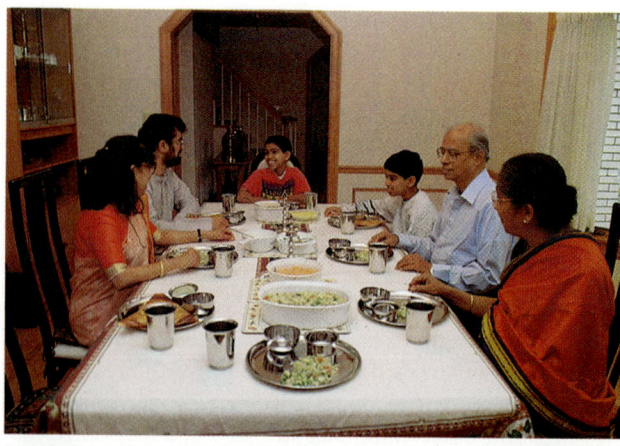

FIGURE 34-9 Family and cultural values often affect diet DELMAR/CENGAGE LEARNING

OTHER FACTORS

Other factors influence the types of foods selected and their nutritional value. Economics is a major influence on food selection; fresh fruits and vegetables and lean meats are expensive and are often substituted with products that tend to be low in protein and high in starch.

Food preferences are an expression of an individual's likes and dislikes. They may be related to the texture of food, how it is prepared, or what was served during childhood. However, preferences can also be an expression of a person's economic, ecological, ethical, or religious beliefs. Vegetarians, for example, follow a diet of plant foods and may include eggs or milk, depending on preference. A vegetarian diet is healthy when it includes a wide variety of foods to ensure adequate amounts of protein, vitamins, and minerals.

Gender may play a role in food selection, owing mainly to stereotyping (for example, the idea that males eat meat and potatoes and females eat salads). Peer pressure often dictates what teenagers eat. Stress, depression, and alcohol abuse alter the appetite. Medications can alter food absorption and excretion and affect the taste of food. GI disorders can cause anorexia, nausea, vomiting, diarrhea, constipation, discomfort, and pain, all of which may influence eating habits and food preferences.

ASSESSMENT

The goals of a nursing assessment are to collect subjective and objective data regarding the client's nutritional status and to determine which type of nutritional support is needed. Nurses are in a unique position to recognize **malnutrition**, or alterations related to inadequate intake, disorders of digestion or absorption, and overeating. Assessment must be performed in a logical fashion and should include three basic components: nutritional history, physical examination with anthropometric measurements, and diagnostic and laboratory data.

NUTRITIONAL HISTORY

The nutritional history of clients experiencing alterations in nutrition and metabolism is of critical importance in the development of the plan of care. Several methods can be used in collecting these subjective data: 24-hour recall, food-frequency questionnaire, food record, and diet history; see Table 34-3 on page 1010 for an example of a nutritional history. Begin the history with a thorough exploration of the client's presenting problems as they relate to onset, duration, nature, pattern, severity, associated symptoms, and efforts made to relieve the symptoms.

24-Hour Recall

The 24-hour recall requires client identification of everything consumed in the previous 24 hours. It is performed easily and quickly by asking pertinent questions. However, clients may be unable to recall their intake accurately or anything

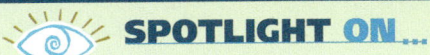

SPOTLIGHT ON...

Caring and Compassion

Personal Biases

Performing a nutritional history requires a questioning, nonjudgmental attitude. Examine your biases to treat the viewpoints of all clients equally. To gain a sincere understanding of clients' perspectives, develop an open mind, and listen with empathy.

atypical for their diet. Family members can often assist with these data, if necessary.

Food-Frequency Questionnaire

The food-frequency method gathers data relative to the number of times per day, week, or month the client eats particular foods. The nurse can tailor the questions to particular nutrients, such as cholesterol and saturated fat. This method helps validate the accuracy of the 24-hour recall and provides a more complete picture of foods consumed.

Food Record

The food record provides quantitative information regarding all foods consumed, with portions weighed and measured for 3 consecutive days. This method requires full client or family member cooperation.

Diet History

The diet history elicits detailed information regarding the client's nutritional status, general health pattern, socioeconomic status, and cultural factors (see Table 34-3). This method incorporates information similar to that collected by the 24-hour recall and food-frequency questionnaire. Inform the client that the history might require more than one interview because of the amount of data to be collected.

Although the history data may indicate adequate nutrition, clients must be reassessed periodically to prevent nutritional problems from occurring. Fear, anxiety, or depression before or during hospitalization may lead to poor food intake, which is the leading cause of malnutrition.

PHYSICAL EXAMINATION

A physical assessment requires decision making, problem solving, and organization; refer to Chapter 27 for a complete discussion of physical assessment. This section presents the physical assessment findings that suggest nutrient imbalance. "The nurse should be aware of rapidly proliferating tissues such as hair, skin, eyes, lips, and tongue that usually show nutrient deficiencies sooner than other tissues" (Hammond, 1999, p. 355). (Refer to Table 34-4 on page 1012 for the assessment findings of clients with nutrient imbalances.) Essential components of anthropometric measurements (height, weight, and skinfolds) are also discussed.

TABLE 34-3 Health History Related to Nutrition and Metabolism

ENVIRONMENT AND LIFESTYLE	POSSIBLE FINDINGS
Employment	• Exposure to heat, toxic chemicals • Extent of physical exertion • Degree of stress
Home environment	• Central air/heat; lives alone or with other family members; ability to shop/cook
Tobacco use	• Use of smokeless tobacco; cigarettes: number of years; packs per day; if quit, how long
Nutritional status	• Weight changes: loss or gain • Fluid consumption for 24 hours: number of glasses of water, cups of coffee or tea, soft drinks; amount of alcohol consumed • Food preferences and restrictions • Dietary restrictions (sodium) • Use of supplements: vitamins, minerals, commercial liquids, herbs
Presenting Problem	**Possible Findings**
Weight loss	• Onset: sudden or gradual duration • Pattern: decreased intake, increased activity • Severity: how much, specific time frame • Associated symptoms: anorexia, nausea, vomiting, diarrhea, dysphagia (difficulty in swallowing), odynophagia (pain in swallowing), polyuria (passage of excessive urine), fatigue, dyspnea, depression, cognitive impairment, motor weakness or paralysis • Efforts to relieve weight loss: increased intake, decreased activity
Anorexia	• Onset: sudden, gradual duration • Pattern: continuous, occasional, related to food intake—specific foods, time of day, activity, drugs, radiation or chemotherapy • Severity: intake for 24 hours • Associated symptoms: weight loss, nausea, vomiting, diarrhea, dysgeusia (distortion of sense of taste), fatigue, depression • Efforts to relieve anorexia: dietary changes—types of foods and preparation, time of day, eating with others or alone
Nausea and vomiting	• Onset: sudden, gradual duration • Nature of emesis: color, consistency, amount • Pattern: continuous, occasional, related to food intake—specific foods, time of day, position or activity • Severity: specific amount in a 24-hour period • Associated symptoms: weight loss, anorexia, dysphagia, diarrhea, fatigue, motor weakness, pain • Efforts to relieve nausea and vomiting: eliminating odors, certain foods, medications; changing position or activity after meals
Diarrhea	• Onset: sudden or gradual duration • Nature of feces: color, consistency, amount • Pattern: frequency, related to food intake • Severity: number of times in 24 hours • Associated symptoms: nausea, vomiting, pain, fatigue, motor weakness, weight loss • Efforts to relieve: decrease fluid intake with meals; identify foods, medications, and other stressors that trigger diarrhea

(Continues)

TABLE 34-3 (Continued)

ENVIRONMENT AND LIFESTYLE	POSSIBLE FINDINGS
Past Health History	**Possible Findings**
Previous or chronic illnesses	• Allergies, anorexia, malnutrition, gastroenteritis, cancer, diabetes mellitus • History of: heart disease, hypertension, renal disease, pulmonary disease • History of trauma: head or crushing injuries
Medications and therapies	• Diuretics, steroids, antacids, antihypertensives, digoxin IV therapy, total parenteral nutrition, chemotherapy
Family History	**Possible Findings**
Illnesses in family members	• Allergies, cancer, anorexia, diabetes mellitus, cardiovascular disease
Knowledge Level	**Possible Findings**
Client's knowledge of disease process	• Ability to name illness • Ability to identify current treatments (e.g., medications)
Coping Ability	**Possible Findings**
Client and family coping strategies	• Client's and family's perceptions of impact of illness on lifestyle • Presence of social support systems

Delmar/Cengage Learning

Intake and Output (I&O)

I&O measurements and daily weights are critical components of a nutritional assessment; refer to Chapter 33, Procedure 34-1, I&O measurements, and Chapter 26 for a complete discussion of weight measurement.

Anthropometric Measurements

Anthropometric measurements (measurements of the size, weight, and proportions of the body) evaluate the client's calorie-energy expenditure balance, muscle mass, body fat, and protein reserves based on height, weight, skinfolds, and limb and girth circumferences. Chapter 26 discusses the assessment of height and weight; refer to Chapter 33 for additional nursing measures relative to daily weights.

The **body mass index (BMI)** determines whether a person's weight is appropriate for height and is calculated using a simple formula:

$$\text{BMI} = \frac{\text{weight (kg)}}{[\text{height (m)}]^2}$$

For example, a person who weighs 65 kg and is 1.6 m tall would have a BMI of $65 \text{ kg}/(1.6 \text{ m})^2$, or 25.4. According to the Centers for Disease Control and Prevention, a healthy BMI for adults is between 18.5 and 24.9. Specific ranges have been established as follows: underweight—BMI less than 18.5; overweight—BMI of 25 to 29; obese—BMI of 30 or more. Height and weight tables are available in most health care settings.

SKINFOLD MEASUREMENTS Skinfold measurement indicates the amount of body fat. This information is beneficial in promoting health and determining risks and treatment modalities associated with chronic illness and surgery. This assessment is usually performed in an outpatient setting when the nurse develops a client's profile.

A special caliper is used to measure skinfolds. The caliper should grasp only the subcutaneous tissue, not the underlying muscle. Measurements can be taken of the triceps, subscapular, biceps, and suprailiac skinfolds.

1. To measure the triceps fold, locate the midpoint of the upper arm. Grasping the skin on the back of the upper arm, place the calipers 1 cm below fingers (see Figure 34-10 on page 1013), and measure the thickness to the nearest millimeter.
2. For a subscapular skinfold measurement, grasp the skin below the scapula with three fingers, angle the fold about 45° laterally to the scapula (see Figure 34-11 on page 1013), place the caliper 1 cm above fingers, and read the measurement.

It is essential to document the skinfold sites, the type of caliper used, and the measurement in millimeters.

TABLE 34-4 Adult Physical Assessment Findings: Nutrient Imbalance

ASSESSMENT FINDINGS	NUTRIENT DEFICIENCIES AND EXCESSES	ASSESSMENT FINDINGS	NUTRIENT DEFICIENCIES AND EXCESSES
Hair		Petechiae and ecchymoses	Vit C and vit K deficiency
Dull, dry brittle	Protein deficiency	Darkening and peeling of sun-exposed areas	Niacin deficiency
Hair loss	Protein, zinc, and biotin deficiency or vit A excess	Poor wound healing	Protein, zinc, and vit C deficiency
Loss of pigment in strips around hair line	Protein and copper deficiency	**Nails**	
Head and neck		Koilonychia (spoon-shaped nails)	Iron deficiency
Headache	Vit A and D excess	Brittle, fragile	Protein deficiency
Epistaxis (nosebleed)	Vit K deficiency	**Heart**	
Thyroid enlargement	Iodine deficiency	Tachycardia	Vit B_1 deficiency
Eyes		Hypertension	Calcium and potassium deficiency or sodium excess
Pale conjunctiva	Iron deficiency	**Abdomen**	
Blue sclerae	Iron deficiency	Ascites	Protein deficiency
Conjunctival and corneal dryness	Vit A deficiency	**Musculoskeletal**	
Corneal vascularization	Vit B_2 deficiency	Muscle wasting	Protein and vit B_1, B_6, and B_{12} deficiency
Mouth		Edema	Protein and vit B_1 deficiency
Lesions at corners of mouth	Vit B_2 deficiency	Calf tenderness	Vit B_1 and C, biotin, and selenium deficiency
Glossitis (red, sore tongue)	Niacin, folate, vit B_{12}, and other vit B deficiencies	Bone tenderness	Vit D, calcium, and phosphorus deficiency or vit A excess
Gingivitis (inflamed gums)	Vit C deficiency	Knock-knees, bowed legs, and fragile bones	Vit D, calcium, phosphorus, and copper deficiency
Hypogeusia (poor sense of taste)	Zinc deficiency	**Neurologic**	
Dysgeusia (bad taste)	Zinc deficiency	Paresthesia	Vit B1, B6, and B12, and biotin deficiency
Dental caries	Fluoride deficiency	Weakness	Vit C, B1, B6, and B12 deficiency
Mottling of teeth	Fluoride excess	Ataxia	Vit B1 and B12 deficiency
Atrophy of papillae on tongue	Iron and vit B deficiency	Tremor	Magnesium deficiency
Skin		Decreased tendon reflexes	Vit B1 deficiency
Dry, scaly	Vit A, zinc, and essential fatty acids deficiency or vit A excess	Disorientation	Vit B1 deficiency
Eczematous lesions	Zinc deficiency	Drowsiness, lethargy	Vit B1 deficiency or vit A and D excess
		Depression	Vit B1 and biotin deficiency

Delmar/Cengage Learning

MID-UPPER-ARM CIRCUMFERENCE The measurement of **mid-upper-arm circumference (MAC)** serves as an index for skeletal muscle mass and protein reserve. Instruct the client to relax and flex the forearm; with a measuring tape, measure the circumference at the midpoint of the upper arm (see Figure 34-12 on page 1013).

ABDOMINAL-GIRTH MEASUREMENT When made repeatedly over a span of time, an abdominal girth measurement serves as an index as to whether abdominal distention is increasing, decreasing, or remaining the same. With an indelible pen, place an X on the client's abdomen at the point of greatest distention. Using a measuring tape, measure the abdomen's circumference.

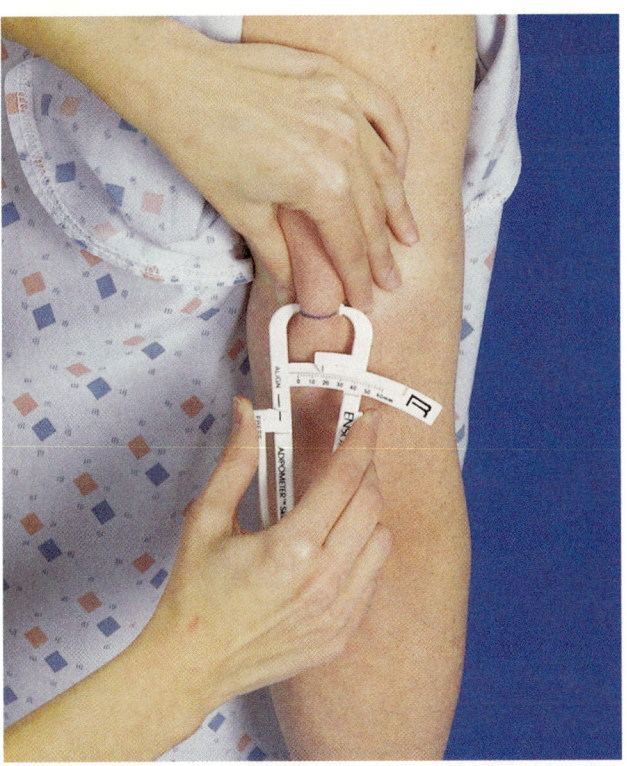

FIGURE 34-10 Measuring Triceps Skinfold, at Midpoint of the Upper Arm DELMAR/CENGAGE LEARNING

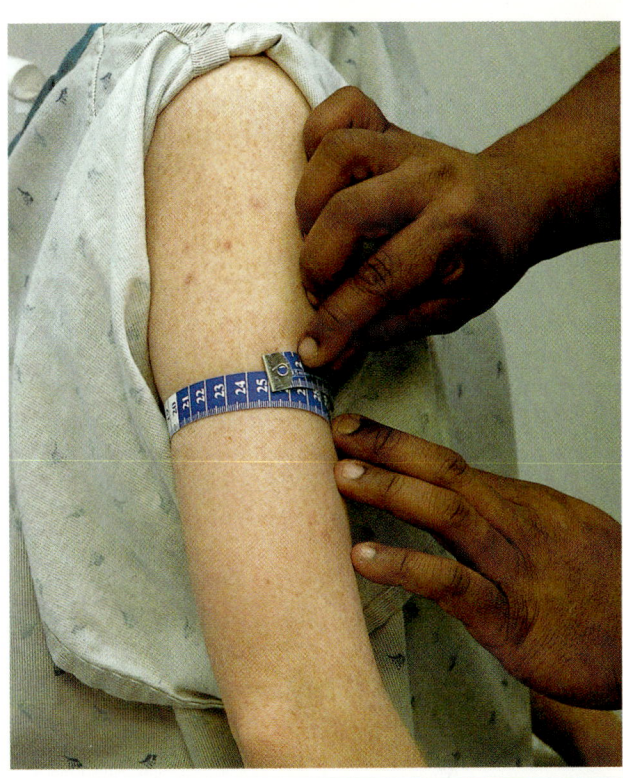

FIGURE 34-12 Measuring the Mid-Upper-Arm Circumference DELMAR/CENGAGE LEARNING

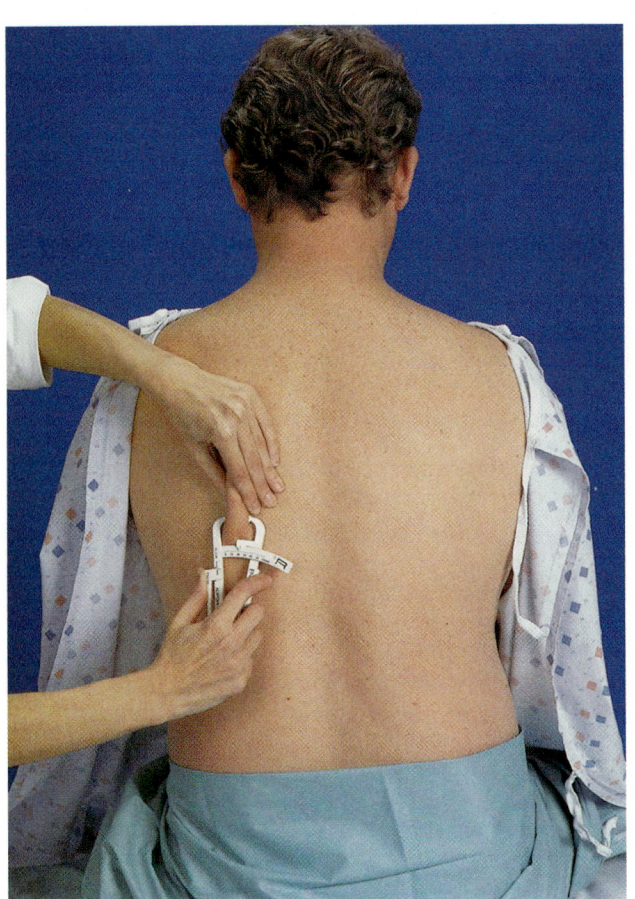

FIGURE 34-11 Measuring the Subscapular Skinfold DELMAR/CENGAGE LEARNING

This measurement should be performed at the same time each day and consistently recorded in either inches or centimeters.

DIAGNOSTIC AND LABORATORY DATA

Biochemical data assessment is another essential source of objective data. Trends revealed in laboratory results can be used to detect alterations in nutrition and metabolism before clinical symptoms are assessed in the examination. Refer to Chapter 28 for a detailed discussion of laboratory testing. No single laboratory test is diagnostic of malnutrition.

Protein Indices

Several tests that reflect protein synthesis can also reflect nutritional status. Serum levels of albumin and transferrin are used to identify protein-calorie malnutrition.

SERUM ALBUMIN Albumin is synthesized in the liver from amino acids. Serum albumin plays an important role in fluid and electrolyte balance and the transport of nutrients, hormones, and drugs. However, serum albumin has a half-life of 21 days and fluctuates according to the level of hydration; therefore, it is not a good indicator of acute alterations in protein status. Clinically, this blood test is used to measure prolonged protein depletion that occurs in chronic malnutrition, liver disease, and nephrosis. Albumin levels below 3.5 g/dL may indicate some degree of malnutrition.

PREALBUMIN Research has provided a newer, more accurate test to evaluate protein status. **Prealbumin** (a precursor of albumin) has a half-life of 2–3 days; it is used to determine protein depletion in acute conditions, such as trauma and inflammation, and serves as a guide for nutritional therapy. Prealbumin levels between 15 mg/dL and 5 mg/dL reflect mild to moderate protein depletion, while levels below 5 mg/dL indicate severe protein depletion.

SERUM TRANSFERRIN Transferrin (nonheme iron) is a blood protein in combination with iron; it is used to transport iron throughout the body to all cells. It is responsive to iron stores, increasing when they are low and decreasing when they are high. This test is considered a sensitive indicator of protein deficiency because it responds promptly to changes in protein intake. Levels below 200 mg/dL may indicate mild to moderate protein depletion, and levels below 100 mg/dL may indicate severe depletion.

Hemoglobin Level

The hemoglobin test measures the oxygen and iron-carrying capacity of the blood; the normal level is 12 to 15 g/100 mL. A decreased hemoglobin may indicate some form of anemia, such as microcytic iron deficiency anemia or blood loss.

Total Lymphocyte Count

Another test that may be used to measure protein depletion is total lymphocyte count. Protein deficiency may cause a depression in the immune system, with a resultant decrease in the total lymphocyte count; this can occur with severe debilitating diseases, such as cancer or renal disease.

Nitrogen Balance

Nitrogen balance studies indicate the degree to which protein is being depleted or replaced in the body. The blood urea nitrogen (BUN) is increased with severe dehydration, malnutrition, starvation, excessive protein intake, and most commonly kidney disease (the kidneys fail to excrete urea). A decreased BUN results from a diet low in protein-rich foods.

Urine Creatinine Excretion

During skeletal muscle metabolism, creatinine is released at a rate in proportion to the total body mass. A 24-hour urine test is done to measure the total amount of creatinine excreted by the kidneys. In malnutrition, the creatinine level is decreased as a result of muscle atrophy.

NURSING DIAGNOSIS

In order to make a nursing diagnosis, the nurse must interpret the subjective and objective data and draw conclusions from the client's assessment data obtained during a comprehensive health history and physical examination. The approved nursing diagnoses are discussed to assist with the appropriate selection of primary and secondary nursing diagnoses for clients with nutritional alterations.

IMBALANCED NUTRITION: LESS THAN BODY REQUIREMENTS

An estimated 30% to 50% of hospitalized clients are at risk for malnutrition; increased morbidity and mortality rates are associated with malnutrition (Bulechek, Butcher, & Dochterman, 2008). The diagnosis *Imbalanced nutrition: less than body requirements* exists when the client fails to ingest or digest food or absorb nutrients. The Nursing Process Highlight lists some possible causes of this nursing diagnosis.

Such clients may experience a weight loss of 20% or more from their ideal weight. The dietary history may reveal inadequate food intake based on the RDAs, a lack of interest in or an aversion to eating, a perceived inability to ingest food, and reduced energy level. Clients have poor muscle tone, with skinfolds less than 60% of standard measurement, and they may experience difficulty in swallowing or masticating food because of muscular weakness. The conjunctive and mucous membranes are usually pale, and the buccal cavity is sore and inflamed.

IMBALANCED NUTRITION: MORE THAN BODY REQUIREMENTS OR RISK FOR IMBALANCED NUTRITION: MORE THAN BODY REQUIREMENTS

Imbalanced nutrition: more than body requirements exists when clients experience or are at risk for an intake of nutrients that exceeds metabolic needs. Clients may be at risk because of one or more of the following factors: hereditary predisposition or obesity in one or both parents; dysfunctional psychological conditioning in relationship to

NURSING PROCESS HIGHLIGHT

Diagnosis

Factors Causing Nutritional Imbalance

Multiple factors can cause *imbalanced nutrition: less than body requirements*:

- **Biological:** Buccal cavity discomfort, pain; difficulty in swallowing; stomach strictures, ulcers; inflammation, obstruction of the biliary or intestinal system; chronic diarrhea; pulmonary disorders; postoperative status; transplantation candidate, pre- and postsurgery; cancer and radiation therapy; immunosuppression
- **Psychological:** Anorexia nervosa; bulimia; severe stress, anxiety, fatigue, or depression; prolonged grieving; lack of knowledge; extreme food fad and dieting practices
- **Economic:** Inadequate finances to purchase protein-rich foods

SECONDARY NURSING DIAGNOSES FOR CLIENTS WITH NUTRITIONAL PROBLEMS

- *Activity intolerance* related to insufficient energy from protein depletion
- *Acute pain* related to lactose intolerance
- *Ineffective health maintenance* related to excessive intake of nutrients
- *Impaired oral mucous membrane* related to dehydration
- *Ineffective breathing pattern* related to decreased energy and fatigue from protein depletion
- *Constipation* related to inadequate dietary intake and fiber
- *Ineffective health maintenance* related to inadequate financial resources to purchase nutritious foods
- *Risk for infection* related to nutrient replacement therapy
- *Deficient knowledge* related to information of normal nutrition
- *Ineffective therapeutic regimen management* related to cultural influences on the client's food preferences
- *Impaired swallowing* related to decreased strength of muscles involved in mastication
- *Chronic low self-esteem* related to obesity
- *Risk for impaired skin integrity* related to inadequate intake of proteins, vitamins, and minerals
- *Nausea* related to gastric irritation or gastric distention
- *Readiness for enhanced nutrition* related to consumption of adequate food and fluid choices

North American Nursing Diagnosis Association. (2009–2011) © 2009, 2007, 2005, 2003, 2001, 1998, 1996, 1994 NANDA International. Used by arrangement with Wiley-Blackwell Publishing, a company of John Wiley & Sons, Inc.

OTHER NURSING DIAGNOSES

The client who is protein-depleted may also experience deficiencies in vitamins (especially A and C) and minerals (especially zinc, magnesium, and iron). Refer to the accompanying display for a list of common secondary nursing diagnoses related to nutritional and metabolic problems. Because the secondary diagnosis is related to the nutritional/metabolic problem, it is written in terms of the etiology of the primary diagnosis, for example, *risk for impaired skin integrity* related to inadequate intake of proteins, vitamins, and minerals.

PLANNING AND OUTCOME IDENTIFICATION

The nurse relies heavily on the data obtained from the nutritional history and collaborates with the client and other health team members in formulating goals and expected outcomes to promote optimal nutritional care. Nursing diagnoses of life-threatening conditions, such as *impaired swallowing* related to decreased or absent gag reflex, are given first priority. Other diagnoses that are actual problems take priority over high-risk problems.

In the planning phase, the nurse identifies and explains to the client the need for and basis of the therapy. The nurse takes into consideration the client's dietary habits, likes, dislikes, needs, readiness for learning, and nutritional assessment data in defining goals and developing outcomes in collaboration with the client. Refer to the accompanying display for samples of NOC nutrition outcomes.

The nurse selects appropriate nursing interventions to match the client's routine patterns, as obtained in the health history, and to support achievement of the goals and outcomes. Proceeding in this fashion facilitates the client's adaptive capabilities through skillful interventions.

COLLABORATION

The management of nutritional problems is usually a long-term process that requires a multidisciplinary approach. For example, obesity management programs often involve clinicians, dietitians, exercise physiologists, health educators, and social workers or psychologists. Family involvement is an essential component in managing obesity.

food, such as using food as a reward or comfort measure; and age-related factors, most notably early infancy, adolescence, and aging.

Clients with more than body requirements experience a weight gain of 10% to 20% over the ideal for height and frame and triceps skinfolds greater than 15 mm in men and 23 mm in women. The client's dietary history may reveal a sedentary activity level and one or more dysfunctional eating patterns: pairing food with other activities, such as watching TV; concentrating the intake of food at night; and eating in response to internal cues (anxiety) or external cues (such as a social event) instead of in response to hunger.

NURSING OUTCOMES CLASSIFICATION (NOC): NUTRITION

- Nutritional Status (1004)
- Nutritional Status: Biochemical Measures (1005)
- Nutritional Status: Energy (1007)
- Nutritional Status: Food & Fluid Intake (1008)
- Nutritional Status: Nutritional Intake (1009)

Moorhead, S., Johnson, M., Swanson, M., & Maas, M. (2008). *Nursing outcomes classification (NOC)* (4th ed.). St. Louis, MO: Mosby.

Since the early 1980s, nutrition support teams (NSTs) were established to reduce the complications of parenteral nutrition (PN). To achieve the expertise required for a consulting service, the teams have become multidisciplinary. The clinical functions of NSTs are:

- Identification of clients who are nutrition impaired or at risk for malnutrition
- Performance of a nutritional assessment to guide nutritional therapy
- Provision of nutritional support that is safe and effective

The nurse is seen as the vital link between the client and other team members to include a prescribing practitioner, nurse, pharmacist, and dietitian. The nurse's role is critical, both for the implementation of nutritional support and for ongoing assessment, because the nurse administers and monitors nutritional therapies.

IMPLEMENTATION

The nurse is responsible for understanding the client's nutritional needs and for making clinical judgments relative to outcomes of therapy. This responsibility includes intervening to prevent the rapid depletion of the body's protein and energy reserves. Performance of nursing interventions to accomplish goals and outcomes includes monitoring the client's weight and intake, diet therapy, and feeding. Client teaching occurs with each intervention to maximize the effectiveness of nutritional therapy.

The Nursing Interventions Classification (NIC) consists of specific interventions for clients with impaired nutrition, such as Behavior Management: Overactivity/Inattention, Eating Disorders Management, Enteral Tube Feeding, Nausea Management, and Nutrition Management. These interventions identify the specific nursing activities for each classification.

MONITORING WEIGHT AND INTAKE

Weight and intake measurements are used to assess the client's nutritional status and to monitor the effectiveness of therapy. Refer to Chapters 26 and 33 for nursing actions relative to daily weights and I&O considerations.

INITIATING DIET THERAPY

Nutritional problems often require dietary modification. Therapeutic nutrition requires consideration of the client's total needs: cultural, socioeconomic, psychological, and physiological. Modified diets should promote effective nutrition within the client's lifestyle; this often requires client teaching regarding the avoidance of certain foods or adding food items to the diet, given the client's sociocultural context, economic restraints, and religious beliefs. See Table 34-5 on page 1017 for the various types of therapeutic diets and examples of food items for each diet; dietary restrictions vary among agencies and in accordance with the client's tolerance. A *diet as tolerated* is prescribed to allow the client to eat whatever foods the client can chew, swallow, and digest and may progress to a *regular diet* without any restrictions. Recent research has changed the nutritional management of clients by introducing dietary support early after surgery, trauma, or acute illness; this change stresses the need for positive nitrogen balance and its role in healing and recovery.

ASSISTANCE WITH FEEDING

Assessment data provide direction regarding how to assist the client with eating. Clients with difficulty in self-feeding, chewing, or swallowing will require assistance to promote safety and adequate intake of nutrients; see the accompanying Nursing Process Highlight on page 1018.

Clients with a neurologic disease such as an acute stroke, Parkinson's disease, or dementia or with a history of prolonged or multiple endotracheal intubations or tracheostomy may need a bedside swallow screen to identify dysphagia and aspiration risk until further studies can be done by a speech-language pathologist (Grams & Spremulli, 2008). If the client is managing oral secretion, offer small pieces of ice or sips of water and observe for cough, drooling, voice change (especially a wet or gurgling quality), and swallowing difficulty. Stop the screen immediately if any of these symptoms occur, and notify the prescribing practitioner.

Because eating is a social activity (see Figure 34-13 on page 1017), it is important to encourage a family member or friend to be present at meals. If this is not possible, assess the availability of other resources to provide social stimulation during meals, such as watching TV, listening to music, or having a staff member remain with the client.

PROVIDING NUTRITION SUPPORT

Proper nutrition in hospitalized clients is necessary for wound healing, recovery, reduction in morbidity, and consequent reductions in length of stay and mortality. The most common nutritional deficiency in hospitalized clients is protein-energy malnutrition. This type of malnutrition depletes body cell mass and impairs tissue and organ function. When protein-energy malnutrition is left untreated, the following client negative outcomes may occur:

- Weakness
- Compromised immunity
- Decreased wound healing
- Increased risk for complications

Nutrition support (NS) is prescribed for those clients at risk for protein-energy malnutrition.

There are two routes for delivery of NS in adult clients: enteral nutrition (EN) and PN. **Enteral nutrition** includes both the ingestion of food orally and the delivery of nutrients through a GI tube. **Parenteral nutrition** refers to nutrients bypassing the small intestine and entering the blood directly. EN is preferred over PN because of decreased bacterial translocation and reduced expense and is usually delivered through a feeding tube (see Figure 34-14 on page 1018).

TABLE 34-5 Therapeutic Diets

TYPE	DESCRIPTION
Clear liquid	Prescribed primarily for surgical clients: water, broth/bouillon, clear fruit juices, gelatin, carbonated beverages, coffee, tea, popsicles
Full liquid	Prescribed mainly for postoperative clients: clear liquids, plus all fruit and vegetable juices, smooth-textured dairy products, custard and pudding
Pureed	Prescribed for clients with dysphagia: full liquids, plus pureed fruits, vegetables, and meats, scrambled eggs
Mechanical soft	Prescribed for clients having difficulty chewing/swallowing: pureed foods that are finely diced or ground, plus cheese, barley, rice, pancakes, and breads
Soft	Prescribed for clients having difficulty chewing/swallowing: mechanical soft foods, plus enriched pasta, broiled seafood, and desserts without nuts and dried fruits
Liberal bland	Prescribed for clients with excessive digestive enzymes: eliminates chemical and mechanical food irritants such as fried foods, alcohol, and caffeine
Low residue	Prescribed for client with mucosal irritation existing with diverticulitis, ulcerative colitis, and Crohn's disease: eliminates raw fruits (except bananas), vegetables, seeds, plant fiber, and whole grains and limits dairy products to two servings a day
High fiber	Prescribed for clients with diverticulosis: raw fruits and vegetables, seeds, plant fiber and whole grains; the opposite of low residue
Fat controlled	Prescribed for clients with atherosclerosis, heart disease, and obesity: decreases saturated fats by restricting animal fats, gravies, sauces, chocolate, and whole-milk products
Sodium restricted	Prescribed for clients with excess fluid volume, hypertension, heart failure, myocardial infarction, and renal failure: restrictions for mild, 2 to 3 g; moderate, 1000 mg; strict, 500 mg; and severe, 250 mg
Lactose intolerant	Prescribed for client who lacks or is deficient in lactase, an enzyme that splits lactose into glucose and galactose: eliminates milk and dairy products, except yogurt
Candidiasis	Prescribed for client with *Candida albicans*, a normal, parasitic yeastlike fungus that may multiply with certain conditions or therapies, such as antibiotics or chemotherapy: eliminates all fruits, sugar, yeast, and fermented foods

Delmar/Cengage Learning

Critical indicators for determining the feeding route and NS formula include GI function, expected duration of therapy, aspiration risk, and the potential for or the actual development of organ dysfunction. For example, the decision to initiate PN or EN support is based on evidence that the client is unable to meet his or her own nutritional needs by oral intake and will therefore experience malnutrition. Refer to Figure 34-15 on page 1019 for a clinical decision algorithm that outlines the selection process for choosing the route of nutritional support in adult clients. The client's NS may be determined by an NST in accordance with American Society for Parenteral and Enteral Nutrition (ASPEN) guidelines.

The nurse is responsible for eliciting the client's or family's continued consent and collaboration with the therapy.

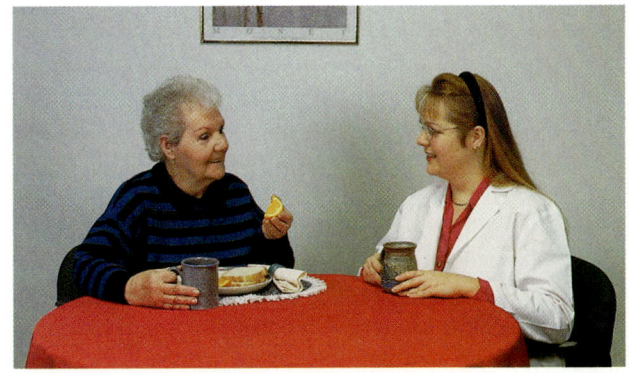

FIGURE 34-13 Eating is a social activity DELMAR/CENGAGE LEARNING

NURSING PROCESS HIGHLIGHT

Implementation

Nursing Measures That Promote Client Feeding

- Before bringing the meal tray into the room, ask whether the client needs to void or have a bowel movement.
- Provide hygiene measures before serving the meal tray.
- Position the client in a comfortable position, preferably in a chair, if not contraindicated.
- Ask about the client's eating habits and the foods he or she prefers to eat first. Ask what help is needed. For instance, older adults may want scrambled eggs placed in a sandwich to make them easier to handle.
- Make sure the foods are being served at the correct temperature.
- Provide assistance if the client is unable to handle eating utensils or to open containers and packages.
- Provide adequate time for the client who has difficulty chewing or swallowing. Make sure that someone is in the room while the client is eating.
- Document the type and amount of food taken at each meal.
- Remove the tray after the meal, and provide hygiene measures.

The prescribing practitioner obtains the client's informed consent for starting the therapy. The nurse teaches the client and family about the nutritional support to restore a sense of independence and self-esteem. Many staff nurses are board certified in NS by the ASPEN.

ENTERAL TUBE FEEDING

Candidates for enteral tube feeding are clients who have a functional GI tract and will not, should not, or cannot eat. Therefore, tube feedings are used for clients who are (or may become) malnourished and in whom oral feedings are insufficient to maintain adequate nutritional status.

Enteral tube feedings maintain the structural and functional integrity of the GI tract, enhance the utilization of nutrients, and provide a safe and an economical method of feeding. Enteral tube feedings are contraindicated in clients with the following:

- Diffused peritonitis
- Intestinal obstruction that prohibits normal bowel functioning
- Intractable vomiting; paralytic ileus
- Severe diarrhea

Feeding Tubes

Most feeding tubes are made of silicone or polyurethane, which are durable and biocompatible with formulas. They vary in diameter (8 to 12 French) and length in accordance with the route and formula. The prescribing practitioner selects the route (see Figure 34-14) and type of feeding tube on the basis of the anticipated duration of feeding, the condition of the GI tract, and the potential for aspiration.

Insertion of Enteral Feeding Tubes

Nasoenteral insertion of a gastric feeding tube is the simplest and most often used method of tube feeding. It is used as a

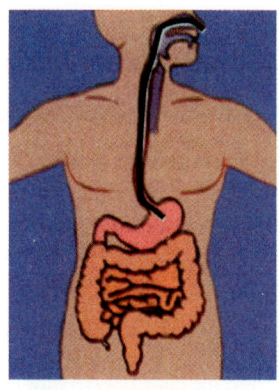

Nasogastric Route

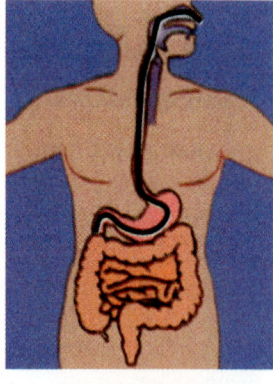

Nasoduodenal Route

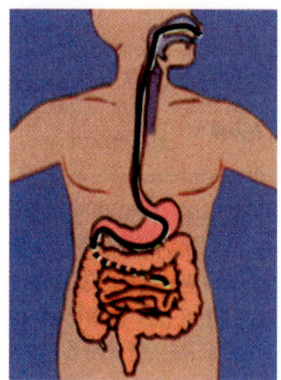

Nasojejunal Route

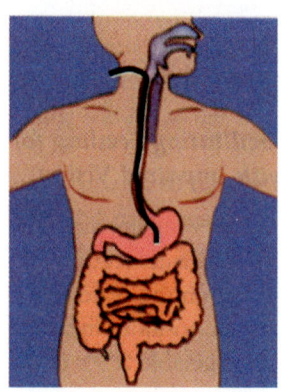

Esophagostomy Route

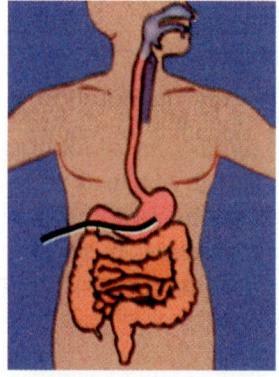

Gastrostomy Route

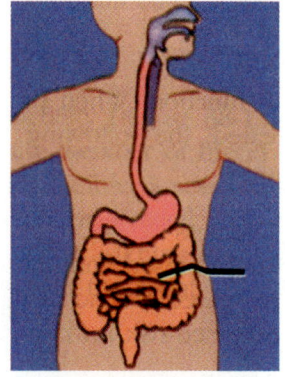

Jejunostomy Route

FIGURE 34-14 Enteral Feeding Routes DELMAR/CENGAGE LEARNING

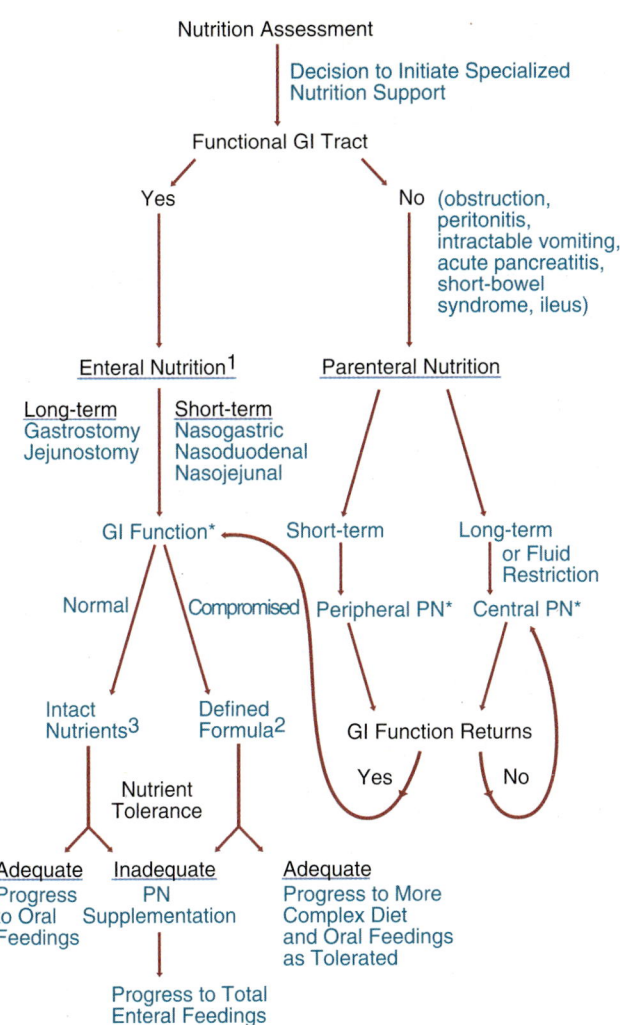

Nutrition Assessment

Decision to Initiate Specialized
Nutrition Support

Functional GI Tract

Yes   No (obstruction,
peritonitis,
intractable vomiting,
acute pancreatitis,
short-bowel
syndrome, ileus)

Enteral Nutrition[1]   Parenteral Nutrition

Long-term   Short-term
Gastrostomy   Nasogastric
Jejunostomy   Nasoduodenal
           Nasojejunal

GI Function*   Short-term   Long-term
                       or Fluid
                       Restriction

Normal   Compromised   Peripheral PN*   Central PN*

Intact   Defined   GI Function Returns
Nutrients[3]   Formula[2]
                          Yes   No

Nutrient
Tolerance

Adequate   Inadequate   Adequate
Progress   PN   Progress to More
to Oral   Supplementation   Complex Diet
Feedings   and Oral Feedings
                           as Tolerated

Progress to Total
Enteral Feedings

FIGURE 34-15 **Clinical Decision Algorithm** REPRINTED FROM THE AMERI-
CAN SOCIETY FOR PARENTERAL AND ENTERAL NUTRITION (ASPEN) (1993). GUIDELINES FOR THE USE OF
PARENTERAL AND ENTERAL NUTRITION IN ADULT AND PEDIATRIC PATIENTS. *JOURNAL OF PARENTERAL AND
ENTERAL NUTRITION, 17,* 1SA-52SA. ASPEN DOES NOT ENDORSE THIS MATERIAL IN ANY FORM OTHER THAN
ITS ENTIRETY. FOR INFORMATION ON ORDERING A COMPLETE SET OF GUIDELINES, CONTACT ASPEN, 8630
FENTON STREET, SUITE 412, SILVER SPRING , MD 20910, (301) 587-6315.

temporary measure for clients who are expected to resume oral feeding. Nasogastric intubation refers to insertion of a tube through the nostril into the stomach (see Procedure 34-1). Nasoduodenal or nasojejunal intubation allows nasal access to the duodenum and jejunum; it is done with a longer tube and decreases the client's risk of vomiting and aspiration. Radiographic visualization is used to confirm tube placement prior to feeding.

Enterostomy is the surgical creation of an artificial fistula (gastrostomy, jejunostomy) in the intestines by an incision through the abdominal wall. Tube enterostomies can be placed at various points along the GI tract and are performed when long-term tube feeding is anticipated or when obstruction makes nasal intubation impossible.

Percutaneous endoscopic gastrostomy (PEG) tube placement is usually performed by the prescribing practitioner at the bedside or in the endoscopy room; *insertion of a PEG tube does not require surgery.* Endoscopy nurses are often trained to assist with PEG placement. PEG has become an

accepted technique to provide enteral access for both children and adults.

Enteral Formulas

Nutrients administered through tubes are liquefied so they can be easily digested and absorbed. Commercially prepared formulas are available and used in most health care settings. Enteral tube feeding is used with caution in clients with severe pancreatitis, enterocutaneous fistulae, and GI ischemia. These feedings are not recommended during the early stages of short-bowel syndrome or in the presence of severe malabsorption. There are three basic types of formulas, which differ in osmolality, digestibility, kilocalories, lactose content, viscosity, and fat content:

- *Isotonic formula* contains proteins, fats, and carbohydrates with a high molecular weight and an osmolality equal to that of the body (300 mOsm). Isocal and Osmolite are isotonic formulas that supply 1 kcal/mL and are lactose free.
- *Elemental (monomeric) formula* contains monosaccharides and amino acids with minimal triglyceride content in hypertonic concentrations. Vivonex and Vivonex HN are elemental formulas that supply 1 kcal/mL; they are started at half strength or less and gradually increased to full strength due to their hypertonic concentration.
- *Fluid restriction formula* contains a highly concentrated source of kilocalories (2 kcal/mL). Magnacal is a fluid restriction formula that is started at half strength or less and gradually increased to full strength due to the hypertonic concentration.

Administration of Enteral Feedings

Once the feeding tube's position has been radiographically verified, the formula can be administered as prescribed (see Procedure 34-2). Most clients with a small-bore tube receive continuous feeding with a formula pump to regulate the rate. One of the advantages of continuous feeding is that it keeps gastric volume small, minimizing residual volume and reducing the risk of aspiration pneumonia; the client is less likely to experience bloating, nausea, abdominal distention, and diarrhea.

Safety Considerations

Clients receiving EN through a feeding tube are at risk for aspiration. Tube feeding aspiration can result from several

▼ SAFETY FIRST ▼

SMALL-BORE FEEDING TUBE
When inserting a small-bore feeding tube with a guide wire or stylet, never attempt to reinsert the guide wire or stylet while the tube is in the client. The guide wire or stylet may perforate the GI mucosa, especially the esophagus, and injure the client.

▼ **SAFETY FIRST** ▼

ALLERGIES
Before administering a tube feeding, determine whether the client has any food allergies. Clients may be lactose intolerant or may have an allergy to the formula.

▼ **SAFETY FIRST** ▼

GASTRIC RESECTION
Never insert, manipulate, or remove a nasogastric tube on gastric resection clients: The suture line could easily be interrupted, causing hemorrhage.

---

factors: displacement of the tube into the esophagus, large amounts of gastric residue, and lowered intestinal motility and delayed gastric emptying, which may occur in clients who are on bed rest or receiving narcotics for pain relief. Auscultate for bowel sounds to determine gastric motility. If the bowel sounds are hypoactive or absent, stop or withhold additional feeding and notify the prescribing practitioner.

Always assess placement of the feeding tube before administering any liquids. Clients who are receiving continuous gastric feeding should be assessed every 4 hours for tube placement and residual gastric contents. Aspirate gastric contents with a syringe. This is done more easily with a large-bore tube rather than a small-bore one. The lumen of a small-bore tube collapses easily, making aspiration difficult and sometimes impossible. Observe and check the pH of the aspirate as explained in Procedure 34-1. Replace stomach contents after checking the residue to prevent fluid and electrolyte imbalance.

Although the literature documents the numerous research studies regarding the various methods to verify feeding tube position, there is no evidence to document 100% accuracy of any one nonradiographic method to verify tube placement. Huffman, Pieper, Jarczk, Bayne, and O'Brien (2004) reviewed the research literature on methods that document proper position of orally or nasally placed feeding tubes and determined that pH testing, combined with visual inspection of the aspirate, is the most reliable bedside method of verifying feeding tube position. Caution should be used when testing the pH aspirate of clients receiving certain drugs that may alter the pH, such as acid-suppressing medications or continuous feedings. The best practice for feeding tube verification is as follows:

- Document pH of aspirate with initial placement. Radiographic confirmation should be obtained for nasointestinal feeding tubes after initial placement.
- Document insertion distance with initial placement and record the external length of the tube in the nursing notes.
- Check the pH of aspirate before administering any medication or feeding.

A pH of 4 or less in adults (5 or less in children) suggests that the tip of the tube is in a gastric location, and the appearance of the aspirate can verify this. The characteristics of aspirates are:

- *Gastric aspirates:* Cloudy and green, tan or off-white, or bloody or brown (fresh or old blood)
- *Intestinal aspirates:* Basically clear and yellow to bile-colored

- *Pleural aspirates:* Tan or off-white mucus, may be pale yellow and serous (indicating blood)

When the nurse has any question regarding proper position, elective replacement and reassessment and/or radiographic confirmation should be considered before the administration of medications or feeding.

Client safety and comfort require daily cleansing of the feeding tube's exit site. Cleanse the skin with a clean washcloth, soap, and water. Nasal feeding tubes require daily removal of the tape from the nose and cleansing and inspection of the skin for irritation, inflammation, and infection and of the nares for erosions, ulcers, or abscesses.

Enterostomy tubes require surgical asepsis of the exit site until the incision heals; rotate the tubes within the stoma to promote healing. Report any observations of redness, irritation, or gastric leakage at the site. Once the stoma has healed, the tube can be removed and reinserted for each feeding. Between feedings, a prosthetic device may be used to cover the ostomy opening.

PEG tubes require daily rotation to relieve pressure on the skin. Notify the prescribing practitioner if the nurse is unable to rotate the PEG; it may be an indication of internal embedding of the tube into the gastric wall. When the tube is internally embedded, it can cause gastric acid reflux, which results in skin breakdown, sepsis, and cellulitis. Care must be taken to avoid dislodgment of the tube. Keep it secured to the client's abdomen with tape, being careful not to use excessive tension. PEG tubes require frequent flushing to prevent clogging. These tubes have small lumens. If a tube becomes clogged, flush it with 60 mL of lukewarm tap water.

Potential Complications

Clients receiving EN need to be monitored closely to prevent complications. The nurse should perform the following actions:

1. Assess the client for signs of gastric retention: nausea, vomiting, and cramping. Palpate the abdomen for distention, auscultate for bowel sounds with a stethoscope, and aspirate the gastric contents every 4 hours. If the aspirate exceeds 100 mL in a 4-hour period or if bowel sounds are absent (indicating an ileus), discontinue the feeding and notify the prescribing practitioner. *Do not remove the feeding tube.*
2. Monitor the feeding tube placement every 4 hours by checking for any coils or kinks in the back of the throat and measuring the length of tubing outside of the body.
3. Assess the client for pulmonary aspiration by checking the gag reflex. If the reflex is absent, suction the client.

Discontinue the feeding and remove the tube if signs of respiratory distress are present, and notify the prescribing practitioner.

4. Keep the client in a high Fowler's position to prevent aspiration if vomiting should occur. If vomiting does occur, suction client immediately and assess the formula amount and rate at which it was given.

5. Dilute feedings to half strength, and slow the feeding time to prevent diarrhea.

6. To maintain or achieve patency of gastric and/or jejunostomy feeding tubes, a medical device called a DeClogger may be used as prescribed by the client's prescribing practitioner to maintain the patency of these tubes (see the accompanying Nursing Checklist).

Teach the client and caregiver how to monitor for complications prior to discharge for home treatment. The client and caregiver should be given the opportunity to practice these assessment measures and demonstrate competency in performing the actual procedures.

Clients with feeding tubes may be discharged to the home. The NST evaluates these clients to determine:

- Ability to meet nutrient requirements orally
- Clinical status relative to home discharge
- Tolerance of prescribed nutritional therapy
- Willingness and ability to perform the necessary tasks of tube feeding
- Benefits of continuing therapy at home

The NST works with the client and caregiver to secure the necessary supplies prior to discharge from the hospital. Clients on home feedings require monitoring by nurses and nutritional support specialists who are familiar with the procedure and complications of enteral tube feeding.

Removal of a Nasogastric Tube

When the prescribing practitioner determines that the client's nutritional status no longer warrants EN therapy or the need to provide decompression of the gastric contents, the nasogastric tube is removed; refer to the accompanying Nursing Checklist on page 1022. If the client is connected to suction for decompression, the prescribing practitioner may prescribe clamping the tubing for several hours prior to removal to ensure a functioning GI tract.

PARENTERAL NUTRITION

PN is the infusion of a solution directly into a vein to meet the client's daily nutritional requirements. Formerly called hyperalimentation, it is frequently referred to as **total parenteral nutrition (TPN)**, the intravenous infusion of a solution containing dextrose, amino acids, fats, essential fatty acids, vitamins, and minerals. Other terms used interchangeably with TPN are 3 in 1 (dextrose, amino acids, and fats) and total nutrient admixtures (TNAs).

PN is used to treat malnourished clients or clients who have the potential for becoming malnourished and who are not candidates for enteral support. PN can be prescribed for either short-term or long-term use, as previously discussed in the decision algorithm (see Figure 34-15).

☑ NURSING CHECKLIST

Use of a DeClogger

1. Gather equipment: towel, receptacle for used items, nonsterile gloves, and appropriate size DeClogger that corresponds to the size of the feeding tube as prescribed by the prescribing practitioner.
2. Verify the prescribing practitioner's prescription.
3. Review the agency's policy.
4. Check the client's armband, and explain the procedure.
5. Provide for privacy.
6. Wash hands.
7. Turn the enteral feeding pump to the pause mode; if feeding to gravity, clamp the tubing.
8. Don nonsterile gloves.
9. Place the clean towel under the tube to protect the bed linens.
10. Disconnect tubing, and place cap on delivery tube to prevent contamination.
11. Attempt to flush tube with 30–60 cc of water.
12. Gently insert the appropriate size DeClogger into the opening of the tube.
13. Slowly rotate the DeClogger in a clockwise fashion until the stop disc meets the opening of the tube.
14. To remove, slowly rotate the DeClogger in a counter-clockwise fashion as you pull back on the device.
15. Flush the feeding tube with 30–60 cc of water.
16. Reconnect the delivery tube, and restart enteral feedings.
17. Discard the DeClogger into the receptacle, remove gloves, place in receptacle, and dispose of receptacle in accordance with agency policy.
18. Wash hands, and document procedure in the client's medical record.

The type of device used for PN therapy is determined by the duration of the therapy and the osmolality of the solution. Peripheral parenteral nutrition (PPN) is used for short-term treatment to deliver isotonic or mildly hypertonic solutions into a peripheral vein; the volume is usually limited to between 2000 and 3000 mL/day, providing a caloric value of about 2000 kcal/day.

Central parenteral nutrition (CPN) is used for long-term therapy to infuse highly hypertonic solutions directly into the superior vena cava. The delivery of highly hypertonic solutions into peripheral veins can cause sclerosis, phlebitis, or swelling; refer to Chapter 33 for a complete discussion of intravenous therapy complications. Malnourished clients are prone to infections because their immune systems have been

✔ NURSINGCHECKLIST

Removal of a Nasogastric Tube

1. Gather equipment: tube plug or clamp, towel, washcloth, paper towel, receptacle for contaminated items, and nonsterile gloves.
2. Verify the prescribing practitioner's prescription.
3. Check the client's armband, and explain the procedure.
4. Provide for privacy.
5. Wash hands and don gloves.
6. Place the client in a high Fowler's position, and adjust the height of the bed to a comfortable working position.
7. Place the towel across the client's chest.
8. Clamp or plug the tube, and unpin the tube from the client's gown.
9. Remove the tape securing the tube from the client's nose.
10. Hold the paper towel open in nondominant hand under the client's chin; with dominant hand, grasp and pinch the tube near the nostril, and remove the tube with a steady, continuous pull, allowing the tube to fall into the paper towel.
11. Dispose of the tube and paper towel in the receptacle.
12. Clean the client's nares, and provide oral hygiene.
13. Position the client comfortably, place call light within easy reach, and return bed to a low position.
14. Remove gloves, place in receptacle, and dispose of receptacle in accordance with agency policy.
15. Wash hands, and document procedure in the client's medical record.

compromised. EN and PN provide a positive medium for the potential growth of microorganisms. To decrease the risk of infection, institute the following nursing measures:

1. Verify placement of feeding line prior to administration of liquids.
2. Administer nutrients in accordance with the prescribed time interval.
3. Add small quantities of enteral formula to the bag.
4. Wash reusable EN feeding bag with warm water and soap after each use, at least every 24 hours.
5. Keep PN refrigerated; remove from refrigerator 30 minutes prior to administration.
6. Change EN and PN tubing every 24 hours.

Specific client populations that benefit from PPN or CPN are described in the accompanying display.

Components of Parenteral Nutrition

PN solutions are predigested or chemically prepared nutrients that can be administered singly or as admixtures. The basic components of PN are:

1. Carbohydrates, primarily in the form of monohydrous glucose, ranging from 5% solution for PPN to 50% to 70% hypertonic solution for CPN; provides client with 60% to 70% of caloric (energy) needs
2. Amino acids, in the form of synthetic crystalline amino acid solutions; provides 5% to 15% of the total calories (CPN solutions contain sufficient amino acids for tissue synthesis)
3. Lipids (fat emulsions), prepared from safflower and soybean oil with egg phospholipids; supply up to 30% of client's caloric (energy) intake; additional lipid emulsions and glucose or amino acids provide for a TNA isotonic solution. Clients with a known egg allergy should not receive TPN with lipid emulsions.

Other ingredients, called admixtures, provide for the client's biochemical needs (electrolytes, vitamins, and trace elements such as zinc, selenium, chromium, magnesium, iodine, copper, iron, and molybdenum).

Medications, such as heparin, may also be added to the TPN solution. Heparin is commonly added to reduce the buildup of a fibrinous clot at the catheter's tip. When the TPN catheter is the only available venous access, TPN may be used to

CANDIDATES FOR PPN OR CPN THERAPY

SHORT-TERM (UP TO 2 WEEKS) PPN

1. Preoperative for severely depleted clients
2. Postoperative for abdominal surgery clients who have been NPO for several days because of an ileus
3. Inflamed or ulcerated bowel needing 1 or more weeks of rest: acute exacerbations of Crohn's disease and colitis, radiation enteritis, acute or necrotizing pancreatitis, or an enterocutaneous or a high-output fistula
4. Congenital anomalies before surgical repair: intestinal obstruction, tracheoesophageal fistula, midgut malrotation, volvulus, and omphalocele
5. Short-bowel syndrome: small-bowel resection of 75% or more to control diarrhea and prevent dehydration and malnutrition
6. Cancer clients receiving chemotherapy or radiation therapy

LONG-TERM (GREATER THAN 2 WEEKS) CPN

1. Hyperemesis gravidarum
2. Low-birth-weight neonates
3. Failure to thrive
4. Intractable diarrhea
5. Severely burned clients

deliver antibiotics. The TPN solution should be prepared only by a pharmacist using sterile technique and a laminar flow hood to reduce the risk of contamination. See the Nursing Checklist on page 1024 on interventions for a client receiving TPN.

Client assessment for home parenteral nutrition (HPN) should consider the physical, psychosocial, and financial resources of the client and the caregiver. Maintaining a client on HPN is challenging because of the expense, technology, and required changes in lifestyle. When the PN is prescribed daily, it is usually administered overnight to minimize disruption to the client's lifestyle. Home health nurses should visit the client daily until the client and caregiver demonstrate proficiency in handling the equipment and maintaining aseptic technique.

Clients receiving PN in the home environment require close monitoring to prevent catheter sepsis and cardiac overload. The PN solution should be administered with a volumetric infusion pump. If the home does not have air conditioning to maintain the proper temperature of the solution during infusion, the solution can be divided into two bags. The second bag can be refrigerated while the first bag is infusing. The same schedule is followed for monitoring the biochemical effectiveness of PN, as discussed earlier for the hospitalized client.

Refeeding Syndrome

Refeeding syndrome is a complication that can occur during the initial phase of EN or PN therapy, oral intake, or dextrose-containing IV fluids. It occurs in severely malnourished clients who experience significant fluid and electrolyte imbalances after aggressive nutritional support is initiated. Malnourished clients adapt to nutritional deprivation and compensate by decreasing basal energy requirements. The initiation of replacement therapy, especially if the PN is undertaken too aggressively, can result in an electrolyte shift from plasma to the intracellular fluid.

Electrolyte disturbances, mainly decreased levels of phosphorus, magnesium, or potassium, occur immediately after the rapid initiation of refeeding, usually within 12 to 72 hours, and can continue for the next 2 to 7 days. Cardiac complications can develop within the first week, often within the first 12 to 48 hours, with neurologic signs and symptoms developing more slowly (Yantis & Velander, 2008). The clinical manifestations include edema, hypernatremia, hypokalemia, hypomagnesemia, and hypophosphatemia. Nursing measures are directed at prevention by initiating EN and PN therapy slowly and monitoring the client's electrolytes to prevent cardiac complications.

ADMINISTERING MEDICATION THROUGH A FEEDING TUBE

Refer to agency protocol regarding medication administration and contraindications. Feeding tubes with a double lumen have two separate ports; read the manufacturer's instructions to determine which port to use to administer the medication. Administering medications through the wrong port may cause the tube to clog.

Check for tube placement, clear the tubing of formula, and check the patency of the tube by flushing it with warm water before administering the medication. It is advisable to use the liquid form of any medications whenever possible. After administering each medication, flush the port to prevent clogging. Measure the aspirates removed, all liquids instilled into the tube, and the water used for flushing and medications, and record on the client's I&O record. Refer to Chapter 30 for additional information on administering medication through a feeding tube.

COMPLEMENTARY AND ALTERNATIVE THERAPY

Holistic nursing recognizes wellness as a state of harmony among mind, body, and spirit. To nourish means to provide that which is necessary for life, health, and growth; to nourish also means to cherish, to strengthen, and to promote. Nourishment encourages expansion and growth, supporting each being as unique, whole, and individual. The following discussion provides a broad perspective regarding the use of nutrients in complementary therapies and how herbal medicine incorporates certain plants for their specific properties in order to treat digestive symptoms and diseases.

Although there are numerous types of complementary therapies, they all integrate, to some degree, nutrition as part of their therapeutic regimen. Diet and nutrition are used by many alternative modalities for the prevention and treatment of chronic diseases:

1. *Ayurvedic medicine,* India's ancient system of healing, treats the whole person with diet, nutrition, and lifestyle recommendations to promote health and spiritual development. For example, diabetes is a complex condition with a multitude of metabolic imbalances involving the regulation of insulin and glucose in the body. Clients with type 2 diabetes mellitus die of cardiovascular disease at rates two to four times higher than nondiabetic populations of similar demographic characteristics; they also experience increased rates of nonfatal myocardial infarction and stroke (ACCORD, 2008). With the growing prevalence of obesity in the United States, diabetes is currently considered an epidemic disease that is largely preventable and treatable through yoga. Yoga's effectiveness at preventing and treating diabetes is due to its emphasis on a healthy diet and lifestyle as well as its ability to balance the endocrine system, massage and tone the abdominal organs, stimulate the nervous and circulatory systems, and reduce stress (Upadhyay, Balkrishna, & Upadhyay, 2008).
2. *Traditional Chinese medicine,* one of the oldest systems of healing, incorporates acupuncture, Chinese herbs, massage, food therapy, exercise, and lifestyle changes into prevention and treatment.
3. *Chiropractic medicine,* an American heritage, relies on a sound nutritional program as adjunct therapy to support the body's inherent ability to heal itself by reestablishing an unobstructed flow of nerve impulses between the brain and the rest of the body.
4. *Naturopathic medicine,* an ancient form of healing that was formalized in America into a system of preventive and restorative treatments around the early 1900s, uses

✓ NURSINGCHECKLIST

Interventions for Client Receiving TPN

1. Monitor weight: baseline and daily weight for 1 week and twice a week thereafter. The ideal weight gain for a client is 1 pound per week. Rapid weight gain may be indicative of fluid overload; monitor such a client for peripheral and pulmonary edema.
2. Monitor I&O: Record daily I&O and compare these data with the client's weight. Closely monitor the infusion rate with an infusion pump (preferably a volumetric pump for the greatest accuracy).
3. Monitor biochemical lab values:
   • Electrolytes, especially magnesium and calcium, if these have been added to the PN solution, on Day 1 and once a week thereafter while on PN. With severely malnourished clients, observe for "refeeding syndrome" (a rapid drop in potassium, magnesium, and phosphate serum levels). Initiate feeding slowly to avoid cardiac overload.
   • Prealbumin serum levels: Check on Day 1 and once a week while on PN. In clients who are severely dehydrated, the albumin levels may drop initially as treatment restores hydration.
   • Glucose (capillary): Check every 6 hours for the first week, then once daily while on PN. Monitor for signs of hyperglycemia (thirst and oliguria), and confirm weekly blood glucose meter levels with laboratory tests.
   • Bleeding indices (prothrombin time [PT]) on Day 1 and once a week while on PN; indicated for clients receiving heparin therapy.
   • Liver function tests, especially enzymes, bilirubin, triglycerides, and cholesterol on Day 1 and once a week for clients on PN with lipids; abnormal values may indicate an intolerance to or an excess in lipid emulsions or problems with the metabolism with glucose and protein.
   • Renal function tests, especially blood urea nitrogen, creatinine, and 24-hour urinary urea nitrogen, on Days 2–5; abnormal values indicate an excess of amino acids.
   • Transferrin should be measured on Day 1 and every 2 weeks thereafter.
4. Administer solution with an IV tubing filter to remove crystals from the solution, vent air, and trap microorganisms.
5. Change IV tubing, using aseptic technique, as indicated by the agency's protocol; most infection control guidelines recommend changing the tubing every 24 hours.
6. Use a volumetric pump to ensure accurate infusion rates.
7. Monitor for common complications of PN therapy:
   • Phlebitis or thrombosis at the IV site, as indicated by tenderness and redness
   • Catheter tip sepsis, as indicated by fever and other signs and symptoms of sepsis
   • Liver, renal, and metabolic complications (as discussed in monitoring the biochemical laboratory values)
8. Wean the client from PN, documenting the dietary intake of total calories and protein.
9. Teach the client and the caregiver about the management of PN therapy, and arrange for a home health care consult; if possible, have the home health nurse consult with the client while the client is still in the hospital to promote continuity of care.

---

clinical nutrition as a main cornerstone of therapy to achieve and maintain health.

5. *Osteopathic medicine,* founded by Dr. Andrew Taylor Still, a medical surgeon for the Union Army during the Civil War, integrates into conventional medicine nutritional recommendations for prevention. For example, to prevent coronary heart disease, a diet low in saturated fats is combined with antioxidants (vitamins C, A, and E) to help prevent free radical formation, thus preventing tissue breakdown as well as the accumulation of plaque in the arteries.

6. *Herbal medicine* recognizes food as medicine, ensuring that the unique healing properties of specific herbs have a direct effect upon tissue. The healing effect is through direct contact with the tissue and the effects

caused by the metabolism and absorption of the chemicals present in the various plants. Based on a holistic context, herbal medicine recognizes that true healing must involve all dimensions of the person to change whatever dietary indiscretions exist as well as to make other adjustments in the person's lifestyle.

Many herbal products are available in various forms such as teas, extracts, capsules, and tablets to provide nutrients that nourish our bodies and relieve digestive symptoms. The following discussion addresses the digestive and nondigestive actions of certain herbs: bitters, chamomile, dandelion, peppermint, rosemary, and slippery elm.

Bitters is a term used to describe a group of herbs that have a bitter taste. The taste of bitterness on the tongue sends a message to the brain through the nervous system to

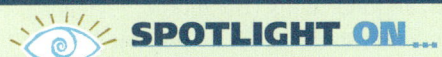

SPOTLIGHT ON...

Legal and Ethical

Withholding Nutritional Support

The obligation to promote the good of the client is basic to being a health care provider and is part of each professional's duty to the client. This obligation underlies the requirement to evaluate the benefits and burdens of a treatment from the client's perspective.

When and by whom should a decision be made to withhold or withdraw nutritional support in the absence of an advance directive? Consider the benefits to the client and the burden that nutritional support places on the client, family, and caregiver.

UNCOVERING THE

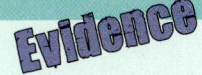

TITLE OF STUDY

"Percutaneous Endoscopic Gastrostomy Feeding in Nursing Homes"

AUTHORS

A. M. Brotherton and B. Carter

PURPOSE

To explore the experiences of relatives of nursing home residents receiving percutaneous endoscopic gastrostomy (PEG) feeding.

METHOD

Qualitative methodology using semistructured interviews explores the experiences and perceptions of eight relatives.

FINDINGS

The relatives expressed four themes: dependence and resulting disempowerment, having minimal or no involvement in the decision-making process for PEG placement, betrayal, and the losses associated with the social aspects of eating.

IMPLICATIONS

There is a need for professional education about the psychosocial implications of feeding and an increased level of support for relatives to assist them to develop coping strategies.

Brotherton, A., & Carter, B. (2007). Percutaneous endoscopic gastrostomy feeding in nursing homes. *Clinical Nursing Research, 16*(4), 350–369.

stimulate the secretion and activity of the esophagus, and the secretions of the stomach, duodenum, and gallbladder, and to stimulate the production of insulin by the pancreas. The bitterness promotes appetite and in a complex way aids digestion. Bitter herbs are considered digestive stimulants because they stimulate various parts of the digestive system to increase or improve digestive activity. The most valuable bitter herbs are barberry, centaury, gentian root, goldenseal, mugwort, white horehound, and wormwood.

Chamomile contains calcium, essential oils, iron, magnesium, manganese, potassium, tannic acid, vitamin A, apigenin (a sedative compound), and other nutritive ingredients. It possesses the following actions: antiinflammatory, appetite stimulant, digestive aid, diuretic, nerve tonic, and sleep aid. Traditionally, chamomile is used for stress and anxiety, indigestion, and insomnia, and it is often used to treat colitis, diverticulosis, fever, headaches, and pain. It is effective as a gargle or mouthwash for treating gingivitis. *Caution:* This herb should not be taken over long periods of time, as it may cause an allergy to ragweed; it should not be used by persons who are allergic to ragweed (Balch, 2006).

Dandelion leaves and roots are high in iron, manganese, phosphorus, protein, aluminum, and vitamin A, with trace amounts of calcium, chromium, niacin, riboflavin, silicon, zinc, and vitamin C. It is a potent digestive tonic that may be used in conditions that affect the GI tract, such as heartburn, gas, gastroesophageal reflux, and constipation. Dandelion has a toning effect on the liver, gallbladder, and pancreas, providing relief from gallstones or gallbladder attacks as well as diabetes and hypoglycemia. Dandelion is considered safe and may be taken as often as needed. *Caution:* Due to its laxative effects, large sudden intake may result in diarrhea; start with smaller doses, and gradually increase over time.

Peppermint contains essential oils, tannic acid, vitamin C, and other ingredients. It is one of the best carminative agents (stimulates and soothes the digestive system, removes gas), and it enhances digestion by increasing stomach acidity. It is

NURSING PROCESS HIGHLIGHT

Implementation

Collaborative Measures to Support Behavioral Change

Planning interventions to assist clients with their nutritional problems requires consideration of the specific contributing factors, food preferences and beliefs, and chronic conditions related to the problem. Changing eating patterns requires client motivation and desire to change. No one can make another person change his or her behavior, but nurses can assist their clients with the "why" and "how" regarding change. Reinforce all positive changes.

often recommended for chills, colic, diarrhea, headache, heart trouble, indigestion, nausea, poor appetite, rheumatism, and spasms. *Caution:* This herb may interfere with iron absorption.

Rosemary is often used as a natural food preservative because of its chemical and nutritive content. It is considered a circulatory and digestive bitter; it fights bacteria, relaxes the stomach, and acts as a decongestant; it also helps prevent liver toxicity, and it has anticancer and antitumor properties. It relieves intestinal colic, flatulent dyspepsia, headaches, high and low blood pressure, circulatory problems, and menstrual cramps, and it is used to treat ulcerative colitis, Crohn's disease, and fevers, especially colds and influenza (Balch, 2006).

Slippery elm bark contains calcium, phosphorus, polysaccharides, starch, tannins, and vitamin K. It soothes inflamed mucous membranes of the stomach, bowels, and urinary tract. It may be used to treat gastritis, gastric or duodenal ulcer, enteritis, colitis, diarrhea, and colds, flu, and sore throat.

Garlic (*Allium sativum*), the second most utilized supplement, has shown antiviral, antibacterial, antifungal, and antioxidant abilities. Garlic's medicinal actions may help or prevent certain diseases such as Alzheimer's disease, cancer, cardiovascular disease, children's conditions, dermatologic applications, stress, and infections (Bongiorno, Fratellone, & LoGiudice, 2008). Some studies indicate possible benefits in diabetes, drug toxicity, and osteoporosis.

EVALUATION

Evaluation of nutritional therapy is ongoing. The nurse uses current data to measure the achievement of goals and outcomes; once they are achieved, the plan of care is revised accordingly. If goals are not met, the nurse should determine whether the nursing diagnosis was accurate or whether the nursing interventions were appropriate and the outcomes achievable.

The plan of care should be modified to maximize the client's response to therapy. For example, if the home health client states compliance with diet therapy to maintain the HDL, LDL, and cholesterol levels within normal limits, but the values are not within normal limits, then institute a food record to monitor cholesterol and fat intake for 3 consecutive days. Visit the client on the fourth day and review the record. Provide teaching as necessary to assist the client in changing eating patterns.

NURSING CARE PLAN

Client with Imbalanced Nutrition: More Than Body Requirements

CASE PRESENTATION
Mrs. Jones, age 55, was diagnosed 2 years ago with type 2 (non–insulin-dependent) diabetes. She is being seen in the clinic for her 6-month visit. She says, "I hardly have the energy to get up and dress in the morning. I am thirsty all day and awaken several times during the night, having to go to the bathroom." She does not work and hasn't been involved in community activities for the past 5 years since her youngest child graduated from high school. Her daily routine involves cooking for her husband and brother, reading, and watching TV for 6–8 hours. She loves to bake fresh breads and pastry. She has a history of obesity and does not exercise. She says, "I eat because I have nothing else to do."

ASSESSMENT
- Weight, 80.6 kg
- Height, 5'4"
- Triceps skinfold, 28 mm
- Elevated blood glucose
- Weight gain, 3.6 kg
- Sedentary lifestyle
- Eats in response to boredom

NURSING DIAGNOSIS: *Imbalanced nutrition: more than body requirements* related to excess intake of high-calorie foods, eating in response to boredom, and sedentary lifestyle
NOC: Motivation, weight control
NIC: Weight management

(Continues)

NURSING CARE PLAN (Continued)

EXPECTED OUTCOMES

The client will

1. Verbalize factors contributing to excess weight.
2. Lose 1–2 lb/week while eating well-balanced meals.
3. Engage in 20–30 minutes of exercise 3 times a week.
4. Explore outside interests to decrease boredom and increase feelings of self-worth.

INTERVENTIONS/RATIONALES

1. Conduct a dietary history, using open-ended statements to assist client in exploring psychological factors that may contribute to eating. Nonjudgmental approach to acquiring information will encourage client trust and honesty.
2. Adapt eating habits to decrease amount of intake (having smaller servings, taking small bites and chewing each bite 12 times, putting the fork on the plate between bites, drinking water with meals, eating only at mealtime, chewing sugar-free gum when watching TV). Healthy eating habits and tips on recognizing fullness during a meal will help the client eat to satisfy hunger, not boredom.
3. Assess client's motivation to lose weight. Having client's support for care plan will influence success.
4. Discuss risk factors and symptoms (thirst and urination) of diabetes. Client's understanding of her disease may increase motivation to manage it.
5. Instruct client to maintain a daily dietary intake log: time, type, and amount. Helps client recognize her eating patterns and note healthy and unhealthy behaviors.
6. Provide client with dietary materials: Review the food pyramid and diabetic exchange list; plan with client an 1800-kilocalorie diet for a week, taking into consideration food preferences. Ensures client has information necessary to plan healthy meals within recommended guidelines.
7. Return visit with nurse in 1 week. Monitor progress and assess plan of care. Review with client age-appropriate exercises; emphasize need for daily walking. Changing sedentary lifestyle will increase self-esteem, burn calories, and increase energy level.
8. Review with client community and church interests outside the home, unrelated to cooking and eating. Helps client focus on activities not involving food to decrease boredom and to increase self-esteem.

EVALUATION

1. The client verbalized boredom as the main reason for eating; she said, "I have nothing else to do with the children gone, except cook and eat."
2. On return visit, the client reported drinking water with meals, chewing her food slowly, and chewing gum while watching TV.
3. Make clinic appointment; client has phone number of the nurse and dietitian to answer questions; 1800-kilocalorie meal plan made for 1 week.
4. On return visit, the client was found to have lost 1.8 lb.
5. On return visit, the client indicated that she now walks to the store 4–5 times a week (40 minutes round trip).
6. The client reported on return visit that she is now volunteering 2 hours three times a week at the church's child care center.

(Continues)

CONCEPT MAP

THE CLIENT WITH IMBALANCED NUTRITION: MORE THAN BODY REQUIREMENTS

Mrs. Jones, age 55, was diagnosed 2 years ago with type II (non-insulin-dependent) diabetes. She is being seen in the clinic for her 6-month visit.

Family dynamics includes

Her daily routine involves cooking for her husband and brother, reading, and watching the TV for 6–8 hours.

Obesity and does not exercise

Assessment findings

Weight: 80.6 kg
Height: 5'4"
Triceps skinfold: 28 mm
Elevated blood glucose
Weight gain: 3.6 kg
Sedentary lifestyle
Eats in response to boredom

Assessment data indicate

Social background includes

She does not work and hasn't been involved in community activities for the past 5 years since her youngest child graduated from high school. She loves to bake fresh breads and pastry.

Holistic and support system assessment findings include

She is a religious and spiritual woman and considered by all to be the "heart" of her family. She has always been generous, and her friends are many.

Analysis of assessment data lead to the priority

①

Nursing Diagnosis 1:
Imbalanced Nutrition More Than Body Requirements related to excess intake of high-calorie foods, eating in response to boredom, and sedentary lifestyle.

Assessment data lead to these conclusions

1. **Discuss risk factors and symptoms (thirst and urination) of diabetes.**

Client understanding of her disease may increase motivation to manage it.

2. **Instruct client to maintain a daily dietary intake log: time, type, and amount.**

Helps client recognize her eating patterns and note healthy and unhealthy behaviors.

3. **Provide with dietary materials, review the Food Pyramid and Diabetic Exchange List; plan with client an 1800 kcal diet for a week, taking into consideration food preferences.**

Ensures client has information necessary to plan healthy meals within recommended guidelines.

4. **Return visit with nurse in one week. Monitor progress and assess plan of care. Review with client age-appropriate exercises; emphasize need for daily walking.**

Changing sedentary lifestyle will increase self-esteem, burn calories, and increase energy level.

Expected Outcomes

Nursing Interventions and *Rationales*

The client will:
Verbalize factors contributing to excess weight
Lose 1–2 lbs/week while eating well-balanced meals
Engage in 20–30 minutes of exercise 3 times a week
Explore outside interests to decrease boredom and increase feeling of self worth

1. **Conduct a dietary history, using open-ended statements to assist client in exploring psychological actors that may contribute to eating.**

Nonjudgmental approach to acquiring information will encourage client trust and honesty.

2. **Adapt eating habits to decrease amount of intake (smaller servings, taking small bites and chewing each bite 12 times, putting the fork on the plate between bites, drinking water with meals, eating only at mealtime, chewing sugar-free gum when watching TV).**

Healthy eating habits and tips on recognizing fullness during a meal will help the client eat to satisfy hunger, not boredom.

3. **Assess client's motivation to lose weight.**

Having client's support for care plan will influence success.

Successful implementation of nursing care is indicated by...

Successful implementation of nursing care is indicated by...

The Client verbalized boredom as the main reason for eating: she said, "I have nothing else to do with the children gone, except cook and eat."

On return visit, the client reported drinking water with meals, chewing her food slowly, and chewing gum while watching TV.

Make clinic appointment; client has phone number of the nurse and dietician to answer questions; 1800 kcal meal plan made for one week.

On return visit, the client was found to have lost 1.8 lbs.

On return visit, the client indicated that she now walks to the store 4–5 times a week (40 minutes round trip).

The client reported on return visit that she is now volunteering 2 hours 3 times a week at the church's child care center.

Key:

☐ Case Scenario

☐ Assessment Data

☐ Nursing Diagnosis *Prioritized as 1, 2, etc.*

⬭ Expected Outcome

☐ Interventions and *Rationales*

☐ Evaluation

Client with Imbalanced Nutrition: Less Than Body Requirements

CASE PRESENTATION
Jim, age 28, has been HIV-positive for 4.5 years. He arrives at the clinic complaining of diarrhea and cramping for 3 weeks and a burn wound on his right forearm that will not heal. He states, "I do not have the energy to eat or get dressed." The past month, he has eaten mainly bread, cereal, milk, and potatoes.

ASSESSMENT
- Weight loss
- Dry, scaly skin
- Pale conjunctiva
- Decreased hgb, HCT, MCV
- Triceps skinfold, 7.2 mm
- Gingivitis
- Decreased Na, K, Fe, zinc
- Decreased serum albumin, prealbumin, transferrin, nitrogen balance, zinc, and total lymphocyte count (TLC); urine creatinine excretion

NURSING DIAGNOSIS: *Imbalanced nutrition: less than body requirements* related to inability to absorb nutrients because of HIV enteropathy

NOC: Nutrient intake.

NIC: Nutrition management.

EXPECTED OUTCOMES
The client will

1. Receive adequate nutrients to meet metabolic needs.
2. Stabilize weight within 24–48 hours after initiation of TPN.
3. Gain 0.25–0.5 kg/wk.
4. Select a diet high in calcium, iron, protein, and calories.

INTERVENTIONS/RATIONALES
1. Weigh in daily; record hourly I&O; monitor qh BP, P, R rate, breath sounds, edema.
   Monitors overall health status for changes, balance of fluid intake and output, and signs of deterioration.
2. NPO until diarrhea subsides; record frequency and consistency of stools (weight and measure).
   As prescribed; monitors progression of diarrhea.
3. Administer TPN as ordered; implement TPN protocol. Maintains caloric intake needs safely.
4. Monitor daily laboratory data: glucose, vitamins, minerals, trace elements, electrolytes; monitor prealbumin and BUN every other day. Assesses nutritional effect of TPN.
5. Mouth care every 2–4 hours to keep mucous membranes moist. Provides for client comfort.
6. Collaborate with the nutritional support team for a progressive diet postdiarrhea, taking into consideration client's food preferences. Outlines appropriate diet; client is most likely to eat foods he prefers.
7. Offer small, frequent feedings. Facilitates digestion and maintains constant energy levels.
8. Provide oral hygiene before and after meals. Enhances taste sensation.
9. Assist the client with meals as needed. Provide rest periods 1 hour before and after meals. Surrounds eating with quiet time to focus; improves digestion.
10. Gradually wean the client off TPN as ordered. Begin return to oral nutrition intake.
11. Monitor daily calorie count for 3 days and stool counts daily. Gives indication of amount eaten versus amount excreted; monitors diarrhea.
12. Allow client to select food high in protein and calories. Involvement in diet planning increases compliance.
13. Administer drugs between meals. Helps avoid nausea at mealtime.
14. Provide positive reinforcement for increased food intake and weight gain. Helps client acknowledge progress; shows support for plan of care.
15. Assess the client's knowledge of the RDAs. Current knowledge levels will determine learning needs.
16. Instruct the client on dietary planning based on the Food Guide Pyramid, as directed by the nutritional support team. Client involvement in dietary planning increases likelihood of success.

(Continues)

NURSING CARE PLAN (Continued)

EVALUATION

1. Fluid intake and output balanced; diarrhea subsided in 24 hours; afebrile.
2. Laboratory values within normal limits 48 hours postadmission.
3. Weight stabilized in 48 hours, with the client tolerating clear liquids.
4. The client is unable to independently select foods to increase body weight; no nausea reported for routine scheduled medications.
5. The client was able to select food items as prescribed by the nutritional support team and gained 0.45 kg in 8 days.

CONCEPT MAP

THE CLIENT WITH IMBALANCED NUTRITION: LESS THAN BODY REQUIREMENTS

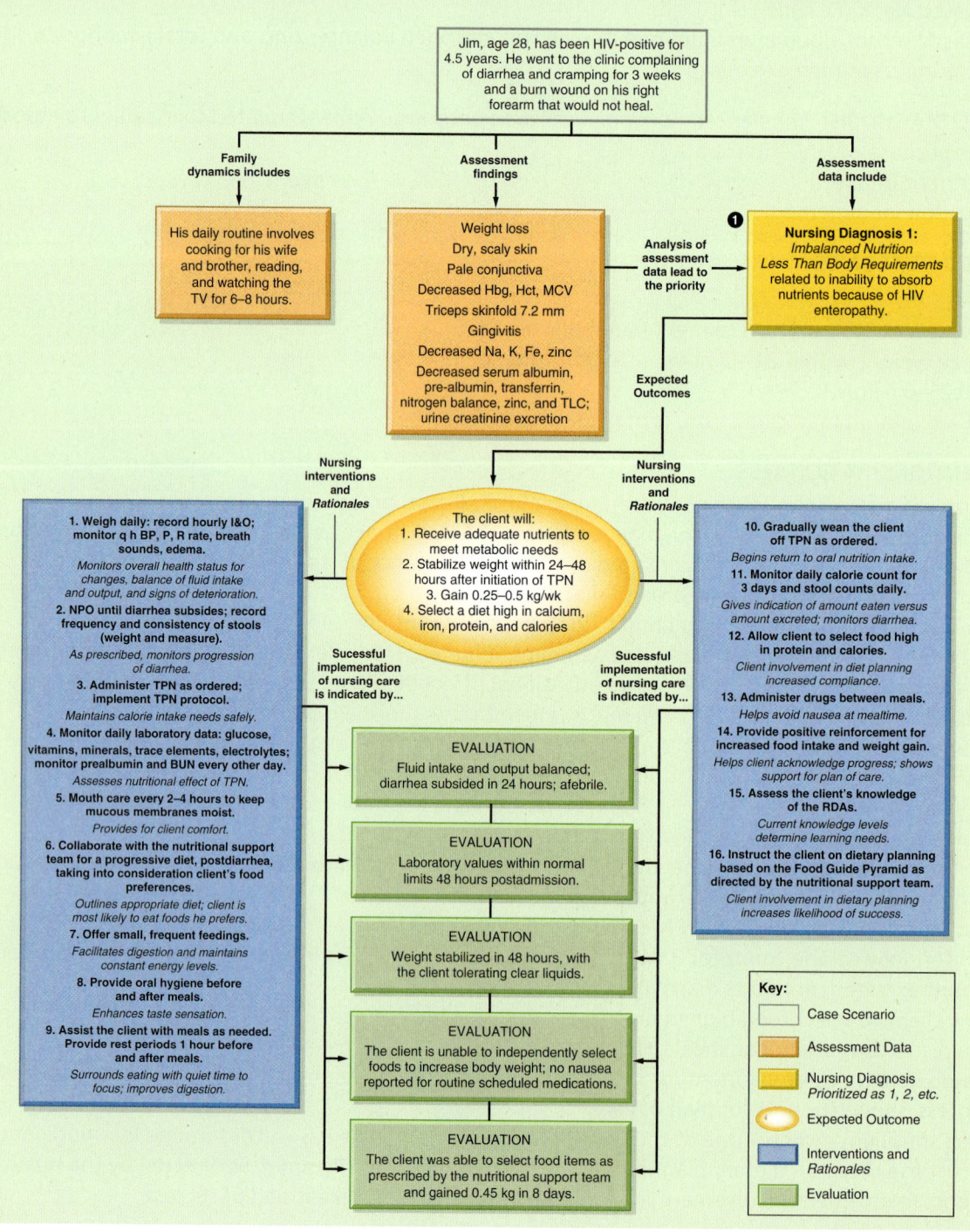

PROCEDURE
34-1

**PROCEDURE
34-1**

Inserting a Nasogastric or Nasointestinal Tube for Suction and Enteral Feedings

EQUIPMENT

- Nonsterile gloves
- Cup of ice or water and straw
- Towel and tissues
- Flashlight or penlight
- Hypoallergenic tape, rubber band, safety pin
- 20-mL syringe or Asepto syringe, 30 mL or larger with small-bore tube
- Disposable irrigation set (optional)
- Wall mount or portable suction equipment as available

- Ice chips in an emesis basin
- Water-soluble lubricant
- Tongue blade
- pH chemstrip
- Number 6, 8, or 12 French tube for gastric suction (Levine, Salem sump, or Anderson) or a small-bore feeding tube, 8 or 12 French tube (Keofeed, Dobbhoff, Moss)
- Administration set with pump or controller for feeding tube

ACTION	RATIONALE
1. Review client's medical record.	1. Confirms prescribing practitioner's prescription for inserting a nasogastric tube; history of nasal or sinus problems.
2. Gather equipment. Wash hands/hand hygiene.	2. Promotes efficiency. Prevents the spread of microorganisms.
3. Check client's armband; explain procedure, showing items.	3. Verifies correct client; reduces anxiety and increases client cooperation.
4. Place client in Fowler's position, at least a 45° angle or higher, with a pillow behind client's shoulders; provide for privacy. *Place comatose clients in semi-Fowler's position.*	4. Facilitates passage of the tube into the esophagus and swallowing.
5. Place towel over chest, with tissues in reach. Don gloves.	5. Prevents soiling of gown and bedding and protects nurse from contamination with bodily fluids; lacrimation can occur during insertion through nasal passages.
6. Examine nostrils and assess as client breathes through each nostril.	6. Determines the most patent nostril to facilitate insertion.

7. Measure length of tubing needed by using tube as a tape measure:
  • Measure from bridge of client's nose to earlobe to xiphoid process of sternum (see Figure 34-16A on page 1032).
  • If tube is to go below stomach (nasoduodenal or nasojejunal), add an additional 15 to 20 cm (see Figure 34-16B).
  • Place a small piece of tape on tube to mark length.
	7. Approximates length of tube needed to reach stomach.

(Continues)

PROCEDURE 34-1
Inserting a Nasogastric or Nasointestinal Tube for Suction and Enteral Feedings (Continued)

ACTION	RATIONALE

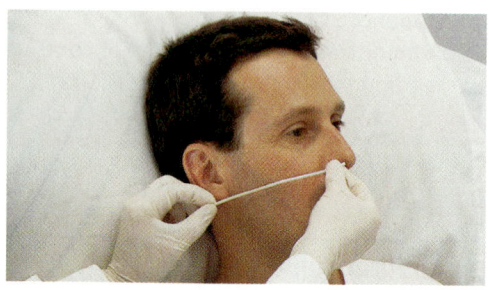

A

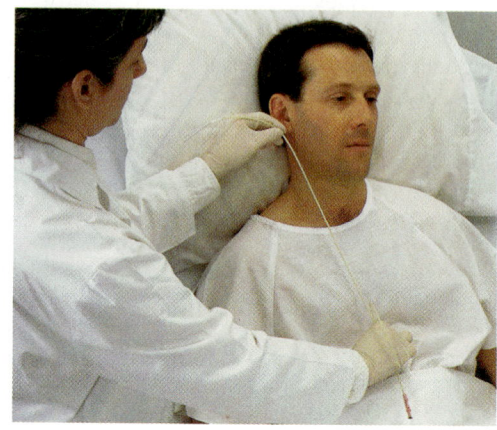

B

FIGURE 34-16 A. Measuring the Length of Nasogastric Tubing; B. Measuring the Length of Nasoduodenal or Nasojejunal Tubing DELMAR/CENGAGE LEARNING

ACTION	RATIONALE
8. Have client blow nose, and encourage swallowing of water if level of consciousness and treatment plan permit.	8. Clears nasal passage without pushing microorganisms into inner ear; facilitates passage of tube.
9. Lubricate first 4 inches of tube with water-soluble lubricant.	9. Facilitates passage into the nares.
10. Insert tube as follows: • Gently pass tube into nostril to back of throat (client may gag); aim tube toward back of throat and down. • When client feels tube in back of throat, use flashlight or penlight to locate tip of tube. • Instruct client to flex head toward chest. • Instruct client to swallow, offer ice chips or water, and advance tube as client swallows. • If resistance is met, rotate tube slowly with downward advancement toward client's closest ear; do not force tube.	10. Promotes passage of tube with minimal trauma to mucosa. • Ensures tip's placement. • Opens esophagus and assists in tube insertion after tube has passed through nasopharynx and reduces risk of tube entering trachea. • Assists in pushing tube past oropharynx. • Tube may be coiled or kinked or in the oropharynx or trachea.
11. Withdraw tube immediately if changes occur in respiratory status.	11. Indicates placement of tube in the bronchus or lung.
12. Advance tube, giving client sips of water, until taped mark is reached.	12. Assists with tube insertion.

(Continues)

PROCEDURE 34-1
Inserting a Nasogastric or Nasointestinal Tube for Suction and Enteral Feedings (Continued)

ACTION	RATIONALE
13. Check placement of tube: • Attach syringe to free end of tube, and aspirate sample of gastric contents. Measure with chemstrip pH (see Figure 34-17). • Leave syringe attached to free end of tube. • If prescribed, obtain x-ray; keep client on right side until x-ray is taken.	13. Ensures proper placement in the stomach; pH below 4, tube is in stomach; pH range of 6 to 7 indicates intestinal sites or pleural fluid from the tracheobronchial tree. • Prevents leakage of gastric contents. • Confirms correct placement; if nasoduodenal or nasojejunal feedings are required, passage through pylorus may require several days.
14. Secure tube with tape (see Figure 34-18), or use a commercially prepared tube holder. • Split a 4-inch piece of tape to a length of 2 inches, and secure tube with tape by placing the intact end of the tape over the bridge of the nose. Wrap split ends around the tube as it exits the nose. • Place a rubber band, using a slip knot, around the exposed tube (12–18 inches from nose toward chest); after x-ray, pin rubber band to client's gown.	14. Prevents tube from becoming dislodged. • Prevents trauma to nasal mucosa by reducing pressure on nares. • Allows client movement without causing friction on nares; metal devices are removed for x-rays to prevent artifacts.
15. Instruct client about movements that can dislodge the tube.	15. Reduces anxiety and teaches client how to prevent tugging on tube with head movement.

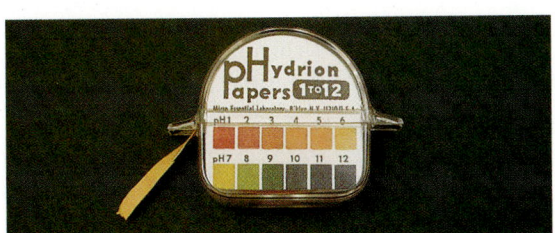

FIGURE 34-17 For Measuring the pH of Aspirate DELMAR/CENGAGE LEARNING

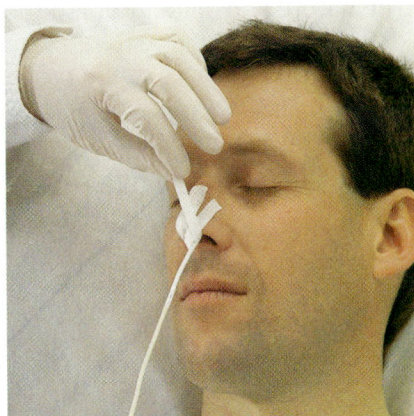

FIGURE 34-18 Securing Tube to the Client's Nose with Tape DELMAR/CENGAGE LEARNING

(Continues)

PROCEDURE 34-1
Inserting a Nasogastric or Nasointestinal Tube for Suction and Enteral Feedings (Continued)

ACTION	RATIONALE
16. Gastric decompression: • Remove syringe from free end of tube, and connect tube to suction tubing; set machine on type of suction and pressure as prescribed. • Levine tubes are connected to intermittent low pressure. • Salem sump or Anderson tube is connected to continuous low suction. • Observe nature and amount of gastric tube drainage. • Assess client for nausea, vomiting, and abdominal distention.	16. Provides for decompression as prescribed by prescribing practitioner; intermittent or continuous suctioning is determined by type of tube inserted. • Provides information about patency of tube and gastric contents. • Indicates effectiveness of intervention.
17. Provide oral hygiene and cleanse nares with a tissue.	17. Promotes comfort.
18. Remove gloves, dispose of contaminated materials in proper container, and wash hands/hand hygiene.	18. Prevents the spread of microorganisms; protects other workers from coming into contact with objects contaminated with body fluids.
19. Position client for comfort, and place call light within easy reach.	19. Promotes comfort and safety.
20. Document: • The reason for the tube insertion • The type of tube inserted • The type (intermittent or continuous) of suctioning and pressure setting • The nature and amount of aspirate and drainage • The client's tolerance of the procedure • The effectiveness of the intervention, such as nausea relieved	20. Promotes continuity of care and shows implementation of intervention.

INSERTION OF A SMALL-BORE FEEDING TUBE

ACTION	RATIONALE
21. Repeat Actions 1 through 8, as stated earlier.	21. See Rationales 1 through 8.
22. Open adapter cap on tube, snap off end of water vial, and inject water into feeding tube adapter.	22. Activates Keolube lubricant in tube's lumen.
23. Close adapter cap.	23. Ensures a tight fit so water does not leak from adapter site.
24. Check that stylet does not protrude through holes in feeding tube; adjust as necessary.	24. Prevents mucosa trauma.
25. Repeat Actions 9 through 12, as stated earlier.	25. See Rationales 9 through 12.
26. Check placement of tube: • Aspirate gastric contents with Luer-Lok syringe (see Figure 34-19 on page 1035). • Measure pH of aspirate with chemstrip pH.	26. Ensures that correct placement has been achieved; provides measurement of pH of secretions, as explained in Rationale 13. *Note:* May not be able to aspirate contents from small-bore tubes.

(Continues)

PROCEDURE 34-1
Inserting a Nasogastric or Nasointestinal Tube for Suction and Enteral Feedings (Continued)

ACTION	RATIONALE

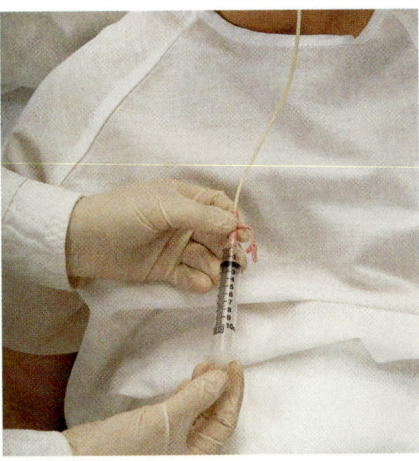

FIGURE 34-19 Aspirating Gastric Contents with Luer-Lok Syringe with Stylet in Place DELMAR/CENGAGE LEARNING

27. Leave stylet in place until x-ray confirms that placement in case tube needs to be advanced into the duodenum or jejunum.	27. Provides a safety measure. See the Safety First display, on page 1019, on small-bore feeding tubes in this chapter (in the Enteral Tube Feeding section).
28. Obtain x-ray. Remove stylet from feeding tube after x-ray, and plug open end of tube until feeding.	28. Confirms placement of tube prior to instilling formula; prevents gastric juices from seeping out of the tube.
29. Repeat Actions 17 through 20.	29. See Rationales 17 through 20.
30. Replace small-bore tube every 3 to 4 weeks.	30. Prevents obstruction and sepsis of small-bore tubes.
31. Wash hands/hand hygiene.	31. Prevents the spread of microorganisms.

delegation tip

Inserting and maintaining a nasogastric tube is the responsibility of the nurse. Oral hygiene for the client may be delegated.

nursing tips

Prepare the split tape before putting on gloves.

Administering Enteral Tube Feedings

EQUIPMENT

- Asepto syringe or 20- to 50-mL syringe
- Emesis basin
- Clean towel
- Disposable gavage bag and tubing
- Formula
- Infusion pump for feeding tube
- Water to follow feeding
- Nonsterile gloves

ACTION	RATIONALE
1. Identify client and review medical record for formula, amount, and time.	1. Verifies health care provider's prescription for appropriate formula and amount.
2. Wash hands/hand hygiene.	2. Prevents the spread of microorganisms.
3. Check client's armband.	3. Verifies correct client.
4. Explain procedure to client.	4. Reduces anxiety and increases client cooperation.
5. Assemble equipment. Add color to formula per institutional policy. If using a bag, fill with prescribed amount of formula.	5. Ensures efficiency when initiating feeding. Color will distinguish formula aspirate.
6. Place client on right side in high Fowler's position.	6. Reduces risk of pulmonary aspiration in the event that the client vomits or regurgitates formula.
7. Wash hands/hand hygiene, and don nonsterile gloves.	7. Reduces transmission of pathogens from gastric contents.
8. Provide privacy.	8. Puts the client at ease.
9. Observe for abdominal distention; auscultate for bowel sounds.	9. Assesses for delayed gastric emptying; indicates presence of peristalsis and ability of GI tract to digest nutrients.
10. Check feeding tube (see Figure 34-20 on page 1037). Insert syringe into adapter port, aspirate stomach contents, and determine amount of gastric residue. If residue is greater than 50 to 100 mL (or in accordance with agency protocol), hold feeding until residue diminishes. Instill aspirated contents back into feeding tube.	10. Indicates whether gastric emptying is delayed. Reduces risk of regurgitation and pulmonary aspiration related to gastric distention. Prevents electrolyte imbalance.
11. Administer tube feeding.	11. Provides nutrients as prescribed.

INTERMITTENT BOLUS

ACTION	RATIONALE
12. Pinch the tubing.	12. Prevents air from entering tubing.
13. Remove plunger from barrel of syringe and attach to adapter.	13. Provides system to deliver feeding.
14. Fill syringe with formula (see Figure 34-21 on page 1037).	14. Allows gravity to control flow rate, reducing risk of diarrhea from bolus feeding.
15. Allow formula to infuse slowly; continue adding formula to syringe until prescribed amount has been administered.	15. Prevents air from entering stomach. Decreases risk of diarrhea.

(Continues)

PROCEDURE 34-2
Administering Enteral Tube Feedings (Continued)

ACTION	RATIONALE

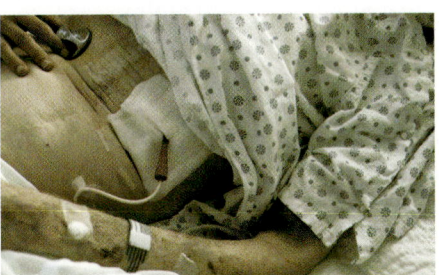

FIGURE 34-20 Check that the feeding tube is intact and in place, auscultate for bowel sounds, and look for abdominal distention DELMAR/CENGAGE LEARNING

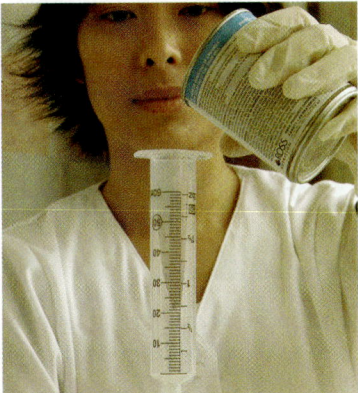

FIGURE 34-21 Administer the prescribed amount of formula DELMAR/CENGAGE LEARNING

16. Flush tubing with 30 to 60 mL or prescribed amount of water.

16. Ensures that remaining formula in tubing is administered and maintains patency of tube; prevents air from entering the stomach.

INTERMITTENT GAVAGE FEEDING

17. Hang bag on IV pole so that it is 18 inches above the client's head (see Figure 34-22).

18. Remove air from bag's tubing.

17. Allows gravity to promote infusion of formula.

18. Prevents air from entering stomach. Decreases risk of diarrhea.

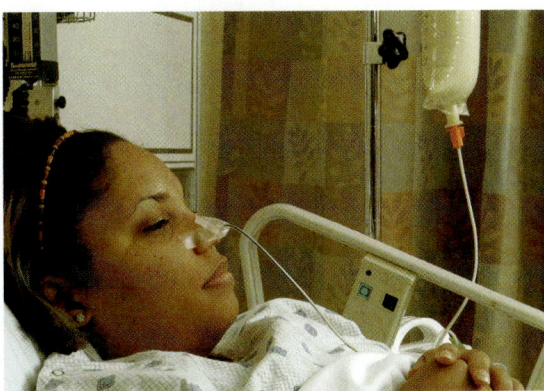

FIGURE 34-22 Hang the formula bag on an IV pole approximately 18 inches above the client's head DELMAR/CENGAGE LEARNING

(Continues)

PROCEDURE 34-2
Administering Enteral Tube Feedings (Continued)

ACTION	RATIONALE
19. Attach distal end of tubing to feeding tube adapter, and adjust drip to infuse over prescribed time.	19. Allows gravity to control flow rate, reducing risk of diarrhea from bolus feeding.
20. When bag empties of formula, add 30 to 60 mL or prescribed amount of water; close clamp.	20. Prevents air from entering stomach and reduces risk for gas accumulation. Maintains patency of feeding tube.
21. Change bags every 24 hours.	21. Decreases risk of multiplication of microorganisms in bag and tubing.

CONTINUOUS GAVAGE

22. Check tube placement at least every 4 hours.	22. Ensures that feeding tube remains in stomach.
23. Check residual at least every 8 hours.	23. Indicates ability of GI tract to digest and absorb nutrients.
24. If residual is above 100 mL, stop feeding.	24. Reduces risk of regurgitation and pulmonary aspiration related to gastric distention.
25. Add prescribed amount of formula to bag for a 4-hour period; dilute with water if prescribed.	25. Provides client with prescribed nutrients and prevents bacterial growth (formula is easily contaminated).
26. Hang gavage bag on IV pole. Prime tubing.	26. Removes air from tubing.
27. Thread tubing through feeding pump (see Figure 34-23), and attach distal end of tubing to feeding tube adapter; keep tubing straight between bag and pump.	27. Provides for controlled flow rate; prevents loops in tubing.

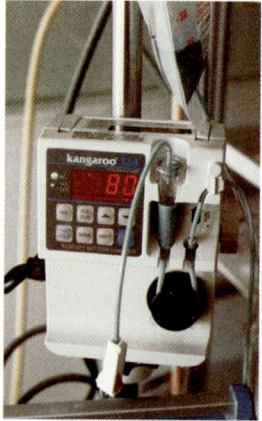

FIGURE 34-23 Thread the gavage bag tubing through the feeding pump DELMAR/CENGAGE LEARNING

28. Adjust drip rate.	28. Infuses formula over prescribed time.
29. Monitor infusion rate and signs of respiratory distress or diarrhea.	29. Prevents complications associated with continuous gavage.
30. Flush tube with water every 4 hours as prescribed or following administration of medications.	30. Maintains patency of tube.

(Continues)

PROCEDURE 34-2
Administering Enteral Tube Feedings (Continued)

ACTION	RATIONALE
31. Replace disposable feeding bag at least every 24 hours, in accordance with institution's protocol.	31. Prevents the spread of microorganisms.
32. Elevate head of bed at least 30° at all times, and turn client every 2 hours.	32. Prevents aspiration, promotes digestion, and reduces skin breakdown.
33. Provide oral hygiene every 2–4 hours.	33. Provides comfort and maintains the integrity of buccal cavity.
34. Administer water as prescribed, with and between feedings.	34. Ensures adequate hydration.
35. Remove gloves and wash hands/hand hygiene.	35. Prevents the spread of microorganisms.
36. Record total amount of formula and water administered on intake and output (I&O) form and client's response to feeding.	36. Documents administration of feeding and achievement of expected outcome; for example, client tolerates feeding and weight is maintained or increased.

delegation tip

Feedings via gastrostomy tubes may be given by LPNs/LVNs if the facility and the state permit. They must be properly trained in assessing tube placement, proper positioning of the client, and administration of the correct type and rate of feeding. All medications must be administered by the nurse.

nursing tips

Formulas can spoil. This is especially true in non-air-conditioned areas in hot, humid weather. Discard them if they have been opened and unused per manufacturers' specifications.

It is the responsibility of the nurse to perform daily equipment quality controls to ensure that the volume is being delivered as indicated by the setting on the infusion pump. If the pump fails and delivers the wrong amount of fluid, the nurse is responsible.

KEY CONCEPTS

- The metabolism of nutrients (carbohydrates, proteins, fats, vitamins, and minerals) plays an essential role in providing the body with the substances necessary for maintaining homeostasis.

- Most nutrients are absorbed in the small intestine through the processes of osmosis, diffusion, and active transport.

- The intracellular productions of energy from carbohydrates, proteins, and fats are interrelated and depend on other physiological processes, such as conversions that take place in the liver, glycolysis, Krebs cycle, and electron transport system.

- A calorie is the quantity of heat required to raise the temperature of 1 gram of water 1°C.

- There are six categories of nutrients: water, carbohydrates, proteins, fats, vitamins, and minerals.

- Carbohydrates have a protein-sparing action, based on a minimum daily ingestion of 50 to 100 grams (200–400 kcal).

- Proteins are essential for almost every bodily function, beginning with the genetic control of protein synthesis, cell function, and cell reproduction.

- Diets high in saturated fats are associated with an increased incidence of coronary heart disease.

- Low-density lipoproteins are responsible for the formation of atherosclerosis, which develops from a high blood plasma level of cholesterol and usually results from a diet high in saturated fats.

- Daily food guides assist healthy persons in meal planning.
- The recommended dietary allowance represents the dietary intake of essential nutrients by age category, inclusive of weight and height.
- The *Dietary Guidelines for Americans 2005* promotes weight management by balancing calories from foods and beverages with calories expended.
- The Food Guide Pyramid outlines the number of servings in each of the six foods groups needed to maintain a healthy weight.
- Peer-group influence, social pressures, and other emotional stressors of adolescence may have a negative effect on eating habits, leading to obesity, fad diets, anorexia nervosa, and bulimia.
- Food preferences are usually developed in childhood, are modified throughout the life span, and are an expression of an individual's likes and dislikes.
- Malnutrition refers to alterations relative to inadequate intake, disorders of digestion or absorption, and overeating.
- Assessment includes three basic components: nutritional history, physical examination with anthropometric measurements, and diagnostic and laboratory data.

- Anthropometric measurements evaluate the client's calorie-energy expenditure balance, muscle mass, body fat, and protein reserves based on height, weight, skinfold, and limb and girth circumferences.
- The blood urea nitrogen (BUN) is increased with severe dehydration, malnutrition, starvation, excessive protein intake, and, most commonly, kidney disease.
- The nurse is responsible for understanding the client's metabolic needs and for making clinical judgments relative to nutritional outcomes.
- Therapeutic nutrition requires consideration of the client's total needs: cultural, socioeconomic, psychological, and physiological.
- Protein-energy malnutrition is the most common nutritional deficiency in hospitalized clients.
- Enteral and parenteral nutrition are two methods of delivering nutrition support in adult clients.
- Clients receiving PN in the home environment require close monitoring to prevent catheter sepsis and cardiac overload.
- Refeeding syndrome occurs during the initial phase of EN or PN and can be averted by starting the therapy gradually and slowly increasing the rate.

REVIEW QUESTIONS

1. Which are considered basic nutrients in the body? Select all that apply.
   a. Water
   b. Vitamins
   c. Minerals
   d. Carbohydrates
   e. Proteins
   f. Lipids
2. The evidence-based guidelines issued by the National Institutes of Health call for weight loss by restricting intake and increasing physical activity. Which food items should be eliminated from a client's diet to achieve these guidelines? Select all that apply.
   a. Saturated fats
   b. Animal fats
   c. Added sugar and salt
   d. Alcohol
   e. Green leafy vegetables
   f. Dark fruits
3. Diet teaching for a postoperative client should include the increase of which nutrient to assist with tissue repair?
   a. Vitamin
   b. Carbohydrate
   c. Protein
   d. Fat

4. Which subjective assessment should the nurse include when assessing a client's gastrointestinal tract?
   a. Rebound tenderness
   b. Diarrhea
   c. Generalized red abdominal rash
   d. Hematuria
5. During an inspection of the abdomen, which abdominal findings should the nurse report as abnormal?
   a. Bilateral symmetrical abdomen
   b. Flat abdominal contour
   c. Strong abdominal pulsations
   d. Depressed umbilicus beneath the abdominal surface
6. Which anthropometric measurement indicates the amount of body fat?
   a. Height
   b. Weight
   c. Body mass index
   d. Skinfold
7. The nurse obtains a pH of 8.0 when aspirating for gastric contents when assessing correct tube placement. The nurse evaluates a pH of 8.0 to be
   _____.
   a. Alkaline, indicating respiratory secretions
   b. A neutral pH

c. Acidic, confirming gastric secretions

d. Indicative of intestinal secretions

8. When assessing a client with a nasogastric tube, the nurse discovers it is set on continuous high suction. Which nursing intervention should the nurse implement?

   a. Clamp the tube for 30 minutes, then reconnect it to continuous high suction.

   b. Call the prescribing practitioner and remove the tube.

   c. Irrigate the tube with 30 mL of warm water and record the drainage characteristics.

   d. Change the suction to low intermittent suction.

9. The type of malnutrition that most commonly occurs in the acutely ill hospitalized client is

   _____.

   a. Anorexia nervosa

   b. Mixed malnutrition

   c. Marasmus

   d. Protein-energy malnutrition

10. Which of the following are the three essential nutrients included in PN required for anabolism and tissue synthesis?

   a. Trace elements, protein, and fats

   b. Protein, carbohydrates, and fats

   c. Fats, electrolytes, and carbohydrates

   d. Vitamins, electrolytes, and protein

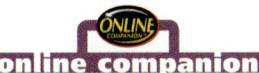

online companion

Visit the DeLaune and Ladner online companion resource at **www.delmar.cengage.com** for additional content and study aids. Click on Online Companions, then select the Nursing discipline.

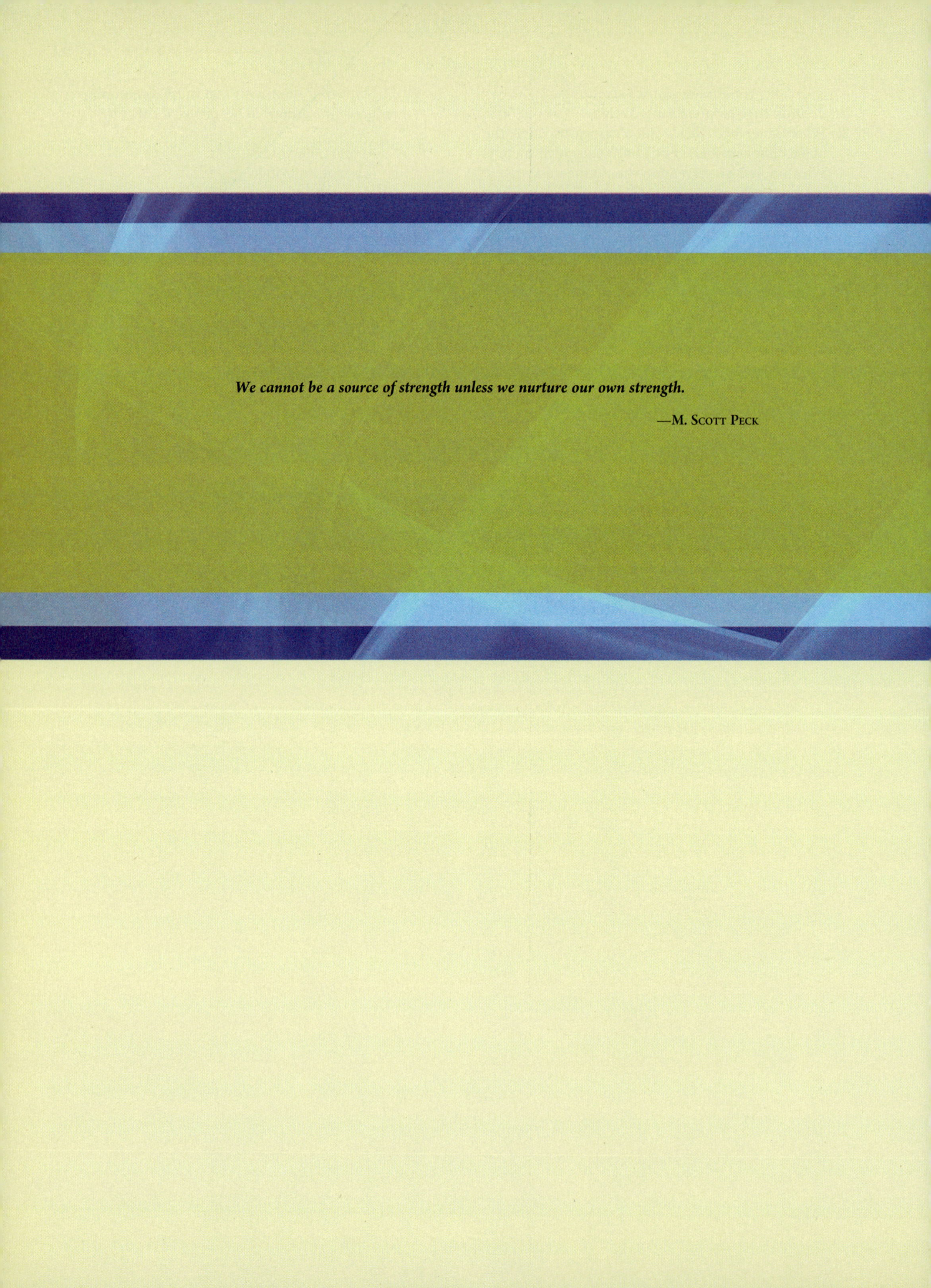

We cannot be a source of strength unless we nurture our own strength.

—M. SCOTT PECK

CHAPTER 35

Comfort and Sleep

COMPETENCIES

1. Describe types of pain.
2. Assess the nature of pain as it relates to onset, intensity, and duration.
3. Discuss the physiology of pain.
4. Describe nonpharmacologic interventions in pain control.
5. Discuss the use of pharmacologic interventions in pain control.
6. Describe the stages of sleep.
7. Discuss age-related sleep variations.
8. Explain how sleep deprivation affects an individual.
9. Discuss nursing interventions that promote comfort, rest, and sleep.

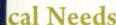
ontrol pain theory
algesia
somnia
ery
nnia
mic pain
nating
d agonist-antagonists
ulation
fascial pain syndromes
lepsy
algia
opathic pain

chronobiology
circadian rhythms
colic
counterstimulation
cutaneous pain
distraction
efferent (descending) pain
   pathway
endorphins

nociception
nociceptors
pain
pain threshold
pain tolerance
parasomnia
paresthesia
patient-controlled analgesia
   (PCA)

perception
phantom limb pain
physical dependence
progressive muscle relaxation
recurrent acute pain
referred pain
reframing
relaxation techniques
rest
sleep
sleep apnea
sleep cycle
sleep deprivation
somatic pain
somnambulism
tolerance
transcutaneous electrical nerve
   stimulation (TENS)
transduction
transmission
trigger point
visceral pain

The experience of pain and the quality of rest and sleep are both factors that can have a significant impact on a client's health. Both are personal experiences that can affect all other aspects of an individual's health, including physical well-being, mental status, and effectiveness of coping mechanisms. Pain is the most common reason that people seek health-related treatment (Jeong & Holden, 2008). This chapter explores the nature of pain, the importance of rest and sleep, and nursing care to help clients maintain their optimal health when the presence of pain or a rest or sleep disturbance threatens to compromise their health status.

PAIN

Pain is a universal human experience; it is defined as "the state in which a person experiences and reports the presence of severe discomfort or an uncomfortable sensation" (Carpenito-Moyet, 2008, p. 126). Pain is a subjective experience that is often difficult for clients to describe and nurses to understand, yet it is among the most common complaints that cause individuals to seek health care. The International Association for the Study of Pain (IASP) (2007) states that pain may be accompanied by sensory and emotional experiences as a result of actual or potential tissue damage. Until recently, pain was viewed as a symptom that required diagnosis and treatment of the underlying cause. It is now clear that pain itself can be detrimental to the health and healing of clients. Pain is a stressor that can trigger both physiological and psychological discomfort. Untreated pain can lead to physical disorders related to undernutrition, immobility, and immune suppression.

Because of a growing national awareness of the undertreatment of pain, clients are regularly being assessed for pain. The Joint Commission offers guidelines regarding clients' rights and standards of care for pain management. The Joint Commission's pain standards mandate pain assessment and management as a priority in daily clinical practice; pain intensity is considered the *fifth vital sign,* along with temperature, pulse, respiration, and blood pressure, and the client has the right to a full pain workup when pain is not easily characterized or treated. These guidelines rely on pain rating scales, discussed later in this chapter, and they are most applicable to acute or postoperative pain.

NATURE OF PAIN

Pain, a response to noxious stimuli, can be a protective mechanism to prevent further injury, as seen in clients who guard or protect an injured body part. The sensation of pain as the warning of potential tissue damage may be absent in people with nerve or spinal cord abnormalities, diabetic neuropathy, multiple sclerosis, and nerve or spinal cord injury.

Common Myths about Pain

Because pain is subjective (dependent on a client's perception) and cannot be objectively measured by another individual through a laboratory test or diagnostic data, it is often misunderstood and misjudged. A client's report about level of pain will vary on the basis of cultural and experiential backgrounds, and the nurse's interpretations of a client's pain will be filtered through the nurse's own biases and expectations. Incongruence between the nurse's view and the client's perception of pain can often lead to undermedication and unnecessary suffering on the client's part. The accompanying Spotlight On display outlines some of the common myths about pain, along with factual statements countering those beliefs.

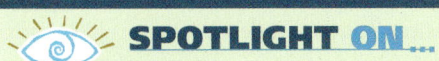

SPOTLIGHT ON...

Compassion

Common Myths about Pain

Myth	Fact
• The nurse is the best judge of a client's pain.	• Pain is a subjective experience; only the client can judge the level and severity of pain.
• If pain is ignored, it will go away.	• Pain is a real experience that can be appropriately treated.
• Clients should not take any measures to relieve their pain until it is unbearable.	• Pain control and relief measures are effective in lowering pain levels and help clients function more normally and comfortably.
• Most complaints of pain are purely psychological (e.g., "it's all in your head"); only "real" pain manifests in obvious physical signs such as moaning or grimacing.	• Most clients honestly report their perception of pain. • Physical responses to pain vary greatly depending on experience and cultural norms. • Visible expressions of pain are not always reliable indicators of its severity.
• Clients with severe tissue damage experience significant pain; those with lesser damage feel less pain.	• Individuals' perceptions of pain are subjective; the extent of tissue damage is not necessarily proportional to the extent of pain experienced.
• Clients taking pain medications will become addicted to the drug.	• Addiction is unlikely when analgesics are carefully administered and closely monitored.

Types of Pain

Pain can be qualified in two basic ways: by its cause or origin and by its description or nature. Pain categorized by its origin is either cutaneous, somatic, or visceral. **Cutaneous pain** is caused by stimulation of the cutaneous nerve endings in the skin and results in a well-localized "burning" or "prickling" sensation; getting a knot in the hair that is pulled out during combing may cause cutaneous pain. **Somatic pain** is nonlocalized and originates in support structures such as tendons, ligaments, and nerves or may be deep pain; jamming a knee or finger will result in somatic pain. **Visceral pain** is discomfort in the internal organs and is less localized and more slowly transmitted than cutaneous pain. Visceral pain is often difficult to assess because the location may not be directly related to the cause. Pain originating from the abdominal organs is often called **referred pain** because the sensation of pain is not felt in the organ itself but instead is perceived at the spot where the organs were located during fetal development. Figure 35-1 on page 1046 shows the cutaneous areas where visceral pain is often referred.

Acute pain is most frequently identified by its sudden onset and relatively short duration, mild to severe intensity, and a steady decrease in intensity over a period of days to weeks. Some forms of acute pain may have a slower onset. Once the noxious stimulus is resolved, the pain usually decreases. Examples of noxious stimuli are needlesticks, surgical incisions, burns, and fractures.

Recurrent acute pain is identified by repetitive painful episodes that may recur over a prolonged period or throughout the client's lifetime. These painful episodes alternate with pain-free intervals. Examples of recurrent pain include migraine headaches, sickle cell pain crises, and the pain of angina pectoris due to myocardial hypoxia.

Chronic persistent pain is identified as long-term (lasting 6 months or longer) nearly constant, or recurrent pain that produces significant negative changes in the client's life. Unlike acute pain, chronic pain may last long after the pathology is resolved. According to the National Center for Health Statistics (2006), more than 76 million Americans have chronic pain; that is more than all Americans with diabetes, heart disease, and cancer combined.

The American Geriatrics Society (AGS, 2009) describes persistent pain as pain that may or may not be associated with disease and states that it is prevalent in older persons. The AGS recommends use of *persistent pain* rather than *chronic pain* because the term *persistent* has a more positive connotation. Many individuals equate the word *chronic* with untreatable and, thus, expect to have no relief from long-term pain.

Chronic acute pain occurs almost daily over a long period, has the potential for lasting months or years, and has a high probability of ending. Severe burn injuries and cancer are examples of pathophysiology leading to chronic acute pain, which may last for long periods before the condition is cured or controlled.

Chronic nonmalignant pain (CNP) occurs almost daily and lasts for at least 6 months, with intensity ranging from mild to severe. Chronic pain, a primary motivator for

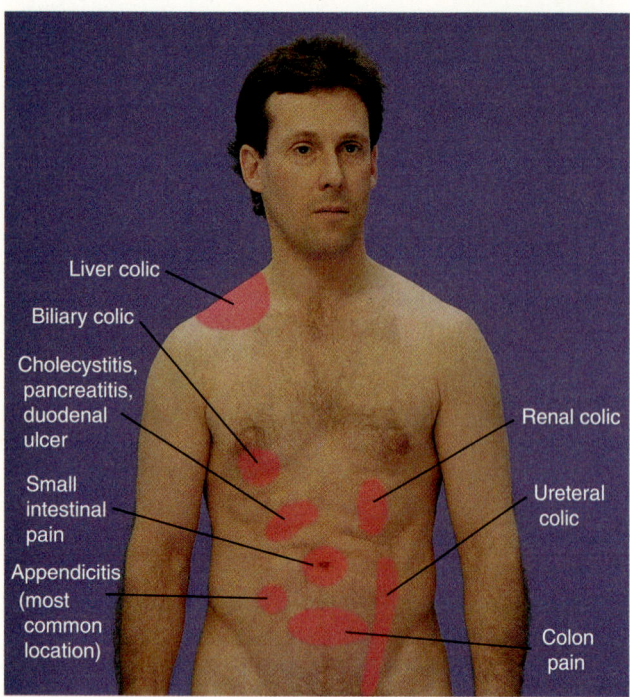

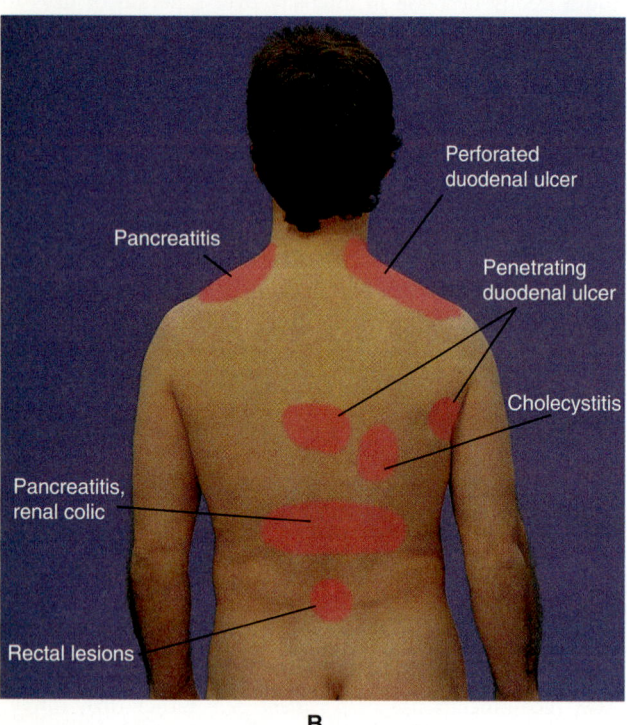

FIGURE 35-1 Areas of Referred Pain. A. Anterior View; B. Posterior View DELMAR/CENGAGE LEARNING

individuals to seek health care intervention, can greatly influence a client's quality of life, including emotional, social, vocational, and financial areas. Examples of pathophysiology leading to CNP include:

- Many forms of **neuralgia** (paroxysmal pain that extends along the course of one or more nerves)

- Low back pain
- Rheumatoid arthritis
- Ankylosing spondylitis
- **Phantom limb pain** (a form of neuropathic pain that occurs after amputation, with pain sensations referred to an area in the missing portion of the limb)
- **Myofascial pain syndromes** (a group of muscle disorders characterized by pain, muscle spasm, tenderness, stiffness, and limited motion)

CNP may be associated with several problems, including:

- Activity intolerance, which leads to physical deconditioning
- Functional impairment with resultant changes in role performance (parent, breadwinner)
- Social isolation, which alters relationships
- Sleep deprivation
- Frustration, anxiety, anger, and depression

When CNP is severe enough to disable the client, nurses understand that pain management becomes a priority in order to improve the client's quality of life.

PHYSIOLOGY OF PAIN

Noxious stimuli activate **nociceptors** (receptive neurons for painful sensations) that, together with the axons of neurons, convey information to the spinal cord where reflexes are activated. The information is simultaneously transmitted to the brain supraspinally. Long-lasting changes in cells within the spinal cord's **afferent (ascending)** and **efferent (descending) pain pathways** may occur after a brief noxious stimulus.

Physiological responses (such as elevated blood pressure, pulse rate, and respiratory rate; dilated pupils; pallor; and perspiration) to even a brief acute pain episode will begin showing adaptation within a short period, possibly minutes to a few hours. Physiologically, the body cannot sustain the extreme stress response for anything other than short periods of time. The body conserves its resources by physiological adaptation (returning to normal or near-normal blood pressure, pulse rate, and respiratory rate; normal pupil size; and dry skin) even in the face of continuing pain of the same intensity. Pain can be categorized into two types, according to its pathophysiology (see Table 35-1 on page 1047).

Nociceptive Pain

The four fundamental processes involved in **nociception**, the process by which an individual becomes consciously aware of pain, are as follows:

- **Transduction**—the changing of noxious stimuli in sensory nerve endings to energy impulses
- **Transmission**—movement of impulses from the site of origin to the brain
- **Perception**—developing conscious awareness of pain
- **Modulation**—the changing of pain impulses

TRANSDUCTION OF PAIN When noxious stimuli occur, tissues are damaged. Cell damage releases the following sensitizing substances:

TABLE 35-1 Pathology-Based Pain Classification

	NOCICEPTIVE PAIN	NEUROPATHIC PAIN
Description	Normal processing of noxious stimuli; may damage tissue if prolonged	Abnormal processing of stimuli by peripheral nervous system (PNS) or central nervous system (CNS)
Examples	Somatic pain, visceral pain	Centrally generated pain: • Phantom pain • Spinal cord injury Peripherally generated pain: • Diabetic neuropathy • Trigeminal neuralgia

Data from Boswell, M. V., & Cole, B. C. (2006). *Weiner's pain management: a practical guide for clinicians* (7th ed.). Boca Raton, FL: CRC Press; McGuire, L. (2010). Pain: the fifth vital sign. In D. D. Ignatavicius & M. L. Workman (Eds.), *Medical-surgical nursing: patient-centered collaborative care* (6th ed.). St. Louis, MO: Elsevier, p. 39.

- Prostaglandins (PG)
- Bradykinin (BK)
- Serotonin (5-HT)
- Substance P (SP)
- Histamine (H)

Release of these substances alters the electrical charge on the neuronal membrane. This change in electrical charge is a result of movement of calcium, sodium, potassium, and chloride ions across cell membranes. The impulse is then ready to be transmitted along the nociceptor fibers (Straud & Spaeth, 2008).

TRANSMISSION OF PAIN The specific action of pain varies depending on the type of pain. In cutaneous pain, cutaneous nerve transmissions travel through a reflex arc from the nerve ending (point of pain) to the brain at a speed of approximately 300 feet per second, with a reflex response causing an almost immediate reaction. This explains why when a hot stove is touched the person's hand jerks back *before* there is conscious awareness that damage is occurring (see Figure 35-2 on page 1048). After a hot stove is touched, a sensory nerve ending in the skin of the finger initiates nerve transmission that travels through the dorsal root ganglion to the dorsal horn in the gray matter of the spinal cord. From there, the impulse travels though an interneuron that synapses with a motor neuron, which exits the spinal cord at the same level. This motor neuron, and the stimulation of the muscle it innervates, is responsible for the swift movement of the hand away from the hot stove.

In the case of the hot stove, the sensory neuron synapses not only with an interneuron but also with an afferent sensory neuron. The impulse travels up the spinal cord to the thalamus, where a final synapse conducts the impulse to the cortex of the brain. The efferent or descending motor neuron response is conducted from the brain through the spinal cord, where it synapses with a motor neuron that exits the spinal cord and innervates the muscle.

In visceral pain, transmission of pain impulses is slower and less localized than in cutaneous pain. The internal organs (including the gastrointestinal [GI] tract) have a minimal number of nociceptors, which explains why visceral pain is poorly localized and is felt as a dull aching or throbbing sensation. However, internal organs have extreme sensitivity to distension. The cramping pain of **colic** (acute abdominal pain), for example, results when:

- Flatus or constipation causes distension of the stomach or intestines.
- There is hyperperistalsis, as in gastroenteritis.
- A substance tries to pass through a lumen (an opening) that is too small.

The physiology of **ischemic pain**, or pain occurring when the blood supply of an area is restricted or cut off completely, also differs from that of cutaneous pain. The restriction of blood flow causes inadequate oxygenation of the tissue supplied by those vessels as well as inadequate metabolic waste product removal. Ischemic pain has the most rapid onset in an active muscle and a much slower onset in a passive muscle. Examples of ischemic pain are muscle cramps, sickle cell pain crisis, angina pectoris, and myocardial infarction. When ischemic pain occurs in a muscle that continues to work, a muscle spasm (cramp) is the outcome. If the blood supply to the heart is severely restricted or completely cut off and is not restored quickly, a myocardial infarction will occur. See the Safety First display on page 1048.

In acute pain episodes, substances released from injured tissue lead to stress hormone responses in the client. This causes an increased metabolic rate, enhanced breakdown of body tissue, impaired immune function, increased blood clotting, and water retention, and it triggers the fight-or-flight reaction, leading to tachycardia and negative emotions.

▼ **SAFETY FIRST** ▼

ISCHEMIC PAIN
Supplemental oxygen and pain medication must be administered quickly to clients with ischemic pain to minimize oxygen deprivation and prevent infarction (tissue death).

PAIN PERCEPTION   When the impulse has been transmitted to the cortex and is interpreted by the brain, the information is available on a conscious level. It is then that the person becomes aware of the intensity, location, and quality of pain. This information is interpreted in light of previous experience, adding the affective component to the pain experience.

MODULATION   Modulation refers to activation of descending neural pathways that inhibit transmission of pain. Descending neurons originate in the brain stem and descend to the dorsal horn of the spinal cord. The descending fibers release substances that produce analgesia by blocking the transmission of noxious stimuli. Pain modulation is a result of the effects of endogenous opioids, also called enkephalins and **endorphins**.

Neuropathic pain arises from damage to portions of the peripheral or central nervous system (CNS). This pain is *not* nociceptive pain, nor that which is due to ongoing tissue injury or inflammation. It is important to differentiate neuropathic pain from other types of pain because the treatment differs significantly. Table 35-2 on page 1049 identifies some of the differences between nociceptive and neuropathic pain.

Neuropathic pain is a result of abnormal processing of sensory input by either the peripheral or CNS. Two types of neuropathic pain are **allodynia** (a nonpainful stimulus is felt as painful in spite of the tissue appearing normal) and **paresthesia** (an abnormal sensation such as burning, prickling, or tingling).

Myofascial pain was first described by Travell and Rinzler (1952) as pain that occurs as a result of a small, hypersensitive region in a muscle ligament, fascia, or joint

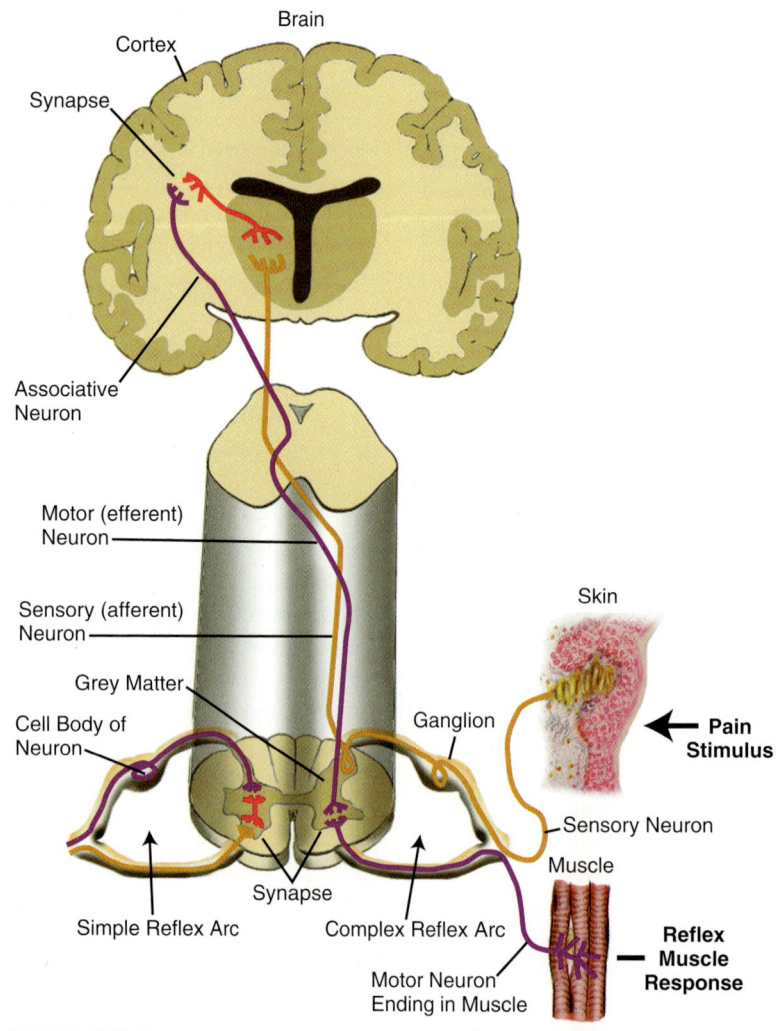

FIGURE 35-2 Reflex Arcs DELMAR/CENGAGE LEARNING

TABLE 35-2 **Differences between Nociceptive Pain and Neuropathic Pain**

	NOCICEPTIVE PAIN	NEUROPATHIC PAIN
Pain descriptors	Varied	Sharp, shooting, lancinating, tingling, pins and needles, strange or dull, aching, burning
Pain pattern	Pain intensity decreases steadily over period of days to weeks in the absence of repeated injury or inflammation	Pain persists or even intensifies during weeks or months after injury
Response to opioids	Generally relieves pain with acceptable margin between comfort and sedation	"Resistant" to opioids, with significant pain remaining even when opioid doses lead to severe sedation
Response to NSAIDs	Generally effective at partial reduction of pain intensity	Rarely relieved by NSAIDs
Response to tricyclic antidepressants, anticonvulsants, local anesthetics	Generally ineffective	Often decreased significantly or relieved

Data from Allen, S. (2005). Pharmacotherapy of neuropathic pain. *Continuing Education in Anaesthesia, Critical Care & Pain, 5*(4): 134–137; Daniel, H. C., Narewska, J., Sherpell, M. Hoggart, B., Johnson, R.I, & Rice, A. S. (2008). Comparison of psychological and physical function in neuropathic and nociceptive pain: implications for cognitive behavioral pain management programs. *European Journal of Pain, 12*(6):734–741.

capsule called a **trigger point**. The trigger point is a hypersensitive point that when stimulated causes a local twitch or "jump" response. Myofascial pain is often accompanied by a localized, deep ache that is surrounded by a referred area of **hyperalgesia**, or extreme sensitivity to pain.

Gate Control Theory of Pain

Theories of pain transmission and interpretation attempt to describe and explain the pain experience. In 1965, Melzack and Wall proposed the **gate control pain theory**, which was the first to recognize that the psychological aspects of pain are as important as the physiological aspects. The gate control theory combines cognitive, sensory, and emotional components—in addition to the physiological aspects—and

proposes that they can act on a gate control system to block the individual's perception of pain. Pain perception is regulated through a gating mechanism at the dorsal horn of the spinal cord. The gating mechanism causes vasoconstriction and decreased nerve conduction velocity, thereby reducing the transmission of noxious stimuli. As a result, the level of conscious awareness of painful sensation is altered.

The gate control theory is based on the premise that pain impulses travel through either small-diameter or large-diameter nerve cells, both of which pass through the same gate. The large-diameter cells have the ability, when properly stimulated, to "close the gate" and thus block transmission of the pain impulse to the brain (see Figure 35-3). Stimulants such as cutaneous massage, opioid release, and

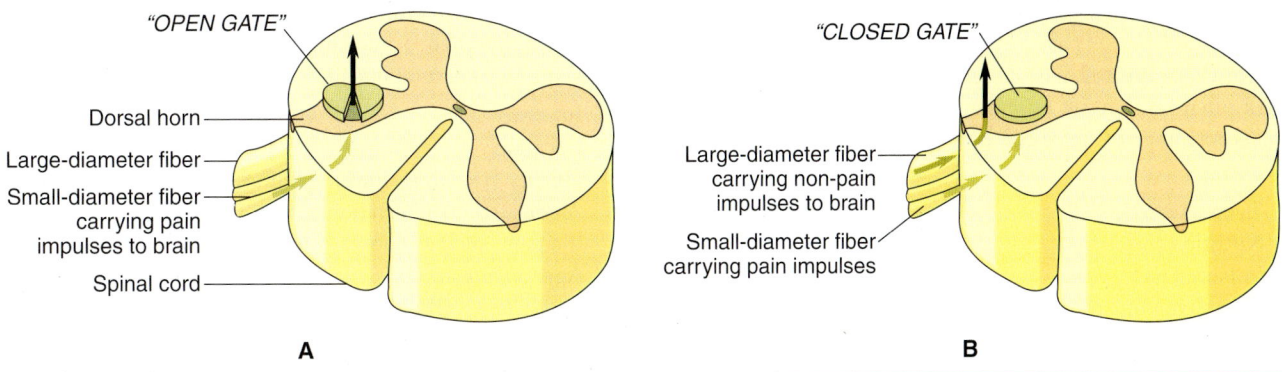

FIGURE 35-3 Gate Control Theory: Blocking Transmission of Pain DELMAR/CENGAGE LEARNING

excessive stimulation all activate the large-diameter cells to close the gate. Clinically, the effectiveness of several non-pharmacologic modalities, such as massage, acupuncture, and acupressure, supports the gate control theory.

FACTORS AFFECTING THE PAIN EXPERIENCE

The subjective nature of pain varies from person to person and is influenced by several variables. Many factors account for the differences in a client's individual response to pain, including age, previous experience with pain, and cultural factors.

Age

Age can greatly influence a client's perception of the pain experience. Infants are sensitive to pain and typically exhibit discomfort through crying or physical movement. Toddlers also use crying and physical movement to indicate pain, and they begin to develop the skills needed to verbally describe pain or point to the area that is hurting. Children often do not understand why pain occurs and can therefore be frightened or resentful of the pain experience; in some cases, children revert to habits of their younger years (regression) as a coping mechanism when faced with pain they cannot otherwise manage.

Adolescents often sense great peer pressure and may be reluctant to admit having pain for fear of being called weak or sensitive. Adults may continue pain behaviors they learned as children and may also be reluctant to admit pain or seek medical care because of fear of the unknown or fear of the impact that treatment may have on their lifestyle.

Older adults may often ignore their pain, viewing it as an unavoidable consequence of aging; family and health care members may inadvertently support this stereotype and be less than responsive to an older client's complaints of pain. Pain may be manifested differently by older individuals. For example, pain may be referred (e.g., gallbladder pain is felt in the shoulder). Also, the intensity of pain in some older clients may not accurately reflect the severity of the underlying pathology (e.g., a myocardial infarction may be felt as a fluttering sensation).

Pain related to chronic disease is prevalent among the elderly population, even those who live in the community (Martinez, 2009). Persistent pain is common in older persons and among nursing home residents (Zwakhalen, Hamers, Abu-Saad, & Berger, 2006). According to Martinez (2009), 73% to 80% of the elderly population have reported pain symptoms. However pain in many elders is not reported and, therefore, is untreated. The undertreatment of pain in the older client often is the result of underreporting and underdetection. Some outcomes of untreated pain in older adults include the following:

- Sleep alterations
- Nutrition problems
- Impaired gait
- Cognitive impairments
- Decreased socialization
- Increased incidence of falls
- Decreased ability to function independently

Previous Experience with Pain

Clients' previous experiences with pain will often influence their reactions. Coping mechanisms that were used in the past may affect clients' judgment as to how the pain will affect their lives and what measures they can use to successfully manage the pain on their own. Client teaching about pain expectations and management methods can often allay clients' fears and lead to more successful pain management, especially in those clients who do not have previous pain experience or who have memories of a previous devastating pain experience that they do not wish to repeat.

Cultural Norms and Attitudes

Cultural diversity in pain responses can easily lead to problems in pain management. There are no significant differences among groups in the level of intensity at which pain becomes appreciable or perceptible. However, cultural values regarding pain can affect the client's beliefs about pain as well as responses to pain, and the level of intensity or duration of pain the client is willing to endure is culturally determined.

Expression of pain is also governed by cultural values. In some cultures, tolerance of pain, and therefore "suffering in silence," is expected; in others, full expression of pain may include animated physical and emotional responses. The nurse must be careful not to equate the level of expression of pain with the level of actual pain experienced but instead to consider cultural influences that affect the expression of pain.

ASSESSMENT

In order for pain to be treated effectively, it must first be assessed accurately. The client's self-report of the existence and intensity of the pain is the most accurate and reliable evidence of the nature of the pain. Assessment of pain includes the collection of subjective and objective data through the use of various assessment tools and the construction of a database to use in developing a pain management plan. Pain assessment should be performed for every client, as recommended by the Joint Commission.

Data Collection

As pain intensity is considered the fifth vital sign, nurses need to assess all clients for pain on admission for any health care service. The client's perception of the pain should cover a description of several qualifiers, including:

- Intensity
- Location
- Quality (radiating, burning, diffuse)
- Associated manifestations (factors that often accompany the pain, such as nausea, constipation, or dizziness)
- Aggravating factors (variables that worsen the pain, such as exercise, certain foods, or stress)
- Alleviating factors (measures the client can take to lessen the effect of the pain, such as lying down, avoiding certain foods, or taking medication)

Nurses must look for nonverbal signs of pain, such as changes in motor activity or facial expression. It is also important to ask family members to share their observations; they may be the first ones to note subtle behavior changes indicative of pain. When assessing a client's report of pain, the nurse should also determine a client's pain threshold and pain tolerance level. **Pain threshold** is the level of intensity at which pain becomes appreciable or perceptible and will vary with each individual and type of pain. **Pain tolerance** is the level of intensity or duration of pain the client is willing or able to endure. A client's perceptions and attitudes about pain are dramatically influenced by many factors, including previous experiences and cultural background.

Clients' behavioral adaptation may yield no report of pain unless questioned specifically. **Distraction** (focusing attention on stimuli other than pain) may also be used by clients. Clients often minimize the pain behaviors they are able to control for a number of reasons, including:

- To be a "good" client and avoid making demands
- To maintain a positive self-image by not appearing to be weak
- By using distraction as a method of making pain more bearable (young children are particularly adept at this)
- Exhaustion

Pain is fatiguing, as a significant amount of energy is used to deal with it. The longer a person suffers pain, the greater the level of fatigue. Although there is no conscious awareness of pain during sleep, there may be a dream-state awareness; see the accompanying Nursing Process Highlight. The stress response continues, and the body, physiologically, pays the price. Clients also wake up with considerably more pain than they had before going to sleep, thereby requiring even more intervention (pharmacologic and nonpharmacologic) to reduce the pain.

Occasionally there is a discrepancy between pain behaviors observed by the nurse and the client's self-report of pain. Client pain behaviors include splinting of the painful area,

distorted posture, impaired mobility, insomnia, anxiety, attention seeking, and depression. Discrepancies between behaviors and the client's self-report can be due to coping skills (e.g., relaxation techniques or distraction), stoicism, anxiety, or cultural differences in expected pain behaviors. Whenever these discrepancies occur, they should be addressed with the client, and the pain management plan should be altered accordingly.

Assessment Tools

Pain assessment tools are the single most effective method of identifying the presence and intensity of pain in clients. Tools used for assessing pain should be appropriate to the client's age and cultural context. When assessing pain, health care professionals should avoid making value judgments. For example, clients who watch the clock for the next pain medication or wake up from sleep requesting the medication should not be labeled as "drug seekers." Research has shown that clients may rest and sleep despite moderate to severe pain, and distractions, especially laughter, is an effective way of coping with pain (Ufema, 2008). See Table 35-3 on page 1052 for sample questions used in pain assessment.

INITIAL PAIN ASSESSMENT TOOL Figure 35-4 on page 1053 is a tool that may be used for initial pain assessment for clients who have complex or persistent pain. The tool assesses location, intensity, and quality, precipitating and alleviating factors, and how the pain affects function and quality of life. Once this tool is completed, another less detailed tool can be used for the ongoing monitoring of the client's pain level; see the accompanying Nursing Process Highlight.

PAIN INTENSITY SCALES Pain intensity scales are another quick, effective method for clients to rate the intensity of their pain (see Figure 35-5 on page 1054). The verbal rating scale (VRS) and the numeric rating scale (NRS) are often used together to collect more accurate client input. The VRS uses adjectives ranging from "no pain" to "excruciating pain"

NURSING PROCESS HIGHLIGHT

Assessment

Assessing the Effect of Pain on Sleep

Questioning clients about the effect that pain has on their sleep habits will help clarify the intensity of the pain and its effect on clients' patterns of daily living. Ask: Does the pain:

- Prevent you from falling asleep?
- Make finding a comfortable sleeping position difficult?
- Wake you up from a sound sleep?
- Keep you from falling back asleep once awakened?
- Leave you feeling tired and unrefreshed after a sleeping session?

NURSING PROCESS HIGHLIGHT

Assessment

The client may exhibit any or all of the following indicators of pain:

- Reporting or complaining of pain
- Focusing on pain
- Crying or moaning
- Frowning or grimacing
- Rubbing or protecting painful areas
- Altering posture or movements to lessen pain
- Splinting painful areas by increasing muscle tension
- Reporting insomnia, fatigue, or depression

TABLE 35-3 Pain Assessment Questions

CHARACTERISTIC	QUESTION	EXPLANATION
Quality	"How do you feel?"	Common descriptors include aching, burning, dull, numb, sharp, and throbbing.
Intensity	"Using this scale, what number best describes your pain?" "Which picture best describes your pain?"	Use the verbal rating scale (VRS) and the numeric rating scale (NRS) in combination. Use the Wong-Baker faces scale.
Location	"Where does it hurt?" "What part of your body is painful?"	Encourage client to point to the affected area. On a printed body outline, have client shade in the areas that correspond to painful areas of his or her body.
Duration	"Is the pain constant?" "Does the pain come and go?"	Instruct client to time painful episodes.
Triggers	"What makes the pain worse?" "What lessens the pain?"	Have client focus on triggers such as positions, activities, or situations.
Effects	"How has the pain affected your life?" "Do you have any symptoms in addition to pain?"	Include effects on work, school, relationships, eating, sleep, energy level, recreation/leisure, and moods. Ask client about presence of confusion, constipation, itching, nausea or vomiting, problems with urination, and sleepiness or drowsiness.
Knowledge level	"What do you understand about your pain and its causes?" "What have you been taught about your pain?" "Have you taken any medicine for pain? If so, what?"	Document the client's responses.

Data adapted from Macintyre, P., Rowbotham, D. & Walker, S. (2008). *Clinical pain management acute pain* (2nd ed.). New York: Oxford University Press, USA; Spies, K., Rehberg, Bl., Schug, S., Jaehnichen, G., & Harper, S, (2008). *Pocket guide pain management*. Warren, IL: Springer.

to describe intensity. Frequent use of these tools will increase understanding of pain severity. When using the NRS, clients are asked to assign their pain a number, with 0 meaning no pain and 10 representing the worst possible pain. "On a scale of 0 to 10, with 0 being no pain at all and 10 being the worst pain you could ever have, how much do you hurt right now?" If there are multiple painful areas, this question can be asked regarding each area.

With the Joint Commission requiring pain assessments for all clients, using behavioral pain scales for clients who cannot self-report has become common practice (D'Arcy, 2008). The assessment tools designed for use by the non-self-reporting client include the Pain Assessment in Advanced Dementia Scale for clients with dementia and the Payen Behavioral Pain Scale for critically ill, sedated, and mechanically ventilated clients. These tools are effective when used consistently by nurses to assess pain in nonverbal clients (D'Arcy, 2008).

PAIN DIARY Client input is essential if accurate assessment data are to be collected. Self-monitoring of symptoms

can be promoted by having clients complete a pain diary. The pain diary should include:

- Date and time
- Intensity
- Situation (What were you doing?)
- How did you feel?
- What were you thinking?
- What did you do to ease the pain?
- How effective was the pain control strategy?

PSYCHOSOCIAL PAIN ASSESSMENT A psychosocial assessment is performed to identify the client's attitudes and beliefs regarding pain and social support. The initial assessment should include an evaluation of the client's mood (depression or anxiety), self-efficacy, coping skills, and concerns. Concerns regarding pain may include feelings of helplessness and fears about using certain types of drugs and addiction. An initial evaluation should include assessment of social support, family or caregiver relationships, work history, cultural environment, spirituality, and accessibility to health care services.

Date_____

Patient's Name_____   Age_____Room_____

Diagnosis_____   Physician_____

Nurse_____

I. Location: Patient or nurse marks drawing.

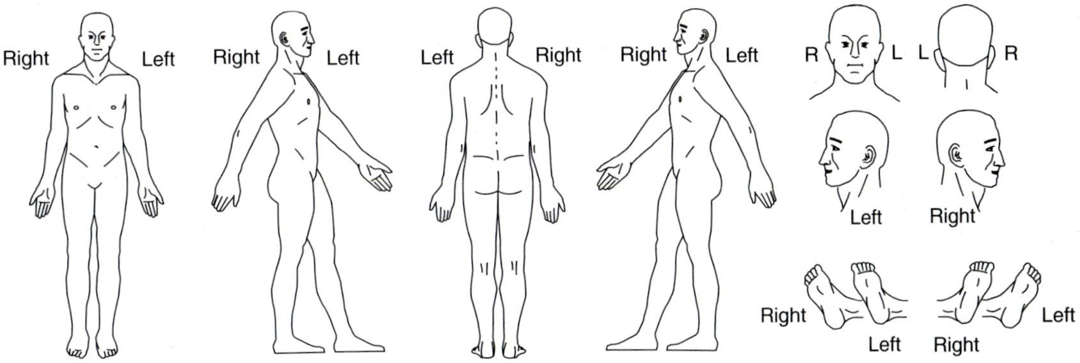

II. Intensity: Patient rates the pain. Scale used_____

       Present: _____

       Worst pain gets:_____

       Best pain gets:_____

       Acceptable level of pain:_____

III. Quality: (Use patient's own words, eg., prick, ache, burn, throb, pull, sharp)_____

IV. Onset, duration, variations, rhythms:_____

V. Manner of expressing pain: _____

VI. What relieves the pain?_____

VII. What causes or increases the pain?_____

VIII. Effects of pain: (Note decreased function, decreased quality of life.)

          Accompanying symptoms (e.g., nausea)_____

          Sleep_____

          Appetite_____

          Physical activity_____

          Relationship with others (e.g., irritability)_____

          Emotions (e.g., anger, suicidal, crying)_____

          Concentration_____

          Other_____

IX. Other comments:_____

X. Plan:_____

FIGURE 35-4 **Initial Pain Assessment Tool** MAY BE DUPLICATED FOR USE IN CLINICAL PRACTICE. REPRINTED WITH PERMISSION FROM MCCAFFERY, M., & PASERO, C. (1999). *PAIN: CLINICAL MANUAL FOR NURSING PRACTICE* (2ND ED.). ST. LOUIS, MO: MOSBY.

Pain Intensity Scales

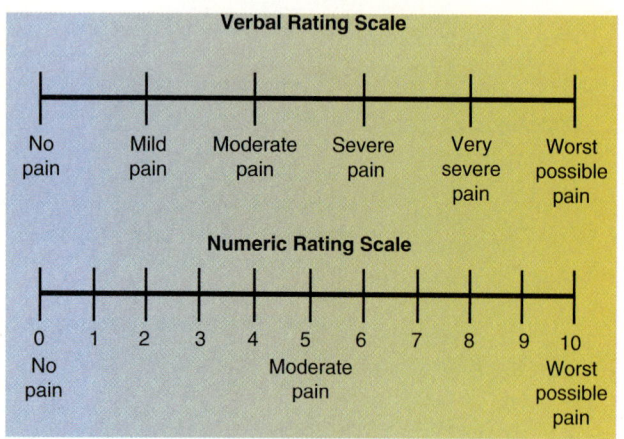

FIGURE 35-5 **Pain Intensity Scales** FROM ACUTE PAIN MANAGEMENT GUIDELINE PANEL. (1992). *ACUTE PAIN MANAGEMENT: OPERATIVE OR MEDICAL PROCEDURES AND TRAUMA. CLINICAL PRACTICE GUIDELINES* (AHRQ PUBLICATION NO. 92-0033). ROCKVILLE, MD: AGENCY FOR HEALTHCARE RESEARCH AND QUALITY.

Developmental Considerations

Because pain experiences and reports can be influenced by age and developmental level, special consideration should be used to factor in those influences. Infants, children, and adolescents provide a special challenge in pain assessment because their pain behaviors often differ from those considered normal in the adult population. Certain myths hinder the accurate assessment and management of pain in children; see Table 35-4.

Two useful tools for assessing pain in children are the Wong-Baker Faces Rating Scale and the Poker Chip Tool. The Wong-Baker Faces Rating Scale can be used with children as young as 3 years, as it helps them express their level of pain by pointing to a cartoon face that most closely resembles how they are feeling (see Figure 35-6).

The Poker Chip Tool consists of four red poker chips that can easily be carried in a pocket and available when needed. The chips are aligned horizontally on a hard surface in front of the child, and they are described as "pieces of hurt." The chips are described from left to right as just a little bit of hurt, a little more hurt, more hurt, and the most hurt you could ever have. The child is then asked, "How many pieces of hurt do you have right now?" This tool can be used with children 4 to 13 years old.

The verbal 0 to 10 scale is also frequently used for school-age and adolescent clients in a number of settings. It is important to remember that any child under stress or with anxiety will regress, and regression may make use of the verbal 0 to 10 scale in children under 8 to 10 years of age of questionable value. See the accompanying Spotlight On display on page 1055 for developmental considerations.

NURSING DIAGNOSIS

The two primary nursing diagnoses used to describe pain are *acute pain* and *chronic pain.* According to NANDA (2009),

TABLE 35-4 Myths about Pain and Children

MISCONCEPTION	FACT
Infants do not feel pain.	Anatomic structures for pain processing reach adult maturity at 36 weeks after conception.
Children tolerate pain better than adults.	Even though children may not express pain as adults do, there are behavioral indicators of pain in children. Children as young as age 3 can use pain scales to communicate the level of pain experienced.
Children become accustomed to pain or painful procedures.	Some children show increased signs of discomfort with repeated painful procedures. Anxiety over impending procedures only exacerbates pain.
Narcotics are more dangerous for children than for adults.	When used appropriately, opioids are not more dangerous for children than for adults.

Delmar/Cengage Learning

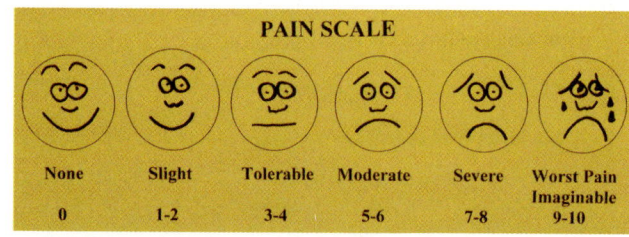

FIGURE 35-6 **Wong-Baker Faces Pain Rating Scale** REPRINTED WITH PERMISSION FROM HOCKENBERRY, M. J., & WILSON, D. (2008). *WONG'S NURSING CARE OF INFANTS AND CHILDREN* (8TH ED.). ST. LOUIS, MO: ELSEVIER.

acute pain is defined as an uncomfortable experience that occurs as a result of actual or potential tissue damage. The onset may be sudden or slow. *Chronic pain* and acute pain are differentiated by the length of time that the unpleasant experiences last; acute pain has lasted less than six months, whereas, chronic pain has a duration of greater than six months. Presenting characteristics of *acute pain* and *chronic pain* are listed in the Nursing Process Highlight on page 1055.

If the client presents with problems in addition to pain, the nurse must be alert to the possibility that the pain may be the *cause* (not the effect) of another problem. For example, a client may be experiencing *impaired physical mobility* or *activity intolerance* related to pain caused by a broken leg, as evidenced by verbal complaint, fatigue, and guarding the affected leg.

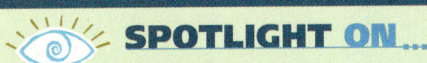

SPOTLIGHT ON...

Professionalism

Pain Assessment Tools

After reviewing these brief case presentations, determine the type of pain assessment tool most appropriate for each:

1. A developmentally normal 42-year-old man during an overnight hospital stay after orthopedic surgery on the ankle
2. A developmentally normal 12-year-old oncology client with severe mucositis (inflammation of the mucous membrane) after chemotherapy for recurrent osteosarcoma (following an above-the-knee amputation) with metastases to multiple ribs and severe phantom limb pain

PLANNING AND OUTCOMES

When planning care for the client experiencing pain, mutual goal setting is of utmost importance. After assessing the client's perception of the problem, work with the client in developing realistic outcomes. Be sure to use both nonpharmacologic and pharmacologic interventions in planning strategies to help the client achieve desired levels of functioning and pain control.

When asking about the client's goal for pain relief, the nurse often has to state, "We can't usually get rid of all your pain, but if we could get it down to a place that it didn't bother you so much, what would that be?" Thus, the family and health care professionals involved will all be aware of a realistic goal for pain relief.

The goal of palliative care is to provide interventions that support the achievement of quality of life for clients and their families. The Hospice and Palliative Nurses Association's (HPNA) position statement on pain addresses "unrelieved pain" as the most feared symptom of those at the end of life. "Unrelieved pain can contribute to unnecessary suffering, as evidenced by sleep disturbances, hopelessness, loss of control, and impaired social interactions. Pain may actually hasten death by increasing physiological stress, decreasing mobility, [and] contributing to pneumonia and thromboemboli" (HPNA, 2008, p. 1). See the accompanying display on page 1056 for the HPNA position statement on pain.

Collaboration

In order to identify all of the potentially treatable contributing factors to pain, management of pain often requires an interdisciplinary team. This is especially true for persistent (chronic) pain that is a multifaceted problem, involving physiological, psychological, and social factors. The treatment of pain requires collaboration between interdisciplinary team members and may require the services of a *pain manager/specialist,* such as a physician or nurse practitioner. Almost all

NURSING PROCESS HIGHLIGHT

Diagnosis

Diagnosis	Selected Defining Characteristics
Acute pain	• Verbalization of severe discomfort • Restlessness • Variations in vital signs indicative of autonomic responses • Guarding behavior • Sleep disturbances • Grimace • Self-focus • Distracted behavior • Changes in appetite and eating
Chronic pain	• Verbalization of pain over an extended period of time • Impaired functional ability • Sleep disturbances • Guarding behavior • Irritability • Self-focus • Restlessness • Depression • Muscle atrophy of affected area • Weight changes • Fatigue • Fear of reinjury

Data from *Nursing Diagnoses—Definitions and Classification 2009-2011* © 2009, 2007, 2005, 2003, 2001, 1998, 1996, 1994 NANDA International. Used by arrangement with Wiley-Blackwell Publishing, a company of John Wiley & Sons, Inc.

health care providers, such as psychologists, pharmacists, spiritual counselors, social workers, and rehabilitation specialists, participate in the management of persistent pain and palliative care.

IMPLEMENTATION

The Nursing Interventions Classification (NIC) system defines those nursing actions regarding pain management, identifies certain measures to relieve pain (e.g., patient-controlled analgesia assistance), and addresses specific pain relief actions within other related intervention sets, such as *client rights protection* and *dying care.* The NIC activities clearly emphasize the need for nurses to listen to clients' description of pain and to respect their right to obtain effective pain management. See the accompanying display on page 1057 for a sample of NIC-defined activities for pain management. Managing pain presents the nurse with many challenges and requires the collaborative efforts of other health care professionals. The NIC system also presents specific interventions for various pharmacological, nonpharmacological, and interpersonal strategies for pain management. These strategies are discussed later in this section.

Nurse-Client Relationship

Pain is a subjective symptom, it is not visible, and only the client knows how it feels. The client's self-report of pain is the most valid assessment data to direct nursing care. Nurses need to assist clients in using the proper language to report pain symptoms.

Establishment of a therapeutic relationship is the foundation for effective nursing care of the client experiencing pain. Clients who trust their nurses to be there, to listen, and to act are the ones who are most likely to be comfortable. See the Uncovering the Evidence display on page 1057.

CLIENT EDUCATION Client education regarding pain management begins with defining pain, identifying the probable causes, introducing clients to pain assessment tools, and allowing clients to choose the tool they would like to use. The importance of talking to health care providers about the client's pain and using a preventive approach to pain management must also be emphasized. Provide written information to reinforce verbal explanations. Teach the importance of around-the-clock dosing instead of prn administration of analgesic medications. Refer to the Client Teaching checklist on page 1058.

When a client is to be discharged from a health care facility, discharge teaching should include pain management information with specific guidelines:
General overview of pain
- Definition
- Cause and contributing factors
- Pain assessment, including use of assessment tools
- Importance of preventive approach
- Family involvement

Pharmacologic pain management

- Overview of drug management
- Addiction, dependence, and tolerance
- Respiratory depression
- Communicating with health care providers about pain
- Controlling accompanying symptoms (e.g., constipation, nausea)

Nonpharmacologic pain management

- Importance of strategies
- Review of past experience with nonpharmacologic methods
- Demonstration of specific techniques

Both nonpharmacologic and pharmacologic interventions can be effective in caring for clients with pain. In some cases of mild pain, nonpharmacologic techniques may be the primary intervention, with medication available as "backup." In cases of moderate to severe pain, nonpharmacologic techniques can be an effective adjunctive or complementary treatment.

HPNA POSITION STATEMENT ON PAIN

The HPNA supports the provision of appropriate pain management for patients in all clinical settings. It is the position of the HPNA board of directors that:

- All people, including vulnerable populations such as cognitively impaired, infants, children, and the elderly, facing progressive, life-limiting illness have the right to optimal pain relief.
- All health care providers have an obligation to believe the patient's report of pain.
- Pain assessment and management should incorporate principles of cultural sensitivity as well as patients' values and beliefs.
- All health care professionals caring for patients with progressive, life-threatening illnesses need to acquire and utilize current knowledge and skills to implement appropriate pain management.
- Health care organizations need to adopt policies and procedures that address the assessment and pharmacologic and nonpharmacologic management of pain.
- Pain management should include, as appropriate, advanced technology.
- Pain assessments and management should be aligned with evidenced-based practice.
- The need for regulatory control of opioids must be balanced with access to opioids for all patients who need them.
- Pain management should be part of the education for all health care providers who are caring for patients with advanced, life-limiting illnesses.
- Health care professionals must advocate for their patients to ensure adequate pain relief.
- Uncontrolled pain should be considered an emergency, with all health care professionals taking responsibility to provide relief.
- Patients have the right to participate actively in decisions about their pain management.
- Families should be supported in their efforts to observe and relieve pain when appropriate.
- Hospice and palliative care programs should share their knowledge of pain management concepts with others in their communities.
- Use of placebos for pain management is inappropriate and unethical.

Reprinted with permission from Hospice and Palliative Nurses Association. (2008). *HPNA position statement: Pain management.* Pittsburgh, PA: Author.

UNCOVERING THE

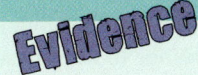

TITLE OF STUDY

"The Quality of Postoperative Pain Management from the Perspectives of Patients, Nurses and Patient Records"

AUTHORS

L. Gunningberg and E. Idvall

PURPOSE

To study the quality of postoperative pain management in a university hospital.

METHOD

This study compared client and nurse data using the Strategic and Clinical Quality Indicators in Postoperative Pain Management questionnaire in two nursing departments.

FINDINGS

Clients in general surgery experienced more pain than clients in thoracic surgery. In general surgery, the clients assessed their worst pain significantly higher than the nurse did. The clients who experienced more pain were less satisfied with the quality of their care and experienced higher pain intensity levels.

IMPLICATIONS

In both departments, areas identified as needing improvement were communication, action, trust, and environment. It is important to discuss what information the client needs as well as how and when it should be given.

Gunningberg, L., & Idvall, E. (2007). The quality of postoperative pain management from the perspectives of patients, nurses and patient records. *Journal of Nursing Management, 15*(7), 756–766.

SAMPLE OF THE NIC SYSTEM'S PAIN MANAGEMENT ACTIVITIES

- Use therapeutic communication strategies to acknowledge the pain experience and to convey acceptance of the client's response to pain.
- Determine the impact of the pain experience on quality of life (e.g., sleep, appetite, activity, cognition, mood, relationships, performance of job, and role responsibilities).
- Evaluate, with the client and the health care team, the effectiveness of past pain control measures that have been used.
- Utilize a developmentally appropriate assessment method that allows monitoring change in pain and assists in identifying actual and potential precipitating factors (e.g., flow sheet, daily diary).
- Consider the client's willingness to participate, ability to participate, preferences, support of significant others for method, and contraindications when selecting a pain relief strategy.
- Select and implement a variety of measures (e.g., pharmacologic; nonpharmacologic, such as biofeedback, TENS, hypnosis, relaxation, guided imagery, music therapy, distraction, play therapy, activity therapy, acupressure, hot and cold application, and massage; and interpersonal) to facilitate pain relief, as appropriate.
- Teach principles of pain management.
- Evaluate the effectiveness of the pain control measures used through ongoing assessment of the pain experience.
- Promote adequate rest and sleep to facilitate pain relief
- Utilize a multidisciplinary approach to pain management, when appropriate.

Bulechek, G., Butcher, H., & Dochterman, J. (2008). *Nursing interventions classification (NIC)* (5th ed.). St. Louis, MO: Elsevier.

Pharmacologic Pain Management

Principles for the care of clients experiencing pain follow:

- Assess the pain.
- Treat the contributing factors (pathology).
- Individualize the client's analgesic therapy.
- Choose the least invasive route of administration.
- Administer analgesics at regularly scheduled intervals (around-the-clock dosing) rather than on an as-needed (prn) basis.
- Keep clients in control of their own analgesia as much as possible.
- Titrate doses to provide maximum pain relief and minimum side effects.

Other general principles that guide practice are discussed in the following sections.

COMBINE ANALGESICS Combining analgesics on the basis of the World Health Organization's three-step analgesic ladder is imperative to provide effective pharmacologic intervention for clients with all types of pain. The use of adjuvant medication is recommended (Management of Cancer Pain Guideline Panel, 1994). **Adjuvant medications** are those drugs used to enhance the analgesic efficacy of opioids, to treat concurrent symptoms that exacerbate pain, and to provide independent analgesia for specific types of pain. Adjuvant medication (medication without intrinsic analgesic properties) is often helpful in treating chronic pain. Adjuvant drugs include anticonvulsants, antidepressants, and sedatives.

✓ CLIENT TEACHING CHECKLIST

Pain Management Information

- Help clients understand the importance of effective pain management. Explain the outcomes of unrelieved pain.
- Teach at the client's level of comprehension. Assess literacy level.
- Respect the client's cultural beliefs related to pain.
- Correct any misconceptions about the use of opioid analgesics. Instruct the client about the low risk for addiction when these medications are used for pain relief.
- Instruct the client on the use of complementary methods for relieving pain, including massage, application of heat and cold, and imagery.

For example, gabapentin (Neurontin) is one anticonvulsant useful in treating older clients experiencing chronic pain (Boswell & Cole, 2006). Education for clients taking adjuvant medication must explain the need to continue to take the analgesic drug with the adjuvant medication. Table 35-5 lists some common adjuvant medications used in pain management.

MAINTAIN THERAPEUTIC SERUM LEVELS Currently, many prescribing practitioners use "as needed" or "prn" range orders for opioid analgesics for the management of acute pain (Boswell & Cole, 2006). Range orders provide safe and flexible dosing adjustments based on the client's response to treatment. Historically, the use of as-needed orders for pain management has caused the undertreatment of pain because prescribers have failed to order adequate doses at frequent intervals, and nurses administer inadequate doses. In an effort to provide clinical guidelines that address the use of as-needed orders, the American Society for Pain Management Nursing (ASPMN) and the APS (2004) issued

TABLE 35-5 Adjuvant Medications for Pain Management

MEDICATION	TYPE OF PAIN	EFFECTS
Tricyclic antidepressants (amitriptyline, doxepin, imipramine, trazodone)	Neuropathic pain frequently described as dull, aching, or throbbing	• Mood elevation, enhancement of opioid analgesia, direct analgesic effects • Anticholinergic side effects: dry mouth, constipation, urinary retention
Anticonvulsants (carbamazepine, clonazepam, phenytoin)	Neuropathic pain frequently described as sharp shooting, burning, or lancinating	• Suppresses the spontaneous neuronal firing, which causes this type of pain
Corticosteroids (dexamethasone, prednisone)	Pain due to cerebral or spinal cord edema or pain in peripheral nerves caused by perineural edema	• Mood elevation, strong anti-inflammatory activity, appetite stimulation
Antihistamine (hydroxyzine)	Pain or nausea in the anxious client	• Relief of complicating symptoms, including anxiety, insomnia, nausea, and pruritus
Neuroleptic (methotrimeprazine)	Alternative analgesic for clients who are opioid-tolerant or have opioid-limiting side effects, especially constipation	• Antiemetic and anxiolytic • This is the one phenothiazine to date that has demonstrated analgesic properties: methotrimeprazine 15 mg IM was found to be equivalent to morphine 10 mg IM
Psychostimulants (dextroamphetamine, methylphenidate)	Continued pain with opioid-induced sedation	• Improves opioid analgesia and decreases sedation

Data from Macintyre, P., & Shug, S. (2007). *Acute pain management: a practical guide* (3rd ed.). St. Louis, MO: Elsevier.

▼ **SAFETY FIRST** ▼

Placebos should not be used by any route of administration in the assessment and management of pain in any client regardless of age or diagnosis.

a consensus statement regarding support for safe medication practice and the appropriate use of prn range opioid analgesic orders in pain management. "Evidence-based clinical practice guidelines support the need for individual titration of the dose of opioid analgesics" (ASPMN & APS, 2004, p. 1); see the Safety First display.

Nurses should base their decisions regarding implementation of range orders on client assessment and knowledge of the prescribed drug, such as time of onset, peak effect, duration of action, and side effects. The client's response to the analgesic dose interval should be evaluated, documented, and communicated by the nurse. An appropriate use of opioids should be individually tailored based on a sound working knowledge of analgesic pharmacology, appropriately timed reassessments and adjustments, and client response.

CHOOSE APPROPRIATE ROUTES OF ADMINISTRATION

Available routes of administration play an important role in the choice of pain management technique. In general, the oral route (PO) of administration is preferred because it is the most convenient and cost-effective. When the oral route is not feasible, other routes (such as rectal or transdermal) can be used to administer analgesics.

The rectal route is effective when clients are nauseated and vomiting or when they are NPO. Suppositories of morphine, hydromorphone, and oxymorphone are available. Contraindications to rectal administration include diarrhea, lesions of the rectum or anus, or an immunosuppressed status. The transdermal route bypasses GI absorption but has a slow onset and a slow decline in blood level after the patch is removed.

With continuing documentation of unreliable absorption of intramuscular (IM) injections of opioids, the prudent approach is to switch to subcutaneous or intravascular administration. Continuous infusions are possible by either intravenous (IV) or subcutaneous methods. See Table 35-6 on page 1060 for an overview of administration routes; see Chapter 30 for a complete discussion of medication administration routes.

NONSTEROIDAL ANTI-INFLAMMATORY DRUGS

The nonopioid class of pharmacologic agents consists of a group of medications classified as nonsteroidal anti-inflammatory drugs (NSAIDs). NSAIDs attenuate prostaglandin production by inhibiting cyclooxygenase (COX) enzymes. Prostaglandin, a chemical present in most body tissue, is released with cell trauma, causing edema and erythema. NSAIDs block COX, an enzyme with two isoforms (COX-1 and COX-2), and prevent the production of prostaglandin and other substances, provid-

ing analgesia, antipyresis, and anti-inflammation. COX-1 is normally present in the GI tract, kidneys, and platelets, and it catalyzes the synthesis of prostaglandins in the GI mucosa and platelets. The GI side effects of oral NSAIDs, addressed in Table 35-6, probably result from the drugs' inhibition of COX-1 activity and the subsequent protective effects of prostaglandins on GI mucosa. NSAIDs are useful in treating mild to moderate pain, especially painful conditions involving inflammation. NSAIDs are usually classified by their chemical structure. See the accompanying display on classes of NSAIDs.

The widespread use of NSAIDs makes them the culprit in many adverse drug effects. Aspirin, an over-the-counter NSAID, is used frequently to treat mild pain; however, some clients such as asthmatics may have aspirin hypersensitivity. Hypertensive clients also may experience adverse effects with some NSAIDs; for example, ibuprofen may cause an intermediate elevation in blood pressure, naproxen may cause a significant elevation in blood pressure, and celecoxib may hamper the healing of broken bones.

NSAIDs are also subject to the **ceiling effect** (as the dose of medication is increased above a certain level, the analgesic effect remains the same), and only the adverse effects continue to increase. For example, acetaminophen is relatively easy on the GI tract and does not affect platelet aggregation, but large doses over time have caused liver damage, with extreme overdoses causing liver failure.

Educate clients and their families regarding the ceiling effect because they may feel that "If a little helps some, then more is better." The risk for significant side effects and adverse reactions is increased by this misunderstanding.

OPIOID ANALGESICS

Opioids remain the gold standard for managing moderate to severe pain (Patterson, 2008). The opioids and NSAIDs offer pain relief through different mechanisms. For example, the opioids act on several sites in the CNS rather than on the peripheral nervous system, as do the NSAIDs. Opioids alter the release of neurotransmitters; therefore, pain transmission is interrupted at several sites in the CNS. The result is an altered perception of and response to pain.

The opioid analgesics fall into three classes: pure opioid agonists, partial agonists, and **mixed agonist-antagonists** (compounds that block opioid effects on one receptor type while producing opioid effects on a second receptor type). Pure agonists are those that produce a maximal response

CLASSES OF NSAIDS

- Propionic: Ibuprofen, naproxen, ketoprofen
- Acetic: Indomethacin, sulindac, tolmetin
- Salicylic: Aspirin, sodium salicylate, salicylamide
- Anthranilic: Phenylbutazone, piroxicam
- Pyrrolopyrroles: Ketorolac, etodolac
- COX-2 inhibitors: Celecoxib, valdecoxib

TABLE 35-6 Advantages and Disadvantages of Selected Medication Administration Routes

INTERVENTION	ADVANTAGES	DISADVANTAGES
Oral NSAIDs	• Useful for a wide variety of mild to moderate pain. • Widely available, some over the counter. • Additive analgesia when combined with opioids and other modalities. • Can be administered by client or family. • Some are inexpensive.	• Ceiling effect to analgesia. • Side effects, especially gastritis and renal toxicity, can be serious. • May risk bleeding in severely thrombocytopenic clients. • Only one NSAID (ketorolac) is available now for parenteral administration. • Many are expensive. • Contraindicated in high-risk clients with congestive heart failure and coronary artery disease. • Drug interactions: β-blockers, loop diuretics, angiotensin-converting enzyme (ACE) inhibitors, anticoagulants.
Oral opioids	• Effective for both localized and generalized pain. • Ceiling to analgesic effectiveness imposed only by side effects. • Multiple drug choices in the class. • Sedative and anxiolytic properties useful in some acute treatment settings. • Can be administered by client or family. • Some are inexpensive. • Long-acting, controlled-release forms are available.	• Side effects may limit analgesic effectiveness. • Prescription of these substances is regulated. • Stigma or fears associated with use.
Transdermal opioids (fentanyl)	• Long duration of action (48–72 h) from single patch. • Allows use of a strong opioid (fentanyl) in outpatient settings for some clients who have not tolerated morphine and related drugs. • Many clients find them easy to use. • Provides continuous administration of an opioid without use of needles or pumps. • Can be administered by client or family.	• Side effects may not be as quickly reversible as in oral administration. • Mild erythema at site. • Difficult to modify dosage rapidly. • Relatively slow onset of action. • Requires additional short-acting medicine for breakthrough pain. • Expensive.
Rectal opioids	• Relatively easy-to-use alternative route when the oral route is unavailable. • Other opioid suppositories available for morphine-intolerant clients. • Can be administered by client or family. • Less expensive than subcutaneous or intravenous (IV) infusions.	• Not widely accepted by clients or families. • Side effects may limit analgesic effectiveness. • Relatively slow onset of action. • Contraindicated if low white blood cell or platelet count (risks of infection, bleeding).
Subcutaneous infusion	• Can provide rapid pain relief without IV access. • Morphine and hydromorphone are the preferred drugs for this route when administered in the home.	• Only a limited volume of infusate can be administered (e.g., 2–4 mL/h). • Induration or irritation at infusion site may be a complication. • Requires skilled nursing and pharmacy support.

(Continues)

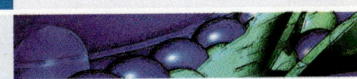

TABLE 35-6 (Continued)

INTERVENTION	ADVANTAGES	DISADVANTAGES
	• When used in patient-controlled analgesia (PCA) mode, allows for rapid individual dose titration and provides sense of control for client.	• Often requires expensive drug infusion pump and recurring charges for disposables.
IV infusion	• Can provide rapid pain relief. • Almost all opioids can be given by this route. • Not limited to infusate volumes. • When used in PCA mode, allows for rapid individual dose titration and provides sense of control for client.	• Infection and infiltration of IV lines are potential complications. • Requires skilled nursing and pharmacy support. • Often requires expensive drug infusion pump and recurring charges for disposables.
Epidural, intrathecal, and intracerebral ventricular routes	• Effective for moderate-to-severe acute pain expected to last 24 hours (e.g., acute post-operative pain). • Usually requires less analgesia and promotes early ambulation following surgery. • Postoperatively better pain relief at rest and after coughing, less nausea and vomiting, and improved bowel function and mental status.	• Tolerance may occur sooner than with oral or rectal administration. • Infection at catheter site can produce meningitis and/or epidural abscess. • Contraindicated in presence of acute spinal cord compression. • Requires careful monitoring, especially when therapy begins and when doses are increased.
Regional neurolytic blocks	• Effective for pain relief with certain diagnoses (e.g., pancreatic cancer). • May be useful for movement-related and abdominal visceral pain that is refractory to drug therapy. • Can allow dosage (and side effect) reduction of systemic drugs for localized pain.	• Risk of postural hypotension, bowel and bladder incontinence, and limb weakness. • Procedure is irreversible. • Requires special expertise. • Expenses for specialized care and operating room costs.

Data from Boswell, M. V., & Cole, B. C. (2006). *Weiner's pain management: a practical guide for clinicians* (7th ed.). Boca Raton, FL: CRC Press; Campbell, W., Nicholas, M., & Breivik, H. (2008). *Clinical pain management practice & procedures* (2nd ed.). New York: Oxford University Press, USA; Spies, K., Rehberg, Bl., Schug, S., Jaehnichen, G., & Harper, S, (2008). *Pocket guide pain management*. Warren, IL: Springer; Stanton-Hicks, M. (2009). *The Cleveland Clinic guide to pain management*. New York: Kaplan.

from cells when they bind to the cells' opioid receptor sites. Morphine (the gold standard against which all other opioids are measured), fentanyl, methadone, hydromorphone, and codeine are pure agonists. Meperidine, although classified as a pure agonist, is not recommended except in clients with a true allergy to all other narcotics, because of its neurotoxicity. Meperidine produces clinical analgesia for only 2.5 to 3.5 hours when given intramuscularly in adults. In pediatric clients receiving intravenous meperidine, analgesia may last for only 1.5 to 2.0 hours. Opioids can be safely administered to an elderly client by starting with a lower dose, monitoring for drug-drug interactions, and titrating doses upward cautiously, depending on the client's response (Patterson, 2008). Caution should be used when administering opioids to elderly clients with decreased blood volume or with renal impairment.

Meperidine should be reserved for very brief courses in otherwise healthy clients who have demonstrated an unusual reaction (e.g., local histamine release at the infusion site) or allergic response during treatment with other opioids such as morphine or hydromorphone (Macintyre & Shug, 2007).

Unlike the NSAIDs, pure agonist opioids are not subject to the ceiling effect. As the dosage is increased, there is increasing pain relief, with the only limiting factor being the degree of side effects, particularly respiratory depression and constipation. Many of the analgesic medications (especially opioids) can cause the unwanted effect of constipation. See the accompanying Client Teaching Checklist on page 1062.

Other side effects that occur frequently in clients on opioid medications are pruritus and nausea, but the degree to which they are present from each medication varies among individuals. Clients must be instructed regarding these *normal* responses to opioids and informed that it does not mean that they are allergic to them. A true allergy to opioids would be indicated by a rash or hives that start after receiving the opioid, a local histamine release at the site of

✓ CLIENT TEACHING CHECKLIST

Preventing Opioid-Induced Constipation

- Eat high-fiber foods.
- Drink 8–10 glasses of fluid per day.
- Eat foods that previously helped relieve constipation.
- Increase physical activity, such as walking.
- Consume a hot beverage about 30 minutes prior to the planned time for a bowel movement.
- Use laxatives or stool softeners only as advised by the health care provider.

infusion, or anaphylaxis. Clients also need to know that the pruritus and nausea generally subside after 4 to 5 days of opioid therapy. In the meantime, an antihistamine such as diphenhydramine or hydroxyzine may be used for pruritus, and an antiemetic such as metoclopramide or trimethobenzamide can be used to treat the nausea. Almost all medications used to treat side effects have their own side effect of sedation; thus, there is the possibility of a cumulative effect of severe sedation.

Mixed agonist-antagonist opioids are believed to be subject to the ceiling effect for pain relief as well as a ceiling effect for respiratory depression. Mixed agonist-antagonist opioids activate one opioid receptor type while simultaneously blocking another type. Butorphanol, pentazocine, and nalbuphine are the most frequently used in pain management.

PATIENT-CONTROLLED ANALGESIA (PCA)
Patient-controlled analgesia (PCA) is a method to relieve pain through self-administration of analgesics (usually opioids, e.g., morphine) by a client using a programmable pump connected to a subcutaneous, intravenous, or epidural catheter. The Joint Commission and the Institute for Safe Medication Practices recommend safe practices for PCA use that include standardized client education on PCA usage; standardized order sets, drugs, and drug concentrations used for PCA; annual competency assessment for nurses; and signatures of two nurses when therapy is initiated and with all dosing changes. See the accompanying display on page 1063 for a sample of NIC activities related to the use of PCA. PCA is used in health care facilities and in the home to manage postoperative or cancer pain. The client is taught how to operate the PCA by pressing the button of the PCA pump to administer the proper bolus (amount of analgesic received when pressing the button) dose of the prescribed analgesic as demanded. A recent study evaluated the effects of analgesic quality provided by a PCA intervention on pain management; the results showed a significant correlation between pain cognition and analgesic quality (Yeh, Yang, Chen, & Tsou, 2007).

The PCA system is designed for client initiation. Although PCA is contraindicated in sedated and confused clients, nurse-activated PCA or PCA by proxy such as a family member or friend is a controversial practice because of the possibility of oversedation. The ASPMN, the Joint Commission, and the Institute for Safe Medication Practices do not support the practice of PCA by proxy; however, the ASPMN does support the practice of authorized agent–controlled analgesia in a variety of client settings when the agency has in place clear guidelines that ensure safe use of the therapy (Wuhrman et al., 2007). The Joint Commission has guidelines that require those health care agencies that allow nurse-activated PCA or PCA by proxy to maintain strict policies, with documented education of family members and other caregivers who administer the PCA by proxy.

Nurses collaborate with the prescribing practitioner, the client, and the client's family members to ensure that PCA orders are clear and complete. Each order must address the analgesic to be used, route of administration, bolus dose, lockout interval, maximum dose limit, the loading dose (first bolus dose), and the basal infusion rate (continuous infusion rate). The lockout interval is the time period during which pressing the button more than once results in only one dose of analgesic received. The maximum dose limit is the amount of analgesic that can be received within a certain period of time (e.g., 1 hour). To safely administer PCA, nurses should maintain a patent catheter, instill the analgesic solution into the PCA chamber, and program the PCA pump according to the prescribed parameters; see Procedure 35-1.

EPIDURAL ANALGESIA
Epidural analgesia has been used traditionally for the administration of opioid analgesics for chronic intractable pain and for chemotherapy. Epidural catheters are placed by anesthesia providers into the epidural space. The epidural space is a *potential* space, without free-flowing fluid, between the walls of the vertebral canal and the dura mater of the spinal cord, and it contains vessels, fat, and nerves. Analgesics are administered through a needle that has been placed into the epidural space; a catheter may be threaded through the needle and taped into place for continuous use to manage acute pain, usually 2 to 4 days (Macintyre, Rowbotham, & Walker, 2008). Epidural analgesic may be administered by bolus, continuous infusion, and patient-controlled epidural analgesia (PCEA).

Nursing management of epidural infusions requires strict aseptic technique to prevent infection; check the external dressing around the catheter site for dampness or discharge and the catheter for breaks. An epidural catheter should be secured carefully to the outside skin (if it is not connected to an implanted reservoir) to prevent displacement of the catheter. To initiate an infusion, connect the catheter to an infusion pump, a port, or a reservoir, or cap it off for bolus injections. Epidural infusions are always administered through electronic infusion devices for proper rate control; the epidural catheter should be clearly labeled to reduce the risk of accidental IV injections, and the infusion tubing should be changed every 24 hours or according to agency policy. Monitor the client for signs of respiratory

NIC SAMPLE ACTIVITIES FOR PATIENT-CONTROLLED ANALGESIA (PCA) ASSISTANCE

- Ensure that the client is not allergic to the analgesic to be administered.
- Teach client and family to monitor pain intensity, quality, and duration; respiration rate; and blood pressure.
- Validate that the client can use a PCA device and is able to communicate, comprehend explanations, and follow directions.
- Teach client and family members how to use the PCA device, to administer an appropriate bolus loading dose of analgesic, and to set an appropriate basal infusion rate on the PCA device.
- Assist the client and family member to set the appropriate lockout interval on the PCA device and demand doses on the PCA device.
- Consult with client, family members, and prescribing practitioner to adjust lockout interval, basal rate, and demand dosage, according to the client's responsiveness.
- Teach client how to titrate doses up or down, depending on the respiratory rate, pain intensity, and pain quality.
- Teach client and family members the action and side effects of pain-relieving agents.
- Document client's pain, amount and frequency of drug dosing, and response to pain treatment on a pain flow sheet.
- Consult with clinical pain experts for a client who is having difficulty achieving pain control.

Bulechek, G., Butcher, H., & Dochterman, J. (2008). *Nursing interventions classification (NIC)* (5th ed.). St. Louis, MO: Elsevier.

depression (see the accompanying display on page 1064) and untoward reactions such as pruritus, nausea, and vomiting. Notify the prescribing practitioner of any signs or symptoms of infection or pain at the insertion site.

Epidural pain management is used for oncology clients when other methods of pain control are insufficient or poorly tolerated (D'Arcy, 2008). An epidural solution usually contains a combination of drugs such as a local anesthetic (bupivacaine) and an opioid (fentanyl or morphine). All drugs administered epidurally should be preservative-free to avoid damage to neural tissue and fluids.

ADDICTION, TOLERANCE, AND PHYSICAL DEPENDENCE
As a result of fears of addiction, family caregivers tend to undermedicate their relative's pain. Family and client

education about addiction and pain medication should be a priority for those receiving opioid therapy. Addiction is a biological and psychosocial dependence on a substance. It is a chronic neurobiologic disease characterized by a craving for the substance, compulsive use, lack of control over the drug, and continued use despite harm (D'Arcy, 2008). Tolerance can occur after repeated administration of an opioid analgesic, when a specific dose loses its effectiveness and the client requires larger and larger doses to produce the same level of analgesia. The first indication of tolerance is decreased duration of action, then decreased analgesia. If this pattern is noted in clients with continuing opioid needs, the analgesic dose needs to be titrated higher immediately. Physical dependence is the reaction of the body, commonly known as withdrawal syndrome, to abrupt discontinuation of an opioid after repeated use.

RESPIRATORY DEPRESSION
Titrating opioid analgesics to obtain optimal pain management with minimal side effects is a difficult task. See the accompanying display for a list of risk factors predisposing to respiratory depression in clients receiving appropriate dosages of sedatives or opioid analgesics. This list should be used to identify clients of all ages who require increased vigilance, possible cardiac and pulse oximetry (determination of oxygen saturation of arterial blood) monitoring, and frequent assessment when taking opioid analgesics. It is not to be construed as a reason for denying the client adequate pain management. When caring for clients receiving opioid analgesics, the nurse should periodically identify the presence and intensity of risk factors.

LOCAL ANESTHESIA
Local anesthetics are effective for pain management in a variety of settings. Topical analgesics produce effective analgesia with reduced systemic drug levels, a factor particularly beneficial to young and older clients. Topical analgesics differ from transdermal delivery systems (see Table 35-6) in that transdermals deliver systemic rather than local effects. Commonly used topical analgesics include capsaicin cream 0.75%, lidocaine/prilocaine (EMLA), and the 5% lidocaine patch. Topical anesthetics are available for teething, sore throats, denture pain, laceration repair, and intravenous catheter insertions. EMLA cream is a mixture of local anesthetics, combining prilocaine and lidocaine. It produces complete anesthesia for at least 60 minutes when topically applied to intact skin.

Another topical anesthetic, TAC, is available for anesthesia during closure of lacerations. It is a combination of tetracaine 0.5%, adrenaline 1:2000, and cocaine 11.8% in a normal saline solution that can be applied directly to the open wound surface in place of local anesthetic infiltration with a needle. This allows pain-free cleansing of the laceration as well as suturing. Because both adrenaline (epinephrine) and cocaine cause vasoconstriction, TAC cannot be used in areas supplied by end-arteriolar blood supply such as digits, the ears, or the nose. It also is contraindicated on burned or abraded skin because this could lead to increased systemic absorption of cocaine and tetracaine, thus placing

RISK FACTORS PREDISPOSING TO RESPIRATORY DEPRESSION WITH USE OF SEDATIVES OR OPIOID ANALGESICS

NEUROLOGICAL IMPAIRMENT
- Cerebral palsy
- Altered level of consciousness

RESPIRATORY COMPROMISE
- Thoracic skeletal deformities (e.g., scoliosis, kyphosis, contracture)
- Neurodegenerative disorders (e.g., muscular dystrophy, tuberous sclerosis, Werdnig-Hoffman disease, myasthenia gravis)
- Pulmonary disease (e.g., cystic fibrosis, reactive airway disease, bronchopulmonary dysplasia, chronic obstructive lung disease)
- Thoracic or high abdominal incision
- Abdominal distension

METABOLIC ALTERATION
- Liver dysfunction or failure
- Metabolic disease
- Sepsis

RENAL COMPROMISE
- Kidney dysfunction or failure
- Single kidney
- Hypovolemia
- Urine output 1 mL/kg/h in children, 30 mL/h in adults, or elevated blood urea nitrogen (BUN) or creatinine

OTHER
- Obesity (when drug is ordered on actual weight rather than estimated lean body weight)
- Increasing sedation
- Agitation
- Preverbal or nonverbal client

CONCURRENT ADMINISTRATION OF OTHER NARCOTICS OR SEDATIVES
- Opioid analgesics
- Sedatives, hypnotics, and tranquilizers
- Anticonvulsants
- Antihistamines
- Psychotropics

the client at risk for seizures. The 5% lidocaine patch reduces pain and may allow tapering of concomitant analgesic therapy in clients with neuropathic pain, such as diabetic polyneuropathy.

Treatment of Neuropathic Pain

Neuropathic pain is often refractory to treatment with NSAIDs and opioids. When increasing doses of opioids are ineffective in controlling postoperative pain, an immediate search for the underlying cause should begin, and the diagnosis of neuropathic pain should be considered. Once diagnosed, the focus of treatment is optimizing functional abilities.

A trial of a tricyclic antidepressant is frequently the first step for a client who describes dull, aching, or throbbing pain. Amitriptyline is often the drug of choice because it has been the most widely studied (Spies et al., 2008). This class of medications is useful in pain management as a result of:

- Mood elevation
- Potentiation of opioid analgesia
- Direct analgesic effects

Clients with neuropathic pain often have significant sleep deprivation. Amitriptyline's action and the side effect of drowsiness improve the client's ability to fall asleep and to sleep for longer periods. Amitriptyline must be started at very low doses, especially in children, the debilitated, or elderly clients, then increased slowly. It should be administered at bedtime to promote sleep and to minimize falls resulting from orthostatic hypotension. The onset of analgesic effects occurs within 1 to 2 weeks, and maximal effect can be seen in 4 to 6 weeks.

Anticonvulsants are often tried first for clients with burning, sharp, shocking, shooting, or lancinating (piercing or stabbing) pain. Carbamazepine is often the drug of choice, with other possibilities being clonazepam or phenytoin. These medications suppress spontaneous neuronal firing that leads to the lancinating pain of nerve injury. Carbamazepine may cause transient bone marrow suppression and requires regular monitoring of serum drug levels, blood counts, and liver function. It should be avoided if possible in clients with any form of bone marrow suppression (e.g., those undergoing chemotherapy, radiation therapy, or taking immunosuppressants posttransplantation).

Corticosteroid effects include mood elevation, antiinflammatory effects, and appetite stimulation. Corticosteroids are effective in reducing the neuropathic pain caused by pressure on nerves both centrally and peripherally.

The two corticosteroids most frequently used in pain management are dexamethasone and prednisone.

If muscle spasms are a major contributor to the client's discomfort, then baclofen can be tried for its antispasmodic effect. This is particularly effective for clients with spinal cord injuries or upper motor neuron dysfunction, including cerebral palsy.

For many individuals, the use of nonpharmacologic methods enhances pain relief. These nonpharmacologic strategies are often used in combination with medication. Complementary and alternative methods are being used with increasing frequency to treat pain. The use of such strategies is often influenced by the client's culture. The accompanying Respecting Our Differences display lists some commonly used complementary and alternative treatment approaches.

In some cases of mild pain, nonpharmacologic techniques may be the primary intervention, with medication available as a backup. In cases of moderate to severe pain, nonpharmacologic techniques can be an effective adjunctive or complementary treatment.

Cognitive-Behavioral Interventions

An effective approach to pain management combines both pharmacologic and nonpharmacologic methods (Zwakhalen et al., 2006). Cognitive-behavioral interventions are designed to educate clients and to modify clients' attitudes and behaviors. These nonpharmacologic approaches are an important part of the multimodal approach to pain management and can be used in conjunction with appropriate analgesics. A major goal of these interventions is to help the client gain a sense of control over the pain. The effectiveness of selected therapies is outlined in Table 35-7 on page 1066.

DISTRACTION Distraction is a pain management strategy that focuses the client's attention on something other than

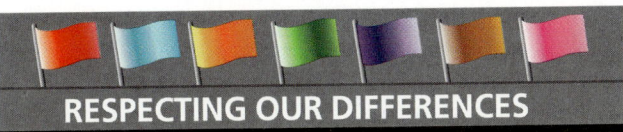

RESPECTING OUR DIFFERENCES

Complementary/Alternative Therapy

- Acupuncture or acupressure
- Application of heat or cold
- Focused breathing
- Herbal remedies
- Humor
- Hypnosis
- Imagery
- Massage
- Meditation
- Music
- Progressive muscle relaxation
- Tai chi
- Therapeutic touch
- Yoga

the pain and associated negative emotions. Children and adolescents seem to be particularly adept at using distraction. As many parents know, interactive games or listening to music can be powerful distraction techniques for children; they can also be effective for adults experiencing pain.

REFRAMING Reframing is a technique that teaches clients to monitor their negative thoughts and replace them with ones that are more positive. Teaching a client to view pain by expressing not "I can't stand this pain, it's never going away" but instead "I've had similar pain before, and it's gotten better" is an example of effective reframing.

RELAXATION TECHNIQUES Relaxation techniques (a variety of methods used to decrease anxiety and muscle tension), imagery (a strategy that uses mental images to assist with relaxation), and progressive muscle relaxation (a strategy in which muscles are alternately tensed and relaxed) are used to achieve both mental and physical relaxation. Physical relaxation leads to reduction of skeletal muscle tension; mental relaxation is used to alleviate anxiety.

BIOFEEDBACK Biofeedback training is another method that may be helpful for the client in pain, especially one who has difficulty relaxing muscles. Biofeedback is a process through which individuals learn to influence their physiological responses. Through biofeedback, clients can alter their pain experience.

CUTANEOUS STIMULATION Counterstimulation is the term used to identify techniques believed to activate the endogenous opioid and monoamine analgesia systems. These interventions are effective by decreasing swelling through cryotherapy (or cold applications), decreasing stiffness (heat applications), and increasing large-diameter nerve fiber input to block small-diameter pain fiber messages (cold, heat, pressure, vibration, or massage). Therapeutic heat and cold are effective pain management tools; they are readily available and easy to use. Both heat and cold can produce analgesia for pain. Heat therapy increases blood flow, increases tissue metabolism, decreases vasomotor tone, and increases the viscoelasticity of connective tissue, making it particularly effective in easing joint stiffness and pain. The use of heat as therapy should be closely monitored, as it can produce increased inflammation and edema.

Cold therapy exerts many benefits, including the following:

- Alleviates edema by reducing vascular flow
- Counteracts inflammation
- Reduces fever
- Diminishes muscle spasms
- Elevates pain threshold as a result of decreasing the velocity of nerve conduction

Application of cold is inappropriate for clients with cold intolerance, vascular insufficiency, and conditions aggravated by cold (e.g., Raynaud's phenomenon).

TRANSCUTANEOUS STIMULATION Transcutaneous stimulation is achieved through the use of transcutaneous

TABLE 35-7 Advantages and Disadvantages of Nonpharmacologic Therapies

INTERVENTION	ADVANTAGES	DISADVANTAGES
Relaxation, imagery, biofeedback, distraction, and reframing	• May decrease pain and anxiety without drug-related side effects. • Can be used as adjuvant therapy with most other modalities. • Can increase client's sense of control. • Most are inexpensive, require no special equipment, and are easily administered.	• Client must be motivated to use self-management strategies. • Requires professional time to teach interventions.
Client education	• Effective in improving ability to follow medical regimen and in decreasing pain. • Multiple teaching aids available. • Promotes self-care in pain treatment and management of side effects.	• Requires professional time to teach pain management regimens.
Psychotherapy, structured support, and hypnosis	• May decrease pain and anxiety for clients who have pain that is difficult to manage. • May increase client's coping skills.	• Requires skilled therapist.
Cutaneous stimulation (superficial heat, cold, and massage)	• May reduce pain, inflammation, or muscle spasm. • Can be used as adjuvant therapy with most other modalities. • Relatively easy to use. • Can be administered by clients or families. • Relatively low cost.	• Heat may increase bleeding and edema after acute injury. • Cold is contraindicated for use over ischemic tissues.
Transcutaneous electrical nerve stimulation (TENS)	• May provide pain relief without drug-related side effects. • Can be used as adjuvant therapy with most other modalities. • Gives client sense of control over pain.	• Requires skilled therapist to initiate therapy. • Potential risk of infection, bleeding.
Acupuncture	• May provide pain relief without side effects. • Can be used as adjuvant therapy with most other modalities.	• Requires skilled therapist.

Data from Boswell, M. V., & Cole, B. C. (2006). *Weiner's pain management: a practical guide for clinicians* (7th ed.). Boca Raton, FL: CRC Press; Campbell, W., Nicholas, M., & Breivik, H. (2008). *Clinical pain management practice & procedures* (2nd ed.). New York: Oxford University Press, USA; Macintyre, P., Rowbotham, D., & Walker, S. (2008). *Clinical pain management acute pain* (2nd ed.). New York: Oxford University Press, USA; Macintyre, P. & Shug, S. (2007). *Acute pain management: a practical guide* (3rd ed.). St. Louis: MO: Elsevier; Zwakhalen, S., Hamers, T., Abu-Saad, H. H., & Berger, M. (2006). Pain in elderly people with severe dementia: a systematic review of behavioural pain assessment tools. *BMC Geriatrics, 6*(3) Retrieved August 28, 2009 from http://www.biomedcentral.com/1471-2318/6/3.

electrical nerve stimulation, acupuncture, and acupressure. **Transcutaneous electrical nerve stimulation (TENS)** is a method of applying minute amounts of electrical stimulation to large-diameter nerve fibers via electrodes placed on the skin. Placement of the electrodes is determined by identifying which nerve innervates the painful area, then determining where that nerve is superficial, or where an anesthetic block would be placed to numb that nerve. Other modalities of pain management should *not* be abandoned while a trial of

TENS occurs. Although TENS can be successful, there are two major contraindications:

1. No electrodes should be placed in the area over or surrounding demand cardiac pacemakers.
2. No electrodes can be placed over the uterus of a pregnant woman.

Meissner (2009) tested the effectiveness of episodic TENS with clients experiencing postoperative pain.

The study suggests that TENS could be used for postoperative clients whose pain does not respond to conventional therapies or who experience adverse reactions to analgesic medications. Refer to Chapter 40 for an additional discussion of the use of TENS.

Acupuncture is another counterstimulation technique; it is performed by a specialist and accomplished by insertion of small solid needles into the skin and musculature at specific sites and at various depths. Acupressure accomplishes the same stimulation through cutaneous pressure over the selected site. Acupressure has been used in traditional Chinese medicine (TCM) since the fifth century BC. Firm pressure is applied by the fingers to specific acupuncture points on the body to unblock the *chi* (energy) (see Figure 35-7). When the client seeks acupressure, acupuncture, or TENS treatment, it is important to determine the efficacy of the present treatment regime.

ENCOURAGE EXERCISE Exercise is an important treatment for chronic pain because it strengthens weak muscles, helps mobilize joints, and helps restore balance and coordi-nation. Passive range of motion should not be used if it increases pain or discomfort. Immobilization is frequently used for clients with episodes of acute pain or to stabilize fractures; however, prolonged immobilization should be avoided whenever possible because it can lead to muscle atrophy and cardiovascular deconditioning. Researchers found that mobilization reduced pain, swelling, and stiffness; allowed clients to return to work sooner; and preserved range of joint motion better than rest (Gevirtz, 2008).

NUTRITION Dietary practices may affect pain by inhibiting biochemical events–associated inflammation. Some foods may actually trigger a painful episode, for example, red wine, cheese, citrus fruits, and cured meats often contribute to the onset of migraine headaches.

Other foods may help alleviate the pain associated with chronic diseases. For example, cherries and berries with red, blue, or black skins have high amounts of bioflavonoids, substances with anti-inflammatory properties. Table 35-8 on page 1068 lists foods with properties that produce a pain-reducing effect.

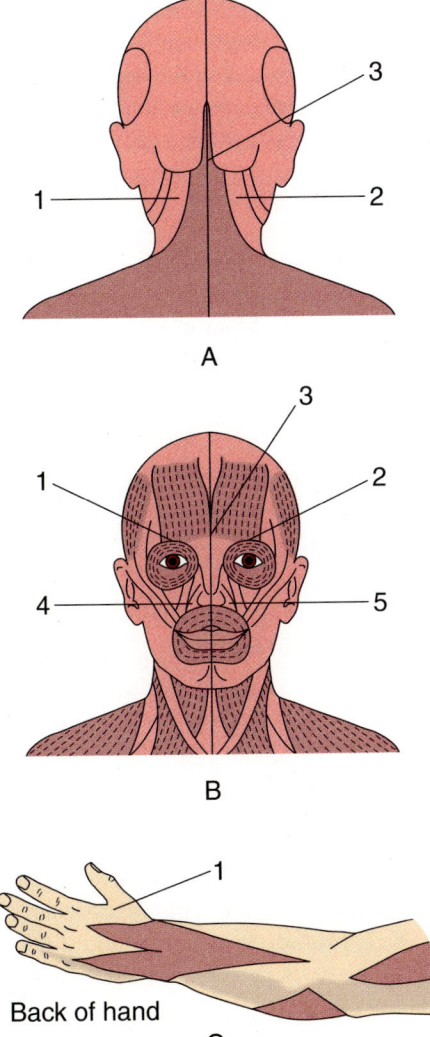

Point Locations

A. Point Location: 1 & 2
In the hollow, approximately 2 to 3 inches wide, between the two large vertical neck muscles below the base of the skull.

A. Point Location: 3
In the large hollow under the base of the skull in the center of the back of the head.

B. Point Location: 1 & 2
Where the bridge of the nose meets the inner ridge of the eyebrows, at the indentation of each inner eye socket.

B. Point Location: 3
Between the eyebrows where the bridge of the nose meets the forehead.

B. Point Location: 4 & 5
At the bottom of each cheekbone adjacent to the nose and in line with the pupil of each eye.

C. Point Location: 1
At the highest spot on the muscle in the webbing between the thumb and index finger. *(Do not press on pregnant individual.)*

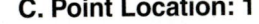

FIGURE 35-7 Acupressure Points for Headache Relief DELMAR/CENGAGE LEARNING

TABLE 35-8 Nutrition and Therapeutic Outcomes

NUTRIENTS	THERAPEUTIC EFFECT
Cherries and berries with black or red-blue skins (raspberries, blackberries)	Rich in bioflavonoids (anti-inflammatory substances); used in pain associated with arthritis and gout
Calcium, magnesium, zinc, and vitamins A, B-complex, C, D, and E (found in fruits, vegetables, legumes, whole grains, sunflower seeds, nuts)	Enhances the effects of analgesics
Fatty acid eicosapentaenoic acid (EPA), a component of certain fish oils (found in cold-water fish)	Inhibits formation of substances associated with inflammation
Amino acids (found in whole grains, starchy vegetables, dairy products, turkey)	Produces mild analgesia

Data from Balch, P. (2008). *Prescription for nutritional healing: The A-to-Z guide to supplements.* New York: Penguin; Nix, S. (2008). *Williams' basic nutrition & diet therapy* (12th ed.). St. Louis: Elsevier. Delmar/Cengage Learning

HERBALS Many herbs may be useful in mediating pain; see Table 35-9 on page 1069. Libster (2002) reports that the topical application of capsaicin cream (0.025%) four times a day for 4 weeks reduced trigger-point pain and increased grip strength in a study of 45 clients with fibromyalgia. As noted in the disclaimer in Table 35-9, nurses should instruct clients to consult with their prescribing practitioners before using any of the herbal remedies because of possible drug interactions.

ENVIRONMENT The environment can influence the perception of pain; therefore, changes in one's environment may reduce pain levels. Pet therapy, consisting of interactive sessions between clients and animals, is helpful for some people experiencing chronic pain. Horticultural therapy (treatment that includes looking at, touching, and growing plants) has several therapeutic benefits, including pain reduction, relaxation, and improved energy level. Participation in gardening can provide distraction from chronic pain. Music therapy may help ease pain by producing relaxation and providing distraction; see Chapter 31 for discussion of music therapy.

Many clients experiencing pain receive health care in their homes. The accompanying Community Considerations display on home care pain management offers recommendations for the home health nurse to use with clients experiencing pain.

EVALUATION

When trying to determine if an intervention works for a particular condition, search the literature and use the best evidence. Use a pain intensity rating scale to determine if the interventions are controlling the pain. Evaluating the efficacy of pain management interventions is ongoing, with client input throughout the process. Evaluation focuses primarily on the client's subjective reports.

Critical to the evaluative process is the complete documentation of pain assessment and client outcomes to facilitate regular reassessment and follow-up. Data should be documented regarding the appropriateness and effectiveness of pain management, including the client's comment, pain location, type of pain, intensity or duration of the pain (pain scale), pain behavior, quality of pain, pain patterns, the factors that increase pain, and the degree of relief due to an intervention within a defined time period.

Regular reassessment is an integral part of effective pain management. In addition to client self-report and nursing observation, family input is a valuable source of information for evaluating the effectiveness of care.

COMMUNITY CONSIDERATIONS

Pain Management Concepts in Home Care

- During each visit, evaluate the client's pain.
- Assess factors influencing effective pain management (e.g., motor, cognitive, and functional alterations).
- Teach clients and family members adjunctive therapies to be used with analgesics to decrease pain (i.e., encourage warm baths or compresses)
- Identify barriers that hinder pain control.
- Encourage the homebound client to use around-the-clock dosing of analgesics.

Data from Clark, M. A. (2008). *Community health nursing: advocacy for population health* (5th ed., p. 533). Upper Saddle River, NJ: Pearson Prentice Hall.

TABLE 35-9 Herbal Pain Management

NAME	PROPERTIES AND USE	CONTRAINDICATIONS AND SIDE EFFECTS
Bromelain (*Ananas comosus*)	• Anti-inflammatory, smooth muscle relaxant • Useful in pain related to oral surgery, sports injury, menstruation	• Nontoxic. • Well tolerated in long-term usage.
Cayenne pepper (*Capsicum frutescens*)	• Depletes substance P • Excites C fibers (repeated application to C fibers kills them) • For pain of osteoarthritis, neuropathy, post-herpetic neuralgia, shingles, fibromyalgia	• Avoid getting into eyes. • May cause brief burning or stinging sensation upon initial use. • Not for use in those allergic to ragweed.
Chamomile (*Matricaria chamomilla*)	• Anti-inflammatory, antispasmodic, analgesic for intestinal spasms • Infants' colic pain, stomachache, gastric ulcers	• Not for use if allergic to ragweed, asters, or chrysanthemums.
Feverfew (*Chrysanthemum parthenium*)	• Prevention of migraines • Rheumatoid arthritis	• Not for use with prescription headache drugs. • Not for use by pregnant and lactating women. • Capsule preferred (chewing leaves may cause mouth ulcers and loss of taste).
Green tea (*Camellia sinensis*)	• Produces antioxidant effects	• Avoid large quantities during pregnancy. • Limit to 1 cup per day for those with anxiety disorders or cardiac arrhythmias.
Kava (*Piper methysticum*)	• Produces relaxation • Treatment of insomnia	• Large amounts may be intoxicating. • Potential for abuse.
Lavender oil (*Lavandula angustifolia*)	• Analgesic, sedative, relaxant • Useful in treating headaches, muscular sprains, arthritis, menstrual cramps	• Warning: May cause extreme drowsiness.
Licorice (*Glycyrrhiza glabra*)	• Anti-inflammatory • Inactivates herpes simplex (for treatment of oral and genital herpes lesions) • Rheumatoid arthritis	• Long-term use can cause hypertension.
Valerian (*Valeriana officinalis*)	• Insomnia, muscle pain, menstrual cramps, intestinal cramps	• Do not use with alcohol or other CNS depressants.

This information is not intended to be a guide for self-medication or the treatment of others. Consult a prescribing practitioner with expertise in the use of herbs before using any herb for medicinal purposes.
Gladstar, R. (2008). *Rosemary Gladstar's herbal recipes for vibrant health*. North Adams, MA: Storey Books; Tierra, M., & Lust, J. (2008). *The natural remedy bible*. New York: Pocket Books.

REST AND SLEEP

Rest and sleep are fundamental components of well-being. All individuals require certain periods of calm and lesser activity so that their bodies can regain energy and rebuild stamina. The need for rest and sleep varies with age, devel- opmental level, health status, activity level, and cultural norms. Pain and impaired sleep are closely related in most people. Sleep disruption and/or deprivation can impair one's ability to think clearly and respond quickly; it can also compromise the cardiovascular and immune systems. Clients can sleep despite pain, especially those who have been living with pain for a long time and are exhausted (D'Arcy, 2008).

Rest refers to a state of relaxation and calmness, both mental and physical. Activity during rest periods can range from lying down to reading a book to taking a quiet walk. When discussing a client's rest patterns, the nurse should try to understand which activities and environments the client defines as restful.

Sleep refers to a state of altered consciousness during which an individual experiences minimal physical activity and a general slowing of the body's physiological processes. Sleep generally occurs in a periodic cycle and usually lasts for several hours at a time; disruptions in the usual sleep routine can be distressing to clients and will most likely impair sleep further. As a restorative function, sleep is necessary for physiological and psychological healing to occur. It is important for clients, their significant others, and health care providers to understand the normal sleep-wake cycle and how sleep affects mood and healing.

PHYSIOLOGY OF REST AND SLEEP

The cycles of wakefulness and sleep are controlled by centers in the brain and influenced by routines and environmental factors. An individual's biological clock also helps determine the specific cycles that will be followed for wakefulness and sleep.

Stages of Sleep

Electroencephalograph (EEG) patterns, eye movements, and muscle activity are used to identify stages of sleep. The stages of sleep are classified in two categories: non–rapid eye movement (NREM) and rapid eye movement (REM) sleep.

NURSING CARE PLAN

The Client with Chronic Pain

CASE PRESENTATION

Sally Atkinson, a 48-year-old woman, injured her back 3 years ago while lifting some boxes of paper at work. Since that time, she has had four epidural steroidal injections for the pain associated with two ruptured discs. Her pain has been intermittent, with some alleviation from the epidural injections. Her last epidural was 3 months ago. She arrives at the clinic stating, "I just don't know how I can go on like this. The pain has been tolerable until last night. I'm hurting so bad!" She is tearful and pacing, saying, "It hurts too much when I sit down."

ASSESSMENT

- Verbalization of pain (9 on a 0 to 10 pain intensity scale)
- Anxious (as evidenced by pacing and tears)
- Blood pressure 148/90
- Pulse strong and regular at 92
- Guarded movement
- History of chronic pain

NURSING DIAGNOSIS 1: *Chronic pain* related to muscle spasm and ruptured discs
NOC: Pain control
NIC: Pain management

EXPECTED OUTCOMES
The client will:

1. Practice selected noninvasive pain relief measures.
2. Report uncontrolled symptoms to health care professionals.
3. Have increased ability to perform daily activities as evidenced by walking 1 mile every day and being able to work.

(Continues)

NURSING CARE PLAN (Continued)

INTERVENTIONS/RATIONALES

1. Assess the client's level of pain, determining the intensity at its best and worst. Determines a baseline for future assessment.
2. Listen to the client while she discusses the pain; acknowledge the presence of pain. Acknowledging the client's pain decreases anxiety by communicating acceptance and validating the client's perceptions.
3. Discuss reasons why pain may be increased or decreased. Helps the client determine a cause-and-effect relationship between pain and specific activities.
4. Teach relaxation techniques such as deep breathing, progressive muscle relaxation, and imagery. Reduces skeletal muscle tension and anxiety, which potentiates the perception of pain.
5. Teach the client and family about treatment approaches (biofeedback, hypnosis, massage therapy, physical therapy, acupuncture, and exercise). Makes the client and family aware of the availability of treatment options.
6. Teach the client about the use of medication for pain relief. Provide accurate information to reduce fear of addiction. Lack of knowledge and fear may prohibit client from taking analgesic medications as prescribed.
7. Encourage the client to rest at intervals during the day. Fatigue increases the perception of pain.
8. Explain the relationship between chronic pain and depression. Knowledge decreases anxiety.

EVALUATION

Ms. Atkinson demonstrates the use of deep breathing and progressive muscle relaxation. After practicing relaxation techniques, she rates her pain as a 2 to 3 on the pain intensity scale. Ms. Atkinson is able to walk for 1 mile, but she still has a backache while sitting at her computer for extended periods of time.

NURSING DIAGNOSIS 2: *Anxiety* related to chronic pain
NOC: Anxiety reduction
NIC: Coping

EXPECTED OUTCOMES
The client will:

1. Verbalize an increase in psychological and physiological comfort level.
2. Demonstrate ability to cope with anxiety as evidenced by normal vital signs and a verbalized reduction in pain intensity.

INTERVENTIONS/RATIONALES

1. Assess the client's level of anxiety. To collect baseline data to be used in measuring a decrease or increase in anxiety level.
2. Speak slowly and calmly. Avoids escalating client's anxiety level and increases the likelihood of client's comprehension.
3. Encourage Ms. Atkinson to verbalize angry feelings. Anger is often a component of chronic conditions because of the prolonged sense of powerlessness. "Stuffing" anger can lead to increased anxiety.

EVALUATION

Ms. Atkinson rates her pain as a 2 to 3 on the pain intensity scale after practicing relaxation techniques. She voices concern that the pain will soon come back. After a relaxation session, her vital signs returned to normal limits. She denies feeling angry.

CONCEPT MAP

THE CLIENT WITH CHRONIC PLAN

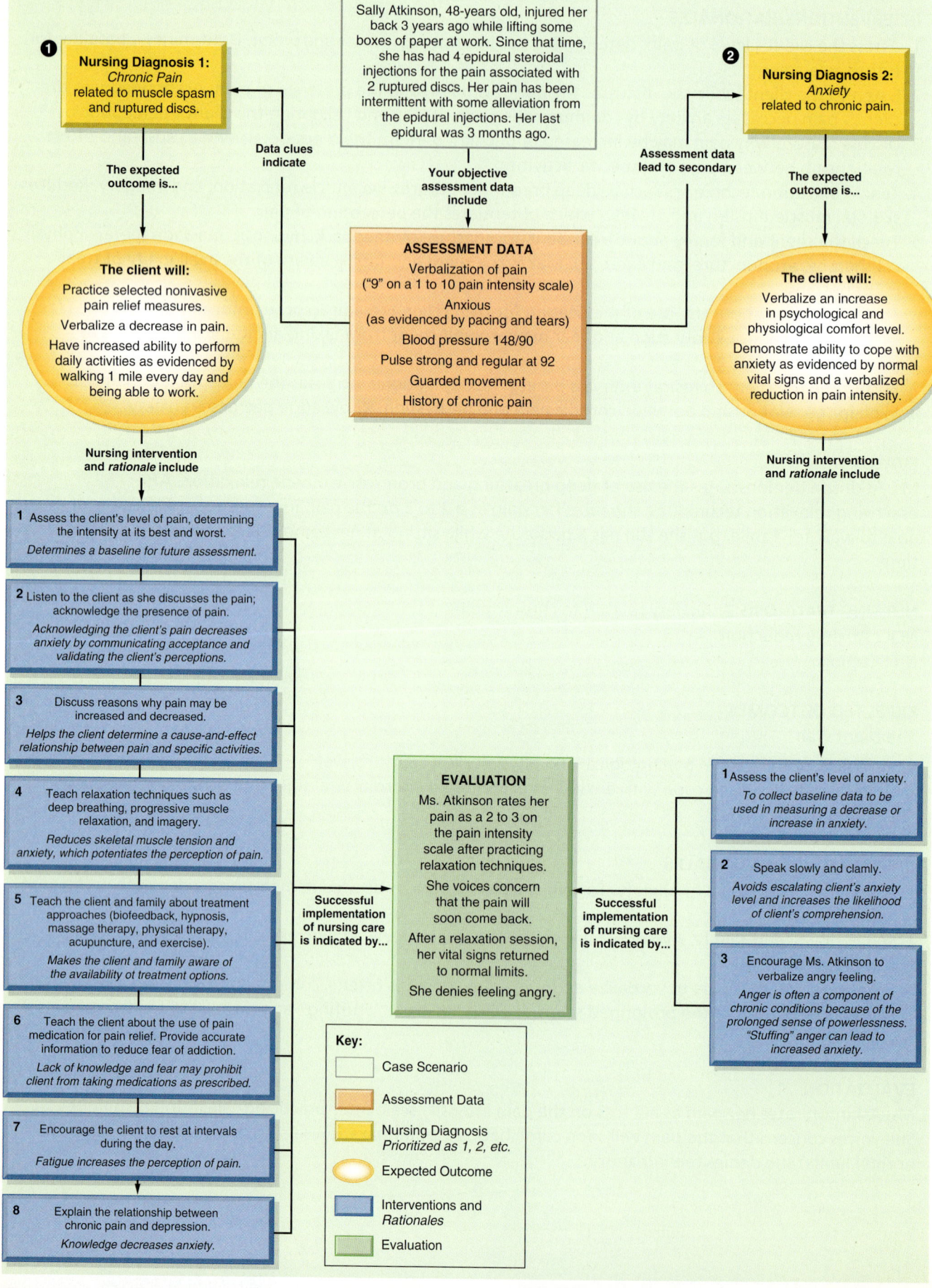

Case Scenario: Sally Atkinson, 48-years old, injured her back 3 years ago while lifting some boxes of paper at work. Since that time, she has had 4 epidural steroidal injections for the pain associated with 2 ruptured discs. Her pain has been intermittent with some alleviation from the epidural injections. Her last epidural was 3 months ago.

❶ Nursing Diagnosis 1: *Chronic Pain* related to muscle spasm and ruptured discs.

❷ Nursing Diagnosis 2: *Anxiety* related to chronic pain.

Data clues indicate

Your objective assessment data include

Assessment data lead to secondary

The expected outcome is...

The client will:
Practice selected nonivasive pain relief measures.
Verbalize a decrease in pain.
Have increased ability to perform daily activities as evidenced by walking 1 mile every day and being able to work.

ASSESSMENT DATA
Verbalization of pain ("9" on a 1 to 10 pain intensity scale)
Anxious (as evidenced by pacing and tears)
Blood pressure 148/90
Pulse strong and regular at 92
Guarded movement
History of chronic pain

The client will:
Verbalize an increase in psychological and physiological comfort level.
Demonstrate ability to cope with anxiety as evidenced by normal vital signs and a verbalized reduction in pain intensity.

Nursing intervention and *rationale* include

1 Assess the client's level of pain, determining the intensity at its best and worst.
Determines a baseline for future assessment.

2 Listen to the client as she discusses the pain; acknowledge the presence of pain.
Acknowledging the client's pain decreases anxiety by communicating acceptance and validating the client's perceptions.

3 Discuss reasons why pain may be increased and decreased.
Helps the client determine a cause-and-effect relationship between pain and specific activities.

4 Teach relaxation techniques such as deep breathing, progressive muscle relaxation, and imagery.
Reduces skeletal muscle tension and anxiety, which potentiates the perception of pain.

5 Teach the client and family about treatment approaches (biofeedback, hypnosis, massage therapy, physical therapy, acupuncture, and exercise).
Makes the client and family aware of the availability ot treatment options.

6 Teach the client about the use of pain medication for pain relief. Provide accurate information to reduce fear of addiction.
Lack of knowledge and fear may prohibit client from taking medications as prescribed.

7 Encourage the client to rest at intervals during the day.
Fatigue increases the perception of pain.

8 Explain the relationship between chronic pain and depression.
Knowledge decreases anxiety.

EVALUATION
Ms. Atkinson rates her pain as a 2 to 3 on the pain intensity scale after practicing relaxation techniques.
She voices concern that the pain will soon come back.
After a relaxation session, her vital signs returned to normal limits.
She denies feeling angry.

Successful implementation of nursing care is indicated by...

Nursing intervention and *rationale* include

1 Assess the client's level of anxiety.
To collect baseline data to be used in measuring a decrease or increase in anxiety.

2 Speak slowly and clamly.
Avoids escalating client's anxiety level and increases the likelihood of client's comprehension.

3 Encourage Ms. Atkinson to verbalize angry feeling.
Anger is often a component of chronic conditions because of the prolonged sense of powerlessness. "Stuffing" anger can lead to increased anxiety.

Key:
- Case Scenario
- Assessment Data
- Nursing Diagnosis *Prioritized as 1, 2, etc.*
- Expected Outcome
- Interventions and *Rationales*
- Evaluation

NREM SLEEP   With the onset of sleep, the heart rate and respiratory rate slow slightly and remain regular. This first phase of sleep is referred to as NREM sleep. NREM sleep consists of four different stages. As the client enters *stage 1 sleep*, there is a general slowing of EEG frequency but an appearance of wave spikes; the eyes tend to roll slowly from side to side, and muscle tension remains absent except in the facial and neck muscles. In adult clients with normal sleep patterns, stage 1 sleep usually lasts only 10 minutes or so. Stage 1 NREM sleep is of a very light quality, which means that during this stage a sleeper can be easily awakened.

Stage 2 sleep is still fairly light sleep, with a further slowing of EEG patterns and loss of slow rolling eye movements. Fifty percent of normal adult sleep may be spent in stage 2. After an initial 20 minutes or so of stage 2 sleep, a deep form of sleep called "stage 3 to 4" is entered.

Stage 3 and *stage 4 sleep* are frequently discussed together because of the difficulty of identifying and separating the two. Stage 3 refers to medium-depth sleep, and stage 4 signals the deepest sleep. During these stages, all cortical brain cells appear to be firing at the same time, resulting in large slow waves on the EEG. When roused from stage 3 to 4 sleep, an adult can take 15 seconds or so to become fully awake. This difficulty in awakening is even more pronounced in children. Stage 3 to 4 sleep is when most sleepwalking, sleeptalking, enuresis, and night terrors occur.

Stage 3 to 4 sleep is felt to have restorative value, necessary for physical recovery. After sleep deprivation studies, stage 3 to 4 sleep is the first to be regained. The majority of growth hormone is secreted at night, peaking during stage 3 to 4 sleep near the beginning of a sleep period. Growth hormone is required not only for growth but also for normal tissue repair in clients of all ages. Stage 3 to 4 sleep accounts for approximately 25% of sleep in children, declines slightly in young adulthood, and then gradually declines in middle age. It may be absent in older clients.

REM SLEEP   After the initial 90 minutes or so of NREM sleep in adults, the client enters REM sleep. The EEG pattern resembles that of the awake state; there are rapid conjugate eye movements; heart rate and respiratory rate are irregular and often higher than when awake; and muscles, including those of the face and neck, are flaccid, leaving the body immobilized. Dreams occur 80% of the time clients are in REM sleep. Unlike stage 3 to 4 sleep, which is most abundant during the early portion of a sleep period, REM sleep periods become longer as the night progresses and the individual becomes more rested. An adult typically has four to six REM sleep periods through the night, accounting for 20% to 25% of sleep. REM sleep makes up 50% of sleep in the newborn, then gradually declines to 20% to 25% of sleep by early childhood. It remains fairly constant throughout the remainder of the life span.

Sleep Cycle

A **sleep cycle** refers to the sequence of sleep that begins with the four stages of NREM sleep in order, with a return

to stage 3, then 2, then passage into the first REM stage (Figure 35-8). The duration of a sleep cycle is generally between 70 and 90 minutes, and the typical sleeper will pass through four to six sleep cycles during an average sleep period of 7 to 8 hours.

The length of the NREM and REM periods of sleep will change as the overall sleep period progresses and the person becomes more relaxed and re-energized. There is less need for stage 3 to 4 sleep and more need for REM sleep as the sleep period progresses, and dreams during the REM phases of later sleep may become more vivid and intense. If the sleep cycle is broken at any point, a new sleep cycle will start, beginning again at stage 1 of NREM sleep and progressing through all of the stages to REM sleep.

BIOLOGICAL CLOCK

The **biological clock** (an endogenous mechanism that measures time) controls the daily fluctuations in hundreds of physiological processes, including body temperature, respiratory rate, performance, alertness, and hormone levels.

Chronobiology is a relatively new branch of science that studies these rhythms that are controlled by our biological clocks. The most widely studied are the **circadian rhythms**, or those that cycle on a daily basis. Other biological rhythms include:

- Ultradian—those much shorter than a day
- Infradian—those lasting a month or more
- Circannual—those requiring about 1 year to complete the cycle

When external time cues such as day-night, sleep-wake, and mealtimes are inconsistent, a desynchronization, or mismatching, of the circadian biological rhythms occurs. This

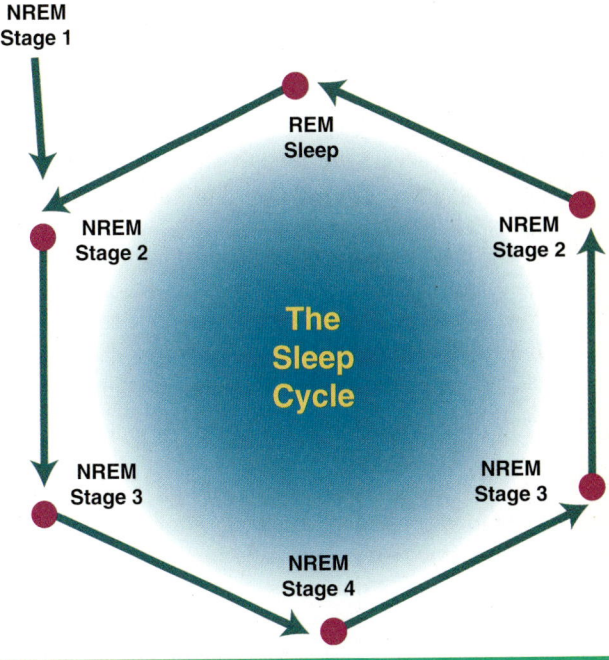

FIGURE 35-8 **The Sleep Cycle** DELMAR/CENGAGE LEARNING

internal desynchronization disrupts the timing of physiological and behavioral activity, which in turn causes chronic fatigue, disrupts sleep patterns, and causes decreased performance and coping abilities. An example of desynchronization is that of the newborn, whose biological rhythms are not established until 3 to 4 months of age. At this point, infants will start to develop longer sleep periods at night and become more predictable in their waking and sleeping patterns.

FACTORS AFFECTING REST AND SLEEP

Several factors can influence the quality and quantity of both sleep and rest. Often, sleep problems result from a combination of many factors.

Degree of Comfort

Comfort is a highly subjective experience. The nurse must assess the degree to which the client's physical and psychological needs have been met. Whenever basic needs are unmet, the person experiences discomfort, which leads to physiological tension, resultant anxiety, and potential impairments in sleep and rest.

Anxiety

A restless body and mind interfere with the ability to sleep. When trying to go to sleep, many individuals often have intrusive thoughts or muscular tension that will interfere with rest and sleep. Anxiety related to work pressures, family demands, and other stressors does not automatically cease when an individual attempts to go to sleep. Anxiety often results in difficulty falling asleep or staying asleep.

Environment

Environmental factors can either enhance or impair sleep. Lighting, temperature, odors, ventilation, and noise level can all interrupt the sleep process when they differ from the norms of the client's usual sleep environment.

Lifestyle

A fast-paced life filled with multiple stressors can result in a person's inability to relax easily or to fall asleep quickly. Relaxation precedes healthy sleep.

Another lifestyle factor that interferes with sleep is having a work schedule that does not coincide with an individual's biological clock (e.g., working at times other than the day shift). Individuals who frequently change work shifts have a real challenge trying to stabilize biological rhythms and rest comfortably.

Diet

The type of food consumed has an impact on the quality and quantity of sleep. Foods high in caffeine, such as coffee, cola, and chocolate, serve as stimulants and often disrupt the normal sleep cycle. Also, consuming a large, heavy, or spicy meal just before bedtime may cause indigestion, which will likely interfere with sleep. Conversely, going to bed when hungry can also result in sleep problems because the individual may be preoccupied with food and hunger pangs instead of concentrating on sleep.

Drugs and Other Substances

Alcohol and nicotine use can impair sleep. Small amounts of alcohol may help some people fall asleep; however, in others alcohol may interfere with REM sleep, causing very restless and nonrefreshing sleep. Nicotine, which is a stimulant, can also impair the sleep cycle by stimulating the body, resulting in difficulty falling and staying asleep. Many medications (both prescription and over the counter) cause fatigue, sleepiness, restlessness, agitation, or insomnia, thus affecting the quality and quantity of rest and sleep.

Cultural Norms

Cultural and societal expectations also affect sleep. Some people perceive sleep as a luxury to be indulged in when they are not too busy with "important" activities. Others view sleep as an absolute necessity. The amount of sleep that a person considers necessary is partially determined by familial and cultural attitudes. See the Respecting Our Differences display.

Life Span Considerations

A person's need for sleep changes with age in a fairly predictable pattern. Although sleep and rest patterns are closely tied to lifestyle and other variables, there are some common variations:

- The *neonate* (birth to 1 month) sleeps in 3- to 4-hour intervals for a total of about 16 to 20 hours a day. The newborn usually is very passive, with little activity during sleep ("sleeping like a baby"), and typically sleeps very soundly. For the first few days or weeks of life, a baby's biological clock is not attuned to regular day-night patterns, so there is often no difference in sleep patterns between day and night.
- The *infant* averages about 12 to 16 hours of sleep a day. As the infant ages, the amount of sleep needed decreases. At approximately 2 months of age, infants can begin to sleep through the night and will typically nap two or three times during the day.

RESPECTING OUR DIFFERENCES

Cultural Norms and Sleep

Which of the two descriptions of sleep (a luxury or a necessity) do you think is most congruent with our society? Which view is closest to your own? Which approach would you take when discussing the rest and sleep needs of a client whose philosophy and views about sleep are in direct contrast to your own?

- During *toddlerhood* the daily average amount of sleep is 12 to 14 hours, which is usually broken down into 10 to 12 hours at night with one or two daytime naps. During this stage, bedtime rituals often develop and assume great importance in providing nighttime security. Repeated and predictable nighttime routines such as baths, brushing teeth, and reading books are helpful in establishing expectations and comfort.
- The *preschool child* sleeps approximately 10 to 12 hours a day. Daytime napping decreases or ceases, unless cultural norms dictate otherwise. Night sleep is often filled with vivid dreams and nightmares that will often awaken children several times during the night.
- A *school-age child* also averages about 10 to 12 hours of sleep daily. Resistance to bedtime and struggles for independence are hallmarks of the school-age child. During this time, the child may develop fear of the dark and will need reassurance and methods to handle this fear.
- *Adolescents* sleep about 8 to 10 hours a day and often decide their bedtime routines and hours. High activity levels often interfere with regular sleep patterns, and irregular sleeping habits often become the norm at this stage.
- The *young adult* averages about 8 hours of sleep a day. During this stage, sleep is often interrupted by young children in the home or work responsibilities. Lifestyle patterns cause many young adults to experience difficulties falling or staying asleep.
- The *middle-age adult* sleeps about 6 to 8 hours a day. Daily stressors may continue to result in insomnia, and the use of sleep-inducing medications is common.
- The sleep requirements for the *older adult* decrease to 5 to 7 hours a day and often include a daytime nap. The quality of sleep often diminishes due to frequent waking, physical pain, and shortened REM sleep. Many older adults misinterpret this decreased need for sleep as insomnia and are thus unduly concerned about not getting "enough" sleep.

ILLNESS OR HOSPITALIZATION

The stress imposed by illness usually disrupts sleep. Sleep is especially disrupted when a person is hospitalized. Some factors associated with hospitalization that lead to sleep impairment include:

- Physical or emotional pain
- Loss of familiar surroundings
- Loss of routine
- Fear of the unknown
- Timing of procedures and treatments
- Noise level (especially unfamiliar noises)
- Loss of privacy

ALTERATION IN SLEEP PATTERNS

Sleep disturbances can take many forms and are quite common. Alterations in sleep patterns are generally viewed as either primary sleep disorders (those in which the sleep alteration is the fundamental problem) or secondary sleep disorders (those in which the alteration has a medical or clinical cause that results in or contributes to the sleep alteration). The most common sleep alterations include insomnia, hypersomnia or narcolepsy, sleep apnea, sleep deprivation, and parasomnias. Problems associated with sleep disturbances are as follows:

- Decreased work productivity (more missed days of work)
- Increased utilization of health care services
- Greater risk of accidents
- Short-term memory problems
- Cognitive and motor performance impairments

Insomnia

Insomnia refers to the chronic inability to sleep or inadequate quality of sleep due to sleep that prematurely ends or is interrupted by periods of wakefulness. Insomnia is *not* a disease, but it may be a manifestation of many illnesses. The person experiencing insomnia often gets caught up in a vicious cycle of not being able to sleep, trying harder to fall asleep, and increasing anxiety about not sleeping, which in turn increases the inability to fall asleep. Perception of sleep quantity can also be important; many insomniacs actually sleep significantly more than they think they do, so there is a discrepancy between perception and reality.

Sleep disturbances are common for individuals experiencing chronic pain. Sleep impairment can exacerbate pain; thus, a vicious cycle is established. The consequences of poor, nonrestorative sleep during the wake time may include change in physical activity, headaches or pain, GI malfunctions, and fibromyalgia. Treatment for insomnia is best directed at modifying those factors or behaviors that are causing it. It is impossible to force sleep.

Hypersomnia or Narcolepsy

Hypersomnia is an alteration in sleep pattern characterized by excessive sleep, especially in the daytime. Persons suffering from hypersomnia often feel that they cannot get enough sleep at night; therefore, they sleep very late into the morning and nap several times throughout the day. Causes of hypersomnia can be physical or psychological; treatment depends on addressing the underlying cause.

Narcolepsy, another sleep alteration, manifests as sudden uncontrollable urges to fall asleep during the daytime. Individuals suffering from narcolepsy often achieve adequate sleep at night but are overwhelmed by sleepiness at unexpected and unpredictable periods during the day. Effective treatments for narcolepsy include avoiding substances or activities that cause sleepiness, taking short daytime naps, or taking prescribed stimulant medications.

Sleep Apnea

Sleep apnea refers to periods of sleep during which airflow stops for 10 seconds or more. Sleep apnea gives rise to complications as a result of oxygen desaturation and carbon dioxide retention. Short-term consequences may include cognitive impairment (including memory changes), personality changes, and impotence. A major problem is daytime sleepiness, which may interfere with functional abilities such as driving and working. If untreated, sleep apnea may contribute to the development of the following cardiovascular disorders: hypertension, coronary heart disease, and heart failure.

The first line of defense against apnea is treating its cause (emotional, cardiac, or respiratory alteration). Use of a nasal continuous positive airway pressure (CPAP) device may also give relief. With some individuals, surgical intervention is required to correct the cause of the apnea.

Sleep Deprivation

Sleep deprivation is a term used to describe prolonged inadequate quality and quantity of sleep, either of the REM or the NREM type. Sleep deprivation can result from age, prolonged hospitalization, drug and substance use, illness, and frequent changes in lifestyle patterns. Sleep and dreaming have a restorative value necessary for mental and emotional recovery and enhance the ability to cope with emotional problems. Therefore, sleep deprivation can cause symptoms ranging from irritability, hypersensitivity, and confusion to apathy, sleepiness, and diminished reflexes. Treating or minimizing the factors that cause the sleep deprivation is the most effective resolution.

Parasomnia

Parasomnia refers to sleep alterations resulting from "an activation of physiological systems at inappropriate times during the sleep-wake cycle" (American Psychiatric Association, 2000, p. 630). **Somnambulism** (sleepwalking), sleep-talking, bedwetting, and **bruxism** (teeth grinding) are the most common parasomnias. Treatment for parasomnias varies, and care should be focused on helping the client and family understand the disorder and its potential safety risks.

ASSESSMENT

Discussion of sleep and activity patterns is included as part of the regular health history. Any client acknowledging a sleep disturbance should be thoroughly assessed to determine sleep routines, sleep alterations, type of disturbances, and impact of sleep problems. Typically the client is a reliable source for this information, but a spouse or partner who shares sleeping arrangements may be able to add valuable information to the client's report. Questions regarding the client's usual sleep patterns should include:

1. Nature of sleep (restful, uninterrupted)
2. Quality of sleep (usual sleep pattern, schedules, hours of sleep, feeling upon awakening)
3. Sleep environment (description of room, temperature, noise level)
4. Associated factors (bedtime routines, use of sleep medications or any other sleep inducers)
5. Opinion of sleep (adequate, restores energy adequately, inadequate, problematic)

Questions regarding altered sleep patterns are intended to reveal such information as:

1. Nature of the problem (inability to fall asleep, difficulty remaining asleep, inability to fall asleep after awakening, restless sleep, daytime sleepiness)
2. Quality of the problem (number of hours of sleep versus number of hours spent trying to sleep, number of hours of sleep a night, duration and frequency of naps or other compensatory measures, number of wakings per sleep period)
3. Environmental factors (lighting, bed, noise level, surrounding stimulation, sleep partner)
4. Associated factors (relation to meals eaten, activity before retiring, life and work stressors, anxiety level, pain, recent illness or surgery)
5. Alleviating factors (mild diet, warm drink before retiring, reading a book, listening to quiet music, taking a hot bath, taking sleeping pills)
6. Effect of problem (fatigue, irritability, confusion)

For clients whose sleep problems do not seem to be well defined, a daily journal of sleep patterns may prove useful. This written account can mirror the preceding outline.

NURSING DIAGNOSIS

After information about the sleep impairment has been collected, data need to be analyzed to formulate appropriate nursing diagnoses. The primary diagnosis for individuals experiencing sleep problems is *insomnia*. According to Carpenito-Moyet (2008), insomnia is defined as "a state in which a person experiences a change in the quantity or quality of his rest pattern that causes discomfort or interferes with desired lifestyle" (p. 387). Alterations in sleep can manifest through verbal complaints of the client, physical signs such as yawning or dark circles under the eyes, or alterations in mood such as apathy or irritability.

If the client presents with problems in addition to the sleep disturbance, the nurse must be alert to the possibility that the sleep disturbance is the *cause* (not the effect) of another problem. For example, a client may be experiencing *activity intolerance* related to lack of sleep as evidenced by verbal complaint, extreme fatigue, disorientation, confusion, and lack of energy.

PLANNING AND OUTCOMES

The plan of care for the sleep-disordered client must be individualized. For the nursing care to be effective, client input should be incorporated when developing expected outcomes. It is important to tailor the outcomes and plan of care to the true cause related to the sleep disturbance or alteration. For example, if the client is experiencing *insomnia* because of bedwetting, then the bedwetting should be targeted for intervention.

Effective outcome identification and planning must consider the fact that many sleep disturbances will require extended periods of time (weeks or months) to correct.

Sleep patterns are by nature habitual and intertwined with lifestyle patterns, and these types of disturbances typically require interventions that have long-term goals. When planning care, the nurse should remember to perform procedures and treatments in a manner that disturbs sleep time and routines as little as possible.

IMPLEMENTATION

Several interventions can promote rest and sleep in clients. The interventions range from simple (e.g., correct bed-making techniques) to complex (teaching clients about necessary lifestyle modifications). The NIC system defines nursing actions that facilitate regular sleep and wake cycles (see the accompanying display on sleep enhancement activities). Several interventions that facilitate sleep are discussed here.

Establish a Trusting Nurse-Client Relationship

The quality of the nurse-client relationship can enhance a client's ability to rest and sleep. Knowing that the nurse is a trustworthy individual allows the client to relax and feel secure. The Nursing Checklist on page 1078 provides guidelines for communicating with the sleep-impaired client. Anxiety can be decreased by the nurse's use of therapeutic communication skills. The *therapeutic use of self* helps allay client anxiety.

Create a Relaxing Environment

Arranging the immediate surroundings to promote sleep is important for the sleep-impaired client. A place to sleep should be inviting. Determine the type of environment the client finds relaxing, then provide this environment in the inpatient setting, or help the client establish this type of environment in the home setting. See the Community Considerations display on page 1078.

Initiate Relaxation Techniques

The client's mood before sleep is of utmost importance. The *belief* that one can—and will—sleep greatly affects sleep quality and quantity. The client who is calm and relaxed is likely to fall asleep quickly and stay asleep all night. Relaxation techniques are useful sleep aids. Progressive muscle relaxation is especially therapeutic for the person who needs to lessen muscular tension and quiet the mind. A recent study (Kim & Sok, 2007) showed a positive response to auricular acupuncture for improving quality of sleep.

See the Respecting Our Differences display on page 1078 for a listing of herbal remedies used in some cultures to promote sleep.

Ensure Appropriate Nutrition

Certain foods can actually enhance sleep. Tryptophan, a substance in milk, promotes sleep by stimulating the brain's production of the neurotransmitter serotonin. The old wives'

NIC SLEEP ENHANCEMENT ACTIVITIES

- Determine the effects of the client's medications on sleep pattern, and adjust medication administration schedule to support client's sleep and wake cycles.
- Monitor and record client's sleep pattern and number of hours of sleep, and note physical (e.g., sleep apnea obstructed airway, pain and discomfort, and urinary frequency) and/or psychological (e.g., fear or anxiety) circumstances that interrupt sleep.
- Adjust environment (e.g., light, noise, temperature, mattress, and bed) to promote sleep.
- Facilitate maintenance of client's usual bedtime routines, presleep cues and props, and familiar objects (e.g., for children, a favorite blanket or toy, rocking, pacifier, or story; for adults, a book to read) as appropriate.
- Assist to eliminate stressful situations before bedtime, and instruct client to avoid bedtime foods and beverages that interfere with sleep.
- Instruct client how to perform autogenic muscle relaxation, and discuss other nonpharmacological forms of sleep inducement, such as massage, positioning, and touch.
- Instruct the client and significant others about factors (e.g., physiological, psychological, lifestyle, frequent work shift changes, rapid time zone changes, excessively long work hours, and other environmental factors) that contribute to sleep pattern disturbances.
- Provide pamphlet with information about sleep enhancement techniques.

Bulechek, G., Butcher, H., & Dochterman, J. (2008). *Nursing interventions classification (NIC)* (5th ed.). St. Louis, MO: Mosby Elsevier Health Sciences.

tale that drinking warm milk promotes sleep is supported by scientific data. Other dietary considerations include avoiding large or heavy meals close to bedtime, refraining from eating spicy or other foods that cause GI distress, and avoiding caffeine after noon.

Initiate Pharmacologic Interventions

If unrelieved pain is a factor in the client's sleep disturbance, then pain management should be the focus of initial interventions. Many of the nonpharmacologic relaxation and imagery interventions can be effective in clients with sleep disturbances.

Pharmacologic agents that may be therapeutic for clients with sleep disturbances include tricyclic antidepressants, antihistamines, and short-acting hypnotics. The tricyclic

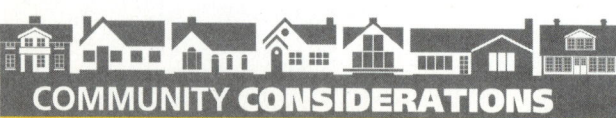

Communicating with the Sleep-Impaired Client

- Thoroughly explain procedures before implementation.
- Encourage client and significant others to verbalize feelings and ask questions.
- Answer questions honestly and completely.
- Identify and support coping mechanisms of client and family.
- Spend adequate time with client to facilitate communication.
- Ascertain and incorporate client preferences as much as possible into plan of care.

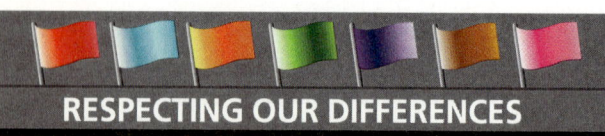

COMMUNITY CONSIDERATIONS

Relaxing Environment

Observe a client care area. Which environmental factors encourage sleep? Which factors interfere with sleep? If you were to design the ideal client care environment, how would you address these variables?

- Colors
- Fabrics
- Lighting
- Noises
- Temperature
- Odors

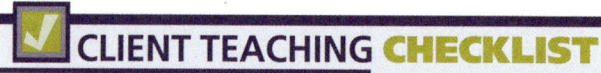

RESPECTING OUR DIFFERENCES

Complementary and Alternative Modalities That Promote Sleep

- Massage
- Imagery
- Meditation
- Herbal: chamomile, hops, lavender, kava, passion flower, skullcap, valerian
- Aromatherapy: chamomile oil, lavender oil

antidepressants of choice are amitriptyline (Elavil) or doxepin (Sinequan). Amitriptyline improves the client's ability to fall asleep and stay asleep by causing sedation when given 1 to 3 hours before bedtime. Doses of amitriptyline for sleep disturbances are significantly lower than doses for treatment of depression, starting at 10 to 25 mg at bedtime and titrating up by 10 to 25 mg every 2 or 3 days until therapeutic effect is achieved.

Antihistamines such as hydroxyzine (Vistaril, Atarax) and diphenhydramine (Benadryl) have mild sedative effects that could promote sleep if given at bedtime. If anxiety throughout the day is of concern, low doses of these medications at regular intervals throughout the day may be effective.

The final group of pharmacologic interventions for sleep disturbances is the short-acting hypnotics. These medications are *not* recommended for routine or long-term use, but they may be effective for short-term intervention. When they are chosen, it is recommended that one with a short half-life be used.

Provide Client Education

Educating clients about sleep-promoting activities is a good investment of the nurse's time. By empowering clients to help themselves relax, the nurse helps them gain a sense of control over their sleep disturbance and boosts their confidence so that they can successfully meet their sleep and rest needs. See the Client Teaching Checklist for managing sleep disturbances.

CLIENT TEACHING CHECKLIST

Managing Sleep Disturbance

To facilitate rest and sleep, the client should be encouraged to:

- Avoid stimulating activities such as strenuous exercise or demanding intellectual activity during the hour before bedtime. Use the time instead to wind down with relaxing activities such as taking a warm bath, reading a book, or sitting by the fire.
- Use bedtime rituals on a consistent basis.
- Practice relaxation techniques such as neck rolls and muscle relaxation to release tensions before going to bed.
- Refrain from watching television, studying, or talking on the phone while lying in bed; use the bed for sleeping only.
- Follow dietary guidelines to avoid caffeine, spicy foods, and heavy meals several hours before bedtime.

NURSING CARE PLAN

The Client Experiencing Altered Sleep Patterns

CASE PRESENTATION
Jacques Porcheron, 6 years old, is brought to your clinic by his father, who states that Jacques has trouble sleeping at night. In the evenings after a dinner of hot dogs, corn or baked beans, and chocolate milk, Jacques reads some books, then watches his favorite superhero video. Afterward, he runs and plays, mimics the actions he sees in the video, and refuses to take a bath or cooperate when getting dressed for bed. Once put to bed at 9:00 p.m., he is up several times for any number of reasons and often is not asleep until midnight. When his father wakes him at 7:00 a.m. for school, Jacques is disagreeable, tired, and difficult to get moving.

ASSESSMENT
Client is experiencing:

- Inability to fall asleep
- Inability to remain asleep
- Inconsistent bedtime rituals that interfere with calm time needed before retiring

NURSING DIAGNOSIS: *Insomnia* related to lack of sleep and disruption in lifestyle as evidenced by parental complaint, ineffective bedtime rituals, and insufficient hours of sleep for developmental age.
NOC: Sleep
NIC: Sleep enhancement

EXPECTED OUTCOMES
The client will:

1. Identify behaviors that are helpful before bedtime.
2. Develop appropriate bedtime rituals to help Jacques wind down from the day.
3. Ensure that Jacques gets 10 to 12 hours of sleep a night.

INTERVENTIONS/RATIONALES
1. Determine from the father and child which sleeping behaviors they would like to achieve. Asking for client input in the desired outcomes will make the plan of care more effective and realistic.
2. Teach family members about effect certain foods can have on digestion and sleep habits, and list with them foods that are good choices for dinners. Educating family members about the potential adverse effects of certain foods will help them plan meals more appropriately.
3. Help client understand which bedtime activities can be detrimental to sleep induction. Understanding which behaviors can interfere with falling asleep will help client and family identify and therefore modify prebedtime behaviors.
4. Explain why overstimulation close to bedtime, such as watching superhero movies and engaging in rowdy play, will prevent the body and mind from slowing down and preparing for sleep. Understanding the psychological and physical implications of overstimulation before bedtime will help clients choose more appropriate bedtime activities.
5. Emphasize the importance of establishing a calming bedtime routine that is followed every night, especially for the school-age child. Children Jacques's age are helped by ritual and knowing what is expected of them, and they need guidance in practicing routines that are appropriate for bedtime.
6. Suggest appropriate bedtime rituals, such as taking a bath, brushing the teeth, reading a book, or listening to calming music. Focusing on quiet activities and routine will help the body and mind prepare for bedtime.
7. Help the family ensure an appropriate sleep environment for Jacques, such as a calm room at a comfortable temperature, lit only by a night light. Promotes sleep and does not interfere with falling back asleep once awake.

(Continues)

NURSING CARE PLAN (Continued)

8. Encourage the family through the preceding steps to work toward having Jacques get at least 10 to 12 hours of sleep a day, which is the normal requirement for a child his age. Helping family members understand which factors may be interfering with Jacques' sleep habits, such as excessive daytime napping or repetitive waking during the night, and also ensuring that they understand his sleep requirements will help them be more effective in their management of his bedtime and sleeping habits.

EVALUATION
After 2 weeks, the father reports that Jacques eats the same type of meals but is no longer allowed to watch stimulating videos after 7:00 p.m. Together they have established bedtime rituals that begin with quiet tablework (reading, arts and crafts, writing) or talks about the day, followed by a warm bath and reading three books together in the recliner in the living room. After this, they put on pajamas and brush teeth, and then Jacques goes up to bed by himself. The father would like to modify Jacques's diet somewhat and is planning this as his goal for the next 2 weeks.

EVALUATION

The plan of care must be individualized for and negotiated with the client. It must be updated on a regular schedule and additional interventions initiated as needed. One of the strongest supportive activities nurses can perform is to make sure clients understand that there is help for sleep problems and that they are not alone in having difficulty successfully managing their sleep patterns. The Nursing Process Highlight lists variables to be considered when evaluating the care of the sleep-disturbed client.

NURSING PROCESS HIGHLIGHT

Evaluation

When evaluating the care of the sleep-disordered client, consider the following variables:

- The client's basic needs were met.
- Client education included the family or significant others.
- An environment conducive to rest was maintained.
- Therapeutic activities were balanced with the client's need for rest and sleep.
- The client's bedtime rituals were followed as closely as possible.
- Anxiety reduction techniques were used appropriately.

PROCEDURE 35-1

Administering Patient-Controlled Analgesia (PCA)

EQUIPMENT
- A patent indwelling subcutaneous (SC), intravenous (IV), or epidural line installed as the prescribed route of administration.
- A PCA pump with manufacturer's instruction guide for operation: PCA pumps usually consist of a programmable infusion pump with syringe inside, a button linked to a timing unit that is activated by the client when demanded, and a tube that can be connected to an indwelling catheter (e.g., IV line).
- Pain medication as ordered by the health care provider
- Label for drug identification
- Adhesive tape
- Disposable gloves
- Naloxone solution (0.4 mg in 10 mL of saline) if giving opioid agonists (e.g., morphine)

(Continues)

PROCEDURE 35-1
Administering Patient-Controlled Analgesia (PCA) (Continued)

ACTION	RATIONALE
1. Wash hands/hand hygiene.	1. Prevents the spread of microorganisms.
2. Assess the client's comfort level: pain location, intensity, characteristics, pattern, and factors that increase or decrease the pain.	2. Identifies pain problem, purpose of pain therapy, and other adjuvant therapies. Establishes baseline to measure improvement.
3. Assess the client's consciousness level and ability to understand the instruction.	3. PCA is contraindicated for sedated and confused clients.
4. Check the PCA (see Figure 35-9) order for drug, concentration, route, basal infusion rate, bolus dose, lockout interval, maximum dose, and any loading dose.	4. Opioid administration requires a prescribing practitioner's order. Dosing parameters are necessary for programming a PCA pump.
5. Check the PCA medication label against the prescribing practitioner's order, and follow the "five rights" principle. PCA medication usually has been placed in the PCA syringe at the pharmacy. Have a second nurse sign when therapy is initiated and with all dosing changes.	5. Minimizes medication error and harm to client.
6. Read the manufacturer's instruction guide before assembling and programming the PCA pump.	6. Different manufacturers or models may require different operation. Follow the manufacturer's instructions to ensure proper operation of the pump.
7. Place the filled PCA syringe into the chamber in the PCA pump, and detect any leaking or damage to the system (see Figure 35-10 and Figures 35-11 and 35-12 on page 1082).	7. Assemble PCA pump and inspect for damage of the system to avoid medication error and harm to client.
8. Program the pump according to the prescribed parameters, usually including basal infusion rate (mg/h), bolus dose (mg), lockout interval (min), and maximum dose limit (mg/h) (see Figure 35-13 on page 1082).	8. Avoids overmedication and ensures accuracy of the medication given.

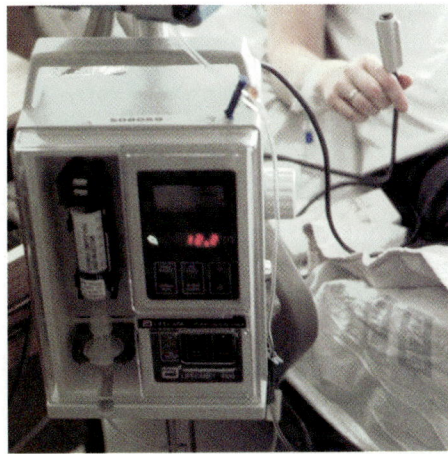

FIGURE 35-9 **PCA Pump** DELMAR/CENGAGE LEARNING

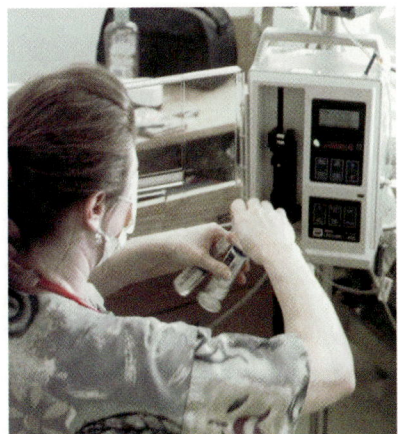

FIGURE 35-10 **Remove the empty PCA syringe** DELMAR/CENGAGE LEARNING

(Continues)

PROCEDURE 35-1
Administering Patient-Controlled Analgesia (PCA) (Continued)

ACTION	RATIONALE

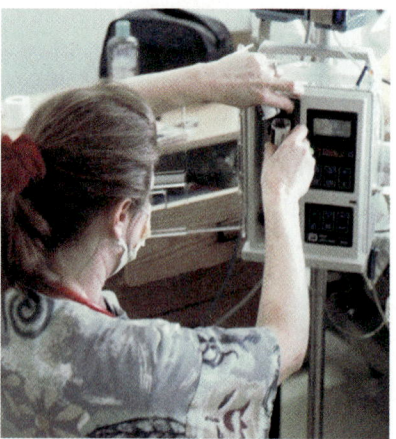

FIGURE 35-11 Place new PCA syringe into the chamber in the PCA pump. DELMAR/CENGAGE LEARNING

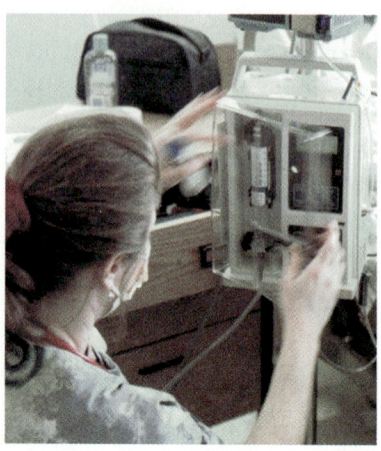

FIGURE 35-12 Check for any leaking or damage to the system, and close the door to the chamber. DELMAR/CENGAGE LEARNING

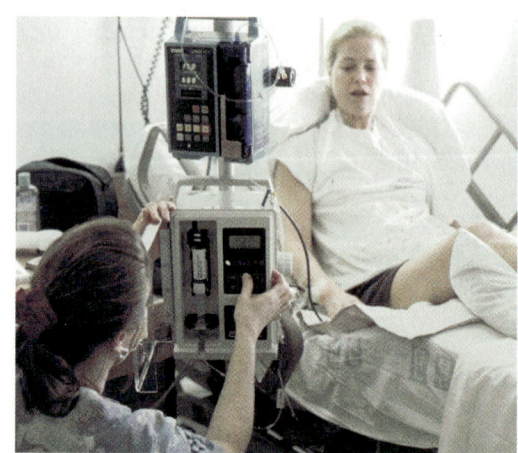

FIGURE 35-13 Program the pump. DELMAR/CENGAGE LEARNING

ACTION	RATIONALE
9. Wear gloves.	9. Sterile technique reduces transmission of microorganisms.
10. Inspect the existing infusion line and puncture site for any inflammatory sign, and check any occlusion or leakage of the infusion line. Check IV catheterization or epidural catheter placement if client needs an infusion line.	10. Avoids skin breakdown and infection for safely administering medication. Infusion line must be patent to deliver medication to vessels.
11. Prime the PCA pump tubing. Connect the PCA pump tubing with the infusion line using aseptic technique, and secure the connection with adhesive tape.	11. Reduces risk of infection and leakage and prevents air embolism.

(Continues)

PROCEDURE 35-1
Administering Patient-Controlled Analgesia (PCA) (Continued)

ACTION	RATIONALE
12. Give the client the control button, and instruct how and when to press the button.	12. Client teaching ensures appropriate use of PCA.

delegation tip

The skill of medication administration is not delegated to ancillary personnel in acute care settings. This may vary in state or federal institutions. Ancillary personnel are generally informed about the medications the client is receiving if adverse effects are anticipated or are being monitored.

nursing tips

- *Periodically assess pain intensity, pain relief, and side effects.*
- *Remember, if the medication is discontinued, any narcotic left in the pump must be wasted. Another nurse must witness the wasting procedure, and the amount, reason, time, and date of the wasting must be documented.*
- *Program the PCA pump with the actual dose; input the drug concentration so that the pump can calculate the volume needed to deliver the dose. The programmed concentration should match what is in the bag or syringe. For example, the client is to receive 1 mg of morphine with each demanded dose from the PCA pump. If the concentration is programmed as 0.1 mg/mL, the pump must deliver 10 mL of solution to achieve the 1 mg dose.*

KEY CONCEPTS

- Pain is a subjective and an individualized experience.
- Pain is defined as whatever the client says it is.
- Pain is increased by anxiety and fatigue.
- Several factors influence the perception of pain, including developmental level, culture, and previous experience.
- The amount of sleep required differs according to developmental stage.

- Nonpharmacologic interventions may be used in managing pain and promoting rest and sleep.
- Pharmacologic agents can be therapeutic for clients experiencing pain or sleep pattern disturbances. However, the medications should not be the only interventions used.

REVIEW QUESTIONS

1. Which of the following is the best way for a nurse to assess for pain in a communicative client?
   a. Note the frequency of pain medication administration.
   b. Observe for changes in the client's vital signs.
   c. Ask the client.
   d. Assess the client's level of anxiety.

2. Which statement regarding IM injections of analgesia is true?
   a. It is the gold standard for relieving acute pain.
   b. It is discouraged in current practice.
   c. It provides for consistent medication absorption.
   d. It rarely causes damage to muscle tissue.

3. Which statement regarding pain and sleep is most correct?
   a. A client may sleep despite being in pain.
   b. A sleeping client is resting comfortably.
   c. The brain shuts down during sleep, and the client does not feel pain.
   d. Clients in pain are not able to fall asleep.

4. Which statement best describes clients with chronic pain?
   a. They become chronic complainers.
   b. They often experience depression.
   c. They rarely become suicide risks.
   d. They have a very high incidence of addiction.

5. The nurse is preparing to teach a class to a group of new graduate nurses on substance use disorders. Which statement should the nurse include in the class?
   a. A client with a substance dependence must take the same drug to relieve withdrawal symptoms.
   b. Substance abuse is both a physical and psychological disorder.

   c. A client who is motivated and has a substance dependence can overcome the addiction by stopping the substance.
   d. A substance must be abused over a long period of time before an addiction develops.

6. Which actions are required to ensure safe use of PCAs? Select all that apply.
   a. Standard order sets are required.
   b. Two nurses must sign when therapy is initiated and with all dosing orders.
   c. PCA solutions and concentrations are standardized.
   d. Competency of all nurses who use PCA in their practice must be documented annually.
   e. A second nurse must witness the wasting of any narcotic left in the pump.
   f. Nurses can activate PCA.

7. When is it appropriate to administer a placebo for pain?
   a. Never
   b. When the prescribing practitioner orders a placebo
   c. When the client is a substance addict and the nurse needs to assess the client's "real" pain
   d. When the client is participating in research and has given informed consent

8. Which factors can impair sleep and rest? Select all that apply.
   a. Discomfort
   b. Anxiety
   c. Noise level
   d. A change in one's normal bedtime
   e. Decaffeinated foods and beverages
   f. Alcohol and nicotine

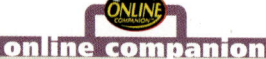

online companion

Visit the DeLaune and Ladner online companion resource at **www.delmar.cengage.com** for additional content and study aids. Click on Online Companions, then select the Nursing discipline.

"Worms will not eat living wood where the vital sap is flowing; rust will not hinder the opening of a gate when the hinges are used each day. Movement gives health and life. Stagnation brings disease and death."

—Ancient proverb in traditional Chinese medicine

CHAPTER 36

Mobility

COMPETENCIES

1. Explain the physiology of mobility.
2. Identify factors affecting mobility.
3. Identify health problems related to immobility.
4. Describe the process of activity and mobility assessment.
5. Discuss nursing diagnoses relevant to clients experiencing mobility impairments.
6. Develop client expected outcomes related to activity and mobility in terms of lifestyle, age, and health promotion.
7. Develop specific nursing interventions that promote mobility and prevent complications due to immobility.
8. Discuss evaluation of client activity and mobility status.

Movement is an activity most people take for granted. The ability to move and be active improves health status, whereas immobility presents a threat to one's physical, mental, and social well-being. This chapter explores nursing responses to individuals with impaired ability to move.

OVERVIEW OF MOBILITY

Mobility refers to the ability to engage in activity and unrestricted movement that includes walking, running, sitting, standing, lifting, pushing, pulling, and performing activities of daily living (ADL). Mobility is often considered an indicator of health status because it influences the correct functioning of many body systems, especially the respiratory, gastrointestinal, and urinary systems. Mobility enhances muscle tone, increases energy level, and is associated with psychological benefits such as independence and freedom.

BODY ALIGNMENT

Body alignment refers to the position of body parts in relation to each other. Proper body alignment results in **balance**, which is an individual's ability to maintain postural equilibrium. When the body is in correct posture, the center of gravity (the center point of an object's mass) is evenly distributed over the foundation points. Correct posture promotes balance, reduces strain and injury to support structures, facilitates respiratory effort, enhances gastrointestinal processes, and gives an appearance of confidence and health. A correct postural stance is maintained by a well-functioning musculoskeletal system. The normal alignment of the spine has a cervical concavity, a thoracic convexity, and a lumbar concavity; see Figure 36-1 on page 1089.

Proper standing body alignment (see Figure 36-2 on page 1089) is characterized by the following:

- Head upright
- Face forward
- Shoulders squared
- Back straight

- Abdominal muscles tucked in
- Arms straight at side
- Hands palm forward
- Legs straight
- Feet forward

The sitting position in proper alignment has similar characteristics; however, the hips and knees are flexed. Figure 36-3 on page 1089 shows proper alignment and posture for the sitting position.

Proper alignment and posture of the client lying in bed appear similar to the standing position; however, the client is supine, as shown in Figure 36-4 on page 1090.

The benefits of proper alignment and posture include (1) client comfort; (2) prevention of contractures; (3) promotion of circulation; (4) less stress on muscles, tendons, nerves, and joints; and (5) prevention of foot drop (plantar flexion).

In a person standing upright, the center of gravity is located in the middle of the pelvis about halfway between the umbilicus and the symphysis pubis. The **line of gravity** (vertical line passing through the center of gravity) is shown in Figures 36-3 and 36-4. The **base of support** is the foundation on which a person or object rests. Stability of one's balance is promoted by a steady base of support and a low center of gravity.

Muscle tone and bone strength allow a person to maintain an erect posture. Muscle contour is affected by the individual's exercise and activity patterns. **Muscle tone** is the normal state of balanced tension present in the body; it allows a muscle to respond quickly to stimuli. Two aberrations of muscle tone include **hypotonicity** (flaccidity), which is a decrease in muscle tone, and **spasticity**, which is an increase in muscle tension and is often noted with extreme flexion or extension.

Muscle shape should be symmetrical. There may be **hypertrophy** (increased muscle size and shape due to an increase in muscle fibers) or **atrophy** (a reduction in muscle size and shape), which manifests as thin, flabby muscles with indistinct contour (see Figure 36-5 on page 1090). Atrophy is usually a result of disuse, whereas hypertrophy occurs when the muscle is overworked.

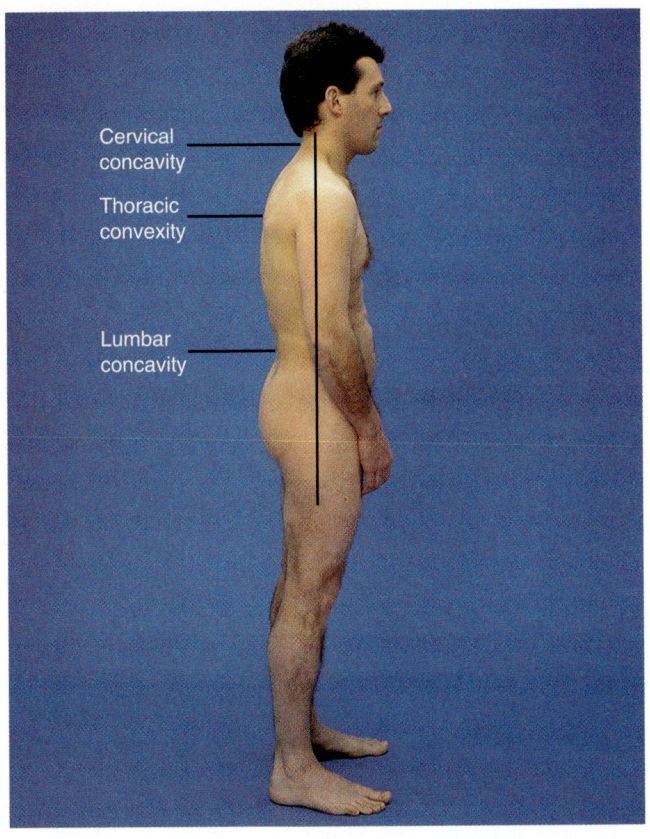

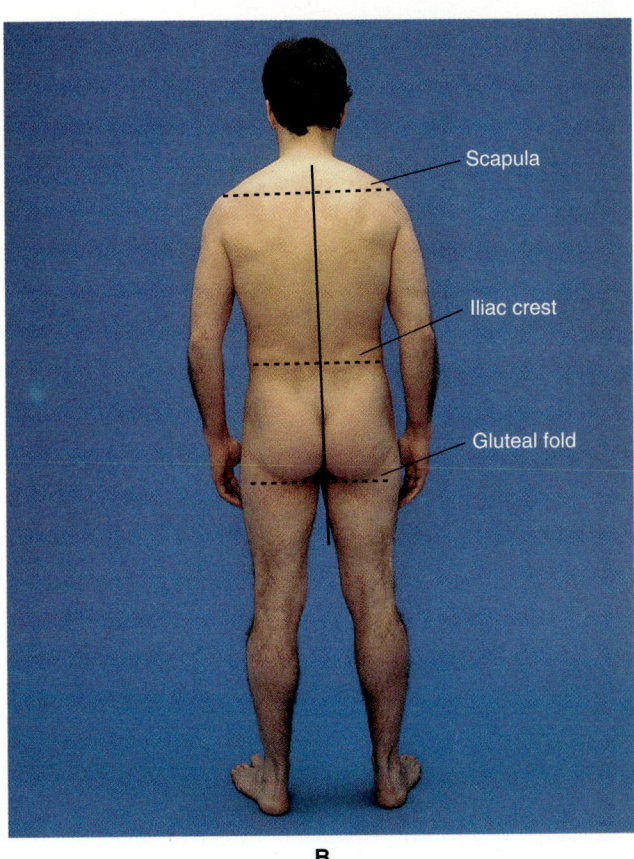

FIGURE 36-1 **Normal Spinal Concavity A.** Lateral View; **B.** Posterior View DELMAR/CENGAGE LEARNING

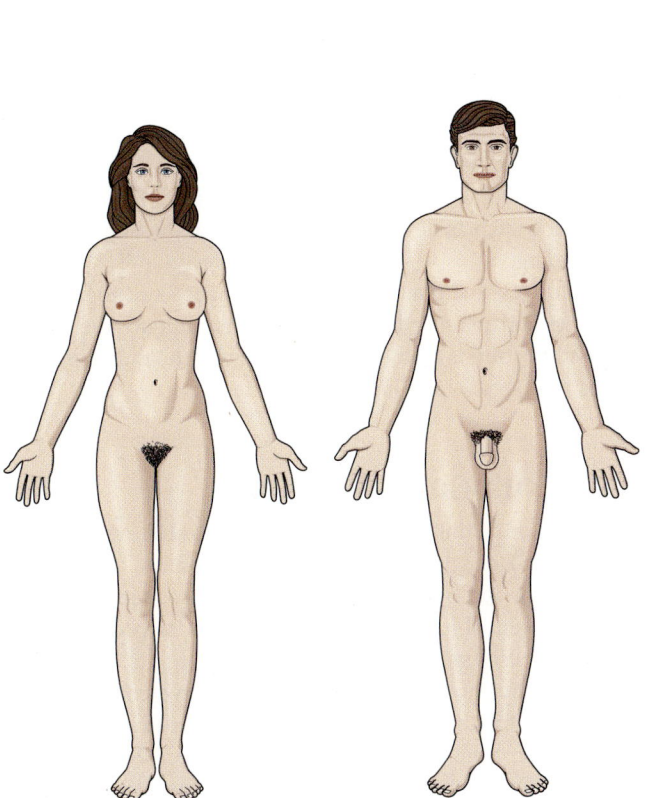

FIGURE 36-2 **Proper Alignment and Posture: Standing Female and Male** DELMAR/CENGAGE LEARNING

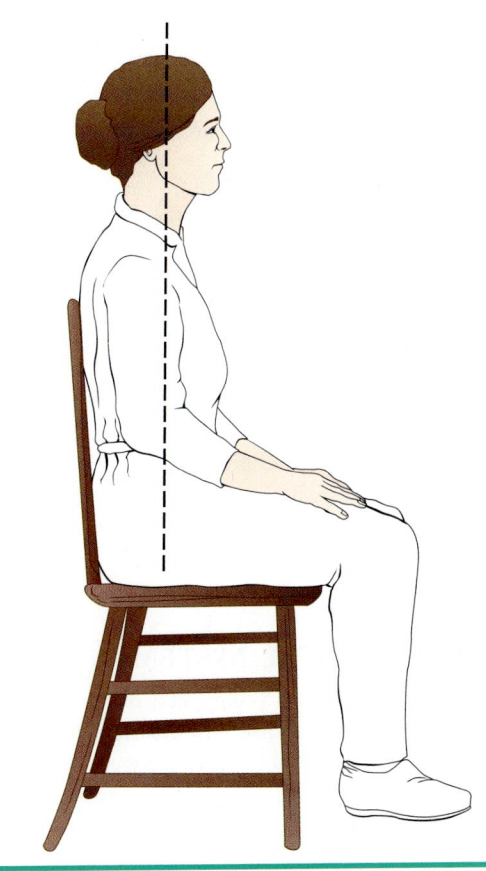

FIGURE 36-3 **Proper Sitting Posture and Line of Gravity** DELMAR/CENGAGE LEARNING

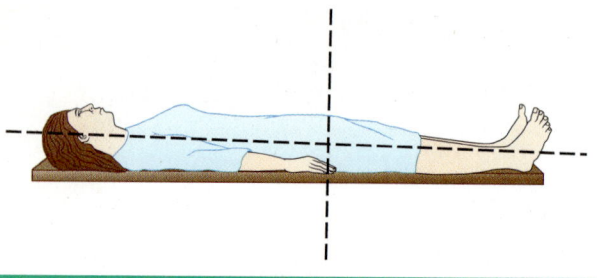

FIGURE 36-4 Proper Supine Posture and Line of Gravity
DELMAR/CENGAGE LEARNING

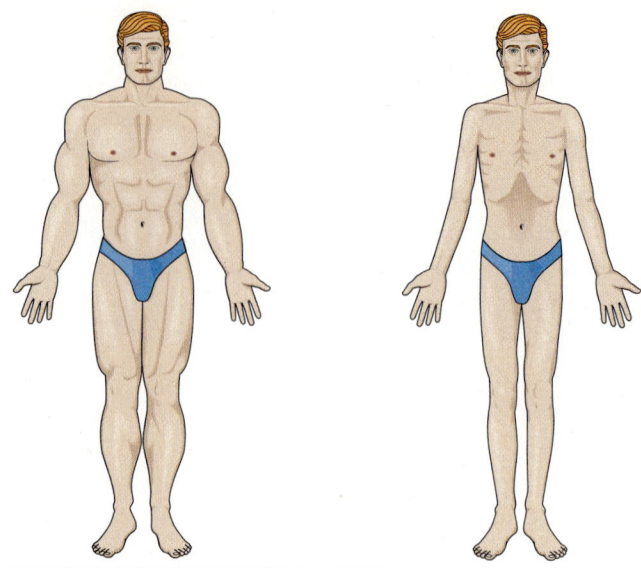

FIGURE 36-5 Variances of Muscle Size and Shape: A. Hypertrophy; B. Atrophy DELMAR/CENGAGE LEARNING

BODY MECHANICS

Functional mobility is governed by body mechanics, the purposeful and coordinated use of body parts and positions during activity. Use of proper body mechanics maximizes the effectiveness of the efforts of the musculoskeletal and neurological systems.

Proper body mechanics are as important to the nurse as to the client. The purpose of proper body mechanics is prevention of strain and injury to the muscles, joints, and tendons. The clinical application of body mechanics is described in the implementation section of this chapter.

Range of motion reflects the extent to which a joint can move. The ranges vary with each joint and are affected by several factors, including age, physical condition, and heredity. When performing ROM exercises, it is important that the nurse put the joint through its complete range. In order to do so, the nurse may place an extremity into abduction (to move a body part away from the midline) or adduction (to move a body part toward the midline). A body part may also be placed in a state of extension (be straightened) or flexion (bending the joint). Opposition (a body part being across from another part at nearly a 180° angle) is also used when performing ROM exercises.

PHYSIOLOGY OF MOBILITY

Mobility is regulated by the coordinated effort of the musculoskeletal and neurological systems. The major functions of the musculoskeletal system are to maintain body alignment and to facilitate mobility.

MUSCULOSKELETAL SYSTEM

The musculoskeletal system (comprised of bones, cartilage, joints, tendons, ligaments, bursa, and muscles) serves several functions, as described in Table 36-1 on page 1091.

Bone is the foundation of the musculoskeletal system. Mobility and weight-bearing capacity are directly related to the bone's size and shape. Joints work with muscles to provide motion and flexibility. Skeletal muscles overlying the joint exert opposing forces and, therefore, cause movement.

Muscles are basically machines that convert energy into mechanical work. Contractility is the common property among the three types of muscles: smooth, cardiac, and skeletal. Skeletal muscle fibers are innervated by somatic nerves and, therefore, are generally under voluntary control.

The muscles work in cooperation with the nervous system to maintain body alignment and cause movement. Muscles act in pairs to perform work. One muscle of the pair produces movement in a single direction. The other muscle of the pair produces movement in the opposite direction. When one muscle of the pair is contracted, the other is relaxed. The opposing actions of contraction and relaxation make motion possible. The position of the tendons upon the bones and the articulation of the bones make possible types of motion such as flexion, extension, circumduction, rotation, and gliding.

Muscles that maintain body alignment work together to stabilize surrounding body parts and to support the body's weight. Posture is maintained primarily by the muscles in the back, neck, trunk, and lower extremities.

NEUROLOGICAL SYSTEM

Muscle contraction is controlled by the central nervous system (CNS) and is influenced by the transport of nutrients and oxygen and by the removal of waste products. An intact CNS is essential for coordinated movement to occur because nerve impulses stimulate the muscles to contract. The myoneural junction is the point at which nerve endings come into contact with muscle cells. The afferent pathway conveys information from sensory receptors to the CNS; these neurons conduct impulses throughout the body. The CNS processes the sensory input and determines a response. The efferent pathway transmits the desired response to skeletal muscles via the somatic nervous system. If the nerve

TABLE 36-1 Musculoskeletal System Components

ANATOMICAL STRUCTURE	DESCRIPTION	FUNCTIONS
Bones	Ossified connective tissue	Facilitates mobility, protects body structures (e.g., brain, spinal cord), and produces blood cells
Joints	The site of a union between two bones	Facilitates motion and allows flexibility
Tendons	Cord or band of inelastic connective tissue	Causes movement of muscles
Ligaments	Band of fibrous tissue connecting bones or cartilages	Supports and strengthens joints, facilitates mobility, and protects structures (e.g., knee, hip)
Bursa	Fluid-filled sac or cavity	Prevents friction between bones and cartilage and facilitates gliding of muscles or tendons over bony surfaces
Cartilage	Dense connective tissue	Facilitates mobility

Delmar/Cengage Learning

impulses are interrupted, the muscle becomes paralyzed and is unable to contract.

Proprioception

Proprioception is the awareness of posture, movement, and changes in equilibrium and the knowledge of position, weight, and resistance of objects in relation to the body. Nerve endings (proprioceptors) in muscles, tendons, and joints continuously provide input to the brain, which, in turn, regulates smooth, coordinated involuntary movement.

Postural Reflexes

Postural tonus is maintained by postural or righting reflexes. Table 36-2 describes the major reflexes involved in maintaining posture.

EXERCISE

Exercise is any physical activity involving muscles that elevates the heart rate above its resting level. Exercise reduces joint pain and stiffness and increases flexibility. Not only does exercise make bones stronger, thereby reducing the risk of osteoporosis and fractures, it also improves muscle strength, coordination, and balance. As a result, overall health status is improved (National Institute of Arthritis and Musculoskeletal and Skin Diseases, 2008). According to the Centers for Disease Control and Prevention (CDC, 2008b), approximately 51% of adults in the United States do not get enough physical exercise to benefit health; 24% of adults are not active in their leisure time.

The U.S. Surgeon General's report *Physical Activity Guidelines for Americans* (U.S. Department of Health and

TABLE 36-2 Reflexes That Maintain Postural Tonus

REFLEX	DESCRIPTION
Labyrinthine sense	Sensory organs in the inner ear activate impulses when the head is turned; impulses are transmitted to cerebellum.
Tonic neck-righting reflexes	Affected by movement of head from side to side; neck muscle tonus is affected most when neck is hyperextended.
Optic reflexes	Visual sensations affect posture by helping the person establish spatial relationships with surrounding objects.
Proprioceptor or kinesthetic sense	Activated when nerve endings in muscles and tendons are stimulated by movements of the joints; informs the brain of the location of a body part.
Antigravity (extensor) reflexes	When extensor muscles are stretched beyond a certain point, their stimulation causes a reflex contraction that counteracts the gravitational pull.
Plantar reflexes	Reflexive contraction of the extensor muscles of the lower legs in response to pressure against the sole of the foot by the floor or ground.

Delmar/Cengage Learning

Human Services, 2008) lists the following health benefits of exercise:

- Lower risk of:
    Early death
    Heart disease
    Stroke
    Type 2 diabetes
    High blood pressure
    Increased lipid levels
    Colon and breast cancers
- Better health function in older adults
- Reduced abdominal obesity
- Weight maintenance after weight loss
- Lower risk of hip fracture
- Increased bone density
- Improved sleep quality

See the Respecting Our Differences display, which lists the CDC's (2008a) recommended amounts of exercise for various age groups.

Vigorous exercise stimulates an increased production of endorphins, which promote a sense of well-being. However, it is important to caution people not to overdo the exercise, especially when first starting a new regimen. The following may be signs of too much exercise: unusual or persistent fatigue, increased weakness, decreased range of motion, joint swelling, or continuing pain (pain that lasts more than 1 hour after exercising). Instruct clients, especially those with sedentary lifestyles or chronic illness, to consult their prescribing practitioner before beginning an exercise program. See the Safety First display on page 1097.

TYPES OF EXERCISE

There are several types of exercise that promote physical and psychological health; see Table 36-3.

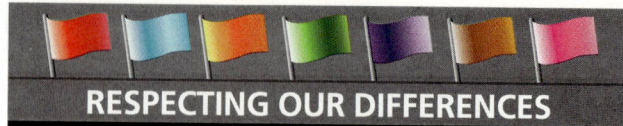

RESPECTING OUR DIFFERENCES

Physical Activity Recommendations for Age Groups

- Children and adolescents: 60 minutes or more of physical activity per day
- Adults: 150 minutes of moderately intense aerobic activity (i.e., brisk walking) each week and muscle-strength activities on 2 or more days per week
- Older adults: same activities and amounts as for other adults

Data from Centers for Disease Control and Prevention. (2008a). *Physical activity for everyone*. Atlanta, GA: Author. Retrieved January 8, 2009, from http://www.cdc.gov/physicalactivity/everyone/guidelines.

Range-of-Motion Exercise

Active range-of-motion (ROM) activities are performed independently by the client; see Table 36-4 on page 1093. During active ROM exercises, the client moves various muscle groups. **Passive ROM** exercises are done by the nurse to help maintain or restore a client's mobility by achieving several outcomes, including the following:

- Prevent contractures
- Improve muscle strength and tone
- Increase circulation
- Decrease vascular complications of immobility
- Facilitate client comfort

TABLE 36-3 Types of Exercise

EXERCISE TYPE	FUNCTION	EXAMPLES
Aerobic	Improve cardiovascular fitness; assist with weight control; improve general functional ability	Rowing, jumping rope, walking, running
Strengthening	Maintain or increase muscle strength	Weight training, calisthenics, physical labor
Isometric	Maintain muscle tone and strength	Quadriceps setting, gluteal setting, triceps setting
Isotonic	Increase and maintain muscle tone and strength; shape muscles; maintain joint mobility; improve cardiovascular fitness	Weight lifting, working with pulleys, ROM exercises, performance of activities of daily living (ADL)
Isokinetic	Condition muscle groups	Exercise equipment and resistive water exercises
Range-of-motion (ROM)	Maintain joint movement; maintain or increase flexibility	Adduction and abduction; flexion and contraction

Delmar/Cengage Learning

TABLE 36-4 Joint Range of Motion

JOINT AND MOVEMENT	EXAMPLE	MUSCLE GROUP(S)	RANGE*
1. Temporomandibular joint (TMJ) (synovial joint) a. Open mouth. b. Close mouth. c. *Protrusion:* Push out lower jaw. d. *Retrusion:* Tuck in lower jaw. e. *Lateral motion:* Slide jaw from side to side.		Masseter, temporalis Pterygoid lateralis Pterygoid lateralis, pterygoid medialis	1–2.5 in. Complete closure 0.5 in. 0.5 in. 0.5 in.
2. Cervical spine (pivot joint) a. *Flexion:* Rest chin on chest. b. *Extension:* Return head to midline. c. *Hyperextension:* Tilt head back.		Sternocleidomastoid Trapezius Trapezius	45° each side 45° 10°
d. *Lateral flexion:* Move head to touch ear to shoulder.		Sternocleidomastoid	45° each side
e. *Rotation:* Turn head to look to side.		Sternocleidomastoid, trapezius	90° each side
3. Shoulder (ball-and-socket joint) a. *Flexion:* Raise straight arm forward to a position above the head. b. *Extension:* Return straight arm forward and down to side of body. c. *Hyperextension:* Move straight arm behind body.		Pectoralis major, coracobrachialis, deltoid, biceps brachii Latissimus dorsi, deltoid, triceps brachii, teres major Latissimus dorsi, deltoid, teres major	180° 180° 50°

(Continues)

TABLE 36-4 (Continued)

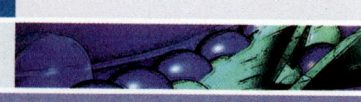

JOINT AND MOVEMENT	EXAMPLE	MUSCLE GROUP(S)	RANGE*
d. *Abduction:* Move straight arm laterally from side to a position above the head, palm facing away from head.	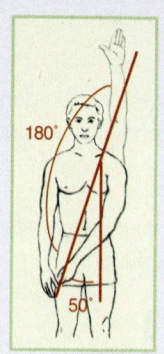	Deltoid, supraspinatus	180°
e. *Adduction:* Move straight arm downward laterally and across front of body as far as possible.		Pectoralis major, teres major	230°
f. *Circumduction:* Move straight arm in a full circle.	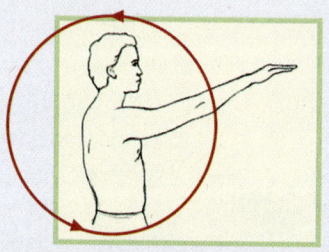	Deltoid, coracobrachialis, latissimus dorsi, teres major	360°
g. *External rotation:* Bent arm lateral, parallel to floor, palm down, rotate shoulder so fingers point up.	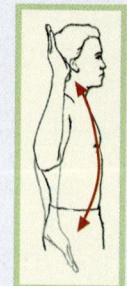	Infraspinatus, teres minor, deltoid	90°
h. *Internal rotation:* Bent arm lateral, parallel to floor, rotate shoulder so fingers point down.		Subscapularis, pectoralis major, latissimus dorsi, teres major	90°
4. Elbow (hinge joint) a. *Flexion:* Bend elbow, move lower arm toward shoulder, palm facing shoulder.	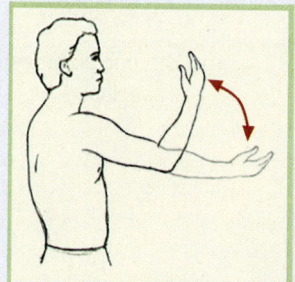	Biceps brachii, brachialis, brachioradialis	150°
b. *Extension:* Straighten lower arm forward and downward.		Triceps brachii	150°
c. *Rotation for supination:* Elbow bent, turn hand and forearm so palm is facing upward.	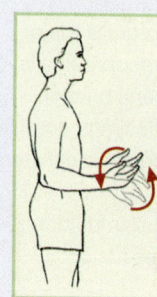	Biceps brachii, supinator	70°–90°
d. *Rotation for pronation:* Elbow bent, turn hand and forearm so palm is facing downward.		Pronator teres, pronator quadrates	70°–90°

(Continues)

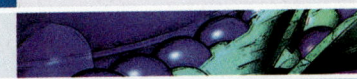

TABLE 36-4 (Continued)

JOINT AND MOVEMENT	EXAMPLE	MUSCLE GROUP(S)	RANGE*
5. Wrist (condyloid joint) a. *Flexion:* Bend wrist so fingers move toward inner aspect of forearm. b. *Extension:* Straighten hand to same plane as arm.		Flexor carpi radialis, flexor carpi ulnaris	80°–90°
		Extensor carpi radialis longus, extensor carpi radialis brevis, extensor carpi ulnaris	80°–90°
c. *Hyperextension:* Bend wrist so fingers move back as far as possible. d. *Radial flexion:* abduction—Bend wrist laterally toward thumb. e. *Ulnar flexion:* adduction—Bend wrist laterally away from thumb.		Extensor carpi radialis longus, extensor carpi radialis brevis, extensor carpi ulnaris	80°–90°
		Extensor carpi radialis longus, extensor carpi radialis brevis, flexor carpi radialis	Up to 20°
		Extensor carpi ulnaris, flexor carpi ulnaris	30°–50°
6. Hand and fingers (condyloid and hinge joints) a. *Flexion:* Make a fist.		Interosseus dorsalis manus, flexor digitorum superficialis	90°
b. *Extension:* Straighten fingers.		Extensor indicis, extensor digiti minimi	90°
c. *Hyperextension:* Bend fingers back as far as possible.		Extensor indicis, extensor digiti minimi	30°–50°
d. *Abduction:* Spread fingers apart.		Interosseus dorsalis manus	25°
e. *Adduction:* Bring fingers together.		Interosseus palmars	25°
7. Thumb (saddle joint) a. *Flexion:* Move thumb across palmar surface of hand.		Flexor pollicis brevis, opponens pollicis	90°
b. *Extension:* Move thumb away from hand.		Extensor pollicis brevis, extensor pollicis longus	90°
c. *Abduction:* Move thumb laterally.		Abductor pollicis brevis, abductor pollicis longus	30°
d. *Adduction:* Move thumb back to hand.		Adductor pollicis transversus, adductor pollicis obliquus	30°
e. *Opposition:* Touch thumb to tip of each finger of same hand.		Opponens pollicis, flexor pollicis brevis	Touching

(Continues)

TABLE 36-4 (Continued)

JOINT AND MOVEMENT	EXAMPLE	MUSCLE GROUP(S)	RANGE*
8. Hip (ball-and-socket joint) a. *Flexion:* Move straight leg forward and upward. b. *Extension:* Move leg back beside the other leg.		Psoas major, iliacus, iliopsoas	90°–120°
		Gluteus maximus, adductor magnus, semitendinosus, semimembranosus	90°–120°
c. *Hyperextension:* Move leg behind body.		Gluteus maximus, semitendinosus, semimembranosus	30°–50°
d. *Abduction:* Move leg laterally from midline.		Gluteus medius, gluteus minimus	40°–50°
e. *Adduction:* Move leg back.		Adductor magnus, adductor brevis, adductor longus	20°–30° past midline
f. *Circumduction:* Move leg backward in a circle.		Psoas major, gluteus maximus, gluteus medius, adductor magnus	360°
g. *Internal rotation:* Turn foot and leg inward, pointing toes toward other leg.		Gluteus minimus, gluteus medius, tensor fasciae latae	90°
h. *External rotation:* Turn foot and leg outward, pointing toes away from other leg.		Obturator externus, obturator internus, quadratus femoris	90°
9. Knee (hinge joint) a. *Flexion:* Bend knee to bring heel back toward thigh.		Biceps femoris, semitendinosus, semimembranosus	120°–130°
b. *Extension:* Straighten each leg, place foot beside other foot.		Rectus femoris, vastus lateralis, vastus medialis, vastus intermedius	120°–130°
10. Ankle (hinge joint) a. *Plantar flexion:* Point toes downward.		Gastrocnemius, soleus	40°–50°
b. *Dorsiflexion:* Point toes upward.		Peroneus tertius, tibialis anterior	20°

(Continues)

TABLE 36-4 (Continued)

JOINT AND MOVEMENT	EXAMPLE	MUSCLE GROUP(S)	RANGE*

11. Foot (gliding joint)
  a. *Eversion:* Turn sole of foot laterally.
  b. *Inversion:* Turn sole of foot medially.
		Peroneus longus, peroneus brevis
		
		Tibialis posterior, tibialis anterior
			5°
			
			5°

12. Toes (condyloid)
  a. *Flexion:* Curve toes downward.
 	
  b. *Extension:* Straighten toes.
 	
  c. *Abduction:* Spread toes apart.
  d. *Adduction:* Bring toes together.
		Flexor hallucis brevis, lumbricales pedis, flexor digitorum brevis
		Extensor digitorum longus, extensor digitorum brevis, extensor hallucis longus
		Interosseus dorsalis pedis, abductor hallucis
		Adductor hallucis, interosseus plantares
			35°–60°
			
			35°–60°
			
			Up to 15°
			
			Up to 15°

*Measurements are approximate.
Delmar/Cengage Learning

▼ SAFETY FIRST ▼

Individuals with cardiovascular problems should be cautioned to exhale when performing isometric exercises in order to avoid increasing blood pressure.

PHYSICAL FITNESS

The goal of regular physical activity is physical fitness that affects an individual's functional ability. There are four components of physical fitness: endurance and strength, joint flexibility, cardiorespiratory fitness, and body composition.

Endurance and Strength

Endurance is the ability to withstand movement in terms of duration and absence of fatigue. A physically fit individual has adequate muscular strength and endurance to accomplish one's goals.

Muscle strength is the amount of force exerted by the muscles against resistance. Good muscle strength allows an individual to lift safely.

Joint Flexibility

The ability to use a muscle through its complete range of motion is referred to as flexibility; see Table 36-4 for a complete description of joint movement. People with limited flexibility are likely to experience shortened muscles and tendons with resulting loss of muscle strength and joint injury. Flexibility can be improved by stretching exercises such as yoga, tai chi, and dancing. Performance of ADL also helps maintain flexibility. Walking, stooping, and lifting activities can promote and maintain flexibility.

Cardiorespiratory Fitness

Exercises that improve cardiorespiratory fitness are discussed in Table 36-3. To improve cardiorespiratory function, physical activity must be maintained for at least 20 minutes in order to raise the heart rate to the target level.

Body Composition

The proportion of fat to lean body tissue is referred to as body composition. Having a body that falls within the normal range of body weight and percentage of body fat depends on balancing caloric intake and expenditure. Any type of physical activity can be useful in developing and maintaining physical fitness; see Table 36-5 on page 1098.

Fitness in Older Adults

Physical fitness is essential for older adults for maintenance of well-being and injury prevention. Muscle strength, coordination, and endurance are affected by the physiological changes of aging. Diminished muscle strength is a result of age-related loss of muscle mass. Muscle coordination and endurance decline due to changes in the CNS and muscles (Miller, 2009).

TABLE 36-5 Steps for Maintaining Ideal Body Weight

ACTION	IMPACT ON ENERGY BALANCE
Decrease amount of time spent in sedentary activities (e.g., watching television), and build physical activity into regular routines.	Increases physical activity; increases calorie consumption
Select foods that are low in fat, calories, and added sugars.	Decreases excessive calorie consumption
Create more opportunities for physical activity in workplaces.	Increases physical activity; increases amount of calories used

Data from National Center for Chronic Disease Prevention and Health Promotion. (2008). *Overweight and obesity: Contributing factors*. Atlanta, GA: Author. Retrieved January 10, 2009, from http://www.cdc.gov/nccdphp/dnpa/obesity/contributing_factors.htm

Such physiological changes can increase the risk of falls. Falls are the greatest cause of injury in people over the age of 70 (Fulmer, Wallace, & Edelman, 2006). Regular exercise, especially weight-bearing exercise (e.g., walking), improves endurance and strengthens bones. Decreased bone density results in osteoporosis, which makes a person more vulnerable to fractures; see the Respecting Our Differences display.

Some benefits of physical exercise in older adults are the following:

- Improves gait and balance
- Improves cardiovascular function
- Increases energy
- Promotes bone density
- Improves mobility
- Promotes weight loss

RESPECTING OUR DIFFERENCES

Osteoporosis in Diverse Groups

Rates of Osteoporosis (listed in groups ranging from highest to lowest risk):

Asians, Alaska Natives, Native Americans

White non-Hispanic women

Hispanic groups

White men

African American men

Miller, C. (2009). *Nursing for wellness in older adults* (5th ed.). Philadelphia: Wolters Kluwer/Lippincott Williams & Wilkins, p. 463.

FACTORS AFFECTING MOBILITY

Mobility and activity level can be influenced by many factors, including overall health status, developmental stage, environment, attitudes, beliefs, and lifestyle.

HEALTH STATUS

An individual's general health status will influence exercise and activity tolerance. Compromised status of any of the body systems may affect an individual's mobility and may, in turn, be affected by a lack of activity. Physical conditioning will also influence mobility and stamina. Physical factors interfering with mobility or exercise include fatigue, muscle cramping, dyspnea, neuromuscular or perceptual deficits, and chest pain.

Mental status is often manifested as changes in mobility or appearance. For instance, a client who shuffles into the room and slumps down into a chair may be sending a message of depression through low activity levels and poor posture.

DEVELOPMENTAL STAGE

An individual's developmental stage will affect mobility and functional ability. See Table 36-6 for examples of common age-related musculoskeletal trauma.

Children

Developmental norms related to mobility have been established for the infant and toddler. Childhood development is monitored through achievement of milestones such as sitting, crawling, walking, running, and hopping. See Chapter 18 for discussion of developmental milestones. For *infants,* mobility involves gross motor behaviors such as posture, head balance, grasping, sitting, creeping, and standing. *Toddlers* are more

TABLE 36-6 Common Age-Related Musculoskeletal Trauma

AGE RANGE	COMMON TRAUMAS
0 to 18 months	Falls
18 months to 6 years	Falls
6 to 20 years	Sports-related injuries, motorcycle accidents, high-impact falls (e.g., cycling, skiing)
20 to 50 years	Sports-related injuries, stress or overuse injuries (e.g., tendonitis), pedestrian injuries
50 to 65 years	Recreation-related injuries, falls, pathological fractures, pedestrian injuries
65+ years	Falls

Delmar/Cengage Learning

active, with walking, running, jumping, kicking, and going up and down stairs. Activity and mobility parameters for the toddler include gross and fine motor behaviors, manual dexterity, and exploration within environmental safety parameters. The *preschooler* increases strength and refines skills by walking, running, and jumping. During *middle childhood* (from 6 to 12 years of age), children have improved posture and locomotion abilities and increased muscle efficiency of the extremities and trunk; these children also have an increase in muscle tissue with a decrease of fat. For both preschool and middle childhood, activity and mobility expectations are centered on development of strength, coordination, and physical capacities.

Adolescents

The *adolescent* years (approximately ages 12 to 18) begin with onset of puberty and end with cessation of somatic growth. Changes are dramatic at this stage, with rapid physical growth and development of secondary sex characteristics. Activity and mobility landmarks are development of muscles plus cardiac, respiratory, and metabolic functions through physical conditioning.

Adults

Adulthood is divided into young, middle, and older age groups. The *young adult* has well-developed musculoskeletal and nervous systems that ideally function at peak efficiency. The *middle-aged* adult has a gradual decrease in muscle mass, strength, and agility. The focus of activity and mobility for both these groups is on maintaining or developing tone, strength, and coordination of the musculoskeletal system.

Older adults experience progressive changes in the physiological systems. The rate of calcium reabsorption, which affects bone density, increases with aging. Bone density loss accelerates in postmenopausal females due to decreased amounts of estrogen. Decreased bone density makes a person more vulnerable to fractures, **kyphosis** (abnormally increased convexity in the curvature of the spine), and a reduction in height.

Aging also negatively affects muscles and connective tissue. The development of muscle atrophy is a gradual process in which muscle fibers deteriorate and are replaced by fibrous connective tissue. Muscle atrophy is accompanied by reduced muscle mass, a loss of muscle strength, and a reduction in overall body mass. The degree of muscle atrophy will be affected by the person's activity level. Staying physically active helps prevent disuse muscle atrophy and helps maximize muscle strength.

Cartilage ages better than bone or muscle; however, some changes occur that do affect joint flexibility. Aging leads to a loss of water content of hyaline cartilage and a reduction in the ability of cartilage to regenerate following trauma. Articulating cartilage may slightly deteriorate as a result of lifetime wear and tear. Aging also affects the health of intervertebral disks. For example, the water content of the disks decreases, which leads to less vertebral flexibility. Thinning of the disks causes older individuals to be more vulnerable to back pain and injury.

As a result of the age-related physical changes, older people often experience some functional alterations in mobility. Ambulation may be altered as a result of joint inflexibility and decreased muscle strength; such alterations are noticed as a reduction in step height and length, as demonstrated in a shuffling gait. Vertebral inflexibility and reduced muscle strength may cause difficulty with client transfers in and out of a sitting position. The elderly client may need assistance in rising from a chair, ambulating, or climbing stairs. Table 36-7 provides an overview of age-related effects on mobility. Aging also affects the cardiovascular and respiratory systems, which directly affect endurance and stamina. Activity and mobility goals focus on maintenance of functional status and safety.

ENVIRONMENT

Environment can influence activity levels in several ways. Home environments, for instance, can be considered safe and "mobility friendly" if they are free of hazards that can disrupt or endanger mobility and activity. Work environments can also affect mobility; repetitive handwork (e.g., keystroking, sewing) can impair mobility and worsen arthritis.

ATTITUDES AND BELIEFS

Influential factors related to exercise are one's attitudes and beliefs, which are greatly affected by culture and family. Leisure activities provide a clue to the person's value system. Individuals who engage in hiking, bicycle riding, or swimming for recreation value an active lifestyle. On the other hand, individuals who consider work to be the dominant area of life may view exercise as "a waste of time." See the Nursing Process Highlight on page 1100. Activities enjoyed by the individual are less likely to produce fatigue than are activities that hold no interest for the person. Thus, individual preferences should be matched with capabilities when planning an exercise program.

LIFESTYLE

Modern lifestyles require little physical activity; thus, few adults in America are naturally fit. The use of many convenience items (e.g., automobiles, fast food, remote controls) encourages little

TABLE 36-7	Effects of Aging on Musculoskeletal System
AGE-RELATED CHANGES	**HEALTH IMPLICATIONS**
Osteoporosis	Risk of fracture
Decreased muscle size and tone	Impaired physical ability
Stiffening of joints	Decreased range of motion leading to: Decreased mobility Increased fall risk
Kyphosis	Shifting center of gravity (fall risk) Decreased self-esteem

Data from Clark, M. J. (2008). *Community health nursing: Advocacy for population health* (5th ed.). Upper Saddle River, NJ: Pearson Prentice Hall.

NURSING PROCESS HIGHLIGHT

Assessment

Assessing Attitudes and Beliefs about Exercise

Asking these questions helps determine the client's perception of physical activity:

Do you routinely climb stairs or use elevators?

Do you usually go everywhere in a car or walk for transportation?

Is exercise a part of your daily routine?

What activities do you enjoy doing in your leisure time?

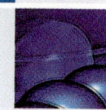

TABLE 36-8 Negative Outcomes of Immobility

Neurologic	Gastrointestinal
Sensory deprivation	Decreased appetite
	Stress ulcers
	Constipation
	Fecal impaction
Cardiovascular	**Urinary**
Increased cardiac workload	Urinary stasis
Orthostatic hypotension	Urinary tract infection
Formation of thrombus	Calculi
Respiratory	**Integumentary**
Increased respiratory effort	Skin shearing
Hypostatic pneumonia	Pressure ulcers
Altered gas exchange	
Musculoskeletal	**Psychological**
Decreased bone density (increased risk of fracture)	Anxiety
Contractures	Depression
Muscle atrophy	Helplessness, hopelessness
Increased pain	Increased dependency

Delmar/Cengage Learning

physical exertion. The sedentary lifestyles of many Americans result in loss of muscle strength, decreased endurance, inadequate cardiorespiratory function, and obesity. A sedentary lifestyle can lead to muscle atrophy, weakened bones, and a lack of motivation and energy to engage in physical activity. Individuals with active lifestyles value exercise and, therefore, are more likely to experience its therapeutic outcomes.

PHYSIOLOGICAL EFFECTS OF MOBILITY AND IMMOBILITY

Maintaining functional mobility and desired activity levels is important for both psychological and physiological reasons. Mobility and lack thereof will both affect the various systems of the body. Table 36-8 summarizes the major complications associated with immobility.

NEUROLOGICAL EFFECTS AND MENTAL STATUS

Mobility and activity can increase an individual's energy levels and sense of well-being. Activity and exercise are excellent means to relieve tension and reduce stress, which result in better sleep patterns and an enhanced sense of well-being.

Client inactivity and immobility are stressors that can lead to frustration, lower self-esteem, anxiety, helplessness, depression, general dissatisfaction, restlessness, unhappiness, and decreased competency self-rating. Immobility affects cognitive abilities, affect, lifestyle, and social and family responsibilities. The fear of falls, pain, and sensory deficits such as visual problems, fatigue, and weakness are compounding factors that increase inactivity and immobility.

CARDIOVASCULAR EFFECTS

The cardiovascular system reaps many benefits from mobility and exercise. The heart becomes more efficient as it adapts to increased demands for oxygen, and cardiac output increases.

A healthy heart muscle leads to a decreased resting heart rate and decreased resting blood pressure. Thus, the heart does not have to work as hard in an individual who exercises regularly as it does in an individual who leads a sedentary lifestyle. Activity increases the oxygen supply to the heart and muscles and thereby benefits overall health.

Immobility increases the workload on the heart as the supine position increases the volume of blood circulating to the heart. This fluid shift increases central venous pressure along with left ventricular diastolic volume and stroke volume, and the cardiac workload increases. The cardiovascular system is prone to form **thrombi** (blood clots) due to venous stasis related to lack of muscle contractions of the legs and pressure on veins, especially the popliteal areas (see Figure 36-6 on page 1101). Thrombi are caused by increased coagulation of the blood due to free calcium from bone demineralization, stasis of venous blood, and intimal damage to veins (as from venipuncture). See the Safety First display on page 1101.

Another cardiovascular problem related to immobility is **orthostatic hypotension**, a decrease in blood pressure resulting from sudden position changes, caused by decreased vessel tone. In orthostatic hypotension, the blood pressure parameters drop at least 25 mm systolic and 10 mm diastolic with postural changes. Orthostatic hypotension is a result of several factors associated with immobility, including:

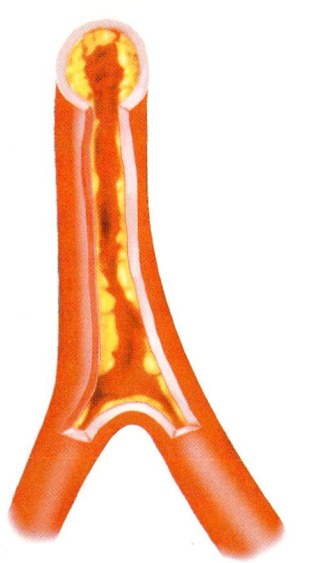

FIGURE 36-6 Effect of Immobility on the Cardiovascular System DELMAR/CENGAGE LEARNING

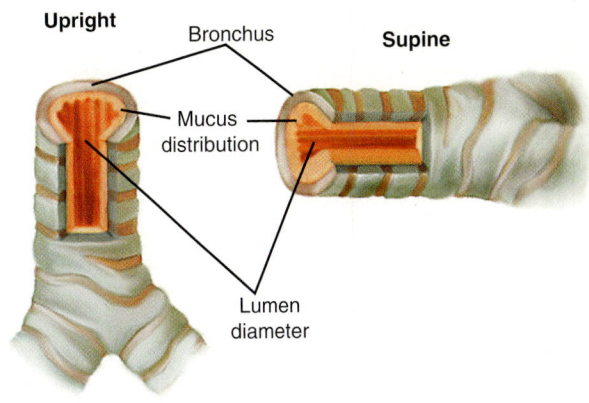

FIGURE 36-7 Effect of Immobility on the Respiratory System
DELMAR/CENGAGE LEARNING

▼ SAFETY FIRST ▼

DEEPVEIN THROMBOSIS (DVT)
Deep vein thrombi have the potential of becoming pulmonary emboli, which are life-threatening. Individuals who are immobile (e.g., on bedrest) are at greater risk of developing DVT.

- Decreased circulating fluid volume
- Decreased autonomic nervous system response
- Blood pooling in lower extremities

These factors lead to decreased venous return, which negatively affects cardiac output; thus, the blood pressure is lowered. Orthostatic hypotension is an indication that the heart is working harder and less efficiently.

Clients who have experienced immobility (e.g., with bed rest) need to have blood pressure checked lying down, sitting, and then standing. This is done to establish baseline parameters to assist in determining the presence of postural-related changes in blood pressure.

RESPIRATORY EFFECTS

The respiratory response to activity is increased intake of oxygen, which results in increased overall respiratory capacity and easier breathing. The effects of oxygenation to the tissues are enhanced, and pooling of secretions in the bronchioles is less likely.

Immobility from sitting or lying limits chest expansion, which is compounded by the effects of respiratory muscle atrophy and ineffective cough (see Figure 36-7). Stasis of respiratory secretions can be worsened by the use of CNS-depressant medications and dehydration and can lead to hypostatic pneumonia and atelectasis.

MUSCULOSKELETAL EFFECTS

Musculoskeletal responses to activity are numerous, including stronger and better-defined muscles, stronger bones, and increased mobility and joint range of motion. Exercise can enhance endurance and tolerance of the muscle groups. Weight-bearing exercises such as walking (as opposed to swimming) are especially beneficial in preventing osteoporosis, or loss of strength and minerals in the bones.

Decreased physical mobility results in gross musculoskeletal impairment, especially when muscular atrophy occurs. Decreased mobilization alters muscle structure by reducing muscle mass and decreasing muscle cell diameter and the actual number of muscle cells. Clients experience rapid fatigue, decreased muscle strength and tone, decreased endurance, decreased mobility of joints, muscle stiffness, joint contracture, and negative nitrogen balance due to protein catabolism. Loss of calcium is a response to immobility and indicates an imbalance between bone formation and breakdown. The lack of pressure (e.g., weight bearing) on bones triggers calcium loss. Bone demineralization occurs as early as 2 or 3 days after onset of immobility and may lead to pathological fractures, renal calculi, and osteoporosis.

DIGESTIVE EFFECTS

Digestive responses to activity include increased appetite and thirst, which indicate that the body's rate of processing nutritional intake is increased. Exercise increases metabolism with resultant absorption of nutrients and excretion of wastes.

Loss of appetite is commonly related to lack of activity, negative nitrogen balance, and altered elimination patterns. Negative nitrogen balance occurs when the nitrogen output exceeds nitrogen intake. The causes of negative nitrogen balance include the increased need for protein in situations of extensive tissue damage, such as surgery and extended immobility. Extended periods of immobility cause muscle atrophy or muscle wasting; thus, there is a need for extra protein intake to provide for muscle repair.

ELIMINATION EFFECTS

Elimination patterns are facilitated by mobility in that retention of wastes is usually prevented and the risk of constipation is reduced or avoided. Activity causes the muscles to become stronger and more efficient, thus enhancing the overall efficiency of elimination.

Constipation and fecal impaction are frequent complications of immobility. Variables contributing to these elimination problems are:

- Lack of activity, which decreases peristalsis
- Lack of privacy
- Inability to sit upright
- Improper diet
- Inadequate fluid intake
- Use of some medications, especially narcotics

Urinary stasis and urinary infections are related to the recumbent position of the immobile person. Decreased peristalsis of the ureters leads to stasis of urine, which is the etiology of urinary calculi (stones) and infection. Bladder distention occurs due to difficult relaxation of the external sphincter and decreased intraabdominal pressure, thus causing overflow incontinence (loss of bladder control) and infection. The combination of increased urinary calcium, urinary stasis, and urinary tract infection leads to calculi formation.

INTEGUMENTARY EFFECTS

The integumentary system benefits from activity and exercise in that increased circulation and blood flow enhance oxygenation of tissues. As a result, the turgor and luster of the skin and hair are maintained.

Pressure ulcers are serious problems related to immobility. Prolonged pressure, shearing force, friction (rubbing), and moisture lead to tissue ischemia (impaired blood circulation), causing skin breakdown and pressure ulcers. Moisture in the form of urine, feces, perspiration, and wound drainage can also lead to skin softening, which increases risk for pressure ulcers. Secondary factors contributing to pressure ulcer development are decreased nutrition, decreased arterial pressure, increased age, and edema. Refer to Chapter 37 for a discussion of pressure ulcers.

ASSESSMENT

During the assessment phase of the nursing process, data regarding activity and mobility of the client are gathered. Assessment data are used to initiate, individualize, plan, evaluate, and modify care on the basis of the client's strengths and limitations. Assessment of mobility status includes a health history and physical examination.

HEALTH HISTORY

Determining a client's health history is the first step in assessing the mobility needs and concerns of a client. Basic information about ADL, exercise patterns (type, frequency),

lifestyle (active, sedentary), activity tolerance, and use of medications should be discussed. If an alteration or recent change in status is noted, then a detailed health history is in order. The nurse should ask what impact the mobility impairment has had on the client's ADL and should have the client describe the exact nature of the problem (onset, duration, associated factors, aggravating factors, alleviating factors). The nurse should ask clients about the use (past and current) of medications, both prescription and over the counter, with the explanation that many drugs negatively affect the musculoskeletal system. It is also important to ask about the use of calcium supplements and estrogen replacement medication.

PHYSICAL EXAMINATION

The physical examination of mobility status typically covers three basic areas: musculoskeletal assessment, neurological assessment, and functional assessment.

Musculoskeletal Assessment

The nurse observes musculoskeletal functioning during every interaction with the client. The accompanying Nursing Process Highlight on page 1103 lists steps in assessing musculoskeletal status. Specific factors for objective assessment include the following:

- Body alignment
- Body mechanics
- Posture (sitting and standing)
- Range of motion
- Strength of muscles
- Endurance
- Muscle tone
- Size and contour of joints
- Inspection of the skin
- Palpation of skin, muscles, and joints

Subjective data include assessment of the client's pain, joint stiffness, muscle cramping, fatigue, weakness, exercise habits, and environmental variables. Children should be evaluated by comparing physical development and abilities with normal values for the age. Older adults should be assessed for functional abilities, strengths, weaknesses, joint limitations, and use of assistive devices such as canes or walkers that are necessary for self-care activities. A complete musculoskeletal assessment includes data related to client weakness, stiffness, and pain related to movement.

Movement and Gait

Gait, the way that one walks, is assessed to determine a baseline. Normal gait is characterized by a smooth, rhythmic movement of muscles when walking. Step height and length are symmetrical for each foot, and the arms swing freely at each side of the torso in opposite movement of the legs. Normally, the lower limbs are able to bear full body weight during standing and ambulation. Gait is described in terms of smoothness, balance, arm movement, effectiveness, and the length and width of the step.

NURSING PROCESS HIGHLIGHT

Assessment

Assessing Musculoskeletal Status

1. Wash hands.
2. Provide an explanation to the client of the assessment procedure.
3. Assist the client to a comfortable position.
4. Use pillows or folded blankets to support painful body parts.
5. Provide assistance with disrobing as needed.
6. Adjust room temperature for client comfort.
7. Provide clear instructions to client (e.g., assuming a certain body position or performing a certain body movement).
8. Inform client before touching or moving a painful body part.
9. Assess skeletal muscles and joints in a cephalocaudal, proximal-to-distal manner. Always compare paired muscles and joints.
10. Examine unaffected body parts before examining affected ones.
11. Avoid unnecessary or excessive manipulation of a painful body part. If the client verbalizes pain, stop the aggravating motion.
12. If needed, assist client in dressing after the physical examination is completed.

Data adapted from Estes, M. E. Z. (2010). *Health assessment and physical examination* (4th ed.). Clifton Park, NY: Delmar/Cengage Learning.

Body Alignment

When assessing body alignment, the nurse seeks to determine whether the movement results in fatigue, muscle stress, or strain. Structural deformities may interfere with body alignment and functional ability; see Table 36-9 on page 1104.

Endurance

When assessing a client's endurance during physical activity, look for reactions such as mood changes, indicators of pain, presence of fatigue, and changes in respiratory and circulatory status. Oxygen consumption increases during muscle activity; thus, assessment of vital signs is essential. The time required for vital signs to return to the normal (baseline) resting values is a significant factor to include in the assessment of mobility.

Pathological Alterations

Assessment to determine the presence of pathological alterations—such as bone disorders, joint impairment, impaired muscle development, postural abnormalities, musculoskeletal trauma, and neurological damage—can offer important data for the determination of mobility limitations.

MUSCLE IMPAIRMENTS Overuse injuries are a common type of musculoskeletal problem, especially in people who exercise too much or incorrectly. Common overuse injuries are listed in Table 36-10 on page 1106.

CONTRACTURES A contracture, a condition of fixed resistance to the passive stretch of a muscle, develops when the muscle fibers become unable to flex; see Figure 36-8 on page 1106. Each muscle has an antagonist that works in the opposite direction. If a muscle group is not moved for a period of time or if proper body alignment is not maintained, the stronger muscle will predominate, causing contracture deformities.

Once a contracture occurs, the only corrective action is surgical release of the fibrous tissue. Prevention of contractures is a major nursing focus with immobile clients. Nursing interventions to prevent a muscle contracture include:

- Encouraging clients to be as active as possible
- Performing ROM exercises
- Positioning to maintain proper body alignment
- Repositioning every 2 hours or more often as needed

MUSCULOSKELETAL TRAUMA Trauma to musculoskeletal tissues can result in many types of impairments (such as those described in Table 36-10). Other common types of musculoskeletal trauma are fractures (broken bones) and surgical amputation.

FRACTURES Hip fractures are disabling injuries that occur in many older people. Hip fractures are usually a result of falls, with complications that lead to the deaths of many of the fallers (Clark, 2008). Hip fracture complications result from immobility and include pressure ulcers, pneumonia, and sepsis from urinary tract infections. When a fracture is suspected, the nurse should assess the area for mobility, pain, color, temperature, pulse, and sensation.

AMPUTATION Any condition in which circulation is inadequate for cellular function may lead to amputation. For example, lower limb amputations are often required as a result of infection, peripheral vascular disease (PVD), neoplasm, and trauma. Pressure ulcers, if inadequately treated, can also lead to the loss of a limb. When pressure ulcers do not heal, infection and gangrene develop. Gangrene first manifests as a blackened area and is often accompanied by pain.

Lower limb amputation is either above or below the knee; the level of amputation depends on the extent of the disease process. Below-the-knee amputation is the most commonly performed type. The goal of the surgery is to preserve the length of the extremity in order to assist with prosthetic fitting. Therefore, as much limb as possible is salvaged.

CENTRAL NERVOUS SYSTEM DAMAGE As movement is a result of coordination between muscles and nerves, an intact CNS is necessary for mobility. Any disruption in the CNS, such as those occurring with spinal cord injury, can impair mobility. Spinal cord injury can lead to partial paralysis or complete loss of mobility.

Spinal Cord Injury (SCI)   Damage to the spinal cord can be a result of hyperextension or compression. With hyperextension, the spinal cord is overstretched, leading to dislocation of the vertebrae or discs and possible compression of the spinal cord. Hyperextension can also completely dissect the spinal cord. In a complete spinal cord injury, voluntary motor activity, sensory function, and proprioception below the level of the injury are absent.

Compression injuries occur when the force of impact fractures the vertebrae or ruptures the discs, forcing bony fragments or discs into the spinal canal. These particles can lacerate or compress the spinal cord, resulting in paralysis below the level of the injury. Prevention of SCI is a major concern of nurses and may be addressed through educating the public on safety precautions related to driving, participation in sports, and leisure activities.

Table 36-9 Spinal Misalignment

ANOMALY	DESCRIPTION	CLINICAL IMPLICATIONS

Scoliosis
• *Postural scoliosis:* no fixed rotation of vertebrae; can be corrected with exercise
• *Structural scoliosis:* fixed rotation of the vertebrae in the direction of the convexity of the curve
	• Lateral deviation in the normally straight vertical line of the spine
	• More common in females, especially during adolescence
	• Some indicators:
	  — One side of body higher than the other or one shoulder blade more prominent
	  — Abnormal waistline tilt with more indentation on one side
	  — Tilting of the hips with one hip more prominent
	  — A prominence of the posterior chest or the shoulder when bending over
		• Can progress to a severe curvature in a short period of time if untreated

Kyphosis	• Abnormally increased convexity in the curvature of the spine
	• Chin tilts downward onto chest with abdominal protrusion
	• Decreased interval between lower rib cage and iliac crests
		• In advanced stages, can interfere with lung expansion
		• Commonly seen in:
		  — Older clients
		  — Osteoporosis

(Continues)

TABLE 36-9 (Continued)

ANOMALY	DESCRIPTION	CLINICAL IMPLICATIONS	
Lordosis	• Forward curvature of the lumbar spine	• More pronounced in obesity and pregnancy (due to change in center of gravity)	
List	• Lateral tilt of the spine • Iliac crests unequal in height • Decreased ROM, usually accompanied by pain	• Commonly present in: — Back injury — Osteoarthritis — Herniated vertebral disc	

Delmar/Cengage Learning

NEUROLOGICAL ASSESSMENT

An intact neurological system is essential for activity and mobility. A complete neurological assessment includes (1) cranial nerves, (2) the motor system, (3) the sensory system, and (4) reflexes. The nurse assesses the motor system for the following variables:

• Size, strength, and tone of muscles
• Presence of involuntary movements
• Balance
• Gait
• Coordination
• Proprioception
• Fine motor function
• Gross motor function

The sensory system is assessed for integrity of peripheral nerves, pain, tactile discrimination (fine touch), and sensation of vibration. Assessment of deep tendon or stretch

TABLE 36-10	Musculoskeletal Trauma and Common Overuse Injuries
Strain	Commonly referred to as "pulled muscles"; caused by overstretching, tearing, or ripping of a muscle or its tendon
Tendonitis	Inflammation of a tendon; caused by chronic, low-grade strain of a muscle-tendon unit
Bursitis	Inflammation of the bursa (lubricating sac surrounding a joint); caused by repeated, low-grade strain of the joint's supporting tissues
Sprain	Overstretching or tearing of ligaments

Delmar/Cengage Learning

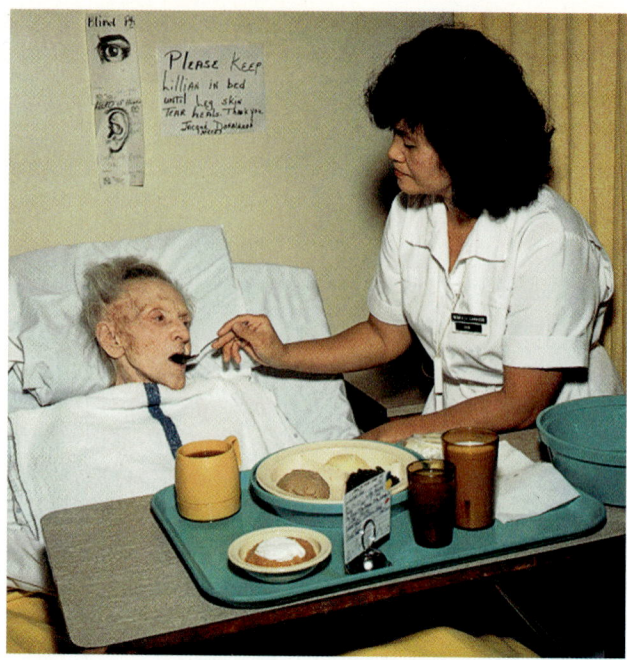

FIGURE 36-9 Some mobility impairments significantly limit a person's ability to perform ADL. DELMAR/CENGAGE LEARNING

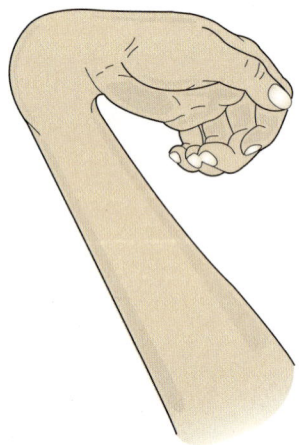

FIGURE 36-8 Hand-Wrist Contracture DELMAR/CENGAGE LEARNING

reflexes focuses on the biceps, triceps, brachioradialis, quadriceps, and Achilles reflexes. Refer to Chapter 27 for further details on physical assessment.

Functional Assessment

Functional assessment focuses on the client's abilities to perform ADL. The client's functional status is assessed in terms of the ability to feed, dress, toilet, move, transfer, and ambulate himself or herself independently or with some degree of required assistance; see Figure 36-9. Functional assessment data are used for initial care planning, for discharge planning, for planning continuity of care in a nursing home or private home, and to provide baseline and ongoing data for rehabilitation.

Clients at high risk for falls include those with prolonged hospitalization, those taking sedatives or tranquilizers, confused clients, and those with a history of physical restraint use. A great majority of falls:

- Occur in the evening
- Occur in the client's room
- Involve wheelchairs
- Involve unattended clients
- Involve clients with poor footwear
- Occur with poor lighting
- Involve clients with poor vision
- Occur with clients experiencing neuromuscular impairment
- Occur when toileting needs arise

Awareness of these risk factors for falls allows the nurse to prevent many client injuries.

The nurse continually evaluates the client's strength and endurance during the entire ambulation process. The Risk Assessment Tool (RAT) for falls was developed to identify clients at high risk for falls and to individualize care (Brians, Alexander, Grota, Chen, & Dumas, 1991). See the accompanying Nursing Checklist on page 1107 for the RAT and Chapter 29 for further discussion of fall prevention.

NURSING DIAGNOSIS

Nursing diagnoses related to mobility focus primarily on activity and mobility levels and the psychosocial impact that alterations in mobility can have on a client and family. Common nursing diagnoses, established by the North American Nursing Diagnosis Association (NANDA, 2009), related to

✓ NURSINGCHECKLIST

Risk Assessment Tool (RAT) for Falls

Directions: Place a check mark in front of elements that apply to your patient. The decision of whether or not a patient is at risk for falls is based on your nursing judgment. GUIDELINE: A patient who has a check mark in front of an element with an asterisk (*) or four or more of the other elements would be identified as at risk for falls.

GENERAL DATA
— Age over 60
— History of falls prior to admission*
— Postoperative/admit for operation
— Smoker

PHYSICAL CONDITION
— Dizziness/imbalance
— Unsteady gait
— Diseases/problems affecting weight-bearing joints
— Weakness
— Paresis
— Seizure disorder
— Impairment of vision
— Impairment of hearing
— Diarrhea
— Urinary frequency

MENTAL STATUS
— Confusion/disorientation*
— Impaired memory or judgment
— Inability to understand or follow directions

MEDICATIONS
— Diuretics or diuretic effects
— Hypotensive or CNS suppressants (narcotic, sedative, psychotropic, hypnotic, tranquilizer, antihypertensive, antidepressant)
— Medication that increases GI motility (laxative, enema)

AMBULATORY DEVICES USED
— Cane
— Crutches
— Walker
— Wheelchair
— Geri chair
— Braces

From Brians, L. K., Alexander, K., Grota, P., Chen, R. W. H., & Dumas, V. (1991). The development of the RISK tool for fall prevention. *Rehabilitation Nursing, 16*(2), 67–69. Reprinted with permission of the Association of Rehabilitation Nurses. Copyright 1991 by the Association of Rehabilitation Nurses.

---

the physical adaptations or risks resulting from altered mobility include:

- *Activity intolerance* related to bed rest and immobility, generalized weakness, sedentary lifestyle, and imbalance between oxygen supply and demand (see Table 36-11 on page 1108)
- *Impaired physical mobility* related to intolerance to activity or decreased strength and endurance, pain, perceptual or cognitive impairment, neuromuscular impairment, musculoskeletal impairment, and depression or severe anxiety (see Table 36-11)
- *Risk for disuse syndrome* per risk factors of paralysis, mechanical immobilization, prescribed immobilization, and severe pain
- *Self-care deficits* related to inability to wash body or body parts, inability to obtain or get to water source, activity intolerance, decreased strength and endurance, pain, or impaired transfer ability
- *Ineffective health maintenance* related to lack of or significant alteration in communication skills (written, nonverbal)
- *Risk for falls* related to impaired mobility

Alterations in family and social processes may also result from immobility and inactivity. Disruption in activity and

mobility leads to impairment of the ability to perform one's usual social, vocational, educational, and family roles. There are often changes in the client's perception of his or her roles. *Disturbed body image* and *Situational low self-esteem* can result from (NANDA, 2009):

1. Changes in physical abilities
2. Changes in family responsibilities
3. Lack of knowledge regarding rehabilitation
4. Denial of abilities and strengths
5. Social insecurity
6. Feelings of worthlessness, hopelessness, or depression

PLANNING AND OUTCOME IDENTIFICATION

Client involvement is essential in the development of outcomes related to mobility needs. Realistic outcomes can be targeted by considering the client's (1) understanding of mobility status; (2) values, thoughts, and concerns regarding mobility problems; (3) general health status; and (4) ability to solve problems.

TABLE 36-11 Nursing Diagnoses and Clients Experiencing Problems with Mobility

NURSING DIAGNOSIS	DEFINING CHARACTERISTICS	RELATED FACTORS
• *Activity intolerance* —a state in which an individual has insufficient physiological or psychological energy to endure or complete required or desired daily activities	• Verbalization of weakness or fatigue • Abnormal physiological responses to activity (e.g., heart rate or blood pressure changes) • Discomfort or dyspnea upon exertion	• Immobility, bed rest • Generalized weakness • Sedentary lifestyle • Imbalance between oxygen supply and demand
• *Impaired physical mobility* —a state in which the person experiences a limitation in independent, purposeful physical movement	• Inability to move purposefully • Hesitant to attempt movement • Limited range of motion • Impaired coordination • Decreased muscle mass, strength, and control	• Decreased strength and endurance • Discomfort or pain • Perceptual or cognitive impairment • Musculoskeletal impairment • Depression, marked anxiety

Data from Carpenito, L. J. (2007). *Handbook of nursing diagnosis* (12th ed.). Philadelphia: Lippincott Williams & Wilkins; North American Nursing Diagnosis Association International (NANDA). (2009). *Nursing diagnoses—Diagnoses and Classification 2009–2011.* © 2009, 2007, 2005, 2003, 2001, 1998, 1996, 1994 NANDA International. Used by arrangement with Wiley-Blackwell Publishing, a company of John Wiley & Sons, Inc.

COLLABORATION

The goal of the interdisciplinary health team during acute hospitalization and rehabilitation is to restore function, thus maximizing the level of the client's independence. Maximal independence includes the ability to perform ADL (eating, dressing, bathing, and moving). Independence in these activities contributes to self-reliance, self-care, self-determination, self-direction, and personal control. Personal client variables that determine the maximal level of independence include extent of disability, competence, age, self-confidence, cognitive ability, knowledge level, and mood state. It is important to develop short-term goals that encourage clients to gain a sense of accomplishment. The nurse should recognize and praise the client's accomplishments that increase mobility.

The level of independence and ability for performance of ADL is enhanced or inhibited by the physical environment. Collaboration of the client, family, caregivers, nurses, physical therapists, and occupational therapists is essential for individualizing the physical environment to permit optimal activity and mobilization. Adaptive devices, such as those that follow, enhance independence for personal activities:

- Eating (e.g., plate guards and hand splints to hold utensils)
- Bathing (e.g., shower chairs and long-handled bath sponges)
- Dressing (e.g., Velcro closures and zipper pulls)
- Toileting (e.g., elevated toilet seats)
- Mobility (e.g., walkers)

Continued practice in self-care activities with adaptive devices promotes confidence. Interdisciplinary cooperation can be used to plan modifications for the home for activity and mobility, especially in the bathroom and kitchen. Physical modifications with adaptive equipment in home environments maximize client activity and mobility.

BED REST

Bed rest is a therapeutic intervention that achieves several objectives, including the following:

- Provides rest for clients who are exhausted
- Decreases the body's oxygen consumption
- Reduces pain and discomfort

The planned duration of bed rest depends on the client's physical condition and ability to move.

Even though implemented for therapeutic reasons, bed rest can be counterproductive to a client's recovery. The inactivity imposed by bed rest causes structural changes in joints and muscles, such as shortening of muscles, decreased range of motion, and contractures. To prevent such complications, bed rest should be avoided as much as possible. For clients whose medical condition necessitates bed rest, ROM exercises must be implemented.

RESTORATIVE NURSING CARE

Being able to move about independently is an important part of the recovery process and can determine whether the client is cared for at home or in a health care facility. Environmental evaluation is particularly important, with the focus on ease and safety of mobility. Promotion of activity through environmental modification increases the quality of life for the client whether injured, ill, or aging. Increased accessibility and mobility can be achieved through planning home modifications such as:

- Ramps
- Wide doorways
- Open-ended door handles replacing doorknobs
- Remote-controlled lighting

- Spacious room arrangements
- Bare floor or low-level pile carpeting
- Grab bars for bathrooms

Efforts by the client and the rehabilitation team to promote activity and mobility can be negated quickly by environmental barriers such as stairs and narrow passageways.

Clients who have limited mobility may be at risk for falls. To decrease the probability of falls at home, client education should focus on creating a safe environment for ambulation; see the Client Teaching Checklist. The accompanying Community Considerations display lists some assistive devices for clients receiving care in the home setting; see Figure 36-10.

HEALTH PROMOTION AND FITNESS

Client expected outcomes include the promotion of activity, mobility, and fitness. Therapeutic exercises maintain flexibility, strength of muscles, range of motion, and energy and increase endurance and the sense of well-being. Factors affecting targeted health promotion outcomes include perceived health status, perceived benefits of exercise, and perceived barriers to exercise as well as attitudes toward exercise. Perceived benefits of exercise and exercise attitudes held by the client have been identified as critical in health promotion and fitness.

IMPLEMENTATION

Interventions for clients with impaired mobility include meeting psychosocial needs, using body mechanics, maintaining body alignment, performing ROM exercises, transferring clients, assisting with ambulation, promoting wellness, using complementary treatment approaches, and documentation.

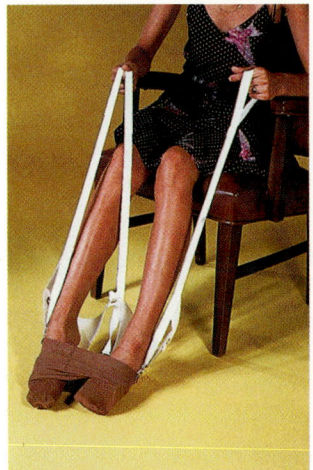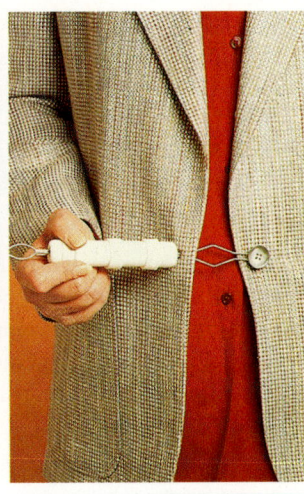

FIGURE 36-10 Assistive devices, such as those shown here, help clients dress independently. DELMAR/CENGAGE LEARNING

MEETING PSYCHOSOCIAL NEEDS

Nursing interventions directed at role changes due to deficits in activity and mobility include (1) fostering open family communication, (2) providing opportunities for family role resumption, (3) prioritizing family roles and responsibilities,

---

✓ CLIENT TEACHING CHECKLIST

Promoting Safety at Home

- Avoid unsecured or loose rugs.
- Use banisters on stairways.
- Install bright lights near steps and stairways.
- Avoid wearing shoes that are ill-fitting, unlaced, or high-heeled or have slippery soles.
- Keep all walkways unobstructed (remove clutter).
- Use caution with telephone lines; use a cordless phone if available to avoid tripping danger.
- Do not walk on wet or waxed floors.
- Use nonskid mats in shower and bathtub.
- Use grab bars near toilet and in shower and bathtub.
- Keep commonly used objects within easy reach.

COMMUNITY CONSIDERATIONS

Home Health Care: Assistive Devices in the Home

The following devices may be rented and may qualify for reimbursement from Medicare or private insurance.

- Electric hospital bed with overhead trapeze (gives client more control of environment)
- Portable commode (extends client's independence)
- Lifting device (assists with transferring dependent client from bed to chair)
- Portable telephone (for client safety and convenience)
- Shower chair and hand-held shower for bathtub (promotes client independence and safety)
- Special mattresses for bed and cushions for chairs (promotes comfort and help maintain skin integrity)
- Overbed table for eating or hand activities (promotes client's ability to perform ADL)
- Comfortable chairs close to the bed (promotes socialization by facilitating visits of family and friends)
- Remote control for client who enjoys television (provides leisure/diversion activity)

and (4) modifying family roles and responsibilities. The accompanying Nursing Process Highlight lists nursing interventions that encourage socialization.

APPLYING PRINCIPLES OF BODY MECHANICS

Often nurses are required to have physical strength in order to assist clients in achieving mobility. Carrying, pulling, pushing, and lifting clients and equipment are all activities involved in the delivery of nursing care. Nurses' implementation of correct body mechanics helps minimize the following:

- Client injury
- Nurse work-related musculoskeletal injury
- Nurse fatigue

The following variables can increase the risk of nurse injury:

- Client weight
- Client weight-bearing ability
- Client combativeness and unpredictability
- Height of bed
- Confined workspace
- Wheelchairs without adjustable arms

Educating staff about the use of proper body mechanics is essential in preventing injury; see Procedure 36-1. The National Institute for Occupational Safety and Health (NIOSH, 2008) is studying methods for reducing injury to health care workers as well as improving client safety. A major recommendation of the NIOSH is to avoid the manual transfer of clients by using mechanical lifts whenever possible. As a result, many health care facilities have implemented no-lift policies and use no-lift teams consisting of those who have been specially trained in the use of transfer devices. "The use of patient-moving equipment appears to reduce the risk of injury and chronic pain ... [and] regular equipment use is associated with a 23% reduction in the incidence of chronic pain and injury in health care professionals" (Hart, 2006). Musculoskeletal disorders (MSD) are injuries and disorders of the muscles, nerves, tendons, ligaments, joints, cartilage, and spinal discs. Examples of MSD include carpal tunnel syndrome, tendonitis, sciatica, herniated disc, and low back pain.

MSD are preventable by educating workers and modifying the work environment, such as providing transfer equipment, and assessing clients. See the Nursing Process Highlight for information that should be assessed prior to moving a client and the Spotlight On display.

MAINTAINING BODY ALIGNMENT: POSITIONING

Clients cannot always move independently and reposition themselves in bed. In such instances, nurses must use proper turning and positioning techniques in order to achieve the following outcomes:

- Increase client comfort
- Prevent contractures
- Prevent pressure sores
- Make portions of the client's body accessible for procedures
- Help clients access their environment

Clients who cannot move independently must be repositioned every 2 hours. Repositioning must be done more often for clients who are uncomfortable or incontinent or who have

---

NURSING PROCESS HIGHLIGHT

Assessment

Factors That Influence Transfer Technique Type

- Client size and weight
- Level of assistance required by client
- Client willingness and ability to cooperate
- Client health status and medical condition

NURSING PROCESS HIGHLIGHT

Implementation

Promoting Socialization

- Foster client autonomy
- Encourage activities in collaboration with recreational therapist
- Involve client with successful role models
- Inform client of vocational, educational, recreational, and social resources
- Involve client and family in support groups
- Facilitate transportation resources

SPOTLIGHT ON...

Professionalism

Preventing MSD Versus Client Needs

A newly hired nursing assistant is assigned to help move a client in order to change the linens. The charge nurse overhears the nursing assistant say that she is not going to move the client because he is too heavy and "I don't want to hurt myself!" What should the nurse do to promote meeting the client's needs and protecting the staff from injury?

fragile skin, poor circulation, decreased sensation, poor nutritional status, or impaired mental status. See Figure 36-11, which provides an algorithm for assistance in planning client repositioning.

Nurses need to be aware of three essential concepts when positioning clients: pressure, friction, and skin shear. A pressure site is any skin surface area on which the client is lying or sitting. The force of the pressure can compromise circulation and lead to skin breakdown and ulceration. Tissue areas over bony prominences are more likely to experience impaired skin integrity. It is important to always inspect the skin under increased pressure areas for signs of irritation (i.e., redness).

Friction is caused when the skin is dragged across a rough surface such as bedsheets or stretcher surfaces. Friction causes heat, which damages the skin and may lead to decreased skin integrity with resultant infection or skin breakdown.

Skin shear is the result of dragging skin across a hard surface. The force of resistance to being dragged tears the deep layers of skin, which can lead to skin ulceration; see the Safety First display.

For clients in bed, limit the number of pillows under the head in order to avoid neck flexion. Arms should be abducted from the body and straight with slight flexion. Hands should rest comfortably in a flat position with fingers open. The knees and hips should be aligned; use sandbags or pillows to prevent external hip rotation. Avoid flexing the knees by the use of pillows placed behind the knees.

Ankles should be flexed at 90°; use pillows or footboard if necessary.

To maintain proper positioning for a client seated in a chair, be sure the head is straight without bending the neck or dangling the head. The trunk should be upright without bending or curving. Arms and hands are to be supported on armrests or the tabletop; avoid dangling the arms. The hands should be in a flat position with the fingers open. Hips and knees should be flexed. The feet are to be flat on the floor or footrest with the ankles at a 90° angle. If the legs are supported on leg rests and are straight, keep the ankles flexed at a 90° angle.

Table 36-12 on page 1112 provides a description of the most commonly used positions: Fowler's (elevated head and trunk), dorsal recumbent (back-lying with slight elevation of head and shoulders), prone (face down), lateral (side-lying), and Sims' (semi-prone).

▼ SAFETY FIRST ▼

To prevent skin shear, avoid dragging a client across the bed or stretcher. Instead, lift the client or use assistive devices such as turn sheets (drawsheets) or transfer boards.

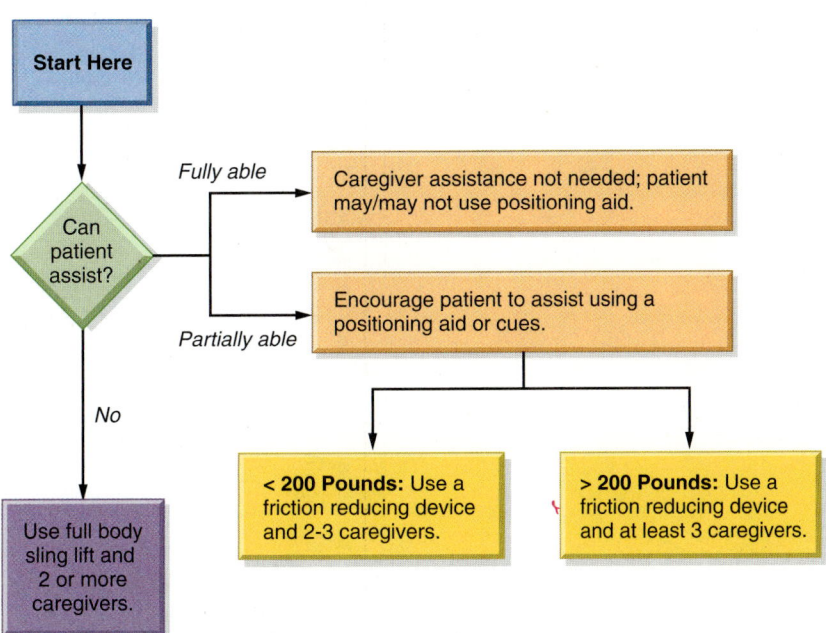

• This is not a one person task: DO NOT PULL FROM HEAD OF BED.
• When pulling a patient up in bed, patient should be flat or in a Trendelenburg position (when tolerated) to aid in gravity, with side rail down.
• For patients with stage III or IV pressure ulcers, care should be taken to avoid shearing force.
• The height of the bed should be appropriate for staff safety (at the elbows).
• If the patient can assist when repositioning "up in bed," ask the patient to flex the knees and push on the count of three.
• During any patient handling task, if the caregiver is required to lift more than 35 lbs. of a patient's weight, then the patient should be considered to be fully dependent and assistive devices should be used.

FIGURE 36-11 **Algorithm: Reposition in Bed, Side-to-Side, Up in Bed** NELSON, A. (2006). *SAFE PATIENT HANDLING AND MOVEMENT ALGORITHMS.* TAMPA, FL: VISN 8 VA SUNSHINE HEALTHCARE NETWORK. RETRIEVED JANUARY 8, 2009, FROM HTTP://WWW.VISN8.MED.VA.GOV/PATIENTSAFETYCENTER.

TABLE 36-12 Positioning

POSITION	DESCRIPTION	INDICATIONS	POTENTIAL COMPLICATIONS	CORRECTIVE MEASURES
Fowler's	Semisitting position; head of bed elevated to 45°–60°; knees slightly elevated.	Promotes comfort; improves respiratory problems (e.g., dyspnea, pneumonia); encourages postoperative drainage.	Flexion contracture of cervical spine	Rest head directly on mattress or support with small pillow only.
			Exaggerated flexion of lumbar spine	Firm support to back; pillow to support lower back.
			Dislocation of shoulder	Elevate forearms on pillows to avoid tension on shoulders.
			Flexion contracture of wrist	Support hands on pillows to maintain natural alignment
			Finger contractures and thumb abduction	Hand-wrist splints.
			External hip rotation	Trochanter roll.
			Hyperextension of knees	Flex knees with small pillow under the thighs.
			Foot drop (plantar flexion)	Maintain dorsal flexion with footboard or high-top tennis shoes.
Dorsal recumbent (supine)	Back-lying position; head and shoulders may be slightly raised.	Promotes comfort. NOTE: Head and shoulders are kept flat after procedures involving spinal anesthetics.	Cervical hyperextension	Maintain correct alignment with pillows under upper shoulders, neck, and head.
			Posterior flexion of lumbar spine	Small pillow or roll under lumbar curvature.
			Clawhand deformities (extension of fingers and abduction of thumbs)	Hand-wrist splints.
			Hyperextension of knees	Pillow under lower legs from below the knees to ankles or small pillow under thighs to slightly flex knees.
			Foot drop (plantar flexion)	Maintain dorsal flexion with footboard or high-top tennis shoes.

(Continues)

TABLE 36-12 (Continued)

Position	Description	Benefits	Potential Problems	Preventive/Supportive Measures
Prone	Face-down position; head is turned to one side.	Helps prevent contractures of hips and knees; promotes drainage from mouth.	Cervical spine flexion	Small pillow under head.
			Hyperextension of spine; respiratory impairment	Small pillow just below the diaphragm.
			Foot drop	Allow feet to dangle over end of mattress, or place lower legs on pillow to keep toes from resting on bed.
Lateral	Side-lying position; lateral aspects of lower scapula and lower ilium support most of body weight.	Promotes comfort; relieves pressure on sacrum and heels.	Lateral flexion of neck	Pillow under head and neck.
			Internal rotation of arm; limited chest expansion leading to respiratory impairment	Maintain alignment of upper arm with pillow underneath. Slightly flex lower arm.
			Extension of fingers and abduction of thumbs	Hand-wrist splints.
			Internal rotation and abduction of femur	Pillows to support leg from groin to foot.
			Twisting of spine	Align both shoulders with both hips.
Sims'	Semi-prone position; upper arm is flexed at shoulder and elbow while lower arm is positioned behind client; both legs flexed in front of client with more flexion in upper leg.	Promotes drainage from mouth; prevents aspiration; reduces pressure on sacrum and greater trochanter of hip; promotes comfort, especially in pregnant clients.	Lateral flexion of cervical spine	Support head with pillow unless drainage from mouth is necessary.
			Damaged nerves and blood vessels of lower arm axillae	Position lower arm behind and away from the back.
			Internal shoulder rotation and abduction	Pillow between chest and upper arm.
			Internal rotation and adduction of hip and leg; lumbar lordosis	Pillow under upper flexed leg from groin to foot.
			Foot drop	Sandbag to dorsiflex lower foot.

Delmar/Cengage Learning

Assisting clients to comfortable therapeutic positions requires much skill. Often the client is unable to assist in repositioning; in such cases, it is best to use two or more staff members to reposition the client in order to prevent injury to clients and staff.

Equipment used for client positioning includes pillows, foam wedges, trochanter rolls, footboards, bed boards, hand-wrist splints, traction, side rails, restraints, and trapeze bars. Table 36-13 describes devices used to help maintain proper positioning.

Hand-wrist splints can facilitate extension of the wrist, hand, and fingers as well as prevent contracture and reduce spasticity. The goal for splint use is to maintain a functional hand. Figure 36-12 shows hand-wrist splints. Clients must be taught the correct way to put on the device, as incorrect use of a splint or brace can cause joint damage, stiffness, or pain.

Side Rails

Falls are common types of injuries in hospitals and long-term care facilities. Side rails, also referred to as bed rails, which are placed on the sides of beds and stretchers to prevent falls, can be raised, lowered, and locked into place; see Figure 36-13 on page 1115. Side rails should not give nurses a sense of security because they increase the likelihood of fall injuries if clients climb over the rails. There have also been incidences in which clients experienced strangulation or death as a result of entrapment in the rails or between the rails and the mattress (Minnick, Mion, Johnson, Catrambone, & Leipzig, 2008). Beds must be placed in the lowest position to reduce the force of a possible fall, should one occur. Also, clients identified as being at risk for falls should be closely monitored.

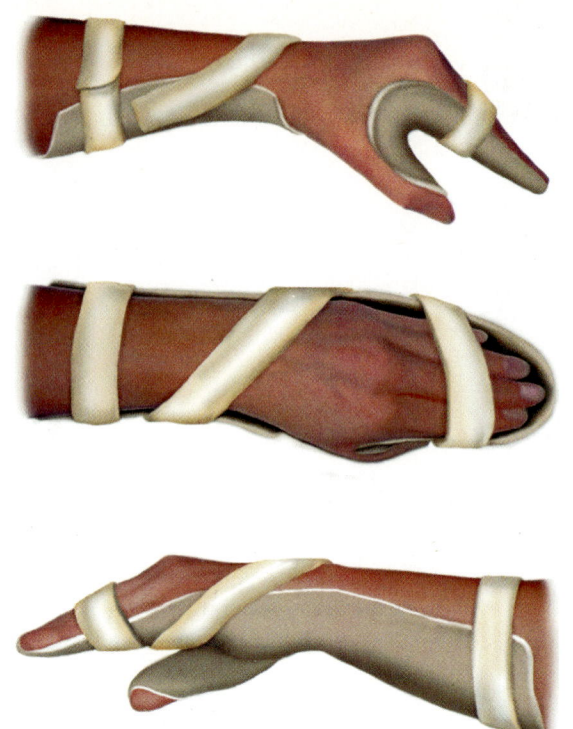

FIGURE 36-12 Hand-Wrist Splints DELMAR/CENGAGE LEARNING

Some clients resist the use of side rails because they feel their independence is altered. It is important that the nurse teach clients and families the purpose of side rails, focusing on safety promotion. Note that some health care agencies require signed notification consenting to the use of raised side rails.

TABLE 36-13 Maintaining Proper Position: Assistive Devices

Bed board	Plywood board placed under entire mattress; improves spinal alignment by providing support
Footboard	Board placed at end of bed to provide support for feet to maintain dorsiflexion; prevents foot drop (dorsiflexion)
Hand-wrist splint	Individually contoured for each client; maintains thumb adduction and opposition to fingers
Pillow	Available in various thicknesses; provides support; elevates body parts
Restraint	Variety of types available (jacket or vest, wrist belt, ankle belt, waist belt); provides immobilization
Side rails	Bars attached to the sides of the bed; assist with mobility and prevent falls
Traction	Used for immobilization and to promote healing of fractures
Trapeze bar	Triangular device hanging from above-bed bar that is secured to bed frame; used by clients with upper extremity function to assist in repositioning and transferring
Trochanter roll	Folded blanket placed under client's buttocks and rolled inward toward client to place thigh in a neutral position; used when client is supine to avoid external rotation of hips and legs

Delmar/Cengage Learning

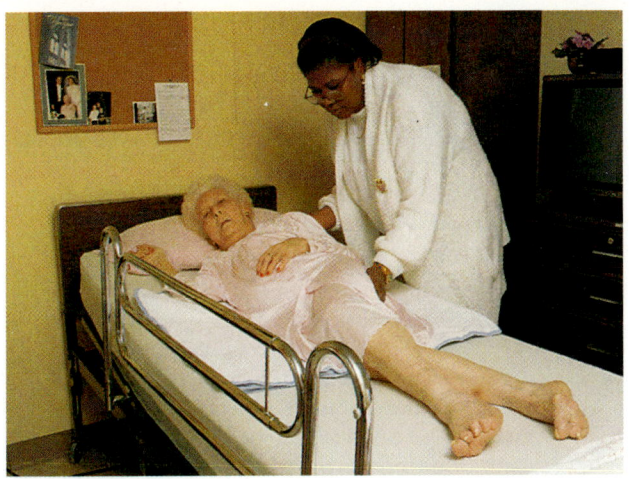

FIGURE 36-13 The use of side rails promotes safety. DELMAR/
CENGAGE LEARNING

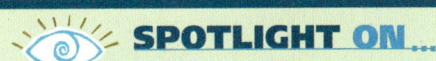

SPOTLIGHT ON...

Legal/Ethical

To Restrain or Not?

You are the charge nurse working nights at a long-term care facility. Two staff members called in sick at the beginning of the shift; therefore, you are very short staffed. Mrs. Ellington, an 84-year-old woman who is very confused, keeps trying to climb out of her bed. She almost fell twice while trying to climb over the bed rails. In an attempt to prevent Mrs. Ellington from falling, you have decided to place her in restraints until you can get more staff to come to work. What are the ethical implications of your actions? The legal ones? Would you change your actions if Mrs. Ellington were your grandmother?

Restraints

Restraints are protective devices used to limit physical activity or to immobilize a client or body part. Restraints are used for the following purposes: to protect the client from falls, to protect a body part, to prevent the client from interfering with therapies (e.g., pulling out tubes or catheters), and to reduce the risk of injury to others. See Chapter 29 for a complete discussion of restraints and the procedure for applying restraints; see the Spotlight On display.

Traction

Traction may be used to maintain body alignment, especially following injury or surgery. There are several traction techniques, including manual, skin, and skeletal; see Figure 36-14. See the accompanying Nursing Process Highlight on page 1116 for a listing of key assessment data for clients using skeletal and skin traction. The nurse must document assessment findings to promote continuity of care.

PERFORMING RANGE-OF-MOTION EXERCISES

ROM exercises are performed several times a day by placing each joint through its full functional motion. The purposes of ROM exercises are to maintain full flexibility, maintain muscle tone and strength, prevent contractures, and improve circulation. See Procedure 36-2 and the Uncovering the Evidence display on page 1116.

TRANSFER TECHNIQUES

Planning plays a major role in safe, effective client transfers; the nurse must determine to what extent the client is able to help with the transfer. If the client is totally dependent or is heavy, the nurse will need other staff members to help. Table 36-14 lists potential hazards involved in client transfers with corresponding nursing interventions to promote safety.

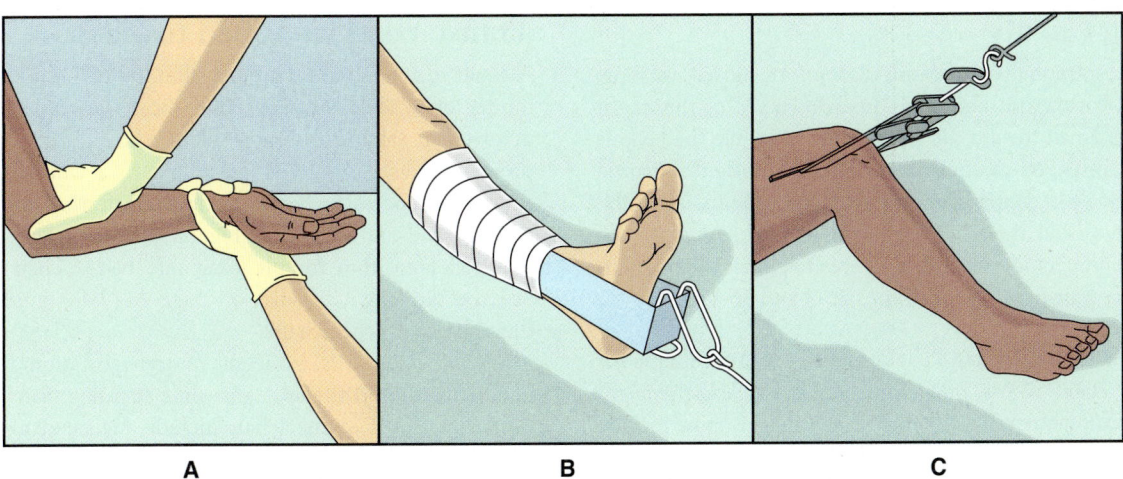

A   B   C

FIGURE 36-14 Traction Techniques: A. Manual; B. Skin; and C. Skeletal DELMAR/CENGAGE LEARNING

UNCOVERING THE

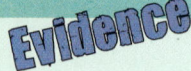

TITLE OF STUDY
"Effects of a Range-of-Motion Exercise Programme"

AUTHORS
C. N. Tseng, C. C. Chen, S. C. Wu, and L. C. Lin

PURPOSE
To examine the effects of a nurse-led range-of-motion (ROM) exercise program on functional abilities of stroke survivors in long-term care facilities.

METHODS
A randomized, controlled trial was conducted with bedridden older stroke survivors in residential care. Participants were randomly assigned to one of three groups: a usual care group, Intervention Group I, or Intervention Group II. Intervention Group I had a registered nurse to supervise participants performing exercises. In Intervention Group II, a registered nurse provided physical assistance for participants in performing ROM exercises.

RESULTS
Both intervention groups had a statistically significant improvement in joint range, activity function, depressive symptoms, and perception of pain compared with the usual care group.

IMPLICATIONS
A nurse-led ROM exercise program can improve the physical and psychological function of bedridden older people with stroke.

Tseng, C. N., Chen, C. C., Wu, S. C., & Lin, L. C. (2007). Effects of a range-of-motion exercise programme. *Journal of Advanced Nursing*, *57*(2), 181–191.

NURSING PROCESS HIGHLIGHT

Assessment

Skeletal and Skin Traction: Assessment Factors

Skeletal Traction

- Location of traction
- Amount of traction being applied
- Countertraction applied
- Body position to be maintained
- Duration of application (continuous, intermittent, or as-needed basis)
- Traction weights free falling
- Traction rope intact, taut, and unobstructed through the pulley
- Immobilized body part in alignment with rest of body
- Appearance of the skeletal pin or wire sites (e.g., dry, encrusted, reddened, edematous)
- Presence of drainage from the skeletal pin or wire sites
- Evidence of skin breakdown

Skin Traction

- Location of traction
- Type of traction (e.g., cervical, Buck's, Russell's)
- Amount of traction weight being applied to the affected body part
- Body position to be maintained
- Duration of application (continuous, intermittent, or as-needed basis)
- Traction weights free falling
- Traction rope intact, taut, and unobstructed through the pulley
- Immobilized body part in alignment with rest of body

Moving Clients

Prolonged immobility can cause discomfort, muscle wasting, thrombus formation, and skin breakdown. Also, the client who slides down toward the foot of the bed while the head is elevated can experience reduced lung capacity and impaired respiratory effort. Nurses often must move clients up in the bed or reposition them. Moving a client may sometimes be done by one person but often requires two staff members to ensure safe transfer; see Procedures 36-3 and 36-4.

LOGROLLING THE CLIENT Logrolling is a technique for moving a client whose body must remain in straight alignment. Situations requiring total alignment of the spine include spinal injury or recovery from spinal surgery. Logrolling is accomplished by two or three nurses working in a coordinated fashion.

Transferring from Bed to Chair

A client may need to be moved from the bed to a chair, commode, or wheelchair. Procedure 36-5 describes the steps involved in safely assisting a client from bed to chair. This procedure discusses moving a client to a wheelchair; however, the process is the same for transferring to a regular chair or bedside commode. Figure 36-15 on page 1118 provides an algorithm for planning safe bed-to-chair transfers. See the Nursing Checklist on page 1117 for guidelines on the safe use of wheelchairs.

A wheelchair is a means of transportation for clients unable to support their weight while standing. Safety instructions for use of a wheelchair include the need to keep the wheels locked when not deliberately moving and to move the footrests out of the way when getting in and out of the wheelchair; see the Safety First display on page 1117.

TABLE 36-14 Client Transfer: Hazards and Safety Measures

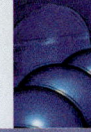

POTENTIAL HAZARD	PREVENTIVE MEASURES
Falling	• Assess client's size and ability to assist. • Ask for help from other staff members if needed. • If client starts to fall, lower gently to the floor while protecting the head. • If client has fallen, assess thoroughly for signs of injury.
Skin damage	• Use a transfer board or drawsheet. • Lift client instead of sliding across surfaces. • Pad surfaces that may cause injury (e.g., bed rails).
Foot injury	• Place nonskid slippers on client. • Do not tuck sheets and blankets tightly over feet. • Ensure that feet do not become tangled in side rails, chair legs, or other equipment.
Dislodging client care equipment	• Assess for presence of all tubes and lines (e.g., catheters, IV lines). • Determine if equipment must be temporarily disconnected during the transfer. • Reconnect equipment promptly when transfer is completed. • Keep the urinary drainage bag at a level lower than the bladder.

Delmar/Cengage Learning

Transferring from Bed to Stretcher

Some clients (e.g., those who are too weak to sit upright, those who are unconscious, or those with injuries prohibiting the erect position) must lie flat during transfers. In such situations, a stretcher (gurney) is used to facilitate client transfer. See Figure 36-16 on page 1119 for an algorithm for bed-to-stretcher transfers. Stretchers have several safety features, including side rails, safety belts and straps, and locking wheels. The nurse should caution clients to move carefully while on the stretcher as it is more narrow than the bed. Reassure the client that side rails will be used to prevent falls. See Procedure 36-6 for instructions on moving clients who need minimal and maximal assistance. See the Nursing Checklist on page 1118 on stretcher transport safety.

Assistive Devices

Nurses must educate clients about the use of assistive devices; see Figure 36-17 on page 1119. There are several devices

✓ NURSING CHECKLIST

Wheelchair Safety

- When moving a client in a wheelchair, back into and out of elevators.
- Back slowly down wheelchair ramps.
- Push the wheelchair ahead of you when going up ramps.
- If going through a self-closing door, back the wheelchair out of the room. You can keep the door open by backing against the door. The wheelchair can then be guided out of the room.
- Lock brakes when the wheelchair is stationary.
- Intravenous infusion bags can be placed on portable IV poles attached to the wheelchair during transport.
- Urinary drainage bags can be placed on the lower body of the wheelchair during transport. Coil the drainage tubing so the catheter is not tugged during transport. Empty bag prior to wheelchair transfer. Keep the bag below the level of the client's urinary bladder.

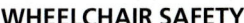

▼ SAFETY FIRST ▼

WHEELCHAIR SAFETY
Caution client to avoid leaning forward in the wheelchair because leaning forward can cause tipping and falling.

available for helping with client transfers. Slide boards (transfer boards) assist the bed-wheelchair transfer by bridging the space between the bed and the wheelchair. Note that specialized wheelchairs with removable armrests are used with slide boards. As the client becomes more independent, the slide board can be used to transfer from the wheelchair to a car. Figure 36-18 on page 1119 shows a slide board transfer to a car.

The hydraulic (mechanical) lift is used for moving immobile clients who are heavy; see Procedure 36-7. A client may be transferred to a chair, wheelchair, bedside commode, stretcher, or scale using a hydraulic lift. The manufacturer's equipment instructions should be followed, and the weight limits must not exceed the manufacturer's specifications. Two staff members are needed to safely operate a hydraulic lift. Hydraulic lifts are not for use with clients who have spinal cord injury, as spinal alignment is not maintained during use of the lift. See the Safety First display on page 1118 for a warning about any type of transfer involving a client with a closed chest drainage system.

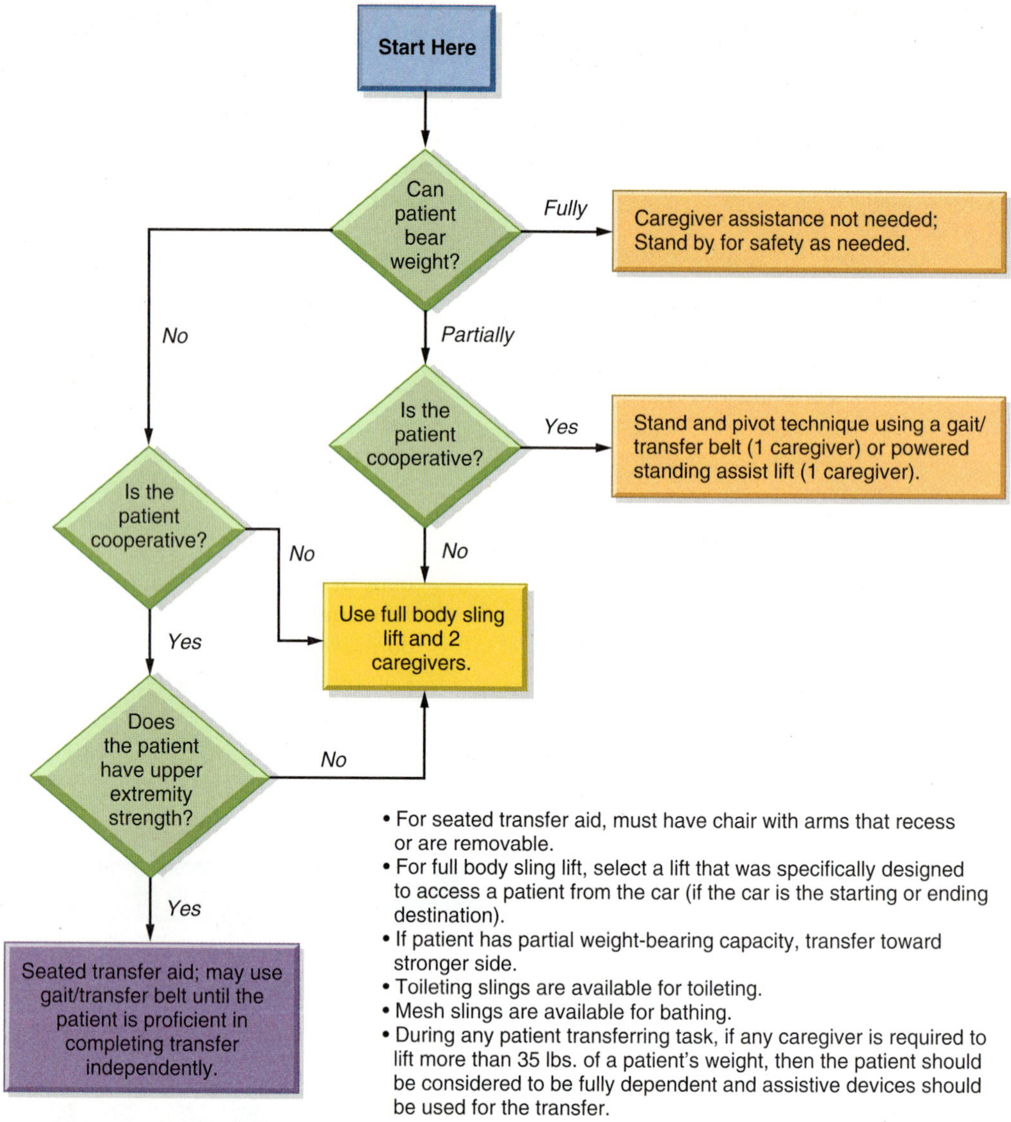

Start Here

Can patient bear weight?

— Fully → Caregiver assistance not needed; Stand by for safety as needed.

— No

— Partially

Is the patient cooperative?

— Yes → Stand and pivot technique using a gait/transfer belt (1 caregiver) or powered standing assist lift (1 caregiver).

— No

Is the patient cooperative?

— No →

— Yes

Use full body sling lift and 2 caregivers.

Does the patient have upper extremity strength?

— No →

— Yes

Seated transfer aid; may use gait/transfer belt until the patient is proficient in completing transfer independently.

- For seated transfer aid, must have chair with arms that recess or are removable.
- For full body sling lift, select a lift that was specifically designed to access a patient from the car (if the car is the starting or ending destination).
- If patient has partial weight-bearing capacity, transfer toward stronger side.
- Toileting slings are available for toileting.
- Mesh slings are available for bathing.
- During any patient transferring task, if any caregiver is required to lift more than 35 lbs. of a patient's weight, then the patient should be considered to be fully dependent and assistive devices should be used for the transfer.

FIGURE 36-15 Algorithm: Transfer to and from Bed to Chair, Chair to Toilet, Chair to Chair, or Car to Chair NELSON, A. (2006). *SAFE PATIENT HANDLING AND MOVEMENT ALGORITHMS.* TAMPA, FL: VISN 8 PATIENT SAFETY CENTER. RETRIEVED JANUARY 8, 2009, FROM HTTP://WWW.VISN8.MED.VA.GOV/PATIENTSAFETYCENTER.

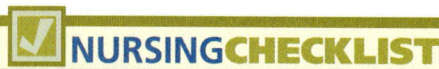

☑ NURSING CHECKLIST

Stretcher Transport Safety

- Use hall ceiling mirrors at intersections before turning corners.
- Lock elevator door open when entering or exiting.
- Stand at head of stretcher to push stretcher up a ramp.
- Back down a steep ramp while positioned at head of stretcher.
- Lock stretcher brakes when standing still.

▼ SAFETY FIRST ▼

TRANSFERS AND CLOSED CHEST DRAINAGE SYSTEM

The closed chest drainage system must remain vertical at all times, including during transfers, to maintain the water seal.

ASSISTING WITH AMBULATION

Client **ambulation** (assisted or unassisted walking) is encouraged soon after the onset of illness, injury, or surgery to prevent the complications of immobility. In planning ambulation, the nurse assesses the client's strength, endurance, and mobility status. Can the client walk alone, or is assistance needed? The presence of equipment (e.g., urinary catheters, IV infusions, drainage tubes) requires assistance; see the accompanying Nursing Checklist on page 1120.

In order to maintain client safety, ambulation must occur in progressive stages. First, the client should be able to tolerate

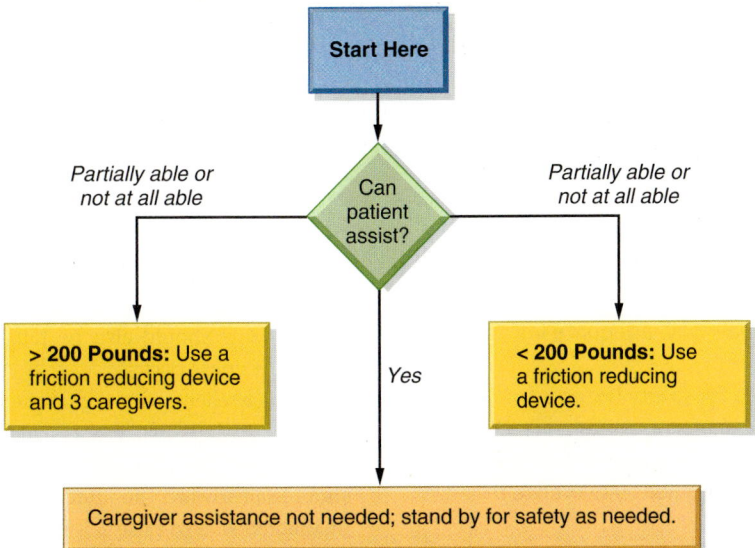

- Surfaces should be even for all laterial patient moves.
- For patients with stage III or IV pressure ulcers, care must be taken to avoid shearing force.
- During any patient transferring task, if any caregiver is required to lift more than 35 lbs. of a patient's weight, then the patient should be considered to be fully dependent and assistive devices should be used for the transfer.

FIGURE 36-16 **Algorithm for Lateral Transfer to and from Bed to Stretcher, Trolley** NELSON, A. (2006). *SAFE PATIENT HANDLING AND MOVEMENT ALGORITHMS.* TAMPA, FL: VISN 8 PATIENT SAFETY CENTER. RETRIEVED JANUARY 8, 2009, FROM HTTP://WWW.VISN8.MED.VA.GOV/PATIENTSAFETYCENTER.

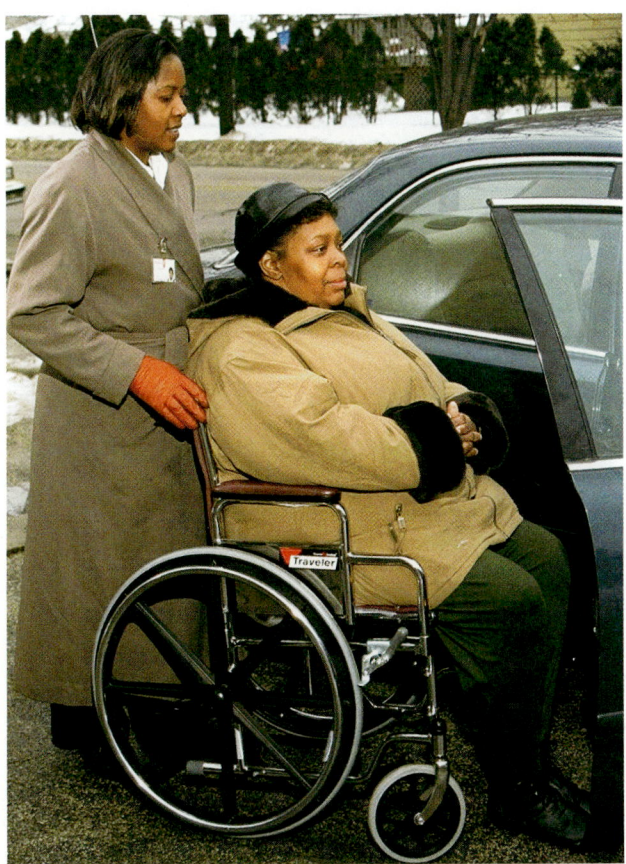

FIGURE 36-17 **Both client and family members need education regarding wheelchair safety.** DELMAR/CENGAGE LEARNING

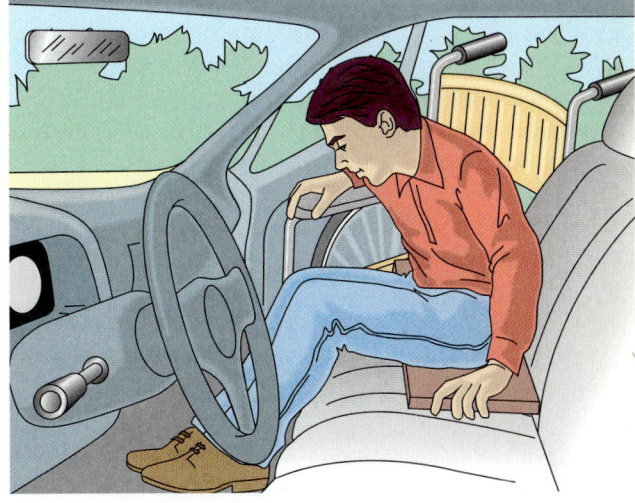

FIGURE 36-18 **Slide Board Transfer** DELMAR/CENGAGE LEARNING

sitting on the bedside and dangling the feet. The next step is client tolerance of standing at the side of the bed. Then progressive ambulation can be initiated; see Procedure 36-8. Sometimes it may be necessary to use a **gait belt** (a two-inch wide webbed belt worn by the client for the purpose of stabilization during transfers and ambulation) to promote client safety.

As ambulation activities are initiated, it is important to assess the client's blood pressure, respiratory rate, pulse, skin

✓ NURSING CHECKLIST

Assisting with Client Ambulation

- Determine the client's activity level and tolerance for physical exertion.
- Assess for factors that may negatively affect ambulation (e.g., mental status, fatigue, pain, medications).
- Evaluate the environment for safety (e.g., presence of obstacles in walkway, adequate lighting, nonslip floor, handrails).
- Check assistive devices for safety hazards.
- Check client's clothing (e.g., nonslip shoes, adequate covering for privacy and warmth).
- During ambulation, assess client's tolerance of activity.
- Postambulation, assess client's recovery from the activity.

color and moisture, and subjective responses. While the client is walking, observe for signs of exertion, including diaphoresis, shortness of breath, or weakness.

It is also important to assess for the presence of orthostatic hypotension in order to prevent falls. Depending on the client's physical conditioning and the effects of orthostatic hypotension, the client may need to slowly progress to independent ambulation. Once the activity is completed, the nurse evaluates the client, focusing on progression of activity. Continuous evaluation of the client's strength and endurance is performed by the nurse.

Preparing the Client to Walk

One of the best ways to encourage ambulation is to help the client become and remain as independent as possible while lying in bed. This includes urging clients to participate in ROM exercises and perform self-care activities as much as possible.

Independent mobility, the goal of most clients, is the ability to walk, run, sit, and turn without mechanical or personal aid. Progressive exercises and activities that promote independent mobility include:

1. *Turning.* The client turns in bed using side rails for stabilization and leverage.
2. *Sitting.* The client raises the head of the bed and lowers the height of the bed. Then the client turns to the side of the bed and swings legs over the side of the bed to assume the dangling position. Arms placed in the tripod position give balance to the sitting position.
3. *Standing.* The client dangles for a few minutes to ensure balance and then bears weight with both feet at the side of the bed. For additional stability and balance, the client can perch on the edge of the bed for several minutes before standing.

4. *Walking.* The client assesses strength and balance while walking, thus allowing a gradual progression of the duration of walking. Instruct clients to rest by sitting or standing still while stabilized with a guide rail if fatigued; see Figure 36-19.

CLIENT EDUCATION Prior to ambulation, clients who have been immobile need to be prepared adequately in order to prevent injury. Listing the therapeutic outcomes of ambulation is one way to teach clients the importance of ambulation. Clients should also be taught to sit down or use side rails if dizziness occurs.

Teach clients the technique for safe falling in order to minimize risk of injury; see Figure 36-20 on page 1121. Clients should be told that if they begin to feel faint, they should fall toward the affected side of the body and use the unaffected side to raise self from the floor or chair.

PREAMBULATORY EXERCISE Helping immobile clients to prepare for ambulation includes instruction of preambulatory exercises in order to strengthen and tone muscles. The quadriceps femoris is the major muscle used for walking; thus, clients should be directed to gently contract and release the leg muscles several times a day. Clients who will be walking with the assistance of walkers and crutches need upper body strength. Instruction in the safe use of ambulatory assistive devices is also necessary for many clients with impaired mobility.

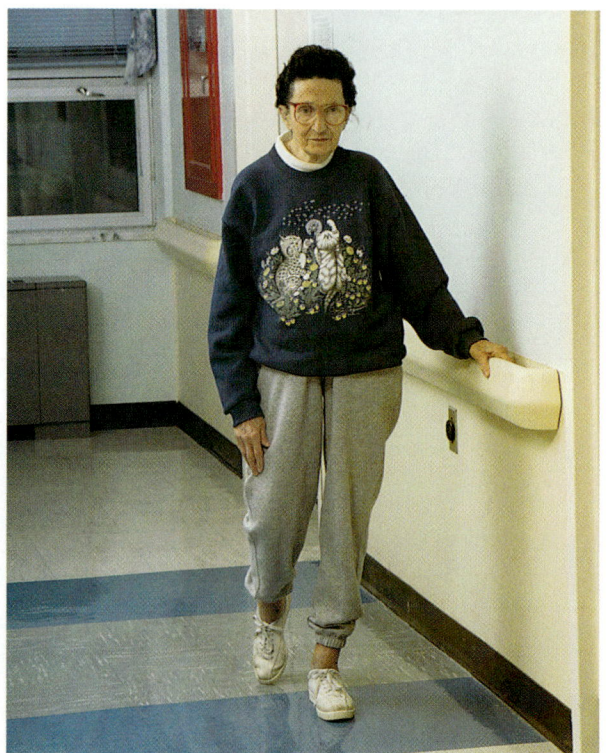

FIGURE 36-19 The use of handrails promotes safety and independence in ambulating. DELMAR/CENGAGE LEARNING

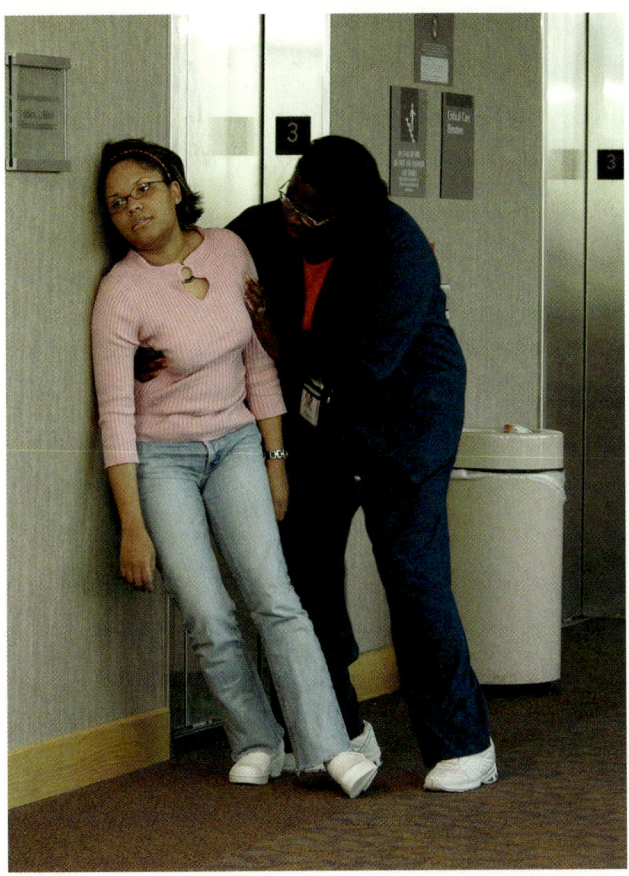

FIGURE 36-20 Support for Falling Client DELMAR/CENGAGE LEARNING

TABLE 36-15 Weight-Bearing Status

DEGREE OF WEIGHT BEARING	DESCRIPTION
Non–weight bearing	Patient does not bear weight on the affected extremity. The affected extremity does not touch the floor.
Touchdown weight bearing	Patient's foot of the affected extremity may rest on the floor, but no weight is distributed through that extremity.
Partial weight bearing	Patient bears 30%–50% of his or her weight on the affected extremity.
Weight bearing as tolerated	Patient bears as much weight as can be tolerated on the affected extremity without undue strain or pain.
Full weight bearing	Patient bears weight fully on the affected extremity.

Reprinted with permission from Maher, A. (1994). *Orthopedic nursing.* Philadelphia: Saunders.

Assistive Devices

Clients who are unable to ambulate independently can use devices designed to help them walk safely. Determination of which device to use is based on the following:

- Upper arm strength
- Endurance (stamina)
- Presence or absence of one-sided weakness
- Weight-bearing ability; see Table 36-15

See Table 36-16 on page 1122 for a comparison of the three most common devices used to assist in walking: canes, walkers, and crutches.

CANES A cane is to be used by the client who can bear weight on both legs but has some weakness in one leg or hip. The straight (standard) cane is used most often; canes with three or four legs are used with clients who need more stability than provided by the straight cane. Quad canes provide more stability but are sometimes more awkward to use than the straight cane; see Figure 36-21 on page 1122, Procedure 36-9, and the Safety First display.

WALKERS A walker is a waist-high, metal, tubular device with a handgrip and four legs. Some walkers have rubber tips on all four legs, whereas others have wheels on the two front legs. The advantages of using a walker include provision of extra support, provision of a sense of security, and independ-

ence. The client first moves the walker forward and then takes a step while balancing his or her weight on the walker; see Procedure 36-9.

A walker is used by clients who need more support than that provided by a cane. Walkers are available with and without wheels. The walker without wheels provides more stability but also requires more client stamina in order to lift the walker. Walkers with wheels are intended for use by clients with limited upper body strength. The nurse should determine the following for clients using walkers:

1. Amount of weight bearing allowed on lower limb
2. Appropriateness for client's height
3. Type of walker (pick-up or rolling)
4. With pick-up walker: client's ability to grip, lift, and propel the walker forward

▼ SAFETY FIRST ▼

To promote safe ambulation using a cane, be sure that:

- The cane is appropriate for the client's height and has suction grips to prevent falls.
- The client is wearing flat shoes with nonskid soles.

TABLE 36-16 Assistive Devices for Ambulation

EQUIPMENT	DESCRIPTION	DIRECTIONS FOR USE
Cane	• Widens base of support • Various styles: (1) regular (straight)—gives minimal support for balance; (2) three-point—provides broader base of support, is more cumbersome; (3) four-point (quad)—broader base of support, more cumbersome	• Use on unaffected side. • Advance cane simultaneously with affected limb. • Hold close to body; do not move cane forward beyond toes of affected foot.
Walker	• Provides more stability than canes due to broader base of support • Various styles: (1) pickup—assists with weight bearing, though lifting may cause some strain for client; (2) rolling—pushed on wheels, which reduces physical strain on client	• For clients with weight-bearing status: Advance walker and step normally. • For partial or non–weight bearing on one limb: Thrust weight forward, then lift walker and replace all four legs on floor.
Crutches	• Less stable than canes and walkers • Requires upper body strength and ability to maintain balance	• Use good posture. • Maintain proper foot position on affected side (foot drop can result from walking on toes or ball of foot). • Eliminate obstacles in ambulatory path.

Data from Miller, C. A. (2009). *Nursing for wellness in older adults* (5th ed.). Philadelphia: Wolters Kluwer/Lippincott Williams & Wilkins; Mincer, A. B. (2007). Assistive devices for the adult patient with orthopaedic dysfunction. *Orthopaedic Nursing*, *26*(4), 226–233.

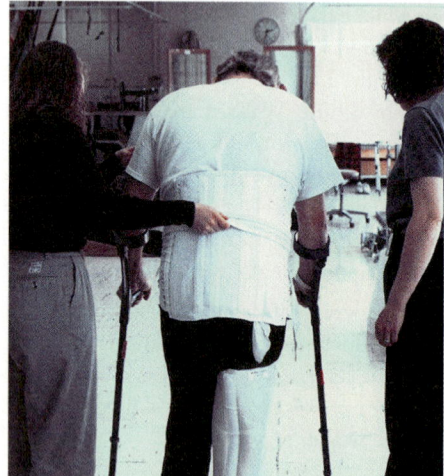

FIGURE 36-21 Nurse promotes safety of a client using a quad cane. Note the use of the gait belt for added safety. DELMAR/CENGAGE LEARNING

5. With rolling walker: client's ability to grip and propel the walker forward

When educating clients about the use of walkers, inform them that when transferring from chair or commode, they should back the walker to the chair or toilet seat and use arms of chair or commode to assist in sitting and standing. Teach clients to always use both hands when using a walker to transfer from standing to sitting; see Figure 36-22.

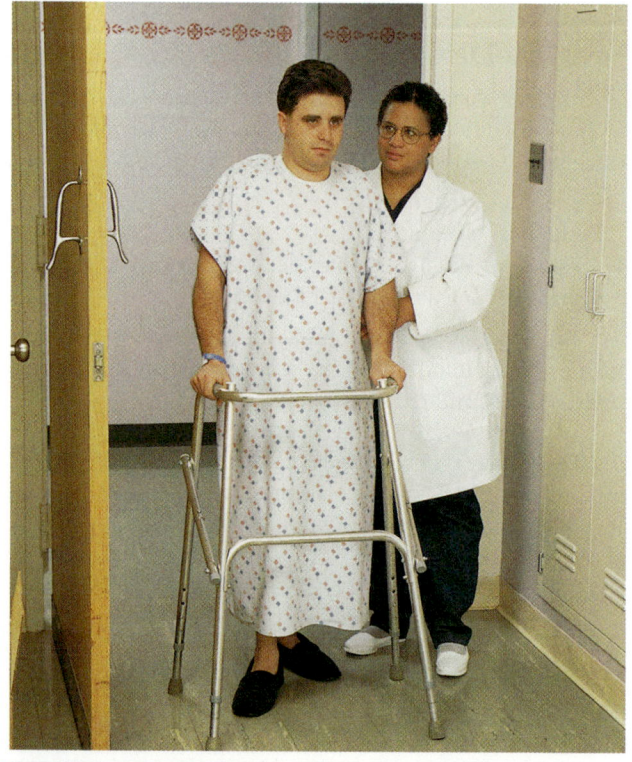

FIGURE 36-22 Client Using a Walker DELMAR/CENGAGE LEARNING

CRUTCHES A crutch is a wooden or metal staff used to increase client mobility. There are two types of crutches: axillary and forearm. The most commonly used type, the axillary crutch, fits under the axilla with the weight being placed on the handgrips. The forearm crutch, which has a handgrip and a metal cuff that fits around the arm, is more convenient but provides less stability than the axillary crutch.

To prevent slipping, crutches have rubber tips, which must be kept dry. If the tips are worn or loose, they must be replaced. The crutch must be regularly inspected because if cracks or bends are present, the person's weight will not be properly supported; see the Client Teaching Checklist.

Crutches can be used by clients who are unable to bear any weight on one leg, clients who can bear partial weight on one leg, and clients who have full weight bearing on both legs. Several gaits are used with crutches: the four-point gait, three-point gait, two-point gait, and swing-through gait.

The *four-point gait* for weight bearing with both legs follows the pattern of right crutch forward, left foot forward, left crutch forward, then right foot forward. The four-point gait with crutches is very stable but slow. The *two-point gait* for weight bearing with both legs has the pattern of right crutch and left foot forward together, then left crutch and right foot forward together. The two-point gait requires more balance but is a faster gait. The *three-point gait* for weight bearing with one leg has the pattern of crutches and weak leg forward together, then weight-bearing leg forward. The *swing-through gait* has the pattern of crutches forward, then legs swing forward together. The swing-through gait has the advantage of speed; however, it requires good balance. See Procedure 36-9 for a description of crutchwalking techniques.

✓ CLIENT TEACHING CHECKLIST

Crutchwalking

Climbing Stairs
This method of climbing stairs provides a broad base of support and stability for the weaker leg:

- Climb stairs using the stronger leg first.
- Bring the crutches to the level of the stronger leg.
- Bring the weaker leg to the level of the crutches and the stronger leg.
- Repeat to climb stairs. This requires time, balance, and strength.

Descending Stairs
This method of descending stairs provides a broad base of support and stability for the weaker leg:

- Support the body with the stronger leg.
- Move the crutches down to the first descending step.
- Move the stronger leg to the first descending step.
- Repeat to descend the staircase. This requires time, balance, and strength.

Sitting in a Chair
The client has greater stability using the stronger leg and chair arm for support:

- Stand in front of a chair.
- Hold the crutches on the side with the weaker leg.
- Grasp the chair arm using the arm on the side of the stronger leg.
- Flex knees and hips to sit in chair.
- Reposition self in chair using arms and stronger leg while sitting.

Rising from the Chair
The client has greater strength using the stronger leg to rise. More stability is provided by the chair arm and crutches for support. Rising requires more strength than sitting:

- Move forward in chair, placing strongest leg on the floor.
- Grasp the chair arm on the same side as the stronger leg.
- Hold the crutches with the hand on the side of the weaker leg.
- Use the chair arm and crutches for support while rising.
- Once standing, place the crutches in the position for ambulation.
- Weak clients may need assistance. The gait belt is useful in such situations.

WELLNESS PROMOTION

Wellness promotion emphasizes the need for physical fitness, which increases well-being, increases sympathetic nervous system activity, improves cardiovascular functioning, and produces and maintains weight loss. The nurse should identify physical activities enjoyed by the client and encourage increased participation. When planning an exercise program, the following elements need to be considered:

* Health status (existing medical conditions)
* Physical condition
* Age
* Preferences for types of activities

See the Safety First display.

COMPLEMENTARY AND ALTERNATIVE TREATMENT MODALITIES

There are numerous complementary and alternative modalities that help improve musculoskeletal health; see the accompanying Respecting Our Differences display. Also, physical activity and relaxation exercises help reduce muscular tension and improve functional abilities. Healing Touch (see Chapter 31) has been shown to reduce pain and inflexibility in muscles and joints, thereby improving mobility for many people (Umbreit, 2006). Therapeutic touch (see Chapter 31) has been found to be effective with clients experiencing musculoskeletal problems, such as sprains, strains, muscle spasms, and fractures (Quinn, 2006). Tai chi (see Chapter 31) has been shown to reduce fall risk by improving balance (Mitty & Flores, 2007).

EVALUATION

A client with activity or mobility deficits must maintain a balance between independence and dependence, which is necessary for positive self-esteem and confidence. This healthy balance can be influenced by support from the client's family and friends. Encouragement, positive acceptance, and affection are ways in which significant others can demonstrate support.

Family members are often unaware of the client's potential to improve. Thus, they may give unnecessary assistance in activities and mobility rather than allow the client to function independently. The client then becomes resentful because there is a loss of self-control. Resentment can also occur with the family who has accepted the heavy responsibilities of

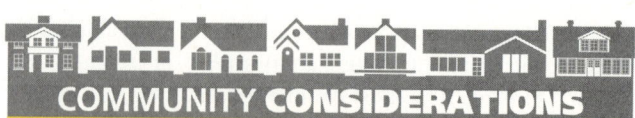

COMMUNITY CONSIDERATIONS

Evaluating Client Activity in the Home Setting

* Mobility status
* Ability to perform ADL
* Use of appropriate adaptive devices
* Use of activities as a basis for building competence and achievement

caregiving. For clients who overestimate their own cognitive and physical capabilities and energy level, safety becomes an important issue.

Long-term activity is the focus of evaluation as the client transfers skills and knowledge from the acute care hospital or rehabilitation facility to home. See the Community Considerations display for areas that need to be evaluated in the home setting. Measures of physical assessment, functional assessment, and performance of ADL are used for follow-up evaluation of the client's status for activity and mobility.

Ongoing assessment of the client's mobility is important because compliance with home exercise programs may lessen over time after discharge. When evaluating long-term activity and mobility goal achievement, the nurse should observe clients in the home setting in order to note their ability to function within their own environment.

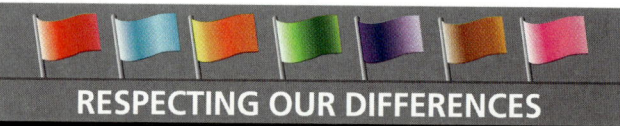

RESPECTING OUR DIFFERENCES

Complementary and Alternative Therapy

* The herb *ginkgo biloba* may be used to promote circulation.
* Acupuncture is a traditional Chinese medicine (TCM) method of pain relief in which a qualified practitioner inserts needles in certain body sites to promote the release of endorphins (i.e., natural painkillers).
* Acupressure is a technique similar to acupuncture; pressure instead of needles is applied to the acupuncture sites to relieve pain.
* Massage protects skin integrity by promoting circulation.
* Moist heat (warm towels, hot packs, bath or shower) promotes circulation.
* Cold (ice bag) helps reduce swelling.
* Transcutaneous electrical nerve stimulation (TENS) is used to decrease pain.
* Biofeedback is used to help clients decrease muscular tension.

▼ SAFETY FIRST ▼

EXERCISE AND CLIMATE

Caution clients to consider the climate when exercising and replenish fluids accordingly. Dehydration affects mobility by increasing joint and back pain and may also lead to client collapse.

NURSING CARE PLAN

The Client with a Fractured Leg

CASE PRESENTATION
Magda Constantin is a 15-year-old high school student recovering from a closed fracture of her right tibia suffered in a soccer game. She states that she is having trouble using crutches and getting around school, especially up and down the stairs. She is unhappy about not being able to play soccer and states, "People stare at me when I walk down the hall."

ASSESSMENT
- Difficulty ambulating due to cast and crutches
- Verbalizations of discomfort about altered mobility and body image

NURSING DIAGNOSIS: *Impaired physical mobility* related to inability to use legs normally and difficulty using crutches.
NOC: Coordinated movement
NIC: Exercise therapy: Ambulation

EXPECTED OUTCOMES
Client will:

1. Understand and demonstrate proper crutch technique.
2. Verbalize a more positive self-image and acceptance of her temporary condition.

INTERVENTIONS/RATIONALES
1. Measure crutch height and fit for client. Determines proper fit, which will relieve pressure, if any, and promotes safe ambulation.
2. Watch client as she walks across the room using the crutches. Provides baseline assessment of crutchwalking skills.
3. Demonstrate correct mechanics of crutch walking using three-point gait. Allows for partial or non–weight-bearing ambulation.
4. Ask client to return demonstrate crutchwalking technique. Shows client's understanding and ability to execute technique.
5. Suggest ways that crutchwalking can be facilitated, such as wearing soft-soled, flat shoes; carrying a backpack strapped over both shoulders; wearing nonbulky shirts to minimize clothing under arms; and taking frequent rest stops while walking. Tips on facilitating crutch gait will help remove barriers to effective walking and increase client comfort and confidence in technique.
6. Help client understand that cast and crutches are a temporary measure to promote proper healing and are not a reflection of overall body health. Client should learn to view situation as temporary and keep in mind that the broken leg is only one part of the whole person and need not detract from other positive qualities.

EVALUATION
Goal met. Magda successfully demonstrates correct crutchwalking technique and decides to purchase a backpack to replace her shoulder bag. She is still somewhat shy about "people staring at me" but seems to be starting to accept the fact that the cast and crutches are temporary. She even jokes that "maybe this is an easy way to get noticed at school."

CONCEPT MAP

The Client with a Fractured Leg

Magda Constantin, a 15-year-old high school student, has a fracture of her right tibia suffered in a soccer game. She states she is having trouble using crutches and getting around school, especially up and down the stairs. She is unhappy about not being able to play soccer and states, "People stare at me when I walk down the hall."

Your assessment data includes

ASSESSMENT DATA
Difficulty ambulating due to cast and crutches
Verbalizations of discomfort about the altered mobility and body image.

Data clues indicate

Nursing Diagnosis:
Risk for Injury related to sensory dysfunction and altered level of consciousness.

The expected outcome is...

The client will: be protected from injury during hospitalization.

Nursing Interventions and *Rationales*

1 Initiate the fall prevention protocol.
Identifies and reduces risk for injury.

2 Reassess the client's injury status every 4 hours.
Identifies changes and highlights need to modify plan of care.

3 Place the client in a room as close as possible to the nurse's station.
Facilitates faster response time to client's needs.

4 Place fall alert signs on the client's door and head of bed.
Alerts other health care workers to client's risk status.

5 Put the bed alarm on.
Helps monitor client status and facilitates prompt response if client tries to get out of bed unassisted.

6 Monitor the client and the environment every 2 hours and whenever a caregiver goes by the client's room.
Provides information on status, progress, and needs of client; encourages team approach to client care.

7 Instruct all caregivers to respond promptly to call light.
Ensures rapid response to client's needs.

8 Teach the client to use the call light; reinforce teaching each time before leaving the client alone.
Ensures that client has means and knowledge to call for assistance if necessary.

Successful implementation of nursing care is indicated by...

Fall prevention protocol implemented; client discharged on third day of hospitalization free from injury.

Key:

☐	Case Scenario
☐	Assessment Data
☐	Nursing Diagnosis *Prioritized as 1, 2, etc.*
⬭	Expected Outcome
☐	Interventions and *Rationales*
☐	Evaluation

PROCEDURE 36-1

Body Mechanics, Lifting, and Transferring

EQUIPMENT
- Transfer or gait belt(s)
- Wheelchair with locks
- Transfer board
- Draw or lift sheet
- Gloves (when contact with body fluids is possible)
- Nonslip shoes or slippers
- Stretcher with locks
- Hydraulic lift

ACTION	RATIONALE
1. Wash hands/hand hygiene. Don gloves if contact with body fluids is possible.	1. Reduces the transmission of microorganisms.
2. Assess the situation for obstacles, heavy clients, poor handholds, or equipment or objects in the way. Reduce or remove safety hazards prior to lifting the client or object. Assess for any tubing or equipment connected to the client.	2. Good planning helps prevent accidental injury.
3. Assess for slippery surfaces, including wet floors; slippery shoes on client, helper, or nurse; and towels, linen, or paper on the floor. Resolve the slippery surface prior to lifting the client or object.	3. Removes the cause of many falls.
4. Assess for hidden risks, including client confusion, combativeness, orthostatic hypotension, medication effects, pain, or fear.	4. Allows the nurse to anticipate and plan for unexpected events.
5. Maintain low center of gravity by bending at the hips and knees, not the waist. Squat down rather than bend over to lift.	5. Provides for the equal distribution of body weight and assists in maintaining safe balance.
6. Establish a wide support base with feet spread apart.	6. Provides stability and lowers the center of gravity.
7. Use feet to move. Avoid twisting or bending from the waist.	7. Assists in maintaining correct body alignment, which increases strength to lift, push, pull, and carry.
8. When pushing or pulling, stand near the object and place one foot partially ahead of the other.	8. Helps avoid back injuries.
9. When pushing a client or an object, lean into the client or object and apply continuous light pressure. When pulling a client or an object, lean away and grasp with light pressure. Never jerk or twist your body to move weight.	9. Firm pressure will provide continuous movement of the object and will avoid abrupt movements that require the expenditure of increased energy.
10. When stooping to move an object, maintain a wide base of support with feet, flex knees to lower body, and maintain straight upper body.	10. Provides the appropriate mechanics for the strength and endurance to achieve the task and to stand up straight upon completion.

(Continues)

PROCEDURE 36-1
Body Mechanics, Lifting, and Transferring (Continued)

ACTION	RATIONALE
11. When lifting or carrying an object, bend the knees in front of the object, take a firm hold, and assume a standing position by using the leg muscles and keeping the back straight.	11. This stance will avoid the use of the back, diminish the potential for spinal twisting, and provide the lifter with a firm center of gravity and strength to lift the required weight.
12. When rising up from a squatting position, arch your back slightly. Keep the buttocks and abdomen tucked in and rise up with your head first.	12. Keeps the back from bowing and increasing the strain on the back muscles.
13. When lifting or carrying heavy objects, keep the weight as close to your center of gravity as possible (see Figure 36-23).	13. Reduces the strain on arm, leg, and back muscles.
14. When reaching for a client or an object, keep the back straight. If the client or object is heavy, do not try to lift the client or object without repositioning yourself closer to the weight (see Figure 36-24).	14. Avoids straining the back and arm muscles.
15. Use safety aids and equipment. Use gait belts, drawsheets, and other transfer assistive devices (see Figure 36-25 on page 1129). Encourage clients to use handrails and grab bars. Wheelchair, cart, and stretcher wheels should be locked when they are stationary.	15. Reduces strain on the nurse and improves safety for the client.
16. Wash hands/hand hygiene.	16. Reduces the transmission of microorganisms.

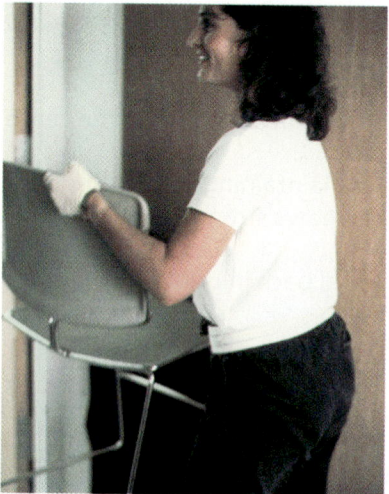

FIGURE 36-23 Hold weight close to your center of gravity.
DELMAR/CENGAGE LEARNING

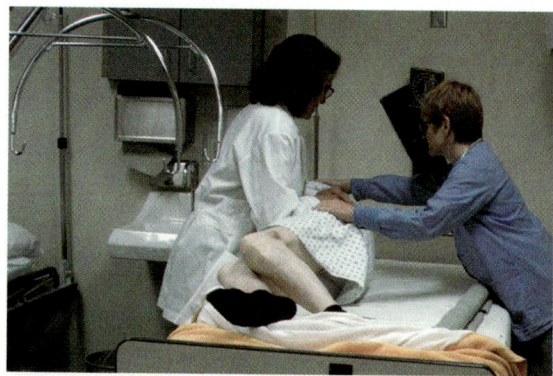

FIGURE 36-24 Keep your back straight when reaching.
DELMAR/CENGAGE LEARNING

(Continues)

PROCEDURE 36-1
Body Mechanics, Lifting, and Transferring (Continued)

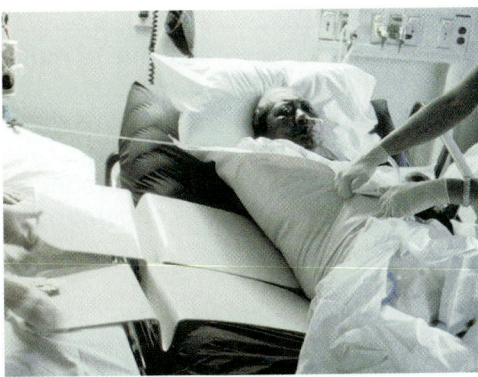

FIGURE 36-25 Use transfer boards to reduce shearing forces and to reduce the effort needed to move the client. DELMAR/CENGAGE LEARNING

delegation tip

- Personnel must be taught how to utilize body mechanics in order to protect themselves as well as clients.

- A professional nurse must supervise ancillary personnel when the client requires complex turning or the use of assistive devices.

nursing tips

- Ancillary personnel must be taught how to safely lift and transfer clients.

- The nurse must verify the ancillary personnel's competency in performing the skills.

PROCEDURE 36-2
Administering Passive Range-of-Motion (ROM) Exercises

EQUIPMENT
- Gloves (when contact with body fluids is possible)

ACTION	RATIONALE
1. Wash hands/hand hygiene. Wear gloves if contact with body fluids is possible.	1. Reduces the transmission of microorganisms.
2. Explain procedure to client, including estimated duration.	2. Decreases anxiety and encourages compliance and participation.
3. Provide for privacy by exposing only the extremity to be exercised.	3. Decreases embarrassment.

(Continues)

PROCEDURE 36-2
Administering Passive Range-of-Motion (ROM) Exercises (Continued)

ACTION	RATIONALE
4. Adjust bed to comfortable height for performing ROM.	4. Prevents muscle strain and discomfort for nurse.
5. Lower bed rail only on the side where you are working.	5. Prevents client falls.
6. Describe the passive ROM exercises you are performing, or verbally cue client to perform ROM exercises with your assistance. When possible, demonstrate movement.	6. Encourages client participation and cooperation.
7. Start at the client's head and perform ROM exercises down each side of the body. Begin exercise on client's stronger (or unaffected) side.	7. Provides a systematic method to ensure that all body parts are exercised. Working on client's unaffected side first promotes comfort and allows nurse to assess limitations or restrictions.
8. Repeat each ROM exercise as the client tolerates, to a maximum of 5 times. Perform each motion in a slow, firm manner. Encourage full joint movement, but do not go beyond the point of pain, resistance, or fatigue.	8. Provides exercise to the client's tolerance or to a level that will maintain the joint function.
9. Head Perform these movements with the client in a sitting position, if possible. • Rotation: Turn the head from side to side. • Flexion and extension: Tilt the head toward the chest and then tilt slightly upward (Figure 36-26). • Lateral flexion: Tilt the head to each side so as to almost touch the ear to the shoulder.	9. • Optimizes the performance of the movements. • Preserves muscle tone and joint flexibility.

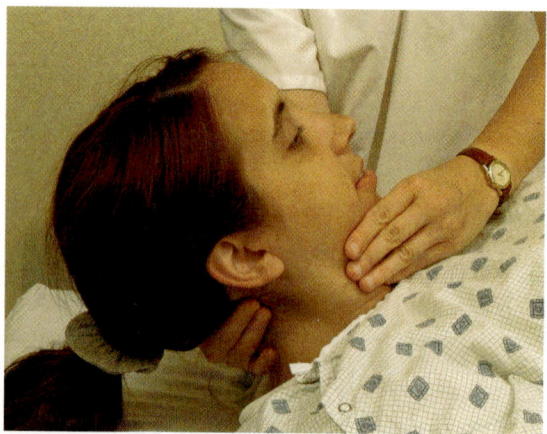
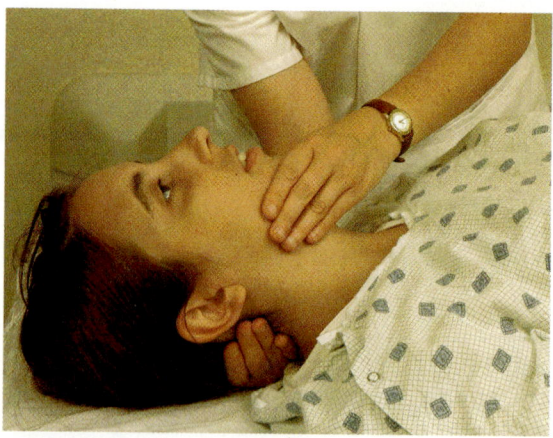

A   B

FIGURE 36-26 Passive ROM Exercises of Head: A. Flexion of Neck; B. Extension of Neck DELMAR/CENGAGE LEARNING

(Continues)

PROCEDURE 36-2
Administering Passive Range-of-Motion (ROM) Exercises *(Continued)*

ACTION	RATIONALE
10. Neck Perform this movement with the client in a sitting position, if possible. • Rotation: Rotate the neck in a semicircle while supporting the head.	10. • Optimizes the performance of the movements. • Preserves muscle tone and joint flexibility.
11. Trunk Perform these movements with the client in a sitting position, if possible. • Flexion and extension: Bend the trunk forward, straighten the trunk, and then extend slightly backward. • Rotation: Turn the shoulders forward and return to normal position. • Lateral flexion: Tilt trunk to the left side, straighten trunk, and tilt to the right side.	11. • Optimizes the performance of the movements. • Preserves muscle tone and joint flexibility.
12. Arm • Flexion and extension: Extend the arm in a straight position upward toward the head, then downward along the side. • Adduction and abduction: Extend the arm in a straight position toward the midline (adduction) and away from the midline (abduction).	12. Preserves muscle tone and joint flexibility.
13. Shoulder • Internal and external rotation: Bend the elbow at a 90° angle with the upper arm parallel to the shoulder; rotate the shoulder by moving the lower arm upward and downward.	13. Preserves muscle tone and joint flexibility.
14. Elbow • Flexion and extension: Supporting the arm, flex and extend the elbow (Figure 36-27).	14. Preserves muscle tone and joint flexibility.

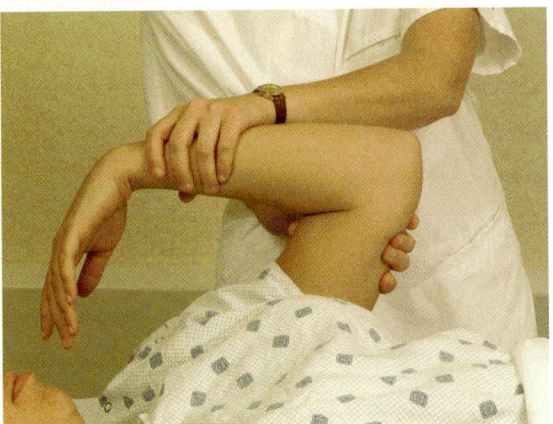
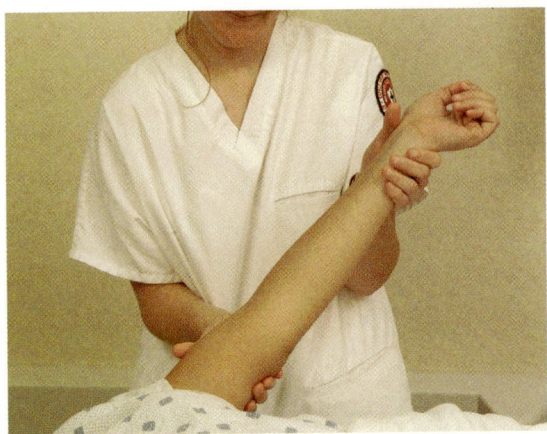

A   B

FIGURE **36-27** Passive ROM Exercises of the Elbow: A. Flexion of Elbow; B. Extension of Elbow DELMAR/CENGAGE LEARNING

(Continues)

PROCEDURE 36-2
Administering Passive Range-of-Motion (ROM) Exercises (Continued)

ACTION	RATIONALE
• Pronation and supination: Extend elbow, and move the hand in palm-up and palm-down positions.	
15. Wrist	15. Preserves muscle tone and joint flexibility.
• Flexion and extension: Supporting the wrist, flex and extend the wrist.	
• Adduction and abduction: Supporting the lower arm, turn wrist right to left, left to right, then rotate the wrist in a circular motion.	
16. Hand	16. Preserves muscle tone and joint flexibility.
• Flexion and extension: Supporting the wrist, flex and extend the fingers.	
• Adduction and abduction: Supporting the wrist, spread fingers apart and then bring them close together.	
• Opposition: Supporting the wrist, touch each finger with the tip of the thumb.	
• Thumb rotation: Supporting the wrist, rotate the thumb in a circular manner.	
17. Hip and leg Perform these movements with the client in a supine position, if possible (Figure 36-28).	17. • Optimizes the performance of the movements. • Preserves muscle tone and joint flexibility.
• Flexion and extension: Supporting the lower leg, flex the leg toward the chest and then extend the leg.	
• Internal and external rotation: Supporting the lower leg, angle the foot inward and outward.	

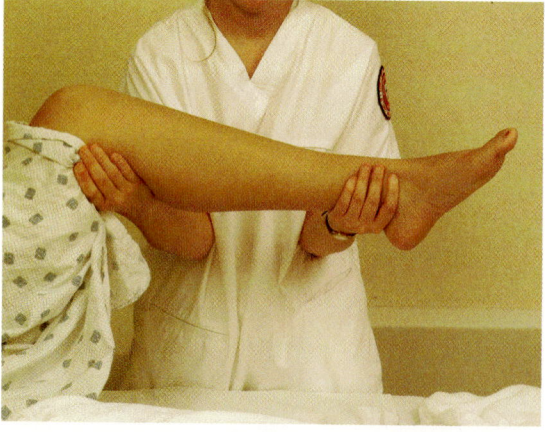
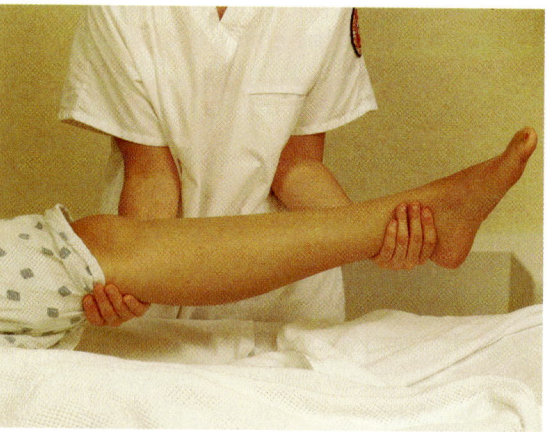

A	B

FIGURE 36-28 Passive ROM Exercises of Hip and Leg: A. Flexion of Hip and Leg; B. Extension of Hip and Leg

DELMAR/CENGAGE LEARNING

(Continues)

PROCEDURE 36-2
Administering Passive Range-of-Motion (ROM) Exercises (Continued)

ACTION	RATIONALE
• Adduction and abduction: Slide the leg away from the client's midline and then back to the midline.	
18. Knee	18. Preserves muscle tone and joint flexibility.
• Flexion and extension: Supporting the lower leg, flex and extend the knee.	
19. Ankle	19. Preserves muscle tone and joint flexibility.
• Flexion and extension: Supporting the lower leg, flex and extend the ankle.	
20. Foot	20. Preserves muscle tone and joint flexibility.
• Adduction and abduction: Supporting the ankle, spread the toes apart and then bring them close together.	
• Flexion and extension: Supporting the ankle, extend the toes upward and then flex the toes downward.	
21. Observe client for signs of exertion, pain, or fatigue during movement.	21. Alerts nurse to discontinue exercise.
22. Replace covers and position client in proper body alignment.	22. Promotes comfort.
23. Place side rails in original position. Adjust bed to lowest position.	23. Prevents falls.
24. Place call light within reach.	24. Facilitates communication.
25. Wash hands/hand hygiene.	25. Reduces the transmission of microorganisms.

delegation tip

- *Administering passive ROM may be delegated to trained ancillary personnel.*
- *Outcomes of the activity must be reported to the nurse.*

nursing tips

- *Continuously assess client's pain level during the ROM exercises.*
- *Do not move a joint beyond the client's comfort level.*
- *Exercise client's unaffected side first.*
- *Document client's ability (e.g., "ROM on left side greater than on right.").*
- *Avoid documenting only client limitations; be sure to record progress in functional abilities.*

PROCEDURE 36-3 Turning and Positioning a Client

EQUIPMENT

- Pillows
- Heel protectors
- Rolled blankets or towels
- Hand rolls
- Footboard
- Gloves (when contact with body fluids is possible)

ACTION	RATIONALE
1. Wash hands/hand hygiene. Don gloves if contact with body fluids is possible.	1. Reduces the transmission of microorganisms.
2. Explain procedure to client.	2. Decreases anxiety. Improves client compliance and cooperation.
3. Gather all necessary equipment. Provide for client privacy.	3. Promotes client dignity and allows for a smooth procedure.
4. Secure adequate assistance to safely complete task.	4. Prevents caregiver muscle strain and provides for client safety.
5. Adjust bed to comfortable working height. Lower side rail on side of bed from which you are assisting client.	5. Prevents caregiver back and muscle strain and promotes client safety.
6. Follow proper body mechanics guidelines:	6. Prevents caregiver back injury and muscle strain and promotes client safety.
• When moving a client in bed, position the bed so that your legs are slightly bent at the knees and hips.	• Spreading feet to create a wide base helps prevent loss of balance.
• Maintain the natural curves in your back while lifting.	• Use of a drawsheet promotes support and control of the client.
• Position one foot slightly in front of the other and spread feet apart to create a wide base for balance.	
• When your arms are placed under the client, slowly lean backward onto your back leg using your body weight to help you lift the client to one side of the bed. Do not extend or rotate your back to move a client in bed.	
• If you cannot move the client easily, always obtain assistance (see Figure 36-29 on page 1135).	
• Be sure the floor is not slippery and that the bed is locked.	
• Always use a turn (draw) sheet when moving a client (see Figure 36-30 on page 1135).	
7. Position drains, tubes, and IVs to accommodate for new client position.	7. Prevents accidental dislodgment or discomfort from movement by reducing mechanical tension.
8. Place or assist client into appropriate starting position. Monitor client status, and provide adequate rest breaks or support as necessary.	8. Prevents client injury.

(Continues)

PROCEDURE 36-3
Turning and Positioning a Client (Continued)

ACTION	RATIONALE

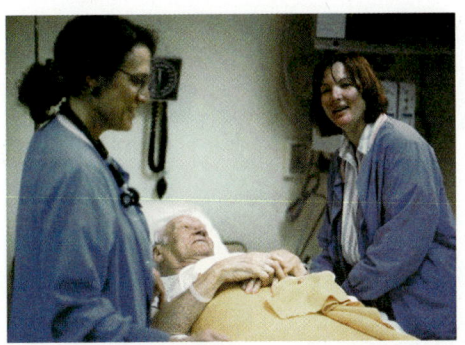

FIGURE 36-29 If the client is heavy or unable to assist, always obtain assistance for both the client's and your safety. DELMAR/CENGAGE LEARNING

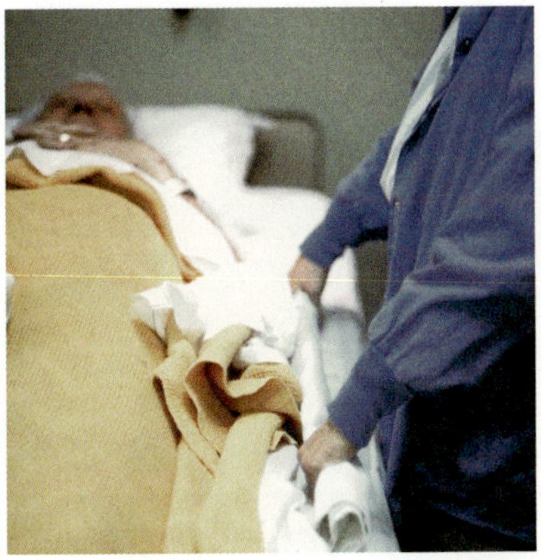

FIGURE 36-30 When moving a client, use a turn (draw) sheet for better support and control. DELMAR/CENGAGE LEARNING

MOVING FROM SUPINE TO SIDE-LYING POSITION

9. Slide your hands underneath the client.
   - Move the client to one side of the bed by lifting the client's body toward you in stages—first the upper trunk, then the lower trunk, and finally the legs.
   - Lift the client's body; do not drag the client across the sheets.
   - Roll the client to side-lying position by placing the client's inside arm next to the client's body with the palm of the hand against the hip.
   - Cross the client's outside arm and leg toward midline and logroll the client toward you using the client's outside shoulder and hip for leverage while maintaining stability and control of top arm and leg.

9. Maintains client body alignment and prevents client injury. Protects caregiver's back and prevents muscle strain.
   - Prevents skin shearing.

MAINTAINING SIDE-LYING POSITION

10. Repeat Actions 1–8.
11. Pillows may be placed to support the client's head and arms (see Figure 36-31 on page 1136). An additional pillow may be used to support the topside leg and fully and equally support the thigh, knee, ankle, and foot (see Figure 36-32 on page 1136). Move the lower arm forward slightly at the shoulder, and bend the elbow for comfort. If the client is unstable, a pillow placed against the back will provide additional support and keep the client from rolling to supine position.

10. See Rationales 1–8.
11. Provides support and comfort.

(Continues)

PROCEDURE 36-3
Turning and Positioning a Client (Continued)

ACTION	RATIONALE

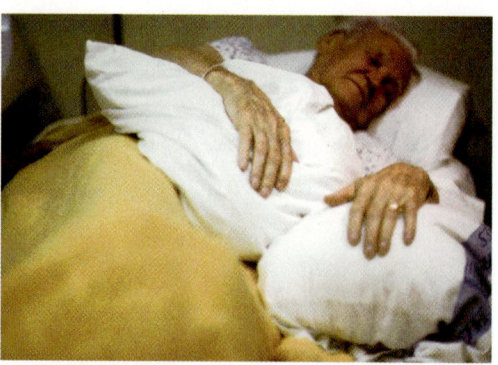

FIGURE 36-31 Place pillows to support the head and arms.
DELMAR/CENGAGE LEARNING

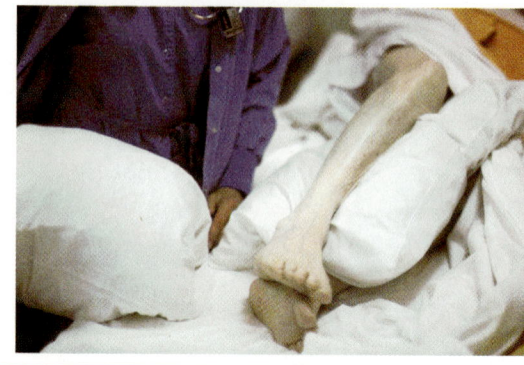

FIGURE 36-32 Place pillows to support the leg, ankle, and foot. DELMAR/CENGAGE LEARNING

MOVING FROM SIDE-LYING TO PRONE POSITION

12. Repeat Actions 1–8.
13. Remove positioning towels, pillows, or other support devices.

   - Assess whether the client's position in bed needs to be adjusted to accommodate the continued movement into prone position.
   - Move the client's inside arm next to the client's body with palm against hip.
   - Roll the client onto the stomach using the shoulder and hip as key points of control.
   - The head must be placed in a comfortable position to one side without excessive pressure to sensitive areas.
   - Pillows under the trunk are placed as needed to relieve pressure and increase comfort.
   - The client's arms are placed comfortably at the client's side, and the legs are uncrossed with the feet approximately a foot apart.

12. See Rationales 1–8.
13. Ensures comfort and safety in movement.

MAINTAINING PRONE POSITION

14. A shallow pillow or a folded towel may be used to support the client's head comfortably as well as a pillow placed under the abdomen to support the back. An additional pillow may be placed under the lower leg to reduce the pressure of the toes and forefoot against the bed.

14. Provides support and comfort.

(Continues)

PROCEDURE 36-3
Turning and Positioning a Client (Continued)

ACTION	RATIONALE
MOVING FROM PRONE TO SUPINE POSITION	
15. Repeat Actions 1–8.	15. See Rationales 1–8.
16. Remove positioning towels, pillows, or other supporting devices.	16. Provides support and comfort.

- Slide your hands underneath the client.
- Move the client segmentally to one side of the bed to accommodate the new position.
- Position the inside arm next to the client's body with the client's palm next to the hip.
- Roll the client to supine by logrolling the client toward you using the client's outside shoulder and hip for leverage.
- Have the client's face positioned away from the direction of the roll to prevent undue pressure to the face or neck.
- When the client reaches supine position, uncross the client's arms and legs and place them in comfortable positions.

ACTION	RATIONALE
MAINTAINING SUPINE POSITION	
17. A footboard may be used to support the foot as well as heel protectors or a pillow placed between the heel and gastrocnemius muscle to reduce the pressure on the heels.	17. Provides support and comfort. Heel protectors and routine assessment of the feet help to prevent pressure sores. Trochanter rolls and pillows help to prevent displacement of the acetabulum (hip joint).

- Assess and compare warmth, sensation, color, and movement of feet.
- To prevent excessive external rotation of the lower extremity, a trochanter roll may be used.
- For comfort, additional pillows may be used to support the client's head, arms, or lower back.

ACTION	RATIONALE
18. Be sure to replace side rails to upright position and lower the bed.	18. Provides for client safety.
19. Place call light within reach of the client.	19. Provides for client safety.
20. Move bedside table close to bed, and place items of frequent use within reach of the client.	20. Provides for client safety.
21. Wash hands/hand hygiene.	21. Reduces the transmission of microorganisms.

delegation tip

- *Turning and positioning are routinely delegated to ancillary personnel who have been appropriately trained.*

- *Ancillary personnel must report the client's response to the activity to the nurse.*

nursing tips

- *Safety is of utmost importance when turning and repositioning the client.*
- *Maintain client comfort as much as possible when moving the client.*

- *Assess the color and integrity of skin at bony prominences.*
- *Provide skin care as needed.*

PROCEDURE
36-4

PROCEDURE 36-4 Moving a Client in Bed

EQUIPMENT

- Hospital bed with side rails
- Turn sheet or drawsheet
- Trapeze if required
- Gloves (when contact with body fluids is possible)

ACTION	RATIONALE
MOVING UP A CLIENT IN BED WITH ONE NURSE	
1. Wash hands/hand hygiene. Don gloves if contact with body fluids is possible.	1. Reduces the transmission of microorganisms.
2. Inform client of reason for the move and how to assist (if able).	2. Reduces anxiety; helps increase comprehension and cooperation; promotes client autonomy.
3. Raise bed to just below waist height. Lower head of bed if tolerated by client. Lower side rails on the side where you are standing.	3. Decreases fall risk. Lessens strain on nurse's back muscles.
4. Remove pillow and place it against the headboard.	4. Prevents having to move against the pillow. Protects client's head.
5. Have the client fold arms across the chest.	5. Prevents getting the client's arms trapped or injured during the move.
6. Have the client hold on to the overhead trapeze, if available (see Figure 36-33).	6. Promotes client autonomy by allowing the client to assist with the move.

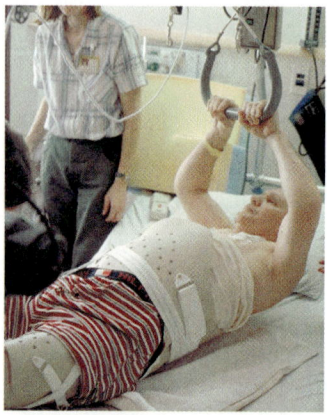

FIGURE 36-33 Have the client hold on to the overhead trapeze to assist in the move. DELMAR/CENGAGE LEARNING

7. Have the client bend the knees and place the feet flat on the bed if able.	7. Allows the client to assist in the move; promotes client autonomy.
8. Stand at an angle to the head of the bed, feet apart, knees bent, feet toward the head of the bed.	8. Promotes good body mechanics.
9. Slide one hand and arm under the client's shoulder, the other under the client's thigh.	9. Distributes the client's weight more evenly. Promotes good lifting technique.

(Continues)

PROCEDURE 36-4
Moving a Client in Bed (Continued)

ACTION	RATIONALE
10. Rock forward toward the head of the bed, lifting the client with you. Simultaneously have the client push with the legs.	10. Allows a smooth motion to lift the client. Client assistance lessens strain on nurse's back muscles; promotes client autonomy.
11. Have the client pull up holding onto the trapeze (if available) as you move the client upward in bed.	11. Client assistance lessens strain on nurse's back muscles; promotes client autonomy.
12. Repeat these steps until the client is moved up high enough in bed.	12. Large or very immobile clients are often not moved far enough in one step.
13. Return the client's pillow under the head.	13. Promotes client comfort.
14. Elevate head of bed, if tolerated by client.	14. Promotes comfort; facilitates eating and drinking; facilitates communication.
15. Assess client for comfort.	15. Comfort is subjective.
16. Adjust the client's bedclothes as needed.	16. Promotes comfort and privacy.
17. Lower bed and elevate side rails.	17. Promotes client safety.
18. Wash hands/hand hygiene.	18. Reduces the transmission of microorganisms.

MOVING UP A CLIENT IN BED WITH TWO OR MORE NURSES

ACTION	RATIONALE
19. Wash hands/hand hygiene. Apply gloves if needed.	19. Reduces the transmission of microorganisms.
20. Inform client of reason for the move and how to assist (if able).	20. Reduces anxiety; helps increase comprehension and cooperation; promotes client autonomy.
21. Elevate bed to just below waist height. Lower head of bed if tolerated by client. Lower side rails.	21. Lessens strain on nurses' back muscles.
22. With two nurses, place turn (draw) sheet under client's back and head.	22. Reduces shearing force, which can precipitate skin breakdown.
23. Roll up the drawsheet on each side until it is next to the client.	23. Provides support under the heavy parts of the body and places the nurses' hands close to the weight to be moved.
24. Follow Actions 4–7.	24. See Rationales 4–7.
25. The nurses stand on either side of the bed, at an angle to the head of the bed. They stand with knees flexed, feet apart in a wide stance.	25. Promotes good body mechanics.
26. The nurses hold their elbows as closely as possible to their bodies.	26. Allows the muscles of the torso to assist the arm muscles in bearing and moving the weight of the client.
27. The lead nurse will give the signal to move: 1-2-3 go. The nurses will lift up (off the bed) on the turn sheet and forward (toward the head of the bed) in one smooth motion. The move is coordinated to transfer the client toward the head of the bed. Simultaneously, have the client push with the legs or pull using the trapeze (see Figure 36-34 on page 1140).	27. Allows a smooth motion to lift the client. Client assistance lessens strain on the nurses' back muscles; promotes client autonomy.
28. Repeat until the client is moved up high enough in bed to be comfortable.	28. Large or very immobile clients are often not moved far enough in one step.
29. Return the client's pillow under the head.	29. Promotes client comfort.
30. Elevate head of bed, if tolerated by client.	30. Promotes comfort; facilitates eating and drinking; facilitates communication.

(Continues)

PROCEDURE 36-4
Moving a Client in Bed (Continued)

ACTION	**RATIONALE**

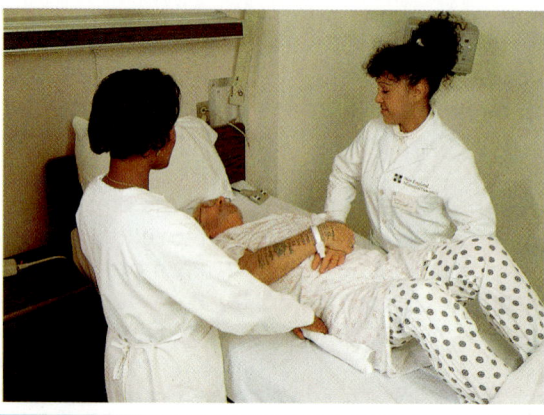

FIGURE 36-34 Moving Client in Bed: Client Positioned with Knees Flexed DELMAR/CENGAGE LEARNING

31. Assess client for comfort.	31. Comfort is subjective.
32. Adjust the client's bedclothes.	32. Promotes comfort and privacy.
33. Lower bed and elevate side rails.	33. Promotes client safety.
34. Wash hands/hand hygiene.	34. Reduces the transmission of microorganisms.

delegation tip

- Moving a client in bed is routinely delegated to ancillary personnel who have received appropriate training.

- Ancillary personnel must report the client's response to the activity to the nurse.

nursing tips

- Safety is of utmost importance when repositioning the client.

- Maintain client comfort as much as possible when moving the client.

PROCEDURE 36-5
Assisting from Bed to Wheelchair, Commode, or Chair

EQUIPMENT

- Bed
- Wheelchair, commode, or chair
- Splints, braces, or other assistive devices needed by the client
- Gloves (when contact with body fluids is possible)
- Shoes or slippers with nonskid soles
- Gait belt
- Transfer board (if needed)

(Continues)

PROCEDURE 36-5
Assisting from Bed to Wheelchair, Commode, or Chair (Continued)

ACTION	RATIONALE
1. Inform client about desired purpose and destination.	1. Reduces client anxiety and increases cooperation.
2. Assess client for ability to assist with the transfer and for presence of cognitive or sensory deficits.	2. Allows planning regarding the amount of assistance and cooperation to expect from the client.
3. Lock the bed in position.	3. Prevents the bed from rolling during the procedure.
4. Wash hands/hand hygiene. Don gloves if contact with body fluids is possible.	4. Reduces the transmission of microorganisms.
5. Place any splints, braces, or other devices on the client.	5. Provides support and prevents injury to the client.
6. Place shoes or slippers on the client's feet.	6. Provides a nonslip surface for stability.
7. Lower the height of the bed to lowest possible position.	7. Reduces distance client has to step down, thus decreasing risk of injury.
8. Slowly raise the head of the bed if not contraindicated by the client's condition.	8. Minimizes lifting.
9. Place one arm under the client's legs and one arm behind the client's back. Slowly pivot the client so the client's legs are dangling over the edge of the bed and the client is in a sitting position on the edge of the bed (see Figure 36-35).	9. Supports client while sitting upright.
10. Allow client to dangle for 2–5 minutes. Help support client if necessary (see Figure 36-36).	10. Allows time for assessing client's response to sitting; reduces possibility of orthostatic hypotension.
11. Bring the chair or wheelchair close to the side of the bed. Place it at a 45° angle to the bed. If the client has a weaker side, place the chair or wheelchair on the client's strong side.	11. Minimizes transfer distance. Allows the client to pivot on the stronger leg.

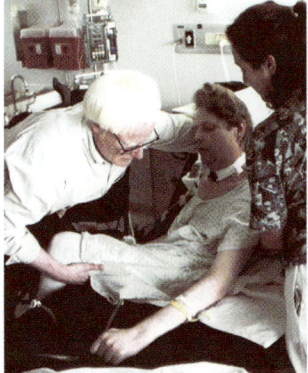

FIGURE 36-35 Pivot the client to a sitting position on the edge of the bed. DELMAR/CENGAGE LEARNING

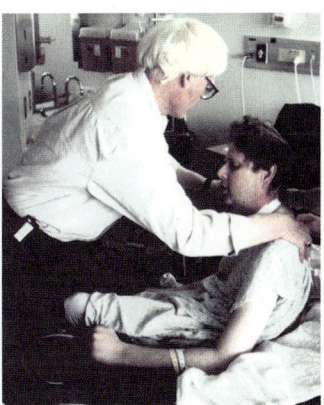

FIGURE 36-36 Support the client, if needed, while the client adjusts to the sitting position. DELMAR/CENGAGE LEARNING

(Continues)

PROCEDURE 36-5
Assisting from Bed to Wheelchair, Commode, or Chair (Continued)

ACTION	RATIONALE
12. Lock wheelchair brakes and elevate the foot pedals. For chairs, lock brakes if available.	12. Provides stability.
13. If you will be using a gait belt to assist the client, place it around the client's waist.	13. Provides a secure handhold for the nurse during the transfer.
14. Assist client to side of bed until feet are firmly on the floor and slightly apart.	14. Moves client into proper position for transfer. Provides stable footing for client.
15. Grasp the sides of the gait belt or place your hands just below the client's axillae. Using a wide stance, bend your knees and assist the client to a standing position.	15. Avoids putting pressure directly on the axillae and risking nerve damage or shoulder subluxation. Wide stance increases nurse stability and minimizes strain on the back.
16. Standing close to the client, pivot until the client's back is toward the chair.	16. Moves client into proper position to be seated.
17. Instruct the client to place hands on the arm supports, or place the client's hands on the arm supports of the chair.	17. Allows client to gain balance and judge distance to seat.
18. Bend at the knees, and ease the client into a sitting position.	18. Increases stability and minimizes strain on back.
19. Assist client to maintain proper posture. Support weak side with pillow if needed.	19. Increases client comfort.
20. Secure the safety belt, place client's feet on feet pedals (see Figure 36-37), and release brakes if you will be moving the client immediately. Make sure tubes and lines, arms, and hands are not pinched or caught between the client and the chair. If the client is sitting in a chair, offer a footstool if available.	20. Ensures client safety; prepares client for movement.
21. Wash hands/hand hygiene.	21. Reduces the transmission of microorganisms.

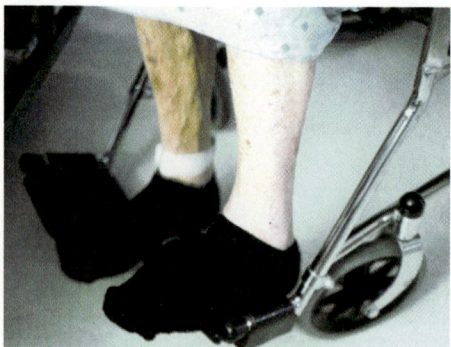

FIGURE 36-37 Position the wheelchair footrests or use a footstool if the client is sitting in a chair. DELMAR/CENGAGE LEARNING

(Continues)

PROCEDURE 36-5
Assisting from Bed to Wheelchair, Commode, or Chair (Continued)

delegation tip

- Moving a client from the bed is routinely delegated to ancillary personnel who have received appropriate training.
- Ancillary personnel must report the client's response to the activity to the nurse.

nursing tips

- Safety is of utmost importance when turning and repositioning the client.
- Maintain client comfort as much as possible when moving the client.
- Place the chair on the client's unaffected, or stronger, side.
- Brace your knees against the client's knees to keep legs from buckling.
- Assess the client's tolerance of the activity.

PROCEDURE 36-6
Assisting from Bed to Stretcher

EQUIPMENT
- Bed
- Transfer or slider boards
- Gloves (when contact with body fluids is possible)
- Stretcher
- Lift sheet
- Pillows
- Other qualified personnel to assist

ACTION	RATIONALE
TRANSFERRING A CLIENT WITH MINIMUM ASSISTANCE	
1. Inform client about desired purpose and destination.	1. Reduces client anxiety and increases cooperation.
2. Wash hands/hand hygiene. Don gloves if contact with body fluids is possible.	2. Reduces the transmission of microorganisms.
3. Raise the height of bed to 1 inch higher than the stretcher and lock brakes of bed.	3. Reduces distance nurse must bend, thus preventing back strain; prevents bed from moving.
4. Instruct client to move to side of bed close to stretcher. Lower side rails of bed and stretcher. Leave side rails on opposite side up.	4. Decreases risk of client falling.
5. Stand at outer side of stretcher and push it toward bed. Lock the stretcher brakes.	5. Diminishes the gap between bed and stretcher; secures the stretcher position.
6. Instruct client to move onto stretcher with assistance as needed.	6. Promotes client independence.
7. Cover client with sheet or bath blanket.	7. Promotes comfort; protects privacy.
8. Elevate side rails on stretcher and secure safety belts about client. Release brakes of stretcher.	8. Prevents falls.

(Continues)

PROCEDURE 36-6
Assisting from Bed to Stretcher (Continued)

ACTION	RATIONALE
9. Stand at head of stretcher to guide it when pushing.	9. Pushing, not pulling, ensures proper body mechanics.
10. Wash hands/hand hygiene.	10. Reduces the transmission of microorganisms.

TRANSFERRING A CLIENT WITH MAXIMUM ASSISTANCE

11. Repeat Actions 1–3.	11. See Rationales 1–3.
12. Assess amount of assistance required for transfer. Usually 2–4 staff members are required for the maximum-assisted transfer.	12. Promotes client independence; ensures that enough staff are present before beginning transfer.
13. Lock wheels of bed and stretcher.	13. Prevents falls.
14. Have one nurse stand close to client's head.	14. Supports client's head during the move.
15. Logroll the client (keep in straight alignment) and place a lift sheet under the client's back, trunk, and upper legs. The lift sheet can extend under the head if client lacks head control abilities.	15. Prevents flexion and rotation of client's hips and spine; maintains correct body alignment.
16. Empty all drainage bags (e.g., T-tube, Hemovac, Jackson-Pratt). Record amounts. Secure drainage system to client's gown prior to transfer.	16. Decreases possibility of spills; prevents dislodging of tubes.
17. Move client to edge of bed near stretcher. Lift up and over to avoid dragging.	17. Prevents dragging, which causes shearing force.
18. Because the client is now on the side of the bed, without the side rail up, the nurse on nonstretcher side of bed holds the stretcher side of the lift sheet up (by reaching across the client's chest) to prevent the client from falling onto the stretcher or off the bed.	18. Protects the client from falling.
19. Place pillow or slider board overlapping the bed and stretcher (see Figure 36-38).	19. Protects head from injury. Slider board eases movement of the client.
20. Have staff members grasp edges of lift sheet. Be sure to use good body mechanics (see Figure 36-39).	20. Provides surface for client to slide on. Prevents dragging and shearing.

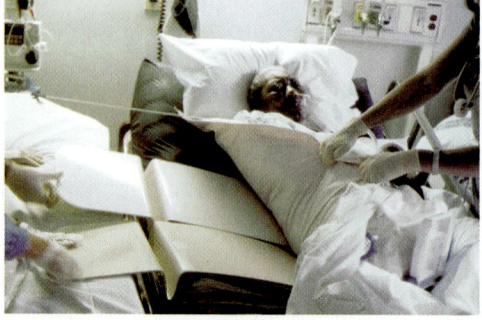

FIGURE 36-38 Place pillow or slider board overlapping the bed and stretcher. DELMAR/CENGAGE LEARNING

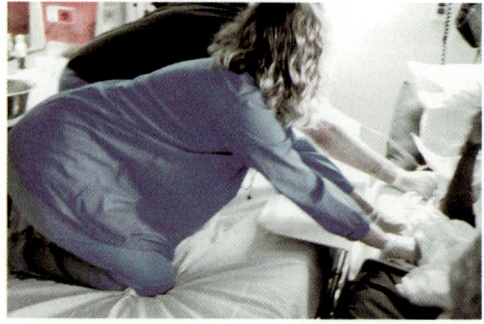

FIGURE 36-39 Firmly grasp edges of lift sheet. DELMAR/CENGAGE LEARNING

(Continues)

PROCEDURE 36-6
Assisting from Bed to Stretcher (Continued)

ACTION	RATIONALE
21. On the count of three, have staff members pull lift sheet and the client onto the stretcher.	21. Working in unison makes the overall job easier and prevents staff injury.
22. Position client on stretcher, place pillow under head, and cover with a sheet or bath blanket.	22. Promotes comfort and provides for privacy.
23. Secure safety belts and elevate side rails of stretcher.	23. Prevents falls.
24. If IV bag is present, move it from bed IV pole to stretcher IV pole after client transfer.	24. Prevents tubing from being pulled and IV from being dislodged.
25. Wash hands/hand hygiene.	25. Reduces the transmission of microorganisms.

delegation tip

- *Moving a client from the bed to a stretcher is routinely delegated to ancillary personnel who have received appropriate training.*
- *The client's response to the activity must be reported to the nurse by ancillary personnel.*

nursing tips

- *Place the stretcher on the client's unaffected or stronger side.*
- *Remind the client that the stretcher is narrow and to move about carefully when on it.*
- *Access which devices can be safely removed and disconnected from the client prior to the transfer.*
- *Be sure to get enough help when transferring clients with complex needs. It may take one or two staff members just to watch the lines and tubes in order to promote a safe transfer.*

PROCEDURE 36-7

Using a Hydraulic Lift

EQUIPMENT
- Mechanical lift
- Equipment should include lift, canvas or mesh sheet, and bars to slide into sheet
- Protective disposable cover or disinfectant to clean canvas
- Gloves (when applicable)

ACTION	RATIONALE
1. Wash hands/hand hygiene. Don gloves if contact with body fluids is possible.	1. Reduces the transmission of microorganisms.
2. Check the prescribing practitioner's order to determine the length of time the client may sit.	2. The prescribing practitioner may want the client to sit only for a specified length of time or for as long as tolerated.
3. Check the client's medical diagnosis and any other medical problems.	3. Assists in determining any problems that sitting may cause or any necessary restrictions.

(Continues)

PROCEDURE 36-7
Using a Hydraulic Lift (Continued)

ACTION	RATIONALE
4. Ask the client how long ago he or she last sat.	4. If the client has been in the bed several days, he or she may complain of dizziness or faintness.
5. Lock the wheels of the bed.	5. Prevents the bed from rolling when the client is moved; helps prevent falls.
6. Position the chair close to the bed.	6. Always transfer the client the shortest possible distance to conserve energy of client and nurse.
7. Position urine drainage, nasogastric (NG), and IV tubing on the side of the bed where the chair will be placed. Allow slack in the tubing.	7. Prevents the tubing from being dislodged when the client is moved.
8. Clamp and disconnect any tubing if condition allows.	8. NG suction tubing and feeding tubing are often allowed to be clamped. This makes moving the client easier.
9. Roll client on side, and position the sling on bed behind the client.	9. The sling is positioned behind the client so the client can be turned in the opposite direction and the sling can be pulled through.
10. Roll client on opposite side, pull the sling through, and position the sling smoothly on the bed.	10. Prevents skin breakdown.
11. Roll the client back onto the sling, and fold the arms over the chest (see Figure 36-40).	11. Prevents injury to the client's arms during the transfer.
12. Make sure the sling is centered under client.	12. Evenly distributes the client's weight.
13. Lower the side rail, and position the lift on the side of the bed with the chair. Be sure to spread the base of the hydraulic lift as indicated in manufacturer's instructions to provide stability (see Figure 36-41). Protect the client from falls while the side rail is down.	13. The side rail must be down to use the lift. Always transfer the client the shortest possible distance. The wheels and base of the lift should be spread to provide a wide, stable base to prevent the lift from tipping.

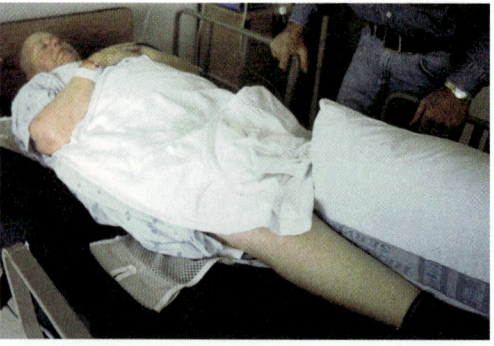

FIGURE 36-40 Roll the client back onto the sling. Position the client's arms across the chest. DELMAR/CENGAGE LEARNING

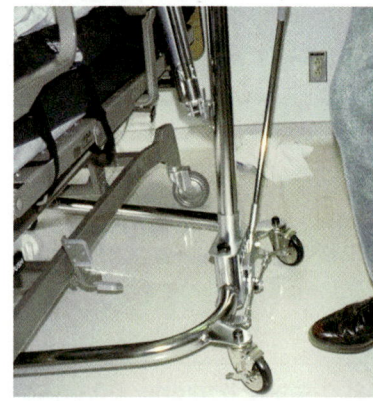

FIGURE 36-41 Spread the base of the hydraulic lift to provide stability. DELMAR/CENGAGE LEARNING

14. Lift the frame, and pass it over the client. Carefully lower the frame, and attach the hooks to the sling (see Figure 36-42 on page 1147).	14. Safely attaches sling to frame.

(Continues)

PROCEDURE 36-7
Using a Hydraulic Lift (Continued)

ACTION	RATIONALE

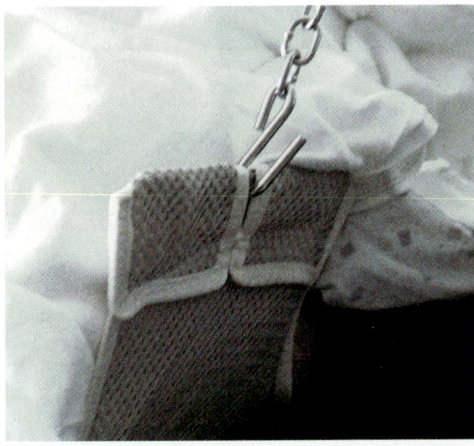

FIGURE 36-42 **Attach the hooks to the sling.** DELMAR/CENGAGE LEARNING

ACTION	RATIONALE
15. Raise the client from the bed by activating the lift.	15. Read the manufacturer's directions to determine the mechanism for raising the particular lift you are using. The various models do not operate in the same manner.
16. Secure the client with a safety belt, and cover the client with a blanket.	16. Provides safety and comfort.
17. Steer the client away from the bed, and slide a chair through the base of the lift.	17. It is safer to slide the chair through the base than to slide the base around the chair.
18. The sling can be disconnected, and the lift can be moved out of the way while the client is sitting in the chair. If the lift will be used to return the client to bed, the sling may be left in place beneath the client.	18. Provides safety and comfort.
19. Reposition and reconnect tubing.	19. Tubing should not be left disconnected. The client may sit for a while and will need all the equipment to function properly.
20. Assess how well the client tolerated the move and whether any dizziness was experienced.	20. The data are necessary for charting whether the client experienced any problems.
21. Place call light, appropriate covers, and padding as needed after transfer. Place protective restraints as needed. Cover feet with slippers if in sitting position.	21. Ensures privacy and protection.
22. Reverse the procedure to return the client to the bed.	22. Transfers client safely and comfortably.
23. Lower the bed, and place the call light within reach.	23. Promotes client safety.
24. Wash hands/hand hygiene.	24. Reduces the transmission of microorganisms.

(Continues)

PROCEDURE 36-7
Using a Hydraulic Lift (Continued)

delegation tip

- Moving a client from the bed to a chair is routinely delegated to ancillary personnel who have received appropriate training.

- Supervision by a professional nurse may be required if the client has multiple devices or invasive lines.

nursing tips

- Provide reassurance to the client to reduce anxiety associated with being temporarily suspended in the air.

- Instruct the client to keep hands crossed over the chest and to sit still during the move.

PROCEDURE 36-8   Assisting with Ambulation

EQUIPMENT
- Gait belt (as needed)
- Gloves (when contact with body fluids is possible)

ACTION	RATIONALE
1. Wash hands/hand hygiene. Don gloves if contact with body fluids is possible.	1. Prevents transmission of microorganisms.
2. Encourage the client to void before ambulating, especially with elderly clients.	2. Prevents need to interrupt ambulation. Restroom may not be readily available.
3. When assisting a client with an intravenous (IV) infusion, place the IV pole with wheels at the head of the bed before having the client dangle the legs so there is room to swing the legs from the bed to the floor. If orders allow, place a saline lock on the IV.	3. Prevents the client's legs from becoming tangled in the IV pole or tubing, causing a fall or causing the tubing to become dislodged. Provides more freedom of movement.
4. Transfer the IV infusion from the bed IV pole to the portable IV pole. The client or the nurse can guide the portable IV pole ahead during ambulation (see Figure 36-43 on page 1149).	4. Supports the IV while the client ambulates.
5. When assisting the client who has a urinary drainage bag, empty the drainage bag prior to ambulation. • Have the client sit on the side of the bed with legs dangling.	5. Emptying the bag reduces the weight of the bag. An empty bag kept below the level of the bladder reduces the risk of urine flowing back into the bladder and, hence, reduces risk of contamination.

(Continues)

PROCEDURE 36-8
Assisting with Ambulation (Continued)

ACTION	RATIONALE
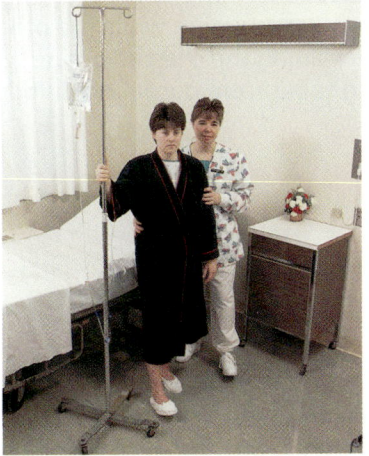	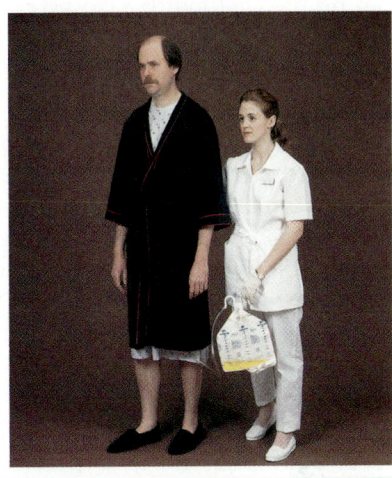

FIGURE 36-43 Ambulating Client with an IV DELMAR/CENGAGE LEARNING

FIGURE 36-44 Ambulating Client with a Urinary Drainage Bag DELMAR/CENGAGE LEARNING

- Remove the urinary drainage bag from the bed. The nurse or client can hold the urinary drainage bag during ambulation.
- Make sure the drainage bag remains below the level of the bladder (see Figure 36-44).

6. When the client has a drainage tube (such as a T-tube, Hemovac, or Jackson-Pratt drainage system), be sure to secure the drainage tube and bag prior to ambulation. Place a rubber band around the drainage tube near the drainage bag. Secure the drainage tube and bag with a safety pin through the rubber band to allow slack. The safety pin can be secured to the client's gown or robe (see Figure 36-45).

6. Prevents the tubing from becoming dislodged or tangled in clothing or other tubes.

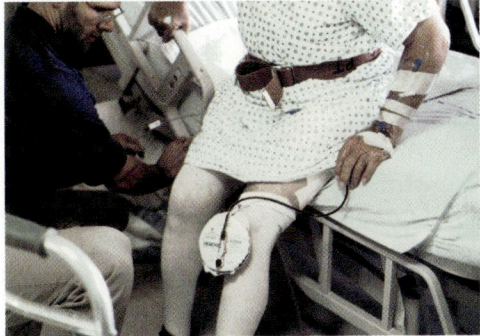

FIGURE 36-45 Secure tubes and drainage bags prior to ambulation so they do not become dislodged. DELMAR/CENGAGE LEARNING

(Continues)

PROCEDURE 36-8
Assisting with Ambulation (Continued)

ACTION	RATIONALE
7. Ambulating the client with a closed chest tube drainage system often requires two nurses, one assisting the client and one nurse managing the closed chest tube drainage system.	7. Two nurses allow one to focus on the client's safety and ambulation while the other focuses on maintaining the chest drainage system and keeping tubes from becoming dislodged.
• While the client is sitting on the edge of the bed with feet dangling, remove the hangers from the drainage system.	
• Hold the closed chest tube drainage system upright at all times to maintain the water seal.	
• Do not pull or tug on the chest tubes; they may not be sutured into place.	
8. Use a transfer belt or gait belt when ambulating a client who is weak (see Figure 36-46). For additional safety, a wheelchair can be pushed alongside the client for ready access if the client feels weak, tired, or faint.	8. The transfer belt is worn by the client for the purposes of stabilization during transfers and ambulation. It provides more support for the client by having the nurse hold the back of the belt.

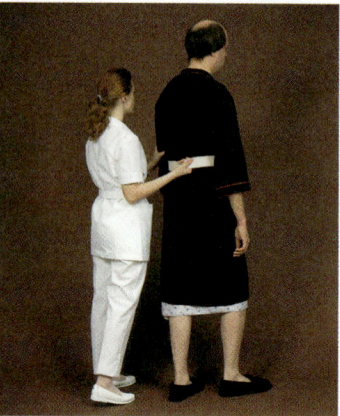

FIGURE 36-46 Ambulating the client using a gait belt for better grip and control. DELMAR/CENGAGE LEARNING

9. If a client feels faint or dizzy during dangling, return the client to a supine position in bed and lower the head of the bed. Monitor the client's blood pressure and pulse.	9. Keeps the client from falling from the bed. Lowering the head of the bed will allow gravity to support blood flow to the brain in the hypotensive client.
10. If the client feels dizzy during ambulation, allow the client to sit in a chair. Stay with the client for safety. Request another staff member to secure a wheelchair, if not already available, to return the client to bed.	10. May stop the client from progressing to full syncope.
11. If the client starts to fall, ease the client to the floor while supporting and protecting the client's head. Position yourself next to and slightly behind the client, and safely ease the client to the floor. Ask other personnel to assist you in returning the client to bed. Assess orthostatic blood pressures.	11. Easing the client to the floor prevents injury to the client.

(Continues)

PROCEDURE 36-8
Assisting with Ambulation (Continued)

delegation tip

- *Assisting a client with ambulation is routinely delegated to ancillary personnel who have received appropriate training.*

- *The client's response to ambulation must be reported to the nurse by ancillary personnel.*

nursing tips

Be sure the client understands the need to have assistance during the first few times of ambulation.

PROCEDURE 36-9   Assisting with Crutches, Cane, or Walker

EQUIPMENT
- Gait belt
- Assistive device: crutches, cane, or walker
- Tape measure
- Nonslip footwear

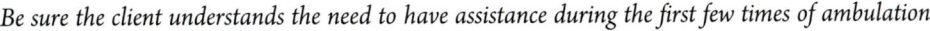

ACTION	RATIONALE
CRUTCHWALKING	
1. Inform client that you will be assisting with ambulation using the device chosen.	1. Reduces anxiety and helps increase comprehension and cooperation.
2. Wash hands/hand hygiene.	2. Reduces the transmission of microorganisms.
3. Assess client for strength, mobility, range of motion, visual acuity, perceptual difficulties, and balance. *Note:* The nurse and physical therapist often work together on assessment and choosing the correct assistive equipment for ambulation.	3. Helps determine the client's capabilities and amount of assistance required.
4. Measure client for size of crutches, and adjust crutches to fit. While supine, measure client from heel to axilla.	4. Correct fit increases client safety and comfort.
5. Provide a robe and nonslip foot coverings or shoes.	5. Provides for privacy and safety.
6. Lower the height of the bed.	6. Allows client to sit with feet on the floor and increases safety.

(Continues)

PROCEDURE 36-9
Assisting with Crutches, Cane, or Walker (Continued)

ACTION	RATIONALE
7. Allow the client to dangle the legs at the side of the bed for several minutes. Assess for vertigo or nausea.	7. Allows for stabilization of blood pressure, thus preventing orthostatic hypotension; also increases client comfort.
8. Apply gait belt around the client's waist if balance is not steady. It is good practice to use a gait belt the first time the client is out of bed.	8. Provides support and promotes safety.
9. Instruct client on method of holding crutches while client remains seated. This should be with elbows bent 30° while hands are on the hand grips and pads 1.5–2 inches below the axillae (see Figure 36-47). Instruct client to position crutches 4–5 inches laterally and 4–6 inches in front of feet. This skill can be demonstrated on yourself.	9. Increases comprehension and cooperation; decreases anxiety.
10. Assist the client to a standing position by placing both crutches in the nondominant hand. Then, using the dominant hand, push off from the bed while using the crutches for balance. Once erect, the extra crutch can be moved into the dominant hand.	10. Allows for stability while promoting independence.

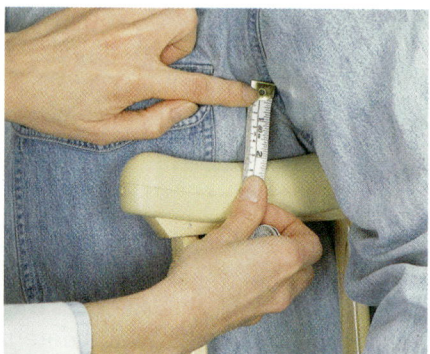

FIGURE 36-47 Adjusting the crutches to fit the client will increase comfort and stability. DELMAR/CENGAGE LEARNING

11. Instruct the client to remain still for a few seconds while assessing for vertigo or nausea. Stand close to the client to support as needed. While client remains standing, check for correct fit of the crutches.	11. Promotes client comfort, support, and safety. If the client becomes dizzy, sit client back down and wait before trying again.

(Continues)

PROCEDURE 36-9
Assisting with Crutches, Cane, or Walker (Continued)

ACTION	RATIONALE

Four-Point Gait (see Figure 36-48)

12. Position the crutches 4.5–6 inches to the side and in front of each foot. Move the right crutch forward 4–6 inches and move the left foot forward, even with the left crutch. Move the left crutch forward 4–6 inches and move the right foot forward, even with the right crutch. Repeat the four-point gait.

12. The four-point gait (used for partial or full weight bearing) provides greater stability. Weight bearing is on three points (two crutches and one foot or two feet and one crutch) at all times. The client must be able to bear weight with both legs.

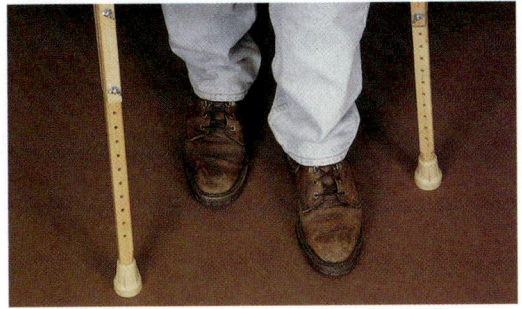
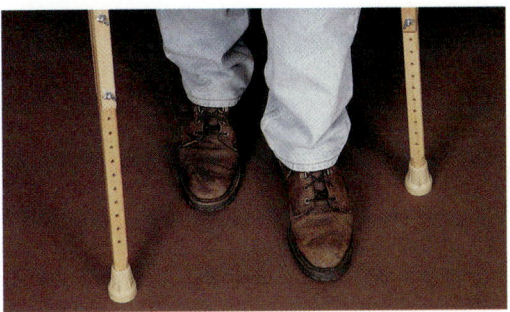

A   B

FIGURE 36-48 Crutchwalking, four-point gait: A. Moving right crutch forward and left foot forward; B. Moving left crutch forward and right foot forward, even with right crutch. DELMAR/CENGAGE LEARNING

Three-Point Gait (see Figure 36-49 on page 1148)

13. Advance both crutches and the weaker leg forward together 4–6 inches. Move the stronger leg forward, even with the crutches. Repeat the three-point gait.

13. The three-point gait (used for partial or non–weight bearing) provides a strong base of support. This gait can be used if the client has a weak or non–weight-bearing leg.

Two-Point Gait

14. Move the left crutch and right leg forward 4–6 inches. Move the right crutch and left leg forward 4–6 inches. Repeat the two-point gait.

14. The two-point gait (used for partial weight bearing) provides a strong base of support. The client must be able to bear weight on both legs.

Swing-Through Gait (see Figure 36-50 on page 1148)

15. This step is basically the same as the three-point gait. The difference is that on the swing, whichever leg is moving will go past the stationary point and set down in front.

15. The swing-through gait permits a faster pace. This gait requires greater balance, strength, and more practice.

(Continues)

PROCEDURE 36-9
Assisting with Crutches, Cane, or Walker (Continued)

ACTION	RATIONALE
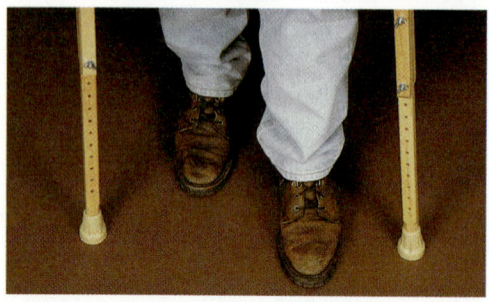	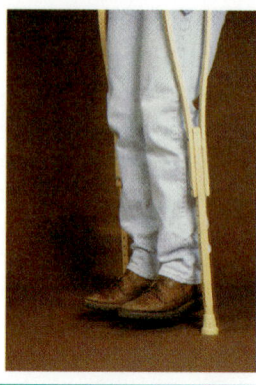

FIGURE 36-49 Crutchwalking, three-point gait: Advancing both crutches and weaker leg forward together. DELMAR/CENGAGE LEARNING

FIGURE 36-50 Crutchwalking: swing-through gait. DELMAR/CENGAGE LEARNING

Walking Upstairs

16. Stand beside and slightly behind client. Instruct client to position the crutches as if walking. Place body weight on hands. Place the strong leg on the first step. Pull the weak leg up and move the crutches up to the first step. Repeat for all steps.

16. Prevents weight bearing on the weaker leg. When ascending stairs, crutches should follow the legs, thereby allowing stability if the client's weight shifts down the stairs while moving. This allows the client to catch himself or herself instead of falling backward.

Walking Downstairs

17. Position the crutches as if walking. Place weight on the strong leg.
   - Move the crutches down to the next lower step.
   - Place partial weight on hands and crutches.
   - Move the weak leg down to the step with the crutches.
   - Put total weight on arms and crutches.
   - Move strong leg to same step as weak leg and crutches.
   - Repeat for all steps.
   - A second caregiver standing behind the client holding on to the gait belt will further decrease the risk of falling.

17. Prevents weight bearing on the weaker leg. Crutches in front of the legs while descending stairs allow the client more forward stability if client's weight shifts down the stairs while moving. This allows client to catch himself or herself before falling forward.

18. Set realistic goals and opportunities for progressive ambulation using crutches.

19. Consult with a physical therapist for clients learning to walk with crutches.

20. Wash hands/hand hygiene.

18. Crutch walking takes up to 10 times the energy required for unassisted ambulation.

19. The physical therapist is the expert for the health care team on crutchwalking techniques.

20. Reduces the transmission of microorganisms.

Sitting with Crutches

21. Instruct client to back up to chair until it is felt with the back of the legs.

22. Place both crutches in the nondominant hand and use the dominant hand to reach back to the chair.

23. Instruct client to lower slowly into the chair.

21. Allows for less turning, better stability, and increased safety.

22. Increases safety by giving client an idea of how far away client is from the seat.

23. Lowering slowly decreases possible injuries.

(Continues)

PROCEDURE 36-9
Assisting with Crutches, Cane, or Walker (Continued)

ACTION	RATIONALE
WALKING WITH A CANE	
24. Repeat Actions 1–10.	24. See Rationales 1–10.
25. Have the client hold the cane in the hand opposite the affected leg. Explain the safety and body mechanics underlying use of a cane on the strong side.	25. Promotes safety and cooperation. Promotes client autonomy. By holding the cane on the stronger side, the client has more control and strength for using it.
26. Have the client push up from the sitting position while pushing down on the bed with arms.	26. Promotes autonomy as well as increases upper body strength.
27. Have the client stand at the bedside for a few moments.	27. Allows the client to gain balance. The nurse can check for strength and balance.
28. Assess the height of the cane. With the cane placed 6 inches ahead of the client's body, the top of the cane should be at wrist level with the arm bent 25%–30% at the elbow.	28. A 25%–30% bend at the elbow provides for better muscle strength and support than if the arm is straight.
29. Walk to the side and slightly behind the client, holding the gait belt if needed for stability.	29. Provides stability or assistance to the client.
The Cane Gait	
30. Move the cane and the weaker leg forward at the same time for the same distance (see Figure 36-51). Place weight on the weaker leg and the cane. Move the strong leg forward. Place weight on the strong leg.	30. The cane helps to provide a wide base of support for the body when the weight is on the weaker leg.
Sitting with a Cane	
31. Have client turn around and back up to the chair. Have client grasp the arm of the chair with the free hand and lower himself or herself into the chair. Be sure to place the cane out of the way but within reach.	31. The cane provides additional support as client lowers himself or herself into the chair.
32. Set realistic goals and opportunities for progressive ambulation using a cane.	32. Walking with a cane takes practice.

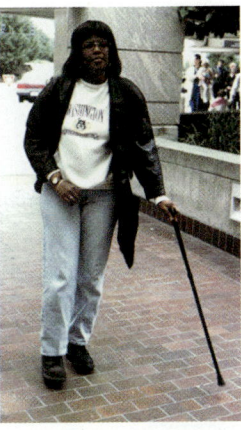

FIGURE 36-51 **Move the cane and the weaker leg forward.** DELMAR/CENGAGE LEARNING

(Continues)

PROCEDURE 36-9
Assisting with Crutches, Cane, or Walker (Continued)

ACTION	RATIONALE
33. Consult with a physical therapist for clients learning to walk with a cane.	33. The physical therapist is the expert for the health care team on cane-walking techniques.
34. Wash hands/hand hygiene.	34. Reduces the transmission of microorganisms.

WALKING WITH A WALKER

ACTION	RATIONALE
35. Repeat Actions 1–10.	35. See Rationales 1–10.
36. Place the walker in front of the client.	36. Positions the walker for use and allows for stability when the client is standing.
37. Have the client put the nondominant hand on the front bar of the walker or on the handgrip for that hand, whichever is more comfortable. Then, using the dominant hand to push off from the bed and the nondominant hand for stabilization, help the client to an erect position.	37. Uses upper body strength and encourages independence.
38. Have the client transfer hand to the walker handgrips.	38. Allows the client to maintain balance while transferring weight.
39. Be sure the walker is adjusted so the handgrips are just below waist level and the client's arms are slightly bent at the elbow.	39. Provides maximum support from the arms while ambulating.
40. Walk to the side and slightly behind the client, holding the gait belt if needed for stability.	40. Allows the nurse to provide stability or assistance if the client needs it.

Walker Gait

ACTION	RATIONALE
41. Move the walker and the weaker leg forward at the same time (see Figure 36-52). Place as much weight as possible or as allowed on the weaker leg, using the arms for supporting the rest of the weight. Move the strong leg forward, and shift the weight to the strong leg (see Figure 36-53).	41. Provides support for a weak or non–weight-bearing leg by using arm and upper body strength.

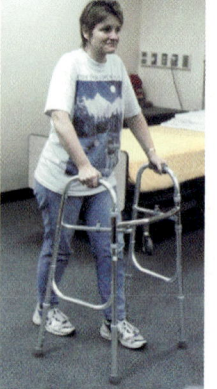

FIGURE 36-52 Move the walker and the weaker leg forward. DELMAR/CENGAGE LEARNING

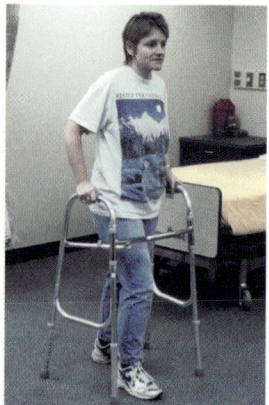

FIGURE 36-53 Use the arms to support the rest of the weight and move the strong leg forward. DELMAR/CENGAGE LEARNING

(Continues)

PROCEDURE 36-9
Assisting with Crutches, Cane, or Walker (Continued)

ACTION	RATIONALE
Sitting with a Walker	
42. Have the client turn around in front of the chair and back up until the back of the legs touch the chair. Have client place hands on the chair armrests, one hand at a time, then lower himself or herself into the chair using the armrests for support.	42. Using the armrests of the chair is a more stable support than using the walker.
43. Set realistic goals and opportunities for progressive ambulation using a walker.	43. Walking with a walker takes practice.
44. Consult with a physical therapist for clients learning to walk with a walker.	44. The physical therapist is the expert for the health care team on walker techniques.
45. Wash hands/hand hygiene.	45. Reduces the transmission of microorganisms.

delegation tip

- *Client ambulation is routinely delegated to ancillary personnel who have received appropriate training.*

- *The initial teaching and the ongoing assessment of proper use of the assistive device are not delegated. The nurse or physical therapist is responsible for observing the client's technique and providing further education as needed.*

nursing tips

Determine client's confidence in ability to use assistive device safely.

KEY CONCEPTS

- The nurse must assess the client's activity and mobility on an ongoing basis during acute hospitalization, rehabilitation, and postdischarge.

- Collaboration between client, family, and members of the interdisciplinary health care team is essential for establishing and modifying goals for activity and mobility.

- Nursing interventions are individualized to maximize client activity, mobility, and independence.

- The nurse should be aware of the home environment and lifestyle of the client.

- The family or caregivers should be included in educational sessions regarding activity and mobility.

- The need for adaptive equipment should be assessed and acquisition of equipment facilitated.

- The client and family should be informed of community resources to maximize activity, mobility, and independence.

- The nurse should be available to assist the client with problem solving after discharge.

REVIEW QUESTIONS

1. Which action should nurses perform to prevent injury when lifting clients?
   a. Keep the client away from the nurse's body.
   b. Lean to one side when lifting with one hand.
   c. Position feet together.
   d. Use legs to lift.

2. Which of the following best explains why the nurse should use a drawsheet when moving a client up in bed with wet linens?
   a. Decrease possible skin shearing
   b. Increase the client's mobility
   c. Keep the bed linens clean
   d. Keep the client's skin dry

3. When assisting a postoperative client to get out of bed the first time, which of the following must the nurse do?
   a. Have the client bend the knees and push up in the bed.
   b. Instruct the client to sit on the side of the bed before standing.
   c. Place the foot of the bed in a high position so it is easier for the client to get out of bed.
   d. Raise all four side rails to assist the client in getting into a seated position.

4. In order to flex the clients' fingers during range-of-motion (ROM) exercises, which of the following should the nurse instruct the client to do?
   a. Straighten the fingers.
   b. Bring the wrist up toward the elbow.
   c. Make a fist.
   d. Gently shake the wrist downward.

5. Which action by the nurse demonstrates inappropriate body mechanics?
   a. Bending from the waist when making a bed
   b. Flexing the knees when lifting an object from the floor
   c. Holding heavy equipment close to the body when walking
   d. Placing the feet apart when transferring a client

6. A client will be ambulating for the first time since surgery. Which of the following should the nurse consider when assisting the client?

   a. Clients who are fearful of walking should be told to look at their feet when walking to ensure correct positioning.
   b. Clients who can lift their legs only 1 to 2 inches off the bed do not have sufficient muscle power to permit walking.
   c. If a client begins to fall, the nurse should slide the client down his or her own body to the floor.
   d. Nurses should have a physical therapist present when ambulating a client for the first time.

7. A client has been bedridden for 5 days. The nurse will expect the client to exhibit which of the following?
   a. Eupnea
   b. High energy level
   c. Hunger
   d. Pressure ulcers

8. Which of the following positions is most likely to contribute to the development of a pressure ulcer in the sacral area?
   a. Fowler's position
   b. Lateral position
   c. Prone position
   d. Sims' position

9. To prevent the formation of pressure ulcers, the bottom sheet on the client's bed should be _____.
   a. changed every day
   b. covered by a drawsheet
   c. kept free of wrinkles
   d. made with mitered corners

10. The nurse is caring for a client who has weakness of the right arm and leg following a cerebrovascular accident (stroke). When setting up the client's hygiene supplies, where should the nurse place the items?
    a. On the bedside table in front of the client
    b. On the client's lap
    c. Within the client's reach on his left side
    d. Within the client's reach on his right side

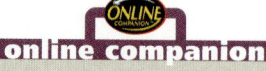

online companion

Visit the DeLaune and Ladner online companion resource at **www.delmar.cengage.com** for additional content and study aids. Click on Online Companions, then select the Nursing discipline.

"In dwelling upon the vital importance of sound observation, it must never be lost sight of what observation is for. It is not for the sake of piling up miscellaneous information or curious facts, but for the sake of saving life and increasing health and comfort."

—Nightingale (in Skretkowicz, 1992)

CHAPTER 37

Skin Integrity and Wound Healing

COMPETENCIES

1. Describe the normal process of tissue healing.
2. Differentiate between primary, secondary, and tertiary wound healing.
3. Discuss factors that may impair or promote wound healing.
4. Discuss common complications of wound healing.
5. Discuss the risk factors and pathogenesis of pressure ulcers.
6. Identify preventive and early treatment measures in clients at risk for pressure ulcer development.
7. Utilize the nursing process for a client with impaired skin integrity by:
   a. Identifying appropriate assessment data
   b. Formulating relevant nursing diagnoses
   c. Developing a plan of care and identifying outcome criteria
   d. Implementing appropriate nursing interventions
   e. Evaluating a plan of care according to outcome criteria
8. Describe the principles of wound assessment and care.
9. Outline dressing products used to treat wounds.
10. Discuss the therapeutic uses of heat and cold therapy and their methods of application.

angiogenesis

black wounds

blanching

clean wounds

clean-contaminated wounds

closed suction drainage systems

collagen

contaminated wounds

debridement

dehiscence

dirty and infected wounds

epithelialization

eschar

evisceration

exudate

friction

full-thickness

hematoma

hemorrhage

hemorrhagic exudate

hemostasis

homeostasis

inflammation

intentional wounds

ischemia

partial-thickness

penrose drains

phagocytosis

pressure ulcer

primary intention healing

purulent exudate

pyogenic bacteria

red wounds

secondary intention healing

serous exudate

shearing

sloughing

superficial

suppuration

sutures

tertiary intention healing

unintentional wounds

vasoconstriction

vasodilation

wound

yellow wounds

Maintaining skin integrity is a primary responsibility of nursing personnel. Impaired skin integrity, such as wounds, may occur as a result of trauma or surgery. The potential for skin breakdown and eventual pressure ulcer formation also exists whenever factors such as prolonged pressure, constant irritation of the skin, and immobility are present. Nurses, through constant and timely observations and interventions, can prevent or minimize skin breakdown. Prevention, early intervention, and treatment programs are essential strategies to decrease the prevalence of pressure ulcers and pain related to inflammation and infection.

WOUNDS

The skin is the body's largest organ and is the primary defense against infection. The body's complex physiological processes promote skin and wound healing, restoring the function and structure of the skin. A disruption in the integrity of body tissue is called a wound.

PHYSIOLOGY OF WOUND HEALING

When an injury is sustained, a complex set of responses is set in motion, and the body begins a three-phase process of wound healing: defensive (hemostasis and inflammatory), reconstructive (proliferative), and maturation. The wound healing process is also defined as having four main phases. When this occurs, the defensive phase is considered two separate phases: hemostasis and inflammation. Regardless of how the healing process is defined, these phases overlap and can take months or years to complete. Understanding these physiological responses will assist the nurse in caring for clients with impaired skin integrity and promoting optimal wound healing.

Defensive (Hemostasis and Inflammatory) Phase

The defensive phase occurs immediately after injury and lasts about 3 to 4 days. The major events that occur in this phase are hemostasis and inflammation. Hemostasis, or cessation of bleeding, occurs by vasoconstriction of large blood vessels in the affected area. Platelets, activated by the injury, aggregate to form a platelet plug and stop the bleeding. Activation of the clotting cascade results in the eventual formation of fibrin and a fibrinous meshwork, which further entraps platelets and other cells. The result is fibrin clot formation, which provides initial wound closure, prevents excessive loss of blood and body fluids, and inhibits contamination of the wound by microorganisms.

Inflammation is the body's defensive adaptation to tissue injury and involves both vascular and cellular responses. During the vascular response, tissue injury and activation of plasma protein systems stimulate the release of various chemical mediators, such as histamine (from mast cells), serotonin (from platelets), complement, and kinins. These vasoactive substances cause blood vessels to dilate and become more permeable, resulting in increased blood flow and leakage of serous fluid into the surrounding tissues. The increased blood supply carries nutrients and oxygen, which are essential for wound healing, and transports leukocytes to the area to participate in phagocytosis, or the envelopment and disposal of microorganisms. The increased blood supply also removes the "debris of battle," which includes dead cells, bacteria, and exudate, or material and cells discharged from blood vessels. The area is red, edematous, and warm to touch, and it has varying amounts of exudate as a result.

During the cellular response, leukocytes move out of the blood vessel into the interstitial space. Neutrophils are the first cells to arrive at the injured site and begin phagocytosis.

They subsequently die and are replaced by macrophages, which arise from blood monocytes. Macrophages perform the same function as neutrophils but remain for a longer time. In addition to being the primary phagocyte of debridement, macrophages are important cells in wound healing because they secrete several factors, including fibroblast activating factor (FAF) and angiogenesis factor (AGF). FAF attracts fibroblasts, which form collagen or collagen precursors. AGF stimulates the formation of new blood vessels. The development of this new microcirculation supports and sustains the wound and the healing process.

Reconstructive (Proliferative) Phase

The reconstructive phase begins on the third or fourth day after injury and lasts 2 to 3 weeks. This phase contains the process of collagen deposition, angiogenesis, granulation tissue development, and wound contraction.

Fibroblasts, normally found in connective tissue, migrate into the wound because of various cellular mediators. They are the most important cells in this phase because they synthesize and secrete collagen. **Collagen** is the most abundant protein in the body and is the material of tissue repair. Initially, collagen is gel-like, but within several months it cross-links to form collagen fibrils and adds tensile strength to the wound. As the wound gains strength, the risk of wound separation or rupture is less likely. The wound can resist normal stress such as tension or twisting after 15 to 20 days. During this time, a raised "healing ridge" may be visible under the injury or suture line.

Angiogenesis, the formation of new blood vessels, begins within hours after the injury. The endothelial cells in preexisting vessels begin to produce enzymes that break down the basement membrane. The membrane opens, and new endothelial cells build a new vessel. These capillaries grow across the wound, increasing blood flow, which increases the supply of nutrients and oxygen needed for wound healing.

Repair begins as granulation tissue, or new tissue, grows inward from surrounding healthy connective tissue. Granulation tissue is filled with new capillaries that are fragile and bleed easily, thus giving the healing area a red, translucent, granular appearance. As granulation tissue is formed, **epithelialization**, or growth of epithelial tissue, begins. Epithelial cells migrate into the wound from the wound margins. Eventually, the migrating cells contact similar cells that have migrated from the outer edges. Contact stops migration. The cells then begin to differentiate into the various cells that compose the different layers of the epidermis.

Wound contraction is the final step of the reconstructive phase of wound healing. Contraction is noticeable 6 to 12 days after injury and is necessary for closure of all wounds. The edges of the wound are drawn together by the action of myofibroblasts, specialized cells that contain bundles of parallel fibers in their cytoplasm. These myofibroblasts bridge across a wound and then contract to pull the wound closed.

Maturation Phase

Maturation, the final stage of healing, begins about the 21st day and may continue for up to 2 years or more, depending on the depth and extent of the wound. During this phase, the scar tissue is remodeled (reshaped or reconstructed by collagen deposition and lysis and debridement of wound edges). Although the scar tissue continues to gain strength, it remains weaker than the tissue it replaces. Capillaries eventually disappear, leaving an avascular scar (a scar that is white because it lacks a blood supply).

Types of Healing

Tissue may heal by one of three methods, which are characterized by the degree of tissue loss. **Primary intention healing** occurs in wounds that have minimal tissue loss and edges that are well approximated (closed). If there are no complications, such as infection, necrosis, or abnormal scar formation, wound healing occurs with minimal granulation tissue and scarring.

Secondary intention healing is seen in wounds with extensive tissue loss and wounds in which the edges cannot be approximated. The wound is left open, and granulation tissue gradually fills in the deficit. Repair time is longer, tissue replacement and scarring are greater, and the susceptibility to infection is increased because of the lack of an epidermal barrier to microorganisms.

Tertiary intention healing, also known as delayed or secondary closure, is indicated when primary closure of a wound is undesirable. Conditions in which healing by tertiary intention may occur include poor circulation or infection. Suturing of the wound is delayed until the problems resolve and more favorable conditions exist for wound healing.

Kinds of Wound Drainage

Chemical mediators released during the inflammatory response cause vascular changes and exudation of fluid and cells from blood vessels into tissues. Exudates may vary in composition but all have similar functions. These functions include:

1. Dilution of toxins produced by bacteria and dying cells
2. Transport of leukocytes and plasma proteins, including antibodies, to the site
3. Transport of bacterial toxins, dead cells, debris, and other products of inflammation away from the site

The nature and amount of exudate vary depending on the tissue involved, the intensity and duration of the inflammation, and the presence of microorganisms.

Serous exudate is composed primarily of serum (the clear portion of blood), is watery in appearance, and has a low protein count. This type of exudate is seen with mild inflammation resulting in minimal capillary permeability changes and minimal protein molecule escape (e.g., seen in blister formation after a burn).

Purulent exudate is also called pus. It generally occurs with severe inflammation accompanied by infection. Purulent exudate is thicker than serous exudate because of the presence of leukocytes (particularly neutrophils), liquefied dead tissue debris, and dead and living bacteria. The process of pus formation is called **suppuration**, and bacteria that produce pus are referred to as **pyogenic bacteria**. Purulent exudates may vary in color (e.g., yellow, green, brown), depending on the causative organism.

Hemorrhagic exudate has a large component of red blood cells (RBCs) due to capillary damage, which allows RBCs to escape. This type of exudate is usually present with severe inflammation. The color of the exudate (bright red versus dark red) reflects whether the bleeding is fresh or old.

Mixed types of exudates may also be seen, depending on the type of wound. For example, a serosanguineous exudate is clear with some blood tinge and is seen with surgical incisions.

FACTORS AFFECTING WOUND HEALING

Wound healing is dependent on multiple influences, both intrinsic and extrinsic. Wounds may fail to heal or may require a longer healing period when unfavorable conditions exist. Factors that may negatively influence healing include age, nutrition, oxygenation, smoking, drug therapy, and diseases such as diabetes. Such factors reduce local blood supply and therefore impair wound healing. Nutrition and diet can also have an impact on the healing process. See Table 37-1

and Table 37-2 (on page 1165) for a summary of factors that affect wound healing.

Hemorrhage

Some bleeding from a wound is normal during and immediately after initial trauma and surgery, but hemostasis usually occurs within a few minutes. **Hemorrhage** (persistent bleeding) is abnormal and may indicate a slipped surgical suture, a dislodged clot, or erosion of a blood vessel. Swelling in the area around the wound or affected body part and the presence of sanguineous drainage from the surgical drain may indicate internal bleeding. Other evidence of bleeding may include the signs and symptoms seen in hypovolemic shock (decreased blood pressure, rapid thready pulse, increased respiratory rate, diaphoresis, restlessness, and cool, clammy skin). A **hematoma**, a localized collection of blood underneath the tissues, may also be seen and appear as a reddish-blue swelling or mass. External hemorrhaging is detected when the surgical dressing becomes saturated with sanguineous drainage. It is also important to assess the linen under the client's wound site because it is possible for blood to seep out from under the sides of the dressing and pool

TABLE 37-1 Factors Affecting Wound Healing

FACTOR	EFFECT
Age	Blood circulation and oxygen delivery to the wound, clotting, inflammatory response, and phagocytosis may be impaired in the very young and in older adults; thus, the risk of infection is greater. Rate of cell growth and epithelialization of open wounds is lower with advancing age, so wound healing is slowed.
Nutrition	A balanced diet with adequate amounts of protein, carbohydrates, fats, vitamins, and minerals is needed to increase the body's resistance to pathogens and to decrease the susceptibility of skin and mucous membranes to infection and trauma. Surgery, severe wounds and infections, stress from burns and trauma, and preexisting nutritional deficits increase nutritional requirements. Malnutrition reduces humoral and cell-mediated factors, leading to immunocompromise, thus impairing wound healing and increasing the risk for infection. Obesity leads to fatty tissue, which has a decreased supply of blood vessels that impairs delivery of nutrients and other elements needed for healing; also, suturing of fatty tissue is more difficult, and complications such as dehiscence or evisceration with subsequent infection may occur.
Oxygenation	Decreased arterial oxygen tension alters the synthesis of collagen and the formation of epithelial cells, causing wounds to heal more slowly. Reduced hemoglobin levels (anemia) decrease oxygen delivery to the tissues and interfere with tissue repair.
Smoking	Functional hemoglobin levels decrease, impairing oxygenation to tissues.
Drug therapy	Steroids reduce the inflammatory response and slow collagen synthesis. Anti-inflammatory drugs suppress protein synthesis, wound contraction, epithelialization, and inflammation. Prolonged antibiotic use, with development of resistant strains of bacteria, may increase the risk of superinfection.
Diabetes mellitus	Small-vessel disease (microvascular changes) can impair tissue perfusion and oxygen delivery. Hemoglobin in poorly controlled diabetes has an increased affinity for oxygen, allowing less to be released to the wound bed. Elevated blood glucose levels impair leukocyte function and phagocytosis. The high-glucose environment is an excellent medium for the growth of bacterial, fungal, and yeast infections.

Adapted from Doughty, D. B. (2007). Wound-healing physiology. In R. A. Bryant & D. P. Nix (Eds.), *Acute and chronic wounds: Current management concepts* (3rd ed.). St. Louis, MO: Mosby Elsevier Health Sciences; and Sussman, C., & Bates-Jensen, B. M. (2005). *Wound care: A collaborative practice manual for physical therapists and nurses* (2nd ed.). Gaithersburg, MD: Lippincott Williams & Wilkins.

under the client. The risk for hemorrhage is greatest during the first 24 to 48 hours after surgery.

Infection

Bacterial wound contamination is one of the most common causes of altered wound healing. A wound can become infected with microorganisms preoperatively, intraoperatively, or postoperatively. During the preoperative period, the wound may become exposed to pathogens because of the manner in which the wound was inflicted, such as in traumatic injuries. Nicks or abrasions created during preoperative shaving may also be a source of pathogens. The risk for intraoperative exposure to pathogens increases when the respiratory, gastrointestinal, genitourinary, and oropharyngeal tracts are opened.

If the amount of bacteria in the wound is sufficient or the client's immune defenses are compromised, clinical infection may result and become apparent 2 to 11 days postoperatively. Infection slows healing by prolonging the inflammatory phase of healing, competing for nutrients, and producing chemicals and enzymes that are damaging to the tissues.

Dehiscence and Evisceration

Wound healing may be disrupted by dehiscence, the partial or complete separation of the wound edges and the layers below the skin. Evisceration occurs when the client's viscera protrude through the disrupted wound. Factors that may predispose a wound to dehiscence include obesity, poor nutrition, problems with suturing, excessive coughing, vomiting, straining, and infection. Wound dehiscence is most likely to occur 4 to 5 days postoperatively, before extensive collagen is deposited in the wound. It may be preceded by sudden straining, such as that associated with coughing, sneezing, or sitting up in bed. Signs of impending dehiscence may include the sensation of "something giving way" and an increased flow of serosanguineous drainage on the wound dressing.

WOUND CLASSIFICATION

Various terms are used to describe and classify wounds. Wounds are usually described based on their etiology, since the treatment for the wound varies depending on the underlying disease process. Wound classification systems describe the cause of the wound, status of skin integrity, extent of tissue damage, cleanliness of the wound, or descriptive qualities of the wound, such as color. Commonly used classification systems follow.

Cause of Wound

- **Intentional wounds** occur during treatment or therapy. These wounds are usually made under aseptic conditions. Examples include surgical incisions and venipunctures.
- **Unintentional wounds** are unanticipated and are often the result of trauma or an accident. These wounds are created in an unsterile environment and therefore pose a greater risk of infection.

TABLE 37-2 Nutrients That Enhance Wound Healing

NUTRIENT	FUNCTION IN WOUND REPAIR
Proteins	
Amino acids	Neovascularization, lymphocyte formation, fibroblast proliferation, collagen synthesis, wound remodeling, and cell-mediated responses (phagocytosis)
Albumin	Osmotic equilibrium control and edema prevention
Carbohydrates	Cellular energy and protein sparing
Fats	Cellular energy, component of cell membrane, and prostaglandin production
Minerals	
Copper	Collagen cross-linking for scar strength
Iron	Collagen synthesis and enhanced leukocytic bacterial activity
Zinc	Cell proliferation and cell membrane stabilization
Vitamins	
A	Collagen synthesis and epithelialization
Pyridoxine, riboflavin, thiamine	Antibody and white blood cell formation; cofactors of enzyme systems
C	Resistance to infection, collagen synthesis, and capillary formation and stabilization
K	Coagulation

Adapted from Doughty, D. B. (2007). Wound-healing physiology. In R. A. Bryant & D. P. Nix (Eds.), *Acute and chronic wounds: Current management concepts* (3rd ed.). St. Louis, MO: Mosby Elsevier Health Sciences; and Sussman, C., & Bates-Jensen, B. M. (2005). *Wound care: A collaborative practice manual for physical therapists and nurses* (2nd ed.). Gaithersburg, MD: Lippincott Williams & Wilkins.

Cleanliness of Wound

This classification system ranks the wound according to its contamination by bacteria and risk for infection (Sussman & Bates-Jensen, 2005).

- **Clean wounds** are intentional wounds that were created under conditions in which no inflammation was encountered, and the respiratory, alimentary, genitourinary, and oropharyngeal tracts were not entered.
- **Clean-contaminated wounds** are intentional wounds that were created by entry into the alimentary, respiratory,

genitourinary, or oropharyngeal tract under controlled conditions.

- **Contaminated wounds** are open, traumatic wounds or intentional wounds in which there was a major break in aseptic technique, spillage from the gastrointestinal tract, or incision into infected urinary or biliary tracts. These wounds have acute nonpurulent inflammation present.
- **Dirty and infected wounds** are traumatic wounds with retained dead tissue or intentional wounds created in situations where purulent drainage was present.

Examples of classification systems that describe wound severity for different wound etiologies are the National Pressure Ulcer Advisory Panel (NPUAP) method, discussed later in this chapter; the Wagner staging system; the partial-thickness and full-thickness skin loss criteria; and Marion Laboratories' red/yellow/black (RYB) color system.

Wagner Ulcer Grade Classification

The Wagner staging system measures the depth and infection in a wound, mainly the dysvascular foot. It is the primary assessment tool used to evaluate diabetic foot ulcers. The classification ranges from 0 to 5, with 0 identifying the predisposing factors that may lead to grades 1 to 3 (superficial ulcer, deep ulcer, abscess osteitis). Grades 4 and 5, respectively, describe gangrene of the forefoot and gangrene of the whole foot.

Classification by Thickness of Skin Loss

The thickness classification system is based on the depth of the wound (see Figure 37-1) and is used for wounds whose etiology is other than pressure wounds, such as skin tears, donor sites, vascular ulcers, surgical wounds, or burns.

Superficial epidermal (first-degree) wounds are confined to the epidermis layer, which comprises the four outermost layers of skin. **Partial-thickness** (first- to second-degree) wounds involve the epidermis and upper dermis, the layer of skin beneath the epidermis. Deep (second-degree) wounds involve the epidermis and deep dermis. **Full-thickness** (third-degree) wounds refer to skin loss that extends through the epidermis and the dermis and into subcutaneous fat and deeper

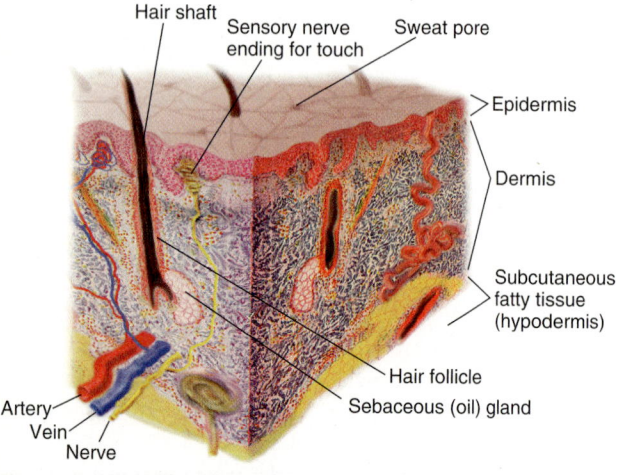

Hair shaft
Sensory nerve ending for touch
Sweat pore
Epidermis
Dermis
Subcutaneous fatty tissue (hypodermis)
Hair follicle
Sebaceous (oil) gland
Artery
Vein
Nerve

FIGURE 37-1 **Structures of the Skin** DELMAR/CENGAGE LEARNING

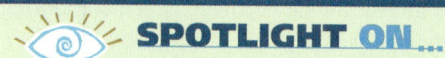

SPOTLIGHT ON...

Legal and Ethical

Impaired Skin Integrity Resulting from Abuse

A woman presents to your clinic with multiple bruises on her breasts, thighs, and abdomen; fresh abrasions on her hands and knees, with gravel mixed in; and two puncture wounds on her left shoulder blade, surrounded by streaks of blue ink. Her injuries are highly suggestive of abuse, especially the puncture wounds, because these could not have been self-inflicted. How do you feel about caring for this client? What are the skin care priorities? What other issues should be addressed with this client once her wounds have been evaluated and any immediate physical needs attended to? What are the procedures for reporting suspected abuse at your clinical agency?

structures. Fourth-degree wounds are deeper than full-thickness loss, extending into the muscle and bone.

Types of wounds are described and illustrated in Figure 37-2 on page 1167, and burns are shown in Figure 37-3 on page 1168.

The RYB Wound Classification System

In 1988, the RYB classification system was introduced for use in conjunction with the other classification systems to assist the nurse in assessing the wound surface color. The three-color system is a tool to direct treatment of open wounds, with each color corresponding to specific therapy needs.

Red wounds are the color of normal granulation tissue and are in the proliferative phase of wound repair. These wounds need to be protected and kept moist and clean. **Yellow wounds** have either fibrinous slough or purulent exudate from bacteria. These wounds need to be cleansed of the purulent exudate, and nonviable slough needs to be removed. **Black wounds** contain necrotic tissue (**eschar**). Eschar may be either black, gray, brown, or tan. These wounds need debridement, which is the removal of nonviable necrotic tissue. Mixed-color wounds often occur. The rule for treatment is to treat the worst color first. For example, a red and black wound would be debrided first, and then moisture and protection would be provided for the red portion.

ASSESSMENT

When it comes to wound care, the nurse is confronted with wounds that are extremely diverse. According to Doughty (2007), accurate assessment of wound healing is a critical component of effective wound management because it drives topical therapy and signals progress or problems in the healing process. The wound may have occurred traumatically just before the client presents to the emergency room, or the

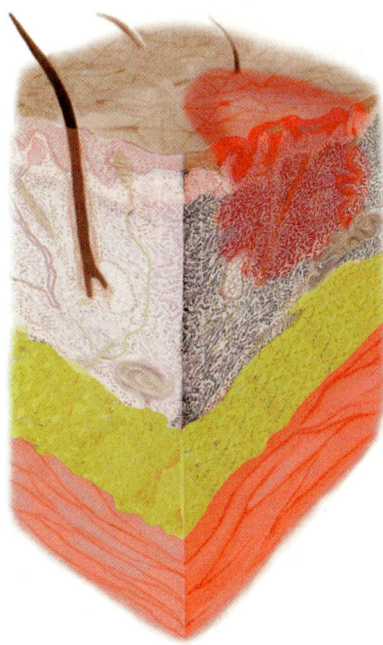

A. **Bruise**, also known as a contusion, results from damage to the soft tissues and blood vessels, which causes bleeding beneath the skin surface. A bruise in a light-skinned individual will change from red to purple to greenish yellow before fading; in a dark-skinned person, the bruise will first look dark red then darker red, brown, or purple, and slowly fade.

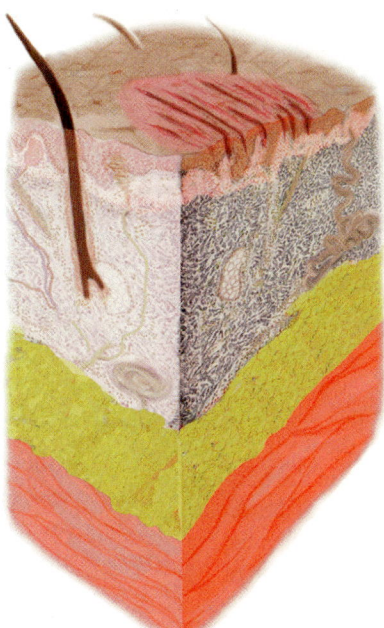

B. **Abrasion**, also known as a scrape or rug burn, results when the outer layer of skin is scraped or rubbed away. Exposure of nerve endings makes this type of wound painful, and the presence of debris from the scraped surface (rug fibers, gravel, sand) makes abrasions highly susceptible to infection.

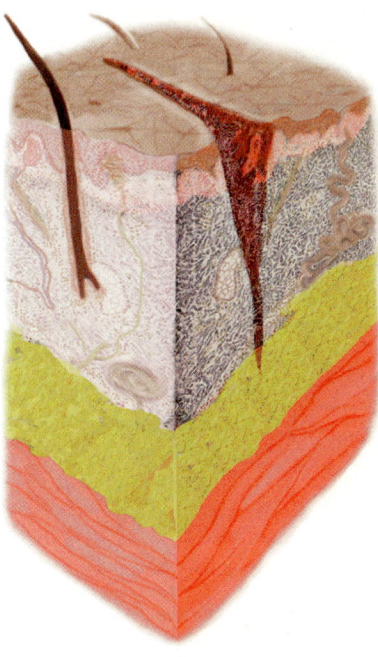

C. **Laceration**, cut, or incision is caused by sharp objects such as knives or glass or from trauma due to a strike from a blunt object that opens the skin, such as a baseball bat. If the wound is deep, the cut may bleed profusely; if nerve endings are exposed, it may also be painful.

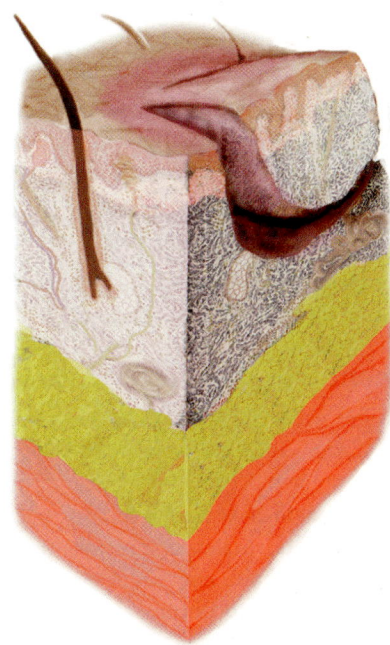

D. **Avulsion** results when the skin or tissue is torn away from the body, either partially or completely. The bleeding and pain will depend on the depth of tissue affected.

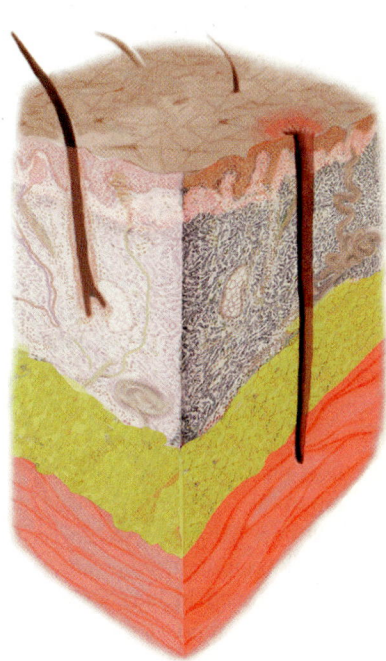

E. **Puncture** results when the skin is pierced by a sharp object such as a pencil, nail, or bullet. If a piece of the object remains in the skin, or if there is little bleeding due to the depth and location of the puncture, infection is likely.

FIGURE 37-2 **Types of Wounds: A.** Bruise; **B.** Abrasion; **C.** Laceration; **D.** Avulsion; **E.** Puncture DELMAR/CENGAGE LEARNING

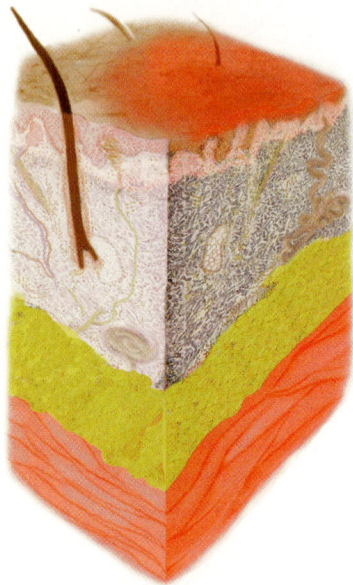

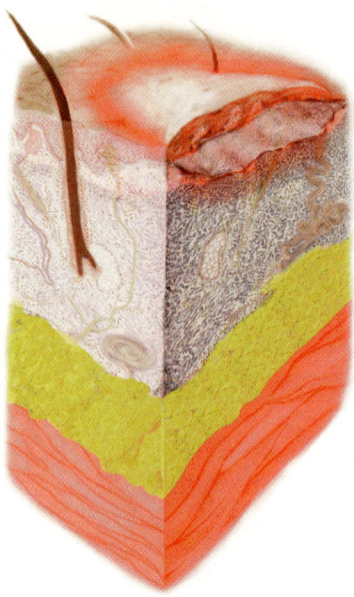

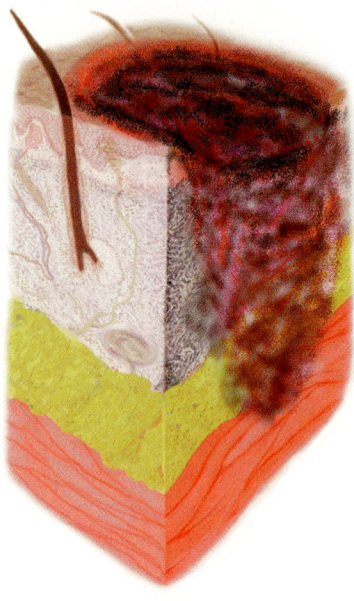

A. **Superficial epidermal** (first-degree burn): Injury to the epidermis; skin is red, dry, and painful.

B. **Deep** (second-degree burn): Injury to the epidermis and upper layers of the dermis; skin is red, is moist or has dry blisters, and is extremely painful; exudate and swelling usually occur.

C. **Full-thickness** (third-degree burn): Injury to the epidermis, dermis, and subcutaneous tissue; skin is dry, pearly white to charred, inelastic, and leathery.

FIGURE 37-3 **Types of Burns** DELMAR/CENGAGE LEARNING

wound may be a slow-healing chronic ulcer. Despite all this diversity, the nurse should approach assessment of the wound in a systematic manner, evaluating the wound's stage in the healing process. The nurse also needs to show sensitivity to the client's pain and tolerance levels during assessment and must always follow Standard Precautions to prevent the transfer of pathogens. Basic criteria for wound assessment follow.

Health History

The health history is conducted to elicit information regarding medical conditions or disease processes that are often associated with delayed or disrupted healing, such as cardiovascular disease, diabetes, renal failure, immunosuppression, gastrointestinal disorders, collagen disorders, malignancy, septic shock, trauma, infection, liver disease, pulmonary disease, musculoskeletal disease, and depression and psychosis. It is important to obtain the data in chronological order: when and how the wound occurred, the initial location and size, and all associated symptoms, such as pain and itching. The history should include aggravating and alleviating factors, such as radiation at the site of the wound, which can influence the healing process. The nurse should document allergies to tape, latex, medications, or other substances. An assessment of the client's nutritional status should evaluate albumin and prealbumin levels, the client's weight trend, and the client's current nutrient intake (Doughty, 2007).

A personal and social history and a functional ability assessment are done to determine the client's ability to provide self-care and to identify support systems present in the home. A risk assessment tool, such as the Braden or Norton scale to assess the risk for pressure ulcers, is a part of the history.

Physical Examination

Although the focus of the assessment will be to accurately describe and/or stage the wound, the physical effects of any existing concurrent condition are evaluated. Three common types of ulcers include:

Vascular ulcers—Evaluate the skin, nails, hair, color, capillary refill, temperature, pulses, edema of the extremity, and hemosiderin (an iron pigment that is a product of RBC hemolysis) in the periulcer area.

Arterial ulcers—Evaluate for weak or absent pulses, thin skin, and lack of hair on the affected extremity.

Neuropathic ulcers—Use the Wagner staging system, previously discussed, to evaluate diabetic ulcers.

Wound Assessment

The following discussion will describe how to assess a wound, documenting location and size and noting length, width, and depth in centimeters. The appearance of the wound bed and surrounding skin is assessed for sinus tracts, undermining, tunneling, exudate, drainage, necrotic tissue, and signs of infection. Some agencies may require a photograph of the wound on admission and documentation of the client's response to therapy.

Location

Assessment begins with a description of the anatomical location of the wound; for example, "5-inch suture line on the right lower quadrant of the abdomen." This task often becomes difficult if the client has multiple wounds close to each other, as is common in burn or multiple-trauma victims. Use of a skin documentation form that incorporates drawings of the body (see Figure 37-4) allows the nurse to draw circles and write numbers to depict the locations of the various wounds.

Size

The length (head to toe), width (side to side), and depth of a wound are measured in centimeters. Single-use measurement guides (tape measures) often come with dressing supplies. To determine the depth of a wound, insert a sterile cotton swab into the deepest point of the wound and mark it at the skin surface level. Then the swab can be measured and the wound depth in centimeters can be documented. Tunneling, also called undermining, can be measured by using a cotton swab to gently probe the wound margins. If tunneling is noted, the location and depth are documented. For clarity in describing the location of the tunneling, refer to the tunnel location using the hands of the clock as a guide, with 12 o'clock pointing at the client's head. Example: "Tunneling occurs at 1 o'clock and its depth is 2 cm."

For extremely irregularly shaped wounds, the wound edges can be traced on a plastic surface. A plastic bag or piece of plastic sheeting folded in half is placed on the wound, and the wound margins are traced. The side of the plastic that has been placed against the skin is cut off and discarded. The rest of the plastic can be placed in the chart.

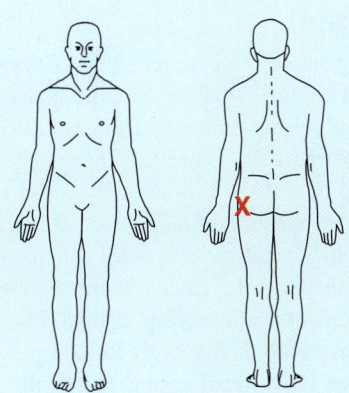

Mark the location of the skin wound, lesions, breakdown, or incision on the above diagram. Describe the character of the wound or lesions below. (If there are multiple wounds, number the areas on figure and provide a description according to the corresponding number.)

X The left trochanter has a stage IV pressure ulcer measuring 4.5 cm X 5.5 cm X 4.6 cm. The wound bed has 20% granulation tissue and 80% loosely attached slough. Undermining is present and extends 3.5 cm from the 2 o'clock to the 6 o'clock position. A large amount of thick, green, foul-smelling exudate is present.

FIGURE 37-4 Documenting the Location and Character of Wounds DELMAR/CENGAGE LEARNING

General Appearance and Drainage

A general description of the color of the wound and surrounding area helps determine the wound's present phase of healing. Gently palpate the edges of the wound for swelling. Document the amount, color, location, odor, and consistency of any drainage.

Nurses who care for the client in the home must demonstrate the need for skilled nursing services by accurately describing all wounds. Document a clear, concise, and accurate picture of the client's wound: size, depth, and location of the wound; nature of drainage; condition and appearance of surrounding skin; and specific individualized instructions for treatment. For example, for Medicare to reimburse for nursing care, the care must be reasonable, be necessary, and reflect a plan of care appropriate for the client's diagnosis, prognosis, and rehabilitative potential.

Pain

Document and notify the prescribing practitioner of any pain or tenderness at the wound site. Pain may indicate infection or bleeding. It is normal to experience pain at the incision site of a surgical wound for approximately 3 days. If there is any sudden increase in pain accompanied by changes in the appearance of the wound, be sure to notify the prescribing practitioner immediately. See Chapter 35 for more information on assessing pain.

Laboratory Data

Cultures of the wound drainage are used to determine the presence of infection and to identify the causative organism. The sensitivity results list the antibiotics that will effectively treat the infection. An elevated white blood cell (WBC) count is indicative of an infectious process. A decreased leukocyte count may indicate that the client is at increased risk for developing an infection related to decreased defense mechanisms. Albumin is a measure of the client's protein reserves; if decreased, there are decreased resources of protein for wound healing. Procedure 37-2 outlines the correct techniques for culturing a wound.

NURSING DIAGNOSES

Nursing diagnoses for clients with wounds focus on prevention of complications and promotion of the healing process through proper wound care and client teaching. The following are NANDA (2009)–approved nursing diagnoses with a partial list of related factors:

1. *Impaired skin integrity* (altered epidermis and/or dermis) related to skeletal prominence; chemical substances; mechanical factors such as shearing forces, pressure, restraint, or physical immobilization; extremes in age; altered nutritional state, such as obesity or emaciation; altered circulation and/or fluid states; alterations in turgor; and medications

2. *Impaired tissue integrity* related to surgical incision; decreased blood flow; immobility; mechanical irritants (pressure, shear, friction); radiation; nutritional deficit

or excess; thermal factors; irritants, including body excretions and secretions; and medications

3. *Risk for infection* related to malnutrition and decreased defense mechanisms

4. *Acute pain* related to inflammation and infection

5. *Disturbed body image* related to changes in body appearance secondary to scars, drains, and removal of body parts

6. *Deficient knowledge* (wound care) related to lack of exposure to information, misinterpretation, and lack of interest in learning (NANDA, 2009)

Nursing diagnoses for clients with wounds must consider the psychosocial aspects of nursing care. Because the skin is a visible organ, variations can cause intense psychological reactions from the client. It is important to remember that in addition to the physical risks of infection and further tissue damage, clients with wounds, pressure ulcers, and burns often have significant psychosocial needs that could benefit from competent nursing attention. *Disturbed body image* is a common reaction to a severe alteration in one's appearance and needs to be managed sensitively and effectively through honest evaluation and prognosis. The nurse may want to encourage a client to look at the wound and learn to accept it as only one part of the body; if that is too upsetting, encourage the client not to look at the wound until it is in more advanced stages of healing.

If *Deficient knowledge* is a primary diagnosis, as is usually the case in first-time wound sufferers, then educating the client about wound care and health promotion is among the nurse's priorities. Make sure the client understands the healing process, the stages of recovery that the wound will go through, and what to expect in terms of pain and regrowth. Encourage the client to follow a healthy diet to provide the body with maximum ammunition for wound repair and to get plenty of rest to allow the body's recuperative elements to do their work.

PLANNING AND OUTCOMES

After identifying the nursing diagnoses, the nurse establishes targeted outcomes for wound healing. When formulating outcomes, the nurse must keep in mind that they should be based on the client's identified needs and should be individualized on the basis of the client's condition. Changes in the health care delivery system have brought about early discharge from the hospital, so clients are often sent home with wounds that need continued care. The *Nursing Outcomes Classification* (NOC) (Moorhead, Johnson, Swanson, & Maas, 2008) addresses two wound healing outcomes in the physiological health (II) domain: Wound Healing: Primary Intention and Wound Healing: Secondary Intention. Wound Healing: Primary Intention ("extent of regeneration of cells and tissues following intentional closure" [Moorhead et al., p. 565]) provides two scales that are used for both Wound Healing outcomes. The first scale (none to extensive) measures the indicators of skin approximation, wound edge approximation, and scar formation. The second scale (extensive to none) is for drainage indicators such as purulent and serosanguineous, surrounding skin (erythema, bruising), periwound edema, skin temperature elevation, and foul wound odor (p. 565).

Wound Healing: Secondary Intention is defined by NOC as the "extent or regeneration of cells and tissues in an open wound" (p. 567); the first set of indicators measures granulation, scar formation, and decreased wound size. The second set of indicators provides for monitoring drainage, surrounding skin erythema, wound inflammation, periwound edema, and other specific wound alterations.

Wound healing is the goal for most clients; however, when wound healing is impossible because of chronic ischemia, malnutrition, or the client's inability to adhere to the treatment regimen, the treatment goal becomes maintenance (e.g., developing an effective system for wound management and transferring responsibility for wound care to the client and caregiver) (Rolstad, Ovington, & Harris, 2007). Based on the client's overall health status and the wound, the nurse should decide with the client and family whether the goal is to promote healing or maintain the wound and the client's comfort. If the client chooses palliative care, then the goal might be to prevent further deterioration of the wound and avoid painful treatments. Ayello and Cuddigan (2004) discuss palliative wound care from the perspective that some palliative care clients may benefit from active treatment to promote healing (e.g., some minimally invasive treatments may reduce wound size, drainage, and pain, thus improving quality of life [p. 13]).

The goals for clients with wounds generally focus on promoting wound healing, preventing infection, and educating the client. An example of a goal for debilitated clients would be demonstrating no signs of infection and preventing pressure to certain skin areas for extended periods of time.

Collaboration

Wound management often requires the collaborative strategies of interdisciplinary teams. Interdisciplinary teams may be composed of a wound ostomy clinician, dietitian, physical therapist, registered nurses, and the client's prescribing practitioner. Doughty (2007) addresses the need for accurately identifying and correcting etiologic factors and working collaboratively with other health team members to ensure appropriate nutrition and glucose control, topical therapy, and management of a nonhealing wound. The challenges in wound care are twofold: the need to incorporate the client and caregiver as active team members and the need to provide both outcomes-oriented and cost-effective care.

In order to achieve client outcomes, each discipline must contribute its unique perspective and knowledge to promote wound healing and prevent wound complications. Nurses must have information regarding their interventions and outcomes to share with other disciplines. The use of NOC and *Nursing Interventions Classification* (NIC) provides for professional nursing language that encourages systemic planning among all of the disciplines.

IMPLEMENTATION

Nursing interventions to promote wound healing and prevent infection include emergency measures to maintain **homeostasis** (state of internal constancy of the body) and cleansing and dressing of the wound. NIC (Bulechek, Butcher,

& Dochterman, 2008) identifies nursing measures regarding the prevention and promotion of wound healing: Skin Care: Donor Site, Skin Care: Graft Site, Skin Care: Topical Treatment, and Skin Surveillance. Wound Healing is the "prevention of wound complications and the promotion of wound healing" (p. 777) and provides for such activities as monitoring the characteristics of the wound, including drainage, color, size, and odor; dressing changes; cleansing the wound; applying an appropriate ointment; referrals; and instruction.

Initiate Emergency Measures

The nurse assesses the type and extent of injury that the client has sustained. If hemorrhage is detected, then sterile dressings and pressure should be applied to stop the bleeding. Standard Precautions are always implemented. The client's vital signs should be monitored frequently and the prescribing practitioner notified immediately.

When dehiscence or evisceration occurs, the client should be instructed to remain quiet and to avoid coughing or straining. The client should be positioned to prevent further stress on the wound. Sterile dressings, such as ABD pads soaked with sterile normal saline, should be used to cover the wound and abdominal contents. This will reduce the risk of bacterial contamination and drying of the viscera. The surgeon should be notified immediately and the client prepared for surgical repair of the area.

Comfort Measures

Depending on the extent of tissue damage, a wound is usually painful. Several nursing measures may be used to minimize discomfort during dressing changes. Tape should be removed by carefully freeing all edges and lifting straight up to prevent stress on sensitive tissue. Position the client to decrease strain on the wound. Administer prescribed analgesics 30 to 60 minutes prior to dressing changes, depending on the drug's time of peak action.

In a large international study, among six symptoms associated with chronic wounds, clients rated pain as the greatest concern. The researchers found that clients with venous, mixed, and arterial leg ulcers reported experiencing more frequent pain during dressing changes than those with other wound types (Price et al., 2008). Sixty-five percent of the participants took some type of analgesic to manage wound-related pain, but 21% reported that it usually was not effective (Price et al., 2008).

Cleanse the Wound

The goal of cleansing the wound is to remove debris and bacteria from the wound bed with as little trauma to the healthy granulation tissue as possible. Choice of cleansing agent depends on the prescribing practitioner as well as agency protocol. It is recommended that isotonic solutions such as normal saline or lactated Ringer's be used to preserve healthy tissue. Much research has been conducted on the proper use of antiseptic solutions in open wounds. The results remain debatable, and continued research is needed to investigate the effects of antiseptic agents on leukocytes and fibroblasts. Studies suggest that some of these antiseptic solutions at dilute concentrations remain bactericidal yet not cytotoxic to healthy fibroblasts.

The major principles to keep in mind when cleansing a wound are:

1. Use Standard Precautions at all times.
2. When using a swab or gauze to cleanse a wound, work from the clean area out toward the dirtier area. For example, when cleaning a surgical incision, start over the incision line, and swab downward from top to bottom. Change the swab and proceed again on either side of the incision, using a new swab each time (see Figure 37-5).
3. When irrigating a wound, warm the solution to room temperature, preferably to body temperature, to prevent lowering of the tissue temperature. Be sure to allow the irrigant to flow from the cleanest area to the contaminated area to avoid spreading pathogens (see Procedure 37-1).

Dressing the Wound

The three purposes of a wound dressing are to:

1. Keep the wound moist and therefore enhance epithelialization
2. Clean the wound or keep it clean
3. Protect the wound from physical trauma or bacterial invasion

Keeping these three purposes in mind, the nurse and prescribing practitioner are confronted with the daunting task of determining the appropriate dressing for the client's wound. Choosing the right dressing depends on the nurse's wound assessment and the characteristics of the wound bed (Baranoski, 2008a, 2008b). In order to make an appropriate dressing choice, the nurse needs to be familiar with the proper use and indications for each dressing category and to select the one that meets the client's wound healing needs (see Table 37-3 on page 1172).

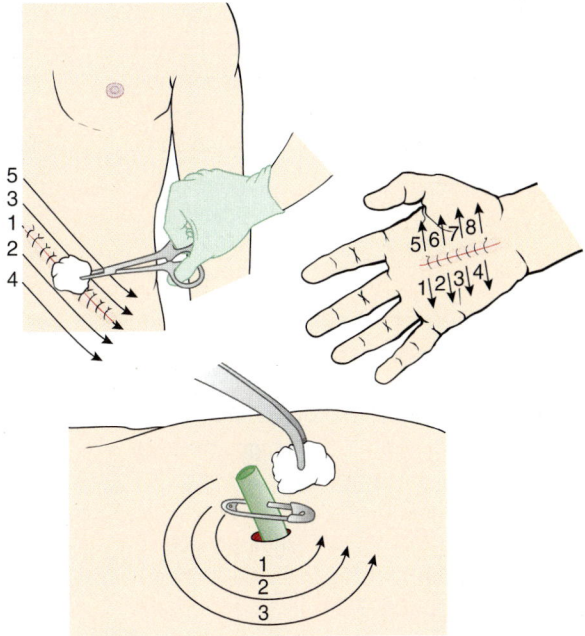

FIGURE 37-5 Cleaning a wound or surgical incision; use a clean sterile swab for each stroke. A. Begin in the center of the wound. **B.** Gently stroke the swab outward, away from the incision line. **C.** Clean around a drain site in a circular motion. DELMAR/CENGAGE LEARNING

TABLE 37-3 Wound Dressing Guidelines

DRESSING TYPE AND EXAMPLES*	INDICATIONS	ADVANTAGES	DISADVANTAGES	TIPS FOR USING
Transparent adhesive films (ACU-Derm, Bioclusive, OpSite, Tegaderm, Transeal, UniFlex, Polyskin)	• Superficial burns, lacerations • Skin donor sites • Pressure ulcers: stage I and some stage II (partial thickness, lightly exuding) • Secondary dressing in certain situations • Dry necrotic wounds that need autolytic debridement	• Impermeable to external fluids and bacteria • Transparent • Conformable • Do not require secondary dressing • Promote autolytic debridement • Reduce surface friction	• Nonabsorptive • Application can be difficult • Cannot be used on wounds with fragile surrounding skin, infected wounds, third-degree burns, or draining wounds	• Allow 1- to 2-inch margin around wound bed • Dressing change schedule varies with wound condition and location
Hydrocolloids (Comfeel, Cutinova Hydro, DuoDERM, IntraSite, Restore, Tegasorb, Hydrocol, Ultec)	• Partial- and full-thickness wounds • Pressure ulcers: stages I–IV • Wounds with necrosis or slough • Wounds with mild to moderate exudate	• Conformable • Impermeable to external bacteria and contaminants • Support autolytic debridement • Minimally to moderately absorptive • Can be used with compression (treatment of venous stasis ulcers) • "Thin" forms diminish friction • Reduce pain	• Not recommended for wounds with heavy exudate, sinus tracts, or infections; full-thickness wounds; or wounds with fragile surrounding skin (check package insert) • Not transparent • May curl or "seep" under edge	• Characteristic odor as well as yellow exudate that looks similar to pus is normal when dressing is removed from wound • Allow 1- to 1½-inch margin of healthy tissue around wound edges • Taping edges will help prevent curling
Collagens (Fibracol, Medifil, particles/gels/pads, skin temp sheets, OASIS)	• Partial- and full-thickness wounds • Pressure ulcers • Stage III and some IV • Dermal ulcers • Donor sites • Surgical wounds	• Comfortable • Absorbent, nonadherent • May be used in combination with topical agents	• Contraindicated: sensitive to bovine and porcine products and third-degree burns • May require rehydration • Not recommended for necrotic wounds	• Requires secondary dressing to secure
Hydrogels (Aquasorb, Carrasyn Hydrogel Wound Dressing, ClearSite, Elasto-Gel, IntraSite Gel, Normlgel, Transorb, Vigilon)	• Stage II–IV ulcers • Wounds with necrosis or slough • Burns and tissue damaged by radiation • Dermal ulcers • Painful wounds	• Soothing, cooling • Fill dead space • Rehydrate dry wound beds • Promote autolytic debridement • Provide minimal to moderate absorption • Conform to wound bed • Can be used when infection is present	• Most require secondary dressing • Not used for heavily exuding wounds • May dry out, then adhere to wound bed (sheet form in particular) • May macerate surrounding skin • Many are nonadherent	• Sheet forms work best on superficial wounds • Dressing change daily • Use skin barrier wipe on surrounding intact skin to decrease risk of maceration • Has variable absorptive properties

(Continues)

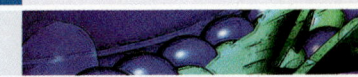

TABLE 37-3 (Continued)

DRESSING TYPE AND EXAMPLES*	INDICATIONS	ADVANTAGES	DISADVANTAGES	TIPS FOR USING
Exudate absorbers (AlgiDERM, Bard Absorption Dressing, Debrisan, DermaSORB Spiral Dressing, Mesalt, Kaltostat, Sorbsan)	• Wounds with moderate to large amounts of exudate • Wounds with combination exudate and necrosis • Wounds that require packing and absorption • Infected, exuding wounds	• Absorb up to 20 times their weight in drainage • Fill dead space • Support debridement in presence of exudate • Easy to apply	• Require secondary dressing • Not recommended for dry or lightly exuding wounds • Can dry wound bed	• Can use gauze pad or transparent film as secondary dressing • Change schedule varies (with type of product used and amount of exudate) from every 8 hours to every 3 to 4 days
Polyurethane foams (Allevyn, Epi-Lock, Hydrasorb, Lyofoam, Mitraflex)	• Stage II–IV ulcers • Secondary dressing for wounds with packing to provide additional absorption • Around draining tubes	• Nonadherent; easy to apply and remove • Conformable; may be used under compression • Manage light to moderate amounts of exudate • Can be used on wounds that have surrounding body hair	• Require secondary dressing, tape, or net to hold in place • Not for use with dry eschar, wounds with no exudate, or wounds with sinus tracts unless package insert so indicates	• Protect intact surrounding skin with skin sealant to prevent maceration • Change schedule varies from 1 to 5 days • Frequency of dressing changes depends on the amount of wound drainage
Alginate (composite of cellulose-like fibers, made from brown seaweed)	• Stages III–IV pressure ulcers • Partial- to full-thickness wounds • Moderate to heavy draining wounds • Dermal wounds • Surgical incisions or dehisced wounds • Sinus tract, tunnel, and cavity wounds • Infected wounds	• Highly absorptive, nonocclusive • Hemostatic properties for minor bleeding • Trauma-free removal • Available in sheets, ropes, and other composite dressings • Can be used on infected wounds	• Contraindicated for dry eschar, third-degree burns, surgical implantation, heavy bleeding • Requires secondary dressing to hold in place	• Forms a soft gel when mixed with wound fluid • Has a distinctive odor noticeable during dressing changes
Nonadherent dressings (Adaptic, Exu-Dry, Sofsorb, Telfa, Vaseline Gauze, Xeroform)	• Skin donor sites • Abrasions, skin tears • Lacerations • Infected wounds, partial- and full-thickness wounds that require packing	• Readily available • Do not adhere • Cover partial- and full-thickness wounds without exudate • Can be used with topical antimicrobials, ointments, or creams	• Limited moisture retention • Require secondary dressing to retain moisture, protect from outside contaminants, and keep in place • May stick to wound if dressing dries out, causing wound damage with removal	• Change schedule varies from 8- to 24-hour intervals

(Continues)

TABLE 37-3 (Continued)

DRESSING TYPE AND EXAMPLES*	INDICATIONS	ADVANTAGES	DISADVANTAGES	TIPS FOR USING
Gauze dressings (numerous products available)	• Exudative wounds • Wounds with dead space, tunneling, or sinus tracts • Wounds with combination exudate or necrotic debris	• Readily available • Can be used with appropriate solutions such as gels, normal saline, or topical antimicrobials to keep wounds moist • Can be used on infected wounds • Effective for packing wounds with tunnels, tracts, or undermining	• Will disrupt wound healing if allowed to dry • Require secondary dressing • Fibers may shed or adhere to wound bed	• Change schedule varies with amount of exudate • Pack loosely into wound; tight packing compromises blood flow and delays wound closure • If too wet, dressing will macerate surrounding skin; protect surrounding skin with moisture barrier ointment or skin sealant as needed

*The products listed are representative of type; this list is not meant to be all-inclusive. Refer to manufacturers' directions for product usage.
Adapted from Baranoski, S. (2008a). Wound & skin care: Choosing a wound dressing, Part I. *Nursing 2008*, 38(1), 60–61. Baranoski, S. (2008b). Wound & skin care: Choosing a wound dressing, Part II. *Nursing 2008*, 38(2), 14–15.

Wounds and ulcers are either granular and partial or full thickness, or stage II; or necrotic and full-thickness, or stages III or IV. Granular wounds that are nondraining usually require one of the following dressings: transparent; hydrocolloid; hydrogel; composite, which is a combination of two or more different products such a foam, hydrocolloid, or hydrogel; growth factor; and moist gauze. For a granular draining wound, one of the following dressings may be used: foam, calcium alginate, hydrocolloid, composite, collagen, and gauze. Necrotic wounds that are nondraining usually require one of the following dressings: transparent, hydrogel, hydrocolloid, and moist gauze. A draining necrotic wound may require one of the following: foam, alginate, collagen, composite, gauze, and contact layer. Besides the different types of dressing, there are other wound products such as lubricating sprays and emollients, which provide moisture to the wound bed and stimulate local circulation, and enzymatic debriders that are used on full-thickness necrotic wounds and infected wounds.

In addition, it is important to remember that the dressing plans must be modified as the wound changes. An excellent guide to help the nurse in the decision-making process is the RYB color code. Procedures 37-3 and 37-4 explain the proper technique for dry sterile dressing and wet-to-damp dressing changes. The properties of the dressing and the wound determine the length of time a dressing is left in place.

Monitor Drainage of Wounds

During the inflammatory response, exudates develop within a wound. When excessive drainage accumulates in the wound bed, tissue healing is delayed. If the outer surface is allowed to heal while the drainage remains entrapped within the wound, infection and abscess formation may occur. To facilitate drainage of any excess fluid, the prescribing practitioner may insert a tube or drain.

When the drain is inserted by the surgeon at the time of surgery, one end of the drain is placed in the operative site and the other end is usually passed through a separate small stab wound near the main incision. Various types of drains exist on the market. Some flexible drains such as **Penrose drains** function by gravity and have an open end that drains onto dressings. **Closed suction drainage systems** commonly have a reservoir that is capable of creating negative pressure or a vacuum. The gentle suction that is created draws exudate from the wound into the reservoir. As fluid enters the reservoir, suction is lost; therefore, the nurse must empty the reservoir when it is half full. Hemovac and Jackson-Pratt drains are examples of closed suction drainage systems (see Figure 37-6 on page 1175).

Nurses are responsible for maintaining the patency of the system and for assessing the amount, type, and color of the drainage. It is important for the nurse to be cautious when changing wound dressings to prevent accidental removal or dislodgement of drains.

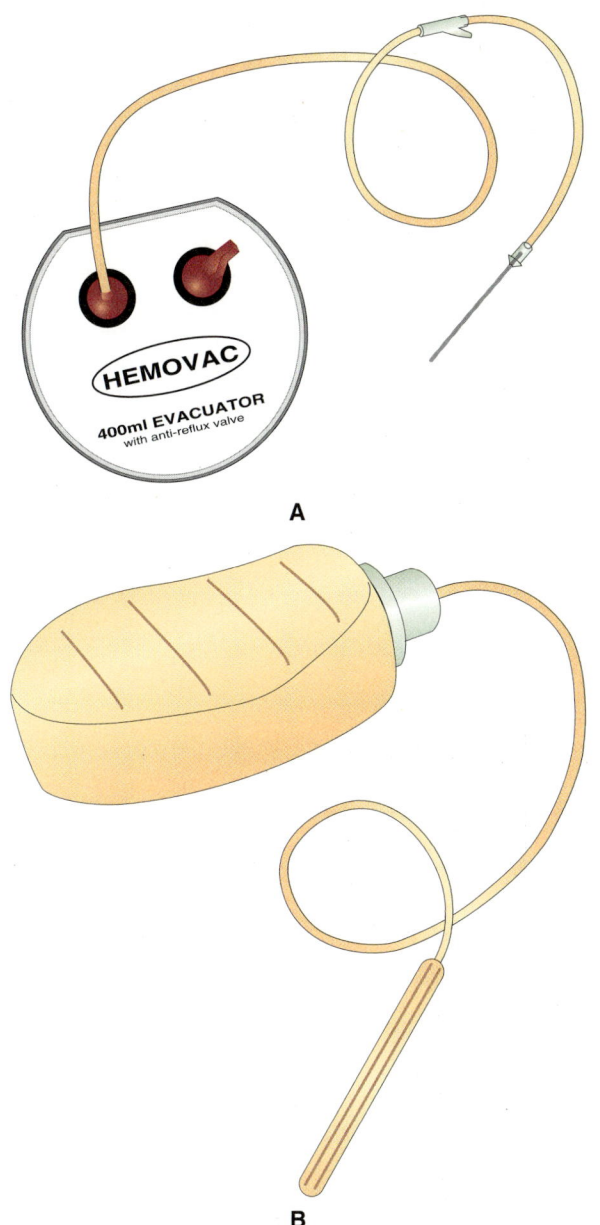

FIGURE 37-6 Drainage Systems: A. Closed System (Hemovac);
B. Tube and Reservoir System (Jackson-Pratt) DELMAR/CENGAGE LEARNING

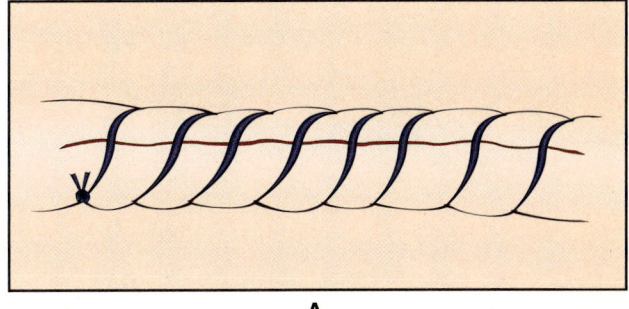

A

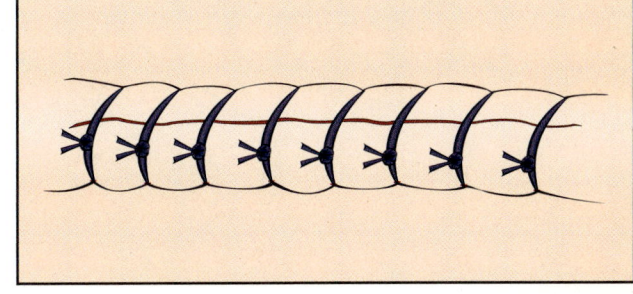

B

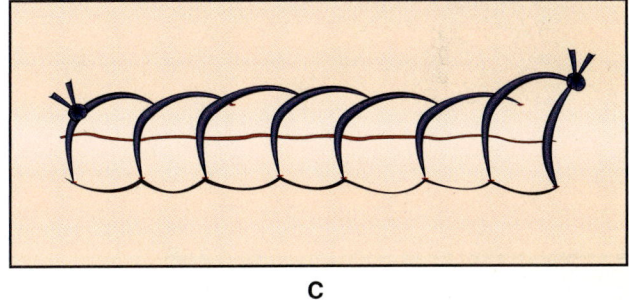

C

FIGURE 37-7 Selected Suturing Methods: A. Continuous;
B. Intermittent; **C.** Blanket Continuous DELMAR/CENGAGE LEARNING

Provide Suture Care

Sutures are a surgical means of closing a wound by sewing, wiring, or stapling the edges of the wound together. When placed deep within the tissue layers, sutures made of absorbable material are used so that the sutures will not need to be removed but rather can dissolve into the tissue. For surface closures, steel staples or sutures made of wire, nylon, cotton, or other materials are used; these need to be removed as the wound heals.

Nurses are often responsible for removing sutures and should therefore be familiar with different suturing methods (see Figure 37-7). Continuous sutures are made with one thread, tied at the beginning and end of the suture line. Intermittent sutures are each tied individually. In blanket continuous sutures,

the single thread is grounded again in the last suture exit. When removing sutures, never pull a suture back through the skin. Sutures beneath tissue are sterile, but those that are visible are considered contaminated, and pulling them through the tissue introduces a risk of infection. Instead, cut the suture as close to the skin as possible on one side, then pull it through the skin from the other side.

To remove staples, the nurse inserts the end tips of the stapler remover under each wire staple. The end tips are placed in the middle of the staple; then the nurse slowly squeezes together the handles of the stapler remover, freeing the staple from the skin.

Checking Bandages, Binders, and Slings

Bandages and binders are applied over wound dressing sites to secure, immobilize, or support a body part; to hold a dressing in place; or to prevent or minimize swelling of a body part. Bandages are long rolls of material, such as gauze, webbing, or muslin, designed to be wrapped around body parts. Figure 37-8 on page 1176 illustrates several different methods of bandaging.

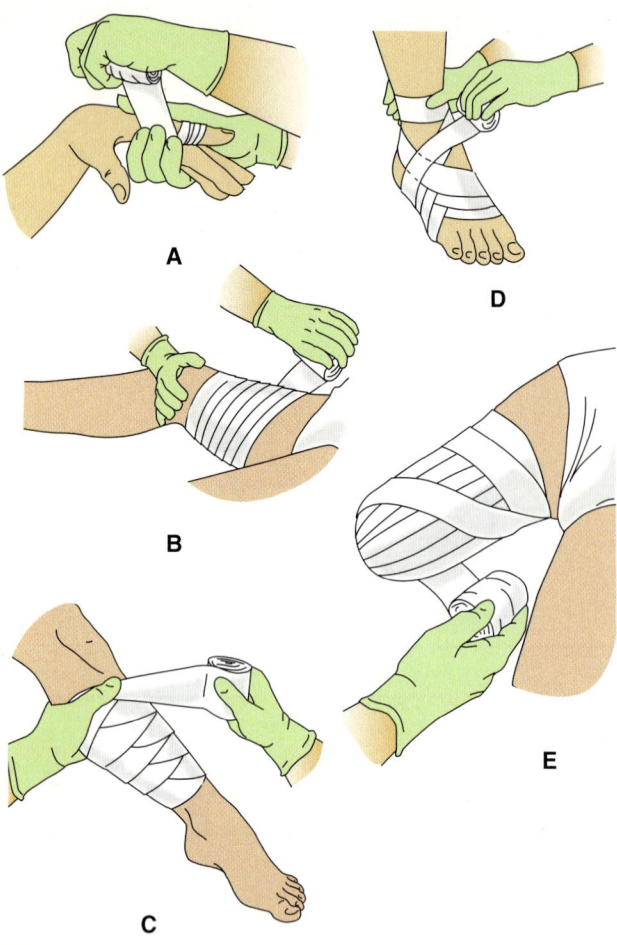

FIGURE 37-8 Common Bandaging Methods: A. Circular turns are wrapped around a body part several times to anchor the bandage or supply support. **B.** Spiral turns begin with two circular turns that anchor the bandage, then proceed up the body part, with each turn covering two-thirds the width of the preceding turn. **C.** Spiral reverse turns begin with a circular turn. Then the bandage is reversed, or twisted, once each turn to accommodate a limb that gets larger as the bandaging progresses. **D.** Figure-eight turns crisscross in the shape of a figure eight and are used on a joint that requires movement. **E.** Recurrent turns are anchored with circular turns and follow a back-and-forth motion, and they are completed with circular turns. They are used to cover a fingertip, head, or amputated stump. DELMAR/CENGAGE LEARNING

CLINICAL APPLICATION

Home Care

Early discharge is one of the latest trends in health care. Clients are often being sent home with wounds that need special dressings. To facilitate an easy transition for the client from the hospital to the home, the nurse begins discharge planning during the admission assessment. At this time, the nurse determines the client's support system and availability to assist as caregivers, the home environment, and resources available to the client. Ongoing assessments provide data for the identification of physical care and home environment needs. At times, a referral for home care nursing is necessary. Common areas for health teaching include:

- Wound care
- Diet therapy
- Medications
- Signs and symptoms of complications of wound healing

Binders are bandages made for specific body parts, usually the abdomen, perineal area, or arm (sling) (see Figure 37-9). Abdominal binders support the abdomen and are used following abdominal surgery or childbirth. Perineal binders, called T binders, are used to hold pads or dressings in the perineal area. Because of the urination and defecation needs of clients, T binders must be changed regularly. A sling is a cloth support for an injured arm that wraps around the back of the neck to maintain the arm in a set position. See the Nursing Checklist on page 1177.

Administer Heat and Cold Therapy

Cells in the hypothalamus act as a thermostat to regulate body temperature. When the hypothalamic thermostat detects that

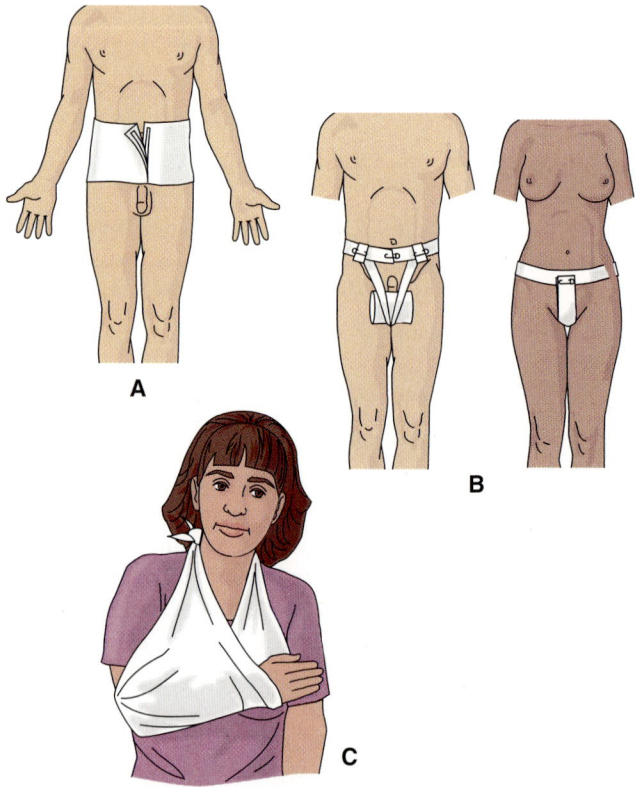

FIGURE 37-9 Common Binders: A. Abdominal; **B.** T Binders: Male and Female; **C.** Arm Sling DELMAR/CENGAGE LEARNING

the body temperature is either too high or too low, it responds systemically by instituting appropriate temperature-decreasing (vasodilation, sweating) or temperature-increasing (vasoconstriction, shivering) mechanisms to restore body temperature to the normal level.

Local responses to heat and cold occur through stimulation of temperature-sensitive receptors in the skin. Impulses travel from the periphery to the hypothalamus and the cerebral cortex. The hypothalamus then initiates heat-producing or heat-reducing reactions of the body. The conscious sensations of temperature are aroused in the cerebral cortex.

Heat and cold receptors adapt to changes in temperature. Upon initial exposure, receptors are strongly stimulated by extremes in temperature, but within a short time, this response declines as the receptors adapt to the new temperature variations. This adaptive ability of the body to temperature variations can be dangerous to clients insensitive to heat and cold extremes and may predispose them to serious injury. Nurses and clients need to understand this adaptive response when applying heat and cold.

Heat is one of the oldest nursing measures used to reduce pain and promote healing. Heat causes **vasodilation** and increases blood flow to the affected area, producing skin redness and warmth. Heat produces maximum vasodilation in 20 to 30 minutes; after this period, reflex vasoconstriction occurs along with tissue congestion. Periodic removal and reapplication of heat will restore vasodilation. Prolonged exposure to heat damages epithelial cells and results in redness, tenderness, and even blister formation.

The application of cold lowers the temperature of the skin and underlying tissues and causes **vasoconstriction**. Vasoconstriction reduces blood flow to the affected area and produces skin pallor or a bluish discoloration and coolness. Maximum vasoconstriction is achieved at 15°C (60°F); at temperatures below 15°C, the vessels begin to dilate. Prolonged exposure to cold results in a reflex vasodilation. Initially the skin is reddened, but later it takes on a bluish-purple, mottled appearance with numbness and pain because of impaired circulation and tissue ischemia. Vasodilation and vasoconstriction of the blood vessels in the skin result primarily from increased sensitivity of the vessels to nerve stimulation but also from a protective reflex response that passes to the spinal cord and then back to the vessels. The therapeutic effects of heat and cold applications are outlined in Table 37-4 on page 1178.

The body's response to the application of heat and cold is influenced by a number of factors. These factors affect tolerance to heat and cold:

- Body part: Certain areas of the skin have a sensitivity to temperature variations. The inner aspect of the wrist and forearm, the neck, and the perineal area are temperature sensitive, while the backs of the hands and the feet are not as sensitive.
- Duration of application: Therapeutic benefits of heat and cold applications are achieved with short periods of exposure to temperature variations. Tolerance increases as the length of exposure increases.
- Area of body exposed: The larger the area exposed to heat and cold, the lower the tolerance to temperature changes.
- Damage to body surface area: Injured skin areas are more sensitive than intact areas to temperature variations.
- Individual tolerance: Tolerance to temperature variations is affected by age and physical condition. The young and older adults are especially susceptible to heat and cold. Neurosensory impairments may interfere with the reception and perception of stimuli, increasing the risk of injury.
- Age: Thinner skin layers in children and older adults increase the risk for burns from heat and cold applications. Older adults have a decreased sensitivity to pain.

The following conditions necessitate precautions in the use of heat and cold applications:

- Neurosensory impairment: Clients with reduced perception of sensory or painful stimuli (e.g., spinal cord injuries) are at an increased risk for tissue injury.
- Impaired mental status: Clients who are confused or unconscious need to be monitored and assessed frequently to ensure safety.
- Impaired circulation: Clients with cardiovascular and peripheral vascular problems or diabetes may not have the ability to dissipate heat through dilation of blood vessels and are at an increased risk for tissue injury.
- Skin and tissue integrity (open wounds, broken skin, scar formation, edema): Subcutaneous tissues are more sensitive to temperature variations than are superficial tissues (e.g., cold can decrease blood flow to an open wound, thereby inhibiting healing).

Heat and cold can be applied in dry and moist forms (see Figure 37-10 on page 1178). The type of wound or injury, location, and presence of drainage or inflammation

✓ NURSING CHECKLIST

Applying Bandages and Binders

When applying bandages and binders:

- Determine which type of support is needed for the wound and dressing.
- Note the appearance and condition of the skin and surrounding area, especially swelling, redness, excessive warmth, exudate, irritation, or uncovered wound areas.
- Ensure that the wound has a fresh sterile dressing before applying a bandage or binder to minimize intrusion and discomfort of the client for unnecessary dressing changes.
- Document the appearance of the skin that will be outside the bandage or binder to monitor changes in circulation, temperature, color, or swelling that occur once the bandage or binder is in place.
- Replace soiled or damp bandages and binders promptly.

TABLE 37-4 Therapeutic Effects of Heat and Cold Applications	
PHYSIOLOGICAL RESPONSES	**THERAPEUTIC BENEFITS**
Heat therapy	
• Promotes vasodilation. • Decreases blood viscosity. • Increases tissue metabolism. • Increases capillary permeability. • Reduces muscle tension.	• Improves blood flow. • Increases delivery of oxygen and nutrients, leukocytes, and antibodies to facilitate the inflammatory process. • Facilitates removal of wastes and toxins. • Produces a local warming effect. • Decreases venous congestion in injured tissues. • Increases absorption of fluid by capillaries and promotes removal of excess fluid from interstitial spaces, thereby reducing edema. • Promotes muscle relaxation and decreases pain from spasm or stiffness.
Cold therapy	
• Promotes vasoconstriction. • Increases blood viscosity. • Decreases tissue metabolism. • Has a local anesthetic effect. • Decreases muscle tension.	• Decreases blood flow to site of injury, thereby decreasing inflammation and edema formation. • Decreases blood flow, facilitating clotting and control of bleeding. • Reduces the tissues' oxygen consumption. • Raises the threshold of pain receptors, thereby decreasing pain.

Delmar/Cengage Learning

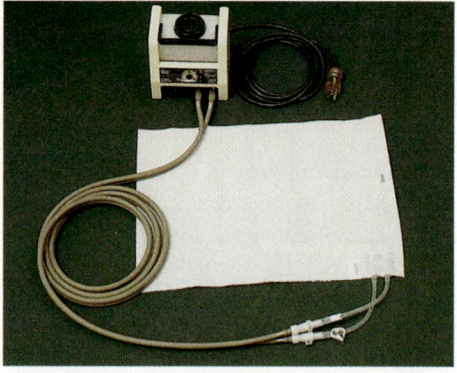

A

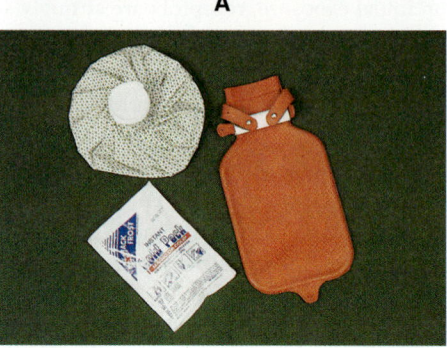

B

FIGURE 37-10 Types of Heat and Cold Applications: **A.** Aquathermal Heating Unit; **B.** Cold Packs DELMAR/CENGAGE LEARNING

maintain skin integrity. Goals for clients with wounds generally focus on wound healing, prevention of infection, and client education. If goals are not achieved, the nurse will need to examine the nursing interventions and strategies that were employed and revise the nursing care plan accordingly. Reviewing techniques and procedures, especially those performed by the client or other caregivers in the client's support system, is especially important.

PRESSURE ULCERS

Pressure ulcer, pressure sore, decubitus ulcer, and bedsore are terms used to describe impaired skin integrity related to mechanical factors such as unrelieved, prolonged pressure; shearing forces; and restraint (NANDA, 2009). The pressure causes **ischemia**, which is a temporary deficiency of blood supply to tissue or an organ. The unrelieved pressure or pressure in combination with shearing and/or friction results in localized damage that causes tissue necrosis when the soft tissue and blood supply are compressed between a bony prominence and an external surface for a prolonged period of time.

Pressure ulcers have plagued the nursing profession for years as a major health care problem in terms of a client's suffering and financial cost and have increased in occurrence by 63% from 1993 to 2003 in hospitalized clients (Wurster, 2007). This increase in occurrence has initiated many actions and regulations by national organizations. The NPUAP (2004) was instrumental in getting the Healthy People

are considered when selecting moist or dry applications. See Table 37-5 on page 1179 for a discussion about the various forms of dry and moist heat and cold, their therapeutic effects, and general guidelines for their application. See the Nursing Checklist on page 1181.

EVALUATION

The nurse needs to evaluate the client's achievement of the goals established during the planning phase to achieve or

TABLE 37-5 Overview of Heat and Cold Applications

DRY HEAT	DRY COLD
Hot water bag • Fill two-thirds full with warm water, and remove air at top so bag is easier to mold over body part. • Cover bag with towel or pillowcase (never apply directly on skin surface). • Keep bag in place 20–30 minutes, then remove. • Do not allow client to lie on hot water bag.	**Ice bag, ice collar** • Fill two-thirds full with crushed ice so bag is easier to mold over body part. • Cover bag with towel or pillowcase, and apply to affected area for 30 minutes. • Provides cold to localized area (e.g., muscle sprain, hematoma) to prevent edema formation, control bleeding, and anesthetize body part.
Hot packs • Commercially prepared, disposable hot packs supply warm dry heat to injured area. • Striking or squeezing the pack releases chemicals that create heat.	**Cold packs** • Commercially prepared single-use ice packs provide cold for designated period of time. • When pack is squeezed or kneaded, an alcohol-based solution is released, creating the cold temperature.
Aquathermia pads • Useful in treating muscle sprains and for areas with mild inflammation or edema. • Unit consists of a waterproof plastic or rubber pad connected by two hoses to an electrical control unit that has a heating element and a motor. The reservoir of the unit is filled two-thirds full with distilled water. • The desired temperature is usually set with a key at 45°C or 113°F for adults. • Cover the pad with a thin cloth or pillowcase prior to application. • Treatment usually continues for 20–30 minutes. • Do not have client lie on pad.	
Electrical heating pads • Provide constant, even heat, are lightweight, and can easily be molded to a body part. • Unit composed of electrical coil enclosed within a waterproof pad covered with cotton or flannel cloth. • Instruct client to avoid using high setting to prevent burns. • Do not insert sharp objects into pad. • Do not allow client to lie directly on the pad because heat will not dissipate and the client may be burned.	

MOIST HEAT	MOIST COLD
Warm compresses (gauze dressing moistened in a prescribed warmed solution) • Applied to improve circulation, relieve edema, and hasten the suppurative process and healing. • For an open wound, use sterile technique. • Solution to moisten gauze can be heated first to 40.5°C (105°F) or according to agency protocol. Procedure is similar to application of a wet-to-dry dressing and the use of a hot water bag or a heating pad to cover the dressing.	**Cold compresses** • Applied to either decrease or prevent bleeding and reduce inflammation. • Procedure similar to that for warm compresses, except cold compresses applied for 20 minutes at a temperature of 15°C (59°F). • Observe for signs and symptoms of burning or numbness, mottling of skin, redness, extreme paleness, or bluish skin discoloration.

(Continues)

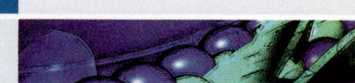

TABLE 37-5 (Continued)

MOIST HEAT	MOIST COLD
• Technique may be clean or sterile. • Remove compress after 20–30 minutes and redress wound.	
Warm soaks • Immersion of body part in warmed solution promotes circulation, decreases edema, increases muscle relaxation, and provides a means to debride wounds and apply medicated solution. • Can also be accomplished by wrapping body parts in dressings and saturating them with warmed solution. • Position client comfortably. Place waterproof pads under area to be treated. • Sterile technique is generally indicated for open wounds, such as a burn. Check agency protocol regarding the temperature of the solution.	**Cold soaks** • Procedure similar to that for warm soaks. • Desired temperature for 20-minute soak is 15°C (59°F). • Take precautions (such as preventing drafts and draping shoulders) to prevent client from chilling.
Sitz bath • Used for clients who have had rectal surgeries, episiotomy during childbirth, painful hemorrhoids, or vaginal inflammation. • Only client's pelvic area is immersed in warm fluid; client sits in a special tub or chair or in a basin placed on toilet seat so legs and feet remain out of water (immersing the entire body causes widespread vasodilation, negating the effect of local heat to perineum or pelvic area). • Water temperature should be from 40°–43°C (105°–110°F). • Duration of bath is usually 15–20 minutes. • Prevent overexposure and chilling by draping a bath blanket over client's shoulders and thighs, and prevent drafts. • Assess client during bath for extensive vasodilation, faintness, dizziness, weakness, increased pulse rate, and pallor.	

Adapted from Lehmann, J. F. (Ed.). (1982). *Therapeutic heat and cold* (3rd ed.). Baltimore, MD: Williams & Wilkins.

Consortium to include an objective that specifically addresses pressure ulcers in the Healthy People 2010 objectives.

The Centers for Medicare and Medicaid Services (CMS, 2008) has instituted ways to reduce or eliminate the occurrence of "never events"; refer to Chapter 29 for a discussion of never events. According to the National Quality Forum, never events are errors in medical care that are clearly identifiable, preventable, and serious in their consequences for clients and that indicate a real problem in the safety and credibility of a health care facility. The CMS has included stage III and IV pressure ulcers acquired after admission to a health care facility as never events.

The Joint Commission (2008) has a broader definition of pressure ulcer that includes decubitus ulcers and any other areas of ulceration associated with pressure such as prosthetic limbs or dental prostheses. Any client experiencing urinary or fecal incontinence, malnutrition, paralysis, or physical deformity is at risk for pressure ulcer development.

PHYSIOLOGY OF PRESSURE ULCERS

The reduction of blood flow causes **blanching** (white color) of the skin when pressure is applied. When pressure is relieved, the skin takes on a brighter color (reactive hyperemia) due to

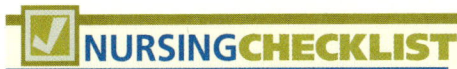

Heat and Cold Applications

General guidelines to follow when using heat and cold applications include:

- Obtain a prescribing practitioner's order that details the site to be treated, the type of therapy, and the frequency and duration of application.
- Select temperature on the basis of client status and agency policy.
- Thoroughly explain procedure and expected benefits to client.
- Assess client's status before, during, and after treatment is performed to prevent injury.
- Document effects of therapy.

vasodilation, the body's normal compensatory response to the absence of blood flow. If this area blanches with fingertip pressure or if the redness disappears within an hour, no tissue damage is anticipated. If, however, the redness persists and no blanching occurs, then tissue damage is present.

Other forces acting in conjunction with pressure contribute to pressure ulcer formation. **Shearing** is the force exerted against the skin when a client is moved or repositioned in bed by being pulled or allowed to slide down in bed. The skin and subcutaneous tissue tend to adhere to the bed surface and remain stationary, while deeper underlying tissues pull away and slide in the direction of movement. This action results in the stretching and tearing of blood vessels, reduced blood flow, and necrosis. Shearing forces account for the high incidence of sacral ulcers.

Friction is the force of two surfaces moving across one another. When a client moves or is pulled up in bed, rubbing of the skin against the sheets creates friction. Friction can remove the superficial layers of the skin, making it more prone to breakdown.

RISK FACTORS FOR PRESSURE ULCERS

Pressure ulcers can be prevented if at-risk individuals and the specific factors placing them at risk can be identified. Many risk factors have been associated with pressure ulcer formation, including immobility and inactivity, incontinence, malnutrition, decreased mental status, diminished sensation, and age-related changes. Validated risk assessment tools such as the Braden scale (Braden, 2001) or the Norton scale (Norton, 1989) can be used to predict who will or will not develop pressure ulcers (see Table 37-6 on page 1182 and Table 37-7 on page 1184).

ASSESSMENT

The Joint Commission (2008) encourages the use of a valid risk assessment tool such as the Braden scale or the Norton scale to be used to identify clients at risk for developing

pressure ulcers upon admission to a facility. All clients admitted to a health care facility should be thoroughly assessed, and the status of any existing pressure ulcers must be clearly documented on admission. The nursing plan of care for clients at risk for pressure ulcers should include skin care; nutritional support; avoidance of skin injury from friction and shearing when repositioning, transferring, and turning; using repositioning devices when appropriate; and maintaining appropriate levels of activity and mobility. The Joint Commission also addresses the need for staff educational programs on the assessment, prevention, and treatment protocols for clients at risk for developing a pressure ulcer.

Pressure ulcers are staged to classify the degree of tissue damage (see Figure 37-11 on page 1184). The revised NPUAP (2007) statement recommends the following staging system:

- **Stage I.** Nonblanchable erythema of intact skin, the heralding lesion of skin ulceration. In individuals with darker skin, discoloration of the skin, warmth, edema, induration, or hardness may also be indicators.
- **Stage II.** Partial-thickness skin loss involving the epidermis, dermis, or both. The ulcer is superficial and presents clinically as an abrasion, a blister, or a shallow crater.
- **Stage III.** Full-thickness skin loss involving damage or necrosis of subcutaneous tissue that may extend down to, but not through, underlying fascia. The ulcer presents clinically as a deep crater with or without undermining of adjacent tissue.
- **Stage IV.** Full-thickness skin loss with extensive destruction, tissue necrosis, or damage to muscle, bone, or supporting structures. Undermining and sinus tracts may also be associated with stage IV pressure ulcers.

When eschar (scab or dry crust that results from death of the skin) is present, it should be described, since accurate staging of the ulcer is not possible until **sloughing** (shedding of dead tissue as a result of skin ulceration) and **debridement** (removal of necrotic tissue to foster the regeneration of healthy tissue) occur (NPUAP, 2007).

NURSING DIAGNOSES

Nursing diagnoses for clients with pressure ulcers will be similar to those for clients with wounds because the type of injury and its consequences are similar. The emphasis is on gentle client care and client teaching to promote healing of the ulcer and to prevent its recurrence. Identifying the client's psychological needs as well, in terms of diagnoses such as *Disturbed body image,* risk for *Social isolation,* alterations in *Self-esteem* related to the body image disturbance, and *Anxiety,* will ensure that the client's symptoms are addressed holistically.

PLANNING AND OUTCOMES

As with nursing diagnoses, the planning and outcomes phase of the nursing process for relieving pressure ulcers is similar to that for clients with wounds. Individualized outcomes based on the client's overall physical condition, the stage of

TABLE 37-6 Braden's Scale for Predicting Pressure Sore Risk

Patient's Name _____ Evaluator's Name _____ Date of Assessment _____

Sensory perception Ability to respond to discomfort	1. Completely limited: Unresponsive to painful stimuli, either because of state of unconsciousness or severe sensory impairment, which limits ability to feel pain over most of body surface.	2. Very limited: Responds only to painful stimuli (but not verbal commands) by opening eyes or flexing extremities. Cannot communicate discomfort verbally, OR has a sensory impairment that limits the ability to feel pain or discomfort over one-half of body surface.	3. Slightly limited: Responds to verbal commands by opening eyes and obeying some commands, but cannot always communicate discomfort or need to be turned, OR has some sensory impairment that limits ability to feel pain or discomfort in one or two extremities.	4. No impairment: Responds to verbal commands by obeying. Can communicate needs accurately. Has no sensory deficit that would limit ability to feel pain or discomfort.		
Moisture Degree to which skin is exposed to moisture	1. Very moist: Skin is kept moist almost constantly by perspiration and urine. Dampness is detected every time patient is moved or turned. Linen must be changed more than one time each shift.	2. Occasionally moist: Skin is frequently, but not always, kept moist; linen must be changed two to three times every 24 hours.	3. Rarely moist: Skin is rarely moist more than three to four times a week, but linen does require changing at that time.	4. Never moist: Perspiration and incontinence are never a problem; linen changed at routine intervals only.		
Activity Degree of physical activity	1. Bedfast: Confined to bed.	2. Chairfast: Ability to walk severely impaired or nonexistent and must be assisted into chair or wheelchair. Is confined to chair or wheelchair when not in bed.	3. Walks occasionally: Walks occasionally during day, but for very short distances, with or without assistance. Spends majority of each shift in bed or chair.	4. Walks frequently: Walks a moderate distance at least once every 1 to 2 hours during waking hours.		
Mobility Ability to change and control body position	1. Completely immobile: Unable to make even slight changes in position without assistance.	2. Very limited: Makes occasional slight changes in position without help but unable to make frequent or significant changes in position independently.	3. Slightly limited: Makes frequent though slight changes in position without assistance but unable to make major changes in or maintain position independently.	4. No limitations: Makes major and frequent changes in position without assistance.		

(Continues)

TABLE 37-6 (Continued)

	1. Very poor:	2. Probably inadequate:	3. Adequate:	4. Excellent:
Nutrition Usual food intake pattern	Never eats a complete meal. Rarely eats more than one-third of any food offered. Intake of protein is negligible. Takes even fluids poorly. Does not take a liquid dietary supplement, OR is NPO and/or maintained on clear liquids or IV for more than 5 days.	Rarely eats a complete meal and generally eats only about one-half of any food offered. Protein intake is poor. Occasionally will take a liquid dietary supplement, OR receiving less than optimum amount of liquid diet or tube feeding.	Eats over half of most meals. Eats moderate amount of protein source one to two times daily. Occasionally will refuse a meal. Will usually take a dietary supplement if offered, OR is on a tube feeding or TPN regimen that probably meets most nutritional needs.	Eats most of every meal. Never refuses a meal. Frequently eats between meals. Does not require a dietary supplementation.
	1. Problem:	2. Potential problem:	3. No apparent problem:	
Friction and shear	Requires moderate to maximum assistance in moving. Complete lifting without sliding against sheets is impossible. Frequently slides down in bed or chair, requiring frequent repositioning with maximum assistance. Either spasticity, contracture, or agitation leads to almost constant friction.	Moves feebly independently or requires minimum assistance. Skin probably slides against bedsheets or chair to some extent when movement occurs. Maintains relatively good position in chair or bed most of time but occasionally slides down.	Moves in bed and in chair independently and has sufficient muscle strength to lift up completely during move. Maintains good position in bed or chair at all times.	
				Total score

Key: 16, minimum risk; 13–14, moderate risk; 12 or less, high risk; NPO, nothing by mouth; IV, intravenously; TPN, total parenteral nutrition.

Braden, B. J. (1989). Clinical utility of the Braden scale for predicting pressure sore risk. *Decubitus*, 2(3), 44–46, 50–51. Copyright 1988 by Barbara Braden and Nancy Bergstrom. Reprinted with permission of the authors.

TABLE 37-7 Norton Scale for Pressure Ulcer Risk

PHYSICAL CONDITION		MENTAL CONDITION		ACTIVITY		MOBILITY		INCONTINENT		TOTAL SCORE
Good	4	Alert	4	Ambulant	4	Full	4	Not	4	
Fair	3	Apathetic	3	Walk/help	3	Slightly limited	3	Occasional	3	
Poor	2	Confused	2	Chairbound	2	Very limited	2	Usually/urine	2	
Very bad	1	Stupor	1	Bed	1	Immobile	1	Doubly	1	
Date										

Adapted from Norton, D., McLaren, R., & Exton-Smith, A. N. (1962). *An investigation of geriatric nursing problems in hospital.* London: National Corporation for the Care of Old People (now the Centre for Policy on Aging).

the wound, and the client's risk factors will help in identifying priority interventions. The outcomes as defined by NOC, previously addressed in the section on wounds, provide indicators that measure size and wound edge approximations, granulation, scar formation, and decreased wound size. Client teaching should be included as an integral part of the planning process; if the client desires, family and support persons should be brought into the learning circle as well.

IMPLEMENTATION

Pressure ulcers can be prevented through a variety of measures. Early identification of high-risk individuals and contributing risk factors and an ongoing assessment of risk factors and skin integrity should be done to decrease the possibility of pressure ulcer formation. NIC (Bulechek et al., 2008) identifies the following nursing measures regarding prevention and

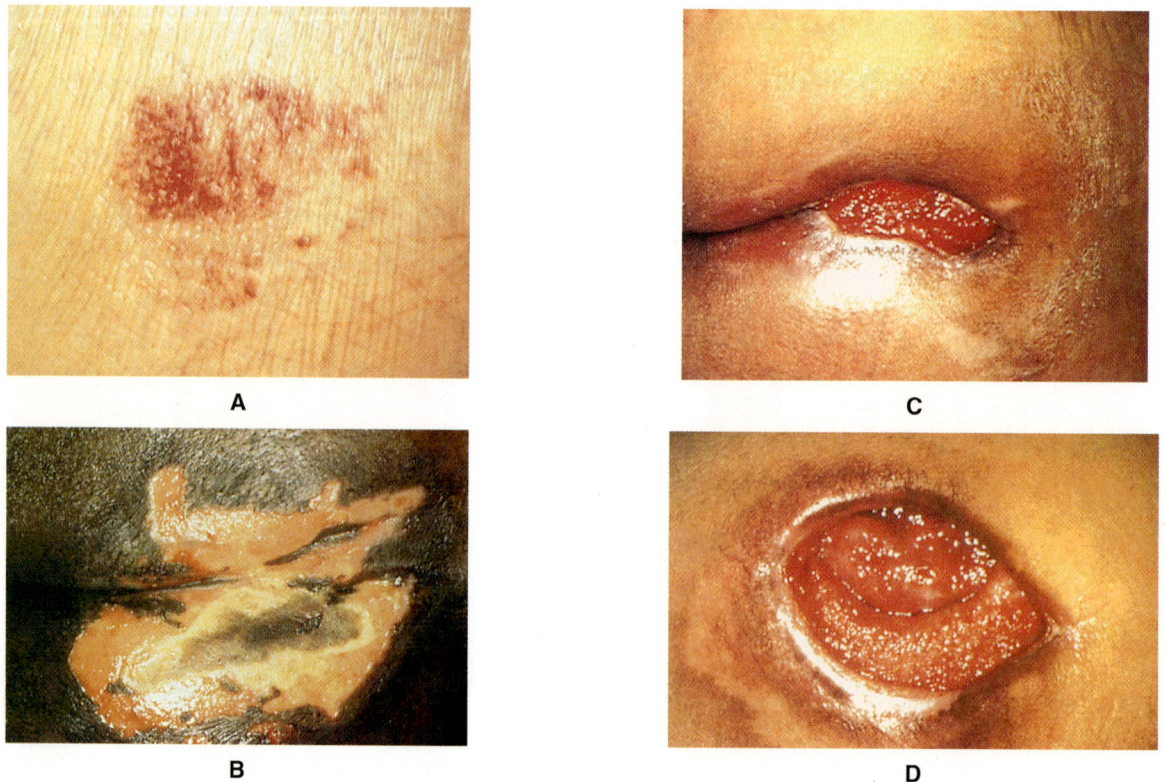

A **B** **C** **D**

FIGURE 37-11 Four Stages of Pressure Ulcers: A. Stage I; **B.** Stage II; **C.** Stage III; **D.** Stage IV PERMISSION TO REPRODUCE THIS COPYRIGHTED MATERIAL HAS BEEN GRANTED BY THE OWNER, HOLLISTER INCORPORATED.

pressure management and care: Pressure Ulcer Prevention, Pressure Management, and Pressure Ulcer Care. Nursing care is focused on preventive measures, such as the application of protective barriers, repositioning and monitoring pressure points, and monitoring the client's nutritional and circulatory status. The management and care of pressure ulcers require many of the aforementioned preventive activities, in addition to keeping the ulcer clean and moist to promote healing and teaching the caregiver wound care procedures.

Other areas to focus on in the prevention of pressure ulcers include nutritional status, hygiene and skin care, positioning, and the use of support surface therapy. The following interventions may be used as guidelines by the nurse in caring for adult clients at risk for pressure ulcer development. They are based on recommendations developed by the Agency for Health Care Policy and Research (AHCPR, 1996).

Monitor Nutritional Status

The nurse should monitor the nutritional status of clients at risk for or who have a pressure ulcer. Nutrients provide the needed substrates for the tissue metabolism that is necessary for healing. Adequate nutrition helps decrease the incidence of pressure ulcers and contributes to the healing process. Clients with a pressure ulcer should have a total caloric intake of at least 30–35 calories/kg/day and a protein intake of 1.25–1.5 g/kg/day, or enough to maintain a positive nitrogen balance; a client with a draining ulcer may require as much as 2.5 g/kg/day of protein (Schmidt, 2002). Fluid intake must be adequate, at a minimum of 30–35 mL/kg/day, with water being the main fluid.

Other recommended nutrients include an intake of vitamin C at 60–120 mg/kg/day and zinc at 12–15 mg/kg/day if the client is deficient in this mineral (Makelbust & Sieggreen, 2001). Zinc must be used with caution. If given in large doses, it can be toxic; also, it should not be taken longer than 2 to 3 weeks. See Chapters 33 and 34 for a complete discussion of fluid and electrolytes and nutrition.

Ensure Proper Hygiene and Skin Care

Proper skin care is essential to preventing skin breakdown. To maintain and improve tissue tolerance to pressure, the nurse should perform the following interventions:

- Assess the skin at least once a day, paying particular attention to bony prominences.
- Cleanse the skin at routine intervals and at time of soiling. Keep the client's skin clean, dry, and free of irritation and maceration by urine, feces, and sweat. A moisture-barrier cream can also be applied to the perineal area to protect the skin from moisture and toxins from urine and stool.
- Use warm water and mild cleansing agents so as not to irritate and dry the skin. Avoid the use of soaps and alcohol-based lotions, which may cause drying and leave an alkaline residue that discourages normal skin bacteria, leading to growth of opportunistic bacteria. Minimize the force and friction applied to the skin during cleansing so as not to disrupt the "natural barrier" to the skin.

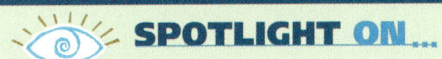

SPOTLIGHT ON...

Caring and Compassion

Caring for Clients with Pressure Ulcers

Advanced-stage pressure ulcers can have extensive necrotic tissue, significant drainage, and a very strong odor. Have you ever seen skin in an advanced stage of tissue deterioration? How would you feel about caring for a client with a stage IV pressure ulcer? Would your opinion be different if the client were an 8-year-old comatose child or an 80-year-old bedridden client?

- If the skin is dry, use moisturizing lotions and minimize exposure to cold and low humidity, which can cause dryness of the skin.
- Avoid massage over bony prominences. Current evidence suggests that massage may be harmful and cause deep tissue trauma (Makelbust & Sieggreen, 2001; U.S. Department of Health and Human Services, 1992).

Debridement

Nursing care for pressure ulcers requires cleansing, debriding, and dressing the wound (see Table 37-3 for wound dressing guidelines). In order to properly assess and stage a wound, the wound must be clean. Wounds that are covered with necrosis or foreign debris prohibiting visual inspection and identification of tissue depth involvement cannot be staged. The AHCPR guidelines do not recommend the debridement of a dry, stable eschar ulcer on the heel without signs of edema, erythema, fluctuance (fluid wave), or drainage because the eschar serves as a natural barrier to infection. Necrotic ulcers on the heel or toe should be wrapped in a soft dressing material to prevent trauma and monitored for signs of infection.

Baranoski and Thimsen (2003) describe eschar as brown to black tissue that covers a wound that may be loose, firmly adherent, hard, soft, or boggy. Wounds deprived of moisture will have eschar that is hard and firmly adhered to the wound bed. Slough is described as a "soft, moist avascular (devitalized) tissue that may be white, yellow-tan, or green [and] may be loose or firmly adherent to the wound base" (Baranoski & Thimsen, 2003, p. 8).

In healthy individuals the body's natural defenses keep a wound debrided; however, in malnourished clients or clients who have medical conditions, such as diabetes, or certain types of wounds, such as pressure ulcers, the accumulation of necrotic tissue cannot keep pace with the body's natural debridement process (Ayello, Cuddigan, & Kerstein, 2002). Debridement is essential to wound healing because necrotic tissue retards healing and is a medium for bacterial growth; removing the necrotic tissue restores circulation to the wound. Failure to remove necrotic tissue from a large open wound causes loss of large amounts of protein and places the client at risk for osteomyelitis, generalized infection, septicemia, and death.

In Europe, maggots or larval therapy and some newer debridement technologies are being used, but four common debridement methods are used in the United States and Canada: surgical or sharp, mechanical, enzymatic, and autolytic (Ayello et al., 2002); see Table 37-8 for debridement methods. In the absence of a severe infection, the prescribing practitioner has time to consider the most appropriate method of debridement. Primary or initial debridement is based on knowledge of wound characteristics, client characteristics, the debridement method, and the biology of chronic wound healing (Baranoski & Thimsen, 2003). "Maintenance debridement should be repeated until the causative agent of the wound is removed or controlled" (Ayello & Cuddigan, 2004, p. 13).

Provide Proper Positioning

Positioning interventions prevent the adverse effects of pressure, friction, and shear. For most clients, maintaining current activity levels, mobility, and range of motion is sufficient to prevent pressure ulcers. For the immobilized client, the following interventions may help prevent the development of pressure ulcers:

- Turn and reposition the client at least every 1 to 2 hours so ischemic areas can recover. If a reddened area does not blanch when pressed, turn the client more often.
- When positioning, pay attention to body alignment. The position shown in Figure 37-12 relieves pressure on the sacrum and trochanters. There should be a 30° angle between the client's trochanters and the surface of the bed. The hips and knees should be flexed. To maintain this position,

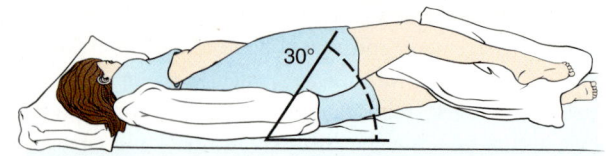

FIGURE 37-12 Avoiding Pressure Points with the 30° Lateral Position DELMAR/CENGAGE LEARNING

support the client's back with a pillow or foam wedge, and put a pillow between the knees.

- When turning the client, remove the pillows and wedges, lower the head of the bed, and use a draw sheet to lift, not drag, the client to a new position. Maintain the head of the bed at 30° or less to prevent shearing.
- If the client is supine, make sure the heels are not resting on the mattress. Suspend them by placing a pillow or foam pad lengthwise under the lower legs.
- Place at-risk clients on pressure-reducing surfaces.
- Have clients who are able to sit up shift their weight every 15 minutes; those who cannot do so need to be repositioned at least every hour.
- Use a pressure-reducing device such as a foam overlay on the seating surface to reduce pressure on the ischial tuberosities by redistributing weight over a much larger surface area. Do not use donut-shaped cushions, which reduce blood supply to the affected area, leading to even more ischemia.

Employ Support Surfaces

Various support surfaces are available to support the entire body and evenly distribute pressure. These devices can be

TABLE 37-8 Debridement Methods

METHOD	DEFINITION
Surgical or sharp debridement	The fastest way to remove dead tissue, used for all levels of bacterial load; first choice in treating worsening cellulitis or wound-related sepsis.
Mechanical debridement	Wet-to-dry dressings, hydrotherapy (whirlpool), and wound irrigation (pulsed lavage); caution should be used when infection is starting to spread.
Enzymatic or chemical debridement	Topical biologic enzyme, such as proteolytics, fibrinolytics, and collagenases, to selectively break down necrotic tissue; can be used in infected wounds but is most effective when used in conjunction with mechanical or surgical debridement.
Autolytic debridement	Enhances the body's own enzymes and moisture to soften and break down necrotic tissue using a semiocclusive or occlusive dressing, such as a transparent or hydrocolloid dressing, to cover the wound; however, it is not a very effective method for removing hard, black necrotic tissue. Used with caution for contaminated, colonized, or critically colonized wounds.

Adapted from Ayello, E., Cuddigan, J., & Kerstein, M. (2002). Skip the knife: Debriding wounds without surgery. *Nursing 2002, 32*(9), 58–64; Ayello, E., & Cuddigan, J. (2004). Conquer chronic wounds with wound bed preparation. *Nurse Practitioner, 29*(3), 8–27.

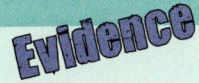

UNCOVERING THE Evidence

TITLE OF STUDY
"Reducing Hospital-Acquired Heel Ulcer Rates in an Acute Care Facility: An Evaluation of a Nurse-Driven Performance Improvement Project"

AUTHORS
M. L. McElhinny and C. Hooper

PURPOSE
To reduce the incidence of hospital-acquired ulcers of the heel in an acute care setting with a nurse-driven performance improvement project.

METHOD
This was a descriptive, evaluative study using secondary data analysis in a 172-bed facility. The prevalence and incidence of heel pressure ulcers were obtained through skin surveys prior to implementation of the prevention program in 2004 and following its implementation in 2006 after introduction of the Braden Scale for Predicting Pressure Sore Risk. Heel pressure ulcers were staged using the National Pressure Ulcer Advisory Panel staging system and recommendations provided by the Agency for Health Care Quality Research clinical practice guidelines.

FINDINGS
The incidence of hospital-acquired heel pressure ulcers in 2004 was 13.5% (4 of 37 clients), compared to 2006, when there was an incidence of hospital-acquired heel pressure ulcers of 13.8% (5 of 36 clients).

IMPLICATIONS
The intervention did not appear to have adequate staff support in the following areas: educational method used; development of organization-approved, evidence-based, standardized protocols for prevention and treatment of heel ulcers; and assistance of facility management in conveying the importance of as well as their support for the project.

McElhinny, M. L., & Hooper, C. (2008). Reducing hospital-acquired ulcer rates in an acute care facility: An evaluation of a nurse-driven performance improvement project. *Journal of Wound Ostomy Continence Nursing, 35*(1), 79–83.

foam, gel, water, or air (e.g., eggcrate mattresses, alternating air-filled mattresses) and replacement mattresses (replace standard mattresses). Pressure-relieving devices include specialty beds that replace hospital beds. Examples are low-air-loss (LAL) beds (e.g., Flexicair), air-fluidized beds (e.g., Clinitron), and beds that provide kinetic therapy. Kinetic beds (e.g., RotoRest) provide continuous passive motion or oscillation to counteract the effects of immobility. See Chapter 36 for a complete discussion of beds used to counteract the effects of immobility. See Table 37-9 on page 1188 for a list of selected support devices.

Complementary Therapies

Nature is rich in plants that promote the healing of cuts, burns, and wounds. Herbalists recognize that skin problems may reflect a variety of internal conditions; therefore, herbs used to treat wounds are selected based on their internal and external actions. Herbs that create the following actions are particularly useful for wound healing: vulneraries (promote healing of wounds and ulcers), alteratives (restore proper bodily function), diaphoretics (promote sweating and capillary dilation), antimicrobials (resist pathogenic microorganisms, usually by strengthening the immune system), and nervines (act on the nervous system as either tonics, relaxants, or stimulants). Some of the vulnerary herbs discussed next also work as astringents (bind to skin and mucous tissue, reduce irritation and inflammation, protect against infections) to arrest bleeding and to condense tissue.

Chickweed, a common garden weed, is a vulnerary and antimicrobial. It may be applied directly to an insect bite to relieve itching and irritation or used as an ointment in combination with marshmallow for cuts and wounds (Tierra & Lust, 2008).

Comfrey contains a chemical, allantoin, that stimulates cell proliferation and promotes wound healing both inside and out. Although it can be used internally to treat gastric and duodenal ulcers, comfrey is often used externally as a compress or poultice to speed the healing of wounds and fractures and reduce scarring. *Caution should be exercised when using comfrey to treat deep wounds, since it can lead to tissue forming over the wound before the wound heals from within, creating a risk for an abscess to form* (Tierra & Lust, 2008). The anticancer action of this herb has been reputed, and the herb should be used with caution in anyone with a family history of cancer.

Aloe vera is a common household plant. The juice from the plant is used externally to treat minor cuts and burns, sunburn, and insect bites. It has been used effectively to decrease the scarring from acne. Aloe is primarily a vulnerary herb that promotes wound healing and has an antimicrobial action. Internally this herb is used as a cathartic and an emmenagogue (normalize and tone the female reproductive system) and *should be used with caution during pregnancy and should be avoided during breastfeeding, since it is excreted in the mother's milk. Caution also should be exercised when taking dieter's teas containing aloe and other substances, as they act as laxatives when consumed in large quantities and*

used as adjunct therapy to help reduce pressure and prevent ulcers, but they are no substitute for frequent positioning, and there is no scientific evidence that any one support surface works consistently better than another.

In addition to pressure reduction or relief, many support surfaces reduce shear and friction and control moisture. Pressure-reducing support surfaces include overlays filled with

TABLE 37-9 Support Surfaces

TYPE	EXAMPLES (MANUFACTURER)	INDICATIONS	ADVANTAGES	DISADVANTAGES
Foam overlay	Biogard (Bio Clinic) Geo-Matt (Span-America) First Wave (Pegasus Airwave)	Pressure reduction, comfort	Low cost, easy to use	Hot; traps moisture; pressure reduction lost with continued use; easily contaminated by body fluids
Static air mattress (air overlay)	Sof-Care (Gaymar Industries) Roho (Roho) First Step (Kinetic Concepts International [KCI])	Pressure relief		Damaged by sharp objects; inflation has to be monitored
Fluid overlay (water mattress)	Medline Water Overlay (Medline) MedRite Water Flotation Mattress (MedRite International)	Pressure reduction, comfort	Easy to clean, multiple-use	Leaks with puncture
Static, low air loss	Flexicair (Support Systems International) Kin Air (KCI) Prime-Air (Hill-Rom) Silk-Air (Hill-Rom)	Pressure relief when repositioning is difficult or contraindicated	Bed adjusts to variety of positions; filter reduces risk of airborne contamination; cushions provide pressure relief	Bed does not absorb fluid
Active, low air loss (oscillating)	Biodyne (KCI) TheraPulse (KCI) TotalCare SpO2RT (Hill-Rom) V-Cue (Hill-Rom)	Clients who are unstable and cannot tolerate sudden changes in position; clients with pneumonia changes to mobilize secretions	Protects skin integrity; promotes removal of pulmonary secretions	Limited motion
Air fluidized	Clinitron (Hill-Rom) Fluid Air (KCI) Rite Hite (Hill-Rom) Clinitron At-Home (Hill-Rom)	Clients who require minimal movement to prevent skin damage by shearing forces; pressure relief	Minimum pressure on bony prominences; fluidization makes turning easy; facilitates drainage and substance in beads reduces risk of infection	Heavy transport difficult; foam backrest provides limited head elevation; drying effect may inhibit cough and may dehydrate
Rotation	Tilt and Turn (SMI Patient Care) RotoRest (KCI)	Clients who require frequent turning but have unstable spines; movement, skeletal stability	Provides skeletal stability; mobilizes secretions; supports traction	Movement increases risk of friction and shearing and may cause motion sickness
Bariatric	Burke (KCI) Barimagnum (Hill-Rom) Total Care Bari Sport (Hill-Rom)	Management of morbidly obese	Supports independence; converts to chair	Not wide enough to facilitate repositioning

Delmar/Cengage Learning

Client with Impaired Skin Integrity

CASE PRESENTATION

Mr. Short is a 48-year-old client who was involved in a motor vehicle accident. Three days after abdominal surgery, he develops fever, tenderness around the incision, and purulent drainage from the wound. The prescribing practitioner opens the incision and orders normal saline wet-to-dry dressing changes three times a day.

ASSESSMENT

- Temperature 38°C or 101.8°F
- Pulse 110
- Respirations 20
- BP 130/70
- Incision—red, tender to touch, yellow, purulent drainage
- Labs—WBC ↑

NURSING DIAGNOSIS: *Impaired skin integrity* related to presence of contaminants
NOC: Wound healing
NIC: Wound care

EXPECTED OUTCOMES

1. Within 1 week the client's wound will be free of infection as evidenced by:
   a. Absence of fever
   b. Absence of redness, exudate
   c. Normal WBC count
2. Within 1–2 weeks the client's wound will exhibit signs of healing as evidenced by:
   a. Presence of granulation tissue
   b. Wound being closed and without drainage

INTERVENTIONS/RATIONALES

1a. Assess and document the wound for presence of redness, pain, and exudate with every dressing change. Exudate indicates infection.
1b. Assess VS q4h. VS reflect client's overall condition.
1c. Assess WBC count. WBC counts show progression of infection.
2a. Apply wet-to-dry dressing changes tid utilizing sterile technique. Promotes clean environment, which encourages wound healing.
2b. Ensure good hand washing before and after all dressing changes. Limits exposure of incision to pathogens.

EVALUATION

The client should be free of infection, with no evidence of fever, redness, or exudate. WBC count and VS should be within normal range within 1 week. The wound should exhibit beefy-red granulation tissue, and the wound's edges should be contracting 1 week after admission.

(Continues)

CONCEPT MAP

THE CLIENT WITH IMPAIRED SKIN INTEGRITY

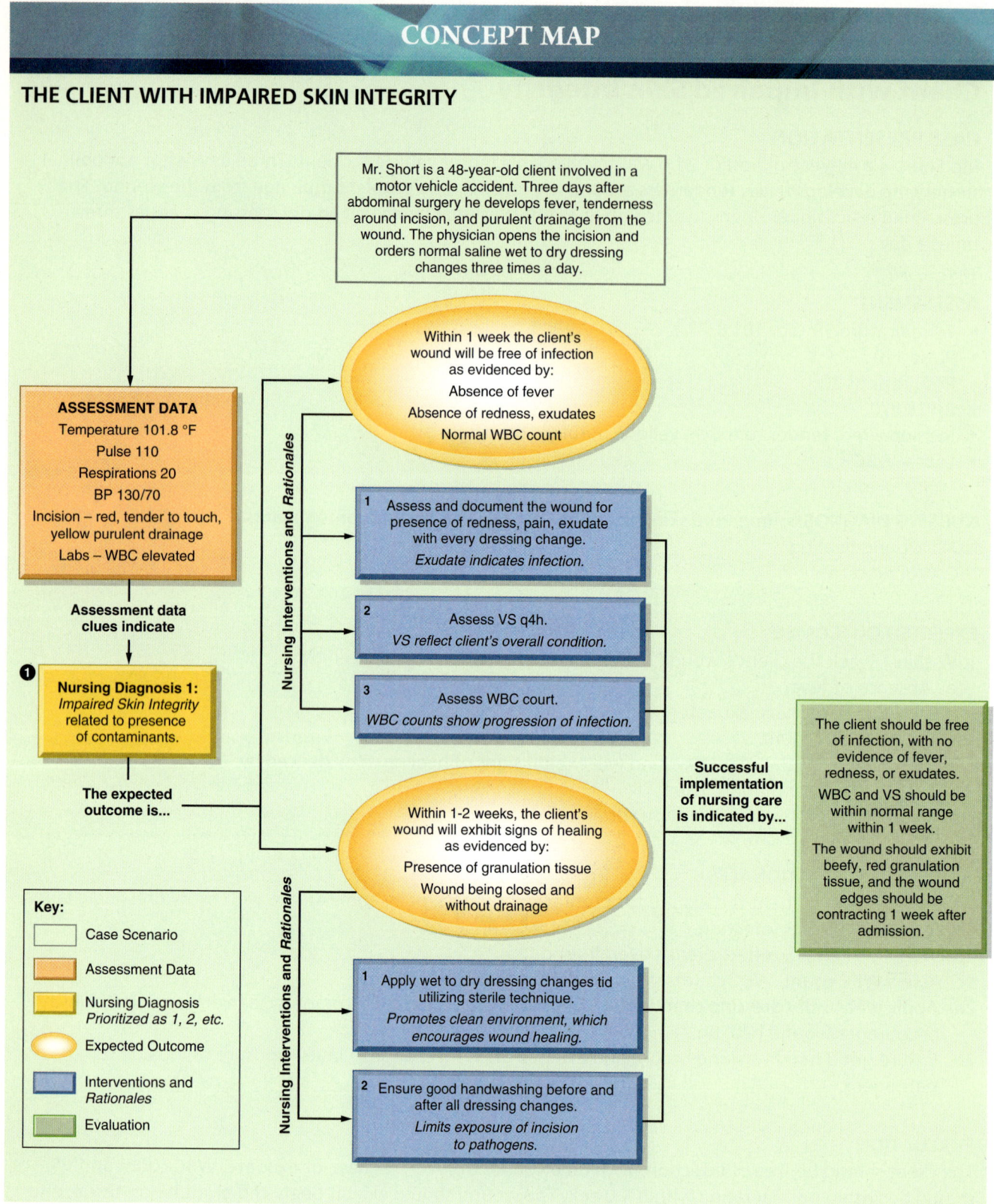

Mr. Short is a 48-year-old client involved in a motor vehicle accident. Three days after abdominal surgery he develops fever, tenderness around incision, and purulent drainage from the wound. The physician opens the incision and orders normal saline wet to dry dressing changes three times a day.

ASSESSMENT DATA
Temperature 101.8 °F
Pulse 110
Respirations 20
BP 130/70
Incision – red, tender to touch, yellow purulent drainage
Labs – WBC elevated

Assessment data clues indicate

❶ Nursing Diagnosis 1:
Impaired Skin Integrity related to presence of contaminants.

The expected outcome is...

Within 1 week the client's wound will be free of infection as evidenced by:
Absence of fever
Absence of redness, exudates
Normal WBC count

Nursing Interventions and Rationales

1 Assess and document the wound for presence of redness, pain, exudate with every dressing change.
Exudate indicates infection.

2 Assess VS q4h.
VS reflect client's overall condition.

3 Assess WBC court.
WBC counts show progression of infection.

Within 1-2 weeks, the client's wound will exhibit signs of healing as evidenced by:
Presence of granulation tissue
Wound being closed and without drainage

Nursing Interventions and Rationales

1 Apply wet to dry dressing changes tid utilizing sterile technique.
Promotes clean environment, which encourages wound healing.

2 Ensure good handwashing before and after all dressing changes.
Limits exposure of incision to pathogens.

Successful implementation of nursing care is indicated by...

The client should be free of infection, with no evidence of fever, redness, or exudates.
WBC and VS should be within normal range within 1 week.
The wound should exhibit beefy, red granulation tissue, and the wound edges should be contracting 1 week after admission.

Key:
Case Scenario
Assessment Data
Nursing Diagnosis *Prioritized as 1, 2, etc.*
Expected Outcome
Interventions and *Rationales*
Evaluation

can disrupt potassium levels and contribute to cardiac arrhythmias (Fontaine, 2000).

Woundwort is a vulnerary, an antiseptic, an antispasmodic, and an astringent used primarily as a wound healer. It is equivalent to comfrey as a wound healer and may be used directly on the wound or as an ointment or a compress (Tierra & Lust, 2008).

Other herbs that may be used to promote wound healing and relieve irritation and pain associated with an ulcer or a wound are tea tree oil, lavender oil, colloid silver, *Echinacea,* golden seal (refer to Chapter 31 for a complete discussion of their antimicrobial action), slippery elm, knitbone, and self-heal.

Although most wounds heal with a well-balanced diet, special attention should be given to the diet when wounds are at risk for infection. Avoid stressor foods such as refined sugars, excess caffeine, and alcoholic beverages because they may decrease the body's immune function and healing. The diet should be rich in essential fatty acids, vitamin A, zinc, and vitamin C to promote the skin's healing. Foods rich in these essential elements are green and yellow vegetables, eggs, cold-water fish, raw seeds and nuts, and oysters.

EVALUATION

Evaluation of the plan of care for a client with a pressure ulcer will consider the physical signs of healing and the status of the pressure ulcer as well as the client's adaptation to the altered skin integrity. Each intervention should be evaluated for its effectiveness and the plan of care revised to reflect those actions that have proven the most beneficial in realizing the expected outcomes of care.

PROCEDURE 37-1

Irrigating a Wound

EQUIPMENT
- Sterile gloves
- Disposable gloves
- Sterile irrigation kit (basin, piston irrigation syringe, solution container)
- Moisture-proof container or bag for use after the irrigation procedure
- Irrigation solution (per health care provider's order)
- Waterproof pad
- Sterile dressing material to redress the wound

ACTION	RATIONALE
1. Confirm the health care provider's order for wound irrigation, and note the type and strength of the ordered irrigation solution.	1. Wound irrigation is a dependent nursing action that requires a medical order stating the type of solution to be used.
2. Assess the client's pain level and medicate if needed with analgesic 30 minutes before procedure if the medication is to be given PO or IM.	2. Allows time for medication to be absorbed to increase the analgesic effect.
3. Explain the procedure to the client. Wash hands/hand hygiene.	3. Helps decrease the client's anxiety and increase the client's cooperation. Prevents the spread of microorganisms.
4. Place a waterproof pad on the bed. Assist the client onto the pad and into a position that will allow the irrigant to flow through the wound and into the basin from the cleanest to dirtiest area of the wound.	4. Positioning of the client and placement of a waterproof pad will decrease contamination of bed linen.
5. Wash hands/hand hygiene, and apply the disposable gloves; remove and discard the old dressing.	5. Prevents the spread of microorganisms.
6. Assess the wound's appearance and note quality, quantity, color, and odor of drainage.	6. Provides assessment of the status of the wound.
7. Remove and discard the disposable gloves. Wash hands/hand hygiene.	7. Prevents the spread of microorganisms.
8. Prepare the sterile irrigation tray and dressing supplies. Pour the room-temperature irrigation solution into the solution container.	8. Aseptic technique is used to prevent introduction of microorganisms into the wound. Room-temperature solution reduces the client's discomfort.
9. Apply sterile gloves (and goggles, if needed).	9. Promotes sterile environment.

(Continues)

PROCEDURE 37-1
Irrigating a Wound (Continued)

ACTION	RATIONALE
10. Position the sterile basin below the wound so the irrigant will flow from the cleanest area to the dirtiest area and into the basin.	10. Decreases possibility of wound contamination.
11. Fill the piston or bulb syringe with irrigant and gently flush the wound. Hold the syringe approximately 1 inch above the wound bed to irrigate. Refill the syringe and continue to flush the wound until the solution returns clear and no exudate is noted or until the prescribed amount of fluid has been used (see Figures 37-13 and 37-14).	11. Gently irrigating the wound decreases trauma to granulation tissue. This provides the ideal pressure for cleansing and removal of debris.
12. Dry the edges of the wound with sterile gauze (see Figure 37-15).	12. Drying the edges of the wound prevents maceration of tissues caused by excess moisture.
13. Assess the wound's appearance and drainage.	13. Provides indication of change in wound status.
14. Apply a sterile dressing. Remove sterile gloves and dispose of properly. Wash hands/hand hygiene.	14. Protects the wound from microorganisms; prevents the spread of microorganisms.
15. Document all assessment findings and actions taken.	15. Records information for evaluation.

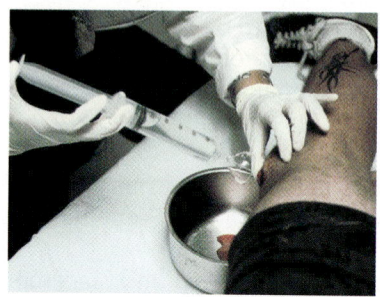

FIGURE 37-13 Gently flush the wound. DELMAR/CENGAGE LEARNING

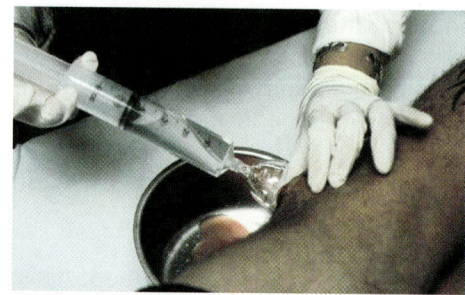

FIGURE 37-14 Hold the syringe close to the wound, but be careful not to touch the wound with the syringe. DELMAR/CENGAGE LEARNING

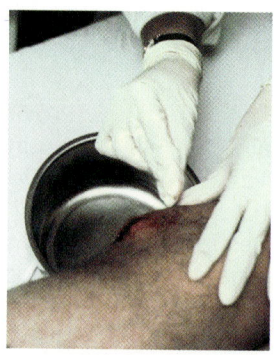

FIGURE 37-15 Dry the edges of the wound with sterile gauze. DELMAR/CENGAGE LEARNING

(Continues)

PROCEDURE 37-1
Irrigating a Wound (Continued)

delegation tip

Wound irrigation requires nursing assessment, aseptic technique, and monitoring of wound healing. This procedure is not delegated to ancillary personnel.

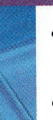

nursing tips

- *Be sure the irrigant is at room temperature, or ideally body temperature, to avoid traumatizing the granulating tissues and to avoid client discomfort.*
- *A small wound can be irrigated with a syringe and solution poured into a sterile specimen cup.*

PROCEDURE 37-2
Obtaining a Wound Drainage Specimen for Culturing

EQUIPMENT
- Disposable gloves
- Sterile gloves and dressing supplies
- Normal saline and irrigation tray
- Culture tube and swab
- Moisture-proof container or bag

ACTION	RATIONALE
1. Wash hands/hand hygiene, apply disposable gloves, and remove old dressing. Place old dressing in moisture-proof container, and remove and discard gloves. Wash hands/hand hygiene again.	1. Prevents the spread of microorganisms. Makes the wound accessible for obtaining the culture.
2. Open the dressing supplies using sterile technique and apply gloves.	2. Maintains sterile environment.
3. Assess the wound's appearance; note quality, quantity, color, and odor of discharge.	3. Provides assessment of the amount and character of the wound's drainage prior to irrigation. Reddened areas and heavy drainage suggest infection.
4. Irrigate the wound with normal saline prior to culturing the wound; do not irrigate with antiseptic.	4. Irrigation decreases the risk of culturing normal flora and other exudates such as protein; irrigating with an antiseptic prior to culturing may destroy the bacteria.
5. Using a sterile gauze pad, absorb the excess saline, and then discard the pad.	5. Removal of excess irrigant prevents maceration of tissue caused by excess moisture.
6. Remove the culture tube from the packaging (see Figure 37-16 on page 1194). Remove the culture swab from the culture tube, and gently roll the swab over the granulation tissue. Avoid eschar and wound edges (see Figure 37-17 on page 1194).	6. Decreases the chance of collecting superficial skin microorganisms.

(Continues)

PROCEDURE 37-2
Obtaining a Wound Drainage Specimen for Culturing (Continued)

ACTION	RATIONALE

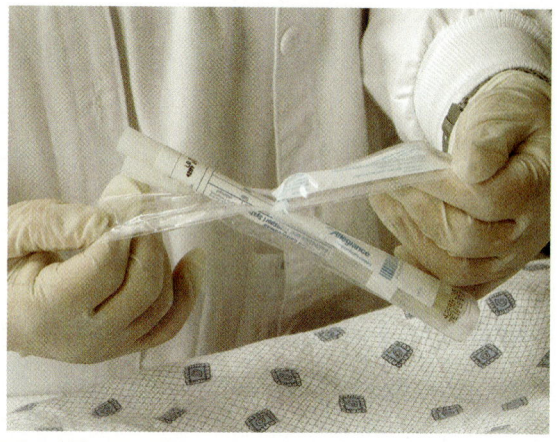

FIGURE 37-16 Remove the culture tube from the packaging. DELMAR/CENGAGE LEARNING

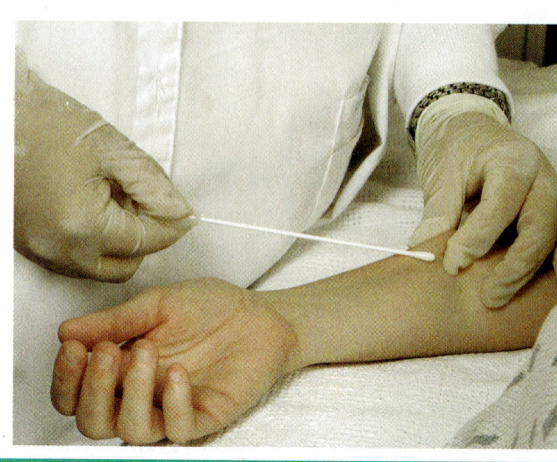

FIGURE 37-17 Roll the swab over the area to be cultured. DELMAR/CENGAGE LEARNING

7. Replace the swab into the culture tube, being careful not to touch the swab to the outside of the tube. Recap the tube. Crush the ampule of medium located in the bottom or cap of the tube (see Figure 37-18).

7. Avoids contamination with microorganisms. Releases the medium to surround the swab.

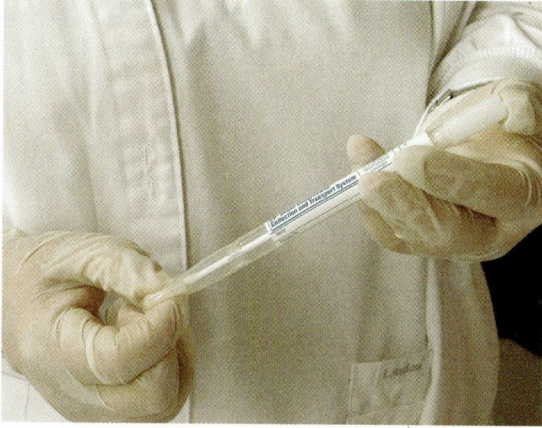

FIGURE 37-18 Crush the ampule to release the medium inside the culture tube. DELMAR/CENGAGE LEARNING

8. Remove gloves, wash hands/hand hygiene, and apply sterile gloves. Dress the wound with sterile dressing.

9. Label the specimen, place in biohazard transport bag, and arrange to transport the specimen to the laboratory according to institutional policy.

8. Prevents the spread of microorganisms and contamination of the wound.

9. Ensures proper handling of specimen.

(Continues)

PROCEDURE 37-2
Obtaining a Wound Drainage Specimen for Culturing (Continued)

ACTION	RATIONALE
10. Remove gloves. Wash hands/hand hygiene.	10. Prevents the spread of microorganisms.
11. Document all assessment findings and actions taken. Document that a specimen was obtained.	11. Records information for evaluation and promotes continuity of care.

delegation tip

Obtaining a wound culture requires nursing assessment and aseptic technique and is potentially an invasive procedure; therefore, delegation to ancillary personnel is not appropriate.

nursing tips

- Do not irrigate the wound with anything except sterile saline or sterile water prior to obtaining the specimen.
- Be aware of what you are doing while holding the culture swab. Touching the swab to anything but the area to be cultured and sterile surfaces contaminates the swab and invalidates the test.
- In anaerobic cultures, be sure the specimen is immersed in the medium at the bottom of the tube.

PROCEDURE 37-3

Applying a Dry Dressing

EQUIPMENT
- Clean exam gloves
- Container for proper disposal of soiled dressing
- Sterile 4 × 4 gauze pads
- Washcloth (optional)
- ABD pads (optional)
- 2-inch tape (foam or paper)

ACTION	RATIONALE
1. Gather supplies (see Figure 37-19 on page 1196).	1. Promotes a smooth work flow.
2. Provide privacy; draw curtains; close door.	2. Maintains client comfort and privacy while body is exposed during procedure.
3. Explain procedure to client.	3. Provides information about the procedure.
4. Wash hands/hand hygiene.	4. Prevents the spread of microorganisms.
5. Apply clean exam gloves.	5. Promotes infection control and protection from body fluids.
6. Remove dressing and place in appropriate receptacle. Remove soiled gloves with contaminated surfaces inward and discard in appropriate receptacle; apply clean gloves.	6. Dressings and gloves soiled with body fluids are considered contaminated and subject to biohazard disposal in the correct manner per institution protocol. It is standard for the surgeon to do the first postoperative dressing change. The initial dressing is maintained for 24 to 48 hours postoperatively, unless conditions of the dressing

(Continues)

PROCEDURE 37-3
Applying a Dry Dressing (Continued)

ACTION	RATIONALE

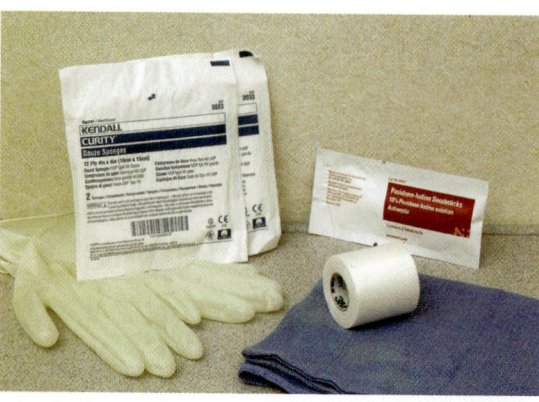

FIGURE 37-19 Gauze sponges, clean gloves, tape, and antiseptic solution are used to change a dry dressing. DELMAR/CENGAGE LEARNING

ACTION	RATIONALE
	call for contacting the health care provider for a dressing change order. Until the removal of the initial dressing, the nurse will reinforce the dressing as needed.
	The frequency of the dressing change depends upon the particular wound and the preference of the health care provider. This will usually be specified in the orders.
7. Assess the appearance of the undressed wound bed for healing.	7. Assess for signs of redness, foul odor, swelling, irritation, drainage, dehiscence, bleeding, or skin breakdown.
8. Cleanse the skin around the incision if necessary with a clean, warm, wet washcloth.	8. Dried blood or drainage on the surrounding skin can be an irritant and a medium for microbes.
• If the suture line requires cleansing, it should be done gently. Use normal saline, half-strength hydrogen peroxide, or Betadine swab (consult orders of health care provider and/or institution policy regarding antiseptic agents) and cotton-tip applicators using a rolling motion.	• The suture line itself should not be disturbed unnecessarily. • Avoid Betadine if client has an iodine allergy.
• Used applicators should not be reintroduced into the sterile solution (see Figure 37-20 on page 1197).	• Reintroduction of the soiled applicator into sterile solution will contaminate the solution.
9. Remove used exam gloves.	9. Exam gloves used to remove the old dressing are considered dirty and should be removed and discarded appropriately.
10. Wash hands/hand hygiene.	10. Hands should be washed prior to setting up dressing supplies to prevent the spread of microorganisms.
11. Set up supplies.	11. Following removal of the dressing, the nurse will have a better idea of which supplies are needed and in what amount.

(Continues)

PROCEDURE 37-3
Applying a Dry Dressing (Continued)

ACTION	RATIONALE

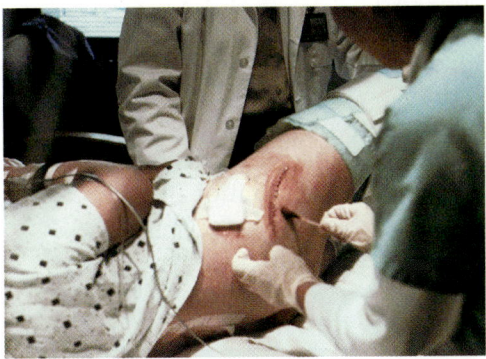

FIGURE 37-20 Clean the suture lines gently, as appropriate.
DELMAR/CENGAGE LEARNING

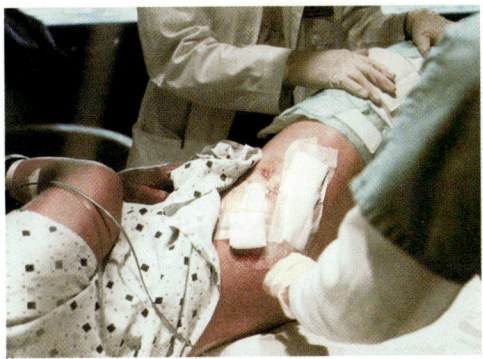

FIGURE 37-21 Apply 4 × 4 gauze pads, folded in half. Tape the gauze in place. DELMAR/CENGAGE LEARNING

12. Apply a new pair of clean exam gloves.

13. Grasping just the edges, apply a new dressing using 4 × 4 gauze pads folded in half to the 2 × 4 size. Place the folded gauze pad lengthwise on wound and tape lightly, or apply tubular mesh for those with sensitive skin (see Figure 37-21). Initial the dressing, citing date and time changed.
    Optional: An ABD pad may be applied on top of the dressing for added protection over sutures or for the client's comfort.
14. Remove gloves and dispose of appropriately, then wash hands/hand hygiene.
15. Conduct client and family education session about the dressing, which may include teaching the dressing technique to the client and family.

12. This is considered a clean procedure after the initial dressing is removed if the skin margins are approximated with the skin closures.
13. A light dressing of 4 × 4 pads may be the only dressing that is needed to protect the incision from clothing or to collect a small amount of tissue drainage. This maintains a record of the dressing change for the next nurse.

14. Prevents the spread of microorganisms.

15. Educates the client and family and prepares for discharge.

delegation tip

The application of bandages to the client is not delegated to ancillary personnel. Family members may be taught this skill prior to the client's discharge. Occasionally, ancillary personnel will be delegated the task of applying a clean dry gauze as skin protection, but the nurse is responsible for the assessment of the integrity of the client's skin.

nursing tips

- *Do not overdress the wound.*
- *Check the room for supplies before bringing more into the room.*
- *Order specially needed supplies in advance of the procedure; do not wait until the last minute.*
- *Client and family education and preparation for discharge begin upon admission.*

PROCEDURE 37-4

Applying a Wet-to-Damp Dressing (Wet-to-Moist Dressing)

EQUIPMENT

- Clean exam gloves
- Container for proper disposal of soiled dressing
- Sterile gloves
- Moisture-proof gown (optional)
- Sterile towel
- Normal saline or ordered solution

- Sterile bowl
- Sterile 4 × 4 gauze pads, multiple
- Cover sponges or fluffs (optional)
- ABD dressing pads
- 2-inch tape (foam or paper)
- Tubular mesh (optional)
- Montgomery straps (optional)

ACTION	RATIONALE
1. Review order of health care provider for wound care and gather supplies.	1. Promotes a smooth work flow.
2. Provide privacy; draw curtains; close door.	2. Maintains client's comfort and privacy while body is exposed during procedure.
3. Assess need for pain medication. Pain is rated on a scale from 0 (lowest) to 10 (greatest). Assess need based on quality, pain pattern, location, and last pain medication received.	3. Removal of a wet-to-damp or moist dressing may be painful to the client, so careful assessment of pain medication needs prior to the dressing change is important.
4. Explain procedure to client.	4. Provides information about the procedure.
5. Wash hands/hand hygiene.	5. Prevents the spread of microorganisms.
6. Apply clean exam gloves, a moisture-proof gown, mask, and eye protection, as appropriate.	6. Provides infection control and protection from body fluids. If there is copious drainage or the wound is infected, a gown, a mask, and eye protection should be worn. A mask will also help the nurse if the drainage is foul smelling.
7. Inform client that the dressing is going to be removed.	7. Helps prepare client and alleviates anxiety.
8. Remove wet-to-damp dressing, noting number of gauze pads used, and place in appropriate receptacle (see Figure 37-22 on page 1199).	8. The dressing should be removed slowly yet deliberately. Moistening the dressing with saline is not recommended because this defeats the purpose of the debriding and cleaning action. If it is found that the dressing is extremely dry and removal will result in injury, a small amount of saline to loosen that portion of the dressing is indicated (see Figure 37-23 on page 1199). To counteract the problem of an extremely dry dressing, increase the wetness of the dressing or increase the frequency of dressing changes. Count the number of gauze pads so you know how many to use when replacing the dressing.
9. Observe the undressed wound for healing (granulation and approximation of edges), signs of infection (inflammation, edema, warmth, pain), and drainage.	9. Allows for evaluation of effectiveness of treatment.

(Continues)

PROCEDURE 37-4
Applying a Wet-to-Damp Dressing (Wet-to-Moist Dressing) (Continued)

ACTION	RATIONALE

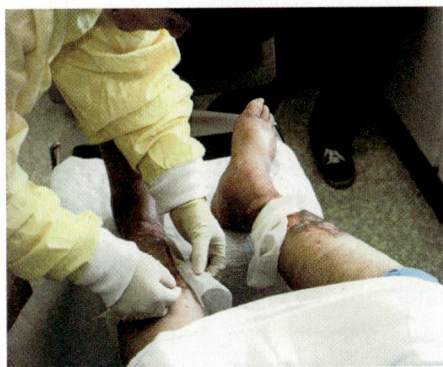

FIGURE 37-22 Carefully remove the old dressing, allowing it to debride the wound as you pull it away. DELMAR/CENGAGE LEARNING

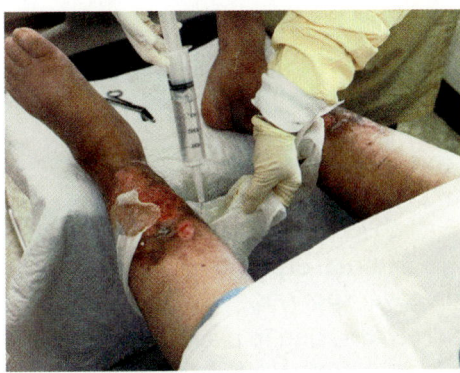

FIGURE 37-23 If the dressing is too dry and removing it will cause injury, use a small amount of saline to loosen the portion of the dressing that adheres too tightly to the wound. DELMAR/CENGAGE LEARNING

10. Cleanse the skin around the incision if necessary with a clean, warm, wet washcloth.	10. Dried blood or drainage on the surrounding skin can be an irritant and a medium for microbes.
11. Remove used exam gloves.	11. Exam gloves used to remove the old dressing are considered dirty and should be removed and discarded appropriately.
12. Wash hands/hand hygiene.	12. Prevents the spread of microorganisms.
13. Set up supplies in a sterile field, including pouring ordered solutions into appropriate containers if indicated for the dressing change (see Figure 37-24).	13. Following removal of the dressing, the nurse will have a better idea of which supplies are needed and in what amount.

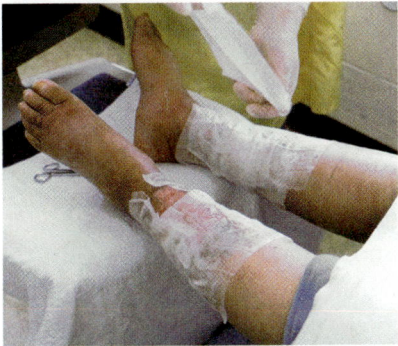

FIGURE 37-24 Place the gauze on the wound. DELMAR/CENGAGE LEARNING

14. Apply sterile gloves.	14. This is a sterile dressing change.
15. Place gauze or packing material to be moistened in the bowl with the normal saline or other solution. • Wring gauze or packing of saline until damp. • Gently place damp gauze over the area (see Figure 37-24).	15. If a solution is not specified, then normal saline is used. Wounds considered dirty or contaminated may call for special solutions ordered by the health care provider to moisten the wound packing. Alternative solutions

(Continues)

PROCEDURE 37-4
Applying a Wet-to-Damp Dressing (Wet-to-Moist Dressing) (Continued)

ACTION	RATIONALE
	include dilute povidone-iodine and dilute acetic acid. Follow institutional guidelines.
	• Avoid overwringing of the dressing to prevent excessive drying. The dressing should be wet to damp, depending upon the depth and size of the wound and the interval of the dressing change.
	• Dresses the wound.
16. Apply external dressing of dry 4 × 4 gauze pads, cover sponges, fluffs, or ABD pads.	16. The external dressing is determined by the size and shape of the wound.
• Secure dressing in place with tape, Montgomery straps, or tubular mesh (see Figure 37-25).	• Tape for short-term dressings in clients who are not sensitive to adhesives is the method of choice for securing dressings. For long-term dressings or for those clients who are sensitive to tape, use Montgomery straps or tubular mesh.
	Tubular mesh is a nice alternative to hold the dressing in place because tape is not involved—the mesh is simply pulled up or down to accommodate the dressing change.

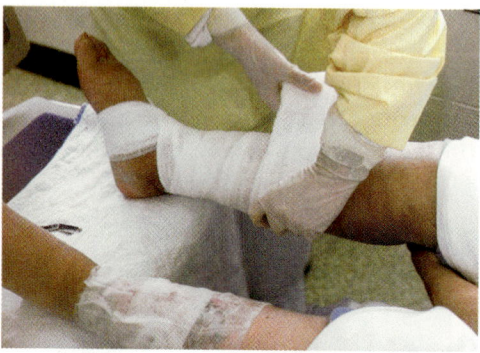

FIGURE 37-25 Wrap the wet gauze with an external dressing of dry gauze bandages. DELMAR/CENGAGE LEARNING

17. Remove gloves and wash hands/hand hygiene.	17. Prevents the spread of microorganisms. Be sure to discard gloves in appropriate receptacle.
18. Mark the dressing with the date and time it was changed, and initial it.	18. This maintains a record of the dressing change for the next nurse and provides for continuity of care.
19. Conduct client and family education session about the dressing, which may include teaching the dressing technique to the client and family.	19. Educates the client and family and prepares for discharge.

(Continues)

PROCEDURE 37-4
Applying a Wet-to-Damp Dressing (Wet-to-Moist Dressing) (Continued)

delegation tip

Applying a wet-to-damp dressing requires sterile technique and professional assessment skills and cannot be delegated to ancillary personnel.

nursing tips

- *Make a list, if necessary, of needed supplies to take into the room.*
- *If you are going to be in a client's room for some time, let others know so that they can cover your call lights and you can devote your attention to the dressing change.*
- *When doing very small wet-to-damp dressing changes, the normal saline can be carefully poured on open packets of sterile 4 × 4 pads, thus bypassing the need for a sterile bowl.*
- *Order specially needed supplies in advance of the procedure; do not wait until the last minute.*
- *Client and family education and preparation for discharge begin upon admission.*
- *Carefully evaluate and communicate client's wound healing response to dressing treatments. Consult wound specialist and change treatment as recommended or as ordered.*

PROCEDURE 37-5

Preventing and Managing the Pressure Ulcer

EQUIPMENT
- Pillows
- Rolled-up blankets or towels
- Egg-crate mattress
- Specialty beds if ordered by prescribing practitioner or qualified practitioner
- Heel and elbow protectors
- Lotion or powder as needed
- Soap and water

ACTION	RATIONALE
1. Check the health care provider's order for specific positioning of client and dressing change instructions.	1. Because of the client's medical condition, the health care provider may want the client in a specific position and/or may have ordered dressing changes for a pressure ulcer.
2. Gather all the equipment you will need.	2. Having all your equipment in the room will increase the consistency of client care.
3. Identify the client and explain the procedure to the client.	3. Providing explanations to the client will employ the client's cooperation and provide time for client education.
4. Wash hands/hand hygiene.	4. Prevents the spread of microorganisms.
5. Provide for client privacy and apply gloves.	5. Shows respect for the client's privacy. Gloves protect both the client and the nurse from potential body fluid contact.

(Continues)

PROCEDURE 37-5
Preventing and Managing the Pressure Ulcer (Continued)

ACTION	RATIONALE
6. Adjust the bed to your level and lower the side rail nearest you without leaving client unattended.	6. Adjusting the bed to your level will make the procedure easier on your back. Lowering the side rails will allow you closer contact with the client to provide care.
7. Assess client's risk for developing pressure ulcers by using the Braden scale or a similar risk chart (see Table 37-6).	7. Informs the nurse about the extent of the client's education of risk factors and the preventive care needs to be instituted immediately.
8. Assess client's skin over all pressure points, such as sacrum (see Figure 37-26), ischial tuberosities, feet, heels (see Figure 37-27), elbows (see Figure 37-28), and back of head.	8. A reddened area in light-skinned clients and a bluish or purple area in dark-skinned clients indicate that the tissue was under pressure.

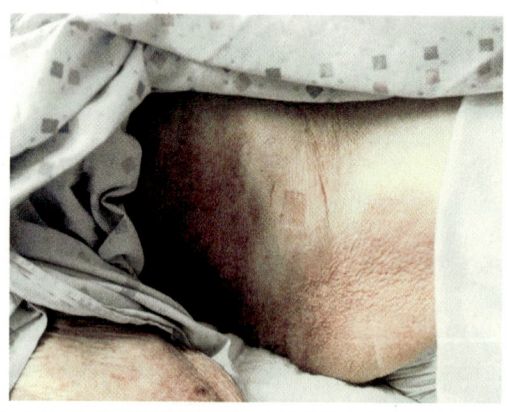

FIGURE 37-26 **Assess the sacrum.** DELMAR/CENGAGE LEARNING

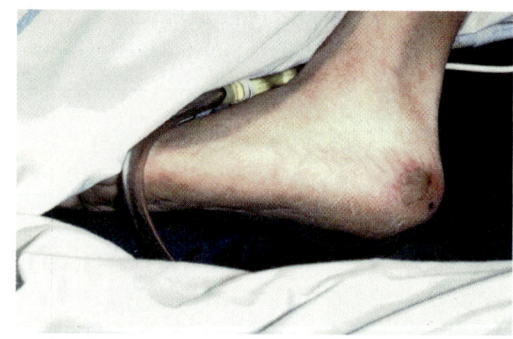

FIGURE 37-27 **Assess the feet and heels.** DELMAR/CENGAGE LEARNING

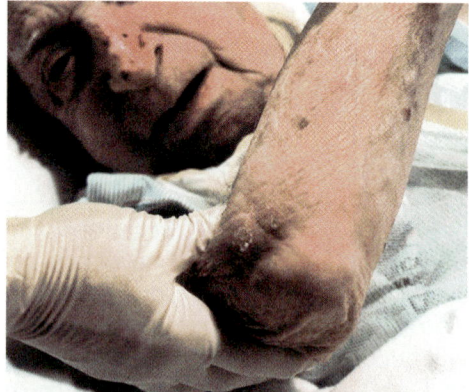

FIGURE 37-28 **Assess the elbows.** DELMAR/CENGAGE LEARNING

9. Assess other sites for potential areas of pressure points.	9. Other potential sites and causes of pressure include the NG tube and tape on the tip of the nose, IV dressing tape, a Foley catheter touching the labia or taped area of skin, endotracheal tube and tape, and side rails touching the skin.

(Continues)

PROCEDURE 37-5
Preventing and Managing the Pressure Ulcer (Continued)

ACTION	RATIONALE
10. Change client's position.	10. Increases client comfort and prevents contractures and decubiti.
11. Keep client's position at 30° or less.	11. A position of 30° or lower will limit the pressure on the sacrum.
12. Provide skin care if area is soiled or sweaty, but do not massage pressure points.	12. Skin care keeps skin clean and dry, and new preliminary evidence documents that massaging bony prominences may actually cause deep tissue trauma.
13. Use support devices such as special beds (see Figure 37-29), egg-crate mattresses, pillows (see Figures 37-30 and 37-31), towels, blankets, and heel protectors (see Figure 37-32) to support the body.	13. Lifting the heels and elbows off of the bed will limit the pressure to these areas. Also, providing support between the legs will limit the pressure.
14. Perform dressing change to a pressure ulcer as ordered or per agency policy (see Figures 37-33 and 37-34 on page 1204), remembering aseptic or sterile technique.	14. Providing wound care to existing pressure ulcers will facilitate wound healing and begin to protect the client from a potential infection.
15. Return side rail to the upright position and lower the bed.	15. Provides for client safety.

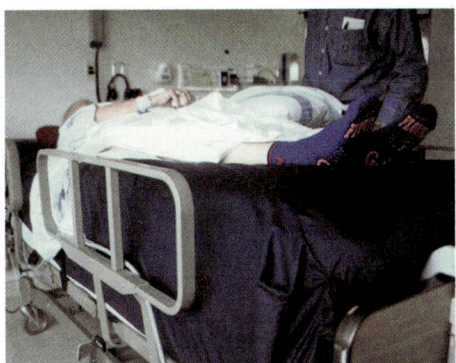

FIGURE 37-29 Special beds have air- or fluid-filled mattresses and are used to reduce the pressure on bony prominences. DELMAR/CENGAGE LEARNING

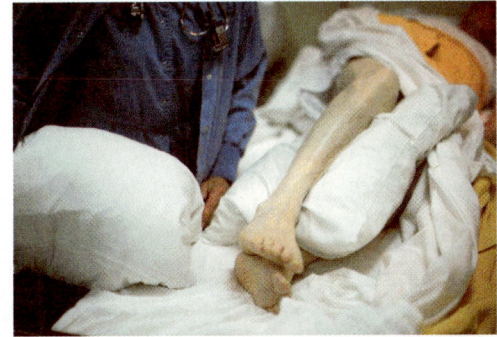

FIGURE 37-30 Pillows are used to take the pressure off the heels and feet. DELMAR/CENGAGE LEARNING

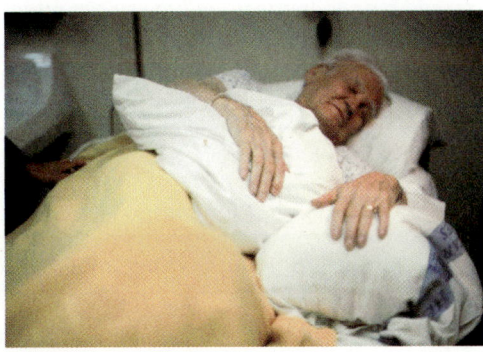

FIGURE 37-31 Pillows are used to support the hands and elbows. DELMAR/CENGAGE LEARNING

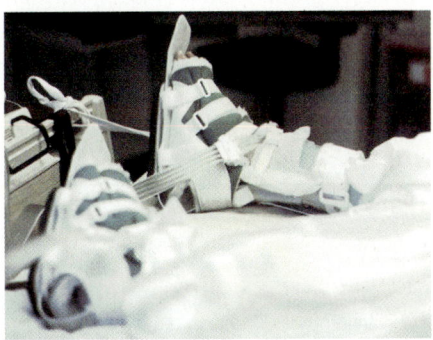

FIGURE 37-32 These heel protectors guard the heels from pressure and friction. DELMAR/CENGAGE LEARNING

(Continues)

PROCEDURE 37-5
Preventing and Managing the Pressure Ulcer (Continued)

ACTION	RATIONALE

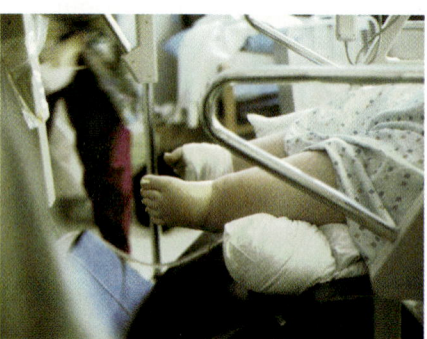

FIGURE 37-33 This client's heels and feet have been protected from pressure with a special bed and pillow support. An existing pressure ulcer wound on the right foot has been cleaned and dressed. DELMAR/CENGAGE LEARNING

16. Remove gloves and wash hands/hand hygiene.
17. Document appearance of pressure points and/or ulcers, including skin care and wound care provided and position changes.
18. Create an every-2-hours turning schedule if one is not available.

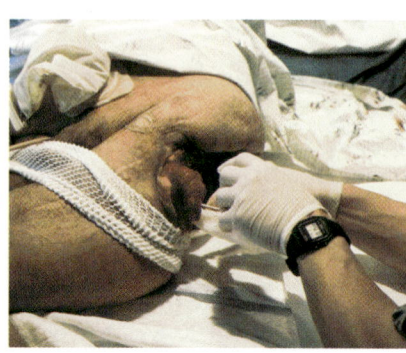

FIGURE 37-34 A dressing change is performed on a large pressure ulcer. DELMAR/CENGAGE LEARNING

16. Prevents the spread of microorganisms.
17. Provides a picture of skin surface and interventions instituted to prevent pressure points and/or to provide for tissue healing.
18. A turning schedule helps promote further compliance with preventive measures for providing care.

delegation tip

Assessment of pressure ulcers is the role of the nurse. Licensed and ancillary personnel may observe the wound for improvement or deterioration during daily care and report that information to the nurse.

nursing tips

- Look at the client's skin, especially the pressure areas, at least every 2 hours, and reposition the client as often as possible.
- Do not massage the skin over the site. Recent research has discouraged massaging the area because of the potential to cause deep tissue trauma.
- Look for pressure ulcers in unexpected places such as under any area that has tape on it, including the nasogastric tube, IV dressing, and wound dressing. Inspect the back of the head, ears, and elbows as well.
- When taking dressings off a pressure ulcer, note the sequence, size, and type of dressings used so you can repeat the sequence when reapplying the dressings. Be familiar with the health care provider's order.
- Avoid elastic bandages if the client has a history of latex allergy.

KEY CONCEPTS

- A wound is a disruption in the integrity of the body tissue that puts an individual at risk for infection.
- Wounds go through a three-step healing process that includes a defensive (inflammatory) phase, a

reconstructive (proliferative) phase, and a maturation phase.
- The type of exudate from a wound can help determine the pathology of the infectious process.

- Wounds are often classified by their cause, level of cleanliness, depth, or color.
- Nursing diagnoses for clients with wounds and pressure ulcers focus on both the physical (*Acute pain, Risk for infection, Chronic pain, Impaired tissue integrity*) and the psychosocial (*Anxiety, Deficient knowledge, Disturbed body image*) aspects.
- A significant nursing intervention in all cases of *Impaired skin integrity* is client education on wound care and promotion of healing; the client's support people are often included in this teaching.

- Heat and cold applications help the body's own systems respond to and therefore relieve the pain that accompanies wounds.
- Pressure ulcers, or bedsores, are a common problem in acute and chronic care settings, resulting in longer stays for clients and increased costs of health care.
- Pressure ulcers are classified into four stages, depending on the depth of tissue damage.
- Proper positioning is the most effective preventive measure for pressure ulcers.

REVIEW QUESTIONS

1. The nurse has to apply a bandage on a joint. Which bandaging method should be used?
   a. Circular turns
   b. Spiral turns
   c. Spiral reverse turns
   d. Figure-eight turns
2. Proper technique for performing a wound culture is to _____.
   a. cleanse the wound with normal saline prior to obtaining the specimen
   b. swab the wound drainage
   c. remove crust from the necrotic tissue and then swab
   d. obtain the specimen from drainage on the dressing
3. Which intervention is most appropriate for a client with a muscle sprain and hematoma?
   a. Binder
   b. Ace bandage
   c. Ice bag
   d. Polyurethane foam
4. The appropriate nursing action for a client with a Braden scale score of 16 is to _____.
   a. assess the client according to agency policy
   b. implement a turning schedule
   c. apply a transparent wound dressing on the coccyx
   d. request an order for physical therapy
5. Which wound care instruction should be given to a client being discharged from the hospital with a skin tear?
   a. Cover the skin tear with a transparent dressing.
   b. Use a nonadherent dressing over the wound.

   c. Eat a high-fat diet to promote wound healing.
   d. Drink 3000 mL of water every day to keep the skin hydrated.
6. Which client is at the greatest risk for a pressure ulcer?
   a. A 52-year-old obese female, 2 days postoperative for a knee replacement, who has an indwelling urinary catheter
   b. A 74-year-old thin male who is awaiting surgery for a fractured hip
   c. A 91-year-old emaciated female with a blood sugar of 160 mg/dL who is sitting in a wheelchair
   d. A 67-year-old obese male who has cellulitis of his right lower leg
7. A superficial abrasion with partial-thickness skin loss involving the epidermis and dermis would be staged as what degree of ulceration?
   a. Stage I
   b. Stage II
   c. Stage III
   d. Stage IV
8. Which nursing activity should the registered nurse delegate to a licensed practical nurse?
   a. Instruct a client on irrigation for a chronic wound.
   b. Develop a plan of care for the irrigation of a skin ulcer.
   c. Obtain a health history from a client admitted with a pressure sore on the coccyx.
   d. Monitor the vital signs of a client with cellulitis for evidence of sepsis.

online companion

Visit the DeLaune and Ladner online companion resource at **www.delmar.cengage.com** for additional content and study aids. Click on Online Companions, then select the Nursing discipline.

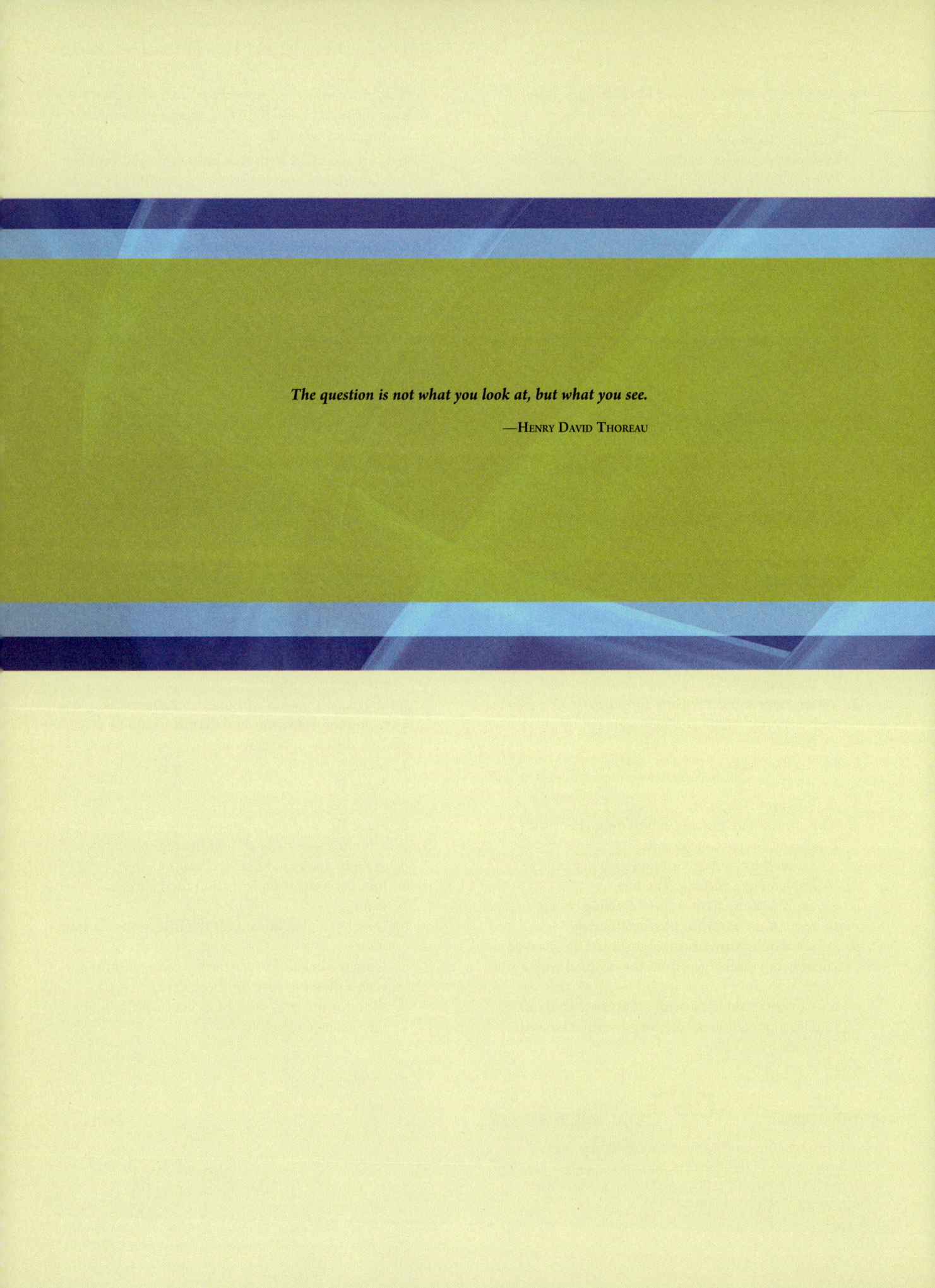

The question is not what you look at, but what you see.

—Henry David Thoreau

CHAPTER 38

Sensation, Perception, and Cognition

COMPETENCIES

1. Describe normal cognitive and sensory perceptual functioning.
2. Describe cognitive development across the life span.
3. Identify responses to sensory deprivation and overload.
4. Describe the learning needs of clients experiencing alterations in cognition and sensory perception.
5. Explain use of the nursing process with clients experiencing alterations in cognition and sensory perception.

Making sense of one's situation, learning new information, and recalling memories of the past are activities that make each person a unique individual. Performance of these activities relies on intact cognition, sensation, and perceptual abilities.

This chapter discusses the physiology of sensation, perception, and cognition and the common alterations in each functional area. Information on the nurse's role in caring for individuals with sensory, perceptual, or cognitive alterations is presented.

PHYSIOLOGY OF SENSATION, PERCEPTION, AND COGNITION

Sensation is the ability to receive and process stimuli through the sensory organs. There are two types of stimuli: external and internal. External stimuli are received and processed through the sight (visual), hearing (auditory), smell (olfactory), taste (gustatory), and touch (tactile) modes. Internal stimuli are received and processed through kinesthetic (an awareness of the position of the body) and visceral (feelings originating from large organs within the body) modes.

Perception is the ability to experience, recognize, organize, and interpret sensory stimuli. **Sensory perception** is the ability to receive sensory impressions and, through cortical association, relate the stimuli to past experiences and to form impressions of the nature of the stimuli.

Perception is closely associated with **cognition**, the intellectual ability to think. The processes of organizing and interpreting stimuli are dependent on a person's level of intellectual functioning. Cognition includes the elements of memory, judgment, and orientation. The well-being of an individual is dependent on the functions of sensation, perception, and cognition because it is through these mechanisms that the person fully experiences and interacts with the environment.

Sensory, perceptual, and cognitive alterations can be either temporary or progressive in their manifestations and can result from disease or trauma. Whatever the cause of the alterations, these conditions usually lead to social isolation and increased dependence on others. In addition, impairment in sensory, perceptual, and cognitive functions can place the individual at risk for injury to himself or herself or to others.

Sensation, perception, and cognition are neurological functions. The nervous system is composed of two major subsystems: the central nervous system (CNS) and the peripheral nervous system (PNS), which consists of the somatic and autonomic nervous systems (see Figure 38-1).

The CNS and PNS act in unison to accomplish three purposes: collection of stimuli from the receptors at the end of the peripheral nerves, transport of the stimuli to the brain for integration and cognitive processing, and conduction of responses to the stimuli from the brain to responsive motor centers in the body.

The CNS is composed of the brain and spinal cord, which are protected by the bony structures of the skull and vertebral column. The brain, the most complex of the body's organs, is composed of three basic structures: the cerebrum (which consists of the temporal, frontal, parietal, and occipital lobes), the cerebellum, and the brain stem (see Figure 38-2 on page 1209). Table 38-1 on page 1209 describes each of these structures. The structures of the brain serve as both receptors and reactors by collecting stimuli and effecting responses to those stimuli. The spinal cord links the advanced neurosensory mechanisms that occur in the brain to the rest of the body via a coordinated pathway of neurons.

Sensory perception involves the function of both the cranial and peripheral nerves. The cranial nerves arise from the three structures of the brain and govern the movement and function of various muscles and nerves throughout the body (see Figure 38-3 on page 1210). The peripheral

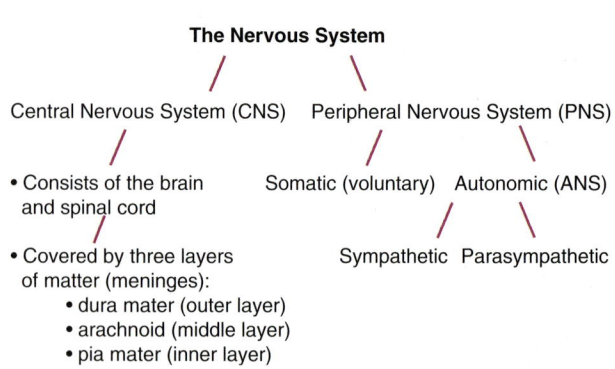

The Nervous System

Central Nervous System (CNS) — Peripheral Nervous System (PNS)

Central Nervous System (CNS):
- Consists of the brain and spinal cord
- Covered by three layers of matter (meninges):
  - dura mater (outer layer)
  - arachnoid (middle layer)
  - pia mater (inner layer)

Peripheral Nervous System (PNS):
- Somatic (voluntary)
- Autonomic (ANS)
  - Sympathetic
  - Parasympathetic

FIGURE 38-1 The Nervous System DELMAR/CENGAGE LEARNING

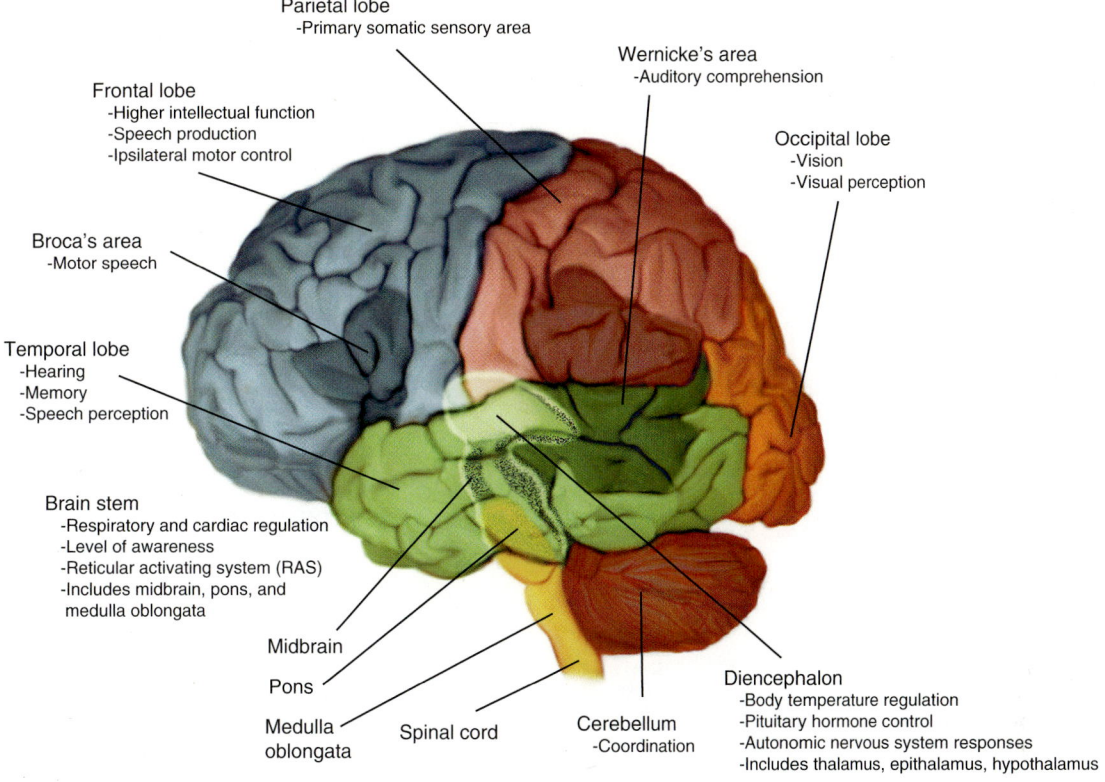

FIGURE 38-2 **Cross-Section of the Brain** DELMAR/CENGAGE LEARNING

TABLE 38-1 Structures and Functions of the Brain

STRUCTURE	DESCRIPTION	PRIMARY FUNCTIONS
Cerebrum	• Composed of gray matter and white matter. • Basal ganglia (masses of gray matter) are part of the extrapyramidal system.	• Is responsible for: — Thinking — Memory — Learning • Receives and interprets sensory input (stimuli); responds to sensory stimuli • Helps control motor function
Cerebellum	• Located behind and under the cerebrum. • Is a fissured mass consisting of a body that includes a narrow middle strip and two lateral lobes.	• Is concerned with unconscious functions • Is responsible for smooth-muscle functioning • Maintains equilibrium
Brain stem	Composed of three structures: • The midbrain • The pons • The medulla oblongata	• Influences visual and auditory senses • Connects the upper and lower levels of the CNS • Affects respiratory rate; prevents coma by maintaining wakefulness • Controls vital functions: — Heart rate — Respiratory rate — Swallowing — Coughing • Processes sensory input from spinal tract

From Guyton, A. C., & Hall, J. (2005). *Textbook of medical physiology* (11th ed.). Philadelphia: Elsevier.

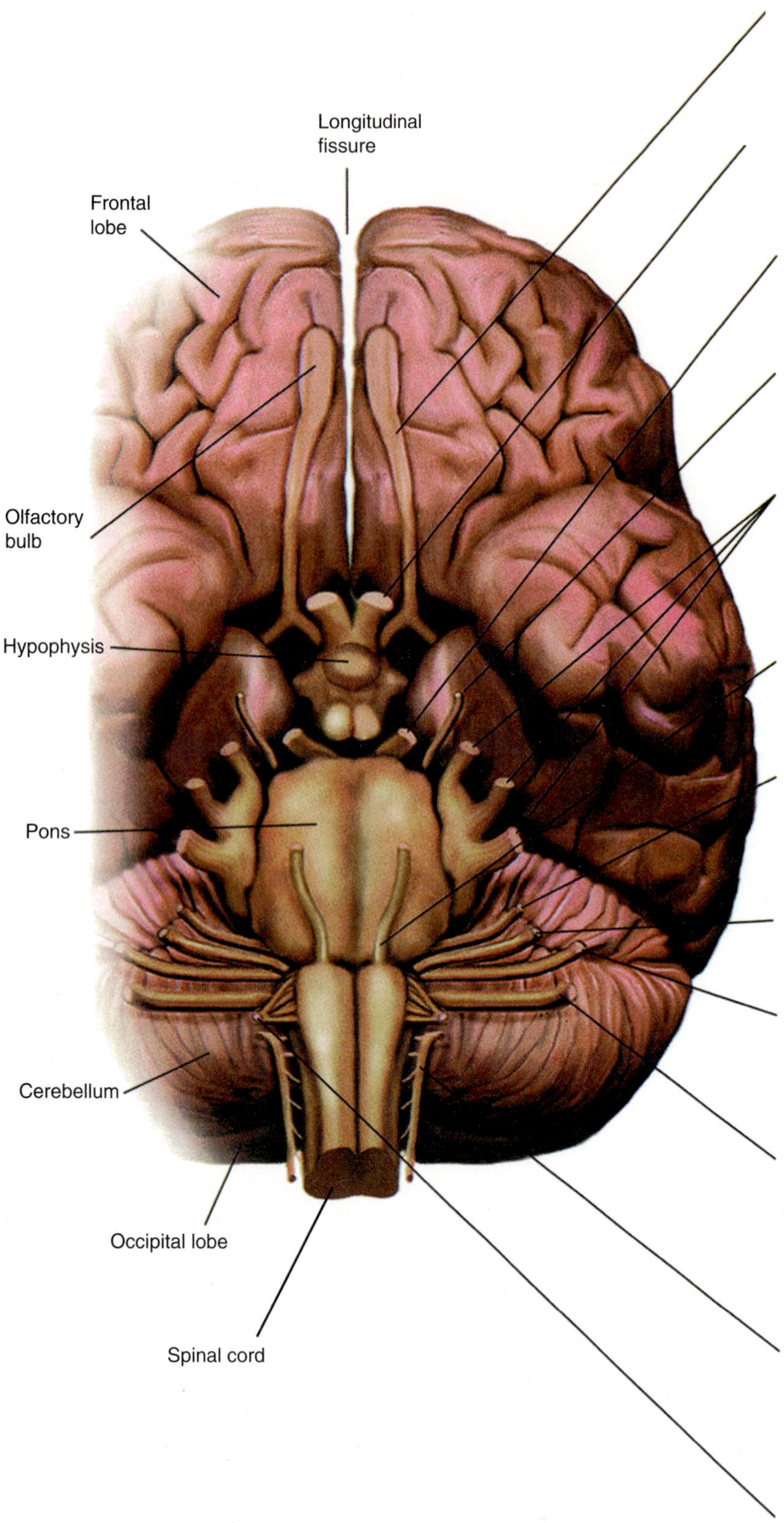

Longitudinal fissure

Frontal lobe

Olfactory bulb

Hypophysis

Pons

Cerebellum

Occipital lobe

Spinal cord

CN I. **Olfactory**
Function: Sense of smell (Sensory)

CN II. **Optic**
Function: Arises from retinas of the eyes and carries impulses associated with vision (Sensory)

CN III. **Oculomotor**
Function: Controls extrinsic eye muscles and regulates pupil size (Motor and Sensory)

CN IV. **Trochlear**
Function: Aids voluntary movements of eyeballs (Motor and Sensory)

CN V. **Trigeminal**
Function: Controls major sensory nerves of the face. Has 3 divisions: ophthalmic, maxillary, and mandibular (Motor and Sensory)

CN VI. **Abducens**
Function: Supplies the lateral rectus muscle of the eyes (Motor and Sensory)

CN VII. **Facial**
Function: Supplies the muscles of the face, scalp, taste buds, and lacrimal glands (Motor and Sensory)

CN VIII. **Vestibulocochlear**
Function: Supplies the ears (Sensory)

CN IX. **Glossopharyngeal**
Function: Supplies the tongue and pharynx, taste buds, and the carotid sinus (Motor and Sensory)

CN X. **Vagus**
Function: Runs close to common carotid arteries and internal jugular veins to the thorax and lower abdomen; has a broad parasympathetic distribution (Motor and Sensory)

CN XI. **Spinal Accessory**
Function: Supplies the trapezius and sternocleidomastoid muscles; responsible for proprioception (Motor and Sensory)

CN XII. **Hypoglossal**
Function: Supplies intrinsic and extrinsic muscles of tongue; involved in proprioception (Motor and Sensory)

FIGURE 38-3 **The Cranial Nerves** DELMAR/CENGAGE LEARNING

nerves connect the CNS to other parts of the body (see Figure 38-4).

COMPONENTS OF SENSATION AND PERCEPTION

The sensory system is a complex network that consists of **afferent nerve pathways** (ascending pathways that transmit sensory impulses to the brain), **efferent nerve pathways** (descending pathways that send sensory impulses from the brain), the spinal cord, the brain stem, and the higher cortex (cerebral lobes). Figure 38-5 shows the major sensory pathways.

COMPONENTS OF COGNITION

Cognition includes the cerebral functions of memory, judgment, and emotion. In order for higher functions (e.g.,

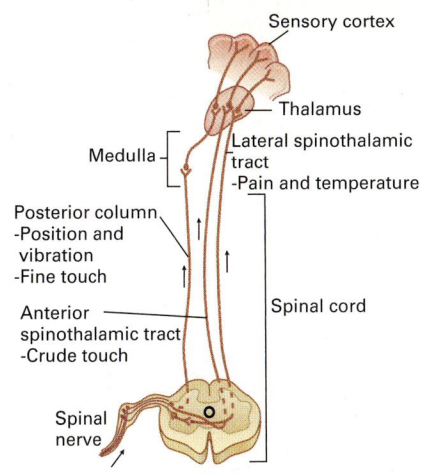

FIGURE 38-5 Major Sensory Pathways DELMAR/CENGAGE LEARNING

memory, affect, judgment, perception, and language) to occur, consciousness must be present.

Consciousness

Consciousness is a state of awareness of self, others, and the surrounding environment. It affects both cognitive (intellectual) and affective (emotional) functions. An alert individual (one who is aware of self and stimuli) is able to perceive reality accurately and to base behavior on those perceptions. The components of consciousness provide a foundation for behavior and emotional expression, thereby contributing to the uniqueness of each individual's personality.

Consciousness depends on the functioning of the reticular activating system (RAS), which is located within the midbrain and thalamus, as well as connective fibers between these structures and areas within the cerebral cortex. The RAS controls activities such as sleep and wakefulness and monitors the selective transmission of stimuli to other parts of the neurosensory system. Consciousness may be altered by various metabolic, traumatic, or other factors such as the pharmacological actions of drugs that affect mental status. The primary components of consciousness are arousal and awareness, both of which must be present before higher cognitive functioning occurs.

AROUSAL   The degree of **arousal**, a component linked closely to the appearance of wakefulness and alertness, is indicated by a person's general response and reaction to the environment. People exhibit arousal, the state of being prepared to act, by behaving in an alert, aware manner and by experiencing periods of wakefulness. The degree of an individual's arousal is indicated by the general response and reaction to the environment. Impaired arousal can exist when a sleep deficit is experienced; there may be an inability to take advantage of opportunities for activity because of limited periods of rest.

AWARENESS   **Awareness** is the capacity to perceive sensory impressions and react appropriately through thoughts and actions. An essential element in awareness is

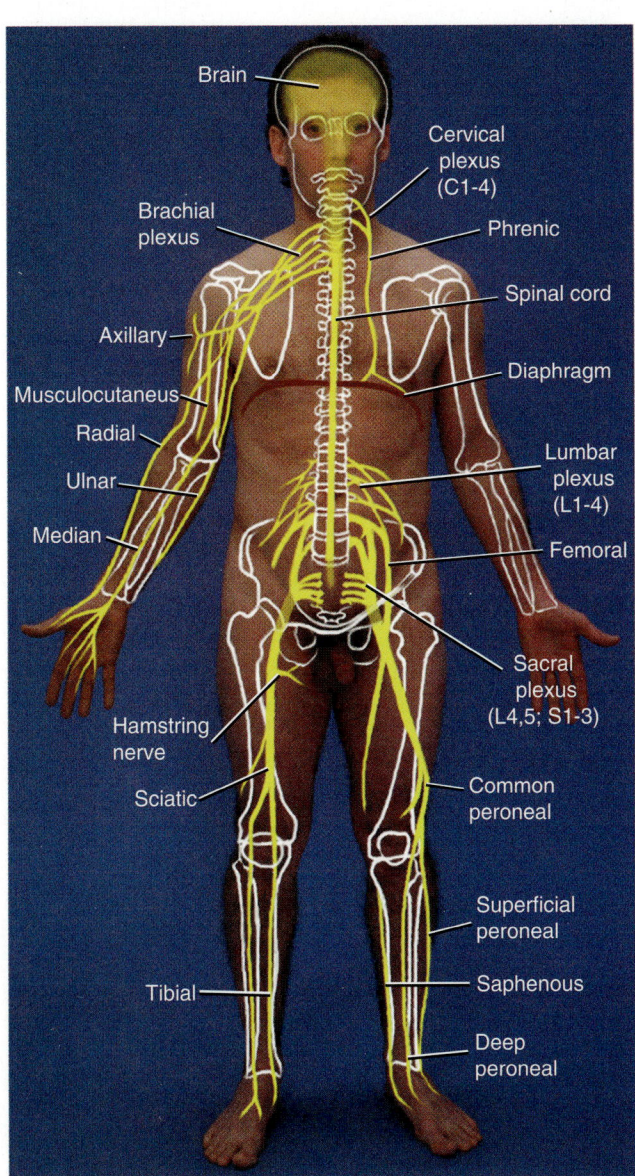

FIGURE 38-4 The Peripheral Nerves DELMAR/CENGAGE LEARNING

orientation, the perception of self in relation to the surrounding environment. When awareness is impaired, orientation to time is frequently the first area affected. The degree of disorientation is worse when the individual loses awareness of place and self (person). Changes in a client's orientation to time, place, and person are often early indicators of an altered level of consciousness (LOC). Several tools have been developed to measure LOC, which includes a measure of orientation.

Memory

There are three types of memory: immediate, recent, and remote. **Immediate memory** is the retention of information for a specified and usually short period of time. An example of this function is the recall of a telephone number long enough to dial it. **Recent memory** is the result of events that have occurred over the past 24 hours. An example of recent memory is the remembrance of foods eaten for dinner the previous night. **Remote memory** is the retention of experiences that occurred during earlier periods of life, such as an adult's memories of childhood. The ability to learn is dependent on remote memory.

Affect

Affect (mood or feeling) is an important component of cognition in that variations of mood can influence one's thinking ability. For example, depression may affect the client's concentration and attention. Also, anxiety narrows the perceptual field and interferes with the ability to concentrate by decreasing attention span.

Judgment

Judgment, the ability to compare or evaluate alternatives to life situations and arrive at an appropriate course of action, is closely related to reality testing and depends on effective cognitive functioning. When assessing logic and judgment, it is important to decide whether the client is answering questions appropriately. The assessment goal is to determine the use of reasoning and decision-making ability. It may be assessed by asking a question such as "What would you do if you were inside a burning building?" Answers that indicate impaired judgment may be given by clients experiencing frontal lobe damage, dementia, mental retardation, or psychosis. Behaviors indicative of impaired judgment include impulsiveness, unrealistic decision making, and inadequate problem-solving ability.

Perception

Cognitive perceptions are considered in the context of the individual's awareness of reality. Misperceptions of reality can occur in the form of an **illusion** (an inaccurate perception or misinterpretation of sensory stimuli) or a **hallucination** (a sensory perception that occurs in the absence of external stimuli and is not based on reality).

Clients who are anxious and fearful or who are taking certain medications may experience misperceptions of environmental stimuli. For example, a postoperative client, after receiving analgesic medication for pain, sees a belt from his

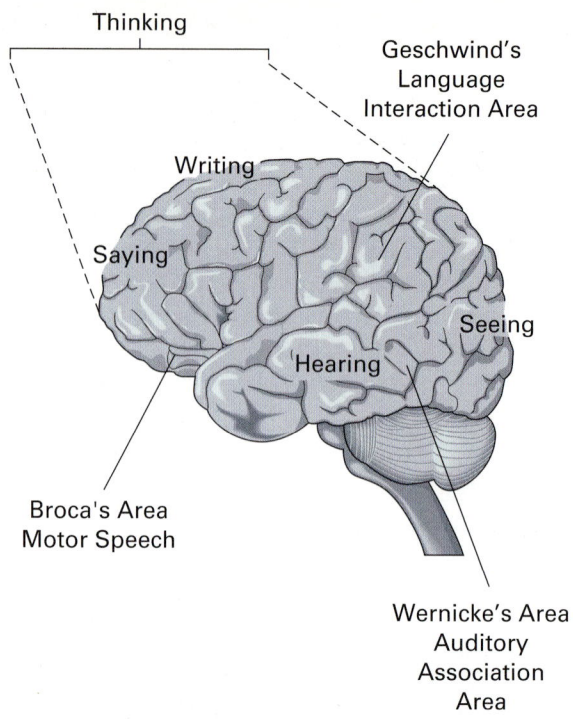

FIGURE 38-6 Language Perception Areas of the Brain. Note Broca's motor speech area in the frontal lobe, Wernicke's auditory association area in the temporal lobe, and Geschwind's language interaction area in the parietal lobe. DELMAR/CENGAGE LEARNING

bathrobe lying on the floor and thinks there is a snake in the room. Once the nurse determines that the client is experiencing an illusion, appropriate reassurance and reality orientation can be implemented to reduce the client's anxiety.

Language

Language is one of the most complex cognitive functions, involving not only the spoken word but also reading, writing, and comprehension. Each of these skills is controlled by specific areas located in the cerebral cortex (see Figure 38-6).

Characteristics of speech are **fluency** (ability to talk in a steady manner), **prosody** (melody of speech that conveys meaning through changes in the tempo, rhythm, and intonation), and content.

FACTORS AFFECTING SENSATION, PERCEPTION, AND COGNITION

The functions of sensation, perception, and cognition are influenced by many factors, including age, environment, lifestyle, stress, illness, and medications.

AGE

Neurosensory pathways in infants and children are immature and do not allow for sophisticated discrimination among stimuli. As children mature they learn to apply their perceptions of the environment to different situations and can thus modify their behaviors accordingly. This process continues throughout the life cycle. For young adults, cognitive functioning is generally more advanced than during adolescence.

Intelligence is difficult to measure; intelligence quotient (IQ) tests, which are intended to predict academic achievement, are not very reliable indicators of adult intelligence. The measurement of intelligence in middle-aged adults is affected by several variables, including motivation, risk taking and caution, and anxiety.

Intellectual functioning is maintained in part by a stimulating environment. **Crystallized intelligence** (acquired knowledge) develops over time as individuals apply life experiences and previously learned skills in order to solve problems. However, **fluid intelligence**, the ability to acquire new concepts in order to adapt to unfamiliar situations, decreases over time (Jaeggi, Buschkuehl, Jonides, & Perrig, 2008).

Cognitive development in older adults shows no decline in intellectual function. Memory loss is an area of concern for many older adults. Research suggests that there is a gradual, age-related reduction in the ability to perform memory tasks (Grady, Springer, Hongwanishkul, McIntosh, & Winocur, 2006). Strategies such as list making and posting reminder notes can be helpful in compensating for minor memory losses. Some activities that encourage cognitive development in older people are reading, studying a new topic (e.g., language, computer skills), solving mathematical problems, and working word puzzles.

ENVIRONMENT

The amount and type of environmental stimuli affect sensation, perception, and cognition. Excessive stimuli in the form of visual impressions and noise can create feelings of anxiety and disorientation within clients. Too few relevant stimuli decrease the client's response to people and the environment, thus leading to isolation.

Crowded living conditions, traffic congestion, and living where sound levels are high are stressors associated with negative physical and psychological health outcomes. Prolonged exposure to loud sounds may impair hearing acuity. Hearing loss affects quality of life and health. In addition to noise-induced hearing loss, which may be permanent, other effects of exposure to noise include tension headaches, lack of concentration, anxiety, hypertension, and insomnia (Belojević, Jakovljević, Stojanov, Slepčevic, & Paunović, 2008; Rhee, Kim, Roh, Kim, & Kwon, 2008; Riethmuller, Muller-Wenk, Knoblauch, & Schoch, 2008).

LIFESTYLE

The amount and quality of sensory information that people feel comfortable in processing are based on their work and leisure habits. Some people may prefer quiet environments in which to think, whereas others derive energy and productivity from the activity around them.

Stress

Stress and anxiety can exert a negative influence on a person's behavior and thought patterns. Depending on the type and degree of stress, the person either finds ways to cope

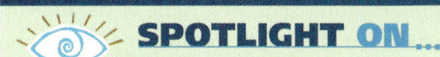

SPOTLIGHT ON...

Caring

Improving Cerebral Blood Flow

It is important for people to maintain an adequate flow of oxygenated blood to the brain. The following activities are helpful: controlling hypertension, monitoring and treating hyperlipidemia and diabetes, and smoking cessation.

with the situation or becomes overwhelmed with the stimuli being received. Individuals experiencing high anxiety levels may become disoriented.

Health Status

Specific conditions, such as diabetes mellitus and atherosclerosis, can impair neurosensory pathways and result in deficits in sensation, perception, and cognition. Diseases of the CNS can result in loss of sensory function and paralysis. Decreased hemoglobin levels generally result in impaired cognition; see the Spotlight On display. Cerebral vascular accidents (strokes) result in cognitive impairments, which may be transient or long term (Lee et al., 2008). "Cognitive impairment is common in the first weeks after stroke … and premorbid moderate alcohol consumption is associated with acute cognitive impairment" (Nys et al., 2007, p. 416). Individuals who experience chronic stress are also at risk of experiencing cognitive impairment (Öhman, Nordin, Bergdahl, Slunga Birgander, & Stigsdotter Neely, 2007).

A person admitted to a health care agency experiences stimuli that are different from those usually encountered in the everyday routine. A change in environment can overwhelm one's ability to perceive and interpret sensory input. As a result, the treatment milieu itself can become a stressor that negatively affects sensory, perceptual, and cognitive functions.

Medications

Certain medications have the potential to alter or depress the neurosensory system. For example, sedatives and narcotics can alter the perception of sensory stimuli. Medications that alter LOC include:

- Analgesics
- Antidepressants
- Antidiuretics
- Antihypertensives
- Benzodiazepines
- Sedatives

SENSORY, PERCEPTUAL, AND COGNITIVE ALTERATIONS

An individual usually experiences discomfort and anxiety when subjected to a change in the type or amount of incoming stimuli. A person can become confused as a result of either overstimulation or understimulation. According to the individual's ability to process the stimuli, confusion (or disorientation) may occur. **Disorientation** is a mentally confused state in which the person's awareness of time, place, self, or situation is impaired; when awareness of these four factors is accurate, a person is said to be "oriented × 4."

Sensory overstimulation and sensory deprivation can lead to cognitive alterations in healthy adults. Such alterations may include physical symptoms (e.g., nausea), altered time perceptions, paranoid ideation, and visual, auditory, and olfactory distortions (similar to hallucinations). The three types of alterations are sensory deficits, sensory deprivation, and sensory overload.

SENSORY DEFICITS

A **sensory deficit** is a change in the perception of sensory stimuli. These deficits can affect all five senses. Examples of sensory deficits are vision and hearing losses such as those caused by cataracts, glaucoma, and presbycusis (steady loss of hearing acuity that occurs with aging).

The client's response to these losses usually depends on the time of onset and severity of the condition. If the problem occurs suddenly and without warning, the client may have difficulty in adjusting to the loss of sensory and perceptual function. If the alteration occurs gradually, the client may be able to accommodate the change and actually compensate for it by strengthening one or more of the other senses.

The effects of illness or intensive medical treatments can exacerbate the problems related to sensory deficits. For example, a client with acute hearing loss can feel alone and vulnerable when faced with an environment that does not provide an effective means (such as interpreters who sign) through which communication can occur. Because of these responses, clients with sensory deficits are at serious risk of experiencing either sensory deprivation or sensory overload.

SENSORY DEPRIVATION

Sensory deprivation is a state of reduced sensory input from the internal or external environment, manifested by alterations in sensory perception. Individuals can experience sensory deprivation as a result of illness, trauma, or isolation. A person experiencing sensory deprivation misinterprets the limited stimuli with a resultant impairment of thoughts and feelings.

The following are factors contributing to sensory deprivation:

- Visual or auditory impairments that limit or prohibit perception of stimuli
- Drugs that produce a sedative effect on the CNS and interfere with the interpretation of stimuli
- Trauma that results in brain damage and decreased cognitive function
- Isolation, either physical or social, that results in the creation of a nonstimulating environment

Some contributing factors (e.g., brain damage or blindness) result in chronic sensory deprivation, whereas others lead to acute, transient states of deprivation (e.g., an individual receiving analgesic medications). Individuals who are sensory deprived may exhibit any of the following characteristics:

- Inability to concentrate
- Poor memory
- Impaired problem-solving ability
- Confusion
- Irritability
- Emotional lability (mood swings)
- Depression
- Boredom and apathy
- Drowsiness
- Hallucinations (see Table 38-2)

TABLE 38-2 Types of Hallucinations

HALLUCINATION	DEFINITION	EXAMPLE
Visual	Perception of sights that are not actually present in the environment	"I see a little pink elephant at the foot of my bed."
Auditory	Perception of sounds that are not present in the environment	"I hear the space aliens telling me that I'll be in outer space soon."
Tactile	Perception of being touched by things not actually present in the environment	"I feel bugs crawling on my skin."
Olfactory	Perception of odors not present in the environment	"I smell old rubber tires burning all the time."
Gustatory	Perception of tastes that do not actually correspond to the foods being eaten	"That bitter taste is in all the food."

Delmar/Cengage Learning

SENSORY OVERLOAD

Sensory overload is a state of excessive and sustained multisensory stimulation manifested by behavioral change and perceptual distortion. The individual experiencing this alteration is unable to process the amount or intensity of stimuli being received. Individuals experiencing sensory overload may exhibit any of the following characteristics:

- Anxiety and restlessness
- Irritability
- Disorientation
- Insomnia
- Fatigue
- Impaired problem-solving ability

Some factors that contribute to sensory overload are:

- Pain originating from a heightened quality or quantity of internal stimuli
- Invasive procedures that result in an increased amount of external stimuli
- Activity-filled, busy environment that contributes to the amount of stimuli being perceived
- Medications that stimulate the CNS and prohibit client from ignoring selective stimuli

- Presence of strangers, both health care professionals and others, who contribute to the quantity of stimuli
- Diseases that affect the CNS and that maximize the perception of stimuli

A common type of stimulus that clients often experience is excessive noise; exposure to high noise levels interferes with the following:

- Ability to shift attention
- Ability to perform complex tasks requiring sustained attention
- Verbal learning and memory
- Ability to make verbal associations

ASSESSMENT

When caring for clients with sensory, perceptual, and cognitive alterations, the nurse must conduct a thorough health history and perform a complete physical examination of the client in order to identify existing or potential problems. See Table 38-3 for an overview of assessing cognition and sensory perception.

TABLE 38-3 Neurological Screening Assessment

ASSESSMENT PARAMETER	ASSESSMENT SKILL	COMMENTS
Mental status, level of consciousness	• Note general appearance, speech content, memory, logic, judgment, and speech patterns during history taking. • Perform Glasgow Coma Scale (GCS) with motor assessment component and pupil assessment.	• If any abnormalities or inconsistencies are evident, perform full mental status assessment. • If GCS is <15, perform full assessment of mental status and consciousness. If motor assessment is abnormal or asymmetrical, perform complete motor and sensory assessment.
Sensation	• Assess pain and vibration in the hands and feet, light touch on the limbs.	• If deficits are identified, perform a complete sensory assessment.
Cranial nerves	• Assess CN II, III, IV, VI: visual acuity, gross visual fields, funduscopic examination, pupillary reactions, and extraocular movements. • Assess CN VII, VIII, IX, X, XII: facial expression, gross hearing, voice, and tongue.	• If any abnormalities exist, perform a complete assessment of all 12 cranial nerves.
Cerebellar function	• Observe the client's initial gait. • Observe the client's ability to (a) walk heel to toe, (b) walk on toes, (c) walk on heels, (d) hop in place, and (e) perform shallow knee bends.	• If any abnormalities exist, perform a complete cerebellar assessment.
Reflexes	• Assess the muscle stretch reflexes and the plantar response.	• If an abnormal response is elicited, perform a complete reflex assessment.

Delmar/Cengage Learning

HEALTH HISTORY

In order to collect data that are used to develop the plan of care, the nurse performs a health history on the client experiencing alterations in sensation, perception, and cognition. Elements of the health history include the client's usual level of functioning, current sensory problems, and potential alterations. The nurse should also explore issues such as the client's current occupation, home environment, and ability to perform both daily routines and self-care activities. The accompanying Nursing Process Highlight presents examples of questions that the nurse can ask the client during the health history.

PHYSICAL EXAMINATION

During the physical examination, the nurse evaluates the client's visual, auditory, gustatory, olfactory, and tactile status. Physical examination focuses specifically on the client's ability to see, hear, taste, smell, perceive heat and cold, and perceive pain. See Chapter 27 for a complete discussion of assessing sensory and neurological status. Table 38-4 provides some guidelines helpful in assessing sensory perceptual status.

NURSING PROCESS HIGHLIGHT

Assessment

Health History: Sample Questions

- Are you experiencing any difficulty in seeing objects, either near or far from you?
- Do you currently wear eyeglasses, bifocals, or contacts?
- Have you recently experienced any changes in your vision—for example, blurred vision, pain, sensitivity to light, or eye fatigue?
- Are you experiencing any changes in your hearing?
- Do you currently wear a hearing aid?
- Have you experienced any unusual sensations in the ears, such as a buzzing or ringing noise?
- Has your appetite or preference for certain foods changed recently?
- Are you experiencing any difficulty in your ability to smell particular odors?
- Do you experience unusual heat or cold in any of your extremities?
- Are you having any problems performing activities such as eating, brushing your hair, bathing, or toileting?
- Have you been exposed to loud noises or chemicals in your work environment or neighborhood?

TABLE 38-4 Assessing Sensory Perceptual Status

SENSATION BEING ASSESSED	ASSESSMENT FOCUS
Visual	• Presence of visual problems, including: — Blurred vision — Double vision — Blind spots — Rainbows or halos around objects — Photosensitivity • Difficulty seeing far or near • Family history of visual problems (such as glaucoma, cataracts) • Use of contact lenses or eyeglasses • Date of last eye examination
Auditory	• Presence of hearing problems • Recent changes in hearing ability • Ability to distinguish sounds (tone and pitch) • Presence of buzzing or ringing noises • Use of a hearing aid
Gustatory	• Changes in ability to taste • Difficulty in differentiating salty, sweet, sour, and bitter tastes • Changes in appetite
Olfactory	• Changes in ability to smell • Ability to distinguish common smells (such as food, perfume, flowers)
Tactile	• Difficulty in feeling temperature changes in extremities • Impairment of pain perception in extremities • Presence of unusual sensations in extremities (such as tingling or numbness)

Delmar/Cengage Learning

Assessment of Cranial Nerves

There are 12 pairs of cranial nerves, most of which have both sensory and motor functions (see Figure 38-3). Assessment of the cranial nerves is done to determine the presence of any neurological deficits. Chapter 27 provides a detailed discussion on assessing the cranial nerves.

MENTAL STATUS ASSESSMENT

A thorough mental status examination includes a systematic assessment of all the emotional and cognitive functions. Changes in LOC provide clues for underlying disorders, which must be identified and treated early; see the Safety First display. Mental status is usually assessed during the health history interview. See the Nursing Checklist for general guidelines on conducting a mental status assessment.

The Mini–Mental Status Examination (MMSE) (Folstein, Folstein, & McHugh, 1975) was developed to determine one's baseline mental status; it includes several questions that assess orientation. The MMSE can be administered as a screening tool for clients in all settings. It is not intended to be used as a diagnostic tool but rather to screen clients for the cognitive aspects of mental functioning: orientation, registration, attention and recall, and language (Folstein et al., 1975). The highest possible score is 30, with a score of 21 or less usually indicating cognitive impairment. A more detailed mental status assessment is warranted if the client presents with any of the following: memory deficit, confusion, aphasia (impairment in language functioning), mood swings, irritability, excessive headaches, behavioral changes, or seizures.

Levels of Consciousness

When assessing clients for sensory, perceptual, and cognitive alterations, the nurse should evaluate the LOC. When describing assessment data relative to LOC, the nurse should include a brief description of the type of stimuli used to test LOC and the client's response. The accompanying Respecting Our Differences display on page 1218 gives a list of terms commonly used in describing LOC.

The Glasgow Coma Scale (GCS) was developed as a standardized tool to assess LOC objectively (Table 38-5). The tool may be used in a variety of clinical situations and is meant to be used in conjunction with a complete neurological assessment. There is a revised version of the GCS for use with children or other individuals who communicate at the preverbal level; see Table 38-6 on page 1218.

FUNCTIONAL ABILITIES

The nurse needs to have an understanding of the client's ability to conduct self-care activities. Any sensory, perceptual, or cognitive impairments may interfere with the client's

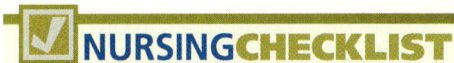

NURSINGCHECKLIST

Assessment of Mental Status

- Assessment begins as the client approaches. Observe gait, posture, mode of dress, involuntary movements, and voice to refine assessment priorities.
- The history should be holistic because neurological disorders can affect all body systems.
- The history should be age-sensitive:
  - Utilize other family members when client is a child.
  - Acknowledge adolescents' ability to speak for themselves.
  - Do not make assumptions regarding older clients' ability to relate their own health history.
- Allow the client to remain clothed during the history and mental status assessment.
- Consider language and cultural norms when obtaining the history and performing the mental status assessment.

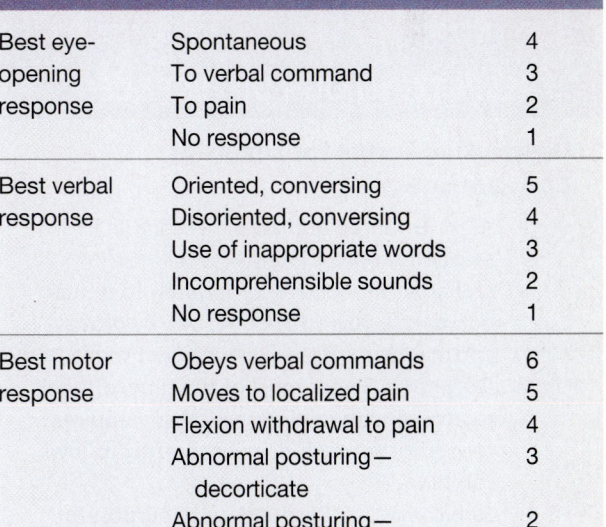

TABLE 38-5 Glasgow Coma Scale

BEHAVIOR	RESPONSE	SCORE
Best eye-opening response	Spontaneous	4
	To verbal command	3
	To pain	2
	No response	1
Best verbal response	Oriented, conversing	5
	Disoriented, conversing	4
	Use of inappropriate words	3
	Incomprehensible sounds	2
	No response	1
Best motor response	Obeys verbal commands	6
	Moves to localized pain	5
	Flexion withdrawal to pain	4
	Abnormal posturing—decorticate	3
	Abnormal posturing—decerebrate	2
	No response	1
Total		3 to 15

Note: With the GCS, a score of 15 indicates a fully oriented person. A score of 7 or less is considered a state of coma. A score of 3 is the lowest possible score and is indicative of deep coma.
Delmar/Cengage Learning

▼ SAFETY FIRST ▼

LEVEL OF CONSCIOUSNESS AND RESPIRATORY FUCNTION

Deterioration in a client's level of consciousness may indicate that intracranial pressure is increasing. This is a life-threatening condition that requires immediate intervention because it depresses respirations.

TABLE 38-6 Pediatric Glasgow Coma Scale

BEHAVIOR	RESPONSE	SCORE
Best eye-opening response	Eyes open spontaneously	4
	Eye opening to speech	3
	Eye opening to pain	2
	No eye opening	1
Best verbal response	Coos or babbles (normal activity)	5
	Is irritable and continually cries	4
	Cries to pain	3
	Moans to pain	2
	No verbal response	1
Best motor response	Spontaneous or purposeful movement	6
	Withdraws from touch	5
	Withdraws from pain	4
	Abnormal flexion to pain—decorticate	3
	Extension to pain—decerebrate	2
	No response	1

Note: Any score of less than 8 represents a significant risk to mortality.
Delmar/Cengage Learning

RESPECTING OUR DIFFERENCES

Descriptive Terms for Levels of Consciousness

- *Alert.* Oriented and aware of stimuli; responds appropriately.
- *Lethargic.* Responds appropriately to stimuli but may be slow to respond; may be drowsy and may drift off to sleep when not stimulated.
- *Obtunded.* Sleeps most of the time; difficult to arouse with minimal response; requires constant stimulation; inconsistently follows commands.
- *Semicomatose.* Responds with purposeful movements when stimulated, but does not follow commands and is nonverbal.
- *Comatose.* Unconscious with no meaningful response to stimuli. Light coma may include reflex motor response to painful stimuli (decorticate or decerebrate posturing); deep coma includes no motor response to any stimuli.

ability to perform activities of daily living (ADL). Functional impairments can interfere with the client's ability to keep the home environment clean and safe. A thorough assessment of self-care abilities includes assessment of skills related to dressing, grooming, bathing, feeding, and toileting. See the accompanying Nursing Process Highlight for hints on assessing potential hearing loss.

ENVIRONMENT

A person's environment can affect sensory, perceptual, and cognitive status in a variety of ways. For example, a nonstimulating environment can lead to sensory deprivation, whereas an environment that is excessively stimulating can result in sensory overload.

People who are at increased risk for sensory perceptual deficits include those who are:

- Older
- Living alone
- Institutionalized
- Homebound
- Experiencing chronic illness or physical handicaps
- Mentally ill
- Affected by a developmental delay

The nurse assesses the type and quantity of stimuli in the client's environment (the health care facility or the home). See the accompanying Community Considerations display on page 1219 for information on assessing the client's home environment.

People with sensory, perceptual, and cognitive alterations are at increased risk of injury. See the Spotlight On display on page 1219. Also see Table 38-7 on page 1219, which lists hazards associated with impairment of sensory, perceptual, and cognitive abilities.

NURSING PROCESS HIGHLIGHT

Assessment

Potential Hearing Loss

Any of the following could be an indicator of hearing loss:

- Experiences tinnitus (ringing in the ears)
- Has a sensation of "stuffiness" or fullness in the ear
- Experiences dullness of hearing (even if temporary)
- Needs to lip-read in order to "hear"
- Fails to respond when spoken to
- Gives inappropriate answers to questions
- Turns head to the side to hear better
- Speaks too loudly or too softly

TABLE 38-7 Safety Hazards Associated with Sensory Perceptual Impairments

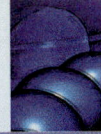

SENSORY IMPAIRMENT	SAFETY RISK
Visual	Tripping, falling
Auditory	Lack of awareness of warning sounds (i.e., automobile horns, sirens, smoke detectors)
Olfactory	Inability to perceive warning odors (i.e., burning food, escaping gas)
Gustatory	Lack of awareness of spoiled or contaminated food or beverages
Tactile	Lack of awareness of excessive pressure on a body part / Risk of exposure to extreme temperature (i.e., frostbite, burns)

Delmar/Cengage Learning

COMMUNITY CONSIDERATIONS

Assessing the Client's Home for Environmental Stimuli

To determine the presence of sensory stimuli, the nurse assesses the presence of the following in the home:

- Adequate lighting
- Clock and calendar
- Odors
- Noise
- Other people (family members or frequency of visitors)
- Television or radio
- Books, magazines, newspapers

DIAGNOSIS

Several nursing diagnoses are applicable to clients experiencing sensory, perceptual, and cognitive alterations. The nurse needs to establish a diagnosis that is most closely related to the client's priority needs. The North American Nursing Diagnosis Association International (NANDA) diagnostic label that is applicable for many clients experiencing altered sensory perception and cognition is *Disturbed sensory perception (specify: visual, auditory, kinesthetic, gustatory, tactile, olfactory).* This condition occurs whenever stimuli are misinterpreted

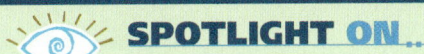

SPOTLIGHT ON...

Legal/Ethical

Safety of the General Public Versus Individual Liberty

Your 72-year-old neighbor, Mrs. Stafford, confides in you one afternoon at her home that she is becoming "more deaf by the minute." She tells you, "Next week when I go in for my driver's license renewal, I am not going to tell them about my little problem." Your neighborhood has several small children who run into and out of the street while playing. How do you respond to Mrs. Stafford?

through exaggeration or distortion (NANDA, 2009). See Table 38-8 on page 1220 for other relevant diagnoses, with defining characteristics and related factors.

PLANNING AND OUTCOME IDENTIFICATION

Nurses understand the importance of promoting optimal sensory stimulation for clients in every practice setting. The following goals will promote supportive, restorative care for clients experiencing sensory, perceptual, or cognitive alterations:

The client will:

- Remain safe and free from injury
- Experience a level of arousal that promotes the meaningful perception of stimuli
- Remain oriented to time, place, person, and situation
- Demonstrate intact functioning of senses (using assistive devices if necessary)
- Perform self-care activities appropriate to own functional capability

The current trend is to provide care for individuals experiencing cognitive deficits at home. See the accompanying Nursing Process Highlight on page 1221 for guidelines on planning the delivery of care in a long-term care facility.

The American Psychiatric Association (2000) has identified the following as skills to be encouraged in order to promote cognitive functioning: stability, consistency, self-identification, and active participation. Table 38-9 on page 1221 lists nursing interventions that enhance the development of these four essential skills.

IMPLEMENTATION

Safety is a major concern of nurses caring for clients with sensory, perceptual, and cognitive alterations. Actions must be taken to ensure that the client's environment is hazard free and, at the same time, that it provides adequate stimulation. This section describes nursing interventions that promote

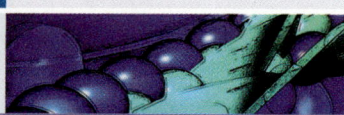

TABLE 38-8 Nursing Diagnoses Related to Sensory, Perceptual, and Cognitive Impairments

DIAGNOSIS	DEFINING CHARACTERISTICS	RELATED FACTORS
Disturbed sensory perception (specify)	**Major** • Inaccurate interpretation of environmental stimuli • Negative change in amount or pattern of incoming stimuli **Minor** • Disoriented to time, place, or people • Impaired problem-solving ability • Changes in behavior or communication pattern • Restlessness • Disturbed sleep patterns • Hallucinations • Fear • Anxiety	• Cerebrovascular accident • Meningitis or encephalitis • Fluid and electrolyte imbalance • Decreased oxygen transport • Medications • Physical isolation • Immobility • Social isolation • Stress
Disturbed thought processes	**Major** • Inaccurate interpretation of stimuli, internal or external **Minor** • Cognitive deficits, including memory deficits • Suspiciousness • Delusions • Hallucinations • Distractibility • Confusion, disorientation • Impulsivity	• Mental disorders or personality changes resulting from biochemical changes • Hormonal changes • Depression • Anxiety • Fear • Loss • Isolation • Ambiguous communication • Abuse • Social isolation
Social isolation	**Major** • Expressed feelings of aloneness and desire for more social contact **Minor** • Verbalization that time is passing slowly • Inability to concentrate • Impaired decision making • Expressed feelings of uselessness • Feelings of rejection • Increased irritability • Restlessness • Failure to interact with others nearby • Feelings of hopelessness	• Communicable disease • Psychiatric illness • Death of a significant other • Divorce • Terminal illness • Hospitalization • Institutionalization • Loss of means of transportation • Unemployment
Risk for injury	**Major** • Developmental age • Altered mobility • Confusion • Disorientation **Minor** • Malnutrition	• Sensory dysfunction (decreased sensation, impaired vision, diminished sense of smell)

From Carpenito-Moyet, L. J. (2007). *Handbook of nursing diagnosis: Application to practice* (12th ed.). Philadelphia: Lippincott Williams & Wilkins; North American Nursing Diagnosis Association International. (2009). *Nursing diagnoses—Definitions and classification 2000–2011* © 2009, 2007, 2005, 2003, 2001, 1998, 1996, 1994 NANDA Interntaional. Used by arrangement with Wiley-Blackwell Publishing, a company of John Wiley & Sons.

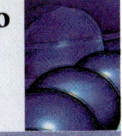

TABLE 38-9 Nursing Interventions to Promote Cognitive Function

INTERVENTION	EXAMPLES
Memory retraining	Supporting reality orientation
Social skills therapy	Reinforcing behaviors to be used when interacting with others
Communication therapy	Improving speech patterns or words to complete a thought
	Minimizing sensory deprivation
Stress management therapy	Identifying and using factors that minimize stress
Reminiscence therapy	Using storytelling and memory recall to identify with past experiences
Behavioral therapy	Maintaining consistency and stability to specify expected behaviors
	Recognizing and controlling environmental stressors
	Using written schedules and directions to assist with activities
Medication administration	Using pharmacologic agents to manage disruptive behaviors

Data from American Psychiatric Association. (2000). *Diagnostic and statistical manual of mental disorders* (4th ed., text rev.). Washington, DC: Author.

appropriate sensory, perceptual, and cognitive functioning. Care of clients with visual and hearing impairments is discussed. Also presented is information on communicating with a confused client and a client who is unconscious.

MANAGING SENSORY DEFICITS

Clients with sensory deficits, including tactile, auditory, and visual impairments, need sensitive nursing care to best adapt to their environments and specific challenges. Safety and appropriate sensory stimulation are major areas of concern; see the Safety First display. Education is very effective in preventing accidents, such as spinal cord injury. In addition to working with clients in the acute phase of illness or injury, nurses also provide restorative care.

Tactile Alterations

The client with impaired tactile sensation is placed at an increased risk for development of skin breakdown. Therefore, it is important to encourage a safe living environment and to educate the individual and significant others in injury preven-

NURSING PROCESS HIGHLIGHT

Planning

Long-Term Care: Promoting Sensory Stimulation

- Call the client by name.
- Introduce yourself by name.
- On every shift, inform the client of the year, month, day of month, day of week, name of facility, and name of health care provider.
- Have a calendar and clock that are easy to see near the client's bed.
- Explain all procedures prior to implementation.
- Name and state the purpose of medications before administration.
- Have all necessary assistive devices (eyeglasses, dentures, hearing aid) accessible.
- Encourage client and family to personalize immediate environment with personal items (clothing, family photos, and personal possessions, such as quilts or furniture from home, if feasible).

tion measures. For more information on preventing tissue and skin breakdown, refer to Chapter 37. See the Client Teaching Checklist on page 1222, which describes therapeutic approaches for maintaining skin integrity of clients with altered touch sensation.

Hearing Deficit

In addition to safety hazards, individuals with impaired hearing are also at risk for social isolation because of the difficulty communicating with others. Nurses must ensure that they spend time with hearing-impaired clients, focus on nonverbal communication, and face the client when speaking. Check all assistive devices used by clients to ensure that they are working properly. Use an interpreter when one is available for signing. If an interpreter is available, the nurse must talk to the *client,* not to the interpreter; see the accompanying Respecting Our Differences display on page 1222 for more information on communicating through an interpreter. Other communication aids include finger spelling, communication boards, and the use of paper and pen for writing messages. Refer to

▼ **SAFETY FIRST** ▼

SENSORY ALTERATIONS AND SAFETY
The client with impaired level of consciousness, weak memory, altered judgment, or confusion is at high risk for injury. It is essential to create a living environment that is safe for people experiencing sensory, perceptual, and cognitive deficits.

✓ CLIENT TEACHING CHECKLIST

The Client with a Tactile Deficit

Teach the client and family that burns can occur not only from heat but also from friction, chemicals, or tape. It is important for the client to inspect skin daily and to avoid the following:

- Sun exposure
- Hot bath water
- Hot water bottles, heating pads
- Placing containers of hot food or liquids in lap
- Eating hot foods or other items that maintain heat for extended periods (e.g., pizza) without first testing the temperature
- Sitting on objects that may be hot (heaters, concrete or rocks in sunlight)
- Walking on hot surfaces (pavement or sand) without shoes
- Contact with items in or on an automobile that are hot from exhaust or sunlight (e.g., tailpipe, heater vents directed at feet, seatbelt buckles, steering wheel, and leather or vinyl upholstery)
- Overexposure to very low temperatures (cold weather or ice packs) without proper protection

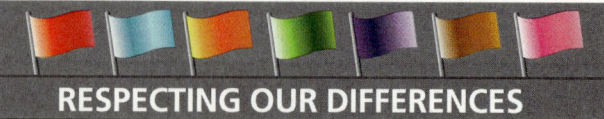

RESPECTING OUR DIFFERENCES

Communicating through an Interpreter

- Plan what you intend to say ahead of time; this avoids confusing the interpreter by having to back up, restate, or revise previous statements.
- Use short sentences and questions.
- Avoid the use of ambiguous statements and questions.
- Avoid the use of technical and medical jargon.

Chapters 15 and 21 for more information on communicating with clients who are hearing impaired.

Visual Impairment

Clients with visual impairments often have developed the other senses to a high degree. The nurse can, therefore, use a variety of ways to enhance communication with such clients. For example, the nurse should do the following:

- Ask the client to explain what is helpful (e.g., preferred means of communicating, usual routine).
- Look directly at the client while speaking.
- Encourage the client to handle items and objects; use objects that can be identified by other senses.
- Keep furniture and other items in their usual places; orient the client to the environment by using clock hours to indicate the position of items in relation to the client.
- Use your normal tone, volume, and rate of speaking.
- Inform the client when you are entering or leaving the room.
- Ask for permission before touching the client.

See Chapters 15 and 21 for discussion of communicating with visually impaired clients.

MANAGING SENSORY DEPRIVATION

It is important to provide an adequate amount of sensory stimulation to those clients who are at risk for developing sensory deprivation. The nurse should provide multisensory stimuli for 5–10-minute intervals throughout the day. Examples of appropriate stimuli are:

- Taped voices of family or friends
- Music (familiar to clients)
- Television
- Touch (applying lotions, different textures to skin)
- Frequent position changes
- Familiar visual stimuli (pictures, personal items)

Allow rest periods with no stimulation (e.g., 30 minutes to 1 hour of uninterrupted sleep every 2–4 hours) to avoid sensory overload.

MANAGING SENSORY OVERLOAD

Caring for clients experiencing sensory overload can be very challenging for nurses, especially in critical care areas (e.g., the emergency department, intensive care unit). It is important to reduce environmental stimuli as much as possible. Reorient clients frequently by talking to them, stating their names, and informing them of the day and time. Also, the nurse should promote social stimulation by encouraging visitors as appropriate to the client's health needs. The accompanying Nursing Checklist on page 1223 provides guidelines for nursing interventions for clients experiencing sensory overload. See also the Uncovering the Evidence display on page 1223.

Assisting the Confused Client

Nurses need to be sensitive and supportive when communicating with a client who is confused because many clients are aware of their cognitive deficit and become frustrated about their inability to process environmental stimuli correctly. The nurse must ask about the client's preferred means of communication and tailor the interaction accordingly. The accompanying Respecting Our Differences display on page 1223 lists some hints for communicating with confused clients.

Sensitive nursing care includes allowing additional time for the client to respond to questions, speaking directly to the client in uncomplicated language, repeating information

UNCOVERING THE

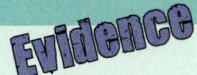

TITLE OF STUDY

"Effects of Intensive Care Unit Noise on Patients: A Study on Coronary Artery Bypass Graft Surgery Patients"

AUTHORS

N. Akansel and S. Kaymakçi

PURPOSE

(1) To measure the noise levels in specific locations of an intensive care unit (ICU) and (2) to determine disturbance levels of clients owing to noise.

METHODS

The study was conducted with 35 clients who had coronary artery bypass graft surgery. The noise level was measured next to the bed of each client. Each client was questioned about disturbance owing to the ICU noise.

FINDINGS

Noises created by other clients who were admitted for the emergency department and operating room, monitor alarms, and conversations among staff members were the most disturbing noise sources for participants. Clients who were located in beds that were closer to the nurses' station were more affected by the noise than other clients.

IMPLICATIONS

Nurses are in key positions to identify stressors that affect clients during hospitalization. Planned nursing activities and proper design of the ICU may help alleviate the negative effects of noise on client well-being.

Akansel, N., & Kaymakçi, S. (2008). Effects of intensive care unit noise on patients: A study on coronary artery bypass graft surgery patients. *Journal of Clinical Nursing, 17*(12), 1581–1590.

NURSING CHECKLIST

Care of the Client Experiencing Sensory Overload

- Address the client by name.
- Provide explanations of all procedures prior to implementation.
- Modify environment to reduce excessive multi-sensory stimulation; reduce distractions, loud noise, and excessive light.
- Use a calm, unhurried manner when communicating with the client.
- Provide a private room whenever feasible.
- Plan the delivery of care to allow for rest periods with no stimulation.
- Use soft background music.
- Keep the environment free of strong odors (including perfume or aftershave lotion).
- Limit the number and frequency of visitors.

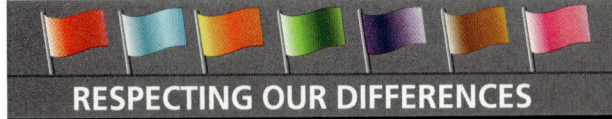

RESPECTING OUR DIFFERENCES

Communicating with the Confused Client

- Choose simple words and short sentences.
- Use a calm tone of voice.
- Avoid talking down to the client.
- Avoid talking about clients as if they were not present.
- Minimize noise and distractions to help the client focus.
- Call the client by name.
- Allow enough time for a response, being careful not to interrupt.

as needed, and using visual clues and body language to reinforce verbal messages. It is also important to address only one topic at a time and to give simple directions in sequence. For example, "First, sit up in bed. Then slide your legs over the edge of the bed." Other interventions that are therapeutic for confused clients include the following:

- Written schedule of activities
- Written checklists for performing ADL
- Written directions for medication self-administration
- Active participation in activities

The accompanying Community Considerations display on page 1224 provides information to share with significant others who are caring for a confused client.

CARING FOR THE UNCONSCIOUS CLIENT

Individuals who are unconscious can often hear what is spoken even though they are unable to respond. Thus, it is important for the nurse to be cautious of what is said in the presence of an unconscious client. Nurses should talk in a normal conversational tone while providing care. Also, remember the value of nonverbal communication, and touch the unconscious client. See the accompanying Nursing Checklist on page 1224 for additional guidelines in communicating with a client who is unconscious.

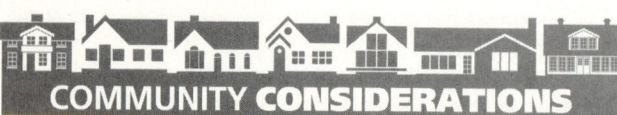

COMMUNITY CONSIDERATIONS

The Confused Client at Home

- Keep clutter in traffic areas at a minimum; remove small rugs that can cause tripping.
- Make sure that bed is low and that there is proper lighting to help prevent falls.
- Keep dangerous objects (e.g., matches, firearms, knives) from client's reach.
- Keep medications out of client's reach.
- Lock doors to areas that could be potentially dangerous if client wandered there.
- Assist in dressing appropriately for the season.
- Do not allow the client to stay alone; have a responsible adult provide supervision.
- Try to keep daily activities as routine as possible.
- Keep activities simple and uncomplicated.
- Provide signs, posters, clocks, and calendars as memory aids.
- Encourage client to be independent while providing assistance as needed.
- Always treat the client with respect and dignity.

USE OF RESTRAINTS

Restraints, both physical and chemical, are sometimes used with clients experiencing cognitive or sensory perceptual alterations. Even though restraints are used to protect cognitively impaired clients from harm, there are some risks of using restraints. Some of the risks associated with the use of restraints include strangulation, impaired circulation, increased risk of falls, and perception that one is being punished.

Therefore, the Centers for Medicare and Medicaid Services and the Joint Commission are mandating the reduced use of restraints in all health care facilities. Minimizing the use of restraints must be done in order to respect client dignity while, at the same time, promoting safety of clients and staff members. See Chapter 29 for guidelines on the safe use of restraints.

COMPLEMENTARY AND ALTERNATIVE THERAPIES

Natural therapies can play an essential role in maintaining a healthy CNS. This section discusses the use of herbs and aromatherapy as methods for enhancing mental well-being. Refer to Chapter 31 for a complete discussion of complementary and alternative treatment approaches.

Herbals

There are four groups of herbs that especially benefit the nervous system: tonics, sedatives, demulcents, and stimulants; see Table 38-10 on page 1225.

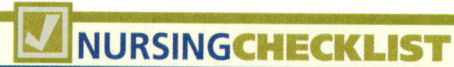

✔ NURSING CHECKLIST

Communicating with an Unconscious Client

- Orient the client to self, situation, place, and time.
- Address the client by name and explain all procedures prior to implementation.
- Maintain a routine to increase the client's sense of security.
- Use touch deliberately.
- Actively listen to significant others.
- Encourage significant others to talk to and touch the client often.
- Treat the client with the same respect and dignity you display to all clients.

Aromatherapy

Aromatherapy can be used to relax or stimulate the CNS. Aromatic molecules emit signals that travel to the limbic system, the emotional switchboard of the brain. The aromas of essential oils serve as catalysts for psychological and physiological changes within the brain. The accompanying Nursing Process Highlight lists some essential oils used to promote a healthy CNS.

EVALUATION

Evaluating the care of the client with sensory, perceptual, and cognitive alterations is dependent on individualized expected outcomes for each client. Evaluation of outcome achievement is performed through the nurse's use of observation and communication skills. An important component of evaluation is determination of clients' ability to meet their own needs. Evaluation of the client's self-care abilities provides information for discharge planning, including follow-up care or placement in a long-term care facility, if necessary.

NURSING PROCESS HIGHLIGHT

Implementation

Essential Oils and CNS Health

- Chamomile (*Anthemis nobilis*): Alleviates physical and mental stress
- Lavender (*Lavandula angustifolia*): Calming, sedative effect
- Mandarin (*Citrus reticulata*): Relieves anxiety
- Peppermint (*Mentha piperita*): Stimulant; strengthens adrenal cortex
- Yarrow (*Achillea millefolium*): Promotes sleep

Data from Gladstar, R. (2008). *Rosemary Gladstar's herbal recipes for vibrant health*. North Adams, MA: Storey Books; Skidmore-Roth, L. (2009). *Mosby's handbook of herbs and natural supplements* (4th ed.). St. Louis, MO: Elsevier.

TABLE 38-10 Effect of Herbs on the CNS

CLASSIFICATION	FUNCTIONS	HERBS
Nerve tonics	• Nourish, tone, and strengthen nerve tissues and cells • High in calcium, magnesium, B vitamins, and protein content • To be most effective, should be taken over long period of time	• Chamomile (*Anthemis nobilis*) • Ginkgo (*Ginkgo biloba*) • St. John's wort (*Hypericum perforatum*) • Skullcap (*Scutellaria lactiflora*)
Nerve demulcents	• Soothe and heal irritated, inflamed nerve endings • Gel-like consistency coats and protects nerve endings	• Barley (*Hordeum vulgare*) • Flax seed • Marshmallow root (*Althaea officinalis*) • Oats (*Avena sativa*) • Slippery elm (*Ulmus rubra*)
Nerve sedatives	• Relax the nervous system • Help reduce pain and tension • Promote sleep • Many exert antispasmodic effects	• Catnip (*Catnip cataria*) • Passion flower (*Passiflora incarnata*) • Hops (*Humulus lupulus*)
Nerve stimulants	• Activate nerve endings by increasing circulation • Provide nutrients • Revitalize the nervous system	• Cayenne (*Capsicum annuum*) • Ginger (*Zingiber officinalis*) • Ginseng (*Panax quinquefolius, Eleuthero-coccus senticosus*) • Lemon balm (*Melissa officinalis*) • Peppermint (*Mentha piperita*) • Rosemary (*Rosmarinus officinalis*) • Sage (*Salvia officinalis*)

Data from Gladstar, R. (2008). *Rosemary Gladstar's herbal recipes for vibrant health*. North Adams, MA: Storey Books; Skidmore-Roth, L. (2009). *Mosby's handbook of herbs and natural supplements* (4th ed.). St. Louis, MO: Elsevier.

NURSING CARE PLAN

The Client with Impaired Memory

CASE PRESENTATION
Mr. Brown, a 53-year-old male, arrives at the clinic with his son, who had found Mr. Brown wandering aimlessly along a road in his community. The son is worried that his father is becoming "more and more forgetful every day." This was first noticed 1 month ago, when Mr. Brown forgot his phone number when completing a job application. Since then, the memory lapses have become more frequent and are now interfering with daily routines (he forgets to take his blood pressure medicine and gets lost returning home). Mr. Brown is currently unemployed and has no health care insurance. He denies that there is any problem and reluctantly agreed to come in today after hearing on the radio about free blood pressure screenings offered by the clinic.

ASSESSMENT
• Impaired memory
• Disorientation (occasionally)

(Continues)

NURSING CARE PLAN (Continued)

- Impaired judgment
- Impaired problem solving or decision making

NURSING DIAGNOSIS 1: *Acute confusion* related to unknown etiology as evidenced by fluctuations in cognition and level of consciousness (LOC) and memory disturbances

NOC: Cognitive orientation
NIC: Reality orientation

EXPECTED OUTCOME
The client will maintain current LOC with no demonstrated deterioration.

INTERVENTIONS/RATIONALES
1. Assess LOC. Establishes a baseline of data in order to intervene quickly if mental status changes.
2. Tell Mr. Brown your name and why you are meeting with him. Keeps client oriented to reality.
3. Talk to Mr. Brown while providing care. Maintains reality orientation.
4. Whenever possible, avoid the use of drugs that may cause drowsiness or sedation. Increased drowsiness or sedation will make it difficult to determine changes in neurological function.
5. Encourage physical and mental activity, daily exercise, and interaction (e.g., with family or friends, newspaper, TV). Improves memory, attention, and orientation.
6. Prepare the client for changes in activity or routines. Reduces confusion and creates a routine to improve orientation.

EVALUATION
Goal partially met. Mr. Brown was oriented to self and place when he arrived at the clinic.

NURSING DIAGNOSIS 2: *Risk for injury* related to cognitive deficits

NOC: Risk control
NIC: Risk identification

EXPECTED OUTCOME
Mr. Brown will remain free of injury.

INTERVENTIONS/RATIONALES
1. Assess environment and make alterations to enhance safety if necessary. Alterations will lessen likelihood of injury.
2. Provide support to significant others and supervision for tasks deemed potentially harmful to client, discouraging tasks as appropriate (e.g., cooking, smoking). Prevents physical injury to client and danger to others.
3. Provide a list of community resources and cost of services (e.g., day treatment centers, home health agencies) and encourage utilization of resources as appropriate. A list will promote access to available resources that offer a safe environment through part- or full-time supervised care.

EVALUATION
Goal partially met. Mr. Brown remained free of injury while at the clinic. He stated he was not interested in the list of community resources.

KEY CONCEPTS

- The well-being of an individual is dependent upon the functions of sensation, perception, and cognition, which are controlled by the central nervous system.

- Primary components of consciousness include arousal and awareness.

- Cognitive and perceptual functioning is inferred through assessment of the client's behaviors (e.g., consciousness, orientation, speech, thought processes, and perceptions).

- The sensory system is made up of a complex network of afferent fibers within the peripheral nerves, efferent tracts located in the spinal cord and brain stem, and the higher cortex (cerebral lobes).

- Consciousness is a state of awareness of one's self, others, and the surrounding environment, and it affects intellect and emotions.

- Consciousness is controlled by the reticular activating system located within the midbrain and thalamus as well as connective fibers between these structures and areas within the cerebral cortex.

- The degree of arousal (alertness) is indicated by a person's general response to the environment.

- Orientation refers to awareness of self in relation to the surrounding environment; an individual who is

- "oriented × 4" is aware of time, place, person, and situation.

- There are three distinct types of memory: immediate, recent, and remote.

- An individual's affect (mood or feeling tone) can influence thinking ability.

- Judgment is the ability to compare or evaluate alternatives to life situations and arrive at an appropriate course of action.

- There are two types of perceptual distortions: illusions and hallucinations.

- Language is one of the most complex of cognitive functions, involving the ability to speak, read, write, and comprehend.

- A person can become confused as a result of either overstimulation or understimulation.

- Sensory deprivation, a state of reduced sensory input, can occur as a result of illness, trauma, or isolation.

- Sensory overload is a state of excessive and sustained multisensory stimulation manifested by behavior change and perceptual distortion.

REVIEW QUESTIONS

1. Which nursing activities are most therapeutic for a client with a visual impairment?
   a. Face the client's interpreter to avoid confusion.
   b. Inform the client when you are entering the room.
   c. Speak in a high-pitched tone of voice.
   d. Talk rapidly to help the client quickly process information.

2. The nurse should be especially alert for the possibility of burns in clients with which sensory perceptual deficits?
   a. Auditory
   b. Olfactory
   c. Tactile
   d. Visual

3. A client is admitted to the intensive care unit following surgery. Which potential problem should be a priority for the nurse who is planning to care for this client?
   a. Decreased anxiety
   b. Impaired mobility
   c. Sensory deprivation
   d. Sensory overload

4. A client has been started on benzodiazepine therapy for treatment of anxiety. When assessing the client,

the nurse will know that the client will most likely exhibit _____.
   a. bloating and flatulence
   b. confusion
   c. headache
   d. nausea

5. A client is admitted to the emergency department following an automobile accident in which he was driving under the influence of alcohol. The client says, "There are ants crawling on my arms!" This client is likely experiencing which type of hallucination?
   a. Auditory
   b. Gustatory
   c. Olfactory
   d. Tactile

6. The nurse must assess a client experiencing a sensory deficit for development of which of the following?
   a. Back pain
   b. Pneumonia
   c. Polyuria
   d. Pressure ulcers

7. A client with an impaired gustatory sensory perception is being treated in the home. When teaching family members how to care for the client, which of the following should have the highest priority?
   a. Buying a hearing aid
   b. Checking expiration dates on food packages
   c. Providing large-print reading materials
   d. Repositioning the client frequently

8. A client is exhibiting signs of confusion. Which nursing actions will promote a safe environment for this client? Select all that apply.
   a. Apply restraints to prevent falls.
   b. Keep the ambient noise level high.
   c. Keep the bed in a low position, and close to the floor.
   d. Keep the room clean and organized.
   e. Perform all ADL for the client in order to conserve his or her energy.
   f. Place the client in a quiet area with no visitors.

9. Which action by the nurse is therapeutic for an unconscious client?
   a. Explain procedures to the client in a normal tone of voice.
   b. Perform nursing tasks quickly and quietly in order not to disturb the client.
   c. Place the client in a quiet room far away from the nurse's station.
   d. Request that family members leave the client alone until consciousness is regained.

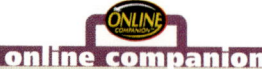
online companion

Visit the DeLaune and Ladner online companion resource at **www.delmar.cengage.com** for additional content and study aids. Click on Online Companions, then select the Nursing discipline.

There are so many things we do, from treatments and antibiotics to laughter, prayer, and collaboration. Our purpose is to facilitate healing.

—Winslow (in Gray, Rayome, & Anson, 1995)

CHAPTER 39

Elimination

COMPETENCIES

1. Describe the normal urinary elimination process.
2. Explain age-related changes that affect elimination.
3. Assess the critical elements of urinary structures.
4. Relate the principles of asepsis to urinary catheterization.
5. Discuss normal bowel elimination.
6. Assess the critical elements of bowel function.
7. Describe the expected outcomes of nursing interventions that promote normal elimination.
8. Discuss nursing interventions for selected alterations in bowel function.

KEY TERMS

bacteriuria	functional incontinence	stoma
constipation	hematuria	stool
defecation	hemorrhoids	stress urinary incontinence
detrusor muscle	impaction	urge urinary incontinence
diarrhea	instability incontinence	urinalysis
dysuria	nocturia	urinary incontinence
extraurethral incontinence	peristalsis	urinary retention
fecal incontinence	pyuria	voiding
flatulence	specific gravity	

Elimination patterns are essential to maintain health. The urinary and gastrointestinal (GI) systems together provide for the elimination of body wastes. The urinary system filters and excretes urine from the body, thereby maintaining fluid, electrolyte, and acid-base balance. Normal bowel function provides for the regular elimination of solid wastes.

During periods of stress and illness, clients experience alterations in elimination patterns. Nurses assess for changes, identify problems, and intervene to assist clients with maintaining proper elimination patterns. The nurse's role encompasses teaching clients self-care activities to promote independence and health.

PHYSIOLOGY OF ELIMINATION

The urinary system is composed of the kidneys, ureters, bladder, and urethra. The kidneys form the urine, the ureters carry urine to the bladder, the bladder acts as a reservoir for the urine, and the urethra is the passageway for the urine to exit the body.

The GI tract is composed of the stomach, small intestine, large intestine, and rectum. The small intestine absorbs nutrients, the large intestine absorbs fluids and the remaining nutrients, and the distal portion of the large intestine collects and stores the remaining solid waste until elimination occurs.

URINARY ELIMINATION

The physiological mechanisms that govern urinary elimination are complex and not yet completely understood. Continence in the adult requires anatomic integrity of the urinary system, nervous control of the detrusor muscle, and a competent sphincter mechanism. Urinary incontinence occurs when abnormalities of one or more of these factors cause an uncontrolled loss of urine that produces social, physiological, or hygienic difficulties for the client.

Structures of the Urinary Tract

The urinary system is typically divided into upper and lower tracts. The upper urinary tract includes the kidneys, renal pelves, and ureters; the lower urinary tract includes the urinary bladder, urethra, and pelvic muscles (see Figure 39-1 on page 1233).

UPPER URINARY TRACT The kidneys are a pair of reddish brown, bean-shaped organs located in the retroperitoneal space, adjacent to vertebral bones T12 to L2. The right kidney lies slightly lower than the left because of the presence of the liver. The periphery of the kidney contains approximately 1 million nephrons; collectively this aspect of the organ is called the parenchyma. The hilus of the kidney (its convex surface) contains the renal pelvis and the ureters, which connect the kidneys and the bladder. The primary function of the kidney is to maintain internal homeostasis through filtration of the blood and production of urine. In addition, the kidney is an endocrine organ (producing erythropoietin, a hormone that aids in the production of red blood cells), and it plays a role in vitamin D synthesis.

After production within the nephron, urine passes through the calyceal system of the kidneys into the renal pelvis. The renal pelvis is shaped like a funnel, holds approximately 15 mL of urine, and serves as a temporary storage area for urine before transport to the lower urinary tract. The ureter is a long tube, shaped like an inverted S, that begins at the renal pelvis, passes under the psoas muscle of the back, and enters the pelvis near the sacroiliac junction. When entering the pelvis, the ureters curve medially to end in the base of the bladder. The union between bladder and ureter is called the ureterovesical junction.

Both the renal pelvis and ureters consist primarily of smooth muscle, and they move urine from the upper to the lower urinary tract by muscular contraction. This process is called peristalsis, and it is similar to the peristaltic waves of the GI system used to digest food and produce fecal waste. The process of peristalsis occurs during the prolonged phases of bladder filling and storage, but it is temporarily interrupted during micturition.

LOWER URINARY TRACT The bladder is a hollow, muscular organ located in the pelvis. It has a fixed base and a distensile upper portion composed of multiple bundles of smooth muscle. Collectively, the smooth muscle bundles are called the detrusor muscle.

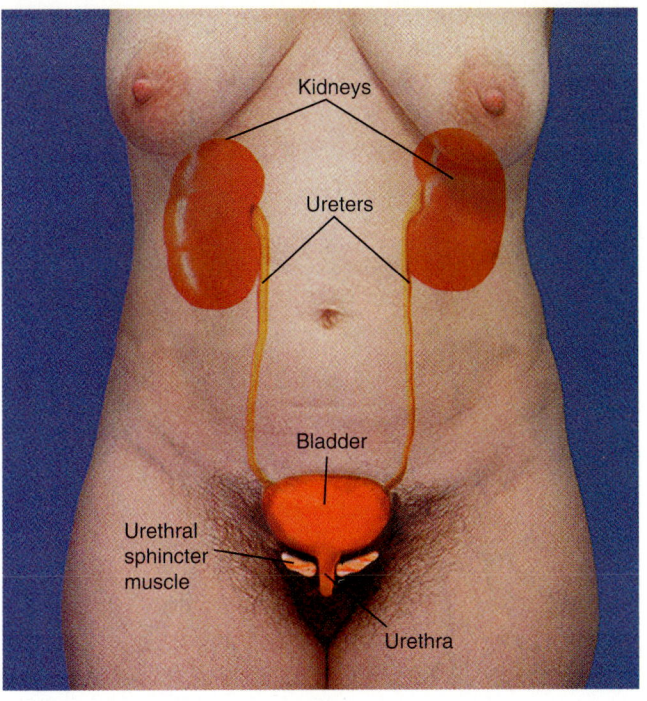

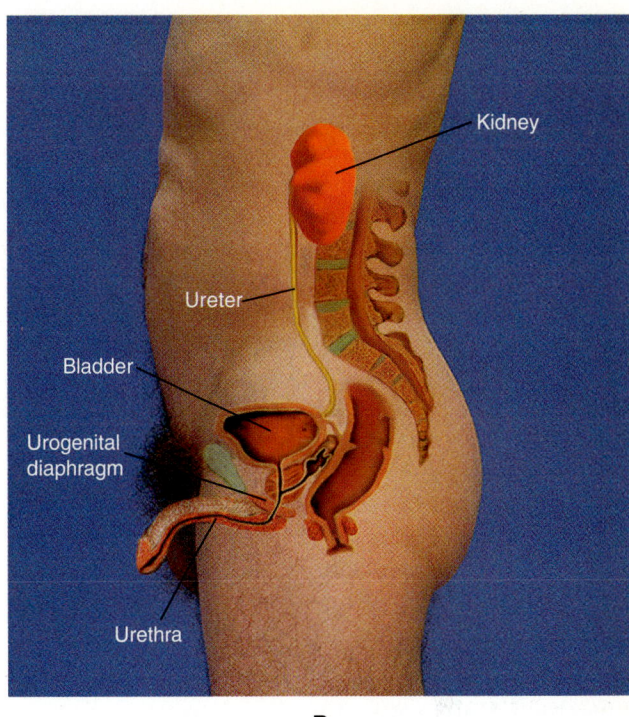

FIGURE 39-1 Urinary Tract: A. Female; B. Male DELMAR/CENGAGE LEARNING

The urethra is a tube that is a conduit for urinary elimination. The urethra differs significantly in women and men. In women, the urethra exits the bladder base and travels at a 16° angle to the external meatus located at the vestibule. The female urethra is approximately 3.5 to 5.5 cm long, and the distal third is histologically fused with the vaginal wall (see Figure 39-1). The entire length of the urethra forms a sphincter mechanism with elements of compression and elements of tension.

In men, the urethra is approximately 23 cm long. It begins at the bladder base, pierces the anterior portion of the prostate, and turns to exit the body through the penis. The proximal third of the male urethra forms a sphincter mechanism comparable to the female urethra. The distal two-thirds is a conduit for the expulsion of urine or semen.

The pelvic muscles connect the anterior and posterior aspects of the bony pelvis, support the organs of the true pelvis, and contribute to the urethral sphincter mechanism in both women and men. The pelvic muscles contain primarily slow-twitch fibers that are physiologically suited for prolonged periods of tone. In addition, fast-twitch fibers within the pelvic muscles respond rapidly to sudden increases in abdominal pressure, although they soon fatigue. Fibers from the pelvic muscles surround the membranous urethra of the male and the proximal two-thirds of the female urethra. In both sexes, the urethra pierces the muscular diaphragm of the pelvic muscles.

Nervous Control of the Detrusor Muscle

The detrusor muscle, the smooth muscle of the bladder, is under indirect voluntary control, allowing the continent adult to postpone urination until a socially appropriate time and location for bladder evacuation is identified. Specific areas of the brain, spinal cord, and peripheral nervous system modulate the reflex activity of the detrusor muscle.

Central nervous control of the bladder begins in several modulatory centers in the brain. A neurologic lesion affecting one or more of these areas causes hyperactive detrusor contractions and a loss of bladder control. The primary areas in the brain that modulate the detrusor muscle are located in the frontal lobes, thalamus, hypothalamus, basal ganglia, and cerebellum. The limbic system, which controls many aspects of autonomic nervous function, also influences continence.

A micturition center, located near the base of the brain, has two groups of neurons that mark the origin of the urination (micturition), the evacuation of urine from the bladder. In the infant, urinary elimination is controlled entirely by the micturition center, which evacuates the bladder when a specific "threshold" volume is reached or when the bladder is stimulated in another way. In the adult, however, the micturition center is controlled by the multiple centers of the brain, and urination usually occurs when the individual wishes to empty the bladder.

Reticulospinal tracts in the spinal cord transmit messages from the brain and brain stem to the peripheral nerves of the bladder. Bladder filling and urinary storage are promoted by excitation of the sympathetic nervous system via efferent, sympathetic spinal nuclei at spinal segments T10 to L2. Excitation of these neurons relaxes the detrusor muscle and contracts the muscular elements of the sphincter mechanism. Urinary evacuation is accomplished through the parasympathetic nervous system. Excitation of neurons located at segments S2 to S4 causes **voiding** (urination) by contraction of the detrusor muscle and relaxation of muscular elements of the sphincter mechanism.

Two peripheral nerves transmit messages from the central nervous system to the detrusor muscle. The pelvic plexus transmits parasympathetic impulses to the smooth muscle of the detrusor. Nervous excitation of the parasympathetic nerves causes release of a neurotransmitter, acetylcholine, which produces contraction of detrusor muscle cells. Other substances also affect contraction of the detrusor muscle, but all act under the influence of the central nervous system.

The inferior hypogastric nerves provide the majority of sympathetic tone to the bladder wall and sphincter mechanism. In the detrusor muscle, excitation of β-adrenergic receptors causes release of norepinephrine, which inhibits detrusor muscle contraction. In addition, stimulation of α-adrenergic (excitatory) receptors at the bladder neck, in the proximal urethra, and in the prostatic urethra in men causes contraction of muscular components of the sphincter mechanism, promoting urethral closure and continence.

Urethral Sphincter Mechanism

The urethral sphincter is traditionally divided into two muscles, an internal (smooth muscle) and external (striated) sphincter. Unfortunately, this schema leads to more confusion than it addresses, and it should be discarded for a conceptualization of the sphincter as a single mechanism, comprising elements of compression and elements of tone, with essential supportive structures.

Urethral compression relies on three components: urethral mucosa softness, mucous secretions, and a vascular cushion. During bladder filling and urinary storage, the epithelium must fill in the gaps of the collapsed (closed) urethral lumen, creating a watertight seal through which no urine can escape. Coaptation requires a pliable, soft, and unscarred urethra, with adequate mucous secretions to reduce surface tension and to fill in the microscopic gaps left by the epithelium. These elements of compression are supplemented by a rich network of vascular connections in the submucosal space. This vascular network promotes urethral closure by nourishing the epithelium and mucous production cells and by serving as a cushion for the transmission of force exerted by the muscular elements of the sphincter mechanism. In women, all the elements of compression are directly influenced by the presence of estrogens.

Elements of urethral tension protect the individual from urinary leakage during physical exercise or exertion. Smooth muscle bundles at the bladder neck and proximal urethra (and prostatic urethra of the male) close the urethra during bladder filling and urinary storage. The urethral wall also contains a set of highly specialized, triple-innervated striated muscle fibers that form a rhabdosphincter. It is crucial for maintaining continence during normal exertion. Striated muscle fibers from the pelvic muscle surround the urethra and contribute to the sphincter. These muscles are particularly needed when abdominal pressure changes from sneezing, coughing, or lifting a heavy object.

The muscular elements of the urethra rely on supportive structures to provide an optimal configuration allowing them to contract and relax efficiently. Loss of support interferes with efficient urethral sphincter function.

BOWEL ELIMINATION

The process of normal fecal elimination is not completely understood. Continence primarily relies on the consistency of the **stool** (fecal material), intestinal motility, compliance and contractility of the rectum, and competence of the anal sphincters.

Structures of the Gastrointestinal Tract

The GI system (alimentary canal) begins at the mouth and ends at the anus. The small intestine in the adult is approximately 22 feet long. The small intestine is primarily responsible for the digestion and absorption of nutrients, vitamins, minerals, fluids, and electrolytes. The digestive chyme (mixture of partially digested food and secretions) travels through the small bowel by a combination of segmental contractions and peristaltic waves. Substances that are well tolerated move through the bowel relatively slowly; foods or drugs that are toxic or irritable to the small bowel are evacuated rapidly. The small intestine joins the large bowel (colon) at the ileocecal valve. This valve works in conjunction with the ileocecal sphincter to control emptying of contents from the small intestine into the colon and to prevent regurgitation of digestive chyme from the large to small bowel (see Figure 39-2).

The colon is approximately 5 to 6 feet long in adults. It is divided into six segments: the cecum, ascending colon, transverse colon, descending colon, sigmoid colon, and anal canal. The primary functions of the colon are to collect, concentrate, transport, and eliminate waste materials (feces). The anal

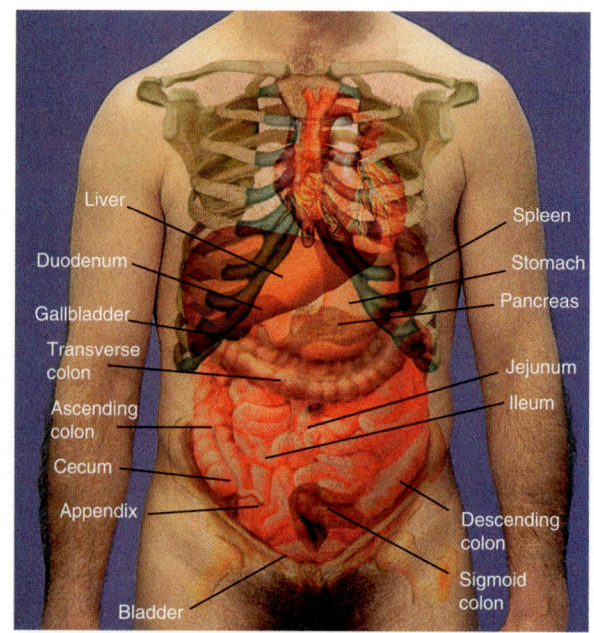

FIGURE 39-2 Gastrointestinal Tract DELMAR/CENGAGE LEARNING

sphincter consists of smooth and skeletal muscles that line the distal portion of the anal canal. It works with the anus to store and to eliminate feces under voluntary control.

Intestinal Motility and Rectal Accommodation

Fecal continence relies on regular delivery of small boluses of stool that are stored in the rectum before elimination. The transit time from ingestion of food to passage of stool from the bowels varies. Typically, at least 80% of intake that is not absorbed by the body is excreted from the bowel within 5 days following ingestion. Transit time is significantly affected by the type of foods ingested, subsequent dietary intake, exercise, and stress-related factors.

Filling of the rectum causes a growing awareness of the presence of stool, which is stored until an appropriate opportunity for defecation, the evacuation of stool from the rectum, is identified. In the continent individual, an initial awareness of stool in the rectum is identified at 150 mL. The desire to defecate is typically transient, diminishing as the rectum accommodates larger volumes of stool. When 400 mL or more of stool is collected in the rectum, this urge becomes strong, and the call to defecate becomes more persistent. Failure to heed the call to defecate may lead to overdistension of the rectum with hardening of the stool and subsequent constipation.

Anal Sphincter Mechanism

The anal sphincter is divided into two mechanisms called the internal and external sphincters (see Figure 39-3). An internal anal sphincter is primarily made up of smooth muscle bundles that are connected to the smooth muscle of the rectum. It begins in the distal portion of the rectum and extends approximately 3 cm into the anal canal. The internal sphincter mechanism is primarily innervated by sympathetic nerves

that promote smooth muscle contraction and by parasympathetic nerves that cause sphincter relaxation.

The external sphincter is composed of striated muscle fibers that are divided into deep and superficial components. The deep portion of the external anal sphincter comprises muscle fibers that encircle the proximal aspect of the anal canal and attach to the symphysis pubis, forming a U shape. The superficial portion of the anal sphincter also encircles the anal canal, forming a U shape; however, it attaches to the coccyx and postanal plate rather than to the anterior aspect of the pelvis. Like the periurethral muscles, the striated component of the external anal sphincter contains both fast- and slow-twitch fibers that allow sustained tone over a period of time before voluntary defecation.

Sensory receptors located at the proximal anal canal affect anal function. These specialized sensory receptors are able to "sample" fecal contents, allowing the individual to differentiate among solid stool, liquid stool, and gas.

Distension of the rectum causes a reflex inhibition of the internal anal sphincter and contraction of the external sphincter. The proximal anal sphincter then samples the contents of the rectum, and the individual perceives the desire to defecate. If the person postpones defecation, rectal accommodation occurs and the desire to defecate is postponed. If the desire to defecate is heeded, the person voluntarily relaxes the external anal sphincter and evacuates the bowel of feces.

The significance of rectal contractions during defecation remains unclear. Many persons strain to defecate, and abdominal force is readily transmitted to the rectum, creating an effective expulsive force. The continent individual is able to simultaneously increase abdominal pressure by straining and maintain external anal sphincter relaxation, allowing effective evacuation of feces from the bowel.

FACTORS AFFECTING ELIMINATION

AGE

A client's age or developmental level will affect control over urinary and bowel patterns. Infants initially lack a pattern to their elimination. Control over bladder and bowel movements can begin as early as 18 months of age but is typically not mastered until age 4. Nighttime control usually takes longer to achieve, and boys typically take longer to develop control over elimination than girls.

Control of elimination is generally constant throughout the adult years, with the exception of illness and pregnancy stages, when temporary loss of control, urgency, and retention may develop. With increasing age comes loss of muscle tone and therefore bladder control; this is usually accompanied by the urge to void more frequently.

DIET

Adequate fluid and fiber intake are critical factors to a client's urinary and bowel health. Inadequate fluid intake is a primary

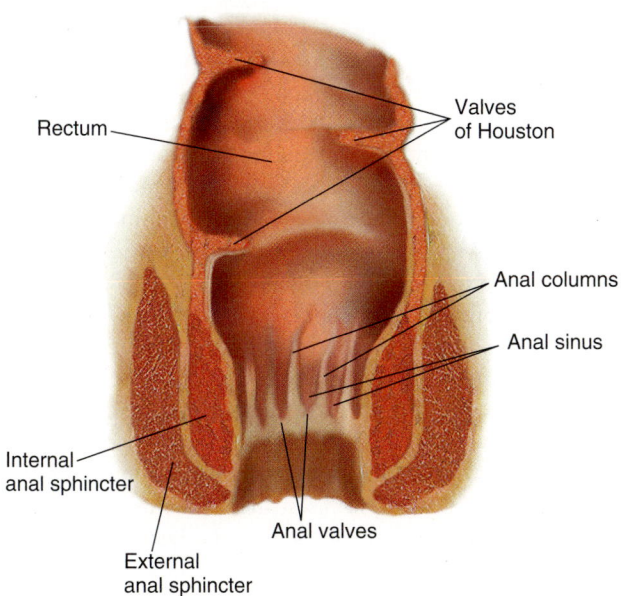

Rectum

Valves of Houston

Anal columns

Anal sinus

Internal anal sphincter

Anal valves

External anal sphincter

FIGURE 39-3 **Anal Sphincter** DELMAR/CENGAGE LEARNING

cause of constipation, as is ingestion of constipating foods such as certain dairy products. Diarrhea and *flatulence* (discharge of gas from the rectum) are a direct result of foods ingested, and clients need to be educated as to which foods and fluids promote healthy elimination and which foods may inhibit it.

EXERCISE

Exercise enhances muscle tone, which leads to better bladder and sphincter control. Peristalsis is also aided by activity, thus promoting healthy bowel elimination patterns.

MEDICATIONS

Medications can have an impact on a client's elimination health and patterns and should be assessed during the health history interview. Cardiac clients, for instance, are commonly prescribed diuretics, which increase urine production. Antidepressants and antihypertensives may lead to urinary retention. Some over-the-counter (OTC) cold remedies, especially antihistamines, may also result in urinary retention. Other OTC medications are designed specifically to promote bowel elimination or to soften stools; the nurse needs to inquire about all medications being taken in order to provide proper care for a client experiencing alterations in elimination patterns.

COMMON ALTERATIONS IN ELIMINATION

URINARY ELIMINATION

Urinary incontinence and urinary retention are the most common causes of altered urinary elimination patterns. Urinary incontinence is the uncontrolled loss of urine that constitutes a social or hygienic problem. Urinary incontinence is

prevalent in men and women across the life span, affecting an estimated 13 million Americans. "It affects approximately 30 percent of the elderly and 50 percent of nursing home residents. Depending on the case mix, rates can be 70 percent and higher in nursing home facilities with a frail, functionally impaired population" (Newman, 2004, p. 17). *Urinary retention* is the inability to completely evacuate urine from the bladder during micturition. There are two primary types of urinary incontinence, acute and chronic. In addition, chronic urinary incontinence can be subdivided into several distinctive types. Because each has its own etiology and management, it is important to determine the type of incontinence before subjecting the client to the expense, potential risks, and rigors of a treatment program.

Acute Urinary Incontinence

Acute urinary incontinence is a transient and reversible loss of urine. It may occur during an acute illness or after an injury. Common causes of acute urinary incontinence include urinary tract infection, atrophic vaginitis, polyuria related to diabetes, acute confusion, immobility, and sedation. Medications that increase or decrease bladder or urethral sphincter tone also may contribute to acute incontinence.

Chronic Urinary Incontinence

Acute incontinence is distinguished from established or chronic incontinence. There are four predominant types of chronic urine loss: stress urinary incontinence, instability incontinence, functional incontinence, and extraurethral incontinence.

STRESS URINARY INCONTINENCE Stress urinary incontinence (SUI) is the uncontrolled loss of urine caused by physical exertion in the absence of a detrusor muscle contraction. SUI is associated with urethral hypermobility or with intrinsic sphincter deficiency. According to Weiss and Newman (2002), there is consistent evidence that the frequency of SUI in women increases with age. The relaxation of the pelvic muscle accelerates rapidly after menopause and may progress with aging. These changes may cause the prolapse of pelvic organs.

Urethral hypermobility is the abnormal movement of the bladder base and urethra during physical exertion. The relationship between urethral hypermobility and SUI is not entirely understood, although several mechanisms have been proposed. Descent of the urethra into the lower portion of the pelvis may cause a loss of abdominal pressure transmission when compared with forces that affect the bladder. In addition, muscular contraction is compromised in the hypermobile urethra. Loss of the normal anatomical relationships between the urethral sphincter and related structures also may contribute to SUI by reducing the efficiency of the muscular elements of the sphincter. The contribution of estrogen deficiency, which compromises the elements of urethral coaptation in the woman, accelerates the rate of atrophy of the mucosal tissue that lines the urethra and vagina. Because of the atrophy and a decline in mucus production within the urethra, the urethra's ability to maintain a tight seal is

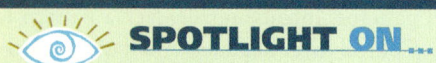
SPOTLIGHT ON...

Caring and Compassion

Sensitivity During the Genital Exam

Assessment of the genital area can produce feelings of anxiety and embarrassment in both clients and nurses. Before beginning the genital examination, consider your client's cultural background and what beliefs or attitudes the client may have about having the examination. Does the client's culture prohibit a female nurse from examining a male client? Does the client's culture prohibit a male nurse from examining a male client? Remember that you are assessing a person, not just a body part.

weakened, especially when intra-abdominal pressure increases with the Valsalva maneuver (Weiss & Newman, 2002). Table 39-1 identifies common factors that contribute to SUI.

Intrinsic sphincter deficiency is a disorder of the muscular components of the urethral sphincter. Sphincter closure is compromised, and urinary leakage is often severe. Severe urine loss caused by intrinsic sphincter deficiency is defined as *total incontinence* by the North American Nursing Diagnosis Association (NANDA, 2009) system. Unlike urethral hypermobility, which is a women's health concern, intrinsic sphincter deficiency occurs in both genders and is related primarily to iatrogenic or neuropathic causes. Table 39-1 identifies common causes of intrinsic sphincter deficiency. It is important to note that intrinsic sphincter deficiency and urethral hypermobility frequently coexist in women.

INSTABILITY INCONTINENCE Instability incontinence is the loss of urine caused by a premature or hyperactive contraction of the detrusor. In the person with normal sensations of the lower urinary tract, these unstable detrusor contractions initially cause a precipitous desire to urinate, followed by urinary leakage unless the opportunity to toilet is immediately available. In those without sensations of bladder filling and impending urination, the contraction is followed by urinary incontinence that is often described as unpredictable. The NANDA (2009) classification schema divides this type of incontinence into two forms: *urge incontinence* and *reflex incontinence*. This distinction is clinically relevant because reflex incontinence is commonly associated with detrusor sphincter dyssynergia, an uncontrolled contraction

of striated muscle of the sphincter mechanism during micturition. Dyssynergia, or a loss of coordination between the bladder and sphincter mechanism, causes a functional obstruction of the bladder outlet and urinary retention. Table 39-2 outlines common causes of instability incontinence of urine.

FUNCTIONAL INCONTINENCE Functional incontinence is the loss of urine caused by altered mobility, dexterity, access to the toilet, or changes in mentation. Altered mobility and dexterity produce incontinence when the individual is unable to reach the toilet within a reasonable time after the onset of the urge to urinate. These conditions are worsened in an unfamiliar environment, such as a hospital, where side rails are raised on beds and sedatives are used to enhance sleep. Difficulty in reaching the toilet due to environmental

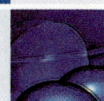

TABLE 39-2 Common Causes of Instability Incontinence

Urge urinary incontinence	Neuropathic (sensations preserved) • Cerebrovascular accident • Brain tumor • Hydrocephalus • Organic brain syndrome (also associated with functional urinary incontinence) • Incomplete spinal lesions (when sensations of bladder filling are preserved) Bladder inflammation • Bladder calculi • Bladder tumor (particularly carcinoma in situ) • Cystitis (may exacerbate subclinical instability) • Atrophic vaginitis
	SUI (39% of women with SUI experience instability and urge incontinence; cause of relationship unclear)
	Bladder outlet obstruction
	Idiopathic (may represent subtle neuropathy or other undiagnosed disorder)
Reflex incontinence	• Spinal lesions above neurologic level S2 • Complete cord injury • Transverse myelitis • Multiple sclerosis

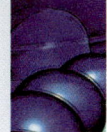

TABLE 39-1 Common Causes of Stress Urinary Incontinence

Urethral hypermobility	• Multiple vaginal deliveries • Forceps-assisted deliveries • Pelvic muscle denervation • Estrogen deficiency • Obesity (exacerbating factor)
Intrinsic sphincter deficiency	Iatrogenic • Multiple bladder suspensions (women) • Radical prostatectomy (men) • Transurethral resection of prostate (men; rare) • Y-V plasty surgery (both genders) Neuropathic • Lesion of lumbosacral spine • Cauda equina syndrome • Pelvic fracture

factors (e.g., stairs, poor lighting, toilet height, narrow doors that are impassable to wheelchairs or walkers) also produces functional incontinence when the obstacles render the person unable to enter the bathroom with reasonable ease. Acute confusion or dementia causes urinary incontinence when the signals to toilet become unclear. Functional incontinence exists as a separate entity from stress or instability urinary leakage. Nonetheless, it is important to remember that functional limitations also exacerbate these forms of urine loss.

Functional incontinence related to dementia may be managed by a prompted voiding technique. Prompted voiding is a technique of providing the opportunity to toilet on the basis of an individualized prompted urge response toileting (PURT) program or using a routine schedule. A PURT program is based on knowledge of the individual's typical voiding pattern. The client's voiding pattern is assessed by the use of a specially designed device to monitor urinary elimination patterns or by routine assessment of containment devices for wetness. The client is then placed on a prompted voiding schedule requiring the nurse or other caregiver to approach the client, offer the opportunity to urinate, and assist with toileting. Voiding is praised, as is dryness during the period before voiding. PURT is limited to clients with adequate cognitive awareness to respond to the prompted voiding and to those with caregivers willing to comply with the demands of this ongoing program. Prompted voiding programs also may be instituted using a more arbitrary schedule for toileting, usually every 2 to 3 hours.

EXTRAURETHRAL INCONTINENCE Extraurethral incontinence is the uncontrolled loss of urine that exists when the sphincter mechanism has been bypassed. According to the NANDA (2007) classification system, extraurethral leakage is termed *total incontinence,* although that term is also applied to severe SUI. The three causes of extraurethral incontinence are ectopia, a congenital defect in which leaks occur from a source outside the urethra; a fistula, an acquired passage allowing urinary leakage; or a surgical bypass of the urinary bladder, such as the ileal conduit. The severity of extraurethral incontinence varies from a dribbling leakage superimposed on an otherwise normal voiding pattern to a continuous urine loss that replaces any recognizable voiding pattern.

Urinary Retention

Urinary retention is caused by two conditions: bladder outlet obstruction and deficient detrusor muscle contraction strength. Bladder outlet obstruction causes incomplete bladder evacuation by blocking the outflow of urine through the sphincter mechanism or the urethra. Deficient detrusor muscle contraction strength occurs when contractions are insufficient to maintain urethral opening long enough for complete emptying of the bladder's contents. Because the management of each condition is different, it is important to differentiate between these disorders during evaluation. Table 39-3 describes common causes of urinary retention.

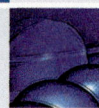

TABLE 39-3	**Common Causes of Urinary Retention**
Bladder outlet obstruction	Prostatic enlargement • Benign prostatic hyperplasia • Prostate cancer • Prostatitis
	Bladder neck dyssynergia (dyssynergia of the smooth muscle of the sphincter mechanism)
	Detrusor sphincter dyssynergia (typically indicates dyssynergia between detrusor and striated muscle of sphincter)
	Urethral stricture
	Urethral tumor (rare)
Deficient detrusor contraction strength	Transient conditions • Fecal impaction • Acute immobility • Side effects of drugs, including anticholinergics, tricyclic antidepressants • Side effect of recreational drugs, including hallucinogens • Herpes zoster of sacral dermatomes
	Established conditions • Lesions of sacral spine • Cauda equina syndrome • Diabetes mellitus (late stages) • Tabes dorsalis • Poliomyelitis

Delmar/Cengage Learning

BOWEL ELIMINATION

Many diseases and conditions affect bowel function. Although many alterations in bowel elimination patterns may be observed, this discussion is limited to three common alterations: constipation, diarrhea, and fecal incontinence.

Constipation

Colonic **constipation** is the infrequent and difficult passage of hardened stool. (Perceived constipation, influenced by psychological and emotional stress, is not included in this discussion.)

Dietary factors may contribute to constipation. Dehydration causes drying of the stool as the body increases the reabsorption of water and sodium from the bowel. Inadequate dietary bulk also dehydrates the stool. Diverticular disease, a common problem in older adults, also reduces colonic transit, further increasing the risk of constipation.

Neuropathic conditions promote constipation by diminishing the efficiency of gastric motility. They also weaken the abdominal muscles, reducing the efficiency of straining and rectal evacuation. Lesions of the brain (e.g., cerebrovascular accident, spinal disorders, disc problems, spinal stenosis) contribute to constipation by reducing mobility, weakening the abdominal muscles, and diminishing the motility of the smooth muscle of the colon and rectum. Functional limitations, particularly impaired mobility, predispose older adult clients to constipation; they perceive a diminished desire to defecate and have a prolonged colonic transit time. Multiple medications, particularly narcotics, sedatives, anticholinergics, antidepressants, antiparkinsonian drugs, and iron, also contribute to constipation.

In women, mechanical factors may exacerbate constipation. A rectocele is the herniation of the rectum and surrounding tissues into the potential space of the vagina (see Figure 39-4). A significant rectocele causes a mechanical obstruction to defecation and subsequent constipation. Both women and men may experience constipation because of incomplete control of the anal sphincter. In this case, failure of complete relaxation of the anal sphincter causes fecal retention, drying of stool, and constipation.

In severe cases, the hardened stool may consolidate into an impaction. This bolus of stool serves as a nidus for bacterial overgrowth and produces an obstruction that further slows colonic transit time and the passage of further fecal contents.

Diarrhea

Diarrhea is the passage of liquefied stool that, because of its increased frequency and consistency, represents a change in the person's bowel habits. The primary causes of diarrhea include infectious agents, malabsorption disorders, inflammatory bowel disease, short bowel syndrome, side effects of drugs, and laxative or enema misuse.

Infectious diarrhea occurs when overgrowth of a pathogen produces osmotic diarrhea via toxins or reduced absorptive ability due to mucosal damage. Common pathogens include *Clostridium difficile (C. difficile),* enterotoxigenic *Escherichia coli, Salmonella, Shigella, Entamoeba histolytica,* and *Giardia* (see Chapter 29 for additional information regarding *C. difficile*).

Malabsorption syndromes produce diarrhea when unabsorbed substances in the diet create an osmotic imbalance and liquefaction of the stool. Lactose intolerance, sorbitol intolerance, and celiac sprue syndrome are examples of common malabsorption syndromes that predispose clients to diarrhea. Persons with inflammatory bowel disease (IBD) or short bowel syndrome are predisposed toward diarrhea because of a reduced surface area for reabsorption. IBD refers to one of two disorders: Crohn's disease or ulcerative colitis. These diseases cause diarrhea, abdominal pain, fever, arthritis of the spine and large joints of the arms and legs, and anorexia, and both can be debilitating and even life threatening (Day, 2008).

Specific drugs may cause diarrhea as a side effect. Administration of multiple antimicrobial agents may indirectly predispose the client to diarrhea by promoting an overgrowth of *C. difficile* in the bowel. Cholinergic drugs increase motility and reduce reabsorption of water and electrolytes from the stool. Other drugs produce osmotic diarrhea, primarily because of the vehicle for delivery, which frequently contains sorbitol and a high osmolality.

Enteral feedings contain a relatively high osmolality that frequently predisposes the client to diarrhea. These formulas may contain lactose, which causes intolerance in some people. The risk of diarrhea is further enhanced in the critically ill who have highly catabolic states and decreased absorptive ability and among those receiving bolus administration of intravenous fluids.

The misuse of laxatives and enemas is frequently associated with diarrhea among clients living at home. Overuse of saline cathartics may produce osmotic diarrhea, and the chronic misuse of laxatives may alter motility patterns and cause an osmotic shift in the bowel.

Secretory diarrhea occurs when the normal mechanisms that produce intestinal fluid are hyperactivated, causing excessive production and movement of food through the intestinal system. Zollinger-Ellison syndrome, pancreatic cholera, carcinoid syndrome, and villous adenoma may produce severe, chronic diarrhea.

Fecal Incontinence

Fecal incontinence is the involuntary loss of stool of sufficient magnitude to create a social or hygienic problem. The primary mechanisms that predispose the adult to incontinence of stool are dysfunction of the anal sphincter, disorders of the delivery of stool to the rectum, disorders of rectal storage, and anatomic defects.

A disorder of stool volume and consistency is typically not enough to produce fecal incontinence in the otherwise normal individual. Instead, the person is likely to perceive a precipitous urgency to defecate, an impulse that is heeded rapidly. However, if the volume of stool is sufficient and the storage capacity of the rectum is compromised or sphincter function is suboptimal, fecal incontinence may result. When severe constipation leads to an impaction of stool, bacteria in the rectum overgrow, producing a liquefied medium. The toxins produced by this liquefied stool are likely to stimulate

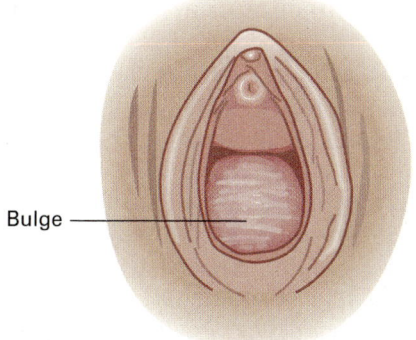

Bulge

FIGURE 39-4 **Rectocele** DELMAR/CENGAGE LEARNING

the bowel and may produce transient seepage of stool in the normally continent client.

Low compliance of the rectum also predisposes the client to fecal incontinence. In the normal individual, the rectum is able to accommodate 400 mL of feces at low pressure. However, clients with radiation proctitis, rectal wall fibrosis due to inflammatory disorders, infectious proctitis, chronic obstruction, or malignancies store lower volumes of stool at higher pressures. Low rectal compliance diminishes storage capacity and causes greater than normal urgency to defecate when stool enters the rectum. When a large volume of stool enters the rectum rapidly, the urgency to defecate is likely to be overwhelming, and the risk of incontinence is significant.

Anal sphincter dysfunction is likely to cause incontinence when both the internal and external mechanisms are compromised. Neurologic lesions are the most common cause of anal sphincter dysfunction. Typically, the client is able to compensate for sphincter weakness, provided the rectum is presented with a normal delivery of solid stool. However, in the presence of diarrhea, significant fecal incontinence may occur.

Sensory disorders also predispose the client to fecal incontinence. Loss of the sensitive epithelium in the proximal anal canal interferes with the client's ability to differentiate gas and solid and liquid contents in the rectum. In addition, loss of proprioception in the rectum disturbs the client's ability to detect rectal fullness. These individuals are particularly prone to incontinence when a large bolus of stool enters the rectum rapidly or when an impaction occurs.

Anatomic disorders also may compromise sphincter function and predispose the individual to fecal incontinence. Among women, the most common risk factor is obstetric trauma. Vaginal deliveries, particularly those requiring the use of forceps and those complicated by third-degree tearing, are likely to damage the anal sphincter mechanism.

ASSESSMENT

The nursing assessment of elimination is based on a client interview and history, evaluation of an objective log or record of urinary or fecal elimination patterns, focused physical examination, and review of diagnostic laboratory data. When altered patterns of elimination indicate a significant health problem, additional diagnostic information is used to formulate a plan of care.

HEALTH HISTORY

Because issues of elimination may produce feelings of anxiety, guilt, or shame among clients, the interview must be instigated by the nurse and conducted in a setting that provides adequate privacy. Clients are asked to describe their usual elimination habits. Table 39-4 on page 1241 presents the typical questions asked when assessing urinary and fecal elimination patterns.

When screening questions concerning altered patterns of elimination reveal significant findings, the interview should be expanded to include specific questions about the nature of the elimination disorder. These questions explore the type of incontinence, complicating factors, and bladder (see Table 39-5 on page 1242) and bowel management strategies currently used by the client. Nurses need to speak freely with clients regarding continence problems since they may have a negative effect on a client's self-image and self-esteem.

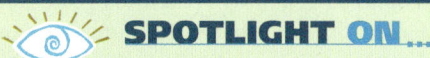

SPOTLIGHT ON...

Caring and Compassion

Assessment of Elimination Patterns

Consider your feelings about urinary and fecal incontinence. Many people, including health care professionals, consider incontinence to be a hygienic rather than a health concern. Parents may view incontinence in children to be a form of misbehavior. Some adults consider incontinence to be a form of childlike or infantile behavior, or they may believe that urinary or fecal leakage is an inevitable consequence of aging. Consider your feelings if you lost control of your bowels or your bladder. Would you not wish your health care providers to consider this a significant problem worthy of aggressive treatment? Would you feel embarrassed about bringing up this problem to a nurse or prescribing practitioner? Would you be relieved when a nurse or prescribing practitioner asked you about this problem? Would you desire privacy when discussing this health care issue?

SPOTLIGHT ON...

Legal and Ethical

Spotting Sexual Abuse

Suspect abuse if you note any of the following during inspection of a client's genital area: bruises, cuts, tears, or bleeding, especially around the genitals, anus, buttocks, hips, and thighs. Emotional signs such as refusing a rectal examination, lack of eye contact during the examination, or extreme anxiety or guarding of body parts during the assessment may all be indicators of abuse. Document all signs of suspected abuse, and know your state's and institution's policies regarding reporting abuse. Remember that no client, regardless of age or gender, should be excluded from evaluation for sexual abuse.

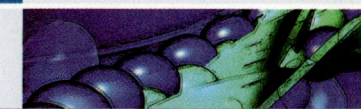

TABLE 39-4 Health History Questions for Clients with Altered Elimination

AREA OF INQUIRY	SAMPLE QUESTION	SIGNIFICANT FINDINGS
Determine duration of problem	• How long have you been bothered with problems controlling your bladder or bowel?	• Association of onset of urinary or fecal incontinence with injury; disorder of central nervous system, brain, or spine; pelvic trauma; vaginal delivery; onset of climacteric.
Determine type of urinary incontinence	• What activities make you leak? • Do you leak when you cough, sneeze, laugh, exercise, or walk? • Do you leak with a strong urge to urinate? • Do you leak with no sensation or warning? • How much do you typically leak? • Is it enough to dampen your underclothing? • Is it enough to saturate your underclothing, dress, or pants? • Is it enough to run down your legs and require a change of clothing?	• Leakage with physical exertion is related to SUI. • Leakage associated with a sudden urge to urinate is related to detrusor hyperactivity (urge incontinence). • Leakage associated with no sensation or warning is generally associated with bypassing of sphincter (extraurethral incontinence). • SUI is typically associated with smaller volumes of leakage with each episode. • Urge incontinence often produces larger-volume leakage.
Determine type of fecal incontinence	• Do you have trouble controlling gas or liquid stool?	• Fecal incontinence associated with motility disorders (dietary intolerance), low compliance of the rectal vault, or rectal urgency is associated with diarrhea. • Intermittent fecal incontinence associated with mild anal sphincter intolerance may cause loss of control only when coping with liquid stool or gas. Regular loss of solid stool is typically associated with central nervous system disorders or significant dysfunction of the anal sphincter mechanism.
Identify complicating factors of urinary incontinence	• Do you ever experience bladder (urine or urinary tract) infections? • Do you feel you completely empty your bladder? • Do you ever lose control of your bowels? • Do you ever seep stool?	• Urinary tract infections are commonly associated with incontinence complicated by obstruction or urinary retention. • Combined fecal and urinary incontinence typically implies neurologic disorders, including altered mentation.
Identify complicating factors of fecal incontinence	• Are there any foods that routinely cause you to experience nausea, vomiting, or diarrhea? • Do you experience constipation? • Do you pass hardened stool? • How frequently do you move your bowels?	• Intolerance of specific dietary elements (e.g., lactose) increases small bowel motility and the subsequent risk of incontinence. • The infrequent, difficult passage of hardened stool (constipation) increases the bacterial load within the rectum, creating a liquid stool around the hardened stool. This bacteria-laden, liquefied stool increases both rectal urgency and the risk of fecal incontinence.

(Continues)

TABLE 39-4 (Continued)

AREA OF INQUIRY	SAMPLE QUESTION	SIGNIFICANT FINDINGS
Identify bladder management program	• How do you manage your leakage?	• Clients often experience complications of urinary incontinence, including altered skin integrity, shame, and humiliation. These can be prevented by using better containment devices.
Identify bowel management program	• How do you evacuate (move) your bowels? • Do you regularly use laxatives, suppositories or other stool softeners, or an enema to assist with a bowel movement?	• The normal individual may move the bowels as frequently as once each day or as little as once every 2–3 days. Clients with perceived or organic constipation frequently use laxatives, stool softeners, or enemas to assist with bowel movements. • Clients with paralyzing neurologic lesions often must use a digital stimulation, an enema, or a suppository to stimulate a bowel movement.

Delmar/Cengage Learning

TABLE 39-5 Questions for Clients with Altered Patterns of Urinary Elimination

AREA OF INQUIRY	SAMPLE QUESTION	SIGNIFICANT FINDINGS
Diurnal voiding habits	• How long can you postpone urination? • Can you postpone urination for 2 hours?	• Diurnal frequency greater than every 2 hours
Nocturia (awakening from sleep to urinate)	• How many times do you wake up at night and urinate? • Does the urge to urinate interrupt your sleep?	• Nocturia greater than once per night in adults younger than 65 years old • Nocturia greater than twice per night in older adults
Urinary incontinence	• Do you leak urine or lose bladder control? • Does this leakage cause any problems for you?	• Any leakage sufficient to be defined as a problem by the client or significant others
Urinary retention	• Do you feel you completely empty your bladder? • Have you ever been unable to urinate at all?	• Any episode of acute urinary retention; suspicion of chronic retention (incomplete emptying) significant when complicated by urinary tract infections or incontinence

Delmar/Cengage Learning

PHYSICAL EXAMINATION

The physical examination for elimination patterns focuses on functional issues associated with urinary or fecal incontinence and assesses the perineal and perianal areas. Functional evaluation begins with the interview and continues throughout the physical examination. Mental status can be evaluated by listening to the client's responses to questions and by observing interactions with others. When mental assessment reveals changes from normal or expected function, a more specific tool, such as the Mini–Mental Status Examination, may be administered (see Chapter 38 for a complete discussion of the Mini–Mental Status Examination).

Mobility and dexterity are evaluated by observation or by asking the client to perform simple tasks. Mobility may be evaluated by observing the client undress or move onto a table, chair, or bed. Dexterity is assessed by observing the client remove clothing; particular attention is paid to the manipulation of zippers, buttons, shoestrings, and snaps.

Inspect all four abdominal quadrants for symmetry, contour, shape, and skin color, noting masses, peristaltic waves, scars, venous patterns, stomas, and lesions. Peristaltic waves are normally not visible; however, observable peristalsis may be a sign of small or large bowel obstruction. Bowel obstructions may be caused by intrinsic or extrinsic compression of the bowel from a tumor, postsurgical adhesions, an ileus (obstruction of the bowel), or a volvulus (twisting of the intestine). Physical assessment findings may also include nausea followed by vomiting when the bowel obstructs, distended abdomen with hyperactive bowel sounds on auscultation above the obstruction, and acute spasms of pain lasting 5 to 15 minutes; with time, bowel sounds become hypoactive (Held-Warmkessel & Schiech, 2008). If the client is experiencing abdominal pain, the client may guard (tighten the abdominal muscles) on palpation; if this occurs, have the client flex the knees to relax the abdomen to provide for a complete palpation of the abdomen. Constipation or obstipation (intractable constipation) develops because the intestinal contents above the obstruction are not being passed.

The perineum is initially inspected for skin integrity. Among clients with severe urinary leakage, the characteristic odor of urine may be present, and the skin may show signs of a monilial rash (maculopapular, red rash with satellite lesions) or an ammonia contact dermatitis (papular rash with saturated, macerated skin). Among clients with severe fecal incontinence, the skin is frequently denuded, red, and painful to touch, particularly if it has been exposed to liquid stool. The integrity of the skin typically remains intact with mild to moderate fecal or urinary incontinence, although a monilial rash may be present. This monilial rash may involve the inner aspect of the thighs, and it frequently extends throughout the skin surface covered by a containment device.

The vaginal vault of the woman is inspected for signs of atrophic vaginitis and for bladder and urethral support. The atrophic vagina has a dry, thin, friable mucosa with a loss of rugae (regular folds of tissue observed in the normal vagina). It is tender to touch, pale, and cracks or bleeds easily. The vaginal introitus and vault may be quite small, and the client may be intolerant of even gentle efforts to distend the vagina for examination. Atrophic vaginal changes are important to assess because they are associated with SUI, irritative voiding symptoms, and urge incontinence.

Pelvic support is assessed in the woman because it is associated with pelvic muscle weakness. Loss of pelvic muscle tone is associated with pelvic descent, increasing the risk of urethral hypermobility or intrinsic sphincter deficiency. Both can lead to SUI or defects of the anal sphincter or rectocele, causing chronic constipation and incomplete evacuation of stool with defecation. Paravaginal support is assessed using a gloved hand or speculum. The posterior vaginal wall is supported using either a Sims speculum or a gloved finger

gently inserted into the vagina. The woman is asked to cough or strain down, and movement of the posterior vaginal wall is evaluated. Bulging of the anterior wall indicates a cystocele or loss of support of the bladder base. This maneuver is repeated, and the posterior vaginal wall is evaluated for the presence of a rectocele. Uterine prolapse is noted when the uterus or cervix migrates toward the vaginal introitus in response to physical exertion.

The sensations of the perineal area are assessed, using a small needle to evaluate sharp versus dull stimuli and using two probes to determine one- versus two-point discrimination. The bulbocavernosus reflex (BCR) is evaluated by gently tapping on the clitoris while observing the anal sphincter. A positive reflex will produce an anal "wink" or contraction of the perianal muscle. A weaker response is assessed by placing a gloved finger at the anus or by pelvic muscle electromyogram using patch or needle electrodes. Loss of sensations or absence of the BCR indicates neurologic damage associated with urinary incontinence or retention.

Careful inspection of the perianal area and a digital rectal examination are particularly important for men and women. The cheeks of the buttocks should be pulled apart and the anus and surrounding area visually inspected. The client may be asked to bear down and the anus inspected for prolapse or for gaping, indicating significant weakness of the anal sphincter. In both genders, the anal sphincter is assessed for tone and symmetry. The gloved, lubricated finger is gently inserted into the anal sphincter. The finger is rotated 360° and the tone of the external sphincter is assessed. In addition, the rectum is palpated for evidence of stool or the hardened, large mass of feces characteristic of fecal impaction. **Hemorrhoids**, perianal varicosities of the hemorrhoidal veins, may also be identified. The prostate is examined for size, consistency, and induration when urinary retention is suspected. Benign prostatic hyperplasia, a common cause of urinary retention in older men, produces a uniform enlargement of the prostate. In contrast, prostate cancer causes asymmetric enlargement or discrete, hard nodules.

When altered patterns of urinary or fecal elimination are suspected from the health history, a log or diary should be completed. The simple bladder log is kept over a long period of time to determine patterns of urinary elimination and patterns of incontinence. A more detailed log allows the nurse to evaluate fluid intake, client responses to prompted toileting, functional bladder capacity, and the estimated volume of an incontinent episode.

DIAGNOSTIC AND LABORATORY DATA

When significant urinary or fecal elimination problems are observed, further testing is needed to evaluate the underlying cause of the condition and to determine treatment options. When urinary incontinence exists, a dipstick **urinalysis** is obtained and evaluated for nitrites, leukocytes, hemoglobin, glucose, and specific gravity. When nitrites or leukocytes are present, a microscopic analysis is completed to determine the presence of white blood cells in the urine (**pyuria**) and bacteria in the urine (**bacteriuria**). Urine culture and

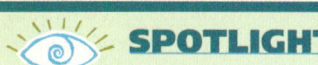

SPOTLIGHT ON...

Professionalism

Professionalism During the Rectal Assessment

The rectal examination may cause the client to feel uncomfortable or embarrassed. How would you handle the following situations if they were to occur during the rectal assessment?

- The client has an erection during the examination.
- The client loses bowel control.
- The client passes flatus during the examination.

sensitivity testing are completed and the client is treated for a urinary tract infection. If glucose is noted in the urine, the client may undergo further evaluation for diabetes mellitus, or methods of glucose control may be reviewed and adjusted in the client with known diabetes. If the specific gravity (the weight of urine compared with the weight of distilled water) of the urine is abnormally low (below 1.010), the volume of fluid consumed by the client over a 24-hour period is evaluated further. Hematuria (blood in the urine) may be noted.

More detailed diagnostic testing of lower urinary tract function may be obtained in cases of complex urinary retention or incontinence. Urodynamics is a set of tests that measure bladder and surrounding abdominal pressures. Pressure data are combined with electromyography of the pelvic muscles and urinary flow rate to determine lower urinary tract function during bladder filling and micturition.

Laboratory tests also may be obtained for select cases of fecal incontinence. A stool culture may be analyzed for ova and parasites, electrolytes, or culture when dietary intolerance or a GI infection is thought to be causing diarrhea and related incontinence. When anal sphincter weakness is suspected as a cause of fecal incontinence, anorectal manometry may be completed to further evaluate anal sphincter and rectal vault function. When pelvic muscle weakness and descent are thought to cause fecal incontinence, defecography (x-ray images of the rectal vault and anal sphincter obtained during defecation) or anorectal ultrasonography may be completed.

Although colonoscopy is the gold standard for colorectal cancer screening, there are several other screening tests available for colorectal cancer, including the fecal occult blood test, the immunochemical fecal occult blood test, flexible sigmoidoscopy, double-contrast barium enema, and computed tomography colonography. The American Cancer Society has developed colorectal screening guidelines based on risk factors; see Chapter 27 for additional information regarding colorectal screening and Chapter 28 for endoscopy procedures.

NURSING DIAGNOSIS

The following nursing diagnoses are frequently encountered in clients experiencing changes in urinary and bowel habits. These nursing diagnoses are based on NANDA's (2009) classification.

IMPAIRED URINARY ELIMINATION

Impaired urinary elimination is the state in which the individual experiences a disturbance in urine elimination. Defining characteristics include dysuria (painful urination), frequency, hesitancy, incontinence, nocturia, retention, and urgency. Altered urinary elimination patterns can result from multiple causes, including anatomic obstruction, sensory motor impairment, and urinary tract infection.

STRESS URINARY INCONTINENCE

Stress urinary incontinence is the state in which an individual experiences a loss of urine less than 50 mL occurring with increased abdominal pressure. Major characteristics include reported or observed dribbling with increased abdominal pressure. Minor characteristics may include urinary urgency and urinary frequency (more often than every 2 hours). The client may also be experiencing related factors such as degenerative changes in pelvic muscles and structural supports associated with increased age, high intra-abdominal pressure (e.g., obesity, gravid uterus), incompetent bladder outlet, overdistension between voidings, or weak pelvic muscles and structural supports.

REFLEX URINARY INCONTINENCE

The state in which an individual experiences an involuntary loss of urine, occurring at somewhat predictable intervals when a specific bladder volume is reached, is known as *Reflex urinary incontinence*. Major characteristics include no awareness of bladder filling, no urge to void or feelings of bladder fullness, and uninhibited bladder contraction or spasm at regular intervals. Related factors include a neurologic impairment (e.g., spinal cord lesion that interferes with conduction of cerebral messages above the level of the reflex arc).

URGE URINARY INCONTINENCE

Urge urinary incontinence is the state in which an individual experiences involuntary passage of urine occurring soon after a strong sense of urgency to void. Major characteristics include urinary urgency, frequency (voiding more often than every 2 hours), and bladder contracture or spasm. Minor characteristics include nocturia (more than two times per night), voiding small amounts (less than 100 mL) or large amounts (more than 550 mL), and inability to reach the toilet in time. Urge incontinence may be related to decreased bladder capacity (e.g., history of pelvic inflammatory disease, abdominal surgeries, indwelling urinary catheter), irritation of bladder stretch receptors causing spasm (e.g., bladder infection), alcohol, caffeine, increased fluids, increased urine concentration, or overdistension of the bladder.

FUNCTIONAL URINARY INCONTINENCE

The state in which an individual experiences an involuntary, unpredictable passage of urine is called *Functional urinary incontinence.* Major characteristics include the urge to void or bladder contractions sufficiently strong to result in loss of urine before reaching an appropriate receptacle. Altered environment and sensory, cognitive, or mobility deficits may contribute to functional incontinence.

TOTAL URINARY INCONTINENCE

Total urinary incontinence is the state in which an individual experiences a continuous and unpredictable loss of urine. Major characteristics include constant flow of urine occurring at unpredictable times without distension, uninhibited bladder contractions or spasms, unsuccessful incontinence refractory treatments, and nocturia. Related factors include neuropathy that prevents transmission of the reflex that indicates bladder fullness; neurologic dysfunction causing triggering of micturition at unpredictable times; independent contraction of the detrusor reflex owing to surgery, trauma, or disease that affects spinal cord nerves; or anatomy (fistula).

URINARY RETENTION

The state in which the individual experiences incomplete emptying of the bladder is known as *Urinary retention.* Major characteristics for urinary retention include bladder distension and small, frequent voiding or absence of urine output. Minor characteristics include sensation of bladder fullness, dribbling, residual urine, dysuria, and overflow incontinence. High urethral pressure caused by a weak detrusor, inhibition of the reflex arc, a strong sphincter, and blockage are related factors for urinary retention.

CONSTIPATION

A state in which an individual experiences a change in normal bowel habits characterized by a decrease in frequency or passage of hard, dry stools is called *Constipation.* Defining characteristics include decreased activity level, frequency of less than the usual pattern, hard-formed stools, a palpable mass, reported feelings of pressure and fullness in rectum, and straining at stool. Other possible characteristics include abdominal pain, appetite impairment, back pain, headache, interference with daily living, and use of laxatives. Related factors for constipation are still under development by NANDA; some possible considerations may be change in daily routine and less than adequate fluid and dietary intake.

PERCEIVED CONSTIPATION

Perceived constipation is the state in which an individual makes a self-diagnosis of constipation and ensures a daily

bowel movement through abuse of laxatives, enemas, and suppositories. Major characteristics include expectation of daily bowel movement, with the resulting overuse of laxatives, enemas, and suppositories, and expected passage of stool at the same time every day. Related factors may include cultural or family health beliefs, faulty appraisal, or impaired thought processes.

DIARRHEA

Diarrhea is the state in which an individual experiences a change in normal bowel habits characterized by the frequent passage of loose, fluid, unformed stools. Defining characteristics include abdominal pain, cramping, increased frequency, increased frequency of bowel sounds, loose or liquid stools, and urgency. Other possible characteristics include change in the color of stools. GI, metabolic, nutritional, or endocrine disorders; infectious processes; tube feedings; fecal impaction; change in dietary intake; adverse affects of medications; and high stress levels may all contribute to diarrhea.

BOWEL INCONTINENCE

A state in which an individual experiences a change in normal bowel habits characterized by involuntary passage of stool is called *Bowel incontinence.* Related factors may include GI and neuromuscular disorders, colostomy, loss of rectal sphincter control, and impaired cognition.

OTHER DIAGNOSES

Other nursing diagnoses that may be important for clients experiencing alterations in elimination patterns include *Situational low self-esteem, Deficient knowledge, Risk for infection, Risk for impaired skin integrity,* and *Toileting self-care deficit.* Nursing diagnoses and the resulting plan of care need to be developed to ensure delivery of thoughtful nursing care for both the physical and psychosocial aspects of altered elimination patterns that may affect a client's well-being.

PLANNING AND OUTCOMES

The targeted outcomes for clients with alterations in elimination patterns center around restoring and maintaining regular elimination habits and preventing potential associated complications such as infections and altered skin integrity. Interventions that respond to the client's physical needs relating to maintaining skin health and fluid volume balance need to be developed, as well as strategies to address the client's psychosocial needs, such as countering deficient knowledge, enhancing self-esteem, and reducing or controlling anxiety.

The Nursing Outcomes Classification (NOC) (Moorhead, Johnson, Swanson, & Mass, 2008) presents nursing sets for *urinary continence, urinary elimination, bowel continence,* and *bowel elimination.* Each of the NOC sets is in the physiological health (I) domain. The primary continence scales span from never demonstrated to consistently demonstrated while the primary elimination scales go from severely compromised to not compromised. *Urinary continence* (control of elimination of urine from the bladder) includes recognizing the urge to void, voiding greater than 150 mL each time in an appropriate receptacle, starting and stopping the stream, and emptying the bladder completely. *Urinary elimination* (collection and discharge of urine) refers to the elimination pattern and the urine odor, amount, color, and clarity. *Bowel continence* (control of passage of stool from the bowel) includes recognizing the urge to defecate, maintaining a predictable pattern of stool evacuation with adequate sphincter tone to control defecation, ingesting an adequate amount of fiber; and toileting independently. *Bowel elimination* (formation and evacuation of stool) refers to the elimination pattern, stool color and amount for the client's diet, and the passage of stool without aids.

The secondary scales go from severe to none to allow for rating the severity of important complications or symptoms. For example, the secondary scale for a urinary tract infection (<100,000 white blood count) refers to visible urine particles, pain with urination, urinary frequency, retention, and incontinence (stress, urge, and functional).

Client teaching is also a critical factor in planning care for clients with urinary and fecal complications. The nurse's role in educating clients concerning proper diet and exercise regimens to maintain urinary and fecal health is an important aspect of planning care. When ostomies are involved, clients and their families will need instruction on and demonstration of proper care and the warning signs of infection.

IMPLEMENTATION

The Nursing Interventions Classification (NIC) (Bulechek, Butcher, & Dochterman, 2008) for clients with alterations in urinary continence and elimination are as follows: bladder and habit training, catheterization, elimination management, incontinence care, retention care, and bladder irrigation. NIC interventions for clients with alterations in bowel continence and elimination include bowel incontinence care, bowel irrigation, management, and training.

MAINTAIN ELIMINATION HEALTH

The nursing management of altered patterns of urinary and bowel elimination begins with an understanding of the principles for general bladder and bowel health and by primary prevention of problems whenever feasible. All clients should be taught basic principles of fluid intake and urinary output, regular bowel evacuation, stool consistency, and altered patterns of elimination. The Client Teaching Checklists offer suggestions for maintaining urinary and bowel elimination patterns.

Fluid Intake

Clients should be taught to drink an adequate volume of fluid each day. The recommended daily allowance (RDA) for fluids is 30 mL/kg body weight, or roughly 1/2 oz/lb

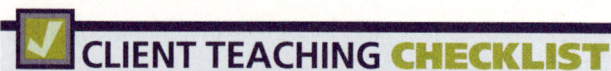

CLIENT TEACHING CHECKLIST

Managing Altered Urinary Elimination

- Ensure adequate daily fluid intake (15 mL/lb body weight).
- Reduce or avoid bladder irritants.
- Reduce alcohol consumption.
- Stop smoking.
- Teach pelvic muscle exercises to women (Kegel exercises).

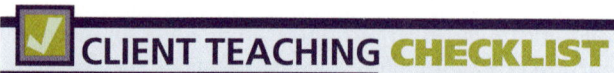

CLIENT TEACHING CHECKLIST

Managing Altered Fecal Elimination

- Understand the relationship between dietary and fluid intake and stool consistency.
- Understand the relationship between altered stool consistency and altered patterns of bowel elimination, including incontinence.
- Ensure adequate daily fluid intake (15 mL/lb body weight).
- Ensure adequate intake of dietary fiber.
- Establish regular schedule of defecation.
- Heed the urge to defecate.

body weight. In the average-sized adult, this equals 1500 to 2000 mL/d, although obese and thin individuals will vary from this range. Manipulation of the volume of fluid intake showed only a weak correlation with voluntary or incontinent episodes in the classical research regarding older women (Wyman, Elswick, Ory, Wilson, & Fantl, 1993). A person who experiences altered patterns of urinary elimination, particularly incontinence, is likely to reduce fluid intake in an attempt to manage the problem. Many clients reason that curtailing fluid intake will reduce urinary output and the risk of incontinence. Unfortunately, it will not. Systematic dehydration may increase rather than diminish the risk of urinary incontinence by promoting bacteriuria and by concentrating the urine, thereby enhancing its irritative properties when stored in the bladder. Dehydration also causes the body to compensate for a shortage of available fluids by reabsorbing fluids and sodium from the bowel, causing drying of the stool and constipation.

Diet

Persons with urinary incontinence or frequent urination associated with urgency should be taught to recognize potential bladder irritants. Specific foods and beverages irritate the bladder and produce frequent urination and bladder discomfort in certain persons, while exerting relatively little effect among others. Foods or substances that may irritate the bladder are:

- Caffeinated beverages, carbonated drinks, and acidic fluids (including coffee and tea)
- Aspartame, particularly when added to a caffeinated or carbonated beverage
- Citrus fruits or juices
- Foods containing tomatoes or tomato-based sauces
- Chocolate
- Greasy or spicy foods

Dietary fiber may prevent constipation and increase the desire to defecate. The client is advised to increase the amount of fiber-rich foods in the diet, including grains, fruits, and vegetables (see Table 39-6). Remind the client that dietary fiber should be increased gradually; a sudden increase in fiber may produce bloating and abdominal discomfort. Clients with either chronic constipation or diarrhea may have to avoid certain foods that trigger symptoms. For example, clients with irritable bowel syndrome (IBS) may benefit from avoiding alcohol, caffeine, high-fat foods, excess fruit, sorbitol, and gas-producing vegetables, which may aggravate IBS symptoms (Brown-Guttovz, 2008).

Lifestyle and Prevention

For many clients, lifestyle and habits affect normal elimination patterns. Individual, social, family, and cultural variables play an important role in elimination. Proper nutrition, adequate rest and sleep, and regular exercise help maintain healthy elimination patterns. Clients with elimination problems can take measures to correct or alter the problem by modifying their lifestyle.

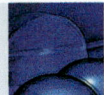

TABLE 39-6	Common Dietary Fiber Sources	
Whole grains	Wheat, rye, oat, millet, buckwheat
	All-Bran cereal
	Shredded wheat cereal
	Popcorn
	Brown rice
Fruits	Apples, pears
	Blackberries, raspberries, strawberries
	Peaches, apricots
	Bananas
Vegetables	Beans
	Asparagus, broccoli, Brussels sprouts
	Carrots
	Garlic
	Acorn squash, zucchini squash

Delmar/Cengage Learning

ALCOHOL AND TOBACCO USE   Consumption of alcohol exerts significant effects on the bladder. Alcohol suppresses antidiuretic hormone (ADH) excretion by the hypothalamus, causing polyuria and increasing the risk of urinary leakage. In addition, the sedative effects of alcohol increase the risk of urinary incontinence, both while awake and during sleep. Alcohol irritates the intestines and bowels, causing inflammation. The irritant effect causes increased elimination of fluid in the stool, resulting in diarrhea. With chronic use of alcohol, inflammation results, causing enteritis or colitis.

Cigarette smoking also may irritate the bladder. Cigarette smoke may increase the risk of SUI because of its association with a chronic cough, and smoking is a significant risk factor for the development of bladder cancer. Smoking stimulates the bowel through the action of nicotine, present in tobacco, causing increased bowel tone and motility. The result is diarrhea.

STRESS MANAGEMENT   Managing stress promotes healthy bowel and urinary elimination patterns. Acute and chronic stress affect both elimination systems. According to Hertig's (2007) study of IBS, stress has been implicated in contributing to the initiation and exacerbation of bowel discomfort symptoms in clients with IBS; in order to reduce GI symptoms, the treatment protocols for IBS should incorporate strategies that decrease stress and psychological distress. The bowel responds by increasing activity when the parasympathetic nervous system is stimulated. However, the longer lasting effect of norepinephrine causes slowing of the GI tract. In response to the effect of ADH, the kidneys retain fluid. The effect of ADH in combination with the effect of norepinephrine and epinephrine elevates the blood pressure. Using education and support, nurses can help clients manage stress.

Elimination Habits

The client is urged to establish a regular schedule of bowel elimination and to answer the desire to defecate. In the normal individual, the desire to move the bowel is transient and lost when avoided or ignored. Although occasional avoidance of the urge to defecate is a useful tool for continence, routine avoidance may predispose the client to constipation and reduce the efficiency of bowel evacuation. The urge to defecate is typically greatest after a meal, and it may be enhanced by dietary stimulants such as fiber or a caffeinated beverage or by light exercise. In an unfamiliar setting, such as the hospital, it is important to provide adequate privacy so that the client can heed the urge to defecate without undue interruption or embarrassment.

Encourage the client to establish a regular elimination pattern to prevent urinary incontinence. This can be successfully accomplished by using techniques such as relaxation and timing. The client, with the assistance of the nurse, establishes a voiding schedule. Once the client has met the goal of staying continent for the established time period, the interval between voidings can be lengthened. Within the interval between urinations, the client can use relaxation exercises to help manage the feelings of urgency.

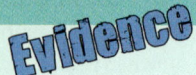

UNCOVERING THE

TITLE OF STUDY
"Daily Stress and Gastrointestinal Symptoms in Women with Irritable Bowel Syndrome"

AUTHOR
Vicky Hertig

PURPOSE
To examine the relationship of daily self-reported stress to gastrointestinal (GI) and psychological distress symptoms both across women and within a woman in a comparison group of women with IBS.

METHODS
Women with IBS were divided into subgroups based on bowel pattern and compared to a group of women without IBS. Self-reported stress measures; abdominal symptoms, bowel pattern, and intestinal gas; and psychological distress symptoms were obtained daily for 1 month. Across-women and within-woman analyses were used.

FINDINGS
There were significant across-women correlations among mean daily stress, psychological distress, and GI symptoms in the total IBS group and IBS bowel pattern subgroups. The across-women relationships between daily stress and GI symptoms were diminished when anxiety and depression were controlled in the analyses. Within-woman analyses showed little evidence of a relationship between day-to-day variations in stress; however, stress was strongly related to anxiety and depression.

IMPLICATIONS
GI symptom distress is associated with self-reported stress in women with IBS. Psychological distress moderates the effects of stress on GI symptoms. IBS treatment protocols that incorporate strategies that decrease stress and psychological distress are likely to reduce GI symptoms.

Hertig, V. (2007). Daily stress and gastrointestinal symptoms in women with irritable bowel syndrome. *Nursing Research, 56*(6), 399–406.

Positioning

Positioning of the client plays an important role in elimination. Sitting is the usual position for both men and women for bowel elimination. Sitting is also the usual position for women to urinate; standing is the position preferred by some men. Clients unable to use the toilet require assistance in accomplishing elimination. Devices such as the bedpan, commode, or urinal can be substituted (see Figures 39-5 and 39-6).

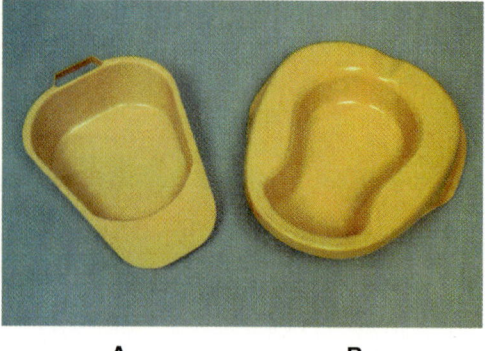

A   **B**

FIGURE 39-5 Types of Bedpans: A. Fracture; B. Regular
DELMAR/CENGAGE LEARNING

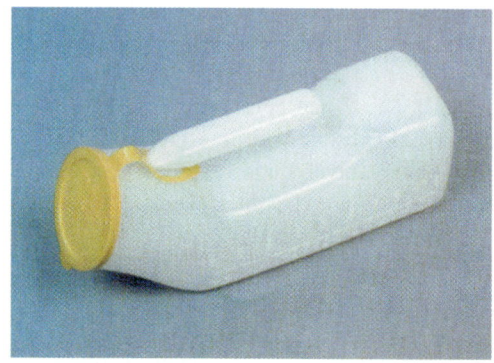

FIGURE 39-6 Male Urinal DELMAR/CENGAGE LEARNING

Clients who use a bedpan need as comfortable a setting as possible; therefore, after placement of the bedpan, the head of the bed should be elevated to a 45° angle, unless contraindicated. The nurse may need to assist the client to cross the legs in order to create somewhat of a sitting position. Male clients who are unable to stand should have the head of the bed elevated to a 45° angle, unless contraindicated, while using the urinal. Procedure 39-1 outlines the steps in positioning and removing a bedpan.

Clients who are able to get out of bed but are unable to ambulate to the toilet can use a bedside commode, which resembles a toilet but is portable. Typically, the client is assisted to stand and pivot to the commode from the bed.

INITIATE EXERCISE REGIMEN

Regular exercise leads to good muscle tone and body metabolism. Exercise also stimulates the bowels to move regularly and leads to good urine production. Poor muscle tone can lead to impaired bladder muscle contraction and poor urination control. Pelvic muscle exercises are taught to manage SUI, and a strength training program is begun using principles of exercise physiology. Clients are taught to identify, isolate, and contract the pelvic muscles and to avoid contraction of distant muscle groups such as the thigh or abdominal muscles. Because clients frequently have difficulty isolating the pelvic muscles, biofeedback may be helpful. The nurse teaches the client to perform a single exercise that combines maximal strength and endurance. The client is asked to perform a maximal strength contraction of the muscles "surrounding the urethra and vagina or rectum" for a count of 10, or approximately 6 seconds, followed by a rest period of equal length. The program begins with few contractions (typically 10 or fewer), and the number of repetitions is increased to a maximum of 35 to 50. The exercise regimen must be integrated into activities of daily living for maximal effectiveness. Pelvic muscle exercises, particularly when combined with biofeedback techniques, are typically taught by a specialty practice or advanced practice nurse with specific education in the management of the client with SUI.

Other management techniques are administered by the advanced practice or specialty practice nurse. These include transvaginal or transrectal electrical stimulation and placement of a vaginal pessary (a supportive device).

Inadequate tone in the abdominal muscles, diaphragm, and perineal muscles can cause difficulty in defecating. If a client is suffering from constipation, a regimen of walking or light recreational exercise should be recommended to promote peristalsis and defecation.

SUGGEST ENVIRONMENTAL MODIFICATIONS

Functional incontinence is managed by removing the barriers to toileting. The environment is manipulated to maximize opportunities for toileting, to minimize the impact of poor mobility, and to remove any environmental barriers. Clothing is carefully evaluated, and buttons, zippers, and multiple layers of clothing are exchanged for items that are simpler to remove. Mobility is maximized by selection of shoes with nonskid soles, and Velcro straps are preferred over strings when dexterity is compromised. The accompanying Community Considerations display on home care describes the effectiveness of environmental modifications in managing functional incontinence.

The nursing management of fecal incontinence begins with measures to normalize stool consistency because constipation and diarrhea increase the risk of incontinent episodes. The environment is also manipulated to minimize functional limitations to bowel elimination. Mobility is enhanced by assistive devices (canes, walkers) as needed and by altering seating and toilets to a height that allows optimal ease when transferring. Clothing is altered to minimize the time required for removal in preparation for defecation. Environmental barriers including poor lighting, narrow doorways, and slippery flooring are removed, or portable toileting facilities are made available.

INITIATE BEHAVIORAL INTERVENTIONS

A scheduled defecation program is used for clients with either a diminished ability to sense rectal distension or altered cognition who are unable to adequately respond to the presence of a bolus of stool in the rectum. The colon is cleansed of any excess stool, using an oral laxative or enema. The diet

COMMUNITY CONSIDERATIONS

Home Care

Mr. M is a 79-year-old with Parkinson's disease and altered cognition. His home health care nurse was consulted for management of his incontinence. A recent medical evaluation showed mild sensory urgency but failed to demonstrate significant urge or SUI. He is cared for primarily by Mrs. M, his 70-year-old wife. She reports using paper towels and baby diapers to contain his urinary leakage. She notes that he is wet every 2 to 3 hours and that he awakens her at night to urinate, but he is unable to postpone voiding long enough to reach the toilet.

On the basis of this health history, his home health care nurse diagnosed functional incontinence. She inspected the home and found that the bathroom was 35 steps from the couch and 15 steps from the bed. Mr. M walks with some difficulty, requiring a walker for assistance. He usually wears slick-soled shoes and trousers with two buttons and a zipper. The home health nurse recommended alterations in clothing and the addition of a handheld urinal for rapid urination. Mr. M has begun to wear stretch-band trousers that can be easily lowered for urination. A handheld urinal was offered when the urge to urinate was perceived, thereby dramatically reducing the number of incontinent episodes. Because of these interventions, no containment device was required for urination, and his incontinent episodes were reduced from two to three per day to fewer than one per week.

is altered to enhance the formation of a soft, solid stool, and supplemental bulk is added if indicated. Patterns of bowel elimination are evaluated, and the client is encouraged to defecate on this schedule if feasible. Otherwise, bowel elimination is scheduled after either a meal or another stimulant, such as a caffeinated beverage or a pharmacologic agent. The importance of heeding the urge to defecate is emphasized, and the client with altered cognition is prompted to defecate.

Clients with significant sensory and motor deficits of the rectum and anus typically require a scheduled defecation program combined with vigorous stimulation of defecation. Persons with a paralyzing neurologic disorder have significant loss of anal sphincter control, poor abdominal muscle control, and altered colonic mobility. As a result, defecation must be scheduled and vigorously stimulated to avoid impaction and fecal incontinence. The colon is cleansed and stool consistency is normalized at the outset of the program. A timetable for bowel elimination is identified. Because of the need for an extensive process for effective defecation, this program must consider the schedule of the client and significant others as well as premorbid defecation patterns. The bowel is stimulated by a pharmacologic device, such as bisacodyl or a mini-enema.

Behavioral interventions play a primary role in the management of urge incontinence. Methods of biofeedback are used to teach the client to perform either a "quick flick" maneuver or a sustained contraction in response to an episode of precipitous urgency. The quick flick is a rapid, maximal contraction of the pelvic muscles held for 3 to 4 seconds, and a sustained contraction is held for 6 to 10 seconds. The client is instructed to stop, rather than rush to the bathroom, thus decreasing the risk of falling. Several quick flicks or a sustained contraction are then performed until the precipitous urge is controlled. At this point, the client is instructed to proceed to the bathroom at a normal pace, but without further delays.

Other techniques, including electrical stimulation and more extensive biofeedback training, also may be used for urge incontinence. These treatment programs are typically managed by the advanced practice or specialty practice continence nurse.

The management of urinary retention is influenced by the underlying cause and the severity of the symptom. Mild urinary retention caused by poor detrusor contractility or obstruction may be managed by timed voiding or by double voiding. Timed voiding is a strategy to reduce overdistension and loss of muscle tone in clients with diminished sensations of urinary urgency. The client is taught to urinate at specific intervals, typically every 3 to 4 hours. Double voiding is an attempt to increase the efficiency of urine evacuation by contracting the detrusor twice during micturition. The client is taught to void, rest on the toilet for 2 to 5 minutes, and void again.

Intermittent catheterization is used for moderate to severe urinary retention, when the residual urine volume is 50% or more of the total bladder capacity. Intermittent self-catheterization is taught using a clean technique. The client is taught to wash the hands and to locate and catheterize the urethra using a water-based soluble lubricant. Catheters may be cleaned and reused, and the client or significant other may catheterize without applying sterile gloves.

MONITOR SKIN INTEGRITY

Because problems with urinary functioning may result in disturbances in hydration and excretion of body wastes, the skin should be carefully assessed for color, texture, turgor, and the excretion of any wastes. The integrity of the skin in the perineal area also should be assessed. Problems with incontinence may result in severe excoriation.

The risk of altered skin integrity is significant. The client is taught to regularly clean and thoroughly dry the skin. Clients with fragile skin are advised to use a skin cleanser; otherwise, use of soap and water is adequate. After cleansing, the skin should be dried thoroughly. A hair dryer set on the low (cool) setting may be recommended.

When monitoring a client with diarrhea, the nurse should assess the perineal skin for altered integrity. After each defecation, the skin is routinely cleansed with tap water or a gentle cleanser specifically designed for incontinence. Soap and water and abrasive cleaning techniques are avoided because they increase discomfort and the risk of altered skin integrity. The skin is then protected by application of a sealant or moisture barrier. Denuded skin is first treated with a pectin-based powder, followed by a skin sealant or moisture barrier.

APPLY A CONTAINMENT DEVICE
Condom Catheter

The condom catheter is a device that resembles a condom with a large-caliber connector at its distal end (see Figure 39-7). This is connected to a drainage bag via a leg bag or bedside container for urinary containment. Procedure 39-2 discusses the application of a condom catheter. Several types of condom catheters are available. The ideal device adheres to the penile skin without producing irritation and has sufficient elasticity to maintain its watertight seal whether the penis is in an erect or a flaccid state. Because of the potential for altered skin integrity, the condom catheter is reserved for severe SUI.

Men without adequate upper extremity dexterity may manage urine containment using a condom catheter. The bladder outlet resistance caused by detrusor sphincter dyssynergia must be managed by pharmacotherapy or by transurethral or laser sphincterotomy. A special device, the UroLume, also may be inserted. This device consists of a wire mesh that is inserted into the urethra via a special cystoscopic device and expanded at the membranous urethra. The wire mesh of the UroLume gently holds the sphincter open, promoting urine evacuation and preventing the deleterious effects of sphincter dyssynergia.

Incontinent and Dribble Pads

Many women attempt to contain urine with feminine hygiene pads. Although these pads effectively contain menstrual flow, they are not designed for urine loss. As a result, they must be changed frequently, and the risk of odor and soiling outer clothing is enhanced. Women with mild SUI typically benefit from a small incontinent pad that adheres to the undergarments. Unlike the feminine hygiene pad, the ideal incontinent pad contains Superabsorbents® that increase the product's absorptive ability. Women with more

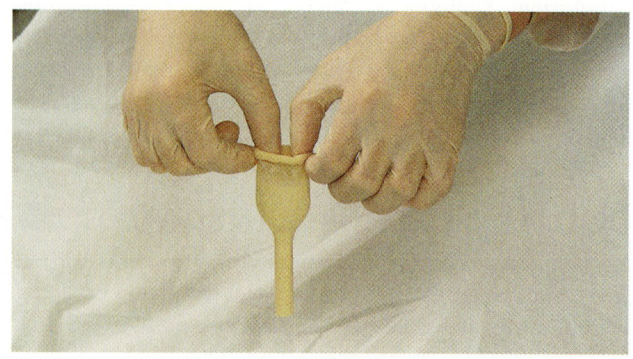

FIGURE 39-7 Condom Catheter DELMAR/CENGAGE LEARNING

severe SUI also may use a device that adheres to the under-garments. However, larger pads that are capable of absorbing up to 500 mL are recommended (see Figure 39-8). Only women with very severe leakage are advised to use an incontinent brief. It is important to remember that containment devices are considered temporary, and the ultimate goal is reduction or ablation of urinary leakage so that pads are not needed.

Men with mild SUI may use a "dribble pad," a device that adheres to the undergarments and holds the penis is a specially designed pouch. More absorptive pads or incontinent briefs are reserved for severe cases. Two additional devices, the penile clamp and condom catheter, are also used for men with SUI. The penile clamp is a constrictive device that mechanically closes the pendulous urethra. The device is worn for a brief period and removed to prevent ischemia to local tissues. Because of the risk of necrosis and discomfort associated with the clamp, its use is limited.

Rectal Pouch and Rectal Tube

Severe diarrhea may justify the use of a rectal pouch or rectal tube to contain leakage and to protect the surrounding skin. The rectal pouch is a drainable pouch attached to an adhesive skin barrier that conforms to the perianal region. The pouch is attached to the perianal area, and any exposed skin

NURSING PROCESS HIGHLIGHT

Implementation

Client Teaching

Teach the client and significant others to remove and reapply the condom. Teach skin inspection and care during routine changes for the hospitalized client. Advise the client to seek care if erosions, rashes, or other lesions are noted on the penis.

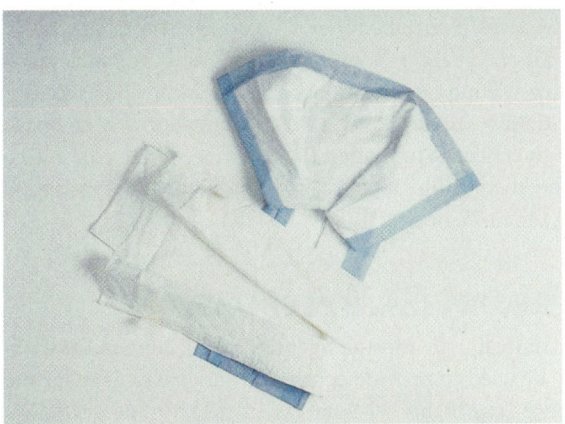

FIGURE 39-8 Incontinent Pads DELMAR/CENGAGE LEARNING

surfaces are carefully protected with a skin sealant. Attachment to intact skin is relatively straightforward; however, application to denuded skin is difficult, and consultation with an enterostomal therapist or incontinence nurse specialist is recommended.

The rectal tube is an alternative to the rectal pouch. A larger catheter (30 French) is passed into the rectum and attached to a large bedside drainage bag. Although the rectal tube is effective for short-term use, its safety when used over longer periods of time is uncertain.

INITIATE DIET AND FLUID THERAPY

It is important to remember that foods and beverages affect each client differently and that a very restrictive diet, designed to remove all potential irritants, is not reasonable for most clients. Therefore, nurses can teach the client to eliminate potential irritants one at a time and to judge the effects on patterns of voiding and urinary leakage.

Dietary fiber and fluid intake can be increased to promote the passage of soft, hydrated stool. The client who is unable or unwilling to obtain adequate fiber from the diet may be given a bulk laxative (such as Metamucil) or a bran mixture as a specific dietary supplement. The nurse should present options for taking this supplement, honoring the client's preferences whenever feasible. Initially, 3 to 6 g of the supplement is administered, and the dosage is gradually increased until a soft, well-formed stool is obtained.

The initial management of diarrhea involves the removal of factors that predispose the individual to the condition and the maintenance of adequate fluid and electrolyte balance. The nurse collaborates with the client, prescribing practitioner, and dietitian to determine foods that contribute to diarrhea by malabsorption or inflammation of the GI tract. These foods are then eliminated from the diet or given with a substance (such as Lactaid) that renders them tolerable to the client. Persons with infectious diarrhea are given antimicrobials to destroy the pathogens that produce diarrhea. Anti-inflammatory drugs are administered as directed for diarrhea caused by inflammatory disorders of the bowel (see the accompanying Nursing Checklist on page 1252 on managing diarrhea).

Bulking agents may be used for clients with watery diarrhea. These agents absorb water in the stool and improve the consistency of feces. Antidiarrheal drugs, including diphenoxylate and loperamide, may be administered to reduce intestinal motility and increase absorption of water from the stool. However, these drugs are contraindicated in clients with infectious diarrhea because the diminished motility would enhance overgrowth of pathogens in the GI tract.

Clients who have significant diarrhea may experience mild to severe dehydration and electrolyte imbalances. Oral fluids are given as tolerated; beverages containing glucose and electrolytes are encouraged. In contrast, beverages that contain caffeine are avoided because they stimulate colonic motility. Individuals with severe fluid volume deficits and large-volume diarrhea may require intravenous fluid and electrolyte support until the diarrhea subsides.

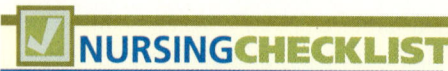

NURSINGCHECKLIST

Managing Diarrhea

- Eliminate from the diet foods and beverages that contain malabsorbed substances.
- Administer antimicrobials for infectious diarrhea.
- Administer anti-inflammatory agents for irritative disorders of the bowel.
- Administer bulking agents for watery stools.
- Provide oral fluids as tolerated; offer fluids rich in electrolytes.
- Administer intravenous fluids and electrolytes as directed for clients unable to tolerate oral fluids.
- Monitor perianal skin for integrity.
- Apply skin barriers for altered integrity.
- Apply a rectal pouch or insert a rectal tube for severe, large-volume diarrhea.

ADMINISTER MEDICATIONS

Constipation is initially managed by assisting the individual to pass hardened stool or by removing any impacted feces (see the accompanying Nursing Checklist on managing constipation). Bowel evacuation is encouraged by an oral laxative, such as psyllium, a bulk-forming agent. Constipation resulting in an impaction requires mechanical disruption and removal, followed by a cleansing enema or an oral laxative. As an alternative, a pulsed irrigation enhanced evacuation (PIEE) system can be used to remove severe impaction. The PIEE uses gravity to deliver intermittent pulses of warmed saline to break up and remove hardened and impacted fecal material.

The medical management of SUI includes both OTC and prescription drugs. OTC medications such as Dexatrim without caffeine and Sudafed contain the α-adrenergic agonists phenylpropanolamine and pseudoephedrine, respectively,

NURSINGCHECKLIST

Managing Constipation

- Remove hardened or impacted stool by mechanical means, cleansing enema, stimulant or laxative, or pulsed irrigation enhanced evacuation (PIEE).
- Increase dietary fiber and fluid until soft, formed stool is obtained.
- Administer supplemental bulk laxative for client intolerant of dietary fiber.
- Encourage light exercise to stimulate defecation.
- Encourage regular pattern of defecation.
- Teach client to stimulate defecation by mini-enema, oral laxative or stimulant, or digital stimulation as needed.

which increase urethral sphincter tone and relieve urinary leakage. Nurses teach the client the specific purpose of these medications, and they advise clients to ignore the dosage and scheduling recommendations on the medication container. Instead, the client is taught to take the medication only during waking hours rather than around the clock to reduce the risk of associated insomnia. Potential side effects associated with these medications, such as restlessness and hypertension, are discussed with the client, and blood pressure is monitored regularly.

SUI also may be managed by prescription medications including imipramine (Tofranil) and topical estrogens, often administered in combination. The client is taught the dosage and administration of each of these agents. Because imipramine has anticholinergic as well as α-adrenergic effects, clients are advised of additional side effects including dry mouth, the potential for constipation, and mydriasis. Women who are placed on topical or systemic estrogens are advised to seek ongoing care from their gynecologist, including routine vaginal examinations and Papanicolaou (Pap) smears.

Medications are often prescribed for urge urinary incontinence. Anticholinergics or antispasmodics relax detrusor muscle contractions by blocking the action of acetylcholine, by a local anesthetic effect, or by a direct effect on the detrusor muscle. Common agents, their actions, and potential side effects are described in Table 39-7 on page 1253. None of these agents will be effective unless the client is taught to adhere to a timed voiding schedule and to identify and limit the intake of bladder irritants.

Several pharmacologic agents may be used in the management of urinary retention. Finasteride, a 5-α-reductase inhibitor, is used to reduce prostatic size and related urinary retention. Men who take finasteride are taught the dosage and administration of the drug and its potential side effects, including impotence and loss of libido. Caregivers are cautioned to refrain from handling the drug without gloves because transdermal absorption and irritation of the skin have been reported.

α-Adrenergic blocking agents also may be used to manage urinary retention caused by prostatic hyperplasia, bladder neck dyssynergia, or detrusor-striated sphincter dyssynergia. Because of the risk of postural hypotension when the medication reaches a peak plasma level, the client is taught to take these drugs before bedtime. Clients are also taught to monitor for medication side effects, including postural dizziness during waking hours, fatigue, and headache. The significance of titrating the dosage of an α-blocking agent is emphasized, and the client is reminded that the dosage must be retitrated if the medication is inadvertently stopped for a period of more than 72 hours.

PERFORM CATHETERIZATION

Occasionally, an indwelling urethral or suprapubic catheter may be used to provide continuous drainage for reflex incontinence (see Figure 39-9 on page 1253). An indwelling catheter may be inserted for an acute episode of urinary retention or when other strategies to manage retention are ineffective.

TABLE 39-7 Common Anticholinergic and Antispasmodic Medications

AGENT	EFFECT	COMMON SIDE EFFECTS
Oxybutynin (Ditropan)	Relaxation of unstable detrusor contractions; reduces urgency; maximal therapeutic response requires 5–7 days	Dry mouth, slightly blurred vision, constipation, nightmares; confusion may occur in older adult clients
Propantheline (Pro-Banthine)	Relaxation of unstable detrusor contractions; maximal therapeutic response requires 3–5 days	Similar to oxybutynin effects
Hyoscyamine (Levsin)	Relaxation of unstable detrusor	Similar to oxybutynin effects, but dry mouth less pronounced

Delmar/Cengage Learning

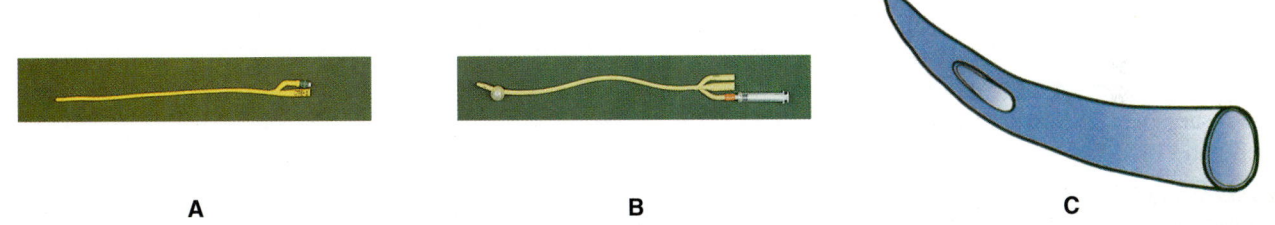

A   **B**   **C**

FIGURE 39-9 Types of Catheters: A. Foley Catheter; B. Three-Way Foley Catheter with Balloon Inflated; C. Coudé Catheter DELMAR/CENGAGE LEARNING

A catheter is chosen that minimizes urethral irritation and maximizes drainage from the bladder. A silicone or other inert-material catheter is preferred over a Silastic catheter coated with Teflon. A Lubricious-coated catheter (Bard Urological, Covington, GA) also may be used because of its hydrophilic nature and its low friction coefficient. The client is provided with a drainage bag with adequate storage capacity for overnight use (typically 2000 mL) and a leg bag with nonlatex straps when indicated.

The use of a coudé catheter is indicated when intermittent catheterization is needed. The coudé catheter works much like the other catheters; however, a distinguishing feature is that the tip of the catheter is more pointed and curved. The coudé catheter does not have a balloon; therefore, it cannot be used for a procedure requiring an indwelling catheter. Procedures 39-3 and 39-4 discuss catheterization. Procedures 39-5 and 39-6 discuss irrigation of catheters.

Intermittent Self-Catheterization

Women with reflex incontinence have more limited options for management because no effective condom device has been designed for women. Intermittent self-catheterization is chosen whenever feasible. This option is typically used in combination with pharmacotherapy for detrusor hyperreflexia. Indwelling catheterization is used only when other means of bladder management are not feasible.

Of the bladder management programs available for the client with a spinal injury or multiple sclerosis and reflex incontinence, intermittent self-catheterization is preferred when feasible. The nurse teaches the client with adequate upper extremity dexterity to perform self-catheterization, and the skill is also taught to significant others. Pharmacotherapy, consisting of an anticholinergic agent, imipramine, or (rarely) a calcium channel blocker, is frequently required to control hyperreflexic detrusor contractions.

ADMINISTER ENEMAS

Enema administration is a procedure used to introduce fluid into the lower bowel. The purpose of an enema is to cleanse the lower bowel, to assist in the evacuation of stool or flatus, or to instill medication. Table 39-8 on page 1254 outlines four types of enemas, along with the solutions and the indications for use of each.

Enemas can be large or small, depending on their purpose. Large-volume enemas, which typically contain 500 to 1000 mL fluid, are administered to cleanse the bowel. Small-volume enemas are used for the purpose of evacuating stool or instilling medications in the lower bowel. These are usually found as prepackaged solutions, which contain 150 to 240 mL fluid. Refer to Procedures 39-7 and 39-8 for guidelines on enema administration.

TABLE 39-8 Types of Enemas

TYPE	SOLUTION	INDICATION
Cleansing	Tap water Soap suds Normal saline	Evacuates lower bowel before diagnostic studies or surgery
Retention (should be retained for at least 30 min)	Emollient (oil)	Softens and lubricates stool for easy evacuation
Carminative (return flow)	Tap water Normal saline	Relieves distension due to flatus
Medication	Normal saline Sterile water mixed with prescribed medication	Depends on what medication is introduced

Delmar/Cengage Learning

TABLE 39-9 Solutions Used for Enemas

SOLUTION	ACTION	CLASS
Tap water	Stimulates and dilates bowel	Hypotonic
Soap suds	Dilates, stimulates, and irritates bowel	Hypotonic
Normal saline	Dilates, stimulates, and irritates bowel	0.9% (isotonic), <0.9% (hypotonic), >0.9% (hypertonic)
Oil	Lubricates, softens	Lubricant
Sodium polystyrene sulfonate (Kayexalate)	Reduces serum potassium	Hypertonic
Antibiotic	Cleansing	Antibacterial; may be hypertonic or hypotonic

Delmar/Cengage Learning

▼ SAFETY FIRST ▼

ENEMA ADMINISTRATION

If "enema till clear" is ordered, no more than 3 L fluid should be administered in any one series of enemas. Repeated enemas produce irritation of the bowel mucosa and perianal area as well as electrolyte loss and exhaustion. If returns are not clear, consult prescribing practitioner for further instructions.

Caution should be used when administering large-volume enemas because fluid and electrolyte imbalance can occur. This is related to the volume, frequency, and type of solution used. Large-volume enemas disrupt the normal flora of the bowel, predisposing the client to diarrhea as the bowels recover from this traumatic event. Provide yogurt with active cultures or buttermilk to help the client restore normal flora. Antibiotic enemas may disrupt vitamin K synthesis by intestinal flora. Supplemental vitamin K may be required until normal intestinal flora is restored. Table 39-9 lists the types of enema solutions and their effects.

INITIATE RECTAL STIMULATION

As an alternative to a scheduled defecation program, digital rectal stimulation may be used to regulate fecal elimination patterns. This process requires circular palpation of the anal sphincter and distal anus for 2 to 3 minutes. This process is repeated in 20 minutes if defecation does not occur. Deep breathing is encouraged during defecation because it drops the diaphragm and partially compensates for the client's inability to effectively strain.

Persons with chronic fecal incontinence due to anal sphincter incompetence may be managed with biofeedback techniques. These techniques are typically taught by a specialty or advanced practice nurse with specific training in the field of GI disorders and biofeedback techniques.

MONITOR ELIMINATION DIVERSIONS

When certain disease conditions cause a disruption to the normal flow of either urine or feces, the treatment is a temporary or permanent artificial opening (stoma) in the abdominal wall. Altered body image is a significant issue for clients with a urinary or bowel diversion. Client teaching should begin as soon as possible. Show the client the stoma and the associated equipment to care for the stoma so that this new situation can be integrated into the client's body image. Nursing care should be provided in an open, accepting manner and encourage the client and family to express their feelings regarding the stoma.

Urinary Diversions

Surgically created extraurethral incontinence is managed by a pouch. The ileal conduit is, by design, an incontinent stoma constructed from a 10-cm segment of ileum. The ileum is isolated from the fecal stream and connected to the ureters using a refluxing end-to-end anastomosis. A small incision is made in the abdominal wall, and a stoma is constructed from the distal portion of the ileal segment. An enterostomal nurse is consulted to advise the surgeon on stoma site selection and to assist the client to adapt to and learn to manage the stoma.

The continent urinary diversion is an alternative to the ileal conduit. It contains a reservoir for urinary storage and gains continence from various mechanisms. The urinary reservoir may be created from small or large bowel. The Kock Indiana and Florida pouches are types of pouches created from intestinal material. Continence is obtained by forming an abdominal reservoir. Continence also may be preserved by the Mitrofanoff technique, which uses a segment of appendix or ureter to create a continent stoma. Evacuation of urine from the reservoir relies on intermittent catheterization of these continent mechanisms. Orthotopic urinary diversions have been described in which the bladder is attached to the urethra, and its sphincter mechanism is relied on for continence. Urine may be evacuated from the urinary reservoir by catheterization of the urethra or by strain voiding.

Bowel Diversions

The fecal stream is diverted when tissue damage from trauma or inflammation necessitates the temporary bypassing of a segment of bowel or when permanent resection of malignant or irreversibly damaged tissue is necessary. Several techniques are used to create a fecal diversion; some require a pouch to contain fecal contents, whereas others maintain continence. Continent diversions rely on catheterization of an abdominal stoma or evacuation of stool from a pouch reservoir reattached to the anal sphincter.

Virtually any portion of the large and small intestine can be diverted or used to form a fecal reservoir. Some diversions rely on a stoma, a surgically created opening, for the evacuation of fecal contents. Stomas are primarily constructed in three ways. An *end stoma* is created by dividing the bowel and bringing the proximal segment to the abdominal wall. The end is rolled and attached to the skin of the abdomen, creating a red rosette of intestinal mucosa. A *double-barrel stoma* is constructed by dividing the bowel and bringing both the proximal and distal ends to the abdominal wall. The proximal end is used to evacuate stool. The distal stoma is typically referred to as a mucous fistula. The double-barrel stoma is designed for temporary diversion of the fecal stream. A *loop stoma* is created by opening the anterior aspect of the bowel either longitudinally or transversely. The resulting stoma has both proximal and distal openings that are separated by the posterior wall of the bowel loop. It is designed for temporary fecal diversion.

The fecal stream is diverted at the most distal point possible to maximize the absorption of food, fluid, and electrolytes and to preserve continence. The *ileostomy,* a diversion of the bowel at the level of the ileum, is more uncommon than it was during earlier decades. A permanent ileostomy is typically reserved for clients with severe Crohn's colitis, familial adenomatous polyposis, or chronic ulcerative colitis. A loop (temporary) ileostomy may be created as one stage in

an ileoanal reservoir procedure or as a staged procedure for the relief of obstruction of the ascending colon.

The colostomy is created as a permanent or temporary fecal diversion (see Figure 39-10). Among adults, it may be created in cases of severe diverticulitis or trauma. The most common indication for a permanent colostomy among adults is an abdominoperineal resection for lower rectal cancer. A temporary colostomy may be created from the transverse colon or (rarely) from the cecum. The descending or sigmoid colon may be temporarily diverted because of radiation proctitis or low rectal carcinoma. "Getting good adhesion of the skin barrier is vital to changing an ostomy pouch" (Kent, 2008). Procedure 39-9 outlines steps for changing a colostomy pouch.

Continent diversions of the bowel may incorporate the anus and sphincter or may be constructed with an abdominal stoma. The ileoanal reservoir is created in a staged approach. In the first stage an abdominal colectomy is completed, followed by a rectal mucosectomy, creation of a J- or S-shaped pouch comprising the anus and ileum, and a temporary end or loop ileostomy. In the second stage the temporary ileostomy is taken down and the ileoanal reservoir is reattached to the rectal stream.

The Kock continent ileostomy is performed as a single procedure. A colectomy and proctectomy are performed, and the distal 45 cm of the ileum is used to form the reservoir for the ileostomy and the abdominal stoma. The abdominal stoma is rendered continent by intussusception of the bowel that is stabilized to the abdominal wall by stapling or suturing the nipple valve. A polyglycolic acid mesh may be incorporated to provide further support if necessary. Effluent gathered in the reservoir is evacuated by catheterization thorough the abdominal stoma.

MONITOR SURGICAL MANAGEMENT

The surgical management for SUI differs for urethral hypermobility as compared with intrinsic sphincter deficiency. Urethral hypermobility is managed by a bladder suspension designed to prevent descent of the bladder base and urine loss during physical exertion. The selection of the procedure depends on the severity of the incontinence and client and surgeon preference.

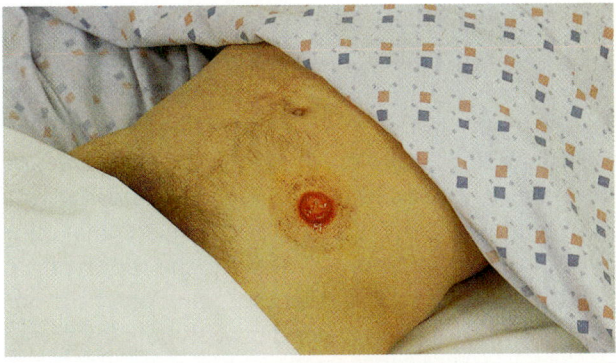

FIGURE 39-10 Colostomy. What are some major nursing implications when caring for this client? DELMAR/CENGAGE LEARNING

Clients with adequate urethral support and intrinsic sphincter deficiency may be managed with a urethral bulking agent, such as Contigen (Bard Urological, Covington, GA). This product is a glutaraldehyde cross-linked collagen that improves continence by enhancing compressive elements of the urethral sphincter mechanism. It is injected transurethrally, and local anesthesia with systemic sedation is often used in preference to general anesthesia. Women with a combination of urethral hypermobility and intrinsic sphincter deficiency may undergo a suburethral sling procedure, in which the proximal third of the urethra is supported with fascia or a synthetic material.

An artificial urinary sphincter device also may be used to manage intrinsic sphincter deficiency. This mechanical device allows the client to mechanically inflate and deflate a cuff that compresses underlying urethral tissues. Each of these procedures requires specific nursing care and instruction. See a urologic nursing text for a detailed discussion of the nursing care for urologic surgery.

Surgery plays only a limited role in the management of urge incontinence. Surgical procedures designed to denervate the bladder (sever nerves needed for contraction of the detrusor muscle) have had little success because of significant complications, including fecal incontinence and impotence among men. A surgically implanted device designed to deliver electrical stimulation to the lower urinary tract has been approved for use in the United States.

The management of reflex incontinence is complicated by the combination of urine leakage and urinary retention caused by detrusor sphincter dyssynergia. A bladder management program is chosen that both protects the upper urinary tracts from serious damage and maximizes continence.

Surgical reconstruction is sometimes used in the long-term management of reflex incontinence. An augmentation enterocystoplasty enlarges bladder capacity and alleviates reflex incontinence by converting the hyperreflexic bladder into a large, atonic bladder with improved storage ability. Unfortunately,

the augmented bladder rarely empties efficiently, and clients are advised that lifelong intermittent self-catheterization will be necessary after augmentation surgery. A continent or incontinent urinary diversion is occasionally used to manage urine elimination in the client with reflex incontinence. However, urinary diversion is completed only when bladder function threatens the normal function of the upper urinary tracts.

Fistulae and ectopia are managed by surgical closure whenever possible. When surgery is not feasible, a fistula may be treated by careful application of a sclerosing agent, such as tetracycline or doxycycline in suspension. The solution is applied monthly, and a skin barrier is used on the area surrounding the fistula to prevent scarring. The fistula that cannot be closed surgically or by sclerosing therapy must be managed by application of a urinary containment device and a preventive skin program.

Surgery or endoscopic procedures alleviate urinary retention caused by bladder outlet obstruction. Transurethral resection of the prostate, open prostatectomy, VaporTrode, visual ablation of the prostate, and other procedures are used to alleviate obstruction caused by benign prostatic hyperplasia. Transurethral incision of the bladder neck or transurethral sphincterotomy may be used for bladder neck or striated sphincter dyssynergia. Refer to a textbook of urologic nursing for the care following these specialized procedures.

COMPLEMENTARY AND ALTERNATIVE THERAPIES

"One of the largest health problems in the western world is in the area of elimination" (Barney, 1996, p. 57). When the body fails to eliminate waste that is full of toxic substances, other systems are compromised and the person becomes prone to illness. Herbalists view the role of the kidneys and the intestines in a holistic manner. The proper function of any part of the body is dependent on the effective elimination of waste products and toxins.

NURSING CARE PLAN

The Client Experiencing Constipation

CASE PRESENTATION

Mrs. M is a 30-year-old woman who sustained a complete spinal cord injury of the seventh cervical vertebra 2 years before this hospital admission. She currently manages her bowels by enemas every 5 to 7 days when she notes pressure and distension of her abdomen. She has frequent episodes of fecal incontinence, described as passage of moderate amounts of black, watery stool. She manages these episodes by administering one or two enemas, followed by passage of a large volume of odorous, dark feces. She denies any problems with bowel control before her spinal injury, stating that she moved her bowels every other day, typically after breakfast. Currently, she reports fluid intake of 3 to 4 glasses per day. She eats primarily meats, white breads, some pastas, and one portion of vegetables per day. She does not routinely eat cereals or fruits or supplement her diet with bulk laxatives.

(Continues)

NURSING CARE PLAN (Continued)

ASSESSMENT
- Inadequate fluid intake
- Inadequate fiber intake
- Presence of large impaction in the rectum

NURSING DIAGNOSIS 1: *Constipation* related to spinal cord injury and neurogenic bowel
NOC: Bowel elimination
NIC: Constipation/impaction management

NURSING DIAGNOSIS 2: *Bowel incontinence* related to fecal impaction, altered stool consistency, and neurogenic bowel
NOC: Bowel continence
NIC: Bowel training

EXPECTED OUTCOME
The rectum will be cleansed of impaction.

INTERVENTION/RATIONALE
1. Administer PIEE until impaction is disrupted. Bowel is clear of impacted stool as assessed by digital examination.

EXPECTED OUTCOME
Stool will be soft and formed.

INTERVENTIONS/RATIONALES
1. Encourage dietary intake of fiber-rich foods, including one serving of cereal per day, one serving of fruit, and two servings of vegetables.
2. Increase fluid intake to 15 mL/lb body weight; encourage water intake to equal at least 50% of fluids.
3. Administer supplemental bulk laxatives (Metamucil) if client is unable to alter diet to meet needs for fiber.

Stool will be soft, formed feces without impacted or dry, hardened material.

EXPECTED OUTCOME
A regular routine for bowel elimination will be established.

INTERVENTIONS/RATIONALES
1. Begin a bowel program every other day.
2. Determine time for evacuation with client; encourage defecation after breakfast, based on premorbid bowel elimination pattern.
3. Encourage bowel evacuation program after meal if premorbid schedule is not feasible with current activities.

Bowel evacuation will occur every other day after a meal, based on client's activities of daily living, preferences, and premorbid bowel elimination patterns.

EXPECTED OUTCOME
Bowel management program will cause completed elimination of feces from rectum.

INTERVENTIONS/RATIONALES
1. Begin stimulated, scheduled bowel evacuation program using an oral laxative, mini-enema, and digital stimulation program.
2. Discuss program with client and significant others, giving description of each stimulation program, time required, cost implications, and advantages and disadvantages.

(Continues)

NURSING CARE PLAN (Continued)

Client will completely evacuate the bowel using a stimulation or timed management program.

EXPECTED OUTCOME
Fecal incontinent episodes will be alleviated.

INTERVENTIONS/RATIONALES
1. Teach client relationship among stool consistency, regularity of evacuation, fecal impaction, and fecal continence.
2. Advise client to consult nurse specialist or gastroenterologist if fecal incontinent episodes persist despite regulation of bowel management program.
3. Warn client that occurrence of diarrhea may predispose to acute transient fecal incontinence.

Fecal incontinent episodes will be reduced by greater than 50%.

Gladstar (2001) states that "longevity herbs are not life extenders; what they will do is increase quality of life, so that you feel better and better as you grow older" (p. 19). Dandelion leaf and nettle are considered longevity herbs that maintain the health and vitality of the kidneys. Herbs that aid the functions of the urinary system are:

- *Diuretics:* dandelion root and leaf (refer to Chapter 34 for a full discussion of this herb) and cleavers
- *Antiseptics:* bearberry, birch, boldo, buchu, celery seed, couch grass, juniper, and yarrow
- *Antimicrobials:* echinacea root (refer to Chapter 32 for a full discussion of this herb) and wild indigo root
- *Demulcents:* corn silk, couch grass, and marshmallow leaf

Herbs that possess other properties may also be used. For example, urinary astringents (Beth root, horsetail, and plantain tormentil) can be used to treat blood in the urine caused by minor problems and to aid the healing of lesions. Antilithics (gravel root, hydrangea, and stone root) can be used to prevent the formation of or aid in the removal of calculi (stones or gravel) in the urinary system.

Both urinary and fecal elimination are reliant upon sufficient amounts of fiber and fluids in the diet. Poor nutrition is the most common cause of chronic constipation (Barney, 1996). These herbs are helpful in relieving constipation: *Cascara sagrada* bark, senna, ginger root, butternut root bark, and burdock root. Also, milk thistle, a cholagogue, may be used to aid liver function and to enhance bile flow to soften stools.

Cascara sagrada bark is an old Indian remedy to encourage peristalsis and tone relaxed muscles of the digestive tract. Senna is the most widely used stimulant laxative when compared to synthetic drugs (Barney, 1996). *Cascara* and senna should be combined with aromatics and carminatives such as

licorice and ginger root to increase palatability and reduce gripping. Ginger root aids in digestion and enhances bile flow from the liver. Burdock root is a mild laxative and an effective diuretic; its cleansing effect goes beyond its diuretic and laxative properties as it promotes perspiration and strengthens the liver.

Psyllium seed and flaxseed are also helpful for constipation. Psyllium seed must be taken with a full glass of water. Mineral oil should not be taken on a regular basis because, if inhaled, it can damage the lungs, and it reduces the absorption of fat-soluble vitamins (Balch, 2006).

EVALUATION

Evaluating the effectiveness of the nursing interventions is an ongoing process. The client's level of maintenance or restoration of elimination patterns and return to an appropriate level of independence are indicators of success. When evaluating these aspects, it is important for the nurse to reassess how realistic the original identified outcomes were, especially for goals that were not met, and to modify the target outcomes accordingly. Prevention of skin breakdown and infection can also be used to determine the appropriateness of the plan of care. Client understanding of procedures and self-care should be evaluated to determine the effectiveness of teaching plans, and modifications should be made to address deficiencies and ongoing learning needs. If support persons were included in the teaching process, their understanding of skills and competence with procedures should also be measured. If additional care or teaching is deemed necessary, clients should be given referrals for community and other resources to support their continuing learning needs.

PROCEDURE 39-1

Assisting with a Bedpan or Urinal

EQUIPMENT
- Bedpan (regular or fracture) or urinal
- Disposable gloves
- Bedpan cover
- Toilet paper
- Washcloth and towel

ACTION	RATIONALE
POSITIONING A BEDPAN	
1. Close curtain or door.	1. Provides for privacy.
2. Wash hands/hand hygiene; apply gloves.	2. Reduces transmission of microorganisms.
3. Lower head of bed so client is in supine position.	3. The supine position will increase ability of client to move to side-lying position.
4. Elevate bed.	4. Ensures proper body mechanics.
5. Assist client to side-lying position using side rail for support.	5. Provides for best position for proper placement of bedpan.
6. Place bedpan under buttocks. Place a fracture pan with the lower end near the client's lower back region. Place large bedpans with the opening near the client's thighs.	6. Ensures proper placement of the bedpan before client rolls on top of bedpan.
7. While holding the bedpan with one hand, help the client roll onto his or her back, while pushing against the bedpan (toward the center of the bed) to hold it in place (see Figure 39-11).	7. Prevents dislocation or misalignment of bedpan.
8. Alternative: Help the client raise the hips using the overbed trapeze, and slide the pan in place. Alternative: If the client is unable to turn or raise hips, use a fracture pan instead of a bedpan. With a fracture pan, the flat side is placed toward the client's head (see Figure 39-12).	8. Provides an alternate way to position the pan. Fracture pan reduces the amount of movement and lift required to place the pan.

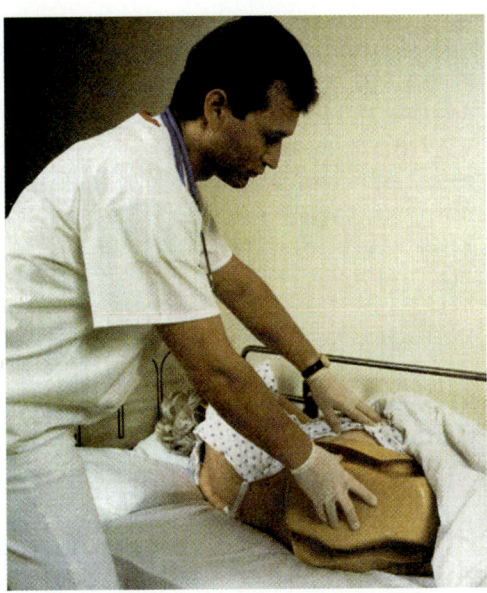

FIGURE 39-11 **Place the bedpan against the client's buttocks while rolling client to side.** DELMAR/CENGAGE LEARNING

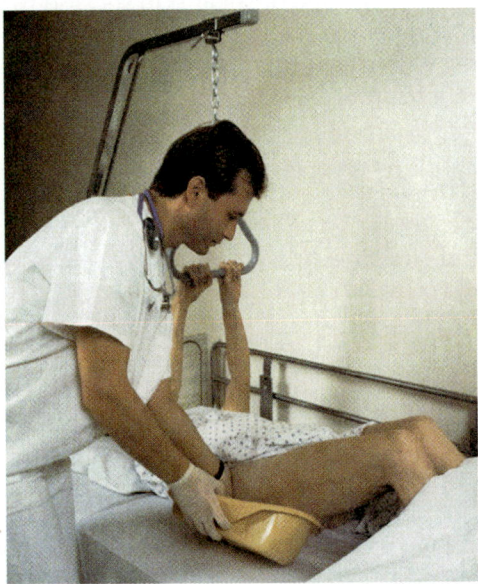

FIGURE 39-12 **Slip the bedpan under the client's buttocks while client lifts himself or herself with the trapeze.** DELMAR/CENGAGE LEARNING

(Continues)

PROCEDURE 39-1
Assisting with a Bedpan or Urinal (Continued)

ACTION	RATIONALE
9. Check placement of bedpan by looking between client's legs.	9. May prevent spillage from misalignment of bedpan.
10. If indicated, elevate head of bed to 45° angle or higher for comfort.	10. Check order of prescribing or qualified practitioner; bed remains flat if client has a spinal cord injury or spinal surgery. Elevating the head of bed creates a more normal elimination position.
11. Place call light within reach of client; place side rails in upright position, lower bed, and provide privacy.	11. Privacy allows for a more comfortable elimination environment; elevated side rails provide for safety.
12. Remove gloves; wash hands/hand hygiene.	12. Reduces transmission of microorganisms.

POSITIONING A URINAL

ACTION	RATIONALE
13. Repeat Actions 1 and 2.	13. See Rationales 1 and 2.
14. Lift the covers and place the urinal so the client may grasp the handle and position it. If the client cannot do this, you must position the urinal and place the penis into the opening (see Figures 39-13 and 39-14).	14. Ensures proper placement of the urinal and reduces the risk of spillage.
15. Remove gloves; wash hands/hand hygiene.	15. Reduces transmission of microorganisms.

REMOVING A BEDPAN

ACTION	RATIONALE
16. Wash hands; apply gloves/hand hygiene.	16. Reduces transmission of microorganisms.
17. Gather toilet paper and washing supplies.	17. Having supplies at the bedside allows smooth and safe completion of the procedure.
18. Lower head of bed to supine position.	18. Increases client's ability to move to side-lying position.
19. While holding bedpan with one hand, roll client to side and remove the pan, being careful not to pull or shear skin sticking to the pan and being careful not to spill contents.	19. Prevents possible spillage of bedpan contents.
20. Assist with cleaning or wiping; always wipe with a front to back motion.	20. Client may not be able to clean self; wiping from front to back decreases chances of cross-contamination from anus to urethra.

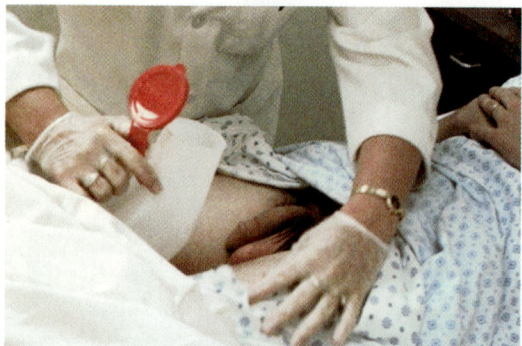

FIGURE 39-13 Lift the covers and place the urinal. Allow the client to adjust the position. DELMAR/CENGAGE LEARNING

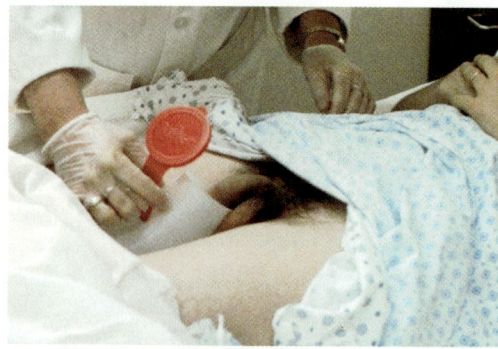

FIGURE 39-14 If the client is unable to assist, place the penis into the opening of the urinal. DELMAR/CENGAGE LEARNING

(Continues)

PROCEDURE 39-1
Assisting with a Bedpan or Urinal (Continued)

ACTION	RATIONALE
21. Empty bedpan (observe and measure urine output and check for occult blood if ordered), clean bedpan, and store it in proper place; if bedpan is to be emptied outside client's room, cover it during transport.	21. Promotes privacy and decreases the chance of spilling contents. Assessment of types of stool evaluates for constipation and diarrhea.
22. Remove soiled gloves; wash hands.	22. Reduces transmission of microorganisms.
23. Allow client to wash hands.	23. Provides for physical hygiene and comfort.
24. Place call light within reach; recheck that side rails are in the upright position.	24. Ensures client safety and comfort.
25. Wash hands/hand hygiene.	25. Reduces transmission of microorganisms.
REMOVING A URINAL	
26. Wash hands/hand hygiene; apply gloves.	26. Reduces transmission of microorganisms.
27. Empty the urinal, measuring urine output if ordered, rinse the urinal, and replace it within client's reach. Observe odor and color of urine before discarding.	27. Provides a way to measure client's output. Keeping the urinal within reach promotes client autonomy. Helps evaluate for concentrated urine, infection, and renal problems.
28. Remove soiled gloves; wash hands.	28. Reduces transmission of microorganisms.
29. Allow client to wash hands.	29. Provides for physical hygiene and comfort.
30. Place call light within reach; recheck that side rails are in the upright position.	30. Ensures client safety and comfort.
31. Wash hands/hand hygiene.	31. Reduces transmission of microorganisms.

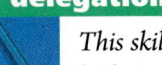

delegation tip

This skill is routinely delegated to ancillary personnel who have been trained in Standard Precautions and proper body positioning and to report color, odor, and amount of output to the nurse.

nursing tips

Elimination is normally a private function done without assistance. However, during periods of immobility and illness, assistance is needed. The main focus of the nurse is to provide maximum comfort and privacy to lessen the client's embarrassment.

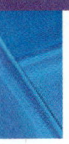

PROCEDURE 39-2

Applying a Condom Catheter

EQUIPMENT
- Condom catheter kit with adhesive strip
- Urinary drainage bag
- Clean gloves
- Basin with warm water and soap
- Towel and washcloth

(Continues)

PROCEDURE 39-2
Applying a Condom Catheter (Continued)

ACTION	RATIONALE
1. Wash hands/hand hygiene.	1. Reduces transmission of microorganisms.
2. Protect the client's privacy by closing the door and pulling curtains around the bed.	2. Allows privacy for the client.
3. Position the client in a comfortable position, preferably a supine position, if tolerated by the client. Raise the bed to a comfortable height for the nurse.	3. The client will be more comfortable and tolerate the procedure more readily; a supine position facilitates the cleaning and application of the catheter. Raising the bed to a comfortable height promotes good body mechanics.
4. Apply latex-free gloves.	4. Gloves should be worn to prevent the possible transmission of microorganisms when there is a chance of coming into contact with any body fluid.
5. Fold the client's gown across the abdomen, and pull the sheet up over the client's legs.	5. Provides minimal exposure of the client, thereby reducing the client's embarrassment.
6. Assess the client's penis for any signs of redness, irritation, or skin breakdown.	6. The client may require an indwelling catheter if there is a significant amount of skin breakdown. Assessment will give baseline data for comparison with future assessments.
7. Clean the client's penis with warm soapy water. Retract the foreskin on the uncircumcised male and clean thoroughly in folds.	7. Removes microorganisms present in any drainage or feces that could enter the urinary meatus and cause a urinary tract infection. Avoids trapping microorganisms in folds around the meatus.
8. Return the client's foreskin to its normal position.	8. Failure to return the foreskin to a normal position can lead to swelling of the penis and possible constriction.
9. Shave any excess hair around the base of the penis if required by institutional policy.	9. Prevents additional discomfort from the adhesive strip when the condom catheter is removed. Also prevents hair from catching on the adhesive strip, causing discomfort.
10. Rinse and dry the area.	10. Moist warm environment can lead to the growth of microorganisms.
11. If a condom kit is used, open the package containing the skin preparation. Wipe and apply skin preparation solution to the shaft of the penis. If the client has an erection, wait for termination of erection before applying the catheter.	11. Preparation solutions protect the client's skin from irritation. An erection may occur from manipulation of the penis while cleaning the area. This is a normal reaction and will terminate in a few minutes.
12. Apply the double-sided adhesive strip around the base of the client's penis in a spiral fashion. The strip is applied 1 inch from the proximal end of the penis. Do not completely encircle the penis or tightly encompass penis.	12. Applying the adhesive in a spiral fashion does not compromise circulation of the penis. Encircling the penis can constrict the penis, impair circulation, and cause edema.
13. Position the rolled condom at the distal portion of the penis and unroll it, covering the penis and the double-sided strip of adhesive. Leave a 1- to 2-inch space between the tip of the penis and the end of the condom (see Figure 39-15 on page 1263).	13. The condom sticks to the adhesive and remains in place. The extra spacing prevents pressure and erosion of the tip of the penis.

(Continues)

PROCEDURE 39-2
Applying a Condom Catheter (Continued)

ACTION	RATIONALE

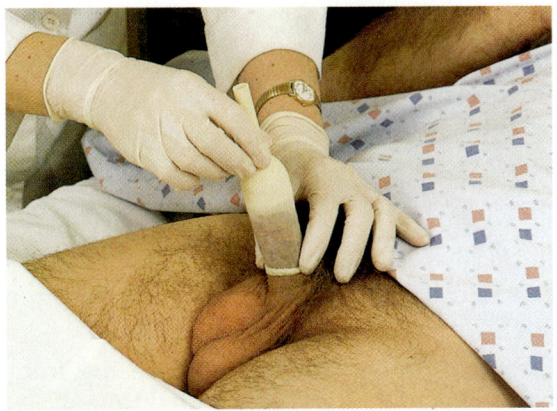

FIGURE 39-15 Unroll condom catheter to the base of the penis. DELMAR/CENGAGE LEARNING

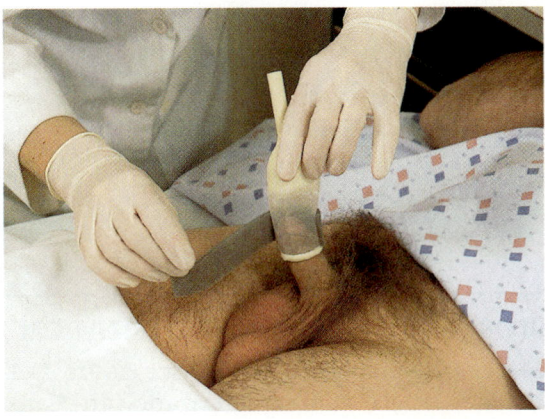

FIGURE 39-16 Secure the condom catheter with the adhesive strip. DELMAR/CENGAGE LEARNING

14. Gently press the condom to the adhesive strip (see Figure 39-16).
15. Attach the drainage bag tubing to the catheter tubing. Make sure the tubing lies over the client's legs, not under. Secure the drainage bag to the side of the bed below the level of the client's bladder or to the client's leg.

16. Determine that the condom and tubing are not twisted.

17. Cover the client.
18. Dispose of the used equipment in appropriate receptacle and wash hands.
19. Return the client's bed to the lowest position, and reposition client to comfortable or appropriate position.
20. Empty the bag, measure the client's urinary output, and record every 4 hours. After procedure, remove gloves; wash hands/hand hygiene.
21. Remove the condom once a day to clean the area and assess the skin for signs of impaired skin integrity.

14. Enables the condom to adhere evenly to the adhesive strip.
15. The drainage bag is positioned below the level of the client's bladder to prevent reflux of the urine onto the penis and microorganisms from entering the penis. The tubing is placed over the leg to promote urine flow away from the client. Constant exposure to urine and moisture can irritate the penis.
16. If the condom or tubing is twisted, the urine cannot flow out and the condom will leak or fall off.
17. Maintains privacy of the client.
18. Reduces transmission of microorganisms.

19. Reduces potential injury from falls.

20. Records output and prevents bag from becoming overly full or too heavy. Reduces transmission of microorganisms.
21. Promotes hygiene and reduces the possibility of skin breakdown.

delegation tip

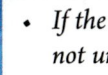

Application of a condom catheter may be delegated to properly trained ancillary personnel. The need for condom drainage and the ongoing assessment of the client's skin condition should be followed up by the nurse.

nursing tips

- *If the client gets an erection, assure him that it is not unusual when applying a condom catheter.*

- *Wrap the adhesive strip in a spiral fashion to avoid constricting the penis and causing skin breakdown.*

Inserting an Indwelling Catheter: Male

EQUIPMENT
- Indwelling or straight catheter with drainage system
- Sterile catheterization kit
- Adequate lighting source
- Disposable gloves
- Blanket or drape
- Soap and washcloth
- Warm water
- Towel
- Forceps

ACTION	RATIONALE

PERFORMING URINARY CATHETERIZATION: MALE CLIENT

ACTION	RATIONALE
1. Gather the equipment needed (see Figure 39-17). Read the label on the catheterization kit. Note if the catheter is included in the kit and, if so, what type it is. Gather any supplies you will need that are not in the prepackaged kit. Wash hands/hand hygiene.	1. Promotes efficiency in the procedure. Kits from various manufacturers come with different equipment. The catheter may or may not be packaged in the kit. Sterile gloves and the urine drainage bag may also need to be gathered separately.
2. Provide for privacy and explain procedure to client.	2. Promotes cooperation and client dignity.
3. Set the bed to a comfortable height to work, and raise the side rail on the side opposite you.	3. Promotes proper body mechanics and ensures client safety.
4. Assist the client to a supine position with legs slightly spread (see Figure 39-18).	4. Relaxes muscles and allows visualization of the area to facilitate insertion of the catheter.
5. Drape the client's abdomen and thighs if needed.	5. Promotes client comfort and warmth.
6. Ensure adequate lighting of the penis and perineal area.	6. Facilitates proper execution of technique.
7. Wash hands/hand hygiene; apply latex-free disposable gloves; and wash perineal area.	7. Reduces transfer of microorganisms. Avoids reaction to latex.
8. Remove gloves and wash hands/hand hygiene.	8. Reduces transfer of microorganisms.
9. Open the catheterization kit, using aseptic technique. Use the wrapper to establish a sterile field (see Figure 39-19 on page 1265).	9. Provides an area for the sterile equipment to be laid out and assembled. Establish the sterile field close to the client. If the client is able to cooperate, the sterile field can sometimes be established in the open area between the client's legs.

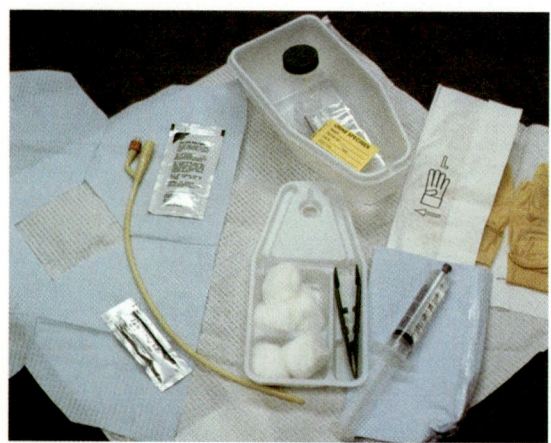

FIGURE 39-17 Catheterization Kit DELMAR/CENGAGE LEARNING

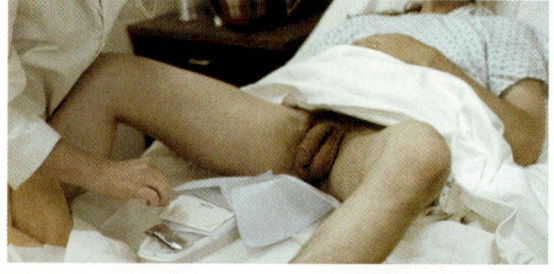

FIGURE 39-18 Assist the client to a supine position with legs spread. This allows visualization of the area and relaxes muscles. DELMAR/CENGAGE LEARNING

(Continues)

PROCEDURE 39-3
Inserting an Indwelling Catheter: Male (Continued)

ACTION	RATIONALE

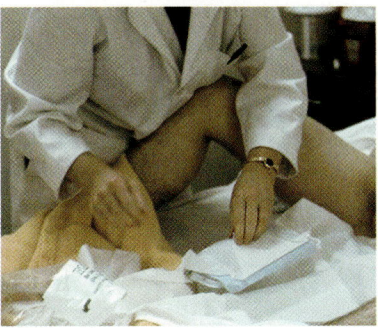

FIGURE 39-19 Open the catheterization kit, using the wrapper to establish a sterile field between the client's legs. DELMAR/CENGAGE LEARNING

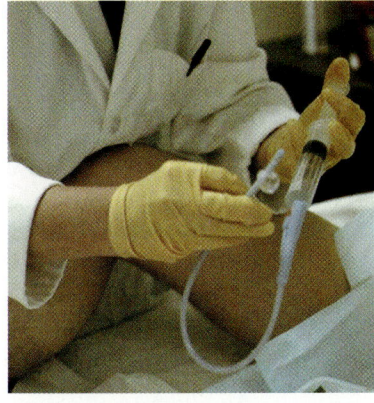

FIGURE 39-20 Inflate and deflate the retention balloon to test its patency. DELMAR/CENGAGE LEARNING

10. If the catheter is not included in the kit, carefully drop the sterile catheter onto the field using aseptic technique. Add any other items needed.

11. Apply sterile gloves. These may be included in the kit.

12. Place the fenestrated drape from the catheterization kit over the client's perineal area with the penis extending through the opening.

13. If inserting a retention catheter, attach the syringe filled with sterile water to the Luer-Lok tail of the catheter. Inflate and deflate the retention balloon. Detach the water-filled syringe (see Figure 39-20).

14. Attach the catheter to the urine drainage bag if it is not preconnected.

15. Generously coat the distal portion of the catheter with water-soluble, sterile lubricant and place it nearby on the sterile field.

16. With your nondominant hand, gently grasp the penis and retract the foreskin (if present). With your dominant hand, cleanse the glans penis with a povidone-iodine solution or other antimicrobial cleanser (see Figure 39-21 on page 1266).

17. Hold the penis perpendicular to the body and pull up gently.

18. Inject 10 mL sterile, water-soluble lubricant (use a 2% Xylocaine lubricant whenever feasible) into the urethra.

10. Prevents contamination of the sterile equipment and the sterile field.

11. Prevents contamination of the sterile equipment and the sterile field.

12. Provides a sterile field at the procedural site. Prevents accidental contamination from adjacent areas.

13. Tests the patency of the retention balloon. Detaching the syringe prevents accidental inflation during catheter insertion.

14. The catheter and drainage system may be preconnected; otherwise, it is connected before catheterization to avoid exposing the client to ascending infection from an open-ended catheter.

15. Facilitates catheter insertion.

16. Removes dirt and minimizes the risk of urinary tract infection by removing surface pathogens.

17. Facilitates catheter insertion by straightening urethra.

18. Avoids urethral trauma and discomfort during catheter insertion and facilitates insertion.

(Continues)

PROCEDURE 39-3
Inserting an Indwelling Catheter: Male (Continued)

ACTION	RATIONALE

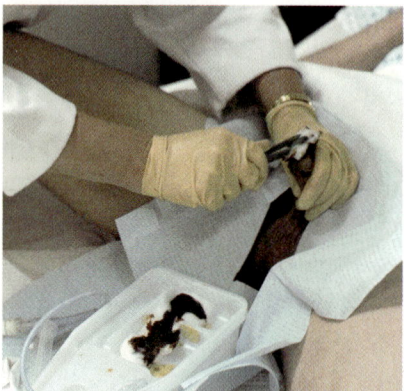

FIGURE 39-21 Cleanse the glans penis with a povidone-iodine solution. DELMAR/CENGAGE LEARNING

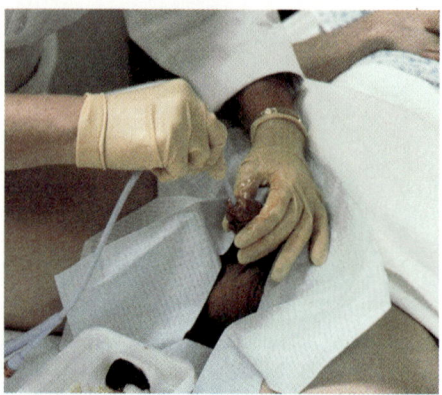

FIGURE 39-22 Steadily insert the catheter. DELMAR/CENGAGE LEARNING

19. Holding the catheter in the dominant hand, steadily insert the catheter about 8 inches, until urine is noted in the drainage bag or tubing (see Figure 39-22).

19. Provides a visual confirmation that the catheter tip is in the bladder.

20. If the catheter will be removed as soon as the client's bladder is empty, insert the catheter another inch, place the penis in a comfortable position, and hold the catheter in place as the bladder drains.

20. The catheter needs to be inserted far enough to allow complete bladder drainage but not so far as to possibly irritate the bladder, causing spasms.

21. If the catheter will be indwelling with a retention balloon, continue inserting until the hub of the catheter (bifurcation between drainage port and retention balloon arm) is met (see Figure 39-23).

21. Ensures adequate catheter insertion before retention balloon is inflated.

22. Reattach the water-filled syringe to the inflation port.

22. Provides a sterile method of inflating the retention balloon.

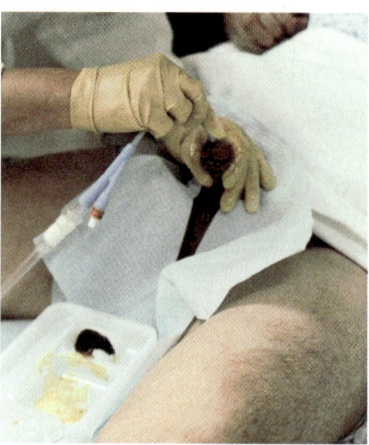

FIGURE 39-23 Continue inserting the catheter until the bifurcation between the drainage port and the retention balloon reaches the end of the penis. This ensures the retention balloon will be fully in the bladder prior to inflation.
DELMAR/CENGAGE LEARNING

(Continues)

PROCEDURE 39-3
Inserting an Indwelling Catheter: Male (Continued)

ACTION	RATIONALE

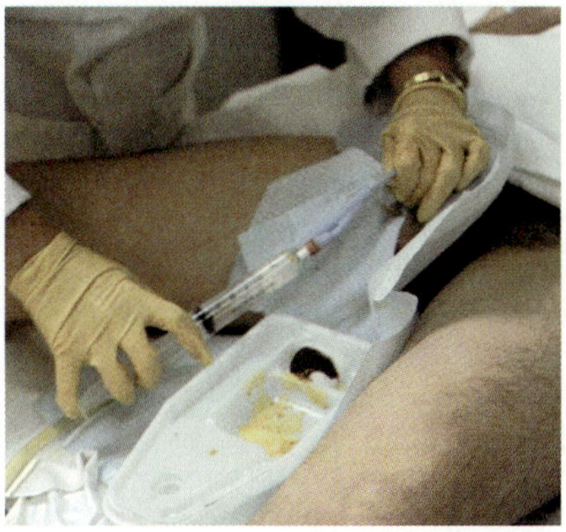

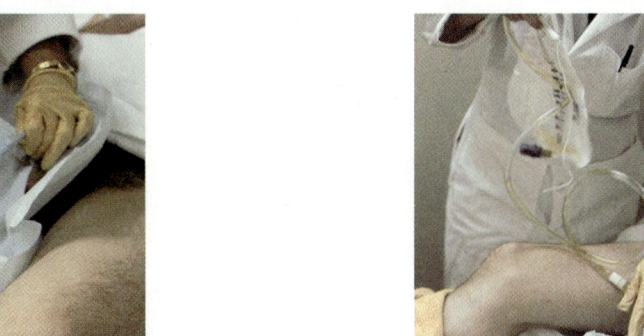

FIGURE 39-24 Inflate the retention balloon. DELMAR/CENGAGE LEARNING

FIGURE 39-25 Place the drainage bag tubing over the leg. DELMAR/CENGAGE LEARNING

23. Inflate the retention balloon with sterile water per manufacturer's recommendations or the prescribing practitioner's orders (see Figure 39-24).
24. Instruct the client to immediately report discomfort or pressure during balloon inflation; if pain occurs, discontinue the procedure, deflate the balloon, and insert the catheter farther into the bladder. If the client continues to complain of pain with balloon inflation, remove the catheter and notify the client's health care provider.
25. Once the balloon has been inflated, gently pull the catheter until the retention balloon is resting snug against the bladder neck (resistance will be felt when the balloon is properly seated).
26. Secure the catheter according to institutional policy. Securing it to either the client's thigh or abdomen is generally acceptable.
27. Place the drainage bag below the level of the bladder. Do not let it rest on the floor (see Figure 39-25 and Figure 39-26 on page 1268). Secure the drainage tubing to prevent pulling on the tubing and the catheter.
28. Remove gloves; dispose of equipment. Wash hands/hand hygiene.
29. Help client adjust position. Lower the bed.
30. Assess and document the amount, color, odor, and quality of urine.

23. Ensures retention of the balloon. Retention catheters are available with a variety of balloon sizes. Use a catheter with the appropriate size balloon.
24. Pain or pressure indicates inflation of the balloon in the urethra; further insertion will prevent misplacement and further pain or bleeding.

25. Maximizes continuous bladder drainage and prevents urine leakage around the catheter.

26. Prevents excessive traction from the balloon rubbing against the bladder neck, inadvertent catheter removal, or urethral erosion.
27. Maximizes continuous drainage of urine from the bladder (drainage is prevented when the drainage bag is placed above the abdomen).

28. Prevents transfer of microorganisms.

29. Promotes client comfort and safety.
30. Monitors urinary status.

(Continues)

PROCEDURE 39-3
Inserting an Indwelling Catheter: Male (Continued)

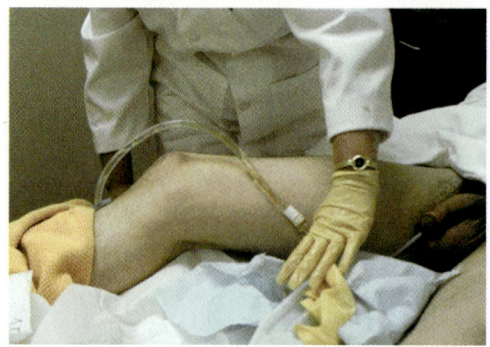

FIGURE 39-26 Place the drainage bag below the level of the bladder, but do not rest it on the floor. DELMAR/CENGAGE LEARNING

delegation tip

The skill of male urinary catheterization may be delegated to properly trained ancillary personnel depending on institution policies. The nurse is responsible to evaluate the client for contraindications to delegating this procedure, such as the risk for a difficult or traumatic insertion. The nurse may then decide to perform the procedure or to defer to the prescribing practitioner.

nursing tips

If the client suddenly complains of sharp pain, pull the catheter back and notify the prescribing practitioner.

PROCEDURE 39-4
Inserting an Indwelling Catheter: Female

EQUIPMENT
- Indwelling or straight catheter with drainage system
- Sterile catheterization kit
- Adequate lighting source
- Disposable gloves
- Blanket or drape
- Soap and washcloth
- Warm water
- Towel

ACTION	RATIONALE
PERFORMING URINARY CATHETERIZATION: FEMALE CLIENT	
1. Gather the equipment needed (see Figure 39-27 on page 1269). Read the label on the catheterization kit. Note if the catheter is included in the kit and, if so, what type it is. Gather any supplies you will need that are not in the prepackaged kit.	1. Promotes efficiency in the procedure. Kits from various manufacturers come with different equipment. The catheter may or may not be packaged in the kit. Sterile gloves and the urine drainage bag may also need to be gathered separately.

(Continues)

PROCEDURE 39-4
Inserting an Indwelling Catheter: Female (Continued)

ACTION	RATIONALE

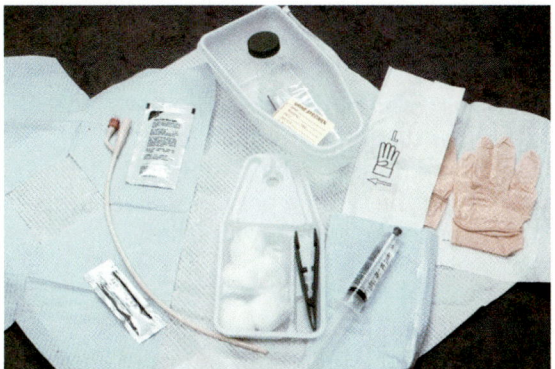

FIGURE 39-27 **Catheterization Kit** DELMAR/CENGAGE LEARNING

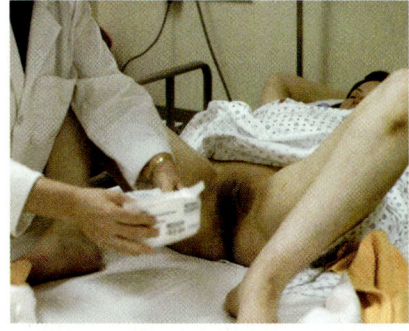

FIGURE 39-28 **Position the client supine with legs spread.**
DELMAR/CENGAGE LEARNING

2. Provide for privacy and explain procedure to client. Assess for allergy to povidone-iodine. Wash hands/hand hygiene.
3. Set the bed to a comfortable height to work, and raise the side rail on the side opposite you.
4. Assist the client to a supine position with legs spread and feet together or to a side-lying position with upper leg flexed (see Figure 39-28).
5. Drape the client's abdomen and thighs for warmth if needed.
6. Ensure adequate lighting of the perineal area.
7. Wash hands/hand hygiene; apply disposable gloves.
8. Wash perineal area.
9. Remove gloves and wash hands.
10. Open the catheterization kit, using aseptic technique. Use the wrapper to establish a sterile field (see Figure 39-29).

2. Promotes cooperation and client dignity.

3. Promotes proper body mechanics and ensures client safety.
4. Relaxes muscles and allows visualization of the area to facilitate insertion of the catheter.

5. Promotes client comfort and warmth.

6. Facilitates proper execution of technique.
7. Reduces transfer of microorganisms.

8. Reduces transfer of microorganisms.
9. Reduces transfer of microorganisms.
10. Provides an area for the sterile equipment to be laid out and assembled. Establish the sterile field close to the client. If the client is able to cooperate, the sterile field can sometimes be established in the open area between the client's legs.

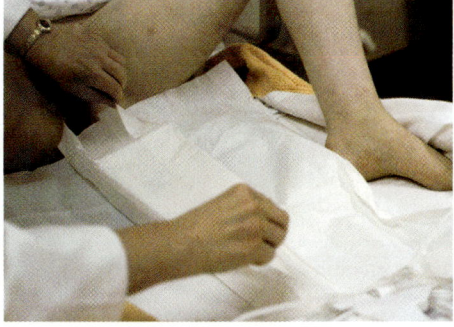

FIGURE 39-29 **Open the catheterization kit, using the wrapper to establish a sterile field between the client's legs.** DELMAR/CENGAGE LEARNING

(Continues)

PROCEDURE 39-4
Inserting an Indwelling Catheter: Female (Continued)

ACTION	RATIONALE
11. If the catheter is not included in the kit, drop the sterile catheter onto the field using aseptic technique. Add any other items needed.	11. Prevents contamination of the sterile equipment and the sterile field.
12. Apply sterile gloves. These may be included in the kit.	12. Prevents contamination of the sterile equipment and the sterile field.
13. If inserting a retention catheter, attach the syringe filled with sterile water to the Luer-Lok tail of the catheter. Inflate and deflate the retention balloon. Detach the water-filled syringe.	13. Tests the patency of the retention balloon. Detaching the syringe prevents accidental inflation during catheter insertion.
14. Attach the catheter to the urine drainage bag if it is not preconnected.	14. The catheter and drainage system may be preconnected; otherwise, connect it before catheterization to avoid exposing the client to ascending infection from an open-ended catheter.
15. Generously coat the distal portion of the catheter with water-soluble, sterile lubricant and place it nearby on the sterile field (see Figure 39-30).	15. Facilitates catheter insertion.
16. Place the fenestrated drape from the catheterization kit over the client's perineal area with the labia visible through the opening.	16. Provides a sterile field at the procedural site. Prevents accidental contamination from adjacent areas.
17. Gently spread the labia minora with the fingers of your nondominant hand and visualize the urinary meatus (see Figure 39-31).	17. Helps locate the meatus, so the catheter can be placed in the correct spot.
18. Holding the labia apart with your nondominant hand, use the forceps to pick up a cotton ball soaked in povidone-iodine, and cleanse the periurethral mucosa. Use one downward stroke for each cotton ball and dispose. Keep the labia separated with your nondominant hand until you insert the catheter (see Figure 39-32 on page 1271).	18. Cleans the area and minimizes the risk of urinary tract infection by removing surface pathogens.

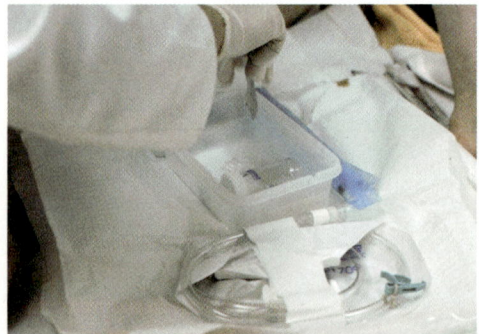

FIGURE 39-30 Open the lubrication package and squeeze lubricant onto the sterile field, where it will be used to lubricate the catheter. DELMAR/CENGAGE LEARNING

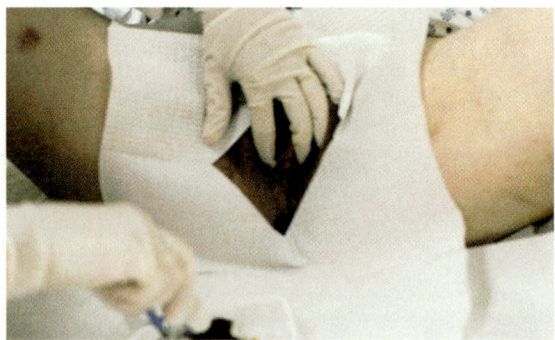

FIGURE 39-31 Spread the labia minora and visualize the urinary meatus. DELMAR/CENGAGE LEARNING

(Continues)

PROCEDURE 39-4
Inserting an Indwelling Catheter: Female (Continued)

ACTION	RATIONALE

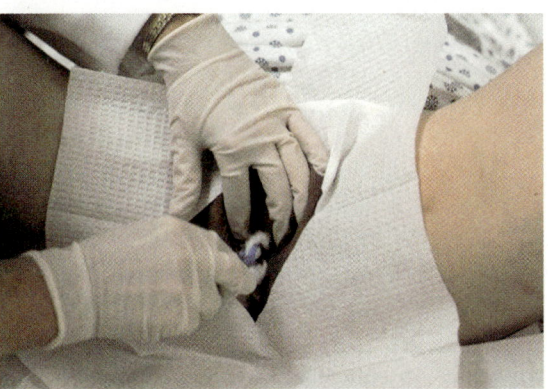

FIGURE 39-32 Using forceps, pick up a cotton ball soaked in povidone-iodine. Cleanse the periurethral mucosa. DELMAR/CENGAGE LEARNING

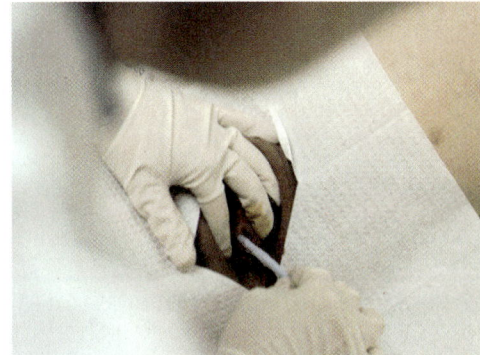

FIGURE 39-33 Steadily insert the catheter into the meatus. DELMAR/CENGAGE LEARNING

19. Holding the catheter in the dominant hand, steadily insert the catheter into the meatus until urine is noted in the drainage bag or tubing (see Figure 39-33).

20. If the catheter will be removed as soon as the client's bladder is empty, insert the catheter another inch and hold the catheter in place as the bladder drains.

21. If the catheter will be indwelling with a retention balloon, continue inserting another 1 to 3 inches.

22. Reattach the water-filled syringe to the inflation port.

23. Inflate the retention balloon using manufacturer's recommendations or according to the prescribing practitioner's orders (see Figure 39-34).

19. Provides a visual confirmation that the catheter tip is in the bladder.

20. The catheter needs to be inserted far enough to allow complete bladder drainage, but not so far as to possibly irritate the bladder, causing spasms.

21. Ensures adequate catheter insertion before retention balloon is inflated.

22. Provides a sterile method of inflating the retention balloon.

23. Ensures retention of the balloon. Retention catheters are available with a variety of balloon sizes. Use a catheter with the appropriate size balloon.

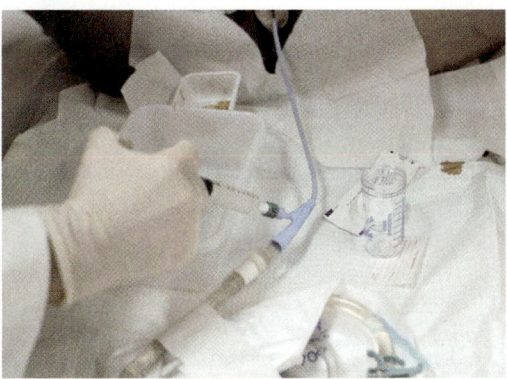

FIGURE 39-34 Inflate the retention balloon. DELMAR/CENGAGE LEARNING

(Continues)

PROCEDURE 39-4
Inserting an Indwelling Catheter: Female (Continued)

ACTION	RATIONALE

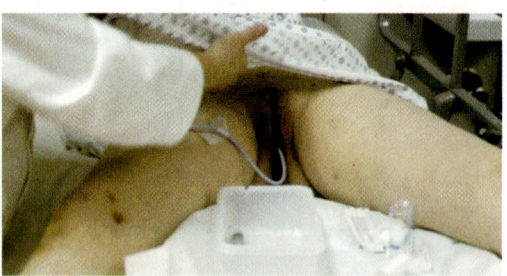

FIGURE 39-35 Tape the catheter to the client's thigh.
DELMAR/CENGAGE LEARNING

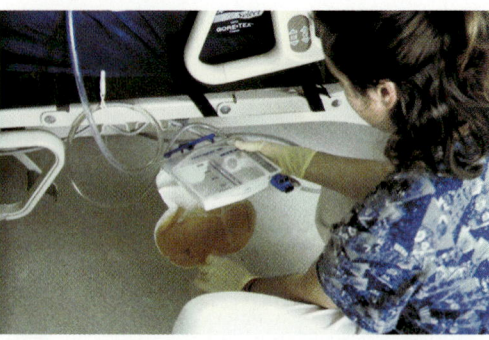

FIGURE 39-36 Monitor the urinary status. Assess and document the amount, color, and quality of urine. DELMAR/CENGAGE LEARNING

24. Instruct the client to immediately report discomfort or pressure during balloon inflation; if pain occurs, discontinue the procedure, deflate the balloon, and insert the catheter farther into the bladder. If the client continues to complain of pain with balloon inflation, remove the catheter and notify the client's health care provider.

24. Pain or pressure indicates inflation of the balloon in the urethra; further insertion will prevent misplacement and further pain or bleeding.

25. Once the balloon has been inflated, gently pull the catheter until the retention balloon is resting snugly against the bladder neck (resistance will be felt when the balloon is properly seated).

25. Maximizes continuous bladder drainage and prevents urine leakage around the catheter.

26. Tape the catheter to the abdomen or thigh snugly, yet with enough slack so it will not pull on the bladder (see Figure 39-35).

26. Prevents excessive traction from the balloon rubbing against the bladder neck, inadvertent catheter removal, or urethral erosion.

27. Place the drainage bag below the level of the bladder. Do not let it rest on the floor. Make sure the tubing lies over, not under, the leg.

27. Maximizes continuous drainage of urine from the bladder (drainage is prevented when the drainage bag is placed above the abdomen).

28. Remove gloves, dispose of equipment, and wash hands.

28. Prevents transfer of microorganisms.

29. Help client adjust position. Lower the bed.

29. Promotes client comfort and safety.

30. Assess and document the amount, color, odor, and quality of urine (see Figure 39-36).

30. Monitors urinary status.

31. Wash hands/hand hygiene.

31. Reduces transmission of microorganisms.

delegation tip

Insertion of an indwelling catheter in a female client is generally not delegated to ancillary personnel. The delegation of this skill depends on institution policy and the availability of licensed staff versus properly trained ancillary personnel.

nursing tips

- *If you miss and insert the catheter in the vagina, leave it there so you can use it as a landmark to find the meatus on the next try.*
- *If the client is unable to tolerate lying supine with her legs spread, attempt to visualize the meatus with the client in the side-lying position.*

- *Be aware that a client with a history of sexual assault or trauma may be anxious or apprehensive about the procedure.*
- *The lithotomy position can be used for women with a history of knee or hip disease or surgery.*

PROCEDURE 39-5	**Irrigating an Open Urinary Catheter**

EQUIPMENT

- Sterile gloves
- Sterile cover for the end of the drainage tubing
- Disposable, water-resistant drape or towel
- Sterile Asepto or Toomey syringe with container for irrigant

- Sterile antiseptic swabs
- Sterile irrigating solution (labeled with date and time of opening, if opened)

ACTION	RATIONALE
1. Verify the need for bladder or catheter irrigation.	1. Ensures that procedure is being applied correctly; reduces unnecessary opening of the system and risk of infection.
2. For prn catheter irrigation, palpate for full bladder and check current output against previous totals.	2. If irrigation is on a prn basis, it may not be needed currently.
3. Verify prescribing practitioner's orders for type of irrigation and irrigant as well as amount.	3. Ensures accuracy in the provision of treatment.
4. If repeat procedure, read previous documentation in the record.	4. Establishes prior client responses to prior teaching done by staff.
5. Assemble all supplies (see Figure 39-37). Wash hands/hand hygiene.	5. Having all supplies in room enables the nurse to maintain sterility of supplies once they are opened and laid out.
6. Premedicate client if ordered or needed.	6. Increases comfort for the procedure.
7. Provide teaching to the client as needed, based on what client already knows.	7. Knowledge will increase client cooperation and decrease anxiety.
8. Assist the client to a dorsal recumbent position.	8. Facilitates the flow of irrigant into the bladder.
9. Wash hands/hand hygiene.	9. Decreases transmission of microorganisms.
10. Provide for client privacy with a closed door or curtain.	10. Decreases client anxiety.
11. Empty the collection bag of urine.	11. Starting with an empty collection bag makes it easier to identify clots or sediment passed as a result of irrigation.

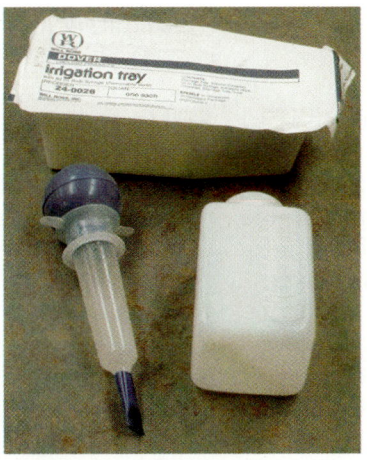

FIGURE 39-37 Irrigation Kit DELMAR/CENGAGE LEARNING

(Continues)

PROCEDURE 39-5
Irrigating an Open Urinary Catheter (Continued)

ACTION	RATIONALE

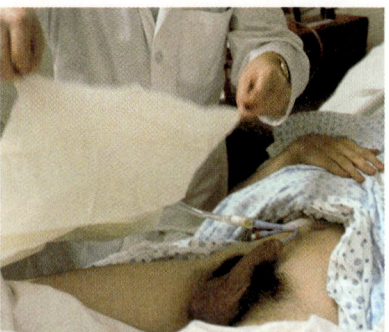

FIGURE 39-38 Expose the retention catheter. DELMAR/CENGAGE LEARNING

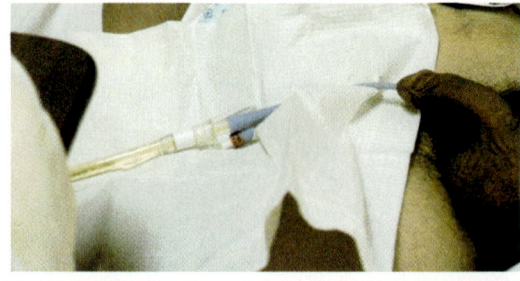

FIGURE 39-39 Place a water-resistant drape under the retention catheter. DELMAR/CENGAGE LEARNING

12. Expose the retention catheter, and place the water-resistant drape underneath it (see Figures 39-38 and 39-39).

12. Protects the bedclothes and client from urine and body fluids.

13. Open the sterile syringe and container. Stand it up carefully in or on the wrapper and add 100 to 200 cc sterile diluent without touching or contaminating the tip of the syringe or the inside of the receptacle.

13. Enables nurse to maintain sterility of gloves once they are applied.

14. Open the end of the antiseptic swab package, exposing the swab sticks.

14. Enables nurse to maintain sterility of gloves once they are applied.

15. Open the sterile cover for drainage tube.

15. Enables nurse to maintain sterility of gloves once they are applied.

16. Apply the sterile gloves.

16. Maintains sterility of the procedure.

17. Disinfect the connection between the catheter and the drainage tubing.

17. Minimizes risk of contaminating the system.

18. After the disinfectant dries, loosen the ends of the connection.

18. Enables the nurse to open the connection without accidently contaminating either end.

19. Grasp the catheter and tubing 1 to 2 inches from their ends, with catheter in the nondominant hand.

19. Maintains sterility of the procedure and allows the nurse to be positioned to use the dominant hand for the syringe.

20. Fold the catheter to pinch it closed between the palm and last three fingers; use the thumb and first finger to hold the sterile cap for the drainage tube.

20. Allows for one nurse to handle all equipment simultaneously, thus maintaining sterility.

21. Separate the catheter and tube, covering the tube tightly with the sterile cap.

21. Maintains sterility of equipment.

22. Fill the syringe with 30 cc for catheter irrigation or 60 cc for bladder irrigation. Insert the tip of the syringe into the catheter and gently instill the solution into the catheter (see Figures 39-40 and 39-41 on page 1275).

22. Catheter can be irrigated with 30 cc of solution, minimizing bladder discomfort, while irrigating a bladder takes 60 cc.

23. Clamp catheter if ordered (medicated solution). If not clamped, irrigant may be released into a collection container or aspirated back into the syringe (see Figure 39-42 on page 1275).

23. Fine sediment or clear irrigant with medication can run freely; material with more solids (sediment or clots) may need gentle aspiration.

24. If the bladder or catheter is being irrigated to clear solid material, repeat irrigation until return is clear.

24. Clearing the catheter completely in this irrigation means a lower total number of irrigations and less opening of the system, thus decreasing the risk of infection.

(Continues)

PROCEDURE 39-5
Irrigating an Open Urinary Catheter (Continued)

ACTION	RATIONALE

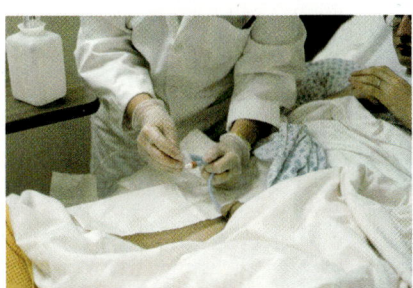

FIGURE 39-40 Separate the catheter and tube. DELMAR/CENGAGE LEARNING

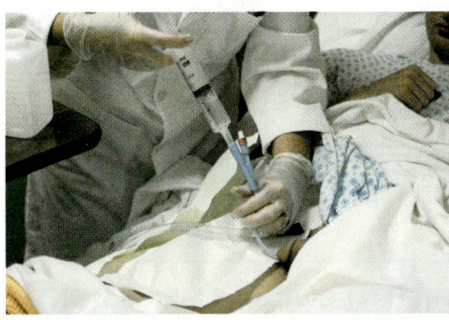

FIGURE 39-41 Insert the tip of the syringe into the catheter, and gently instill the solution. DELMAR/CENGAGE LEARNING

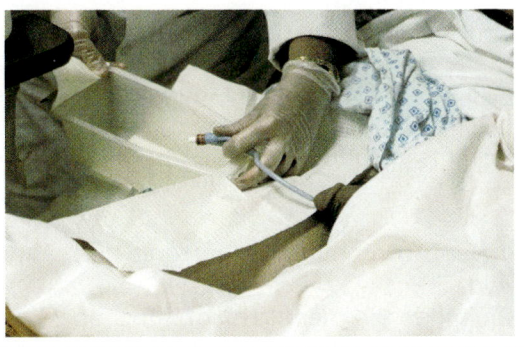

FIGURE 39-42 Irrigant is released into a collection container. DELMAR/CENGAGE LEARNING

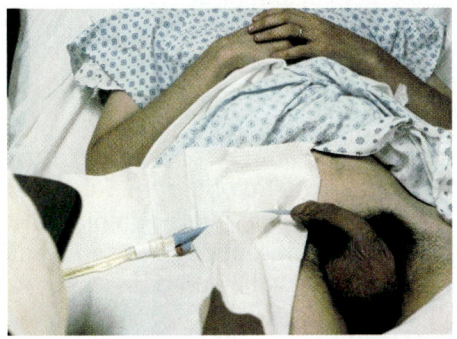

FIGURE 39-43 Reconnect the tubing to the catheter. DELMAR/CENGAGE LEARNING

25. Reconnect system and remove sterile gloves. Wash hands (see Figure 39-43).

26. When irrigation is finished, record type of returns and total amount of irrigation fluid used.

27. Monitor client for pain, urine color and clarity, any solid material passed, and total intake and output.

28. Wash hands/hand hygiene.

25. Maintains sterility of system and reduces transmission of microorganisms.

26. This information can be compared to evaluate status of the urinary tract and catheter. A catheter that is being frequently irrigated for sediment, for instance, may need to be changed, or medications may need to be adjusted.

27. Monitoring output after irrigation evaluates the efficacy of the treatment.

28. Reduces transmission of microorganisms.

delegation tip

The task of irrigating a urinary catheter cannot be delegated, as it requires the skills and problem-solving abilities of a nurse.

nursing tips

Never try to force irrigation of any tube. If the tube does not irrigate smoothly, stop and assess the situation.

PROCEDURE
39-6

PROCEDURE 39-6 Irrigating the Bladder Using a Closed-System Catheter

EQUIPMENT
- Three-way indwelling catheter or Y adapter
- IV pole
- Ordered irrigation solution
- Sterile gloves
- Closed-irrigation tubing
- Large urine collection bag
- Antiseptic swabs

ACTION	RATIONALE
INTERMITTENT BLADDER IRRIGATION USING A STANDARD RETENTION CATHETER AND A Y ADAPTER	
1. Wash hands/hand hygiene.	1. Prevents spread of microorganisms.
2. Close privacy curtain or door.	2. Provides privacy.
3. Hang the prescribed irrigation solution from an IV pole.	3. Different solutions may be ordered depending on the results the prescribing practitioner desires. Bladder irrigant is generally packaged in 2000- to 4000-mL bottles.
4. Insert the clamped irrigation tubing into the bottle of irrigant and prime the tubing with fluid, expelling all air and reclamping the tube.	4. Prevents introduction of air into the bladder.
5. Prepare sterile antiseptic swabs and sterile Y connector if one will be used.	5. Prevents contamination of sterile gloves and field.
6. Apply sterile gloves.	6. Minimizes the client's risk of infection when connecting the irrigant to the catheter and drainage system.
7. Clamp the urinary catheter.	7. Prevents urine leakage onto the bed linens.
8. Unhook the drainage bag from the retention catheter.	8. Allows the Y adapter to be inserted into the system.
9. While holding the drainage tubing and the drainage port of the catheter in your nondominant hand, cleanse both the tubing and the port with antiseptic swabs.	9. Reduces risk of contamination and infection.
10. Connect one port of the Y connector to the drainage port of the retention catheter.	10. Provides a bifurcation for irrigant to instill as well as urine to drain.
11. Connect another port of the Y adapter to the drainage tubing and bag.	11. Collects the urine and drained irrigant. This may be the established urine collection bag or a new sterile bag that is large enough to hold the increased volume of drainage.
12. Attach the third port of the Y adapter to the irrigant tubing.	12. Instills the irrigant into the closed system.
13. Unclamp the urinary catheter and establish that urine is draining through the catheter into the drainage bag.	13. If the urine does not flow freely after unclamping, the catheter may have become clogged with a clot or debris. Notify the client's prescribing practitioner of the lack of urine drainage.
14. To irrigate the catheter and bladder, clamp the drainage tubing distal to the Y adapter.	14. Prevents the irrigant from bypassing the bladder and flowing directly into the drainage bag.

(Continues)

PROCEDURE 39-6
Irrigating the Bladder Using a Closed-System Catheter (Continued)

ACTION	RATIONALE

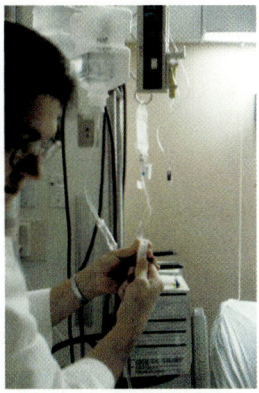

FIGURE 39-44 Clamp the irrigant tubing. DELMAR/CENGAGE LEARNING

ACTION	RATIONALE
15. Instill the prescribed amount of irrigant.	15. The bladder normally feels full when it contains approximately 300 cc of urine. If a prescribed amount of irrigant was not ordered, do not instill more than 150 cc of irrigant. If the client has undergone bladder surgery, do not instill irrigant without knowing the specific amount ordered.
16. Clamp the irrigant tubing (see Figure 39-44).	16. Prevents further instillation of irrigant.
17. If the prescribing practitioner has ordered the irrigant to remain in the bladder for a measured length of time, wait the prescribed length of time.	17. Some irrigation solutions contain medication and are meant to remain in contact with the bladder wall for a prescribed length of time.
18. Unclamp the drainage tubing and monitor the drainage as it flows into the drainage bag.	18. Assess the drainage for volume, color, clarity, and the presence of any clots or debris.

CLOSED BLADDER IRRIGATION USING A THREE-WAY CATHETER

ACTION	RATIONALE
19. Wash hands/hand hygiene.	19. Reduces transmission of microorganisms.
20. Close privacy curtain or door.	20. Provides privacy.
21. Explain procedure to the client. Answer questions and provide support.	21. Reduces anxiety and uncertainty associated with the procedure.
22. Hang prescribed irrigation solution from an IV pole.	22. Different solutions may be ordered depending on the results desired. Bladder irrigant is generally packaged in 2000- to 4000-mL bottles.
23. Insert the clamped irrigation tubing into the bottle of irrigant and prime the tubing with fluid, expelling all air and reclamping the tube (see Figure 39-45 on page 1278).	23. Prevents introduction of air into the bladder.
24. Prepare sterile antiseptic swabs and any other sterile equipment needed.	24. Prevents contamination of sterile gloves and field.
25. Apply sterile gloves (see Figure 39-46 on page 1278).	25. Minimizes the client's risk of infection when connecting the irrigant to the catheter and drainage system.

(Continues)

PROCEDURE 39-6
Irrigating the Bladder Using a Closed-System Catheter (Continued)

ACTION	RATIONALE

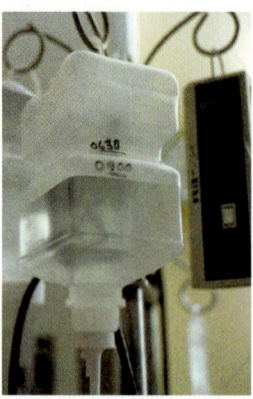

FIGURE 39-45 **Insert the clamped irrigation tubing into the bottle of irrigant.** DELMAR/CENGAGE LEARNING

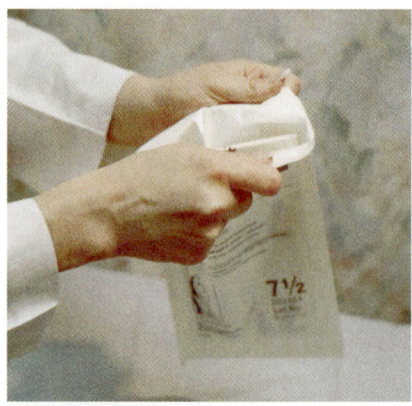

FIGURE 39-46 **Apply sterile gloves.** DELMAR/CENGAGE LEARNING

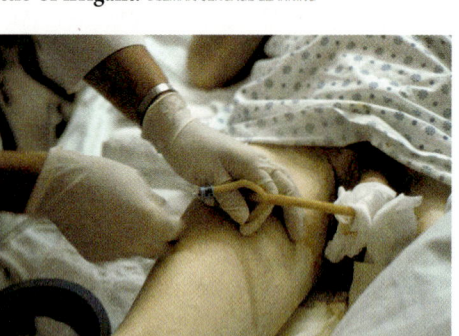

FIGURE 39-47 **Remove the cap from the irrigation port of the three-way catheter.** DELMAR/CENGAGE LEARNING

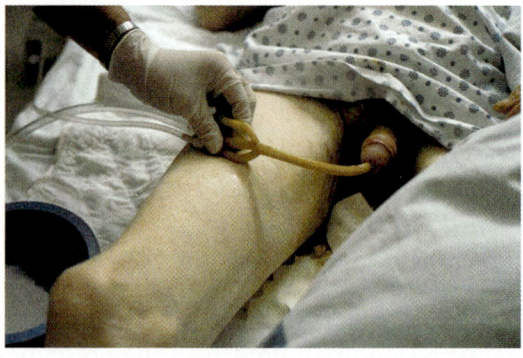

FIGURE 39-48 **Attach the irrigation tubing, remove the clamp from the catheter, and observe for urine drainage. Carefully observe the drainage for color, clarity, and the presence of debris.** DELMAR/CENGAGE LEARNING

ACTION	RATIONALE
26. Clamp the urinary catheter.	26. Prevents leakage of urine onto the bedclothes.
27. Remove the cap from the irrigation port of the three-way catheter (see Figure 39-47).	27. Allows access for the irrigant tubing.
28. Cleanse the irrigation port with the sterile antiseptic swabs.	28. Minimizes the risk of infection.
29. Attach the irrigation tubing to the irrigation port of the three-way catheter.	29. Introduces the irrigant into the system.
30. Remove the clamp from the catheter and observe for urine drainage (see Figure 39-48).	30. Ensures catheter remains patent after being clamped. Some surgical procedures can cause bleeding and clotting of the catheter.

IF INTERMITTENT IRRIGATION HAS BEEN ORDERED

31. Instill the prescribed amount of irrigant.	31. The bladder normally feels full when it contains approximately 300 cc of urine. If a prescribed amount of irrigant was not ordered, do not instill more than 150 cc of irrigant. If the client has undergone bladder surgery, do not instill irrigant without knowing the specific amount ordered.
32. Clamp the irrigant tubing.	32. Prevents further instillation of irrigant.

(Continues)

PROCEDURE 39-6
Irrigating the Bladder Using a Closed-System Catheter (Continued)

ACTION	RATIONALE

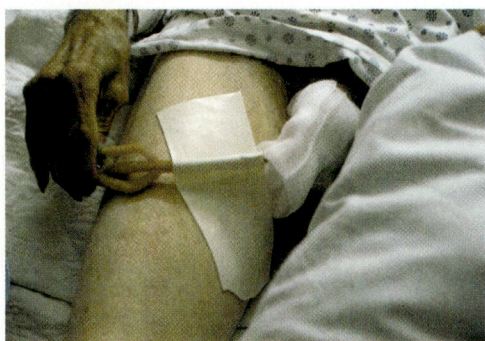

FIGURE 39-49 Securely tape the catheter to the thigh to prevent it from becoming dislodged. DELMAR/CENGAGE LEARNING

ACTION	RATIONALE
33. If the prescribing practitioner has ordered the irrigant to remain in the bladder for a measured length of time, clamp the drainage tube prior to instilling the irrigant and wait the prescribed length of time.	33. Some irrigation solutions contain medication and are meant to remain in contact with the bladder wall for a prescribed length of time.
34. Monitor the drainage as it flows into the drainage bag.	34. Assesses the drainage for volume, color, clarity, and the presence of any clots or debris.
35. Tape the catheter securely to the thigh (see Figure 39-49).	35. Prevents the catheter from becoming dislodged.
36. Wash hands/hand hygiene.	36. Reduces transmission of microorganisms.

If Continuous Bladder Irrigation Has Been Ordered

ACTION	RATIONALE
37. Adjust the clamp on the irrigation tubing to allow the prescribed rate of irrigant to flow into the catheter and bladder.	37. Regulates the amount of irrigant flowing in and out of the bladder to prevent distention or damage to any surgical site.
38. Monitor the drainage for color, clarity, debris, and volume as it flows back into the drainage bag.	38. Assesses for bleeding, clotting, and blockage of urine drainage or other complications.
39. Tape the catheter securely to the thigh (see Figure 39-49).	39. Prevents the catheter from becoming dislodged.
40. Wash hands/hand hygiene.	40. Reduces transmission of microorganisms.

delegation tip

This task cannot be delegated. Bladder irrigation using a closed-system catheter requires the skills of a nurse.

nursing tips

- *Do not slow a continuous irrigation without specific orders from the client's prescribing practitioner, obvious signs of bladder distention, or a plugged catheter.*
- *Be sure to track the amount of irrigant instilled and the amount of drainage. The drainage must always equal or exceed the amount instilled.*
- *Be sure to note the amount of irrigant instilled in the intake and output record so the amount instilled can be subtracted from the output to determine the urine output. Negative amounts must be reported.*

<table>
<tr><td>PROCEDURE
39-7</td><td>**Administering an Enema**</td></tr>
</table>

EQUIPMENT

Large-Volume Cleansing Enema

- Absorbent pad for the bed
- Disposable gloves
- Bedside commode or bedpan if client will not be able to ambulate to bathroom
- Lubricant
- Enema container

- Tubing with clamp and nozzle
- Thermometer for enema solution
- Toilet tissue
- IV pole
- Washcloth, towel, and basin

Small-Volume Prepackaged Enema

- Prescribed prepackaged enema
- Lubricant if the tip is not prelubricated
- Toilet tissue

- Bedpan or commode if the client cannot use the bathroom
- Absorbent pad for bed
- Gloves

Return-Flow Enema

- Absorbent pad for the bed
- Disposable gloves
- Bedside commode or bedpan if client will not be able to ambulate to bathroom
- Prescribed solution

- Lubricant
- Enema container
- Tubing with clamp and nozzle
- Thermometer
- Toilet tissue

ACTION	RATIONALE

LARGE-VOLUME CLEANSING ENEMA

1. Wash hands/hand hygiene.
2. Assess client's understanding of procedure and provide privacy.
3. Apply gloves.
4. Prepare equipment (see Figure 39-50).
5. Place absorbent pad on bed under client. Assist client in attaining left lateral position with right leg flexed as sharply as possible. If there is a question regarding the client's ability to hold the solution, place a bedpan on the bed nearby (see Figure 39-51).

1. Reduces transmission of microorganisms.
2. Prepares client for procedure.

3. Prevents contact with feces.
4. Ensures a smooth procedure.
5. Facilitates flow of solution into the rectum and colon. The flexed leg provides the best exposure of the anus.

FIGURE 39-50 Assemble the equipment at the bedside.
DELMAR/CENGAGE LEARNING

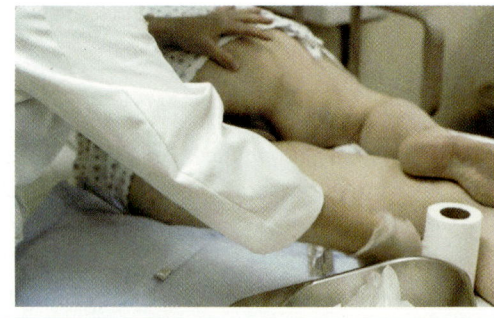

FIGURE 39-51 Position the client in the left lateral position with the right leg sharply flexed. DELMAR/CENGAGE LEARNING

(Continues)

PROCEDURE 39-7
Administering an Enema (Continued)

ACTION	RATIONALE
6. If specified, heat solution to desired temperature using thermometer to measure. Enemas administered to adults are usually given at 105°F to 110°F (40.5°F to 43°C), and those administered to children are usually administered at 100°F (37.7°C). Solution should be at least body temperature to prevent cramping and discomfort.	6. Enemas work best when solution is warm. If enemas are too hot, damage can be done to the bowel mucosa. If enemas are too cold, spasms may occur.
7. Pour solution into the bag or bucket; add water if needed (see Figure 39-52). Open clamp and allow solution to prime tubing. Clamp tubing when primed.	7. Expels air from the tubing, which could cause intestinal distention and discomfort.
8. Lubricate 5 cm (2 in) of the rectal tube unless the tube is part of a prelubricated enema set (see Figure 39-53).	8. Minimizes trauma to the anal sphincter during insertion of the rectal tube.
9. Holding the enema container level with the rectum, have the client take a deep breath. Slowly and smoothly insert rectal tube into rectum approximately 7 to 10 cm in an adult. The rectum of an adult is usually 10 to 20 cm (4 to 6 in). The tube should be inserted beyond the internal sphincter. Aim the rectal tube toward the client's umbilicus (see Figure 39-54).	9. A deep breath helps to relax the sphincter. Insertion of rectal tube toward the umbilicus guides tube along rectum.

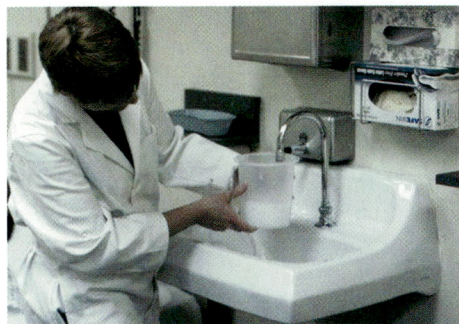

FIGURE 39-52 Place solution into the bucket and add water as needed. DELMAR/CENGAGE LEARNING

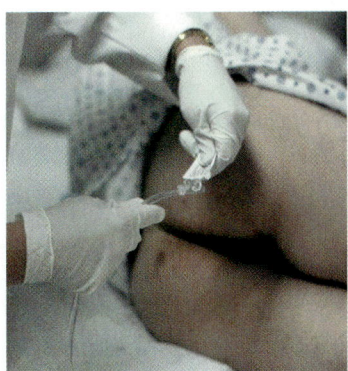

FIGURE 39-53 Lubricate 2 inches of the rectal tube with lubricant. DELMAR/CENGAGE LEARNING

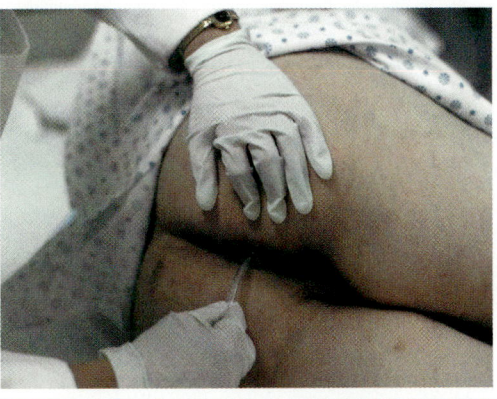

FIGURE 39-54 Gently and smoothly insert the rectal tube into the rectum. DELMAR/CENGAGE LEARNING

(Continues)

PROCEDURE 39-7
Administering an Enema (Continued)

ACTION	RATIONALE
10. Raise the container holding the solution and open clamp. (If using an enema set, squeeze the container holding solution.) The solution should be 30 to 45 cm (12 to 18 in) above the rectum for an adult, and 7.5 cm (3 in) above the rectum for an infant. The solution may be placed on an IV pole at the proper height.	10. Solution should be at a height above rectum that allows gravity flow of solution into the rectum but does not cause damage to the rectal lining because of a too rapid increase in rectal pressure.
11. Slowly administer the fluid.	11. Administering enema slowly with momentary pauses decreases the incidence of intestinal spasms and cramps.
12. When solution has been completely administered or when the client cannot hold any more fluid, clamp the tubing, remove the rectal tube, and dispose of it properly.	12. The urge to defecate indicates that a sufficient amount of fluid has been administered.
13. Clean lubricant, any solution, and any feces from the anus with toilet tissue (see Figure 39-55).	13. Minimizes skin irritation.
14. Have the client continue to lie on the left side for the prescribed length of time.	14. Certain types of enemas are more effective when retained for a specified amount of time. It is easier for the client to retain the enema in a lying position, where gravity can be resisted.
15. When the client has retained the enema for the prescribed amount of time, assist to the bedside commode or toilet or onto the bedpan. If the client is using the bathroom, instruct not to flush the toilet when finished.	15. Client will be prepared to expel fluid and feces.
16. When the client is finished expelling the enema, assist to clean the perineal area if needed.	16. Prevents skin breakdown and excoriation.
17. Return the client to a comfortable position. Place a clean, dry protective pad under the client to catch any solution or feces that may continue to be expelled.	17. Provides comfort for the client and protects the linen from potential soiling.
18. Observe feces and document data.	18. Provides a record of the results.
19. Remove gloves; wash hands/hand hygiene.	19. Reduces transmission of microorganisms.

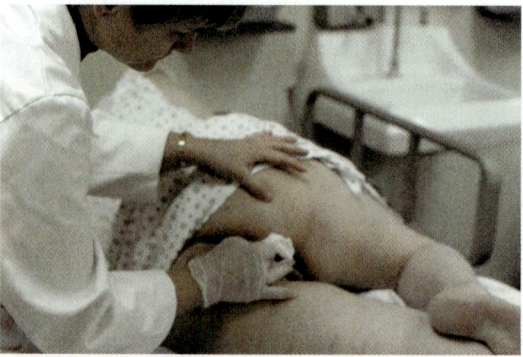

FIGURE 39-55 Clean the anal area to remove excess lubricant. DELMAR/CENGAGE LEARNING

(Continues)

PROCEDURE 39-7
Administering an Enema (Continued)

ACTION	RATIONALE

SMALL-VOLUME PREPACKAGED ENEMA

20. Wash hands/hand hygiene.
21. Remove prepackaged enema from packaging. Be familiar with any special instructions included with the enema. The packaged enema may be stood in a basin of warm water to warm the fluid prior to use (see Figure 39-56).
22. Apply gloves.
23. Place absorbent pad on bed under client. Assist client in attaining left lateral position with right leg flexed as sharply as possible (see Figure 39-57), or you may use the knee-chest position (see Figure 39-58). If there is a question regarding the client's ability to hold the solution, place a bedpan on the bed nearby.
24. Remove the protective cap from the nozzle, and inspect the nozzle for lubrication. If the lubrication is not adequate, add more.

20. Reduces transmission of microorganisms.
21. Prepares the enema for use.

22. Protects hands from exposure to feces.
23. Facilitates flow of solution into the rectum and colon. The flexed leg provides the best exposure of the anus. The knee-chest position provides good exposure and allows gravity to aid in retention of the enema.

24. Prevents trauma to the rectal mucosa.

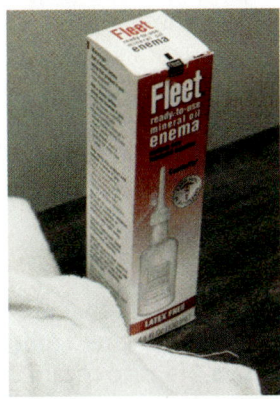

FIGURE 39-56 A Commercial Enema DELMAR/CENGAGE LEARNING

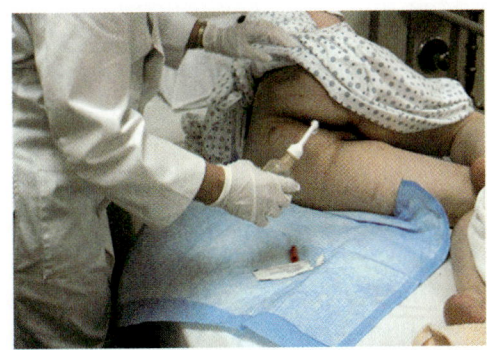

FIGURE 39-57 Position the client in the left lateral position with the right leg sharply flexed. DELMAR/CENGAGE LEARNING

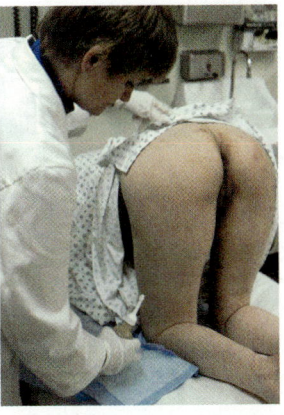

FIGURE 39-58 Alternately, you may position the client in the knee-chest position. DELMAR/CENGAGE LEARNING

(Continues)

PROCEDURE 39-7
Administering an Enema (Continued)

ACTION	RATIONALE
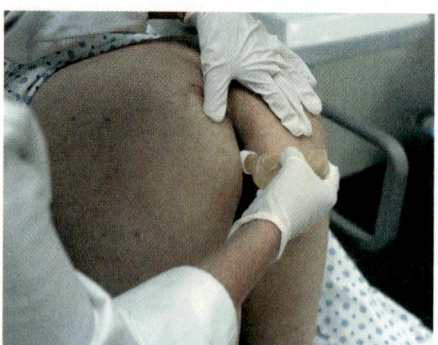	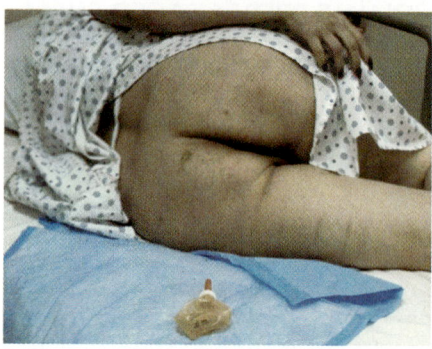

FIGURE 39-59 After inserting the nozzle into the anus, squeeze the container until all the solution is instilled. DELMAR/CENGAGE LEARNING

FIGURE 39-60 Remove the nozzle and container, and have the client continue to lie on the left side for the prescribed length of time. Dispose of the empty container in a trash receptacle. DELMAR/CENGAGE LEARNING

25. Squeeze the container gently to remove any air, and prime the nozzle.

25. Reduces introduction of air into the rectum.

26. Have the client take a deep breath. Simultaneously gently insert the enema nozzle into the anus, pointing the nozzle toward the umbilicus.

26. Relaxes the rectal sphincter. Pointing the nozzle toward the umbilicus positions the nozzle away from the rectal walls.

27. Squeeze the container until all the solution is instilled (see Figure 39-59).

27. Allows the client to get the full benefit of the solution.

28. Remove the nozzle from the anus, and dispose of the empty container in a trash receptacle (see Figure 39-60).

28. Prevents the spread of microorganisms.

29. Clean lubricant, any solution, and any feces from the anus with toilet tissue.

29. Minimizes skin irritation.

30. Have the client continue to lie on the left side for the prescribed length of time.

30. Certain types of enemas are more effective when retained for a specified amount of time. It is easier for the client to retain the enema in a lying position, where gravity can be resisted.

31. When the client has retained the enema for the prescribed amount of time, assist to the bedside commode or toilet or onto the bedpan. If the client is using the bathroom, instruct not to flush the toilet when finished.

31. Client will be prepared to expel fluid and feces.

32. When the client is finished expelling the enema, assist to clean the perineal area if needed.

32. Prevents skin breakdown and excoriation.

33. Return the client to a comfortable position. Place a clean, dry protective pad under the client to catch any solution or feces that may continue to be expelled.

33. Provides comfort for the client and protects the linen from potential soiling.

34. Observe feces and document data.

34. Provides a record of the results.

35. Remove gloves; wash hands/hand hygiene.

35. Reduces transmission of microorganisms.

RETURN-FLOW ENEMA
36. Wash hands/hand hygiene.
37. Assess if client understands procedure.

36. Practices clean technique.
37. Prepares client for procedure.

(Continues)

PROCEDURE 39-7
Administering an Enema (Continued)

ACTION	RATIONALE
38. Apply gloves.	38. Prevents contact with feces.
39. Place absorbent pad on bed under client. Assist client in attaining left lateral position with right leg flexed as sharply as possible.	39. Facilitates flow of solution into the rectum and colon. The flexed leg provides the best exposure of the anus.
40. If specified, heat solution to desired temperature using thermometer to measure. Enemas administered to adults are usually given at 105°F to 110°F (40.5°C to 43°C), and those administered to children are usually administered at 100°F (37.7°C). Solution should be at least body temperature to prevent cramping and discomfort.	40. Enemas work best when solution is warm. If enemas are too hot, damage can be done to the bowel mucosa. If enemas are too cold, spasms may occur.
41. Pour solution into the bag or bucket, open clamp, and allow solution to prime tubing. Clamp tubing when primed.	41. Expels air from the tubing that could cause intestinal distention and discomfort.
42. Lubricate 5 cm (2 in) of the rectal tube unless the tube is part of a prelubricated enema set.	42. Minimizes trauma to the anal sphincter during insertion of the rectal tube.
43. Holding the enema container level with the rectum, have the client take a deep breath. Simultaneously, slowly and smoothly insert rectal tube into rectum approximately 7 to 10 cm in an adult. Rectum of an adult is usually 10 to 20 cm (4 to 6 in). The tube should be inserted beyond the internal sphincter. Aim the rectal tube toward the client's umbilicus.	43. A deep breath helps to relax the sphincter. Insertion of rectal tube toward the umbilicus guides tube along rectum.
44. Raise the container holding the solution and open clamp. The solution should be 30 to 45 cm (12 to 18 in) above the rectum for an adult and 7.5 cm (3 in) above the rectum for an infant (see Figure 39-61).	44. Solution should be at a height that allows gravity flow of solution into the rectum but does not cause damage to the rectal lining because of a too rapid increase in rectal pressure.
45. Slowly administer approximately 200 cc of solution.	45. Administering enema slowly with momentary pauses decreases the incidence of intestinal spasms and cramps.
46. Clamp the tubing and lower the enema container 12 to 18 inches below the client's rectum. Open the clamp (see Figure 39-62).	46. Allows the solution to flow back out of the rectum.

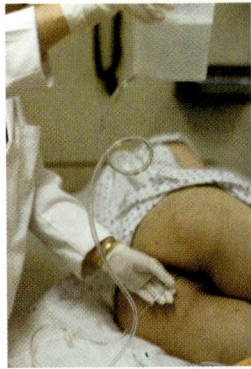

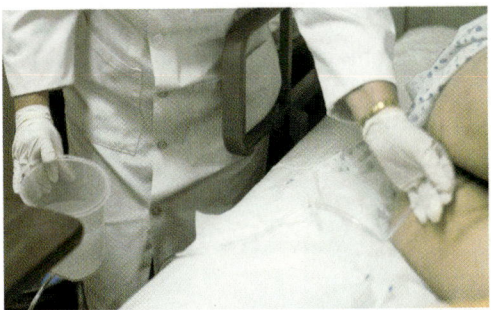

FIGURE 39-61 Raise the container 12 to 18 inches above the rectum and instill 200 cc of solution. DELMAR/CENGAGE LEARNING

FIGURE 39-62 Lower the container 12 to 18 inches below the client's rectum. Observe for air bubbles as the solution returns. DELMAR/CENGAGE LEARNING

(Continues)

PROCEDURE 39-7
Administering an Enema (Continued)

ACTION	RATIONALE
47. Observe the solution container for air bubbles as the solution returns. Note any fecal particles that may be returned.	47. Assesses the effectiveness of the procedure. Air bubbles in the container indicate flatus being passed from the rectum.
48. When no further solution is returned to the container, clamp the tubing and raise the enema container 12 to 18 inches above the client's rectum. Open the clamp and instill approximately 200 cc of fluid.	48. Continues to stimulate peristalsis and remove flatus.
49. Repeat raising and lowering the solution container until no further flatus is seen. Most institutions have guidelines regarding the number of returns to perform. A good rule of thumb is not more than 3 times.	49. Limiting the number of returns prevents unduly tiring or stressing the client.
50. After the final return of fluid, clamp the tubing and gently remove it from the client's anus. Clean the anus with tissue to remove any lubricant or solution.	50. Prevents skin irritation.
51. If the client feels the need to empty rectum, assist onto the bedpan or up to the bathroom or commode.	51. Allows any retained solution to be expelled. Stimulates peristalsis.
52. When the client is finished expelling any retained solution, assist to clean the perineal area if needed.	52. Prevents skin breakdown and excoriation.
53. Return client to a comfortable position. Place a clean, dry protective pad under the client to catch any solution or feces that may continue to be expelled.	53. Provides comfort for the client and protects the linen from potential soiling.
54. Observe any expelled solution, and document the results of the enema.	54. Provides a record of the results.
55. Remove gloves; wash hands/hand hygiene.	55. Reduces transmission of microorganisms.

delegation tip

Administering an enema is a procedure that ancillary personnel are able to perform after proper instruction and supervision. Instruct ancillary personnel to notify the nurse if any difficulty in administering or negative reactions such as severe cramping or inability to retain the enema occur. Results should be documented and reported to the nurse.

nursing tips

Instruct the client that lying on the back with knees and hips flexed toward the chest may make it easier to self-administer an enema.

PROCEDURE 39-8
Irrigating and Cleaning a Stoma

EQUIPMENT
- Colostomy irrigation kit
- 4 × 4 gauze or stoma cover
- Tape, if gauze is used
- Clean gloves
- Ostomy odor eliminator
- Bedpan, toilet, or basin

(Continues)

PROCEDURE 39-8
Irrigating and Cleaning a Stoma (Continued)

ACTION	RATIONALE

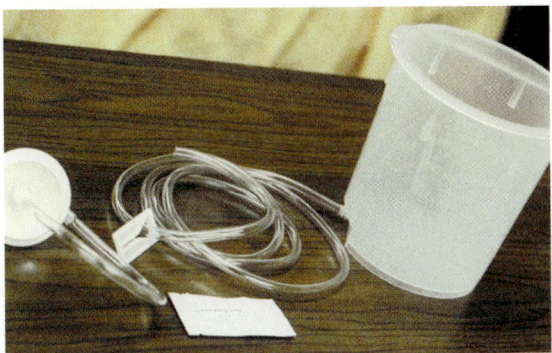

FIGURE 39-63 Colostomy Irrigation Kit DELMAR/CENGAGE LEARNING

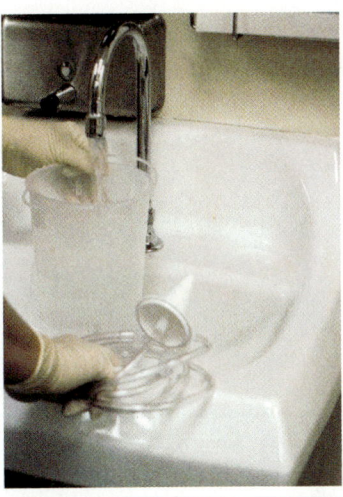

FIGURE 39-64 Colostomy irrigation solution may be administered using a bag or bucket. Fill with tepid tap water. DELMAR/CENGAGE LEARNING

1. Wash hands/hand hygiene.
2. Apply clean gloves.
3. Assemble irrigation kit (see Figure 39-63): Attach cone or catheter to irrigation bag tubing.
4. Fill irrigation bag with 1000 cc tepid tap water (see Figure 39-64).
5. Open clamp and let water from the irrigation bag fill the tubing.
6. Hang bottom of irrigation bag at height of client's shoulder, or 18 inches above the stoma if the client is supine.

7. Check direction of intestine by inserting a gloved finger into orifice of stoma.

8. Place irrigation sleeve over stoma and hold in place with belt (see Figure 39-65 on page 1288).
9. Spray inside of irrigation sleeve and bathroom with odor eliminator (usual dose is 2 sprays).
10. Cuff end of irrigation sleeve and place into toilet bowl (if client is in bathroom) or bedpan (if client is in bed or on chair) (see Figure 39-66 on page 1288).
11. Lubricate the cone end of the irrigation tubing (see Figure 39-67 on page 1288) and insert into orifice of stoma through the top opening of irrigation sleeve (see Figure 39-68 on page 1288).
12. Close top of irrigation sleeve over the tubing.

1. Reduces transmission of microorganisms.
2. Practices clean technique.
3. Ensures that all equipment is ready to use.

4. The colon is already filled with microorganisms, so the use of sterile water is not necessary.
5. This eliminates any air bubbles, which can cause intestinal cramping.
6. Hanging the irrigation bag too high will cause increased intestinal cramping, and hanging the irrigation bag below shoulder level will cause poor results. This height provides resistance of back pressure from flatus.
7. Determining direction of stoma prior to irrigation of colostomy prevents trauma to mucosa and conduit.
8. Irrigant and stool need a vehicle for containment.
9. Helps to decrease or eliminate odor from stool as it is passed from the bowel.
10. Facilitates drainage of water and stool into a suitable container.

11. Prevents cone from causing trauma to intestinal lumen.

12. Prevents water and stool from splashing outside the irrigation sleeve.

(Continues)

PROCEDURE 39-8
Irrigating and Cleaning a Stoma (Continued)

ACTION	RATIONALE

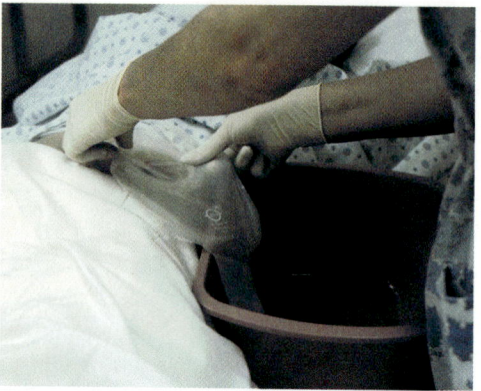

FIGURE 39-65 Place the irrigation sleeve over the stoma.
DELMAR/CENGAGE LEARNING

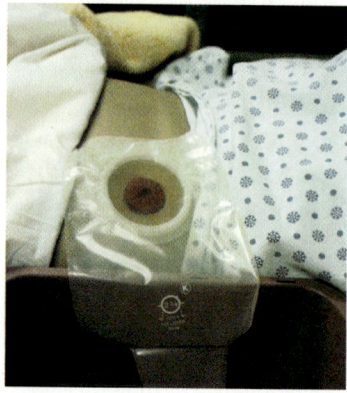

FIGURE 39-66 Place the end of the irrigation sleeve into a basin, bedpan, or toilet bowl. DELMAR/CENGAGE LEARNING

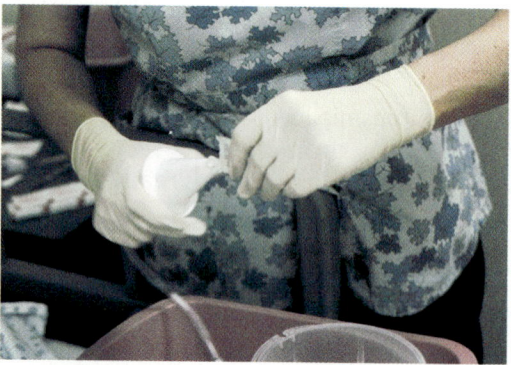

FIGURE 39-67 Lubricate the cone end of the irrigation tubing. DELMAR/CENGAGE LEARNING

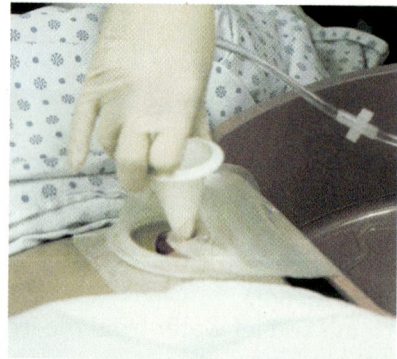

FIGURE 39-68 Insert the cone into the orifice of the stoma.
DELMAR/CENGAGE LEARNING

13. Slowly run water through tubing into colon (see Figure 39-69).

14. Remove cone after all water has emptied out of irrigation bag.

13. Alleviates intestinal cramping. If cramping should start, immediately stop and allow client to rest for a few minutes.
14. Irrigation of colostomy has been completed.

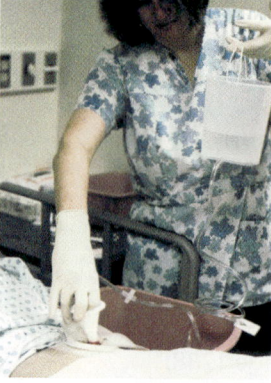

FIGURE 39-69 Gently instill 500 to 1000 cc of tepid water. DELMAR/CENGAGE LEARNING

(Continues)

PROCEDURE 39-8
Irrigating and Cleaning a Stoma (Continued)

ACTION	RATIONALE
15. Close end of irrigation sleeve by attaching it to the top of the sleeve.	15. This maintains a closed system for any remaining stool and irrigant to empty into.
16. Encourage client to ambulate to facilitate emptying of remaining stool from colon.	16. Ambulating influences peristalsis.
17. Remove irrigation sleeve after 20 to 30 minutes or when stool is no longer emptying from colon.	17. Practices clean technique.
18. Cleanse stoma and skin with warm tap water. Pat dry.	18. Gentle care of the stoma prevents injury to the mucosa, which has no nerve endings and is very friable.
19. Place gauze pad over stoma to absorb mucus from stoma.	19. Protects both the client's clothing and the stoma from irritation.
20. Secure gauze with hypoallergenic tape.	20. Ensures that the gauze remains in place.
21. Remove gloves and wash hands/hand hygiene.	21. Reduces transmission of microorganisms.

delegation tip

This task cannot be delegated to ancillary personnel. Colostomy irrigation and cleaning require the skills of a nurse.

nursing tips

- *Assess skin integrity when performing stoma care. A healthy stoma should be red and moist but not painful; a dusky appearance, cyanosis, or pallor indicates a compromised blood supply. Document any sign of skin breakdown.*

- *Change the stoma pouch frequently if the skin underneath the appliance appears irritated.*

PROCEDURE 39-9
Changing a Colostomy Pouch

EQUIPMENT
- Appropriate pouch
- Skin barrier
- Pouch clip or rubber band
- Skin paste
- Disposable gloves
- Soap and washcloth
- Warm water

ACTION	RATIONALE
1. Gather equipment (see Figure 39-70 on page 1290). Explain the procedure to client and provide for privacy. Include caregivers in instruction if indicated.	1. Promotes cooperation and boosts caregiver confidence in ability to perform procedure.
2. Assist client to a standing (preferable) or sitting position.	2. Facilitates application of pouch by reducing wrinkles.

(Continues)

PROCEDURE 39-9
Changing a Colostomy Pouch (Continued)

ACTION	RATIONALE

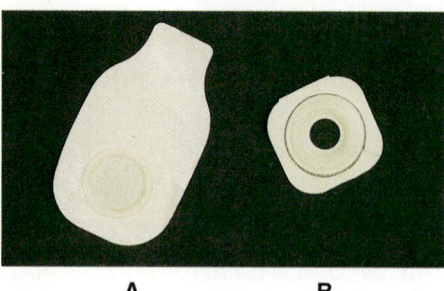

FIGURE 39-70 A. Colostomy Pouch; B. Skin Barrier DELMAR/ CENGAGE LEARNING

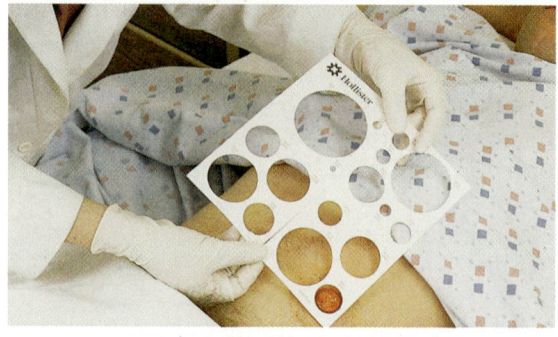

FIGURE 39-71 Measure the stoma for the colostomy pouch. DELMAR/CENGAGE LEARNING

3. Wash hands/hand hygiene; don gloves.
4. Remove the soiled pouch by gently pressing on the skin while pulling the pouch.
5. Dispose of the pouch in a plastic bag after removing the clip used to seal the pouch.
6. Cleanse the skin with soap and water.

7. Inspect the peristomal skin for redness, altered skin integrity, or rashes; consult the enterostomal nurse if lesions of the peristomal skin are observed.
8. Remove excessive hair with a safety razor or electric razor.
9. Inspect the pouch opening and ensure that it fits the stoma; use a pouch pattern to customize the fit if indicated (see Figure 39-71).
10. Apply a skin sealant or skin paste if indicated; apply skin barrier (see Figure 39-72).
11. Gently apply the pouch and press into place (see Figure 39-73). Seal the inferior opening with the clip or a rubber band.

3. Reduces risk of contamination.
4. Avoids trauma to the peristomal skin.

5. Minimizes odor associated with the pouch change.
6. Removes fecal material and pathogens and prepares the skin for pouch reapplication.
7. Peristomal skin conditions cause morbidity and problems with pouch application unless managed promptly.

8. Promotes the seal between pouch adhesive and peristomal skin.
9. Ensures appropriate-sized pouch and protects the peristomal skin.

10. Promotes an effective seal and protects the peristomal skin.
11. Prevents leakage of effluent from the pouch.

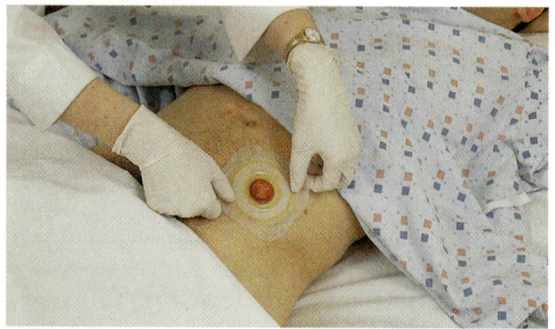

FIGURE 39-72 Apply the skin barrier to the stoma. DELMAR/ CENGAGE LEARNING

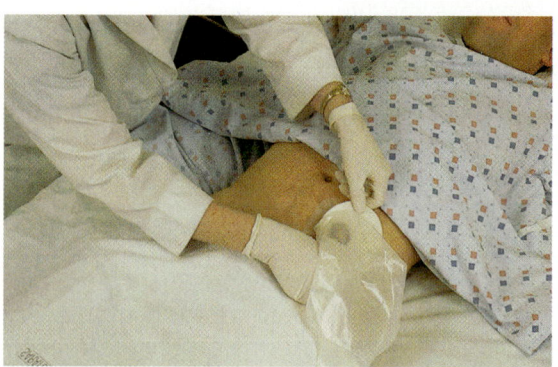

FIGURE 39-73 Press the pouch into place. DELMAR/CENGAGE LEARNING

(Continues)

PROCEDURE 39-9
Changing a Colostomy Pouch (Continued)

ACTION	RATIONALE
12. Remove gloves and discard; wash hands/hand hygiene.	12. Reduces risk of transfer of microorganisms.
13. Note type and size of pouch, condition of stoma (drainage amount and odor; surrounding skin), and client response.	13. Documents client status and condition of stoma.

delegation tip

This task cannot be delegated to ancillary personnel. Changing a colostomy pouch requires the skills of a nurse.

nursing tips

- *Assess skin integrity when performing stoma care. Document any sign of skin breakdown. An ischemic stoma usually appears dark red or black.*
- *Use latex-free gloves and pouches if history of allergy or contact dermatitis.*

- *Change the stoma pouch frequently if the skin underneath the appliance appears irritated.*

KEY CONCEPTS

- Normal urination requires anatomic integrity of the lower urinary tract, nervous control of the detrusor muscle, and competence of the urethral sphincter mechanism.
- Normal bowel evacuation relies on motility factors, the storage abilities of the rectum, and competence of the internal and external sphincter mechanisms.
- Common alterations in urinary elimination include SUI, instability incontinence (urge and reflex incontinence), functional urinary incontinence, extraurethral incontinence, and urinary retention.
- Constipation and diarrhea are common alterations in stool consistency that cause changes in fecal elimination patterns and predispose clients to bowel incontinence.
- Clients with altered patterns of urinary and bowel elimination are evaluated with a detailed historical

interview, focused physical examination, record of bladder and bowel elimination patterns, and review of laboratory values.

- Multiple options, including behavioral management strategies, pharmacotherapy, and surgical interventions, are used to manage clients with altered patterns of elimination.
- Altered stool consistency is prevented or alleviated by managing malabsorption syndromes, maintaining a regular pattern of elimination, ensuring dietary intake of adequate fluid and fiber, and heeding the urge to defecate.
- Bowel incontinence is managed by normalization of stool consistency, maximization of rectal storage abilities, and management of anal sphincter incompetence.

REVIEW QUESTIONS

1. Anticholinergic and antispasmodic medications, such as oxybutynin and propantheline, may be used to treat _____.
   a. stress urinary incontinence
   b. reflex urinary incontinence
   c. urge urinary incontinence
   d. urinary retention

2. When assessing the abdomen of a client with abdominal guarding, _____.
   a. stop the assessment and report the findings
   b. flex the client's knees
   c. position the client on the left side
   d. position the client on the right side

3. A permanent colostomy is usually performed to treat _____.
   a. lower rectal cancer
   b. Crohn's colitis
   c. prostate cancer
   d. urinary retention

4. Dandelion root and leaf are considered _____.
   a. diuretics
   b. antiseptics
   c. antimicrobials
   d. demulcents

5. A healthy stoma should appear _____.
   a. dusky
   b. moist
   c. pale
   d. cyanotic

6. Which of the following procedures may not be delegated to trained ancillary personnel?
   a. Assisting a client with a bedpan or urinal
   b. Application of a condom catheter
   c. Inserting an indwelling catheter in a male
   d. Irrigating and cleaning a stoma

7. Which of the following should the nurse include in the procedure for female urinary catheterization?
   a. Expose the urinary meatus with the dominant hand.
   b. Lubricate 2 inches of the catheter.
   c. Insert the catheter 8 inches with the sterile, gloved hand.
   d. Allow the labia to relax after the meatus is cleansed.

online companion

Visit the DeLaune and Ladner online companion resource at **www.delmar.cengage.com** for additional content and study aids. Click on Online Companions, then select the Nursing discipline.

Life's not just living, it's living in health.

—Guterman (1960)

CHAPTER 40

Nursing Care of the Perioperative Client

COMPETENCIES

1. Discuss the three phases of the perioperative experience in relation to the client's expected outcomes and the major functional roles of the nurse.

2. Assess the physiological, psychological, social, cultural, spiritual, and age-related aspects of the perioperative client's health status.

3. Recognize sociocultural and ethical factors that affect decision making in planning care with the perioperative client.

4. Demonstrate an awareness of age-related functions and values when assessing and teaching clients.

5. Plan, implement, and evaluate the nursing care outcomes for perioperative clients in various health care settings.

6. Document nursing interventions that achieve the individualized expected outcomes for perioperative clients.

7. Describe essential components of discharge teaching for the perioperative client.

ds

postoperative
preoperative
pulse oximeter
transcutaneous electrical nerve
    stimulation (TENS)
urgency

...val
...erthermia
...lled analgesia

...mpression device

before surgery is performed to ensure that Medicare and other third-party payers will reimburse the facility for incurred surgical costs.

SURGICAL INTERVENTIONS

Surgery is performed to correct anatomical or physiological defects and to provide therapeutic interventions. Surgeries are categorized according to the degree of **urgency** (timely intervention of surgery):

1. Emergency surgery requires immediate intervention to sustain life. Emergency cases take precedence over urgent and electively scheduled procedures.
2. Urgent surgery dictates intervention as necessary to maintain health in situations that are not life threatening. These cases are usually added to the surgical schedule rather than replacing a previously scheduled procedure.
3. Elective cases are nonemergent, nonurgent procedures, prescheduled at the convenience of the client and the surgeon because the delay presents no physiological harm. The procedure usually occurs within days or months of the diagnosis.

Once the degree of urgency is established, the reason for performing the surgical intervention is categorized according to the expected outcome (see Table 40-1 on page 1297).

In a true emergency, saving the client's life is the primary goal. Stat blood work, including a type and crossmatch, is performed while the client and the OR are prepared for the surgery. Urgent and elective surgeries allow the client and prescribing practitioner time to discuss the setting and scheduling of the surgery.

SETTING

Ambulatory care centers and prescribing practitioner offices are the usual settings for minor surgical procedures, such as removal of skin lesions and laparoscopy for inspection and biopsy. Outpatient surgery areas (1-day surgery centers or free-standing ambulatory clinics) provide the client and prescribing practitioner with alternative services for urgent and elective surgeries.

surgery until the client is transferred to the operating room (OR). The **intraoperative** (during surgery) phase begins when the client is transferred to the OR and ends with client transfer to a postanesthesia care unit (PACU). When the client leaves the OR and is taken to a PACU, the **postoperative** (after surgery) phase begins; this phase continues until the client is discharged from the care of the surgeon. The perioperative nurse manages, teaches, and studies the care of clients undergoing operative and other invasive procedures.

Changes have occurred in perioperative services as a result of advances in technology (such as lasers), laparoscopic and minimally invasive endoscopic surgeries, and limited resources such as cost-containment measures in health care. These changes have challenged health care providers to be more responsive and cost-effective in delivering perioperative services. Wherever procedures occur, all clients deserve to be treated with the same standard of care.

Surgery is a major source of a hospital's income. Although major surgical interventions still occur in the hospital setting, the 1980s introduced a trend to perform surgery in ambulatory settings. Many of the services of the hospital's perioperative departments are now performed in outpatient settings. This change has had a positive impact on decreasing health care costs related to surgery. At the same time, health care providers are challenged to work in greater collaboration to decrease the client's length of stay in the hospital, increase satisfaction with the services, and prevent complications.

Ambulatory surgery clinics (free-standing facilities) also began in the 1980s as an outgrowth of federally regulated reforms from the Health Care Financing Administration (HCFA). The HCFA's goal in health care reform was to decrease inpatient costs of services. Except for inpatient hospitalization, ambulatory surgery clinics provide all the services offered by hospitals.

In 1989, the HCFA developed a listing of urgent and elective surgeries that require preauthorization for Medicare clients. Preauthorization means the surgery must be approved

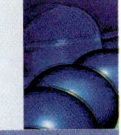

TABLE 40-1	Surgical Interventions Based on Expected Outcomes
INTERVENTION	**EXPECTED OUTCOME**
Diagnostic/ exploratory	Determine the origin of presenting symptoms and extent of a disease process (e.g., biopsy)
Reconstructive	Correct a disease process or improve cosmetic appearance (e.g., arthroplasty and rhinoplasty)
Curative	Repair or remove a diseased organ or restore normal physiological functioning (e.g., amputation or aneurysm repair)
Palliative	Decrease the spread of the disease process to prolong life or to alleviate pain (e.g., colostomy or partial tumor removal)
Transplant	Remove diseased tissue or organ and replace with functioning tissue or organ (e.g., kidney)

Delmar/Cengage Learning

Outpatient surgical units focus on the needs of the client and strive to expedite the rendering of services with a preadmission visit. Preauthorization documents for Medicare or third-party insurance payers should be processed and approved before the preadmission visit.

During the preadmission visit, the circulating nurse and anesthesia provider perform the preoperative assessment and initiate teaching. Diagnostic tests are performed in the outpatient surgical unit as opposed to the traditional process of having a client go to the various hospital departments for testing. Performing diagnostic testing in this fashion promotes a sense of caring for the client's needs and decreases the preadmission time.

On the day of surgery, clients who have been preadmitted go directly to an outpatient surgical unit, where they are prepared for surgery. Family members are encouraged to remain with the client while the client awaits transfer to the operative area.

Perioperative care is initiated for the hospitalized client when the decision is made for surgery. The client is reassessed and the nurse collaborates with the client in planning the care. Client and family teaching is begun as soon as possible to allow time to reinforce the teaching.

Preparing a client for a surgical procedure requires the collaboration of many professionals. Specific role responsibilities focus on assessment, client and family teaching, and interventions to promote client achievement of expected outcomes.

CLIENT SAFETY

Safety is a major concern for the surgical client. Surgeries and procedures involving the wrong site, client, and procedure continue despite national efforts by regulators and professional organizations (Michaels, 2007). In support of the national effort to create a safe health care environment and to prevent surgical errors, the Joint Commission established its National Patient Safety Goals (NPSGs) program in 2002, and the first set of goals was effective in 2003. The NPSGs were established to help accredited organizations address specific areas of concern regarding client safety. The development and annual updating of the NPSGs and requirements are overseen by an expert panel of widely recognized safety experts as well as nurses, prescribing practitioners, pharmacists, risk managers, and other professionals who have hands-on experience in addressing client safety issues in a wide variety of health care settings. The Joint Commission's 2009 NPSGs (2008) for all procedures and surgeries are summarized as follows:

1. Implement best practices for preventing surgical infections, to be phased in during 2009 with full implementation in 2010:
   - Prior to all surgical procedures, the hospital educates clients and their families, implements policies and practices, and conducts periodic risk assessments regarding surgical site infection prevention.
   - Antimicrobial agents for prophylaxis used for specific procedures or diseases are administered according to evidence-based standards and best practice guidelines.
   - The appropriate method of hair removal is by clippers or depilatories; shaving is an inappropriate method of hair removal.
2. Clearly identify the intended site for the procedure:
   - The practitioner performing the procedure marks the procedure site while the client is awake and aware of the marking, if possible.
   - The site marking has the following characteristics:
     - It is made near the site.
     - It includes the practitioner's initials.
     - It is made with a marker that remains visible after the skin prep, final positioning, and sterile draping (adhesive site markers are not acceptable).
   - In addition to preoperative skin marking for spinal procedures, special intraoperative radiographic techniques are used for marking the exact vertebral level.
   - Have in place an alternative process for clients who refuse site marking or who cannot easily be marked under the following conditions:
     - Cases in which it is technically or anatomically impossible to mark the site, such as the perineum or with premature infants
     - Minimal access procedures that intend to treat a lateralized internal organ, for which the intended site is indicated by a mark at or near the insertion site and remains visible after completion of skin prep and sterile draping

- Interventional procedures such as cardiac catheterization, in which the catheter/instrument insertion site is not predetermined
- Tooth extraction, for which the site is documented on the dental radiographs or dental diagram and is available in the procedure room prior to the start of the procedure
- Premature infants, for whom the mark may cause a permanent tattoo

3. Time-out is performed immediately prior to staring the procedure to conduct a final assessment that the correct client, site, positioning, and procedure are identified and that all relevant documents, related information, and necessary equipment are available.

- The time-out has the following characteristics:
  - It is standardized, as defined by the hospital.
  - It is initiated by a designated member of the team.
  - It involves the immediate members of the procedure team.
  - It involves interactive verbal communication between all team members, with all members having the opportunity to express concerns about the procedure verification.
  - It includes a defined process for reconciling differences in responses.
- During the time-out, all other activities are suspended without compromising client safety.
- When two or more procedures are being performed on the same client, a time-out is called to confirm each subsequent procedure before it is initiated.
- The time-out addresses the following:
  - Correct client identity
  - Confirmation of the correct site and site marking
  - An accurate procedure consent form
  - An agreement of the procedure to be performed
  - Correct client position
  - Proper labeling and display of relevant images and results
  - The need to administer antibiotics or fluids for irrigation purposes
  - Safety precautions based on client history or medication use
- The completed components of the Universal Protocol and time-out are documented.

The Joint Commission goals require the collaborative efforts of all surgical personnel and the client to ensure a safe experience.

To facilitate the implementation of its safety goals, the Joint Commission also issued in 2004 the *Universal Protocol for Preventing Wrong Site, Wrong Procedure, Wrong Person Surgery*. The universal protocol is based on the consensus of clinical experts and endorsed by more than 40 professional health care associations and organizations. The Association of periOperative Registered Nurses (AORN), formerly called the Association of Operating Room Nurses, has a position statement regarding "Correct Site Surgery" that endorses the Joint Commission's *Universal Protocol for Preventing Wrong Site, Wrong Procedure, Wrong Person Surgery*.

ANESTHESIA

Anesthesia means the absence of pain. Anesthetic agents render a person insensible to pain during surgical, obstetric, and therapeutic or diagnostic procedures. Anesthesia requires a balancing of several agents to provide sedation, analgesia, muscle relaxation, and anesthesia for procedures of varying complexity. The types of anesthesia and their effects are listed in Table 40-2 on page 1299.

GENERAL ANESTHESIA

General anesthesia refers to the drug-induced state of analgesia, amnesia, muscle relaxation, and unconsciousness. General anesthesia represents a critical experience for surgical clients. The needs of these clients require that perioperative nurses possess knowledge of the basic principles of general anesthesia.

The common routes for administering general anesthetics are inhalation and parenteral; other routes used less frequently are oral and rectal. Inhalation agents are administered in the form of gases or as vapors of volatile liquids through an anesthesia delivery system and a face mask, endotracheal tube, or laryngeal mask airway (LMA) that may be inserted without a muscle relaxant. Commonly used inhalation agents that can produce all of the elements of general anesthesia are listed in the accompanying display on page 1299; these agents are absorbed by the lungs. Nitrous oxide (compressed gas) is both absorbed and eliminated by the lungs, whereas percentages of different volatile liquids vary in excretion between the lungs and kidneys.

Although anesthesia is administered parenterally, it takes several intravenous drugs to produce all the elements of general anesthesia. Injectable agents used for induction or maintenance of anesthesia are from one of the following drug classifications: barbiturates, benzodiazepines, narcotics, and neuromuscular blocking agents. See the accompanying display on page 1300 for common drugs in each of these classifications.

Barbiturates provide a rapid induction of short duration and are therefore used for invasive diagnostic and obstetric procedures and minor surgery. When barbiturates are contraindicated, other short-acting agents are used: ketamine or a nonbarbiturate drug (etomidate or propofol). Neuromuscular blocking agents produce muscle relaxation required for select surgical procedures; these drugs vary in their duration of action.

The client's individualized plan for balanced anesthesia may involve the concurrent or sequential use of many agents. For instance, thoracic muscle relaxation that is required for lung surgery can be provided by intravenous administration of a neuromuscular blocking agent. During the surgery, various types of vapors and gases may also be administered with oxygen to provide anesthesia. For abdominal surgery, muscle relaxation can be achieved by injecting a local anesthetic into the cerebrospinal fluid; after the abdominal anesthesia level

TABLE 40-2 Effects of Anesthetic Agents

TYPE OF ANESTHESIA	EXPECTED RESULT	TECHNIQUE	RISKS
General anesthesia	Total unconscious state, placement of a tube into the trachea	Drug injected into the bloodstream, breathed into the lungs, or administered by other routes	Mouth or throat pain, hoarseness, injury to mouth or teeth, awareness under anesthesia, injury to blood vessels, aspiration, pneumonia
Spinal or epidural analgesic/ anesthesia (with and without sedation)	Temporary decreased sensation or loss of feeling and movement to lower part of the body	Drug injected through a needle/catheter placed either directly into the spinal canal (spinal or subarachnoid) or immediately outside the spinal canal (epidural)	Headache, backache, buzzing in the ears, convulsions, infection, persistent weakness, numbness, residual pain, injury to blood vessels, "total spinal"
Major/minor nerve block (with and without sedation)	Temporary loss of feeling or movement of a specific limb or area	Drug injected near multiple nerves or a plexus (major) or into or around a nerve or small nerve group (minor), providing loss of sensation to the area of the operation	Infection, convulsions, weakness, persistent numbness, residual pain, injury to blood vessels
Intravenous regional anesthesia (with and without sedation)	Temporary loss of feeling and/ or movement of an extremity	Drug injected into veins of arms or legs while using a tourniquet	Infection, convulsions, persistent numbness, residual pain, injury to blood vessels
Monitored anesthesia care (with sedation)	Reduced anxiety and pain, partial or total anesthesia	Drug injected into the bloodstream, breathed into the lungs, or administered by other routes, producing a semiconscious state	Unconscious state, depressed breathing, injury to blood vessels
Monitored anesthesia care (without sedation)	Measurement of vital signs, availability of anesthesia provider for further intervention	None	Increased awareness, anxiety, and/or discomfort

Adapted with permission from the American Association of Nurse Anesthetists. (2004). *Informed consent in anesthesia*. Park Ridge, IL: Author.

INHALATION GENERAL ANESTHETIC AGENTS

VOLATILE LIQUIDS

- Halothane (Fluothane, Somnothane)
- Methoxyflurane (Penthrane)
- Enflurane (Ethrane)
- Isoflurane (Forane)

is established, a short-acting barbiturate may be infused to provide general anesthesia during the surgical procedure. Although the incidence of drug toxicity in anesthesia is rare, clients need to be informed about these inherent risk factors.

REGIONAL ANESTHESIA

The increased use of balanced anesthesia for surgical procedures has made it increasingly important for perioperative nurses to be knowledgeable about regional and local anesthetic agents. Regional anesthesia blocks nerve impulse conduction to a specific area or region of the body to decrease intractable pain or to produce an anesthetic field without the loss of consciousness.

An analgesic or anesthetic state is obtained by injecting a local anesthetic solution along a specific nerve path (see the accompanying display for a list of commonly used local anesthetic agents). Regional anesthesia can be administered with or without sedation (see Table 40-2 for the various techniques used in administering regional anesthesia).

LOCAL ANESTHESIA

Local anesthesia refers to use of an anesthetic agent that disrupts sensation at the nerve endings. The two techniques used for administering local anesthesia are topical and infiltration. Topical anesthesia is the direct application of local anesthetics to tissues in the form of ointments, lotions, solutions, or sprays. After the use of oral anesthetic solutions (e.g., viscous lidocaine), *fluids and foods must be withheld until the gag reflex returns.*

Infiltrate anesthesia refers to intradermal, subcutaneous, or submucosal injection to provide a circumscribed area of anesthesia. This technique provides a local nerve block that is used for suturing lacerations or extracting teeth.

COMMON INTRAVENOUS AGENTS USED FOR GENERAL ANESTHESIA

- Barbiturates: methohexital sodium, thiamylal sodium, thiopental sodium propofol
- Benzodiazepines: diazepam and midazolam
- Narcotics: alfentanil hydrochloride, fentanyl, and sufentanil citrate
- Neuromuscular blocking agents: atracurium besylate, doxacurium chloride, gallamine triethiodide, metocurine iodide, mivacurium chloride, pancuronium bromide, pipecuronium bromide, succinylcholine chloride, tubocurarine chloride, and vecuronium bromide

---

COMMONLY USED LOCAL ANESTHETIC AGENTS

- Bupivacaine hydrochloride (Marcaine, Sensorcaine)
- Chloroprocaine (Nesacaine, Nesacaine-MPF)
- Etidocaine hydrochloride (Duranest)
- Lidocaine hydrochloride (Xylocaine)
- Mepivacaine hydrochloride (Carbocaine, Polocaine)
- Procaine hydrochloride (Novocain)
- Tetracaine hydrochloride (Pontocaine)

PREOPERATIVE PHASE

The primary goal of preoperative nursing care is to place the client in the best possible condition for surgery through careful assessment and thorough preparation. Assessment of the client's status before surgery establishes baseline data to direct interventions throughout the perioperative phases. Each member of the health care team has identified functions relating to the assessment of the client's physiological, psychological, social, cultural, and spiritual status. *The findings from the client's assessment must be documented throughout the surgical experience.*

ASSESSMENT

Assessment of the perioperative client includes a nursing history and physical examination. A complete assessment is performed at the outpatient clinic during the preadmission visit. On the day of surgery, the nurse conducts a focused assessment to ensure current, accurate data.

During the assessment process, the nurse evaluates the client's level of anxiety and fear. Bulechek, Butcher, and Dochterman (2008) describe these feelings:

- Anxiety is a vague, uneasy feeling whose source is often nonspecific or unknown to the client.
- Fear is a feeling of dread related to an identifiable source that the client validates.

Anxiety is accompanied by well-defined physiological changes, such as an increased heart rate, clammy hands, muscular tension (especially in the neck muscles), and behavioral manifestations, such as rapid speech and irritability.

Nursing History

The perioperative nursing history provides information relative to factors that can increase a client's risk or influence the expected surgical outcomes. Pertinent data are obtained from the client interview: medical history, including family history of anesthesia complications (malignant hypertension); medications; allergies; age-related factors; social, cultural, and spiritual concerns; and psychological status. See Chapter 6 for more details.

Nurses should conduct the interview in a quiet room, free from background noise. Many older adult clients have some degree of high-tone hearing loss, so it is necessary to speak in a strong, clear voice.

Clients who have difficulty comprehending the surgical procedure should have a responsible family member present during the interview. A third person can help clarify precisely what the nurse said and can interpret such instructions for other family members.

Medical History

The nurse reviews the client's medical record. The surgeon's history and physical findings provide pertinent data regarding the reasons for surgery. If the client was previously hospitalized, the nurse obtains the previous medical records to have available on the nursing unit. Hospitalization records are reviewed to gain an overview of the client's health status because preexisting medical conditions can increase the client's surgical risks.

During the preoperative interview, the registered nurse (RN) (or circulating nurse) reviews the client's information regarding past illnesses and the main reason for seeking surgical treatment. The surgeon's history and physical findings provide a comprehensive review of the client's current information within a prescribed period of time (usually within 7 days) and pertinent data regarding the reasons for the surgery. Any complications from a previous surgery or anesthesia should be recorded.

It is important to note if the client has had prior blood transfusions or reactions. At this time the nurse can ascertain whether the client has objections to receiving blood or blood products or has made arrangements for blood replacement. Some clients prefer to donate their own blood in advance so that it can be held in reserve if the need for it arises during surgery. Family members or friends may also donate blood to decrease the cost to the client.

Medications

During the nursing history, the nurse needs to assess exactly what drugs the client has been taking. The client's response to questions about the use of alcohol, tobacco, "street drugs," prescriptions, over-the-counter (OTC) drugs, and herbs should be documented because these substances have surgical implications.

Certain prescription drugs (antihypertensives, tranquilizers, steroids, and diuretics), as well as certain OTC medications and herbal preparations, can increase the client's anesthesia risks. Some medications must be stopped at least 2 weeks prior to surgery, or the surgery may be canceled. Clients with chronic diseases are likely to be taking numerous medications that can cause complications during the perioperative period (see the accompanying display on drugs that place surgical clients at risk).

HERBS Question clients regarding their use of herbal products and supplements as part of the preoperative assessment. Certain herbal products and supplements (e.g., *Ephedra sinica,* or Chinese ephedra or ma huang; St. John's wort; feverfew) may place the client at risk if taken before surgery.

Ephedra can produce the same side effects as ephedrine (e.g., increased blood pressure and heart rate, insomnia, anxiety). St. John's wort is used widely as a mild to moderate antidepressant because of its ability to inhibit monoamine oxidase (MAO). MAO inhibitors may interact with various types of anesthetic agents. Feverfew inhibits platelet aggregation and may affect the client's clotting time.

Although some herbal products may place the client at risk during surgery, other herbs, such as *bromelain,* can reduce healing time and pain following various surgical procedures. Bromelain is obtained from the pineapple plant and refers to a group of sulfur-containing enzymes that digest protein (proteolytic enzymes or proteases). Bromelain reduces edema, inflammation, and pain when taken preoperatively.

DRUGS THAT PLACE SURGICAL CLIENTS AT RISK

- Aspirin: May increase bleeding
- Antidepressants: May lower blood pressure during anesthesia
- Bromide in medications (e.g., Sominex): Can accumulate and produce signs and symptoms of dementia
- Drugs with anticholinergic effects: Increase the potential for confusion
- Steroids: Suppress immunity
- Nonsteroidal anti-inflammatory medications: Increase the risk of stress ulcers and displace other drugs from blood proteins

ALLERGIES Allergies and sensitivities to foods, drugs, or other substances should be documented on the assessment record. Of special importance is questioning the client about allergies to iodine. Povidone-iodine, a common antiseptic, is used to prepare the skin for surgery. The nurse places a note regarding the client's allergies on the front of the chart to alert perioperative team members.

Age-Related Considerations

Age-related considerations are critical aspects of assessment. The client's age and developmental stage can influence the ability to cope with surgery. Age-related factors can also influence existing health care problems and the client's response to surgery. For instance, infants are at risk during surgical interventions because their physiological functions are immature. The infant's ability to respond to stress is also altered.

Morbidity and mortality rates for surgical clients over the age of 90 are much higher than for those in the 70 to 75 age group. Older clients may be fearful of death, especially if this is their first hospitalization or surgery. The risk of surgery for many older clients is complicated by chronic disease processes. Age-related risk factors for the older adult should be assessed on an individual basis. When older adult clients are adequately prepared for a noncomplicated surgical procedure, they can tolerate many types of surgeries as well as younger clients. However, studies have shown that when older adult clients are subjected to emergency surgeries or long, complicated surgeries, their decreased ability to adapt to physical and psychological stress may have a negative surgical outcome.

Social and Cultural Considerations

Data relative to the client's social and cultural orientation are incorporated into care. In our multicultural world, our communities are diverse, requiring that the nurse incorporate these data into the plan of care and utilize appropriate teaching methods. Many facilities provide interpreters to prevent language from being a communication barrier.

Cultural beliefs can influence a client's perception of surgery. Listen to the concerns a client expresses during the interview. Surgeries that cause changes in body image can alter self-esteem. The client may worry about being sexually attractive or active after surgery. The nurse may initiate discussion regarding sexual outcomes of surgery; encourage the client to verbalize fears in order to increase adaptive coping. As always, the nurse is cognizant of the client's comfort level when broaching any topic that could be considered sensitive in nature.

Spiritual Considerations

Clients must be provided the opportunity to express their spiritual values and beliefs. Religious beliefs are discussed and incorporated into the client's plan of care. A client may ask to see a member of the clergy before surgery. The beliefs of the client should be respected. The client has the right to refuse certain types of interventions. For example, some religions do not allow the administration of blood products as treatment. When the client indicates that religious beliefs prevent blood administration, the health care team should identify alternative methods of treatment and discuss these with the client during the preoperative phase. Collaborating with the client preoperatively helps prevent ethical dilemmas from arising during the other perioperative phases in the event that the client loses a large quantity of blood.

Psychosocial Status

A psychosocial evaluation is conducted with the client and family by assessing their degree of understanding and anxiety regarding the surgical procedure (see the accompanying display on assessment questions). Assess the client's knowledge of the surgical procedure and the expected surgical outcomes. It is important that the client express agreement with the surgical plan of care.

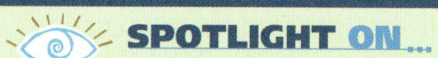

SPOTLIGHT ON...

Caring and Compassion

Responding to a Client's Alterd Self-Image

As a student nurse, how can you assist the client in verbalizing fears about alterations in body image that have sexual implications? A 30-year-old woman is admitted for removal of a cancerous breast. Her mother died at age 30 from breast cancer. The client has been married for 5 years and has a 3-week-old infant. Her husband is with her. You have to admit and interview the client for the nursing history. How would you approach the medical diagnosis? Would you feel comfortable helping this client verbalize her fears?

ASSESSMENT QUESTIONS: PSYCHOSOCIAL STATUS

- Why are you having surgery?
- When did this problem start?
- What do you think caused this problem?
- Has this caused any problems with your relationships with others?
- Has your problem prevented you from working?
- Are you able to take care of your own needs?
- Are you experiencing any discomfort or pain?
- What are you expecting from this surgery?
- Is there anything that you do not understand regarding your surgery?
- Are you worried about anything?
- Will someone be available to assist you when you return home?

Physical Assessment

The perioperative nursing assessment includes the review of medical records, a client interview, and a partial or complete physical examination. Key points include, but are not limited to, the following: age, height, weight, skin condition, preexisting conditions, nutritional status, and physical or mobility limitations. The decision to conduct a partial or complete physical depends on the client's health status relative to the surgical procedure, the setting, and the amount of time available to gather pertinent data.

The nurse in an outpatient setting, on the day of surgery, usually performs a partial examination. The client's medical record should be reviewed to ensure that a complete nursing physical was conducted during the preadmission visit. The nurse should focus on obtaining pertinent assessment data to establish baseline parameters for prioritizing the client's care. The client's neurologic assessment is integrated throughout the interview and physical examination.

GENERAL SURVEY Observe the client's condition starting with the initial contact. For instance, if the client walks into the unit, observe and note the client's gait; note if assistance is needed with ambulation. Does the client need assistance when transferred to a bed? When shaking the client's hand, note the strength and sensation of the hand grasp and the skin temperature. Coldness of the hand may indicate impaired circulation.

During the interview, assess the level of consciousness and orientation. Does the client respond appropriately to questions? Observe for signs of hearing impairment or loss of vision. Note if the client is wearing glasses.

HEAD AND NECK While talking with the client, assess if eye contact is maintained. Note the color of the sclera and inspect for drainage from the eyes. Inspect the general condition of the scalp, noting alopecia or seborrheic dermatitis. Inspect the oral cavity, check for any loose teeth, and assess the tongue and mucous membranes (note color and moisture). Observe the client's lips and tongue, especially if client has a history of cardiac disease. Note if the client has dentures.

Inspect the neck and verify the strength of the carotid pulses, one at a time; palpate jugular veins for distension. If the client is a child or has cancer, palpate the cervical lymph nodes. Assess for range of motion.

UPPER EXTREMITIES   Palpate the client's brachial and radial pulses bilaterally; note the rate and character of each pulse. Check the capillary refill. Assess the skin; note the temperature, texture, and integrity. Assess for range of motion. For instance, if the client is scheduled for a neurosurgical procedure, the perioperative RN (or circulating nurse) assesses the strength and character of the client's handgrips and dorsal/plantar flexion ("push-pulls") with resistance.

ANTERIOR AND POSTERIOR CHEST AND ABDOMEN
Inspect and palpate the chest wall, noting the breathing pattern and expansion of the chest wall. Auscultate heart sounds, and listen to anterior and posterior breath sounds; note crackles, gurgles, or wheezing.

Inspect the abdomen for distension, and listen for bowel sounds in all four quadrants. Palpate the abdomen for rigidity, enlarged organs, or rebound tenderness.

LOWER EXTREMITIES   Assess the length and position of each leg. Palpate the bilateral strength of femoral, popliteal, and pedal pulses, noting the rate and character of each pulse. Assess the skin; note the temperature, texture, integrity, and presence of edema. Check the capillary refill. Inspect the bony prominences of the ankles and feet. Assess for strength and sensation by having the client bend the leg and push the foot against the nurse's hand. Assess for range of motion. Clients scheduled for spinal anesthesia should be assessed for gross motor function and strength.

The nurse documents on the medical record and communicates to the health care team all significant assessment data. This information establishes baseline parameters to direct decision making throughout the perioperative phases. Spinal anesthesia causes temporary paralysis of the lower extremities. Preoperative weakness or impaired movement of the lower extremities should be reported to nurses caring for clients recovering from spinal anesthesia; postoperatively this report prevents the recovery nurse from making the wrong decisions when full motor function fails to return.

DIAGNOSIS

The nursing diagnosis is a concise clinical judgment of a client problem formulated to direct nursing actions to achieve the expected outcome (AORN, 2007). The nurse formulates nursing diagnoses based on an analysis of assessment data and the nature of surgery. Physical assessment findings are compared against diagnostic test results; for example, cardiovascular

findings are analyzed with blood chemistry and electrocardiogram (ECG) results.

Selection of the most appropriate nursing diagnosis should focus on the specific perioperative phase (see Table 40-3 on page 1304). The diagnosis may be pertinent to all three perioperative phases or to one or more phases.

For instance, as described in the Nursing Process Highlight, Mrs. Broussard is experiencing pain that is caused by the degenerative changes in the hip joint as a result of arthritis. Although the surgeon will remove the diseased joint, Mrs. Broussard will continue to experience pain. In fact, the pain may worsen for several weeks postoperatively. The most appropriate diagnosis for Mrs. Broussard is *Pain*. Preoperatively, the pain is related to the degeneration of the hip joint; postoperatively, the pain is related to swelling at the surgery site.

Common nursing diagnoses for the preoperative client are *Deficient knowledge* related to the surgery, *Anxiety*, and *Fear*. Clients and families view the perioperative experience differently on the basis of prior experiences and coping skills. Some clients are threatened; others consider the experience to be a challenge. Some clients are highly anxious, whereas others experience a moderate degree of anxiety. Besides the primary threat of surgery, clients also have to deal with separation from family and loss of independence.

Associated nursing diagnoses address the client's preexisting health condition. For instance, an associated diagnosis for Mrs. Broussard is *Impaired physical mobility* related to musculoskeletal impairment. This nursing diagnosis would be initiated preoperatively and throughout the perioperative experience.

NURSING PROCESS HIGHLIGHT

Assessment

Mrs. Broussard, 69, was admitted to an outpatient surgical unit for a total hip replacement (arthroplasty). The surgeon explained the surgical procedure during her last office visit. Preauthorization has been granted for the surgery. Diagnostic testing, a comprehensive history and physical examination, and postoperative exercise instructions were performed during the preadmission visit. Mrs. Broussard has been suffering for 10 years with chronic degenerative arthritis. She has experienced increasing pain and loss of mobility in her left hip for the past 6 months.

- In collecting data from Mrs. Broussard during the focused assessment, what types of information are essential for the development of a plan of care for her on the day of surgery?
- Which baseline data should be obtained from Mrs. Broussard during the partial physical examination?
- What further data should be collected at this time?

TABLE 40-3 Perioperative Nursing Diagnoses

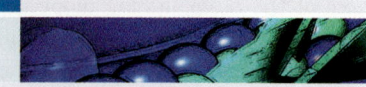

Preoperative phase	*Deficient knowledge* related to: • Nature and purpose of the surgical procedure • Preoperative preparation to decrease postoperative risks		• Impaired skin integrity • Risk of impaired skin integrity • Impaired tissue integrity • Latex allergy response • Risk for latex allergy
	Anxiety related to: • Deficient knowledge of a new experience • Inherent risk factors of the surgical procedure and anesthesia		*Hypothermia* related to: • Exposure to cool environment • Decreased metabolic rate • Ineffective thermoregulation • Excess fluid volume • Deficient fluid volume
	Fear related to: • The unknown • Effects of surgery on economic and employment status • Pain • Body image disturbance • Sexual dysfunction • Disturbed sleep pattern	Postoperative phase	*Ineffective airway clearance* related to: • Anesthesia (diminished cough reflex) • Increased pulmonary congestion
			Ineffective breathing pattern related to: • Pain • Decreased energy or fatigue
Intraoperative phase	*Risk for perioperative positioning injury* related to: • Sensory and perceptual disturbances due to anesthesia • Edema • Ineffective protection • Ineffective tissue perfusion • Impaired physical mobility • Disturbed sensory perception • Impaired skin integrity • Risk for peripheral neurovascular dysfunction		*Ineffective tissue perfusion (cardiopulmonary)* related to: • Anesthesia • Position or immobility
			Deficient fluid volume related to: • Active fluid volume loss • Inadequate fluid intake
			Imbalanced nutrition: Less than body requirements related to: • Anesthesia • Surgical manipulation of intestines
	Risk for injury related to: • Physical (equipment or sponge count) • Environmental • Positional • Deficient fluid volume • Risk for imbalance fluid volume • Risk for aspiration • Decreased cardiac output • Transport (AORN, 2007) • Electrical (AORN, 2007) • Chemical (AORN, 2007) • Laser (AORN, 2007) • Radiation (AORN, 2007) • Hyperthermia (AORN, 2007)		*Urinary retention* related to: • Anesthesia • Surgical manipulation of the bladder
			Acute pain related to surgical incision
			Risk for infection related to: • Impaired skin integrity from surgical wound • Deficient knowledge of wound or drainage tube care
	Risk for infection related to: • Invasive procedure • Imbalanced nutrition		*Situational low self-esteem* related to: • Altered body image, effects of surgery • Dependence on others during recuperation from surgery

From *North American Nursing Diagnosis Association. (2009). Nursing diagnoses—Diagnoses and classification 2009–2011.* © 2009, 2007, 2005, 2003, 2001, 1998, 1996, 1994 NANDA International. Used by arrangement with Wiley-Blackwell Publishing, a company of John Wiley & Sons, Inc.

PLANNING AND OUTCOMES

Outcomes are positive statements, the anticipated goals that clients are expected to achieve at the close of the perioperative experience based on the nursing diagnoses. The nurse develops goals with client-focused expected outcomes based on the relevant nursing diagnoses. Nurses collaborate with other health care team members and the client in establishing the goals and outcomes. The overall goal is to protect the client from injury related to anesthesia and surgery. The plan of care directs the selection of specific nursing interventions that promote the client's achievement of expected outcomes, for example, client teaching.

The current health care system challenges the perioperative nurse to be responsible to surgical clients who may enter and exit the diverse health care settings at various points along the continuum of care with different experiences. Some clients are admitted to the hospital the day of surgery and some the evening before; some have surgery as an outpatient and some in the prescribing practitioner's office. Some clients with general anesthesia may be discharged the day of surgery.

Discharge planning needs are incorporated into the plan of care on admission and ideally include family and client education. The following considerations are included in discharge planning:

- Psychosocial and spiritual support systems and community resources
- Financial aspects of the illness
- The degree of illness or disability
- Rehabilitation
- Preventive care
- Client teaching needs

Some clients need the services of a home health agency on discharge. The perioperative nurse usually coordinates home care with the social worker.

Collaboration

Effective perioperative management is directed by a multidisciplinary team in accordance with recognized standards of care and individualized expected client outcomes. Institutional protocol, which defines how procedures will be performed, is initiated in the preoperative phase and continues throughout the other phases.

Each member of the health care team (surgeon, anesthesia provider, and nurse) has a specific role and responsibility toward the perioperative client. Collaboration between all health care providers is essential in planning client care. "Collaboration means that people with different areas of expertise are working as equals to define issues, design solutions, and achieve high quality outcome" (Rubenfeld & Scheffer, 1999, p. 352).

SURGEON Prescribing practitioners are credentialed by health care facilities to perform surgery. The surgeon is the primary prescribing practitioner the nurse communicates with regarding client care needs. Before surgery, the surgeon:

- Determines the need for the surgical intervention on the basis of the client's medical diagnosis and findings from the medical history and physical examination
- Determines the surgical setting in collaboration with the client
- Orders diagnostic tests only if directly correlated to the procedure or client diagnosis (see the accompanying display on common preoperative diagnostic tests)
- Obtains client's consent for the surgical procedure
- Teaches the client about the outcomes and risks of the procedure

A major role function of the surgeon is *explaining and documenting evidence that the client understands the nature of the surgical procedure, the risk factors, and expected outcomes of the surgery.* This is done with a surgical consent form, the client's written permission to allow the surgeon to provide surgery. Many states, through statutory provisions, require prescribing practitioners to perform and document client teaching. Once the client demonstrates understanding, the client signs the form, giving permission for the specific surgical intervention.

ANESTHESIA PROVIDER The anesthesia provider (anesthesiologist or certified RN anesthetist) actively participates in each perioperative phase. The main role of the anesthesia provider is to ensure client safety relative to the administration of anesthesia. The anesthesia provider:

- Obtains informed consent for anesthesia services
- Performs a preanesthesia evaluation that includes a thorough history, such as complications from previous anesthesia, and physical examination
- Selects anesthetic agents

COMMON PREOPERATIVE DIAGNOSTIC TESTS

- Urinalysis
- Complete blood count (CBC)
- Prothrombin time (PT) and partial thromboplastin time (PTT): Clients with known or suspected coagulation defects or to establish baseline information
- Chemistry profile: Clients with diseases that can alter electrolytes
- Electrocardiogram (ECG)
- Human immunodeficiency virus (HIV) testing: In accordance with agency policy
- Chest x-ray films: Clients over 60 years of age, smokers, or those scheduled for general anesthesia

- Teaches the client regarding the anesthetic medications, their side effects, and risk factors
- Performs intubation (the insertion of an endotracheal tube into the bronchus through the nose or mouth to ensure an airway) and extubation (the removal of an endotracheal tube)

Most surgical procedures have predetermined anesthetic agents based on policy; if there is a variance from the norm, the anesthesia provider seeks agreement with the surgeon. The decision to use particular anesthetic agents is based on the client's health status, the surgical procedure, and the anticipated duration of the surgery.

During the client interview, the anesthesiologist inquires about previous anesthesia experiences that can place the client at risk, such as connective tissue abnormalities that suggest the presence of the autosomal dominant malignant hyperthermia (MH) gene. Malignant hyperthermia is a potentially lethal syndrome caused by a hypermetabolic state that is precipitated by the administration of certain anesthetic agents, for example, succinylcholine. When appropriate and feasible, medical records from previous surgeries are reviewed as part of the preanesthesia examination.

REGISTERED NURSE The AORN promotes client care through the development of standards, guidelines, and recommended practices of perioperative nursing. The AORN has also developed the Perioperative Nursing Data Set (PNDS) to standardize nursing terminology regarding the perioperative client experience from preadmission until discharge to promote evidence-based practice. The PNDS is the first nursing language developed by a specialty organization that has been recognized by the American Nurses Association. The PNDS is composed of 4 domains, 74 nursing diagnoses, 133 interventions, and 28 outcomes unique to the role of the perioperative nurse.

Perioperative nurses perform critical functions that vary with specific surgical procedures and the unique needs of individual clients to achieve positive client outcomes (Parker, Mimick, & Kee, 1999). Rubenfeld and Scheffer (1999) identified three guiding principles for implementing care based on professional standards: maintain client safety; provide effective care; and provide care as efficiently as possible. These principles are incorporated into each phase of the perioperative standards of nursing practice.

The nurse coordinates the client's care in a timely fashion to ensure safety and avoid surgical delays. Activities include:

- Scheduling the diagnostic tests.
- Verifying that all the necessary documents (e.g., signed consent form) are in the client's medical record.
- Reporting abnormal diagnostic results to the surgeon. Depending on the test results, treatment may be instituted to correct any abnormalities, or the surgery may be canceled.

A major part of the nurse's time is spent in preparing and teaching the client. Preoperative teaching is structured to provide planned educational activities to presurgical clients and

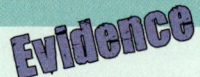

UNCOVERING THE Evidence

TITLE OF STUDY
"Operating Theater Culture: Implications for Nurse Retention"

AUTHORS
Bridget Gillespie, Marianne Wallis, and Wendy Chaboyer

PURPOSE
To explore characteristics of the organizational culture of the operating theater and how this culture is communicated and sustained.

METHODS
This study was a mini-ethnography of three themes related to primacy of knowledge and competence, social order, and situational control, which are important cultural indicators in the operating theater.

FINDINGS
The level to which members are able to assimilate and meet role expectations depends on the amount of knowledge and experience they possess.

IMPLICATIONS
A lack of acceptance has the potential to affect members' willingness to continue working in the operating theater and, consequently, may contribute to existing nursing shortages in this specialty.

Gillespie, B., Wallis, M., & Chaboyer, W. (2008). Operating theater culture: Implications for nurse retention. *Western Journal of Nursing Research*, 30(2), 259–277.

family (significant others) according to assessed anxiety and fear levels, as discussed later in this chapter. See Table 40-4 on page 1307 for the roles of the RN in the perioperative environment.

As technology becomes more sophisticated and health care resources become more limited, ethical issues have become more complex (Schroeter, 1999). Ethical dilemmas are inherent in perioperative nursing; for example, lack of respect for the client's dignity, withholding information or lying to clients, inadequate consents, incompetent health care providers, and do-not-resuscitate (DNR) orders are all issues that have implications for the management of care in perioperative settings. Schroeter (1999) studied the aspects of informed consent and the impaired or incompetent colleague in the perioperative practice setting and determined that perioperative nurses can accurately identify ethical situations occurring in the environment and that the majority of the participants reported that they would take action. The ethical competency of perioperative nurses is paramount to ensure that safe, competent, and ethical care is provided to all surgical clients.

TABLE 40-4 Roles for the RN in the Perioperative Environment

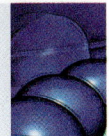

Scrub person (Phillips, 2004)	Staff member of the sterile team. The RN, licensed vocational nurse (LVN), or surgical technologist is responsible for establishing and maintaining the safety, efficiency, and integrity of the sterile field throughout the surgical or invasive procedure.
Circulating nurse (Phillips, 2004)	Registered nurse member of the nonsterile team who coordinates and directs the activities of the intraoperative environment during the surgical procedure. The RN continually assesses and manages client safety needs and the sterile team utilizing critical thinking skills.
RN first assistant (RNFA) (Rothrock, 1999)	As an expanded perioperative role, the RN who has received additional educational preparation assists the surgeon in performing the surgical procedure throughout the perioperative course of client care. The RNFA is prescribing practitioner based, hospital based, or entrepreneurial in practice and is credentialed by the facility in which the RNFA performs first-assisting duties.

Delmar/Cengage Learning

IMPLEMENTATION

Preparing the client for surgery requires the nurse to perform multiple interventions within specific time constraints. However, the nurse must remain responsive to the client's needs, demonstrating a caring attitude (see Figure 40-1). Documentation tools (e.g., consent form, preoperative checklist) are available to assist the nurse in providing safe, timely preoperative care. Throughout the perioperative experience, active planning, intervention, and evaluation are essential elements to reduce the risk of complication. See the accompanying display for the *Nursing Interventions Classification* (NIC) recommendations regarding preoperative coordination for facilitating preadmission diagnostic testing and preparation of the surgical client.

Surgical Consent Form

Although surgeons are responsible for obtaining informed consent, nurses should verify that consent has been obtained before treatment begins. Consent is given only for the extent

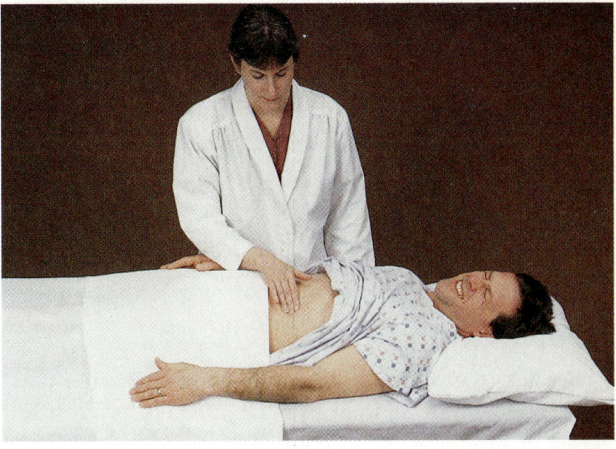

FIGURE 40-1 The nurse prepares a client for surgery. While the nurse was performing preoperative assessment, the client demonstrated pain through facial expression. What implications might the client's pain have for the surgery? What actions should the nurse take, considering the potential effects on the client's perioperative experience? DELMAR/CENGAGE LEARNING

of action documented on the informed consent. Nurses can identify problems with consent when the client:

- Cannot explain the procedure or identify the risks
- Signed the form more than 30 days before surgery
- Had an unauthorized person sign the consent form
- Did not sign the consent form
- Signed a consent form that identified an incorrect surgical site
- Signed a consent form that identified a procedure incongruent with that now identified

NIC: PREOPERATIVE COORDINATION

- Review planned surgery and prescribing practitioner orders.
- Obtain client history, physical assessment, and blood and urine specimens; notify prescribing practitioner of abnormal diagnostic test results, as appropriate.
- Describe and explain preadmission treatments and diagnostic tests; inform client and significant others of the date and time of surgery, time of arrival, admission procedure, and locations of receiving unit, surgery area, and waiting area; and allow time for client and significant others to ask questions and voice concerns.
- Discuss postoperative discharge plans and determine ability of caretakers.

Adapted from Bulechek, G., Butcher, H., & Dochterman, J. (2008). *Nursing interventions classification (NIC)* (5th ed., p. 578). St. Louis, MO: Mosby Elsevier Health Sciences.

The nurse should notify the surgeon in the event that any problems with consent are identified.

If the surgeon proceeds without appropriate consent, nursing administration should be notified and the nurse should make personal notations outside the medical record. This practice protects the nurse should the situation be brought to court. If the client reverses a decision and decides against surgery, the nurse is obligated to inform the surgeon in order to prevent unwanted treatment.

Preoperative Checklist

A checklist is a form that allows the nurse to insert a check mark ($\sqrt{}$) beside symptoms or to fill in one or two words in answer to a cue or a question. Although some variations exist in how agencies format the preoperative checklist, the forms usually have similar content. Nursing activities are usually designated by time intervals: "night before surgery" and "day of surgery." Time designations help to prevent surgical delays that can increase the client's anxiety and the agency's costs. Table 40-5 on page 1309 presents a sample preoperative checklist that incorporates most of the intervention activities described in NIC—Surgical Preparation (2930).

Although clients in outpatient settings arrive the day of surgery, the nurse prepares the client's medical record the day before for necessary documentation as itemized in Table 40-5. This preparation ensures that assessment, diagnostic tests, and teaching were done on the preadmission visit and allows time to obtain missing information and to assess the need for reinforcement or reevaluation as necessary.

On the day of surgery, the nurse focuses on the immediate physical interventions to prepare the client for surgery. While admitting and preparing the client for surgery, the nurse uses this time to encourage the client to verbalize any concerns. Allowance should be made for family members or significant others to remain with the client as the client awaits transfer to the OR.

Client Teaching

Most clients view surgery as a threatening and anxiety-provoking event. Client teaching reduces anxiety. The risks of surgical complications are decreased when the client knows what to expect and receives instruction in postoperative exercises (Bulechek et al., 2008; Lindeman & Van Aernam, 1971).

Teaching the client and family members (significant others) is the responsibility of the multidisciplinary team. The nurse verifies that the client or family member is able to describe, in his or her own words, the reason for the surgery, what will be done during the surgical procedure, the side effects of the anesthetic agents, and the possible complications of both the surgery and the anesthesia.

The nurse plays a major role in relieving the client's anxiety by facilitating communication between prescribing practitioners and the client and family and by reinforcing teaching regarding preoperative care. The client's family should be involved in the teaching sessions. Table 40-6 on page 1311 presents an overview to perioperative teaching activities with the client's expected outcomes.

Teaching aids (videotapes and pamphlets) are resources for client instruction during the perioperative processes. The nurse selects teaching materials based on the client's ability to read and understand. The nurse provides accurate, consistent information throughout the teaching process. The teaching aids must reinforce the verbal instructions of the nurse, anesthesia provider, and surgeon. Informational materials should explain what will happen in each of the perioperative areas (such as the holding area) to foster client cooperation. Refer to Chapter 21 for additional information on client teaching and NIC intervention, Teaching: Preoperative (5610).

TYPES OF SURGICAL INCISIONS Nurses need to be knowledgeable about common surgical incisions to reinforce the surgeon's teaching and to answer the client's questions. Two main factors govern incisions: direction and location. Incisions may be vertical, horizontal, transverse, or oblique. For minimally invasive surgeries, such as laparoscopic cholecystectomy, small incisions are strategically placed to facilitate access to the gall bladder utilizing laparoscopic instrumentation and video equipment. Placement of trocars will vary in size and placement according to the procedure to be performed. Figure 40-2 on page 1312 illustrates and describes the location of common surgical incisions.

POSTOPERATIVE EXERCISE INSTRUCTION As early as 1941, nurses were challenged to participate in preoperative instruction. In 1983, Leventhal and his colleagues suggested that the effectiveness of existing preoperative instruction could be increased by assisting clients to assume self-regulation after surgery.

Preoperative teaching of postoperative exercises prepares the client physically and emotionally for the impending surgery. Language barriers, identified during assessment, are considered when teaching the client. The goal of instruction is to have the client demonstrate the performance of exercises while verbalizing why the exercises are used during the postoperative phase (see Procedure 40-1).

Clients may experience their worst postoperative pain while coughing, deep breathing, and exercising. Clients with abdominal or chest surgery may avoid using muscles in the affected areas to take deep breaths or to cough effectively. Deep breathing and coughing facilitate removal of accumulated pulmonary secretions. Certain anesthetic agents depress the central nervous system, causing some clients to experience shallow respirations. Inhaled gases and oxygen have a direct drying effect on the respiratory mucosa, which increases the viscosity of mucus, making the secretions difficult to raise with coughing. These factors place the client at risk for respiratory complications (see the accompanying display on common respiratory complications after surgery on page 1310).

To prevent respiratory complications, the nurse teaches clients to use a breathing technique in which the client turns, coughs, and deep breathes to achieve sustained maximum inspiration (SMI). SMI promotes the reinflation of the alveoli and the removal of mucus secretions.

Several devices help encourage clients to perform SMI exercises. The breathing devices, called **incentive spirometers**,

TABLE 40-5 Preoperative Checklist

	CK (✓)	COMMENTS	NURSE CK (✓)
Complete Night before Surgery			
List of allergies			
Procedure scheduled			
Surgical permit signed/witnessed			
Surgical site marked for procedures; right/left distinction, multiple structures, or multiple levels			
History/physical on chart and/or dictated			
Preanesthetic evaluation done			
Client's level of anxiety/fear regarding procedure assessed			
Able to state type and purpose of surgery			
Demonstrates ability to perform: Deep breathing, turning, and coughing exercises			
Leg exercises			
PM care with shower or bath given			
Nail polish and makeup removed			
Old chart requested and obtained			
Type and cross-match for _____ units of blood			
Blood consent signed and witnessed			
Lab work a. CBC _____ b. UA _____			
Tonsillectomy and adenoidectomy clients: a. _____ PTT b. _____ PT c. _____ Platelets			
If ordered by MD: a. ECG _____ b. Chest x-ray _____			
Add other lab work ordered (specify)			
Notify surgeon of abnormal lab work			
New progress note and prescribing practitioner order sheet on chart			
Weight			
NPO after midnight (if applicable)			
Signature of Nurse _____		Date _____	
Complete Day of Surgery			
Jewelry removed and secured with responsible party			
Dental prosthesis and contact lenses removed			
Hospital gown/cap on and undergarments removed			
Voided on call to surgery			
Indwelling catheter ordered and inserted			

(Continues)

TABLE 40-5 (Continued)

	CK (✓)	COMMENTS	NURSE CK (✓)
Tampon removed			
IdentiBand and/or blood band on and checked for accuracy			
Time _____ P _____ R _____ BP _____ T _____			
Pre-op medicine given: Medication _____ Time _____ AM PM			
Side rails up and bed to lowest level			
Client instructed not to get out of bed without nursing assistance			
Addressograph plate/MAR on chart			
VS 30 minutes after preop (if remains on unit)			
BP _____ P _____ R _____ T _____			
Old chart sent to surgery per request			
Surgical prep done and checked			
To surgery: Time _____ Via _____			
Signature of Nurse _____		Date_____	
Holding Room Nurse Signature _____		Date_____	

BP, blood pressure; CBC, complete blood count; ECG, electrocardiogram; MAR, medication administration record; NPO, nothing by mouth; P, pulse; PT, prothrombin time; PTT, partial thromboplastin time; R, respirations; T, temperature; UA, urinalysis; VS, vitals signs.

Delmar/Cengage Learning

---

measure the client's ventilatory volume and provide the user with a tangible reward for generating an adequate respiratory flow. Devices range from simple types, such as a Ping-Pong ball in a plastic tube, to sophisticated models. When the client takes a deep breath, the ball moves upward and the amount of air is measured, making the results visible to the client.

Turning, deep breathing, coughing, and using spirometry prevent respiratory complications by:

- Promoting pulmonary circulation
- Promoting the exchange of gases by increasing lung compliance
- Facilitating the removal of mucus secretions from the tracheobronchial tree

Postoperatively the client is encouraged to move in bed and perform leg exercises as explained in Procedure 40-1. These exercises assist in preventing circulatory complications that can arise from anesthetic agents that depress the metabolic and heart rates; see the accompanying display on page 1311. Early ambulation also increases respiratory function and the return of peristalsis.

COMMON RESPIRATORY COMPLICATIONS AFTER SURGERY AND ANESTHESIA

- Pulmonary embolism: A blood clot that has moved to the lungs, causing pulmonary obstruction
- Atelectasis: Decreased ventilation caused by the pooling of secretions in dependent areas of the bronchiole
- Pneumonia: Inflammation of lung tissue
- Hypoxemia: Lowered oxygen level in the blood

OTHER DEVICES Besides exercises, other devices are used to prevent postoperative circulatory complications, namely, antiembolism stockings and pneumatic compression. Another device, continuous passive motion, increases range of motion for immobilized clients after surgery. The CPM device also

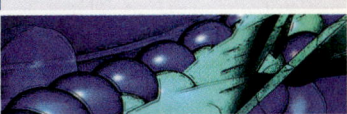

TABLE 40-6 Preoperative Teaching Interventions and Expected Client Outcomes

INTERVENTION	EXPECTED CLIENT OUTCOMES
Preparation activities	The client can: • Describe in own terms the purpose, risk factors, and outcomes of surgery and anesthesia. • Explain restrictions on food the evening before, identifying the time frame (6–8 h) of NPO, when no food and drink are allowed by mouth. • Explain the meaning and purpose of skin and bowel preps. • Identify medications to be taken or omitted the day of surgery. • Describe activities that will occur in each perioperative area: holding area, fluids will be started in a vein; position on the operating room table; stay in recovery until awake, then be transferred to an intensive care unit.
Postoperative exercise instructions	The client can demonstrate on two consecutive occasions postoperative exercises: deep breathing, coughing and pillow splinting, turning and proper body alignment; leg and foot exercises; and out-of-bed transfers.
Proper application and usage of medical devices	For example, the client can demonstrate proper use of incentive spirometer, application of TED hose, and self-medicating pain infusion pump.
Physical or environmental changes following surgery	The client can demonstrate knowledge of the rehabilitation process: daily physical therapy for 2 weeks and a home health nurse for 10 days to administer prophylactic antibiotics and to monitor and refill the patient-controlled analgesia pump.

TED, thromboembolic disorder.

Delmar/Cengage Learning

COMMON CIRCULATORY COMPLICATIONS AFTER SURGERY AND ANESTHESIA

- Thrombophlebitis: Inflammation of a vein with the formation of a blood clot
- Thrombus: A blood clot in the circulatory system
- Embolus: A blood clot or air that moves in the circulatory system from its place of origin

stimulates healing of articular cartilage by reducing swelling and adhesions.

Pain is managed with devices such as transcutaneous electrical nerve stimulation and patient-controlled analgesia. The client needs to be informed about the use of such devices preoperatively to promote achievement of postoperative pain outcomes. All medical devices require a prescribing practitioner's order.

Antiembolism stockings are elastic hose that compress leg veins to facilitate the return of venous blood. Depending on the surgical site, these stockings can be applied preoperatively (e.g., abdominal surgery) and utilized throughout the perioperative course at the direction of the surgeon.

Elastic stockings are available in a variety of lengths, colors, and sizes to accommodate specific needs. One type of hose goes from the foot to the knee; another type goes from the foot to midthigh. Some stockings have partial openings on the foot to expose either the toes or heel so that the nurse can assess circulation.

The prescribing practitioner usually specifies the size and style of the hose and the frequency of application. If the prescribing practitioner does not indicate the size, the nurse uses a tape to measure the circumference of the calf and thigh and the length of the client's leg from the heel to the gluteal furrow. Stockings are removed for 20 to 30 minutes three times a day to allow for assessment and hygienic care. Assessment should include inspection for redness, palpation for tenderness or increased temperature, and testing for Homans' sign. (See the Nursing Checklist on application of antiembolism stockings on page 1313.)

A **pneumatic compression device** provides intermittent compression cycles to the veins of the extremities to promote circulation. The device consists of either vinyl surgical sleeves that slide over each calf or Velcro-secured vinyl compression hoses that are applied under the thigh and leg with a knee-opening site that is placed over each popliteal area (see Figure 40-3 on page 1312). Both types of vinyl appliances have tube connectors that attach to an air pump machine. Observe the client applying the stockings, connecting the tubes to the air pump, and setting the correct pressure.

The air pump has an on-off switch and a dial to set the desired pressure. Turning on the pump initiates compression cycles, which cause the vinyl sleeves to inflate and deflate automatically. The nurse assesses the circulation to the extremities

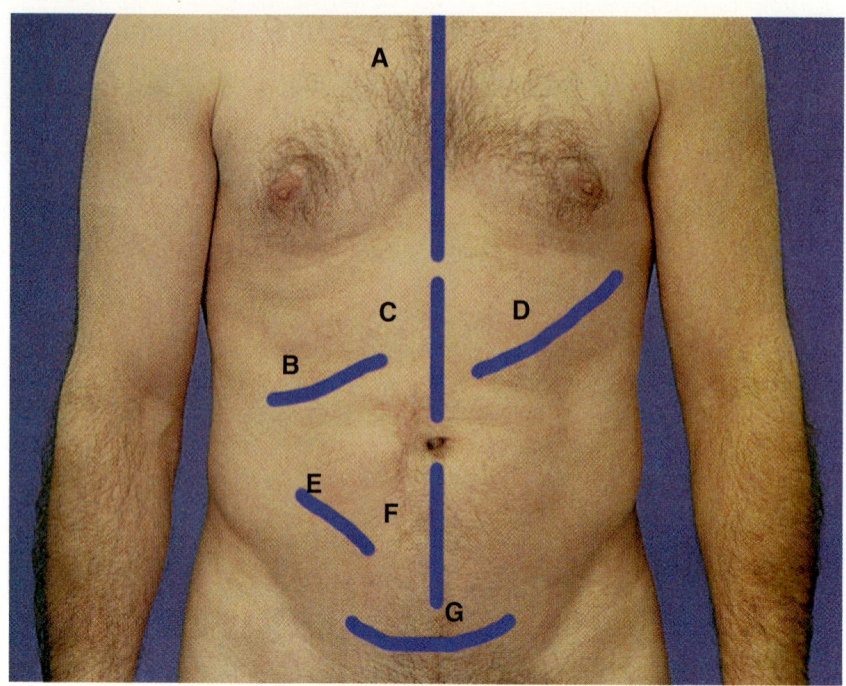

INCISION	LOCATION	ORGAN
A. Sternal split	Begins at the top of the sternum and extends downward to the sternal notch	Heart
B. Oblique subcostal	Begins in the epigastric area and extends laterally and obliquely below the lower costal margin	Right side: Gallbladder, biliary
		Left side: Spleen
C. Upper vertical midline	Begins below the sternal notch and extends distally around the umbilicus	Stomach, duodenum, pancreas
D. Thoracoabdominal	Begins midway between the xiphoid process and the umbilicus and extends across the seventh or eighth intercostal space to the midscapular line	Thorax, heart
E. McBurney	Begins below the umbilicus, goes through McBurney's point, and extends toward the right flank	Appendix
F. Lower vertical midline	Begins below the umbilicus and extends downward toward the symphysis pubis	Bladder, uterus
G. Pfannenstiel	Begins 1.5 inches above the symphysis pubis with a curved transverse cut across the lower abdomen	Uterus, fallopian tubes, ovaries

FIGURE 40-2 Location of Common Surgical Incisions DELMAR/CENGAGE LEARNING

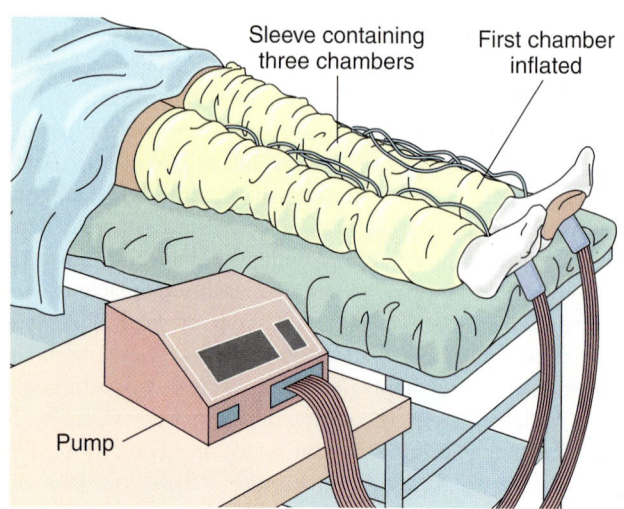

Sleeve containing three chambers

First chamber inflated

Pump

FIGURE 40-3 Pneumatic Compression Device DELMAR/CENGAGE LEARNING

and placement of the stockings every 2 to 3 hours. The stockings are removed three times a day for 20- to 30-minute intervals to allow for hygiene care. Instruct the client on how to clean the vinyl stockings by disconnecting the stockings from the air pump and wiping off with tepid, soapy water.

The **continuous passive motion (CPM) device** increases range of motion and stimulates healing of the articular cartilage by decreasing swelling and the formation of adhesions. It is used for clients with a nursing diagnosis of either *Impaired physical mobility* related to the surgical intervention or *Altered tissue perfusion* related to surgical intervention and immobility. The goal is to increase tolerance of the CPM device. The expected client outcome is to maintain maximum mobility of the joint.

Before initiating CPM, the nurse:

- Assesses the neurovascular status (skin color and temperature, pulses, capillary refill, sensation, and movement) of the client's extremity

✓ NURSINGCHECKLIST

Application of Antiembolism Stockings

- Wash hands and obtain the stockings, making sure the type and size are correct.
- Check the client's identification band.
- Show the client the stockings and explain the procedure to elicit cooperation. Make sure the client knows that the stockings are to be removed routinely and washed daily according to package directions.
- Provide for privacy. The client should be in a comfortable position to observe your technique while you apply one of the stockings.
- Wash, rinse, and dry the legs; stockings should be applied only to clean, dry skin.
- Talcum powder can be applied to the feet and legs to allow the stocking to move more easily over the skin.
- Turn the stocking inside out, except the foot portion.
- Place the foot of the stocking over the client's toes and on the foot; with your nondominant hand supporting the client's ankle, use your dominant hand to pull the heel pocket over the client's heel (see Figure 40-4).

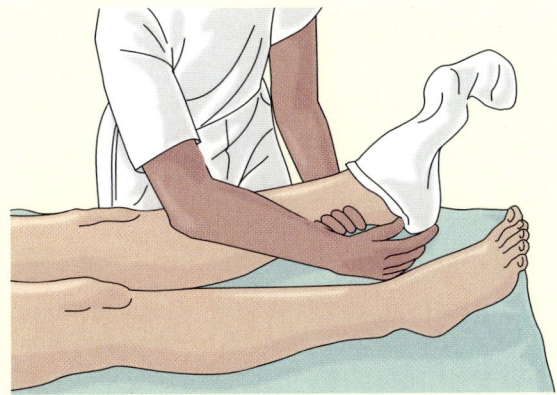

FIGURE 40-4 When applying antiembolism stockings, support client's ankle while pulling stocking up. DELMAR/CENGAGE LEARNING

- Slide the stocking up the leg, straightening as you apply; make sure that kinks and wrinkles are smoothed out to provide even pressure.
- Knee-length stockings should end 1 in (2.5 cm) below the knees.
- If the stocking goes to midthigh, have the client flex the knee while you pull the stocking over the knee and thigh; the stocking should be 1 to 3 in (2.5 to 7.5 cm) from the groin.
- The top of the stockings should not be folded over because additional constriction can occur.
- Have the client apply the other stocking, and assess the client's learning.
- Document client learning.

✓ NURSINGCHECKLIST

Instructing the Client on the Use of the TENS Device

- Place electrodes on the skin in the area of pain (e.g., on both sides of an incision).
- Connect the lead wires to the electrodes and portable battery-powered transmitter.
- Turn on and regulate for comfort by working with one lead at a time, beginning with a zero setting.
- Gradually increase the level of stimulation until the client feels discomfort, indicating that maximum stimulation has been achieved to block pain sensation; then reduce the volume slightly to prevent continued contraction of muscles.
- Repeat the same process with the other lead; this time allow the client to perform the actions.
- Ensure that the client knows to apply the electrodes to clean, unbroken skin.

- Applies the disposable soft goods to the CPM device according to the manufacturer's instructions
- Sets the machine to provide the degree of flexion and extension according to the prescribing practitioner's orders (e.g., 0° extension and 35° flexion)
- Adjusts the speed to control movement

When the device is readied, the client is positioned in the middle of the bed to accommodate the CPM unit. The nurse places the client's legs in the padded CPM device, making sure that the knees are at the hinged joint of the machine. The nurse measures the angle of flexion with a goniometer when the device has reached its greatest height. The client is taught how to operate the "go/stop" button and is instructed to report any discomfort or pain that occurs with motion.

Postprocedure, clients experience pain, a subjective experience that may or may not be verbalized. Postoperative pain should be discussed with the client preoperatively so that clinical practice guidelines can be used to assess the severity of pain using either a verbal rating scale or a visual analog scale; refer to Chapter 35 for a discussion of pain scales. It is important to understand that all clients respond to pain in a different manner.

A **transcutaneous electrical nerve stimulation (TENS)** unit controls pain by delivering electrical impulses to nerve endings that block the passage of pain signals from entering the dorsal spinal root. (See the Nursing Checklist on instructing a client on the use of the TENS device.) The TENS unit is effective in reducing pain and the amount of pain medication required to maintain comfort after surgery. The unit consists of a transmitter, lead wires, and electrodes (see Figure 40-5 on page 1314).

The **patient-controlled analgesia (PCA)** pump is a device that allows the client to control the delivery of

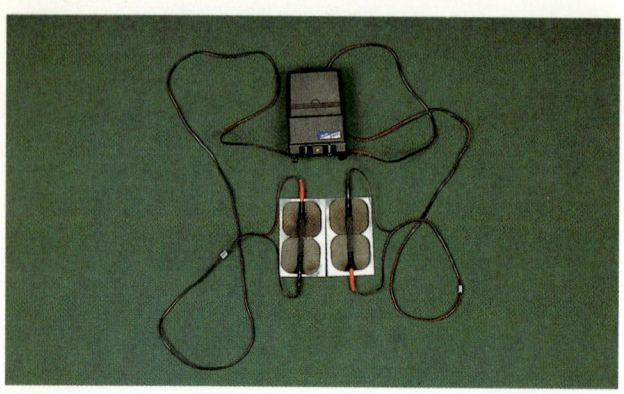

FIGURE 40-5 **Transcutaneous Electrical Nerve Stimulation (TENS) Unit** DELMAR/CENGAGE LEARNING

intravenous or subcutaneous pain medication in a safe, effective manner. The client self-regulates the delivery of the medication. Several different types of PCA devices are available; the manufacturers provide instructions for setting up the infusion pump. The pain medication is contained within an infusion pump and set according to the prescribing practitioner's order: type and concentration of pain medication, loading dosage, and **lock-out interval** (minimum time allowed between doses for the client to self-medicate).

Before initiating the PCA pump, the nurse assesses the client's level of consciousness, orientation, reading ability, and ability to learn and comprehend. PCA is used most frequently in adolescents and adults. Family members are also taught how to recognize the signs of drug overdose in home-bound clients. Instruct the client on the PCA unit:

- To self-administer the medication as needed
- That the amount of the drug the machine delivers within a particular time frame is regulated to prevent overdose
- On the use of the control button

The advantages of a PCA unit are rapid pain relief, increased client satisfaction, and often the use of less medication than with the traditional intramuscular analgesia method.

Physical Preparation

Physical preparation should be discussed with the client to ensure that the client is mentally and physically prepared for surgery. These nursing functions are individualized to the client's needs as determined by health status and the type of surgical procedure scheduled. Activities such as restricting fluids, bowel preparation, or the removal of nail polish are done the evening before, regardless of the setting. Other activities occur the day of surgery in various perioperative settings.

SKIN PREPARATION The skin and hair follicles harbor microorganisms that can contaminate a surgical wound. The skin around the operative site is prepared to reduce the number of organisms present and to inhibit rebound growth. Preparation of the skin to reduce contamination of the surgical wound occurs in two phases. The evening before or the day of surgery, the client washes the area involved in the surgical procedure with an antimicrobial soap. The client is

usually instructed to wash the surgical area vigorously several times to decrease the chance of wound infection.

Most agencies follow the recommendations of the Centers for Disease Control and Prevention (CDC), the Joint Commission, and AORN regarding the second phase. During the second phase, the skin is surgically prepared by removing hair in the operative site. The CDC and AORN recommend that this be done in the OR. Prior to the Joint Commission's 2009 NPSGs, shaving with a razor was done in the OR immediately before surgery; however, this technique for preparing the skin is no longer acceptable because of the increased risk for infection caused by razor cuts and nicks in the skin. As stated earlier in this chapter, effective January 1, 2010, when hair removal is necessary, the appropriate method is clippers or depilatories. Methods used to prep the skin are discussed in the section on the intraoperative phase later in this chapter.

NUTRITION Nutrition and fluid considerations are determined by the client's health status and the nature of the surgical procedure and anesthesia. Clients scheduled for surgical procedures requiring only local anesthetic agents may be allowed a light breakfast or clear liquids the day of surgery. However, clients scheduled for regional or general anesthesia are instructed not to eat or drink (NPO) for 6 to 8 hours before surgery. Restricting food and fluids decreases the risk of aspiration of gastric contents into the lungs during anesthesia.

Clients at risk for dehydration are infants, older adults, those with preexisting nutritional imbalances, and those having surgical procedures that cause extensive loss of blood and other body fluids. These clients are usually given intravenous fluids preoperatively to maintain fluid and electrolyte balances. Measurement of intake and output allows the nurse to monitor the client's fluid and electrolyte status.

GASTROINTESTINAL PREPARATION Gastrointestinal surgeries may require special procedures to prepare the stomach or intestines. These special procedures are performed to decrease the risk of complications such as aspiration or infection.

Nasogastric Tube Some clients may require a nasogastric tube to facilitate stomach decompression to prevent postoperative abdominal distension. Insertion of a nasogastric tube causes client discomfort and can increase apprehension regarding surgery; therefore, the tube is usually inserted during the intraoperative phase when the client is under anesthesia (see Chapter 34). Inform clients that the tube can cause irritation to the nasal mucosa and may result in a sore throat.

Bowel Preparation The surgeon prescribes the type of bowel preparation on the basis of the surgical procedure. Enemas and laxatives are not routinely administered unless the client is having abdominal surgery. Intestinal surgeries require a bowel preparation to cleanse the intestines of fecal material by administering either a cathartic or enema to empty the bowel (see Chapter 39). Antibiotics are given to reduce the bacterial content. Cleansing the bowel is necessary because surgical manipulation of the intestines interrupts normal peristalsis. Also, incision of any portion of the gastrointestinal tract places the client at risk for peritonitis if fecal material enters the abdominal cavity.

The client is usually instructed to eat a light meal the evening before, avoiding high-fat foods, and is given a laxative. The morning of surgery, enemas may be given. If the surgeon orders "enemas until clear" (no fecal return), refer to the agency's policy. Administering enemas until clear can place the NPO client at risk for fluid and electrolyte imbalances. The client's stress response may already be compromised by the fear of surgery; administering repeated enemas may further decrease the client's coping mechanisms.

URINARY ELIMINATION The client is instructed to void before receiving the preoperative medication or being transferred to the OR. The bladder needs to be empty to prevent distension and incontinence during the surgery.

Some surgeries can require continuous decompression of the bladder; the OR nurse usually inserts a Foley catheter before or during surgery. See Chapter 39 for details on catheterization. If this occurs, the client should be informed about the catheter and how long the catheter will be left in place. Inform the client that a Foley catheter causes a sensation of pressure and an urge to urinate.

SAFETY PRECAUTIONS Outpatient clients are instructed to leave their jewelry at home and to avoid the use of makeup the day of surgery for safety reasons. Jewelry and other metal objects can cause burns when electrocautery is used during surgery. Rings can compromise circulation. Hairpins can injure the scalp when the head is positioned for anesthesia. Makeup and nail polish can interfere with the practitioner's assessment of oxygenation.

Unnecessary prosthetic devices should also be left at home to prevent client injury or loss. Outpatient areas have limited space to secure valuables. Contact lenses should always be removed and stored before surgery to avoid corneal ulceration and displacement. Partial dentures and other orthodontic devices must be removed to prevent displacement into the throat during anesthesia.

If the client feels helpless without certain devices, such as glasses and hearing aids, it should be documented on the preoperative checklist that the client is wearing such devices. The OR nurse removes such devices immediately before or after anesthesia induction.

Hospitalized clients are usually instructed to give their valuables to a family member before surgery. Otherwise, these items are removed from the client's room and placed in a safe area according to hospital policy. The nurse documents on the preoperative checklist the disposition of valuables and prosthetic devices.

MEDICATIONS Efforts are made to continue routine medications throughout the perioperative experience. The surgeon instructs outpatient clients on which medications to take the day of surgery. The nurse is responsible on the day of surgery to document which medications were taken and to notify the surgeon when drugs were omitted.

Clients scheduled to receive only local anesthesia are usually instructed to wait until after the procedure to take their medications unless there may be a time delay that could have a negative effect on the client. The following medications that increase client risk are withheld:

- Anticoagulants, ibuprofen, and aspirin: May increase blood loss. Clients routinely taking oral anticoagulants are given subcutaneous heparin to ensure prompt reversal with intravenous protamine sulfate should the need arise; oral anticoagulants are not reversed by protamine sulfate.
- MAO inhibitors: May interact with anesthetic agents and are discontinued 2 weeks before surgery.
- Aminoglycosides: Potentiate the effect of neuromuscular blockers.
- Oral hypoglycemic agents: Are continued until the evening before surgery except for chlorpropamide, which is discontinued 48 hours before surgery. To prevent intraoperative fluctuations in blood sugar, an intravenous infusion of glucose and insulin is begun before surgery.
- OTC medications and herbal preparations that are contraindicated for anesthesia are ceased as long as 2 weeks prior to surgery.

The client should always disclose all medications currently in use to the prescribing practitioner when a surgical procedure is scheduled. The medication dosage can be adjusted preoperatively for certain drugs. For instance, corticosteroid therapy should be continued when clients have been maintained on the drug for 2 months or more; the dose to be given on the day of surgery depends on the client's daily therapy.

Medications to reduce anxiety and facilitate the induction of anesthesia are administered as prescribed. To prevent client discomfort with traditional intramuscular preanesthetic injections, facilities with a holding area use this setting to initiate intravenous therapy and administer the preanesthetic drugs intravenously.

SPOTLIGHT ON...

Legal and Ethical

Nursing Intervention

What should a nurse do if a client refuses a treatment? You are caring for a 16-year-old boy who was in an automobile accident and is scheduled for bladder surgery. The parents are present for perioperative teaching. You explain what will happen during the surgical procedure and that the boy will have a catheter after surgery. The boy gets upset, saying he does not want a tube. What type of age-related teaching materials might you use in this situation?

EVALUATION

Evaluation of actual and expected outcomes of the perioperative client is done over the three phases. Preoperative evaluation focuses on the client's ability to verbalize and demonstrate the exercises. The outcome is evaluated when the client successfully performs the exercises after surgery. Measurement of the client's ability to perform postoperative exercises should first be assessed during the teaching session and again an hour later to evaluate learning. If the client needs coaching to perform the exercises, reinforce teaching until the client demonstrates the exercises appropriately.

Assessment of the client's knowledge regarding the nature, purpose, and risks of the surgical procedure is measured preoperatively. Likewise, the nurse listens to the client's comments and monitors physiological indicators (e.g., vital signs) to measure fears and anxieties regarding the surgery.

The evaluation of a client's preoperative preparation for surgery should include understanding of the procedure, verbalization and return demonstration of postoperative exercises, and postoperative expectations resulting from the surgery. Refer to the accompanying Nursing Process Highlight to understand how the nurse evaluates achievement of client expected outcomes.

Documentation

Documentation of preoperative activities must be entered in the client's medical record on the appropriate forms. The preoperative checklist is used to document accurate comple-

tion of preoperative activities. Documentation on this form means that all aspects of care have been performed as ordered. When the OR personnel come to transfer the client, the preoperative nurse signs the checklist, entering the time and mode of transportation to the OR (e.g., by stretcher).

INTRAOPERATIVE PHASE

The intraoperative phase begins when the client is transferred to the OR and ends with the client's discharge from the OR. The goal of nursing care during this phase is to ensure client safety. Maintaining a safe environment includes protecting the client from injury, infection, and complications arising from anesthetic agents, hazards, and the surgical procedure. The nursing interventions are based on the AORN's (2008) preoperative standards and recommended practices.

SURGICAL ENVIRONMENT

The surgical area usually consists of three zones: unrestricted, semirestricted, and restricted. The unrestricted area is designed for personnel to enter in street clothes: receiving desk, holding area, and locker rooms. Surgical attire (scrub clothes, disposable shoe covers, and caps) is required in the semirestricted and restricted zones. Personal protective equipment (PPE) (e.g., goggles, gloves, gowns) is utilized as part of the Occupational Safety and Health Administration (OSHA) and Joint Commission guidelines. Evidence-based practice has shown that shoe covers are no longer required as a conduction precaution; however, OR personnel may still wear shoe covers to keep their shoes clean. Hallways and storage areas constitute the semirestricted area. Restricted zones (controlled and germ-free areas) include the OR and rooms where sterile instruments are prepared.

Holding Area

The holding area is a unit where the surgical team prepares the client for surgery (see Figure 40-6 on page 1317). The anesthesia provider usually starts the intravenous infusion and administers the preoperative intravenous medication. The nurse confirms that aspects of care on the preoperative checklist have been performed. A family member is usually encouraged to remain with the client while the client awaits transfer to the OR.

Occupational Hazards

Perioperative personnel are at risk of exposure to harmful pathogens and other dangers. Dangers of a particular concern to perioperative nurses are latex allergies, needlesticks, eye splashes, back injuries, and indoor pollution. Precautions should be in place that are in compliance with OSHA standards regarding bloodborne pathogens, medical waste and hazards materials (including personal protection devices), disposal of needles and syringes, and contaminated supplies.

NURSING PROCESS HIGHLIGHT

Evaluation

Achievement of Expected Outcomes

In evaluating the nursing care of Mrs. Broussard during the preoperative phase of her total hip replacement surgery, the following questions should be considered:

- What methods can be used to determine whether Mrs. Broussard understands the events that will occur during the surgery?
- What postoperative exercises should Mrs. Broussard be asked to demonstrate for the evaluation of her ability to perform these measures?
- What types of information should Mrs. Broussard be able to share about the postoperative course of treatment?
- What methods can be implemented to elicit Mrs. Broussard's concern or anxiety about the surgery itself or the expectations for her recovery?

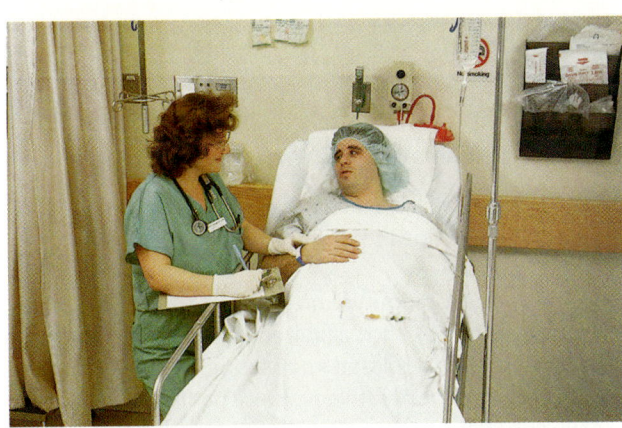

FIGURE 40-6 Holding Area. What is this nurse doing to prepare this client for surgery? DELMAR/CENGAGE LEARNING

See Chapter 29 for a complete discussion of latex allergy and OSHA's standards.

Health care agencies need to have a process in place to document compliance with OSHA requirements. Akduman et al. (1999) studied the compliance of OR personnel with universal precautions during surgical procedures in four subspecialties: orthopedic, gynecologic, cardiothoracic, and general surgery. Personnel were informed in advance about data collection regarding the use of protective equipment. The study revealed that only 39% of the personnel wore protective goggles, 5% wore face shields, 32% wore regular glasses, and nearly 25% wore no eye protection. Although double-gloving was higher in orthopedics than other areas, only 28% of the observed personnel double-gloved. A 22% rate of exposure was observed during 76 cases, with 3 percutaneous injuries (2 scalpel, 1 needlestick) and 14 cutaneous blood and bodily fluid exposures. The study proposed the need for consistent training in and reinforcement of OSHA's guidelines.

Slattery (1998) refers to the hospital environment as a "chemical soup" and addresses the agents that compromise the quality of indoor air. Pollution in the OR is caused by fumes from high levels of disinfectants; surgical smoke from tissue being cut, vaporized, or coagulated; and waste gases from anesthetic agents. Disinfectants such as glutaraldehyde used to sterilize instruments are not regulated, and the fumes may cause serious respiratory and dermatologic problems. OR nurses are also at risk with respect to laser plume or surgical smoke, which can lead to respiratory problems, burning, watery eyes, nausea, and viral contamination and regrowth. To decrease the exposure to these dangerous pollutants, agencies should have policies in place that require clients and personnel to wear high-filtration masks and should provide rooms with smoke evacuators.

ASSESSMENT

The first activity of assessment for the OR nurse is to check the client's identification band and confirm the surgical site. Agency protocol and standards of care from the AORN establish the focus areas of assessment for the client and the environment.

Assessment of proper positioning to ensure comfort and safety includes:

- Checking for client alterations that can affect positioning during the procedure, such as previous skeletal or joint surgery, presence of a joint or vascular prothesis, poor nutrition, and compromised skin integrity
- Making sure the OR bed is prepared to receive the client: for example, warming mattress on bed, proper orientation of bed, bed wheels locked
- Ensuring that accessories are clean and readily available for a specific position: for example, Wilson frame, chest rolls, pillows, headrest

Throughout the surgical procedure, the nurse assesses for pressure areas of the extremities, joints, or any body surface; skin discoloration; and temperature. Whenever the client's position is changed during surgery, the nurse reassesses for signs of circulatory impairment from positioning and equipment in contact with the skin.

NURSING DIAGNOSES

Common intraoperative nursing diagnoses promote client comfort, safety, and support during the surgical procedure. See the previous Table 40-3 on perioperative nursing diagnoses.

PLANNING AND OUTCOMES

The focus of intraoperative care planning is on nursing activities that promote the client's achievement of expected intraoperative outcomes (see the accompanying display on page 1318). These outcomes are directed at placing the client in a safe environment free from injury. The OR team monitors the client throughout the surgical procedure for complications.

Specific nursing care is planned to encompass the surgeon's specifications for positioning and to alleviate or prevent any individual client problem. Surgeons have preference cards that identify the type of equipment and instruments for various surgical procedures (e.g., indications and use of electrical equipment). Planning also involves determining the appropriate mode of client transfer, equipment and positioning aids, and need for ancillary personnel to accomplish the positioning. The plan of care should be individualized to include needs relative to the client's health status such as diabetes, malnourishment, or paralysis.

Collaboration

The surgical team consists of the surgeon, anesthesia provider, RN, surgical technologist, RN first assistant (RNFA) or physician assistant (PA), and other members of the health care team.

The roles and responsibilities of the surgeon and anesthesia provider have already been discussed. The OR team usually consists of:

- Surgeon: Scrubbed and in surgical attire to perform the surgery

COMMON INTRAOPERATIVE CLIENT OUTCOMES

- The client demonstrates knowledge related to the physical environment and surgical intervention.
- The client's needs are met while in a dependent state from the anesthesia.
- The client is maintained in a safe, germ-free environment during the surgical procedure.
- The client is free from infection 72 hours postoperatively.
- The client's skin integrity is maintained by proper positioning on the operating room table.
- The client is maintained in proper body alignment to prevent injury from positioning.
- The client is free from injury related to exposure from heat loss.
- The client is free from injury related to chemical, electrical, and physical hazards.
- The client's fluid and electrolyte balance is maintained.

- Anesthesia provider: Masked and in clean scrub attire to administer the anesthesia
- Surgical assistant (first assistant): Can be another prescribing practitioner, RNFA, or PA who is scrubbed, is in sterile attire, and assists the surgeon to ligate, suction, and suture
- Scrub nurse or technologist: Scrubbed and in sterile attire; prepares the instrument tray and passes the instruments, sponges, needles, and sutures to the surgeon
- Circulating nurse: In clean scrub attire and mask; obtains supplies, delivers materials, pours solutions, handles specimens, positions the client and surgical drapes, disposes of soiled items, and coordinates care of the client

Both the scrub and circulating nurses are responsible for counting the number of used instruments, needles, and sponges. Before the surgeon closes the incision, these items are counted to ensure that nothing is being left in the operative site.

INTERVENTIONS

Nursing interventions are selected to facilitate caring and to achieve the expected outcomes, such as the client is free from infection 72 hours postoperatively. Because anesthesia inhibits the client's ability to protect himself or herself, the OR staff implements surgical asepsis, safe positioning, and other interventions that promote client safety (e.g., the client is never left unattended).

Nursing care includes communication skills to reduce the client's anxiety. The OR staff communicates a caring

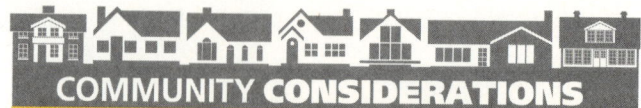

COMMUNITY CONSIDERATIONS

Nursing Care and Client Populations

What options are available to nurses who have personal objections to caring for certain client populations?

The Special Committee on Ethics of the AORN conducted a study to elicit acquired immunodeficiency syndrome (AIDS)–related knowledge, attitudes, and practices of perioperative nurses. The findings revealed that:

Nurses continue to be reluctant to provide care to HIV-positive clients if given a choice. Sixty percent of perioperative nurse respondents said they "somewhat agreed" or "strongly agreed" with this sentiment compared with 62% of the respondents in the original study. One AORN respondent said, "I don't believe anyone should be legally required to care for any patient with any illness/disease" (Reeder, Hamlet, Killen, King, & Uruburu, 1994, p. 456).

What is your reaction to the AORN respondent? Read the American Nurses Association Code of Ethics in reviewing your own values toward HIV-positive clients.

attitude, functioning under the assumption that anesthetized clients will be able to recall comments made during surgery.

Surgical Asepsis

Surgical asepsis is used to decrease the client's risk for an infection. Surgical asepsis refers to handwashing, wearing surgical attire, handling sterile instruments and equipment, and establishing and maintaining sterile fields. The sterile field is free of microorganisms, and only sterile items can be placed inside the field.

Surgical handwashing is performed to remove soil and microorganisms from the skin. The skin on the hands and arms should be intact (free of lesions). Agency policy determines how the scrub is to be performed (e.g., method and timing); see Chapter 29.

Once the scrub nurse is properly attired for surgery, strict adherence to aseptic principles guides all actions. The hands and arms are held above the waist at all times. Only attire from the waist to the gown's collar and the anterior surface of the sleeves is considered sterile. The scrub nurse sets up the instrument table, using sterile drapes and instruments. Only the tops of instrument tables are considered sterile. Items placed within a sterile field are opened, dispensed, and transferred using techniques to maintain their sterility. Soiled or contaminated articles are removed immediately from the room by the circulating nurse.

Skin Preparation

Skin preparation (prep) is performed to decrease the risk for infection by reducing the resident microbial count on the skin and inhibiting rebound growth of microbes when the skin is incised during surgery. The second phase of the surgical skin prep is usually done by OR personnel before surgery to prevent the growth of microorganisms.

Guidelines for when and where the skin is to be prepped for the surgical procedure differ according to agency policy, surgeon preference, and incision site. The preference card usually indicates the type of preparation. The OR nurse ensures that the operative site is clean.

The skin prep should comply with the CDC and Joint Commission recommendations to avoid unnecessary hair removal. Hair can be removed by clipping and depilatory. A dry shave refers to the removal of hair by clipping or the use of a depilatory. Figure 40-7 designates the body surfaces to be prepared for surgical procedures involving the head, neck, ear, and upper thorax. Preparation of the upper extremities, chest, and abdomen are illustrated in Figure 40-8 on page 1320.

When performing a skin prep, the nurse should provide the client with an explanation of the procedure, privacy, comfort, and safety. Common agents for prepping the skin include povidone-iodine, chlorhexidine, alcohol, and hexachlorophene. If the client has any adverse reactions to the prep, the nature of the reaction should be documented and the prescribing practitioner notified.

Positioning and Draping

The surgical client is usually sedated or anesthetized and therefore is unable to communicate any discomfort. Proper positioning ensures client comfort and safety, preserves vascular supply, and prevents neuromuscular damage to tissue; refer to NIC, Positioning: Intraoperative (0842). At the same time, positioning also provides access to the surgical site, airway, intravenous lines, and all monitoring devices.

All sharp surfaces in contact with the client's skin are padded to prevent injury from positioning. Bony prominences (e.g., sacrum, elbows, and heels) are padded to avoid excessive pressure on these points. The nurse ensures that skin surfaces are insulated from metal bed attachments (e.g., padded arm boards, headrest, stirrups). Appropriate devices

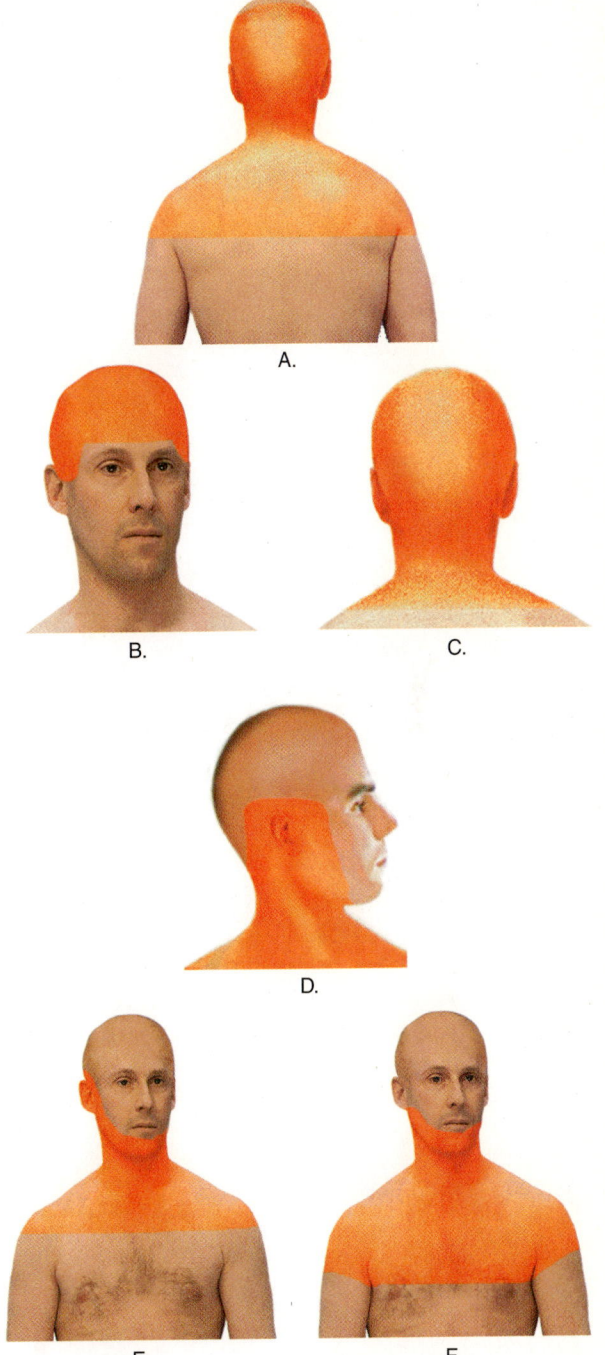

FIGURE 40-7 Preparation of the Head for Surgery: A–C. Head for a Craniotomy; D. Neck for Otological Surgery; E., F. Upper Thorax for Thyroidectomy DELMAR/CENGAGE LEARNING

are made available to support extremities to prevent compression of vital structures, such as the ulnar nerve or Achilles tendons.

The circulating nurse ensures that at least four persons are available for positioning clients under general anesthesia. Restraints (or belts) are available to secure the client to the operating bed; sufficient soft padding is used to maintain anatomical alignment of the head and neck with the spine.

▼ SAFETY FIRST ▼

CHEMICAL BURNS

After the skin preparation, remove all solution that has pooled under the client; chemical skin burns can result from prolonged exposure to antiseptic solutions.

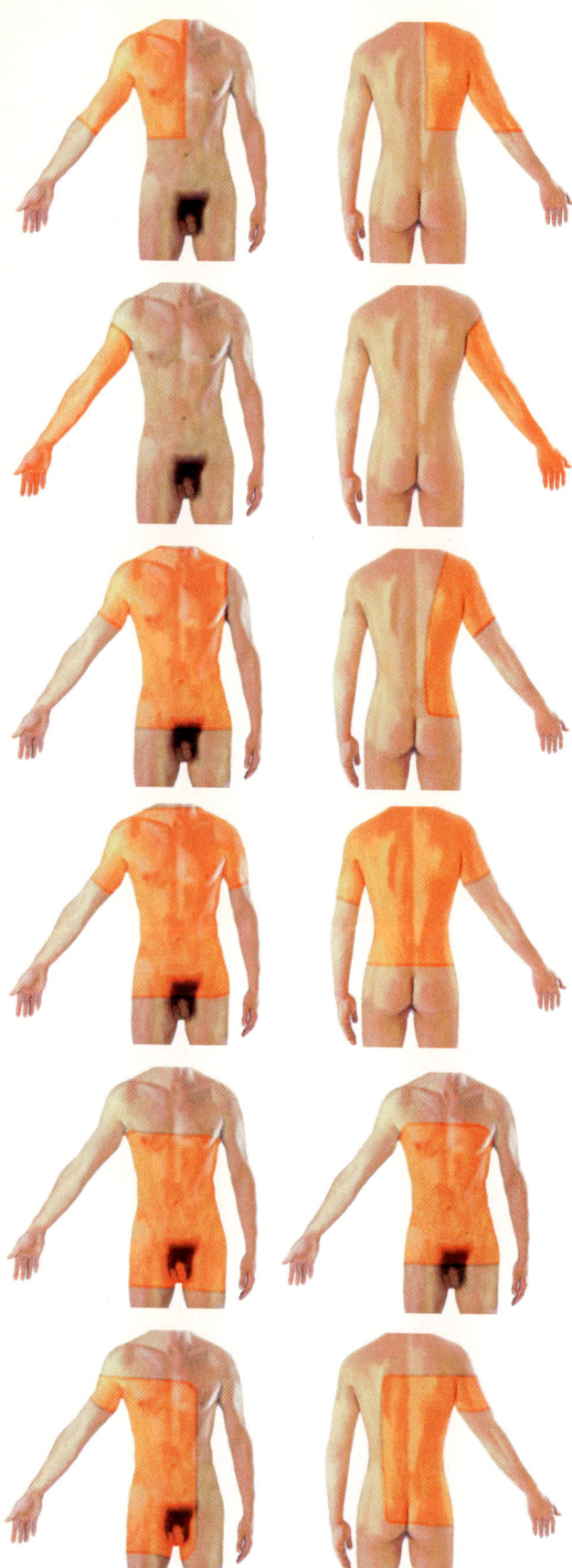

FIGURE 40-8 **Surgical Preparation of Upper Extremities and Trunk for Surgery, Anterior and Posterior Views** DELMAR/CENGAGE LEARNING

Once the client is positioned properly and the site has been prepped, the sterile team applies the sterile drapes. OR drapes are designed to expose specific operative sites. The staff keeps the sterile drapes dry and in place.

Electrical Hazards

During surgery the client can be exposed to an electrical surgical generator (electrocautery device to eliminate bleeding and reduce contamination); refer to NIC, Surgical Precautions (2920). Electricity cannot flow unless a circuit is complete; thus, electricity introduced into the body has to find a pathway back to the generator. A ground pad is provided for that purpose.

Proper grounding technique is essential for the safe and effective use of the generator. The circulating nurse ensures that the selected ground site is free of skinfolds, scar tissue, erythema, skin lesions, or bony protuberances. The site should be as close as possible to the operative area. Throughout the surgery, the circulating nurse monitors the electrocautery for signs of improper function. At the end of the procedure, when drapes are removed, the circulating nurse inspects the ground site for any unusual skin discoloration, burns, or skin reaction.

Lasers provide another method for cutting and coagulating tissue during surgical procedures. Lasers deliver high-energy beams directly onto the tissue and reduce tissue damage and scarring that can inhibit healing. To prevent injury to the skin and eyes, the conscious client and staff wear special high-filtration masks to protect them from surgical smoke. All wear protective eyewear dependent upon the type of laser in use during the procedure. Appropriate signage designating the proper attire and precautions needed to safely enter the OR is posted to inform staff that the laser is in use.

Heat Loss

Injury from hypothermia is prevented by measures implemented to minimize heat loss. During surgery, body heat is lost by positioning on a cold OR table (conduction); administration of cold gases (convection); exposure of large operative sites, such as thoracic and abdominal areas (evaporation); and exposure to cold OR temperatures (radiation). Anesthetic agents can also alter thermoregulation and lower metabolism. Body temperature is maintained by applying warming mattresses or warmed blankets, warming and humidifying inhaled gases, warming irrigating and intravenous solutions, and increasing room temperature when the client is exposed (e.g., during skin prep and positioning).

Monitoring Physiological Functioning

After intubation and induction of anesthesia, the client is monitored for:

- Ventilation and circulation
- ECG and oxygen analyzer alterations
- Fluid intake, urinary output, and calculated blood loss

- Behavioral changes
- Body temperature
- Diagnostic testing (collection of specimens and cultures, x-rays, and fluoroscopy)
- Placement of medical devices (ground pad, position support, drains, catheters, implants, packings, and dressings)

These measures assist in identifying and correcting any serious problems before they can result in client injury.

EVALUATION

Before the client is transferred to the PACU, the circulating nurse evaluates and documents achievement of client outcomes. Evaluation is based on reassessment of findings for the client during and after surgery. The circulating nurse documents the specific data on the OR record, which usually reflects AORN standards of intraoperative care and other direct care issues pertinent to client outcomes.

TRANSFER TO POSTANESTHESIA CARE UNIT

While the surgeon is closing the incision, the circulating nurse gives a telephone report to a recovery room or PACU nurse regarding the client's health status, surgical outcomes, special equipment needs, and nursing interventions. This information allows the PACU staff time to prepare to receive the client.

Planning for personnel and equipment needed to safely transfer the client is usually handled by the circulating nurse. Moving the semianesthetized client from the OR table to the PACU stretcher for transport requires the coordinated effort of at least four persons. Assurance is made that a sufficient number of staff are available to move the client while maintaining proper body alignment and preventing the dislodgement of any tubes, drains, or monitoring devices.

Safety measures are implemented to prevent injury to both client and staff members. The staff uses good body mechanics and assistive devices, such as drawsheets or body rollers, to allow proper weight distribution of the client. The stretcher wheels are locked to prevent movement. The client is always lifted from the table, as opposed to being dragged or pulled with drawsheets, to prevent skin irritation or shearing. The nurse applies stretcher belts (restraints) prior to transport. Also, the head of the stretcher is elevated, side rails are raised, and the placement of tubes and drains is confirmed.

Once on the stretcher, the client is quickly transported by the circulating nurse and the anesthesia provider to the PACU. The client at this time is at high risk for injury related to the effects of residual anesthesia: airway distress, vomiting and aspiration, and circulatory alterations. The anesthesia provider stays with the client while the circulating nurse gives a report to the PACU nurse assigned to the client. The report should include all pertinent anesthesia and surgery information (see the Nursing Checklist).

After giving the report, the circulating nurse documents the time of discharge, method and disposition of transfer, and

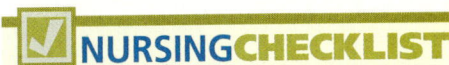

NURSING CHECKLIST

Preparing the Postanesthesia Report

- Brief history of client's health status: preexisting conditions and medical diagnoses requiring surgery
- Baseline and OR vital signs
- Results of diagnostic testing (e.g., blood gases)
- Administration of anesthetic agents and other medications
- Estimated blood loss
- Total volume of output from all tubes and drains
- Total volume of infused intravenous fluids and blood products
- Presence and status of devices (e.g., tubes, drains, antiembolism hose)
- Any other problems treated during the surgery or other special nursing interventions

a general statement regarding the client's status. The client usually remains on the same PACU stretcher throughout the stay in the unit.

POSTOPERATIVE PHASE

The primary goal of nursing care during the immediate postoperative phase is to maintain the "A-B-Cs": airway, breathing, and circulation. Ongoing care is directed toward restoring the client to the preoperative health status. Clients receiving local anesthetics, without sedation, are usually transferred to the outpatient ambulatory care setting for observation while awaiting discharge. Their postoperative care is usually nonemergent in nature and is discussed later in the section titled Ongoing Postoperative Care.

General anesthesia requires intubation. Extubation is performed by the anesthesia provider before the client leaves the OR or in the PACU when assessment data confirm adequate gas perfusion. Clients with heart and other major surgeries are not extubated immediately. The endotracheal tube is usually removed on the first postoperative day. Intubated clients are usually transferred to intensive care units for 2 or 3 days.

ASSESSMENT

Following the initial assessment of the client's respiratory status, the nurse performs a total assessment (see Table 40-7 on page 1322). The postoperative nursing care protocol, based on AORN standards of care and guidelines from the American Society of PeriAnesthesia Nurses (ASPAN), is initiated. The protocol identifies those areas requiring immediate assessment and reassessment as discussed in Table 40-7.

TABLE 40-7 Initial Postoperative Assessment: Normal and Abnormal Findings

AREA OF ASSESSMENT	NORMAL FINDINGS	ABNORMAL FINDINGS
Airway and respiratory status • Adequacy of airway and return of gag, cough, and swallowing reflexes • Type of artificial airway • Rate, rhythm, and depth of respirations • Symmetry of chest wall movements and use of accessory muscles • Breath sounds • Color of mucous membranes • Pulse oximeter readings • Amount and method of oxygen administration • If awake, ability to breathe deeply and cough	The client is able to: • Expel an oral airway; exhibit return of gag reflex • Breathe deeply and cough freely with normal rate for age, even without use of accessory muscles, and exhibit chest wall symmetry; show breath sounds present in all lobes; show pink mucous membranes • Show pulse oximeter reading between 95% and 100% • Demonstrate proper use of incentive spirometer, if awake	• Upper airway obstruction: stridor, retractions, asymmetrical chest movement • Laryngospasm: high-pitched squeaky sounds • Dyspnea: shortness of breath or difficulty in breathing • Diminished breath sounds, wheezing, rales, or rhonchi • Residual neuromuscular blockage: weak inspiratory effort, inability to lift head, or inadequate muscle strength
Circulatory status • Apical and peripheral pulses • Blood pressure (BP) • Nail bed and skin color and temperature • Capillary refill • Homans' sign Monitoring devices: • Cardiac monitor (ECG) • Pressure readings (arterial BP or central venous pressure)	The client has: • Normal apical rate and peripheral pulses • BP within 20 mm HG of baseline measurements • Pink nail beds; warm and dry skin • Capillary refill < 3 s • Negative Homans' sign • Normal ECG rhythm	• Hypotension: BP < 20 mm of baseline; rapid, weak pulse; bluish nail beds; capillary refill < 3 s • Hemorrhage/hypovolemic shock: rapid, weak pulse; increasing respirations; restlessness hypotension; cold, clammy skin; pallor; urinary output < 30 mL/h • Positive Homans' sign (calf pain present on dorsiflexion of foot) • ECG pattern: dysrhythmias; signs of cardiac ischemia
Neurologic status • Level of consciousness (Glasgow Coma Scale) • Eye opening • Verbal response • Motor response	The client: • Spontaneously opens eyes • Is orientated • Obeys commands (Glasgow Coma Scale of 15, highest rating)	Glasgow Coma Scale score of 15 indicates some alteration in consciousness; a score of 7 is considered coma
Fluid and metabolic status • Intake and output • Palpate for bladder distention • Patency of intravenous (IV) infusion (type, rate, and amount) • Signs of dehydration (skin integrity and turgor) or overload (edema) • Patency, amount, and character of drainage (catheters, drains, or tubes) • Inspect operative dressing (type, color, and amount of drainage) • Auscultate for bowel tones in all four quadrants and inspect for abdominal distension	Fluid intake balanced with total output and electrolytes within normal limits, considering replacement of blood volume lost during surgery: • IV fluids infusing per surgeon's order • Absence of bladder distension • Good skin turgor • Absence of edema • Drains and other tubing patent and intact • Dressing dry and intact • Bowel tones faint or absent during the immediate recovery phase • Absence of nausea and vomiting	• Signs of deficient fluid volume (thirst, poor skin turgor, low-grade temperature, tachycardia, respirations $\geq$ 30, a 10–15 mm Hg decrease in systolic BP, slow venous filling, urinary output < 25 mL/h) • Bright red blood on operative dressing • Signs of excess fluid volume (increased central venous pressure and edema, pulmonary or peripheral)

(Continues)

TABLE 40-7 Continued

AREA OF ASSESSMENT	NORMAL FINDINGS	ABNORMAL FINDINGS
Level of discomfort or pain • Location, intensity, and duration • Type, amount of analgesia administered and client's response	Client free from pain	Pain not relieved by analgesia
Wound management • Inspect the dressing • Type and amount of analgesia administered and client's response • If drainage is present, reassess in 15-min intervals	Dressing dry and intact	Clot dislodged: bright red drainage on the dressing

Delmar/Cengage Learning

Focused assessment is performed relative to the surgical procedure as discussed in the Nursing Process Highlight.

NURSING DIAGNOSIS

Refer to the earlier Table 40-3 listing perioperative nursing diagnoses. Clients with preexisting conditions, identified during the preoperative period, will continue to require special nursing care. Depending on the individual client's needs, other nursing diagnoses can be included in the plan of care.

Some surgeries have unpleasant outcomes. The loss of an extremity or other body part or function can cause the client and family to experience ineffective coping. These situations require compassion and consideration to assist those involved to work through and express their feelings. Support needs to be given not only to the client but also to the family. Physical healing can occur before emotional or spiritual healing does. Learning to cope with a loss sometimes extends beyond the postoperative phase. See Chapters 14 and 25 for more information.

PLANNING AND OUTCOMES

Planning the care for postanesthesia clients addresses the development of nursing interventions to achieve the client's expected outcomes during recovery from anesthesia and surgery. Care planning is done in two parts: immediate care rendered in the PACU area and ongoing post-PACU care. Nursing care in the PACU usually lasts 1 to 3 hours and is directed toward returning the client to a safe physiological level of functioning after anesthesia. Care is prioritized according to the type of anesthesia and surgical interventions through the assistance of appropriate agency protocols (e.g., care of the client following extubation). See the accompanying

display on page 1324 for a sample of *Nursing Outcomes Classification* (NOC) measurements regarding postanesthesia care.

After discharge from the PACU, the nurse ensures that the client is knowledgeable about home care. Post-PACU care is begun for outpatients in the ambulatory setting. The

NURSING PROCESS HIGHLIGHT

Assessment

Client Specific (Focused)

During surgery Mrs. Broussard was placed in a lateral position and given a general anesthetic. She was extubated before leaving the OR with an oral airway in place on arrival to the PACU. Following assessment and management of the "A-B-Cs," the nurse assessed alignment of the left hip; the client's level of pain; incision dressing for drainage, inspecting posteriorly where drainage can pool; and circulatory, motor, and sensory status below the site of surgery.

- What immediate assessment parameters must the nurse address to ascertain the status of the postoperative client?
- What priority areas must the nurse assess?
- What measures should be implemented to determine the client's level of pain?
- What are the nurse's priorities when inspecting the incision?
- What signs or manifestations should the nurse be alert for regarding the incision?

NOC: POSTPROCEDURE RECOVERY STATUS

- Definition: Extent to which an individual returns to baseline function following a procedure requiring anesthesia or sedation
- Scales: Severe deviation from normal range to no deviation from normal range, and severe to none
- Indicators: Patent airway; spontaneous respirations; forceful cough; systolic blood pressure within 20 mm Hg of baseline; gag reflex; retaining oral fluids; fully awake; moving extremities on command; thermoregulation; urine output; voiding; drainage from tube or drain; drainage on dressing; nausea; vomiting; shivering; pain

Adapted from Moorhead, S., Johnson, M., Swanson, M., & Maas, M. (2008). *Nursing outcomes classification (NOC)* (4th ed., p. 448). St. Louis, MO: Mosby Elsevier Health Sciences.

nursing interventions reinforce client safety and teaching for discharge. For clients who are hospitalized postoperatively, the nursing care plan encompasses both inpatient and discharge needs.

INTERVENTIONS

Care in the recovery unit is directed by standards of care and protocols. These tools assist the nurse in determining the most effective interventions for specific client populations, type of anesthesia, and surgical procedure. Postoperative nursing interventions are based on assessment and reassessment findings.

Safety measures are initiated immediately on arrival into the recovery unit (see Figure 40-9). Intubated clients require the constant attendance of a nurse at the bedside. The head of

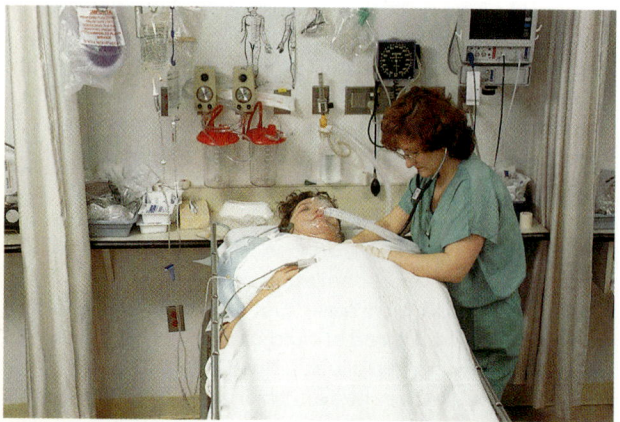

FIGURE 40-9 Postanesthesia care unit (PACU). **What is the most essential action the nurse should implement with the client in this situation?** DELMAR/CENGAGE LEARNING

the stretcher is maintained in a high Fowler's position. Stretcher belts and side rails are left in place from transfer; wheels on the stretcher are locked. Lifesaving equipment is at the client's bedside. The following is a discussion of nursing interventions for the postoperative client that incorporates nursing activities as defined by NIC, Postanesthesia Care (2870).

Monitor Respiratory Status

On arrival in the recovery area, the client is placed on high-humidity oxygen and attached to a **pulse oximeter**, a sensor device to measure the oxygen saturation level of the blood; see Procedure 40-2. The client is at risk for ineffective breathing patterns resulting from the anesthesia. At least every 15 minutes the nurse monitors the reading on the pulse oximeter along with respirations. A patent airway can be maintained with an endotracheal tube, nasal or oral airways, and suctioning when needed. See Chapter 32 for a complete discussion of airway devices.

If the client is extubated and experiences difficulty in breathing, reestablish the upper airway: Bring the chin forward, hyperextend the neck, and turn the head to the side. If the obstruction is unrelieved, insert either a nasal or an oral airway and suction. If these measures fail to relieve the obstruction, notify the anesthesia provider. The anesthesia provider is responsible for treating any physiological impairments related to anesthesia.

The nurse tapes the endotracheal tube on intubated clients to ensure proper placement. The client is maintained in a high Fowler's position to optimize breathing and lung expansion, unless contraindicated. Bronchial secretions are removed by suctioning the intubated client. Suctioning is performed on the basis of assessment findings:

- Rhonchi (low-pitched gurgling sounds in large airways)
- Low-pitched, musical wheezes despite bronchodilator therapy
- Increased peak airway pressure in clients receiving mechanical ventilation

The lungs are usually hyperinflated and hyperoxygenated before, between, and after suctioning to prevent hypoxemia and cardiac dysrhythmias. The nurse observes the ECG monitor while suctioning to observe for signs of hypoxemia.

Hypoxemia can be caused by inadequate lung ventilation from the depressant effects of anesthesia or narcotics. The PACU client is at risk for hypoxemia from the effects of general anesthesia, which reduces the inspiratory effort, and the presence of pain, which reduces ventilatory effort. Older or obese clients are especially vulnerable to postoperative hypoxemia.

The early symptoms of hypoxemia are drowsiness and confusion. These symptoms are usually present in PACU clients recovering from anesthesia. A blood oxygen level measurement less than 95% is an indication of hypoxemia.

EXTUBATION The agency's protocol is implemented to determine the parameters for extubation, such as the client being able to lift the head for 5 seconds and produce strong bilateral hand grasps. The nurse obtains a tidal volume, negative inspiratory force, and vital capacity (if the client can cooperate) before extubation. See Chapter 32 for further discussion. The anesthesia provider is notified when the oxygen saturation percentage is within safe limits to allow extubation.

The nurse confirms the presence of bilateral breath sounds immediately before and after extubation by auscultation. The procedure is explained to elicit client cooperation and to allay anxiety. Before extubation, the pharynx and trachea are suctioned. The client is instructed to inhale deeply while the anesthesia provider deflates the cuff and removes the endotracheal tube at maximal lung inflation to encourage initial gas flux outward, allowing the forceful exhaling of secretions.

The client is placed immediately on humidified oxygen for at least 30 minutes and monitored with a pulse oximeter for an hour after extubation. Ventilation is maintained by encouraging deep breathing, coughing, turning, and taking deep breaths every 5 to 10 minutes.

Monitor Circulatory Status

The client is monitored carefully for the signs of hypotension (see Table 40-7), which can occur from the myocardial depressant effects of residual anesthesia or hypovolemia. The cardiac monitor displays the client's heart rhythm; it is used to detect and treat tachycardia, bradycardia, dysrhythmias, and cardiac ischemia.

Hypovolemic shock, the marked reduction in circulating blood volume, is caused by hemorrhage. The symptoms of hemorrhage are presented in Table 40-7. A rapid pulse rate can indicate pain, bleeding, dehydration, or shock. Impaired capillary refill indicates inadequate tissue perfusion to extremities.

Passive range of motion and the application of antiembolism hose or other devices promote circulation of the intubated or semiconscious client. Postoperative leg exercises are begun as soon as the client recovers from the effects of anesthesia. These measures prevent circulatory complications such as thrombophlebitis, thrombus, and embolus formation.

Monitor Neurologic Status

Monitoring the client's level of consciousness is done in relation to how the airway is maintained:

- The unconscious client with an absence of the cough and gag reflex will have an endotracheal tube or airway.
- The semiconscious client with partial return of all reflexes will have an oral or nasal airway.
- The conscious client with full return of all reflexes will breathe without assistance from an artificial airway.

The Glasgow Coma Scale is used to measure the client's level of response. See Chapter 38 for a description of the Glasgow Coma Scale.

The nurse monitors clients who had spinal anesthesia for return of reflexes, sensation, and movement of extremities below the level of anesthesia. Extremities are assessed for color, temperature, and pedal pulses.

Nursing care of clients with spinal anesthesia includes the prevention of a postspinal headache. The postspinal headache is thought to be caused by the leakage of cerebrospinal fluid from the puncture site in the dura. Measures to prevent a headache include strict bed rest for 24 to 48 hours, adequate hydration with intravenous saline, and injection of 5 to 20 mL autologous blood into the epidural space at the puncture site.

Monitor Fluid and Metabolic Status

During the immediate postoperative phase, gastrointestinal and genitourinary assessment and interventions are considered from a fluid and metabolic perspective. The client is maintained on intravenous infusions as prescribed by the surgeon. The goal of intravenous therapy is to maintain the circulating fluid volume. Infusion sites are inspected for patency immediately when the client arrives in the PACU. Frequent inspection of these sites is necessary throughout recovery; intravenous access must be maintained in the event of complications (e.g., hemorrhage) that warrant emergency administration of intravenous fluids or medications. Secretions from tubes, drains, and the incision site are measured to determine output. The client's total output is compared against the volume of intravenous replacement fluids.

After surgery, the muscle tone of the bladder is compromised by analgesic or anesthetic agents. Assess for bladder distension by palpating the contour of the lower abdomen for a rounded mass above the symphysis pubis. When clients cannot void within 8 hours, the surgeon is notified for an order to catheterize. If the client has a Foley catheter, it should flow freely with urine.

Postoperative nausea and vomiting can be caused by multiple factors. Anesthetic agents and opiates can stimulate the chemoreceptors of the inner ear and the vomiting center in the brain. Deficient fluid volume, electrolyte imbalances, drugs, and general anesthesia by mask technique can also cause nausea and vomiting. Nausea and vomiting are treated with antiemetics.

Anesthetic agents can decrease peristalsis, resulting in diminished or absent bowel tones. Manipulation of the intestines further decreases the loss of bowel tones. The nurse auscultates for bowel tones and inspects for abdominal distension. A nasogastric tube is usually in place for clients with abdominal surgery and clients at risk for nausea and vomiting postoperatively.

With abdominal surgery, the nurse also monitors for abdominal distension to detect internal hemorrhage. When clients with abdominal surgery develop abdominal distension, inspect the tape over the incision dressing; tension on the tape can cause disruption of skin integrity (irritation and blisters). This can also increase the client's risk for a wound infection. **Cullen's sign,** a bluish discoloration around the umbilicus in postoperative clients, can indicate intra-abdominal or perineal bleeding.

Clients are kept on an NPO status until the gag reflex returns, they are free from nausea, and the presence of bowel tones is detected. Certain drugs, such as analgesic and anesthetic agents, have a drying effect on the oral mucous membranes. Dehydration from loss of body fluids also causes dryness and thirst. Oral hygiene is performed frequently to promote comfort and prevent infections.

Manage Pain

Nurses assess for pain by allowing the client to rate the intensity of pain. Studies comparing nurses' and clients' ratings of pain have found little similarity between the two (Pasero, 2008). One study compared the pain ratings of 119 postoperative clients and their nurses. The ratings matched only 35% of the time; nurses underassessed pain in 45% of the cases and overassessed pain in 20% of the cases.

Pain management is monitored and treated by intravenous narcotics in titrated doses until the client is fully conscious. Once the client is fully conscious, pain is managed according to prescribing practitioner order: PCA, continuous epidural anesthesia, intravenous or intramuscular injection, or TENS. See Chapter 35 for a complete discussion of pain management.

The nurse should institute comfort measures such as splinting the incision line and positional changes to decrease the client's pain response. Besides incisional pain, the client can experience pain for other reasons, such as positioning during surgery, presence of tubes (endotracheal, nasogastric, chest, or Foley), and tight dressings or casts. Skin care and back rubs are done to promote comfort and circulation.

The Agency for Healthcare Research and Quality has clinically relevant practice guidelines for the management of postoperative pain. Three interdisciplinary panels, chaired by nurses, developed guidelines to inform the public on pain management:

- The provider should anticipate the pain.
- It is least therapeutic to be medicated when in pain.
- There are alternatives to pharmacologic management of pain.

Relaxation techniques, distraction, environmental manipulation, massage, and positioning are optional therapies. See Chapter 31 for additional information on complementary therapies for pain management.

EVALUATION AND DISCHARGE FROM THE PACU

The anesthesia provider is responsible for releasing the client from the PACU. Agencies have specific standards of care that have to be met before discharge. These standards address achievement of specific client outcomes with inherent parameters for evaluation, such as:

- The client is conscious, oriented, and can move all extremities.
- The client demonstrates full return of reflexes.
- The client can clear the airway and cough effectively.
- Vital signs have been stable or within baseline ranges for 30 minutes.
- Intake and urinary output are adequate to maintain the circulating blood volume.

- The client is afebrile, or a febrile condition has been treated accordingly.
- Dressings are dry or have only minimal drainage.

The surgeon manages the client's treatment throughout the remainder of the postoperative phase.

ONGOING POSTOPERATIVE CARE

The postoperative phase continues until the client is released from the surgeon's care. The primary goal during this phase is to restore physiological functioning, promote healing, and prevent complications. When the client is discharged from the PACU, the client goes either directly to an inpatient hospital bed or to the outpatient ambulatory unit for observation. The surgeon will later decide whether to admit the client to an inpatient 24-hour observation room or to discharge the client. When clients are discharged to their residence, they often require the services of a home health nurse to assist with their postoperative care. The home health nurse will continue to assess and provide necessary care until the client achieves the expected outcomes.

Postoperative nursing care after discharge is based on the nursing diagnoses and expected outcomes that still have not been met (see the accompanying display on discharge teaching). Clients who are discharged without the services of a home health agency assume their own care or have a family member or significant other serve as the care provider. In this situation, specific written discharge instructions are explained to the client or care provider.

Ineffective Airway Clearance

Ineffective airway clearance during this phase can result from a diminished cough reflex or increased pulmonary congestion. The nurse monitors skin color and respiratory rate and depth and auscultates breath sounds to determine the adequacy of

---

DISCHARGE TEACHING

CLIENT EXPECTED OUTCOMES
Before discharge, the client can:

- List the symptoms to be reported to the prescribing practitioner on occurrence.
- Describe limitations in activity.
- Explain dietary limitations.
- Explain the meaning and purpose of medications.
- Explain potential food or drug interactions.
- Describe the use of Standard Precautions as appropriate.
- Demonstrate aseptic technique in changing dressings.
- Demonstrate use or application of prescribed medical devices (identify appropriate device).

oxygenation and to identify complications (e.g., atelectasis). Deep breathing, coughing, and the use of the incentive spirometer are continued until the client demonstrates achievement of respiratory outcomes.

Ineffective Tissue Perfusion

Ineffective tissue perfusion (cardiopulmonary) related to inadequate circulation is a possible nursing diagnosis. The nurse monitors pulse rate and quality, blood pressure, skin and nail bed color and condition, and temperature for indications of decreased oxygenation at the cellular level. Capillary refill and peripheral pulses are checked for adequate circulation to the extremities. The nurse monitors the lower extremities for signs of superficial vein thrombosis (local warmth, swelling, pain, redness) and deep vein thrombosis (a positive Homans' sign).

Postoperative leg exercises are performed until the client is able to ambulate and resume activities of daily living. Antiembolism hose are usually worn until the client returns for the first office visit. At that time the surgeon assesses the need to continue use of the hose.

Other devices, pneumatic compression, and CPM are maintained according to the prescribing practitioner's order. Clients are encouraged to ambulate while these devices are in place to promote respiratory, circulatory, and gastrointestinal functions. The CPM device is used until signs of incision swelling have decreased, healing is evident, and range of motion is achieved.

Deficient Fluid Volume

Deficient fluid volume can be related to active fluid volume loss, inadequate fluid intake from being NPO, or nausea and vomiting. The client is monitored for intake and output that includes secretions from drainage tubes, drains, and dressings. If oral fluids are restricted, the client is maintained on intravenous infusions as ordered by the surgeon. The nurse monitors the patency of the intravenous line, observes for signs of infiltration, and records the amount and type of fluids infused. The nurse assesses for signs of dehydration or fluid overload. See Chapter 33 for a discussion of fluid balance.

Home health clients with continuous intravenous therapy are maintained on an infusion pump. The caregiver is taught how to add infusions to the line under sterile technique. The home health nurse visits the client daily to assess for intravenous patency. A nurse is usually on call 24 hours for clients receiving continuous infusions.

Imbalanced Nutrition

Imbalanced nutrition: less than body requirements is usually related to anesthesia or surgical manipulation of the intestines. Until peristalsis returns and nausea, anorexia, or vomiting subsides, the client is maintained on intravenous therapy to preserve fluid and electrolyte balance. Nasogastric tube drainage is measured, and color and consistency are documented. See Chapter 34 for more information.

Clients with abdominal surgery can take up to 2 to 3 days or longer for return of normal gastrointestinal function. The nurse auscultates the abdomen for gurgling and rumbling sounds in all four quadrants to indicate return of peristalsis.

Early ambulation promotes the return of peristalsis. When bowel tones return and nausea subsides, the client's diet is progressive: First, ice chips are offered, then clear to full liquids; if tolerated, the diet is progressed to soft or regular. Some clients are on a regular diet within hours after surgery. See Chapter 34 for a discussion of types of modified diets.

Urinary Retention

Urinary retention is related to anesthesia or surgical manipulation that causes temporary loss of bladder tone. Efforts are made to promote urination (e.g., male clients are more prone to void if they can stand). If the client does not void within 8 hours after surgery, assess for bladder distension and notify the surgeon. The surgeon can order a straight or Foley catheter. *Clients must void before they can be released from the ambulatory setting.*

Acute Pain

Position changes and splinting are continued to relieve pain. Clients can be discharged to home with a PCA pump. Before discharge the nurse ensures that the client is able to correctly self-administer using the PCA. Efforts are made to provide adequate rest by scheduling procedures that do not interfere with sleep.

Risk for Infection

The client with a surgical incision is at risk for infection. Wound healing begins as early as 2 hours after surgery. The nurse ensures that the dressing is clean, dry, and intact; dressings promote rapid reepithelialization and protect against infection. Various types of dressings are used: conventional absorbent nonocclusive, semiocclusive hydroactive, and occlusive hydrocolloid.

Nurses use Standard Precautions while caring for clients and sterile technique when changing a dressing. The incision line is assessed when the nurse changes the dressing. For some clients, the surgeon usually orders prophylactic antibiotics and removes any catheters or drains as soon as possible to prevent an infection. If the client were to develop a deep wound infection, it could necessitate prosthesis removal.

To monitor for signs of an infection, the nurse notes the type and amount of drainage on the dressing and the stage of wound healing. Vital signs are measured, recorded, and analyzed against laboratory results, especially the white blood cell count and differential. The client is taught to care for the wound and to observe for the complications of wound healing: hemorrhage, hematoma formation, infection, dehiscence, and evisceration. See Chapter 37 for a discussion of these complications.

EVALUATION

Evaluation is based on client-specific postoperative nursing diagnoses and achievement of outcomes. The time frame for the client's achieving the outcomes can vary with the client's health status, surgical procedure, and other factors, such as age. The nurse documents achievement of outcome criteria data (see the Nursing Checklist on postoperative documentation on page 1328).

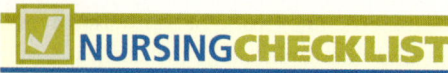

NURSINGCHECKLIST

Postoperative Documentation

- The client's respiratory function has returned to baseline level within 1 week after surgery as demonstrated by respirations 16 to 20/minute, deep and regular; skin color pink; lungs sounds clear on auscultation; and oxygen saturation greater than 95%.
- The client's cardiopulmonary function has returned to baseline level within 1 week after surgery as demonstrated by blood pressure with 10 to 20 mm Hg of baseline measurement; absence of dysrhythmias; pulse rate 60 to 90 beats per minute; skin pink, warm, and dry; capillary refill less than 3 seconds; peripheral pulses present; negative Homans' sign; and output within 500 mL of intake.
- The client is free from signs of a wound infection within 72 hours after surgery as demonstrated by normal temperature; pulse and respirations at baseline level; sutures intact; incision line without swelling, redness, or purulent exudate; and scab sloughing.

PROCEDURE 40-1

Postoperative Exercise Instruction

EQUIPMENT

- Educational materials
- Tissues
- Pillow
- Nonsterile gloves
- Disposable volume-oriented incentive spirometer

ACTION	RATIONALE
1. Wash hands/hand hygiene; organize equipment.	1. Reduces transmission of microorganisms and promotes efficiency.
2. Check the client's identification band.	2. Facilitates proper identification of client.
3. Place client in a sitting position.	3. Promotes full chest expansion.
4. Demonstrate deep breathing exercise.	4. Shows client how to breathe deeply.
5. Have client return demonstrate deep breathing:	5. Fosters learning.
• Place one hand on abdomen (umbilical area) during inhalation.	• Exerts counterpressure during inhalation.
• Expand the abdomen and rib cage on inspiration.	• Promotes maximum chest expansion.
• Inhale slowly and evenly through your nose until you achieve maximum chest expansion.	• Maintains full expansion of the alveoli.
• Hold breath for 2 to 3 seconds.	• Increases the pressure, preventing immediate collapse of the alveoli.
• Slowly exhale through your mouth until maximum chest contraction has been achieved.	• Promotes maximum chest contraction.
• Repeat the exercise three or four times; allow client to rest.	• Enforces learning.
6. The nurse demonstrates splinting and coughing.	6. Shows the client how to raise mucus secretions from the tracheobronchial tree.
7. Don gloves.	7. Reduces transmission of microorganisms.
8. Keep the client in a sitting position, head slightly flexed, shoulders relaxed and slightly forward, and feet supported on the floor.	8. Promotes full expansion of chest cage and use of accessory muscles to produce a deep, productive cough.

(Continues)

PROCEDURE 40-1
Postoperative Exercise Instruction (Continued)

ACTION	RATIONALE
9. Have the client return demonstrate splinting and coughing:	9. Fosters learning.
• Have the client slowly raise head and sniff the air.	• Increases the amount of air and helps to aerate the base of the lungs.
• Have the client slowly bend forward and exhale slowly through pursed lips.	• Dries the tracheal mucosa as air flows over it; there is a slight increase in the carbon dioxide level, which stimulates deeper breathing.
• Repeat breathing two to three times.	
• When the client is ready to cough, have client place a folded pillow against the abdomen; have the client grasp the pillow against the abdomen with clasped hands (see Figure 40-10).	• Loosens mucus plugs and moves secretions to the main bronchus.
• Have client take a deep breath and begin coughing immediately after inspiration is completed by bending forward slightly and producing a series of soft, staccato coughs.	• Elevates the diaphragm and expels air in a more forceful cough; supports the abdominal muscles and reduces pain when coughing if the client has an abdominal incision.
• Have a tissue ready.	• Removes secretions from the main bronchus.
	• Provides a tissue for sputum disposal.
10. Instruct the client on the use of an incentive spirometer (see Figure 40-11). Have the client:	10. Reinflates the alveoli and removes mucous secretions.
• Hold a volume-oriented incentive spirometer upright.	• Promotes proper functioning of the device.

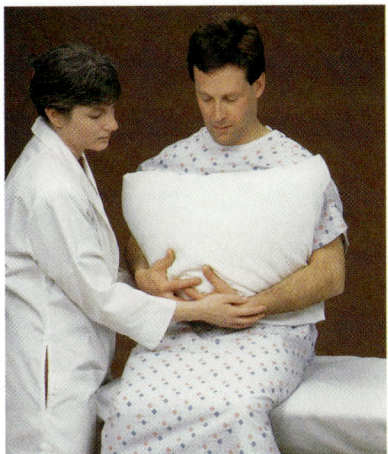

FIGURE 40-10 Splinting DELMAR/CENGAGE LEARNING

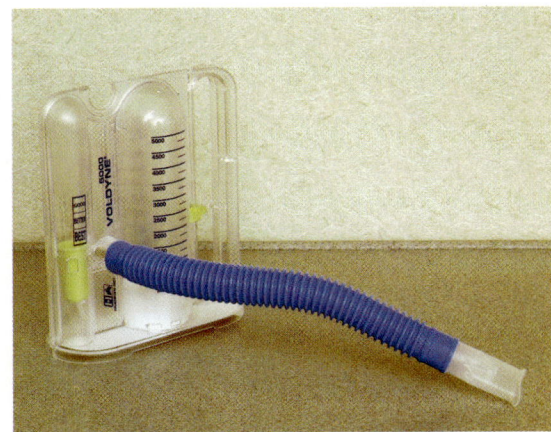

FIGURE 40-11 Incentive Spirometer DELMAR/CENGAGE LEARNING

• Take a normal breath and exhale, then seal lips tightly around the mouthpiece; take a slow, deep breath to elevate the balls in the plastic tube, and hold the inspiration for at least 3 seconds.	• Allows for greater lung expansion; holding the inspiration increases the pressure, preventing immediate collapse of the alveoli.
	• Encourages the client to do respiratory exercises.
• The client simultaneously measures the amount of inspired air volume on the calibrated plastic tube.	• Allows normal expiration.
	• Provides client the opportunity to relax.
	• Encourages sustained maximal inspiration and loosens secretions. *(Continues)*

PROCEDURE 40-1
Postoperative Exercise Instruction (Continued)

ACTION	RATIONALE
• Remove the mouthpiece, and exhale normally.	• Facilitates removal of secretions.
• Take several normal breaths.	• Prevents transmission of microorganisms.
• Repeat the procedure four to five times.	
• Have the client cough after the incentive effort; repeat Action 9. Have a tissue ready.	
• Have client clean mouthpiece under running water and place in clean container (disposable mouthpiece changed every 24 hours).	
11. The nurse explains leg and foot exercises (see Figure 40-12).	11. Elicits client cooperation.
12. Instruct client to return demonstrate in bed:	12. Fosters learning of how to improve venous blood return:
• Have the client, with heels on bed, push the toes of both feet toward the foot of the bed until the calf muscles tighten; then relax feet. Pull the toes toward the chin until calf muscles tighten; then relax feet (see Figure 40-12B).	• Causes contraction and relaxation of the calf muscles.
• With heels on bed, lift and circle both ankles, first to the right and then to the left; repeat three times, and relax.	• Causes contraction and relaxation of the quadriceps muscles.
• Flex and extend each knee alternately, sliding foot up along the bed; relax (see Figure 40-12C).	• Causes contraction and relaxation of the quadriceps muscles.

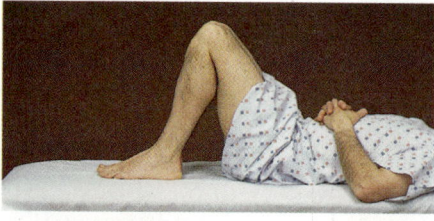

A

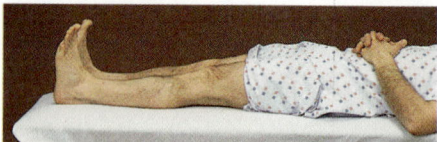

B

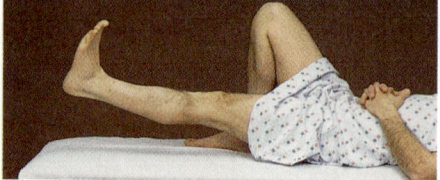

C

FIGURE 40-12 Leg Exercises DELMAR/CENGAGE LEARNING

(Continues)

PROCEDURE 40-1
Postoperative Exercise Instruction (Continued)

ACTION	RATIONALE
13. The nurse shows the client how to turn in bed and get out of bed.	13. Elicits client cooperation.
14. Instruct the client who will have a left-sided abdominal or chest incision to turn to the right side of bed and sit up as follows:	14. Fosters learning how to turn and get out of bed without putting pressure on the incision line.

- Flex the knees.
- With the right hand, splint the incision with hand or small pillow.
- Turn toward right side by pushing with the left foot and grasping the shoulder of the nurse or partial foot rail of the bed with the left hand.
- Raise up to a sitting position on the side of the bed by using the left arm and hand to push down against the mattress (see Figure 40-13).

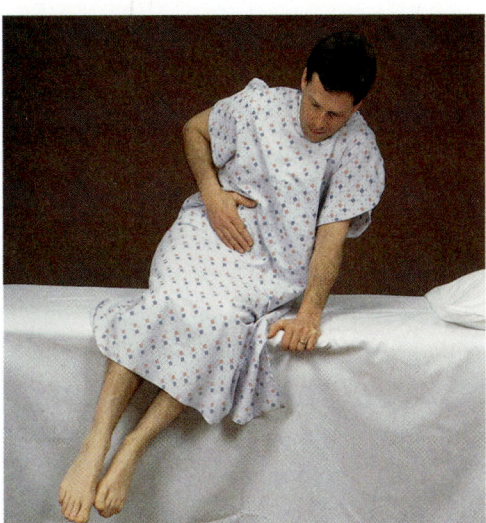

FIGURE 40-13 Out-of-Bed Transfers DELMAR/CENGAGE LEARNING

ACTION	RATIONALE
15. Reverse instructions (use left side instead of right) for the client with a right-sided incision according to Action 14.	15. Same as Rationale 14.
16. Instruct clients with orthopedic surgery (e.g., hip surgery) how to use a trapeze bar.	16. Facilitates movement in bed without putting pressure on a leg or hip joint.

(Continues)

PROCEDURE 40-1
Postoperative Exercise Instruction (Continued)

delegation tip

It is the registered nurse's responsibility to initiate client teaching after completing an assessment that validates the need for the intervention. Follow-up assessment regarding the effectiveness of these exercises is also the registered nurse's responsibility; however, ancillary personnel should be instructed to encourage these activities, to assist clients into the proper positions, and to report results. Ancillary personnel may assist clients to perform coughing and deep breathing exercises, incentive spirometer exercises, and leg exercises.

nursing tips

- *The best time to teach postoperative exercises is before surgery. Remember to assess the client's motivation to learn and ability to pay attention.*
- *Encourage the client to use a pillow or other splinting method to ease the discomfort of coughing, turning, and deep breathing.*
- *Keep the incentive spirometer close to the client to encourage its use.*

PROCEDURE 40-2

Administering Pulse Oximetry

EQUIPMENT
- Pulse oximeter
- Proper sensor
- Alcohol wipe or soap and water
- Nail polish remover if necessary

ACTION	RATIONALE
1. Wash hands/hand hygiene.	1. Reduces transmission of microorganisms.
2. Select an appropriate sensor. Sensors are commonly used for the fingertips.	2. The sensor should be selected based on the size of the person and the site to be used.
3. Select an appropriate site for the sensor. Fingers are most commonly used; however, toes (see Figure 40-14 on page 1333), ear lobes, nose, forehead (see Figure 40-15 on page 1333), hands, and feet can be used. Assess for capillary refill and proximal pulse. If the client has poor circulation, use an earlobe, forehead, or nasal sensor instead. In children, sensors may be used on the hand, foot, or trunk. If older adult clients have thickened nails, pick another site.	3. Decreased circulation alters the O_2 saturation measurement.
4. Clean the site with an alcohol wipe. Remove artificial nails or nail polish if present, or select another site. Clean any tape adhesive. Use soap and water if necessary to clean the site.	4. Polish and artificial fingernails alter the results.

(Continues)

PROCEDURE 40-2
Administering Pulse Oximetry (Continued)

ACTION	RATIONALE

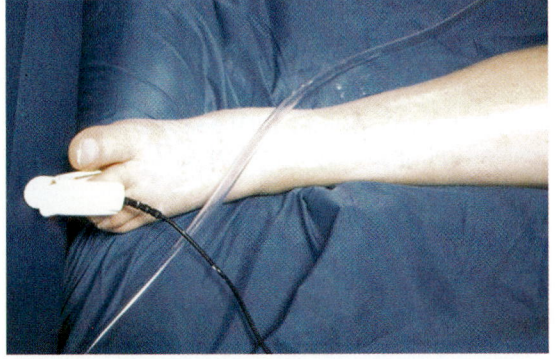

FIGURE 40-14 Pulse Oximeter Sensor Placed on a Toe DELMAR/CENGAGE LEARNING

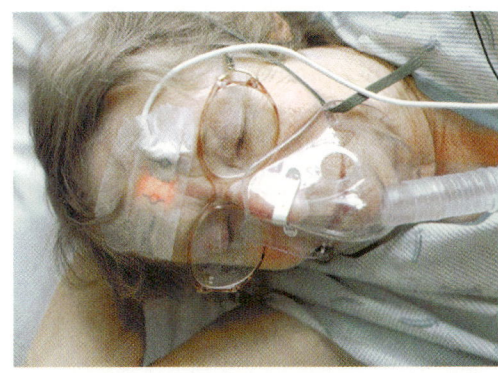

FIGURE 40-15 Pulse Oximeter Sensor Placed on the Forehead DELMAR/CENGAGE LEARNING

5. Apply the sensor. Make sure the photon detectors are aligned on opposite sides of the selected site (see Figure 40-16).

6. Connect the sensor to the oximeter with a sensor cable. Turn on the machine. Initially a tone can be heard, followed by an arterial wave-form fluctuation with each arterial pulse. In most oximeters if the battery is low, a low-battery light illuminates when 15 minutes of battery life are remaining. Oximeters should remain plugged in even when not in use (see Figure 40-17).

5. Proper application is necessary for accurate results.

6. The tone and wave-form fluctuation indicate that the machine is detecting blood flow with each arterial pulsation.

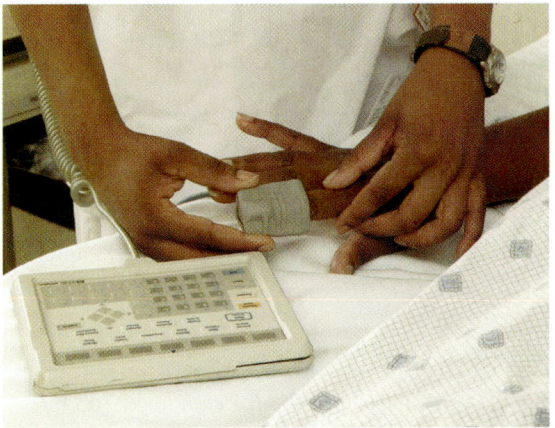

FIGURE 40-16 Apply the sensor to the selected site. DELMAR/CENGAGE LEARNING

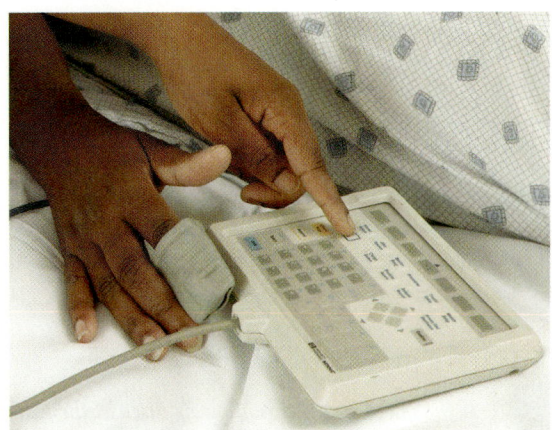

FIGURE 40-17 Follow the manufacturer's instructions when taking an oximetry reading. DELMAR/CENGAGE LEARNING

7. Adjust the alarm limits for high and low O_2 saturation levels according to the manufacturer's directions. Pulse rate limits most often can also be set. Adjust volume.

7. The alarms indicate that the saturation levels or pulse rates are outside the designated levels and alert the nurse of abnormal O_2 saturation levels and pulse rates.

(Continues)

PROCEDURE 40-2
Administering Pulse Oximetry (Continued)

ACTION	RATIONALE
8. If taking a reading, note the results (see Figure 40-18). If the oximeter is being used for constant monitoring, move the site of spring sensors every 2 hours and adhesive sensors every 4 hours.	8. Prevents skin breakdown from pressure and skin irritation from the adhesive.
9. Cover the sensor with a sheet or towel to protect it from exposure to bright light.	9. Ambient light sources such as sunlight or warming lights may interfere with the sensor and alter the Sao_2 results.
10. Notify the prescribing practitioner of abnormal results.	10. Low Sao_2 levels require medical attention because permanent tissue damage may result from low oxygen saturation.
11. Record the results of O_2 saturation measurements according to prescribing practitioner's order or protocol. Include in the documentation the type of sensor used, the site of application, the hemoglobin levels, and your assessment of the client's skin at the sensor site.	11. Communicates the findings to the other members of the health care team and contributes to the legal record by documenting the care given to the client.

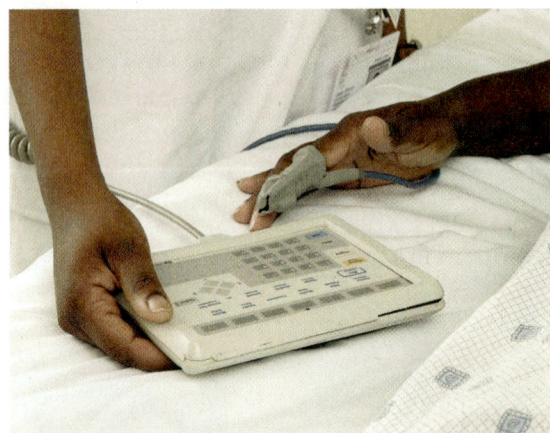

FIGURE 40-18 Note the results on the oximeter. DELMAR/CENGAGE LEARNING

delegation tip

Ancillary personnel routinely perform pulse oximetry. They should be instructed on acceptable parameters and to report any abnormal findings to the nurse.

nursing tips

- *If the client has a chronic lung disease, then the highest attainable value might be 90% (or even lower [65% to 80%]) instead of 92% to 100%. Know the client's normal values and carefully evaluate changes in respiratory, cardiac, and mental status.*
- *The client with diabetes, peripheral vascular disease, or hypothyroidism may have thickened or discolored nail beds. Assess the client and move the sensor to an alternate site if required.*
- *Always remember to treat the client and not the machine. If the alarm goes off frequently, yet the client is asymptomatic, then move or secure the sensor, or change the machine.*

KEY CONCEPTS

- The major role of nursing functions in caring for the perioperative client is to foster the achievement of expected outcomes of care.

- Outpatient surgical clinics decrease the client's length of stay in the hospital and health care costs.

- Management of the perioperative client occurs in various health care settings.

- Ensuring the safety of the surgical client requires the collaborative efforts of all surgical personnel.

- Effective perioperative management is directed by a multidisciplinary team on the basis of recognized standards of care, protocols, and individualized expected client outcomes.

- Assessment of the client's status before surgery establishes baseline data to direct interventions throughout the perioperative phases.

- The NIC identifies one of the major preoperative roles of the registered nurse as coordinator, ensuring the obtainment of baseline data and communication among the surgical team members.

- Interventions of the health care team focus on decreasing the perioperative client's risks for complications.

- The first intervention for the OR nurse is to check the client's identification band and confirm the surgical site.

- Prior to release from the OR, the circulating nurse evaluates and documents the achievement of client outcomes during the intraoperative phase.

- NOC indicators provide an inclusive listing of identifiers to monitor the postoperative client's return to normal (baseline) function.

- Documentation of the client's response to interventions and achievement of expected outcomes provides the framework for evaluation.

- Coordination of discharge care begins in the preoperative phase and is reinforced throughout the other two phases.

REVIEW QUESTIONS

1. Which drugs place the surgical client at risk for perioperative complications? Select all that apply.
   a. Acetaminophen (Tylenol)
   b. Acetylsalicylic acid (aspirin)
   c. Omeprazole (Prilosec)
   d. Diphenhydramine (Sominex)
   e. Ibuprofen (Motrin)
   f. Sertraline (Zoloft)

2. Preoperative client teaching regarding an upcoming outpatient surgery should include _____.
   a. postoperative nursing interventions
   b. risk for postoperative complications
   c. risks and benefits of the proposed surgical procedure
   d. risks and benefits of anesthesia choices

3. Which is the greatest risk factor for a client scheduled for general anesthesia?
   a. Expresses concern about the scheduled procedure
   b. Ate a pack of cookies within the last 2 hours
   c. Has a history of smoking and had the last cigarette 24 hours ago
   d. Has a history of hypertension that is controlled by diet and exercise

4. Which is a priority nursing intervention used to prevent infection in the perioperative client?

   a. Preparation of the skin overlying the surgical site
   b. Maintenance of hemodynamic status
   c. Maintenance of client's temperature
   d. Determination of estimated blood loss

5. During assessment of a client scheduled for a procedure to rule out cancer, the nurse observes tears in the client's eyes. Which response by the nurse is the most therapeutic intervention?
   a. Contact the surgeon to speak with the client.
   b. Ask the client to describe his or her feelings.
   c. Medicate the client with a preoperative analgesic.
   d. Reassure the client that there is nothing to worry about.

6. Which is the priority nursing intervention to be performed by the nurse for a client during the postoperative phase?
   a. Establish a patent airway.
   b. Maintain adequate blood pressure.
   c. Establish level of consciousness.
   d. Assess level of pain.

7. A postoperative client is experiencing impaired capillary refill to the lower extremities. The most appropriate nursing diagnosis is _____.
   a. *Ineffective breathing pattern*
   b. *Ineffective airway clearance*
   c. *Ineffective tissue perfusion*
   d. *Infection*

8. The postoperative phase begins when the client is transferred from the operating room and ends when
   _____ .
   a. the client's vital signs are stable
   b. the client is fully alert and responsive
   c. the client is discharged from the agency
   d. the client is discharged from the surgeon's care

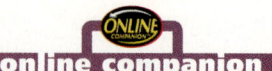
online companion

Visit the DeLaune and Ladner online companion resource at **www.delmar.cengage.com** for additional content and study aids. Click on Online Companions, then select the Nursing discipline.

GLOSSARY

A

abduction To move a body part away from the midline.

absorption Process by which the end products of digestion pass through the epithelial membranes in the small and large intestines into the blood or lymph system; passage of a drug from the site of administration into the bloodstream.

abstract Summary statement of a research article that identifies the purpose, methodology, findings, and conclusions.

accommodation Component of cognitive development that allows for readjustment of the cognitive structure (mind-set) in order to take in new information.

accountability Process that mandates that individuals are answerable for their actions and have an obligation (or duty) to act.

accreditation Process by which a voluntary, nongovernmental agency or organization appraises and grants accredited status to institutions and programs or services that meet predetermined structure, process, and outcome criteria.

acculturation Process that consists of learning norms, beliefs, and behavioral expectations of a group through which people of a subculture assume the characteristics of the dominant culture.

acid A molecule or an ion that can function as a hydrogen ion donor.

acid-base balance Regulation of hydrogen ion concentration.

acid-base buffer system A solution containing two or more chemical compounds that prevents marked changes in the hydrogen ion concentration when either an acid or a base is added to a solution.

acidosis A condition that occurs when there is an excessive number of hydrogen ions in a solution.

acquired immunity Formation of antibodies that protect the individual against invading agents such as lethal bacteria, viruses, toxins, and foreign tissues from other animals.

active euthanasia Process of taking deliberate action that will hasten the client's death.

active listening Listening that focuses on the feelings of the individual who is speaking.

active range of motion Range-of-motion exercises performed independently by the client.

actual nursing diagnosis Nursing diagnosis that indicates that a problem exists; composed of the diagnostic label, related factors, and signs and symptoms.

acupressure The use of finger pressure applied to specific points (energy pathways) on the body to promote healing.

acupuncture The use of needles inserted at specific points on the body (energy pathways) to promote healing.

acute illness Disruption (usually reversible) in functional ability characterized by a rapid onset, intense manifestations, and a relatively short duration.

acute pain Discomfort identified by sudden onset and relatively short duration, mild to severe intensity, and a steady decrease in intensity over several days or weeks.

adaptation Component of cognitive development that refers to the changes that occur as a result of assimilation and accommodation; ongoing process by which an individual adjusts to stressors in order to achieve homeostasis.

addiction Physiological and psychological dependence upon a substance.

adduction To move a body part toward the midline.

adjuvant medication Drugs used to enhance the analgesic efficacy of opioids, treat concurrent symptoms that exacerbate pain, and provide independent analgesia for specific types of pain.

administrative law Laws developed by groups that are appointed to governmental administrative agencies and entrusted with enforcing the statutory laws passed by the legislature.

adolescence Developmental stage from the ages of 12 to 20 years that begins with the appearance of the secondary sex characteristics (puberty).

advance care medical directive Document in which an individual, in consultation with the prescribing practitioner, relatives, or other personal advisers, provides precise instructions for the type of health care the client wants or does not want in a number of scenarios (e.g., end-of-life decisions).

advance directive Written instruction for health care that is recognized under state law and is related to the provision of such care when the individual is incapacitated.

advanced practice nursing Practice of nursing at a level requiring an expanded knowledge base and clinical expertise in a specialty area.

adventitious breath sounds Superimposed sounds on the normal vesicular, bronchovesicular, and bronchial breath sounds.

adverse reaction Any drug effect other than what is therapeutically intended.

aerobic metabolism Metabolism of nutrients in the presence of oxygen; a metabolic pathway that uses oxygen to convert glucose into cellular energy.

affect Mood or feeling.

affective domain Area of learning that involves attitudes, beliefs, and emotions.

afferent nerve pathway Ascending pathways that transmit sensory impulses to the brain.

afferent pain pathway Ascending the spinal cord.

ageism Imposition of age stereotypes and discrimination.

agent An entity that is capable of causing disease.

agglutination Clumping together of red blood cells.

agglutinin A specific kind of antibody whose interaction with antigens is manifested as agglutination.

agglutinogen Any antigenic substance that causes agglutination by the production of agglutinin.

aggregates Individuals, families, and other subgroupings of people who are associated because of similar social, personal, or health care needs; a defined group or population.

airborne transmission Occurs when a susceptible host contacts droplet nuclei or dust particles that are suspended in the air.

algor mortis Lack of skin elasticity as a result of death.

alkalosis Excessive removal of hydrogen ions from a solution.

Allen test Assessment procedure that measures the collateral circulation to the radial artery.

allodynia Pain caused by a stimulus that does not normally evoke pain.

allopathic That which is recognized by a specific culture as being traditional, conventional, or mainstream (e.g., Western medicine).

alternative therapies Treatment approaches that are not accepted by mainstream medical practice.

ambulation Assisted or unassisted walking.

amniocentesis Withdrawal of amniotic fluid to obtain a sample for specimen examination.

anabolism Constructive phase of metabolism.

anaerobic metabolism Metabolism of nutrients in the absence of oxygen; a metabolic pathway that converts glucose into energy in the absence of oxygen.

analysis Breaking the whole down into parts that can be examined.

analyte A substance dissolved in a solution; also called a solute.

anemia Reduction in the amount of hemoglobin in the blood, thus decreasing the oxygen-carrying capacity of the blood.

anesthesia Absence of pain.

aneurysm Weakness in the wall of a blood vessel.

angina Pain in the chest, neck, or arm resulting from myocardial ischemia.

angina pectoris Pain caused by tissue ischemia in the heart.

angiocatheter An intracatheter with a metal stylet.

angiogenesis The formation of new blood vessels.

angiography Visualization of the vascular structures through the use of fluoroscopy with a contrast medium.

anions Ions with a negative charge.

anorexia nervosa Self-imposed starvation that results in a 15% or more loss of body weight.

anthropogenic Reflecting changes in the relationship between humans and their environments.

anthropometric measurements Measurement of the size, weight, and proportions of the body.

antibody An immunoglobulin produced by the body in response to bacteria, viruses, or other antigenetic substances; counteracts and neutralizes the effects of antigens and destroys bacteria and other cells. Agglutinin is one type of antibody.

anticipatory grief Occurrence of grief work before an expected loss.

antigens A substance, usually a protein, that causes the formation of an antibody and reacts specifically with that antibody (e.g., agglutinogen).

antioxidants Substances that block or inhibit destructive oxidation reactions.

antiseptic hand rub Applying an antiseptic hand cleanser to the hands in order to reduce the number of microorganisms

antiseptic handwash "Washing hands with water and soap or other detergents containing an antiseptic agent" (CDC, 2002, p. 4).

anxiety Subjective response that occurs when a person experiences a threat to well-being; a diverse feeling of dread or apprehension.

aphasia Impairment or absence of language function.

apnea monitor Machine with chest leads that monitors the movement of the chest.

appetite Desire for specific foods instead of food in general (hunger); involves a psychological desire or craving.

aromatherapy Therapeutic use of concentrated essences or essential oils that have been extracted from plants and flowers.

arousal A component linked closely to the appearance of wakefulness and alertness.

arterial blood gases (ABGs) Measurement of levels of oxygen and carbon dioxide, as well as pH and bicarbonate ion, in arterial blood.

arthritis Inflammation of the joints that causes pain and swelling.

arthroplasty Total hip replacement.

artifact Specific type of nonverbal message that includes items in the client's environment, grooming, or use of clothing and jewelry.

ascites Accumulation of fluid in the abdomen.

asepsis Absence of microorganisms.

aseptic technique Infection control practice used to prevent the transmission of pathogens.

aspiration Procedure performed to withdraw fluid that has abnormally collected or to obtain a specimen.

assault Intentional and unlawful offer to touch a person in an offensive, insulting, or physically intimidating manner.

assessment First step in the nursing process; includes collection, verification, organization, interpretation, and documentation of data.

assessment model Framework that provides a systematic method for organizing data.

assimilation Component of cognitive development that involves taking in new experiences or information.

assisted suicide Situation in which a health care professional provides a client with the means to end his or her own life.

atelectasis Collapsed alveoli.

atherosclerosis Disease characterized by narrowing and eventual occlusion of the lumen (opening of the arteries) by deposits of lipids, fibrin, and calcium on the interior walls of the arteries.

atherosclerotic plaque A thick, hard deposit on the walls of the inner arteries that can clog the arteries in the heart and the brain.

atrophy Thinning of skin surface and loss of markings; thin, flabby muscles due to a reduction in muscle size and shape.

attending behaviors A set of nonverbal listening skills that conveys interest in what the other person is saying.

auditory channel Transmission of messages through spoken words and by cues.

auditory learner Style of learning in which an individual learns by hearing.

auscultation Physical examination technique that involves listening to sounds in the body that are created by movement of air or fluid.

auscultatory gap The temporary disappearance of sounds at the end of Korotkoff phase I and beginning of phase II.

autocratic leadership style Style of leadership in which the leader maintains strong control, makes the decisions, and solves all the problems.

autoimmune disorder A malfunction of the body's immune system that causes the body to attack its own tissues.

autonomy Being self-directed and taking initiative instead of waiting for direction from others; ethical principle that refers to the individual's right to choose for oneself and the ability to act on that choice.

autopsy Postmortem examination to determine the cause of death.

autoregulation Redistribution of blood flow to areas of greatest need.

awareness The capacity to perceive sensory impressions and react appropriately through thoughts and actions.

Ayurveda A healing system based on Hindu philosophy and Indian philosophy that embraces the concept of an energy force in the body that seeks to maintain balance or harmony.

B

bacteriuria Bacteria in the urine.

balance The body's ability to maintain postural equilibrium.

basal metabolic rate (BMR) Energy needed to maintain essential physiological functions when a person is at complete rest both physically and mentally.

base A molecule or an ion that will combine with hydrogen ions.

baseline values Establish the norm against which subsequent vital sign measurements can be compared.

base of support Foundation on which a person or object rests.

basic human need Need that must be met for survival.
battery Touching another person without consent.
behavior Observable response of an individual to external stimuli.
beneficence Ethical principle regarding the duty to promote good and prevent harm.
bereavement Period of grieving following the death of a loved one.
bioavailability Readiness to produce a drug effect.
bioethics Application of general ethical principles to health care.
biofeedback Measurement of physiological responses that yields information about the relationship between the mind and body and helps clients learn how to manipulate these responses through mental activity.
biological agent Living organisms that invade the host, such as bacteria, viruses, fungi, and protozoa.
biological clock Endogenous mechanism capable of measuring time in a living organism.
biopsy Excision of a small amount of tissue.
bisexuality Having an equal or almost equal preference for sexual partners of either gender.
black wound Contains necrotic tissue (eschar).
blanching Reduction of blood flow causing the skin to turn white when pressure is applied.
blood pressure Measurement of pressure pulsations exerted against the blood vessel walls during systole and diastole.
body alignment Position of body parts in relation to each other.
body image Individual's perception of physical self, including appearance, function, and ability.
body mass index (BMI) Determines whether a person's weight is appropriate for height by dividing the weight in kilograms by the height in meters squared.
body mechanics Purposeful and coordinated use of body parts and positions during activity.
bodymind Inseparable connection and operation of thoughts, feelings, and physiological functions.
bonding Formation of attachment between parent and child.
bradycardia A heart rate less than 60 beats per minute in an adult.
bradypnea Respiratory rate of 10 or fewer breaths per minute.
bronchial sounds Loud and high-pitched sounds with a hollow quality heard longer on expiration than inspiration from air moving through the trachea.
bronchovesicular sounds Medium-pitched and blowing sounds heard equally on inspiration and expiration from air moving through the large airways, posteriorly between the scapula and anteriorly over bronchioles lateral to the sternum at the first and second intercostal spaces.

bruits Blowing sounds that are heard when the blood flow becomes turbulent as it rushes past an obstruction.
bruxism Teeth grinding during sleep.
buccal Pertaining to the inside cheek.
bulimia Insatiable appetite.
bulimia nervosa An eating disorder characterized by episodic binge eating followed by purging.
burnout State of physical and emotional exhaustion that occurs when caregivers deplete their adaptive energy; characterized by fatigue, depersonalization, and decreased feelings of personal accomplishment.
butterfly needle Winged-tipped needle.

C

cachexia Weight loss marked by weakness and emaciation that usually occurs with a chronic illness such as tuberculosis or cancer.
calorie Quantity of heat required to raise the temperature of 1 g of water 1°C.
capitated rate Preset fees based on membership, not services provided; payment system used in managed care.
carbohydrate Organic compound composed of carbon, hydrogen, and oxygen.
cardiac catheterization Radiographic study with the use of a contrast medium injected into a vascular catheter that is threaded into the heart, coronary, or pulmonary vessels.
cardiac conduction system Specialized cells in the heart that generate and conduct electrical impulses; consists of the sinoatrial node, internodal pathways, atrioventricular node, bundle of His, right and left bundle branches, and Purkinje fibers.
cardiac cycle Series of electrical and mechanical events resulting in a cycle of atrial and ventricular contraction and relaxation.
cardiac output Measurement of blood pumped by the heart in 1 minute; measured by multiplying the heart rate by the ventricle's stroke volume.
cardiopulmonary resuscitation (CPR) Technique of applying respiration and chest compressions to support oxygenation in the event of cardiac and respiratory arrest.
case management Methodology for organizing client care through an episode of illnesses so that specific clinical and financial outcomes are achieved within an allotted time frame.
catabolism Destructive phase of metabolism.
categorical imperative Concept that states that one should act only if the action is based on a principle that is universal.
catharsis Process of talking out one's feelings; "getting things off the chest" through verbalization.
cations Ions with a positive charge.
cavities Dental caries.

ceiling effect As the dose of medication is increased above a certain level, the analgesic effect remains the same.

centering Process of bringing oneself to an inward focus of serenity that is done before beginning an energetic touch therapy treatment.

central line Venous catheter inserted into the superior vena cava through the subclavian, internal, or external jugular vein.

certification Process by which a nongovernmental agency or association certifies that an individual licensed to practice a profession has met predetermined standards specified by that profession for specialty practice.

chain of infection Phenomenon of developing an infectious process.

chakra A concentrated area of energy that influences the physical body, emotions, mental patterns, and spiritual awareness.

change Dynamic process in which an individual's response to a stressor leads to an alteration in behavior.

change agent Individual who intentionally creates and implements change.

channel Medium through which a message is transmitted.

charting by exception (CBE) Charting method that requires the nurse to document only deviations from preestablished norms.

chemical agent Substances that can interact with the body, such as pesticides, food additives, medications, and industrial chemicals.

chemical restraint Medications used to control the client's behavior.

chest physiotherapy (CPT) Technique of percussing or vibrating the chest wall in an effort to mobilize pulmonary secretions; usually accompanies postural drainage.

chiropractic Promotion of healing through manipulation of the spinal column.

cholesterol Lipid that is produced by the body and used in the synthesis of steroid hormones. Cholesterol is excreted in bile.

cholinesterase Enzyme manufactured in the liver that is responsible for the breakdown of acetylcholine and other choline esters.

chronemics Study of the effects of time on the communication process.

chronic acute pain Discomfort that occurs almost daily over a long period, has the potential for lasting months or years, and has a high probability of ending.

chronic illness Disruption in functional ability usually characterized by a gradual, insidious onset with lifelong changes that are usually irreversible.

chronic nonmalignant pain Discomfort that occurs almost daily and lasts for at least 6 months, with intensity ranging from mild to severe.

chronic obstructive pulmonary disease (COPD) Category of alterations in ventilation including emphysema, asthma, and chronic bronchitis.

chronic persistent pain Discomfort that is persistent, nearly constant, and long lasting (6 months or longer); or recurrent pain that produces significant negative changes in a person's life.

chronobiology A relatively new branch of science that studies rhythms that are controlled by our biological clocks.

chronological age Exact age of a person from birth.

chylomicrons Lipoproteins synthesized in the intestines that transport triglycerides to the liver.

circadian rhythms Biological rhythms that cycle on a daily basis.

civil law Law that deals with relations between individuals.

clean-contaminated wound Intentional wound created by entry into the alimentary, respiratory, genitourinary, or oropharyngeal tract under controlled conditions.

clean object Object considered to have the presence of some microorganisms that are usually not pathogenic.

cleansing Removal of soil or organic material from instruments and equipment used in providing client care.

clean wound Intentional wound created under conditions in which no inflammation was encountered, and the respiratory, alimentary, genitourinary, and oropharyngeal tracts were not entered.

client advocate Person who speaks up or acts on behalf of the client.

client behavior accident When the client's behavior or actions precipitate the incident, for example, poisonings, burns, and self-inflicted cuts and bruises.

closed question Interviewing technique that consists of questions that can be answered briefly with one-word responses.

closed suction drainage system Fluid-draining method that commonly has a reservoir capable of creating negative pressure or a vacuum.

cluster Set of data cues in which relationships between and among cues are established to identify a specific health state or condition.

cognition The intellectual ability to think.

cognitive domain Area of learning that involves intellectual understanding.

cognitive reframing Stress management technique in which the individual changes his or her own negative perception of a situation or event to a more positive, less threatening perspective.

cohesiveness Bonding of group members with one another.

colic Acute abdominal pain.

collaboration A partnership in which all parties are valued for their contribution.

collaborative problems Certain physiological complications that nurses monitor to detect onset of changes in status.

collagen The most abundant protein in the body and the material of tissue repair.

colloid Nondiffusible substances.

colonization Multiplication of microorganisms on or within a host that does not result in cellular injury.

communicable agent Infectious agents that are capable of being transmitted to a client by direct or indirect contact through a vehicle (or vector) or airborne route.

communicable disease Diseases produced by infectious agents.

communication Dynamic, continuous, and multidimensional process for sharing information as determined by standards or policies.

community Group of people united by some common element or shared interest.

community health nursing Nursing specialty that is divided into two sections: public health and home health care nursing.

comorbidity Existence of simultaneous disease processes within an individual.

competency Ability, qualities, and capacity to function in a particular way.

complementary therapies Treatment approaches that can be used in conjunction with conventional medical therapies.

complicated grief Associated with traumatic death such as death by homicide, suicide, or an accident.

comprehensive assessment Type of assessment that provides baseline client data, including a complete health history and current needs assessment.

compromised host Person whose normal defense mechanisms are impaired and who is therefore susceptible to infection.

computed tomography Radiological scanning of the body with x-ray beams and radiation detectors that transmit data to a computer that transcribes the data into quantitative measurement and multidimensional images of the internal structures.

computer literacy Familiarity with the use of personal computers, including the use of software tools.

concept Vehicle of thought.

conceptual framework Structure that links global concepts together to form a unified whole.

conceptualization Process of developing and refining abstract ideas.

conduction Loss of heat to an object in contact with the body.

consciousness State of awareness of self, others, and the surrounding environment.

conscious procedural sedation Minimally depressed level of consciousness during which the client retains the ability to maintain a continuously patent airway and to respond appropriately to physical stimulation or verbal commands.

constipation Infrequent and difficult passage of hard stool.

construct Abstraction or mental representation inferred from situations, events, or behaviors.

consultation Method of soliciting help from a specialist in order to resolve diagnoses.

contact transmission Direct physical transfer of an agent from an infected person to a host through direct contact with a contaminated object or close contact with contaminated secretions.

contaminated wound Open, traumatic wound or intentional wound in which there was a major break in aseptic technique, spillage from the gastrointestinal tract, or incision into infected urinary or biliary tracts.

continuous passive motion device (CPM) Device that increases range of motion and stimulates healing of the articular cartilage by decreasing swelling and the formation of adhesions.

continuous quality improvement Approach to quality management in which scientific, data-driven approaches are used to study work processes that lead to long-term system improvements.

contract law Enforcement of agreements among private individuals.

contracture A condition of fixed resistance to the passive stretch of a muscle.

contrast medium Radiopaque substance that facilitates roentgen imaging of the body's internal structures.

convalescent stage Period of time from the beginning of the disappearance of acute symptoms until the client returns to the previous state of health.

convection Movement of heat away from the body's surface.

costal (thoracic) breathing Occurs when the external intercostal muscles are used to move the chest upward and outward.

counterstimulation Techniques believed to activate the endogenous opioid and monoamine analgesia systems.

crackles Heard predominantly on inspiration over the base of the lungs as an interrupted fine crackle (dry, high-pitched crackling, popping sound of short duration) that sounds like a piece of hair being rolled between the fingers in front of the ear or a coarse crackle (moist, low-pitched crackling, gurgling sound of long duration) that sounds like water going down the drain after the plug has been pulled on a full tub of water.

crepitus Grating or crackling sensation caused by two rough surfaces rubbing together.

criminal law Acts or offenses against the welfare or safety of the public.

crisis Acute state of disorganization that occurs when the individual's usual coping mechanisms are no longer effective.

crisis intervention Specific technique used to assist clients in regaining equilibrium.

criteria Standards that are used to evaluate whether the behavior demonstrated indicates accomplishment of the goal.

critical pathway Abbreviated summary of key elements from the case management plan.

critical period Time of the most rapid growth or development in a particular stage of the life cycle in which an individual is most vulnerable to stressors of any type.

critical thinking Disciplined, deliberate method of thinking used to search for meaning; employs strategies such as asking questions, evaluating evidence, identifying assumptions, examining alternatives, and seeking to understand various points of view.

cross-functional team Interdepartmental, multidisciplinary group that is assigned to study an organization-wide process.

crystallized intelligence The application of life experiences and learned skills to solve problems.

crystalloid Electrolyte solution with the potential to form crystals.

cues Small amounts of data that are applied to the decision-making process.

Cullen's sign Bluish discoloration around the umbilicus in postoperative clients; can indicate intra-abdominal or perineal bleeding.

cultural assimilation Process by which individuals from a minority group are absorbed by the dominant culture and take on the characteristics of the dominant culture.

cultural competence Process through which the nurse provides care that is appropriate to the client's cultural context.

cultural diversity Individual differences among people that result from racial, ethnic, and cultural variables.

culture Dynamic and integrated structures of knowledge, beliefs, behaviors, ideas, attitudes, values, habits, customs, languages, symbols, rituals, ceremonies, and practices that are unique to a particular group of people; growing microorganisms to identify a pathogen.

customer Anyone who uses the products, services, or processes provided by an organization.

cutaneous pain Caused by stimulation of the cutaneous nerve endings in the skin and results in a well-localized "burning" or "prickling" sensation.

cyanosis Blue or gray discoloration of the skin resulting from reduced oxygen levels in the arterial blood.

cystocele Protrusion of the urinary bladder through the wall of the vagina.

cytomegalovirus (CMV) DNA virus that causes intranuclear and intracytoplasmic changes in infected cells.

D

data clustering Process of grouping significant cues together according to a specific assessment model to establish a nursing diagnosis.

data interpretation Recognition of patterns in data to determine nursing diagnoses.

data verification Process through which data are validated as being complete and accurate.

deadspace Condition in which lung tissue is well ventilated but poorly perfused.

deamination Removal of the amino groups from the amino acids.

debridement Removal of necrotic tissue to foster the regeneration of healthy tissue.

decision making The consideration and selection of interventions that facilitate the achievement of a desired outcome.

declarative knowledge Specific facts or information and an understanding of the nature of that knowledge.

defamation Act that occurs when information that damages an individual's reputation is communicated to a third party either in writing (libel) or verbally (slander).

defecation Evacuation of feces from the rectum.

defendant Person being sued in a lawsuit.

defense mechanisms Unconscious operations that protect the mind from anxiety.

defining characteristics Observable cues/inferences that cluster as manifestations of an actual or wellness diagnosis.

definition Clear description of diagnosis that differentiates it from other similar diagnoses.

deglutition Swallowing of food.

degrees Units that measure the heat of the body.

dehiscence Partial or complete separation of a wound's edges and the layers below the skin.

delegation Process of transferring a selected nursing task in a situation to an individual who is competent to perform that task.

democratic leadership style Style of leadership that is based on the belief that every group member should have input into the development of goals and problem solving; also called participative leadership.

deontology Ethical theory that considers the intrinsic moral significance of an act itself as the criterion for determination of good.

dependence Reliance on or need to take a drug.

dependent nursing intervention Nursing action that requires an order from a prescribing practitioner or other health care professional.

dependent variable Outcome variable of interest.

depersonalization Treating an individual as an object rather than as a person.

dermatome map Cutaneous area whose sensory receptors and axons feed into a single dorsal root of the spinal cord.

detrusor muscle Smooth muscle of the bladder wall.

development Behavioral changes in functional abilities and skills.

developmental tasks Certain goals that must be achieved during each developmental stage of the life cycle.

diabetes mellitus A disease in which the pancreas fails to secrete adequate levels of insulin to accommodate blood glucose levels.

diagnosis Science and art of identifying problems or conditions.

diagnostic label (concept) One or more nouns (may also include an adjective) that name the diagnosis; can be a word or a phrase that describes the pattern or related cues.

diaphragmatic (abdominal) breathing Occurs when the diaphragm contracts and relaxes, as observed by the movement of the abdomen.

diarrhea Passage of liquified stool (increased frequency and decreased consistency of stool sufficient to represent a change in bowel habits).

diastole Process of cardiac chamber filling.

dietary fiber The part of food that body enzymes cannot digest and absorb.

diffusion Movement of molecules in a solution or a gas from an area of high concentration to one of low concentration.

diffusion defect Decrease in efficiency of gas diffusion from the alveolar space into the pulmonary capillary blood.

digestion Mechanical and chemical processes that convert nutrients into a physically absorbable state.

digital subtraction angiography Computerized imaging of the vasculature with visualization on a monitor screen following the intravenous injection of iodine through a catheter.

dirty and infected wound Traumatic wound with retained dead tissue or intentional wound created in situations where purulent drainage was present.

dirty object Object considered to have a high number of microorganisms, with some that are potentially pathogenic.

disaccharide Double sugar.

disaster Any event (human-made or natural) that causes destruction that cannot be relieved without assistance.

discharge planning Planning that involves critical anticipation and planning for the client's needs after discharge; the client begins to resume self-care activities before leaving the health care environment.

discipline Field of study.

disinfectant Chemical solutions used to clean inanimate objects.

disinfection Elimination of pathogens, except spores, from inanimate objects.

disorientation A mentally confused state in which the person's awareness of time, place, self, and situation is impaired.

disseminated intravascular coagulation (DIC) An acquired hemorrhagic syndrome characterized by uncontrollable formation and deposition of thrombi.

dissolution Rate at which a drug becomes a solution.

distraction Focusing attention on stimuli other than pain.

distress Experienced when stressors evoke an ineffective response.

distribution Movement of drugs from the blood into various body fluids and tissues.

documentation Written evidence of the interactions between and among health care professionals, clients and their families, and health care organizations; the administration of tests, procedures, treatments, and client education; the result or client's response to these diagnostic tests and interventions.

dominant culture Group whose values prevail within a society.

Doppler Handheld transducer.

drug allergy Hypersensitivity to a drug.

drug incompatibility Undesired chemical or physical reaction between a drug and a solution, between two drugs, or between a drug and the container or tubing.

drug tolerance Reaction that occurs when the body becomes accustomed to a specific drug and requires larger doses of the drug to produce the desired therapeutic effect.

dullness A muffled thudlike sound that occurs over dense tissue.

durable power of attorney Document or legal status that enables any competent individual to name someone to exercise health-related decision-making authority, under specific circumstances, on the individual's behalf when the client is incapable of making decisions for himself or herself.

duration The time a drug remains in the system in a concentration great enough to have a therapeutic effect.

duty Obligation created either by law, contract, or any voluntary action.

dysfunctional grief Failure to progress through the stages of overwhelming emotions associated with grief or failure to demonstrate any behaviors commonly associated with grief.

dyspnea Difficulty in breathing as observed by labored or forced respirations through the use of accessory muscles in the chest and neck to breathe.

dysrhythmia Irregular heartbeat.

dysuria Painful urination.

E

echocardiogram Ultrasonic procedure used to reveal abnormal structure or motion of the heart wall and thrombi.

edema Detectable accumulation of increased interstitial fluid.

efferent nerve pathway Descending pathways that send sensory impulses from the brain.

efferent pain pathway Descending the spinal cord.

effleurage Massage technique consisting of long, smooth strokes used at the beginning and end of treatment and between other movements.

electrocardiogram Graphic recording of the heart's electrical activity.

electrochemical gradient Sum of all the diffusion forces acting on the membrane.

electroencephalogram Graphic recording of the brain's electrical activity.

electrolyte Element or compound that, when dissolved in water or another solvent, dissociates (separates) into ions (electrically charged particles) and provides for cellular reactions.

embryonic stage Developmental stage that occurs during the first 2–8 weeks after fertilization of a human egg.

empathy Understanding another person's perception of a situation.

empowerment Process of enabling others to do for themselves.

encoding Use of language and other specific signs and symbols for sending messages.

endorphins Group of opiate-like substances produced naturally by the brain; these substances raise the pain threshold, produce sedation and euphoria, and promote a sense of well-being.

endoscopy Visualization of a body organ or cavity through a scope.

energetic-touch therapies Techniques in which the hands are used to direct or redirect the flow of the body's energy fields to enhance balance within the fields.

enmeshment Overinvolvement or lack of separateness of family members; occurs as a result of unhealthy boundaries within the family unit.

enteral instillation Administration of drugs through a gastrointestinal tube.

enteral nutrition The nonvolitional delivery of nutrients through a gastrointestinal tube.

enzyme Protein produced in the body that catalyzes chemical reactions in organic matter.

epidemiology The study of the distribution and determinants of health-related states or events in populations.

epithelialization Growth of epithelial tissue.

e-prescribing The electronic transmission of drug prescriptions to a pharmacy from a hospital-based inpatient ordering system, personal digital assistants, wireless computers, or other handheld devices.

equipment accident Results from the malfunction or improper use of medical equipment, for example, electrocution and fire.

erythema Increased blood flow to an inflamed area.

erythrocytes Red blood cells.

eschar The scab or dry crust resulting from death of the skin.

essential amino acids Amino acids that are required for growth and development and must be obtained from food.

ethical dilemma Situation that occurs when there is a conflict between two or more ethical principles.

ethical principles Beliefs that govern actions.

ethical reasoning Process of thinking through what one ought to do in an orderly, systematic manner in order to provide justification of actions based on principles.

ethics Branch of philosophy concerned with determining right from wrong on the basis of a body of knowledge.

ethnicity Cultural group members' perception of themselves (group identity) and others' perception of them.

ethnocentrism Assumption of cultural superiority and an inability to accept other cultures' ways of organizing reality.

etiology Related cause of or contributor to a problem.

eupnea Easy respirations with a normal breath rate of breaths per minute that are age specific.

eustress Type of stress that results in positive outcomes.

euthanasia Intentional action or lack of action causing the merciful death of someone suffering from a terminal illness or incurable condition; derived from the Greek word *euthanatos,* which literally means "good or gentle death."

evaluation Fifth step in the nursing process; involves determining whether client goals have been met, partially met, or not met.

evaporation Continuous insensible heat loss from the skin and lungs when water is converted from a liquid to a gas.

evidence-based practice The application of the best available empirical evidence, including recent research findings, to clinical practice in order to aid clinical decision making.

evisceration Occurs when the client's viscera protrude through the disrupted wound.

exclusive provider organization Organization in which care must be delivered by the plan in order for clients to receive reimbursement for health care services.

excretion Elimination of drugs from the body.

existentialism Movement that is centered on individual existence in an incomprehensible world and the role that free will plays in it.

expected outcome Detailed, specific statement that describes the methods through which a goal will be achieved and includes aspects such as direct nursing care, client teaching, and continuity of care.

expert witness Person called by parties in a malpractice suit who is a member of the same profession as the party being sued and who is qualified to testify to the expected behaviors usually employed by members of the profession when in a similar situation.

expiration (exhalation) Movement of gases from the lungs to the atmosphere.

expressed contract Conditions and terms of a contract given in writing by the concerned parties.

extension To straighten a joint.

external respiration See *oxygen uptake.*

extinction Ability to discriminate the points of distance when two body parts are simultaneously touched.

extraurethral incontinence Uncontrolled loss of urine caused when the sphincter mechanism has been bypassed.

extubation Removal of an endotracheal tube.

exudate Material and cells discharged from blood vessels.

F

faith Belief in and relationship with a higher power.

false imprisonment Situation that occurs when clients are made to wrongfully believe they cannot leave a place.

family A dynamic system of people living together who are united by significant emotional bonds.

family functions Roles that allow family members to adapt in order to develop as individuals and as members of the family unit.

family roles Behaviors expected of family members.

family structure Form a family takes in adapting and maintaining itself as a dynamic system of people living together who are united by significant emotional bonds.

fat-soluble vitamins Vitamins that require the presence of fats for their absorption from the gastrointestinal tract and for cellular metabolism.

fatty acids Basic structural units of most lipids that contain carbon chains and hydrogen.

fecal incontinence Involuntary loss of stool of sufficient duration and volume to create a social or hygienic problem.

feedback Information the sender receives about the receiver's reaction to a message.

fee-for-service Health care recipient directly pays the provider for services as they are provided.

felony Crime of a serious nature usually punishable by imprisonment in a state penitentiary or by death.

fetal alcohol syndrome Condition in which fetal development is impaired by maternal consumption of alcohol.

fetal stage Intrauterine developmental period from 8 weeks to birth.

fidelity Ethical concept that means faithfulness and keeping promises.

fight-or-flight response State in which the body becomes physiologically ready to respond to a stressor by either fighting or running away from the danger (which may be actual or perceived).

fixation Inadequate mastery or failure to achieve a developmental task that inhibits healthy progression through subsequent stages.

flashback Rush of blood back into intravenous tubing when a negative pressure is created on the tubing.

flatulence Discharge of gas from the rectum.

flexion To bend a joint.

floras Microorganisms on the human body.

flow rate Volume of fluid to infuse over a set period of time.

fluency Ability to talk in a steady manner.

fluid intelligence Ability to acquire new concepts and adapt to unfamiliar situations; mental activities based on organizing information.

focus charting Documentation method using a columnar format to chart data, action, and response.

focused assessment Type of assessment that is limited in scope in order to focus on a particular need, health care problem, or potential health care risk.

formal contract Written contract that cannot be changed legally by an oral agreement.

fraud Wrong that results from a deliberate deception intended to produce unlawful gain.

free radicals Atoms or groups of atoms that can cause damage to cells.

free radical scavengers Substances that remove or destroy free radicals.

friction Force of two surfaces moving against one another; massage technique whereby the heels of the hands or the thumb pads are used to apply deep penetrating pressure on knotted muscles.

full disclosure Communication of complete information to potential research subjects regarding the nature of the study, the subject's right to refuse participation, and the likely risks and benefits that will be incurred.

full-thickness wound Skin loss that extends through the epidermis and dermis and into subcutaneous fat and deeper structures.

functional assessment Assessment of the client's ability to perform activities of daily living.

functional incontinence Loss of urine caused by altered mobility or dexterity, access to the toilet, or changes in mentation.

functional nursing Type of care delivery system in which nursing care is divided into tasks to be completed; various levels of personnel provide care depending on the complexity of the task.

functional team Departmental or unit-specific group whose scope is limited to departmental or work area processes.

G

gait or transfer belt Two-inch wide webbed belt worn by the client for the purpose of stabilization during transfers and ambulation.

gallop Extra heart sounds.

gate control pain theory Combines cognitive, sensory, and emotional components—in addition to the physiological aspects—and proposes that they can act on a gate control system to block the individual's perception of pain.

gender identity View of one's self as male or female in relationship to others.

general adaptation syndrome Physiological response that occurs when a person experiences a stressor.

general anesthesia Anesthesia that causes the client to lose all sensation and consciousness; used for major surgical procedures.

germicide Chemical that can be applied to both animate and inanimate objects to eliminate pathogens.

germinal stage Developmental stage that begins with conception and lasts approximately 10 to 14 days.

gingivitis Inflammation of the gums.

Glasgow Coma Scale International scale used in grading neurologic responses to determine the client's level of consciousness.

gluconeogenesis Conversion of amino acids into glucose or glycogen.

glycolysis Breakdown of glucose by enzymes located inside the cell's cytoplasm.

goal Aim, intent, or end.

goniometer Protractor with two movable arms used to measure the angle of a skeletal joint during range of motion.

Good Samaritan acts Laws that provide protection to health care providers by ensuring immunity from civil liability when the caregiver provides assistance at the scene of an emergency and does not intentionally or recklessly cause the client injury.

grand theory Theory composed of concepts representing global and complex phenomena.

graphesthesia Ability to identify numbers, letters, or shapes drawn on the skin.

grief Series of intense physical and psychological responses that occur following a loss.

grief work Phrase coined from Lindemann; it describes the process experienced by the bereaved. It consists of freedom from attachment to the deceased, becoming reoriented to the environment in which the deceased is no longer present, and establishing new relationships.

group communication A complex level of communication that occurs when three or more people meet in face-to-face encounters or through another communication medium, such as a conference call.

group dynamics Study of the events that take place during small-group interaction and the development of subgroups.

groupthink Going along with the majority opinion while personally having another viewpoint.

growth Quantitative (measurable) changes in the physical size of the body and its parts.

guided imagery A process in which the person uses all the senses to experience the sensation of relaxation.

H

half-life Time it takes the body to eliminate half of the blood concentration level of the original drug dose.

halitosis Bad breath.

hallucination A sensory perception that occurs in the absence of external stimuli and is not based on reality.

hand hygiene "A general term that applies to either handwashing, antiseptic handwash, antiseptic hand rub or surgical antiseptic handwash" (CDC. [2002]. *Guideline for hand hygiene in healthcare settings*. Retrieved November 10, 2005, from http://www.cdc.gov/handhygiene)

handwashing "Washing hands with plain (i.e., nonantimicrobial) soap and water" (CDC, 2002, p. 4).

healing Process of recovery from illness, accident, or disability.

healing touch Energy-based therapeutic modality that alters the energy fields through the use of touch, thereby affecting physical, mental, emotional, and spiritual health.

health Process through which the person seeks to maintain an equilibrium that promotes stability and comfort; includes physiological, psychological, sociocultural, intellectual, and spiritual well-being.

health care–associated infections Infections acquired in the hospital or other health care facilities that were not present or incubating at the time of admission.

health care delivery system Mechanism for providing services that meet the health-related needs of individuals.

health history Review of the client's functional health patterns prior to the current contact with a health care agency.

health maintenance organization Prepaid health plan that provides primary health care services for a preset fee and focuses on cost-effective treatment methods.

health-promoting behaviors Actions that increase well-being or quality of life.

health promotion Process undertaken to increase levels of wellness in individuals, families, and communities.

health-seeking behaviors Activities that are directed toward attaining and maintaining a state of well-being.

heart failure Inability of the heart to pump enough blood to meet the metabolic needs of the body; often accompanied by a backup of blood in the venous circuits (congestive heart failure).

heaves Lifting of the cardiac area secondary to an increased workload and force of left ventricular contraction.

Heimlich maneuver Application of sharp, upward thrusts to the abdomen in order to remove an airway obstruction.

hematoma Localized collection of blood underneath the tissues that may appear as a reddish-blue swelling or mass.

hematuria Blood in the urine; *microscopic hematuria* is the presence of blood noted on microscopic examination of the urine; *gross hematuria* is the presence of blood visible to the naked eye.

hemoconcentration Reduced volume of plasma water and the increased concentration of blood cells, plasma proteins, and protein-bound constituents; occurs with increased capillary hydrostatic pressure, which causes water to shift from the intravascular into the interstitial space.

hemodynamic regulation Physiological function of blood circulating to maintain an appropriate environment in tissue fluids.

hemoglobin electrophoresis A laboratory test that uses an electromagnetic field to identify various types of hemolytic anemia.

hemolysis A breakdown of red cells and the release of hemoglobin.

hemorrhage Persistent bleeding.

hemorrhagic exudate Has a large component of red blood cells due to capillary damage, which allows red blood cells to escape.

hemorrhoids Perianal varicosity of the hemorrhoidal veins.

hemostasis Cessation of bleeding that occurs by vasoconstriction of large blood vessels in the affected area.

heterosexuality Sexual activity between a man and a woman.

high-biological-value proteins (complete proteins) Proteins that contain all of the essential amino acids.

high-level wellness State in which individuals function at their maximum health potential while remaining in balance with the environment.

history Study of the past, including events, situations, and individuals.

homeostasis Equilibrium (balance) between physiological, psychological, sociocultural, intellectual, and spiritual needs.

homosexuality Sexual activity between two members of the same sex.

hope Factor that enables one to cope with distressing events.

hospice Type of care for the terminally ill founded on the concept of allowing individuals to die with dignity and surrounded by those who love them.

hospital-acquired condition Also called a "never event" because it is an event that should never happen in a hospital, such as a pressure ulcer or fall.

humoral immunity Stimulation of B cells and antibody production.

hydrostatic pressure Pressure that a liquid exerts on the sides of the container that holds it; also called filtration force.

hygiene The science of health.

hyperalgesia Extreme sensitivity to pain.

hypercalcemia Excess in the extracellular level of calcium.

hypercapnia Elevation of carbon dioxide levels in the blood indicating inadequate alveolar ventilation.

hyperchloremia Excess in the extracellular level of chloride.

hyperglycemia Condition characterized by a blood glucose level greater than 110 mg/dL.

hyperkalemia Excess in the extracellular level of potassium.

hypermagnesemia Excess in the extracellular level of magnesium.

hypernatremia Excess in the extracellular level of sodium.

hyperphosphatemia Excess in the extracellular level of phosphorus.

hypersomnia An alteration in sleep pattern characterized by excessive sleep, especially in the daytime.

hypertension Refers to a persistent systolic pressure greater than 135 to 140 mm Hg and a diastolic pressure greater than 90 mm Hg.

hyperthyroidism Increased secretion of thyroid hormones, which increases the rate of metabolism.

hypertonic Solution with more solutes in proportion to the volume of body water; also called a hyperosmolar solution.

hypertonicity Increased muscle tone.

hypertrophy Increase in muscle size and shape due to an increase in muscle fiber.

hyperventilation Characterized by deep, rapid ventilations.

hypervolemia Increased circulating fluid volume.

hypocalcemia Deficit in the extracellular level of calcium.

hypochloremia Deficit in the extracellular level of chloride.

hypoglycemia Condition characterized by a blood glucose level less than 80 mg/dL.

hypokalemia Deficit in the extracellular level of potassium.

hypomagnesemia Deficit in the extracellular level of magnesium.

hyponatremia Deficit in the extracellular level of sodium.

hypophosphatemia Deficit in the extracellular level of phosphorus.

hypotension A systolic blood pressure less than 90 mm Hg or 20 to 30 mm Hg below the client's normal blood pressure.

hypothesis Statement of an asserted relationship between dependent variables.

hypothyroidism Decreased secretion of thyroid hormones, which decreases the metabolic rate.

hypotonic Solution with less solute in proportion to the volume of water; also called a hypo-osmolar solution.

hypotonicity Flabby muscle with poor tone.

hypoventilation Characterized by shallow respirations.

hypoxemia Decreased oxygen level in the blood.

hypoxia Oxygen deprivation of the body's cells.

I

identity What sets one person apart as a unique individual; may include a person's name, gender, ethnic identity, family status, occupation, and various roles.

idiosyncratic reaction Reaction of overresponse, underresponse, or an atypical response.

illness Inability of an individual's adaptive responses to maintain physical and emotional balance that subsequently results in an impairment in functional abilities.

illness stage When the client is manifesting specific symptoms of an infectious process.

illusion An inaccurate perception or misinterpretation of sensory stimuli.

imagery Relaxation technique in which the individual uses the imagination to visualize a pleasant, soothing image.

immediate memory The retention of information for a specified and usually short period of time.

impaction Hard bolus of stool that obstructs the fecal stream.

impaired nurse Nurse who is habitually intemperate or is addicted to the use of alcohol or habit-forming drugs.

implantable port Device with a radiopaque silicone catheter and a plastic or stainless steel injection port with a self-sealing silicone-rubber septum.

implementation Fourth step in the nursing process; involves the execution of the nursing plan of care formulated during the planning phase of the nursing process.

implied contract Contract that recognizes a relationship between parties for services.

incentive spirometers Breathing devices that measure the client's ventilatory volumes.

incidence Refers to the prevalence of a disease in a population or community. The predictive value of the same test can be different when applied to people of differing ages, genders, and geographic locations.

incident report Documentation of an unusual occurrence or an accident in delivery of client care.

incontinence Loss of the ability to initiate, control, or inhibit elimination.

independent nursing intervention Nursing action initiated by the nurse that does not require direction or an order from another health care professional.

independent variable Variable that is believed to cause or influence the dependent variable.

infancy Developmental stage from the first month to the first year of life.

infarction Death (necrosis) of an area of tissue caused by oxygen deprivation.

infection Invasion and a multiplication of microorganisms in body tissue that result in cellular injury.

infectious agent Microorganism that causes infections.

infiltration Seepage of foreign substances into the interstitial tissue.

inflammation Nonspecific cellular response to tissue injury or infection.

informatics The science of turning data into information.

information technology The management and processing of information with the assistance of computers.

informed consent Client understands the reason for the proposed intervention, knows its benefits and risks, and agrees to the treatment by signing a consent form.

initial planning Development of the beginning of care by the nurse who performs the admission assessment and gathers the comprehensive admission assessment data.

insensible heat loss Heat that is lost through the continuous, unnoticed water loss that occurs with evaporation.

insomnia Refers to the chronic inability to sleep or inadequate quality of sleep due to sleep that prematurely ends or is interrupted by periods of wakefulness.

inspection Physical examination technique that involves careful visual observation.

inspiration (inhalation) Intake of air into the lungs.

instability incontinence Loss of urine caused by a premature or hyperactive contraction of the detrusor.

insulin Pancreatic hormone that aids in the diffusion of glucose into the liver and muscle cells and the synthesis of glycogen.

integrative therapy A clinical approach that combines Western technological medicine with techniques from Eastern medicine.

integumentary system Skin, hair, scalp, and nails.

intentional wound Occurs during treatment or therapy, usually under aseptic conditions, such as surgical incisions and venipunctures.

interdependent nursing intervention Actions that are implemented in a collaborative manner by the nurse with other health care professionals.

intermittent claudication Ischemia to the extremities usually brought on by activity and relieved by rest.

internal respiration Process of gas exchange between capillary blood and the body's cells, in which the cells receive oxygen and carbon dioxide is removed.

interpersonal communication Process that occurs between two people either in face-to-face encounters, over the telephone, or through other communication media.

interview Therapeutic interaction that has a specific purpose.

intracath Plastic tube for insertion into a vein.

intradermal (ID) Injection into the dermis.

intramuscular (IM) Injection into the muscle.

intraoperative (during surgery) Phase that begins when the client is transferred to the operating room and ends when the client is transferred to a postanesthesia care unit.

intrapersonal communication Messages one sends to oneself, including "self-talk," or communication with oneself.

intrapsychic theory Theory that focuses on an individual's unconscious processes. Feelings, needs, conflicts, and drives are considered to be motivators of behavior.

intravenous (IV) Injection into a vein.

intravenous (IV) therapy Administration of nutrients, fluids, electrolytes, or medications by the venous route.

intubation Insertion of an endotracheal tube into the bronchus through the nose or mouth to ensure an airway.

invasive Accessing the body tissues, organs, or cavities through some type of instrumentation procedure.

ischemia Oxygen deprivation, usually caused by poor perfusion, that is usually temporary and localized.

ischemic pain Pain occurring when the blood supply of an area is restricted or cut off completely.

isotonic Solution with body water and solutes (sodium) in equal amounts; also called an isosmolar solution.

J

judgment The ability to compare or evaluate alternatives to life situations and arrive at an appropriate course of action.

jurisprudence Body of judge-made law.

justice Ethical principle based on the concept of fairness that is extended to each individual.

K

Kardex Summary worksheet reference of basic client care information.

ketogenesis Conversion of amino acids into keto acids or fatty acids.

ketones Products of incomplete fat metabolism.

kilocalorie Equivalent to 1000 calories.

kinesthetic channel Transmission of messages through sensation of touch.

kinesthetic learner Learning style in which a person processes information by experiencing the information or by touching and feeling.

kyphosis Abnormally increased convexity in the curvature of the spine.

L

laissez-faire leadership style Style of leadership in which the leader assumes a passive, nondirective, and inactive style.

lancinating Piercing or stabbing pain.

late potentials Electrical activity that occurs after normal depolarization of the ventricles.

laws Rules or regulations that are enacted by legal entities.

leadership Interpersonal process that involves motivating and guiding others to achieve goals.

learning Process of assimilating information, with a resultant change in behavior.

learning plateau Peak in effectiveness of teaching and depth of learning.

learning style Way in which an individual incorporates new information.

legal regulation Process by which the state attests to the public that the individual licensed to practice is competent to do so.

lentigo senilis Benign brown-pigmented areas on the face, hands, and arms of older people.

leukocytes White blood cells.

liability Obligation one has incurred or might incur through any act or failure to act.

licensure Method by which a state holds the nurse accountable for safe practice to citizens of that state.

licensure by endorsement Process by which an individual who is duly licensed as a registered nurse under the laws of one state or country has his or her credentials accepted and approved by another state or country.

licensure by examination Process by which an individual who has completed an approved program of studies leading to registered nurse licensure seeks initial licensure by successfully passing a standardized competency examination.

line of gravity Vertical line passing through the center of gravity.

lipids Organic compounds that are insoluble in water but soluble in organic solvents such as ether and alcohol; also known as fats.

lipoproteins Blood lipids bound to protein.

liver mortis Bluish purple discoloration that is a by-product of red blood cell destruction.

living will Document prepared by a competent adult that provides direction regarding medical care should the person become incapacitated or otherwise unable to make decisions personally.

local adaptation syndrome Physiological response to a stressor (e.g., trauma, illness) affecting a specific part of the body.

local anesthesia Anesthesia that causes the client to lose sensation to a localized body part (e.g., spraying the back of the throat with lidocaine decreases the gag reflex).

localized infection Limited to a defined area or single organ with symptoms that resemble inflammation (redness, tenderness, and swelling).

lock-out interval Minimum time allowed between doses for the client to self-medicate; feature found in infusion pumps used for patient-controlled analgesia.

locus of control A person's perception of the source of control over events and situations affecting the person's life.

logrolling Technique for moving a client whose cervical spine must stay in alignment with the entire vertebral column.

long-term goal Statement written in objective format demonstrating an expectation to be achieved in resolution of the nursing diagnosis over a long period of time, usually over weeks or months.

lordosis Abnormal forward curvature of the lumbar spine.

loss Any situation in which a valued object is changed or is no longer accessible to an individual.

low-biological-value proteins (incomplete proteins) Proteins lacking in one or more of the essential amino acids.

lumbar puncture Aspiration of cerebrospinal fluid from the subarachnoid space.

lymphokine A substance of low molecular weight that is not an antibody, is secreted by T cells in response to stimulation by antigens, and has a role in cell-mediated immunity.

M

magnetic resonance imaging An imaging technique that uses radio waves and a strong magnetic field to make continuous cross-sectional images of the body.

maladaptation Process of ineffective coping with stressors.

malignant hyperthermia (MH) A potentially lethal syndrome caused by a hypermetabolic state that is precipitated by the administration of certain anesthetic agents.

malnutrition Nutritional alterations related to inadequate intake, disorders of digestion or absorption, or overeating.

malpractice Professional person's wrongful conduct, improper discharge of professional duties, or failure to meet the standards of acceptable care that results in harm to another person.

mammography A low-dose radiographic study of the breast tissue.

managed care System of providing and monitoring care in which access, cost, and quality are controlled before or during delivery of services. These networks "manage" or control costs in many ways (e.g., by limiting referrals to costly specialists). HMOs are a common form of managed care.

management Accomplishment of tasks either by oneself or by directing others.

mandatory licensure laws Legislation that prohibits any individual from practicing as a registered nurse without a current license.

mastication Chewing into fine particles and then mixing the food with enzymes in saliva.

material principle of justice Rationale for determining when there can be unequal allocation of scarce resources.

maturation Process of becoming fully grown and developed; involves physiological and behavioral aspects.

maturational loss Adolescent who loses the younger child's freedom from responsibility.

medical asepsis Practices to reduce the number, growth, and spread of microorganisms.

medical diagnosis Clinical judgment by the prescribing practitioner that identifies or determines a specific disease, condition, or pathologic state.

meditation Quieting the mind by focusing one's attention.

menarche Onset of the first menstrual period.

message Stimulus produced by a sender and responded to by a receiver.

metabolic rate Rate of heat liberated during chemical reactions.

metabolism Aggregate of all chemical reactions in every body cell.

metacommunication Relationship aspect of communication that refers to the message about the message.

metaparadigm Unifying force in a discipline that names the phenomena of concern to that discipline.

micro-range theory Theory that explains a specific phenomenon of concern to a discipline.

middle adulthood Developmental stage from the ages of 40 to 65 years.

middle-range theory Theory that addresses more concrete and more narrowly defined phenomena than a grand theory but does not cover the full range of phenomena of concern to a discipline.

mid-upper-arm circumference (MAC) Measures skeletal muscle mass and serves as an indicator of protein reserve.

mindfulness Form of meditation in which one focuses only on the present moment.

minerals Inorganic elements.

minority group Group of people who constitute less than a numerical majority of the population and who, because of their cultural or physical characteristics, are labeled and treated differently than others in the society.

misdemeanor Offense less serious than a felony that may be punished by a fine or sentence to a local prison for less than 1 year.

mixed agonist-antagonist Compound that blocks opioid effects on one receptor type while producing opioid effects on a second receptor type.

mobility Ability to engage in activity and free movement.

mode of transmission Process that bridges the gap between the portal of exit of the biological agent from the reservoir or source and the portal of entry of the susceptible "new" host.

modular nursing Care delivery system in which caregivers are assigned to a small segment of clients in close geographical proximity.

modulation The changing of pain impulses.

monosaccharides Simple sugars.

monounsaturated fatty acids Fatty acids with one double or triple bond.

morality Behavior in accordance with custom or tradition that usually reflects personal or religious beliefs.

moral maturity Ability to decide for oneself what is "right."

mourning Period of time during which grief is expressed and resolution and integration of the loss occur.

multidimensionality Acting based on the belief that we live at many realms of the universe all at once.

murmur Swishing or blowing sounds of long duration heard during the systolic and diastolic phases created by turbulent blood flow through a valve.

muscle tone Normal state of balanced tension present in the body that allows muscles to respond quickly to stimuli.

music-thanatology Holistic and palliative method for use of music with dying clients; solely concerned with dissipating any obstacle to a peaceful passage.

myocardial infarction Necrosis of the heart muscle.

myofascial pain syndromes A group of muscle disorders characterized by pain, muscle spasm, tenderness, stiffness, and limited motion.

myoneural junction Point at which nerve endings come in contact with muscle cells.

N

narcolepsy A sleep alteration that manifests as sudden uncontrollable urges to fall asleep during the daytime.

narrative charting A story format of documentation that describes the client's status, interventions and treatments, and the response to treatments.

necrosis Tissue death as the result of disease or injury.

need Anything that is absolutely essential for existence.

negative nitrogen balance Condition that exists when nitrogen output exceeds intake and protein catabolism exceeds anabolism.

negligence Failure of an individual to provide the care in a situation that a reasonable person would ordinarily provide in a similar circumstance.

neonatal period First 28 days of life following birth.

networking Process of building connections with others.

neuralgia Paroxysmal pain that extends along the course of one or more nerves.

neurogenic fever Long-term elevation of body temperature thought to result from a disruption of the normal body temperature set point as a result of damage to the hypothalamus.

neuropathic pain Arises from damage to portions of the peripheral or central nervous system.

neuropeptides Amino acids produced in the brain and other sites in the body that act as chemical communicators.

neurotransmitters Chemical substances produced by the body that facilitate nerve impulse transmission.

nitrogen balance Net result of intake and loss of nitrogen that measures protein anabolism and catabolism.

nociception The process by which an individual becomes consciously aware of pain.

nociceptors Receptive neurons for painful sensations that, together with the axons of neurons, convey information to the spinal cord where reflexes are activated.

nocturia Awakening from sleep to urinate.

nonessential amino acids Amino acids that can be synthesized in the adult body.

noninvasive The body is not entered with any type of instrument.

nonmaleficence Ethical principle that means the duty to cause no harm to others.

nonverbal message Message communicated without words.

nurse Stems from the Latin word *nutrix,* or *nutrio,* which means to nourish.

nurse-client relationship One-to-one interactive process between client and nurse that is directed at improving the client's health status or assisting in problem solving.

nurse practice act Law determined by each state governing the practice of nursing.

nursing audit Process of collecting and analyzing data to evaluate the effectiveness of nursing interventions.

nursing diagnosis Second step in the nursing process and includes clinical judgments made about wellness states, illness states and syndromes, and the readiness to enhance current states of wellness experienced by individuals, families, and aggregate populations (communities).

nursing informatics The use of information and computer technology to support all aspects of nursing practice.

nursing intervention Action performed by a nurse that helps the client achieve the results specified by the goals and expected outcomes.

Nursing Interventions Classification (NIC) Standardized language for nursing interventions.

Nursing Minimum Data Set (NMDS) Elements contained in clinical records and abstracted for studies on the effectiveness and costs of nursing care.

nursing order Statement written by the nurse that is within the scope of nursing practice to plan and initiate.

Nursing Outcomes Classification (NOC) Classification system of nurse-sensitive outcomes.

nursing process Systematic method of providing care to clients; consists of five steps: assessment, diagnosis, outcome identification and planning, implementation, and evaluation.

nursing research Systematic application of formalized methods for generating valid and dependable information about the phenomena of concern to the discipline of nursing.

nutraceuticals Natural substances found in plant or animal foods that act as protective or healing agents.

nutrition Process by which the body metabolizes and utilizes nutrients.

nystagmus Involuntary rhythmical oscillation of eyes.

O

obesity Weight that is 20% or more above the ideal body weight.

objective data Observable and measurable data that are obtained through both standard assessment techniques performed during the physical examination and laboratory and diagnostic tests.

obligatory loss of proteins Degradation of the body's own proteins into amino acids in response to inadequate protein intake.

observation Skill of watching carefully and attentively.

obstructive pulmonary disease Category of lung diseases characterized by obstruction of the airways and trapping of air distal to the obstruction.

occult Blood in the stool that can be detected only through a microscope or by chemical means.

older adulthood Developmental stage occurring from the age of 65 and beyond.

ongoing assessment Type of assessment that includes systematic monitoring and observation related to specific problems.

ongoing planning Planning that entails continuous updating of the client's plan of care.

onset of action Time it takes the body to respond to a drug after administration.

open-ended questions Interview technique that encourages the client to elaborate about a particular concern or problem.

operative knowledge An understanding of the nature of knowledge (knowing the "how" or "why").

opposition One body part being across from another part at nearly 180°.

oppression Condition in which the rules, modes, and ideals of one group are imposed on another group.

organization Means by which members of a profession join together to promote and protect the profession as a valuable service to society.

organizational culture Commonly held beliefs, values, norms, and expectations that drive the workforce.

orientation Perception of self in relation to the surrounding environment.

orientation phase First stage of the therapeutic relationship, in which the nurse and client become acquainted, establish trust, and determine the expectations of each other.

orthostatic hypotension (postural hypotension) Refers to a sudden drop of 25 mm Hg in systolic pressure and 10 mm Hg in diastolic pressure when the client moves from a lying to a sitting or a sitting to a standing position.

osmolality Measurement of the total concentration of dissolved particles (solutes) per kilogram of water.

osmolarity Concentration of solutes per liter of cellular fluid.

osmole Unit of measure of osmotic pressure.

osmosis Process caused by a concentration difference of water.

osmotic pressure Force that develops when two solutions of different strengths are separated by a selectively permeable membrane.

osteoarthritis Most common type of degenerative arthritis, in which the joints become stiff and tender to touch.

osteoporosis Process in which reabsorption exceeds accretion of bone.

outcome evaluation Process of comparing the client's current status with the expected outcomes.

oximeter Machine that measures the oxygen saturation of the blood through a probe clipped to the fingernail or earlobe.

oxygen uptake Process of oxygen diffusing from the alveolar space into the pulmonary capillary blood; also called external respiration.

oxyhemoglobin dissociation curve Graphic representation of the relationship between partial pressure of oxygen and oxygen saturation.

P

pain A universal human experience defined as "a state in which an individual experiences and reports the presence of severe discomfort or an uncomfortable sensation" (Carpenito, 2003, p. 58).

pain threshold The level of intensity at which pain becomes appreciable or perceptible; varies with each individual and type of pain.

pain tolerance The level of intensity or duration of pain the client is willing or able to endure.

palliative care Control of the symptoms rather than cure.

palpation Physical examination technique that uses the sense of touch to assess texture, temperature, moisture, organ location and size, vibrations and pulsations, swelling, masses, and tenderness.

Papanicolaou test Smear method of examining stained exfoliative cells.

paracentesis Aspiration of fluid from the abdominal cavity.

paradigm Pattern, model, or mind-set that strongly influences one's decisions and behaviors.

paradigm revolution Turmoil experienced by a discipline when a competing paradigm gains acceptance over the dominant, prevailing paradigm.

paradigm shift Acceptance of a competing paradigm over the prevailing paradigm.

parasomnia Refers to sleep alterations resulting from "an activation of physiological systems at inappropriate times during the sleep-wake cycle" (American Psychiatric Association, 1994, p. 579).

paraverbal communication The way in which a person speaks, including voice tone, pitch, and inflection.

paraverbal cues Verbal messages accompanied by cues, such as tone and pitch of voice, speed, inflection, volume, and other nonlanguage vocalizations.

parenteral Introducing a medication into the system by any route other than the oral-gastrointestinal tract.

parenteral nutrition Nutrients bypass the small intestine and enter the blood directly.

paresthesia Abnormal sensation such as burning, prickling, or tingling.

paroxysmal nocturnal dyspnea Episode of sudden shortness of breath occurring during sleep.

partial-thickness wound Involves the epidermis and upper dermis, the layer of skin beneath the epidermis.

passive euthanasia Process of cooperating with the client's dying process.

passive range of motion Range-of-motion exercises performed by the nurse for the dependent client.

patency Openness of tube lock or bodily passageway.

paternalism Practice by which health care providers decide what is "best" for clients and then attempt to coerce clients to act against their own choices.

pathogen Microorganisms that cause diseases in humans.

pathogenicity Ability of a microorganism to produce disease.

patient-controlled analgesia (PCA) Device that allows the client to control the delivery of intravenous or subcutaneous pain medication in a safe, effective manner through a programmable pump.

peak plasma level Achievement of the highest blood concentration of a single drug dose until the elimination rate equals the rate of absorption.

peer evaluation Process by which professionals provide critical performance appraisal and feedback that is geared toward corrective action.

Penrose drain Functions by gravity and has an open end that drains onto dressings.

perception Person's sense and understanding of the world; conscious awareness of pain.

percussion Physical examination technique that uses short, tapping strokes on the surface of the skin to create vibrations of underlying organs.

performance improvement Activities and behaviors that each individual does to meet customers' expectations.

perineal care Cleansing of the external genitalia, perineum, and surrounding area.

perioperative Refers to the management and treatment of the surgical client during the three phases of surgery: preoperative, intraoperative, and postoperative.

peristalsis Coordinated, rhythmic, serial contraction of the smooth muscles of the gastrointestinal tract.

permeability Capability of a substance, molecule, or ion to diffuse through a membrane.

petrissage Massage technique using squeezing, kneading, and rolling movements to release muscle tension and stimulate circulation.

phagocytosis Process by which certain cells engulf and dispose of foreign bodies.

phantom limb pain Neuropathic pain in which pain sensations are referred to an area from which an extremity has been amputated.

pharmacognosy The study of the biochemical aspects of natural products.

pharmacokinetics Study of the absorption, distribution, metabolism, and excretion of drugs.

phenomenon Observable fact or event that can be perceived through the senses and is susceptible to description and explanation.

philosophy Statement of beliefs that is the foundation for one's thoughts and actions.

phlebitis Inflammation of a vein.

phlebotomist Individual who performs venipuncture.

phospholipids Composed of one or more fatty acid molecules and one phosphoric acid radical and usually contain a nitrogenous base.

physical agents Factors in the environment that are capable of causing disease, such as heat, light, noise, radiation, and machinery.

physical dependence Reaction of the body, commonly known as withdrawal syndrome, to abrupt discontinuation of an opioid after repeated use.

physical restraints Reduce the client's movement through the application of a device.

phytonutrients Chemicals found in plants.

PIE charting Documentation method using problem, intervention, evaluation (PIE) format.

piggybacked Addition of an intravenous solution to infuse concurrently with another infusion.

piloerection Hairs standing on end as a result of the body's decrease in body temperature.

plaintiff Party who initiates a lawsuit that seeks damages or other relief.

planning Third step of the nursing process; includes the formulation of guidelines that establish the proposed course of nursing action in the resolution of nursing diagnoses and the development of the client's plan of care.

plan of care Written guide that organizes data about a client's care into a formal statement of the strategies that will be implemented to help the client achieve optimal health.

plateau Level at which a drug's blood concentration is maintained.

pleura Lining of the chest cavity.

pleural friction rub Heard on either inspiration or expiration over the anterior lateral lungs as a continuous creaking, grating sound.

pneumatic compression device Device that provides intermittent compression cycles to the veins of the extremities to promote circulation.

pneumothorax Collection of air or gas in the pleural space, causing the lungs to collapse.

point-of-care charting Documentation system that allows health care providers to gain immediate access to client information at the bedside.

poison Any substance that causes an alteration in the client's health, such as injury or death, when inhaled, injected, ingested, or absorbed by the body.

politics Way in which people try to influence decision making, especially decisions about the use of resources.

polyp A small, abnormal growth of tissue.

polypharmacy Concurrent use of several different medications.

polysaccharide Complex sugar.

polyunsaturated fatty acids Fatty acids that have many carbons unbonded to hydrogen atoms.

Port-a-Cath A port that has been implanted under the skin with a catheter inserted into the superior vena cava or right atrium through the subclavian or internal jugular vein.

positive nitrogen balance Condition that exists when nitrogen intake exceeds output and protein anabolism exceeds catabolism.

possible nursing diagnosis Nursing diagnosis that indicates a situation exists in which a problem could arise unless preventive action is taken or a "hunch" or intuition by the nurse that cannot be confirmed or eliminated until more data have been collected. It is composed of the diagnostic label and related factors.

postoperative (after surgery) Begins when the client leaves the operating room and is taken to a postanesthesia care unit; this phase continues until the client is discharged from the care of the surgeon.

postural drainage A technique of positioning that promotes gravitational drainage of specific lung lobes.

power Ability to do or act, resulting in the achievement of desired results.

preadolescence Developmental stage from the ages of approximately 10 to 12 years.

prealbumin Precursor of albumin.

precapillary sphincters Smooth muscles surrounding the smallest arterioles that control blood flow through the capillary beds.

predictive value The ability of screening test results to correctly identify the disease state, such as a true positive correctly identifies persons who actually have the disease, whereas a true negative correctly identifies persons who do not actually have the disease (Fischbach, 2000).

preferred provider organization Type of managed care model in which member choice is limited to providers within the system.

prenatal period Developmental stage beginning with conception and ending with birth.

preoperative (before surgery) Refers to the time interval that begins when the decision is made for surgery until the client is transferred to the operating room.

presbycusis Hearing loss associated with old age.

preschool stage Developmental stage from the ages of 3 to 6 years.

presence The process of just being with another; a therapeutic nursing intervention.

pressure ulcer Impaired skin integrity related to mechanical factors such as unrelieved, prolonged pressure; shearing forces; and restraint.

primary care provider Health care provider whom a client sees first for health care; typically, a family practitioner (prescribing practitioner/nurse), internist, or pediatrician.

primary health care Client's point of entry into the health care system; includes assessment, diagnosis, treatment, coordination of care, education, preventive services, and surveillance.

primary intention healing Occurs in wounds that have minimal tissue loss and edges that are well approximated (closed).

primary nursing Nursing management system in which the professional nurse assumes complete responsibility for total care for a small number of clients.

primary source Major provider of information about a client; research article written by one or more researchers.

prn orders Drug orders that are administered as needed.

proactive Initiating change rather than responding to change imposed by others.

problem-oriented medical record (POMR) Documentation focused on the client's problem with a structured, logical format to narrative charting called SOAP (subjective and objective data, assessment, plan).

process Series of steps or acts that lead to accomplishment of a goal or purpose.

process evaluation Measurement of nursing actions by examination of each phase of the nursing process.

process improvement Process that examines the flow of client care between departments in order to ensure that the processes work as they were designed and that acceptable levels of performance are achieved.

prodromal stage Time interval from the onset of nonspecific symptoms until specific symptoms of the infectious process begin to manifest.

profession Group (vocational or occupational) that requires specialized education and intellectual knowledge.

professional regulation Process by which nursing ensures that its members act in the public interest by providing a unique service that society has entrusted to them.

professional standards Authoritative statements developed by the profession by which quality of practice, service, and education can be judged.

progressive muscle relaxation Stress management technique involving tensing and relaxing muscles.

proposition Statement that proposes a relationship between concepts.

proprioception Awareness of posture, movement, and changes in equilibrium and knowledge of position, weight, and resistance of objects in relation to the body.

prosody Melody of speech that conveys meaning through changes in the tempo, rhythm, and intonation.

proteins Organic compounds of amino acid polymers connected by peptide bonds that contain carbon, hydrogen, oxygen, and nitrogen.

protocol Series of standing orders or procedures that should be followed under certain specific conditions.

proxemics Study of the distance between people and objects.

psychomotor domain Area of learning that involves performance of motor skills.

psychoneuroimmunology Study of the complex relationship between the cognitive, affective, and physical aspects of humans.

puberty Appearance of secondary sex characteristics that signals the beginning of adolescence.

public law Law that deals with an individual's relationship to the state.

pulse Bounding of blood flow in an artery that is palpable at various points on the body.

pulse deficit Condition in which the apical pulse rate is greater than the radial pulse rate.

pulse oximeter Sensor device used to measure the oxygen saturation level of the blood.

pulse pressure Measurement of the ratio of stroke volume to compliance (total distensibility) of the arterial system.

pulse quality Refers to the "feel" of the pulse, its rhythm and forcefulness.

pulse rate Indirect measurement of cardiac output obtained by counting the number of apical or peripheral pulse waves over a pulse point.

pulse rhythm Regularity of the heartbeat.

pulse volume Measurement of the strength or amplitude of the force exerted by the ejected blood against the arterial wall with each contraction.

purulent exudate Pus, generally occurring with severe inflammation accompanied by infection.

pyogenic bacteria Bacteria that produce pus.

pyorrhea Periodontal disease.

pyrexia When heat production exceeds heat loss and body temperature rises above the normal range.

pyrogens Bacteria, viruses, fungi, and some antigens.

pyuria Pus (white blood cells) in the urine.

Q

qualitative analysis Integration and synthesis of narrative, nonnumerical data.

qualitative research Systematic collection and analysis of subjective narrative materials, using procedures for which there tends to be a minimum of research-imposed control.

quality Meeting or exceeding requirements of the client.

quality assurance Traditional approach to quality management in which monitoring and evaluation focus on individual performance, deviation from standards, and problem solving.

quantitative research Systematic collection of numerical information, often under conditions of considerable control.

R

race Grouping of people based on biological similarities such as physical characteristics.

racism Discrimination directed toward individuals who are misperceived to be inferior because of biological factors.

radiation Loss of heat in the form of infrared rays.

radiofrequency ablation The delivery of low-voltage, high-frequency alternating electrical current to cauterize the abnormal myocardial tissue.

radiography Study of x-rays or gamma ray–exposed film through the action of ionizing radiation.

range of motion Extent to which a joint can move.

rapport Bond or connection between two people that is based on mutual trust.

rationale Explanation based on the theories and scientific principles of natural and behavioral sciences and the humanities.

readiness for learning Evidence of willingness to learn.

receiver Person who intercepts the sender's message.

recent memory The result of events that have occurred over the past 24 hours.

recommended dietary allowances (RDA) Recommended allowances of essential nutrients

established by the Food and Nutrition Board of the Academy of Sciences–National Research Council.

reconstitution Adaptation to a stressor.

recontextualizing Exploration of a developed theory in terms of its applicability to other settings or groups.

recurrent acute pain Identified by repetitive painful episodes that may recur over a prolonged period or throughout the client's lifetime.

red cell indices Laboratory measurement of the size and hemoglobin content of the red cells.

red wound Wound that is the color of normal granulation tissue and in the proliferative phase of wound repair.

referred pain The sensation of pain is not felt in the organ itself but instead is perceived at the spot where the organs were located during fetal development.

reframing A technique that teaches clients to monitor their negative thoughts and replace them with ones that are more positive.

regional anesthesia Anesthesia that causes the client to lose sensation in a particular area of the body (e.g., laparoscopy for a tubal sterilization).

regurgitation Backward flow of blood through a diseased heart valve, also known as insufficiency.

related factors Elements that can precede, be associated with, contribute to, or be related to nursing diagnoses in some type of patterned relationship.

relaxation response State of increased arousal of the parasympathetic nervous system that leads to a relaxed physiological state.

relaxation techniques A variety of methods used to decrease anxiety and muscle tension.

religion Set of beliefs associated with a formal organized group, such as a church, synagogue, mosque, or temple.

remote memory The retention of experiences that occurred during earlier periods of life.

research Systematic method of exploring, describing, explaining, relating, or establishing the existence of a phenomenon, the factors that cause changes in the phenomenon, and how the phenomenon influences other phenomena.

research design Overall plan used to conduct research.

resident floras Microorganisms that are always present, usually without altering the client's health.

respiration The act of breathing.

rest A state of relaxation and calmness, both mental and physical.

restorative nursing care Nursing care provided to clients who have residual impairment as a result of disease or injury; seeks to increase the client's independence and ability to perform self-care.

restraints Protective devices used to limit the physical activity of a client or to immobilize a client or extremity.

restrictive pulmonary disease A category of lung diseases characterized by impaired mobility or elasticity of the lungs or chest wall.

review of systems A brief account of any recent signs or symptoms related to any body system.

rhonchi Heard predominantly on expiration over the trachea and bronchi as a continuous, low-pitched musical sound.

rigor mortis Stiffening of the body after death caused by contraction of the skeletal and smooth muscles.

risk factors Elements that increase the chances of an individual, family, or community being susceptible to a disease state or life event affecting health.

risk for infection State in which an individual is at increased risk for being invaded by pathogenic organisms.

risk nursing diagnosis Nursing diagnosis that indicates that a problem does not yet exist but specific risk factors are present; composed of the diagnostic label preceded by the phrase "risk for" with the specific risk factors listed.

role Set of expected behaviors associated with a person's status or position.

role conflict When the expectations of one role compete with the expectations of other roles.

S

saccharides Sugar units.

satiety Feeling of fulfillment from food.

saturated fatty acids Glycerol esters of organic acids whose atoms are joined by a single-valence bond.

school-age period Developmental stage from the ages of 6 to 12 years.

scoliosis Lateral deviation of the vertical line of the spine.

scope of practice Legal boundaries of practice for health care providers as defined in state statutes.

sebum Produced by the skin and contains fatty acids that kill some bacteria.

secondary gain Outcomes of the sick role other than alleviation of anxiety (primary gain); examples include gaining attention and sympathy, avoiding responsibilities, and receiving financial compensation or reward.

secondary intention healing Seen in wounds with extensive tissue loss and wounds in which the edges cannot be approximated.

secondary source Source of data other than the client, such as family members, other health care providers, or medical records; article in which an author addresses the research of someone else.

self-care Learned behavior and a deliberate action in response to a need.

self-care deficit Exists when the client is not able to perform one or more of the activities of daily living.

self-concept Individual's perception of self; includes self-esteem, body image, and ideal self.

self-efficacy Belief in one's ability to succeed; according to social cognitive theory of learning, serves as an internal motivator for change.

self-esteem Individual's perception of self-worth; includes judgments about one's self and one's capabilities.

semipermeable Selective permeability of membranes.

sender Person who generates a message.

sensation The ability to receive and process stimuli received through the sensory organs.

sensitivity Determines the susceptibility of a pathogen to an antibiotic; the ability of a test to correctly identify those individuals who have the disease.

sensory deficit A change in the perception of sensory stimuli.

sensory deprivation A state of reduced sensory input from the internal or external environment, manifested by alterations in sensory perceptions.

sensory overload Increased perception of the intensity of auditory and visual stimuli.

sensory perception The ability to receive sensory impressions and, through cortical association, relate the stimuli to past experiences to form an impression of the nature of the stimulus.

serous exudate Exudate that is composed primarily of serum (the clear portion of blood), is watery in appearance, and has a low protein count.

sex roles Culturally determined patterns associated with being male or female.

sexuality Human characteristic that refers not just to gender but to all the aspects of being male or female, including feelings, attitudes, beliefs, and behavior.

sexual orientation Individual's preference for ways of expressing sexual feelings.

shaman Folk healer–priest who uses natural and supernatural forces to help others.

shamanism Practice of entering altered states of consciousness with the intent of helping others.

shearing The force exerted against the skin when a client is moved or repositioned in bed by being pulled or allowed to slide down in bed.

short-term goal Statement written in objective format demonstrating an expectation to be achieved in resolution of the nursing diagnosis in a short period of time, usually a few hours or days.

shunting Condition in which alveolar regions are well perfused but not adequately ventilated.

side effects Mild nontherapeutic drug effects.

signal-averaged ECG Surface electrocardiogram that amplifies late potentials.

simultaneity paradigm Nursing viewpoint that focuses on the quality of life from the client's perspective and conceptualizes the interaction between person and environment as mutual and simultaneous.

single-payer system Health care delivery model in which the government is the only entity to reimburse.

single point of entry Entry into the health care system is required through a point designated by the plan.

situational leadership Style of leadership in which there is a blending of styles based on current circumstances and events.

situational loss Occurs in response to external events, usually beyond the individual's control (e.g., death of a significant other).

skinfold measurement Measures the amount of body fat.

skin shear Result of dragging skin across a hard surface.

skin turgor Normal resiliency of the skin.

sleep A state of altered consciousness during which an individual experiences minimal physical activity and a general slowing of the body's physiological processes.

sleep apnea A syndrome in which breathing periodically ceases during sleep, often associated with heavy snoring.

sleep cycle The sequence of sleep that begins with the four stages of non–rapid eye movement sleep in order, with a return to stage 3, then 2, then passage into the first rapid eye movement stage.

sleep deprivation A term used to describe prolonged inadequate quality and quantity of sleep, either of the rapid eye movement or the non–rapid eye movement type.

sloughing Shedding of dead tissue as a result of skin ulceration.

small-group ecology Study of proxemics in small-group situations.

Snellen chart Chart that contains various-sized letters with standardized numbers at the end of each line of letters.

SOAP charting Documentation method using subjective data, objective data, assessment, and plan.

solute A substance dissolved in a solution; also called an analyte.

solvent A liquid with a substance in solution.

somatic pain Nonlocalized pain originating in support structures such as tendons, ligaments, and nerves; may be a deep pain.

somnambulism Sleepwalking.

source-oriented (SO) charting Narrative recording by each member (source) of the health care team on a separate record.

spasticity Increase in muscle tension.

specific gravity Weight of urine compared with weight of distilled water; a specific gravity greater than 1.0 indicates solutes in the urine.

specificity The ability of a test to correctly identify those individuals who do not have the disease.

spherocytes Small, thick red cells.

spiritual distress State experienced when an individual perceives that his or her belief system, or that person's place within it, is threatened.

spirituality Multidimensional aspect of self that refers to one's relationship with oneself, a sense of connection with others, and a relationship with a higher power or divine source.

spiritual well-being Sense of connectedness between the self, others, nature, and a higher power that can be accessed through prayer or other means.

spores Single-celled microorganisms or microorganisms in the resting or inactive stage.

standing order Standardized intervention written, approved, and signed by a prescribing practitioner that is kept on file within health care agencies to be used in predictable situations or in circumstances requiring immediate attention.

stat order An order for a single dose of medication to be given immediately.

statutory law Laws enacted by legislative bodies.

stenosis Narrowing or constriction of a blood vessel or valve.

stereognosis Ability to identify objects by manipulation and touch.

stereotyping Belief that all people within the same racial, ethnic, or cultural group act alike and share the same beliefs and attitudes.

sterilization The total elimination of all microorganisms, including spores.

stock supply Medications dispensed and labeled in large quantities for storage in the medication room or nursing unit.

stoma Surgically created opening.

stomatitis Inflammation of the oral mucosa.

stool Fecal material.

stress Body's reaction to any stimulus.

stressor Any stimulus encountered by an individual; leads to the need to adapt.

stress test Measures the client's cardiovascular response to exercise tolerance.

stress urinary incontinence Uncontrolled loss of urine caused by physical exertion in the absence of a bladder contraction.

striae Red or silvery-white streaks due to rapid stretching of skin with resultant damage to elastic fibers of dermis.

stridor Heard predominantly on inspiration as a continuous crowing sound.

stroke volume Measurement of blood that enters the aorta with each ventricular contraction.

structure evaluation Determination of the health care agency's ability to provide the services offered to its client population.

subcutaneous Injection into the subcutaneous tissue.

subjective data Data from the client's point of view, including feelings, perceptions, and concerns.

sublingual Under the tongue.

superficial wound Confined to the epidermis layer, which comprises the four outermost layers of skin.

supernumerary nipples Extra nipples that appear as pigmented moles along the "milk line" of the breast.

suppression Conscious defense mechanism whereby a person decides to avoid dealing with a stressor at the present time.

suppuration The process of pus formation.

surfactant Phospholipid secreted by type II alveolar cells that reduces the alveolar surface tension and thus helps prevent alveolar collapse.

surgical asepsis Sterile technique; consists of those practices that eliminate all microorganisms and spores from an object or area.

surgical hand antisepsis "Antiseptic handwash or antiseptic hand rub performed preoperatively by surgical personnel to eliminate transient and reduce resident hand flora. Antiseptic detergent preparations often have persistent antimicrobial activity" (CDC. [2002]. *Guideline for hand hygiene in healthcare settings.* Retrieved November 10, 2005, from http://www.cdc.gov/Handhygiene)

susceptible host Person who lacks resistance to an agent and is thus vulnerable to disease.

suture Surgical means of closing a wound by sewing, wiring, or stapling the edges of the wound together.

synergy Combined power of many people.

synthesis Putting data together in a new way.

systemic infection Affects the entire body and involves multiple organs.

systole Process of cardiac chamber emptying or ejecting blood.

T

tachycardia A heart rate in excess of 100 beats per minute in an adult.

tachypnea Respiratory rate greater than 24 breaths per minute.

tactile fremitus Vibrations created by sound waves.

tapotement Massage technique using a light tapping of the fingers that stimulates movement in tired muscles.

taxonomy of nursing diagnoses Classifies diagnostic labels based on which human responses the client is demonstrating in response to the actual or perceived stressor.

teaching Active process in which one individual shares information with another as a means to facilitate behavioral changes.

teaching-learning process Planned interaction that promotes a behavioral change that is not a result of maturation or coincidence.

teaching strategies Techniques employed by the teacher to promote learning.

team Group of individuals who work together to achieve a common goal.

team nursing Type of nursing care delivery system in which a variety of personnel (professional, technical, and unlicensed) provide care.

teleology Ethical theory that states that the moral value of a situation is determined by its consequences.

teratogenic substance Substance that can cross the placental barrier and impair normal growth and development.

termination phase Third and final stage of the therapeutic relationship; focuses on evaluation of goal achievement and effectiveness of treatment.

tertiary intention healing Also known as delayed or secondary closure, it is indicated when primary closure of a wound is undesirable.

testimony Written or verbal evidence given by a qualified expert in an area.

thallium Radionuclide that is the physiological analogue of potassium.

theory Set of concepts and propositions that provide an orderly way to view phenomena.

therapeutic Describes actions that are beneficial to the client.

therapeutic communication Use of communication for the purpose of creating a beneficial outcome for the client.

therapeutic massage Application of pressure and motion by the hands with the intent of improving the recipient's well-being.

therapeutic procedure accidents Occur during the delivery of medical or nursing interventions.

therapeutic range Achievement of a constant therapeutic blood level of a medication within a safe range.

therapeutic relationship A relationship that benefits the client's health status.

therapeutic touch Holistic technique that consists of assessing alterations in a person's energy fields and using the hands to direct energy to achieve a balanced state.

therapeutic use of self Process in which nurses deliberately plan their actions and approach the relationship with a specific goal in mind before interacting with the client.

thermoregulation Body's physiological function of heat regulation to maintain a constant internal body temperature.

thoracentesis The aspiration of fluids from the pleural cavity.

thrills Vibrations that feel similar to a purring cat.

thrombus Blood clot.

toddler Developmental stage beginning at approximately 12 to 18 months of age, when a child begins to walk, and ending at approximately age 3.

tolerance Can occur after repeated administration of an opioid analgesic, when a specific dose loses its effectiveness and the client requires larger and larger doses to produce the same level of analgesia.

tort Civil wrong committed upon a person or property stemming from a direct invasion of some legal right of the person, the infraction of some public duty, or the violation of some private obligation by which damages accrue to the person.

tort law Enforcement of duties and rights among individuals independent of contractual agreements.

total client care Variation of the primary nursing management system in which responsibility for client care changes from shift to shift with the assigned caregiver.

totality paradigm Nursing viewpoint that conceptualizes the interaction between person and environment as constant in order to accomplish goals and maintain balance.

total parenteral nutrition (TPN) Intravenous infusion of a solution containing dextrose, amino acids, fats, essential fatty acids, vitamins, and minerals.

total quality management Method of management and system operation that is used to achieve continuous quality improvement.

touch Means of perceiving or experiencing through tactile sensation.

toxic effect Reaction that occurs when the body cannot metabolize a drug, causing the drug to accumulate in the blood.

tracheotomy A surgical procedure in which an opening (stoma) is made through the anterior neck into the trachea; an artificial airway (tracheostomy tube) is placed into the stoma.

transcultural nursing Formal area of study and practice focused on comparative analysis of different cultures and subcultures with respect to cultural care, health and illness beliefs, values, and practices, with the goal of providing health care within the context of the client's culture.

transcutaneous electrical nerve stimulation (TENS) Method of applying minute amounts of electrical stimulation to large-diameter nerve fibers via electrodes placed on the skin to block the passage of pain to the dorsal spinal root.

transducer Instrument that converts electrical energy to sound waves.

transduction The changing of noxious stimuli in sensory nerve endings to energy impulses.

transferrin (nonheme iron) Combination of a blood protein and iron.

transient floras Microorganisms that are episodic.

transmission Movement of impulses from the site of origin to the brain.

transsexuality Belief that one is psychologically of the sex opposite one's anatomic gender.

trigger point A hypersensitive point that when stimulated causes a local twitch or "jump" response.

triglycerides Lipid compounds consisting of three fatty acids and a glycerol molecule.

trocar Large-bored abdominal paracentesis needle.

trough The lowest blood serum concentration of a drug in a person's system.

tympany Musical drumlike sound that occurs over air-filled cavities.

type and cross-match Laboratory test that identifies the client's blood type (e.g., A or B) and determines the compatibility of the blood between potential donor and recipient.

U

ultrasound Use of high-frequency sound waves instead of x-ray film to visualize deep body structures; also called an echogram.

uncomplicated grief A fairly predictable grief reaction following a significant loss, ending with the relinquishing of the lost object and resumption of the previous life.

unintentional wound Unanticipated wound and often the result of trauma or an accident.

unit dose form System of packaging and labeling each dose of medication, usually for a 24-hour period.

unprofessional conduct Conduct that could adversely affect the health and welfare of the public.

unsaturated fatty acids Glycerol esters of organic acids whose atoms are joined by double- or triple-valence bonds.

urgency Timely intervention of surgery.

urge urinary incontinence Uncontrolled discharge of urine caused by hyperactive (unstable) contractions of the detrusor muscle.

urinalysis Laboratory analysis of the urine.

urinary incontinence Uncontrolled loss of urine of sufficient duration and volume to create a social or hygienic problem.

urinary retention Inability to completely evacuate the bladder.

urobilinogen Derived from the normal bacterial action of intestinal floras on bilirubin.

utility Ethical principle that states that an act must result in the greatest amount of good for the greatest number of people involved in a situation.

V

vaccination Provides acquired immunity against specific diseases.

value Variation of the variable.

values Principles that influence the development of beliefs and attitudes.

values clarification Process of analyzing one's own values to better understand what is truly important to oneself.

variable Anything that may differ from the norm.

variations Goals not met or interventions not performed according to the time frame; also called variance.

vasoconstriction The narrowing of the vessels, usually leading to reduced blood flow.

vasodilation The widening of the vessels, usually leading to increased blood flow.

vectorborne transmission Occurs when an agent is transferred to a susceptible host by animate means such as mosquitoes, fleas, ticks, lice, and other animals.

vehicle transmission Occurs when an agent is transferred to a susceptible host by contaminated inanimate objects such as water, food, milk, drugs, and blood.

venipuncture Puncturing of a vein with a needle to aspirate blood.

ventilation Movement of air into and out of the lungs for the purpose of delivering fresh air to the alveoli.

ventilation-perfusion (V/Q) mismatching Condition in which perfusion and ventilation of the lung areas are not adequately balanced.

veracity Ethical principle that means that one should be truthful, neither lying nor deceiving others.

verbal message Message communicated through words or language, both spoken and written.

vesicant Medication that causes blisters and tissue injury when it escapes into surrounding tissue.

vesicular sounds Soft, breezy, and low-pitched sounds heard longer on inspiration than expiration that result from air moving through the smaller airways over the lung's periphery, with the exception of the scapular area.

vibration Massage technique using rapid movements that stimulate or relax muscles.

virulence Degree of pathogenicity of an infectious microorganism (pathogen).

visceral pain Discomfort in the internal organs that is less localized and more slowly transmitted than cutaneous pain.

visual channel Transmission of messages through sight, observation, and perception.

visual learner Style of learning in which people learn by processing information by seeing.

vital capacity Amount of air exhaled from the lungs after a minimal full inspiration.

vital signs Measurement of the client's body temperature (T), pulse (P) and respiratory (R) rates, and blood pressure (BP).

vitamins Organic compounds.

voiding Process of urine evacuation.

W

walking rounds Reporting method used when the members of the care team walk to each client's room and discuss care and progress with each other and the client.

water-soluble vitamins Vitamins that require daily ingestion in normal quantities because they are not stored in the body.

wellness Condition in which an individual functions at optimal levels.

wellness nursing diagnosis Nursing diagnosis that indicates the client's expression of a desire to obtain a higher level of wellness in some area of function. It is composed of the diagnostic label preceded by the phrase "potential for enhanced."

wheezes Heard predominantly on expiration all over the lungs as a continuous sonorous wheeze (low-pitched snoring) or sibilant wheeze (high-pitched musical sound).

whistle-blowing Calling attention to the unethical, illegal, or incompetent actions of others.

working phase Second stage of the therapeutic relationship in which problems are identified, goals are established, and problem-solving methods are selected.

work of breathing Amount of muscular energy (work) required to accomplish ventilation.

wound Disruption in the integrity of body tissue.

Y

yellow wound Has either fibrinous slough or purulent exudate from bacteria.

young adulthood Developmental stage from the ages of 21 to approximately 40 years.

Z

Z-track (zigzag) technique Method of intramuscular injection to seal the medication in the muscle, preventing the drug from irritating the subcutaneous tissue.

REFERENCES

CHAPTER 1

American Association of Colleges of Nursing. (1995). *The essentials of baccalaureate education.* Washington, DC: Author.

American Association of Colleges of Nursing. (1996). *Position statement: The baccalaureate degree in nursing as minimal preparation for professional practice.* Washington, DC: Author.

American Association of Colleges of Nursing. (1998). *The essentials of baccalaureate education for professional nursing practice.* Washington, DC: Author.

American Nurses Association. (1990). *Standards for nursing staff development.* Kansas City, MO: Author.

American Nurses Association. (1991). *Nursing's agenda for health care reform.* Washington, DC: Author.

Association of Academic Health Centers. (1994). *Proceedings from the Second Congress of Health Professions Educators.* Washington, DC: Author.

Bellack, J. P., & O'Neal, E. H. (2000). Recreating nursing practice for a new century. *Nursing and Health Care Perspectives, 21*(1), 14–21.

Chinn, P. L. (1994). *Developing the discipline: Critical studies in nursing history and professional issues.* Gaithersburg, MD: Aspen.

Coxwell, G., & Gillerman, H. (2000). *National League for Nursing educational competencies for graduates of associate degree nursing programs.* Sudbury, MA: Jones & Bartlett and National League for Nursing.

Donahue, M. P. (1985). *Nursing, the finest art: An illustrated history.* St. Louis, MO: Mosby.

Dossey, B. (1995). Endnote: Florence Nightingale today. *Critical Care Nursing, 15*(4), 98.

Institute of Medicine. (1998). *Leading health indicators for Healthy People 2010: Second interim report.* Washington, DC: National Academies Press.

Nightingale, F. (1969). *Nursing: What it is and what it is not.* New York: Dover Publications.

O'Neil, E. H. (1993). *Health professions education for the future: Schools in service to the nation.* San Francisco: Pew Health Professions Commission.

Pew Health Professions Commission. (1995). *Critical challenges: Revitalizing the health professions for the twenty-first century.* San Francisco: University of California Center for the Health Professions.

Secretary's Commission on Nursing. (1988). *Final report.* Washington, DC: Department of Health and Human Services.

Shugars, D. A., O'Neil, E. H., & Bader, J. D. (Eds.). (1991). *Healthy America: Practitioners for 2005: An agenda for action for U.S. health professional schools.* Durham, NC: Pew Health Professions Commission.

CHAPTER 2

Andrews, H., & Roy, C. (1991). *The Roy adaptation model: The definitive statement.* East Norwalk, CT: Appleton & Lange.

Barnum, B. (1994). *Nursing theory: Analysis, application, evaluation.* Philadelphia: Lippincott.

Barrett, M. (2002). What is nursing science? *Nursing Science Quarterly, 15*(1), 51–60.

Catalano, J. (2006). *Nursing now! Today's issues, tomorrow's trends* (4th ed.). Philadelphia: F. A. Davis.

Chinn, P., & Kramer, M. (1999). *Theory and nursing: Integrated knowledge development* (5th ed.). St. Louis, MO: Mosby.

Fawcett, J. (1993). *Analysis and evaluation of nursing theories.* Philadelphia: F. A. Davis.

Fawcett, J. (2000). *Analysis and evaluation of contemporary nursing knowledge: Nursing models and theories.* Philadelphia: F. A. Davis.

Fawcett, J. (2002a). The nurse theorists: 21st-century updates—Jean Watson. *Nursing Science Quarterly, 15*(3), 214–219.

Fawcett, J. (2002b). The nurse theorists: 21st-century updates—Madeleine M. Leininger. *Nursing Science Quarterly, 15*(2), 131–136.

Fawcett, J. (2003). The nurse theorists: 21st-century updates—Martha E. Rogers. *Nursing Science Quarterly, 16*(1), 44–51.

Fawcett, J. (2005). *Contemporary nursing knowledge: Analysis and evaluation of conceptual models of nursing* (2nd ed.). Philadelphia: F. A. Davis.

Fawcett, J., & Gigliotti, E. (2001). Using conceptual models of nursing to guide nursing research: The case of the Neuman systems model. *Nursing Science Quarterly, 14*(4), 339–345.

Felgen, J. (2003). Caring: Core value, currency, and commodity ... is it time to get tough about "soft"? *Nursing Administration Quarterly, 27*(3), 208–214.

Henderson, V. (1966). *The nature of nursing: A definition and its implication for practice, research, and education.* New York: Macmillan.

Kuhn, T. (1970). *The structure of scientific revolutions* (2nd ed.). Chicago: University of Chicago Press.

Leininger, M. (1991). The theory of culture care diversity and universality. In M. Leininger (Ed.), *Cultural care diversity and universality: A theory of nursing* (pp. 5–65). New York: National League for Nursing.

Leininger, M. (1996). Cultural care theory, research, and practice. *Nursing Science Quarterly, 9*(1), 71–78.

Leininger, M., & McFarland, M. (2002). *Transcultural nursing: Concepts, theories, research, and practices* (3rd ed.). New York: McGraw-Hill.

Levine, M. (1989). The four conservation principles: 20 years later. In J. Riehl-Sisca (Ed.), *Conceptual models for nursing practice* (3rd ed.). Stamford, CT: Appleton & Lange.

Levine, M. (1990). Conservation and integrity. In M. Parker (Ed.), *Nursing theories in practice.* New York: National League for Nursing.

Levine, M. (1995). The rhetoric of nursing theory. *Image: Journal of Nursing Scholarship, 27*(1), 14.

McEwen, M., & Willis, E. M. (2007). *Theoretical basis for nursing* (2nd ed.). Philadelphia: Lippincott.

Meleis, A. (1997). *Theoretical nursing: Development and progress* (3rd ed.). Philadelphia: Lippincott.

Neuman, B. (1995). *The Neuman systems model* (3rd ed.). Norwalk, CT: Appleton & Lange.

Newman, M. (1986). *Health as expanding consciousness.* St. Louis, MO: Mosby.

Nightingale, F. (1946). *Notes on nursing: What it is and what it is not.* London: Harrison & Sons. (Original work published 1859)

Orem, D. (1991). *Nursing concepts of practice* (4th ed.). New York: McGraw-Hill.

Parker, M. (2001). *Nursing theories and nursing practice.* Philadelphia: F. A. Davis.

Parse, R. (1987). *Nursing science: Major paradigms, theories, and critiques.* Philadelphia: Saunders.

Parse, R. (1998). *The human becoming school of thought: A perspective for nurses and other health professionals.* Thousand Oaks, CA: Sage.

Parse, R. (2000). Paradigms: A reprise. *Nursing Science Quarterly, 13*(3), 275–276.

Parse, R. R. (2006). Rosemarie Rizzo Parse's human becoming school of thought. In M. Parker (Ed.), *Nursing theories and nursing practice* (2nd ed., pp. 187–193). Philadelphia: F. A. Davis.

Rogers, M. (1970). *An introduction to the theoretical basis of nursing.* Philadelphia: F. A. Davis.

Rogers, M. (1990). Nursing: Science of unitary, irreducible human beings: Update 1990. In E. Barrett (Ed.), *Visions of Rogers' science based nursing.* New York: National League for Nursing.

Rogers, M. (1992). Nursing science and the space age. *Nursing Science Quarterly, 5*(1), 27–34.

Roy, S. C., & Andrews, H. (1999). *The Roy adaptation model* (2nd ed.). Norwalk, CT: Appleton & Lange.

Watson, J. (1985). *Nursing: Human science and human care.* Norwalk, CT: Appleton-Century-Crofts.

Woodward, W. (2003). Preparing a new workforce. *Nursing Administration Quarterly, 27*(3), 215–222.

CHAPTER 3

Benefield, L. E. (2002). Evidence-based practice: Basic strategies for success. *Home Healthcare Nurse, 20*(12), 803–807.

Boswell, C. (2007). *Introduction to nursing research: Incorporating evidence-based practice.* Sudbury, MA: Jones & Bartlett.

Brockopp, D., & Hastings-Tolsma, M. (2003). *Fundamentals of nursing research* (3rd ed.). Sudbury, MA: Jones & Bartlett.

Burns, N., & Grove, S. K. (2004). *The practice of nursing research: Conduct, critique, and utilization* (5th ed.). Philadelphia: W. B. Saunders.

Cacchione, P. (2008). Interprofessional nursing research. *Clinical Nursing Research, 17*(1), 30–40.

Carper, B. A. (1978). Fundamental patterns of knowing in nursing. *Advances in Nursing Science, 1,* 13–23.

Carper, B. A. (1992). Philosophical inquiry in nursing: An application. In J. F. Kikuchi & H. Simmons (Eds.), *Philosophic inquiry in nursing.* Newbury Park, CA: Sage.

Houser, J. (2008). *Nursing research: Reading, using, and creating evidence,* Sudbury, MA: Jones & Bartlett.

Morse, W., Oleson, M., Duffy, L., Patek, A., & Sohr, G. (1996). Connecting the research and nursing processes: Making a difference in baccalaureate students' attitudes and abilities. *Journal of Nursing Education, 35*(4), 148–151.

National Institute of Nursing Research. (2003). *NINA research themes for the future.* Bethesda, MD National Institutes of Health. Retrieved from http://www.nih.gov/ninr/NINR/2003.

National Institute of Nursing Research. (2008). *The NIH Public Trust Initiative launches the "Partners in Research" program.* Bethesda, MD National Institutes of Health. Retrieved July 18, 2008, from http://www.gov/ninr.

Nokes, K., & Nwakeze, P. (2007). Assessing cognitive capacity for participation in a research study. *Clinical Journal of Nursing Research, 16*(4), 336–349.

Polit, D., & Beck, C. (2006). *Essentials of nursing research appraising evidence for nursing practice* (6th ed.). Philadelphia: Lippincott Williams & Wilkins.

Polit, D. F., Beck, C. T., & Hungler, B. P. (2005). *Essentials of nursing research: Methods, appraisal, and utilization* (6th ed.). Philadelphia: Lippincott.

Rutledge, D. N., & Donaldson, N. E. (1995). Building organizational capacity to engage in research utilization. *Journal of Nursing Administration, 25,* 12–16.

CHAPTER 4

American Nurses Association. (2004). *Nursing: Scope and standards of practice.* Washington, DC: Author.

American Nurses Association. (2005). *Nursing's agenda for health care reform.* Washington, DC: Author.

Buerhaus, P. I., Staiger, D. O., & Aeurbach, D. I. (2009). *The future of the workforce in the United States: Data, trends, and implications.* Boston: Jones & Bartlett.

Bureau of Labor Statistics, U.S. Department of Labor. (2007). *Occupational outlook handbook, 2009–2009 edition.* Retrieved August 8, 2008, from http://www.bls.gov/oco/ocos083.htm.

Duderstadt, K. G., Hughes, D. C., Soobader, M. J., & Newacheck, P. W. (2006). The impact of public insurance expansions on children's access and use of care. *Pediatrics, 118,* 1676–1682.

Edelman, C. L., & Mandle, C. L. (2006). *Health promotion throughout the life span* (6th ed.). St. Louis: Mosby Elsevier.

Gordon, S., Buchanan, J., & Bretherton, T. (2008). *Safety in numbers: Nurse-to-patient ratios and the future of health care.* Ithaca, NY: Cornell University Press.

Heinrich, J., & Thompson, T. M. (2007). Organization and delivery of health care in the United States: A patchwork system. In D. J. Mason, J. K. Leavitt, & M. W. Chaffee (Eds.), *Policy and politics in nursing and health care* (5th ed., pp. 201–213). Philadelphia: Saunders.

Hicks, L. L., & Boles, K. E. (2008). Why health economics? In C. Harrington & C. L. Estes (Eds.), *Health policy* (5th ed.). Boston: Jones & Bartlett.

Hunt, R. (2009). *Introduction to community-based nursing* (4th ed.). Philadelphia: Wolters Kluwer/Lippincott.

Joint Commission. (2008). *2009 accreditation manual for hospitals.* Oakbrook Terrace, IL: Author.

Kane, R. L., Shamliyan, T. A., Mueller, C., Duval, S., & Wilt, T. J. (2007). The association of registered nurse staffing levels and patient outcomes: Systematic review and meta-analysis. *Medical Care, 45*(12), 1126–1128.

Kilduff, M., & Krackhardt, D. (2008). *Interpersonal networks in organizations: Cognition, personality, dynamics and culture.* New York: Cambridge University Press.

Mark, B. A., & Harless, D. W. (2007). Nurse staffing, mortality, and length of stay in for-profit and not-for-profit hospitals. *Inquiry, 44*(2), 167–186.

McCallion, P. (2007). *Housing for the elderly: Policies and practice issues.* New York: Taylor & Francis.

Michel, M., & Wortham, S. (2008). *Bullish on uncertainty: How organized cultures transform participants.* New York: Cambridge University Press

National Coalition on Health Care. (2008). *Health insurance costs.* Retrieved August 7, 2008, from http://www.nchc.org/facts/costs.html.

Price, M., Fitzgerald, L., & Kinsman, L. (2007). Quality improvement: The divergent views of managers and clinicians. *Journal of Nursing Management, 15*(1), 43–50.

Pulcini, J. A., Neary, S. R., & Mahoney, D. F. (2007). Health care financing. In D. J. Mason, J. K. Leavitt, & M. W. Chaffee (Eds.), *Policy and politics in nursing and health care* (5th ed., pp. 241–264). Philadelphia: Saunders.

Thungjaroenkul, P., Cummings, G. G., & Embleton, A. (2007). The impact of nurse staffing on hospital costs and patient length of stay: A systematic review. *Nursing Economics, 25*(5), 155–165.

CHAPTER 5

Alfaro-LeFevre, R. (2008). *Critical thinking and clinical judgment: A practical approach* (4th ed.). Philadelphia: Saunders.

American Nurses Association. (2004). *Nursing: Scope and standards of practice.* Washington, DC: Author.

Bandman, E. L., & Bandman, B. (1995). *Critical thinking in nursing.* Norwalk, CT: Appleton & Lange.

Billay, D., Myrick, F., Luhanga, F., & Yonge, O. (2007). A pragmatic view of intuitive knowledge in nursing practice. *Nursing Forum, 42*(3), 147–155.

Carpenito, L. J. (2007). *Nursing diagnosis: Application to clinical practice* (12th ed.). Philadelphia: Lippincott Williams & Wilkins.

Chitty, K. K. (2007). *Professional nursing: Concepts and challenges* (5th ed.). Philadelphia: W. B. Saunders.

Edelman, C. L., & Mandle, C. L. (2006). *Health promotion throughout the life span* (6th ed.). St. Louis, MO: Mosby.

Eisenhauer, L. A., Hurley, A. C., & Dolan, N. (2007). Nurses' reported thinking during medication administration. *Journal of Nursing Scholarship, 39*(1), 83–87.

Ennis, R. H. (1987). A taxonomy of critical thinking dispositions and abilities. In J. B. Baron & R. J. Sternberg (Eds.), *Teaching thinking skills: Theory and practice* (pp. 119–128). New York: W. H. Freeman.

Ennis, R. H. (1989). Critical thinking and subject specificity: Clarification and needed research. *Educational Researcher, 18,* 4–10.

Facione, P. A. (1990). Critical thinking: A statement of expert consensus for purposes of educational assessment and instruction (executive summary). In *The Delphi Report* (pp. 1–19). Millbrae, CA: California Academic Press.

Forehand, M. (2005). Bloom's taxonomy: Original and revised. In M. Orey (Ed.), *Emerging perspectives on learning, teaching, and technology.* Retrieved August 6, 2008, from http://projects.coe.uga.edu/epltt/index.phy?title+Bloom%27s_Taxonomy.

Fry, V. S. (1953). The creative approach to nursing. *American Journal of Nursing, 53*(3), 301–302.

Johnson, D. (1959). A philosophy for nursing diagnosis. *Nursing Outlook, 7,* 198–200.

Moorhead, S., Johnson, M., Maas, M., & Swanson, E. (2007). *Nursing outcomes classification* (4th ed.). St. Louis, MO: Mosby.

National League for Nursing. (1997). *Interpretive guidelines for standards and criteria 1997: Baccalaureate and higher degree.* New York: National League for Nursing Accrediting Commission.

Orlando, I. (1961). *The dynamic nurse-patient relationship.* New York: G. P. Putnam & Sons.

Paul, R. (1992). *Critical thinking: What every person needs to survive in a rapidly changing world.* Santa Rosa, CA: Foundation for Critical Thinking.

Perry, W. G. (1970). *Forms of intellectual and ethical development in the college years.* New York: Holt, Rinehart, & Winston.

Pesut, D. J., & Herman, J. (1999). *Clinical reasoning: The art and science of critical and creative thinking.* Clifton Park, NY: Thomson Delmar Learning.

Shin, K. R., Lee, J. H., Ha, J. Y., & Kim, Y. H. (2006). Critical thinking dispositions in baccalaureate nursing students. *Journal of Advanced Nursing, 56*(2), 182–189.

Standing, M. (2007). Clinical decision-making skills on the developmental journey from student to registered nurse: A longitudinal inquiry. *Journal of Advanced Nursing, 60*(3), 257–269.

Watson, G., & Glaser, E. M. (1964). *Critical thinking appraisal.* Orlando, FL: Harcourt Brace Jovanovich.

Wiedenbach, E. (1963). The helping art of nursing. *American Journal of Nursing, 63*(11), 54–57.

Wilkinson, J. M. (2006). *Nursing process and critical thinking* (4th ed.). Redwood City, CA: Addison-Wesley Nursing.

Yura, H., & Walsh, M. B. (1967). *The nursing process.* Washington, DC: Catholic University of America Press.

CHAPTER 6

Andrews, H. A., & Roy, C. (2008). *The Roy adaptation model* (3rd ed.). Upper Saddle River, NJ: Pearson.

Edwards, B., & Sines, D. (2008). Passing the audition—The appraisal of client credibility and assessment by nurses at triage. *Journal of Clinical Nursing, 17*(18), 2444–2451.

Gordon, M. (2002). *Manual of nursing diagnoses* (10th ed.). St. Louis, MO: Mosby.

Maslow, A. (1971). *The farther reaches of human nature.* New York: Viking Press.

North American Nursing Diagnosis Association International. (2009). *Nursing diagnoses—Definitions and classification 2009–2011.* Philadelphia: John Wiley & Sons, Inc.

Orem, D. E. (2001). *Nursing: Concepts of practice* (6th ed.). St. Louis, MO: Mosby.

CHAPTER 7

American Nurses Association. (2004). *Nursing: Scope and standards of practice.* Washington, DC: Author.

American Nurses Association. (2008). *Nursing informatics: Scope and standards of practice.* Washington, DC: Author.

Bevis, E. M. (1978). *Curriculum building in nursing: A process.* St. Louis, MO: Mosby.

Carpenito-Moyet, L. J. (2007). *Nursing diagnosis: Application to clinical practice* (12th ed.). Philadelphia: Lippincott Williams & Wilkins.

da Cruz, D. A. L. M., de Mattos Pimenta, C. A., & Lunney, M. (2006). Teaching how to make accurate nurses' diagnoses using an evidence-based practice model. In R. F. Levin & H. R. Feldman (Eds.), *Teaching evidence-based practice in nursing* (pp. 229–246). New York: Springer.

Fry, V. S. (1953). The creative approach to nursing. *American Journal of Nursing, 53,* 301–302.

Muller-Staub, M., Needham, I., Odenbreit, M., Lavin, M. A., & van Achterberg, T. (2007). Improved quality of nursing documentation: Results of a nursing diagnoses, interventions, and outcomes implementation study. *International Journal of Nursing Terminologies & Classifications: The Official Journal of NANDA International, 18*(1), 1–2.

North American Nursing Diagnosis Association International. (2009). *Nursing diagnoses—Definitions and classification 2009–2011.* Philadelphia: John Wiley & Sons, Inc.

Ralph, S. S., & Taylor, C. M. (2008). *Sparks & Taylor's Nursing diagnosis reference manual* (7th ed.). Philadelphia: Lippincott Williams & Wilkins.

CHAPTER 8

Alfaro-LeFevre, R. (2005). *Applying nursing process: A tool for critical thinking* (5th ed. rev.). Philadelphia: Lippincott Williams & Wilkins.

Alfaro-LeFevre, R. (2008). *Critical thinking in nursing: A practical approach* (4th ed.). Philadelphia: Saunders.

American Nurses Association. (2004). *Nursing: Scope and standards of practice.* Washington, DC: Author.

Carpenito-Moyet, L. J. (2007). *Handbook of nursing diagnosis* (12th ed.). Philadelphia: Lippincott Williams & Wilkins.

Doenges, M. E., Moorhouse, M. F., & Geissler, A. C. (2006). *Nursing care plans: Guidelines for planning and documenting patient care* (7th ed.). Philadelphia: Davis.

Moorhead, S., Johnson, M., Maas, M., & Swanson, E. (2007). *Nursing outcomes classification (NOC)* (4th ed.). St. Louis, MO: Mosby.

O'Conner, J., Seeto, C., Saini, B., Bosnic-Anticevich, B. S., Krass, I., Armour, C., et al. (2008). Healthcare professional versus patient goal setting in intermittent allergic rhinitis. *Patient Education and Counseling, 70*(1), 111–117.

Ralph, S. S., & Taylor, C. M. (2008). *Nursing diagnosis reference manual* (7th ed.). Philadelphia: Lippincott Williams & Wilkins.

Wilkinson, J. M. (2006). *Nursing process and critical thinking* (4th ed.). Upper Saddle River, NJ: Prentice-Hall.

CHAPTER 9

American Nurses Association. (2004). *Nursing: Scope & standards of practice* (2nd ed.). Washington, DC: Author.

Bulechek, G. M., Dochterman, J. M., & Butcher, H. K. (2007). *Nursing interventions classification (NIC)* (5th ed.). St. Louis, MO: Elsevier.

Chitty, K. K., & Black, B. P. (2007). *Professional nursing: Concepts and challenges* (5th ed.). St. Louis, MO: Elsevier.

Shever, L. L., Titler, M., Dochterman, J., Fei, Q., & Picone, D. M. (2007). Patterns of nursing intervention use across 6 days of acute care hospitalization for three older patient populations. *International Journal of Nursing Terminologies and Classifications, 18*(1), 18–29.

CHAPTER 10

Alfaro-LeFevre, R. (2008). *Critical thinking in nursing: A practical approach* (4th ed.). Philadelphia: Saunders.

American Nurses Association. (2004). *Nursing: Scope and standards of practice.* Washington, DC: Author.

Bulechek, G. M., Dochterman, J. M., & Butcher, H. K. (2007). *Nursing interventions classifications (NIC)* (5th ed.). St. Louis, MO: Elsevier.

Li, H. C. (2007). Evaluating the effectiveness of preoperative interventions: The appropriateness of using the Children's Emotional Manifestation Scale. *Journal of Clinical Nursing, 16*(10), 1919–1926.

Moorhead, S., Johnson, M., Maas, M., & Swanson, E. (2007). *Nursing outcomes classification (NOC)* (4th ed.). St. Louis, MO: Elsevier.

North American Nursing Diagnosis Association. (2009). Nursing diagnoses—Definitions and classification 2009–2011. Philadelphia: John Wiley & Sons, Inc.

Wilkinson, J. M. (2008). *Nursing diagnosis handbook* (9th ed.). Upper Saddle River, NJ: Prentice-Hall.

CHAPTER 11

Alfaro-LeFevre, R. (2008). *Critical thinking and clinical judgment: A practical approach* (4th ed.). Philadelphia: Saunders.

American Nurses Association. (1976). *One strong voice.* Kansas City: Author.

American Nurses Association. (2004). *Nursing: Scope and standards of practice.* Washington, DC: Author.

American Nurses Association. (2005). *Principles for delegation.* Retrieved December 2, 2008, from http://www.safestaffingsaveslives.org//WhatisSafeStaffingPrinciples/PrinciplesforDelegationhtml.aspx.

American Nurses Association. (2008). *American Nurses Association bylaws.* Retrieved December 2, 2008, from http://www.nursingworld.org/FunctionalMenuCategories/AboutANA/WhoWeAre/ANABylaws.aspx.

Canadian Nurses Association. (2007). *CNA: Canadian Nurses Association 2007 report.* Ottawa: Author.

Canadian Nurses Association. (2008). *Code of ethics for registered nursing* (Centennial ed.). Ottawa: Author.

Chitty, K. K., & Black, B. P. (2007). *Professional nursing: Concepts and challenges* (5th ed.). St. Louis: Elsevier.

Covey, S. (2006). *Habit 3: Put first things first.* Salt Lake City, UT: Franklin Covey.

Ellis, J. R., & Hartley, C. L. (2007). *Nursing in today's world: Trends, issues, and management* (9th ed.). Philadelphia: Lippincott Williams & Wilkins.

Hansten, R. I., & Jackson, M. (2008). *Clinical delegation skills* (4th ed.). Boston: Jones & Bartlett.

International Council of Nurses. (2001). *Constitution and regulations.* Geneva, Switzerland: Author.

Kelly, P. (2008). *Nursing leadership & management* (2nd ed.). Clifton Park, NY: Cengage Delmar.

Mastal, M. R., Joshi, M., & Schulke, K. (2007). Nursing leadership: Championing quality and patient safety in the boardroom. *Nursing Economics, 25*(6), 323–330.

National Council of State Boards of Nursing. (2004). *Frequently asked questions regarding the National Council of State Boards of Nursing (NCSBN) Nurse Licensure Compact (NLC).* Retrieved December 2, 2008, from http://www.ncsbn.org/158.htm.

National Council of State Boards of Nursing. (2006). *Joint statement on delegation: American Nurses Association (ANA) and the National Council of State Boards of Nursing (NCSBN)*. Retrieved December 2, 2008, from https://www.ncsbn.org/joint_statement.pdf.

National Council of State Boards of Nursing. (2007). *NCLEX-RN: Test plan for the National Council Licensure examination for Registered Nurses*. Retrieved December 2, 2008, from https://ncsbn.org/1287.htm.

National Council of State Boards of Nursing. (2008). *Participating states in the NLC*. Retrieved December 2, 2008, from http://www.ncsbn.org/158.htm.

National League for Nursing. (2008). *Bylaws*. New York: Author.

National Student Nurses Association. (2008). *Getting the pieces to fit 2008–2009: A handbook for state associations and school chapters*. New York: Author.

U.S. Department of Health and Human Services, Health Resources & Services Administration. (2008). *Practitioner data banks*. Retrieved December 2, 2008, from http://bhpr.hrsa.gov/dqa.

Zerwekh, J., & Claborn, J. C. (2008). Reality shock. In *Nursing today: Transition and trends* (6th ed.). Philadelphia: Saunders, pp. 3–24.

CHAPTER 12

Aiken, T. D. (2008). *Legal and ethical issues in health occupations* (2nd ed.). St. Louis, MO: Elsevier.

American Hospital Association. (2003). *The patient care partnership: Understanding rights, expectations, and responsibilities*. Chicago: Author.

American Nurses Association. (1994). *Position statement: Active euthanasia*. Washington, DC: Author.

American Nurses Association. (2001). *Code for nurses with interpretative statements*. Washington, DC: Author.

American Nurses Association. (2008a). *Guide to the code of ethics for nurses: Interpretation and application*. Washington, DC: Author.

American Nurses Association. (2008b). *Scope and standards of forensic nursing practice*. Washington, DC: Author.

Austin, S. (2008). Seven legal tips for safe nursing practice. *Nursing 2008, 38*(3), 34–40.

Burkhardt, M. A., & Nathaniel, A. K. (2007). *Ethics and issues in contemporary nursing* (3rd ed.) Clifton Park, NY: Cengage Delmar Learning.

Canadian Nurses Association. (2008). *Code of ethics for nursing: Centennial edition*. Ottawa: Author.

Centers for Medicare and Medicaid Services. (2003). Fraud report form. Retrieved June 30, 2004, from http://cms.hhs.gov/forms.

Ellis, J. R., & Hartley, C. L. (2007). *Nursing in today's world: Trends, issues, and management* (9th ed.). Philadelphia: Lippincott Williams & Wilkins.

International Council of Nurses. (2006). *ICN code for nurses: Ethical concepts applied to nursing*. Geneva: Imprimeries Populaires.

Occupational Safety & Health Administration. (2008). *Safety and health topics: Healthcare facilities*. Retrieved December 11, 2008, from http://www.osha.gov/SLTC/healthcarefacilities/index.html.

O'Donnell, L. T. (2007). Ethical dilemmas among nurses as they transition to hospital case management: Implications for organizational ethics, Part II. *Professional Case Management, 12*(4), 219–231.

Raths, L., Harmin, M., & Simon, S. (1978). *Values and teaching* (2nd ed.). Columbus, OH: Merrill.

U.S. Department of Health and Human Services. (2002). *HHS fact sheet: Modifications to the standards for privacy of individually identifiable health information—Final rule*. Retrieved August 27, 2002, from http://www.hhs.gov/news/press/2002press/20020809.html.

Westra, B. L., Delaney, C. W., Konicek, D., & Kennan, G. (2008). Nursing standards to support the electronic health record. *Nursing Outlook, 56*(5), 258–266.

Willson, B. (2007). Legal issues. *Nursing BC, 39*(3), 11.

Zerwekh, J., & Claborn, J. C. (2008). *Nursing today: Transition and trends* (6th ed.). Philadelphia: Saunders.

CHAPTER 13

American Nurses Association. (1985). *Code for nurses with interpretive statements*. Kansas City, MO: Author.

American Nurses Association. (1997). *Standards of clinical nursing practice*. Kansas City, MO: Author.

American Nurses Association. (2007). *Scope and standards of nursing informatics practice*. Washington, DC: American Nurses Publishing.

Androwick, I., Kraft, M., & Haas, S. (2008). Information technology core competencies: From now to tomorrow. *Nursing Outlook, 56*(4), 189–190.

Association of College and Research Libraries. (2008). *Information literacy competency standards for higher education*. Retrieved November 9, 2008, from http://www.ala.org/acrl/ilintro.html#ildef.

DeMilliano, M. (2009). *8 common charting mistakes to avoid*. Hatboro, PA: Nurses Service Organization. Retrieved March 5, 2009, from http://www.nso.com/nursing-resources/article/223.jsp.

Hakes, B., & Whittington, J. (2008). Assessing the impact of an electronic medical record on nurse documentation time. *CIN: Computers, Informatics, Nursing, 26*(4), 234–241.

Heathcare Information and Management Systems Society. (2008). *HIMSS'PHR, ePHR definition*. Retrieved November 17, 2008, from http://www.himss.org/asp/topics_FocusDynamic.asp?faid=228.

Hebda, T., & Czar, P. (2009). *Handbook of informatics for nurses & healthcare professionals*. Upper Saddle River, NJ: Pearson Prentice Hall.

Institute of Medicine. (2007). *The learning healthcare system: Workshop summary*. Washington, DC: National Academies Press.

Kossman, S., & Scheidenhelm, S. (2008). Nurses' perceptions of the impact of electronic health records on work and patient outcomes. *CIN: Computers, Informatics, Nursing, 26*(2), 69–77.

Kuruzovich, J., Angst, C., Faraj, S., & Agarwal, R. (2008). Wireless communication role in patient response time: A study of Vocera integration with a nurse call system. *CIN: Computers, Informatics, Nursing, 26*(3), 159–166.

Milo, D., & Carlton, K. (2008). A collaborative model to ensure graduating nurses are ready to use electronic health records. *CIN: Computers, Informatics, Nursing, 26*(1), 2–3.

Newhouse, R. (2008). Evidence synthesis: The good, the bad, and the ugly. *Journal of Nursing Administration, 38*(3), 107–109.

Ozbolt, J., & Saba, V. (2008). A brief history of nursing informatics in the United States of America. *Nursing Outlook, 56*(5), 199–205.

Prinz, L., Cramer, M., & Englund, A. (2008). Telehealth: A policy analysis for quality, impact on patient outcomes, and political feasibility. *Nursing Outlook, 56*(4), 152–158.

Salmond, S. (2007). Advancing evidence-based practice: A primer. *Orthopaedic Nursing, 26*(2), 114–125.

Simpson, R. (2008). Chief nurse executives: Creating nursing's future with IT. *Nursing Administration Quarterly, 32*(3), 253–256.

Skretkowicz, V. (Ed.). (1992). *Florence Nightingale's notes on nursing*. London: Scutari Press.

Stevens, K. (2008). Evidence and the executive expert opinion: Dr. Kathleen Stevens. *Journal of Nursing Administration, 38*(3), 109–111.

Straight, M. (2008). One strategy to reduce medication errors: The effect of an online continuing education module on nurses' use of the Lexi-Comp feature of the Pyxis MedStation 2000. *CIN: Computers, Informatics, Nursing, 26*(1), 23–30.

Thede, L. (2008). CIN Plus. *CIN: Computers, Informatics, Nursing, 26*(1), 2.

The Joint Commission (JC). National Patient Safety Goals. Retrieved November 17, 2008, from http://www.jc.org/accredited+organizations/patient+safety.

CHAPTER 14

Almerud, S., Alapack, R. J., Fridlund, B., & Ekebergh, M. (2008). Caught in an artificial split: A phenomenological study of being a caregiver in the technologically intense environment. *Intensive & Critical Care Nursing, 24*(2), 130–136.

American Nurses Association. (2004). *Nursing: Scope and standards of practice.* Washington, DC: Author.

Benner, P. (2001). *From novice to expert: Excellence and power in clinical nursing practice* (comm. ed.). Upper Saddle River, NJ: Prentice-Hall.

Canadian Nurses Association. (1986). *A definition of nursing practice. Standards for nursing practice.* Ottawa: Author.

Diers, D. (1986). To profess—To be a professional. *Journal of Nursing Administration, 16,* 27.

Dossey, B., Keegan, L., & Guzzetta, C. (2008). *Holistic nursing: A handbook for practice* (5th ed.). Boston: Jones & Bartlett.

Kirk, T. W. (2007). Beyond empathy: Clinical intimacy in nursing practice. *Nursing Philosophy, 8*(4), 233–243.

Leininger, M., & McFarland, M. R. (2002). *Transcultural nursing: Concepts, theories, research, and practice.* New York: McGraw-Hill.

McGrath, M. (2008). The challenges of caring in a technological environment: Critical care nurses' experiences. *Journal of Clinical Nursing, 17*(8), 1096–1104.

Nightingale, F. (1969). *Nursing: What it is and what it is not.* New York: Dover Publications.

O'Connell, E. (2008). Therapeutic relationships in critical care nursing: A reflection on practice. *Nursing in Critical Care, 13*(3), 138–143.

Oudshoorn, A., Ward-Griffin, C., & McWilliam, C. (2007). Client-nurse relationships in home-based palliative care: A critical analysis of power relations. *Journal of Clinical Nursing, 16*(8), 1435–1443.

Peplau, H. (1952). *Interpersonal relations in nursing.* New York: Putnam.

Reb, A. (2007). The experience of hope in women with advanced ovarian cancer. *Oncology Nursing Forum, 34*(2), 487.

Warelow, P., Edward, K. L., & Vinek, J. (2008). Care: What nurses say and what nurses do. *Holistic Nursing Practice, 22*(3), 146–153.

Watson, J. (2007). *Nursing: Human science and human care* (rev. ed.). Boston: Jones & Bartlett.

Watson, J. (2008). *The philosophy and science of caring* (rev. ed.). Denver: University Press of Colorado.

Williams, A. M., Dawson, S., & Kristjanson, L. J. (2008). Exploring the relationship between personal control and the hospital environment. *Journal of Clinical Nursing, 17*(12), 1601–1609.

CHAPTER 15

American Nurses Association. (2004). *Statement on the scope and standards of psychiatric–mental health clinical nursing practice.* Washington, DC: Author.

Antai-Otong, D., & Wasserman, F. (2007). Therapeutic communication. In D. Antai-Otong & P. Hawkins (Eds.), *Psychiatric nursing: Biological and behavioral concepts* (2nd ed.). Clifton Park, NY: Delmar Learning, pp. 149–175.

Bartlett, G., Blais, R., Tamblyn, R., Clermont, R. J., & MacGibbon, B. (2008). Impact of patient communication problems on the risk of

preventable adverse events in acute care settings. *Canadian Medical Association Journal, 178*(12), 1573–1574.

Boggs, K. (2006). Developing therapeutic communication. In K. Boggs & E. Arnold (Eds.), *Interpersonal relationships: Professional communication skills for nurses* (5th ed.). Philadelphia: Saunders, pp. 216–231.

Edelman, C. L., & Mandle, C. L. (2006). *Health promotion throughout the lifespan* (6th ed.). St. Louis, MO: Mosby Elsevier.

Kneisl, C. R. (2009). Communicating and relating. In C. R. Kneisl & E. Trigoboff, *Contemporary psychiatric mental health nursing* (2nd ed.). Upper Saddle River, NJ: Pearson, pp. 194–214.

North American Nursing Diagnosis Association International. (2009). *Nursing diagnoses—Definitions and classification 2009–2011.* Philadelphia: John Wiley & Sons, Inc.

Peplau, H. (1960). Talking with patients. *American Journal of Nursing, 60*(7), 964.

Ruesch, J. (1961). *Therapeutic communication.* New York: Norton.

Spector, R. E. (2008). *Cultural diversity in health and illness* (7th ed.). Upper Saddle River, NJ: Pearson.

Stuart, G. W., & Laraia, M. T. (2004). Therapeutic nurse-patient relationship. In G. W. Stuart & M. T. Laraia (Eds.), *Principles and practice of psychiatric nursing* (8th ed.). St. Louis, MO: Mosby, pp. 15–49.

CHAPTER 16

Bandura, A. (1977). *A social learning theory.* Englewood Cliffs, NJ: Prentice-Hall.

Bandura, A. (1986). *Social foundation of thought and action: A social, cognitive theory.* Englewood Cliffs, NJ: Prentice-Hall.

Becker, M. H. (1974). The health belief model and sick role behavior. *Health Education Monogram, 2,* 409–419.

Cagle, C. S. (2006). School-age child. In C. L. Edelman & C. L. Mandle (Eds.), *Health promotion throughout the life span* (6th ed.). St. Louis, MO: Mosby Elsevier, pp 467–501.

Costanzo, C., & Walker, S. N. (2008). Incorporating self-efficacy and interpersonal support in an intervention to increase physical activity in older women. *Women & Health, 47*(4), 91–108.

Dossey, B. M., & Guzzetta, C. E. (2008). *Holistic nursing: A handbook for practice* (5th ed.). Boston: Jones & Bartlett.

Dunn, H. (1961). *High-level wellness.* Arlington, VA: R. W. Beatty.

Edelman, C., & Mandle, C. L. (2006). *Health promotion throughout the life span* (6th ed.). St. Louis, MO: Mosby.

Fontaine, K. L. (2009). Gender identity and sexual disorders. In C. R. Kneisl & E. Trigoboff (Eds.), *Contemporary psychiatric-mental health nursing* (2nd ed.). Upper Saddle River, NJ: Prentice-Hall, pp. 521–548.

Go, G. V. (2006). Changing populations and health. In C. L. Edelman & C. L. Mandle (Eds.), *Health promotion throughout the life span* (6th ed.). St. Louis, MO: Mosby, pp. 23–49.

Guyton, A. C., & Hall, J. E. (2005). *Textbook of medical physiology* (11th ed.). Philadelphia: Elsevier.

Leavell, H., & Clark, A. E. (1965). *Preventive medicine for doctors in the community.* New York: McGraw-Hill.

Maslow, A. (1970). *Motivation and personality* (2nd ed.). New York: Harper & Row.

Masters, W., & Johnson, V. (1966). *The human sexual response.* Boston: Little, Brown.

Maville, J. A., & Huerta, C. G. (2007). Theoretical foundations of health promotion. InJ. A. Maville & C. G. Huerta (Eds.), *Health promotion in nursing* (2nd ed.). Clifton Park, NY: Delmar Learning, pp. 40–56.

North American Nursing Diagnosis Association International. (2009). *Nursing diagnoses—Definitions and classification 2009–2011.* Philadelphia: John Wiley & Sons, Inc.

Pender, N. J. (1987). *Health promotion in nursing practice.* East Norwalk, CT: Appleton & Lange.

Price, K. (2006). Health promotion and some implications of consumer choice. *Journal of Nursing Management, 14*(6), 494–501.

Rosenstock, I. (1974). Historical origin of the health belief model. In M. H. Becker (Ed.), *The health belief model and personal health behavior.* Thorofare, NJ: Charles B. Slack, pp. 3–24.

U.S. Department of Health and Human Services, Office of Disease Prevention and Health Promotion. (2005). *Healthy people 2010.* Retrieved November 17, 2008, from http://www.healthypeople.gov.

CHAPTER 17

Administration for Children and Families, U.S. Department of Health and Human Services. (2008). *Child maltreatment 2006.* Washington, DC: Author. Retrieved July 22, 2008, from http://www.acf.hhs.gov/programs/cb/pubs/cm06/index.htm.

American Nurses Association. (2008). *Adapting standards of care under extreme conditions: Guidance for professionals during disasters, pandemics, and other extreme emergencies.* Washington, DC: Author.

Antai-Otong, D. (2007). *Psychiatric nursing: Biological and behavioral concepts* (2nd ed.). Clifton Park, NY: Cengage Delmar Learning.

Binder, E. B., Bradley, R. G., Liu, W., Epstein, M. P., Deveau, T. C., Mercer, K. B., et al. (2008). Association of FKBP5 polymorphisms and childhood abuse with risk of posttraumatic stress disorder symptoms in adults. *Journal of the American Medical Association, 299*(11), 1291–1305.

Bradley, R. G., Binder, E. B., Epstein, M. P., Tang, Y., Nair, H. P., Liu, W., et al. (2008). Influence of child abuse on adult depression: Moderation by the corticotrophin-releasing hormone receptor gene. *Archives of General Psychiatry, 65*(2), 190–200.

Carter, B., & McGoldrick, M. (2004). *The expanded life cycle: Individual, family, and societal perspectives* (3rd ed.). Boston: Allyn & Bacon.

Dreher, M., Shapiro, D., & Asselin, M. (2006). *Healthy places, healthy people: A handbook for culturally competent community nursing practice.* Indianapolis, IN: Sigma Theta Tau International.

Duvall, E. M., & Miller, B. C. (1985). *Marriage and family development* (6th ed.). New York: Harper & Row.

Economic Research Service, U.S. Department of Agriculture. (2006). *Briefing rooms: Food security in the United States: Measuring household food security.* Washington, DC: Author. Retrieved July 20, 2008, from http://www.ers.usda.gov/Briefing/FoodSecurity/measurement.htm.

Eggenberger, S. K., & Nelms, T. P. (2007). Being family: The family experience when an adult member is hospitalized with a critical illness. *Journal of Clinical Nursing, 16*(9), 1618–1628.

Fontaine, K. L. (2009). Persons at risk for abuse or violence. In C. R. Kneisl & E. Trigoboff (Eds.), *Contemporary psychiatric-mental health nursing* (2nd ed.). Upper Saddle River, NJ: Prentice Hall, pp. 638–669.

Hitchcock, J. E. (2003). Frameworks for assessing families. In J. E. Hitchcock, P. E. Schubert, & S. A. Thomas (Eds.), *Community health nursing: Caring in action* (2nd ed.). Clifton Park, NY: Delmar, pp. 589–622.

Holley, U. A. (2007). Social isolation: A practical guide for nurses assisting clients with chronic illness. *Rehabilitation Nursing, 32*(2), 51–56.

Hota, B., Ellenbogen, C., Hayden, M. K., Aroutcheva, A., Rice, T. W., & Weinsten, R. (2007). Community-associated methicillin-resistant *Staphylococcus aureus* skin and soft tissue infections at a public hospital: Do public housing and incarceration amplify transmission? *Archives of Internal Medicine, 167*(10), 1026–1033.

Hunt, R. (2009). *Introduction to community-based nursing* (4th ed.). Philadelphia: Wolters Kluwer Lippincott Williams & Wilkins.

Kaakien, J. R., Hanson, S. M., & Birenbaum, L. K. (2009). Family development and family nursing assessment. In M. Stanhope & J. Lancaster (Eds.), *Foundations of nursing in the community: Community-oriented practice* (3rd ed.). St. Louis, MO: Elsevier, pp. 321–340.

Klevens, R. M., Morrison, M. A., Nadie, J., Petit, S., Gershman, K., Ray, S., et al. (2007). Invasive methicillin-resistant *Staphylococcus aureus* infections in the United States. *Journal of the American Medical Association, 298*(15), 1763–1771.

Moore, C. G., Probst, J. C., Tompkins, M., Cuffe, S., & Martin, A. B. (2007). The prevalence of violent disagreements in U.S. families: Effects of residence, race/ethnicity, and parental stress. *Pediatrics, 119*(Suppl. 1), S68–76.

Whitaker, R. C., Phillips, S. M., & Orzol, S. M. (2006). Food insecurity and the risks of depression and anxiety in mothers and behavior problems in their preschool-aged children. *Pediatrics, 118*(3), e859–868.

Widom, C. S., DuMont, K., & Czaja, S. J. (2007). A prospective investigation of major depressive disorder and comorbidity in abused and neglected children grown up. *Archives of General Psychiatry, 64*(1), 49–56.

CHAPTER 18

Centers for Disease Control and Prevention. (2007a). *Health protection goals.* Atlanta, GA: Author. Retrieved May 12, 2009, from http://www.cdc.gov/osi/goals/people/index.html.

Centers for Disease Control and Prevention. (2007b). *Recommended adult immunization schedule—United States, October 2007–September 2008.* Atlanta, GA: Author. Retrieved May 12, 2009, from http://www.cdc.gov/vaccines/pubs/acip-list.htm.

Centers for Disease Control and Prevention. (2007c). *Recommended immunization schedule for persons aged 0–6 years—United States, 2008.* Atlanta, GA: Author. Retrieved May 12, 2009, from http://www.cdc.gov/vaccines/pubs/acip-list.htm.

Centers for Disease Control and Prevention. (2007d). *Recommended immunization schedule for persons aged 7–18 years—United States, 2008.* Retrieved May 12, 2009, from http://www.cdc.gov/vaccines/pubs/acip-list.htm.

Clawson, B., Selden, M., Lacks, M., Deaton, A. V., Hall, B., & Bach, R. (2008). Complex pediatric feeding disorders: Using teleconferencing technology to improve access to a treatment program. *Pediatric Nursing, 34*(3), 213–216.

Ebersole, P., Hess, P., Luggen, A. S., Touhy, T., & Jett, K. (2007). *Toward healthy aging: Human needs and nursing response* (7th ed.). St. Louis, MO: Elsevier.

Edelman, C. L., & Mandle, C. L. (2006). *Health promotion throughout the lifespan* (6th ed.). St. Louis, MO: Mosby.

Erikson, E. (1968). *Childhood and society.* New York: Norton.

Estes, M. E. Z. (2010). *Health assessment and physical examination* (4th ed.). Clifton Park, NY: Delmar/Cengage Learning.

Fowler, J. W. (1981). *Stages of faith: The psychology of human development and the quest for meaning.* New York: Harper & Row.

Freud, S. (1961). *Civilization and its discontents.* New York: Norton.

Gilligan, C. (1982). *In a different voice: Psychologic theory and women's development.* Cambridge, MA: Harvard University Press.

Gilligan, C., & Attanucci, D. (1988). Two moral orientations: Gender differences and similarities. *Merrill-Palmer Quarterly, 34*(3), 332–333.

Guyton, A. C., & Hall, J. E. (2005). *Textbook of medical physiology* (11th ed.). Philadelphia: Elsevier.

Hale, P. J. (2006). HIV, hepatitis, and sexually transmitted diseases. In M. Stanhope & J. Lancaster (Eds.), *Foundations of community health nursing* (2nd ed.). St. Louis, MO: Mosby, pp. 535–560.

Havighurst, R. J. (1972). *Developmental tasks and education.* New York: Longman.

Herrmann, N. (1990). *The creative brain* (2nd ed.). Lake Lure, NC: Ned Herrmann Group.

Hockenberry, M. J., Wilson, D., & Jackson, C. (2006). *Wong's nursing care of infants and children* (8th ed.). St. Louis, MO: Elsevier.

Ignatavicius, D. D., & Workman, M. L. (2009). *Medical-surgical nursing: Critical thinking for collaborative care* (6th ed.). St. Louis, MO: Elsevier.

Kneisl, C. R., & Trigoboff, E. (2009). *Contemporary psychiatric mental health nursing* (2nd ed.). Upper Saddle River, NJ: Pearson.

Kohlberg, L. (1977). *Recent research in moral development.* New York: Holt, Rinehart, & Winston.

Leung, A. K. C., & Robson, W. L. M. (2008). Premature adrenarche. *Journal of Pediatric Healthcare, 22*(4), 230–233.

Levinson, D. (1978). *The seasons of a man's life.* New York: Knopf.

Mainstone, A. (2008). Essential nutrition for babies. *British Journal of Midwifery, 16*(9), 612–616.

Murray, R. B., Zentner, J. P., & Yakimo, R. (2008). *Nursing assessment and health promotion through the lifespan* (8th ed.). Upper Saddle River, NJ: Prentice-Hall.

Piaget, J. (1963). *The origins of intelligence in children.* New York: Norton.

Piaget, J., & Inhelder, B. (1969). *The psychology of the child.* New York: Basic Books.

Sullivan, H. S. (1953). *Interpersonal theory of psychiatry.* New York: Norton.

Varcarolis, E., & Halter, M. J. (2008). *Essentials of psychiatric mental health nursing: A communication approach to evidence-based practice.* St. Louis, MO: Elsevier.

CHAPTER 19

American Association of Retired Persons Foundation. (2007). State fact sheets for grandparents and other relatives raising children. Retrieved November 26, 2008, from http://aarp.org/family/grand-parenting/articles.

American Nurses Association. (2001). *Scope and standards of gerontological nursing practice* (2nd ed.). Washington, DC: Author.

Ayalon, L. (2008). Volunteering as a predictor of all-cause mortality: What aspects of volunteering really matter? *International Psychogeriatics, 20*(5), 1000–1013.

Belsky, J. (2007). *Experiencing the lifespan.* New York: Worth.

Carpenito, J. L. (2007). *Handbook of nursing diagnosis* (12th ed.). Philadelphia: Lippincott Williams & Wilkins.

Centers for Medicare and Medicaid Services. (2008). Alternatives to nursing home care. Retrieved November 22, 2008, from http://www.cms.hhs.gov.

Counsell, S. R., Callahan, C. M., Clark, D. O., Tu, W., Buttar, A. B., Stump, T. E., et al. (2007). Geriatric care management for low-income seniors: A randomized controlled trial. *Journal of the American Medical Association, 298*(22), 2673–2674.

Cowely, J., Diebold, C., Gross, J. C., & Hardin-Fanning, F. (2006). Management of common problems. In K. L. Mauk (Ed.), *Gerontological nursing: Competencies for care.* Boston: Jones & Bartlett, pp. 475–562.

Doenges, M. E., Moorhouse, M. F., & Geissler, A. C. (2006). *Nursing care plans: Guidelines for individualizing patient care* (7th ed.). Philadelphia: F. A. Davis.

Dowdall, S. M., Taplay, K., Flores-Vela, A., & Maville, J. A. (2007). The older adult. In J. A. Maville & C. G. Huerta (Eds.), *Health promotion in nursing* (2nd ed.). Clifton Park, NY: Delmar Cengage Learning, pp. 267–291.

Ebersole, P., Hess, P., Luggen, A. S., Touhy, T., & Jett, K. (2007). *Toward healthy aging: Human needs and nursing response* (7th ed.). St. Louis, MO: Mosby Elsevier.

Erikson, E. (1968). *Childhood and society.* New York: Norton.

Federal Interagency Forum on Aging Related Statistics. (2007). *Older Americans 2008.* Retrieved November 22, 2008, from http://aging-stats.gov/agingstatsdotnet/main_site/data/2008_documents/population.pdf.

Fontaine, K. L. (2009). Persons at risk for violence. In C. R. Kneisl & E. Trigoboff (Eds.), *Contemporary psychiatric-mental health nursing* (2nd ed.). Upper Saddle River, NJ: Pearson Prentice Hall. pp. 638–669.

Hao, Y. (2008). Productive activities and psychological well-being among older adults. *Journals of Gerontology. Series B, Psychological Sciences and Social Sciences, 63*(2), S64–72.

Kautz, D. D. (2006). Appreciating diversity and enhancing intimacy. In K. L. Mauk (Ed.), *Gerontological nursing: Competencies for cure.* Boston: Jones & Bartlett, pp. 619–646.

Lindau, S. T., Schumm, L. P., Laumann, E. O., Levinson, W., O'Muircheartaigh, C. A., & Waite, L. J. (2007). A study of sexuality and health among older adults in the U.S. *New England Journal of Medicine, 357*(8), 762–774.

Matsui, M., & Capezuti, E. (2008). Perceived autonomy and self-care resources among senior center users. *Geriatric Nursing, 29*(2), 141–147.

Mauk, K. L. (2006). Introduction to gerontological nursing. In K. L. Mauk (Ed.), *Gerontological nursing: Competencies for care.* Boston: Jones & Bartlett, pp. 5–28.

Murray, R. B., Zentner, J. P., & Yakimo, R. (2008). *Nursing assessment and health promotion strategies through the life span* (8th ed.). Norwalk, CT: Appleton & Lange.

North American Nursing Diagnosis Association International. (2009). *Nursing diagnoses—Definitions and classification 2009–2011.* Philadelphia: John Wiley & Sons, Inc.

Piliavin, J. A., & Siegl, E. (2008). Health benefits of volunteering in the Wisconsin longitudinal study. *Journal of Health and Social Behavior, 48*(4), 450–464.

Radina, M. E., Lynch, A., Stalp, M. C., & Manning, L. K. (2008). "When I am an old woman, I shall wear purple": Red Hatters cope with getting old. *Journal of Women & Aging, 20*(1-2), 99–114.

Trigoboff, E. (2009). Elders. In C. R. Kneisl & E. Trigoboff (Eds.), *Contemporary psychiatric-mental health nursing* (2nd ed.). Upper Saddle River, NJ: Pearson Prentice-Hall, pp. 749–772.

U.S. Census Bureau. (2008). *Current population survey, annual social and economic supplement, 1960–2007.* Retrieved November 22, 2008, from http://www.census.gov.

U.S. Department of Justice. (2008). *Victim characteristics, summary findings.* Retrieved November 26, 2008, from http://www.ojp.usdoj.gov/bjs/cvict_v.htm.

van Solinge, H., & Henkens, K. (2008). Adjustment to and satisfaction with retirement: Two of a kind? *Psychology and Aging, 23*(2), 422–434.

Wallace, M. (2006). Older adult. In C. L. Edelman & C. L. Mandle (Eds.), *Health promotion throughout the lifespan* (6th ed.). St. Louis, MO: Mosby, pp. 571–598.

Windsor, T. D., Anstey, K. J., & Rodgers, B. (2008). Volunteering and psychological well-being among young-old adults: How much is too much? *Gerontologist, 48*(1), 59–70.

CHAPTER 20

Berry-Caban, C. S., & Crespo, H. (2008). Cultural competency as a skill for health care providers. *Hispanic Health Care International, 6*(3), 115–121.

College of Nurses of Ontario. (2008). *Culturally sensitive care: Practice guideline.* Retrieved August 1, 2009, from http://www.cno.org/docs/qa/44027_PRguide.pdf.

Degazon, C. (2006). Cultural influences in nursing in community health. In M. Stanhope & J. Lancaster (Eds.), *Foundations of community health nursing* (2nd ed.). St. Louis, MO: Mosby, pp. 73–92.

Edelman, C. L., & Mandle, C. L. (2006). *Health promotion throughout the life span* (6th ed.). St. Louis, MO: Mosby.

Fralic, M. F. (1995). Leading a diverse healthcare workforce [Comment]. *Capsules & Comments in Nursing Leadership & Management, 2*(4), 31.

Hall, J. M., Robinson, C. H., & Broyles, T. J. (2007). Environmental health. In M. A. Nies & M. McEwen (Eds.), *Community/public health nursing: Promoting health of populations* (4th ed., p. 237). Philadelphia: Saunders Elsevier, pp. 196–209.

Leininger, A. M. (2005). *Culture care diversity and universality: A worldwide nursing theory* (2nd ed.). Boston: Jones & Bartlett.

Munoz, C., & Luckmann, J. (2005). *Transcultural communication in nursing* (2nd ed.). Clifton Park, NY: Thomson Delmar Learning.

National Center for Health Statistics. (2007). *Chartbook on trends in the health of Americans/Health, United States, 2007.* Hyattsville, MD: Author. Retrieved December 19, 2008, from http://www.cdc.gov/nchs.

National Conference of State Legislatures. (2008). *Children's health reforms and 2008 federal poverty guidelines.* Retrieved December 19, 2008, from http://www.ncsl.org/programs/health/kidsins.htm.

North American Nursing Diagnosis Association International. (2009). *Nursing diagnoses—Definitions and classification 2009–2011.* Philadelphia: John Wiley & Sons, Inc.

Peguero, A. A. (2008). Is immigrant status relevant in school violence research? An analysis with Latino students. *Journal of School Health, 78*(7), 397–404.

Smith, W. R., Betancourt, J. R., Wynia, M. K., Bussey-Jones, J., Stone, V. E., Phillips, C. O., et al. (2007). Recommendations for teaching about racial and ethnic disparities in health and health care. *Annals of Internal Medicine, 147*(9), 654–665.

Spector, R. E. (2008). *Cultural diversity in health and illness* (7th ed.). Upper Saddle River, NJ: Prentice-Hall.

Stanhope, M., & Lancaster, J. (2006). *Foundations of community health nursing* (2nd ed.). St. Louis, MO: Mosby.

U.S. Census Bureau. (2008). *Income, poverty, and health insurance coverage in the United States: 2007.* Retrieved August 1, 2009, from http://www.census.gov/www/prod/2008pubs/p60-235.pdf.

U.S. Department of Human Services. (n.d.). *Healthy people 2010.* Retrieved December 19, 2008, from http://www.healthypeople.gov.

Warren, B. J. (2008). Ethnopharmacology: The effect on patients, health care professionals, and systems. *Urologic Nursing, 28*(4), 292–295.

Weidel, J. J., Provencio-Vasquez, E., Watson, S. D., & Gonzales-Guarda, R. (2008). Cultural consideration for intimate partner violence and HIV risk in Hispanics. *Journal of the Association for Nurses in AIDS Care, 19*(4), 247–251.

CHAPTER 21

American Hospital Association. (2003). *The patient care partnership: Understanding rights, expectations, and responsibilities.* Chicago: Author.

American Nurses Association. (2003). *Nursing: A social policy statement* (2nd ed.). Washington, DC: Author.

American Psychiatric Association. (2000). *Diagnostic and statistical manual of mental disorders* (4th ed., text rev.). Washington, DC: Author.

Bandura, A. (1977). *Social learning theory.* Englewood Cliffs, NJ: Prentice-Hall.

Bloom, B. S. (1977). *Taxonomy of educational objectives: The classification of educational goals, Handbook I: Cognitive domain.* New York: Longman.

Ebersole, P., Hess, P., Luggen, A. S., Touhy, T., & Jett, K. (2007). *Toward healthy aging: Human needs and nursing response* (7th ed.). St. Louis, MO: Elsevier, pp. 438–475.

Edelman, C. L., & Mandle, C. L. (2006). *Health promotion throughout the life span* (6th ed.). St. Louis, MO: Elsevier Mosby.

Hunt, R. (2009). *Introduction to community-based nursing* (4th ed.). Philadelphia: Lippincott Williams & Wilkins.

Knowles, M. S. (1984). *The adult learner: A neglected species* (3rd ed.). Houston: Gulf Publishing.

Louisiana State Board of Nursing. (2004). *Law governing the practice of nursing.* New Orleans: Author.

Mauk, K. L. (2010). Teaching older adults. In K. L. Mauk (Ed.), *Gerontological nursing: Competencies for care.* Boston: Jones & Bartlett, pp. 284–299.

Pieper, B., Sieggreen, M., Nordstrom, C. K., Freeland, B., Kulwicki, P., Frattaroli, M., et al. (2007). Discharge knowledge and concerns of patients going home with a wound. *Journal of Wound and Ostomy Continence Nursing, 34*(3), 245–253.

Schaefer, C. T. (2008). Integrated review of health literacy interventions. *Orthopaedic Nursing, 27*(5), 301–317.

Weld, K. K., Padden, D., Ramsey, G., & Bibb, S. C. G. (2008). A framework for guiding health literacy research in populations with universal access to healthcare. *Advances in Nursing Science, 31*(4), 308–318.

CHAPTER 22

Edelman, C. L., & Mandle, C. L. (2006). *Health promotion throughout the life span* (6th ed.). St. Louis, MO: Mosby Elsevier.

Evans, R. R., Roy, J., Geiger, B. F., Werner, K. A., & Burnett, D. (2008). Ecological strategies to promote healthy body image among children. *Journal of School Health, 78*(7), 359–367.

McWilliams, J. R., & McWilliams, P. (1991). *Life 101.* Los Angeles: Prelude Press.

North American Nursing Diagnosis Association International. (2009). *Nursing diagnoses—Definitions and classification 2009–2011.* Philadelphia: John Wiley & Sons, Inc.

Peplau, H. E. (1959). *Interpersonal relations in nursing.* New York: Putnam.

Rushton, C. H. (2007). Respect in critical care: A foundational ethical principle. *AACN Advanced Critical Care, 18*(2), 149–156.

Stuart, G. W., & Laraia, M. T. (2008). *Stuart & Sundeen's principles and practices of psychiatric nursing* (9th ed.). St. Louis, MO: Mosby Elsevier.

Sullivan, H. S. (1953). *The interpersonal theory of psychiatry.* New York: Norton.

CHAPTER 23

Aguilera, D. C. (1997). *Crisis intervention: Theory and methodology* (8th ed.). St. Louis, MO: Mosby.

Alfaro-LeFevre, R. (2008). *Critical thinking in nursing: A practical approach* (4th ed.). Philadelphia: Saunders.

Beck, A. (1976). *Cognitive therapy and emotional disorders.* New York: International Universities Press.

Carpenito, L. J. (2007). *Handbook of nursing diagnosis* (12th ed.). Philadelphia: Lippincott Williams & Wilkins.

Centers for Disease Control and Prevention. (2008). *Overweight and obesity.* Retrieved December 28, 2008, from http://www.cdc.gov/nccdphp/dnpa/obesity.

DeLaune, S. C. (2009). Anxiety and dissociative disorders. In C. R. Kneisl & E. Trigoboff (Eds.), *Contemporary psychiatric-mental health nursing* (2nd ed.). Upper Saddle River, NJ: Prentice-Hall, pp. 443–477.

Doenges, M. E., Moorhouse, M. F., & Murr, A. C. (2006). *Nursing care plans: Guidelines for individualizing patient care* (7th ed.). Philadelphia: F. A. Davis.

Fontaine, K. L. (2004). *Healing practices: Alternative therapies for nursing.* Upper Saddle River, NJ: Prentice-Hall.

Freud, S. (1959). Inhibitions, symptoms and anxiety. In J. Strachey (Trans.), *The standard edition of the complete psychological works of Sigmund Freud* (Vol. 20). London: Hogarth Press.

Keegan, L. (2008). Nutrition, exercise, and movement. In B. M. Dossey & L. Keegan (Eds.), *Holistic nursing: A handbook for practice* (5th ed.). Boston: Jones & Bartlett, pp. 257–287.

Kobasa, S. C. (1979). Stressful life events, personality and health. An inquiry into hardiness. *Journal of Personality and Social Psychology, 37*(1), 1–11.

Kobasa, S. C., Maddi, S. R., & Kahn, S. (1982). Hardiness and health: A prospective study. *Journal of Personality and Social Psychology, 45*(4), 839–850.

Lewin, K. (1951). *Field theory in social science.* New York: Harper.

Lippitt, R., Watson, J., & Westley, B. (1958). *The dynamics of planned change.* New York: Harcourt Brace.

Nemcek, M. A., & James, G. D. (2007). Relationships among the nurse work environment, self-nurturance and life satisfaction. *Journal of Advanced Nursing, 59*(3), 240–247.

North American Nursing Diagnosis Association International. (2009). *Nursing diagnoses—Definitions and classification 2009–2011.* Philadelphia: John Wiley & Sons, Inc.

Peplau, H. E. (1952). *Interpersonal relations in nursing.* New York: Putnam.

Rentfro, A. R. (2006). Health promotion and the individual. In C. L. Edelman & C. L. Mandle (Eds.), *Health promotion throughout the life span* (6th ed., pp. 129–151). St. Louis, MO: Mosby.

Selye, H. (1974). *Stress without distress.* New York: New American Library.

Selye, H. (1976). *Stress in health and disease* (Rev. ed.). Boston: Butterworths.

Shirley, M. R. (2006). Authentic leaders creating healthy work environments for nursing practice. *American Journal of Critical Care, 15*(3), 256–267.

Stuart, G. W., & Laraia, M. T. (2008). *Stuart & Sundeen's principles and practice of psychiatric nursing* (9th ed.). St. Louis, MO: Elsevier.

Sullivan, H. S. (1953). *The interpersonal theory of psychiatry.* New York: Norton.

CHAPTER 24

Burkhardt, M. A., & Nagai-Jacobson, M. G. (2008). Transcultural and spiritual issues. In M. A. Burkhardt & A. K. Nathaniel (Eds.), *Ethics & issues in contemporary nursing* (3rd ed.). Clifton Park, NY: Thomson Delmar Learning.

Carpenito-Moyet, L. J. (2007). *Nursing diagnosis: Application to clinical practice* (12th ed.). Philadelphia: Lippincott Williams & Wilkins.

Davis, L. (2006). Hospitalized patients' expectations of spiritual care from nurses. In S. D. Ambrose (Ed.), *Religion and psychology: New research.* Hauppague, NY: Nova Science Publishers.

Dew, R. E., Daniel, S. S., Goldston, D. B., & Koenig, H. G. (2008). Religion, spirituality, and depression in adolescent psychiatric outpatients. *Journal of Nervous and Mental Disease, 196*(3), 247–251.

Dossey, B. M., & Keegan, L. (2008). *Holistic nursing: A handbook for practice* (5th ed.). Boston: Jones & Bartlett.

Estes, M. E. Z. (2010). *Health assessment and physical examination* (4th ed.). Clifton Park, NY: Delmar/Cengage Learning.

Frankl, V. (1985). *Man's search for meaning.* New York: Washington Square Press.

Giger, J. N., & Davidhizar, R. E. (2007). *Transcultural nursing: Assessment and intervention* (5th ed.). St. Louis, MO: Mosby.

Griffin, M. T. Q., Salman, A., Lee, Y., Seo, Y., & Fitzpatrick, J. J. (2008). A beginning look at the spiritual practices of older adults. *Journal of Cardiovascular Nursing, 25*(2), 100–102.

Hockenberry, M. L., Wilson, D., & Jackson, C. (2006). *Wong's nursing care of infants and children* (8th ed.). St. Louis, MO: Elsevier Science.

Hoffert, D., Henshaw, C., & Nvududu, N. (2007). Enhancing the ability of nursing students to perform a spiritual assessment. *Nurse Educator, 32*(2), 66–72.

International Council of Nurses. (2006). *ICN code of ethics for nurses.* Geneva, Switzerland: Author.

Koenig, H. G. (2007). Religion and remission of depression in medical inpatients with heart failure/pulmonary disease. *Journal of Nervous and Mental Disease, 195*(5), 389–395.

Loustalot, F. (2008). Assessing patients' spiritual needs. *Kai Tiaki Nursing New Zealand, 14*(8), 21–22.

Newlin, K., Melkus, G. D., Tappen, R., Chyun, D., & Koenig, H. G. (2008). Relationships of religion and spirituality to glycemic control in black women with type 2 diabetes. *Nursing Research, 57*(5), 331–339.

North American Nursing Diagnosis Association International. (2009). *Nursing diagnoses—Definitions and classification 2009–2011.* Philadelphia: John Wiley & Sons, Inc.

Pipe, T. B., Kelly, A., LeBrun, G., Schmidt, D., Atherton, P., & Robinson, C. (2008). A prospective descriptive study exploring hope, spiritual well-being, and quality of life in hospitalized patients. *MEDSURG Nursing, 17*(4), 247–257.

Reyes-Ortiz, C. A., Gerges, I. M., Raji, M. A., Koenig, H. G., Kuo, Y. F., & Markides, K. S. (2008). Church attendance mediates the association between depressive symptoms and cognitive functioning among older Mexican Americans. *Journals of Gerontology. Series A, Biological Sciences and Medical Sciences, 63*(5), 480–486.

Vivat, B. (2008). Measures of spiritual issues for palliative care patients: A literature review. *Palliative Medicine, 22,* 859–868.

CHAPTER 25

American Association of Colleges of Nursing. (2004). *Peaceful death: Recommended competencies and curricular guidelines for end-of-life nursing care.* Retrieved July 2004 from http://www.aacn.nche.edu.

American Association of Colleges of Nursing. (2008). *Fact sheet. End-of-Life Nursing Education Consortium (ELNEC).* Retrieved January 2, 2009, from http://www.aacn.nche/edu/ELNEC/factsheet.htm.

American Nurses Association. (1997). *Statement by the American Nurses Association on measuring the quality of care at the end of life.* Retrieved June 2004 from http://www.nursingworld.org.

Bowlby, J. (1961). The process of mourning. *International Journal of Psychoanalysis, 42*(33), 4–5.

Bowlby, J. (1982). *Attachment and loss: Vol. 2. Separation anxiety and anger.* New York: Basic Books.

Carpenito, L. J. (2007). *Handbook of nursing diagnosis* (12th ed.). Philadelphia: Lippincott Williams & Wilkins.

Center to Advance Palliative Care. (2009). *What is palliative care?* Retrieved January 2, 2009, from http://www.getpalliativecare.org/whatis.

Engle, G. L. (1961). Is grief a disease? *Psychosomatic Medicine, 23,* 18–22.

Engle, G. L. (1964). Grief and grieving. *American Journal of Nursing, 64*(9), 93–98.

Hospice Foundation of America. (2008). *Choosing hospice.* Retrieved January 2, 2009, from http://www.hospicefoundation.org.

International Council of Nurses. (1997). *Basic principles of nursing care.* Washington, DC: American Nurses Publishing.

Kübler-Ross, E. (1969). *On death and dying.* New York: Macmillan.

Kübler-Ross, E. (1974). *Questions and answers on death and dying.* New York: Macmillan.

Levin, B. (1998). Grief counseling. *American Journal of Nursing, 98*(5), 69–72.

Lindemann, E. (1944). Symptomatology and management of acute grief. *American Journal of Psychiatry, 101,* 141–148.

North American Nursing Diagnosis Association International. (2009). *Nursing diagnoses—Definitions and classification 2009–2011.* Philadelphia: John Wiley & Sons, Inc.

Robichaux, C. M., & Clark, A. P. (2006). Practic of expert critical care nurses in situations of prognostic conflict at the end of life. *American Journal of Critical Care, 15*(5), 480–490.

Spector, R. E. (2008). *Cultural diversity in health and illness* (7th ed.). Upper Saddle River, NJ: Prentice-Hall.

U.S. Census Bureau. (2008). *American community survey, 2005–2007.* Retrieved January 2, 2009, from http://www.census.gov/acs.

Worden, J. W. (1982). *Grief counseling and grief therapy: A handbook for the mental health practitioner.* New York: Springer.

Worden, J. W. (1991). *Grief counseling and grief therapy* (2nd ed.). New York: Springer.

CHAPTER 26

Beard, R., & Day, M. (2008). Fever and hyperthermia: Learn to beat the heat. *Nursing, 38*(6), 28–31.

Edelman, C. L., & Mandle, C. L. (2006). *Health promotion throughout the life span* (6th ed.). St. Louis, MO: Elsevier Health Sciences.

Exergen Corporation. (2008). *TemporalScanner temporal artery thermometry.* Watertown, MA: Author. Retrieved September 9, 2008, from http://www.exergen.com/medical/eductr/technology.htm.

Giger, J. N., & Davidhizar, R. E. (2008). *Transcultural nursing assessment and intervention* (5th ed.). St. Louis, MO: Elsevier Health Sciences.

Gray, B. B. (1995, June). What heals? What do nurses do that makes a difference? *Critical Care Nurse, 15*(3, Suppl.), 3–16.

Guyton, A. C., & Hall, J. E. (2007). *Textbook of medical physiology* (11th ed.). St. Louis, MO: Elsevier Health Sciences.

Ma, G., Sabin, N., & Dawes, M. (2008). A comparison of blood pressure measurement over a sleeved arm versus a bare arm. *Canadian Medical Association Journal, 178*(5), 585–589.

Moorhead, S., Johnson, M., & Maas, M. (2008). *Nursing outcomes classification (NOC)* (4th ed.). St. Louis, MO: Elsevier Health Sciences.

National High Blood Pressure Education Program, National Institutes of Health. (2003). *The Seventh Report of the Joint National Committee on Prevention, Detection, Evaluation, and Treatment of High Blood Pressure.* Bethesda, MD: Author. Retrieved September 8, 2008, from http://www.nhlbi.nih.gov/guidelines/hypertension/jnc7full.pdf.

North American Nursing Diagnosis Association International. (2007). *Nursing diagnoses: Definitions and classification 2007-2008.* Philadelphia: Author.

Schulman, C. (2005). The effect of antipyretic therapy upon outcomes in critically ill patients: A randomized, prospective study *Surgical Infections, 6*(4), 368–375.

CHAPTER 27

American Cancer Society. (2009). *Cancer facts and figures, 2009.* Retrieved August 18, 2009, from http://www.cancer.org/docwnloads/STT.500809web.pdf.

D'Amico, D., & Barbarito, C. (2007). *Health & physical assessment in nursing.* Upper Saddle River, NJ: Pearson Prentice Hall.

Estes, M. E. Z. (2010). *Health assessment and physical examination* (4th ed.). Clifton Park, NY: Delmar/Cengage Learning.

Giddens, J. F. (2007). A survey of physical assessment techniques performed by RNs: Lessons for nursing education. *Journal of Nursing Education, 46*(2), 83–87.

Jarvis, C. (2007). *Physical examination & health assessment* (5th ed.). Philadelphia: Elsevier.

Krebs, L. U. (2007). Sexual assessment: Research and clinical. *Nursing Clinics of North America, 42*(4), 525–529.

National Cancer Institute. (2008). *Surveillance epidemiology and end results.* Retrieved January 26, 2009, from http://seer.cancer.gov/statfacts/html/prost.html.

CHAPTER 28

Advice P.R.N. Venipuncture: Armed with the facts. (2008). *Nursing2008, 38*(6), 10.

American Cancer Society. (2008). *Blood test may spot people at risk for colorectal cancer.* Retrieved August 2008 from http://www.cancer.org.

Fischbach, F., & Dunning, M. (2008). *A manual of laboratory and diagnostic tests* (8th ed.). Philadelphia: Lippincott Williams & Wilkins.

Flasar, C. (2008). What is urine specific gravity? *Nursing2008, 37*(7), 14.

Joint Commission. (2008). *2009 hospitals' national patient safety goals.* Retrieved August 2008 from http://www.jcaho.org.

King, J. (2004). Cardiac stress tests: Which one, why, and when? *Nursing2004, 34*(3), 28.

McConnell, E. A. (1999). Hold the lab in the palm of your hand. *Nursing Management, 30*(5), 57–59.

National Center for Health Statistics. (1999). Deaths: Final data for 1997 (PHS 99–1120). *National Vital Statistics Reports, 47*(19).

Pagana, K. D., & Pagana, T. J. (2006). *Mosby's manual of diagnostic and laboratory tests* (3rd ed.). St. Louis, MO: Elsevier Health Science.

Pagana, K. D., & Pagana, T. J. (2009). *Mosby's diagnostic and laboratory test reference* (9th ed.). St. Louis, MO: Elsevier Health Science.

Rose, K., Rosamond, W., Huston, S., Murphy, C., & Tegeler, C. (2008). Predictors of time from hospital arrival to initial brain-imaging among suspected stroke patients. The North Carolina Collaborative Stroke Registry. *Stroke, 39*(12), 3262–3267.

Schallom, L. (1999). Point of care testing in critical care. *Critical Care Nursing Clinics of North America, 11*(1), 99–106.

Skretkowicz, V. (Ed.). (1992). *Florence Nightingale's notes on nursing* (2nd ed.). London: Scutari Press.

CHAPTER 29

Advice, P.R.N. Hand hygiene: Rubbing out *C. difficile. Nursing2008, 38*(4), 12.

American Nurses Association. (2008). *Workplace safety and needlestick injuries are top concerns for nurses.* Retrieved September 14, 2008, from http://www.nursingworld.org/HomepageCategory/NursingInsider/Archive_1/2008NI/Jun.

Association of periOperative Registered Nurses. (2004). *Standards, recommended practices, and guidelines.* Denver, CO: Author.

Badiaga, S., Raoult, D., & Brouqui, P. (2008). Preventing and controlling emerging and reemerging transmissible diseases in the homeless. *Emerging Infectious Diseases, 14*(9). Retrieved September 12, 2008, from http://www.cdc.gov/EID/content/14/9/1353.htm.

Capezuti, E., Wagner, L., Brush, B., Boltz, M., Renz, S., & Secic, M. (2008). Bed and toilet height as potential environmental risk factors. *Clinical Nursing Research, 17*(1), 50–66.

Cassels, C. (2008). Falls in the elderly: A major cause of TBI death, injury. *Journal of Safety Research, 39*, 269–272.

Centers for Disease Control and Prevention. (2002). *Guidelines for hand hygiene in health-care settings.* Retrieved November 10, 2005, from www.cdc.gov/mmwr/preview/mmwrhtml/rr5116a1.htm.

Centers for Disease Control and Prevention. (2007). *Invasive MRSA.* Retrieved September 12, 2008, from http://www.cdc.gov/ncidod/dhqp/ar_mrsa_Invasive_FS.html.

Centers for Disease Control and Prevention. (2008). *Healthcare-associated infections (HAIs).* Retrieved September 12, 2008, from http://www.cdc.gov?ncidod/dhqp/healthDis.html.

Centers for Medicare & Medicaid Services. (2008). *Medicare takes new steps to help make your hospital stay safer.* Retrieved August 11, 2008, from http://www.cms.hhs.gov/pf/printpage.asp.

Ferris, M. (2008). Fall prevention in long-term care: Practical advice to improve care. *Topics in Advanced Practice Nursing eJournal.* Retrieved September 17, 2008, from http://www.medscape.com/viewarticle/579951.

Harris, H. (2006). *C. difficile*: Attack of the killer diarrhea. *Nursing Made Incredibly Easy, 4*(3), 12–19.

Hinshaw, A. (2008). Navigating the perfect storm: Balancing a culture of safety with workforce challenges. *Nursing Research, 57*(1S), S4–10.

Holcomb, S. (2008). MRSA infections. *Nursing2008, 38*(6), 33.

Joint Commission. (1999). *Introduction to the restraint standards in acute medical and surgical (nonpsychiatric) care. Comprehensive accreditation manual for hospitals.* Oakbrook Terrace, IL: Author.

Joint Commission. (2008). *2009 hospital national patient safety goals.* Retrieved September 12, 2008, from http://www.jointcommission.org/NR/rdonlyres/40A7233C-C4F7_4680_9861_80CDFD5F62C6/0/09_NPSG_HAP_gp_pdf.

Klevens, R., Morrison, M., Nadle, J., Petit, S., Gershman, K., Ray, S., et al. (2007). Invasive methicillin-resistant *Staphylococcus aureus* infections in the United States. *Journal of the American Medical Association, 298*(15), 1763–1771.

Kohn, L., Corrigan, J., & Donaldson, M. (Eds.). (1999). *To err is human: Building a safer health care system.* Washington, DC:

National Academies Press. Retrieved May 6, 2004, from http://bob.nap/edu/html/to_err_is_human.

National Institute for Occupational Safety and Health Centers for Disease Control and Prevention. (1997). *Preventing allergic reactions to natural rubber latex in the workplace.* (DHHS [NIOSH] Publication No. 97-135U). Washington, DC: U.S. Department of Health and Human Services, Public Health Service, Centers for Disease Control and Prevention, National Institute for Occupational Safety and Health.

North American Nursing Diagnosis Association. (2007). *Nursing diagnoses: Definitions and classification 2007–2008.* Philadelphia: Author.

Patient Safety and Quality Improvement Act of 2005, Pub. L. No. 109-41, 119 Stat. 424 (2005).

Ricci, A. (2008). Latex allergy. *Medicine & Health/Rhode Island, 91*(6), 183–186.

Shojania, D., Duncan, B., McDonald, K., & Wachter, R. M. (Eds.). (2001). *Making health care safer: A critical analysis of patient safety practices* (Evidence Report/Technology Assessment No. 43. Prepared by the University of California at San Francisco-Stanford Evidence-Based Practice Center under Contract No. 290-97-0013. AJRO [lib]; ocatopm Mp/01-E058). Rockville, MD: Agency for Healthcare Research and Quality. Retrieved May 6, 2004, from http://www.ahrq.gov/clinic/patsafety/pdf/ptsafety.pdf.

Taylor-Ford, R., Catlin, A., LaPlante, M., & Weinke, C. (2008). Effect of a noise reduction program on a medical-surgical unit. *Clinical Nursing Research, 17*(2), 74–88.

Tinetti, M., Baker, D., King, M., Gottschalk, M., Murphy, T., Acampora, D., et al. (2008). Effect of dissemination of evidence in reducing injuries from falls. *New England Journal of Medicine, 359*(3), 252–261.

Todd, B. (2006). *Clostridium difficile*: Familiar pathogen, changing epidemiology. *American Journal of Nursing, 106*(5), 33.

CHAPTER 30

American Nurses Association. (1997, March/April). ANA, other groups succeed in push for improved prescription information. *American Nurse, 29*(2), 11.

American Nurses Association. (2008). *2007 study of injectable medication errors.* Retrieved September 29, 2008, from http://www.nursingworld.org/HomepageCategory/NursingInsider/Archive-1/2008NI/Jun0.

Beyea, S. C., & Nicoll, L. H. (1995). Administration of medication via intramuscular route: An integrative review of the literature and research-based protocol for the procedure. *Applied Nursing Research, 8*(1), 23–33.

Beyea, S. C., & Nicoll, L. H. (1996). Back to basics: Administering IM injections the right way. *American Journal of Nursing, 96*(1), 34–35.

Brooke, P. (2008). Reporting medication errors: Who needs to know? *Nursing2008, 38*(7), 11.

Bulechek, G., Butcher, H., McCloskey, J., & Dochterman, J. (2008). *Nursing interventions classification (NIC)* (5th ed.). St. Louis, MO: Elsevier Health Science.

Centers for Disease Control and Prevention. (2007). *Standard precautions.* Retrieved September 13, 2008, from http://www.cdc.gov./ncidod/dhqp/gl_isolation_standard.html.

Cohen, M. (2008). Unlabeled syringe: Risky imposter. *Nursing2008, 38*(5), 20.

Crosby, L. R., & Bissell, L. (1989). *To care enough: Intervention with chemically dependent colleagues, a guide for healthcare & other professionals.* Edina, MN: Johnson Institute.

Dasgupta, A. (2003). Review of abnormal laboratory test results and toxic effects due to use of herbal medicines. *American Journal of Clinical Pathology, 120*(1), 127–137.

Dossey, B. M., & Keegan, L. (2008). *Holistic nursing: A handbook for practice* (5th ed.). Sudbury, MA: Jones & Bartlett.

Edlin, G., & Golanty, E. (1988). *Health and wellness* (3rd ed.). Boston: Jones & Bartlett.

Hunt, C. (2008). Which site is best for an I.M. injection? *Nursing2008, 38*(11), 62.

Institute for Safe Medication Practices. (2003). *Preventing medication errors. Medication safety alert! Cultural diversity and medication safety.* Retrieved March 1, 2004, from http://ismp.org/MSAarticles/diversityPrint.htm.

Moore, T. (2007). Serious adverse drug events reported to the Food and Drug Administration, 1998–2005. *Archives of Internal Medicine, 167*(16), 1752–1859.

Moorhead, S., Johnson, M., Maas, M., & Swanson, E. (2008). *Nursing outcomes classification (NOC)* (4th ed.). St. Louis, MO: Elsevier Health Sciences.

National Coordinating Council for Medication Error Reporting and Prevention. (2008). *What is a medication error?* Retrieved September 28, 2008, from http://www.nccmerp.org/about_ MedErrors. html.

North American Nursing Diagnosis Association International. (2009). *Nursing diagnoses—Definitions and classification 2009–2011.* Philadelphia: John Wiley & Sons, Inc.

White, L. B., & Foster, S. (2007). *The herbal drugstore* (2nd ed.). Emmaus, PA: Rodale.

CHAPTER 31

Balch, P. (2008). *Prescription for nutritional healing: The A-to-Z guide to supplements.* New York: Penguin.

Benson, H. (1975). *The relaxation response.* New York: William Morrow.

Benson, H. (2008). *Research overview of Benson-Henry Institute for Mind-Body Medicine, Massachusetts General Hospital.* Retrieved January 2, 2009, from http://www.mbmi.org/research/default.asp.

Bowlby, J. (1984). *Attachment and loss: Vol. 1. Attachment* (2nd ed.). London: Penguin Books.

Briones, T. L. (2007). Psychoneuroimmunology and related mechanisms in understanding health disparities in vulnerable populations. *Annual Review of Nursing Research, 25*, 219–256.

Brown, C. A., & Lido, C. (2008). Reflexology treatment for patients with lower limb amputations and phantom limb—An exploratory pilot study. *Complementary Therapies in Clinical Practice, 14*(2), 124–131.

Buckle, J. (2007). Literature review: Should nursing take aromatherapy more seriously? *British Journal of Nursing, 16*(2), 116–120.

Can Gurkan, O., & Arslan, H. (2008). Effect of acupressure on nausea and vomiting during pregnancy. *Complementary Therapies in Clinical Practice, 14*(1), 46–52.

Choi, A. N., Lee, M. S., & Lim, H. J. (2008). Effects of group music intervention on depression, anxiety, and relationships in psychiatric patients: A pilot study. *Journal of Alternative & Complementary Medicine, 14*(5), 567–570.

Cooke, M., Holzhauser, K., Jones, M., Davis, C., & Finucane, J. (2007). The effect of aromatherapy massage with music on the stress and anxiety levels of emergency nurses: Comparison between summer and winter. *Journal of Clinical Nursing, 16*(9), 695–703.

Cousins, N. (1979). *Anatomy of an illness.* New York: Norton.

Csordas, T. J., Storck, M. J., & Strauss, M. (2008). Diagnosis and distress in Navajo healing. *Journal of Nervous & Mental Disorders, 196*(8), 586–596.

Cuellar, N. G. (2008). Mindfulness meditation for veterans—Implications for occupational health providers. *AAOHN Journal, 56*(8), 357–363.

Eliopoulos, C. (2009). *An invitation to holistic health: A guide to living a balanced life.* Boston: Jones & Bartlett.

Fontaine, K. L. (2004). *Complementary and alternative therapies for nursing practice* (2nd ed.). Upper Saddle River, NJ: Prentice-Hall.

Fyffe, D. C., Brown, E. L., Sirey, J. A., Hill, E. G., & Bruce, M. L. (2008). Older home-care patients' preferred approaches to depression care: A pilot study. *Journal of Gerontological Nursing, 34*(8), 17–22.

Garran, T. A. (2008). *Westerns herbs according to traditional Chinese medicine.* Rochester, VT: Inner Traditions/Bear.

Gladstar, R. (2008). *Rosemary Gladstar's herbal recipes for vibrant health.* North Adams, MA: Storey Books.

Good, M., & Ahn, S. (2008). Korean and American music reduce pain in Korean women after gynecologic surgery. *Pain Management Nursing, 9*(3), 96–103.

Hoffman, D. (2007). *Herbal prescriptions after 50: Everything you need to know to maintain vibrant health* (2nd ed.). Rochester, VT: Inner Traditions International.

Hughes, D., Ladas, E., Rooney, D., & Kelly, K. (2008). Massage therapy as supportive care intervention for children with cancer. *Oncology Nursing Forum, 35*(3), 431–442.

Ikedo, F., Gangahar, D. M., Quader, M. A., & Smith, L. M. (2007). The effects of prayer, relaxation technique during general anesthesia on recovery outcomes following cardiac surgery. *Complementary Therapies in Clinical Practice, 13*(2), 85–94.

Jackson, E., Kelly, M., McNeil, P., Meyer, E., Schlegel, L., & Eaton, M. (2008). Does therapeutic touch help reduce pain and anxiety in patients with cancer? *Clinical Journal of Oncology Nursing, 12*(1), 113–120.

Kalavapalli, R., & Singareddy, R. (2007). Role of acupuncture in the treatment of insomnia: A comprehensive review. *Complementary Therapies in Clinical Practice, 13*(3), 184–193.

Khalsa, K. P. S., & Tierra, M. (2009). *The way of Ayurvedic herbs: A contemporary introduction and useful manual for the world's oldest healing system.* Twin Lakes, WI: Lotus Press.

Kim, K. B., & Sok, S. R. (2007). Auricular acupuncture for insomnia: Duration and effects in Korean older adults. *Journal of Gerontological Nursing, 33*(8), 23–31.

Kim, S. S., Erlen, J. A., Kim, K. B., & Sok, S. R. (2006). Nursing students' and faculty members' knowledge of, experience with, and attitudes toward complementary and alternative therapies. *Journal of Nursing Education, 45*(9), 375–378.

Kunz, D., & Krieger, D. (2004). *The spiritual dimension of therapeutic touch.* Rochester, VT: Inner Traditions International.

Leddy, S. K. (2006). *Integrative health promotion: Conceptual bases for nursing practice* (2nd ed.). Boston: Jones & Bartlett.

Lukan, N., Racz, O., Mocnejova, I., & Tkac, I. (2008). Monitoring antioxidant enzymes in red cells during allergen immunotherapy. *Journal of Physiology & Biochemistry, 64*(2), 143–148.

Maa, S. H., Sun, M. F., & Wu, C. C. (2008). The effectiveness of acupuncture on pain and mobility in patients with osteoarthritis of the knee: A pilot study. *Journal of Nursing Research, 16*(2), 1401–1448.

MacIntyre, B., Hamilton, J., Fricke, T., Ma, W., Mehle, S., & Michel, M. (2008). The efficacy of healing touch in coronary artery bypass surgery recovery: A randomized clinical trial. *Alternative Therapies in Health & Medicine, 14*(4), 24–32.

Macrae, J. (2005). *Therapeutic touch: A practical guide.* New York: Alfred A. Knopf.

Magill, L., & Berenson, S. (2008). The conjoint use of music therapy and reflexology with hospitalized advanced stage cancer patients and their families. *Palliative & Supportive Care, 6*(3), 289–296.

Mayo Clinic. (2007). Relaxation techniques: Learn ways to calm your stress. Retrieved January 3, 2009 from http://www.mayoclinic.com/health/relaxationtechnique/SR00007.

McVicar, A. J., Greenwood, C. R., Fewell, F., D'Arcy, V., Chandrase-kharan, S., & Alldridge, L. C. (2007). Evaluation of anxiety, salivary cortisol and melatonin secretion following reflexology treatment: A pilot study in healthy individuals. *Complementary Therapies in Clinical Practice, 13*(3), 137–145.

Mehl-Madrona, L. (2008). Narratives of exceptional survivors who work with aboriginal healers. *Journal of Alternative & Complementary Medicine, 14*(5), 497–504.

Montague, A. (1986). *Touching: The human significance of the skin* (3rd ed.). New York: Perennial Library.

National Cancer Institute. (2007). *Cancer trends progress report – 2007 update.* Retrieved January 3, 2009, from http://progressreport.cancer.gov/highlights.asp.

National Center for Complementary and Alternative Medicine. (2007a). *Prayer and spirituality in health: Ancient practices, modern science.* Retrieved January 3, 2009, from http://nccam.nih.gov/news/newsletter.

National Center for Complementary and Alternative Medicine. (2007b). *What is complementary and alternative medicine (CAM)?* Retrieved December 29, 2008, from http://nccam.nih.gov/health/whatiscam.

National Center for Complementary and Alternative Medicine. (2008). *2007 statistics on CAM use in the United States.* Retrieved December 29, 2008, from http://nccam.nih.gov/news/camstats.htm.

National Center for Complementary and Alternative Medicine. (2009). *Get the facts: 10 things to know about evaluating medical resources on the Web.* Retrieved August 12, 2009, from http://nccam.nih.gov/health/webresoruces.

Nightingale, F. (1860). *Notes on nursing: What it is and what it is not.* London: Harrison & Sons.

North American Nursing Diagnosis Association International. (2009). *Nursing diagnoses—Definitions and classification 2009–2011.* Philadelphia: John Wiley & Sons, Inc.

Raglio, A., Bellelli, G., Traficante, D., Gianotti, M., Ubezio, M. C., Villani, D., et al. (2008). Efficacy of music therapy in the treatment of behavioral and psychiatric symptoms of dementia. *Alzheimer Disease & Associated Disorders, 22*(2), 158–162.

Reed, T. (2007). Imagery in the clinical setting: A tool for healing. *Nursing Clinics of North America, 42*(2), 261–277.

Rezaei, M., Adib-Hajbaghery, M., Seyedfatemi, N., & Hoseini, F. (2008). Prayer in Iranian cancer patients undergoing chemotherapy. *Complementary Therapies in Clinical Practice, 14*(2), 90–97.

Rheingans, J. I. (2007). A systematic review of nonpharmacologic adjunctive therapies for symptom management in children with cancer. *Journal of Pediatric Oncology Nursing, 24*(2), 81–94.

Shin, H. S., Song, Y. A., & Seo, S. (2007). Effect of Nei-Guan point (P6) acupressure on ketonuria levels, nausea and vomiting in women with hyperemesis gravidarum. *Journal of Advanced Nursing, 59*(5), 510–519.

Skidmore-Roth, L. (2009). *Mosby's handbook of herbs and natural supplements* (4th ed.). St. Louis, MO: Elsevier.

Snyder, M. (2006). Prayer. In M. Snyder & R. Lindquist (Eds.), *Complementary/alternative therapies in nursing* (pp. 143–152). New York: Springer.

Standish, L. J., Kozak, L., & Congdon, S. (2008). Acupuncture is underutilized in hospice and palliative medicine. *American Journal of Hospice & Palliative Care, 25*(4), 298–308.

Tanyi, R. A., & Werner, J. S. (2007). Spirituality in African American and Caucasian women with end-stage renal disease on hemodialysis treatment. *Health Care for Women International, 28*(2), 141–154.

Walker, G., de Valois, B., Davies, R., Young, T., & Maher, J. (2007). Ear acupuncture for hot flushes—The perceptions of women with breast cancer. *Complementary Therapies in Clinical Practice, 13*(4), 250–257.

Weil, A. (2007). *8 weeks to optimum health: A proven program for taking full advantage of your body's natural healing power* (rev. ed.). New York: Random House.

Yang, M. H., Wu, S. C., Lin, J. G., & Lin, L. C. (2007). The efficacy of acupressure for decreasing agitated behaviour in dementia: A pilot study. *Journal of Clinical Nursing, 16*(2), 308–315.

CHAPTER 32

American Heart Association. (2005). Highlights of the 2005 American Heart Association guidelines for cardiopulmonary resuscitation and emergency cardiovascular care. *Currents in Emergency Cardiovascular Care, 16*(4), 1–27.

Arnold, E., Clark, C., Lasserson, T., & Wu, T. (2008). Herbal interventions for chronic asthma in adults and children. *Cochrane Database of Systematic Reviews, 1,* CD005989. Retrieved August 13, 2008, from http://mrw.interscience.wiley.com/cochrane/clsysrev/articles/CD005989/frame.html.

Gaillard, T. (2007). Importance of aerobic fitness in cardiovascular risks in sedentary overweight and obese African-American women. *Nursing Research, 56*(6), 407–415.

Hoffmann, D. (1998). *The new holistic herbal* (3rd ed.). Boston: Element.

Skretkowicz, V. (Ed.). (1992). *Florence Nightingale's notes on nursing.* London: Scutari Press.

CHAPTER 33

Arslan, S., & Karadag, A. (2008). The determination of record-keeping behavior of nurses regarding intravenous fluid treatment: The case of Turkey. *Journal of Infusion Nursing, 31*(5), 287–294.

Bulechek, G., Butcher, H., & Dochterman, J. (2008). *Nursing interventions classification (NIC)* (5th ed.). St. Louis, MO: Mosby Elsevier Health Sciences.

Fischbach, F. (2008). *A manual of laboratory and diagnostic tests* (8th ed.). Philadelphia: Lippincott Williams & Wilkins.

Hadaway, L. (2008). Targeting therapy with central venous access devices. *Nursing2008, 38*(6), 34–40.

Health Care Without Harm. (1999, February 22). *Vinyl IV bags leach toxic chemicals.* Retrieved from http://www.noharm.org.

Hockenberry, M., & Wong, D. (2007). *Wong's nursing care of infants and children* (8th ed.). St. Louis, MO: Mosby Elsevier Health Sciences.

Holcomb, S. (2008). Third-spacing: When body fluid shifts. *Nursing2008, 38*(7), 50–53.

Infusion Nurses Society. (2006). Intravenous nursing standards of practice. *Journal of Intravenous Nursing, 29*(1S), S1–S90.

Kee, J., Paulanka, B., & Polek, C. (2010). *Fluids and electrolytes with clinical applications: A programmed approach* (8th ed.). Clifton Park, NY: Delmar/Cengage Learning.

Macklin, D. (2000). Removing PICC. *American Journal of Nursing, 100*(1), 52–54.

Moorehead, S., Johnson, M., Swanson, M., & Mass, M. (2008). *Nursing outcomes classification (NOC)* (4th ed.). St. Louis, MO: Mosby Elsevier Health Sciences.

Moureau, N. (2008). Using ultrasound to guide PICC and peripheral cannula insertion. *Nursing2008, 38*(10), 20–21.

Oseland, S., & Querciagrossa, A. (2003). Collaboration of nursing and pharmacy in home infusion therapy. *Home Healthcare Nurse, 21*(12), 818–825.

Skretkowicz, V. (Ed.). (1992). *Florence Nightingale's notes on nursing.* London: Scutari Press.

Smeltzer, S., Bare, B., Hinkle, J., & Cheevee, K. (2008). *Brunner & Suddarth's textbook on medical-surgical nursing* (11th ed.). Philadelphia: Lippincott Williams & Wilkins.

Stewart, M. (1999, March/April). IV bags pose patient risk. *American Nurse, 31*(2), 12.

Tierra, M., & Lust, J. (2008). *The natural remedy bible.* New York: Pocket Books.

CHAPTER 34

ACCORD. (2008). *Action to control cardiovascular risk in diabetes.* Retrieved August 26, 2008, from http://www.accordtrial.org/public/index.cfm.

American Society for Parenteral and Enteral Nutrition (1993). Guidelines for the use of parenteral and enteral nutrition in adult and pediatric patients. *Journal of Parenteral and Enteral Nutrition, 17,* 1SA–52SA.

Balch, P. (2006). *Prescription for nutritional healing* (4th ed.). Garden City Park, NY: Penguin.

Bongiorno, P., Fratellone, P., & LoGiudice, P. (2008). Potential health benefits of garlic (*Allium sativum*): A narrative review. *Journal of Complementary and Integrative Medicine, 5*(1), Article 1. Retrieved August 13, 2008, from http://www.bepress.com/jcim/vol5/iss1/1.

Brotherton, A., & Carter, B. (2007). Percutaneous endoscopic gastrostomy feeding in nursing homes. *Clinical Nursing Research, 16*(4), 350–369.

Bulechek, G., Butcher, H., & Dochterman, J. (2008). *Nursing interventions classification (NIC)* (5th ed.). St. Louis, MO: Mosby Elsevier Health Sciences.

Campaign for Food Safety. (1999). *Campaign for food safety news.* Retrieved from http://www.organicconsumers.org.

Genetically altering the world's food. (1999, February 25). *Rachel's Environment & Health News, 639.* Retrieved July 29, 2005, from http://www.rachel.org/en/node/4600.

Gillespie, H. (2006). Exercise. In C. L. Edelman & C. L. Mandle (Eds.), *Health promotion throughout the life span* (6th ed.). St. Louis, MO: Mosby Elsevier Health Sciences.

Grams, L., & Spremulli, M. (2008). Assessing a patient for dysphagia. *Nursing2008, 38*(8), 15.

Hammond, L. (1999). Nutrition-focused physical assessment. *Home Healthcare Nurse, 17*(6), 354–355.

Huffman, S., Pieper, P., Jarczk, K., Bayne, A., & O'Brien, E. (2004). Methods to confirm tube placement: Application of research in practice. *Pediatric Nursing, 30*(1), 10–13.

James, K., & Kohlbry, P. (2004). Adult obesity. *Advance for Nurses, 2*(3), 19–23.

Long, C. (1999). Certified organic. *Organic Gardening, 46*(6), 44–45.

Minister of Supply and Services of Canada. (2001). *Canada's food guide to healthy eating* (Cat. No. H39-252/1992E). Ottawa, ON: Author.

Moorhead, S., Johnson, M., Swanson, M., & Maas, M. (2008). *Nursing outcomes classification (NOC)* (4th ed.). St. Louis, MO: Mosby Elsevier Health Sciences.

Morris, M. (2004). Diet and Alzheimer's disease: What the evidence shows. *Medscape General Medicine, 6*(1). Retrieved January 22, 2004, from http://www.medscape.com/viewarticle/466037.

North American Nursing Diagnosis Association International. (2009). *Nursing diagnoses—Definitions and classification 2009–2011.* Philadelphia: John Wiley & Sons, Inc.

Roth, R. (2007). *Nutrition and diet therapy* (9th ed.). Clifton Park, NY: Delmar/Cengage Learning.

Upadhyay, A., Balkrishna, A., & Upadhyay, R. (2008). Effect of pranayama [voluntary regulated yoga breathing], and yogasana [yoga postures] in diabetes mellitus (DM): A scientific review. *Journal of Complementary and Integrative Medicine, 15*(1), Article 3. Retrieved August 13, 2008, from http://www.bepress.com/jcim/vol5/iss1/3.

U.S. Departments of Agriculture and Health and Human Services. (1992, August). *The food guide pyramid: A guide to daily food choices* (Leaflet No. 572). Washington, DC: Author.

U.S. Departments of Health and Human Services and Agriculture. (2005). *Dietary guidelines for Americans, 2005* (6th ed.). Washington, DC: Government Printing Office.

Yantis, M., & Velander, R. (2008). How to recognize and respond to refeeding syndrome. *Nursing2008, 38*(5), 34–39.

CHAPTER 35

Acute Pain Management Guideline Panel. (1992). *Acute pain management: Operative or medical procedures and trauma. Clinical practice guideline* (AHRQ Publication No. 92-0033). Rockville, MD: Agency for Healthcare Research and Quality.

AGS Panel on Persistent Pain in Older Persons. (2009). Pharmacological management of persistent pain in older persons. American Geriatric Society. *Journal of the American Geriatric Society.* Retrieved August 2009 from http://www.americangeriatrics.org/education/executive_summary/.shtml.

Allen, S. (2005). Pharmacotherapy of neuropathic pain. *Continuing Education in Anaesthesia, Critical Care & Pain, 5*(4), 134–137.

American Psychiatric Association. (2000). *Diagnostic and statistical manual of mental disorders: DSM-IV* (4th ed., text rev.). Washington, DC: Author.

American Society for Pain Management Nursing & the American Pain Society. (2004). *The use of "as-needed" range orders for opioid analgesics in the management of acute pain: A consensus statement of the American Society for Pain Management Nursing and the American Pain Society.* Pensacola, FL: Author.

Balch, P. (2008). *Prescription for nutritional healing: The A-to-Z guide to supplements.* New York: Penguin.

Boswell, M. V., & Cole, B. C. (2006). *Weiner's pain management: A practical guide for clinicians* (7th ed.). Boca Raton, FL: CRC Press.

Bulechek, G., Butcher, H., & Dochterman, J. (2008). *Nursing interventions classification (NIC)* (5th ed.). St. Louis, MO: Elsevier.

Campbell, W., Nicholas, M., & Breivik, H. (2008). Clinical pain management practice & procedures (2nd ed.). New York: Oxford University Press, USA.

Carpenito-Moyet, L. J. (2008). *Nursing diagnosis: Application to clinical practice* (12th ed.). Philadelphia: Wolters Kluwer Lippincott Williams & Wilkins.

Clark, M.A. (*2008*). *Community health nursing: Advocacy for population health* (5th ed., p. 533). Upper Saddle River, NJ: Pearson Prentice Hall.

D'Arcy, Y. (2008). Pain management survey report. *Nursing2008, 38*(6), 42–49.

Daniel, H. C., Narewska, J., Sherpell, M. Hoggart, B., Johnson, R. L., & Rice, A. S. (2008). Comparison of psychological and physical function in neuropathic and nociceptive pain: Implications for cognitive behavioral pain management programs. *European Journal of Pain, 12*(6), 734–741.

Gevirtz, C. (2008). Bracing and splinting to manage pain. *Nursing2008, 38*(5), 58.

Gladstar, R. (2008). *Rosemary Gladstar's herbal recipes for vibrant health.* North Adams, MA: Storey Books.

Gunningberg, L., & Idvall, E. (2007). The quality of postoperative pain management from the perspectives of patients, nurses and patient records. *Journal of Nursing Management, 15*(7), 756–766.

Hockenberry, M. J., & Wilson, D. (2007). *Wong's nursing care of infants and children* (8th ed.). St. Louis, MO: Elsevier.

Hospice and Palliative Nurses Association. (2008). *HPNA position statement on pain.* Pittsburgh, PA: Author.

International Association for the Study of Pain. (2007). IASP pain terminology. Retrieved August 28, 2009, from http://www.iasp-pain.org/AM/Template/cfm?Section+Pain_Definitions&Template+/CM/HTMLDisplay.cfm&ContentID+1728.

Jeong, Y., & Holden, J. (2008). Commonly used preclinical models of pain. *Western Journal of Nursing Research, 30*(3), 350–364.

Kim, K., & Sok, S. (2007). Auricular acupuncture for insomnia: Duration and effects in Korean older adults. *Journal of Gerontology Nursing, 33*(8), 23–28.

Macintyre, P., Rowbotham, D., & Walker, S. (2008). *Clinical pain management acute pain* (2nd ed.). New York: Oxford University Press, USA.

Macintyre, P., & Shug, S. (2007). *Acute pain management: A practical guide* (3rd ed.). St. Louis: MO: Elsevier.

Martinez, E. (2009). Pain and age: The older adult. Retrieved August 29, 2009, from http://www.nationalpainfoundation.org/articles/161/pain/pain-and-age—the-older-adult.

McCaffery, M., & Pasero, C. (1999). *Pain: Clinical manual for nursing practice* (2nd ed.). St. Louis, MO: Mosby.

McGuire, L. (2010). Pain: The fifth vital sign. In D. D. Ignatavicius & M. L. Workman (Eds.) *Medical-surgical nursing: Patient-centered collaborative care* (6th ed.). St. Louis, MO: Elsevier.

Meissner, W. (2009). The role of acupuncture and transcutaneous-electrical nerve stimulation for postoperative pain control. *Current Opinion in Anaesthesiology.* Epub ahead of print. Retrieved August 29, 2009, from http://www.ncbi.nlm.nih.gov/sites/entrez.

National Center for Health Statistics. (2006). *Health, United States, 2006 with chartbook on trends in the health of Americans.* Hyattsville, MD: Author. Retrieved January 10, 2009, from http://www.cdc.gov/nchs/data/hus/hus06.pdf.

Nix, S. (2008). *Williams' basic nutrition & diet therapy* (12th ed.). St. Louis: Elsevier.

North American Nursing Diagnosis Association International. (2009). *Nursing diagnoses—Definitions and classification 2009–2011.* Philadelphia: John Wiley & Sons, Inc.

Patterson, C. (2008). Six myths about opioid use. *Nursing2008, 38*(11), 60–61.

Spies, K., Rehberg, B., Schug, S., Jaehnichen, G., & Harper, S, (2008). *Pocket guide pain management.* Warren, IL: Springer.

Stanton-Hicks, M. (2009). *The Cleveland Clinic guide to pain management.* New York: Kaplan.

Straud, R., & Spaeth, M. (2008), Psychophysical and neurochemical abnoramalities in pain processing in fibromyalgia. *CNS Spectrums: The International Journal of Neuropsychiatric Medicine, 13*(3, Suppl 5), 12–17.

Tierra, M., & Lust, J. (*2008*). *The natural remedy Bible.* New York: Pocket Books.

Travell, J., & Rinzler, S. H. (1952). The myofascial genesis of pain. *Postgraduate Medicine, 11*, 425.

Ufema, J. (2008). Judgmental attitudes: Seeing is believing. *Nursing2008, 38*(3), 17–18.

Wuhrman, E., Cooney, M., Dunwoody, C., Eksterowicz, N., Merkel, S., Oakes, L., et al. (2007). Authorized and unauthorized ("PCA by proxy") dosing of analgesic infusion pumps: Position statement with clinical practice recommendations. *Pain Management Nursing, 8*(1), 4–11.

Yeh, M., Yang, H., Chen, H., & Tsou, M. (2007). Using a patient-controlled analgesia multimedia intervention for improving analgesia quality. *Journal of Clinical Nursing, 16*(11), 2039–2046.

Zwakhalen, S., Hamers, T., Abu-Saad, H. H., & Berger, M. (2006). Pain in elderly people with severe dementia: A systematic review of behavioural pain assessment tools. *BMC Geriatrics, 6*(3). Retrieved August 28, 2009, from http://www.biomedcentral.com/1471-2318/6/3.

CHAPTER 36

Brians, L. K., Alexander, K., Grota, P., Chen, R. W. H., & Dumas, V. (1991). The development of the RISK tool for fall prevention. *Rehabilitation Nursing, 16*(2), 67–69.

Carpenito, L. J. (2007). *Handbook of nursing diagnosis* (12th ed.). Philadelphia: Lippincott Williams & Wilkins.

Centers for Disease Control and Prevention. (2008a). *Physical activity for everyone.* Atlanta, GA: Author. Retrieved January 8, 2009, from http://www.cdc.gov/physicalactivity/everyone/guidelines.

Centers for Disease Control and Prevention. (2008b). *U.S. physical activity statistics.* Atlanta, GA: Author. Retrieved January 7, 2009, from http://apps.nccd.cdc.gov/PASurveillance/StateSumV.asp.

Clark, M. J. (2008). *Community health nursing: Advocacy for population health* (5th ed.). Upper Saddle River, NJ: Pearson Prentice Hall.

Estes, M. E. Z. (2010). *Health assessment and physical examination* (4th ed.). Clifton Park, NY: Thomson Delmar Learning.

Fulmer, T., Wallace, M., & Edelman, C. L. (2006). Older adult. In C. L. Edelman & C. L. Mandle (Eds.), *Health promotion throughout the lifespan* (6th ed.). St. Louis, MO: Elsevier Mosby.

Hart, P. (2006). *Safe patient handling: A report.* Washington, DC: AFT Healthcare. Retrieved January 9, 2009, from http://www.aft.org/topics/no-lift/download/PeterHartSurvey-final-03-16-06.pdf.

Maher, A. (1994). *Orthopedic nursing.* Philadelphia: Saunders.

Miller, C. A. (2009). *Nursing for wellness in older adults* (5th ed.). Phildelphia: Wolters Kluwer/Lippincott Williams & Wilkins.

Mincer, A. B. (2007). Assistive devices for the adult patient with orthopaedic dysfunction. *Orthopaedic Nursing, 26*(4), 226–233.

Minnick, A. F., Mion, L. C., Johnson, M. E., Catrambone, C., & Leipzig, R. (2008). The who and why's of side rail use. *Nursing Management, 39*(5), 36–44.

Mitty, E., & Flores, S. (2007). Fall prevention in assisted living: Assessment and strategies. *Geriatric Nursing, 28*(6), 349–357.

National Center for Chronic Disease Prevention and Health Promotion. (2008). *Overweight and obesity: Contributing factors.* Atlanta, GA: Author. Retrieved January 10, 2009, from http://www.cdc.gov/nccdphp/dnpa/obesity/contributing_factors.htm.

National Institute of Arthritis and Musculoskeletal and Skin Diseases. (2008). *Exercise and bone health.* Bethesda, MD: Author. Retrieved January 7, 2009, from http://www.niams.nih.gov/Health_Info/Bone/Bone_Health/Exercise.

National Institute for Occupational Safety and Health. (2008). *Preventing back injuries in healthcare settings: NIOSH science blog.* Atlanta, GA: Author. Retrieved January 9, 2009, from http://www.cdc.gov/niosh/blog/nsb092208_lifting.html.

Nelson, A. (2006). *Safe patient handling and movement algorithms.* Tampa, FL: VISN 8 VA Sunshine Healthcare Network. Retrieved

January 10, 2009, from http://www.visn8.med.va.gov/patientsafety-center.

North American Nursing Diagnosis Association International. (2009). *Nursing diagnoses—Definitions and classification 2009–2011.* Philadelphia: John Wiley & Sons, Inc.

Quinn, J. F. (2006). Therapeutic touch. In M. Snyder & R. Lindquist (Eds.), *Complementary/alternative therapies in nursing.* New York: Springer.

Tseng, C. N., Chen, C. C., Wu, S. C., & Lin, L. C. (2007). Effects of a range-of-motion exercise programme. *Journal of Advanced Nursing, 57*(2), 181–191.

Umbreit, A. W. (2006). Healing touch. In M. Snyder & R. Lindquist (Eds.), *Complementary/alternative therapies in nursing.* New York: Springer.

U.S. Department of Health & Human Services. (2008). *Physical activity guidelines for Americans. At-a-glance: A fact sheet for professionals.* Washington, DC: Author. Retrieved January 7, 2009, from http://www.health.gov/paguidelines/factsheetprof.aspx.

CHAPTER 37

Agency for Health Care Policy and Research. Panel for Treatment of Pressure Ulcers in Adults. (1996). *Treatment of pressure ulcers. Clinical Practice Guidelines No. 15* (AHCPR Publication No. 95-0653). Rockville, MD: Agency for Health Care Policy and Research, Public Health Service, U.S. Department of Health and Human Services.

Ayello, E., & Cuddigan, J. (2004). Conquer chronic wounds with wound bed preparation. *Nurse Practitioner, 29*(3), 8–25.

Ayello, E., Cuddigan, J., & Kerstein, M. (2002). Skip the knife: Debriding wounds without surgery. *Nursing 2002, 32*(9), 58–64.

Baranoski, S. (2008a). Wound & skin care: Choosing a wound dressing, Part I. *Nursing 2008, 38*(1), 60–61.

Baranoski, S. (2008b). Wound & skin care: Choosing a wound dressing, Part II. *Nursing 2008, 38*(2), 14–15.

Baranoski, S., & Thimsen, K. (2003, March). OASIS skin and wound integumentary assessment items: Applying the WOCN Guidance Document. *Home Healthcare Nurse* (Suppl. 1), 3–13.

Braden, B. J. (1989). Clinical utility of the Braden Scale for Predicting Pressure Sore Risk. *Decubitus, 2*(3), 44–46, 50–51.

Braden, B. J. (2001). Risk assessment in pressure ulcer prevention. In D. L. Krasner, G. T. Rodeheaver, & R. G. Sibbald (Eds.), *Chronic wound care: A clinical source book for healthcare professionals.* Wayne, PA: HMP Communications.

Bulechek, G., Butcher, H., & Dochterman, J. (2008). *Nursing interventions classification (NIC)* (5th ed.). St. Louis, MO: Mosby Elsevier Health Sciences.

Centers for Medicare and Medicaid Services. (2008). *Medicare takes new steps to help make your hospital stay safer.* Baltimore, MD: Author. Retrieved October 28, 2008, from http://cms.hhs.gov.

Doughty, D. B. (2007). Wound-healing physiology. In R. A. Bryant & D. P. Nix (Eds.), *Acute and chronic wounds: Current management concepts* (3rd ed.). St. Louis, MO: Mosby Elsevier Health Sciences.

Fontaine, K. L. (2000). *Healing practices: Alternative therapies for nursing.* Upper Saddle River, NJ: Prentice-Hall.

Joint Commission. (2008). *2009 hospital national patient safety goals.* Oakbrook Terrace, IL: Author. Retrieved October 28, 2008, from http://www.jointcommission.org/PatientSafety/NationalPatient SafetyGoals/09_hap_npsgs.htm.

Lehmann, J. F. (Ed.). (1982). *Therapeutic heat and cold* (3rd ed.). Baltimore, MD: Williams & Wilkins.

Makelbust, J., & Sieggreen, M. (Eds.). (2001). *Pressure ulcers: Guidelines for prevention and management* (3rd ed.). Springhouse, PA: Springhouse.

McElhinny, M. L., & Hooper, C. (2008). Reducing hospital-acquired heel ulcer rates in an acute care facility: An evaluation of a nurse-driven performance improvement project. *Journal of Wound Ostomy Continence Nursing, 35*(1), 79–83.

Moorhead, S., Johnson, M., Swanson, E., & Maas, M. (2007). *Nursing outcomes classification* (4th ed.). St. Louis, MO: Mosby.

National Pressure Ulcer Advisory Panel. (2004). *Healthy People 2010: Pressure ulcer objective.* Washington, DC: Author. Retrieved May 10, 2004, from http://www.npuap.org/HP2010.htm.

National Pressure Ulcer Advisory Panel. (2007). *Terms and definitions related to support surface.* Washington, DC: Author. Retrieved October 26, 2008, from http://www.npuap.org/NPUAP_S3I_TD.pdf.

North American Nursing Diagnosis Association International. (2009). *Nursing diagnoses—Definitions and classification 2009–2011.* Philadelphia: John Wiley & Sons, Inc.

Norton, D. (1989). Calculating the risk: Reflections on the Norton scale. *Decubitus, 2*(3), 24–31.

Norton, D., McLaren, R., & Exton-Smith, A. N. (1962). *An investigation of geriatric nursing problems in hospital.* London: National Corporation for the Care of Old People (now the Centre for Policy on Aging).

Price, P., Fagervik-Morton, H., Mudge, E., Beele, H., Ruiz, J., Nystrom, T., et al. (2008). Dressing-related pain in patients with chronic wounds: An international patient perspective. *International Wound Care, 5*(2), 159–171.

Rolstad, B., Ovington, L., & Harris, A. (2007). Principles of wound management. In R. Bryant (Ed.), *Acute and chronic wounds: Nursing management* (3rd ed.). St. Louis, MO: Mosby.

Schmidt, T. (2002). Pressure ulcers: Nutrition strategies that make a difference. *Caring, 21*(6), 18.

Skretkowicz, V. (Ed.). (1992). *Florence Nightingale's notes on nursing.* London: Scutari Press.

Sussman, C., & Bates-Jensen, B. M. (2005). *Wound care: A collaborative practice manual for physical therapists and nurses* (2nd ed.). Gaithersburg, MD: Lippincott Williams & Wilkins.

Tierra, M., & Lust, J. (2008). *The natural remedy bible.* New York: Pocket Books.

U.S. Department of Health and Human Services. (1992). *Pressure ulcers in adults: Prediction and prevention* (Publication No. 92–0047 and 92–0050). Rockville, MD: Public Health Service, Agency for Health Care Policy and Research.

Wurster, J. (2007). What role can nurse leaders play in reducing the incidence of pressure sores? *Nursing Economics, 5*, 267–269.

CHAPTER 38

Akansel, N., & Kaymakçi, S. (2008). Effects of intensive care unit noise on patients: A study on coronary artery bypass graft surgery patients. *Journal of Clinical Nursing, 17*(12), 1581–1590.

American Psychiatric Association. (2000). *Diagnostic and statistical manual of mental disorders* (4th ed., Text Revised). Washington, DC: Author.

Belojević, G. A., Jakovljević, B. D., Stojanov, V. J., Slepčevic, V. Z., & Paunović, K. Z. (2008). Nighttime road-traffic noise and arterial hypertension in an urban population. *Hypertension Research, 31*(4), 775–781.

Carpenito-Moyet, L. J. (2007). *Handbook of nursing diagnosis: Application to practice* (11th ed.). Philadelphia: Lippincott Williams & Wilkins.

Folstein, M. F., Folstein, S. E., & McHugh, P. R. (1975). Mini-mental state: A practical method for grading the cognitive state of patients for the clinician. *Journal of Psychiatric Research, 12*, 189–198.

Gladstar, R. (2008). *Rosemary Gladstar's herbal recipes for vibrant health.* North Adams, MA: Storey Books.

Grady, C. L., Springer, M. V., Hongwanishkul, D., McIntosh, A. R., & Winocur, G. (2006). Age-related changes in brain activity across the adult lifespan. *Journal of Cognitive Neuroscience, 18,* 227–241.

Guyton, A. C., & Hall, J. (2005). *Textbook of medical physiology* (11th ed.). Philadelphia: Saunders.

Jaeggi, S. M., Buschkuehl, M., Jonides, J., & Perrig, W. J. (2008). Improving fluid intelligence with training on working memory. *Proceedings of the National Academy of Sciences of the United States of America, 105,* 6791–6792.

Lee, B. H., Kim, E. J., Ku, B. D., Choi, K. M., Seo, S. W., Kim, G. M., et al. (2008). Cognitive impairments in patients with hemispatial neglect from acute right hemisphere stroke. *Cognitive & Behavioral Neurology, 21*(2), 73–76.

North American Nursing Diagnosis Association International. (2009). *Nursing diagnoses—Definitions and classification 2009–2011.* Philadelphia: John Wiley & Sons, Inc.

Nys, G. M., van Zandvoort, M. J., de Kort, P. L., Jansen, B. P., de Haan, E. H., & Kappelle, L. J. (2007). Cognitive disorders in acute stroke: Prevalence and clinical determinants. *Cerebrovascular Diseases, 23*(5/6), 408–416.

Öhman, L., Nordin, S., Bergdahl, J., Slunga B.L., & Stigsdotter Neely, A. (2007). Cognitive function in outpatients with perceived chronic stress. *Scandinavian Journal of Work, Environment, & Health, 33*(3), 223–232.

Rhee, M. Y., Kim, H. Y., Roh, S. C., Kim, H. J., & Kwon, H. J. (2008). The effects of chronic exposure to aircraft noise on the prevalence of hypertension. *Hypertension Research, 31*(4), 641–647.

Riethmuller, S., Muller-Wenk, R., Knoblauch, A., & Schoch, O. D. (2008). Monetary value of undisturbed sleep. *Noise Health, 10*(39), 46–54.

Skidmore-Roth, L. (2009). *Mosby's handbook of herbs and natural supplements* (4th ed.). St. Louis, MO: Elsevier.

CHAPTER 39

Balch, P. (2006). *Prescription for nutritional healing* (4th ed.). Garden City Park, NY: Penguin.

Barney, D. P. (1996). *Clinical applications of herbal medicine.* Pleasant Grove, UT: Woodland.

Brown-Guttovz, H. (2008). Myths & facts about irritable bowel syndrome. *Nursing2008, 38*(2), 28.

Bulechek, G., Butcher, H., & Dochterman, J. (2008). *Nursing interventions classification (NIC)* (5th ed.). St. Louis, MO: Mosby Elsevier Health Sciences.

Day, M. (2008). Fight back against inflammatory bowel disease. *Nursing2008, 38*(11), 34–41.

Gladstar, R. (2001). *Family herbal: A guide to living life with energy, health, and vitality.* North Adams, MA: Storey Books.

Gray, M., Rayome, R., & Anson, C. (1995). Incontinence and clean intermittent catherization following spinal cord injury … including commentary by Dean, K. P. *Clinical Nursing Research 4*(1), 6–21.

Held-Warmkessel, J., & Schiech, L. (2008). Responding to 4 gastrointestinal complications in cancer patients. *Nursing2008, 38*(7), 32–38.

Hertig, V. (2007). Daily stress and gastrointestinal symptoms in women with irritable bowel syndrome. *Nursing Research, 56*(6), 399–406.

Kent, D. (2008). Changing an ostomy pouching system. *Nursing2008, 38*(12), 50–54.

Moorhead, S., Johnson, M., Swanson, E., & Maas, M. (2008). *Nursing outcomes classification* (4th ed.). St. Louis, MO: Mosby Elsevier Health Sciences.

Newman, D. (2004). Urinary incontinence. *Advance for Nurses, 2*(2), 17–22.

North American Nursing Diagnosis Association International. (2009). *Nursing diagnoses—Definitions and classification 2009–2011.* Philadelphia: John Wiley & Sons, Inc.

Weiss, B., & Newman, D. (2002). *New insight into urinary stress incontinence: Advice for the primary care clinician.* Retrieved July 16, 2002, from http://www.medscape.com.

Wyman, J. F., Elswick, R. K., Jr., Ory, M. G., Wilson, M. S., & Fantl, J. A. (1993). Influence of functional, urological, and environmental characteristics on urinary incontinence in community-dwelling older women. *Nursing Research, 42*(5), 270–275.

CHAPTER 40

Akduman, D., Kim, L. E., Parks, R. L., L'Ecuyer, P. B., Mutha, S., Jeffe, D. B., et al. (1999). Use of personal protective equipment and operating room behaviors in four surgical subspecialties: Personal protective equipment and behaviors in surgery. *Infection Control and Hospital Epidemiology, 20*(2), 110–114.

American Association of Nurse Anesthetists. (2004). *Informed consent in anesthesia.* Park Ridge, IL: Author.

Association of periOperative Nurses. (2007). *PNDS: Perioperative nursing data set* (2nd ed., text rev.). Denver, CO: Author.

Association of periOperative Nurses. (2008). *Perioperative standards and recommended practices.* Denver, CO: Author.

Bulechek, G., Butcher, H., & Dochterman, J. (2008). *Nursing interventions classification (NIC)* (5th ed.). St. Louis, MO: Mosby Elsevier Health Sciences.

Gillespie, B., Wallis, M., & Chaboyer, W. (2008). Operating theater culture: Implications for nurse retention. *Western Journal of Nursing Research, 30*(2), 259–277.

Guterman, N. G. (1960). *The Anchor book of Latin quotations.* New York: Anchor Books.

Joint Commission. (2008). *2009 National patient safety goals.* Oakbrook Terrace, IL: Author. Retrieved December 12, 2008, from http://www.jointcommission.org/patientsafety/nationalpatientsafetygoals.

Lindeman, C., & Van Aernam, B. (1971). Nursing intervention with the presurgical patient: The effects of structured and unstructured preoperative teaching. *Nursing Research, 20,* 319–332.

Michaels, R. (2007). Achieving the National Quality Forum's "never event": Prevention of wrong site, wrong procedure, and wrong patient operation. *Annals of Surgery, 245*(4), 526–532.

Moorhead, S., Johnson, M., Swanson, M., & Maas, M. (2008). *Nursing outcomes classification (NOC)* (4th ed.). St. Louis, MO: Mosby Elsevier Health Sciences.

North American Nursing Diagnosis Association International. (2009). *Nursing diagnoses—Definitions and classification 2009–2011.* Philadelphia: John Wiley & Sons, Inc.

Parker, C., Mimick, P., & Kee, C. (1999). Clinical decision-making process in perioperative nursing. *AORN Journal, 70*(1), 45–62.

Pasero, C. (2008). *Intravenous patient-controlled analgesia for acute pain management.* Pensacola, FL: American Society of Pain Management Nursing.

Phillips, N. F. (2004). *Berry and Kohn's operating room techniques* (10th ed.). St. Louis, MO: Mosby.

Reeder, J., Hamlet, J., Killen, A., King, C., & Uruburu, A. (1994). Nurses' knowledge, attitudes about HIV, AIDS. *AORN Journal, 59*(2), 450–466.

Rothrock, J. C. (1999). *The RN first assistant* (3rd ed.). Philadelphia: Lippincott Williams & Wilkins.

Rubenfeld, A. G., & Scheffer, B. K. (1999). *Critical thinking in nursing: An interactive approach* (2nd ed.). Philadelphia: Lippincott.

Schroeter, K. (1999). Ethical perception and resulting action in perioperative nurses. *AORN Journal, 69*(5), 991–1003.

Slattery, M. (1998). The epidemic hazards of nursing. *American Journal of Nursing, 98*(11), 50–53.

INDEX

Page numbers followed by f indicate figure; those followed by t indicate table; those followed by p indicate procedure.

J

StudyWare™ to Accompany Fundamentals of Nursing: Standards and Practice, Fourth Edition

MINIMUM SYSTEM REQUIREMENTS

- Operating systems: Microsoft Windows XP w/SP 2, Windows Vista w/SP 1, Windows 7
- Processor: Minimum required by Operating System
- Memory: Minimum required by Operating System
- Hard Drive Space: 500MB
- Screen resolution: 1024 × 768 pixels
- CD-ROM drive
- Sound card & listening device required for audio features
- Flash Player 10. The Adobe Flash Player is free, and can be downloaded from http://www.adobe.com/products/flashplayer/

SETUP INSTRUCTIONS

1. Insert disc into CD-ROM drive. The StudyWare™ installation program should start automatically. If it does not, go to step 2.
2. From My Computer, double-click the icon for the CD drive.
3. Double-click the *setup.exe* file to start the program.

TECHNICAL SUPPORT

Telephone: 1-800-648-7450
8:30 A.M.–6:30 P.M. Eastern Time
E-mail: delmar.help@cengage.com

StudyWare™ is a trademark used herein under license.

Microsoft® and Windows® are registered trademarks of the Microsoft Corporation.

Pentium® is a registered trademark of the Intel Corporation.